TEXTBOOK OF
Hepatology
From Basic Science to Clinical Practice

Textbook of Hepatology – Third Edition – Companion CD

A companion CD is included at the back of Volume Two. It contains:
- All chapters in PDF format
- A full text search facility, with search words highlighted in the text.

TEXTBOOK OF
Hepatology
From Basic Science to Clinical Practice

THIRD EDITION

SECTIONS 1–10 AND INDEX

EDITORS

Juan Rodés MD
Director General, Hospital Clinic; Professor of Medicine,
University of Barcelona, Barcelona, Spain

Jean-Pierre Benhamou MD
Professor of Hepatology, Université Denis Diderot Paris 7,
Assistance Publique – Hôpitaux de Paris and Inserm U773,
Service d'Hépatologie, Hôpital Beaujon, Clichy, France

Andres T. Blei MD
Professor of Medicine and Surgery, Northwestern University
Feinberg School of Medicine, Chicago, IL, USA

Jürg Reichen MD
Professor of Medicine, University of Bern; Chief of Hepatology,
University Hospital, Bern, Switzerland

Mario Rizzetto MD
Professor of Gastroenterology, University of Turin, Turin, Italy

ASSOCIATE EDITORS

Jean-François Dufour MD
Professor of Hepatology, University of Bern, Bern, Switzerland

Scott L. Friedman MD
Fishberg Professor of Medicine, Chief, Division of Liver Diseases,
Mount Sinai School of Medicine, New York, NY, USA

Pere Ginès MD
Professor of Medicine, University of Barcelona, Chief, Liver Unit,
Hospital Clinic, Barcelona, Spain

Dominique-Charles Valla MD
Professor of Hepatology, Université Denis Diderot Paris 7,
Assistance Publique – Hôpitaux de Paris and Inserm U773,
Chief, Service d'Hépatologie, Hôpital Beaujon, Clichy, France

Fabien Zoulim MD PhD
Professor of Medicine, Université Lyon 1, Liver Department,
Hospices Civils de Lyon, Head, Inserm U8712, Lyon, France

FOREWORD

Neil McIntyre MD
Emeritus Professor of Medicine, Royal Free and University College
School of Medicine, London, UK

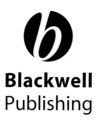

Blackwell
Publishing

© 2007 by Blackwell Publishing Ltd

Blackwell Publishing, Inc., 350 Main Street, Malden, Massachusetts 02148-5020, USA
Blackwell Publishing Ltd, 9600 Garsington Road, Oxford OX4 2DQ, UK
Blackwell Publishing Asia Pty Ltd, 550 Swanston Street, Carlton, Victoria 3053, Australia

First published 1991 by Oxford University Press
Second edition 1999 by Oxford University Press

2007   1

Library of Congress Cataloging-in-Publication Data
Textbook of hepatology : from basic science to clinical practice. — 3rd ed. / edited by
Juan Rodés . . . [et al.].
     p. ; cm.
   Rev. ed. of: Oxford textbook of clinical hepatology. 2nd ed. 1999.
   Includes bibliographical references and indexes.
   ISBN: 978-1-4051-2741-7 (alk. paper)
   1. Liver—Diseases.   I. Rodés, Juan.   II. Oxford textbook of clinical hepatology.
III. Title: Hepatology.
   [DNLM: 1. Liver Diseases. WI 700 T355 2007]

   RC845.O93 2007
   616.3′62—dc22

                                                                2006101699

ISBN: 978-1-4051-2741-7

A catalogue record for this title is available from the British Library

Set in Minion/Frutiger by Graphicraft Limited, Hong Kong
Printed and bound in Singapore by Markono Print Media Pte Ltd

Commissioning Editor: Alison Brown
Development Editor: Rebecca Huxley, Blackwell Publishing Ltd
Development Editor: Nicki van Berckel, University of Barcelona
Production Controller: Debbie Wyer
Project Manager: Gillian Whytock, Prepress Projects Ltd
CD produced by: Meg Barton, Nathan Harris

For further information on Blackwell Publishing, visit our website:
http://www.blackwellpublishing.com

Contents

A companion CD containing all chapters in PDF format with a full text search is included at the back of Volume Two.

Contributors

Juan Miguel Abdo MD
Chief, Clinical Gastroenterology Unit
Mexico General Hospital
Mexico City, Mexico

Juan G. Abraldes MD
Specialist in Hepatology
Liver Unit, Hospital Clinic
Barcelona, Spain

Rakesh Aggarwal MD DM
Professor, Department of Gastroenterology
All India Institute of Medical Sciences
New Delhi, India

Armin Akhavan MD
California Pacific Medical Center
San Francisco, CA, USA

Alfredo Alberti MD
Professor of Clinical and Experimental Medicine
University of Padua
Padua, Italy

Thomas A. Aloia MD
Assistant Professor of Surgery
Baylor College of Medicine
Houston, TX, USA

Pedro L. Alonso MD
Jefe del Servicio
Centro de Salud Internacional
Hospital Clinic
Barcelona, Spain

Peter W. Angus MB BS MD FRACP
Director of Gastroentrology and Hepatology
Austin Hospital
Melbourne, Vic, Australia

Vicente Arroyo MD
Professor of Medicine
Director of the Institute of Digestive and Metobolic
   Diseases
University of Barcelona
Barcelona, Spain

Fred K. Askari MD PhD
Clinical Assistant Professor, Department of Internal

Medicine
University of Michigan Health System
Ann Arbor, MI, USA

Carmen Ayuso MD
Consultant Radiologist
Hospital Clinic
Barcelona, Spain

Charles Balabaud MD
Hepatologist
Hôpital St André
Bordeaux, France

M. Baraitser MD
Consultant in Clinical Genetics
Great Ormond Street Hospital for
   Children
London, UK

Pablo Barreiro MD
Department of Infectious Diseases
Hospital Carlos III
Madrid, Spain

Ralf Bartenschlager PhD
Head of Department of Molecular Virology
University of Heidelberg
Heidelberg, Germany

Pierre Bédossa MD
Professor of Pathology, Université Denis Diderot
   Paris 7;
Assistance Publique – Hôpitaux de Paris and Inserm
   U773;
Department of Pathology, Hôpital Beaujon
Clichy, France

Jacques Belghiti MD
Hôpital Beaujon
Clichy, France

Jean-Pierre Benhamou MD
Professor of Hepatology, Université Denis Diderot
   Paris 7;
Assistance Publique – Hôpitaux de Paris and Inserm
   U773;
Service d'Hépatologie, Hôpital Beaujon
Clichy, France

Luisa Benvegnù MD
Department of Clinical and Experimental
   Medicine
University of Padua
Padua, Italy

Jacques Bernuau MD
Service d'Hépatologie
Hôpital Beaujon
Clichy, France

Ulrich Beuers MD
Professor, Department of Gastroenterology and
   Hepatology
Academic Medical Center
Amsterdam, The Netherlands

Philippe Beutels BSc MSc PhD
Lecturer in Health Economics
Faculty of Medicine
University of Antwerp
Antwerp, Belgium

H.L.C. Beynon MD
Consultant Physician and Rheumatologist
Royal Free Hospital
London, UK

Mayank Bhandari MB BS MS
Flinders Medical Centre
Bedford Park, SA, Australia

Alberto Biglino MD
Associate Professor of Infectious Diseases
University of Turin;
Head, Infectious Diseases Unit
Cardinal Massaja Hospital
Asti, Italy

**José Ignacio Bilbao Jaureguízar
MD**
Department of Radiology
Clínica Universitaria de Navarra
Pamplona, Spain

Paulette Bioulac-Sage MD
Professor of Pathology
Université Bordeaux
Bordeaux, France

Andres T. Blei MD
Professor of Medicine and Surgery
Northwestern University Feinberg School of
   Medicine
Chicago, IL, USA

Guenther Boden MD
Laura H. Carnell Professor of Medicine
Chief, Division of Endocrinology, Diabetes and
   Metabolism
Temple University
Philadelphia, PA, USA

J. van den Bogaerde MD
Royal Free Hospital
London, UK

Luigi Bolondi MD
Department of Internal Medicine and
   Gastroenterology
University of Bologna
Bologna, Italy

Jaime Bosch MD
Senior Consultant
Liver Unit, Hospital Clinic;
Professor of Medicine
University of Barcelona
Barcelona, Spain

Pierre M. Bouloux MD
Department of Medicine
Royal Free Hospital
London, UK

Holger Bourquain MD
MeVis Research GmbH
Bremen, Germany

S. Bresson-Hadni MD PhD
Professor, Department of Hepatology and Liver
   Diseases
Hôpital Jean-Minjoz
Besançon, France

George J. Brewer MD
Active Emeritus Professor of Human Genetics and
   Internal Medicine
University of Michigan Medical School
Ann Arbor, MI, USA

John T. Brosnan DPhil DSc
Professor, Department of Biochemistry
Memorial University of Newfoundland
St. John's, NL, Canada

Margaret E. Brosnan PhD
Professor, Department of Biochemistry
Memorial University of Newfoundland
St. John's, NL, Canada

Kyle E. Brown MD MSc
Assistant Professor, University of Iowa Carver
   College of Medicine;
Staff Physician, Iowa City Veterans Administration
   Medical Center
Iowa City, IA, USA

Concepció Bru MD
Senior Consultant Radiologist
Hospital Clinic
Barcelona, Spain

Miguel Bruguera MD
Senior Consultant
Liver Unit, Hospital Clinic
Barcelona, Spain

Jordi Bruix MD
Senior Consultant and BCLC Director
Liver Unit, Hospital Clinic
Barcelona, Spain

Alan L. Buchman MD MSPH FACP FACG FACN AGAF
Associate Professor
Northwestern University Feinberg School of
   Medicine
Chicago, IL, USA

Christophe Bureau MD
Praticien Hospitalier
CHU Purpan and Inserm U531
Toulouse, France

Andrew K. Burroughs MB ChB FRCP
Professor of Hepatology
University College School of Medicine;
Consultant Physician
Royal Free Hospital
London, UK

Juan Caballeria MD PhD
Senior Consultant
Liver Unit, Hospital Clinic
Barcelona, Spain

Jean-François Cadranel MD
Associate Professor, Collège Médical des Hôpitaux
   de Paris;
Chief, Liver Unit, Hôpital Laennec
Creil, France

Stephen H. Caldwell MD
Director of Hepatology
University of Virginia
Charlottesville, VA, USA

Valeria Camaggi MD
Department of Internal Medicine and
   Gastroenterology
University of Bologna
Bologna, Italy

Bernard Campillo MD
Service de Rééducation Digestive
Hôpital Albert Chenevier
Créteil, France

Enric Carreras MD PhD
Senior Consultant
Director of the Stem Cell Transplantation Program
Hospital Clinic
Barcelona, Spain

Flair José Carrilho MD PhD
Full Professor of Gastroenterology
University of São Paulo School of Medicine
São Paulo, Brazil

Antoni Castells MD
Department of Gastroenterology
Hospital Clinic
Barcelona, Spain

C. Ritchie Chalmers MD
MRC Clinical Training Fellow
Hepatobiliary Department
St James's University Hospital
Leeds, UK

Roger W. Chapman BSc MD MB BS FRCP
Consultant Hepatologist
John Radcliffe Hospital
Oxford, UK

Ramón Charco MD PhD
Consultant, Liver Transplant Unit
IMDiM, Hospital Clinic
Barcelona, Spain

Michael R. Charlton MD
Professor of Medicine
Director of Hepatology
Mayo Clinic College of Medicine
Rochester, MN, USA

Dipankar Chattopadhyay MB BS MS MRCS
Clinical Research Associate
Northern Institute of Cancer Research
Newcastle upon Tyne, UK

Oliver Chazouillères MD PhD
Professor of Hepatology
Université Pierre et Marie Curie Paris 6;
Director, Digestive Department, Hôpital
   Saint-Antoine
Paris, France

Ramsey Cheung MD
Associate Professor
Stanford University School of Medicine
Stanford, CA, USA

Pedro Paulo Chieffi MD PhD
Associate Professor, Department of
   Gastroenterology
University of São Paulo School of
   Medicine
São Paulo, Brazil

Evangelos Cholongitas MD
Hepatologist
Royal Free Hospital
London, UK

Haithem Chtioui MD
Department of Clinical Pharmacology
University of Bern
Bern, Switzerland

Pierre A. Clavien MD
Multiorgan Transplant Program
Toronto General Hospital
Toronto, ON, Canada

Daniel T. Cohen MD
Radiology Resident, Department of Radiology
Massachusetts General Hospital
Boston, MA, USA

David E. Cohen MD PhD
Director of Hepatology
Brigham and Women's Hospital;
Associate Professor of Medicine
Harvard Medical School;
Associate Professor of Health Sciences and Technology
Harvard–MIT Division of Health Sciences and
 Technology
Boston, MA, USA

Massimo Colombo MD
Professor of Gastroenterology
University of Milan
Milan, Italy

Juliet Compston FRCPath FRCP
Professor of Bone Medicine
University of Cambridge;
Honorary Consultant Physician
Addenbrooke's Hospital
Cambridge, UK

Manuel Corachan MD
Senior Consultant in Tropical Medicine
Center for International Health
University Hospital
Barcelona, Spain

Markus Cornberg MD
Department of Gastroenterology
Hanover Medical School
Hanover, Germany

Paulo Renato A.V. Correa MD
Resident, Department of Psychiatry
Yale University School of Medicine
New Haven, CT, USA

Patrick A. Couglin MB ChB MRCS MD
Higher Surgical Trainee, Yorkshire Deanery
Department of Hepatobiliary Surgery
St James's University Hospital
Leeds, UK

Charles S. Cox Jr MD PhD
Director, Pediatric Trauma Program
Distinguished Professor of Surgery and Pediatrics
University of Texas Medical School
Houston, TX, USA

Christopher H. Crane MD
Associate Professor
Program Director and Section Chief,
 Gastrointestinal Section
University of Texas M.D. Anderson Cancer Center
Houston, TX, USA

James M. Crawford MD PhD
Professor and Chair
Department of Pathology, Immunology and
 Laboratory Medicine
University of Florida College of Medicine
Gainesville, FL, USA

Luiz Caetano Da Silva MD
Department of Gastroenterology
University of São Paulo School of Medicine
São Paulo, Brazil

Christopher P. Day MD
Centre for Liver Research
University of Newcastle upon Tyne
Newcastle upon Tyne, UK

Maria T. DeSancho MD
Associate Professor of Clinical Medicine
New York Presbyterian Hospital
New York, NY, USA

Anthony J. DeSantis MD
Assistant Professor of Medicine
Northwestern University Feinberg School of
 Medicine
Chicago, IL, USA

Valeer J. Desmet MD
Emeritus Professor of Pathology
Catholic University of Leuven
Leuven, Belgium

Jean-Charles Deybach MD PhD
President of the French Porphyria Center
Professor of Biochemistry and Molecular Biology
Head of Department of Molecular Genetics and
 Biochemistry
Hôpital Louis Mourier
Colombes, France

Anna Mae Diehl MD
Florence McAlister Professor
Chief, Division of Gastroenterology
Duke University School of Medicine
Durham, NC, USA

Jules L. Dienstag MD
Carl W. Walter Professor of Medicine
Harvard Medical School;
Physician, Massachusetts General Hospital
Boston, MA, USA

Loriana Di Giammarino MD
Division of Gastroenterology and Hepatology
Center Hospitalier Universitaire Vaudois
University of Lausanne
Lausanne, Switzerland

Tom Doherty MD FRCP DTM&H
Hospital for Tropical Diseases
London, UK

Peter T. Donaldson BSc PhD
Lecturer in Molecular Genetics
University of Newcastle upon Tyne
Newcastle upon Tyne, UK

Lluís Donoso MD
Head, Diagnostic Imaging Centre
Hospital Clinic
Barcelona, Spain

James S. Dooley MD FRCP
Reader and Consultant Hepatologist, Centre for
 Hepatology
Royal Free and University College School of
 Medicine
London, UK

Jean-François Dufour MD
Professor of Hepatology
University of Bern
Bern, Switzerland

Franz-Ludwig Dumoulin MD
Professor of Medicine
University of Bonn;
Head, Department of Internal Medicine
St Agnes Hospital
Bocholt, Germany

François Durand MD
Professor of Hepatology, Université Denis Diderot
 Paris 7;
Assistance Publique – Hôpitaux de Paris and Inserm
 U773;
Service d'Hépatologie, Hôpital Beaujon
Clichy, France

Geoffrey M. Dusheiko MB BCh FCPSA FRCP FRCP(Ed)
Professor of Medicine, Centre for Hepatology
Royal Free and University College School of
 Medicine
London, UK

Gregory T. Everson MD
Professor of Medicine and Director of
 Hepatology
University of Colorado Health Sciences Center
Denver, CO, USA

Klaas N. Faber MD
Academic Medical Center
Amsterdam, The Netherlands

Joan Falcó Fages MD
Senior Consultant Radiologist
UDIAT-CD Hospital Parc Taulí
Sabadell, Spain

Geoffrey C. Farrell MD FRACP
Director, Gastroenterology and Hepatology
 Unit
The Canberra Hospital;
Professor of Hepatic Medicine
Australian National University
Garran, ACT, Australia

Jean H.D. Fasel MD
Professor and Head of Clinical Anatomy Research
 Group, Geneva
Centre Médical Universitaire
Geneva, Switzerland

Andrew P. Feranchak MD
Assistant Professor of Pediatrics
University of Texas Southwestern Medical School
Dallas, TX, USA

Javier Fernández MD
Intensive Care Unit, Hepatology
Hospital Clinic
Barcelona, Spain

José C. Fernández-Checa PhD
Professor, Spanish Research Council
Liver Unit, Hospital Clinic
Barcelona, Spain

Peter Fickert MD
Laboratory of Experimental and Molecular
   Hepatology
Medical University of Graz
Graz, Austria

Stefano Fiorucci MD
Associate Professor of Gastroenterology
Universita Degli Studi di Perugia
Perugia, Italy

Constantino Fondevila MD PhD
Transplant Surgeon
Liver Unit, Hospital Clinic;
Digestive Disease Institute, University of Barcelona
Barcelona, Spain

Alejandro Forner MD
Research Fellow
University of Barcelona
Barcelona, Spain

Xavier Forns MD PhD
Senior Specialist
Liver Unit, Hospital Clinic
Barcelona, Spain

Ira J. Fox MD
Charles W. McLaughlin Professor of Surgery
University of Nebraska Medical Center
Omaha, NB, USA

Nader K. Francis MB ChB FRCS PhD
Consultant Surgeon
Yeovil District Hospital
Somerset, UK

Scott L. Friedman MD
Fishberg Professor of Medicine
Chief, Division of Liver Diseases
Mount Sinai School of Medicine
New York, NY, USA

Josep Fuster Obregón MD
Profesor Titular de Cirugía
Universidad de Barcelona;
Jefe de Sección de Cirugia Hépatica y Trasplante
Hospital Clinic
Barcelona, Spain

Michelle C. Gallagher BSc MB BS MRCP
Consultant Gastroenterologist
The Royal Surrey County Hospital
Guildford, UK

Peter R. Galle MD PhD
Professor of Medicine
Johannes Gutenberg University;
Chief Medical Officer
University Hospital of Mainz
Mainz, Germany

Juan Carlos García-Pagán MD
Consultant in Hepatology
Liver Unit, Hospital Clinic
Barcelona, Spain

Carmen García-Ruiz MD
Del Consejo Superior de Investgaciones
   Cientificas
Instituto de Investigación Biomedica de
   Barcelona
Barcelona, Spain

Javier García-Samaniego MD
Department of Infectious Diseases
Hospital Carlos III
Madrid, Spain

Guadalupe García-Tsao MD
Professor of Medicine
Yale University School of Medicine
New Haven, CT, USA

Juan Carlos García-Valdecasas MD
Jefe de Cirugía
Hospital Clinic;
Catedratic de Cirugía
Universidad de Barcelona
Barcelona, Spain

Wolfram H. Gerlich PhD
Professor of Medical Virology
Justus-Liebig University
Giessen, Germany

André P. Geubel MD
Professor, Department of Gastroenterology
Universitaires Saint-Luc
Université Catholique de Louvain
Brussels, Belgium

Dominique P. Germain MD PhD
Professor of Medical Genetics
Centre de Référence de la Maladie de Fabry et des
   Maladies Héréditaires du Tissu Conjonctif;
Assistance Publique – Hôpitaux de Paris
Paris, France

Mihai Gheorghiade MD
Professor of Medicine and Associate Chief of
   Cardiology
Northwestern University Feinberg School of
   Medicine
Chicago, IL, USA

Pere Ginès MD
Professor of Medicine, University of Barcelona;
Chief, Liver Unit, Hospital Clinic
Barcelona, Spain

Daniel Glass MB ChB MRCP
Specialist Registrar in Dermatology
West Hertfordshire Hospitals Trust
Hemel Hempstead, UK

Christian Gluud MD DrMedSci
Head of Copenhagen Trial Unit
Centre for Clinical Intervention Research
Copenhagen University Hospital
Copenhagen, Denmark

Mark D. Gorrell MD PhD
Principal Research Fellow, Faculty of Medicine
University of Sydney;
Principal Scientist, Royal Prince Alfred Hospital
Sydney, NSW, Australia

Roberto J. Groszmann MD
Yale University School of Medicine
New Haven, CT, USA

Frank Grünhage MD
Head, Department of Medicine
University of Bonn
Bonn, Germany

Mónica Guevara MD
Associate Invesitgator
IDIBAPS, Hospital Clinic
Barcelona, Spain

I. Neil Guha MB BS MRCP
Specialist Registrar in Hepatology
Southampton General Hospital
Southampton, UK

Basuki Gunawan MD
Fellow, Gastrointestinal and Liver Division
Keck School of Medicine
University of Southern California
Los Angeles, CA, USA

N. Guañabens MD
Department of Rheumatology, Hospital Clinic
Barcelona, Spain

Dominique Guyader MD PhD
Professor of Hepatology
University of Rennes
Rennes, France

Paul S. Haber MD
Centenary Institute of Cancer Medicine and Cell
   Biology
Royal Prince Alfred Hospital and The University of
   Sydney
Sydney, NSW, Australia

Antoine Hadengue MD
Professeur de Médecine et Chef de Service
Service de Gastroentérologie et Hépatologie
Hôpitaux Universitaires de Genève
Geneva, Switzerland

Edward D. Harris PhD
Professor, Department of Nutrition and Food Science
Texas A&M University
College Station, TX, USA

Dieter Häussinger MD
Professor of Internal Medicine
Heinrich Heine University
Dusseldorf, Germany

Philip N. Hawkins MB PhD FRCP FRCPath FMedSci
Professor of Medicine
University College London;
Consultant, National Amyloidosis Centre
Royal Free Hospital
London, UK

William G. Hawkins MD
Assistant Professor
Washington University in St. Louis
Section of Hepatopancreatobiliary Surgery
Barnes-Jewish Hospital
St. Louis, MO, USA

Roderick J. Hay
Head of School, Medicine and Dentistry
Queen's University Belfast
Belfast, UK

Peter C. Hayes BMSc MB ChB MD PhD
Professor of Hepatology
University of Edinburgh;
Consultant, Liver Unit
Royal Infirmary of Edinburgh
Edinburgh, UK

John Cijiang He MD
Department of Pharmacology and Biological
    Chemistry
Mount Sinai School of Medicine
New York, NY, USA

E. Jenny Heathcote MB BS MD FRCP FRCPC
Professor of Medicine
University of Toronto
Toronto, ON, Canada

J. Michael Henderson MD
Department of General Surgery
The Cleveland Clinic Foundation
Cleveland, OH, USA

Jens H. Henriksen MD
Professor of Clinical Physiology
University of Copenhagen and Hvidovre
    Hospital
Hvidovre, Denmark

Manuel Hernández-Guerra MD
Liver Unit, Hospital Clinic
Barcelona, Spain

Humphrey J.F. Hodgson FMedSci
Sheila Sherlock Chair of Medicine
Director, The UCL Institute of Hepatology,
    Hampstead Campus
Vice Dean and Campus Director
Royal Free and University College School of
    Medicine
London, UK

Chantal Housset MD PhD
Professor of Cell Biology
Université Pierre et Marie Curie Paris 6;
Director, Inserm U680, Hôpital Tenon;
Service de Biochimie–Hormonologie, Hôpital
    Saint-Antoine
Paris, France

Hongjin Huang PhD
Associate Director, Liver Diseases, Celera
Alameda, CA, USA

Harriet Hughes MD
Hospital for Tropical Diseases
London, UK

Alvin B. Imaeda MD PhD
Yale University School of Medicine
New Haven, CT, USA

John P. Iredale BM DM FRCP FMedSci
Professor of Medicine
University of Edinburgh
Edinburgh, UK

Yoshiya Ito MD PhD
Research Associate
University of Arizona College of Medicine
Tucson, AZ, USA

Ravi Iyengar MD
Department of Pharmacology and Biological
    Chemistry
Mount Sinai School of Medicine
New York, NY, USA

Elmar Jaeckel MD
Department of Gastroenterology, Hepatology and
    Endocrinology
Hanover Medical School
Hanover, Germany

Hartmut Jaeschke MD
Department of Pharmacology
University of Arizona
Tucson, AZ, USA

Rajiv Jalan MB BS MD FRCP PhD
Senior Lecturer and Honorary Consultant in
    Hepatology
The UCL Institute of Hepatology
London, UK

Oliver F.W. James BM FRCP
Professor, Centre for Liver Research
University of Newcastle upon Tyne
Newcastle upon Tyne, UK

Peter L.M. Jansen MD
Professor of Medicine
Academic Medical Center
Amsterdam, The Netherlands

Regine Kahl MD
Professor and Head of Institute of Toxicology
University of Dusseldorf
Dusseldorf, Germany

Sanjeeva P. Kalva MD DNB
Assistant Radiologist
Massachusetts General Hospital;
Clinical Instructor
Harvard Medical School
Boston, MA, USA

Igal Kam MD
Chief of Transplant Surgery
University of Colorado Health Sciences
    Centre
Denver, CO, USA

Keishi Kanno MD PhD
Research Fellow, Division of Gastroenterology
Brigham and Women's Hospital and Harvard
    Medical School
Boston, MA, USA

Neil Kaplowitz MD
Professor of Medicine
Keck School of Medicine
University of Southern California
Los Angeles, CA, USA

Saul J. Karpen MD PhD
Associate Professor of Pediatrics
Director, Texas Children's Liver Center
Baylor College of Medicine,
Houston, TX, USA

Mark T. Keegan MB BCh BAO BA MRCPI
Associate Professor of Anesthesia
Consultant in Anesthesia and Critical Care
Mayo Clinic College of Medicine
Rochester, MN, USA

Susanne Keiding MD DSc
Professor, Department of Medicine V
Aarhus University Hospital
Aarhus, Denmark

David Kershenobich MD PhD
Department of Experimental Medicine
National Autonomous University of Mexico
Mexico City, Mexico

Zahida Khan PhD
Department of Pathology
University of Pittsburgh School of Medicine
Pittsburgh, PA, USA

W. Ray Kim MD
Associate Professor of Medicine
Mayo Clinic College of Medicine
Rochester, MN, USA

Raymond S. Koff MD
Clinical Professor of Medicine
University of Connecticut School of
    Medicine
Farmington, CT, USA

Soichi Kojima PhD
Molecular Cellular Pathology Research Unit
RIKEN
Wako, Japan

Masamichi Kojiro MD
Department of Pathology
Kurume University School of Medicine
Kurume, Japan

Sean W.P. Koppe MD
Fellow in Gastroenterology and Hepatology
Northwestern University Feinberg School of
  Medicine
Chicago, IL, USA

Krzysztof Krawczynski MD PhD
Distinguished Consultant, Division of Viral Hepatitis
Centers for Disease Control and Prevention
Atlanta, GA, USA

Michael J. Krowka MD
Professor of Medicine
Mayo Clinic College of Medicine
Rochester, MN, USA

Yolanta T. Kruszynska MD
Associate Professor of Medicine
University of California at San Diego
La Jolla, CA, USA

Thomas G. Ksiazek DVM PhD
Branch Chief, Special Pathogens Branch
Centers for Disease Control and Prevention
Atlanta, GA, USA

Laura M. Kulik MD
Transplant Hepatologist
Northwestern Memorial Hospital
Chicago, IL, USA

Philippe Labrune MD PhD
Professor and Head of Department of Paediatric and
  Medical Genetics
Hôpital Antoine Béclère
Clamart, France

Antonio Lacy MD
Jefe de Sección, Cirugía Gastrointestinal
Institut Clínic de Malaties Digestives i Metaboliques
Hospital Clinic
Barcelona, Spain

Glen A. Laine MD PhD
Wiseman-Lewie-Worth Chair in Cardiology
Director, Michael E. DeBakey Institute
Texas A&M University
College Station, TX, USA

Frank Lammert MD
Professor of Medicine
University of Bonn;
Department of Internal Medicine I
University Hospital Bonn
Bonn, Germany

Dominique Larrey MD PhD
Professor of Hepatology
Montpellier School of Medicine;
Head, Department of Hepatogastroenterology and
  Transplantation
CHU Saint-Eloi
Montpellier, France

Nicholas F. LaRusso MD
Chair, Department of Internal Medicine
Professor of Medicine and Biochemistry/Molecular
  Biology
Mayo Clinic College of Medicine
Rochester, MN, USA

Bernhard H. Lauterburg MD
Department of Clinical Pharmacology
University of Bern
Bern, Switzerland

Daniel Lavanchy MD MHEM
Department of Epidemic and Pandemic Alert and
  Response
World Health Organization
Geneva, Switzerland

Konstantinos N. Lazaridis MD
Assistant Professor of Medicine
Mayo Clinic College of Medicine
Rochester, MN, USA

Brigitte Le Bail MD
Professor of Pathology
Université Bordeaux
Bordeaux, France

Gioacchino Leandro MD
Consultant Gastroenterologist
IRCCS De Bellis
Castellana Grotte, Italy

Didier Lebrec MD
Service d'Hépatologie
Hôpital Beaujon
Clichy, France

Frédéric P. Lemaigre MD PhD
Professor, Christian de Duve Institute of Cellular
  Pathology
Université Catholique de Louvain
Brussels, Belgium

Riccardo Lencioni MD
Associate Professor of Radiology
University of Pisa
Pisa, Italy

Chris Liddle BSc (Med) MB BS PhD FRACP
Associate Dean, Information Technology
Professor of Clinical Pharmacology and Hepatology
University of Sydney
Sydney, NSW, Australia

Vishwanath R. Lingappa MD
California Pacific Medical Center
San Francisco, CA, USA

Josep María Llovet MD
Professor of Research – ICREA
Liver Unit, Hospital Clinic
Barcelona, Spain

Yang Lu MD
Department of Medicine
Albert Einstein College of Medicine
Bronx, NY, USA

Tom Luedde MD PhD
Institute of Genetics
University of Cologne
Cologne, Germany

Geoffrey W. McCaughan MB BS PhD FRACP
A.W. Morrow Professor of Medicine
  (Gastroenterology and Hepatology)
The University of Sydney and Royal Prince Alfred
  Hospital Centenary Research Institute
Sydney, NSW, Australia

P. Aiden McCormick MD
Newman Clinical Research Professor
University College Dublin;
Consultant Hepatologist, Liver Unit
St Vincent's Hospital
Dublin, Ireland

Robert S. McCuskey PhD
Professor of Cell Biology, Pediatrics and
  Physiology
University of Arizona
Tucson, AZ, USA

Pietro E. Majno MD FRCS
Transplantation Unit
Hôpitaux Universitaires de Genève
Geneva, Switzerland

Nisar P. Malek MD
Consultant in Internal Medicine and
  Gastroenterology
Hanover Medical School
Hanover, Germany

Susan V. Mallett MB BS FRCA
Consultant Anaesthetist
The Royal Free Hospital
London, UK

Michael P. Manns MD
Department of Gastroenterology
Hanover Medical School
Hanover, Germany

G.A. Mantion MD
Department of Hepatology and Liver
  Diseases
Hôpital Jean-Minjoz
Besançon, France

Luz Martín-Carbonero MD
Department of Infectious Diseases
Hospital Carlos III
Madrid, Spain

Carmen Martínez MD
Hematology Department
Hospital Clinic
Barcelona, Spain

Rie Matsushima-Nishiwaki MD
First Department of Internal Medicine
Gifu University School of Medicine
Gifu, Japan

Wajahat Z. Mehal MD DPhil
Yale University School of Medicine
New Haven, CT, USA

**Fernando E. Membreno
MD MSc**
Director of Hepatology and Liver Transplantation
Methodist Specialty and Transplant Hospital
San Antonio, TX, USA

**Giorgina Mieli-Vergani MD PhD
FRCP FRCPCH**
Alex Mowat Professor of Paediatric Hepatology
King's College London School of Medicine
London, UK

J.P. Miguet MD
Department of Hepatology and Liver Diseases
Hôpital Jean-Minjoz
Besançon, France

Piotr Milkiewicz MD PhD MRCP
Associate Professor and Reader in Hepatology
Pomeranian Medical School
Szczecin, Poland

**Elisabeth Irene Minder
ProfDrMed**
Chefärztin, Zentrallabor
Stadtspital Triemli
Zurich, Switzerland

Rosa Miquel MD
Servicio de Anatomia Patologica
Hospital Clinic
Barcelona, Spain

Søren Møller MD DMSc
Chief Physician and Associate Professor
Department Clinical Physiology
Hvidovre Hospital
Hvidovre, Denmark

Richard Moreau MD
Service d'Hépatologie
Hôpital Beaujon
Clichy, France

**Michael H. Nathanson MD
PhD**
Professor of Medicine and Cell Biology
Chief, Section of Digestive Diseases
Yale University School of Medicine
New Haven, CT, USA

Miguel Navasa MD
Liver Unit, Hospital Clinic
Barcelona, Spain

James Neuberger DM FRCP
Consultant Physician
Queen Elizabeth Hospital
Birmingham, UK

Peter Neuhaus MD
Professor of Surgery
Charite Campus Virchow Clinic
Berlin, Germany

**Brent A. Neuschwander-Tetri MD
FACP**
Professor of Internal Medicine
Saint Louis University School of Medicine
St. Louis, MO, USA

Susana Neves MD
Department of Pharmacology and Biological
    Chemistry
Mount Sinai School of Medicine
New York, NY, USA

Patrick G. Northup MD MHES
Assistant Professor, Gastroenterology and
    Hepatology
University of Virginia
Charlottesville, VA, USA

Phyllis M. Novikoff PhD
Associate Professor
Albert Einstein College of Medicine
Bronx, NY, USA

Marina Nuñez MD
Department of Infectious Diseases
Hospital Carlos III
Madrid, Spain

Satoshi Ogata MD
Hôpital Beaujon
Clichy, France

Masataka Okuno MD
First Department of Internal Medicine
Gifu University School of Medicine
Gifu, Japan

J. Donald Ostrow MD
Affiliated Professor of Medicine
Gastrointestinal and Hepatology Division
University of Washington School of
    Medicine
Seattle, WA, USA

Ronald P.J. Oude Elferink
Professor of Experimental Hepatology
AMC Liver Center
Amsterdam, The Netherlands

Mario Pagano MD
Department of Pharmacology and Biological
    Chemistry
Mount Sinai School of Medicine
New York, NY, USA

**Georges-Philippe Pageaux
MD PhD**
Professor of Hepatology
CHU Saint-Eloi
Montpellier, France

Valérie Paradis MD PhD
Professor of Pathology, Université Denis Diderot
    Paris 7;
Assistance Publique – Hôpitaux de Paris and Inserm
    U773;
Department of Pathology, Hôpital Beaujon
Clichy, France

Stephen M. Pastores MD
Associate Attending Physician
Memorial Sloan-Kettering Cancer Center
New York, NY, USA

Heinz-Otto Peitgen PhD
Professor and President of MeVis Research
MeVis Research GmbH
Bremen, Germany

Pascal Perney MD
Professor of Internal Medicine
CHU Saint-Eloi
Montpellier, France

Jean-Marie Péron MD PhD
Professor of Hepatogastroenterology
Service d'Hépatogastroenterologie
Toulouse, France

Dominique Pessayre MD
Director of Research
Université Paris 7
Paris, France

Antonello Pietrangelo MD PhD
Professor of Medicine
Center for Hemochromatosis
University of Modena and Reggio Emilia
Modena, Italy

Massimo Pinzani MD PhD
Professor of Medicine
Dipartmento di Medicina Interna
Università delgi Studi di Firenze
Florence, Italy

Fabio Piscaglia MD
Department of Internal Medicine and Gastroenterology
University of Bologna
Bologna, Italy

David J. Plevak MD
Professor of Anesthesiology
Mayo Clinic College of Medicine
Rochester, MN, USA

K. Raj Prasad MS MCh FRCS
Consultant Surgeon
St James's University Hospital
Leeds, UK

Gerhard P. Püschel MD
Full Professor and Head, Department of
    Biochemistry of Nutrition
Institute of Nutrition Science
University of Potsdam
Potsdam, Germany

Hervé Puy MD PhD
Professor of Biochemistry and Molecular Biology
Vice President of the French Porphyria Center
Hôpital Louis Mourier
Colombes, France

Alberto Queiroz Farias MD PhD
Department of Gastroenterology
University of São Paulo School of Medicine
São Paulo, Brazil

Montse Renom MD
Centro de Salud Internacional
Hospital Clinic
Barcelona, Spain

Kalpana Reddy MB BS FRCA
Specialist Registrar in Anaesthesia and Intensive Care
    Medicine
Royal London Hospital
London, UK

Helen L. Reeves BM BS BMedSci MRCP FRCP(Ed) PhD
Senior Lecturer and Honorary Consultant
    Gastroenterologist
University of Newcastle upon Tyne
Newcastle upon Tyne, UK

Jürg Reichen MD
Professor of Medicine
University of Bern;
Chief of Hepatology
University Hospital
Bern, Switzerland

Igino Rigato MD
Liver Research Center
University of Trieste
Trieste, Italy

Antoni Rimola MD PhD
Senior Consultant
Liver Unit, Hospital Clinic
Barcelona, Spain

Mario Rizzetto MD
Professor of Gastroenterology
University of Turin
Turin, Italy

Guillermo Robles-Diaz MD
Department of Experimental Medicine
National Autonomous University of Mexico
Mexico City, Mexico

Juan Rodés MD
Director General
Hospital Clinic;
Professor of Medicine
University of Barcelona
Barcelona, Spain

Pierre E. Rollin MD
Team Leader, Disease Assessment Section
Centers for Disease Control and Prevention
Atlanta, GA, USA

Tania Roskams MD
Professor of Pathology
University of Leuven
Leuven, Belgium

Jayanta Roy-Chowdhury MD MRCP
Professor, Departments of Medicine and Molecular
    Genetics
Albert Einstein College of Medicine
Bronx, NY, USA

Namita Roy-Chowdhury MD PhD
Professor, Departments of Medicine and Molecular
    Genetics
Albert Einstein College of Medicine
Bronx, NY, USA

Antoni Rimola MD PhD
Senior Consultant
Liver Unit, Hospital Clinic
Barcelona, Spain

K. Lenhard Rudolph MD
Heisenberg Professor for Regenerative Medicine and
    Ageing
Hanover Medical School
Hanover, Germany

Luis Ruiz-del-Arbol MD
Associate Professor
Universidad de Alcala and Hospital Ramón y Cajal
Madrid, Spain

Malcolm Rustin BSc MD FRCP
Consultant Dermatologist
The Royal Free Hospital
London, UK

Pierre Rustin PhD
CNRS Research Director
Hôpital Robert Debré
Paris, France

Dushyant V. Sahani MD
Department of Radiology
Massachusetts General Hospital
Boston, MA, USA

Faouzi Saliba MD
Associate Professor
Hôpital Paul Brousse
Villejuif, France

Didier Samuel MD PhD
Professor
Hôpital Paul Brousse
Villejuif, France

Marianne Samyn MD FRCPCH
Consultant Paediatric Hepatologist
King's College London School of Medicine
London, UK

José M. Sánchez-Tapias MD PhD
Senior Consultant
Liver Unit, Hospital Clinic
Barcelona, Spain

Giorgio Saracco MD
Associate Professor of Gastroenterology
University of Turin
Turin, Italy

Tilman Sauerbruch MD
Professor of Medicine
University of Bonn;
Head, Department of Medicine
University Hospital Bonn
Bonn, Germany

Erez F. Scapa MD
Research Fellow, Division of Gastroenterology
Harvard Medical School
Boston, MA, USA

Stephan Schaefer PD DrMed
Provisional Head, Institut für Medizinische
    Mikrobiologie, Virologie und Hygiene
Universität Rostock
Rostock, Germany

Michael Schilsky MD
Associate Professor of Clinical Medicine
Weill Medical College of Cornell University;
Medical Director, Center for Liver Disease and
    Transplantation
Weill Cornell Medical Center
New York, NY, USA

Xiaoye Schneider-Yin PhD
Biochemikerin, Zentrallabor
Stadtspital Triemli
Zurich, Switzerland

Henning Schulze-Bergkamen MD
1st Medical Department
University of Mainz
Mainz, Germany

Marcus Schuchmann MD
1st Medical Department
University of Mainz
Mainz, Germany

Detlef Schuppan MD PhD
Professor of Medicine
Harvard Medical School;
Consultant Hepatologist
Beth Israel Deaconess Medical Center
Boston, MA, USA

Nazia Selzner MD PhD
Transplant Hepatology Fellow
Multiorgan Transplant Program
Toronto General Hospital
Toronto, ON, Canada

David Semela MD
Instructor in Medicine
Mayo Clinic College of Medicine
Rochester, MN, USA

Marco Senzolo MD PhD
Consultant Physician in Gastroenterology
University Hospital of Padua
Padua, Italy

Devanshi Seth BSc MSc PhD
Senior Scientist, Royal Prince Alfred Hospital
Sydney, NSW, Australia

Nicholas A. Shackel MD
Centenary Institute of Cancer Medicine and Cell
    Biology
Royal Prince Alfred Hospital and The University of
    Sydney
Sydney, NSW, Australia

Vijay H. Shah MD
Associate Professor of Medicine, Physiology and
    Cancer Cell Biology
Mayo Clinic College of Medicine
Rochester, MN, USA

Marcelo Simão Ferreira MD
University of São Paulo School of Medicine
São Paulo, Brazil

Antonella Smedile MD
Department of Gastroenterology
Molinette Hospital
Turin, Italy

Michael Sørensen MD
Department of Medicine V
Aarhus University Hospital
Aarhus, Denmark

Vincent Soriano MD PhD
Section Chief, Department of Infectious Diseases
Hospital Carlos III
Madrid, Spain

Laurent Spahr MD
Médecin Adjoint Agrégé et Chargé de Cours
Service de Gastroentérologie et Hépatologie
Hôpitaux Universitaires de Genève
Geneva, Switzerland

Vanessa Stadlbauer MD
Clinical Research Fellow
The UCL Institute of Hepatology
London, UK

Peter Starkel MD PhD
Professor, Department of Gastroenterology
Universitaires Saint-Luc
Université Catholique de Louvain
Brussels, Belgium

**Catherine A.M. Stedman MB ChB
FRACP PhD**
Consultant Gastroenterologist and Clinical
    Pharmacologist
Christchurch Hospital
Christchurch, New Zealand

Stephen F. Stewart MB ChB PhD
Consultant Hepatologist
Freeman Hospital
Newcastle upon Tyne, UK

Felix Stickel MD
Assistant Professor and Consultant Hepatologist
Institute of Clinical Pharmacology
University of Bern
Bern, Switzerland

Bruno Stieger PhD
Department of Medicine
University Hospital
Zurich, Switzerland

Donna B. Stolz PhD
Assistant Director, Center for Biologic Imaging
University of Pittsburgh
Pittsburgh, MA, USA

Christoforos Stoupis MD
Radiologist, Kreisspital
Maennedorf, Switzerland

**Steven M. Strasberg MD FRCSC
FACS FRCS(Ed)**
Pruett Professor of Surgery
Washington University in St. Louis;
Head of Hepatopancreatobiliary Surgery
Barnes-Jewish Hospital
St. Louis, MO, USA

Edna Strauss MD PhD
Professor, School of Medicine
University of São Paulo School of Medicine
São Paulo, Brazil

Vinay Sundaram MD
Senior Resident, Department of Internal
    Medicine
University of Virginia
Charlottesville, VA, USA

Jacob I. Sznajder MD PhD
Professor of Medicine
Chief, Division of Pulmonary and Critical
    Medicine
Northwestern University Feinberg School of
    Medicine
Chicago, IL, USA

Jeffrey H. Teckman MD
Associate Professor of Pediatrics and Biochemistry
Saint Louis University School of Medicine
St. Louis, MO, USA

Carlos Terra MD
Department of Medicine, Hospital Clinic
Barcelona, Spain

**Sundararajah Thevananther
PhD**
Assistant Professor
Texas Children's Liver Center
Baylor College of Medicine
Houston, TX, USA

Claudio Tiribelli MD PhD
Professor of Medicine
Director, Liver Research Center
University of Trieste
Trieste, Italy

Susan Tiukinhoy-Laing MD
Division of Cardiology
Northwestern University Feinberg School of
    Medicine
Chicago, IL, USA

Giles J. Toogood MD
Consultant in Hepatobiliary Transplantation
St. James's University Hospital
Leeds, UK

James Toouli MB BS FRACS PhD
Professor of Surgery
Flinders University
Adelaide, SA, Australia

Michael Trauner MD
Professor of Medicine
Medical University Graz
Graz, Austria

Christian Trautwein MD
Professor, Medizinische Klinik III
University Hospital
Aachen, Germany

James Trotter MD
Associate Professor, Division of Gastroenterology
    and Hepatology
University of Colorado Health Sciences Center
Denver, CO, USA

Juan Turnes MD
Research Associate
Liver Unit, Hospital Clinic
Barcelona, Spain

Dominique-Charles Valla MD
Professor of Hepatology, Université Denis Diderot
    Paris 7;
Assistance Publique – Hôpitaux de Paris and Inserm
    U773;
Chief, Service d'Hépatologie, Hôpital Beaujon
Clichy, France

Pierre Van Damme MD PhD
Professor, Faculty of Medicine
University of Antwerp;
Director, WHO Collaborating Centre for the Control
    and Prevention of Viral Hepatitis
Antwerp, Belgium

Koen Van Herck MD
Research Assistant, Department of Epidemiology
    and Social Medicine
University of Antwerp
Wilrijk, Belgium

María Varela MD
Research Fellow
Liver Unit, Hospital Clinic
Barcelona, Spain

Jean-Nicolas Vauthey MD FACS
Professor of Surgery and Chief of Liver Service
University of Texas M.D. Anderson Cancer
    Center
Houston, TX, USA

**Diego Vergani MD PhD FRCP
FRCPath**
Professor and Director of the Alex Mowat
    Immunopathology Laboratory
King's College London School of Medicine
London, UK

Valérie Vilgrain MD
Professor of Radiology, Université Denis Diderot
    Paris 7;
Assistance Publique – Hôpitaux de Paris;
Chief, Department of Radiology, Hôpital
    Beaujon
Clichy, France

Jean-Pierre Vinel MD
Professor of Hepatogastroenterology
Service d'Hépatogastroenterologie
Toulouse, France

D.A. Vuitton MD PhD
Emeritus Professor of Clinical Immunology
Université de Franch-Comté
Besançon, France

Martin Wagner MD
Fellow, Medical University Graz
Graz, Austria

Wim Wätjen PhD
Institute of Toxicology
University of Dusseldorf
Dusseldorf, Germany

Heiner Wedemeyer MD
Department of Gastroenterology
Hanover Medical School
Hanover, Germany

Richard A. Weisiger MD PhD
Professor of Medicine
University of California
San Francisco, CA, USA

Rebecca G. Wells MD
Assistant Professor of Medicine and of Pathology and
    Laboratory Medicine
The University of Pennsylvania School of
    Medicine
Philadelphia, PA, USA

Alan J. Wigg MB BS FRACP PhD
Consultant Gastroenterology and Hepatologist
Flinders Medical Centre
Adelaide, SA, Australia

Rohan B.H. Williams PhD
School of Biotechnology and Biomolecular
    Sciences
University of New South Wales
Sydney, NSW, Australia

R.M. Winter MD
Professor of Dysmorphlogy and Clinical
    Genetics
Institute of Child Health
London, UK

Allan W. Wolkoff MD
Professor, Department of Medicine
Albert Einstein College of Medicine
Bronx, NY, USA

John B. Wong MD
Chief, Division of Clinical Decision Making
Tufts-New England Medical Center;
Professor of Medicine
Tufts University School of Medicine
Boston, MA, USA

Govardhana Rao Yannam MD MRCS
Postdoctoral Research Associate
University of Nebraska Medical Center
Omaha, NE, USA

Elie Serge Zafrani MD
Professor of Pathology
Hôpital Henri Mondor
Creteil, France

Arthur Zimmermann MD
Professor of Pathology
University of Bern
Bern, Switzerland

Fabien Zoulim MD PhD
Professor of Medicine, Université Lyon 1;
Liver Department, Hospices Civils de Lyon;
Head, Inserm U8712
Lyon, France

Foreword

Juan Rodés and I conceived the idea of this book at his summer house in Montferri in the late 1980s, envisaging it as a predominantly European text. We had both been active in the organization of the European Association for the Study of the Liver (EASL) so, not surprisingly, we chose as fellow editors our friends Jean-Pierre Benhamou (France), Johannes Bircher (Switzerland) and Mario Rizzetto (Italy), all past secretaries of EASL. The five of us met several times in different cities to plan the book.

In the preface to the first edition, which appeared in 1991, we noted our wish to produce a comprehensive account of clinical hepatology, covering not only common liver problems but also the rare conditions seen from time to time by gastroenterologists, and general physicians and surgeons, as well as by hepatologists. We felt it important to cover the effects of liver disease on other parts of the body, and to describe how diseases of other systems affected the liver, interactions which often cause confusing clinical pictures. We added some appendices: one listed non-drug chemicals and toxins causing liver damage, another gave the geographical distribution of infectious diseases, and a third listed some rare diseases in which the liver may be involved, particularly in children. These appendices have been retained.

As we noted in the preface to the second edition, the first enjoyed considerable success and achieved much critical acclaim. I certainly found it useful in my own practice. In the second edition the focus on clinical medicine was strengthened, as it has been in this edition, and the emphasis in the basic science sections was placed on new concepts and techniques. As a result of these changes some material has had to be left out so, as is the case with some other reference books, the hungry reader of this edition may well find pearls by returning to some of the chapters in the second edition.

The present edition, which I am delighted to see is accompanied by a CD, has retained the general format of the two earlier editions, but several topics have been greatly expanded. Clinicians will welcome the increased number of subsections on liver transplantation, imaging and the complex area of congenital and acquired non-infectious conditions which cause fibrosis or cystic change in the liver or biliary tract. In the basic science sections there are more contributions dealing with molecular and cell biology, genetic aspects of liver disease and immunology. One interesting innovation is the introduction of a section on mathematics in hepatology, which I suspect will lead to some interesting developments in future editions.

The number of individual contributions has risen from 146 in the first edition to 209 in this one; the number in the basic science sections has doubled – from 25 to 51. The first edition involved 193 authors; 333 have contributed to this one. Based on past experience, the editors' problems in getting manuscripts in on time must have been formidable. Although the book still has a distinctly European flavour there are contributions from many other countries. The proportion coming from the USA has risen from 9% in the first edition to 24% in this one; the American influence is particularly evident in the coverage of molecular and cell biology.

Johannes Bircher and I stepped down as editors for this edition. That our former editorial colleagues enrolled seven others to join them, two of them based in the USA, reflects the increasing complexity of our knowledge of the liver and its diseases. This book is an attempt to clarify the field for others. I wish Juan, Jean-Pierre and Mario and their new colleagues, and their new publisher, Blackwell Publishing Ltd, every success with this splendid third edition.

Neil McIntyre

Preface to the third edition

This is now the third edition of a textbook the first edition of which was conceived and published back in 1992. In this edition, important changes have been introduced to bring the style of the book more up to date under the guidance of Blackwell Publishing Ltd. Their professionalism, management skills and hard work has helped us to produce this new and exciting edition. The editors, Juan Rodés, Jean-Pierre Benhamou, Andres Blei, Jürg Reichen, Mario Rizzetto, and associate editors, Jean-François Dufour, Scott Friedman, Pere Ginès, Dominique-Charles Valla and Fabien Zoulim, would like to express their deepest gratitude, especially to Alison Brown (Publisher) and Rebecca Huxley (Senior Development Editor).

When this book was first published, there were five editors: Neil McIntyre, Johannes Bircher, Jean-Pierre Benhamou, Mario Rizzetto and Juan Rodés. In this edition, two of the former editors have retired but we are honoured that one has continued his involvement by writing the foreword to the book. Their collaboration on the first two editions deserves our grateful recognition as it set the *Textbook of Hepatology* in process. This third edition has brought about significant changes to the editorial team, which now includes friends and colleagues from the other side of the Atlantic, Andres Blei and Scott Friedman. This has achieved our objective of making the *Textbook* more international.

At the first meeting of the editors and associate editors, it was quickly agreed that the *Textbook* should present the substantial scientific progress that has taken place over the last few years: concepts such as genomics, proteomics, gene arrays, metabolomics, bioinformatics, stem cells, molecular and cell biology, and genetics are now extensively covered throughout the book.

The most significant changes can probably be seen in the sections on functions of the liver, basic concepts of pathobiology, assessment of hepatobiliary disease, portal hypertension and its complications, congenital hepatic fibrosis and non-parasitic cystic diseases of the liver, hepatic non-alcoholic steatosis, tumours of the liver, liver transplantation, and mathematics in hepatology. We have encouraged the use of tables and figures to aid interpretation and understanding. The scientific information is current and exhaustive and is essential for clinical decision making whether diagnostic or therapeutic. We also believe that this book fulfils the requisites necessary for it to be highly useful for translational research.

On this occasion the book has over 200 chapters, contributed by authors from five continents. Our objective of delivering an excellent book has been achieved with the help of everyone who has participated in the book. We fully understand the pressures of time on everyone and for this reason we are very grateful to all of them. Our thanks in particular go to Nicki van Berckel, who also found time to have her second baby, Dylan, and the Senior Development Editor at Blackwell Publishing Ltd, Rebecca Huxley, whose experience has been invaluable. Sincerest thanks to all involved in taking this project to completion.

Juan Rodés
Jean-Pierre Benhamou
Andres T. Blei
Jürg Reichen
Mario Rizzetto
Jean-François Dufour
Scott L. Friedman
Pere Ginès
Dominique-Charles Valla
Fabien Zoulim

Preface to the first edition

We all met several times, in different cities, to plan this book. We wanted to produce a comprehensive account of clinical hepatology, covering not only the common hepatological problems but also the rare conditions which are seen from time to time by hepatologists, gastroenterologists, and general physicians. We thought it important to consider how the liver may be affected in diseases of other systems, and to describe the effects of diseases of the liver on other parts of the body, as these interactions often create a confusing clinical picture; these topics occupy two large sections of the book which should be of particular value to general physicians and specialists in other diseases. We felt a need for a fuller than usual account of the effect of infections on the liver; patients with bacterial, fungal and parasitic infections, and those with viral infections other than the classical viral hepatitides, often have abnormal liver function tests, or symptoms or signs suggesting liver disease.

There are chapters on other topics which have received little attention in other texts, such as symptoms and signs, diagnostic strategy, general management, and prescribing and anaesthesia in liver disease. There are chapters on liver disease in children, in the elderly, and in drug addicts and homosexual men, and one on the history of liver disease.

We also thought it would be helpful to have some appendices: listing non-drug chemicals and toxins causing liver damage, the geographical distribution of infectious diseases, and the rare diseases in which the liver may be involved (particularly in children). Another appendix contains the excellent handouts produced for patients by the American Liver Foundation.

Colleagues often remark that it is irritating, when reading chapters with many references, to have to search at the end of the chapter to find the original sources. We therefore decided to use mainly short 'text references' to enable readers to decide quickly if they are already familiar with the source and, if not, to allow them to jot the reference down with the minimum of effort. We consider this experiment to have been worthwhile, but we hope that readers will tell us if they prefer the conventional approach.

More than 200 authors have contributed to this book; nearly all are acknowledged internationally as experts in their field(s) of interest. We are grateful to all of them. We believe that their expertise is reflected in their contributions, many of which we consider to be quite outstanding.

Our major purpose was to provide a book for practising clinicians. We hope this text will prove useful not only to hepatologists, gastroenterologists, and general physicians, but also to specialists in other fields. It was for this reason that we chose the title 'clinical hepatology'. We believe that this book will provide solutions to many of the hepatological problems which arise in clinical practice, but only our readers can tell whether our belief is justified. If, when using this book, you fail to find the information you are seeking, we would be grateful if you could draw these omissions to our attention (using the cards enclosed), so that they can be corrected in the next edition.

Our book is being brought out in English, French, and Spanish. We would like to thank the staff of the Oxford University Press, Flammarion, and Salvat, not only for their willingness to publish it but for their help and enthusiasm during the long gestation period. We are particularly grateful to the executive editor for the book, Irene Butcher, who dealt initially with all the manuscripts, and later with the galleys and page proofs of this English edition.

Neil McIntyre
Jean-Pierre Benhamou
Johannes Bircher
Mario Rizetto
Juan Rodés

1 Architecture of the liver

1.1 Macroscopic anatomy of the liver

Jean H.D. Fasel, Holger Bourquain, Heinz-Otto Peitgen and Pietro E. Majno

External anatomy

Naturally enough, the human liver was first described according to its external appearance. Under this heading, four traditional anatomical lobes can regularly be distinguished that are demarcated by peritoneal folds, hepatic fissures, extrahepatic blood vessels and extrahepatic bile ducts (Fig. 1).

In an anterior view, the liver appears to be unequally divided into a large right and a small left anatomical lobe by the attachment of the falciform ligament, which reaches the liver by extending obliquely to the right from the midline of the anterior body wall and the caudal surface of the anterior portion of the diaphragm. Lying in the free edge of the falciform ligament, from the umbilicus to the notch between the two lobes, is the round ligament (ligamentum teres hepatis), the remains of the left umbilical vein. The round ligament, normally avascular, is accompanied by paraumbilical veins, which connect the portal vein to veins of the anterior abdominal wall and form part of the potential portocaval collateral circulation. On the visceral surface of the liver, the round ligament runs in the fissure for that ligament and joins the lower end of the umbilical part of the left branch of the portal vein. The left lobe regularly ends in a fibrous appendix.

Although the apparent division of the liver on its anterior surface is into the right and left anatomical lobes, the inferoposterior surface shows the liver hilus (also called porta hepatis or transverse fissure) and four longitudinal markings that delimit additional lobes. These landmarks together are customarily considered to form the letter H, and the parts of the liver between the uprights of the letter are the quadrate and caudate (spigelian) lobe. The fossa of the gallbladder separates the quadrate lobe from the remainder of the right lobe; the left boundary of the quadrate lobe is the fissure that lodges the round ligament (also called the umbilical sulcus). The posterior boundary of the quadrate lobe is the porta hepatis, where the hepatoduodenal ligament attaches to the liver, and through which the portal vein, hepatic arteries and bile ducts enter or leave the liver. The porta hepatis is also the anterior margin of the caudate lobe, which cannot easily be seen in the normally attached liver, as it lies above and behind the lesser omentum, its posteroinferior surface forming the anterior wall of the superior recess of the omental bursa. The caudate lobe is largely separated from the remainder of the right anatomical lobe by the fossa of the vena cava. However, a bridge of liver tissue – the caudate process – connects the caudate and the right lobes between the inferior vena cava and the porta hepatis. The inferior end of the caudate lobe sometimes forms a papillary process. The fissures of the round and venous ligaments are usually continuous with each other and are therefore sometimes referred to as the left sagittal fissure.

The ligamentum venosum is a fibrous cord passing from the left branch of the portal vein to the left hepatic vein just before this enters the inferior vena cava. It represents the remains of a venous shunt, the ductus venosus, established in prenatal life to allow blood returning from the placenta to reach the heart

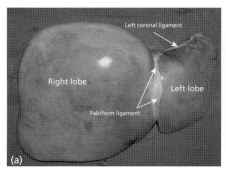
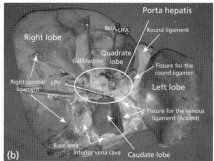

Fig. 1 External aspect of the liver in an anterior (a) and an inferior view (b). Cannulas have been inserted into the right and left branches of the portal vein (RPV, LPV), the right and left branches of the proper hepatic artery (RHA, LHA) and the common bile duct.

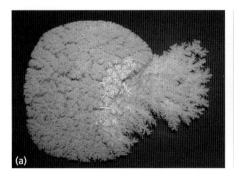 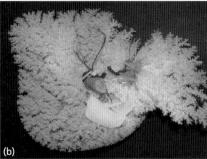

Fig. 2 Internal architecture of the same liver as in Fig. 1, seen as a corrosion cast, reproduced in an anterior (a) and an inferior view (b).

without the necessity of passing through the liver. The portal end of the ductus venosus closes within the first 2 days of postnatal life; the hepatic end, however, may remain patent throughout life, and may then receive tributaries from the liver and the hepatogastric ligament, so that it may function as a hepatic vein in the adult [1].

As it passes behind the liver, the inferior vena cava is embedded in a sulcus on the posterior surface of the liver. It is typically attached in the sulcus not only by loose connective tissue and a variable number of smaller hepatic veins that enter it, but also by more dense tissue which forms a transverse band posterior to the vena cava. Sometimes, also, hepatic parenchyma extends posterior to the vena cava, so that the vessel is partly embedded in the liver.

As far as the peritoneal attachments of the liver are concerned, its chief attachment to the diaphragm is by the right and left coronary ligament. These peritoneal bridges consist of an anterior and a posterior layer that bound the bare area (area nuda). In this area, the liver connects to the diaphragm mostly by fibrous attachments and by the hepatic veins. The right and left coronary ligaments extend laterally and form the triangular ligaments. The posterior layer of the right coronary ligament is sometimes called the hepatorenal ligament, because it is in continuity with the posterior parietal peritoneum lying in front of the right kidney. The liver is connected to the stomach and duodenal bulb by the lesser omentum. This extends to the porta hepatis and the fissure for the ligamentum venosum; it is continuous with the posterior coronary ligaments. The portion attaching to the stomach is also called the hepatogastric ligament, and that attaching to the duodenum, the hepatoduodenal ligament. In addition, peritoneal folds can extend from the liver to the right colic flexure.

This basic description of external features of the liver should not be mistaken for a comprehensive presentation. It has particularly to be remembered that the anatomical appearance of the liver, as for every organ, is subject to wide variability.

Internal anatomy

Although the external aspect of the human liver has been known for centuries, comprehensive and systematic investigations regarding the internal architecture of the organ began around 1880. Naturally enough, these studies were undertaken by anatomists [2–4]. Fifty years later, the question was raised again, particularly by surgeons willing to develop hepatic resectional techniques [5–10]. In the past 20 years, we have witnessed a third wave of interest, spurred by the dramatic developments in imaging techniques. These investigations were brought about principally by radiologists and the need for accurate preoperative localization of focal hepatic lesions [11–14].

Summarizing these investigations, the internal architecture of the human liver can be described with reference to several structures, such as the intrahepatic branches of the portal vein, hepatic arteries, bile ducts and hepatic veins (Fig. 2). The branches of the first three entities are densely interwoven within connective tissue sheaths and form the triad credited to Glisson [15]. The dual supply of the liver is taken over by the hepatic artery and the portal vein.

Arterial supply

The most frequently observed pattern of arterial blood supply to the liver consists of a purely coeliac origin, and is by a common hepatic artery. After it has branched off the gastroduodenal artery, it becomes the proper hepatic artery, which further divides into a right and a left hepatic artery. This pattern is considered to occur in between 44% and 88% of cases. The very different frequencies reported in the literature must be considered with caution, particularly because the terminologies and classifications used are of the utmost variability and have led to confusion, as demonstrated by Feigl and colleagues [16].

Variations from the standard pattern above are common. The two most frequent variants are the right hepatic artery originating from the superior mesenteric artery (11–21%) and the left hepatic artery arising from the left gastric artery (10–30%). It has to be remembered that such variant arteries, even when labelled as accessory in the literature, represent the sole supply of a specific territory of the liver [17,18]. Their ligation could produce hepatic ischaemia of the area they supply. Arterial distribution to different hepatic territories is generally assumed to be identical to the distribution of the portal vein [19].

Portal venous supply

In its prevailing pattern, the portal vein is formed from the convergence of the superior mesenteric and splenic veins. It is about 8 cm long and lies anterior to the inferior vena cava and posterior to the neck of the pancreas. It runs obliquely to the right and ascends behind the first part of the duodenum, the common bile duct and the gastroduodenal artery. At this point, it is directly anterior to the inferior vena cava. It enters the right border of the lesser omentum and ascends anterior to the epiploic foramen to reach the right end of the porta hepatis. In the hepatoduodenal ligament, it lies, in general, posterior to both the common bile duct and the hepatic artery. It is surrounded by the hepatic nerve plexus and accompanied by many lymph vessels. It regularly bifurcates into a right and a left portal branch. The right branch is located anterior to the caudate process and enters the right lobe. It gives rise to one to eight branches before dividing, in general, into two major trunks of almost the same diameter [20–22]. The left branch has a longer extrahepatic course and lies more horizontal than the right branch, and is often of smaller calibre. Two portions can regularly be distinguished, the transverse and the umbilical part of the left portal vein. Two to six branches arise from the transverse portion, the transition from the transverse to the umbilical portion regularly gives off one major branch, and the umbilical portion is the origin of 3–26 branches [20–23].

Venous drainage

Many studies have confirmed large variability in hepatic vein anatomy [e.g. 24–26]. In the predominant pattern, most of the hepatic venous effluent drains into the inferior vena cava by means of three major hepatic veins, right, middle and left. These veins have an extrahepatic length of about 1 cm. Within the liver, the main trunks are considered to run between the Glissonian territories (i.e. within the planes that lie between the areas supplied by a given portovenous, arterial and biliary branch) as the intertwining fingers of two hands. They drain adjacent Glissonian territories. In about 70% of individuals, the middle and left hepatic veins join each other to form a common trunk before entering the inferior vena cava. In addition, 10–20 small inferior hepatic veins (not only from the caudate lobe) drain directly into the inferior vena cava at its retrohepatic portion [19,25]. In about 20% of cases, a significant inferior right hepatic vein has been observed. However, these inferior hepatic veins also vary in the extent of their distribution. According to van Leeuwen [27], the area drained by right accessory veins is inversely proportional to the area drained by the conventional right hepatic vein. Sometimes (8% in the study by Masselot and Leborgne [24]), the right hepatic vein is reduced to an accessory vein, with a larger part of the right dorsal area of the liver being drained by right inferior veins and branches of the middle hepatic vein. In the era of increasing surgical demand for anatomical details, Mehran et al. [28] emphasized the value of the minor hepatic veins.

Biliary drainage

Hjortsö [5] introduced the concept that the intrahepatic branching of the biliary ducts follows a segmental pattern, in the sense that each region of the liver has its specific type of bile drainage. This view was supported by investigations focusing on the biliary system within the human liver [7,29]. Because it is generally agreed that the intrahepatic bile ducts follow an essentially similar type of branching to the corresponding branches of the portal vein and hepatic artery, the biliary territories are considered to be identical to the portalvenous and arterial territories [30]. In contrast to the portal vein branches, which may communicate, no communications have been observed in biliary branches [31].

Lymphatics

The hepatic lymphatic network – not seen at a macroscopic level – is traditionally subdivided into a superficial and a deep system. The superficial vessels are mainly situated in the liver capsule. The deep ones follow the Glissonian triads or the efferent hepatic veins and are said to drain adjacent Glissonian territories [19,32,33]. Lymphatic vessels may thus leave the liver at the inferior and superior liver hilus (porta hepatis or together with the hepatic veins respectively), or run within the peritoneal attachments of the liver mentioned above [34]. The existence of afferent lymph vessels is controversial [33]. Examples of regional lymph nodes are thus situated at the porta hepatis, at the junction between the hepatic veins and the inferior vena cava or in the anterior mediastinum. Further lymphatic drainage reaches nodes both below and above the diaphragm, the greatest outflow being attributed to the thoracic duct.

Innervation

The liver has a dual innervation. The area nuda and adjacent capsule are supplied by somatoafferent branches of the right phrenic nerve, which also supply the parietal peritoneum of the region. The parenchyma is supplied by vegetative plexus originating from the coeliac plexus and the vagal nerves. They surround the branches of the portal vein, hepatic arteries and biliary ducts or run within the cranial part of the lesser omentum [35]. They are considered to carry sympathetic, parasympathetic and visceroafferent fibres.

Divisions of the liver

The liver has been subdivided on the basis of both its external aspect and its internal architecture. As mentioned, the classical anatomical subdivision is based on external landmarks and discerns four lobes (Fig. 1). This partition has been largely extended, particularly since the 1950s, by surgical classifications based on internal hepatic architecture. Among these, the one most commonly used originates from the work of the French

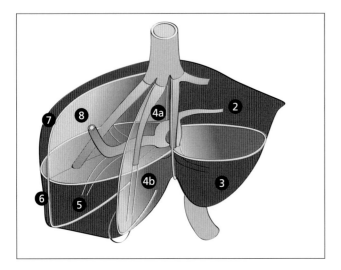

Fig. 3 Schematic subdivision of the liver into eight segments according to Couinaud [9]. From ref. 13, with kind permission of the American Roentgen Ray Society.

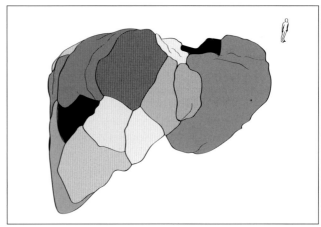

Fig. 4 Anatomical territories at the level of second-order portal venous branches. In the liver under consideration, there are 19 territories, of which 14 are visible in the anterior view illustrated. It becomes apparent that there are many more territories than generally assumed and than suggested by Couinaud's 'eight-segment scheme' [9]. It is this large number of individual vascular territories that has not been considered yet, but which corresponds to anatomical reality. Taking into account this fact explains the seemingly inconsistent observations reported in the literature of different associations of the second-order territories.

surgeon Couinaud [9], which recognized a constant, idealized subdivision of the liver into eight portal segments (Fig. 3). This concept has been adopted worldwide by radiologists and surgeons [36–38]. It has the advantage of offering a scheme that can be easily applied as a very useful referential framework for communication between radiologists, hepatologists and liver surgeons to describe the localization of focal hepatic lesions and the most common types of liver resections. Couinaud's concept can be summarized as follows. The liver is divided into eight territories by means of three vertical and one transverse scissures. The vertical planes contain the inferior vena cava and the right, middle and left hepatic veins. The transverse plane passes through the right and left branches of the portal vein. The liver tissue behind the portal bifurcation is considered as a separate segment, from which the numbering starts in a clockwise pattern, reproduced in Figure 3.

Despite the general acceptance of this eight-segment scheme, an increasing number of anatomical and clinical observations call the concept into question. The *anatomical* literature shows that Couinaud's subdivision is largely contested [5,6,10,22], even by Couinaud himself [39–41]. Publications from the field of *radiology* also challenge Couinaud's concept [42–45]. *Surgeons* have reported discrepancies between Couinaud's concept and intraoperative reality [46–50].

Against this background, our group has reinvestigated the question of vascular territories within the human liver [23]. A systematic analysis of the different levels of the portal venous branching pattern in anatomical corrosion casts allows the following statements to be made. The portal vein irrigates the entire liver. At this level, the liver thus corresponds to *one* territory. The portal vein then bifurcates, in general, into two branches. At the level of these first-order vessels, the liver can thus mostly be subdivided into *two* territories (the right and left hemilivers). There

are three territories in cases of portal trifurcation. As far as the next level of branches is concerned (i.e. vessels of the second order), the human liver in fact consists of many more than the eight segments generally assumed. In accordance with the observations mentioned above with regard to the detailed portal venous branching pattern [20–23], 9–43 territories per liver can be observed, with an average of 20 (Fig. 4). It is this large number of territories at second-order level that has not been considered yet. The reader may find this statement surprising, given the attention that anatomists, surgeons and radiologists have given to the organ for centuries and even in the recent past. But we should quote the observation made by Skandalakis and colleagues: 'Despite its multiple vital functions and its regenerative abilities, the liver has been misunderstood at nearly all levels of organization and in almost every period of time since Galen. The most paradoxical aspect of the understanding of hepatic anatomy has not been lack of knowledge but questions of interpretation; there is a tendency to ignore details that do not fit preconceived ideas. Furthermore, mistaken ideas about the liver seem to have taken longer to correct than misconceptions about most of the other organs of the body, with the exception of the brain' [19].

Taking into account the systematic hierarchical organization of intrahepatic branching patterns explains the seemingly inconsistent observations reported in the literature of different associations of the numerous second-order territories [23]. We have therefore submitted a '1–2–20 principle' for discussion (by analogy with Couinaud's 'eight-segment scheme'). This new working concept is intended to contribute to a better understanding of liver anatomy, increased exactness in radiological localization of hepatic lesions and improved transectional techniques in liver surgery.

Conclusion

Surprisingly enough, the macroscopic anatomy of the liver is far from being definitely described and understood. This statement applies in particular to the concepts evoked for vascular and biliary territories within the organ. The authors suggest using the commonly accepted eight-segment scheme of Couinaud to describe the radiological localization of liver lesions and common hepatectomies, while considering a more loose 1–2–20 concept that allows a more precise description of the anatomy of each individual liver to be given.

References

1 Hollinshead H (1971) *Anatomy for Surgeons*, vol. 2, 2nd edn. New York: Harper & Row, pp. 314–318.

2 Rex H (1888) Beiträge zur Morphologie der Säugerleber. *Morph Jahrb* 14, 517–616.

3 Cantlie J (1898) On a new arrangement of the right and left lobes of the liver. *J Anat Physiol* 32, 4–9.

4 Melnikoff A (1924) Architektur der intrahepatischen Gefässe und Gallengänge des Menschen. *Z Anat Entw Gesch* 70, 411–465.

5 Hjortsö CH (1951) The topography of the intrahepatic duct systems. *Acta Anat* 11, 599–615.

6 Elias H, Petty D (1952) Gross anatomy of the blood vessels and ducts within the human liver. *Am J Anat* 90, 59–111.

7 Healey JE, Schroy PC (1953) Anatomy of the biliary ducts within the human liver. *Arch Surg* 66, 599–616.

8 Gans HG (1955) *Introduction to Hepatic Surgery*. Amsterdam: Elsevier, pp. 1–265.

9 Couinaud C (1957) *Le Foie: Etudes Anatomiques et Chirurgicales*. Paris: Masson.

10 Goldsmith NA, Woodburne RT (1957) The surgical anatomy pertaining to liver resection. *Surg Gynecol Obstet* 105, 310–318.

11 Mukai JK, Stack CM, Turner DA (1987) Imaging of surgically relevant hepatic vascular and segmental anatomy. 1. Normal anatomy. *Am J Roentgenol AJR* 149, 287–292.

12 Soyer P, Roche A, Gad M *et al.* (1991) Preoperative segmental localization of hepatic metastases: utility of three-dimensional CT during arterial portography. *Radiology* 180, 653–658.

13 Soyer P, Bluemke DA, Bliss DF *et al.* (1994) Surgical segmental anatomy of the liver: demonstration with spiral CT during arterial portography and multiplanar reconstruction. *Am J Roentgenol AJR* 163, 99–103.

14 Nelson RC, Chezmar JL, Sugarbaker PH *et al.* (1990) Preoperative localisation of focal liver lesions to specific liver segments: utility of CT during arterial portography. *Radiology* 176, 89–94.

15 Glisson F (1654) *Anatomia Hepatis*. Pullein, London. Cited in: Gans H (1955) *Hepatic Surgery*. Amsterdam: Elsevier, p. 244.

16 Feigl W, Firbas W, Sinzinger H (1973) Ueber das Vorkommen akzessorischer Leberarterien und ihre Genese sowie eine Diskussion ihrer Nomenklatur. *Anat Anz* 134, 139–171.

17 Gupta SC, Gupta SC, Gupta SB (1979) Intrahepatic supply patterns in cases of double hepatic arteries: a study by corrosion casts. *Anat Anz* 146, 166–170.

18 Miyaki TS, Sakagami S, Ito H (1989) Intrahepatic territory of the accessory hepatic artery in the human. *Acta Anat* 136, 34–37.

19 Skandalakis JE, Skandalakis LJ, Skandalakis PN *et al.* (2004) Hepatic surgical anatomy. *Surg Clin North Am* 84, 413–435.

20 Couinaud C (1953) Etude de la veine porte intra-hépatique. *Presse Med* 61, 1434–1438.

21 Laux G, Rapp PE (1953) Le dispositif veineux du lobe de Spigel. *Bull Assoc Anat* 40, 264–271.

22 Platzer W, Maurer H (1966) Zur Segmenteinteilung der Leber. *Acta Anat* 63, 8–31.

23 Fasel JHD, Majno PE, Peitgen HO (2006) Vascular territories in the human liver: a conceptual reappraisal. *Am Surg* (in press).

24 Masselot R, Leborgne J (1978) Etude anatomique des veines sus-hépatiques. *Anat Clin* 1, 109–125.

25 Nakamura S, Tsuzuki T (1981) Surgical anatomy of the hepatic veins and the inferior vena cava. *Surg Gynecol Obstet* 152, 43–50.

26 Van Leeuwen MS, Fernandez A, van Es HW *et al.* (1994) Variations in venous and segmental anatomy of the liver: two- and three-dimensional MR imaging in healthy volunteers. *Am J Roentgenol AJR* 162, 1337–1345.

27 Van Leeuwen MS (1994) Triphasic spiral CT of the liver and 3D liver imaging. Medical thesis, University of Utrecht, Netherlands.

28 Mehran R, Schneider R, Franchebois P (2000) The minor hepatic veins: anatomy and classification. *Clin Anat* 13, 416–421.

29 Faisinger M (1950) The radiology of the intrahepatic biliary tract. *South Afr J Med Sci* 15, 51.

30 Champetier J (1994) Les voies biliaires. In: Chevrel JP (ed.) *Anatomie Clinique*, vol. 2. Paris: Springer, pp. 407–420.

31 Anderhuber F, Lechner P (1986) Occurrence of anastomoses of the intrahepatic bile ducts. *Acta Anat* 125, 42–49.

32 Wolodjko WP (1967) Das Lymphsystem der menschlichen Leber in Beziehung zu ihrer Segmentgliederung. *Z Anat Entw Gesch* 126, 154–171.

33 Trutmann M, Sasse D (1994) The lymphatics of the liver. *Anat Embryol* 190, 201–209.

34 Golab B (1972) Lymphatic vessels of the hepatic ligaments in man. *Folia Morphol (Warsz)* 31, 260–263.

35 Loeweneck H, Feifel G (2004) Bauch. In: Lanz Tv, Wachsmuth W (Begründer) *Praktische Anatomie*, 2 Bd, 6 Teil. Berlin: Springer, p. 262.

36 Bismuth H (1982) Surgical anatomy and anatomical surgery of the liver. *World J Surg* 6, 3–9.

37 Dodd GD III (1993) An American guide to Couinaud's numbering system. *Am J Roentgenol AJR* 161, 574–575.

38 Blumgart LH, Hann LE (2000) Surgical and radiologic anatomy of the liver and biliary tract. In: Blumgart LH, Fong Y (eds) *Surgery of the Liver and the Biliary Tract*, 3rd edn. London: Saunders, pp. 5–10.

39 Couinaud C (1998) Secteur dorsal du foie. *Chirurgie* 123, 8–15.

40 Filipponi F, Romagnoli P, Mosca F *et al.* (2000) The dorsal sector of human liver: embryological, anatomical and clinical relevance. *Hepatogastroenterology* 47, 1726–1731.

41 Abdalla EK, Vauthey JN, Couinaud C (2002) The caudate lobe of the liver: implications of embryology and anatomy for surgery. *Surg Oncol Clin North Am* 11, 835–848.

42 Ohashi I, Ina H, Okada Y *et al.* (1996) Segmental anatomy of the liver under the right diaphragmatic dome: evaluation with axial CT. *Radiology* 200, 779–783.

43 Fasel JHD, Selle D, Evertsz CJ *et al.* (1998) Segmental anatomy of the liver: poor correlation with CT. *Radiology* 206, 151–156.

44 Rieker O, Mildenberger P, Hintze C *et al.* (2000) Segmental anatomy of the liver in computed tomography: do we localize the lesion accurately? *Rofo Fortschr Geb Rontgenstr Neuen Bildgeb Verfahr* 172, 147–152.

45 Fischer L, Cardenas C, Thorn M *et al.* (2002) Limits of Couinaud's liver segment classification: a quantitative computer-based three-dimensional analysis. *J Comput Assist Tomogr* 26, 962–967.

46 Makuuchi M, Hasegawa H, Yamazaki S (1985) Ultrasonically guided subsegmentectomy. *Surg Gynecol Obstet* 161, 346–350.

47 Blumgart LH, Fong Y (2000) *Surgery of the Liver and Biliary Tract*, 3rd edn. London: Saunders, CD-ROM.

48 Cervone A, Sardi A, Conaway GL (2000) Intraoperative ultrasound (IOUS) is essential in the management of metastatic colorectal liver lesions. *Am Surg* 66, 611–615.

49 Scheele J (2001) Anatomiegerechte und atypische Leberresektionen. *Chirurgie* 72, 113–124.

50 Ko S, Murakami G, Kanamura T *et al.* (2004) Cantlie's plane in major variations of the primary portal vein ramification at the porta hepatis: cutting experiment using cadaveric livers. *World J Surg* 28, 13–18.

1.2 Liver and biliary tract histology

Paulette Bioulac-Sage, Brigitte Le Bail and Charles Balabaud

General features

Liver and biliary tract histology, the study of hepatic function, the relation between the structure and function of cells and their organelles and of the extracellular matrix have recently been reviewed in specialized textbooks on pathology [1], biology and pathobiology [2,3] and liver disease [4].

The liver is a voluminous organ (1200–1500 g) that is highly vascularized. It is surrounded by a thin capsule (Glisson's capsule) composed of collagen fibres, scattered fibroblasts, myofibroblasts, small blood vessels and lymphatics. The capsule is thickest around the hilus (or porta hepatis) where blood vessels enter and bile ducts leave the liver. In the parenchyma, the capsule merges with the connective tissue surrounding the portal tracts.

Between the incoming vessels of the portal tracts and the central veins lie the hepatic sinusoids, which allow exchange between blood and unicellular sheets of hepatocytes. In histological sections, portal tracts (which contain branches of the hepatic artery and portal vein, one or two bile ducts, lymphatics, nerves, a few lymphocytes and fibroblasts in loose connective tissue), centrolobular veins (also called the terminal hepatic venule) and the lobular parenchyma are identified (Figs 1 and 2). The apparent structural unit of the liver is the lobule, a polyhedral prism (0.7 × 2 mm), the boundaries of which are limited by four to five portal triads prolonged by connective tissue septa. The centre of the lobule contains the centrolobular vein (Figs 1 and 3). The lobular parenchyma represents approximately 93% of the hepatic parenchyma, portal triads 3% and hepatic veins 4% [5]. At least 15 different cell types can be found in normal liver [6].

Human liver biopsy material (needle or surgical) is usually fixed by immersion for a few hours in 10% neutral formalin. For detailed study of the hepatic parenchyma and sinusoidal cells by electron microscopy (transmission and scanning), it is better to use *in situ* perfusion–fixation of the liver through the portal vein or the hepatic artery. For the localization of antigens (immunocytochemistry) fixed material can be used in many instances. For the performance of *in situ* hybridization and some immunostaining, it can be necessary to use frozen material.

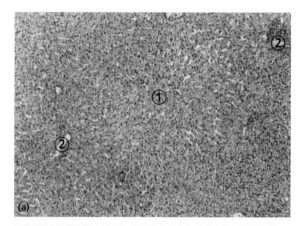

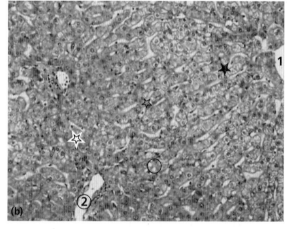

Fig. 1 Hepatic parenchyma: paraffin embedding (5-μm-thick section); haematein eosin saffron; (a) low (× 50) and (b) high (× 230) magnification. The classic lobule cannot easily be seen. Sinusoids lie, from portal tracts (2) to centrolobular veins (1), in between the unicellular sheets of hepatocytes. In medio- and centrolobular zones (black star), sinusoids are larger and radial; in the periportal zone (white star), they are narrower.

The functional unit of the liver

An adequate description of the liver unit should provide not only structural but also secretory and microcirculatory unity [7]. Based on the lobular organization proposed by Matsumoto

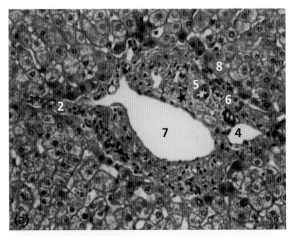

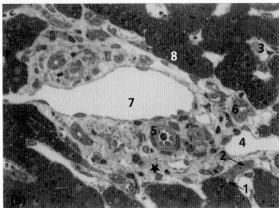

Fig. 2 Small portal tract: (a) paraffin embedding (5-μm-thick section); haematein eosin saffron, × 300; (b) Epon embedding (1-μm-thick section); toluidine blue, × 340. At the periphery of the portal tract, several canals of Hering (1), cholangioles (2) and sinusoids (3), with or without Kupffer cells, can be seen close to venules (4). In the portal tract, arterioles (5) are close to interlobular bile ducts (6), which are lined by a single layer of cuboidal epithelial cells; some inflammatory cells are present in the stroma (*). (7) Portal vein; (8) hepatocytes forming the periportal limiting plate.

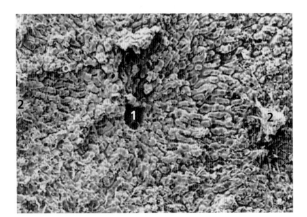

Fig. 3 Hepatic lobule: scanning electron microscopy, × 170. A centrolobular vein (1) is visible at the centre of the lobule limited by two portal tracts (2).

[8] the liver microarchitecture is composed of primary lobules (or modules, a term coined to ascribe considerable degrees of variability in the shape and size of primary units as well as in the number of primary units) [9]. Primary modules are structural elements that are responsible for directing and the timing of blood flow: (i) portal veins and their septal branches (and hepatic arteries); (ii) vascular septa, which connect portal veins and septal branches to a continuous supplying surface and act as a 'watershed' between adjacent primary modules; (iii) long portal sinusoids, which originate directly from and in the vicinity of the portal vessels, with an initial tortuous segment and a subsequent straight radially oriented segment; (iv) short septal sinusoids, which are straight radial and lacking the initial tortuous segment that originates from the vascular septum, where inflow-fronts from neighboring portal vessels meet; and (v) a central venular branch located in the centre of the primary module, draining the sinusoids. Reconstruction reveals a group of primary modules integrated into a secondary module. Integration results from a common drainage by the branches of a central venular tree and from the arrangement of portal venular branches and vascular septa, which form a continuous vascular surface over the entire module and separate it from adjacent modules. Reconstructed primary modules are polyhedral, with seven to nine facets, which are either plane, convex or concave. In addition to variable shapes, the primary modules also vary in size (i.e., height, surface area, volume, number and area of vascular septa). Such morphogenetic plasticity is considered an important part of the modular microarchitecture of the liver. Figure 4 illustrates the classic but oversimplified representation of a primary lobule and Figure 5 a more realistic representation of primary modules integrated into a secondary module. This interpretation should permit a better interpretation of histological sections of normal and pathological liver and provide a basis for understanding the metabolic heterogeneity of liver cells and their functional integration into parenchymal units.

Hepatocytes

Hepatocytes are arranged in unicellular plates or laminae (Remak's plates). These hepatic laminae branch and anastomose with one another to form a complicated walling system, the hepatic muralium, a maze-like arrangement of partitions between which the sinusoids interweave and interconnect in a continuous labyrinth [1,2] (Figs 3 and 6). Hepatocytes surrounding the portal tract, which constitute an interface between the connective tissue of the tract and the hepatic parenchyma, form the limiting plate (Fig. 2).

The plates are composed of about 20 large, polyhedral epithelial cells, approximately 30 μm long and 20 μm wide. The mean volume density is 5000 μm^3. These cells (100 billion) make up approximately 80% of the cell population. The hepatocyte is limited by a membrane in which three domains can be distinguished.

The sinusoidal membrane (70% of the total cell surface area)

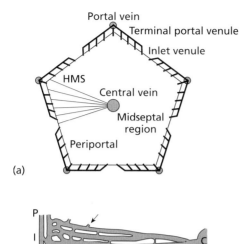

(a)

(b)

Fig. 4 (a) Two-dimensional view of a pentagonal hepatic lobule. In each corner, there is a portal tract. On each side of the lobule, in the septum, there are two opposite-running terminal portal venules (accompanied by an arterial branch and a ductule). The hepatic lobule is divisible into elementary sectors: the hepatic microcirculatory subunits fed by the inlet venules derived from the portal vein (in the portal tract) and the terminal portal venules. Compared with the periportal region, the mid-septal region is remote from the portal supply. (b) A typical hepatic microcirculatory subunit shaped like a cone with a portal inlet venule (I) at the base, where one afferent vessel spreads into many sinusoids. The cross-connecting sinusoids (arrows) reduce, or drop out, while approaching the centrolobular vein (C). From ref. 10, with permission.

is covered with microvilli (0.5 μm long), which increase the surface area sixfold. This membrane burrows in between hepatocytes, delimiting the interhepatocytic space (Figs 7 and 8). Exchange of materials between the blood and hepatocytes (exo- and endocytosis) through the Disse space is a function solely of the sinusoidal plasma membrane.

The canalicular membrane is the biliary pole of the hepatocyte. It is an intercellular space, formed by the opposition of the edges of gutter-like hemicanals (15% of the total cell surface area; 0.4% of the lobular parenchyma) on the surfaces of neighbouring hepatocytes (average diameter, 0.5–1 μm internal diameter in portal area and 1–1.25 μm in centrolobular area (Figs 6, 7 and 8). The surface is covered by microvilli. The canalicular surface is isolated from the Disse space by tight junctions. Using light microscopy, bile canaliculi are not visible in normal liver; but they can be immunostained with anti-CEA polyclonal and anti-CD10 antibodies. They become visible when distended in cholestatic liver. Tone is provided by an encircling mesh of contractile microfilaments fixed on the zonula adherens, which follow the outline of the microvilli.

The lateral membrane (15% of the cell surface area) is more or less straight, separated from the adjacent lateral membranes by an intercellular space of 15 nm. The junctional complexes – desmosomes, gap junctions, intermediate junctions (zonula adherens) and tight junctions – are special membrane differentiations that fix the liver cells together.

Fig. 5 Schematic distribution of alkaline phosphatase activity in the portal and centrolobular area delineating primary and secondary modules. Portal venular branches and vascular septa form a continuum in which blood is distributed over the surface of the modules and from which the sinusoids originate. From portal vessels, blood flows toward the centre and along the vascular septa. Enzyme activity is highest in endothelial cells at the beginning of the 'portal' sinusoids. From there, activity decreases towards the central venule and is higher at the end of the sinusoids. Staining also decreases from both sides along the vascular septum and is faintest where the 'septal' sinusoids originate. Along the septal sinusoids, alkaline phosphatase activity first decreases and then increases towards the end of the sinusoids. Alkaline phosphatase activity in portal areas (dark red), and in central areas (light red). Adapted from ref. 9, with permission.

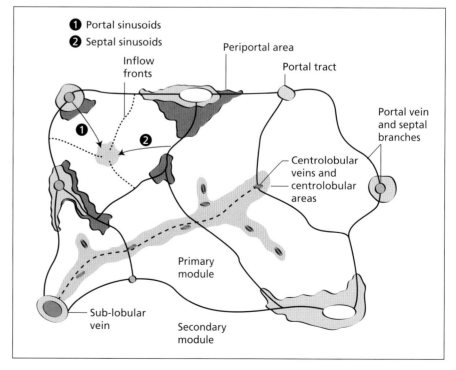

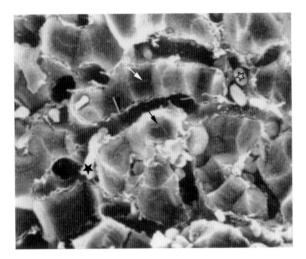

Fig. 6 Hepatic parenchyma: scanning electron microscopy, × 1300. Unicellular sheets of hepatocytes are separated by sinusoids from different planes of sectioning. The block often breaks in between the lateral surface of hepatocytes, allowing visualization of the biliary hemicanaliculi (arrow). In sinusoids, some Kupffer cells (black star) and red blood cells (white star) can be seen. The Disse space can also be identified (arrowhead).

The nucleus is spherical and voluminous, occupying 5–10% of the cell volume, with one or more prominent nucleoli and scattered chromatin. About 25% of the cells are binucleate. There appears to be a clear correlation between nuclear size and ploidy. As many as 15% can be tetraploid nuclei. The adult liver has a very low mitotic index, with estimates ranging from 2 mitoses per 1000 cells to 1 per 10 000 cells.

Light microscopy of the liver shows a pale-staining, eosinophilic cytoplasm containing granular clumps of basophilic material. This material corresponds to rough endoplasmic reticulum. Near the bile canaliculi, there are fine brown granules of lipofuchsin pigment. These are more abundant with age, particularly in the centrolobular zone. A few hepatocytes may contain fat vacuoles. Histochemical procedures are essential to identify components such as glycogen, haemosiderin and lipids. Electron microscopy is necessary to visualize organelles: there is an abundant rough and smooth endoplasmic reticulum, a Golgi apparatus close to the biliary pole, numerous mitochondria (1000–1500 per cell) and peroxisomes. The hepatocyte is rich in glycogen, with the quantity depending on the time of the last meal. The cytoskeleton of the cell comprises microfilaments, intermediate filaments and microtubules, which correspond by immunocytochemistry to actin, cytokeratin and tubulin.

The main morphometric data concerning organelles are presented in Figure 9 [11,12]. The whole cellular machinery performs many functions: uptake, transport, synthesis, biotransformation and degradation (proteins, lipids, carbohydrates, hormones, xenobiotics and bile).

With age the number of hepatocytes decreases and hypertrophy, polyploidy, lysosomes, and smooth endoplasmic reticulum increases. The mitochondria and microbodies remain unchanged with age and the microsomal drug-metabolizing capabilities decrease.

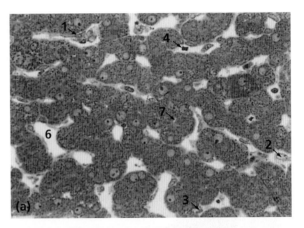

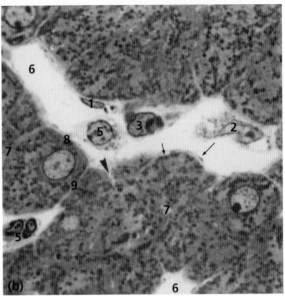

Fig. 7 Sinusoids and sheets of hepatocytes: Epon embedding (1-μm-thick section); toluidine blue (a) × 340; (b) × 1250 magnification. It is possible to identify the sinusoidal cells: endothelial cells with the cell body (1) and the barrier (large arrow), Kupffer cells (2) and stellate cells (3); blood cells, red (4) and white (5), in the sinusoidal lumen (6); the Disse space (small arrow) with the interhepatocytic recess (arrowhead); bile canaliculi (7); the sinusoidal surface (8) and lateral (9) surface of hepatocytes.

Sinusoids

Sinusoids are special capillaries with: (i) a fenestrated endothelial barrier; (ii) resident macrophages (Kupffer cells) 'guarding' the entrance of sinusoids; (iii) liver-associated lymphocytes, some of which are large, granular lymphocytes; and (iv) stellate cells (considered as pericytes) that store vitamin A [13,14] (Fig. 10). Sinusoids have no genuine basement membrane: this facilitates exchange between incoming blood and hepatocytes through the Disse space, as well as immunological defence mechanisms.

In zone 1, sinusoids are tortuous, narrow and anastomotic, but tend to become more parallel and larger in zone 3. The mean diameter (between 7 and 15 μm) is occasionally less than the mean diameter of the red blood cells, which adapt their shape to

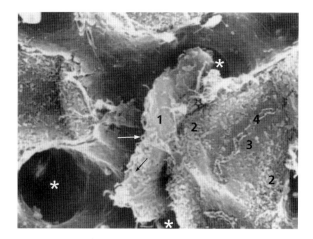

Fig. 8 Kupffer cells: scanning electron microscopy, × 4260. The Kupffer cell (1) with its filipodia (arrow) is located at the branching of several sinusoids (*). The different plasma membranes of the hepatocytes are easily recognizable: the sinusoidal with their microvilli (2), the fairly smooth lateral (3) and canalicular (4) membranes. It is not easy to differentiate collagen bundles from the perisinusoidal cell processes in the Disse space (star).

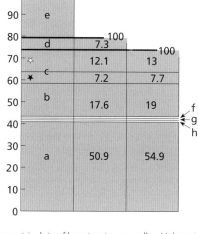

Fig. 9 Morphometric data of hepatocyte organelles. Volumetric composition of the liver expressed as a percentage of the lobular parenchyma (left column), an average hepatocyte (middle column) and hepatocytic cytoplasm (right column). (a) Hyaloplasm; (b) mitochondria; (c) endoplasmic reticulum, rough (white star), smooth (black star); (d) nucleus; (e) extrahepatocytic space (sinusoids and bile canaliculi); (f) lysosomes; (g) lipids; (h) peroxisomes. Lysosomes, lipids and peroxisome volume densities, expressed as a percentage of the cytoplasm, are 2%, 2.1% and 1.3% respectively.

Fig. 10 Diagrammatic representation of sinusoids, sinusoidal cells and Disse space. (a) All four sinusoidal cells are represented in this sinusoid (A) (it is exceptional to see all four, with their nuclei, in the same plane of section) – the Kupffer cell (1), the endothelial cell: cell body (2), processes (3) and fenestrations (arrow); the stellate cell (4) with its lipids (black star) and processes (5); the liver-associated lymphocytes (6). In the Disse space (white star) containing some collagen fibres (7), interhepatocytic recesses (8), sinusoidal membrane microvilli (9) and the lateral membrane (10) of the hepatocyte (B) can be seen. (b) Schema of the sinusoidal wall. Arrows indicate tunnels formed by the processes of the stellate cells and hepatocyte. CF, collagen fibres; H, hepatocyte; HCP, hepatocyte-contacting process of the stellate cell; SP, subendothelial process of the stellate cell; N, nerve fibre; * space of Disse. From ref. 14, with permission.

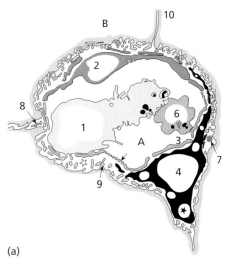

(a)

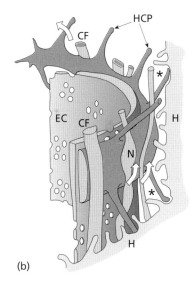

(b)

size differences [15]. The diameter can increase if necessary (up to 180 μm). The mean length is 220–480 μm. The sinusoidal lumina occupy approximately 9–10% of the lobular parenchyma [16].

Sinusoidal cells

These represent about 6% of the lobular parenchyma (2.5%, 2% and 1.4% for endothelial, Kupffer and stellate cells respectively) and 26.5% of all the plasma membranes of the liver. Observation by light microscopy is difficult. Only transmission and scanning electron microscopy and immunocytochemical methods allow correct identification [17].

Endothelial cells

These form the barrier of the sinusoid [18,19]. Their main characteristics are: (i) very thin processes covering a large area (15% of all the plasma membranes of the liver); (ii) fenestrations with a mean diameter of 100 nm, grouped in clusters (sieve plates), which allow the passage of molecules of smaller diameters (Fig. 11) [20]; (iii) numerous pinocytotic vesicles, indicating a high endocytic capacity. They show immunoreactivity with monoclonal antibody MS-1 and express the scavenger receptor, Fc IgG receptor, and also the CD4 molecule. In capillarized sinusoids, where sinusoidal endothelial cells have lost their

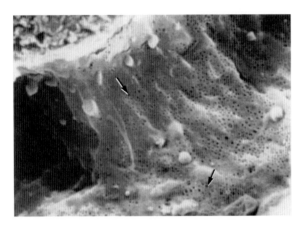

Fig. 11 Endothelial cell: scanning electron microscopy, × 13 440. The endothelial cell processes form the wall of the sinusoid. Fenestrations (arrow) are grouped in clusters, forming so-called sieve plates.

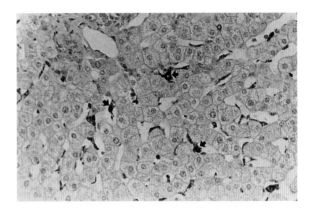

Fig. 13 Kupffer cell identification: paraffin embedding (5-μm-thick section); immunocytochemistry (KP1), × 330. Large Kupffer cells (arrow) are seen in this periportal area.

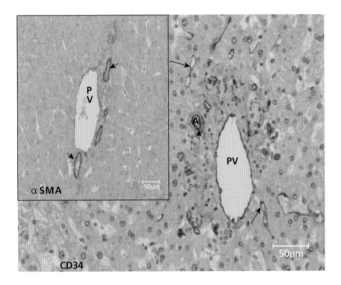

Fig. 12 CD34 immunostaining: all vascular endothelial cells are stained in the portal tract (short black arrow), but not in the sinusoidal endothelial cells, except in a few periportal sinusoids (long black arrow). α-SMA immunostaining (upper left corner): smooth muscle cells of vascular walls are stained but not the hepatic stellate cells in sinusoids.

fenestrations, there is a phenotypic shift towards that of vascular-type endothelium: expression of factor VIII-related antigen, *Ulex europaeus* lectin, CD34 and CD31 molecules. In the normal liver, antibodies such as anti-CD34 stains endothelial cells of vessels but not sinusoidal endothelial cells, except at the immediate periphery of portal tracts (Fig. 12).

Kupffer cells

Attached over a (more or less) large area of the endothelial wall, these cells are located within the sinusoidal lumen [21] (Figs 7 and 8). They are more numerous in zone 1 than in zone 3.

They contain numerous lysosomes (almost a quarter of all the lysosomes of the liver). Kupffer cells can be identified with monoclonal antibodies such as KP1 (anti-CD68) (Fig. 13). They phagocytose many substances, such as latex particles, denatured albumin, bacteria and immune complexes. The extent to which Kupffer cells fail to take up colloids in patients with chronic hepatocellular diseases correlates best with indices of the magnitude of portal–systemic blood shunting. Upon stimulation by immunomodulators, Kupffer cells release mediators and cytotoxic agents.

Liver-associated lymphocytes

Far fewer in number (1:10 Kupffer cells), they comprise different types of lymphocytes, among which are large, granular lymphocytes (also named pit cells) [22]. They are resident luminal cells in contact with Kupffer and/or endothelial cells. Liver-associated lymphocytes differ from peripheral blood lymphocytes (phenotype, cytotoxic activity) [19]. They play a role in defence against tumours and viruses.

Hepatic stellate cells

Previously called perisinusoidal or Ito cells, they can be identified by [23]: (i) their cell body, which is often located in an interhepatocytic recess and contains lipids (Fig. 10) including vitamin A in most (but 20% of the cells do not contain lipids); (ii) their long, thin, cytoplasmic processes, surrounding endothelial cell processes; and (iii) their spines, which establish contact with hepatocyte microvilli [14]. No basement membrane surrounds the hepatic stellate cell. This cell, which belongs to the myofibroblast family, can be identified immunocytochemically in human liver by the presence of cellular retinol binding protein (Fig. 14) which stains this cell in its quiescent or activated phenotype [24]. There are approximately 5 to 20 of these cells per 100 hepatocytes. They store vitamin A and

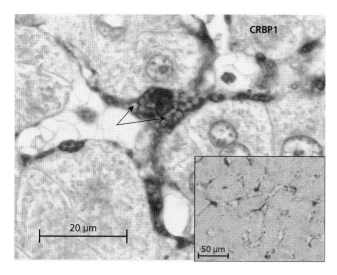

Fig. 14 CRBP 1 immunostaining: at low magnification (right lower corner). Many sinusoids are surrounded by cell bodies and/or processes of hepatic stellate cells. At high magnification lipids are underlined (arrow).

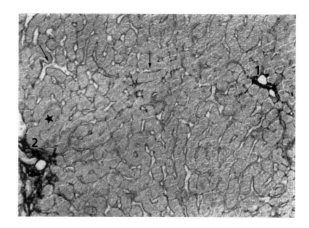

Fig. 15 Identification of the extracellular matrix: paraffin embedding (5-μm-thick section); Sirius red, × 130. This stain allows identification of the thin, perisinusoidal, matricial network (arrow) in between the unicellular, unstained sheets of hepatocytes (star), and of the fibrous tissue around the centrolobular vein (1) and the portal tract (2).

participate in the regulation of microvascular tonus and in the synthesis of the extracellular matrix. This latter function increases when they are activated and transformed into α-smooth muscle actin-positive cells. α smooth muscle actin antibodies (α-SMA) stain smooth muscle cells of the vessel walls, whereas hepatic stellate cells are usually negative in normal liver (Fig. 12).

The Disse space

This lies primarily between the stellate cell sheet and the sinusoidal membrane of the hepatocyte, and represents 2–4% of the hepatic parenchyma [25]. The relatively low porosity of the endothelial barrier (9% of the surface) is compensated for by the presence of a great number of hepatocytic microvilli in the Disse space, and particularly since the endothelial cell lacks a genuine basement membrane. In this space, which is not normally discernible in biopsy material by standard light microscopy, one can observe the different components of the extracellular matrix, which can be identified by immunocytochemistry [26]: these are different types of collagens (mainly type 3 but also types 1 and 4), proteoglycans and fibronectin. The presence of laminin is much debated. This whole network can be visualized by silver or Sirius red staining (Fig. 15).The role of the extracellular matrix is complex: it serves to cement the cells, allows intercellular communication and affects cellular differentiation.

Microcirculation

Blood flows unidirectionally in sinusoids from zone 1 to zone 3. Microcirculation through individual sinusoids is variable [27, 28]. This irregularity is linked to: (i) the presence of inlet, sinusoidal and outlet sphincters composed of sinusoidal lining cells bulging into the lumen; (ii) transient leukocyte plugging; (iii) variations in the morphology of sinusoids in the different zones;

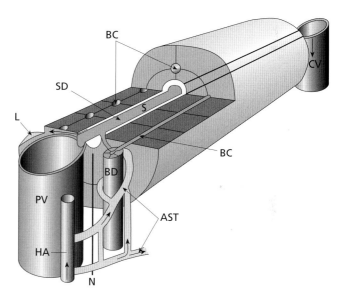

Fig. 16 Diagrammatic representation of the microcirculation and of biliary drainage in the lobule. PV, portal venule; HA, hepatic arteriole; BD, bile ductule; L, lymphatic; N, nerve; AST, arteriosinous twig; S, sinusoid; SD, space of Disse; BC, bile canaliculus; CV, central venule. Arrows indicate direction of flow. Note that the capillaries surrounding the bile duct constitute the peribiliary plexus. From ref. 27, with permission.

(iv) the contribution of arterial flow at the beginning of the sinusoid's pathway (Fig. 16) [27].

The average velocity of erythrocyte flow in sinusoids ranges between 270 and 410 μm/s. There are considerable interactions between blood cells and the sinusoidal wall. Soft, fast-moving red blood cells could help fluid- or solid-phase droplets or particles to penetrate into the Disse space (forced sieving). Compression of the Disse space by less plastic and larger cells such as white blood cells could displace fluids within this space in a downstream direction, promoting the transport of particles and fluids into and out of the space through the fenestrations (endothelial massage) [15]. Average blood pressure is about 4.8 mmHg in terminal portal branches, 30–35 mmHg in arterial blood and 1.7 mmHg in collecting veins.

The hepatic artery

In the portal tract , the artery feeds the bile duct as the peribiliary vascular plexus, the portal tract interstitium including nerve, and the wall of portal vein. Drainage of these vascular beds is collected as an artery-derived portal system which joins the portal vein in the tract or at the inlet venule on entering the lobule. The hepatic artery therefore can resume the portal flow via the artery-derived portal system. Outside the portal tract, the artery dissociates itself to supply the Glisson's capsule which drains into subcapsular lobules, and the walls of central sublobular and hepatic veins. The latter is the pathway by which arterial blood can bypass the hepatic parenchyma into the hepatic vein [29].

Lymphatics (see also Chapter 2.1.3)

Lymph is collected in lymphatics present in portal triads. Liver lymph is first formed in the perisinusoidal Disse space. The fluid then enters the periportal tissue of the Mall space, which lies between the portal connective tissue and the limiting plate, and then the lymphatic capillaries. Lymph is then conveyed by increasingly large lymphatic vessels to the collecting vessels, which leave the liver at the hilus to reach the thoracic duct. The liver's capsule and portal stroma contain numerous lymphatic vessels, which form loose plexuses that connect at intervals with underlying lymphatic vessels. The antibody D2-40 stains specifically endothelial cells of lymphatics (Fig. 17) [30].

Nerves (see also Chapter 2.2.5)

Extrinsic innervation of the liver is constituted by McCuskey [31]:

1 efferent sympathetic nerve fibres (preganglionic splanchnic fibres and postganglionic fibres after synapse in the coeliac ganglion) and parasympathetic nerve fibres (preganglionic fibres from the vagus); these play a part in the metabolism of hepatocytes (carbohydrate and perhaps lipid metabolism), haemodynamic regulation and biliary motility;

2 afferent fibres, which are thought to be involved in osmo- and chemoreception; at the hilus, amyelinic fibres form the anterior and posterior plexuses, which communicate with each other, and these enter the liver mainly around the hepatic artery.

Intrinsic innervation is composed of fibres mainly associated with vascular and biliary structures in the portal spaces (Fig. 18). Certain fibres enter the liver lobule, where they form a network around hepatocytes and extend into the sinusoidal wall, sometimes reaching the centrolobular vein. Fluorescence histochemistry and immunohistochemistry have revealed different types of nerve fibres: adrenergic (the most numerous in man), cholinergic and peptidergic. Some neuropeptides have been identified: vasoactive intestinal peptide (in the pathway of cholinergic fibres), neuropeptide Y (in that of adrenergic fibres), substance P, glucagon and calcitonin gene-related peptide [32].

Functional aspects of liver morphology

Consideration of gradient differences in cell and matrix composition (i.e., enzyme activities) of the liver are important when evaluating gene and protein changes as measured by genomic and proteomic methods. Furthermore, these different functional properties between periportal and centrilobular cells and matrix can also help to explain the regional distribution of lesions and susceptibility of cells to certain hepatotoxicants. Not only do hepatocytes have gradients of gene and protein activity that varies from the periportal region to the centrilobular region,

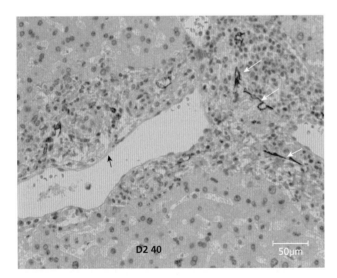

Fig. 17 D2-40 immunostaining: only endothelial cells of lymphatics (black arrow) are stained in this portal tract; vascular endothelial cells (white arrows) are negative.

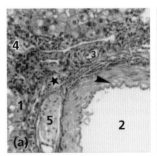
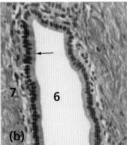

Fig. 18 Large portal tract (partial view): paraffin embedding (5-μm-thick section); haematein eosin saffron; (a) × 115; (b) × 170. (a) A nerve (5) can be seen inside the connective tissue, not far from the limiting plate of hepatocytes (1), a large artery (2), which is easily identifiable by its internal elastic lamina (arrowhead), an arteriole (3) and biliary ducts (4). (b) This large bile duct (6), which is surrounded by a thick fibrous envelope (7), is limited by a cylindrical epithelium (arrow).

but gradients also exist for sinusoidal endothelial, Kupffer and hepatic stellate cells, and for the matrix in the space of Disse [36].

The biliary tract

Intrahepatic biliary tract

The biliary tree contributes to the formation of bile and assures its delivery into the duodenum. It consists of the intrahepatic and extrahepatic biliary tract. In its first and short intrahepatic part, the biliary tree is lined by hepatocytes; it is followed by a series of biliary canals of growing diameter lined by biliary epithelial cells or cholangiocytes. These cells present two distinct poles: an apical pole facing the bile duct lumen, equipped with a variable number of short microvilli, and a basolateral pole in relation to adjacent epithelial cells and the basement membrane. They express high-molecular-weight cytokeratins, and specifically contain CK7 and CK19, in addition to CK8 and CK18 expressed by hepatocytes. Normally, they express class I MHC antigens but not class II, more numerous cell-matrix adhesion molecules than hepatocytes ($\alpha2\beta1$, $\alpha3\beta1$, $\alpha5\beta1$, $\alpha6\beta4$), as well as glutamyl transpeptidase, epithelial membran antigen, carcinoembryonic antigen (cross-reaction at the apex with poly-clonal antibody), and various membrane receptors/transporters involved in bile secretion [33]. Recent research has focused on the expression of different types of mucins in normal and neoplastic biliary epithelium. In the intrahepatic and extrahep-atic bile ducts MUC1 (detected by Mb DF3) is not expressed, nor are MUC2 or MUC4. MUC5AC and MUC6 are expressed in a minority of cases (13% and 30% respectively), the latter being expressed in peribiliary glands in most cases [34].

Bile flows in the opposite direction to that of plasma flow in the canaliculi along the hepatocyte plates, and next enters small ductules or cholangioles in the periportal area. The junction between the last hepatocyte and the first spindle-shaped biliary cells is called the canal of Hering.

The canals of Hering begin in the lobules, are lined partially by cholangiocytes and partly by hepatocytes, and conduct bile from bile canaliculi to terminal bile ducts in portal tracts. They are not readily apparent on routine histological staining but are highlighted by the biliary cytokeratins CK19 and CK7. There is on average one canal of Hering per 10 µm of bile duct length. The canals represent the true hepatocytic–biliary interface that thus lies within the lobule and not at the limiting plate. The canals of Hering consist of, or harbour, facultative hepatic stem cells in humans (Fig. 19) [35].

In cross-section, cholangioles (or ductules) are lined by three or four cells that become cuboidal and stay on a basement mem-brane; they usually have an internal diameter of less than 15 µm. Like the canals of Hering they are not usually apparent by light microscopy in normal livers. On occasion, and in cholestatic livers, they become visible at the periphery of the portal triad, lying in the vascular axis of the septal zone (Fig. 2). They drain the bile into the interlobular bile ducts located in portal triads.

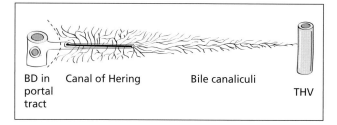

BD in portal tract   Canal of Hering   Bile canaliculi   THV

Fig. 19 Proposed relationships of the canal of Hering to the hepatic parenchyma. The terminal bile duct in the portal tract may give rise to a bile ductule (BD), and then a canal of Hering that penetrates directly into the parenchyma and extends on average one-third of the way to the THV. Because the canal of Hering is by definition made up partially by bile duct epithelial cells and hepatocytes (not shown), it can act as a 'trough' for the collection of bile from hepatocellular bile canaliculi. THV, terminal hepatic vein.

Interlobular bile ducts (< 100 µm diameter), lined by a cuboidal epithelium, are accompanied by arteries in the portal tract; their external diameter is quite similar to that of the adjacent artery (ratio 0.7–0.8).

The confluence of two or more interlobular bile ducts forms the septal ducts (> 100 µm diameter), which are lined by a cylindrical epithelium.

Segmental ducts (between 400 and 800 µm diameter), as well as left and right bile ducts, are histologically similar. Like septal ducts, they are lined by columnar cholangiocytes, and situated on a PAS-diastase-positive basement membrane; they are surrounded by dense, irregular and circumferential, but not concentric, fibrous tissue containing many elastic fibres. A peribiliary plexus of capillaries (branches of the hepatic artery) supplies all the intrahepatic bile ducts. This plexus drains prin-cipally into hepatic sinusoids. In addition to the enterohepatic cycle, a cholehepatic cycle for mono- and dihydroxyl bile acids has been proposed.

Extrahepatic biliary tract

At the exit from the liver, the biliary tract is composed of three portions with many anatomical variations (in size, position and orientation), particularly at the different confluences [36]:
1 the left and right hepatic ducts (diameter 3–4 mm) emerge from the corresponding lobes and after about 1 cm in the hilus, their confluence gives rise to the common hepatic duct;
2 the accessory biliary apparatus comprises the gallbladder and the cystic duct which joins the common hepatic duct to form the common bile duct;
3 the terminal part of the common bile duct enters the duodenum at the papilla of Vater after traversing the sphincter of Oddi.

Hepatic, cystic and common ducts

The diameter of these ducts is less than 15 mm and their walls are very thin (0.5–1.0 mm). The mucosa is relatively flat or pleated with some short folds; it is composed of a single layer of tall, columnar cholangiocytes resting on a dense collagenous connective tissue, rich in elastic fibres and containing some small mucous glands. The surface epithelium forms some pits (sacculi of Beale) which are conspicuous in the extraduodenal portion of the common bile duct and the hepatic duct. Entrerochromaffin, serotonin-containing cells have been described in the cystic duct epithelium. Smooth muscle fibres, circular or oblique, are scant and variable in quantity around the common bile duct; this muscularis is reinforced near the duodenum by circular fibres forming the sphincter of Oddi and is most prominent near the cystic duct, in the axis of mucosa folds, where they form the Heister valve (which controls bile flow). The subserosa is a connective tissue, less dense in periphery than in the inner portion, containing collagen and elastic fibres, blood vessels, nerve fibres and occasionnal ganglion cells. Around the common hepatic ducts, the hilar ducts (and a portion of the larger septal ducts) it also contains some tubular and branched mucous glands [37] which share similarities with the Brunner glands of the duodenum.

The gallbladder

Located within a fossa (on the undersurface) of the right lobe of the liver, the gallbladder is a pear-shapped pocket firmly attached to the liver, which stores and evacuates bile. Occasionally, the gallbladder is freely suspended from the liver by a mesentery. This spindle-shaped bag, measuring 6–12 cm in length and 2.5–5 cm in width, may contain 30–50 mL of bile and consists of a fundus, a body, an infundibulum and a neck; the neck forms an 'S' shape that represents its transition with the cystic duct.

The wall is composed of a mucosa (made of a surface epithelium and underlying lamina propria which forms primary and secondary folds when the gallbladder is empty) lying on a plexiform muscularis and an adventitia (or subserosa; Fig. 20) and a serosa. It lacks a muscularis mucosae and a submucosae. The villosities of the mucosa are separated by herniations of the epithelium sometimes extending through the entire width of the muscular layer (Rokitansky–Aschoff sinuses); in normal tissues, they are few and superficial. The mucosa is lined by a single layer of tall (15–25 μm) 'clear' columnar cells supported by a basement membrane. These cells (Fig. 20) have an ovoid basal nucleus and a pale cytoplasm with microvilli at the apex, filamentous glycocalix and core rootlest, only visible by electron microscopy. Mucosecretion can be found in small amounts, without goblet cells. Some basal cells, quite inconspicuous, rounder and smaller (10–15 μm) than columnar cells, are located immediately above the basement membrane, with their nuclei parallel to it; they should not be confused with intraepithelial lymphocytes, which are more common. Rare pencil-like (dark) columnar cells can be seen, consisting of retracted clear columnar cells. No endocrine cells are present within the fundus and body. Within villosities there is little connective tissue with capillaries. A few tubulo-alveolar mucous glands can be found in the lamina propria but only near the neck. Ganglion cells are rare in the lamina propria. The muscularis is not a well-developed layer of variable thickness

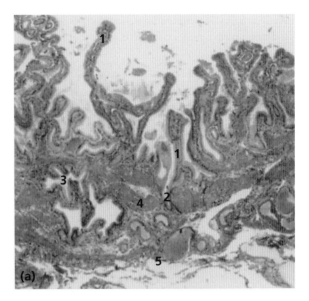

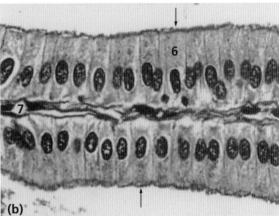

Fig. 20 Gallbladder: paraffin embedding (5-μm-thick section); haematein eosin saffron; (a) low magnification (× 36) and (b) high magnification (× 560). (a) The whole gallbladder wall can be seen: the mucosa with its numerous villosities (1) separated by crypts (2) extending into the connective tissue forming Rokitansky sinuses (3), the muscularis (4) and the adventitia (5). (b) The villosities are limited by a single columnar epithelium (6) with an ovoid nucleus near the basal pole of the cell and a striated apical pole (arrow); their axes are of delicate connective tissue (7).

composed of circular, longitudinal, and oblique smooth-muscle bundles in an elastic loose connective tissue. The adventitia is a connective tissue containing lipocytes, vessels, nerve fibres, ganglion cells, lymphocytes, and Luschka's ducts, which are minor bile ducts that lie in the subserosa connective tissue on the hepatic side; they could be embryonic remnants. On rare occasions, ectopic hepatic, pancreatic, adrenal, gastric and even thyroid tissues have been found in the gallbladder wall. The gallbladder is richly vascularized by blood and lymphatic plexuses located in the lamina propria and in the adventitia; it is innervated by sympathetic motor fibres and numerous sensory nerve endings [38].

The transport properties of biliary epithelial cells and their regulation vary between the various anatomical compartments of the biliary tract. It is usually assumed that intrahepatic ducts are mainly committed to fluid and electrolyte secretion, whereas extrahepatic bile ducts and gallbladder are considered to be specialized in absorption and mucin synthesis. The plasticity of the biliary epithelium is important.

References

1 MacSween RNM, Scothorne RJ (1994) Developmental anatomy and normal structure. In: MacSween RNM, Anthony PP, Scheuer PJ et al. (eds) Pathology of the Liver. Edinburgh: Churchill Livingstone, pp. 1–49.

2 Desmet V (2001) Organizational principles in the liver. In: Arias IM, Boyer JL, Chisari FV et al. (eds) The Liver. Biology and Pathobiology, 4th edn. New York: Raven Press, pp. 3–15.

3 Arias IM, Jakoby WB, Boyer JL et al. (eds) (1994) The Liver. Biology and Pathobiology. New York: Raven Press.

4 Saxena R, Zucker SD, Crawford JM (2003) Anatomy and physiology of the liver. In: Zakim D and Boyer TD (eds) Hepatology: A Textbook of Liver Disease, 4th edn. Philadelphia: Saunders, pp. 3–30.

5 Schroder R, Muller O, Bircher J (1985) The portacaval and splenocaval shunt in the normal rat. A morphometric and functional reevaluation. J Hepatol 1, 107–123.

6 Malarkey DE, Johnson K, Ryan L et al. (2005) New insights into functional aspects of liver morphology. Toxicol Pathol 33, 27–34.

7 Saxena R, Theise ND, Crawford JM (1999) Microanatomy of the human liver – exploring the hidden interfaces. Hepatology 30, 1339–1346.

8 Matsumoto T, Kawakami M (1982) The unit-concept of hepatic parenchym: a re-examination based on angioarchitectural studies. Acta Pathol Jpn 32, 285–314.

9 Teutsch HF (2005) The modular microarchitecture of human liver. Hepatology 42, 317–325.

10 Ekataksin W, Wake K (1997) New concepts in biliary and vascular anatomy of the liver. Prog Liv Dis 15, 1–30.

11 Roessner A, Kolde G, Stahl K et al. (1978) Ultrastructural morphometric investigations on normal human liver biopies. Acta Hepato Gastroenterol 25, 119–123.

12 Rohr HP, Luthy J, Gudat F et al. (1976) Stereology of liver biopsies from healthy volunteers. Virch Arch 371, 261–263.

13 Bioulac-Sage P, Balabaud C (eds) (1988) Sinusoids in Human Liver: Health and Disease. Rijswijk: Kupffer Cell Foundation.

14 Wake K (1995) Structure of the sinusoidal wall in the liver. In Wisse E, Knook DL, Wake K (eds) Cells of the Hepatic Sinusoid. Leiden: Kupffer Cell Foundation, pp. 241–246.

15 Wisse E, de Zanger RB, Charels K et al. (1985) The liver sieve: considerations concerning the structure and function of endothelial fenestrae, the sinusoidal wall and the space of Disse. Hepatology 5, 683–692.

16 Blouin A, Bolender RP, Weibel ER (1977) Distribution of organelles and membranes between hepatocytes and nonhepatocytes in the rat liver parenchyma. A stereological study. J Cell Biol 72, 441–455.

17 Burt AD, Le Bail B, Balabaud C et al. (1993) Morphologic investigation of sinusoidal cells. Semin Liver Disease 13, 21–38.

18 Enomoto K, Nishikawa Y, Omori Y et al. (2004) Cell biology and pathology of liver sinusoidal endothelial cells. Med Electron Microsc 37, 208–215.

19 Braet F, Luo D, Spector I et al. (2001) Endothelial and pit cells in the liver. In: Arias IM, Boyer JL, Chisari FV et al. (eds) The Liver. Biology and Pathobiology, 4th edn. New York: Raven Press, pp. 437–453.

20 Braet F, Wisse E (2002) Structural and functional aspects of liver sinusoidal endothelial cell fenestrae: a review. Comp Hepatol 1, 1.

21 Naito M, Hasegawa G, Ebe Y et al. (2004) Differentiation and function of Kupffer cells. Med Electron Microsc 37, 16–28.

22 Nakatani K, Kaneda K, Seki S et al. (2004) Pit cells as liver-associated natural killer cells: morphology and function. Med Electron Microsc 37, 29–36.

23 Li D, Friedman S (2001) Hepatic stellate cells: morphology, function, and regulation in the liver. In: Arias IM, Boyer JL, Chisari FV et al. (eds) The Liver. Biology and Pathobiology, 4th edn. New York: Raven. Press, pp. 455–473.

24 Lepreux S, Bioulac-Sage P, Gabbiani G et al. (2004) Cellular retinol-binding protein-1 expression in normal and fibrotic/cirrhotic human liver: different patterns of expression in hepatic stellate cells and (myo)fibroblast populations. J Hepatol 40, 774–780.

25 Greenwel P, Rojkind M (2001) The extracellular matrix of the liver. In: Arias IM, Boyer JL, Chisari FV et al. (eds) The Liver. Biology and Pathobiology, 4th edn. New York: Raven Press, pp. 469–473.

26 Dubuisson L, Lepreux S, Bioulac-Sage P et al. (2001) Expression and cellular localization of fibrillin-1 in normal and pathological human liver. J Hepatol 34, 514–522.

27 McCuskey RS (1994) The hepatic microvascular system. In: Arias IM, Boyer JL, Chisari FV et al. (eds) The Liver. Biology and Pathobiology, 4th edn. New York: Raven Press, pp. 1089–1106.

28 Oda M, Yokomori H, Han JY (2003) Regulatory mechanisms of hepatic microcirculation. Clin Hemorheal Microcirc 29, 167–182.

29 Ekataksin W (2000) The isolated artery: an intrahepatic arterial pathway that can bypass the lobular parenchyma in mammalian livers. Hepatology 31, 269–279.

30 Evangelou E, Kyzas PE, Trikalinos TA (2005) Comparison of the diagnostic accuracy of lymphatic endothelium markers: Bayesian approach. Mod Pathol 18, 1490–1497.

31 McCuskey RS (2004) Anatomy of efferent hepatic nerves. Anat Rec A Discov Mol Cell Evol Biol 280, 821–826.

32 Ueno T, Bioulac-Sage P, Balabaud C et al. (2004) Innervation of the sinusoidal wall: regulation of the sinusoidal diameter. Anat Rec Discov Mol Cell Evol Biol 280, 868–873.

33 Alpini G, McGill JM, Larusso NF (2002) The pathobiology of biliary epithelia. Hepatology 35, 1256–1268.

34 Shibahara H, Tamada S, Goto M et al. (2004) Pathologic features of mucin-producing bile duct tumors: two histopathologic categories as counterparts of pancreatic intraductal papillary-mucinous neoplasms. Am J Surg Pathol 28, 327–328.

35 Theise ND, Saxena R, Portmann BC et al. (1999) The canals of Hering and hepatic stem cells in humans. Hepatology 30, 1425–1433.

36 Rosai J (2004) Gallbladder and extrahepatic bile ducts. Normal anatomy. In: Rosai J (ed.) Rosai and Akerman's Surgical Pathology, 9th edn. Edinburgh: Mosby, Edinburgh, pp. 1035–1036.

37 Terada T, Takanuma Y, Ohta G (1987) Glandular elements around the intrahepatic bile ducts in man; their morphology and distribution in normal livers. Liver 7, 1–8.

38 Balemba OB, Salter MJ, Mawe GM (2004) Innervation of the extrahepatic biliary tract. Anat Rec A Discov Mol Cell Evol Biol 280, 836–847.

1.3 Ultrastructure of the hepatocyte

Zahida Khan, James M. Crawford and Donna B. Stolz

Introduction to the hepatocyte

The hepatocyte is the chief parenchymal cell of the liver, and is responsible for maintaining a wide range of specialized functions. In mature male rat liver, hepatocytes comprise approximately 87% of the volume of intralobular liver tissue, with the remainder consisting of vascular space and non-parenchymal cells (Fig. 1, Table 1) [1]. Hepatocytes are large, multifaceted, polyhedral cells, with an approximate volume of 6800 μm^3 and a diameter between 10 and 30 μm. They are arranged in anastomosing plate-like cords separated by adjacent vascular sinusoids. Within the hepatic cords, between adjacent hepatocytes, lies a network of bile canaliculi, allowing passage of bile through intercellular channels, which drain into the nearest branch of the bile duct system.

This specialized architecture optimizes the liver's parallel functions as an exocrine gland, an endocrine gland as well as a blood filter. Owing to the liver's unique vascular organization, whereby blood percolates through the sinusoids from the place of inflow (the portal tract) to outflow (the terminal hepatic vein system), hepatocytes are exposed to a lobular gradient of oxygen, nutrients, toxins and other biologically active molecules. As a result, hepatocytes are not a metabolically homogeneous population of cells, and considerable zonal heterogeneity exists

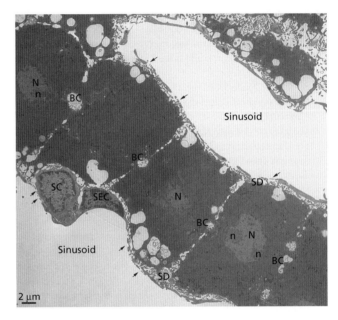

Fig. 1 Low-magnification transmission electron micrograph of a rat hepatic plate. Hepatocytes are aligned as a single layer of cells between the vascular capillaries called sinusoids. Hepatocyte apical membrane domains encircle the bile canaliculus (BC), basal membranes line the space of Disse (SD), while the lateral membranes occupy the remaining plasma membrane, between the BC and the SD. Sinusoidal endothelial cells (SECs) are highly fenestrated (arrows) and abut the hepatocytes along the SD. A stellate cell (SC) is visible within the SD, situated between the SEC and the hepatocyte. The hepatocyte nucleus (N) is centrally located and contains one or two nucleoli (n).

in both structure and function. Nevertheless, the hepatocyte cytoplasm throughout the lobule is packed with the requisite variety of organelles, and what follows is a brief description of each organelle or inclusion.

Hepatocytes maintain a particular organization with respect to other non-parenchymal cells residing in the sinusoid (Fig. 2). While fenestrated sinusoidal endothelial cells (SECs) abut most of the basal hepatocyte surface, stellate cells (SCs, also called cells of Ito or fat-storing cells) integrate between the SECs and the hepatocyte and can serve as contractile cells (Chapter 1.6).

Table 1 Volumes of mononuclear rat hepatocyte organelles and inclusions (from ref. [1]).

Compartment	Volume (μm^3/cell)	Percentage of hepatocyte
Hepatocyte	6791	100
Nucleus	556	8
Cytoplasm	6215	92
Ground substance	4720	69
Lipid droplets	8	1
Mitochondria	1363	20
Peroxisomes	101	1–2
Dense bodies	32	0.5–1

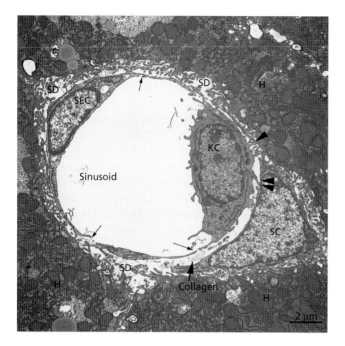

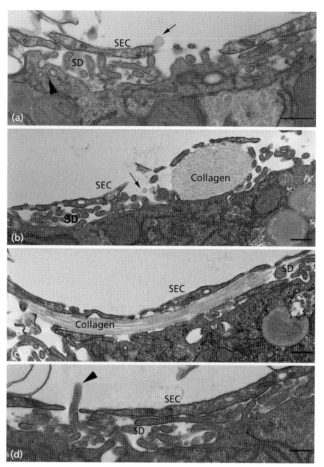

Fig. 2 Non-parenchymal cell organization within the sinusoid with respect to hepatic parenchyma. The sinusoidal endothelial cell (SEC) is fenestrated (arrows) and interacts with the hepatocyte (H) along the space of Disse (SD). Stellate cells (SC) occupy the area within the space of Disse between the SEC and the hepatocytes, often under collagen bundles. The resident macrophage, the Kupffer cell (KC), is adherent to the SEC luminal surface, but cell extensions can protrude through the SEC fenestrations and gaps to interact directly with hepatocytes (arrowhead) or stellate cells (double arrowhead).

Fig. 3 Ultrastructure of the space of Disse. The space of Disse (SD) occupies the area between the sinusoidal endothelial cell (SEC) and the hepatocyte. The SD is filled with numerous microvilli originating from the hepatocyte (a–d). The basal surface of the hepatocyte has many vesicular structures (a, arrowhead), indicating its capacity for trafficking proteins and other molecules in and out of the cell (see also Fig. 13). Chylomicron remnants (a and b, arrows) are often found in SEC fenestrations and within the SD. Collagen bundles are scattered within the SD (b and c). Microvilli have been observed to protrude through the fenestrations of the SEC (d, arrowhead). Bars: 100 nm.

Plasma membrane

Hepatocytes are polarized epithelial cells, yet they do not exhibit the typical basolateral-to-apical axis observed in simple bipolar epithelial cells [2]. On account of their polygonal shape, the hepatocyte's plasma membrane contains domains of subspecialization, which are localized to sinusoidal (basal), lateral, junctional and canalicular (apical) regions (see also Chapter 1.2). Approximately 40% of the hepatocyte surface is exposed to the vascular sinusoids [3]. The fenestrated endothelium lining the sinusoids is intimately associated with at least two faces of a hepatocyte, with no basement membrane in between them, such that each hepatocyte is bathed in plasma on both sides (Figs 1 and 5a). The basal sinusoidal membrane surface of hepatocytes, which delineates the perisinusoidal space (space of Disse), is populated by numerous finger-like projections (microvilli) that greatly enhance the surface area and the hepatocyte's capacity for receptor and transport functions (Fig. 3). Consequently, both coated and uncoated pits can be found at the base of

microvilli, along with caveolae and clathrin-coated endocytic vesicles in the adjoining cytoplasm. On rare occasions, a microvillus may protrude through the fenestrae of a SEC and into the sinusoidal lumen (Fig. 3d); however, the functional significance of this finding is unknown. Other components of the space of Disse include chylomicron remnants, scattered collagen bundles and nerve processes.

In contrast, the hepatocyte's lateral membrane surface does not contain microvilli; it does contain Na^+/K^+-dependent ATPase transport activity, and is therefore capable of generating ion gradients that influence the transport function of the entire 'basolateral' domain of the hepatocyte plasma membrane [4]. In general, the lateral membranes of adjacent hepatocytes are relatively straight and separated by an intercellular space of 10 nm [5]. A number of membrane specializations are also present

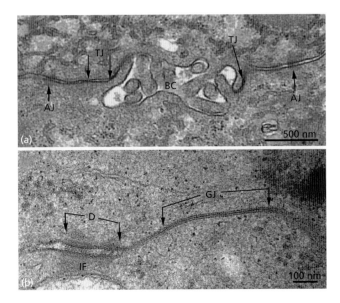

Fig. 4 Junctional components of the hepatocyte lateral membrane.
(a) The tight junctions (TJ) surround the bile canaliculus (BC) and physically
delineate the BC components from the lateral membrane space. Adherent
junctions (AJ) are distal to the TJ and provide cytoskeletal support via
microfilament connections. Together, the TJ and AJ are called the apical
junctional complex. (b) Within the lateral membrane, desmosomes (D) serve
as spot welds between adjacent hepatocytes and stabilize the connection by
attachments with intermediate filaments. Gap junctions (GJ) allow for direct
communication between cells. Located at areas of closely apposed
membrane, gap junctions are composed of plasma membrane-spanning
channels. These channels allow for the passage of small molecules such as
ions, sugars, amino acids, etc. between cells.

along this region, mainly in the form of intercellular junctions.
Saccular unions are simply interdigitating cytoplasmic protrusions of neighbouring plasma membranes. Junctional complexes
are also present, consisting of tight junctions, adherent junctions, desmosomes and gap junctions (Fig. 4). Tight junctions,
also called zonula occludens, are crucial for limiting the lateral
movement of membrane proteins between apical and basolateral domains and maintaining the blood–bile barrier, but do
demonstrate a degree of 'leakiness', as observed in the paracellular pathway of bile secretion [6]. Adherent junctions serve in
an anchoring capacity and convey physical stability to the junction via actin cytoskeletal attachments. Together with the tight
junction, these two components comprise the apical junction
complex. Desmosomes, far less numerous in hepatocytes than
the other components of the apical junction complexes, are
analogous to strong 'spot welds' between neighbouring hepatocytes and are anchored by intermediate filaments. Gap junctions
are composed predominantly of connexins and are involved in
intercellular communication between hepatocytes in each cord,
via exchange of small molecules < 1000 Da, including ions and
metabolites.

Unlike the surrounding lateral membrane intercellular junctional region, the bile canalicular region is surrounded by a
pericanalicular actin microfilament web integrated within
and around the luminal microvilli [5]. The bile canaliculus is
a highly specialized intercellular junction formed by plasma
membranes of contiguous hepatocytes (Fig. 5). Bile canalicular
membranes account for 15% of the hepatocyte's total plasma
membrane surface [7]. They measure approximately 1 μm in

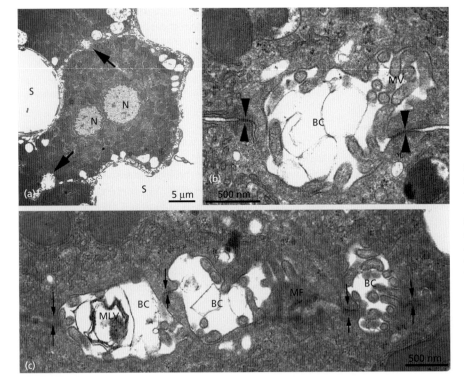

Fig. 5 Ultrastructure of bile canaliculus.
(a) Localization of the bile canaliculus within
the hepatic plate (arrows); S, sinusoid; N,
nucleus (in binucleate hepatocyte). (b) Typical
simple bile canaliculus (BC) bounded on either
side by tight junctions (between arrowheads).
Apical membrane contains many microvilli
(MV). Individual lipid vesicles are present within
the lumen. (c) Compound bile canaliculi (BC)
between adjacent hepatocytes. Each BC is
bounded by separate apical junctional
complexes (arrows). Areas around the BC
are concentrated with microfilaments (MF).
A multilamellar vesicle (MLV) is present within
one of the BC, the result of secondary
transformations of intraluminal biliary lipid.

diameter and constitute the smallest passages of the proximal biliary system, collecting bile that is apically secreted from hepatocytes and channelling it towards the distal biliary tree [5]. The canalicular diameter of periportal hepatocytes is greater than that observed in centrolobular regions; however, structural alterations in canalicular size and morphology are also dependent on hepatocyte exposure to and secretion of bile acids, such as taurocholate [8]. Unilamellar lipid vesicles (~ 60–70 nm in diameter) can be found within the canalicular lumen and adherent to the luminal hemileaflet of the canalicular plasma membrane; their role in the release of phospholipids into the bile canalicular lumen is debated (Fig. 5) [9]. In addition, each bile canaliculus is surrounded by the pericanalicular cytoplasm. This zone (1 μm in radius) is dense in microfilaments, and it may function in canalicular contractility, a normal and spontaneous process that promotes the movement of bile through the canalicular network. Eventually, the bile canaliculus leads to the canals of Hering, which link the intralobular canalicular system to the biliary tree [10,11] (Fig. 6). Canals of Hering contain the purported resident hepatic stem cell, called the oval cell (see Chapter 1.9),

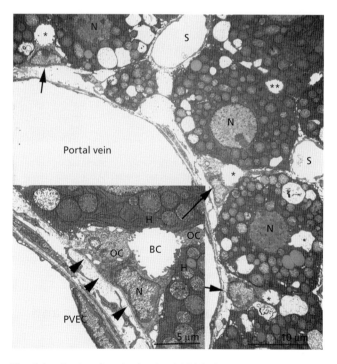

Fig. 6 Localization of canals of Hering (with bile duct epithelial cells and bipotential oval cells) in the periportal region of the mouse liver. The lumina of canals of Hering (*) constitute the terminal channels of the formal biliary tree, and have heterotypical cellular interactions between canal of Hering epithelial cells (arrows) and hepatocytes. These lumina are clearly distinct from homotypical hepatic cellular interactions of upstream bile canaliculi (BC, **). S, sinusoid; N, hepatocyte nucleus. Inset: high magnification of a canal of Hering. Oval cells (OC) are ultrastructurally distinct from mature bile duct epithelial cells or hepatocytes (H), with greatly reduced cytoplasm and a much smaller, oval nucleus. Unlike hepatocytes, oval cells have a basement membrane lining the basal membrane domain (arrowheads). PVEC, portal vein endothelial cell.

Table 2 Surface areas of the major intracytoplasmic organelles in mononuclear rat hepatocytes (from [1]).

Compartment	Surface (μm²/cell)	Percentage of total membrane
Total intracytoplasmic membrane	120 298	100
Rough ER	23 228	19
Smooth ER	51 682	43
Golgi	3138	3
Mitochondria		
Outer envelope	7450	6
Inner membrane and cristae	34 800	29

which has the ability to differentiate into either a hepatocyte or a biliary epithelial cell (cholangiocyte). The oval cell is specifically associated with the bile canaliculus continuum and forms heterogeneous cell interactions with hepatocytes [12].

Other organelles found in the pericanalicular cytoplasm include Golgi, lysosomes and clear vesicles thought to be involved in the transport of apoproteins and ligands for biliary secretion (see Chapter 2.6) [13,14].

Endoplasmic reticulum

In general, hepatocytes contain a substantial amount of both rough and smooth endoplasmic reticulum (ER) (Table 2). Individual distribution patterns can vary based on lobular differences. The most rough ER is found in zone 1 hepatocytes. Rough ER tends to form a perinuclear network of convoluted, parallel, flattened sacs (cisternae) that are actually continuous with each other, the smooth ER and the nuclear envelope (Fig. 7) [5]. A close association of rough ER with mitochondria has been observed, but there is no evidence of a direct communication between them [1].

Rough ER is the site of synthesis of secreted proteins. Protein synthesis involves translation of mRNA on ribosomes. Ultrastructurally, ribosomes are electron-dense granules measuring 15–30 nm in diameter [15]. It is estimated that a single hepatocyte contains over 10 million membrane-bound ribosomes, which cover the outer surface of rough ER (Fig. 7). In addition, a dynamic pool of free ribosomes and polyribosomes also exists in the cytoplasm, and these are responsible for synthesizing cytoplasmic and organellar proteins for the cell.

In continuity with the rough ER, the smooth ER forms an elaborate meshwork of small, smooth-surfaced tubules that are devoid of ribosomes and can communicate directly with the Golgi complex. Zone 3 hepatocytes contain the most smooth ER, which is often distributed in cytoplasmic regions rich in particulate glycogen (Fig. 7). In hepatocytes, smooth ER is specialized for several important metabolic functions, including the synthesis of lipids and bile acids, the storage of calcium and the glucuronidation of bilirubin. The enzyme glucose-6-phosphatase is localized primarily in the smooth ER, thereby permitting

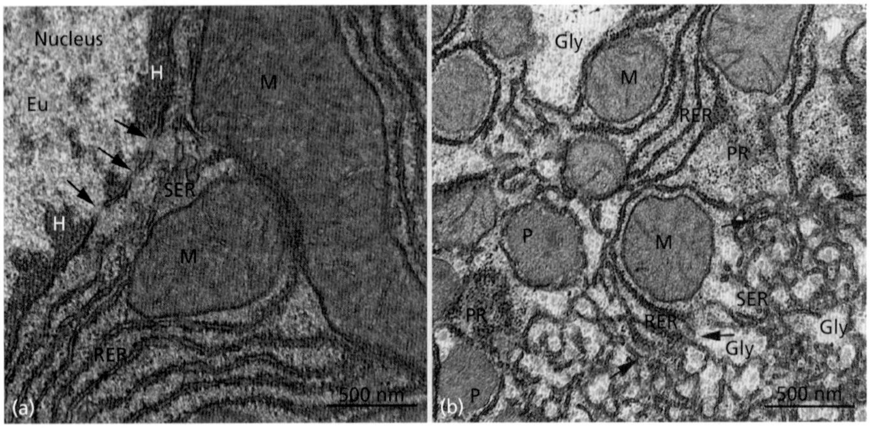

Fig. 7 (a) Hepatocyte nucleus showing euchromatin (Eu), heterochromatin (H) and nuclear pores (arrows) within the nuclear membrane. Smooth endoplasmic reticulum (SER) and rough endoplasmic reticulum (RER) are in close proximity with both the nuclear membrane and mitochondria (M). (b) SER is contiguous with RER as this transition can be seen (between arrows). Peroxisomes (P) and mitochondria (M) are found in close association with both SER and RER. Polyribosomes (PR) can be observed within the cytoplasm as well as particulate glycogen (Gly).

compartmentalization of glucose dephosphorylation from the major glucose-metabolizing systems in the cytoplasm (glycolysis, gluconeogenesis, glycogen synthesis and degradation).

The most crucial function of this organelle in the liver is drug detoxification. Smooth ER houses a number of microsomal mono-oxygenases, including cytochrome P450 enzymes, which are involved in hepatic phase I drug metabolism [16]. In fact, a variety of drugs and xenobiotics, such as phenobarbital, can lead to a massive proliferation of smooth ER, and this is reversed after drug withdrawal via autophagic vacuoles [17]. Of growing concern is the increased susceptibility of zone 3 hepatocytes to toxic injury, as their abundant smooth ER can convert harmless compounds, such as paracetamol and carbon tetrachloride, into damaging free radicals, resulting in liver damage.

Golgi complex

The Golgi apparatus is a highly compartmentalized complex of three to five flattened, parallel cisternae with smooth surfaces, and each layer is separated by a narrow space (20 nm) [5]. These closely packed saccules have dilated peripheral rims and are associated with secretory vesicles. The primary function of the Golgi is to accurately process and sort newly synthesized proteins. This involves posttranslational modifications (e.g. glycosylation, sulphation, phosphorylation), followed by packaging into vesicles that are targeted to the appropriate organelle or plasma membrane. Consequently, the Golgi complex is highly polarized, containing both *cis* and *trans* cisternae (Fig. 8). The convex *cis* surface (forming face) is fenestrated and receives macromolecules delivered by vesicular transport from the ER. Secretory vesicles arise from the concave *trans* surface, which has thicker membranes and forms a *trans*-Golgi network (TGN). In this respect, the Golgi is composed of a dynamic steady-state system of ER-derived membranes [18]. The secretory vesicles vary in size, number and content. In hepatocytes, a large number of Golgi secretory vesicles contain very-low-density lipoproteins (VLDLs), which appear ultrastructurally as spheres 50–70 nm in diameter (Fig. 8) [1]. VLDLs are rich in triglycerides and

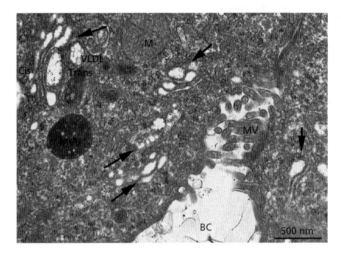

Fig. 8 Golgi apparatuses (arrows) are observed in close proximity to the bile canaliculus (BC). *Cis* and *trans* sides are labelled for one Golgi. Newly synthesized very-low-density lipoproteins (VLDL) are observed within the *trans* Golgi secretory vesicles. A multivesicular body (MVB) is observed in this field.

function in systemic lipid transport. Other vesicles can target acid hydrolases to lysosomes (described below).

Lysosomes, multivesicular bodies and autophagosomes

In general, lysosomes are electron-dense organelles surrounded by a single membrane. They exhibit a high degree of pleomorphism on account of their heterogeneous cargo and variable levels of maturation (Fig. 9). Lysosomes contain an impressive complement of luminal acid hydrolases, including proteases, nucleases, glucosidases, lipases, phospholipases, phosphatases and sulphatases. These hydrolytic enzymes enable the lysosome to degrade the vast majority of biological materials. Consequently, lysosomes can be difficult to identify, as their size and shape, as well as the contents of the individual vesicles, may be either homogenous or heterogeneous, electron dense or

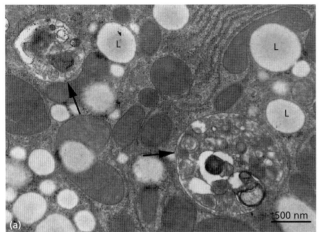

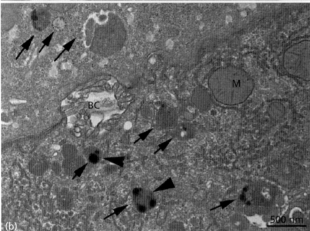

Fig. 9 (a) Lysosomes (arrows) are bounded by a single membrane and are extremely heterogeneous with respect to size, shape and contents. (b) Secondary lysosomes are common within the bile canalicular region of the hepatocyte. These more mature lysosomes are more electron dense (arrows) and often contain lipofuscin granules (arrowheads). BC, bile canaliculus; M, mitochondria; L, lipid.

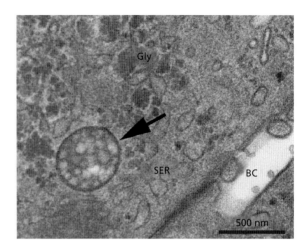

Fig. 10 Multivesicular body (arrowed) close to the bile canaliculus (BC). Glycogen (Gly) and smooth endoplasmic reticulum (SER) are also visible in the field) (see also Fig. 8).

finely granular, and may contain any number of inclusions [1]. Zone 1 hepatocytes contain the greatest amount of both lysosomes and their associated phosphatase activity.

Primary lysosomes that bud off the TGN are acid phosphatase positive and 25–50 nm in diameter [5]. Primary lysosomes fuse with late endosomes, whose contents are bound for degradation. The acid hydrolases donated by the primary lysosomes are activated by the acidic pH of late endosomes, thus forming a secondary (mature) lysosome. These can form residual bodies that often localize in the cytoplasm surrounding the canalicular region of hepatocytes [1,5]. A variety of secondary lysosomes have been described. Multivesicular bodies (MVB) contain multiple small endocytic vesicles that have turned 'inside-out' and have fused with larger vesicles (Figs 8 and 10) [19]. Eventually, MVB become increasingly electron dense as their contents are degraded. Alternatively, in many epithelial cells, MVB are known to fuse with the plasma membrane and expel the vesicular

contents into the extracellular space. In keeping with the pericanalicular localization of a portion of hepatocellular lysosomes, lysosomal contents can be discharged across the canalicular membrane of hepatocytes into bile [20]. Autophagosomes are involved in turnover and contain intact or partially digested organelles (Fig. 11). Lipofuscin granules, which are associated with ageing, are actually electron-dense lysosomes containing lipids and a heterogeneous matrix. Interestingly, hepatic lysosomes also appear to function as iron-storage vacuoles (siderosomes) that contain ferritin-like substances [21].

Mitochondria

Mitochondria are the most abundant organelles in hepatocytes (approximately 800 per cell), and they function in generating energy in the form of adenosine triphosphate (ATP) via oxidative phosphorylation. Mitochondria are large organelles, with an average diameter of up to 0.6 μm and an average length of up to 1.0 μm [22] (Fig. 7). They are actually highly mobile organelles, which closely associate with microtubules and constantly change their shape and position in the cell [5]. Mitochondria undergo turnover, with a half-life of 10.5 days, and their remnants are often identifiable in autophagosomes (Fig. 11). Furthermore, although the number of mitochondria decreases with age, mitochondrial volume remains constant because of increases in the size of the remaining organelles.

Ultrastructurally, mitochondria consist of a double membrane surrounding the mitochondrial matrix (Figs 7 and 12). An intermembrane space exists within the double membrane, where apoptosis-related proteins are confined (and subject to release into the cytoplasm if the 'mitochondrial phase transition' is activated). The outer membrane (OM) is smooth and helps to maintain shape. A number of enzymes are localized to the OM [5]. The inner membrane (IM) has numerous shelf-like

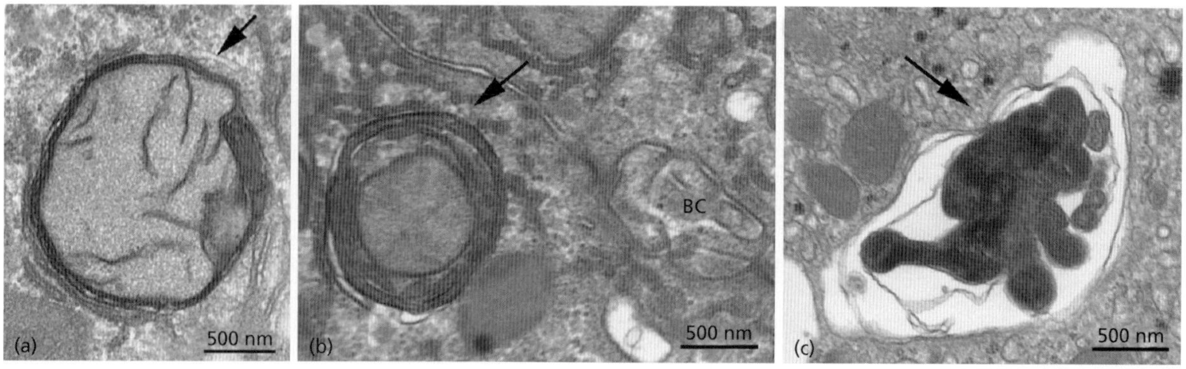

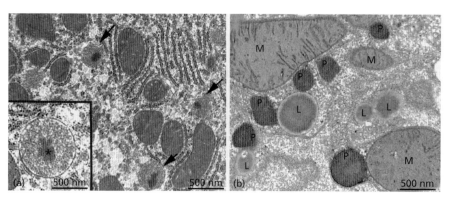

Fig. 11 Mitochondria at various stages of autophagy (arrows) in hepatocytes. (a) Early autophagosome, in which the mitochondrial ultrastructure (cristae) is still visible inside the double-membrane vesicle. (b) More mature mitochondrial autophagosome, in which the cristae structure is less apparent, but more layers of membrane within the autophagosome are visible. (c) More mature autophagosome with mitochondrial components highly condensed within the autophagosome.

Fig. 12 (a) Peroxisomes (arrows), also called microbodies, are approximately 500 nm in diameter in hepatocytes. They are single membrane-bound organelles and, in rodents when viewed by transmission electron micrography (TEM), a dense core of crystalline urate oxidase is visible (inset, *). (b) Peroxisome (P) morphology can be enzymatically enhanced for light micrography and TEM by staining lightly fixed cells or tissues with 3,3'-diaminobenzidine hydrochloride using the method described by Fahimi [29]. M, mitochondria; L, lipids.

invaginations (cristae), which project into the matrix and greatly increase the IM's surface area for housing the electron transport chain and ATP synthases. The electron-dense mitochondrial matrix contains numerous metabolic enzymes involved in the urea cycle, fatty acid oxidation and the tricarboxylic acid (TCA) or Krebs cycle. Mitochondria are self-replicating, deriving proteins both from nuclear somatic genes and about 30 genes of mitochondrial DNA (mtDNA). In the latter instance, the mitochondrial matrix contains circular mtDNA, RNA and ribosomes, all of which are necessary for synthesizing mitochondria-encoded proteins. Mitochondria also contain electron-dense inclusions, representing calcium stores, which disappear rapidly during hypoxia [1]. Occasionally, other crystalloid structures may be apparent in both normal and diseased liver [23].

Peroxisomes (microbodies)

Unlike mitochondria, peroxisomes contain a fine granular, homogeneous matrix surrounded by a single membrane and are approximately 0.2–1.0 μm in diameter [1] (Figs 7 and 12). There are approximately 200 peroxisomes per hepatocyte, making the liver the organ with the most peroxisomes. These organelles are most abundant in zone 3 hepatocytes [5]. In contrast to the large peroxisomes found in liver and kidney, the peroxisomes of most other mammalian cells are much smaller (only 0.15–0.25 μm in diameter).

The peroxisomal matrix in rats contains a laminated crystalloid core, which is thought to represent the enzyme urate oxidase (Fig. 12). In contrast, peroxisomes from human livers very rarely exhibit this nucleoid core [1]. A vast repertoire of peroxisomal enzymes (e.g. oxidases, hydroxylases) has been identified, and these are involved in the synthesis of bile acids, cholesterol, carbohydrates and plasmalogen (an ether lipid), as well as in the metabolism of amino acids and purines. The initial steps in β-oxidation of very-long-chain fatty acids (VLCFAs) also occur in the peroxisome. Most importantly, the enzyme catalase, which detoxifies cellular H_2O_2, accounts for as much as 40% of total peroxisomal protein [5]. In hepatocytes, non-conventional peroxisomal enzymes have also been described, such as inducible nitric oxide synthase (iNOS, NOS2) [24,25].

The biogenesis of peroxisomes has been studied extensively in yeast [26]. Peroxisomes are continuously turned over and, in hepatocytes, their lifespan is only about 1 day. Of particular interest in liver is the phenomenon of peroxisome proliferation, in which certain stimuli can increase peroxisomal volume and density. This is observed in embryonic and postnatal liver development, in recovery following partial hepatectomy and in response to various diseases. Specifically, the fibrate class of anti-hyperlipidaemic drugs (ethyl-α-p-chlorophenoxyisobutyrate, Clofibrate) and salicylates, as well as endogenous fatty acids, can induce peroxisome proliferation by activating the peroxisome proliferator-activated receptor (PPAR) family of transcription factors in rodents, but not in humans (discussed in later sections).

Intracellular vesicles

Casual inspection of almost any ultrastructural image of the hepatocyte cytoplasm will reveal countless intracellular vesicles approximately 100–200 nm in diameter (Fig. 13). These vesicles enable the endocytosis of extracellular proteins as well as trafficking of membrane proteins and sequestered luminal contents between the many organelles of the hepatocyte. In the first instance, a key mechanism for endocytic internalization of receptor-bound macromolecular ligands from the basolateral plasma membrane is via a highly coordinated coalescence of membrane protein receptors and recruitment of intracellular cytoskeletal and chaperone proteins (including especially the 'cage' molecule, clathrin), engendering first 'clathrin-coated pits' (invaginations of the plasma membrane) and then 'clathrin-coated vesicles' (in the cellular space directly beneath the plasma membrane). In the second instance, the magnitude of the

trafficking between organelles such as the ER, Golgi apparatus and plasma membrane is staggering. Overall, the estimated internalization of basolateral plasma membrane area by endocytosis is about 2%/min [14]. The estimated delivery of plasma membrane lipid to the apical (canalicular) membrane of the hepatocyte is 9% of apical membrane area per minute. In order for the hepatocyte to remain at structural steady state, it is therefore necessary for the delivery of membrane lipid to the basolateral plasma membrane at a similar rate of 2%/min. In the case of the canalicular membrane, 8% of the canalicular membrane phospholipid is extruded into bile per minute, as part of normal bile secretion [14]. The remainder of the lipid mass of the canalicular membrane is retrieved back into the hepatocyte via apical endocytosis [27]. Hence, although attention is largely given to defined organelles in discussing the ultrastructure of the hepatocyte, one must acknowledge the profound dynamic contributions of intracellular vesicular traffic.

Additionally, caveolae are small invaginations found on the surface of most cells, including hepatocytes [28]. Latin for 'little caves', caveolae are small (50–100 nm), vessel-shaped invaginations that mediate various aspects of endocytosis including potocytosis, transcytosis and general membrane trafficking.

Nucleus

The nucleus in hepatocytes is round or oval and approximately 6–7 μm in diameter (Figs 1, 5 and 7) [1]. Interestingly, hepatocytes can exhibit one or more centrally localized nuclei, each containing at least one nucleolus (Fig. 5). Within the nucleoplasm, clumps of electron-dense heterochromatin, often closely apposed to the nuclear membrane, can be observed, indicating tightly coiled, inactive chromosomes. Mitotic figures are rare in resting hepatocytes. The double membrane nuclear envelope fuses periodically to form nuclear pores, which are similar to those of other cell types (Fig. 7). The hepatocyte nucleus can also contain a number of inclusions. The most common inclusion is monoparticulate glycogen (30-nm particles), which can accumulate in large or small amounts [5]. Nuclear bodies are also frequent, consisting of 5- to 7-nm filamentous inclusions surrounded by a clear halo [5]. Lipid droplets are rare inclusions in normal hepatocyte nuclei.

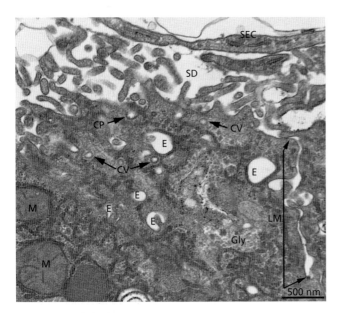

Fig. 13 Intracellular vesicle populations in close proximity to the hepatocyte basolateral membrane. Clathrin-coated pits (CP) regulate receptor-mediated endocytosis of ligands from the basal membrane abutting the space of Disse (SD) and are internalized to form coated vesicles (CV) within the cytoplasm. Coated vesicles can then fuse with endosomes (E), which tightly regulate intracellular trafficking of their contents to other destinations, as well as route contents for recycling or destruction. LM, lateral membrane; SEC, sinusoidal endothelial cell; M, mitochondria; Gly, glycogen.

References

1 Weibel ER, Staubli W, Gnagi HR *et al.* (1969) Correlated morphometric and biochemical studies on the liver cell. I. Morphometric model, stereologic methods, and normal morphometric data for rat liver. *J Cell Biol* 42, 68–91.

2 Tuma PE, Hubbard AL (2001) The hepatocyte surface: dynamic polarity. In: Arias IM, Boyer JL, Chisari FV *et al.* (eds) *The Liver: Biology and Pathobiology*, 4th edn. Philadelphia: Lippincott Williams & Wilkins, pp. 97–117.

3 Schaffner F, Popper H (1985) Structure of the liver. In: Berk JE (ed.) *Bockus Gastroenterology*. Philadelphia: W.B. Saunders, pp. 2625–2658.

4 Boyer JL, Allen RM, Ng OC (1983) Biochemical separation of Na+,K+-ATPase from a 'purified' light density, 'canalicular'-enriched plasma membrane fraction from rat liver. *Hepatology* 3, 18–28.

5 Phillips MJ, Poucell S, Patterson J *et al.* (1987) *The Liver: an Atlas and Text of Ultrastructural Pathology.* New York: Raven Press.

6 Boyer JL (1983) Tight junctions in normal and cholestatic liver: does the paracellular pathway have functional significance? *Hepatology* 3, 614–617.

7 Rohr HP, Luthy J, Gudat F *et al.* (1976) Stereology of liver biopsies from healthy volunteers. *Virchows Arch A Pathol Anat Histol* 371, 251–263.

8 Layden TJ, Boyer JL (1978) Influence of bile acids on bile canalicular membrane morphology and the lobular gradient in canalicular size. *Lab Invest* 39, 110–119.

9 Oude Elferink RP, Paulusma CC, Groen AK (2006) Hepatocanicular transport defects: pathophysiologic mechanisms of rare diseases. *Gastroenterology* 130, 908–925.

10 Oshio C, Phillips MJ (1981) Contractility of bile canaliculi: implications for liver function. *Science* 212, 1041–1042.

11 Ujhazy P, Kipp H, Misra S *et al.* (2001) The biology of the bile canaliculus. In: Arias IM, Boyer JL, Chisari FV *et al.* (eds) *The Liver: Biology and Pathobiology.* Philadelphia: Lippincott Williams & Wilkins, pp. 362–372.

12 Saxena R, Theise ND, Crawford JM (1999) Microanatomy of the human liver: exploring the hidden interfaces. *Hepatology* 30, 1339–1346.

13 Jones AL, Schmucker DL, Mooney JS *et al.* (1979) Alterations in hepatic pericanalicular cytoplasm during enhanced bile secretory activity. *Lab Invest* 40, 512–517.

14 Crawford JM (1996) The role of vesicle-mediated transport pathways in hepatocellular bile secretion. *Semin Liver Dis* 16, 169–189.

15 Tanikawa K (1979) *Ultrastructural Aspects of the Liver and its Disorders.* Tokyo: Igaku-Shoin.

16 Fouts JR, Rogers LA, Gram TE (1966) The metabolism of drugs by hepatic microsomal enzymes. Studies on intramicrosomal distribution of enzymes and relationships between enzyme activity and structure of the hepatic endoplasmic reticulum. *Exp Mol Pathol* 5, 475–490.

17 Feldman D, Swarm RL, Becker J (1980) Elimination of excess smooth endoplasmic reticulum after phenobarbital administration. *J Histochem Cytochem* 28, 997–1006.

18 Lippincott-Schwartz J (2001) The endoplasmic reticulum and golgi complex in secretory membrane transport. In: Arias IM, Boyer JL, Chisari FV *et al.* (eds) *The Liver: Biology and Pathobiology.* Philadelphia: Lippincott Williams & Wilkins, pp. 119–131.

19 Cohen JH, Bouic P, Schmitt D *et al.* (1983) Endocytosis of class II histocompatibility antigens and formation of intracytoplasmic granules at the final differentiation stage of human B lymphocytes. *Immunol Lett* 7, 123–127.

20 Nakano A, Marks DL, Tietz PS *et al.* (1995) Quantitative importance of biliary excretion to the turnover of hepatic lysosomal enzymes. *Hepatology* 22, 262–266.

21 Selden C, Owen M, Hopkins JM *et al.* (1980) Studies on the concentration and intracellular localization of iron proteins in liver biopsy specimens from patients with iron overload with special reference to their role in lysosomal disruption. *Br J Haematol* 44, 593–603.

22 Ma MH, Biempica L (1971) The normal human liver cell. Cytochemical and ultrastructural studies. *Am J Pathol* 62, 353–390.

23 Ma MH, Goldfisher S, Biempica L (1972) Morphology of the normal liver cell. *Prog Liver Dis* 4, 1–17.

24 Stolz DB, Zamora R, Vodovotz Y *et al.* (2002) Peroxisomal localization of inducible nitric oxide synthase in hepatocytes. *Hepatology* 36, 81–93.

25 Loughran PA, Stolz DB, Vodovotz Y *et al.* (2005) Monomeric inducible nitric oxide synthase localizes to peroxisomes in hepatocytes. *Proc Natl Acad Sci USA* 102, 13837–13842.

26 Heiland I, Erdmann R (2005) Biogenesis of peroxisomes. Topogenesis of the peroxisomal membrane and matrix proteins. *FEBS J* 272, 2362–2372.

27 Rahner C, Stieger B, Landmann L (2000) Apical endocytosis in hepatocytes in situ involves clathrin, traverses a subapical compartment, and leads to lysosomes. *Gastroenterology* 199, 1692–1707.

28 Calvo M, Tebar F, Opez-Iglesias C *et al.* (2001) Morphologic and functional characterization of caveolae in rat liver hepatocytes. *Hepatology* 33, 1259–1269.

29 Fahimi HD (1969) Cytochemical localization of peroxidatic activity of catalase in rat hepatic microbodies (peroxisomes). *J Cell Biol* 43, 275–288.

1.4 Liver sinusoidal endothelial cells

David Semela and Vijay H. Shah

Introduction

Liver sinusoidal endothelial cells (LSEC) form a highly specialized layer of cells lining the plates of hepatocytes. LSEC constitute a mechanical filter and a metabolic organ that is critically involved in multiple physiological and pathological processes such as liver organogenesis, liver regeneration, chronic inflammatory liver disease and hepatocarcinogenesis. This chapter will review the current knowledge of LSEC and their role in specific liver conditions.

Role of LSEC in liver homeostasis

It is estimated that 1×10^8 (20%) of all cells in the liver are LSEC, which is the most frequent cell type in the liver after hepatocytes. LSEC form the hepatic microvasculature called liver sinusoids, which consist of LSEC plates between plates of hepatocytes. In comparison to the microvasculature of most other organs and large liver blood vessels, liver sinusoids lack an underlying basement membrane [1]. The vascular bed in the liver is characterized by a discontinuous endothelial cell lining and sieve-like endothelial cells with fenestrae (pores) (Fig. 1). These plates filter the fluids that are exchanged between the sinusoidal lumen and the space of Disse, defined as the perisinusoidal space separating the sinusoids from the adjacent hepatocytes (see Chapter 2.1.2) [2]. Endothelial fenestrae measure 150–175 nm, occur at a frequency of 9–13/µm² and occupy 6–8% of the total endothelial surface in scanning electron microscopy preparations [3]. Endothelial fenestrae have a lobular gradient in diameter and frequency along a portal to central axis [3], resulting in a higher porosity in centrolobular regions. The diameter of fenestrae can be influenced by different agents, such as serotonin, CCl_4, alcohol, nicotine, pantetheine and pressure [2,4–6]. Because of the limited porosity (< 10%) of the endothelial cells, they constitute a barrier that protects the parenchymal cells from direct contact with the blood. The fenestrated lining blocks the passage of particles larger than about 200 nm, such as chylomicrons [7,8]. Chylomicron remnants, which, after being metabolized by lipoprotein lipase, are smaller (30–80 nm) than

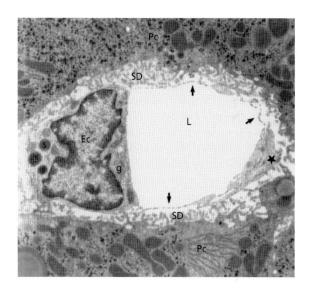

Fig. 1 Endothelial cell surrounding the sinusoidal lumen. The endothelial cell lining is fenestrated and separates the space of Disse from the lumen. It is thought that all transport between the lumen and the parenchymal cells has to pass through this filter. The endothelial lining seems to be supported by processes of fat-storing cells (asterisk). Endothelial cells of the sinusoids have a high endocytotic and digestive capacity, reflected here by the presence of lysosomes, which are quite abundant in these cells. Ec, endothelial cell; g, Golgi apparatus; L, sinusoidal lumen; SD, space of Disse; Pc, parenchymal cell.

chylomicrons, can enter the space of Disse and can be metabolized further by hepatocytes [9]. Fenestrae are surrounded by an intracellular filamentous, fenestrae-associated cytoskeleton ring composed of microfilaments, intermediate filaments and microtubules [10]. The diameter of this ring can increase or decrease, and reorganization of the cytoskeleton can form additional fenestrae within minutes upon stimulation [10–12]. The contraction of fenestrae after serotonin administration is associated with an increase in calcium [10]. Vascular endothelial growth factor (VEGF) induces fenestration in LSEC, possibly through caveolin-1 protein [12].

LSEC represent an important blood clearance system and possess specialized endocytotic mechanisms for uptake of various substances (i.e. transferrin, ceruloplasmin, transcobal-amine II, heparin, albumin, lipoproteins and hyaluronate) and antigens. Hyaluronate is a high-molecular-mass polysaccharide that is cleared from the circulation by LSEC through receptor-mediated endocytosis. The ability of LSEC to take up hyaluronate is used as a functional marker of sinusoidal endothelial cells [13,14]. Rising serum hyaluronate levels corre-late with decreased endocytotic capabilities of LSEC and have been used as an adjunctive test in the assessment of patients with alcoholic liver disease [15]. The mannose receptor has been well studied for its role in binding and internalizing compounds or antigens that contain specific terminal glycoproteins [16, 17]. Ligands are delivered to endosomes and lysosomes after internalization for degradation, and receptors are recycled by returning to the cell surface [17].

LSEC play an important role in immunity and inflammation [18,19]. LSEC facilitate adhesion of leukocytes and lymphocytes by secreting chemokines and expressing molecules such as vas-cular cell adhesion molecule 1 (VCAM-1), vascular adhesion protein (VAP-1) and intercellular adhesion molecule 1 (ICAM-1) [20–22]. LSEC are in direct contact with bloodborne antigens that traverse the bowel mucosa and enter the portal circulation intact. They are very efficient at antigen uptake through their scavenging receptors [18]. Besides major histocompatibility complex (MHC) class I molecules, they also express MHC class II molecules and can act as antigen-presenting cells to T cells [23,24]. They have been shown to prime naive CD4+ T cells [25]. LSEC can cross-present exogenous antigens and render CD8+ T cells tolerant, possibly explaining the phenomenon of immunological tolerance in liver transplant patients and of avoidance of unwanted autoimmune reactions against food antigens [24,26].

LSEC are key players in angiogenesis and vasculogenesis of the liver, which are defined as the formation of new blood vessels from pre-existing vascular beds and *de novo* organization of endothelial cells into vascular structures respectively. Formation of new blood vessels starts with activation of LSEC, which will then proliferate, migrate and, finally, assemble into vascular structures. As described below, this process requires a complex interplay of cells and angiogenic factors and is found in virtually all physiological and pathological hepatic processes.

Molecular biology and signalling in LSEC

In the past decade, tremendous insight has been gained into the molecular biology and signalling pathways of endothelial cells. Numerous receptors and ligands [i.e. VEGF/VEGF receptors (VEGFR), hepatocyte growth factor (HGF)/c-MET, angiopoietins/Tie, fibroblast growth factor (FGF)/FGF receptor, nitric oxide (NO)/integrins] and their role in proliferation, migration, sur-vival and apoptosis of endothelial cells have been identified. VEGF (VEGF-A), a 45-kDa homodimeric glycoprotein that can be produced and secreted by most mammalian cells is the most important growth and survival factor for LSEC and endothelial

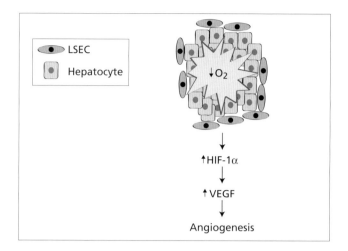

Fig. 2 Hypoxia is a potent stimulator of VEGF expression and angiogenesis. Hypoxia-inducible factor (HIF)-1α is the key transcription factor in hypoxic states in the liver, and it induces the expression of several hypoxia response genes such as *VEGF* and *VEGFR1*. LSEC, liver sinusoidal endothelial cells; HIF-1α, hypoxia-inducible factor 1α; VEGF, vascular endothelial growth factor.

cells in general [27]. VEGF expression is upregulated through different cytokines, growth factors and hypoxia-inducible factor (HIF)-1α (Fig. 2) [27]. Its effects are mediated mainly through the cell surface tyrosine kinase receptors VEGFR-1 [also known as fms-like tyrosine kinase (Flt)-1 or FLT-1 in humans] and VEGFR-2 [also known as mouse fetal liver kinase (Flk)-1 or kinase domain region (KDR) in humans] [27]. VEGFR-1 is highly expressed in LSEC and in endothelial cells of hepatic arterioles [28,29]. VEGFR-2 expression in resting liver is limited to endothelial cells of the larger hepatic vessels, whereas LSEC upregulate VEGFR-2 during liver regeneration [28]. VEGFR-3 [fms-like tyrosine kinase (Flt)-4] has not been detected on LSEC in resting or regenerating liver [28]. Most of the endothelial cell signalling studies have used human umbilical vein endothelial cells, so-called HUVECs, rather than LSEC. However, liver-specific data are emerging, especially from studies using partial hepatectomy in rodents as a model for studying LSEC and their cross-talk with hepatocytes during hepatic regeneration [28–32]. The differential effects of VEGFR-1 and -2 in LSEC are summarized in Table 1. It is now well established that VEGF

Table 1 Differential effects of VEGF receptors 1 and 2 in liver sinusoidal endothelial cells [27].

VEGF receptor 1	VEGF receptor 2
Release of HGF and IL-6	Migration
Cross-talk with VEGF receptor 2	Proliferation
Induction of MMP-9	Survival
Decoy for VEGF	Angiogenesis

VEGF, vascular endothelial growth factor; HGF, hepatocyte growth factor; IL-6, interleukin-6; MMP-9, matrix metalloproteinase 9.

Fig. 3 Paracrine signalling between LSEC and hepatocytes. During liver regeneration, VEGF is produced by hepatocytes and induces the secretion of growth factors such as hepatocyte growth factor (HGF) and interleukin-6 (IL-6) from LSEC, which in turn stimulate hepatocyte proliferation. Activation of VEGFR-2 on LSEC stimulates proliferation, whereas growth and survival are mediated through VEGFR-1. LSEC, liver sinusoidal endothelial cells; VEGF, vascular endothelial growth factor; VEGFR-1, vascular endothelial growth factor receptor 1; VEGFR-2, vascular endothelial growth factor receptor 2; c-Met, hepatocyte growth factor receptor.

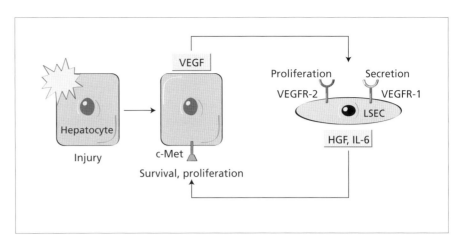

secreted by hepatocytes stimulates LSEC proliferation and liver angiogenesis by signalling through VEGFR-2, whereas activation of VEGFR-1 on LSEC induces the secretion of liver-specific growth factors such as HGF and interleukin (IL)-6, which will promote survival and proliferation of hepatocytes during liver regeneration (Fig. 3). Many of the over 70 activated genes during liver regeneration encode angiogenic growth factors and receptors other than the VEGF and HGF/c-Met signalling pathways [i.e. angiopoietins, platelet-derived growth factor (PDGF), fibroblast growth factor (FGF)] (reviewed in [32]). Similar interactions between endothelial cells and hepatocytes are at play during liver organogenesis (see below).

NO is another key signalling pathway in LSEC. Production of NO via endothelial NO synthase (eNOS) is limited to endothelial cells among all liver cell types [21]. LSEC-derived NO regulates blood flow through sinusoids via paracrine effects on hepatic stellate cells [33]. Shear stress is a key regulator of LSEC NO production, a characteristic that may autoregulate hepatic blood flow [34]. For example, if sinusoidal blood flow is high, eNOS-mediated production of NO dilates the vascular bed, thereby decreasing resistance [34]. In cirrhosis, eNOS-derived production in liver is decreased [35]. Other important agonists that activate eNOS include endothelin (via the ET-B receptor), VEGF, estrogen and others [33,36–38]. Inducible NO synthase (iNOS) is induced upon stimulation by liver injury or cytokine induction [39,40]. LSEC produce NO via iNOS in response to interferon (IFN)-γ and lipopolysaccharide (LPS) [41]. In contrast, tumour necrosis factor (TNF)-α and IL-1β, which stimulates the induction of iNOS in hepatocytes, does not induce iNOS in LSEC [41]. Thus, both eNOS and iNOS are important regulators of NO generation in LSEC depending on the haemodynamic/pathophysiological circumstance.

VEGF and NO have recently been shown to be necessary to maintain the phenotype of LSEC [42]. Inhibition of VEGF or NO signalling causes dedifferentiation of LSEC with loss of fenestrae and the appearance of CD31 on the cell surface. Dedifferentiation is also called capillarization and occurs in various liver pathologies.

Recent advances in large-scale screening technologies for genes and proteins and in the isolation of LSEC allow the investigation of different expression patterns between normal LSEC and activated LSEC in diseased liver tissue. These techniques can identify functional genes using cDNA expression libraries from human LSEC isolated, for example, from hepatocellular carcinoma (HCC) or endothelial surface markers using subtractive proteomic mapping [43–45].

LSEC in specific liver conditions

Liver organogenesis

Liver sinusoids form during liver organogenesis by vasculogenesis, which is defined as *de novo* organization of endothelial cells and/or angioblasts into blood vessels in the absence of any pre-existing vascular system. Liver sinusoids develop between gestational weeks 4 and 12 and are accompanied by recruitment of haematopoietic cells to fulfil the intrahepatic haematopoietic function, which begins by week 7 of gestation and reaches a maximum by week 12 of gestation [46,47]. The differentiation of LSEC during liver organogenesis has been studied in human fetuses, and two phases of differentiation have been identified [47]. In an early phase of structural differentiation (gestational weeks 5–12), LSEC lose markers of continuous endothelium (i.e. CD31, CD34, 1F10). The composition of the subendothelial matrix shifts during this phase from a typical vascular basement membrane (rich in laminin, devoid of tenascin) to that of an adult perisinusoidal matrix (low in laminin and rich in tenascin) [47]. A later structural differentiation (gestational weeks 10–20) is characterized by the acquisition of the markers of adult sinusoidal endothelial cells (CD4, ICAM-1, FcR IgG II, CD14) [47].

Endothelial cells are also critical for normal development of the liver parenchyma and induce the outgrowth of the liver bud into the mesenchyme [46]. Cross-talk between LSEC and hepatocytes through VEGF and HGF signalling has been shown to be crucial during liver organogenesis. Knockout mice for *VEGF* [48,49], *VEGFR1* [50,51] or *VEGFR2* [46] result in embryonic lethality at embryonic (E) days E11–E12, E8.5 and E9.5–E10.5 respectively. *VEGFR2*-deficient mice lack mature endothelial cells and blood vessels and fail to develop a liver bud [46]. Knockout mice for *HGF* [52,53] or the HGF receptor c-Met [54] fail to complete development and also die *in utero* between days E13.5 and E16.5. The livers of these mice are small and show extensive loss of parenchymal cells.

Liver regeneration

LSEC are key players in the process of liver regeneration and have been studied extensively in animal models after partial hepatectomy. Regrowth of liver after resection or liver injury is angiogenesis dependent and can be accelerated by proangiogenic growth factors such as VEGF [29,55–57] or inhibited by LSEC-inhibiting factors such as angiostatin or TNP-470 [58,59]. Detailed studies have shown that, following hepatectomy, LSEC are activated and start to proliferate after hepatocytes, which initially form avascular clusters of 10–14 cells [28,60]. Attracted by chemotactic stimuli, LSEC will migrate and finally revascularize these islands [28,60]. In a final step, the normal architecture of liver sinusoids with fenestrated LSEC is reconstituted [28,60]. Endothelial progenitor cells, mobilized from bone marrow by systemically circulating growth factors and chemokines produced in the regenerating liver, contribute by homing to these sites of neovascularization in the liver and by committing to sinusoidal endothelial cells [61].

On a molecular level, it has been shown that hepatocyte production of VEGF reaches a peak 2–3 days after hepatectomy and is detected mainly in periportal hepatocytes [56,60]. At the same time, LSEC increase the expression of VEGFR-1 and VEGFR-2 and release HGF, which is the most potent stimulator of hepatocyte proliferation (see above and Fig. 3) [28,29]. Neutralizing antibodies against VEGF inhibit LSEC and hepatocyte proliferation, whereas administration of additional VEGF in hepatectomized rodents increases their proliferation [55,56], accelerates gain in liver mass [29] and improves functional hepatic recovery [57].

Hepatocellular carcinoma

Growth of solid tumours such as HCC is dependent on angiogenesis for vascular supply of the malignant tissue [62]. Proliferation of local LSEC and possibly incorporation of circulating endothelial progenitor cells contribute to the formation of new blood vessels in HCC, which is a hypervascular tumour characterized by blood supply derived exclusively from the hepatic artery [62]. This process is regulated by a well-coordinated interplay of various growth factors secreted by hepatocytes, neoplastic cells, hepatic stellate cells and tumour-infiltrating inflammatory cells [63–66]: tumour hypoxia leads to stabilization of HIF-1α with subsequent upregulation of proangiogenic growth factors such as VEGF, which stimulate LSEC proliferation, migration and survival. In addition, genetic mutations

in neoplastic hepatocytes lead to secretion of proangiogenic growth factors and LSEC stimulation. Multiple studies have shown the overexpression of VEGF and other endothelial cell growth factors in HCC [67–76]. Various growth factors [i.e. basic FGF, transforming growth factor (TGF)-α, epidermal growth factor (EGF), PDGF] and cytokines (i.e. IL-1β, TNF-α, IFN-α and -γ) increase the secretion of VEGF in HCC cell lines [68]. Expression of VEGF increases gradually during hepatocarcinogenesis from low-grade dysplastic nodules to high-grade dysplastic nodules to early HCC, and correlates with LSEC microvessel density and sinusoidal capillarization, characterized by loss of fenestrae and development of a basement membrane [66,77]. Serum VEGF levels in patients with HCC correlate with tumour expression of VEGF, stage of HCC, absence of tumour capsule, presence of intrahepatic metastasis, presence of microscopic venous invasion and postoperative recurrence [78–81]. The pretreatment serum VEGF level is a significant inverse predictor of survival in HCC patients undergoing resection and in patients with unresectable HCC undergoing transcatheter arterial chemoembolization [75,82].

Antiangiogenic therapies targeting VEGF and other signalling pathways in LSEC are currently being evaluated in patients with HCC [62]. Genomic and proteomic analysis of isolated LSEC from HCC are promising new strategies for the identification of novel markers and LSEC targets for antiangiogenic therapy in HCC [43–45].

Chronic liver disease

Chronic liver disease with fibrosis and cirrhosis leads to the formation of an abundant vascular network and abnormal hepatic microcirculation [83–86]. The deposited matrix proteins of fibrosis contain and sequester different angiogenic factors such as VEGF, which are liberated during remodelling of the connective tissue framework by proteolytic enzymes such as matrix metalloproteinases [87,88]. Additionally, hypoxia-driven hepatocyte production of VEGF is upregulated during fibrogenesis leading to LSEC proliferation and angiogenesis [89,90]. Hypoxia and VEGF induce the expression of type 1 collagen in activated hepatic stellate cells [90,91]. Neutralizing antibodies against VEGFR-1 and VEGFR-2 in murine CCl$_4$-induced liver fibrosis both suppressed neovascularization in the liver and significantly attenuated the development of fibrosis and the increase in fibrosis markers [92]. Other studies have demonstrated that LSEC are also able to produce extracellular matrix components such as fibronectin, laminin and type 4 collagen when stimulated with TGF-β [93,94].

Development of portal–systemic collateral vessels in portal hypertension is a mechanical consequence of high vascular resistance and increased portal pressure with subsequent opening of collateral vessels [95]. However, recent evidence suggests that active, VEGF-dependent angiogenesis also contributes to this process as the expression of VEGF and VEGFR-2 increases in splanchnic organs after partial portal vein ligation in mice in a time-dependent fashion during the evolution of portal hypertension [96]. Antibodies against VEGFR-2 and VEGFR-2-specific tyrosine kinase inhibitor, given to these animals after ligation, inhibit the formation of portal–systemic collateral vessels [96]. In liver cirrhosis, NO production from LSEC is diminished, whereas production of the constrictor ET-1 is increased, which contributes to the high vascular resistance in portal hypertension [33,35]. This most likely occurs through defects in posttranslational processing of eNOS [38,39].

LSEC in the ageing liver

With ageing, a decrease in the number of fenestrae in LSEC has been described (pseudocapillarization) [97]. It has been hypothesized that this process may lead to disordered lipid metabolism and enhance atherosclerosis as chylomicron remnants are less and less able to traverse the liver sieve [97,98]. The cause of these age-related changes is unclear, although chronic exposure to oxidants and alcohol have been shown to induce changes in LSEC [9,99].

It is beyond the scope of this chapter to cover all diseases affecting LSEC. Veno-occlusive disease (VOD), drug toxicity, ischaemic–reperfusion injury and rejection after liver transplantation will be discussed in other chapters.

References

1 Braet F, Wisse E (2002) Structural and functional aspects of liver sinusoidal endothelial cell fenestrae: a review. *Comp Hepatol* 1 (1), 1.

2 Horn T, Christoffersen P, Henriksen JH (1987) Alcoholic liver injury: defenestration in noncirrhotic livers – a scanning electron microscopic study. *Hepatology* 7 (1), 77–82.

3 Wisse E, De Zanger RB, Charels K et al. (1985) The liver sieve: considerations concerning the structure and function of endothelial fenestrae, the sinusoidal wall and the space of Disse. *Hepatology* 5 (4), 683–692.

4 Fraser R, Clark SA, Day WA et al. (1988) Nicotine decreases the porosity of the rat liver sieve: a possible mechanism for hypercholesterolaemia. *Br J Exp Pathol* 69 (3), 345–350.

5 Braet F, De Zanger R, Sasaoki T et al. (1994) Assessment of a method of isolation, purification, and cultivation of rat liver sinusoidal endothelial cells. *Lab Invest* 70 (6), 944–952.

6 Braet F, Kalle WH, De Zanger RB et al. (1996) Comparative atomic force and scanning electron microscopy: an investigation on fenestrated endothelial cells in vitro. *J Microsc* 181 (1), 10–17.

7 Naito M, Wisse E (1978) Filtration effect of endothelial fenestrations on chylomicron transport in neonatal rat liver sinusoids. *Cell Tissue Res* 190 (3), 371–382.

8 Fraser R, Bosanquet AG, Day WA (1978) Filtration of chylomicrons by the liver may influence cholesterol metabolism and atherosclerosis. *Atherosclerosis* 29 (2), 113–123.

9 Fraser R, Dobbs BR, Rogers GW (1995) Lipoproteins and the liver sieve: the role of the fenestrated sinusoidal endothelium in lipoprotein metabolism, atherosclerosis, and cirrhosis. *Hepatology* 21(3), 863–874.

10 Braet F, De Zanger R, Baekeland M et al. (1995) Structure and dynamics of the fenestrae-associated cytoskeleton of rat liver sinusoidal endothelial cells. *Hepatology* 21(1), 180–189.

11 Braet F, Spector I, De Zanger R et al. (1998) A novel structure involved in the formation of liver endothelial cell fenestrae revealed by using the actin inhibitor misakinolide. *Proc Natl Acad Sci USA* 95 (23), 13635–13640.

12 Yokomori H, Oda M, Yoshimura K et al. (2003) Vascular endothelial growth factor increases fenestral permeability in hepatic sinusoidal endothelial cells. *Liver Int* 23 (6), 467–475.

13 Smedsrod B, Pertoft H, Eriksson S et al. (1984) Studies in vitro on the uptake and degradation of sodium hyaluronate in rat liver endothelial cells. *Biochem J* 223 (3), 617–626.

14 Deaciuc IV, Bagby GJ, Lang CH et al. (1993) Hyaluronic acid uptake by the isolated, perfused rat liver: an index of hepatic sinusoidal endothelial cell function. *Hepatology* 17 (2), 266–272.

15 Phillips MG, Preedy VR, Hughes RD (2003) Assessment of prognosis in alcoholic liver disease: can serum hyaluronate replace liver biopsy? *Eur J Gastroenterol Hepatol* 15 (9), 941–944.

16 Smedsrod B, Pertoft H, Gustafson S et al. (1990) Scavenger functions of the liver endothelial cell. *Biochem J* 266 (2), 313–327.

17 Magnusson S, Berg T (1989) Extremely rapid endocytosis mediated by the mannose receptor of sinusoidal endothelial rat liver cells. *Biochem J* 257 (3), 651–656.

18 Knolle PA, Limmer A (2003) Control of immune responses by scavenger liver endothelial cells. *Swiss Med Wkly* 133 (37–38), 501–506.

19 Jaeschke H (1996) Chemokines, neutrophils, and inflammatory liver injury. *Shock* 6 (6), 403–404.

20 Steinhoff G, Behrend M, Schrader B et al. (1993) Expression patterns of leukocyte adhesion ligand molecules on human liver endothelia. Lack of ELAM-1 and CD62 inducibility on sinusoidal endothelia and distinct distribution of VCAM-1, ICAM-1, ICAM-2, and LFA-3. *Am J Pathol* 142 (2), 481–488.

21 Lalor PF, Adams DH (1999) Adhesion of lymphocytes to hepatic endothelium. *Mol Pathol* 52 (4), 214–219.

22 Bird IN, Spragg JH, Ager A et al. (1993) Studies of lymphocyte transendothelial migration: analysis of migrated cell phenotypes with regard to CD31 (PECAM-1), CD45RA and CD45RO. *Immunology* 80 (4), 553–560.

23 Lohse AW, Knolle PA, Bilo K et al. (1996) Antigen-presenting function and B7 expression of murine sinusoidal endothelial cells and Kupffer cells. *Gastroenterology* 110 (4), 1175–1181.

24 Limmer A, Ohl J, Kurts C et al. (2000) Efficient presentation of exogenous antigen by liver endothelial cells to CD8+ T cells results in antigen-specific T-cell tolerance. *Nature Med* 6 (12), 1348–1354.

25 Knolle PA, Schmitt E, Jin S et al. (1999) Induction of cytokine production in naive CD4(+) T cells by antigen-presenting murine liver sinusoidal endothelial cells but failure to induce differentiation toward Th1 cells. *Gastroenterology* 116 (6), 1428–1440.

26 Onoe T, Ohdan H, Tokita D et al. (2005) Liver sinusoidal endothelial cells have a capacity for inducing nonresponsiveness of T cells across major histocompatibility complex barriers. *Transpl Int* 18 (2), 206–214.

27 Ferrara N, Gerber HP, LeCouter J (2003) The biology of VEGF and its receptors. *Nature Med* 9 (6), 669–676.

28 Ross MA, Sander CM, Kleeb TB et al. (2001) Spatiotemporal expression of angiogenesis growth factor receptors during the revascularization of regenerating rat liver. *Hepatology* 34 (6), 1135–1148.

29 LeCouter J, Moritz DR, Li B et al. (2003) Angiogenesis-independent endothelial protection of liver: role of VEGFR-1. *Science* 299 (5608), 890–893.

30 Yamane A, Seetharam L, Yamaguchi S *et al.* (1994) A new communication system between hepatocytes and sinusoidal endothelial cells in liver through vascular endothelial growth factor and Flt tyrosine kinase receptor family (Flt-1 and KDR/Flk-1). *Oncogene* 9 (9), 2683–2690.

31 Mochida S, Ishikawa K, Inao M *et al.* (1996) Increased expressions of vascular endothelial growth factor and its receptors, flt-1 and KDR/flk-1, in regenerating rat liver. *Biochem Biophys Res Commun* 226 (1), 176–179.

32 Medina J, Arroyo AG, Sanchez-Madrid F *et al.* (2004) Angiogenesis in chronic inflammatory liver disease. *Hepatology* 39 (5), 1185–1195.

33 Shah V (2001) Cellular and molecular basis of portal hypertension. *Clin Liver Dis* 5 (3), 629–644.

34 Shah V, Haddad FG, Garcia-Cardena G *et al.* (1997) Liver sinusoidal endothelial cells are responsible for nitric oxide modulation of resistance in the hepatic sinusoids. *J Clin Invest* 100 (11), 2923–2930.

35 Rockey DC, Chung JJ (1998) Reduced nitric oxide production by endothelial cells in cirrhotic rat liver: endothelial dysfunction in portal hypertension. *Gastroenterology* 114 (2), 344–351.

36 Sakamoto S, Okanoue T, Itoh Y *et al.* (1997) Intercellular adhesion molecule-1 and CD18 are involved in neutrophil adhesion and its cytotoxicity to cultured sinusoidal endothelial cells in rats. *Hepatology* 26 (3), 658–663.

37 Bauer M, Bauer I, Sonin NV *et al.* (2000) Functional significance of endothelin B receptors in mediating sinusoidal and extrasinusoidal effects of endothelins in the intact rat liver. *Hepatology* 31 (4), 937–947.

38 Fulton D, Gratton JP, Sessa WC (2001) Post-translational control of endothelial nitric oxide synthase: why isn't calcium/calmodulin enough? *J Pharmacol Exp Ther* 299 (3), 818–824.

39 Shah V, Kamath PS (2003) Nitric oxide in liver transplantation: pathobiology and clinical implications. *Liver Transpl* 9 (1), 1–11.

40 Rockey DC, Chung JJ (1997) Regulation of inducible nitric oxide synthase and nitric oxide during hepatic injury and fibrogenesis. *Am J Physiol* 273 (1 Pt 1), G124–G130.

41 Rockey DC, Chung JJ (1996) Regulation of inducible nitric oxide synthase in hepatic sinusoidal endothelial cells. *Am J Physiol* 271 (2 Pt 1), G260–G267.

42 DeLeve LD, Wang X, Hu L *et al.* (2004) Rat liver sinusoidal endothelial cell phenotype is maintained by paracrine and autocrine regulation. *Am J Physiol Gastrointest Liver Physiol* 287 (4), G757–G763.

43 Chen X, Higgins J, Cheung ST *et al.* (2004) Novel endothelial cell markers in hepatocellular carcinoma. *Mod Pathol* 17 (10), 1198–1210.

44 Zhong X, Ran YL, Lou JN *et al.* (2004) Construction of human liver cancer vascular endothelium cDNA expression library and screening of the endothelium-associated antigen genes. *World J Gastroenterol* 10 (10), 1402–1408.

45 Oh P, Li Y, Yu J *et al.* (2004) Subtractive proteomic mapping of the endothelial surface in lung and solid tumours for tissue-specific therapy. *Nature* 429 (6992), 629–635.

46 Matsumoto K, Yoshitomi H, Rossant J *et al.* (2001) Liver organogenesis promoted by endothelial cells prior to vascular function. *Science* 294 (5542), 559–563.

47 Couvelard A, Scoazec JY, Dauge MC *et al.* (1996) Structural and functional differentiation of sinusoidal endothelial cells during liver organogenesis in humans. *Blood* 87 (11), 4568–4580.

48 Carmeliet P, Ferreira V, Breier G *et al.* (1996) Abnormal blood vessel development and lethality in embryos lacking a single VEGF allele. *Nature* 380 (6573), 435–439.

49 Ferrara N, Carver-Moore K, Chen H *et al.* (1996) Heterozygous embryonic lethality induced by targeted inactivation of the VEGF gene. *Nature* 380 (6573), 439–442.

50 Fong GH, Rossant J, Gertsenstein M *et al.* (1995) Role of the Flt-1 receptor tyrosine kinase in regulating the assembly of vascular endothelium. *Nature* 376 (6535), 66–70.

51 Fong GH, Zhang L, Bryce DM *et al.* (1999) Increased haemangioblast commitment, not vascular disorganization, is the primary defect in flt-1 knock-out mice. *Development* 126 (13), 3015–3025.

52 Schmidt C, Bladt F, Goedecke S *et al.* (1995) Scatter factor/hepatocyte growth factor is essential for liver development. *Nature* 373 (6516), 699–702.

53 Uehara Y, Minowa O, Mori C *et al.* (1995) Placental defect and embryonic lethality in mice lacking hepatocyte growth factor/scatter factor. *Nature* 373 (6516), 702–705.

54 Bladt F, Riethmacher D, Isenmann S *et al.* (1995) Essential role for the c-met receptor in the migration of myogenic precursor cells into the limb bud. *Nature* 376 (6543), 768–771.

55 Assy N, Spira G, Paizi M *et al.* (1999) Effect of vascular endothelial growth factor on hepatic regenerative activity following partial hepatectomy in rats. *J Hepatol* 30 (5), 911–915.

56 Taniguchi E, Sakisaka S, Matsuo K *et al.* (2001) Expression and role of vascular endothelial growth factor in liver regeneration after partial hepatectomy in rats. *J Histochem Cytochem* 49 (1), 121–130.

57 Redaelli CA, Semela D, Carrick FE *et al.* (2004) Effect of vascular endothelial growth factor on functional recovery after hepatectomy in lean and obese mice. *J Hepatol* 40 (2), 305–312.

58 Drixler TA, Vogten MJ, Ritchie ED *et al.* (2002) Liver regeneration is an angiogenesis- associated phenomenon. *Ann Surg* 236 (6), 703–712.

59 Greene AK, Wiener S, Puder M *et al.* (2003) Endothelial-directed hepatic regeneration after partial hepatectomy. *Ann Surg* 237 (4), 530–535.

60 Martinez-Hernandez A, Amenta PS (1995) The extracellular matrix in hepatic regeneration. *FASEB J* 9 (14), 1401–1410.

61 Fujii H, Hirose T, Oe S *et al.* (2002) Contribution of bone marrow cells to liver regeneration after partial hepatectomy in mice. *J Hepatol* 36 (5), 653–659.

62 Semela D, Dufour JF (2004) Angiogenesis and hepatocellular carcinoma. *J Hepatol* 41 (5), 864–880.

63 Hanahan D, Folkman J (1996) Patterns and emerging mechanisms of the angiogenic switch during tumorigenesis. *Cell* 86 (3), 353–364.

64 Fukumura D, Xavier R, Sugiura T *et al.* (1998) Tumor induction of VEGF promoter activity in stromal cells. *Cell* 94 (6), 715–725.

65 Jung JO, Gwak GY, Lim YS *et al.* (2003) [Role of hepatic stellate cells in the angiogenesis of hepatoma]. *Kor J Gastroenterol* 42 (2), 142–148.

66 Park YN, Kim YB, Yang KM *et al.* (2000) Increased expression of vascular endothelial growth factor and angiogenesis in the early stage of multistep hepatocarcinogenesis. *Arch Pathol Lab Med* 124 (7), 1061–1065.

67 Yoshiji H, Kuriyama S, Yoshii J *et al.* (2002) Synergistic effect of basic fibroblast growth factor and vascular endothelial growth factor in murine hepatocellular carcinoma. *Hepatology* 35 (4), 834–842.

68 Yamaguchi R, Yano H, Iemura A *et al.* (1998) Expression of vascular endothelial growth factor in human hepatocellular carcinoma. *Hepatology* 28 (1), 68–77.

69 Yamaguchi R, Yano H, Nakashima Y *et al.* (2000) Expression and localization of vascular endothelial growth factor receptors in human hepatocellular carcinoma and non-HCC tissues. *Oncol Rep* 7 (4), 725–729.

70 Mise M, Arii S, Higashituji H *et al.* (1996) Clinical significance of vascular endothelial growth factor and basic fibroblast growth factor gene expression in liver tumor. *Hepatology* 23 (3), 455–464.

71 Nakashima Y, Nakashima O, Hsia CC *et al.* (1999) Vascularization of small hepatocellular carcinomas: correlation with differentiation. *Liver* 19 (1), 12–18.

72 Moon E-J, Jeong C-H, Jeong J-W *et al.* (2003) Hepatitis B virus X protein induces angiogenesis by stabilizing hypoxia-inducible factor-1alpha. *FASEB J* 18(2), 382–384.

73 Miura H, Miyazaki T, Kuroda M *et al.* (1997) Increased expression of vascular endothelial growth factor in human hepatocellular carcinoma. *J Hepatol* 27 (5), 854–861.

74 Chow NH, Hsu PI, Lin XZ *et al.* (1997) Expression of vascular endothelial growth factor in normal liver and hepatocellular carcinoma: an immunohistochemical study. *Hum Pathol* 28 (6), 698–703.

75 Chao Y, Li CP, Chau GY *et al.* (2003) Prognostic significance of vascular endothelial growth factor, basic fibroblast growth factor, and angiogenin in patients with resectable hepatocellular carcinoma after surgery. *Ann Surg Oncol* 10 (4), 355–362.

76 Zhou XD (2002) Recurrence and metastasis of hepatocellular carcinoma: progress and prospects. *Hepatobiliary Pancreat Dis Int* 1 (1), 35–41.

77 Kin M, Torimura T, Ueno T *et al.* (1994) Sinusoidal capillarization in small hepatocellular carcinoma. *Pathol Int* 44 (10–11), 771–778.

78 Poon RT-P, Lau CP-Y, Cheung S-T *et al.* (2003) Quantitative correlation of serum levels and tumor expression of vascular endothelial growth factor in patients with hepatocellular carcinoma. *Cancer Res* 63 (12), 3121–3126.

79 Jinno K, Tanimizu M, Hyodo I *et al.* (1998) Circulating vascular endothelial growth factor (VEGF) is a possible tumor marker for metastasis in human hepatocellular carcinoma. *J Gastroenterol* 33 (3), 376–382.

80 Poon RT, Ng IO, Lau C *et al.* (2001) Serum vascular endothelial growth factor predicts venous invasion in hepatocellular carcinoma: a prospective study. *Ann Surg* 233 (2), 227–235.

81 Kim SJ, Choi IK, Park KH *et al.* (2004) Serum vascular endothelial growth factor per platelet count in hepatocellular carcinoma: correlations with clinical parameters and survival. *Jpn J Clin Oncol* 34 (4), 184–190.

82 Poon R, Lau C, Yu W *et al.* (2004) High serum levels of vascular endothelial growth factor predict poor response to transarterial chemoembolization in hepatocellular carcinoma: a prospective study. *Oncol Rep* 11 (5), 1077–1084.

83 Yamamoto T, Kobayashi T, Phillips MJ (1984) Perinodular arteriolar plexus in liver cirrhosis. Scanning electron microscopy of microvascular casts. *Liver* 4 (1), 50–54.

84 Haratake J, Hisaoka M, Yamamoto O *et al.* (1991) Morphological changes of hepatic microcirculation in experimental rat cirrhosis: a scanning electron microscopic study. *Hepatology* 13 (5), 952–956.

85 Huet PM, Goresky CA, Villeneuve JP *et al.* (1982) Assessment of liver microcirculation in human cirrhosis. *J Clin Invest* 70 (6), 1234–1244.

86 Villeneuve JP, Dagenais M, Huet PM *et al.* (1996) The hepatic microcirculation in the isolated perfused human liver. *Hepatology* 23 (1), 24–31.

87 Kalluri R, Sukhatme VP (2000) Fibrosis and angiogenesis. *Curr Opin Nephrol Hypertens* 9 (4), 413–418.

88 Kalluri R (2003) Basement membranes: structure, assembly and role in tumour angiogenesis. *Nature Rev Cancer* 3 (6), 422–433.

89 Rosmorduc O, Wendum D, Corpechot C *et al.* (1999) Hepatocellular hypoxia-induced vascular endothelial growth factor expression and angiogenesis in experimental biliary cirrhosis. *Am J Pathol* 155 (4), 1065–1073.

90 Corpechot C, Barbu V, Wendum D *et al.* (2002) Hypoxia-induced VEGF and collagen I expressions are associated with angiogenesis and fibrogenesis in experimental cirrhosis. *Hepatology* 35 (5), 1010–1021.

91 Wang Y, Luk J, Ikeda K *et al.* (2004) Regulatory role of vHL/HIF-1alpha in hypoxia-induced VEGF production in hepatic stellate cells. *Biochem Biophys Res Commun* 317 (2), 358–362.

92 Yoshiji H, Kuriyama S, Yoshii J *et al.* (2003) Vascular endothelial growth factor and receptor interaction is a prerequisite for murine hepatic fibrogenesis. *Gut* 52 (9), 1347–1354.

93 Xu B, Broome U, Uzunel M *et al.* (2003) Capillarization of hepatic sinusoid by liver endothelial cell-reactive autoantibodies in patients with cirrhosis and chronic hepatitis. *Am J Pathol* 163 (4), 1275–1289.

94 Rieder H, Armbrust T, Meyer zum Buschenfelde KH *et al.* (1993) Contribution of sinusoidal endothelial liver cells to liver fibrosis: expression of transforming growth factor-beta 1 receptors and modulation of plasmin-generating enzymes by transforming growth factor-beta 1. *Hepatology* 18 (4), 937–944.

95 Bosch J, Pizcueta P, Feu F *et al.* (1992) Pathophysiology of portal hypertension. *Gastroenterol Clin North Am* 21 (1), 1–14.

96 Fernandez M, Vizzutti F, Garcia-Pagan JC *et al.* (2004) Anti-VEGF receptor-2 monoclonal antibody prevents portal-systemic collateral vessel formation in portal hypertensive mice. *Gastroenterology* 126 (3), 886–894.

97 Le Couteur DG, Fraser R, Cogger VC *et al.* (2002) Hepatic pseudo-capillarisation and atherosclerosis in ageing. *Lancet* 359 (9317), 1612–1615.

98 Clark SA, Angus HB, Cook HB *et al.* (1988) Defenestration of hepatic sinusoids as a cause of hyperlipoproteinaemia in alcoholics. *Lancet* 2 (8622), 1225–1227.

99 Cogger VC, Mross PE, Hosie MJ *et al.* (2001) The effect of acute oxidative stress on the ultrastructure of the perfused rat liver. *Pharmacol Toxicol* 89 (6), 306–311.

1.5 Kupffer cells

Hartmut Jaeschke

Morphological characteristics and localization of Kupffer cells

Kupffer cells (KC), the largest fixed tissue macrophage population in the body, are located in hepatic sinusoids. They are anchored to the luminal surface of sinusoidal endothelial cells through cytoplasmic processes, some of which can also reach through the fenestrae of the endothelial cells and contact stellate cells and parenchymal cells [1,2]. Other processes can reach across the lumen of the sinusoids to anchor the cell to other endothelial cells [1]. Thus, in contrast to other tissue macrophages, KC are continuously in contact with blood. KC have the typical morphology of macrophages with microvilli, lamellopodia and filopodia on the surface and large numbers of lysosomes and pinocytotic vesicles in the body of the cell (Fig. 1) [1]. In addition, KC show characteristic 'worm-like structures', which represent invaginations of plasma membranes (Fig. 1). The location and the morphological characteristics reflect the main function of KC, which is effectively to remove all foreign material from the blood by phagocytosis or pinocytosis and to eliminate it by lysosomal degradation.

Based on cell number, KC represent approximately 30% of the non-parenchymal cell fraction and about 15% of all liver cells. However, KC account for only 2.5% of the total protein content of the liver [2,3]. The distribution of KC within the sinusoid is variable. The periportal area contains 43% of the cells, the midzonal region about 32%, and the remaining 25% of KC are located in the centrolobular area [4]. The periportal KC are the largest cells, have the highest content of lysosomal enzymes and show the most active phagocytosis [4]. Furthermore, they also generate more superoxide in response to most stimuli [5]. Destruction of predominantly periportal KC reduced hepatic tumour necrosis factor (TNF)α formation during endotoxaemia *in vivo* by 90%, suggesting that the large, periportal KC are also the most active cytokine-producing cells [6].

The origin of KC in the liver is controversial [7–9]. In normal livers, KC have a half-life of several months, which correlates with the small mitotic index [8]. Even when the liver was stressed with partial hepatectomy or zymosan, mitosis

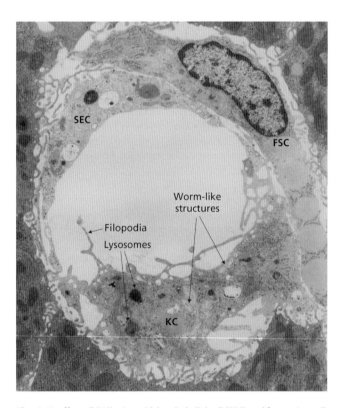

Fig. 1 Kupffer cell (KC), sinusoidal endothelial cell (SEC) and fat-storing cell (FSC) in a sinusoid of rat liver. The Kupffer cell shows characteristic features of macrophages including filopodia, 'worm-like structures' (invaginations of cell membranes) and a high content of lysosomes. Magnification × 5000 (picture courtesy of Dr Robert McCuskey, University of Arizona).

accounted for almost all cell recovery during the initial phase [9]. Mononuclear cell recruitment from blood and bone marrow became more important at later time points [9]. On the other hand, it was suggested that KC do not proliferate and are always replaced by blood-derived monocytes with a half-life of 21 days [7]. Furthermore, KC have the sex karyotype of the donor after bone marrow transplantation, supporting the hypothesis that KC are derived from bone marrow cells [10].

Together, the data indicate that KC can proliferate and can be recruited from the bone marrow. The relative contribution of each pathway depends on the experimental conditions.

Functions of Kupffer cells in the liver

KC, as the resident macrophages, have many functions that are essential for homeostasis in the liver and the innate immune response including phagocytosis, pinocytosis (receptor-mediated endocytosis) and mediator formation [2,11,12]. KC and sinusoidal endothelial cells (SEC) express several receptors, e.g. scavenger receptors and mannose receptors, which can bind endogenous soluble waste molecules (e.g. fibronectin, chondroitin sulphate, collagen) and even viruses, lipopolysaccharide (LPS) and other pathogenic substances. However, internalization and degradation of these soluble molecules by receptor-mediated endocytosis occurs mainly in SEC [11,13]. The main function of KC is to bind and remove particles (> 1 μm in diameter) from blood by phagocytosis, which does not occur in SEC [11].

Phagocytosis

KC *in vivo* phagocytose mainly opsonized particles, which bind to specific receptors [2]. Similar to SEC, KC express Fc-γ receptors [14]. These receptors interact with the Fc domain of immunoglobulin G (IgG) and bind IgG-coated particles and soluble bloodborne IgG–immune complexes. KC phagocytose IgG-coated particles and potentially larger aggregates of immune complexes. Although KC can take up soluble IgG–immune complexes [14], SEC remove them more effectively through endocytosis [11]. KC express scavenger receptors, which are a group of receptors that recognize negatively charged ligands [15]. Oxidized lipoproteins from blood, apoptotic bodies and a variety of pathogens are taken up into KC through scavenger receptors [15,16]. Similarly, scavenger receptors can bind LPS and internalize it without inflammatory mediator formation [17]. Complement is a major host defence system in plasma, and its activation leads to opsonization of pathogens, immunoglobulins and DNA, with larger fragments derived from complement factors C3 and C4, i.e. C3b and C4b. KC express a number of complement receptors, including CR1, CR3 (CD11b/CD18) and CR4 (CD11c/CD18) [18–20]. KC bind, internalize and degrade complement-coated pathogens through receptor-mediated endocytosis or phagocytosis [20]. Fibronectin in plasma is also able to opsonize various endogenous and exogenous substances, which are then bound to fibronectin-specific receptors on KC and internalized through phagocytosis [21]. Although it was generally assumed that KC with their receptors are mainly responsible for the clearance of pathogens from the blood [18], more recent evidence suggests that some bacteria are bound to the surface of KC, where they are internalized and destroyed by infiltrating neutrophils [22]. KC ingest the neutrophils, thus preventing the release of toxic mediators from dying neutrophils [22].

Formation of inflammatory mediators

Upon activation, KC can generate a large amount of inflammatory mediators including cytokines [e.g. TNFα, interleukin (IL)-1, IL-6, IL-10], chemokines (e.g. IL-8), nitric oxide, superoxide and prostanoids [12]. In turn, some of the mediators can bind to KC in an autocrine fashion and either further activate these macrophages (e.g. TNFα) or downregulate proinflammatory mediator formation (e.g. IL-10, IL-13 or prostaglandin E2) [12,23]. Two pathophysiologically important activating pathways in KC will be discussed.

One of the most relevant activators of KC is LPS, a wall component of gut-derived Gram-negative bacteria. LPS activation involves LPS-binding protein (LBP), CD14 and the Toll-like receptor 4 (TLR4) [24]. LBP binds the lipid A portion of LPS with high affinity and can mediate the transfer of LPS to the cell surface receptor CD14 on KC. This activity decreases the amount of LPS necessary to activate KC *in vitro* [25]. On the other hand, LBP can also facilitate the transfer of LPS to lipoproteins [24]. Functional studies in LBP gene knockout mice *in vivo* showed that TNFα formation in response to LPS is unaffected [26]. In addition, administration of recombinant LBP to mice attenuated LPS-induced cytokine formation and protected against LPS-induced liver injury [27]. Thus, the main function of LBP *in vivo* appears to be more to protect against the deleterious effect of LPS and other pathogens rather than being an obligatory mediator for LPS signalling in KC [24,28].

Although rodent or human KC show a low baseline expression of CD14, LPS-induced TNFα formation is still dependent on CD14 [29]. In support of this finding, CD14-deficient mice are insensitive to LPS *in vivo* [30]. CD14 can be upregulated in KC by LPS; increased expression of CD14 was observed in human and rodent livers with inflammatory diseases [24]. The functional significance of CD14 induction could be demonstrated by the reduced inflammatory response and attenuated liver injury in CD14-deficient mice after chronic alcohol treatment [31]. As CD14 is a protein without a transmembrane component, it requires interaction with other proteins, i.e. Toll-like receptors (TLRs), to induce KC activation. Among the 10 currently identified TLRs, TLR2 and TLR4 are highly expressed on macrophages [32]. However, natural mutants of TLR4 and TLR4 gene knockout mice but not animals deficient in TLR2 are completely resistant to LPS [24,32]. TLR4 is specific for LPS [24]. Signalling through TLR4 requires the presence of MD-2 on the cell surface (Fig. 2) [33]. In addition, the cytoplasmic tail of TLR4, which has similarities to the IL-1 receptor family, recruits adapter molecules including MyD88, which binds the serine/threonine kinase IL-1 receptor-associated kinase (IRAK)-1 and -4 [32]. IRAK-4 phosphorylates IRAK-1, which then recruits TNFα receptor-associated factor-6 (TRAF6) to the complex. The IRAK-1/TRAF6 complex dissociates from the receptor and binds transforming growth factor-beta-activated kinase 1 (TAK1) and TAK1-binding proteins (TAB1 and TAB2) (Fig. 2). Whereas IRAK-1 remains at the membrane, the complex of

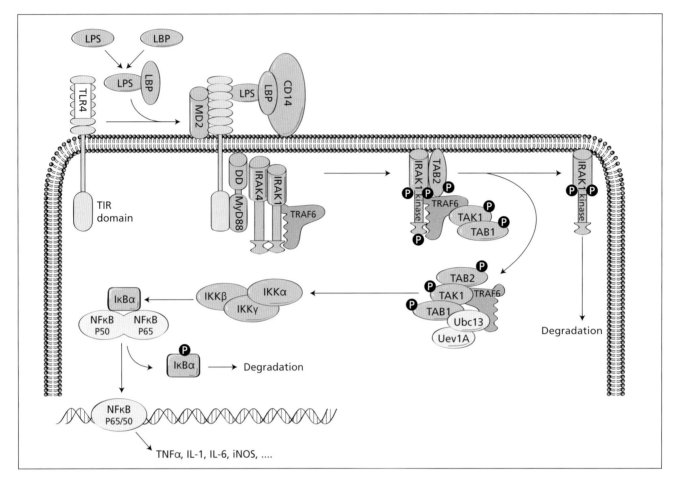

Fig. 2 Toll-like receptor 4 (TLR4) signalling in Kupffer cells (see text for details). Figure adapted from [32]. iNOS, inducible nitric oxide synthase; IRAK, interleukin (IL)-1 receptor-associated kinase; LBP, LPS-binding protein; LPS, lipopolysaccharide, TIR, Toll/IL-1 receptor; TAB, TAK-binding protein; TAK1, transforming growth factor-beta-activated kinase 1; TRAF6, TNF receptor-associated factor 6.

TRAF6/TAK1/TAB1/TAB2 moves into the cytosol and binds additional proteins such as Ubc13 and Uev1A [32], which induces the activation of TAK1 and eventually causes NF-κB activation, its translocation to the nucleus and subsequent formation of various proinflammatory cytokines (Fig. 2) [32]. The critical role of these adapter molecules for LPS signalling in KC is supported by reduced TNFα formation in mice deficient in MD-2 [35], MyD88 [36], IRAK [37] or TAK1 [38]. Despite the importance of the MyD88-dependent signalling pathway for cytokine formation in response to TLR4 activation, MyD88-independent signalling also occurs in macrophages [32,34]. Animals with mutations or a deficiency in the TLR4 receptor are protected against various liver pathogenesis including LPS hepatotoxicity, alcohol-induced liver damage and ischaemia–reperfusion injury [24,34].

Other important stimulators for KC are components of the complement cascade, which can be activated by immune complexes through the classical pathway or by LPS and other microbial surfaces through the alternative pathway [20]. The larger complement fragments C3b and C4b are involved in the opsonization of pathogens, which leads to binding to the complement receptors CR1, CR3 and CR4 on KC and subsequent phagocytosis [20]. On the other hand, the smaller fragments (anaphylatoxins), e.g. C5a, bind to specific high-affinity receptors, e.g. C5aR/CD88, which are members of the rhodopsin subfamily of G protein-coupled receptors [39]. C5aR is constitutively expressed on human and rodent KC [39]. Activation of KC with C5a leads to activation of phospholipases with release of intracellular messengers [40]. Although the detailed intracellular signalling mechanisms for activation of nicotinamide adenine dinucleotide phosphate dehydrogenase (NADPH) oxidase, especially in KC, are not well established, it involves a number of kinases, including protein kinase C, which phosphorylate components such as p40[phox] and p47[phox] [40]. These phosphorylation steps trigger translocation of individual components to the cell membrane and induce the assembly of the active enzyme [40].

Pathophysiological role of Kupffer cells

KC activation has been implicated in a growing number of liver diseases with both detrimental and beneficial impacts. The

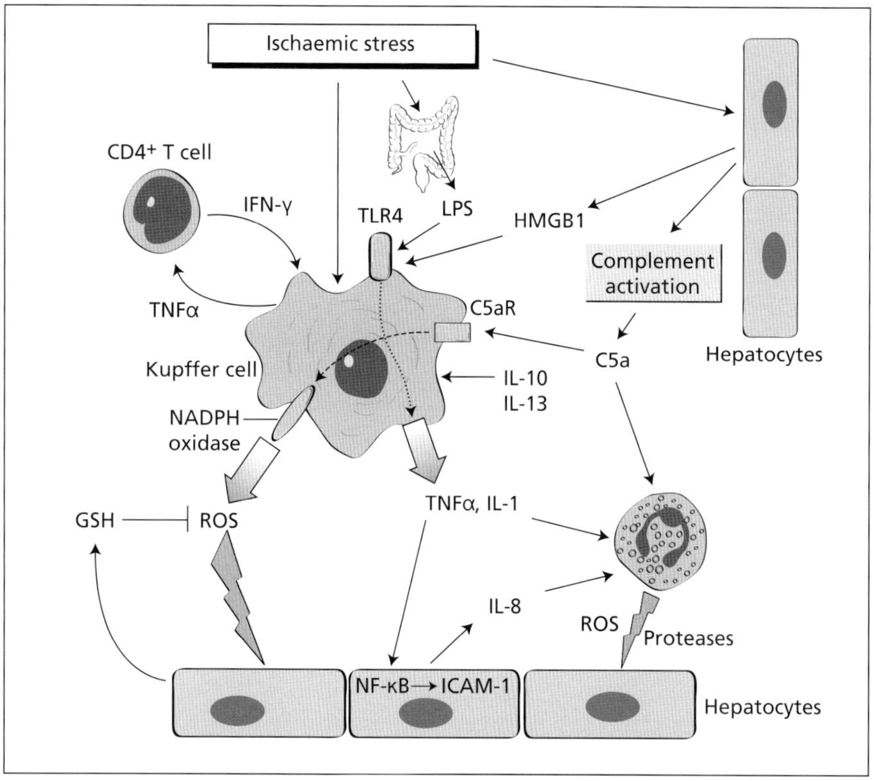

Fig. 3 Central role of Kupffer cells in the pathogenesis of hepatic ischaemia–reperfusion injury (see text for details). Figure adapted from ref. 41. C5aR, C5a receptor; GSH, reduced glutathione; HMGB1, high-mobility group Box 1; ICAM-1, intercellular adhesion molecule-1; IL, interleukin; IFN-γ, interferon-γ; LPS, lipopolysaccharide; ROS, reactive oxygen species; TLR4, toll-like receptor 4.

specific involvement of KC in three relevant injury mechanisms will be highlighted.

Hepatic ischaemia–reperfusion injury

Periods of warm and cold ischaemia can activate KC [41]. Whereas the larger KC of the periportal region are fully activated and generate reactive oxygen, the smaller KC are mainly primed [41,42]. Functional inactivation of KC with gadolinium chloride and other intervention strategies attenuated this oxidant stress and reduced the early reperfusion injury phase [41,42]. Further support for the critical role of a KC-derived vascular oxidant stress in the pathophysiology comes from the observation that reduced glutathione (GSH) released into the sinusoid can detoxify these reactive oxygen species and attenuate reperfusion injury (Fig. 3) [42]. In fact, the enhanced release of GSH from hepatocytes under inflammatory conditions appears to be a general endogenous mechanism to limit a potential detrimental effect of KC-mediated vascular oxidant stress [41]. Consequently, intravenous infusion of GSH attenuated hepatic reperfusion injury by scavenging reactive oxygen in sinusoids [41–43]. Although KC generate mainly superoxide through NADPH oxidase, the major oxidant for GSH in plasma is hydrogen peroxide (H_2O_2) [42]. In addition, H_2O_2 can diffuse into nearby hepatocytes and trigger an intracellular oxidant stress, which is responsible for parenchymal cell damage [44]. Thus, in addition to the interception of vascular reactive oxygen species, strengthening of intracellular defence mechanisms against

oxidant stress is a second important intervention strategy to limit tissue injury due to KC activation [45].

Activated KC also generate cytokines and chemokines, which enhance the inflammatory response and promote the infiltration of neutrophils [23,41]. Although more cell death occurs during the later, neutrophil-mediated injury phase, cytotoxic and proinflammatory mediators derived from activated KC determine the severity of the overall inflammatory response and tissue damage. Thus, limiting early KC activation could be an effective intervention strategy. However, KC are activated through multiple mechanisms during ischaemia–reperfusion (Fig. 3). Exposure of isolated KC to hypoxia leads to reactive oxygen formation during reoxygenation [42]. Although this effect is short-lived *in vitro*, the prolonged oxidant stress *in vivo* suggests additional stimuli. The early cell content release during reperfusion induces activation of complement in plasma [46]. Complement factors such as C5a bind to C5aR on KC and induce superoxide formation [42,46]. More recently, it was shown that high-mobility group Box 1 (HMGB1), a nuclear protein, is released from necrotic cells during hepatic ischaemia–reperfusion and triggers cytokine formation [47]. This effect is mediated through binding of HMGB1 to the TLR4 receptor [48]. Thus, KC can be activated through cellular stress during ischaemia and through mediators generated during reperfusion triggering a non-microbial inflammatory response, which is a critical determinant of the overall tissue injury and potential organ failure (Fig. 3).

Although the overall effect of KC activation is in part direct tissue injury and in part the promotion of the inflammatory response, endogenous IL-13 derived from KC can limit the formation of TNFα during reperfusion [49]. In addition, pharmacological doses of IL-10 or IL-13 suppress the inflammatory response during ischaemia–reperfusion by inhibiting cytokine and chemokine formation [23]. On the other hand, cytokines such as IL-6 were shown to be critical for a regenerative response after reperfusion and, therefore, also have beneficial effects [50]. Thus, KC activation is a critical event in the pathophysiology of hepatic ischaemia–reperfusion injury with both pro- as well as anti-inflammatory mediators being generated by these macrophages (Fig. 3). However, the majority of the literature supports the view that inactivation of KC has an overall beneficial effect in the pathogenesis of this condition.

Alcohol-induced liver disease

Acute and chronic exposure to alcohol (ethanol) causes activation of KC, as indicated by enhanced cytokine and chemokine formation and increased generation of reactive oxygen species [51–53]. However, under certain circumstances, chronic ethanol consumption can also induce tolerance in KC [53]. As alcohol increases the permeability of the mucosal barrier to intestinal microbes and toxins, it is generally accepted that, in animal models of chronic ethanol exposure, e.g. the intragastric feeding model, LPS is one of the key activators of KC and tissue macrophages in alcoholic liver disease (ALD) [54]. The importance of LPS in ALD was demonstrated by reduced liver injury in animals treated with antibiotics [55].

The molecular mechanism of KC activation during alcohol exposure starts with the binding of endotoxin to LBP in plasma. The LPS/LBP complex binds to the CD14 receptor and TLR4, which then transmits the signal intracellularly (Fig. 2). Increasing the expression of CD14 can enhance the sensitivity of ethanol-exposed KC to LPS [52]. Activation of the TLR4 receptor by LPS through CD14 induces the activation of the transcription factors NF-κB and AP-1, which leads to the formation of pro- and anti-inflammatory cytokines, including TNFα, IL-1 and IL-10, CC and CXC chemokines, and priming for reactive oxygen formation [56]. Reduced cytokine formation together with reduced tissue injury in mouse strains deficient in CD14, TLR4 or LBP supports the importance of these signalling events in the development of ALD [51,52]. NF-κB activation together with cytokine and chemokine formation was shown during ALD [56], and inhibition of NF-κB activation with an I-κB superrepressor reduced pathological changes [52]. In addition, enhanced NF-κB activation and cytokine formation in hepatic macrophages isolated from alcohol-fed rats was attenuated after treatment with an iron chelator, suggesting that a labile iron pool within the cell is critical for NF-κB activation and cytokine formation in macrophages [57]. However, LPS may not be the only factor involved in KC activation during ALD [58]. In KC isolated from chronically ethanol-fed rats, LPS-induced TNFα mRNA and protein formation is increased compared with cells from control animals [58]. However, a similar priming effect was also observed when macrophages were exposed to ethanol in culture, indicating that the changes in TNFα formation in vivo may not be entirely due to LPS but could at least in part result from a direct effect of ethanol on KC [59]. Interestingly, exposure of KC to ethanol in vitro had no effect on TNFα transcription, but prolonged the half-life of the mRNA through a p38 MAP kinase-dependent mechanism [59]. In addition, treatment of hepatic macrophages with retinoic acid inhibited LPS-induced mRNA formation of TNFα and other cytokines [60]. Thus, retinoic acid deficiency during chronic alcohol consumption can contribute to TNFα mRNA stability and promote increased cytokine formation [60].

Acute and chronic ethanol exposure leads to the increased formation of reactive oxygen by KC [51]. Priming and activation of KC for superoxide formation by NADPH oxidase can be triggered in vivo by endotoxin, cytokines such as TNFα or complement factors [5,46]. Despite the importance of KC as a source of the oxidant stress during the development of ALD, KC are only one of several critical sources of reactive oxygen formation [51]. Nevertheless, rats treated with inhibitors of NADPH oxidase or mice deficient in p47phox, a component of the NADPH oxidase complex, showed less oxidant stress and reduced injury after chronic alcohol exposure [51]. These data suggest that superoxide derived from NADPH oxidase (KC and neutrophils) is critically involved in the injury process. This may be caused by tissue damage by oxidants, e.g. peroxynitrite and hypochlorous acid, or indirectly by promoting cytokine and chemokine formation with recruitment of mononuclear cells and neutrophils [51,58,61]. Taken together, there is clear evidence that hyperactivation of KC after ethanol exposure contributes to the development of inflammatory tissue injury during ALD. On the other hand, KC-derived anti-inflammatory cytokines such as IL-10 exert a beneficial effect in the pathophysiology [62]. Nevertheless, the majority of evidence mainly suggests a detrimental effect of KC activation during ALD.

Drug-induced liver failure

A variety of drugs and chemicals can induce liver injury involving an inflammatory component in the pathogenesis [63,64]. The clinically most relevant drug hepatotoxicity is caused by paracetamol overdose. Within 24–48 h after a toxic dose of paracetamol in rats, liver macrophages are activated [63]. These liver macrophages consist of the resident KC population and newly recruited monocyte-derived cells [63]. The activated macrophages can generate reactive oxygen, cytokines and chemokines [63–66]. As treatment with gadolinium chloride attenuated paracetamol-induced liver injury, it was concluded that liver macrophages contributed to the injury by generating peroxynitrite, as indicated by the formation of nitrotyrosine protein adducts in necrotic hepatocytes [63]. However, more recent experimental evidence suggests that peroxynitrite is actually formed in the mitochondria of centrolobular hepatocytes [67]. Because at least some of the nitric oxide (NO) generated in hepatocytes is formed by the inducible NO synthase (iNOS), which can be transcriptionally induced by KC-derived cytokines, KC activation may be a critical factor in the pathogenesis. However, formation of IL-10 by KC limits TNFα formation after paracetamol overdose and therefore reduces iNOS induction and peroxynitrite-mediated injury [68]. Complete elimination of KC with liposomally encaspulated chlodronate or the deficiency of the IL-10 gene enhances iNOS induction and aggravates paracetamol-induced liver injury [68,69]. These data suggest that activation of KC during the early phase of paracetamol hepatotoxicity is more beneficial than detrimental [69].

Cytokine formation by activated KC occurs early during paracetamol administration [63,64]. Initially, it was thought that these cytokines contributed to the injury, but the mechanisms remained unclear [64]. As paracetamol toxicity does not involve relevant apoptotic cell death [70], indirect mechanisms such as neutrophil activation may be an explanation. However, although recruited into the liver after paracetamol-induced liver injury, no significant contribution of neutrophils was found [64]. On the other hand, more recent data suggest that TNFα may be important in the regenerative response after paracetamol-induced cell death [71]. In addition, cytokines promote the formation of chemokines responsible for mononuclear cell recruitment in the liver [72]. These macrophages do not appear to cause additional damage, but are involved in removing cell debris and in cell cycle activation and regeneration [72].

References

1 McCuskey RS, McCuskey PA (1990) Fine structure and function of Kupffer cells. *J Electron Microsc Tech* 14, 237–246.

2 Kuiper J, Brouwer A, Knook DL *et al.* (1994) Kupffer and sinusoidal endothelial cells. In: Arias IM, Boyer JL, Fausto N *et al.* (eds) *The Liver: Biology and Pathobiology*, 3rd edn. New York: Raven Press, pp. 791–818.

3 Blouin A, Bolender RP, Weibel ER (1977) Distribution of organelles and membranes between hepatocytes and nonhepatocytes in the rat liver parenchyma. A stereological study. *J Cell Biol* 72, 441–455.

4 Sleyster EC, Knook DL (1982) Relation between localization and function of rat liver Kupffer cells. *Lab Invest* 47, 484–490.

5 Bautista AP, Meszaros K, Bojta J *et al.* (1990) Superoxide anion generation in the liver during the early stage of endotoxemia in rats. *J Leukoc Biol* 48, 123–128.

6 Bautista AP, Skrepnik N, Niesman MR *et al.* (1994) Elimination of macrophages by liposome-encapsulated dichloromethylene diphosphonate suppresses the endotoxin-induced priming of Kupffer cells. *J Leukoc Biol* 55, 321–327.

7 Crofton RW, Diesselhoff-Den Dulk MM, van Furth R (1978) The origin, kinetics, and characteristics of the Kupffer cells in the normal steady state. *J Exp Med* 148, 1–17.

8 Bouwens L, Baekeland M, De Zanger R *et al.* (1986) Quantitation, tissue distribution and proliferation kinetics of Kupffer cells in normal rat liver. *Hepatology* 6, 718–722.

9 Bouwens L, Baekeland M, Wisse E (1984) Importance of local proliferation in the expanding Kupffer cell population of rat liver after zymosan stimulation and partial hepatectomy. *Hepatology* 4, 213–219.

10 Gale RP, Sparkes RS, Golde DW (1978) Bone marrow origin of hepatic macrophages (Kupffer cells) in humans. *Science* 201, 937–938.

11 Smedsrod B (2004) Clearance function of scavenger endothelial cells. *Comp Hepatol* 3 (Suppl. 1), S22.

12 Decker K (1990) Biologically active products of stimulated liver macrophages (Kupffer cells). *Eur J Biochem* 192, 245–261.

13 Seternes T, Sorensen K, Smedsrod B (2002) Scavenger endothelial cells of vertebrates: a nonperipheral leukocyte system for high-capacity elimination of waste macromolecules. *Proc Natl Acad Sci USA* 99, 7594–7597.

14 Lovdal T, Brech A, Kjeken R *et al.* (2001) Receptor-mediated and fluid phase endocytosis in hepatic sinusoidal cells. In: Wisse E, Knook DL, de Zanger R *et al.* (eds) *Cells of the Hepatic Sinusoid*, Vol. 8. Leiden: Kupffer Cell Foundation, pp. 125–131.

15 Pearson AM (1996) Scavenger receptors in innate immunity. *Curr Opin Immunol* 8, 20–28.

16 Van Berkel TJ, De Rijke YB, Kruijt JK (1991) Different fate *in vivo* of oxidatively modified low density lipoprotein and acetylated low density lipoprotein in rats. Recognition by various scavenger receptors on Kupffer and endothelial liver cells. *J Biol Chem* 266, 2282–2289.

17 Haworth R, Platt N, Keshav S *et al.* (1997) The macrophage scavenger receptor type A is expressed by activated macrophages and protects the host against lethal endotoxic shock. *J Exp Med* 186, 1431–1439.

18 Loegering DJ (1986) Kupffer cell complement receptor clearance function and host defense. *Circ Shock* 20, 321–333.

19 Hinglais N, Kazatchkine MD, Mandet C *et al.* (1989) Human liver Kupffer cells express CR1, CR3, and CR4 complement receptor antigens. An immunohistochemical study. *Lab Invest* 61, 509–514.

20 Ember JA, Hugli TE (1997) Complement factors and their receptors. *Immunopharmacology* 38, 3–15.

21 Cardarelli PM, Blumenstock FA, McKeown-Longo PJ *et al.* (1990) High-affinity binding of fibronectin to cultured Kupffer cells. *J Leukoc Biol* 48, 426–437.

22 Gregory SH, Wing EJ (2002) Neutrophil-Kupffer cell interaction: a critical component of host defenses to systemic bacterial infections. *J Leukoc Biol* 72, 239–248.

23 Okaya T, Lentsch AB (2003) Cytokine cascades and the hepatic inflammatory response to ischemia and reperfusion. *J Invest Surg* 16, 141–147.

24 Su GL (2002) Lipopolysaccharides in liver injury: molecular mechanisms of Kupffer cell activation. *Am J Physiol Gastrointest Liver Physiol* 283, G256–G265.

25 Su GL, Klein RD, Aminlari A *et al.* (2000) Kupffer cell activation by lipopolysaccharide in rats: role for lipopolysaccharide binding protein and toll-like receptor 4. *Hepatology* 31, 932–936.

26 Wurfel MM, Monks BG, Ingalls RR *et al.* (1997) Targeted deletion of the lipopolysaccharide (LPS)-binding protein gene leads to profound suppression of LPS responses ex vivo, whereas *in vivo* responses remain intact. *J Exp Med* 186, 2051–2056.

27 Lamping N, Dettmer R, Schroder NW *et al.* (1998) LPS-binding protein protects mice from septic shock caused by LPS or gram-negative bacteria. *J Clin Invest* 101, 2065–2071.

28 Schroder NW, Schumann RR (2005) Non-LPS targets and actions of LPS binding protein (LBP). *J Endotoxin Res* 11, 237–242.

29 Su GL, Goyert SM, Fan MH *et al.* (2002) Activation of human and mouse Kupffer cells by lipopolysaccharide is mediated by CD14. *Am J Physiol Gastrointest Liver Physiol* 283, G640–G645.

30 Haziot A, Ferrero E, Lin XY *et al.* (1995) CD14-deficient mice are

exquisitely insensitive to the effects of LPS. *Prog Clin Biol Res* 392, 349–351.

31 Yin M, Bradford BU, Wheeler MD *et al.* (2001) Reduced early alcohol-induced liver injury in CD14-deficient mice. *J Immunol* 166, 4737–4742.

32 Takeda K, Akira S (2004) TLR signaling pathways. *Semin Immunol* 16, 3–9.

33 Shimazu R, Akashi S, Ogata H *et al.* (1999) MD-2, a molecule that confers lipopolysaccharide responsiveness on Toll-like receptor 4. *J Exp Med* 189, 1777–1782.

34 Schwabe RF, Seki E, Brenner DA (2006) Toll-like receptor signaling in the liver. *Gastroenterology* 130, 1886–1890.

35 Nagai Y, Akashi S, Nagafuku M *et al.* (2002) Essential role of MD-2 in LPS responsiveness and TLR4 distribution. *Nature Immunol* 3, 667–672.

36 Kawai T, Adachi O, Ogawa T *et al.* (1999) Unresponsiveness of MyD88-deficient mice to endotoxin. *Immunity* 11, 115–122.

37 Swantek JL, Tsen MF, Cobb MH *et al.* (2000) IL-1 receptor-associated kinase modulates host responsiveness to endotoxin. *J Immunol* 164, 4301–4306.

38 Sato S, Sanjo H, Takeda K *et al.* (2005) Essential function for the kinase TAK1 in innate and adaptive immune responses. *Nature Immunol* 6, 1087–1095.

39 Zwirner J, Fayyazi A, Gotze O (1999) Expression of the anaphylatoxin C5a receptor in non-myeloid cells. *Mol Immunol* 36, 877–884.

40 El-Benna J, Dang PM, Gougerot-Pocidalo MA *et al.* (2005) Phagocyte NADPH oxidase: a multicomponent enzyme essential for host defenses. *Arch Immunol Ther Exp (Warsz)* 53, 199–206.

41 Jaeschke H (2003) Molecular mechanisms of hepatic ischemia-reperfusion injury and preconditioning. *Am J Physiol Gastrointest Liver Physiol* 284, G15–G26.

42 Jaeschke H (2003) Role of reactive oxygen species in hepatic ischemia-reperfusion injury and preconditioning. *J Invest Surg* 16, 127–140.

43 Bilzer M, Gerbes AL (2000) Preservation injury of the liver: mechanisms and novel therapeutic strategies. *J Hepatol* 32, 508–515.

44 Bilzer M, Jaeschke H, Vollmar AM *et al.* (1999) Prevention of Kupffer cell-induced oxidant injury in rat liver by atrial natriuretic peptide. *Am J Physiol* 276, G1137–G1144.

45 Schauer RJ, Gerbes AL, Vonier D *et al.* (2003) Induction of cellular resistance against Kupffer cell-derived oxidant stress: a novel concept of hepatoprotection by ischemic preconditioning. *Hepatology* 37, 286–295.

46 Jaeschke H, Farhood A, Bautista AP *et al.* (1993) Complement activates Kupffer cells and neutrophils during reperfusion after hepatic ischemia. *Am J Physiol* 264, G801–G809.

47 Tsung A, Sahai R, Tanaka H *et al.* (2005) The nuclear factor HMGB1 mediates hepatic injury after murine liver ischemia–reperfusion. *J Exp Med* 201, 1135–1143.

48 Tsung A, Hoffman RA, Izuishi K *et al.* (2005) Hepatic ischemia/reperfusion injury involves functional TLR4 signaling in non-parenchymal cells. *J Immunol* 175, 7661–7668.

49 Kato A, Okaya T, Lentsch AB (2003) Endogenous IL-13 protects hepatocytes and vascular endothelial cells during ischemia/reperfusion injury. *Hepatology* 37, 304–312.

50 Selzner N, Rudiger H, Graf R *et al.* (2003) Protective strategies against ischemic injury of the liver. *Gastroenterology* 125, 917–936.

51 Arteel GE (2003) Oxidants and antioxidants in alcohol-induced liver disease. *Gastroenterology* 124, 778–790.

52 Hines IN, Wheeler MD (2004) Recent advances in alcoholic liver disease III. Role of the innate immune response in alcoholic hepatitis. *Am J Physiol Gastrointest Liver Physiol* 287, G310–G314.

53 Spitzer JJ, Bautista AP (1998) Tolerance and sensitivity: ethanol and Kupffer cells. *Gastroenterology* 115, 494–496.

54 Bode C, Bode JC (2005) Activation of the innate immune system and alcoholic liver disease: effects of ethanol per se or enhanced intestinal translocation of bacterial toxins induced by ethanol? *Alcohol Clin Exp Res* 29 (11 Suppl.), 166S–171S.

55 Adachi Y, Moore LE, Bradford BU *et al.* (1995) Antibiotics prevent liver injury in rats following long-term exposure to ethanol. *Gastroenterology* 108, 218–224.

56 Nanji AA, Jokelainen K, Rahemtulla A *et al.* (1999) Activation of nuclear factor kappa B and cytokine imbalance in experimental alcoholic liver disease in the rat. *Hepatology* 30, 934–943.

57 Tsukamoto H, Lin M, Ohata M *et al.* (1999) Iron primes hepatic macrophages for NF-kappaB activation in alcoholic liver injury. *Am J Physiol* 277, G1240–G1250.

58 Nagy LE (2003) Recent insights into the role of the innate immune system in the development of alcoholic liver disease. *Exp Biol Med* 228, 882–890.

59 Kishore R, McMullen MR, Cocuzzi E *et al.* (2004) Lipopolysaccharide-mediated signal transduction: stabilization of TNF-alpha mRNA contributes to increased lipopolysaccharide-stimulated TNF-alpha production by Kupffer cells after chronic ethanol feeding. *Comp Hepatol* 3 (Suppl. 1), S31.

60 Motomura K, Ohata M, Satre M *et al.* (2001) Destabilization of TNF-alpha mRNA by retinoic acid in hepatic macrophages: implications for alcoholic liver disease. *Am J Physiol Endocrinol Metab* 281, E420–E429.

61 Jaeschke H (2002) Neutrophil-mediated tissue injury in alcoholic-hepatitis. *Alcohol* 27, 23–27.

62 Grove J, Daly AK, Bassendine MF *et al.* (2000) Interleukin 10 promoter region polymorphisms and susceptibility to advanced alcoholic liver disease. *Gut* 46, 540–545.

63 Laskin DL (1997) Xenobiotic-induced inflammation and injury in the liver. In: McCuskey RS, Earnest DL (eds) *Comprehensive Toxicology*, Vol. 9. New York: Elsevier Science, pp. 151–164.

64 Jaeschke H (2005) Role of inflammation in the mechanism of acetaminophen hepatotoxicity. *Exp Opin Drug Metab Toxicol* 1, 389–397.

65 Jaeschke H, Gores GJ, Cederbaum AI *et al.* (2002) Mechanisms of hepatotoxicity. *Toxicol Sci* 65, 166–176.

66 Jaeschke H, Knight TR, Bajt ML (2003) The role of oxidant stress and reactive nitrogen species in acetaminophen hepatotoxicity. *Toxicol Lett* 144, 279–288.

67 Jaeschke H, Bajt ML (2006) Intracellular signaling mechanisms of acetaminophen-induced liver cell death. *Toxicol Sci* 89, 31–41.

68 Bourdi M, Masubuchi Y, Reilly TP *et al.* (2002) Protection against acetaminophen-induced liver injury and lethality by interleukin 10: role of inducible nitric oxide synthase. *Hepatology* 35, 289–298.

69 Ju C, Reilly TP, Bourdi M *et al.* (2002) Protective role of Kupffer cells in acetaminophen-induced hepatic injury in mice. *Chem Res Toxicol* 15, 1504–1513.

70 Gujral JS, Knight TR, Farhood A *et al.* (2002) Mode of cell death after acetaminophen overdose in mice: apoptosis or oncotic necrosis? *Toxicol Sci* 67, 322–328.

71 Chiu H, Gardner CR, Dambach DM *et al.* (2003) Role of tumor necrosis factor receptor 1 (p55) in hepatocyte proliferation during acetaminophen-induced toxicity in mice. *Toxicol Appl Pharmacol* 193, 218–227.

72 Dambach DM, Watson LM, Gray KR *et al.* (2002) Role of CCR2 in macrophage migration into the liver during acetaminophen-induced hepatotoxicity in the mouse. *Hepatology* 35, 1093–1103.

1.6 The hepatic stellate cell

Massimo Pinzani

Historical notes and nomenclature

The history of hepatic stellate cells (HSC) has not been an easy one. The first trace of their recognition is in a letter that Carl Von Kupffer wrote to the anatomist Waldeyer in 1876 [1]. Von Kupffer, who was studying the hepatic nervous system, observed perisinusoidal star-shaped cells that stained dark with a gold chloride technique used to reveal nerves (Fig. 1). Accordingly, Von Kupffer's first interpretation was that these cells were part of the perivascular nervous network of Waldeyer. In later studies, Von Kupffer changed his view and concluded that HSC were rather a type of phagocyte (as they shared the same distribution of gold particles with true phagocytic cells, today correctly defined as 'Kupffer cells') or, more generally, a 'special endothelial cell of the sinusoids'. Following this brief and confused moment of glory, the concept of HSC fell into limbo for several decades. Between 1928 and the late 1950s, additional key features of HSC (still defined as 'Kupffer cells') were reported: the morphology of a pericyte [2], the presence of intracytoplasmic lipid droplets (i.e. 'fat-storing cells') [3] and the close relation-

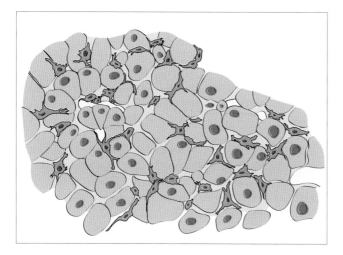

Fig. 1 Reproduction of Kupffer's drawing of the hepatic stellate cells (Sterzellen) in dog liver. Adapted from ref. 4.

ship with branches of the autonomic nervous system [4]. In the early 1970s, work by Kenjiro Wake led to the conclusion that the star-shaped phagocytes described by Kupffer were identical to the fat-storing cells described by Ito, and that the lipid droplets were largely composed of retinoid esters. During the same period, several morphological studies suggested that this cell type could play a role in the pathogenesis of hepatic fibrosis [5–7]. Regardless, liver researchers and clinicians were rather refractory to this concept, in an era in which very little was known about the aetiology and pathogenesis of liver diseases, and the hepatocyte was considered the only relevant liver cell type. The real physiological and pathophysiological relevance of HSC has emerged only in the last 20 years, and there are still many potential issues concerning their role to be resolved. In these years, the knowledge about HSC and, particularly, their profibrogenic role has grown exponentially, and their glory is finally established to the point at which any area of liver disease can now be revisited with respect to the role of HSC. It is quite remarkable that, as for many things, history does not follow a straight line. Although the first intuition of Von Kupffer proved to be misleading, the possible relationship between HSC and the autonomic nervous system has now in fact been validated: nerve endings in the intralobular spaces are localized mainly in the Disse spaces and are oriented towards HSC [3,8]; they express neural cell markers [9], secrete norepinephrine and express a variety of neuroadrenergic receptors [10].

Because of this rather controversial and tortuous history, HSC have been referred to by many different names (the most famous being Ito cells, lipocytes, fat-storing cells, perisinusoidal stellate cells). Each of these names bore sources of potential misunderstanding and, finally, in 1996, an international group of investigators actively working on this topic made the recommendation to refer to this cell type as 'hepatic stellate cell' [11].

Anatomy and ultrastructure

Hepatic stellate cells are located in the space of Disse in close contact with hepatocytes and sinusoidal endothelial cells. In human liver, HSC are disposed along the sinusoids with a

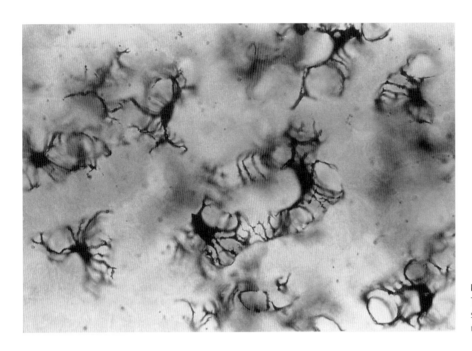

Fig. 2 Stellate cells in the porcine liver. The long cytoplasmic processes encompass sinusoids at regular intervals. Golgi's silver method (× 840). From ref. 72.

nucleus-to-nucleus distance of 40 μm, indicating that the sinusoids are equipped with HSC at certain fixed distances [12] (Fig. 2). Therefore, although the total number of HSC constitutes a small percentage of the total number of liver cells (approximately 5–8%), their spatial disposition and spatial extension may be sufficient to cover the entire hepatic sinusoidal microcirculatory network.

The three-dimensional structure of HSC consists of the cell body and several long and branching cytoplasmic processes (Fig. 3). Two main types of cytoplasmic processes are recognized according to their spatial disposition: the *intersinusoidal* or *interhepatocellular* processes and the *perisinusoidal* or *subendothelial* processes. The interhepatocellular processes penetrate the hepatic cell plates and extend to nearby sinusoids [12]. A single HSC may provide interhepatocellular processes to two or more neighbouring sinusoids. The perisinusoidal processes

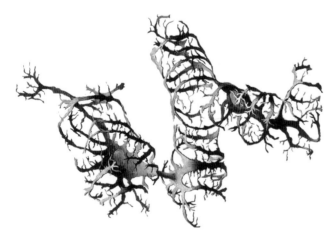

Fig. 3 Drawing of the three-dimensional structure of two hepatic stellate cells of porcine liver. The drawing was made according to the findings obtained by Golgi's silver method. From [73].

encircle the sinusoid located on the same cell plate by means of a series of adjacent periodic side-branches extending subendothelially. In general, the subendothelial processes appear to adhere to the sinusoidal wall by narrow strands of material resembling a basement membrane. These latter structures, although not continuously distributed, seem to ensure a strong connection between HSC and the sinusoidal endothelium [13]. The minute thorn-like microprojections or spines, termed *hepatocyte-contacting* processes [14], are an important and distinctive element of this cell type. These spines face the microvillous facet of hepatocytes and establish close intercellular contacts between HSC and parenchymal cells [15]. Although the functions of these microprojections are presently unknown, several lines of evidence suggest that they may play a role in epithelial–mesenchymal interactions that promote cell differentiation [15,16]. Another possible function of these processes is to serve as part of a mechanism of contact inhibition of HSC [17].

The most relevant ultrastructural feature of HSC in adult normal liver is the presence of cytoplasmic lipid droplets ranging in diameter from 1 to 2 μm (Fig. 4). This feature is related to one of the main known physiological functions of HSC, i.e. the hepatic storage of retinyl esters. However, in both rat and human liver, the number of HSC-containing evident lipid droplets varies up to 75% [4,18]; these are mainly located in lobular zone 2. Two types of lipid droplets have been identified: membrane-bound (type 1) and non-membrane-bound (type 2). Membrane-bound lipid droplets appear to derive from multivesicular bodies [4]. The nucleus of HSC in normal liver is oval and frequently indented by lipid droplets in the cytoplasm. One or more nucleoli and, in general, a tendency to a clumped heterochromatin pattern are often observed. Another important ultrastructural feature of these cells is a well-developed rough endoplasmic reticulum, suggesting active protein synthesis. Numerous microtubular structures are present in the cytoplasm together

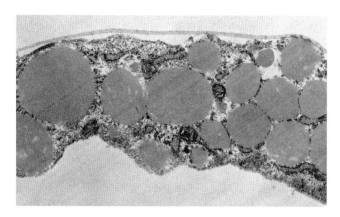

Fig. 4 Transmission electron microphotographs of hepatic stellate cells. Rat hepatic stellate cell in primary culture 3 days after plating. The cell contains numerous large lipid droplets (× 9600). From ref. 74.

with bundles of microfilaments (5 nm thick), particularly along the subsurface cytoplasmic matrix apposed to the neighbouring sinusoidal endothelial cell. Other 10-nm-thick filaments are widely distributed in the cytoplasm, especially around the nucleus and among the rough endoplasmic reticulum area. These microtubules and microfilaments may function as the cytoskeleton of dendritic processes and play a role in lipid synthesis and/or transport. Finally, ultrastructural analysis of the subendothelial processes revealed that these peculiar structures are equipped with massive 5-nm actin-like filaments, thus raising the hypothesis that they may contribute to reinforcing the endothelial lining and/or enhancing the efficiency of contraction of sinusoidal capillaries [4].

Retinoid storage and metabolism
(see also Chapter 2.3.11, Vitamins and the liver)

HSC play a key role in the metabolism and storage of retinoids [19]. In mammals, some 50–80% of total retinol is stored in the liver under normal circumstances. Retinyl esters, derived from esterification of retinol in the intestine, are transported to the liver via the lymphatic route in chylomicrons. Several studies have shown that chylomicron remnant retinyl esters are taken up by hepatocytes. After binding of the newly endocytosed retinoids with specific retinoid-binding proteins (RBP), these compounds are transferred to the neighbouring HSC [20]. In these cells, the uptake as well as the storage and the mobilization of retinoids are mainly regulated by intracellular retinol-binding proteins (CRBP), whose concentration in HSC is 20 times higher than that found in parenchymal cells [21,22]. In addition, *in vitro* experiments have shown that retinol and retinyl acetate can be taken up by HSC through a concentration-dependent gradient [23,24]. In adults, about 80% of total liver retinoids are stored as retinyl esters in HSC [21]. Retinyl esters are a major component of the total lipid mass present in the lipid droplets of HSC. However, the relative percentage of this compound is also dependent on the vitamin A status of the animal. Triacylgly-

cerol is another main component, and its concentration in the droplets does not seem to reflect the nutritional and/or the vitamin A status of the animal. Minor components of the lipid droplets are unesterified retinol, cholesteryl esters, cholesterol, free fatty acids and various phospholipids [25]. Any physiological condition that requires an increased utilization of retinoids at the periphery will result in the mobilization of these compounds from HSC through unknown mechanisms. Several retinoid-related proteins have been identified in stellate cells, including CRBP, retinol palmitate hydrolase, cellular retinoic acid-binding protein (CRABP), bile salt-dependent and -independent retinol ester hydrolase and acyl coenzyme A:retinal acyltransferase [26,27]. Whether stellate cells produce RBP is still in question, because of contradictory reports on the presence of RBP mRNA in stellate cells from different studies [27,28]. Stellate cells also express nuclear retinoid receptors [30], including retinoic acid receptors (RAR)α, β and γ [27,29] and retinoid X receptors (RXR)α and β, but not γ [31].

Intralobular heterogeneity of HSC

Several characteristics of HSC vary according to their location within the liver lobule [32–34]. Considering the classic division of the liver lobule into three zones (zone 1: periportal; zone 2: intermediate; zone 3: pericentral), HSC located in zone 1 appear to be small and contain minute vitamin A–lipid droplets. Perisinusoidal branching processes are short and smoothly contoured with few hepatocyte-contacting processes (Fig. 5), whereas desmin immunoreactivity is present but not particularly intense. HSC located in lobular zone 2 store abundant vitamin A–lipid droplets and extend encompassing processes that show intense desmin immunoreactivity (in the rat). These processes display conspicuous branching and abundant hepatocyte-contacting spines. Proceeding towards the centrilobular vein, HSC become more elongated, assuming a dendritic appearance, whereas their desmin immunoreactivity and vitamin A storage are progressively reduced becoming virtually absent around the centre of the lobule (Fig. 5). It has been reported that the administration of excess vitamin A to rats induces a progressive increase in the number and size of vitamin A–lipid droplets in HSC located in the central zone. Therefore, the intralobular heterogeneity of HSC may reflect, at least, differences in the metabolic handling of vitamin A and in the regulation of sinusoidal blood pressure in different areas of the liver lobule.

Isolation and culture of HSC

HSC isolated from normal liver and activated in culture represent an excellent model for investigating their profibrogenic properties. Nearly all isolation procedures include a first step aimed at obtaining a suspension of non-parenchymal liver cells. For this purpose, adult rat liver is perfused, through the portal vein, with a combination of collagenase (type 4) and pronase. Different technical approaches have been proposed for further purification of a homogeneous population of HSC [35–37].

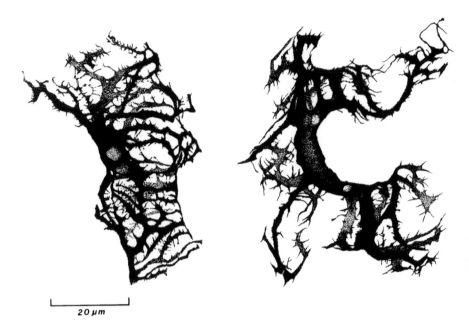

20 µm

Fig. 5 Camera lucida drawings of Golgi-stained hepatic stellate cells in zone 3 (left) and in the terminal region of the sinusoids (right). Note the spine-like microprojections from the lateral edges of subendothelial processes. Porcine liver (× 1200). From ref. 72.

However, all these purification procedures are based on the low buoyant density of these cells as a result of their large fat content. Accordingly, the final yield of HSC obtained from a single rat liver will vary according to the age, body weight and nutritional status of the animal. The highest yield is usually obtained by employing older rats maintained on a normal diet or younger rats fed on a vitamin A-supplemented diet. Modifications of the methods used to isolate HSC from rat liver have been introduced for the isolation of HSC from mice [38] or from wedge sections of normal human liver [39,40]. In particular, concerning the isolation of HSC from human liver, the use of wedge sections obtained at surgery does not offer the possibility of performing an adequate perfusion of the tissue. Therefore, the total yield/g of tissue and the purity of the cell preparation are generally lower than those obtainable from rat liver. However, a virtually 100% pure HSC culture is obtained from the first subculture (passage 1) by plating the cells on plastic substrata and supplementing the culture medium with rather high concentrations of fetal bovine serum (10–20%). These culture conditions appear to be quite selective for HSC and tend to eliminate contaminating endothelial and Kupffer cells [40]. In case higher cell purity is required (i.e. to obtain a pure population of 'freshly isolated' HSC), it is possible to perform further purification by centrifugal elutriation [41] or cell sorting [42].

Identification of HSC and related hepatic fibrogenic cells

The original method for the identification of HSC isolated from liver tissue was based on the detection of their distinctive morphological features and, particularly, the presence of intracytoplasmic lipid droplets [35]. In addition, the effective presence of vitamin A in the lipid droplets could be verified with additional techniques such as the demonstration of quick-fading green autofluorescence at 330 nm and the demonstration of intense cathodoluminescence on frozen section by electron microscopy [43]. However, as described above, the presence of lipid droplets depends on the nutritional status and, more importantly, is a key feature of only a portion of the total HSC population present in the liver lobule. It has become increasingly apparent that HSC are one subtype within a continuum of related mesenchymal cells that collectively comprise the population of fibrogenic cells in normal and diseased liver. Therefore, the identification of cytoskeletal or surface markers able to differentiate HSC from other liver non-parenchymal cells represents an important issue. The first step should be directed towards the identification of vimentin-positive and cytokeratin/factor VIII/monocyte–macrophage cell marker-negative cells. This approach can enable investigators to restrict their analysis to a subclass of mesenchymal cells including HSC, smooth muscle cells, myofibroblasts and fibroblasts [44]. Further steps are then aimed at differentiating HSC from the other subtypes. Among other cytoskeletal constituents, the intermediate filament desmin, characteristic of cells of muscle origin, is considered as a selective marker for the identification of HSC [45]. Desmin is definitively a reliable marker for the identification of HSC in rat or mouse liver tissue, although, as noted above, some intralobular heterogeneity in the intensity of the immunostaining is present. Unfortunately, none of the commercially available antibodies against desmin permits the reliable staining of desmin in human HSC cultures as well as in human liver tissue. The results range from no staining when using monoclonal antibodies to diffuse cytoplasmic staining (not adequate for intermediate filaments) when employing polyclonal antibodies [39,40]. As the majority of these antibodies produce positive immunostaining in human vascular smooth muscle cells, it is possible that human HSC are either desmin negative or their desmin possesses specific epitopes not recognized by the available antibodies.

Consolidated evidence indicates that the smooth muscle isoform of α-actin (α-SMA) represents an additional cytoskeletal marker for the identification of HSC [46,47]. However, α-SMA is not expressed in HSC early after isolation but only after some time in culture. Consequently, α-SMA is commonly employed as a marker of HSC activation.

While these and other markers are still largely employed [45], the problem of HSC identification in both liver tissue and cell isolates has grown remarkably complex in recent years. As noted above, this is related to increasing evidence for the profibrogenic role of other extracellular matrix (ECM)-producing cells, each with a distinct localization and a characteristic immunohistochemical and/or electron microscopic phenotype [9]. These include fibroblasts and myofibroblasts (MF) of the portal tract, smooth muscle cells localized in vessel walls and MF localized around the centrilobular vein. It is also increasingly evident that the relative participation of these different cell types is dependent on the development of distinct patterns of fibrosis [48]. An important advancement in the identification of HSC and other ECM-producing cells (particularly portal MF) in normal and fibrotic liver (rat and human) was provided by Cassiman and Roskams [9]. In an extensive study of the immunohistochemical expression profiles of mesenchymal (myo)fibroblast-like subpopulations in fibrotic/cirrhotic human and rat liver, these authors confirmed the existence of distinct lineages, with the addition of a new entity defined as 'interface' MF [49]; whether these lineages actually derive from different developmental sources is uncertain. The main cell population present in the perisinusoidal space of liver lobules, defined as 'HSC', stained with all tested markers (Table 1) and showed most intense and most widespread staining with α-SMA and neural cell adhesion molecule (N-CAM) antibodies in human liver, while in rat liver, the largest proportion of HSC was stained by glial fibrillary acidic protein (GFAP) and desmin antibodies. The second

subpopulation identified was the 'interface MF', (myo)fibroblast-like cells located at the interface between the portal tract and the parenchyma, or at the interface between the fibrotic septa and the parenchyma. When compared with HSC, interface MF showed no expression of synaptophysin (SYN), neurotrophin receptor tyrosine kinases Trk-B or Trk-C, low-affinity nerve growth factor receptor p75 or neurotrophin (NT) 3, but they did express GFAP, N-CAM, α-SMA, nerve growth factor (NGF), brain-derived nerve growth factor (BDNF), NT-4 and alpha B-crystallin (ABCRYS) in a varying proportion of cells [50,51]. The third subpopulation was the 'septal MF', the (myo)fibroblast-like cells populating the fibrotic septa. They only stained with α-SMA, GFAP, BDNF, ABCRYS, N-CAM and desmin (the last two only in rat) in a varying proportion of cells. This expression profile was identical to that seen in (myo)fibroblast-like cells populating the portal tracts of cirrhotic livers. It is therefore likely that septal MF derive from the expansion of the MF population of the portal tract. On the other hand, interface MF, present in areas of piecemeal necrosis and active fibrogenesis, are likely to derive from the recruitment and activation of HSC. The information derived from this detailed analysis performed in liver tissue can be employed for the identification of HSC and other ECM-producing cells in isolates from human and rat liver [9].

The embryonic origin of HSC

The embryonic origin of HSC still constitutes a rather mysterious issue, which is closely related to the discovery of cell markers able to identify HSC and to differentiate them from other liver ECM-producing cells. In addition, identification of the embryonic origin of stellate cells will improve our understanding of their relationship to other fibrogenic liver cells and will also raise the possibility of using cell lineage-specific promoters to drive transgene expression selectively in stellate cells in vivo with a view to applying gene therapy. Based on morphological similarities and positivity for desmin, vimentin and α-SMA, HSC have been considered for many years to be of mesenchymal origin, derived embryologically from septum transversum (in turn arising from cardiac mesenchyme) as it invades the endoderm-derived hepatic bud. However, when HSC were found to contain a host of neural marker proteins, it was speculated that HSC could be of neuroectodermal origin [52]. Other studies have suggested the possibility that hepatocytes and stellate cells may derive from a common endodermal precursor [53]. Finally, recent studies in humans and animal models suggest that HSC may also derive from bone marrow precursors [54–56].

Rodent, human and HSC lines: differences and similarities

Most of the established experience with HSC cultures derives from cells isolated from normal rat or human liver and activated by culture on plastic substrata. It is not possible to make a clearcut distinction in the behaviour of rat, mouse and human

Table 1 Immunohistochemical expression profile of subpopulations of mesenchymal myofibroblast-like cells in fibrotic human and rat liver (from [42]).

	HSC	Interface MF	Septal MF	Portal MF
Desmin (human/rat)	–/+	–/+	–/±	–/±
α-SMA	+	+	+	+
GFAP	+	+	±	±
BDNF	+	±	±	±
ABCRYS	+	+	±	±
N-CAM (human/rat)	+/+	±/+	±/+	±/+
NGF	+	±	–	–
NT-4	+	±	–	–
NT-3	+	–	–	–
Trk-B	+	–	–	–
Trk-C	+	–	–	–
p75	+	–	–	–
Synaptophysin	+	–	–	–

HSC preparations, although it is likely that there are several differences. As a general rule, observations based on rodent HSC cultures are not necessarily true for human HSC and vice versa, and findings must be validated directly between species. There is still quite a lot of uncertainty about the fate of rat HSC after the first culture on plastic, with some authors supporting the possibility of their extinction by apoptosis [57] and others supporting their final differentiation into MF-like cells. On the other hand, human HSC seem to progress to their activated phenotype without showing signs of apparent apoptosis (actually being very resistant to proapoptotic stimuli) and showing cell markers of the so-called 'interface' MF [9]. It is also relevant that human HSC preparations derived from the liver of different individuals show quantitative differences in gene/protein expression and in response to profibrogenic cytokines. It is therefore very much recommended to perform experiments on more than one human HSC preparation to account for these interindividual differences when describing features of this cell type or its response to specific stimuli.

Several groups have proposed the use of HSC lines as an alternative to working with primary cells (for a review see [45]). The use of HSC lines allow easier manipulation, sharing of cells to validate results and transfectability. However, HSC lines always derive from spontaneously or artificially immortalized HSC, and any specific observation needs to be carefully interpreted and not transferred to the biology of primary cells without validation of key findings. Four human HSC lines have been introduced and characterized recently. The LX-1 and LX-2 lines were generated by either SV40 T-antigen immortalization (LX-1) or spontaneous immortalization in low serum conditions (LX-2) [58]. Both lines express α-SMA, vimentin and GFAP. Similar to primary HSCs, both lines express key receptors regulating hepatic fibrosis and also proteins involved in matrix remodelling. Transforming growth factor β1 stimulation increased their α1(I) procollagen mRNA expression. LX-2, but not LX-1, cells are highly transfectable. The human HSC line TWNT-4 was immortalized by retrovirally introducing human telomerase reverse transcriptase (hTERT) into LI 90 cells established from a human liver mesenchymal tumour [59]. TWNT-4 express platelet-derived growth factor receptor β (PDGF-Rβ), α-SMA and type 1 collagen (α1). Another human HSC line was obtained by infecting human HSC with a retrovirus expressing hTERT [60]. When compared with control human HSC, telomerase-positive HSC did not show signs of senescence and could be cultured for at least 69 passages. Telomerase-positive HSC did not undergo oncogenic transformation and exhibited morphological and functional characteristics of activated HSC.

Extrahepatic HSC and the 'stellate cell system'

Stellate cells also exist in extrahepatic organs such as pancreas, lung, kidney, intestine, spleen, adrenal gland, ductus deferens and vocal cords. Hepatic and extrahepatic stellate cells form what has been defined as the 'stellate cell system'. In recent years, particular attention has been given to pancreatic stellate cells and their potential pathogenic role in chronic pancreatitis and pancreatic cancer [61]. Considering the current uncertainty on the origin of HSC, it is even more difficult to know whether or not all these stellate cells derive from a common precursor.

HSC and extracellular matrix homeostasis

In normal liver, the ECM constitutes about 0.5% of liver wet weight. This specialized tissue component can be subdivided into the pericellular matrix interacting with cell membrane components, the classic interstitial matrix structuring the interstitial spaces and basement membranes supporting epithelial, endothelial and mesenchymal cells. In addition to collagens, ECM is made up of minor amounts of several non-collagenous components. These include large glycoproteins such as fibronectin, laminin, nidogen (entactin), tenascin and undulin, several types of sulphated proteoglycans and, as a pure carbohydrate polymer, hyaluronic acid. The space of Disse, where HSC are located, is a virtual space constituted by an ECM network composed of type 4 collagen, associated with non-collagenous components such as laminin and nidogen. In this context, the presence of collagen I and III, although quantitatively relevant, is limited to large-diameter bundles of fibres reinforcing the architecture of the perisinusoidal space. The resulting complex, defined as 'non-fibrillar', ensures an optimal diffusion between hepatocytes and the bloodstream. In normal liver, all the cellular components delimiting the space of Disse, including hepatocytes, appear to be involved in the synthesis of the main ECM components [62,63]. However, the large majority of collagen III, IV and laminin is synthesized by HSC (III > IV > laminin > I) and sinusoidal endothelial cells (IV > III > laminin > I), whereas all cell types synthesize small amounts of collagen I, supporting the concept that, in normal liver, synthesis of this type of collagen is minimally active. In addition, sinusoidal endothelial cells appear to synthesize collagen IV and laminin in much higher amounts than HSC [64]. These observations are fundamental when considering that, during active liver fibrogenesis, HSC become the major ECM-producing cell type, with a predominant production of collagen I [62–64]. Normal ECM turnover implies that the synthesis of new individual components is associated with their continuous slow degradation. In normal liver, HSC and possibly other sinusoidal cells may contribute to the continuous remodelling of the ECM of the space of Disse by producing matrix metalloproteinase 2 (gelatinase or type 4 collagenase) [65] (see also Chapter 6, Cirrhosis).

HSC as liver-specific pericytes

The possible role of HSC as liver-specific pericytes is suggested by their anatomical location, ultrastructural features and close relationship with the autonomous nervous system (Fig. 6).

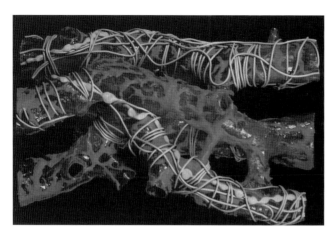

Fig. 6 A three-dimensional model of hepatic sinusoids. Hepatic stellate cells (red) adhere directly to the fenestrated endothelium to make stellate cell–endothelial cell complexes. Nerve fibres (yellow) and collagen fibres (grey) are distributed outside the cell complex, i.e. in the space of Disse. Figure courtesy of Professor K. Wake.

Studies performed over the past decade have shown that HSC isolated from rat or human liver and maintained in culture contract in response to several vasoconstricting stimuli [66]. Contraction of HSC in response to these stimuli has been demonstrated independently from the cell attachment substrata (glass, plastic, silicone membranes or collagen lattices). Importantly, at least after stimulation with thrombin, endothelin-1 and angiotensin II, cell contraction is coupled with an increase in intracellular calcium concentration [67]. These observations contribute greatly to the central issue of considering HSC as pericytes. It should be noted, however, that cultured HSC are characterized by an activated phenotype resembling transitional or MF-like cells rather than quiescent HSC. Therefore, the contractile properties demonstrated in these experiments are likely to be more representative of HSC contractile status in fibrotic liver. Whether or not HSC contract in normal liver tissue still represents a matter for discussion. From the morphological standpoint, some observations argue against the role of HSC in the regulation of sinusoidal blood flow [68]. First, in their *in vivo* tridimensional orientation, HSC do not have a stellate form (typical of their aspect in bidimensional culture on plastic) but rather a 'spider-like' appearance ('arachnocytes') with a small cell body and a series of radiating and parallel slender processes. According to the authors of these observations, cells with this tridimensional appearance are not likely to be 'contraction ready'. Additional limitations to effective cell contraction are offered by the spatial constraints of the space of Disse, by the intracytoplasmic presence of lipid droplets that prevent microfilaments from assembling in a long span and by the ultrastructural evidence of a limited development of contractile filaments in quiescent HSC. Regardless, studies evaluating the hepatic microcirculation by intravital microscopy techniques have suggested that HSC could be involved in the regulation of sinusoidal tone in normal liver [69,70]. An additional matter

of debate is provided by studies aimed at quantifying HSC contraction with techniques able to detect the development of contractile forces in response to vasoconstrictors [71]. The results of these studies indicate that the magnitude and kinetics of contraction and relaxation are consistent with the hypothesis that HSC may affect sinusoidal resistance. However, for understandable technical reasons, these data were obtained in rat HSC in primary culture 7 days after isolation, when a certain degree of activation in culture has already occurred. In conclusion, although HSC could be proposed as liver-specific pericytes based on their location, spatial distribution, relationship with the peripheral nervous system and ultrastructural features, no conclusive evidence establishes a role in regulating normal sinusoidal blood flow.

References

1 Kupffer K (1876) Uber Sternzellen der Leber. Briefliche Mitteilung an Professor Waldeyer. *Arch Mikr Anat* 12, 353–358.

2 Zimmerman K (1928) Uber das Verhaltniss der 'Kupfferschen Sternzellen' zum Endothel der Leberkapillaren beim Menschen. *Ztsch Mikr Anat Forsch* 14, 528–548.

3 Ito T, Nemoto M (1952) Uber die Kupfferschen Sternzellen und die 'Fettspeicherungzellen' (fat storing cells) in der Blutkapillarenwand der menschlichen Leber. *Okajima Folia Anat Jpn* 24, 243–258.

4 Wake K (1980) Perisinusoidal stellate cells (fat-storing cells, interstitial cells, lipocytes), their related structure in and around the liver sinusoids, and vitamin A-storing cells in extrahepatic organs. *Int Rev Cytol* 66, 303–353.

5 McGee JO, Patrick RS (1972) The role of perisinusoidal cells in hepatic fibrogenesis. An electron microscopic study of acute carbon tetrachloride liver injury. *Lab Invest* 26, 429–440.

6 McGee JO, Patrick RS (1972) The role of perisinusoidal cells in experimental hepatic fibrogenesis. *J Pathol* 106 (1), vi.

7 Kent G, Gay S, Inouye T *et al.* (1976) Vitamin A-containing lipocytes and formation of type III collagen in liver injury. *Proc Natl Acad Sci USA* 73, 3719–3722.

8 Ueno T, Bioulac-Sage P, Balabaud C *et al.* (2004) Innervation of the sinusoidal wall: regulation of the sinusoidal diameter. *Anat Rec A Discov Mol Cell Evol Biol* 280, 868–873.

9 Cassiman D, Roskams T (2002) Beauty is in the eye of the beholder: emerging concepts and pitfalls in hepatic stellate cell research. *J Hepatol* 37, 527–535.

10 Oben JA, Diehl AM (2004) Sympathetic nervous system regulation of liver repair. *Anat Rec A Discov Mol Cell Evol Biol* 280, 874–883.

11 Letter to the editor (1996) Hepatic stellate cell nomenclature (letter). *Hepatology* 23, 193.

12 Wake K (1988) Liver perivascular cells revealed by gold and silver impregnation methods and electron microscopy. In: Motta P (ed.) *Biopathology of the Liver, an Ultrastructural Approach.* Dordrecht: Kluwer, pp. 23–26.

13 Wake K (1999) Hepatic stellate cells. In: Tanikawa K, Ueno T (eds) *Liver Diseases and Hepatic Sinusoidal Cells.* Tokyo: Springer-Verlag, pp. 56–65.

14 Wake K (1995) Structure of the sinusoidal wall in the liver. In: Wisse E, Knook DL, Wake K (eds) *Cells of the Hepatic Sinusoid.* Leiden: The Kupffer Cell Foundation, pp. 241–246.

15 Wake K, Motomatsu K, Ekataksin W (1991) Postnatal development of the perisinusoidal stellate cells in the rat liver. In: Wisse E, Knook DL, McCuskey RS (eds) *Cells of the Hepatic Sinusoid*. Leiden: The Kupffer Cell Foundation, pp. 269–275.

16 Gressner AM, Lofti S, Gressner G *et al.* (1992) Identification and partial characterization of a hepatocyte-derived factor promoting proliferation of cultured fat-storing cells (parasinusoidal lipocytes). *Hepatology* 16, 1250–1266.

17 Wanson JC, Mosselmans R (1980) Coculture of adult rat hepatocytes and sinusoidal cells: a new experimental model for the study of ultra-structural and functional properties of liver cells. In: Popper H, Bianchi L, Gudat F *et al.* (eds) *Communications of Liver Cells*. Lancaster: MTP Press, pp. 239–251.

18 Sztark F, Dubroca J, Latry P *et al.* (1986) Perisinusoidal cells in patients with normal liver histology. A morphometric study. *J Hepatol* 2, 358–369.

19 Blomhoff R, Wake K (1991) Perisinusoidal stellate cells of the liver: important roles in retinol metabolism and fibrosis. *FASEB J* 5, 271–277.

20 Blomhoff R, Berg T, Norum KR (1988) Transfer of retinol from parenchymal to stellate cells in liver is mediated by retinol-binding protein. *Proc Natl Acad Sci USA* 85, 3455–3458.

21 Blomhoff R, Rasmussen M, Nilsson A *et al.* (1985) Hepatic retinol metabolism. Distribution of retinoids, enzymes, and binding proteins in isolated rat liver cells. *J Biol Chem* 260, 13560–13565.

22 Uchio K, Tuchweber B, Manabe N *et al.* (2002) Cellular retinol-binding protein-1 expression and modulation during in vivo and in vitro myofibroblastic differentiation of rat hepatic stellate cells and portal fibroblasts. *Lab Invest* 82, 619–628.

23 Matsuura T, Nagamori S, Fujise K *et al.* (1989) Retinol transport in cultured fat-storing cells of rat liver. Quantitative analysis by anchored cell analysis and sorting system. *Lab Invest* 61, 107–115.

24 Pinzani M, Gentilini P, Abboud HE (1992) Phenotypical modulation of liver fat-storing cells by retinoids. Influence on unstimulated and growth factor-induced cell proliferation. *J Hepatol* 14, 211–220.

25 Moriwaki K, Blaner WS, Piantedosi R *et al.* (1988) Effects of dietary retinoids and triglyceride on the lipid composition of rat liver stellate cells and stellate cell lipid droplets. *J Lipid Res* 29, 1523–1534.

26 Blaner WS, Hendriks HF, Brouwer A *et al.* (1985) Retinoids, retinoid binding proteins and retinyl palmitate hydrolase distributions in different types of rat liver cells. *J Lipid Res* 26, 1241–1251.

27 Friedman SL, Wei S, Blaner WS (1993) Retinol release by activated rat hepatic lipocytes: regulation by Kupffer cell-conditioned medium and PDGF. *Am J Physiol* 264, G947–952.

28 Blomhoff R, Norum KR, Berg T (1985) Hepatic uptake of [3H]retinol bound to the serum retinol binding protein involves both parenchymal and perisinusoidal stellate cells. *J Biol Chem* 260, 13571–13575.

29 Weiner FR, Blaner WS, Czaja MJ *et al.* (1992) Ito cell expression of a nuclear retinoic acid receptor. *Hepatology* 15, 336–342.

30 Mangelsdorf DJ, Thummel C, Beato M *et al.* (1995) The nuclear receptor superfamily: the second decade. *Cell* 83, 835–839.

31 Ulven SM, Natarajan V, Holven KB *et al.* (1998) Expression of retinoic acid receptor and retinoid X receptor subtypes in rat liver cells: implications for retinoid signalling in parenchymal, endothelial, Kupffer and stellate cells. *Eur J Cell Biol* 77, 111–116.

32 Ballardini G, Groff P, Badiali de Giorgi L *et al.* (1994) Ito cell heterogeneity: desmin-negative Ito cells in normal rat liver. *Hepatology* 19, 440–446.

33 Zou Z, Ekataksin W, Wake K (1998) Zonal and regional differences identified from precision mapping of vitamin A-storing lipid droplets of the hepatic stellate cells in pig liver: a novel concept of addressing the intralobular area of heterogeneity. *Hepatology* 27, 1098–1108.

34 Higashi N, Senoo H (2003) Distribution of vitamin A-storing lipid droplets in hepatic stellate cells in liver lobules – a comparative study. *Anat Rec A Discov Mol Cell Evol Biol* 271, 240–248.

35 Knook DL, Seffelaar AM, De Leuw AM (1982) Fat-storing cells of rat liver. Their isolation and purification. *Exp Cell Res* 139, 468–471.

36 Friedman SL, Roll FJ (1987) Isolation and culture of hepatic lipocytes, Kupffer cells and sinusoidal endothelial cells by density gradient centrifugation with stractan. *Anal Biochem* 161, 207–218.

37 Mantovaara T, Norlinder H, Pertof H (1990) Isolation of the perisinusoidal vitamin A storing cells from rat liver on Ca²⁺ immobilized glass surfaces. *Exp Cell Res* 187, 170–173.

38 Pinzani M, Abboud HE, Gesualdo L *et al.* (1992) Regulation of macrophage-colony stimulating factor in liver fat-storing cells by peptide growth factors. *Am J Physiol Cell Physiol* 262, C876–C881.

39 Friedman SL, Rockey DC, McGuire RF *et al.* (1992) Isolated hepatic lipocytes and Kupffer cells from normal human liver: morphological and functional characteristics in primary culture. *Hepatology* 15, 234–243.

40 Casini A, Pinzani M, Milani S *et al.* (1993) Regulation of transforming growth factor-β1 in human fat-storing cells. *Gastroenterology* 105, 245–253.

41 Maher JJ, Bissell DM, Friedman SL *et al.* (1988) Collagen measured in primary cultures of normal rat hepatocytes derives from lipocytes within the monolayer. *J Clin Invest* 82, 450–459.

42 Geerts A, Niki T, Hellemans K *et al.* (1998) Purification of rat hepatic stellate cells by side scatter-activated cell sorting. *Hepatology* 27, 590–598.

43 Bioulac-Sage P, Balabaud C (1992) Proliferation and phenotypic expression of perisinusoidal cells. *J Hepatol* 15, 284–287.

44 Pinzani M, Gesualdo L, Sabbah GM *et al.* (1989) Effects of platelet-derived growth factor and other polypeptide mitogens on DNA synthesis and growth of cultured rat liver fat-storing cells. *J Clin Invest* 84, 1786–1793.

45 Geerts A (2001) History, heterogeneity, developmental biology, and functions of quiescent hepatic stellate cells. *Semin Liver Dis* 21, 311–335.

46 Ramadori G, Veit T, Schwogler S *et al.* (1990) Expression of the gene of the alpha-smooth muscle-actin isoform in rat liver and in rat fat-storing (Ito) cells. *Virchows Arch B Cell Pathol Incl Mol Pathol* 59, 349–357.

47 Rockey DC, Boyles JK, Gabbiani G *et al.* (1992) Rat hepatic lipocytes express smooth muscle actin upon activation in vivo and in culture. *J Submicrosc Cytol Pathol* 24, 193–203.

48 Pinzani M, Rombouts K (2004) Liver fibrosis: from the bench to clinical targets. *Dig Liver Dis* 36, 231–242.

49 Cassiman D, Libbrecht L, Desmet V *et al.* (2002) Hepatic stellate cell/myofibroblast subpopulations in fibrotic human and rat livers. *J Hepatol* 36, 200–209.

50 Cassiman D, van Pelt J, De Vos R *et al.* (1999) Synaptophysin: a novel marker for human and rat hepatic stellate cells. *Am J Pathol* 155, 1831–1839.

51 Cassiman D, Denef C, Desmet V *et al.* (2001) Human and rat hepatic stellate cells express neurotrophins and neurotrophin receptors. *Hepatology* 33, 148–158.

52 Geerts A (2004) On the origin of stellate cells: mesodermal, endodermal or neuro-ectodermal? *J Hepatol* 40, 331–334.

53 Kiassov AP, Van Eyken P, van Pelt JF *et al.* (1995) Desmin expressing nonhematopoietic liver cells during rat liver development: an

immunohistochemical and morphometric study. *Differentiation* 59, 253–258.

54 Forbes SJ, Russo FP, Rey V *et al.* (2004) A significant proportion of myofibroblasts are of bone marrow origin in human liver fibrosis. *Gastroenterology* 126, 955–963.

55 Baba S, Fujii H, Hirose T *et al.* (2004) Commitment of bone marrow cells to hepatic stellate cells in mouse. *J Hepatol* 40, 255–260.

56 Suskind DL, Muench MO (2004) Searching for common stem cells of the hepatic and hematopoietic systems in the human fetal liver: CD34+ cytokeratin 7/8+ cells express markers for stellate cells. *J Hepatol* 40, 261–268.

57 Saile B, Matthes N, Neubauer K *et al.* (2002) Rat liver myofibroblasts and hepatic stellate cells differ in CD95-mediated apoptosis and response to TNF-alpha. *Am J Physiol Gastrointest Liver Physiol* 283, G435–G444.

58 Xu L, Hui AY, Albanis E *et al.* (2005) Human hepatic stellate cell lines, LX-1 and LX-2: new tools for analysis of hepatic fibrosis. *Gut* 54, 142–151.

59 Shibata N, Watanabe T, Okitsu T *et al.* (2003) Establishment of an immortalized human hepatic stellate cell line to develop antifibrotic therapies. *Cell Transplant* 12, 499–507.

60 Schnabl B, Choi YH, Olsen JC *et al.* (2002) Immortal activated human hepatic stellate cells generated by ectopic telomerase expression. *Lab Invest* 82, 323–333.

61 Apte MV, Wilson JS (2004) Mechanisms of pancreatic fibrosis. *Dig Dis* 22, 273–279.

62 Milani S, Herbst H, Schuppan D *et al.* (1989) In situ hybridization for procollagen types I, III and IV mRNA in normal and fibrotic rat liver: evidence for predominant expression in nonparenchymal liver cells. *Hepatology* 10, 84–92.

63 Milani S, Herbst H, Schuppan D *et al.* (1989) Cellular localization of laminin gene transcripts in normal and fibrotic human liver. *Am J Pathol* 134, 1175–1182.

64 Maher JJ, McGuire RF (1990) Extracellular matrix gene expression increases preferentially in rat lipocytes and sinusoidal endothelial cells during hepatic fibrosis in vivo. *J Clin Invest* 86, 1641–1648.

65 Milani S, Herbst H, Schuppan D *et al.* (1994) Differential expression of matrix-metalloproteinase-1 and -2 genes in normal and fibrotic human liver. *Am J Pathol* 144, 528–537.

66 Pinzani M, Gentilini P (1999) Biology of hepatic stellate cells and their possible relevance in the pathogenesis of portal hypertension in cirrhosis. *Semin Liver Dis* 19, 397–410.

67 Pinzani M, Failli P, Ruocco C *et al.* (1992) Fat-storing cells as liver-specific pericytes. Spatial dynamics of agonist-stimulated intracellular calcium transients. *J Clin Invest* 90, 642–646.

68 Ekataksin W, Kaneda K (1999) Liver microvascular architecture: an insight into the pathophysiology of portal hypertension. *Semin Liver Dis* 19, 359–382.

69 Zhang JX, Pegoli W, Jr, Clemens MG (1994) Endothelin-1 induces direct constriction of hepatic sinusoids. *Am J Physiol* 266, G624–632.

70 Zhang JX, Bauer M, Clemens MG (1995) Vessel- and target cell-specific actions of endothelin-1 and endothelin-3 in rat liver. *Am J Physiol* 269, G269–277.

71 Thimgan MS, Yee HF, Jr (1999) Quantitation of rat hepatic stellate cell contraction: stellate cells' contribution to sinusoidal tone. *Am J Physiol* 277, G137–G143.

72 Wake K, Sato T (1993) Intralobalar heterogeneity of perisinusoidal stellate cells in porcine liver. *Cell Tissue Res* 273, 227–237.

73 Wake K (1977) Chapter in: Vidal-Vanaclocha F (ed.) *Functional Heterogeneity of Liver Tissue*. Austin, TX: RG Landes Co.

74 Pinzani M (1995) Novel insights into the biology and physiology of the Ito cell. *Pharmac Ther* 66, 387–412.

1.7 Biliary epithelial cells

Jean-François Dufour

An important minority

The bile duct epithelial cells, also called cholangiocytes, are the cells that cover the biliary tree. At the level of the canal of Hering, they appose to hepatocytes and/or oval cells to collect the bile from the bile canaliculi, which are themselves a space between hepatocytes where the primitive bile is formed. The bile circulates through a maze of conduits that progressively merge into larger ductules and bile ducts lined by cholangiocytes to finally reach the extrahepatic duct, the gallbladder and the choledochus, which are also covered by cholangiocytes. Morphometric studies revealed that biliary epithelial cells represent only 3–5% of the cells present in the liver.

Cholangiocytes are polarized cells with a side facing the bile, which comes from the hepatocytes, and a side facing the portal space and its nourishing peribiliary plexus, whose blood arises from the hepatic artery and flows thereafter in hepatic sinusoids. Not surprisingly, cholangiocytes have important vectorial transport functions secreting and resorbing solutes. Cholangiocytes also possess immunological properties by participating in the immune response and being the target of this response in several important liver diseases such as primary biliary cirrhosis, primary sclerosing cholangitis and chronic rejection after liver transplantation. In this sense, cholangiocytes can be seen as the Achilles' heel of the liver.

Transporters and polarity

The biliary epithelium modifies the primitive bile, which has been secreted by hepatocytes at their bile canalicular membrane. In humans, the contribution of the biliary epithelium to the bile flow is estimated to represent 40% of the bile flow. In contrast to hepatocellular secretion, which accumulates in bile complex molecules such as bile acids, phospholipids, cholesterol and glutathione, cholangiocellular secretion transports essentially water and electrolytes. This secretion relies on the correct arrangement of numerous transporters at the apical and at the basolateral sides of the cholangiocytes. Transepithelial transport of Cl^- ions forms the primary driving force for this secretion. Cl^- ions accumulate in cholangiocytes at the basolateral side through $Na^+/K^+/2Cl^-$ transporters. At the apical pole, opening of the cystic fibrosis transmembrane regulator (CFTR) channel lets Cl^- out of the cell into the lumen [1]. This activity is coupled with the activity of an anion exchanger, which exchanges Cl^- for HCO_3^-. This net release of HCO_3^- carries along water. Bile consisting of more than 98% water and aquaporins (AQP), which form water channels, plays an important role in cholangiocellular bile formation. AQP4 is constitutively expressed on the basolateral membrane, whereas AQP1 is targeted to the apical side of the cholangiocytes. Other proteins support these movements of Cl^- and HCO_3^-: on the basal side, a symporter takes up Na^+ and HCO_3^- and an exchanger takes up Na^+ against H^+ (NHE-1); on the apical side, another exchanger takes up Na^+ against H^+ (NHE-2). Apical Cl^- channels form the principal method of regulation of cholangiocellular secretion. Phosphorylation of CFTR by cyclic adenosine monophosphate (cAMP)-dependent protein kinase (PKA) increases the open permeability of this Cl^- channel. Moreover, cAMP translocates subapical vesicles sequestering CFTR, Cl^-/HCO_3^- anion exchanger and AQP1 to the apical plasma membrane [2,3]. In contrast, ATP depletion, as is the case during ischaemia, results in internalization of these apical membrane proteins [4]. Cl^- channels other than CFTR have been discovered. Among these additional Cl^- channels, CIC2 is regulated by cell volume and protein kinase C (PKC) [5], and another is calcium activated [6]. The importance of these Cl^- channels in liver pathobiology is demonstrated by cystic fibrosis, a disease characterized by mutations in the CFTR gene and with clinical liver disease occurring in only about 30% of the patients (see Chapter 16.4).

Cholangiocytes not only secrete solutes into the biliary lumen, but also reabsorb bile components. The same transporters that reuptake bile acids in the terminal ileum (ASBT) retrieve conjugated bile acids from the bile [7]. It has been found that an alternatively spliced form of ASBT (t-ASBT) is targeted to the basolateral membrane and functions as a bile acid efflux protein [8]. The heteromeric organic solute transporter OSTalpha–OSTbeta, which is also localized in the basolateral membrane of cholangiocytes, may play a similar role in the vectorial transport of conjugated bile acids and sterols [9]. Translocation of ASBT to the apical membrane increases bile acid absorption by bile ducts, which amplifies bile acid-induced choleresis via cholehepatic shunting [10]. Bile ductular epithelium reabsorbs glucose by the coordinated expression of SGLT1 on the apical domain and GLUT1 on the basolateral domain [11]. SGLT1 has been implicated in invasion of cholangiocytes by *Cryptosporidium parvum*. *C. parvum* recruits SGLT1 and AQP1 to generate a localized water influx near its attachment site [12]. Cholangiocytes can also retrieve glutamate, which is produced by the luminal degradation of glutathione [13].

The cytoskeleton plays an important role in establishing and maintaining polarity by directing integral proteins to specific locations. Scaffolding proteins tether transporters to the underlying cytoskeleton. The ezrin–EBP50 complex accumulates at the apical pole of cholangiocytes. Ezrin concurrently binds actin, EBP50 and PKA. EBP50 is a PSD95-Dlg-ZO1 (PDZ) domain-containing protein that interacts with the carboxy tail of CFTR. This scaffold not only anchors CFTR to the cytoskeleton, but also fixes PKA near CFTR. Disruption of this association ablates cAMP-activated Cl⁻ channel activity [14]. On the lateral sides of the cholangiocytes, tight junctions restrict the movement of solutes between adjacent cells, maintaining the blood–bile barrier and preventing the apicobasal diffusion of integral membrane proteins. Permeability of the tight junctions in bile ducts is increased by tumour necrosis factor (TNF)α [15]. On their lateral side, cholangiocytes establish contacts through gap junctions. In contrast to hepatocytes, which form gap junctions with connexin 32 and connexin 26, cholangiocellular gap junctions are made of connexin 43 [16]. Finally, biliary epithelial cells are equipped with non-motile cilia. This important structural feature protrudes into the lumen and functions as a mechanoreceptor bent by bile flow. It is now established that polycystic liver and kidney diseases are ciliary diseases (see Chapter 8.1). Polycystin-1 and polycystin-2, which are defective in autosomal dominant polycystic kidney disease, localize to cilia. Loss of fibrocystin, as occurs in autosomal recessive polycystic kidney disease, results in distorted biliary cilia [17].

Regulation of cholangiocyte secretion

Several hormones regulate cholangiocellular secretion. Receptors for secretin, somatostatin, bombesin, vasoactive intestinal polypeptide (VIP), acetylcholine, dopamine and nucleotides are localized on the basolateral membrane of cholangiocytes. Secretin receptors are coupled with G proteins, which activate adenylyl cyclase to produce cAMP, resulting in increased activity of PKA [18]. By favouring the opening of CFTR and by mobilizing subapical vesicles containing CFTR, Cl⁻/HCO$_3^-$ exchanger and AQP1, secretin is the principal choleretic hormone; in humans, it more than doubles bile flow. The stimulation of biliary secretion by secretin is inhibited by other hormones linked to G protein-coupled receptors, such as somatostatin

[19], gastrin [20] and endothelin-1 [21], which interfere with the production of cAMP. Insulin activates PKC in a calcium-dependent manner, and this inhibits the secretin-induced ductal secretion [22]. The neuropeptides bombesin and VIP stimulate fluid and HCO$_3^-$ secretion from rat cholangiocytes by activating the luminal Cl⁻/HCO$_3^-$ exchanger [23,24]. Cholangiocytes express cholinergic M3 receptors, and administration of acetylcholine to rats through the hepatic artery increased HCO$_3^-$ biliary secretion [25]. Using bile duct-ligated rats, it was found that an agonist of the D2 receptor inhibited PKA activity and secretin-induced choleresis via calcium-dependent PKC [26]. Exposure of human cholangiocytes to natriuretic peptide elicits the formation of cGMP, which in turn stimulated Cl⁻ efflux [27], suggesting a role for this second messenger in biliary physiology.

Nucleotides can be secreted into bile by either hepatocytes or cholangiocytes [28]. Bile contains ATP in micromolar concentrations. Exposure of cholangiocytes to ATP elicits cytosolic calcium oscillations [16]. These signals may be mediated through purinergic P2X receptors [29], which are ATP-gated cation channels, and P2Y receptors [30], which are G protein-coupled receptors linked to phospholipase C and the production of inositol trisphosphate. Stimulation of purinergic receptors enhances ductular secretion via the stimulation of calcium-dependent Cl⁻ efflux channels and basolateral NHE-1 [31,32]. Importantly, the P2Y receptors are localized in the apical membrane of biliary epithelial cells [31]. Then, nucleotides secreted into the bile canaliculus by hepatocytes modulate, in a paracrine manner downstream, the secretion of biliary epithelial cells.

Inositol trisphosphate elicits complex calcium signals such as calcium oscillations and calcium waves. These signals rely on inositol trisphosphate receptors, which are intracellular channels releasing calcium from the endoplasmic reticulum. Similarly to gap junctions, it appears that biliary epithelial cells use different isoforms from hepatocytes. In contrast to hepatocytes, which express mostly the inositol trisphosphate receptor isoform 2, biliary epithelial cells abundantly express inositol trisphosphate receptor isoform 3 [33]. Cholestasis has been associated with loss of inositol trisphosphate receptors in cholangiocytes and, consequently, impaired calcium signalling [34].

Portal inflammation may participate directly in cholestasis by impairing ductal secretion. A combination of cytokines [interleukin (IL)-6, interferon (IFN)-gamma, IL-1 and TNFα] inhibits cAMP formation and cyclic AMP-dependent Cl⁻ efflux in isolated bile duct units, but does not affect purinergic/calcium-dependent Cl⁻ efflux [35].

Cholangiocyte proliferation

Cholangiocyte proliferation is not proportionate to cell death in chronic cholestatic liver leading to the progressive disappearance of intrahepatic bile ducts, which is the hallmark of late-stage cholangiopathies. Most of the *in vivo* studies investigating cholangiocyte proliferation have been performed in rodents with the bile duct ligation model. Humoral factors are at play, and pressure is not the only trigger in this model as, after selective ligation of lobar ducts, proliferation also occurs in non-ligated lobes [36]. The same second messenger cAMP that plays a central role in stimulating ductular secretion stimulates cholangiocyte proliferation [37]. The density of secretin receptor is increased fivefold on cholangiocytes after bile duct ligation [38], but this seems to have more of a choleretic effect than a proliferative one. The parasympathetic and sympathetic nervous systems both promote cholangiocyte proliferation. Vagotomy markedly impaired expression of cholinergic M3 receptors and cholangiocyte proliferation after bile duct ligation [39]. Chemical adrenergic denervation also decreased cholangiocyte growth, and this effect could be rescued by stimulating adenylyl cyclase with forskolin [40]. This trophic effect of the nervous system on the biliary epithelium is lacking after liver transplantation. Factors counter-regulating adenylyl cyclase, such as gastrin via the CCK-B/gastrin receptor and somatostatin via the SSTR2 receptor, inhibit cholangiocyte hyperplasic reaction in bile duct-ligated rats [19,41]. Biliary epithelium is a target for growth hormone. Activation of growth hormone receptor stimulates the production of insulin-like growth factor (IGF)1, which has an autocrine proliferative effect on cholangiocytes [42]. Hepatocyte growth factor has also been reported to stimulate the proliferation of human cholangiocytes [43].

Bile acids are trophic substances for the biliary epithelium. Taurocholic acid and taurolithocholic acid, which increase cAMP in cholangiocytes, support their proliferative capacity [44,45]. Deoxycholic acid can transactivate epidermal growth factor via a transforming growth factor (TGF)-α-dependent mechanism and induces cell growth [46]. A diet enriched in ursodeoxycholic acid enhanced cholangiocyte proliferation after partial bile duct ligation [47]; the opposite effect has also been reported [48].

In addition, cholangiocytes possess intracellular steroid hormone receptors. Estrogen receptor alpha and beta are expressed in cholangiocytes, whereas only the alpha subtype is expressed in hepatocytes. Estrogens stimulate *in vitro* cholangiocyte proliferation, and *in vivo* administration of the estrogen antagonist, tamoxifen, inhibited cholangiocyte proliferation after bile duct ligation [49]. Nerve growth factor was found to have an additive proliferative effect to estrogens. Nerve growth factor is secreted by cholangiocytes and acts in an autocrine manner to stimulate the ERK pathway [50].

Besides the typical cholangiocyte proliferation, which is a hyperplasic reaction increasing the number and length of the intrahepatic bile ducts, cholangiocytes from the terminal cholangioles show impressive proliferation ability in cases of severe hepatic necrosis. This ductular reaction occurs at the periphery of the portal tracts. It recruits precursor cells and may even leads to hepatocyte metaplasia. It is better visualized on liver biopsies by specific immunohistochemistry (cytokeratin 7 for example) and correlates with the severity of liver damage. These reactive cholangiocytes display specific phenotypical features. They express neuroendocrine markers (chromogranin A, glycolipid A2-B4, S-100 protein, neural cell adhesion molecule [51]), acquire a multidrug-resistant phenotype by upregulating efflux proteins such as MDR1, MRP1 and MRP3 [52] and have been claimed to produce numerous proinflammatory and chemotactic factors (TNFα, IL-6, IL-8 and monocyte chemotactic protein-1) as well as growth factors [hepatocyte growth factor, platelet-derived growth factor-BB, vascular endothelial growth factor (VEGF) and endothelin-1] but, for some of these factors, definitive evidence has not yet been published. Among these factors, some, such as IL-6, may act in an autocrine manner to stimulate further cholangiocytes [53]. Other mediators enable reactive cholangiocytes to influence neighbouring cells, especially portal fibroblasts and endothelial cells [21], and to attract inflammatory cells, in particular polymorphonuclear cells [54]. Human cholangiocytes in cases of polycystic liver disease produce VEGF and angiopoietin-1; these factors have an autocrine proliferative effect on cholangiocytes that express cognate receptors (VEGF receptors 1, 2 and Tie-2), as well as a paracrine effect on the portal vasculature, thus promoting growth of the cysts [55].

Cholangiocyte apoptosis

Cholangiocyte apoptosis is an important physiological and pathophysiological process in the maintenance of tissue homeostasis. In fetal liver, cholangiocyte apoptosis occurs normally during ductal plate remodelling (see Chapter 1.9). After relief of a biliary obstruction, the hyperplasic biliary tree is subjected to remodelling by apoptosis to eliminate superfluous cholangiocytes [56]. In the bile duct ligation model, vagotomy or administration of tamoxifen deprives cholangiocytes of growth stimuli and leads to apoptosis. Pathophysiologically, excessive cholangiocyte apoptosis is an important feature of immune and ischaemic cholangiopathies resulting in ductopenia (a decrease in the number of bile ducts per portal tract). Human cholangiocytes express the Fas receptor, and IFN-gamma and TNFα upregulate its expression, making cholangiocytes a target of T-cytotoxic lymphocytes bearing Fas ligand [57]. In primary biliary cirrhosis, antimitochondrial antibodies of the IgA type translocate through cholangiocytes, and it has been suggested that these antibodies could intracellularly trigger apoptosis by activating caspases [58]. Conjugated bile acids, which are secreted by hepatocytes, may also affect the sensitivity of cholangiocytes to apoptosis. The taurine conjugate of the widely prescribed ursodeoxycholic acid, tauroursodeoxycholic acid, was found to activate the transcription factor CREB in cholangiocytes, protecting these cells from apoptotic stress [59]. Resistance to apoptosis is equally important as it is a central feature of cholangiocyte transformation in cholangiocarcinogenesis (see below).

Cholangiocyte transformation

Cholangiocarcinoma complicates the course of cholangiopathies characterized by inflammation of the bile ducts. Chronic inflammation induces inducible nitric oxide synthase (iNOS) expression in cholangiocytes. This has several consequences: it causes ductular cholestasis by inhibiting cAMP-dependent HCO_3^- and Cl^- secretory mechanisms [60]; it potentiates DNA damage by inhibiting 8-oxodeo-oxyguanine repair [61]; it nitrosylates caspase-9, blocking apoptosis [62]; and, finally, it contributes to cyclo-oxygenase type 2 (COX-2) overexpression [63]. Cholangiocellular expression of COX-2 is also upregulated by deoxycholic acid via transactivation of the epidermal growth factor receptor [64]. This is relevant because COX-2 has been implicated in cholangiocarcinogenesis and is a potential target for oncological therapy. Prostaglandin E2 prevents Fas-mediated apoptosis of cholangiocytes by increasing the expression of the antiapoptotic factor myeloid cell leukaemia-1 (Mcl-1) [65]. This factor can also be upregulated by the inflammatory mediator IL-6, which has been implicated in cholangiocarcinogenesis [66]. Several other antiapoptotic proteins, such as FLIP, Bcl-2 and $Bcl-X_L$, are overexpressed in malignant biliary epithelium, providing these cells with a survival advantage by evading apoptosis [67].

Immunological aspects

The biliary epithelium is a frontier separating the hepatic parenchyma from a lumen which is in continuity with the intestinal content. Even if this continuity is with the relatively sterile small intestine and even if the bile is an inhospitable milieu for microorganisms with its low glucose concentration, biliary epithelial cells participate in the defence of the organism against invaders. The principal protein in bile is IgA, which binds to pathogens in the biliary and intestinal lumen. In humans, IgAs transit through biliary epithelial cells. Cholangiocytes endocytose IgAs via a specific receptor expressed in their basal membrane. These complexes are transported through the cell to be dispersed into the bile. Peribiliary glands secrete additional mucosal defence factors such as lactoferrin and lysozyme [68].

Toll-like receptors are central to the innate immune response by recognizing pathogen-associated molecular patterns. Normal human cholangiocytes express Toll-like receptors, which mediate the upregulation of beta-defensin-2 via activation of nuclear factor kappaB [69]. Cholangiocytes maintain close cooperation with cells of the immune system. They express adhesion molecules to engage interactions with lymphocytes (ICAM-1, LFA-3). Cytokines such as IFN-gamma and TNFα upregulate the expression of major histocompatibility complex (MHC) class II in biliary epithelial cells [70], but it is unclear to what extent cholangiocytes act as antigen-presenting cells, as they are lacking the co-stimulatory molecules B7-1 (CD80) and B7-2 (CD86). Biliary epithelial cells do not normally express CD40, a member of the TNF receptor superfamily, but do express it in cases of primary biliary cirrhosis [57]. Portal mononuclear cell infiltrate in this disease contains T cells and macrophages positive for CD40 ligand [57]. Immunohistochemistry on biopsies from patients with primary biliary cirrhosis revealed an induction of the expression of MHC II as well as of ICAM-1, the ligand for LFA-1, on biliary epithelial cells, whereas portal lymphocytes stained positive for LFA-1 [71,72].

Cholangiocyte heterogeneity

Not all cholangiocytes are the same. Cells lining small ductules are different from cells lining large ducts. By isolating cholangiocytes according to size, Alpini and co-workers were able to characterize two populations of cholangiocytes with specific functional properties. Small cholangiocytes, which are found in small ducts (15–300 μm), have a diameter around 8 μm, whereas large cholangiocytes, which populate larger ducts (300–800 μm), have a diameter of 15 μm. Both cell types express markers defining biliary epithelial cells: cytokeratins 7 and 19 and γ-glutamyl-transpeptidase. However, in many aspects, these cells appear to be different. The small cholangiocytes are devoid of secretin receptors (SR) and somatostatin receptors ($SSTR_2$), in contrast to the large cholangiocytes whose bile secretion is regulated by these hormones. Consequently, large cholangiocytes express CFTR and Cl^-/HCO_3^- exchanger. The cytochrome P4502E1, an enzyme that participates in redox stress, is expressed only in large cholangiocytes [73]. It is likely that the distribution of the phase I and phase II drug-metabolizing enzymes, which is heterogeneous among cholangiocytes, segregates preferentially between the two populations, explaining why small and large ducts are differently affected by injury and toxins. The proliferative response of small and large cholangiocytes is different. Clinical extrahepatic obstruction such as the experimental model of bile duct ligation results in preferential multiplication of large cholangiocytes. In humans, most of the cholangiocarcinomas arise in large ducts and are probably derived from large cholangiocytes. In contrast, small cholangiocytes display considerable phenotypical plasticity and form a compartment with an important proliferative reserve. Immunological diseases of the biliary epithelium such as primary biliary cirrhosis and autoimmune cholangiopathy primarily affect small cholangiocytes.

References

1 Cohn JA, Strong TV, Picciotto MR *et al.* (1993) Localization of the cystic fibrosis transmembrane conductance regulator in human bile duct epithelial cells. *Gastroenterology* 105, 1857–1864.

2 Doctor RB, Dahl R, Fouassier L *et al.* (2002) Cholangiocytes exhibit dynamic, actin-dependent apical membrane turnover. *Am J Physiol Cell Physiol* 282, C1042–1052.

3 Tietz PS, Marinelli RA, Chen XM *et al.* (2003) Agonist-induced coordinated trafficking of functionally-related transport proteins for water and ions in cholangiocytes. *J Biol Chem* 278, 20413–20419.

4   Doctor RB, Dahl RH, Salter KD et al. (2000) ATP depletion in rat cholangiocytes leads to marked internalization of membrane proteins. Hepatology 31, 1045–1054.

5   Roman RM, Smith RL, Feranchak AP et al. (2001) ClC-2 chloride channels contribute to HTC cell volume homeostasis. Am J Physiol 280, G344–353.

6   Schlenker T, Fitz JG (1996) Ca(2+)-activated Cl– channels in a human biliary cell line: regulation by Ca2+/calmodulin-dependent protein kinase. Am J Physiol 271, G304–310.

7   Lazaridis KN, Pham L, Tietz P et al. (1997) At cholangiocytes absorb bile acids at their apical domain via the ileal sodium-dependent bile acid transporter. J Clin Invest 100, 2714–2721.

8   Lazaridis KN, Tietz P, Wu T et al. (2000) Alternative splicing of the rat sodium/bile acid transporter changes its cellular localization and transport properties. Proc Natl Acad Sci USA 97, 11092–11097.

9   Ballatori N, Christian WV, Lee JY et al. (2005) OSTalpha-OSTbeta: a major basolateral bile acid and steroid transporter in human intestinal, renal, and biliary epithelia. Hepatology 42, 1270–1279.

10 Alpini G, Glaser S, Baiocchi L et al. (2005) Secretin activation of the apical Na+-dependent bile acid transporter is associated with chole-hepatic shunting in rats. Hepatology 41, 1037–1045.

11 Lazaridis KN, Pham L, Vroman B et al. (1997) Kinetic and molecular identification of sodium-dependent glucose transporter in normal rat cholangiocytes. Am J Physiol 272, G1168–1174.

12 Chen XM, O'Hara SP, Huang BQ et al. (2005) Localized glucose and water influx facilitates Cryptosporidium parvum cellular invasion by means of modulation of host-cell membrane protrusion. Proc Natl Acad Sci USA 102, 6338–6343.

13 Eisenmann-Tappe I, Wizigmann S, Gebhardt R (1991) Glutamate uptake in primary cultures of biliary epithelial cells from normal rat liver. Cell Biol Toxicol 7, 315–325.

14 Fouassier L, Duan CY, Feranchak AP et al. (2001) Ezrin-radixin-moesin-binding phosphoprotein 50 is expressed at the apical membrane of rat liver epithelia. Hepatology 33, 166–176.

15 Mano Y, Ishii M, Okamoto H et al. (1996) Effect of tumor necrosis factor alpha on intrahepatic bile duct epithelial cell of rat liver. Hepatology 23, 1602–1607.

16 Bode HP, Wang L, Cassio D et al. (2002) Expression and regulation of gap junctions in rat cholangiocytes. Hepatology 36, 631–640.

17 Masyuk TV, Huang BQ, Ward CJ et al. (2003) Defects in cholangiocyte fibrocystin expression and ciliary structure in the PCK rat. Gastroenterology 125, 1303–1310.

18 Lenzen R, Alpini G, Tavoloni N (1992) Secretin stimulates bile ductular secretory activity through the cAMP system. Am J Physiol 263, G527–532.

19 Tietz PS, Alpini G, Pham LD et al. (1995) Somatostatin inhibits secretin-induced ductal hypercholeresis and exocytosis by cholangiocytes. Am J Physiol 269, G110–118.

20 Glaser SS, Rodgers RE, Phinizy JL et al. (1997) Gastrin inhibits secretin-induced ductal secretion by interaction with specific receptors on rat cholangiocytes. Am J Physiol 273, G1061–1070.

21 Fouassier L, Chinet T, Robert B et al. (1998) Endothelin-1 is synthesized and inhibits cyclic adenosine monophosphate-dependent anion secretion by an autocrine/paracrine mechanism in gallbladder epithelial cells. J Clin Invest 101, 2881–2888.

22 Lesage GD, Marucci L, Alvaro D et al. (2002) Insulin inhibits secretin-induced ductal secretion by activation of PKC alpha and inhibition of PKA activity. Hepatology 36, 641–651.

23 Cho WK, Mennone A, Boyer JL (1998) Intracellular pH regulation in bombesin-stimulated secretion in isolated bile duct units from rat liver. Am J Physiol 275, G1028–1036.

24 Cho WK, Boyer JL (1999) Vasoactive intestinal polypeptide is a potent regulator of bile secretion from rat cholangiocytes. Gastroenterology 117, 420–428.

25 Hirata K, Nathanson MH (2001) Bile duct epithelia regulate biliary bicarbonate excretion in normal rat liver. Gastroenterology 121, 396–406.

26 Glaser S, Alvaro D, Roskams T et al. (2003) Dopaminergic inhibition of secretin-stimulated choleresis by increased PKC-gamma expression and decrease of PKA activity. Am J Physiol Gastrointest Liver Physiol 284, G683–694.

27 St Pierre MV, Schlenker T, Dufour JF et al. (1998) Stimulation of cyclic guanosine monophosphate production by natriuretic peptide in human biliary cells. Gastroenterology 114, 782–790.

28 Chari RS, Schutz SM, Haebig JE et al. (1996) Adenosine nucleotides in bile. Am J Physiol 270, G246–252.

29 Doctor RB, Matzakos T, McWilliams R et al. (2005) Purinergic regulation of cholangiocyte secretion: identification of a novel role for P2X receptors. Am J Physiol Gastrointest Liver Physiol 288, G779–786.

30 Roman RM, Feranchak AP, Salter KD et al. (1999) Endogenous ATP release regulates Cl– secretion in cultured human and rat biliary epithelial cells. Am J Physiol 276, G1391–1400.

31 Dranoff JA, Masyuk AI, Kruglov EA et al. (2001) Polarized expression and function of P2Y ATP receptors in rat bile duct epithelia. Am J Physiol 281, G1059–1067.

32 Zsembery A, Spirli C, Granato A et al. (1998) Purinergic regulation of acid/base transport in human and rat biliary epithelial cell lines. Hepatology 28, 914–920.

33 Dufour JF, Luthi M, Forestier M et al. (1999) Expression of inositol 1,4,5-trisphosphate receptor isoforms in rat cirrhosis. Hepatology 30, 1018–1026.

34 Shibao K, Hirata K, Robert ME et al. (2003) Loss of inositol 1,4,5-trisphosphate receptors from bile duct epithelia is a common event in cholestasis. Gastroenterology 125, 1175–1187.

35 Spirli C, Nathanson MH, Fiorotto R et al. (2001) Proinflammatory cytokines inhibit secretion in rat bile duct epithelium. Gastroenterology 121, 156–169.

36 Polimeno L, Azzarone A, Zeng QH et al. (1995) Cell proliferation and oncogene expression after bile duct ligation in the rat: evidence of a specific growth effect on bile duct cells. Hepatology 21, 1070–1078.

37 Leite MF, Nathanson MH (2005) Signaling pathways in biliary epithelial cells. In: Dufour J-F, Clavien PA (eds) Signaling Pathways in Liver Diseases. Berlin: Springer, pp. 17–26.

38 Tietz PS, Hadac EM, Miller LJ et al. (2001) Upregulation of secretin receptors on cholangiocytes after bile duct ligation. Regul Pept 97, 1–6.

39 LeSage EG, Alvaro D, Benedetti A et al. (1999) Cholinergic system modulates growth, apoptosis, and secretion of cholangiocytes from bile duct-ligated rats. Gastroenterology 117, 191–199.

40 Glaser S, Alvaro D, Francis H et al. (2006) Adrenergic receptor agonists prevent bile duct injury induced by adrenergic denervation by increased cAMP levels and activation of Akt. Am J Physiol Gastrointest Liver Physiol 290, G813–826.

41 Glaser S, Benedetti A, Marucci L et al. (2000) Gastrin inhibits cholangiocyte growth in bile duct-ligated rats by interaction with cholecystokinin-B/gastrin receptors via D-myo-inositol 1,4,5-trisphosphate-, Ca(2+)-, and protein kinase C alpha-dependent mechanisms. Hepatology 32, 17–25.

42 Alvaro D, Metalli VD, Alpini G *et al.* (2005) The intrahepatic biliary epithelium is a target of the growth hormone/insulin-like growth factor 1 axis. *J Hepatol* 43, 875–883.

43 Joplin R, Hishida T, Tsubouchi H *et al.* (1992) Human intrahepatic biliary epithelial cells proliferate *in vitro* in response to human hepatocyte growth factor. *J Clin Invest* 90, 1284–1289.

44 Alpini G, Glaser S, Alvaro D *et al.* (2002) Bile acid depletion and repletion regulate cholangiocyte growth and secretion by a phosphatidylinositol 3-kinase-dependent pathway in rats. *Gastroenterology* 123, 1226–1237.

45 Alpini G, Glaser SS, Ueno Y *et al.* (1999) Bile acid feeding induces cholangiocyte proliferation and secretion: evidence for bile acid-regulated ductal secretion. *Gastroenterology* 116, 179–186.

46 Werneburg NW, Yoon JH, Higuchi H *et al.* (2003) Bile acids activate EGF receptor via a TGF-alpha-dependent mechanism in human cholangiocyte cell lines. *Am J Physiol Gastrointest Liver Physiol* 285, G31–36.

47 Barone M, Maiorano E, Ladisa R *et al.* (2004) Ursodeoxycholate further increases bile-duct cell proliferative response induced by partial bile-duct ligation in rats. *Virchows Arch* 444, 554–560.

48 Alpini G, Baiocchi L, Glaser S *et al.* (2002) Ursodeoxycholate and tauroursodeoxycholate inhibit cholangiocyte growth and secretion of BDL rats through activation of PKC alpha. *Hepatology* 35, 1041–1052.

49 Alvaro D, Alpini G, Onori P *et al.* (2000) Estrogens stimulate proliferation of intrahepatic biliary epithelium in rats. *Gastroenterology* 119, 1681–1691.

50 Gigliozzi A, Alpini G, Baroni GS *et al.* (2004) Nerve growth factor modulates the proliferative capacity of the intrahepatic biliary epithelium in experimental cholestasis. *Gastroenterology* 127, 1198–1209.

51 Roskams T, van den Oord JJ, De Vos R *et al.* (1990) Neuroendocrine features of reactive bile ductules in cholestatic liver disease. *Am J Pathol* 137, 1019–1025.

52 Ros JE, Libbrecht L, Geuken M *et al.* (2003) High expression of MDR1, MRP1, and MRP3 in the hepatic progenitor cell compartment and hepatocytes in severe human liver disease. *J Pathol* 200, 553–560.

53 Park J, Gores GJ, Patel T (1999) Lipopolysaccharide induces cholangiocyte proliferation via an interleukin-6-mediated activation of p44/p42 mitogen-activated protein kinase. *Hepatology* 29, 1037–1043.

54 Morland CM, Fear J, Joplin R *et al.* (1997) Inflammatory cytokines stimulate human biliary epithelial cells to express interleukin-8 and monocyte chemotactic protein-1. *Biochem Soc Trans* 25, 232S.

55 Fabris L, Cadamuro M, Fiorotto R *et al.* (2006) Effects of angiogenic factor overexpression by human and rodent cholangiocytes in polycystic liver diseases. *Hepatology* 43, 1001–1012.

56 Bhathal PS, Gall JA (1985) Deletion of hyperplastic biliary epithelial cells by apoptosis following removal of the proliferative stimulus. *Liver* 5, 311–325.

57 Afford SC, Ahmed-Choudhury J, Randhawa S *et al.* (2001) CD40 activation-induced, Fas-dependent apoptosis and NF-kappaB/AP-1 signaling in human intrahepatic biliary epithelial cells. *FASEB J* 15, 2345–2354.

58 Matsumura S, Van De Water J, Leung P *et al.* (2004) Caspase induction by IgA antimitochondrial antibody: IgA-mediated biliary injury in primary biliary cirrhosis. *Hepatology* 39, 1415–1422.

59 Wang L, Piguet AC, Schmidt K *et al.* (2005) Activation of CREB by tauroursodeoxycholic acid protects cholangiocytes from apoptosis induced by mTOR inhibition. *Hepatology* 41, 1241–1251.

60 Spirli C, Fabris L, Duner E *et al.* (2003) Cytokine-stimulated nitric oxide production inhibits adenylyl cyclase and cAMP-dependent secretion in cholangiocytes. *Gastroenterology* 124, 737–753.

61 Jaiswal M, LaRusso NF, Shapiro RA *et al.* (2001) Nitric oxide-mediated inhibition of DNA repair potentiates oxidative DNA damage in cholangiocytes. *Gastroenterology* 120, 190–199.

62 Torok NJ, Higuchi H, Bronk S *et al.* (2002) Nitric oxide inhibits apoptosis downstream of cytochrome C release by nitrosylating caspase 9. *Cancer Res* 62, 1648–1653.

63 Ishimura N, Bronk SF, Gores GJ (2004) Inducible nitric oxide synthase upregulates cyclooxygenase-2 in mouse cholangiocytes promoting cell growth. *Am J Physiol Gastrointest Liver Physiol* 287, G88–G95.

64 Yoon JH, Higuchi H, Werneburg NW *et al.* (2002) Bile acids induce cyclooxygenase-2 expression via the epidermal growth factor receptor in a human cholangiocarcinoma cell line. *Gastroenterology* 122, 985–993.

65 Nzeako UC, Guicciardi ME, Yoon JH *et al.* (2002) COX-2 inhibits Fas-mediated apoptosis in cholangiocarcinoma cells. *Hepatology* 35, 552–559.

66 Isomoto H, Kobayashi S, Werneburg NW *et al.* (2005) Interleukin 6 upregulates myeloid cell leukemia-1 expression through a STAT3 pathway in cholangiocarcinoma cells. *Hepatology* 42, 1329–1338.

67 Okaro AC, Deery AR, Hutchins RR *et al.* (2001) The expression of antiapoptotic proteins Bcl-2, Bcl-X(L), and Mcl-1 in benign, dysplastic, and malignant biliary epithelium. *J Clin Pathol* 54, 927–932.

68 Saito K, Nakanuma Y (1992) Lactoferrin and lysozyme in the intrahepatic bile duct of normal livers and hepatolithiasis. An immunohistochemical study. *J Hepatol* 15, 147–153.

69 Chen XM, O'Hara SP, Nelson JB *et al.* (2005) Multiple TLRs are expressed in human cholangiocytes and mediate host epithelial defense responses to *Cryptosporidium parvum* via activation of NF-kappaB. *J Immunol* 175, 7447–7456.

70 Cruickshank SM, Southgate J, Selby PJ *et al.* (1998) Expression and cytokine regulation of immune recognition elements by normal human biliary epithelial and established liver cell lines *in vitro*. *J Hepatol* 29, 550–558.

71 Bloom S, Fleming K, Chapman R (1995) Adhesion molecule expression in primary sclerosing cholangitis and primary biliary cirrhosis. *Gut* 36, 604–609.

72 Yasoshima M, Nakanuma Y, Tsuneyama K *et al.* (1995) Immunohistochemical analysis of adhesion molecules in the microenvironment of portal tracts in relation to aberrant expression of PDC-E2 and HLA-DR on the bile ducts in primary biliary cirrhosis. *J Pathol* 175, 319–325.

73 LeSage GD, Benedetti A, Glaser S *et al.* (1999) Acute carbon tetrachloride feeding selectively damages large, but not small, cholangiocytes from normal rat liver. *Hepatology* 29, 307–319.

1.8 Hepatic stem cells

Tania Roskams

Introduction

Professor Bizzozero, a pupil of Professor Golgi, linked the presence of mitotic figures in a given cell type to the cell's capacity to regenerate. He classified cells into three types. *Labile* cells divide so as to continually renew the tissue. Typical examples are epidermis and the epithelium of the gastrointestinal tract. *Stable* cells normally do not divide, but under certain stimuli they still have the capacity to do so. A typical example is the liver, which normally is a silent organ, but which harbours an enormous regenerative capacity after injuries like partial hepatectomy or toxic injury. *Permanent* cells like neurones or muscle cells 'never' divide. In biology, however, 'never' does not exist and in the 1990s, *in vitro* experiments showed that almost all tissues and organs, even the brain and muscle, contain cells with a huge growth potential: tissue-specific stem cells.

Different types of stem cells and their niches

What is a stem cell? A stem cell is an undifferentiated cell capable throughout life of renewing itself as well as of generating one or more types of differentiated cells [1–3]. Every adult cell has a 'mother' (who may have parted from her years ago), and a line of ancestors – stem cells – of increasing differentiation potential. The ultimate stem cells are those of the early embryo, which are totipotential. Further down the line, in the fetus and also in the adult, we find multipotential (pluripotential) stem cells. Those closer to final differentiation are called progenitor, committed or transit cells. This nomenclature is still changing.

In continuously renewing lining epithelia, such as the epidermis, stem cells are easy to find because they squat against the basement membrane. In other tissues, such as the liver, the search is frustrating because, by definition, stem cells look bland and undifferentiated. However, they can be visualized by immunohistochemistry, which reveals distinctive proteins (antigens) on their surface or in their cytoplasm (see Plate 1.8.1, facing p. 72).

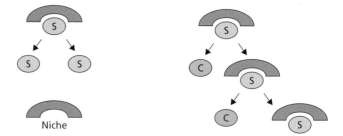

Fig. 1 Schematic representation of symmetrical versus asymmetrical division of stem cells. In symmetrical stem cell division (left), a stem cell (S) generates two stem cells. This happens early in embryonic life. Later on (right), a stem cell generates a stem cell and a committed, somewhat differentiated cell (C). The stem cell niche keeps the stem cell in an undifferentiated state.

When a stem cell replicates, its mitosis can be *symmetrical* (producing two stem cells) or *asymmetrical* (producing one stem cell and one progenitor cell or differentiated cell) (Fig. 1).

A good model to study stem cells is provided by the cells of the blood-forming line; knowledge in this field is so far advanced that therapeutic applications of stem cells are already standard medical practice in haematology [4]. This has happened because the blood's stem cells are relatively easy to find: they have a specific marker, the surface protein CD34, and can be harvested from adult blood, where they represent about 0.01% of the mononuclear cells, and from blood in the umbilical cord and placenta (neonatal blood), where they are more abundant and more prolific [5]. After they have been expanded *ex vivo*, they can be reinjected intravenously, because they know how to home into the bone marrow where they are needed, for example to repopulate a bone marrow destroyed by chemotherapy [6].

This 'sympathy' between blood stem cells and bone marrow runs deeply, and it has taught us something about stem cell biology in general. *In vitro*, blood stem cells totally deprived of a bone marrow-like environment will not survive very long: they need the company of endothelial cells, fat cells, fibroblasts, macrophages, osteoblasts and even some matrix. Normally, in the bone marrow, each haematopoietic stem cell lives in a

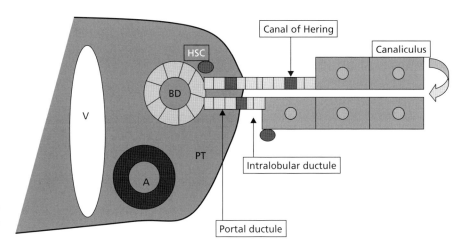

Fig. 2 Anatomy and terminology in human liver. The left side of the figure illustrates the portal tract (PT), containing a branch of the portal vein (V), the hepatic artery (A) and accompanying bile duct (BD). The smallest, most peripheral branches of the biliary tree, the ductules, consist of a portal part (portal ductule) and an intralobular part (intralobular ductule). The canal of Hering is lined partially by hepatocytes and partially by cholangiocytes and forms the connecting piece between the ductules and the canaliculi in between hepatocytes. The progenitor cells are located in the most peripheral branches of the biliary tree, the ductules and the canal of Hering.

microscopic 'niche' of stromal cells that nurse it and provide it with the proper instructions [4,7,8]. Stem cell niches probably also exist in other tissues, but have not been characterized yet.

In the following paragraphs, stem cell properties of hepatocytes and the local progenitor cell compartment in the liver, called 'oval cells' in rodents and the canal of Hering/ductules in human liver, will be discussed (Fig. 2).

Hepatocytes have 'stem cell' properties

In normal circumstances, the liver hardly proliferates and was therefore classified as a 'stable' organ. Hepatocytes in normal adult liver have a lifespan of over a year. After partial hepatectomy, however, proliferation of the main epithelial compartments (hepatocytes and cholangiocytes), followed by proliferation of the mesenchymal cells (hepatic stellate cells and endothelial cells), quickly restores the liver. In rodents, the liver can restore its original volume after two-thirds hepatectomy in approximately 10 days [9,10]. Serial transplantation experiments have shown that hepatocytes have a near infinite capacity to proliferate [11,12]. Since at least 69 doublings can occur, the clonogenic potential of hepatocytes, one of the crucial properties of a stem cell, is confirmed.

Hepatic progenitor cells: localization and activation

When the mature epithelial cell compartments of the liver, hepatocytes and/or cholangiocytes, are damaged or inhibited in their replication, a reserve cell compartment is activated [13]. This compartment, in humans called the progenitor cell compartment and in rodents the oval cell compartment, resides in the smallest and most peripheral branches of the biliary tree, the ductules and canals of Hering [14] (Fig. 2). The *canal of Hering* is a channel lined partly by hepatocytes and partly by cholangio-

cytes. It represents the anatomical and physiological link between the intralobular canalicular system and the biliary tree. Cells of morphology and immunophenotype intermediate between hepatocytes and cholangiocytes ('intermediate cells', see below) are not recognized in normal tissue. A corollary is that the true interface of hepatocytes and the biliary tree does not reside, as has been assumed, at the 'limiting plate', but rather along an array of sites that project starlike from the portal tracts, along the canals of Hering.

Wilson and Leduc were the first to describe this activation of a 'reserve cell compartment' in mouse after severe dietary injury [15]. Subsequently, several models of so-called oval cell reaction in rodents have been described. Mostly, these models employed potential carcinogenic agents to inhibit the proliferation of mature hepatocytes after a regenerative stimulus: for example, acetaminofluorene intoxication of rats after partial hepatectomy or after administration of a necrogenic dose of carbon tetrachloride [16] or ethionine intoxication in mice. Also, models of fatty liver disease like Ob/Ob mice or PARP-1(−/−) mice are characterized by inhibition of the replication of mature hepatocytes, caused by oxidative stress, and show a striking oval cell response [17,18].

The activation of oval cells, or in human liver the 'ductular reaction', comprises expansion of a transit-amplifying cell compartment of small biliary cells that can differentiate into at least biliary epithelial cells and hepatocytes. The progenitor cells are labelled by biliary type cytokeratins (CK) CK7 and 19, oval cell markers OV6 and OV1, neuroendocrine markers chromogranin A, neural cell adhesion molecule and parathyroid hormone-related peptide, and connexin 43. A subpopulation of ductular/progenitor cells express markers of haematopoietic cells (CD34, c-kit, flt-3, Thy-1), which raised the question of whether progenitor cells could be directly derived from bone marrow stem cells. Most studies, however, are concordant with a progenitor cell niche in the ductules/canals of Hering, at the interface between the parenchyma and the portal tract mesenchyme. This is also the location where, during embryonic development, bipotential hepatoblasts form the primitive ductal plate, which has the same phenotype as progenitor cells in adult life: ductal plate cells express biliary markers and (immature) hepatocytic markers like alpha-fetoprotein and also haematopoietic markers like CD34.

Progenitor cell activation or ductular reaction is seen in the majority of chronic human liver diseases. Reactive ductules form strands of small cholangiocytes with an oval nucleus and a small rim of cytoplasm [19]. The degree of progenitor cell activation increases with the severity of the disease [20]. In chronic hepatitis, progenitor cell activation correlates with the degree of inflammation [21]. In a variety of chronic liver diseases like chronic hepatitis C, haemochromatosis and (non)alcoholic steatohepatitis, the degree of progenitor cell activation also correlates with the degree of fibrosis and the stage of the disease [17,20]. In moderate and severe degrees of inflammation, intermediate hepatocytes occur, having a phenotype intermediate between progenitor cells/ductular cells and mature hepatocytes (see Plate 1.8.1, facing p. 72). The number of these intermediate hepatocytes gradually increases with greater degrees of inflammation, and also with increasing necrosis in necrotizing hepatitis and with more advanced stages of (non)alcoholic steatohepatitis [17,20,21] (see Plate 1.8.1, facing p. 72). This strongly suggests a greater degree of differentiation of progenitor cells into hepatocytes when there is more hepatocyte damage. In cirrhotic livers, especially in (non)alcoholic steatohepatitis, whole cirrhotic nodules can be composed of intermediate hepatocytes, which ultrastructurally look strikingly 'normal', without Mallory body formation and without fatty change. This suggests that these intermediate hepatocyte-nodules originate from progenitor cells [17]. In parallel, Falkowski et al. showed, in a three-dimensional reconstruction study, that sequestered hepatocyte 'buds' in cirrhosis are always in continuity with reactive ductules, strongly suggesting a progenitor cell origin [22].

A trigger for progenitor cell activation is certainly a lack of ability of the mature cell compartments to proliferate. Alongside what we know from rodent models, human liver diseases also exhibit inhibition of replication of mature hepatocytes. Recently, it has been shown that hepatocytes are senescent in the cirrhotic stage of a wide variety of chronic human liver diseases because of telomere shortening. Intriguingly, mesenchymal cells, like endothelial cells and hepatic stellate cells, do not show this replicative senescence [23,24]. Probably, this hepatocyte replicative senescence is in part the result of ongoing proliferation during 20–30 years of chronic liver disease. Chronic inflammation, the presence of growth factors and DNA-damaging agents like reactive oxygen species and nitrogen species also play a role. So, similar to rodent models, replicative senescence of hepatocytes triggers progenitor cell activation in humans as well [13,25].

There have been a number of papers illustrating the role of bone marrow stem cells in producing hepatocytes, both in animal models and in humans. The precise role of these stem cells is not clear, because in several models it has been shown that cell fusion of bone marrow stem cells with damaged hepatocytes took place [26].

The society of liver cells and the surrounding stroma; the liver stem cell niche

The liver consists of epithelial cell types (hepatocytes, cholangiocytes and progenitor cells), mesenchymal cell types (Kupffer cells, endothelial cells, hepatic stellate cells) and stroma. Stroma is present in the portal tracts and in the Disse space (Fig. 3).

The importance of this 'society' of cells and the stroma is illustrated by the fact that hepatocytes, which have a huge growth potential in vivo, are very hard to keep alive and differentiated when isolated and placed in culture. When hepatocytes are injured, Kupffer cells secrete interleukin (IL)-6 and transforming growth factor α (TGF-α), which activate hepatic stellate cells. Hepatic stellate cells produce growth factors for hepatocytes and progenitor cells (e.g. hepatocyte growth factor). They also produce matrix components and transforming growth factor β (TGF-β), which inhibits the growth of hepatocytes. Growth factors like hepatocyte growth factor and epidermal growth factor also come from the circulation. The matrix harbours growth factors for hepatocytes and progenitor cells bound to, for example, proteoglycans, which can be quickly released when needed. Release of hepatocyte growth factor by the matrix is in turn inhibited by tissue inhibitor of metalloproteinase (TIMP). Hepatocytes and progenitor cells produce growth factors for endothelial cells, like vascular endothelial growth factor, in order to maintain their vascularization. Recently, a specific growth factor for 'oval cells', TWEAK (transforming growth factor-like weak inhibitor of apoptosis), was described, which does not act on hepatocytes [27]. This is an important step in our understanding of the regulation of oval cell reaction versus hepatocyte proliferation. This growth factor is produced by sinusoidal lining cells. Sinusoidal lining cells, like hepatic stellate cells, proliferate in close anatomical relationship with progenitor cells; in addition, stellate cells produce growth factors for which progenitor cells have the receptors, suggesting a true interaction between these cell compartments [13]. We also know that there are different subtypes of hepatic stellate cells/myofibroblasts [28] (see also Chapter 1.6). Studies identifying the stellate cell subtypes that surround the progenitor cells are underway. In general, defining the so-called 'stem cell niche' for adult human liver progenitor cells will be an important goal for the near future.

Progenitor cells seem to be able to survive when hepatocytes are lost as a result of toxic damage or viral infections. Adenosine triphosphate binding cassette (ABC) transporters play both a secretory and a protective role, and a strong upregulation of apical MDR1 and basolateral multidrug resistance protein (MRP)1 and MRP3 in human hepatocytes and in progenitor cell-related bile ductules was observed [29,30]. We hypothesized

Fig. 3 Society of liver cells. When hepatocytes are injured, Kupffer cells secrete interleukin 6 (IL-6) and transforming growth factor α (TGF-α), which activate hepatic stellate cells. Hepatic stellate cells produce growth factors for hepatocytes and progenitor cells (e.g. hepatocyte growth factor, HGF), matrix components and transforming growth factor β (TGF-β), which inhibits the growth of hepatocytes. Growth factors, such as hepatocyte growth factor and epidermal growth factor (EGF), also come from the circulation. The matrix harbours growth factors for hepatocytes and progenitor cells bound to, e.g. proteoglycans, which can be quickly released when needed. Release of hepatocyte growth factor by the matrix is in turn inhibited by tissue inhibitor of metalloproteinase (TIMP). Hepatocytes and progenitor cells produce growth factors for endothelial cells, such as vascular endothelial growth factor (VEGF), in order to maintain their vascularization. A, hepatic artery; BD, bile duct; PT, portal tract; PV, portal vein.

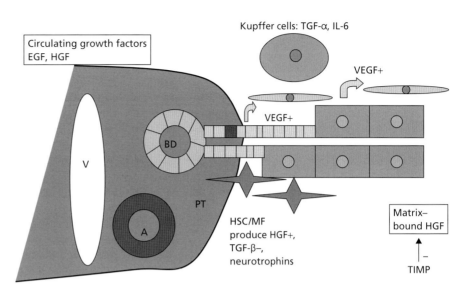

that this change in expression offers protection against the accumulation of toxic bile constituents and may render these cells resistant to oxidative stress.

The possible role of progenitor cells in liver cancer

In the 19th century, pathologists like Virchow observed that some tumours exhibit features of a range of different organs (teratocarcinoma) and hypothesized that these tumours originated from embryonal rests [31]. Today's stem cells are the modern equivalent of embryonal rests: tumours can originate from malignant transformation of a stem cell on its way to a differentiated mature cell type in a given organ (maturation arrest). In continuously renewing systems like the epidermis, gut and haematopoietic tissue, it is widely accepted that cancer arises from stem cells, because stem cells are the only cells that have a lifespan long enough to acquire the requisite number of genetic changes for neoplastic development. The liver, however, is a silent organ in which several cell types have longevity: hepatocytes and cholangiocytes, but also bipotential progenitor cells residing in the most terminal branches of the biliary tree, the ductules and/or canals of Hering [14]. This implies that, in the liver, several cell types can be carcinogen targets. We know from animal experiments that cell proliferation during carcinogen exposure is a prerequisite to 'fix' any genotypic injury into a heritable form.

Animal models show that hepatocytes are implicated in some models of hepatocellular carcinoma (HCC), while other models, using direct injury to the essentially unipotent cholangiocytes,

induce cholangiocarcinoma (CC). Progenitor cells (oval cells in rodents) are activated in many animal models, just like in many instances of human liver damage, irrespective of aetiology, making such cells very likely carcinogen targets. If progenitor cells do give rise to cancer during their maturation/differentiation process (maturation arrest theory), one would expect a range of neoplastic phenotypes, recapitulating stages in normal development, a prediction supported experimentally [32], as well as in human liver tumours (see below). Direct evidence for the involvement of oval cells (progenitor cells) in the histogenesis of HCC was obtained by Dumble *et al.* [33], who isolated oval cells from p53-null mice. When these cells were transplanted into athymic nude mice they produced HCCs.

In *humans*, chronic viral hepatitis B and C, alcoholic and nonalcoholic steatohepatitis, metabolic diseases and mutagens like aflatoxins (toxic metabolites of the food mould *Aspergillus*) are the most important risk factors for the development of HCC (Fig. 4). Chronic inflammatory biliary diseases like primary sclerosing cholangitis, hepatolithiasis (gallstones) and infestation by the liver flukes *Opisthorchis viverrini* and *Clonorchis sinensis* are known risk factors for the development of CC. This underscores the point that oxidative stress and chronic inflammation are common carcinogenic risk factors in all primary liver cancers.

As in rodents, HCC and CC in humans evolve from focal precursor lesions that reflect the stages of multistep carcinogenesis [34] (Fig. 4). Because progenitor cells are activated in most chronic liver diseases that are known risk factors for the development of HCC as well as CC, progenitor cells are potential target cells for carcinogenesis.

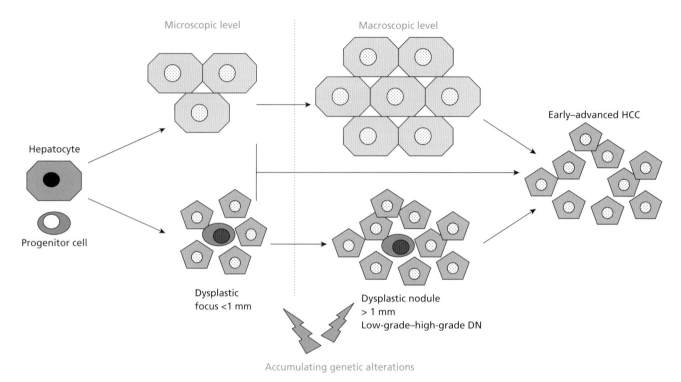

Fig. 4 Hepatocarcinogenesis is a multistep process. The different steps towards malignancy include the microscopically small large-cell and small-cell dysplastic foci (<1 mm). At the macroscopic level, these lesions can evolve into dysplastic nodules (low-grade and high-grade dysplastic nodules). Most of the high-grade dysplastic nodules evolve into cancer (early-advanced stage). The cells of origin can be either hepatocytes or progenitor cells. If progenitor cells give rise to cancer, the earliest premalignant lesions should consist of progenitor cells and their progeny. Indeed about half of the small-cell dysplastic foci, the smallest premalignant lesions known to date, consist of progenitor cells and intermediate cells. DN, dysplastic nodule.

Most tumours still show phenotypical features of their cell of origin and the histopathological classification of tumours is largely based on this. Several studies using detailed immunophenotyping of HCCs showed that a substantial number (28–50%) of human HCCs express markers of progenitor/biliary cells like cytokeratins (CK) 7 and 19, and OV6 [35–38].

Morphologically, these tumours consist of cells with a very immature phenotype and a range of cells with phenotypes intermediate between progenitor cells and hepatocytes. CK19 expression in HCC especially has been associated with a worse prognosis and faster and more recurrence after surgical treatment. Wu et al. [39] observed a significantly shorter survival in patients with HCCs expressing cytokeratin antibody AE1–AE3 and CK19 without any treatment. Uenishi et al. recently reported that HCCs expressing CK19 and CK7 have a lower tumour-free survival rate after curative resection and demonstrated that CK19 expression was an independent predictor of postoperative recurrence [40]. A recent study by Ding et al. [41] correlated overexpression of CK19 with HCC metastasis. In our own consecutive series of 109 HCCs, CK19-positive tumours (in more than 5% of tumour cells) had a higher rate of tumour recurrence after liver transplantation, compared with CK-negative HCCs.

CK19 expression was significantly associated with elevated serum alpha-fetoprotein (>400 ng/mL) and expression of alpha-fetoprotein by the tumour. The association with alpha-fetoprotein, which is also a marker of progenitor cells, is compatible with a progenitor cell origin of these tumours.

Of course, the presence of progenitor cell features in a tumour can be explained in two ways: either the cell of origin is a progenitor cell (maturation arrest theory) or alternatively, tumours dedifferentiate and acquire progenitor cell features during carcinogenesis (dedifferentiation theory). When progenitor cells are the cell of origin of a subtype of primary liver tumours, one would expect that the earliest premalignant precursor lesions would also consist of progenitor cells and their progeny. This is indeed the case: 55% of small-cell dysplastic foci (smaller than 1 mm), the earliest premalignant lesions known to date in humans, consist of progenitor cells and intermediate hepatocytes. This is a very strong argument in favour of the progenitor cell origin of at least part of the HCCs. Large-cell 'dysplastic' foci, on the other hand, consist of mature senescent hepatocytes, being a result of continuous proliferation in chronic liver diseases and not the true precursor lesions of HCC [42].

Moreover, in hepatoblastomas, the most common liver tumour in childhood, cells resembling progenitor cells have been noted [43–45]. This tumour is widely believed to be of stem cell origin, because it can comprise both epithelial and mesenchymal tissue components.

Aberrant expression of p63, a marker for basal/stem cells in several organs including prostate and skin, and of c-kit, a stem cell marker, has been described in CCs, also suggesting a progenitor cell origin of part of these tumours [46].

In many human tumours, it has become apparent that only tumour stem cells are capable of transferring the disease to NOD/SCID mice, so it would not be surprising if hepatic progenitor cells in HCCs are the only cells capable of propagating the tumour in immunodeficient mice [47].

Conclusions

In a wide variety of acute and chronic human liver diseases, progenitor cells proliferate, whereas hepatocytes become senescent in the cirrhotic stage of chronic liver diseases. Because of their bipotential differentiation capacity, progenitor cells are ideal candidates for cell therapy. Alternatively, this cell compartment can be stimulated *in vivo* to stimulate liver regeneration. Better knowledge of the mechanisms of progenitor cell activation and differentiation is needed before these cells can be exploited for regeneration therapy.

References

1 Watt FM, Hogan BL (2000) Out of Eden: stem cells and their niches. *Science* 287, 1427–1430.

2 Alison M, Sarraf C (1998) Hepatic stem cells. *J Hepatol* 29, 676–682.

3 Hall PA (1989) What are stem cells and how are they controlled? *J Pathol* 158, 275–277.

4 Orlic D, Bock TA, Kanz L (eds) (1999) *Hematopoietic Stem Cells. Biology and Transplantation.* New York: New York Academy of Science.

5 Rubinstein P, Carrier C, Caradavou A *et al.* (1998) Outcomes among 562 recipients of placental-blood transplants from unrelated donors. *N Engl J Med* 339, 1565–1577.

6 Levitt DMR (ed.) (1995) *Hematopoietic Stem Cells.* New York: Marcel Dekker.

7 He XC, Zhang J, Li L (2005) Cellular and molecular regulation of hematopoietic and intestinal stem cell behavior. *Ann NY Acad Sci* 1049, 28–38.

8 Zhang J, Niu C, Ye L *et al.* (2003) Identification of the haematopoietic stem cell niche and control of the niche size. *Nature* 425, 836–841.

9 Michalopoulos GK, DeFrances MC (1997) Liver regeneration. *Science* 276, 60–66.

10 Fausto N (2004) Liver regeneration and repair: hepatocytes, progenitor cells, and stem cells. *Hepatology* 39, 1477–1487.

11 Overturf K, Al-Dhalimy M, Finegold M *et al.* (1999) The repopulation potential of hepatocyte populations differing in size and prior mitotic expansion. *Am J Pathol* 155, 2135–2143.

12 Overturf K, Al-Dhalimy M, Manning K *et al.* (1998) Ex vivo hepatic gene therapy of a mouse model of hereditary tyrosinemia type I. *Hum Gene Ther* 9, 295–304.

13 Roskams T, Libbrecht L, Desmet V (2003) Progenitor cells in diseased human liver. *Semin Liver Dis* 23, 385–396.

14 Roskams TA, Thiese ND, Balabaud C *et al.* (2004) Nomenclature of the finer branches of the biliary tree: canals, ductules, and ductular reactions in human livers. *Hepatology* 39, 1739–1745.

15 Wilson JW, Leduc EH (1958) Role of cholangioles in restoration of the liver of the mouse after dietary injury. *J Pathol Bacteriol* 76, 441–449.

16 Alison MR, Golding M, Scarraf CE *et al.* (1996) Liver damage in the rat induces hepatocyte stem cells from biliary epithelial cells. *Gastroenterology* 110, 1182–1190.

17 Roskams T, Yang SQ, Koteish A *et al.* (2003) Oxidative stress and oval cell accumulation in mice and humans with alcoholic and nonalcoholic fatty liver disease. *Am J Pathol* 163, 1301–1311.

18 Yang S, Koteish A, Lin H *et al.* (2004) Oval cells compensate for damage and replicative senescence of mature hepatocytes in mice with fatty liver disease. *Hepatology* 39, 403–411.

19 Roskams T, Desmet V (1998) Ductular reaction and its diagnostic significance. *Semin Diagn Pathol* 15, 259–269.

20 Lowes KN, Brennan BA, Yeoh GC *et al.* (1999) Oval cell numbers in human chronic liver diseases are directly related to disease severity. *Am J Pathol* 154, 537–541.

21 Libbrecht L *et al.* (2000) Deep intralobular extension of human hepatic 'progenitor cells' correlates with parenchymal inflammation in chronic viral hepatitis: can 'progenitor cells' migrate? *J Pathol* 192, 373–378.

22 Falkowski O, Desmet V, Roskams T *et al.* (2003) Regeneration of hepatocyte 'buds' in cirrhosis from intrabiliary stem cells. *J Hepatol* 39, 357–364.

23 Wiemann SU, Desmet V, Roskams T *et al.* (2002) Hepatocyte telomere shortening and senescence are general markers of human liver cirrhosis. *FASEB J* 16, 935–942.

24 Marshall A *et al.* (2005) Relation between hepatocyte G1 arrest, impaired hepatic regeneration, and fibrosis in chronic hepatitis C virus infection. *Gastroenterology* 128, 33–42.

25 Roskams T (2003) Progenitor cell involvement in cirrhotic human liver diseases: from controversy to consensus. *J Hepatol* 39, 431–434.

26 Thorgeirsson SS, Grisham JW (2006) Hematopoietic cells as hepatocyte stem cells: a critical review of the evidence. *Hepatology* 43, 2–8.

27 Jakubowski A, Ambrose C, Parr M *et al.* (2005) TWEAK induces liver progenitor cell proliferation. *J Clin Invest* 115, 2330–2340.

28 Cassiman D, Libbrecht L, Desmet V *et al.* (2002) Hepatic stellate cell/myofibroblast subpopulations in fibrotic human and rat livers. *J Hepatol* 36, 200–209.

29 Ros JE, Roskams T, Geuken M *et al.* (2003) High expression of MDR1, MRP1, and MRP3 in the hepatic progenitor cell compartment and hepatocytes in severe human liver disease. *J Pathol* 200, 553–560.

30 Ros JE, Libbrecht L, Geuken M *et al.* (2003) ATP binding cassette transporter gene expression in rat liver progenitor cells. *Gut* 52, 1060–1067.

31 Sell S (2004) Stem cell origin of cancer and differentiation therapy. *Crit Rev Oncol Hematol* 51, 1–28.

32 Hixson DC, Brown J, McBride AC *et al.* (2000) Differentiation status of rat ductal cells and ethionine-induced hepatic carcinomas defined with surface-reactive monoclonal antibodies. *Exp Mol Pathol* 68, 152–169.

33 Dumble ML, Croager EJ, Yeoh GC *et al.* (2002) Generation and characterization of p53 null transformed hepatic progenitor cells: oval cells give rise to hepatocellular carcinoma. *Carcinogenesis* 23, 435–445.

34 Libbrecht L, Desmet V, Roskams T (2005) Preneoplastic changes in human hepatocarcinogenesis. *Liver Int* 25, 1–12.

35 Yoon DS, Jeong J, Park YN *et al.* (1999) Expression of biliary antigen and its clinical significance in hepatocellular carcinoma. *Yonsei Med J* 40, 472–477.

36 Van Eyken P *et al.* (1988) Cytokeratin expression in hepatocellular carcinoma: an immunohistochemical study. *Hum Pathol* 12, 562–568.

37 Hsia CC, Evarts RP, Natatsukasa H *et al.* (1992) Occurrence of oval-type cells in hepatitis B virus-associated human hepatocarcinogenesis. *Hepatology* 16, 1327–1633.

38 Durnez A (2006) The clinicopathological and prognostic relevance of cytokeratin 7 and 19 expression in hepatocellular carcinoma. A possible progenitor cell organ. *Histopathology* 49, 138–151.

39 Wu PC, Lai VC, Fang JW *et al.* (1999) Hepatocellular carcinoma expressing both hepatocellular and biliary markers also expresses cytokeratin 14, a marker of bipotential progenitor cells. *J Hepatol* 31, 965–966.

40 Uenishi T, Kubo S, Yamamoto T *et al.* (2003) Cytokeratin 19 expression in hepatocellular carcinoma predicts early postoperative recurrence. *Cancer Sci* 94, 851–857.

41 Ding SJ, Li Y, Tan YX *et al.* (2004) From proteomic analysis to clinical significance: overexpression of cytokeratin 19 correlates with hepatocellular carcinoma metastasis. *Mol Cell Proteomics* 3, 73–81.

42 Libbrecht L, Desmet V, Van Damme B *et al.* (2000) The immunohistochemical phenotype of dysplastic foci in human liver: correlation with putative progenitor cells. *J Hepatol* 33, 76–84.

43 Fiegel HC, Gluer S, Roth B *et al.* (2004) Stem-like cells in human hepatoblastoma. *J Histochem Cytochem* 52, 1495–1501.

44 Xiao JC, Ruck P, Adam A *et al.* (2003) Small epithelial cells in human liver cirrhosis exhibit features of hepatic stem-like cells: immunohistochemical, electron microscopic and immunoelectron microscopic findings. *Histopathology* 42, 141–149.

45 Ruck P, Xiao J-C, Kaiserling E (1996) Small epithelial cells and the histogenesis of hepatoblastoma. Electron microscopic, immunoelectron microscopic, and immunohistochemical findings. *Am J Pathol* 148, 321–329.

46 Nomoto K, Tsuneyama K, Abdel Aziz HO *et al.* (2006) Intrahepatic cholangiocarcinoma arising in cirrhotic liver frequently expressed p63-positive basal/stem-cell phenotype. *Pathol Res Pract* 202, 71–76.

47 Alison MR, Lovell MJ (2005) Liver cancer: the role of stem cells. *Cell Prolif* 38, 407–421.

1.9 Embryology of the liver and intrahepatic biliary tract

Frédéric P. Lemaigre

In the embryo, the liver develops from the endoderm, one of the three germ layers formed during gastrulation [1]. The endoderm is constituted of a single cell-layered epithelium that delineates the primitive gut, and shows a regionalized, antero-posterior (cephalocaudal) gene expression profile [2]. Indeed, the endoderm gives rise to a number of organs, such as the lungs, the thyroid gland, the liver, the intestine and the pancreas, and genes that are specifically active in these organs become expressed in the endoderm before organ morphogenesis is initiated. Thus, endodermal domains are specified, that is they are committed to a differentiation fate, before organ morphogenesis proceeds.

The outgrowth of the liver from the ventral wall of the endoderm gives rise to a bud consisting mainly of liver pre-cursor cells called hepatoblasts [3]. Proliferation of these cells is dependent on interactions with blood vessels, mesenchymal cells and extracellular matrix, and is followed by invasion of the hepatoblasts into the nearby septum transversum mesenchyme.

Further growth of the liver is associated with differentiation of the hepatoblasts into either hepatocytes or biliary cells [4,5]. The hepatocytes progressively acquire their mature morphology and line up to adopt the typical cord-like architecture that is established in concert with the development of the hepatic sinusoids (see Chapter 1.2). The biliary cells differentiate around the branches of the portal vein and, after a multistep morphogenic process, give rise to the intrahepatic bile ducts, which are located in the portal tracts and drain the bile from the bile canaliculi to the extrahepatic biliary tract [6,7]. Development of the hepatocytes and biliary cells is tightly controlled by a network of transcription factors [5,8–10] and by interactions with the extracellular matrix and with non-parenchymal cells such as the haematopoietic cells, which infiltrate the liver during development.

In this chapter, the various steps leading from endoderm specification to the acquisition of a mature liver architecture will be described, and the focus will be on mammalian liver development with specific reference to the mouse as a mammalian model organism.

From endoderm to hepatoblast

Hepatic specification of the endoderm is evidenced by the expression of albumin and α-fetoprotein, which starts in the ventral endoderm region that is adjacent to the developing heart and to the septum transversum mesenchyme. Transcription factors of the FoxA (forkhead-box factors, formerly HNF-3) and GATA families bind to regulatory regions of the albumin gene in the endoderm, at a stage preceding the onset of albumin mRNA synthesis [11,12]. As FoxA and GATA factors are able to bind to condensed chromatin and to induce its decompaction [13], it is likely that FoxA and GATA factors decondense endoderm chromatin to give access to another set of transcription factors, which subsequently allow transcription of the albumin gene to be initiated, and so contribute to hepatic specification of the endoderm [3].

Pioneering tissue transplantation experiments performed by LeDouarin [14], and more recent experiments addressing the molecular mechanisms of early hepatogenesis, revealed that fibroblast growth factors (FGF)-1 and -2, which are expressed by the cardiogenic mesoderm, can induce hepatic gene expression in cultured endoderm, provided that threshold concentrations of FGFs are reached [15,16]. The septum transversum mesenchyme, which is located caudally to the cardiogenic mesoderm and in the vicinity of the prehepatic endoderm at the time of hepatic induction, is a source of bone morphogenic proteins (BMP)-2 and -4. BMPs act cooperatively with FGFs in hepatic induction [17]. Interestingly, BMPs induce expression of the transcription factor GATA4 in cultured endoderm [17], thereby establishing a link between BMP signalling from the septum transversum and GATA-mediated chromatin remodelling in the endoderm.

Expansion of the liver bud

The liver bud, which becomes detectable around the 20th day of gestation in humans or at embryonic (E) day 9 in the mouse, mainly consists of a population of hepatoblasts that is delineated by a continuous basement membrane, and is separated from the

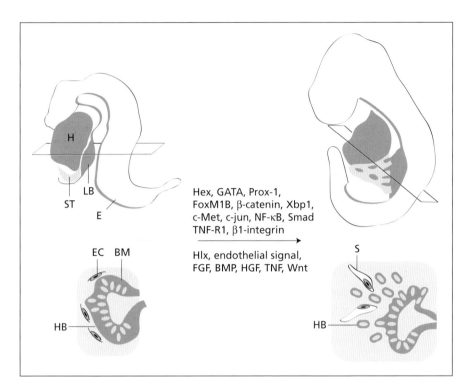

Hex, GATA, Prox-1,
FoxM1B, β-catenin, Xbp1,
c-Met, c-jun, NF-κB, Smad
TNF-R1, β1-integrin

Hlx, endothelial signal,
FGF, BMP, HGF, TNF, Wnt

Fig. 1 Expansion of the liver bud is controlled by cell-autonomous and cell-extrinsic mechanisms. When the liver bud (LB) emerges from the endoderm (E) in the vicinity of the developing heart (H), the hepatoblasts (HB) invade the septum transversum (ST). The liver bud is initially delineated by a continuous basement membrane (BM) and is surrounded by an irregular layer of endothelial cells (EC). Cell-autonomous (above the arrow) and cell-extrinsic (below the arrow) regulators modulate differentiation, proliferation and apoptosis of the hepatoblasts. Sinusoids (S) start to develop within the septum transversum.

septum transversum mesenchyme by an irregular layer of endothelial cells (Fig. 1). The hepatoblasts proliferate, the basement membrane is disrupted, and the cells invade the septum transversum. Expansion of the liver bud requires the activity of the proteins Hex, GATA6 and Prox-1, which are transcription factors expressed in the hepatoblasts [18–21]. Hex and GATA6 control cell proliferation and differentiation, respectively, and Prox-1 regulates cell adhesion. The role of Prox-1 was revealed by the analysis of *Prox1–/–* knockout embryos, which display a phenotype characterized by a lack of delamination of the hepatoblasts from the liver bud. The *Prox1–/–* cells fail to migrate through the basement membrane and remain clustered together, most probably as a result of the overexpression of the cell adhesion protein E-cadherin.

Interactions between hepatoblasts and mesoderm-derived cells also regulate liver bud expansion. As yet unidentified signals from the endothelial cells are required to stimulate hepatoblast proliferation, as evidenced by the lack of expansion of the liver bud in *Flk1–/–* embryos, which lack endothelial cells [22]. Septum transversum cells continue to play a role in liver development beyond the endoderm specification stage, as shown by the stimulation of hepatoblast proliferation by BMPs and FGFs [15,17]. How these factors control proliferation is not well understood, but the identification of BMP-responsive *cis*-acting sequences within regulatory sequences of the *Hex* gene suggests that signalling factors control hepatoblast proliferation by regulating the expression of liver-specific transcription factors.

At later stages of liver development, beyond the stage of bud formation, proliferation and survival of the hepatic cells persistently require the activity of a number of transcription factors in hepatoblasts as well as tight control mechanisms orchestrated by interactions involving the mesenchymal cells, the extracellular matrix and the hepatoblasts. FoxM1B , Xbp1 and β-catenin are transcriptional regulators that stimulate hepatoblast proliferation [23–25]. Another transcription factor, Hlx, which is expressed in mesenchymal cells, indirectly stimulates hepatoblast proliferation [26], most probably by controlling the activity or production of growth factors.

Growth factors secreted by the mesenchymal cells include scatter factor/hepatocyte growth factor (HGF). HGF binds to its receptor c-Met at the hepatoblast cell surface and activates a cascade involving the transcription factor c-jun. Mutations in the genes coding for HGF, c-Met or c-jun induce severe liver hypoplasia leading to embryonic lethality [27–30]. Moreover, HGF can stimulate hepatoblast proliferation cooperatively with Wnt-3a, a growth factor involved in a host of developmental processes, which controls gene expression by activating β-catenin [31]. Another growth factor, namely transforming growth factor (TGF)-β, also controls hepatoblast proliferation, as evidenced by the reduced proliferation rate observed in livers of mouse embryos doubly heterozygous for the TGF-β mediators Smad2 and Smad3 [32]. Moreover, deficiency in Smad2 and Smad3 activity is associated with strongly decreased expression of β1-integrin, a receptor for extracellular matrix components. β1-integrin is needed to allow normal hepatogenesis, as β1-integrin-deficient cells fail to colonize the liver [33].

Liver growth also depends on a balance between proliferation and apoptosis. Cell survival relies on the integrity of NF-κB-mediated signalling pathways, as shown by the fact that disruption of the *RelA* or *IκB* kinase genes is associated with intense apoptosis and liver failure [34–37]. When the *NfκB* gene is disrupted in the absence of tumour necrosis factor (TNF) or of TNF receptor-1, apoptosis is no longer observed, indicating that NF-κB is protective against TNF-induced apoptosis [38,39]. β-catenin, besides its role as a mediator of Wnt in stimulating proliferation of hepatoblasts, is also protective against apoptosis, as evidenced by the high number of apoptotic cells in embryonic liver explants in which β-catenin expression is inhibited [25].

Taken together, the above data indicate that a complex integration of cell-autonomous and cell-extrinsic cues allow the liver to emerge from the endoderm and to grow until it reaches the stage at which the bipotent hepatoblasts enter the hepatocytic or biliary differentiation programme.

Differentiation of hepatoblasts into hepatocytes or biliary cells

Around the eighth week of gestation in humans or around E14 in mouse embryos, the hepatoblasts start to differentiate into either hepatocytes or biliary cells (Fig. 2). The biliary cells are first detected around the branches of the portal vein (see below), while the hepatocytes differentiate in the rest of the parenchyma. Despite intense investigations, this process of cell fate decision remains poorly understood. Hepatocyte differentiation largely depends on the transcription factor HNF-4α [40]. The absence of HNF-4α at the stage when hepatocytes should enter the differentiation programme is associated with a failure to express numerous hepatocytic functions. Another transcription factor, FoxM1B, is critical for biliary differentiation because, in its absence, no biliary cells become detectable [23]. A different role is played by the transcription factor HNF-6, which prevents the premature appearance of biliary markers in the liver and so determines the timing of biliary differentiation [41]. Genes that are controlled by HNF-6 include those coding for HNF-1β, a transcription factor involved in bile duct morphogenesis [42], as well as mediators and regulators of TGF-β signalling [43,44].

Hepatoblast differentiation into either hepatocytes or biliary cells does not exclusively rely on cell-autonomous mechanisms. The Jagged/Notch signalling pathway, which implicates cell–cell regulatory events, is a candidate regulator of hepatoblast fate decisions in the developing liver. This hypothesis stems from the observations that, in patients affected by mutations in the *JAGGED1* gene and suffering from Alagille syndrome (see Chapters 16.10 and 22.1), the liver presents with bile duct paucity (OMIM #118450). Also, mice doubly heterozygous for a *Jagged1* null allele and a hypomorphic *Notch2* allele show lack of bile ducts at birth [45], but it is not yet known what stage of biliary differentiation is affected in these mutant mice. Work with cultured cells revealed that activation of the Notch pathway in isolated mouse hepatoblasts results in repression of hepatocytic differentiation and stimulation of biliary differentiation [46]. There is good evidence that Jagged-1, a Notch ligand, is expressed in the portal mesenchyme when biliary cells start to differentiate. Therefore, a plausible model proposes that hepatoblasts expressing Notch2 interact with the portal mesenchyme cells expressing Jagged-1, and that this triggers biliary

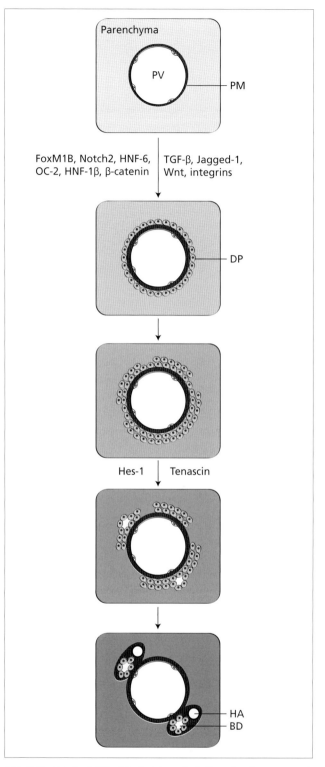

Fig. 2 Development of the bile ducts is controlled by cell-autonomous and cell-extrinsic mechanisms. The hepatoblasts differentiate into biliary cells around the portal mesenchyme (PM) surrounding the branches of the portal vein (PV). The biliary cells form the ductal plate (DP), which becomes bilayered and gives rise to the bile ducts (BD). The branches of the hepatic artery (HA) are associated with the bile ducts. Cell-autonomous (above the arrows) and cell-extrinsic (below the arrows) regulators modulate differentiation and morphogenesis of the bile ducts. The progressive darkening of the parenchyma illustrates the maturation of the hepatocytes.

differentiation of the hepatoblasts while repressing hepatocytic differentiation. However, whether Jagged/Notch signalling is involved in modulating hepatoblast fate decisions *in vivo* awaits further confirmation.

The hepatoblasts express high levels of the Wnt signalling mediator β-catenin [25], which, as mentioned above, promotes proliferation and protects against apoptosis. Experiments with embryonic liver explants revealed that Wnt-3a and β-catenin stimulate expression of the biliary marker cytokeratin 19 (CK19), implicating Wnt/β-catenin signalling in hepatoblast fate decisions [31]. This hypothesis is supported by the observation that liver explants treated with Wnt-3a show a reduced expression of the stem cell marker c-kit, suggesting that Wnt signalling induces the hepatoblasts to exit their bipotential status to enter the biliary differentiation programme. However, this model still needs to be validated by *in vivo* data.

Around the time of hepatoblast cell fate decision, TGF-β signalling occurs as a gradient of activity, which peaks in the hepatoblasts adjacent to the branches of the portal vein. Lower signalling activity is detected at a distance from the portal vein [44]. Increasing TGF-β signalling throughout the parenchyma, as is the case in knockout mice for the Onecut transcription factors HNF-6 or OC-2, induces the expression of biliary markers in all the hepatic cells. The cells then coexpress hepatocyte and biliary markers and are hybrid 'hepatobiliary' cells. In addition, blocking TGF-β signalling inhibits biliary differentiation of the hepatoblasts [44]. Therefore, the intensity, the timing and the location of TGF-β signalling activity are key determinants of hepatoblast fate decision. It is not yet clear how the gradient of TGF-β activity is established and how this gradient interacts with other cell signalling pathways involved in hepatoblast differentiation.

As biliary differentiation occurs around the branches of the portal vein (see below), the portal mesenchyme may promote biliary differentiation, not only by Wnt, Jagged/Notch or TGF-β-mediated signalling, but also via interactions with the extracellular matrix. When the hepatoblasts differentiate into biliary cells, a switch in the expression of integrins is observed. Indeed, hepatoblasts express integrin dimers α1β1, α5β1, α6β1 and α9β1, while the biliary cells show a progressive increase in α6β1 and a decrease in α1β1. In addition, the ductal plate cells start to express the α2β1, α3β1, αVβ1 and α6β4 integrins, which are absent from the hepatoblasts. The increase in α6β1 expression and the biliary-specific expression of α2β1, α3β1 and α6β4, which are laminin receptors, correlate well with the presence of laminin in the portal mesenchyme, suggesting that laminin may be involved in biliary cell development [47].

Maturation of hepatocytes

When the hepatocyte lineage becomes separated from the biliary lineage, the hepatocytes enter a maturation phase that extends beyond birth and consists of the acquisition of a proper morphology and of hepatocyte functions such as urea synthesis,

production of apolipoproteins or gluconeogenesis. A set of liver-enriched transcription factors, organized in a dynamic network of auto- and cross-regulatory loops [48], is instrumental in hepatocyte maturation. These factors include those from the HNF-1, FoxA, HNF-4, C/EBP and Onecut families [8–10]. Much is known about the function of these factors as a result of the analysis of mutant mice and from the identification of the factor binding sites in target genes. In some cases, human patients with mutations in genes coding for liver-enriched transcription factors were found. For instance, mutations in the *HNF1a*, *HNF1b* and *HNF4a* genes are associated with maturity-onset diabetes of the young. HNF-1α and HNF-4α control the expression of glucose metabolism-regulating proteins, but they also control a host of liver functions that include amino acid and lipid metabolism. HNF-4α also determines the epithelial morphology of hepatocytes, as a lack of HNF-4α in mice is associated with major alterations in liver architecture [49]. HNF-1β is a regulator of bile duct development (see below), but is also essential for bile acid sensing and fatty acid oxidation [42]. The three FoxA factors (FoxA-1, -2 and -3) have overlapping DNA-binding properties and functions and, like the other liver-enriched transcription factors, they regulate numerous hepatic functions. C/EBP factors also constitute a family of proteins with overlapping functions (reviewed in [50]). C/EBPα is a regulator of glucose and glycogen metabolism, of lipid homeostasis and hepatocyte proliferation. In addition, lack of C/EBPα perturbs the epithelial organization of the liver, but much less so than the absence of HNF-4α. C/EBPβ is a regulator of gluconeogenesis and a critical stimulator of phosphoenolpyruvate carboxykinase gene expression. Finally, with regard to Onecut factors, the function of HNF-6 has been determined mainly by the analysis of *Hnf6* knockout mice, which show abnormal glucose metabolism and major alterations in biliary development [41,51,52]. The Onecut factor OC-2 regulates biliary development [44].

Liver-enriched transcription factors form a regulatory network that is modulated by signalling from the environment. Starting around E12 in the mouse, hepatocytes are in close contact with haematopoietic cells. These cells persist in the liver until birth and exert a paracrine control on hepatocyte maturation (reviewed in ref. 53). Oncostatin M, an interleukin (IL)-6-related cytokine secreted by the haematopoietic cells, synergizes with glucocorticoid hormones to induce liver-specific functions and to control the morphology and cell adhesion properties of hepatocytes [54,55]. The response induced by oncostatin M requires the integrity of the *Jumonji* gene, which codes for a transcription factor expressed in hepatocytes [56]. Conversely, the integrity of hepatocytic functions is required to allow haematopoietic cell differentiation to proceed, as evidenced by the fact that hepatic B lymphopoiesis is impaired when hepatocytes are devoid of HNF-6 [57]. Also, when hepatocytes have matured, they no longer support differentiation of haematopoietic cells [55], indicating that haematopoietic cells and hepatocytes cross-regulate each other dynamically.

Development of the intrahepatic bile ducts

The biliary cells differentiate all around the branches of the portal vein, closely apposed to the portal mesenchyme (Fig. 2). Around the eighth week of gestation in humans, or E15 in mice, biliary cells form a monolayered and nearly continuous ring of cells, called the ductal plate. The ductal plate then becomes bilayered, and it enters a phase of remodelling around the 12th week of gestation in humans (E16 in mice). Lumina start to form between the two cell layers, giving rise to tubular structures that will develop into the intrahepatic bile ducts. Those portions of the ductal plate that are not involved in duct formation progressively disappear, and the ducts become surrounded by portal mesenchyme.

As stated above, transcription factors, cell signalling and cell–matrix interactions promote differentiation of hepatoblasts into biliary cells. Further steps in bile duct morphogenesis are regulated by the transcription factors HNF-6, OC-2, HNF-1β and Hes-1. Indeed, in *Hnf6–/–* and *Hnf1b–/–* mice, biliary cells are present, but the ductal plates fail to develop properly; transient biliary cysts are formed and, at birth, biliary cells surround the portal tracts without giving rise to ducts [41,42]. The biliary histology in these mice is similar to that described in human ductal plate malformations (see Chapter 8.1). In *Oc2–/–* mice, the ductal plate presents with premature dilations [44]. Hes-1, a transcription factor and target of Notch signalling, is dispensable for ductal plate formation, but is critically required for the development of tubular structures from the ductal plate [58].

The identification of transcription factors regulating bile duct morphogenesis has not yet allowed the characterization of several key aspects of duct formation. For instance, the mechanism promoting the formation of the second layer of cells forming the ductal plate is unknown. This most probably occurs by differentiation rather than proliferation, as very few proliferating cells are found in the ductal plate [41,59]. Another unresolved issue is what triggers the regression of those ductal plate portions that are not implicated in duct formation. Apoptosis is involved [60], but the rather low amount of apoptosing cells may not suffice to explain the regression of the ductal plate. Tube formation from the ductal plate requires the activity of the transcription factor Hes-1, but may also be controlled by extracellular matrix components. Indeed, tenascin is specifically found at the interface between the portal mesenchyme and the biliary cells of the developing ducts, but is absent near the ductal plate cells not involved in duct formation [61]. In addition, tubulogenesis is controlled by soluble factors, and there is *in vitro* evidence that HGF, insulin and EGF may participate in this process in the liver, but these results need to be confirmed *in vivo*.

Finally, novel insights into the mechanisms of bile duct morphogenesis may derive from the understanding of diseases that present with biliary cysts in the liver. Biliary cells have a primary cilium at their apical surface, and deficiencies in cilium formation or function are associated with bile duct anomalies [62].

Such diseases include the autosomal recessive form of polycystic kidney disease (ARPKD). ARPKD patients have mutations in the *PKHD1* gene, which codes for polyductin/fibrocystin, a protein associated with the primary cilium. The function of the cilium is not well understood, but some data favour the hypothesis that they sense fluid flow and induce a cellular response that controls tubulogenesis. Animal models such as the PCK rat [62] or transgenic mice with a targeted mutation of the *Pkhd1* gene [63] show biliary cysts and ductal plate malformations. The study of these animals should provide more insight into the role of the cilium in bile duct morphogenesis.

Vascular development in the liver

The right vitelline vein gives rise to the portal vein, which ramifies into several branches that connect with the hepatic sinusoids [64]. The precursors of the hepatic sinusoids become detectable around the fourth week of gestation in humans, i.e. during liver bud expansion [65,66]. They form sinusoid-like vessels that separate the hepatoblasts. At this stage, the endothelial cells express markers of continuous endothelia. Later, when the hepatocytes become organized in cords, the sinusoidal endothelium expresses markers of adult sinusoids, indicating that sinusoids undergo a process of maturation [66]. Interestingly, morphogenesis of the hepatic sinusoids depends on interactions with hepatocytes. This was concluded from the analysis of *Hnf4a–/–* mouse livers, in which abnormal differentiation of hepatocytes is associated with profound malformations of the hepatic sinusoids [49].

Sinusoids are separated from hepatocytes by the space of Disse, within which the hepatic stellate cells are found. These cells become detectable in the prenatal period, namely around the 12th week of gestation in humans or E13.5 in mice [67]. Their embryological origin is not well established but, on the basis of their gene expression profile, it has been suggested that they originate from the mesenchyme or from the neuroectoderm [68].

The hepatic artery usually arises from the coeliac trunk and ramifies in the portal tracts of the liver. There are differences between rodents and humans as to the timing of hepatic artery branch formation. In mice, the hepatic artery branches develop within a few days of birth in the vicinity of well-formed bile ducts [69], while in humans they become detectable around the 20th week of gestation, adjacent to the ductal plate [70]. Interestingly, hepatic artery branch development is dependent on the integrity of the biliary structures. Indeed, treatment of rats with a drug that promotes cholangiocyte proliferation induces a parallel remodelling of the hepatic artery branches [71]. In *Hnf6–/–* or *Hnf1b–/–* mouse livers, the bile ducts fail to form, and hepatic artery branches are either hyperplastic or absent [69]. Moreover, in humans, the ductal plate malformations found in Meckel syndrome or in Jeune syndrome are associated with anomalies of the hepatic artery branches [69].

It can be concluded that, throughout liver development, differentiation and morphogenesis of the hepatocytes, bile ducts and blood vessels depends on cross-regulations involving dynamic cell-intrinsic and cell-extrinsic mechanisms. The characterization of these mechanisms is ongoing and is a prerequisite for the full understanding of the pathophysiology of liver diseases.

References

1 Wells JM, Melton DA (1999) Vertebrate endoderm development. *Annu Rev Cell Dev Biol* 15, 393–410.

2 Grapin-Botton A, Melton DA (2000) Endoderm development: from patterning to organogenesis. *Trends Genet* 16, 124–130.

3 Zaret KS (2002) Regulatory phases of early liver development: paradigms of organogenesis. *Nature Rev Genet* 3, 499–512.

4 Lemaigre F, Zaret KS (2004) Liver development update: new embryo models, cell lineage control, and morphogenesis. *Curr Opin Genet Dev* 14, 582–590.

5 Zhao R, Duncan SA (2005) Embryonic development of the liver. *Hepatology* 41, 956–967.

6 Shiojiri N (1997) Development and differentiation of bile ducts in the mammalian liver. *Microsc Res Tech* 39, 328–335.

7 Lemaigre FP (2003) Development of the biliary tract. *Mech Dev* 20, 81–87.

8 Costa RH, Kalinichenko VV, Holterman AX *et al.* (2003) Transcription factors in liver development, differentiation, and regeneration. *Hepatology* 38, 1331–1347.

9 Schrem H, Klempnauer J, Borlak J (2002) Liver-enriched transcription factors in liver function and development. Part I: the hepatocyte nuclear factor network and liver-specific gene expression. *Pharmacol Rev* 54, 129–158.

10 Schrem H, Klempnauer J, Borlak J (2004) Liver-enriched transcription factors in liver function and development. Part II: the C/EBPs and D site-binding protein in cell cycle control, carcinogenesis, circadian gene regulation, liver regeneration, apoptosis, and liver-specific gene regulation. *Pharmacol Rev* 56, 291–330.

11 Gualdi R, Bossard P, Zheng M *et al.* (1996) Hepatic specification of the gut endoderm in vitro: cell signaling and transcriptional control. *Genes Dev* 10, 1670–1682.

12 Bossard P, Zaret KS (1998) GATA transcription factors as potentiators of gut endoderm differentiation. *Development* 125, 4909–4917.

13 Cirillo LA, Lin FR, Cuesta I *et al.* (2002) Opening of compacted chromatin by early developmental transcription factors HNF3 (FoxA) and GATA-4. *Mol Cell* 9, 279–289.

14 LeDouarin NM (1975) An experimental analysis of liver development. *Med Biol* 53, 427–455.

15 Jung J, Zheng M, Goldfarb M *et al.* (1999) Initiation of mammalian liver development from endoderm by fibroblast growth factors. *Science* 284, 1998–2003.

16 Serls AE, Doherty S, Parvatiyar P *et al.* (2005) Different thresholds of fibroblast growth factors pattern the ventral foregut into liver and lung. *Development* 132, 35–47.

17 Rossi JM, Dunn NR, Hogan BL *et al.* (2001) Distinct mesodermal signals, including BMPs from the septum transversum mesenchyme, are required in combination for hepatogenesis from the endoderm. *Genes Dev* 15, 1998–2009.

18 Keng VW, Yagi H, Ikawa M *et al.* (2000) Homeobox gene Hex is essential for onset of mouse embryonic liver development and differentiation of the monocyte lineage. *Biochem Biophys Res Commun* 276, 1155–1161.

19 Martinez Barbera JP, Clements M, Thomas P *et al.* (2000) The homeobox gene Hex is required in definitive endodermal tissues for normal forebrain, liver and thyroid formation. *Development* 127, 2433–2445.

20 Sosa-Pineda B, Wigle JT, Oliver G (2000) Hepatocyte migration during liver development requires Prox1. *Nature Genet* 25, 254–255.

21 Zhao R, Watt AJ, Li J *et al.* (2005) GATA6 is essential for embryonic development of the liver but dispensable for early heart formation. *Mol Cell Biol* 25, 2622–2631.

22 Matsumoto K, Yoshitomi H, Rossant J *et al.* (2001) Liver organogenesis promoted by endothelial cells prior to vascular function. *Science* 294, 559–563.

23 Krupczak-Hollis K, Wang X, Kalinichenko VV *et al.* (2004) The mouse Forkhead Box m1 transcription factor is essential for hepatoblast mitosis and development of intrahepatic bile ducts and vessels during liver morphogenesis. *Dev Biol* 276, 74–88.

24 Reimold AM, Etkin A, Clauss I *et al.* (2000) An essential role in liver development for transcription factor XBP-1. *Genes Dev* 14, 152–157.

25 Monga SP, Monga HK, Tan X *et al.* (2003) Beta-catenin antisense studies in embryonic liver cultures: role in proliferation, apoptosis, and lineage specification. *Gastroenterology* 124, 202–216.

26 Hentsch B, Lyons I, Li R *et al.* (1996) Hlx homeo box gene is essential for an inductive tissue interaction that drives expansion of embryonic liver and gut. *Genes Dev* 10, 70–79.

27 Schmidt C, Bladt F, Goedecke S *et al.* (1995) Scatter factor/hepatocyte growth factor is essential for liver development. *Nature* 373, 699–702.

28 Uehara Y, Minowa O, Mori C *et al.* (1995) Placental defect and embryonic lethality in mice lacking hepatocyte growth factor/scatter factor. *Nature* 373, 702–705.

29 Bladt F, Riethmacher D, Isenmann S *et al.* (1995) Essential role for the c-met receptor in the migration of myogenic precursor cells into the limb bud. *Nature* 376, 768–771.

30 Hilberg F, Aguzzi A, Howells N *et al.* (1993) c-jun is essential for normal mouse development and hepatogenesis. *Nature* 365, 179–181.

31 Hussain SZ, Sneddon T, Tan X *et al.* (2004) Wnt impacts growth and differentiation in ex vivo liver development. *Exp Cell Res* 292, 157–169.

32 Weinstein M, Monga SP, Liu Y *et al.* (2001) Smad proteins and hepatocyte growth factor control parallel regulatory pathways that converge on beta1-integrin to promote normal liver development. *Mol Cell Biol* 21, 5122–5131

33 Fassler R, Meyer M (1995) Consequences of lack of beta 1 integrin gene expression in mice. *Genes Dev* 9, 1896–1908.

34 Beg AA, Sha WC, Bronson RT *et al.* (1995) Embryonic lethality and liver degeneration in mice lacking the RelA component of NF-κB. *Nature* 376, 167–170.

35 Li Q, Van Antwerp D, Mercurio F *et al.* (1999) Severe liver degeneration in mice lacking the IkappaB kinase 2 gene. *Science* 284, 321–325.

36 Li ZW, Chu W, Hu Y *et al.* (1999) The IKKbeta subunit of IkappaB kinase (IKK) is essential for nuclear factor kappaB activation and prevention of apoptosis. *J Exp Med* 189, 1839–1845.

37 Rudolph D, Yeh WC, Wakeham A *et al.* (2000) Severe liver degeneration and lack of NF-kappaB activation in NEMO/IKKgamma-deficient mice. *Genes Dev* 14, 854–862.

38 Doi TS, Marino MW, Takahashi T *et al.* (1999) Absence of tumor necrosis factor rescues RelA-deficient mice from embryonic lethality. *Proc Natl Acad Sci USA* 96, 2994–2999.

39 Rosenfeld ME, Prichard L, Shiojiri N *et al.* (2000) Prevention of hepatic apoptosis and embryonic lethality in RelA/TNFR-1 double knockout mice. *Am J Pathol* 156, 997–1007.

40 Li J, Ning G, Duncan SA (2000) Mammalian hepatocyte differentiation requires the transcription factor HNF-4alpha. *Genes Dev* 14, 464–474.

41 Clotman F, Lannoy VJ, Reber M *et al.* (2002) The onecut transcription factor HNF6 is required for normal development of the biliary tract. *Development* 129, 1819–1828.

42 Coffinier C, Gresh L, Fiette L *et al.* (2002) Bile system morphogenesis defects and liver dysfunction upon targeted deletion of HNF1beta. *Development* 129, 1829–1838.

43 Plumb-Rudewiez N, Clotman F, Strick-Marchand H *et al.* (2004) The transcription factor HNF-6/OC-1 inhibits the stimulation of the HNF-3α/Foxa1 gene by TGFβ in mouse liver. *Hepatology* 40, 1266–1274.

44 Clotman F, Jacquemin P, Plumb-Rudewiez N *et al.* (2005) Control of liver cell fate decision by a gradient of TGFβ signaling modulated by Onecut transcription factors. *Genes Dev* 19, 1849–1854.

45 McCright B, Lozier J, Gridley T (2002) A mouse model of Alagille syndromeP: Notch2 as a genetic modifier of Jag1 haploinsufficiency. *Development* 129, 1075–1082.

46 Tanimizu N, Miyajima A (2004) Notch signaling controls hepatoblast differentiation by altering the expression of liver-enriched transcription factors. *J Cell Sci* 117, 3165–3174.

47 Couvelard A, Bringuier AF, Dauge MC *et al.* (1998) Expression of integrins during liver organogenesis in humans. *Hepatology* 27, 839–847.

48 Odom DT, Zizlsperger N, Gordon DB *et al.* (2004) Control of pancreas and liver gene expression by HNF transcription factors. *Science* 303, 1378–1381.

49 Parviz F, Matullo C, Garrison WD *et al.* (2003) Hepatocyte nuclear factor 4alpha controls the development of a hepatic epithelium and liver morphogenesis. *Nature Genet* 34, 292–296.

50 Lekstrom-Himes J, Xanthopoulos KG (1998) Biological role of the CCAAT/enhancer-binding protein family of transcription factors. *J Biol Chem* 273, 28545–28548.

51 Jacquemin P, Durviaux SM, Jensen J *et al.* (2000) Transcription factor hepatocyte nuclear factor 6 regulates pancreatic endocrine cell differentiation and controls expression of the proendocrine gene ngn3. *Mol Cell Biol* 20, 4445–4454.

52 Lannoy VJ, Decaux JF, Pierreux CE *et al.* (2002) Liver glucokinase gene expression is controlled by the onecut transcription factor hepatocyte nuclear factor-6. *Diabetologia* 45, 1136–1141.

53 Kinoshita T, Miyajima A (2002) Cytokine regulation of liver development. *Biochim Biophys Acta* 1592, 303–312.

54 Kamiya A, Kinoshita T, Ito Y *et al.* (1999) Fetal liver development requires a paracrine action of oncostatin M through the gp130 signal transducer. *EMBO J* 18, 2127–2136.

55 Kinoshita T, Sekiguchi T, Xu MJ *et al.* (1999) Hepatic differentiation induced by oncostatin M attenuates fetal liver haematopoiesis. *Proc Natl Acad Sci USA* 96, 7265–7270.

56 Anzai H, Kamiya A, Shirato H *et al.* (2003) Impaired differentiation of fetal hepatocytes in homozygous jumonji mice. *Mech Dev* 120, 791–800.

57 Bouzin C, Clotman F, Renauld JC *et al.* (2003) The onecut transcription factor hepatocyte nuclear factor-6 controls B lymphopoiesis in fetal liver. *J Immunol* 171, 1297–1303.

58 Kodama Y, Hijikata M, Kageyama R *et al.* (2004) The role of notch signaling in the development of intrahepatic bile ducts. *Gastroenterology* 127, 1775–1786.

59 Fabris L, Strazzabosco M, Crosby HA *et al.* (2000) Characterization and isolation of ductular cells coexpressing neural cell adhesion molecule and Bcl-2 from primary cholangiopathies and ductal plate malformations. *Am J Pathol* 156, 1599–1612.

60 Terada T, Nakanuma Y (1995) Detection of apoptosis and expression of apoptosis-related proteins during human intrahepatic bile duct development. *Am J Pathol* 146, 67–74.

61 Terada T, Nakanuma Y (1994) Expression of tenascin, type IV collagen and laminin during human intrahepatic bile duct development and in intrahepatic cholangiocarcinoma. *Histopathology* 25, 143–150.

62 Masyuk TV, Huang BQ, Ward CJ *et al.* (2003) Defects in cholangiocyte fibrocystin expression and ciliary structure in the PCK rat. *Gastroenterology* 125, 1303–1310.

63 Moser M, Matthiesen S, Kirfel J *et al.* (2005) A mouse model for cystic biliary dysgenesis in autosomal recessive polycystic kidney disease (ARPKD). *Hepatology* 41, 1113–1121.

64 Lassau JP, Bastian D (1983) Organogenesis of the venous structures of the human liver: a hemodynamic theory. *Anat Clin* 5, 97–102.

65 Gouysse G, Couvelard A, Frachon S *et al.* (2002) Relationship between vascular development and vascular differentiation during liver organogenesis in humans. *J Hepatol* 37, 730–740.

66 Couvelard A, Scoazec JY, Dauge MC *et al.* (1996) Structural and functional differentiation of sinusoidal endothelial cells during liver organogenesis in humans. *Blood* 87, 4568–4580.

67 Wandzioch E, Kolterud A, Jacobsson M *et al.* (2004) Lhx2–/– mice develop liver fibrosis. *Proc Natl Acad Sci USA* 101, 16549–16554.

68 Geerts A (2001) History, heterogeneity, developmental biology, and functions of quiescent hepatic stellate cells. *Semin Liver Dis* 21, 311–335

69 Clotman F, Libbrecht L, Gresh L *et al.* (2003) Hepatic artery malformations associated with a primary defect in intrahepatic bile duct development. *J Hepatol* 39, 686–692.

70 Libbrecht L, Cassiman D, Desmet V *et al.* (2002) The correlation between portal myofibroblasts and development of intrahepatic bile ducts and arterial branches in human liver. *Liver* 22, 252–258.

71 Masyuk TV, Ritman EL, LaRusso NF (2003) Hepatic artery and portal vein remodeling in rat liver: vascular response to selective cholangiocyte proliferation. *Am J Pathol* 162, 1175–1182.

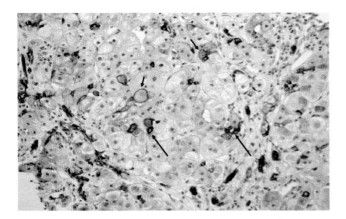

Plate 1.8.1 Cytokeratin 7 immunohistochemical stain illustrating liver progenitor cells (long arrows) and intermediate hepatocytes (short arrows) in a liver after severe hepatocyte damage.

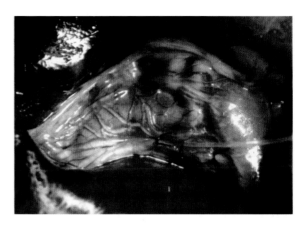

Plate 2.1.3.1 Photograph of the liver (on the left) covered with ascites fluid. The portal vein runs across the field flowing from right to left into the liver. A large number of translucent lymphatics are seen exiting the liver at the hilus, coursing over the portal vein and flowing from left to right in the photograph. Lymphatic valves can be seen as points of constriction in some of lymphatic vessels. One of the large lymphatics in the photograph has been cannulated for the purposes of lymph collection. The lymphatic catheter is tied in place with lengths of black suture. A large lymph node can be seen at the right of the photograph.

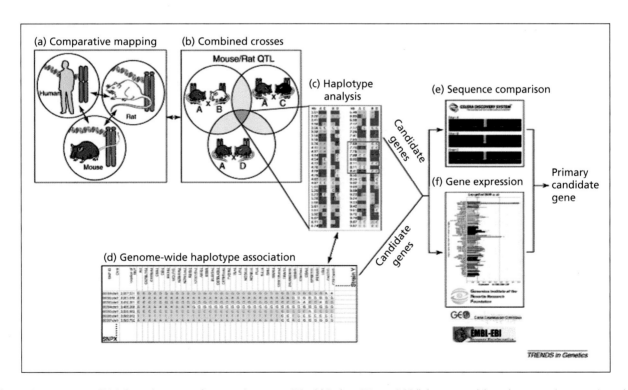

Plate 3.3.3.1 Integrated bioinformatics strategy for narrowing mouse QTLs. (a) Rodent QTLs can initially be narrowed through comparative genomics and (b) combined cross-analysis. (c) Those QTLs identified in multiple crosses can be narrowed by haplotype analysis. Combining experimental QTLs narrowed using steps a–c with results from genomewide haplotype association (d) can further narrow the QTL to a region < 5 Mb. (e) The number of candidate genes can be reduced further using sequence databases (f) and expression databases to identify primary candidate genes that are differentially expressed in liver or contain a coding sequence polymorphism. Reproduced with permission from ref. 45.

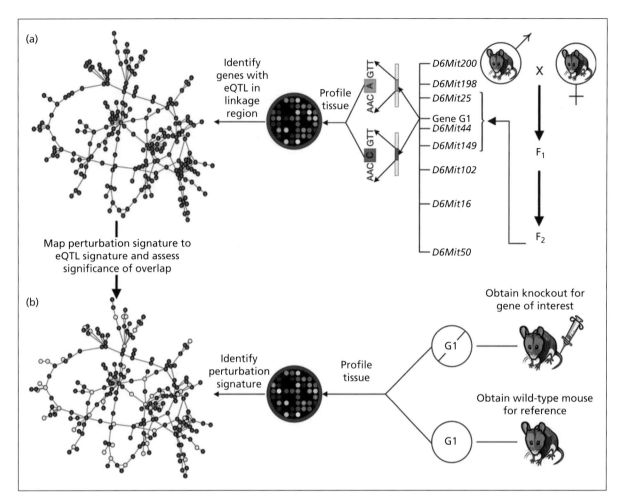

Plate 3.3.3.2 Intersecting perturbation signatures in gene expression data to map genes for complex traits. (a) QTLs for complex traits are mapped in an experimental cross. A genetic locus at G1 is highlighted as being linked to a trait of interest in the F2 population. An SNP in G1 highlighted as the causal variant underlying the complex trait. Hepatic expression levels are monitored using microarrays. Expression traits found to be genetically linked to the G1 locus are determined. The transcriptional network on the left highlights expression traits linked to the G1 locus (blue nodes), in addition to expression traits interacting with genes linked to the G1 locus (white nodes), with G1 denoted by the red node. (b) Livers from mice genetically engineered with respect to G1 are profiled (e.g. knockout mice in this case). Genes that are differentially regulated between the perturbed and unperturbed system are identified. Highlighted to the left is the portion of the network that is observed to change when gene G1 is perturbed. This signature is compared with the eQTL signature defined in (a). If expression traits controlled by the G1 locus are enriched for expression traits that are differentially regulated as described in (b) (blue nodes), then this matched pattern of expression provides direct experimental support that G1 is the gene underlying the linkage to the complex trait in the F2 population. Reproduced with permission from ref. 58.

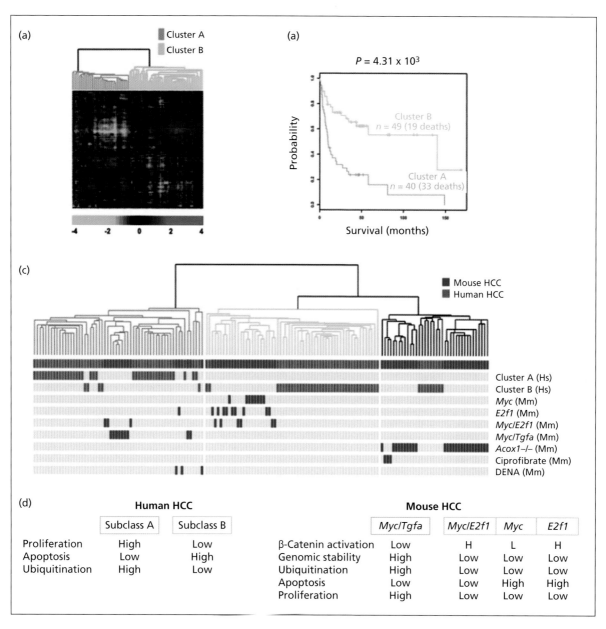

Plate 3.3.3.3 Gene expression profiling of human HCCs and comparative functional genomics to identify best-fit mouse models for the study of human cancer. (a) Hierarchical cluster analysis of human HCCs. The data are presented in matrix format in which rows represent the individual gene and columns represent individual tissue. The red and green colours in cells reflect high and low expression levels, respectively, as indicated in the scale bar ($\log_2$ transformed scale). (b) Significant association of gene expression patterns with patient survival. Kaplan–Meier plot of overall survival of HCC patients grouped on the basis of gene expression profiling shown in (a). (c) Hierarchical cluster analysis of integrated human and mouse HCCs. The data are presented as a dendrogram. Red and blue bars represent human and mouse HCCs respectively. The identity of each HCC tissue is shown at the end of each row (see ref. 59 for details). (d) Phenotypical similarities between HCCs generated in the transgenic mouse models and subclass A and B of human HCCs. These models should be particularly valuable for both testing potential therapeutic targets and preclinical trials of drugs. Reproduced with permission from ref. 60.

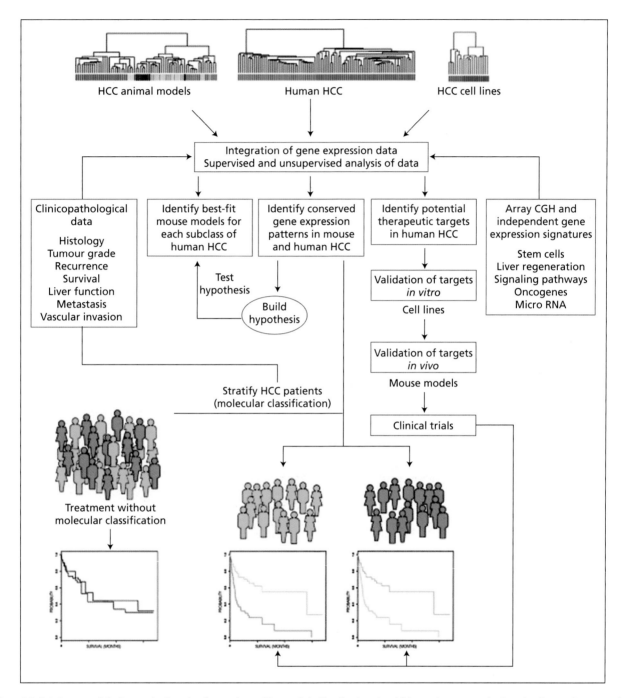

Plate 3.3.3.4 Framework for integrative functional genomics and future clinical implications. In addition to the comparative functional genomics approach that combines gene expression data from primary human HCCs and mouse HCC models, gene expression signatures unique for different physiological condition such as liver development and liver regeneration as well as hepatic stem cells are collected and integrated into the gene expression patterns from human HCCs. This approach will further help not only to uncover the molecular pathways involved in HCC pathogenesis but also to stratify patients for the most beneficial target-specific therapies. Reproduced with permission from ref. 60.

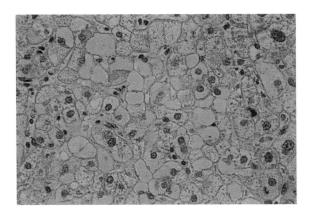

Plate 4.1.1 Liver biopsy from a patient with chronic hepatitis B. Numerous ground-glass hepatocytes with homogeneous, pale pink cytoplasm can be seen [haematoxylin and eosin (H&E) × 65].

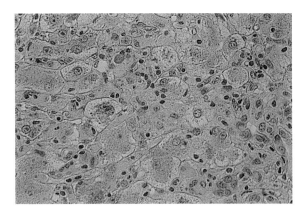

Plate 4.1.2 Liver biopsy from a patient with acute hepatitis B, characterized by liver cell pleomorphism and parenchymal inflammation. Pleomorphism of hepatocytes is reflected in unequal size and staining quality. Ballooned hepatocytes appear swollen and pale, especially in the peripheral part of their cytoplasm. Two small eosinophilic apoptotic cell fragments lie close to lymphocytes (H&E × 104).

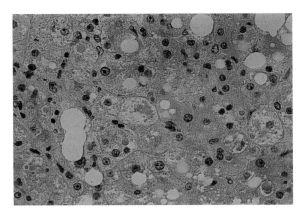

Plate 4.1.3 Liver biopsy from a patient with alcoholic liver disease. The picture shows some steatosis vacuoles, two pale, swollen hepatocytes containing an irregularly shaped Mallory body, and several parenchymal cells with one or more round, eosinophilic inclusions: megamitochondria (H&E × 104).

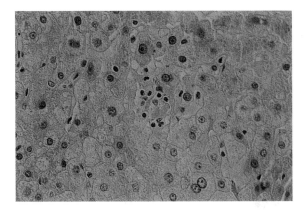

Plate 4.1.4 Liver biopsy from a patient with chronic persistent hepatitis B. Small focus of focal (or 'spotty') necrosis, with accumulation of lymphocytes and mononuclear cells around a dying liver cell, of which only two small eosinophilic fragments (apoptotic bodies) are recognizable (H&E × 104).

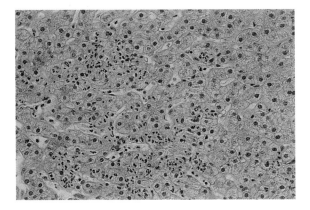

Plate 4.1.5 Surgical liver biopsy. 'Surgical necroses' are represented by clusters of accumulating polymorphonuclear neutrophils (H&E × 65).

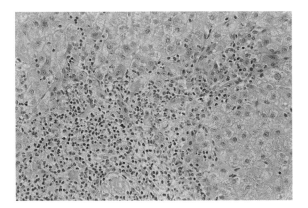

Plate 4.1.6 Liver biopsy from a patient with chronic active hepatitis B, characterized by piecemeal necrosis. The portal tract (lower left corner) shows dense mononuclear cell infiltration, which extends into the surrounding parenchyma, creating an irregular connective tissue–parenchymal interphase. A longer extension (up to right upper corner) represents an early stage of active septum formation (H&E × 65).

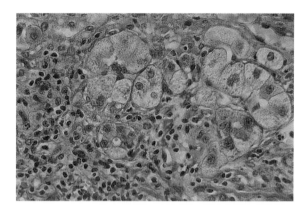

Plate 4.1.7 Liver biopsy from a patient with post-hepatitic cirrhosis. Hepatitic liver cell rosettes represent small groups of sequestrated hepatocytes, surrounded by fibrosis and inflammatory infiltration [Masson's trichrome (collagen appears blue) × 104].

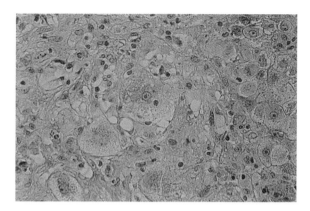

Plate 4.1.8 Liver biopsy from a patient with acute hepatitis B. The picture shows liver cell pleomorphism and ballooning, and interrupted continuity of liver cell plates. Note the presence (centre) of a lymphocyte, surrounded by a narrow clear halo, in the cytoplasm of a ballooned hepatocyte: emperipolesis (H&E × 104).

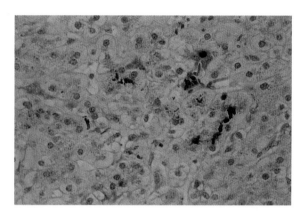

Plate 4.1.9 Liver biopsy from an infant with biliary atresia. The picture shows bilirubin granules in a couple of hepatocytes (hepatocellular bilirubinostasis), coarse bilirubin-stained casts in dilated canaliculi (canalicular bilirubinostasis), and coarse bilirubin deposits in hypertrophic, red-stained (PAS-positive) Kupffer (Kupffer cell bilirubinostasis (PAS–Schiff after diastase digestion (PAS-D) × 104).

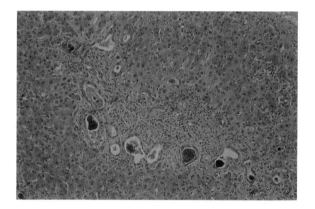

Plate 4.1.10 Liver biopsy from a severely jaundiced patient with monilia sepsis. The picture shows an obliquely cut portal tract, extending from the upper left to lower right corner. The upper and lower border is lined by a large number of extremely dilated ductules containing bile concrements in varying degree of inspissation (ductular bilirubinostasis) (H&E × 26).

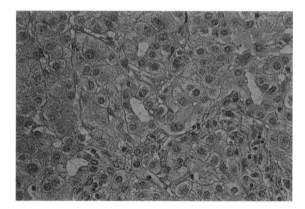

Plate 4.1.11 Liver biopsy from a 9-year-old child with incomplete obstruction of the common bile duct by annular pancreas. Chronic cholestasis is reflected in the appearance of cholestatic liver cell rosettes: groups of hepatocytes arranged around a central lumen. In this instance, there are no obvious bile concrements in the lumina (H&E × 104).

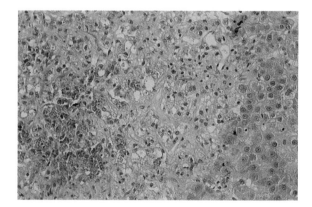

Plate 4.1.12 Liver biopsy from a patient with long-standing extrahepatic bile-duct obstruction. The picture shows part of a large paraportal bile infarct (compare with the appearance of relatively normal parenchyma on the right side). The central part of the necrotizing area (left side of picture) is most heavily impregnated with bilirubin pigment (H&E × 65).

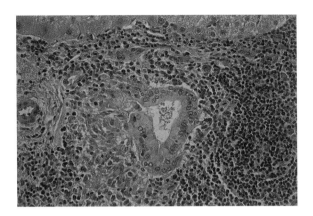

Plate 4.1.13 Liver biopsy from a patient with primary biliary cirrhosis. The picture shows a cross-sectioned interlobular bile duct, lying amidst a densely lymphoplasmocytic infiltrate. Note the focal rupture of the bile duct lining (near 10'clock) and the development of an epithelioid granuloma on the rupture side of the duct (H&E × 65).

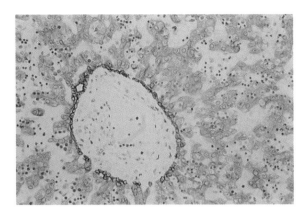

Plate 4.1.14 Liver specimen from a 16-week-old human fetus. The picture shows a portal vein branch surrounded with mesenchyme. Adjacent to the latter lies a partly double layer of smaller and darker stainng cells (the ductal plate). A tubular lumen has formed in one of the double layered segments (upper left). The primitive hepatocytes are weakly stained, with stronger positivity near the cell periphery. Interspersed haematopoietic cells are keratin negative (immunoperoxidase stain for cytokeratins (antibody CAM 5.2, which stains cytokeratins -8, -18, and -19): counterstain with Harris haematoxylin × 65).

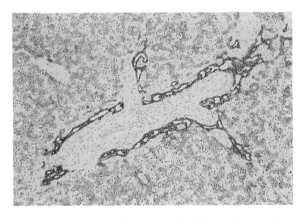

Plate 4.1.15 Liver specimen from a 20-week-old human fetus with Meckel syndrome. The picture shows a portal vein with two short side branches surrounded with mesenchyme. Adjacent to the latter lies a double layer of small, darkly-staining cells which form numerous cross-sectioned tubular structures. Persistence of these structures indicates lack of remodelling of the ductal plate, i.e. the ductal plate malformation. The primitive hepatocytes are weakly stained, with stronger positivity near the cell periphery. Interspersed haematopoietic cells are negative for keratin (immunoperoxidase stain for cytokeratins (antibody CAM 5.2, which stains cytokeratins -8, -18, and -19): counterstain with Harris haematoxylin, × 65).

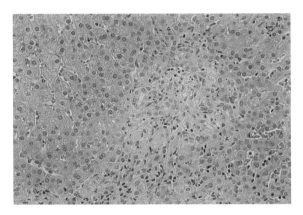

Plate 4.1.16 Liver biopsy from a patient with primary sclerosing cholangitis. The portal tract in the centre appears oedematous; an increased number of ductular profiles can be seen extending into the surrounding parenchyma, with a sprinkling of polymorphonuclear and mononuclear inflammatory cells (cholangiolitis) (H&E × 65).

Plate 4.1.17 Liver biopsy from a patient with inactive macronodular cirrhosis. A passive septum appears as a sharply delineated blue-stained line. Note the presence of vessels and the absence of inflammatory cells in the septum. The nodular parenchyma appears hyperplastic, with plates of thickness of two or more cells (Masson's trichrome stain × 65).

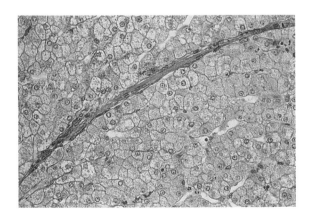

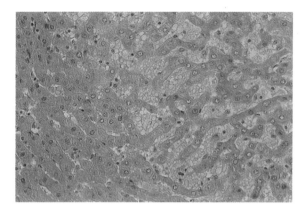

Plate 4.1.18 Liver biopsy from a patient with venous outflow block (heart decompensation). Note the dilatation of the sinusoids, engorged with erythrocytes, and the thinning of the liver cell plates in acinar zone 3 (right side of picture) (H&E × 65).

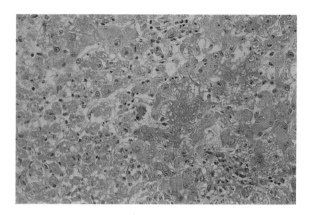

Plate 4.1.19 Liver biopsy from a pregnant patient with eclampsia. A small portal tract is located near the lower right corner. Several paraportal sinusoids are blocked with pink fibrin clots (centre and upper right). Note the early stage of ischaemic necrosis of parts of the parenchyma (left side), with increased eosinophilia of the cytoplasm and pyknosis of the nuclei (H&E × 65).

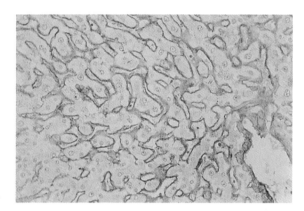

Plate 4.1.20 Liver biopsy from a patient with light chain deposit disease. A terminal hepatic venule (centre vein) is located in the lower right corner. The Disse space between sinusoidal lumina and liver cell plates contains material which is immunoreactive for kappa light chains of immunoglobulin (immunoperoxidase stain for kappa light chains: counterstain of nuclei with H&E × 65).

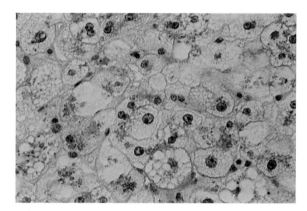

Plate 4.1.21 Liver biopsy from a patient with tetracycline intoxication. The picture shows part of the parenchyma, characterized by small droplet steatosis. The hepatocytes contain numerous small fat droplets, and retain their nucleus in central poition. Granular bilirubin pigment also accumulates between the fat vacuoles (hepatocellular bilirubinostasis) H&E × 104).

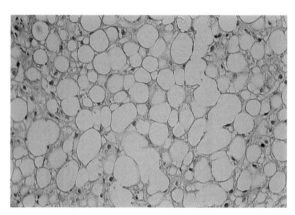

Plate 4.1.22 Liver biopsy from a patient with alcohol abuse. Most hepatocytes contain single, large fat vacuoles, pushing the nucleus to the periphery of the cell. Some adjacent vacuoles fuse to larger 'fatty cysts' (H&E × 65).

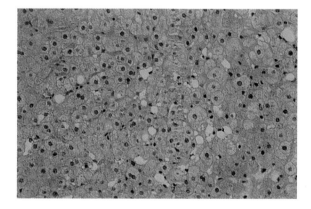

Plate 4.1.23 Liver biopsy from a patient with vitamin A intoxication. Numerous clear spaces occur between the hepatocytes: they correspond to hyperplastic Ito cells (so-called fat storing cells); they contain fat droplets in their cytoplasm which indent the contour of their nucleus (H&E × 65).

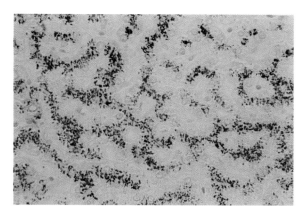

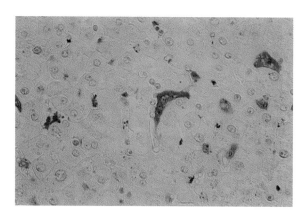

Plate 4.1.24 Liver biopsy from a patient with idiopathic (genetic) haemochromatosis. Blue-stained haemosiderin granules accumulate in the pericanalicular region of the hepatocytes (which is a typical localization of lysosomes) (Prussian blue stain for iron; neutral red counterstain × 104).

Plate 4.1.25 Liver biopsy from a patient under chemotherapy for leukaemia. Reticulendothelial siderosis: blue-stained haemosiderin granules accumulate in hyperplastic Kupffer cells; the parenchymal cells are negative (Prussian blue stain for iron; neutral red counterstain × 104).

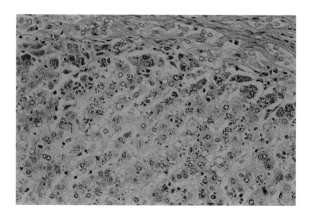

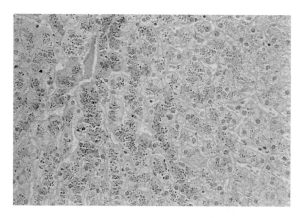

Plate 4.1.26 Liver biopsy from a patient with liver cirrhosis and α_1-antitryspsin deficiency. Part of a cirrhotic nodule is shown; red-stained (PAS-positive) inclusions of variable size are present in hepatocytes, especially in the nodular periphery near a connective tissue septum (upper part) (PAS-D × 65).

Plate 4.1.27 Liver biopsy from a patient with Dubin–Johnson syndrome. A terminal hepatic venule (central vein) is located near the upper left corner. The hepatocytes contain numerous brown pigment granules, especially in acinar zone 3 (H&E × 65).

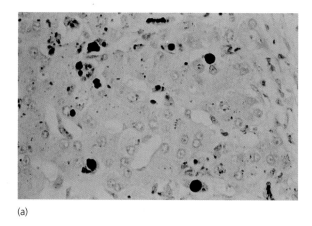

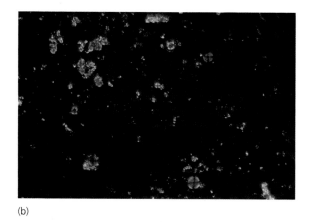

(a)

(b)

Plate 4.1.28 Liver specimen from a patient with erythropoietic protoporphyria. Brown–black deposits of variable size are seen in hepatocytes, canaliculi, and hyperplastic Kupffer cells. (a) H&E × 104. (b) The same area under polarized light: the deposits show birefringence, in Maltese cross configuration in the larger deposits. (Specimen courtesy of Dr B. Portmann, London.)

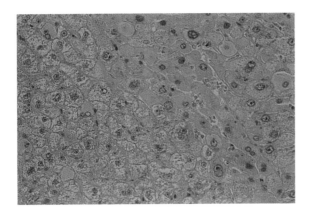

Plate 4.1.29 Liver biopsy from a patient with hepatitis B virus-positive liver cirrhosis. The upper right half of the picture shows hepatocytes with enlarged cytoplasmic and nuclear size (dysplastic cells). Ground-glass change of the cytoplasm is seen in some of the dysplastic and non-dysplastic cells (H&E × 104).

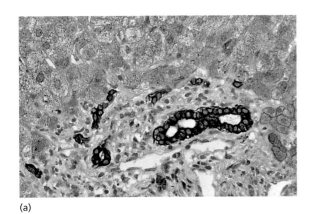

(a)

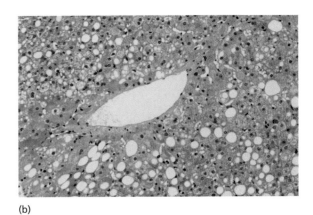

(b)

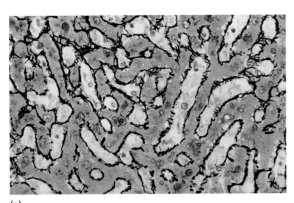

(a)

Plate 5.5.1 Examples of normal hepatic structures. (a) Part of a portal tract (bottom) and the adjacent periportal parenchyma (top). Cholangiocytes are selectively stained (brown) by use of cytokeratin-19 staining. The normal portal tract space usually contains one interlobular bile duct, an artery (not shown) and small portal vein branches (the triad). The figure also shows few ductules. Close to the latter, a rim of hepatocytes forms the transition between lobular parenchyma and the portal tract. This is the limiting plate, a crucial structural and functional compartment border. (b) Centre of the lobule. The ovoid space is the terminal or central vein. The identification of this vein, together with portal tracts, serves to estimate the normal or abnormal geometry of the liver lobule. (c) Silver stain of normal parenchyma. The black structures are reticulin fibres located to the perisinusoidal space. This stain is best suited to show the normal configuration of hepatocyte plates and the geometry of sinusoids.

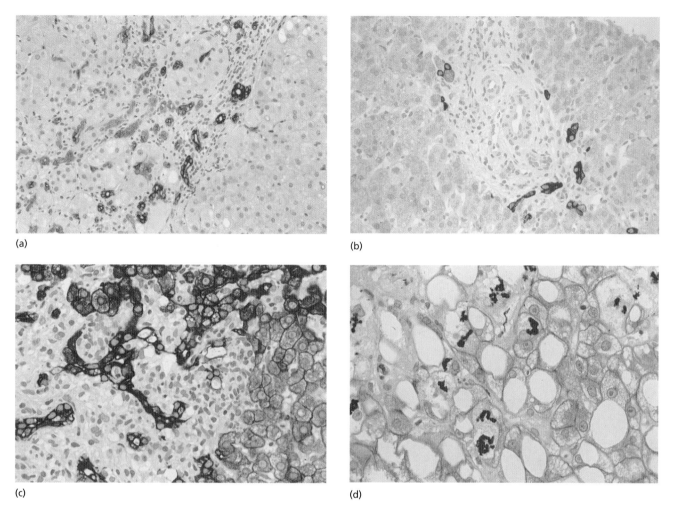

(a)

(b)

(c)

(d)

Plate 5.5.2 Immunohistochemistry in liver biopsies. (a) Selective immunohistochemical demonstration of bile ducts and ductules (cytokeratin-19). This is an example of ductular proliferation (ductular reaction) preferentially seen in bile duct obstruction and hepatic remodelling. The amount and distribution of ductules are not reliably detectable in H&E stains. (b) In this cytokeratin-19 preparation, few ductules are visualized, but an interlobular bile duct is absent. This represents a ductopenic state, in this case Alagille syndrome. (c) Although less important than the cytokeratin-19 immunostain, demonstration of cytokeratin-8 expression may be useful for the identification of parenchymal cell damage – in the present example piecemeal necrosis (interface lesions). (d) This ubiquitin immunostain depicts several fully developed Mallory bodies in ballooned hepatocytes.

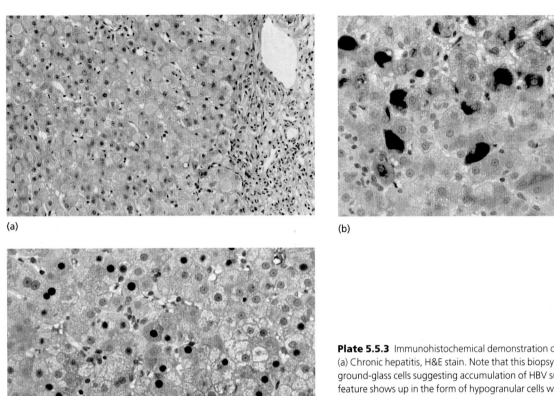

(a)

(b)

(c)

Plate 5.5.3 Immunohistochemical demonstration of viral antigens. (a) Chronic hepatitis, H&E stain. Note that this biopsy exhibits several ground-glass cells suggesting accumulation of HBV surface antigen. This feature shows up in the form of hypogranular cells with a displaced nucleus. (b) Immunohistochemistry for HBV surface antigen. The hypogranular part of the hepatocyte cytoplasm seen in ground-glass cells (a) is markedly reactive for this antigen (in red). (c) Immunohistochemistry for HBV core antigen. Numerous hepatocyte nuclei are markedly positive (in red), and there is also some staining of the cytoplasm in a minority of the cells.

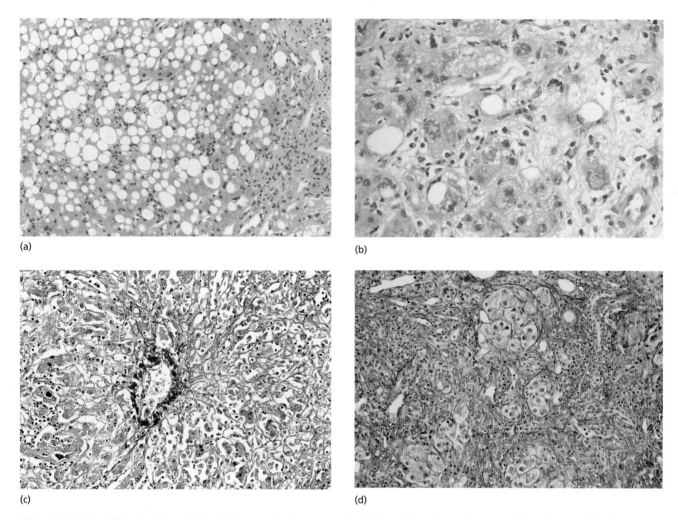

Plate 5.5.4 Alcoholic fatty liver disease. (a) In addition to marked macrosteatosis, this biopsy shows intralobular accumulations of neutrophils, indicating acute alcoholic steatohepatitis (H&E stain). (b) Ballooned hepatocytes with numerous Mallory bodies, visualized as markedly dense and eosinophilic structures in a pale cytoplasm. In this case, Mallory bodies are easily identifiable, and there will be no need of immunohistochemsitry (H&E stain). (c) Alcoholic liver disease. This collagen stain (sirius red) shows a pathological accumulation of collagen fibres around hepatocyte cords. This is perisinusoidal fibrosis. The lattice seen in this section is called chicken fence fibrosis. (d) In advanced alcoholic liver fibrosis, the hepatic lobular architecture is effaced, and only spheroid remnants of the former lobule (yellow) are noted (sirius red stain).

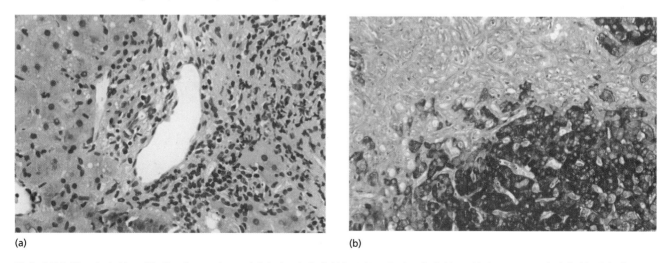

Plate 5.5.5 Chronic viral hepatitis: the piecemeal necrosis (interface lesion). (a) Portal tract in chronic viral hepatitis. In contrast to the left side of the figure, the adjacent parenchyma to the right of the portal tract is partially destroyed, and the limiting plate is no longer seen. This interface lesion is an important feature for assessing inflammatory activity (H&E stain). (b) The geometry of an interface lesion is depicted here by use of a PAS stain. Note the atrophy of former zone 1 cells.

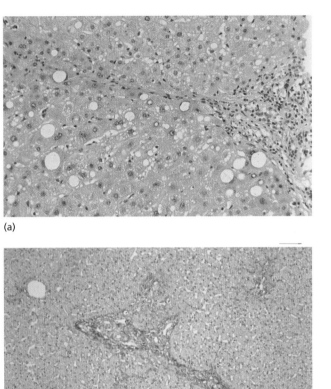

(a)

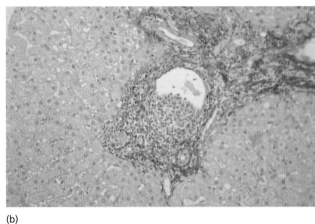

(b)

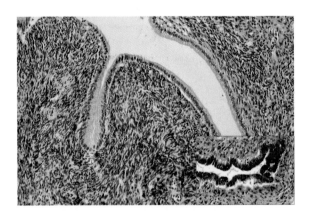

(c)

Plate 5.5.6 Chronic viral hepatitis: staging. (a) Chronic hepatitis with slighty activity. A thin fibrous septum extends from the portal tract seen to the right, but its precise geometry is not clearly seen in this H&E stain. (b) Portal tract in chronic hepatitis; sirius red stain. The portal tract is enlarged and deformed, caused by incipient septal fibrosis. (c) Portal tract in chronic hepatitis, chromoaniline blue stain. In this stain, blue septa, both incomplete and complete, are noted.

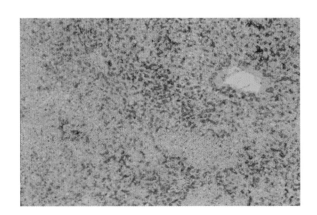

Plate 8.2.2.1(b) Cystadenoma: periodic acid–Schiff (PAS) mucus staining is shown in the lower right corner. See Fig. 1, p. 813 for part (a).

Plate 9.4.1 Dengue virus antigen in liver tissue visualized by immunohistochemical staining with anti-DEN polyclonal antibodies.

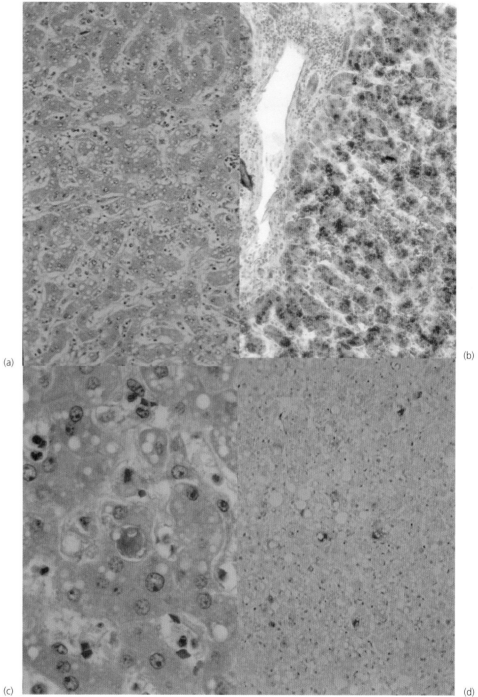

Plate 9.4.2 YF histological findings in the liver. (A) Midzonal necrosis, (B) oil-red positive staining for steatosis, (C) Councilman bodies and microvesicular steatosis, and (D) immunohistochemical staining of YF antigen.

(a)

(b)

(c)

(d)

2 Functions of the liver

2.1 Hepatic circulation

2.1.1 Regulation of hepatic blood flow

Christophe Bureau, Jean-Marie Péron and Jean-Pierre Vinel

Approximately 100 mL of blood passes through 100 g of liver every minute, which represents 25–30% of the cardiac output (CO). This very large flow is brought from two different sources:
• the hepatic artery provides roughly one-third of the blood and 50% of the oxygen delivered to the liver;
• the portal vein accounts for two-thirds of total hepatic blood flow (HBF) and 50% of hepatic oxygen supply. It drains blood from the spleen, the omentum and splanchnic organs, carrying to the liver most substances absorbed through the gut.

Significant changes in HBF are observed under physiological conditions. Thus, HBF decreases during sleeping and during exercise [1]; it increases after a meal [1]; it is enhanced during expiration and reduced by inspiration [2,3]. Finally, it diminishes as age increases [4].

In the normal liver, resistance to blood flow is low, with a pressure gradient below 5 mmHg between the portal vein and the hepatic veins. HBF is regulated through three different sites of resistance:
• terminal hepatic arterioles, richly supplied in smooth muscle cells, for arterial flow;
• arterioles of splanchnic organs for portal venous flow;
• sinusoids and terminal hepatic venules [5,6] for intrahepatic resistance, which influences both total HBF and flow distribution within the liver.

Changes in resistances, hence in HBF, are under the command of so-called 'intrinsic mechanisms', neural and humoral factors, and can be caused by drugs.

Intrinsic mechanisms

Pressure flow autoregulation

Within the physiological range of pressures, resistance is adapted so that blood flow through a vascular bed remains constant. This autoregulatory mechanism has been demonstrated in the hepatic artery, but not in the portal venous vascular bed. It has been suggested that perivascular smooth muscle cell tone changes as a response to stretching. This response could be mediated by adenosine [7].

Hepatic arterial buffer response

It has been shown almost a century ago [8] that occlusion of the portal vein induces an immediate increase in the blood flow to the hepatic artery. The hepatic artery is almost fully dilated at low portal flows, as evidenced by the inability of adenosine infusion to induce further dilatation; it is almost fully constricted at high portal flows, as shown by lack of further constriction to norepinephrine [9]. Such a compensatory mechanism cannot maintain total liver blood flow, but oxygenation of the liver parenchyma is generally considered to be improved by an increased efficiency of oxygen extraction [10,11]. Using different models of blood flow reduction in pigs, Bracht *et al.* [12] observed a 52% reduction in portal venous flow, which was associated with a 100% increase in hepatic arterial flow. However, hepatic oxygen extraction changed with the cause of decreased blood flow: it increased in a model of tamponade, but did not when abdominal flow was reduced [12]. In such conditions, hepatic oxygenation could therefore be compromised.

Several mechanisms could account for this autoregulation:
• changes in resistance in the terminal vessels in response to changes in sinusoidal pressure;
• changes in po_2, which might in turn change vascular resistance through a direct action on perivascular smooth muscle cells;
• changes in the concentration of vasoactive molecules secondary to changes in blood flow.

Accordingly, a fall in portal blood flow would induce an increase in the local concentration of vasodilators, which would in turn increase arterial blood flow. Conversely, an increase in portal flow would remove vasodilators, causing arterial vasoconstriction.

Experimental data support the role of adenosine in mediating this autoregulation. Intraportal injections of adenosine elicit hepatic arterial vasodilatation. Adenosine is released at a constant rate in the space of Mall, which contains the hepatic arterioles and portal venules, and its concentration is regulated by washout into these vessels, principally the portal vein. If flow in the portal vein is reduced, the concentration of adenosine rises, causing dilatation of the hepatic arteriole [13–15]. It has been shown in the rabbit [16] that 8-phenyltheophylline, an adenosine receptor antagonist, inhibited this response which, on the contrary, was potentiated by dipyridamole, an adenosine uptake inhibitor. Adenosine triphosphate (ATP) is also able to dilate the hepatic arterial vascular bed [16], at least in part through nitric oxide (NO) production [17]. A non-selective P_1-purinoreceptor antagonist [8-(p-sulphophenyl)-theophylline] has been found to inhibit the ATP-mediated arterial buffer response. These results suggest that hepatic artery dilatation induced by ATP is partly mediated through activation of P_1-purinoreceptors after catabolism of ATP to adenosine [16].

In patients with cirrhosis, hepatic artery vascular responsiveness to altered portal blood flow seems to be blunted [18]. However, this impairment in acute hepatic arterial buffer response (HABR) could be accounted for by the continuous activation of HABR, which has been observed in cirrhotic patients [19]. Accordingly, HABR seems to be preserved in cirrhosis and could play a protective role in hepatic circulation [20].

Such a buffer response has not been found in the portal vein. Actually, changes in hepatic arterial flow do not cause significant changes in the portal venous flow [14].

Veno-arterial response

Elevation of hepatic vein pressure induces an increase in hepatic arterial resistance and a decrease in arterial blood flow [21]. The precise mechanism of this response remains unknown.

It has also been shown that an increase in portal pressure increases resistance in the splanchnic vascular bed [22] which, in turn, tends to decrease portal venous inflow.

After a meal, total HBF increases, owing to enhanced mesenteric (hence portal) blood flow, but also hepatic arterial blood flow [23]. This suggests that autoregulation can be overcome by mechanisms as yet unknown. It could be due to the presence in the portal blood of substances with vasodilating properties on the hepatic artery, for example bile salts [24] and hormones such as glucagon or vasoactive inhibitory polypeptide (VIP) [25]. Furthermore, after a meal, po_2 tends to decrease, and pco_2, pH and osmolarity to increase in portal blood. All these changes have been shown to augment hepatic arterial blood flow [26].

Neural regulation

Hepatic denervation after liver transplantation has no major deleterious effects on HBF [27], which suggests that, in normal subjects, neural regulation probably plays little role in the regulation of HBF.

Parasympathetic nerves

Parasympathetic nerves play no major role in the regulation of HBF as neither denervation nor electrical stimulation of parasympathetic nerves nor drugs with anticholinesterase activity affect HBF [28]. However, hepatic vagal nerves could play a role in the distribution of blood flow within the liver by dilating sinusoids [29], thereby increasing the ratio of perfused to non-perfused sinusoids.

Sympathetic nerves

Denervation of the hepatic sympathetic nerves in urethane-anaesthetized rats has no influence on HBF, indicating that the sympathetic nerves have no tonic influence on HBF [28]. Their stimulation induces constriction of both arteries and, to a lesser extent, portal vessels [30]. This results in a decrease in HBF through activation of α-adrenergic receptors, as it can be prevented by treatment with phentolamine, an α-adrenoceptor antagonist [28].

Carneiro and Donald [31] showed an inverse relationship between carotid sinus pressure, on the one hand, and resistance in liver vessels, on the other hand, so that hypotension induces vasoconstriction of the hepatic arterial and portal systems. The maximum increase in resistance was 45% and 22% for the arterial and portal beds respectively. Because of vasoconstriction mediated through activation of both α_2-adrenergic receptors and the renin–angiotensin system, up to 40% of blood volume can be expelled from the liver into the systemic circulation without compromising liver function [32]. This phenomenon may play an important role in the control of haemodynamics because about 30% of the liver volume is blood, making this organ the major blood reservoir of the body.

The importance of liver innervation in the regulation of systemic haemodynamics is further exemplified by the interactions between portal blood flow and renal function. Actually, it has been shown in rats that a 50% decrease in intrahepatic portal flow decreased urine flow by 38% and sodium excretion by 44%, although systemic arterial blood pressure was not significantly changed [33]. This so-called 'hepatorenal reflex' (HRR) is mediated through activation of hepatic afferent nerves by adenosine, which results in a sympathetic reflex to the kidneys causing fluid retention. HRR is abolished by hepatic denervation. In cirrhotic rats exhibiting water and sodium retention, renal dysfunction was partially corrected by intrahepatic administration of 8-phenyltheophylline, an adenosine receptor antagonist [34]. HRR could therefore play a role in water and sodium retention observed in cirrhosis.

Humoral regulation

Secretin, cholecystokinin-pancreozymin (CCK-PZ) and glucagon [35] have a vasodilator effect on the hepatic artery and increase arterial blood flow. Furthermore, glucagon, at a dose too low to induce vasodilatation, antagonizes the vasoconstrictor response to several stimuli (such as sympathetic nerve stimulation or vasopressin infusion) [36]. It could therefore play a protective role in hepatic blood flow, when systemic conditions induce reduction of blood flow in most other territories [37]. Prostacyclin [38] and epinephrine at low doses [39] also have a vasodilator effect. In contrast, epinephrine at high doses [39], dopamine [40], norepinephrine [38], angiotensin [36] and vasopressin [41] reduce liver blood flow through vasoconstriction of splanchnic and hepatic arteries. The role of these humoral factors under physiological conditions remains to be determined. Animal studies suggest that histamine, angiotensin II as well as hepatic nerve stimulation induce constriction of hepatic venous sphincters, which could contribute to flow regulation and protect the liver from changes in central venous pressure.

NO plays a key role in the regulation of HBF. It increases splanchnic blood flow by its vasodilating action at the level of the mesenteric arterioles [42]. Furthermore, it increases flow within the sinusoids, and regulation of intrahepatic resistance is ascribed to a precise equilibrium between the production of NO, a potent vasodilator [43], and endothelin, a powerful vasoconstrictor [44]. This is achieved by contraction or relaxation of perisinusoidal stellate cells [43,45]. Carbon monoxide (CO), a byproduct of the breakdown of haem by haem oxygenase, could also play a role in smooth muscle relaxation [46]. In the normal rat, NO has been shown to be a potent vasodilatory mediator in the hepatic arterial circulation, although it had little effect in the portal venous vascular bed [47]. In the same set of experiments, CO was shown to have no effect on the hepatic artery, whereas it maintained portal venous vascular tone in a relaxed state [47].

An imbalance between increased endothelin production and a decrease in NO production, added to an exaggerated contractility of stellate cells, is considered to play a major role in the increased hepatic resistance that characterizes portal hypertension [48].

Effects of drugs

Several factors determine the effects of drugs on HBF:
- their action on blood pressure elicits baroreflex constriction or dilatation in the hepatic arterial bed, which tends to mask any direct effect on hepatic vasculature;
- interactions between arterial and portal flow regulation may hinder the specific effect of a drug on one of these flows;
- in human subjects, only total hepatic blood flow is measured, which may further obscure different changes in the hepatic arterial and the portal venous vascular beds.

Volatile anaesthetics can significantly alter hepatic perfusion. Halothane causes a dose-dependent decrease in portal venous blood flow, and hepatic arterial flow may decrease simultaneously [49].

β-Adrenergic stimulants such as isoproterenol, salbutamol and terbutaline cause intrahepatic arterial vasodilatation [50,51]. Dopamine has been found to induce hepatic arterial

vasodilatation and to increase HBF [52]. Angiotensin-converting enzyme (ACE) inhibitors, such as captopril, reduce HBF [53]. Calcium antagonists, such as nifedipine [54] or verapamil [55], have a direct vasodilating effect on the hepatic arterial bed, so that, in spite of a reduction in systemic arterial pressure, HBF is increased. Glyceryl trinitrate reduces HBF [54], probably through a reflex vasoconstrictor response to a decrease in blood pressure.

Finally, it is to be noted that ethanol has been shown to increase portal blood flow without changing hepatic arterial blood flow [56].

References

1 Hopkinson BR, Schenk WG Jr (1968) The electromagnetic measurement of liver blood flow and cardiac output in conscious dogs during feeding and exercise. *Surgery* 63, 970–975.
2 Horvath SM, Kelly T, Folk GE Jr *et al.* (1957) Measurement of blood volumes in the splanchnic bed of the dog. *Am J Physiol* 189, 573–575.
3 Moreno AH, Burchell AR, Van der Woude R *et al.* (1967) Respiratory regulation of splanchnic and systemic venous return. *Am J Physiol* 213, 455–465.
4 Wynne HA, Cope LH, Mutch E *et al.* (1989) The effect of age upon liver volume and apparent liver blood flow in healthy man. *Hepatology* 9, 297–301.
5 Lautt WW, Greenway CV, Legare DJ *et al.* (1986) Localization of intrahepatic portal vascular resistance. *Am J Physiol* 251, G375–G381.
6 Shah V, Haddad FG, Garcia-Cardena G *et al.* (1997) Liver sinusoidal endothelial cells are responsible for nitric oxide modulation of resistance in the hepatic sinusoids. *J Clin Invest* 100, 2923–2930.
7 Ezzat WR, Lautt WW (1987) Hepatic arterial pressure-flow autoregulation is adenosine mediated. *Am J Physiol* 252, H836–H845.
8 Burton-Opitz R (1911) The vascularity of the liver: the influence of the portal blood flow upon the flow in the hepatic artery. *Q J Exp Physiol* 4, 93–102.
9 Lautt MM, Dallas JL, Waleed RE (1990) Quantitation of the hepatic arterial buffer response to graded changes in portal blood flow. *Gastroenterology* 98, 1024–1028.
10 Llautt WW (1977) Hepatic vasculature: a conceptual review. *Gastroenterology* 73, 1163–1169.
11 Mathie RT, Blumgart LH (1983) The hepatic haemodynamic response to acute portal venous blood flow reductions in the dog. *Pflugers Arch* 399, 223–227.
12 Bracht H, Takala J, Tenhunen JJ *et al.* (2005) Hepatosplanchnic blood flow control and oxygen extraction are modified by the underlying mechanism of impaired perfusion. *Crit Care Med* 33, 645–653.
13 Lautt WW (1983) Relationship between hepatic blood flow and overall metabolism: the hepatic arterial buffer response. *Fed Proc* 42, 1662–1666.
14 Lautt WW, Legare DJ, d'Almeida MS (1985) Adenosine as putative regulator of hepatic arterial flow (the buffer response). *Am J Physiol* 248, H331–H338.
15 Lautt WW (1985) Mechanism and role of intrinsic regulation of hepatic arterial blood flow: hepatic arterial buffer response. *Am J Physiol* 249, G549–G556.
16 Browse DJ, Mathie RT, Benjamin IS *et al.* (2003) The role of ATP and adenosine in the control of hepatic blood flow in the rabbit liver in vivo. *Comp Hepatol* 2, 9.

17 Mathie RT, Ralevic V, Alexander B et al. (1991) Nitric oxide is the mediator of ATP-induced dilatation of the rabbit hepatic arterial vascular bed. Br J Pharmacol 103, 1602–1606.

18 Iwao T, Toyonaga A, Shigemori H et al. (1996) Hepatic artery hemodynamic responsiveness to altered portal blood flow in normal and cirrhotic livers. Radiology 200, 793–798.

19 Aoki T, Imamura H, Kaneko J et al. (2005) Intraoperative direct measurement of hepatic arterial buffer response in patients with or without cirrhosis. Liver Transpl 11, 684–691.

20 Richter S, Mucke I, Menger MD et al. (2000) Impact of intrinsic blood flow regulation in cirrhosis: maintenance of hepatic arterial buffer response. Am J Physiol Gastrointest Liver Physiol 279, G454–G462.

21 Hanson KM, Johnson PC (1966) Local control of hepatic arterial and portal venous flow in the dog. Am J Physiol 211, 712–720.

22 Mitzner W (1974) Effect of portal venous pressure on portal venous inflow and splanchnic resistance. J Appl Physiol 37, 706–711.

23 Katz ML, Bergman EN (1969) Simultaneous measurements of hepatic and portal venous blood flow in the sheep and dog. Am J Physiol 216, 946–952.

24 Mitchell GG, Torrance HB (1966) The effects of a bile-salt sodium dehydrocholate upon liver blood-flow in man. Br J Surg 53, 807–808.

25 Eriksson LS, Hagenfeldt L, Mutt V et al. (1989) Influence of vasoactive intestinal polypeptide (VIP) on splanchnic and central hemodynamics in healthy subjects. Peptides 10, 481–484.

26 Gelman S, Ernst EA (1977) Role of pH, PCO2 and O2 content of portal blood in hepatic circulatory autoregulation. Am J Physiol 233, E255–E262.

27 Colle I, Van Lierberghe H, Troisi R et al. (2004) Transplanted liver: consequence of denervation for liver functions. Anat Rec A Discov Mol Cell Evol Biol 280, 924–931.

28 Kurosawa M, Unno T, Aikawa Y et al. (2002) Neural regulation of hepatic blood flow in rats: an in vivo study. Neurosci Lett 321, 145–148.

29 Koo A, Liang IY (1979) Parasympathetic cholinergic vasodilator mechanism in the terminal liver microcirculation in rats. Q J Exp Physiol Cogn Med Sci 64, 149–159.

30 Greenway CV, Lawson AE, Mellander S (1967) The effects of stimulation of the hepatic nerves, infusions of noradrenaline and occlusion of the carotid arteries on liver blood flow in the anaesthetized cat. J Physiol 192, 21–41.

31 Carneiro JJ, Donald DE (1977) Change in liver blood flow and blood content in dogs during direct and reflex alteration of hepatic sympathetic nerve activity. Circ Res 40, 150–158.

32 Carneiro JJ, Donald DE (1977) Blood reservoir function of dog spleen, liver, and intestine. Am J Physiol 232, H67–H72.

33 Ming Z, Smyth DD, Lautt WW (2002) Decreases in portal flow trigger a hepatorenal reflex to inhibit renal sodium and water excretion in rats: role of adenosine. Hepatology 35, 167–175.

34 Ming Z, Lautt WW (2004) Reflex regulation by portal blood flow on renal function in healthy and cirrhotic rats: role of adenosine-A conceptual review. Proc West Pharmacol Soc 47, 33–34.

35 Richardson PD, Withrington PG (1977) The effects of glucagon, secretin, pancreozymin and pentagastrin on the hepatic arterial vascular bed of the dog. Br J Pharmacol 59, 147–156.

36 Richardson PD, Withrington PG (1976) The inhibition by glucagon of the vasoconstrictor actions of noradrenaline, angiotensin and vasopressin on the hepatic arterial vascular bed of the dog. Br J Pharmacol 57, 93–102.

37 Richardson PD, Withrington PG (1982) Physiological regulation of the hepatic circulation. Annu Rev Physiol 44, 57–69.

38 Hassan S, Pickles H (1983) Epoprostenol (prostacyclin, PGI2) increases apparent liver blood flow in man. Prostaglandins Leukotr Med 10, 449–454.

39 Richardson PD, Withrington PG (1979) Responses of the hepatic arterial and portal venous vascular beds of the dog to intra-arterial infusions of noradrenaline and adrenaline: inhibition of the hepatic arterial vasoconstrictor responses by intraportal infusions of glucagon. Br J Pharmacol 66, 82P.

40 Richardson PD, Withrington PG (1978) Responses of the canine hepatic arterial and portal venous vascular beds to dopamine. Eur J Pharmacol 48, 337–349.

41 Hanson KM (1970) Vascular response of intestine and liver to intravenous infusion of vasopressin. Am J Physiol 219, 779–784.

42 Kusayama T, Yamazaki J, Nagao T (1996) Flow dependence of nitric oxide-mediated pressure change in rat mesenteric beds with different tonus. Eur J Pharmacol 312, 301–307.

43 Mittal MK, Gupta TK, Lee FY et al. (1994) Nitric oxide modulates hepatic vascular tone in normal rat liver. Am J Physiol 26, G416–G422.

44 Zhang JX, Pegoli W Jr, Clemens MG (1994) Endothelin-1 induces direct constriction of hepatic sinusoids. Am J Physiol 266, G624–G632.

45 Kawada N, Tran-Thi TA, Klein H et al. (1993) The contraction of hepatic stellate (Ito) cells stimulated with vasoactive substances. Possible involvement of endothelin 1 and nitric oxide in the regulation of the sinusoidal tonus. Eur J Biochem 213, 815–823.

46 Suematsu M, Goda N, Sano T et al. (1995) Carbon monoxide: an endogenous modulator of sinusoidal tone in the perfused rat liver. J Clin Invest 96, 2431–2437.

47 Pannen BHJ, Bauer M (1998) Differential regulation of hepatic arterial and portal venous vascular resistance by nitric oxide and carbon monoxide in rats. Life Sci 62, 2025–2033.

48 Rockey DC (2003) Vascular mediators in the injured liver. Hepatology 37, 4–12.

49 Gatecel C, Losser MR, Payen D (2003) The postoperative effects of halothane versus isoflurane on hepatic artery and portal vein blood flow in humans. Anesth Analg 96, 740–745.

50 Hirsch LJ, Ayabe T, Glisk G (1976) Direct effects of various catecholamines on liver circulation in dogs. Am J Physiol 230, 1394–1399.

51 Richardson PDI, Withrington PG (1978) Pressure-flow relationships and effects of noradrenaline and isoprenaline on the hepatic arterial and portal venous vascular beds of the dog. J Physiol 282, 451–470.

52 Richardson PDI, Withrington PG (1978) Responses of the canine hepatic arterial and portal venous vascular beds to dopamine. Eur J Pharmacol 48, 337–349.

53 Crossley IR, Bihari D, Gimson AE et al. (1984) Effects of converting enzyme inhibitor on hepatic blood flow in man. Am J Med 76, 62–65.

54 Feely J (1984) Nifedipine increases and glyceryl trinitrate decreases apparent liver blood flow in normal subjects. Br J Pharmacol 17, 83–85.

55 Meredith PA, Elliot HL, Pasanisi F et al. (1985) Verapamil pharmacokinetics and apparent hepatic and renal blood flow. Br J Pharmacol 20, 101–106.

56 Kawasaki T, Carmichael FJ, Salvidia V et al. (1990) Relationship between portal venous and hepatic arterial blood flows: spectrum of response. Am J Physiol 259, G1010–G1018.

2.1.2 Hepatic microcirculation

Yoshiya Ito and Robert S. McCuskey

Hepatic circulation (see also Chapter 2.1.1)

The mammalian liver has a dual blood supply. Approximately 80% of the blood entering the liver is poorly oxygenated venous blood supplied by the portal vein, whereas the remainder is well oxygenated and supplied by the hepatic artery. These blood vessels enter at the hilus (porta hepatic), where efferent bile ducts as well as lymphatics also exit the organ. The venous drainage of the liver courses independently of the above structures to drain into the inferior vena cava near the diaphragm.

Within the liver, distributing branches of the portal vein and hepatic artery course in parallel and, after repeated branching, terminal branches of these vessels (portal venules and hepatic arterioles) supply blood to the hepatic sinusoids (Fig. 1). The sinusoids are the principal vessels involved in transvascular exchange between the blood and the parenchymal cells. Branches of hepatic arterioles also supply the capsule of the liver as well as the bile ducts, where they feed a peribiliary plexus of capillaries which, in turn, drains into the sinusoids. Portal and arterial blood flowing through the sinusoids is collected in small branches of the hepatic veins (central or terminal hepatic venules) through which the blood is returned through larger hepatic veins to the inferior vena cava (Fig. 1). Lymphatic vessels originate as blind-ending capillaries in the connective tissue spaces (portal tracts) associated with the portal veins and hepatic arteries (Fig. 1). The fluid contained in these lymphatics flows toward the hepatic hilus and eventually into the cisternae chyli.

Hepatic microvascular system

The hepatic microvascular system comprises all the intrahepatic vessels with internal diameters < 300 μm. It thus includes all blood and lymphatic vessels immediately involved in the delivery and removal of fluids to and from the hepatic parenchyma, namely portal venules, hepatic arterioles, sinusoids, central venules and lymphatics. The principal sites for regulating blood flow and solute exchange are in the sinusoidal network, which exhibits structural and functional heterogeneity. Although the factors that regulate blood flow through the hepatic microvascular system and their relation to hepatic structure and function are incompletely understood, perturbations of the hepatic microcirculation in many disease states results in alterations in the perfusion of the sinusoids, hepatic oxygenation and the exchange processes between the blood contained in the sinusoids and surrounding parenchymal cells [1–3].

Figure 1 illustrates the hepatic microvascular system: afferent and efferent microvascular connections to the sinusoids within a single hepatic lobule as determined principally by *in vivo* microscopic studies. Most blood enters the sinusoids from portal venules. These inlets are reported to be guarded by sphincters composed of sinusoidal lining cells termed the afferent or inlet sphincters (Fig. 1) [4–6]. Arterial blood enters some of the sinusoids, principally through branches of hepatic arterioles, arteriosinus twigs that terminate in sinusoids near their origins from portal venules (Fig. 1) [6–8]. In addition, occasional

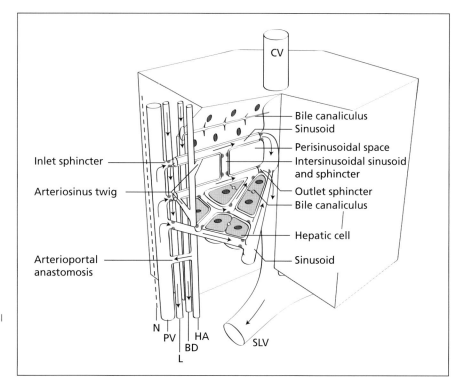

Fig. 1 Hepatic microvasculature as determined by *in vivo* microscopic studies over a period of more than 50 years [4–7]. PV, portal venule; HA, hepatic arteriole; L, lymphatic; BD, bile ductile; N, nerve; CV; central venule; SLV, sublobular hepatic venule. Arrows indicate direction of flow.

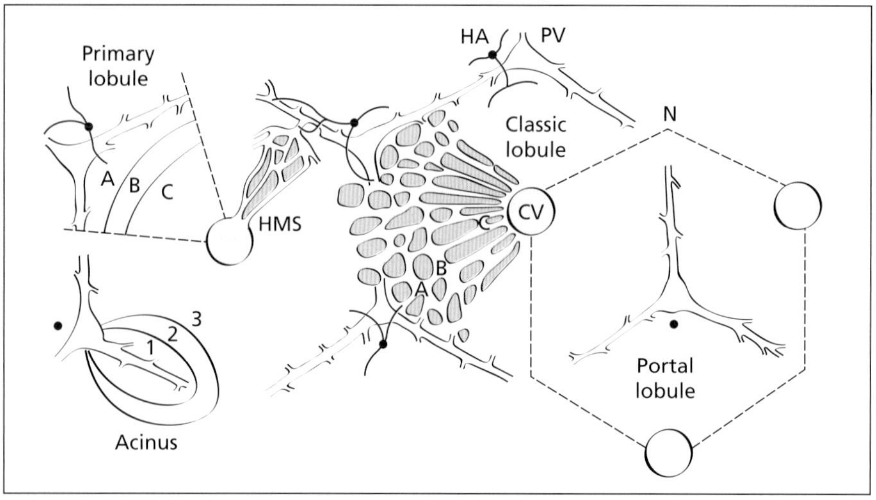

Fig. 2 Contiguous hepatic lobules illustrating the interconnecting network of sinusoids derived from two portal venules (PV). Note that the sinusoids become more parallel as they course towards the central venule (CV), which forms the axis of the classic lobule (centre). Hepatic arterioles (HA) supply blood to sinusoids near the periphery of the lobule, usually by terminating in inlet venules or terminal portal venules. As a result, three zones (1,2,3) of differing oxygenation and metabolism have been postulated by Rappaport [20] to comprise a hepatic acinus, with its axis being the portal tract (lower left). Several acini would comprise the portal lobule (lower right) described by Mall [61]. Matsumoto and Kawakami [14] proposed that each classic lobule contains several cone-shaped subunits with convex surfaces fed by portal and arterial blood at the periphery and with their apices at the central venule (upper left). A, B and C represent haemodynamically equipotential lines in a 'primary lobule'. Recently, a modification by Ekataksin *et al.* [15] further subdivided lobules into conical hepatic microcirculatory subunits (HMS), each being supplied by a single inlet venule.

direct connections (arterioportal anastomoses, APA) have been observed within the terminal portal venules [6,8]. The frequency of these APAs appears to be species dependent [8]. As all these structures are independently contractile, the sinusoids receive a varying mixture of portal venous and hepatic arterial blood [6,8]. Some evidence suggests that, between the hilus and periphery of hepatic lobes, the fraction of blood delivered to the sinusoids by the hepatic artery differs [9]. Finally, occasional branches of hepatic arterioles cross the lobule to supply capillaries in the walls of large hepatic veins [10].

The organization of the sinusoid network exhibits heterogeneity. Near portal venules and hepatic arterioles, sinusoids are arranged in interconnecting polygonal networks; further away from the portal venules, the sinusoids become organized as parallel vessels that terminate in central venules (terminal hepatic venules) (Fig. 2) [11–13]. Short intersinusoidal sinusoids connect adjacent parallel sinusoids (Figs 1 and 2) [6].

Blood leaving the sinusoids and flowing into the central venules passes through outlet or efferent sphincters composed of sinusoidal lining cells (Fig. 1) [6]. Sinusoidal lining cells are also reported to serve as sphincters within the sinusoid network and to regulate the distribution of blood flow in short segments of sinusoids [6].

Hepatic microvascular functional units

The organization of the hepatic microvasculature into structural or functional units related to liver function and disease has been the subject of some debate during the past century (Fig. 2) [2].

It should be noted, however, that none of the proposed concepts is mutually exclusive. Studies using three-dimensional reconstruction of sectioned livers, scanning electron microscopic examination of corrosion casts and *in vivo* microscopy of several species support the concept of the functional unit being a conical microvascular subunit of the classic lobule [14] (Fig. 2). Recently, these 'primary lobules' were renamed 'hepatic microvascular subunits (HMS)' and were demonstrated to consist of a group of sinusoids supplied by a single inlet venule and its associated termination of a branch of the hepatic arteriole from the adjacent portal space (Fig. 2) [15].

Morphological sites for regulating the hepatic microcirculation

There are several potential morphological sites for regulating blood flow through the sinusoids. These include the various segments of the afferent portal venules and hepatic arterioles, the sinusoids themselves, as well as central venules. These vessels contain several types of contractile cells.

Portal venules and central venules contain in their walls limited amounts of smooth muscle relative to their luminal size but, nevertheless, they are contractile and responsive to pharmacological agents. Hepatic arterioles are more responsive because of a complete investment of smooth muscle and relatively small lumina. The principal site of regulation of blood flow through the sinusoids, however, is thought to reside in the sinusoid itself, where the major blood pressure fall occurs in the liver [6,16]. *In vitro* primary culture studies and *in vivo* microscopic studies of the hepatic microcirculation have also identified the sinusoid as a principal site of regulation within normal and injured livers [3,17,18].

The structure of the hepatic sinusoids is mainly composed of endothelial cells, Kupffer cells and hepatic stellate cells. The sinusoidal endothelial and Kupffer cells are responsive to a wide variety of pharmacodynamic substances. By contracting (or swelling), they may selectively reduce the patency of the sinusoid lumen, thereby altering the rate and distribution of blood flow [6,19]. Evidence for sphincters at the inlet of sinusoids from portal venules and at the outlets of sinusoids into central venules was initially reported by a number of investigators using *in vivo* microscopy [4,5,7], but others failed to find any evidence for such sphincters [20]. Most methods, including electron microscopy, have failed to demonstrate either smooth muscle fibres or other contractile cells at these locations in healthy animals. Sinusoidal endothelial cells were subsequently identified by high-resolution *in vivo* microscopy to act as sphincters by swelling or contracting in response to vasoactive substances, thereby narrowing the sinusoidal lumen and limiting blood flow [6]. The relative role of Kupffer vs. endothelial cells in this process is not resolved, but both appear to be involved.

Recently, attention has focused on the hepatic stellate cell as the cell responsible for controlling sinusoidal diameter, being located in the space of Disse. Hepatic stellate cells possess extensively long, branching cytoplasmic processes, surrounding the sinusoidal wall [21]. These structural features of hepatic stellate cells are similar to pericytes in other organs, indicating that hepatic stellate cells are specialized pericytes in the liver. Hepatic stellate cells exhibit contractile properties, which have been demonstrated in *in vitro* primary culture systems [22–24] and in the perfused liver [17,18]. Both their anatomical location and contractility or relaxation in response to various vasoactive substances have led to the proposal that hepatic stellate cells serve to regulate the diameters and blood flow at the sinusoidal level.

As a result of these structures, blood flow through individual sinusoids is variable. At sites where the lumen is narrowed by the bulging, nuclear regions of sinusoidal lining cells, flow may be impeded by leukocytes that transiently plug the vessel and obstruct flow [25]. Transient leukocyte plugging is more frequent in the periportal sinusoids, which are narrower and more tortuous than those in the centrolobular region. The more plastic erythrocytes usually flow easily through such sites unless the lumen is reduced or near zero. Some sinusoids, however, may act as thoroughfare channels and have relatively constant rates of blood flow, while others have more intermittent flow [26]. This may depend not only on the distribution of intrasinusoidal sphincter cells but also on the distribution of arteriosinus twigs (AST) and the contribution of arterial blood flowing to individual sinusoids. For example, arterial blood flowing into an individual sinusoid through a dilated AST may increase the rate of sinusoidal blood flow [27]. Because of the delivery of arterial blood at higher pressure, some arterial blood may even reverse the entry of portal blood into the sinusoids. As a result, the AST,

in concert with the initial segment of the sinusoid in which it terminates, may form a 'functional' arterioportal anastomosis so that arterial blood is delivered into the portal venules [6,28]. In the anaesthetized healthy animal, however, terminal branches of the hepatic arteriole containing flow are seen infrequently so that most blood delivered to the sinusoids is derived from the portal venules [28]. Consistent with this is the *in vivo* microscopic observation that the velocity of flow in sinusoids as well as in portal and central venules located near the capsule of the liver is not significantly altered by hepatic arterial occlusion in healthy anaesthetized rats [29]. However, arterial inflow to the sinusoids may be more significant in regions near the hepatic hilum [9].

The frequency distribution of the wide variations in blood flow in the sinusoids exhibits a polymodal pattern composed of several Gaussian distributions [26]. These wide variations in flow are due to the structural features previously described for the sinusoids and also to intermittent arterial inflow into the sinusoids [6,27]. Blood pressure in portal and central venules has been measured to be about 6–7 cm H_2O and 1.5–3.0 cm H_2O respectively [16,17]. Arterial blood enters the sinusoid at pressures ranging from 12 to 25 cm H_2O [27].

Regulation of sinusoidal perfusion by vasoactive mediators

As mentioned previously, various sinusoidal lining cells including sinusoidal endothelial cells, Kupffer cells and hepatic stellate cells play a role in regulating the diameters of sinusoids and influencing the distribution and velocity of blood flow in these vessels [2,3,30]. Recently, hepatic stellate cells have received the most attention in the liver as the cell responsible for controlling the diameters of sinusoids [31,32]. A number of vasoactive substances have been reported to change intrahepatic vascular resistance by affecting the hepatic stellate cells. Among them are three vasoactive mediators, endothelin, nitric oxide and carbon monoxide, which contribute to the regulation of sinusoidal blood flow and will be discussed in this section. With respect to other mediators, including eicosanoids, cytokines and neural and humoral elements, see Chapter 2.2.5 and other reviews [2,32,33].

Endothelins (ETs)

Endothelin is a potent and longlasting vasoconstrictor. Hepatic stellate cell contractility in response to ET has been established in primary culture system [20–22]. *In vivo* microscopic studies have demonstrated that ET-1 narrows the lumens of sinusoids in isolated perfused livers [17], as well as in livers with intact afferent and efferent vessels [34]. The constricted sites of the sinusoids elicited by ET-1 are colocalized with the sites of hepatic stellate cells [17]. The active constriction of the sinusoids in response to ET-1 contributes to the reduction in sinusoidal perfusion and results in insufficient hepatic tissue oxygenation [34].

Two classes of ET receptors have been identified, namely the ET_A receptor subtype and ET_B receptor subtype. ET_A receptor, which is expressed on the vascular smooth muscle cells, mediates vasoconstriction. On the other hand, ET_B receptor, which is expressed on the endothelial cells, mediates vasodilatation through nitric oxide (NO) production. In the sinusoids of the liver, both ET_A and ET_B receptors are expressed. The ET_A receptor is expressed only on hepatic stellate cells and hepatocytes, whereas the ET_B receptor is expressed on all hepatic cell types including Kupffer cells, endothelial cells, hepatic stellate cells and hepatocytes. Of particular interest is that both ET_A and ET_B receptors are predominantly identified in the hepatic stellate cells [35]. In the intact liver, ET-1-induced vasoconstriction of the sinusoids is mediated by ET_A receptors, but not by ET_B receptors [36]. However, sinusoidal constriction in response to ET_B receptor agonist is revealed when endothelial nitric oxide synthase (eNOS) is inhibited simultaneously [37]. A critical balance between ETs and NO may be a determinant that regulates sinusoidal perfusion.

Some controversy exists regarding the principal site of ET-1-induced vasoconstriction within the normal liver, because ETs act not only on hepatic stellate cells but also on upstream preterminal portal venular smooth muscles and portal venular actin filaments [38]. In fact, the preterminal portal venules [39] or portal venules [40–42] constrict in response to ETs. This raises the question of whether or not the diameters of sinusoids may decrease as a result of passive recoil when inflow is reduced or eliminated and intrasinusoidal pressure falls. An in vivo microscopic study reported that clamping of the portal vein dramatically reduced sinusoidal blood flow in most sinusoids to near zero [30]. Then, the lumina of these vessels rapidly returned to their initial diameters upon restoration of portal blood flow. Thus, it appears that sinusoidal blood pressure normally distends the sinusoidal wall, which can recoil when the pressure drops. In the absence of elastic fibres in the space of Disse, it is likely that hepatic stellate cells are responsible for this reaction given the nature of their attachment to parenchymal cells by obliquely oriented microprojections from the lateral edges of their subendothelial processes [43].

In chronic liver diseases including fibrosis and cirrhosis, hepatic stellate cells are activated to transform into myofibroblasts, which are characterized by the expression of smooth muscle-type contractile proteins such as α-actin. The phenotypical changes in hepatic stellate cells as well as upregulation of a contractile intracellular signalling pathway enhance the contractile response of hepatic stellate cells to ETs [31,44]. In addition, upregulated expression of ET receptors [45] as well as decreased activity of eNOS [46] also contribute to the exacerbated response of hepatic stellate cells to ETs. Therefore, during chronic liver injury, hepatic stellate cells are thought to be responsible for the pathogenesis of increased intrahepatic vascular resistance.

In acute liver injury elicited by endotoxaemia and hepatic ischaemia/reperfusion [47,48], sinusoidal constriction in response to ET-1 is increased despite no evidence of phenotypical transformation of hepatic stellate cells. The mechanisms of increased response to ET during acute liver injury appear to be dependent on an increased expression of ET_B receptor together with disassociation of the ET_B receptor from activation of eNOS [3,37]. This disassociation is, at least in part, the result of over-expression and binding of caveolin-1 to eNOS. Increased response to ET occurring in the hepatic microcirculation reduces sinusoidal blood flow, leading to the development of ischaemia and the progression of injury.

Nitric oxide (NO)

The main biological effect of NO is relaxation of vascular smooth muscle cells, thereby reducing the vascular tone, through activation of soluble guanylate cyclase (sGC). In the liver, sinusoidal endothelial cells constitutively produce NO, which is synthesized by eNOS [46]. NO causes relaxation of isolated hepatic stellate cells in vitro [23]. Endogenous NO production in sinusoidal endothelial cells modulates the intrahepatic vascular resistance in the perfused liver [49,50] and regulates the sinusoidal diameters in the intact liver [51]. In addition to the vasodilative effect of NO, it also exerts a protective role in liver microcirculation by preventing leukocyte and platelet adhesion to the sinusoidal endothelium. However, several studies have shown that NO exhibits a minor vasodilatory effect on the sinusoids in the perfused liver [18] as well as in the intact liver [52]. The low level of biologically active NO in and around the sinusoids might not serve as a major endogenous modulator of sinusoidal vascular resistance in the normal liver [53]. Haemoglobulin in erythrocytes flowing through the sinusoids would rapidly trap NO released from the sinusoidal endothelial cells [54]. Rather, NO is thought to play an important role in regulating the sinusoidal vascular tone within the normal liver by counterbalancing the local vasoconstrictors such as ETs [37] and norepinephrine [49]. Thus, sinusoidal vascular tone appears to be maintained under the fine balance between vasoconstrictors and vasodilators. Conversely, an imbalance of NO and ETs contributes to changes in vascular tone characteristic of the disease process. In the cirrhotic liver, decreased activity of eNOS results in reduced generation of NO [46,50], and the vasodilative response to NO is impaired [55]. As a result, reduced bioavailability of hepatic NO in liver cirrhosis contributes to sinusoidal constriction and increased intrahepatic vascular tone [50]. The reduced production of hepatic NO in cirrhotic livers is attributed not only to upregulated expression of caveolin-1, an NOS inhibitory protein [56], but also to a decrease in eNOS activator, Akt, and phosphorylation of eNOS [57].

Carbon monoxide (CO)

CO has been considered a gaseous mediator analogous to NO. Like NO, CO serves as an endogenous factor that keeps sinusoids in a relaxed state [58]. In the perfused liver, endogenously generated CO from the haem oxygenase (HO) reaction serves as a vasorelaxant to the hepatic sinusoids. The principal sites of action of CO in the hepatic sinusoids colocalize with the hepatic stellate cells [18]. Isolated hepatic stellate cells are relaxed by CO *in vitro* [18]. The mechanism by which CO maintains the low vascular tone of the sinusoids appears to involve sGC-mediated relaxation of hepatic stellate cells.

CO is produced by HO, which is an enzyme responsible for the degradation of protohaem IX to form biliverdin, free divalent ion (Fe^{2+}) and CO. HO mainly exists as two isoforms, HO-1 and HO-2. In the liver, HO-1 is induced ubiquitously among all types of hepatic cells by stressors, but prominently in Kupffer cells, whereas HO-2 is constitutively expressed on hepatocytes [54]. It is likely that CO constitutively generated by HO-2 in hepatocytes maintains sinusoidal blood flow under ordinary conditions. Considering the anatomical orientation of the hepatic parenchymal cells in and around the sinusoids, HO-2 in parenchymal cells is positioned where CO released by HO-2 can directly access the hepatic stellate cells to modulate their contractility without being captured by haemoglobulin in the circulation [54]. However, in the innervated liver *in vivo*, CO appears to exhibit a minimal vasodilatory effect on the sinusoids [59]. The sinusoidal blood flow *in vivo* is finely regulated and is affected by various factors including neural and humoral regulation, the hepatic arteriolar inflowing and the haemodynamics from the splanchnic circulation. Instead, in the stressed liver, CO overproduced by HO-1 appears to be necessary to protect the liver microcirculation [48,59,60]. Under stressed conditions in the liver, the HO/CO system counterbalances the vasoconstrictive effect of ET-1 to regulate sinusoidal vascular tone [59,60].

References

1 McCuskey RS (1993) Functional morphology of the liver with emphasis on microvasculature. In: Tavoloni N, Berk PD (eds) *Hepatic Transport and Bile Secretion*. New York: Raven Press, pp. 1–10.

2 McCuskey RS (1994) The hepatic microvascular system. In: Arias IM, Boyer JL, Fausto N *et al.* (eds) *The Liver: Biology and Pathobiology*, 3rd edn. New York: Raven Press, pp. 1089–1106.

3 Clemens MG, Zhang JX (1999) Regulation of sinusoidal perfusion: in vivo methodology and control by endothelins. *Semin Liver Dis* 19, 383–396.

4 Bloch EH (1955) The *in vivo* microscopic vascular anatomy and physiology of the liver as determined by the quartz-rod method of transillumination. *Angiology* 6, 340–349.

5 Knisely MH, Harding F, Debacker H (1957) Hepatic sphincters. *Science* 125, 1023–1026.

6 McCuskey RS (1966) A dynamic and static study of hepatic arterioles and hepatic sphincters. *Am J Anat* 119, 455–487.

7 Irwin JW, MacDonald J (1953) Microscopic observation of the intrahepatic circulation in the guinea pigs. *Anat Rec* 117, 1–15.

8 Bloch EH (1970) The termination of hepatic arterioles and the functional unit of the liver as determined by microscopy of the living organ. *Ann NY Acad Sci* 170, 78–87.

9 Conway JG, Popp JA, Thurman RG (1985) Microcirculation in periportal and pericentral regions of lobule in perfused rat liver. *Am J Physiol* 249, G449–G456.

10 Ekataksin W (2000) The isolated artery: an intrahepatic arterial pathway that can bypass the lobular parenchyma in mammalian livers. *Hepatology* 31, 269–279.

11 Hase T, Brim J (1966) Observation of the microcirculatory architecture of the rat liver. *Anat Rec* 156, 157–174.

12 Kardon RH, Kessel RG (1980) Three-dimensional organization of the hepatic microcirculation in the rodent as observed by scanning electron microscopy of corrosion casts. *Gastroenterology* 79, 72–81.

13 Wisse E, DeZanger RB, Jacobs R *et al.* (1983) Scanning electron microscopic observations on the structure of portal veins, sinusoids, and central veins. *Scanning Electron Microsc* 3, 1441–1452.

14 Matsumoto T, Kawakami M (1982) The unit-concept of hepatic parenchyma – a re-examination based on angio architectural studies. *Acta Pathol Jap* 32, 285–314.

15 Ekataksin W, Zou Z, Wake K *et al.* (1995) HMS, hepatic microcirculatory subunits in mammalian species: intralobular 'grouping' of liver tissue with definition enhanced by the 'drop-out' sinusoids. In: Wisse E, Knook DL, Wake K (eds) *Cells of the Hepatic Sinusoids*, Vol. 5. Leiden: Kupffer Cell Foundation, pp. 247–251.

16 Nakata K, Leong GF, Brauer RW (1960) Direct measurement of blood pressures in minute vessels of the liver. *Am J Physiol* 199, 1181–1188.

17 Zhang JX, Pegoli W, Clemens MG (1994) Endothelin-1 induced direct constriction of hepatic sinusoids. *Am J Physiol* 266, G624–G632.

18 Suematsu M, Goda N, Sano T *et al.* (1995) Carbon monoxide: an endogenous modulator of sinusoidal tone in the perfused rat liver. *J Clin Invest* 96, 2431–2437.

19 Nakata K (1967) Microcirculation and hemodynamical analysis of the blood circulation in the liver. *Acta Pathol Jap* 17, 361–376.

20 Rappaport AM (1973) The microcirculatory hepatic unit. *Microvasc Res* 6, 212–228.

21 Wake K (1980) Peri-sinusoidal stellate cells (fat-storing cells, interstitial cells, lipocytes), their related structure in and around the liver sinusoids, and vitamin A-storing cells in extrahepatic organs. *Int Rev Cytol* 66, 303–353.

22 Pinzani M, Failli P, Ruocco C *et al.* (1992) Fat-storing cells as liver-specific pericytes: special dynamics of agonist-stimulated intracellular calcium transients. *J Clin Invest* 90, 642–646.

23 Kawada N, Tran-Thi TA, Klein H *et al.* (1993) The contraction of hepatic stellate (Ito) cells stimulated with vasoactive substances. Possible involvement of endothelin 1 and nitric oxide in the regulation of the sinusoidal tonus. *Eur J Biochem* 213, 815–822.

24 Rockey DC, Housset CN, Friedman SL (1993) Activation-dependant contractility of rat hepatic lipocytes in culture and *in vivo*. *J Clin Invest* 92, 1795–1804.

25 Wisse E, DeZanger RB, Jacobs R *et al.* (1985) The liver sieve: consideration concerning the structure and function of endothelial fenestrae, the sinusoid wall and the space of Disse. *Hepatology* 5, 683–692.

26 Koo A (1987) Nervous control of the hepatic microcirculation. In: Tsuchiya M, Asano M, Mishima Y (eds) *Microcirculation – an Update*, Vol. 2. Amsterdam: Excerpta Medica, pp. 335–338.

27 Rappaport AM (1977) Microcirculatory units in the mammalian liver. *Bibl Anat* 16, 116–120.

28 McCuskey RS, Vonnahme FJ, Grun M (1983) In vivo microscopic and electron microscopic observations of the hepatic microvascular system following portacaval anastomosis. *Hepatology* 3, 96–104.

29 Koo A, Liang IYS, Cheng K (1976) Effect of the ligation of the hepatic artery on the microcirculation in the cirrhotic liver in the rat. *Aust J Exp Biol Med Sci* 54, 287–295.

30 McCuskey RS (2000) Morphological mechanisms for regulating blood flow through hepatic sinusoids. *Liver* 20, 3–7.

31 Reynaert H, Thompson MG, Thomas T *et al.* (2002) Hepatic stellate cells: role in microcirculation and pathophysiology of portal hypertension. *Gut* 50, 571–581.

32 Rockey DC (2003) Vascular mediators in the injured liver. *Hepatology* 37, 4–12.

33 Ueno T, Bioulac-Sage P, Balabaud C *et al.* (2004) Innervation of the sinusoidal wall: regulation of the sinusoidal diameter. *Anat Rec* 280A, 868–873.

34 Okumura S, Takei Y, Kawano S *et al.* (1994) Vasoactive effect of endtothelin-1 on rat liver *in vivo. Hepatology* 19, 155–161.

35 Housset C, Rockey DC, Bissell DM (1993) Endothelin receptors in rat liver: lipocytes as a contractile target for endothelin 1. *Proc Natl Acad Sci USA* 90, 9266–9270.

36 Zhang JX, Bauer M, Clemens MG (1995) Vessel and target cell specific actions of endothelin-1 and endothelin-3 in rat liver. *Am J Physiol* 269, G269–G277.

37 Bauer M, Bauer I, Sonin NV *et al.* (2000) Functional significance of endothelin B receptors in mediating sinusoidal and extrasinusoidal effects of endothelins in the intact rat liver. *Hepatology* 31, 937–947.

38 Oda M, Tsukada N, Honda K *et al.* (1987) Hepatic sinusoidal endothelium – its functional implications in the regulation of sinusoidal blood flow. In: Tsuchiya M, Asano M, Mishima Y *et al.* (eds) *Microcirculation – an Update*, Vol. 2. Amsterdam: Excerpta Medica, pp. 317–320.

39 Kaneda K, Ekataksin W, Sogawa M *et al.* (1998) Endothelin-1-induced vasoconstriction causes a significant increase in portal pressure of rat liver: localized constrictive effect on the distal segment of preterminal portal venules as revealed by light and electron microscopy and serial reconstruction. *Hepatology* 27, 735–747.

40 Bauer M, Zhang JX, Bauer I *et al.* (1994) ET-1 induced changes in the hepatic microcirculation: sinusoidal and extrasinusoidal sites of action. *Am J Physiol* 267, G143–G149.

41 Ito Y, Katori M, Majima M *et al.* (1996) Constriction of mouse hepatic venules and sinusoids by endothelins through ETB receptor subtype. *Int J Microcirc Clin Exp* 16, 250–258.

42 Oda M, Yokomori H, Han JY (2003) Regulatory mechanisms of hepatic microcirculation. *Clin Hemorheol Microcirc* 29, 167–182.

43 Wake K (1996) Sinusoidal structure and dynamics. In: Vidal-Vanaclocha F (ed.) *Functional Heterogeneity of Liver Tissue: from Cell Lineage Diversity to Sublobular Compartment-specific Pathogenesis.* Austin, TX: R.G. Landes Co., pp. 57–67.

44 Rockey DC, Weisiger RA (1996) Endothelin induced contractility of stellate cells from normal and cirrhotic rat liver: implication for regulation of portal pressure and resistance. *Hepatology* 24, 233–240.

45 Leivas A, Jimenez W, Bruix J *et al.* (1998) Gene expression of endothelin-1 and ET(A) and ET(B) receptors in human cirrhosis: relationship with hepatic hemodynamics. *J Vasc Res* 35, 186–193.

46 Rockey DC, Chung JJ (1998) Reduced nitric oxide production by endothelial cells in cirrhotic rat liver: endothelial dysfunction in portal hypertension. *Gastroenterology* 114, 344–351.

47 Pannen BH, Bauer M, Zhang JX *et al.* (1996) A time-dependent balance between endothelins and nitric oxide regulating portal resistance after endotoxin. *Am J Physiol* 271, H1953–H1961.

48 Pannen BH, Al-Adili F, Bauer M *et al.* (1998) Role of endothelins and nitric oxide in hepatic reperfusion injury in the rat. *Hepatology* 27, 755–764.

49 Mittal MK, Gupta TK, Lee FY *et al.* (1994) Nitric oxide modulates hepatic vascular tone in normal rat liver. *Am J Physiol* 267, G416–G422.

50 Shah V, Haddad FG, Garcia-Caidena G *et al.* (1997) Liver sinusoidal endothelial cells are responsible for nitric oxide modulation of resistance in the hepatic sinusoids. *J Clin Invest* 100, 2923–2930.

51 Bauer C, Walcher F, Kalweit U *et al.* (1997) Role of nitric oxide in the regulation of the hepatic microcirculation *in vivo. J Hepatol* 27, 1089–1095.

52 Nishida J, McCuskey RS, McDonnell D *et al.* (1994) Protective role of NO in hepatic microcirculatory dysfunction during endotoxemia. *Am J Physiol* 267, G1135–G1141.

53 Suematsu M, Wakabayashi Y, Ishimura Y (1996) Gaseous monoxides: a new class of microvascular regulator in the liver. *Cardiovasc Res* 32, 679–686.

54 Goda N, Suzuki K, Naito M *et al.* (1998) Distribution of heme oxygenase isoforms in rat liver. Topographic basis for carbon monoxide-mediated microvascular relaxation. *J Clin Invest* 101, 604–612.

55 Dudenhoefer AA, Loureiro-Silva MR, Cadelina GW *et al.* (2002) Bioactivation of nitroglycerin and vasomotor response to nitric oxide are impaired in cirrhotic rat livers. *Hepatology* 36, 381–385.

56 Shah V, Toruner M, Haddad F *et al.* (1999) Impaired endothelial nitric oxide synthase activity associated with enhanced caveolin binding in experimental cirrhosis in the rat. *Gastroenterology* 117, 1222–1228.

57 Morales-Ruiz M, Cejudo-Martn P, Fernandez-Varo G *et al.* (2003) Transduction of the liver with activated Akt normalizes portal pressure in cirrhotic rats. *Gastroenterology* 125, 522–531.

58 Suematsu M, Kashiwagi S, Sano T *et al.* (1994) Carbon monoxide as an endogenous modulator of hepatic vascular perfusion. *Biochem Biophys Res Commun* 205, 1333–1337.

59 Rensing H, Bauer I, Zhang JX *et al.* (2002) Endothelin-1 and heme oxygenase-1 as modulators of sinusoidal tone in the stress-exposed rat liver. *Hepatology* 36, 1453–1465.

60 Wakabayashi Y, Takamiya R, Mizuki A *et al.* (1998) Carbon monoxide overproduced by heme oxygenase-1 causes a reduction of vascular resistance in perfused rat liver. *Am J Physiol* 277, G1088–G1096.

61 Mall FP (1906) A study of the structural unit of the liver. *Am J Anat* 5, 227–308.

2.1.3 Hepatic lymph and lymphatics

Glen A. Laine and Charles S. Cox Jr

Basic lymphatic biophysics

Lymphatic vessels are found throughout the body, developing embryologically from the venous system. Lymphatics are thin-walled vessels lined by endothelium and, with the exception of initial or collecting lymphatics, they are surrounded by lymphatic smooth muscle. A series of valves divides segments of lymphatic vessels into 'lymphangions', the operational unit of the lymphatic system. Lymphatic valves ensure unidirectional flow of lymph from the periphery of the body and organ systems

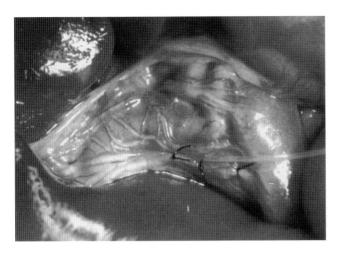

Fig. 1 Photograph of the liver (on the left) covered with ascites fluid The portal vein runs across the field flowing from right to left into the liver. A large number of translucent lymphatics are seen exiting the liver at the hilus, coursing over the portal vein and flowing from left to right in the photograph. Lymphatic valves can be seen as points of constriction in some of lymphatic vessels. One of the large lymphatics in the photograph has been cannulated for the purposes of lymph collection. The lymphatic catheter is tied in place with lengths of black suture. A large lymph node can be seen at the right of the photograph. See also Plate 2.1.3.1, facing p. 72.

to the central venous circulation. Lymph nodes are located at various points along lymphatic vessels. Lymphatics serve three major functions: (i) removal of oedema fluid from all body systems; (ii) transport of lipids from the gastrointestinal lacteals to the central venous circulation; and (iii) transportation of antigens to lymph nodes for processing and formation of sensitized lymphocytes, which are also returned to the central venous circulation. Lymphatics serve to maintain normal interstitial fluid volume, normal fat metabolism and a normal immune system.

Figure 1 (see also Plate 2.1.3.1, facing p. 72) shows a photograph of the liver (on the left) covered by ascites fluid. The portal vein runs across the field flowing from right to left into the liver. A large number of translucent lymphatics are seen exiting the liver at the hilus, coursing over the portal vein and flowing from left to right in the photograph. Lymphatic valves can be seen as points of constriction in some of the lymphatic vessels. One of the large lymphatics in this photograph has been cannulated for the purposes of lymph collection. The lymphatic catheter is tied in place with lengths of black suture. A large lymph node can be seen at the right of the photograph.

The hepatic lymphatic system is quite unique, generating approximately 75% of total body lymph. Approximately 80% of hepatic lymph exits the liver via the hilar lymphatics, then enters the cisterna chyli. The remaining 20% of lymph flows through lymphatics along the hepatic veins. The hepatic sinusoids (also referred to as hepatic capillaries) are very permeable to plasma proteins with pores of approximately 100–200 μm or larger opening from the sinusoids into the hepatic interstitium or 'space of Disse' [1]. The 'reflection coefficient' is a term used to describe the permeability of capillaries to plasma proteins.

The reflection coefficient ranges from 0 to 1, with 0 describing a system totally permeable to plasma proteins (e.g. the liver) and a reflection coefficient of 1 being a capillary bed totally impermeable to protein (e.g. the brain). As the hepatic sinusoids or capillaries have a reflection coefficient of near 0, plasma, along with a full complement of plasma proteins and clotting factors, moves freely from the hepatic vasculature into the space of Disse and is collected by the hepatic lymphatics [2]. This also explains the well-documented ability of hepatic lymph to clot.

Should the liver develop excess interstitial fluid volume, it is one of the few organs that can move this excess fluid across the Glisson's capsule as a transudate, resulting in ascites. As plasma proteins cross the sinusoids without restriction, there is some controversy as to why hepatic lymph and hepatic ascites fluid is not identical to circulating plasma. Sieving of proteins at another barrier such as the hepatic interstitium or Glisson's capsule could explain this phenomenon.

In pathological conditions causing increased sinusoidal pressures and overproduction of interstitial fluid, the liver can alter sinusoidal permeability, increasing the sinusoidal reflection coefficient by decreasing the size of sinusoidal openings into the space of Disse. This change in hepatic sinusoidal permeability is secondary to collagen deposition or fibrosis, i.e. sinusoidal capillarization [3,4]. Unfortunately, decreasing the size of pores from the sinusoids into the hepatic interstitium limits the movement of antigenic material into the hepatic interstitium and, ultimately, into the lymphatic system, thus minimizing exposure of the lymph nodes to antigens and compromising the immune response. This is of particular importance in the liver because the portal blood from the intestine may carry pathogens or other antigenic material from the intestine, which can be caught by Kupffer cells and broken down for potential delivery to lymph nodes, thus stimulating lymphocyte production. It should be pointed out that pathogens or toxic substances may also reach the circulation via the lymphatic system. New techniques for cannulating the lymphatics from various organs, particularly the intestine, and shunting the lymph to the outside of the body removes these toxic substances, particularly in trauma patients, thus minimizing secondary organ damage [5]. These cannulation techniques should be applied with caution as shunting lymph to the exterior of the body can have several negative consequences. In particular, excessive fluid volume may be lost, plasma proteins can be depleted, thus reducing plasma colloid osmotic pressure, and patients may become immunologically compromised secondary to removal of lymphocytes. Mechanically separating and reinfusing lymphocytes can overcome immune issues, while intravenous volume infusion, including concentrated albumin, will address fluid volume and colloid osmotic pressure issues.

Lymphatic contractions

Lymphatics throughout the body and in the liver have additional unique characteristics not found in other vessels. Lymphatics are

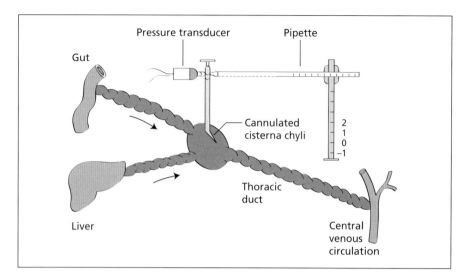

Fig. 2 Schematic representation of the liver and gut lymphatic system. Liver and gut lymph both flow into the cisterna chyli, through the thoracic duct and into the central venous circulation. Lymphatic valves prevent retrograde lymph flow.

capable of rhythmic contractions similar to the heart, yet respond to preload or stretch like smooth muscle. Lymph can thus be propelled forwards by either external compression or rhythmic contractions of the lymphatics, with valves ensuring unidirectional flow. The lymphatic pump has finite capabilities: much as the heart cannot overcome very high afterloads, the lymphatic system cannot overcome central venous pressures at their physiological extremes. The importance of lymph being able to respond to elevated outflow pressures including lymphatic obstructions or elevated central venous pressure cannot be overemphasized. Lymphatics can employ the standard mechanisms or techniques used by muscles to generate greater force of contraction and more flow, including hypertrophy and increasing contraction frequency. Bypassing lymphatic obstructions by growing new lymphatic vessels is often observed. When central venous pressure is elevated throughout the body, growing new lymphatics or 'lymphangiogenesis' is of no significant value as all new lymphatic vessels will be presented with elevated outflow pressures no matter where they enter the venous circulation.

Importance of central venous pressure

To demonstrate the importance of maintaining a low central venous pressure to ensure normal lymph flow and decrease the chances of oedema formation and organ dysfunction, a simple experiment was performed. As seen in the schematic Figure 2, lymph from both the liver and the gut flows into the cisterna chyli. Lymph then enters the thoracic duct and returns to the subclavian vein or central venous circulation. Introducing a fluid-filled catheter into a lymphatic – taking care not to cause obstruction – we can measure fluid flow into or out of the cisterna chyli. The fluid-filled and calibrated pipette may be raised or lowered to adjust the outflow pressure experienced by the lymphatic system. The hydrostatic zero is set at the point of cisterna chyli cannulation. In Figure 3, flow from the cisterna chyli

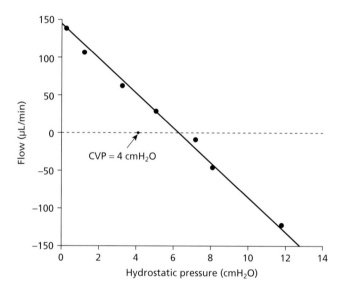

Fig. 3 Flow through the calibrated pipette (μL/min) plotted as a function of the hydrostatic pressure head (cmH$_2$O) developed by elevating the pipette connected to the cisterna chyli. Low central venous pressure (CVP) model, 4 cmH$_2$O.

through the pipette (μL/min) was recorded as hydrostatic pressure was increased (cmH$_2$O). As pipette height – and thereby outflow pressure – is increased, flow from the lymphatic system decreases. When the hydrostatic pressure head in the elevated pipette overcomes cisterna chyli pressure, flow in the pipette reverses direction and begins flowing into the lymphatic system. The contents of the pipette along with lymph from the liver and intestine then flow together into the thoracic duct and central veins. This is a scenario for a normal or low central venous pressure of approximately 4 cmH$_2$O. Figure 4 presents data from the same system in which central venous pressure has been elevated to 14 cmH$_2$O. Again, as pipette height is elevated, flow into the pipette from the cisterna chyli decreases until flow stops. At this

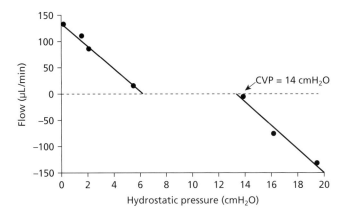

Fig. 4 Flow through the calibrated pipette (μL/min) plotted as a function of hydrostatic pressure head (cmH$_2$O) generated secondary to pipette elevation with an elevated central venous pressure (CVP) of 14 cmH$_2$O. Note the decrease and then cessation of flow prior to elevated driving pressure becoming greater than CVP. Decreased or arrested lymph flow must accumulate as oedema or ascites fluid.

point, the force driving lymph from the liver and gut cannot overcome the hydrostatic pressurehead of the catheter and pipette and cannot overcome central venous pressure. Further elevation of the pipette results in a state of no lymph flow until the hydrostatic pressure within the catheter and pipette reaches the same level as the central venous pressure, in this case 14 cmH$_2$O. At this time, flow from the pipette into the cisterna chyli, thoracic duct and central venous circulation begins. Retrograde flow into the liver and the gut is prevented by unidirectional valves. This experiment was performed to demonstrate the critical role that central venous pressure plays in maintaining lymph flow and minimizing oedema and ascites formation. This is particularly important in patients receiving large-volume fluid resuscitations or vasoactive drugs, which can increase central venous pressure. It should be pointed out that the hepatic vasculature is also highly sensitive to central venous pressure elevation as there is no restriction for fluid movement from the sinusoids into the hepatic interstitium. Any change in venous outflow pressure results in large fluid fluxes from the hepatic circulation into the hepatic interstitium and lymphatic vessels.

We should also point out the concept of 'lymphatic interaction'. When lymphatics from two or more organs converge, lymphatic interaction takes place. Some organs are capable of producing larger lymph flows at higher driving pressures, while others produce small volumes of lymph at low driving pressures. For example, the lymph from the liver and gut converges in the cisterna chyli. As the liver can generate a greater lymph driving pressure and volume lymph flow, lymph flow from the intestine can be compromised because of its lower driving pressure. A study by Stewart and Laine [6] clearly demonstrated that an increase in liver lymph flow can reduce gut lymph flow, through hepatic lymphatic interaction, thus potentiating gut oedema. This mechanism could potentially potentiate oedema in the

spleen, pancreas and gallbladder or any other organ system with lymph entering the cisterna chyli when the liver is producing large volumes of lymph.

Clinical conditions impacting on hepatic fluid balance and lymphatic function

Factors that affect fluid balance within the hepatoportal circulation include intra- and extrahepatic venous outflow obstruction. Intrahepatic diseases/conditions such as cirrhosis and schistosomiasis cause portal venous hypertension and an alteration in intestinal microvascular fluid balance. Extrahepatic processes include the Budd–Chiari syndrome, constrictive pericarditis/right heart failure and the abdominal compartment syndrome (which is both a cause and an effect of altered hepatoportal fluid flux). To discuss these specific entities, it is useful to consider how intra-abdominal physical forces affect hepatoportal lymph flow.

Extrahepatic causes of increased hepatoportal microvascular fluid flux

Budd–Chiari syndrome

The Budd–Chiari syndrome can be the cause of hepatoportal venous hypertension resulting from hepatic vein obstruction. Hepatic venous obstruction leaves no route for egress of hepatic arterial and portal venous inflow. Hepatic congestion, ascites and portal hypertension result. The extent and rapidity of occlusion determine the clinical presentation.

Abdominal compartment syndrome

The abdominal compartment syndrome (ACS) is defined as the combination of (i) intra-abdominal pressure greater than 25 mmHg, (ii) progressive organ dysfunction and (iii) improved organ dysfunction after decompression. Primary ACS is a complication of damage control laparotomy for trauma. The space-occupying nature of abdominal packs together with ongoing bleeding and progressive bowel oedema all contribute to increased intra-abdominal pressure (IAP). Primary ACS can occur in patients who fail non-operative management of abdominal solid organ injuries because of ongoing bleeding either within the abdominal cavity or into the retroperitoneum. Secondary ACS is the development of increased IAP due to resuscitation-induced bowel oedema and ascites. We have shown that alterations in hepatoportal lymph flow are critical in the pathophysiology of both syndromes. In a series of experiments, we demonstrated that abrupt elevation in IAP, as with primary ACS, stopped lymph flow through the cisterna chyli. In contrast, with secondary ACS, lymph flow via the cisterna chyli is increased as the result of an increased lymph driving pressure that exceeds the lymphatic outflow (intra-abdominal) pressure. However, the increase in lymph flow is not sufficient to prevent the development of gut oedema and ascites.

Pathophysiology of extrahepatic causes of increased hepatoportal fluid flux

Internal occlusion of the hepatic veins/suprahepatic inferior vena cava or external compression of the abdominal venous outflow due to ACS serve to increase microvascular filtration across the liver and intestinal microcirculation. Elk *et al.* [7] studied lymphatic function in the liver after hepatic venous pressure elevation. Using a model that measured lymph flow and lymphatic driving pressure, the effects of venous pressure elevation could be studied. Their studies showed that small increases in hepatic venous pressure substantially increased liver lymph flow. The increased liver lymph flow was associated with both increased effective lymphatic driving pressure and decreased effective resistance to lymph flow. One reason why the liver is exceptionally sensitive to any increase in venous pressure is that the hepatic sinusoids are almost freely permeable to protein. Therefore, the plasma protein osmotic pressure opposing fluid filtration from the microvessels is ineffective in opposing fluid filtration from the sinusoids. Two other considerations affect hepatoportal lymph flow/fluid flux: ascites formation and hepatic–intestinal lymphatic interactions. Microvascular fluid flux that overwhelms the ability to maintain fluid balance in the liver results not only in organ congestion/oedema but also in transudation of fluid into the abdominal cavity as ascites. When this occurs in large volumes, further extrahepatic compression of the venous outflow may occur. The lymphatic vessels that drain the intestine and liver empty into the cisterna chyli and, from there, into the thoracic duct. Therefore, pressure within the cisterna chyli is outflow pressure for both hepatic and intestinal lymphatics. The finding that elevating lymphatic outflow pressure to an organ undergoing increased microvascular filtration has a marked oedemagenic effect is important. Increasing hepatic lymph flow serves to increase pressure within the cisterna chyli to 6 mmHg. With moderately increased portal vein pressures, intestinal lymph flow increased, but the elevated cisterna chyli pressure results in a marked increase in intestinal oedema and intestinal ascites formation. The interaction between intestinal and hepatic lymphatics becomes significant because extrahepatic causes of increased hepatoportal lymph flow often increase intestinal microvascular fluid flux and lymph flow as well.

Intrahepatic causes of increased hepatoportal fluid flux

The main clinical problem associated with portal hypertension – most commonly due to alcoholic or postviral cirrhosis – is variceal haemorrhage. However, the focus of this section is on the effects of disease processes on microvascular and lymphatic function. The increased resistance to portal flow is caused by deposition of collagen in the space of Disse (sinusoidal) and by regenerating nodules that distort the small hepatic veins (postsinusoidal). Thus, in cirrhosis, there is both sinusoidal hypertension and splanchnic portal venous hypertension. As noted above, small increases in hepatic microvascular pressures drastically increase hepatic lymph flow on account of the unique nature of the sinusoidal microvasculature. If hepatic microvascular pressures rise high enough, the amount of trans-sinusoidal fluid flux overwhelms the lymphatic flow capacity, and ascitic fluid (hepatic lymph) passes through the hepatic capsule into the peritoneal cavity. Over time, as collagen is laid down in the space of Disse, the microvasculature undergoes a process termed capillarization. This results in a reduction in the hydraulic conductivity and permeability to proteins across the sinusoidal microvascular barrier. Ultimately, the protein concentration of hepatic lymph (and ascitic fluid) decreases. Both the liver and the intestine are important sites of ascites formation. Clinically significant ascites is uncommon in patients with prehepatic portal hypertension. Reasons for this clinical phenomenon include the lack of increased hepatic lymph flow and maintained hepatic protein synthesis.

References

1 Granger HJ, Barrowman JA (1984) Gastrointestinal and liver edema. In: Staub NC, Taylor AE (eds) *Edema*. New York: Raven Press, pp. 615–656.

2 Laine GA, Hall GT, Laine SH *et al.* (1979) Transinusoidal fluid dynamics in canine liver during venous hypertension. *Circ Res* 45, 317–323.

3 Schaffner F, Popper H (1963) Capillarization of hepatic sinusoids. *Gastroenterology* 44, 239–242.

4 Reichen J, Le M (1986) Verapamil favorably influences hepatic microvascular exchange and function in rats with cirrhosis of the liver. *J Clin Invest* 78(2), 448–455.

5 Cox CS Jr, Fisher U, Allen S *et al.* (2004) Lymphatic diversion prevents myocardial edema following mesenteric ischemia/reperfusion. *Microcirculation* 11, 1–8.

6 Stewart R, Laine G (2001) Flow and lymphatic networks: Interaction between hepatic and intestinal lymph vessels. *Microcirculation* 8, 221–227.

7 Elk JR, Drake RE, Williams JP *et al.* (1988) Lymphatic function in the liver after hepatic venous pressure elevation. *Am J Physiol* 254(17), G748–G752.

2.2 Functions of the liver

2.2.1 Functional organization of the liver

Paulo Renato A. V. Correa and Michael H. Nathanson

Introduction

Liver architecture is characterized by a few key anatomical features: the portal triad, the central vein and the sinusoids. This apparent simplicity is in contrast to the vast number of functions performed by the liver. Considered one of the central organs of metabolism, the liver is able to synthesize or degrade a wide variety of molecules in a regulated way. This includes substances as different as carbohydrates, lipids, amino acids, bile acids and exogenous compounds. In addition, the liver produces most of the circulating plasma proteins, including its most abundant component, albumin. It may seem paradoxical that this basic structure is associated with such complex functions. However, with the development of more sophisticated experimental methods, the molecular heterogeneity of hepatocytes is now appreciated, and a much more subtle organization of the liver has been revealed, which in fact shows an intricate pattern of distribution for the different liver functions. In this chapter, the ideas regarding the relationship between structure and function in the liver will be reviewed.

Liver structure, circulation and microcirculation

Liver cells

The liver contains a number of cell types including hepatocytes, cholangiocytes, stellate cells, portal fibroblasts, endothelial cells, macrophages, pit cells and oval cells. Nevertheless, a single cell type, the hepatocyte, accounts for two-thirds of the liver mass [1]. The importance of hepatocytes results not only from the fact that they are the principal constituent of liver, but also from the number, variety and complexity of biological processes that they perform. They synthesize and secrete plasma proteins, including albumin, coagulation factors, lipoproteins and acute phase reactants. It is in the hepatocytes that the metabolism of carbohydrates, lipids, amino acids, bilirubin and xenobiotics takes place. Finally, bile, the main exocrine secretory product of liver, is produced by hepatocytes.

Liver cell plates

The portal triad is composed of terminal branches of the two blood vessels that perfuse the liver, the portal vein and the hepatic artery, plus a bile duct, which drains the bile produced by hepatocytes. The central veins drain the blood from the sinusoids towards the hepatic vein and inferior vena cava [2]. The sinusoids are special vessels lined by fenestrated and discontinuous endothelial cells [3]. In cross-sectional view, the hepatocytes form cords of cells oriented as if radiating from the central vein. Each of these cords of hepatocytes forms a plate of cells in three dimensions (Fig. 1). The cell plate is formed in such a way that each hepatocyte has its apical or canalicular border facing other hepatocytes, where they form a bile canaliculus. The basolateral region of each hepatocyte is separated from the sinusoidal endothelium by the space of Disse. The cell plates anastomose extensively, although each cell plate is typically one hepatocyte in thickness. The plates are limited on both sides by sinusoids [4].

Functional unit of hepatic parenchyma

A functional unit should represent the simplest element into which the organ can be divided that still reflects the organ function as a whole. In the case of the liver, several structures have been proposed as the functional unit, including the hepatic lobule and the hepatic acinus. However, on a cell and molecular level, the cell plate can be seen as the functional unit of the liver [5].

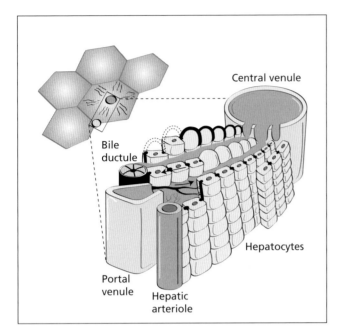

Fig. 1 The liver cell plate. The basic structural and functional unit of the liver is the liver cell plate, which is the sheet or plate of hepatocytes extending from the portal triad (portal venule, hepatic arteriole and bile ductule) to the central venule. Note that blood flows through the sinusoids, from the portal triad to the central venule, while bile (dark red) flows through bile canaliculi, in the opposite direction to the bile ductule. Gradients in protein expression along the liver cell plate result in zonal differences in biochemical, metabolic and signalling pathways.

Protein synthesis and gene expression

Gene expression in the cell plate

The liver secretes 1.2 g of albumin per kg of body weight per day [6]. In addition, the enzymatic machinery necessary to maintain metabolic processes has to be modified constantly, as the hormonal stimuli change to reflect the metabolic demands of the body. This ongoing, adaptive process of protein synthesis means that the expression of numerous genes has to be tightly regulated in hepatocytes. This matching of functional demand and protein synthesis is controlled by both hormonal and metabolic signals. It also creates the opportunity for the differential expression of genes across the liver cell plate and, therefore, the compartmentalization of the various metabolic and synthetic pathways to specific regions along the cell plate. This concept has been called the 'metabolic zonation' of the liver [7]. The main idea for this model was derived from studies on carbohydrate metabolism, in which it was demonstrated that two physiologically opposite metabolic processes, gluconeogenesis and glycolysis, could be performed simultaneously by hepatocytes in the periportal and pericentral regions respectively [8]. Further research, including of other metabolic pathways, confirmed that the concept of metabolic zonation is applicable to many liver functions and reflects an important level of metabolic control [7]. This

compartmentalized expression of proteins has been demonstrated for a number of enzymes and receptors, including hydroxymethylglutaryl (HMG)-CoA reductase [9], cholesterol 7α-hydroxylase [10], glutamine synthetase [11], the glucose transporter GLUT-1 [12], carbamoylphosphate synthetase [13], the epidermal growth factor (EGF) receptor [14] and the V_{1a} vasopressin receptor [15].

Regulation of compartmentalized gene expression in the cell plate

Identification of the stimuli responsible for the differential transcription of genes across the liver cell plate has been an area of interest, in order to understand how metabolic zonation is generated. This differential gene expression that results in zonation can be understood in part by analysing the microcirculation of the liver. The liver structure creates a specific pattern of blood circulation. Blood arrives through the hepatic artery and portal vein, spreads through the sinusoids and is drained by the central vein. In this trajectory from the portal pole of the cell plate to the central vein, the composition of blood changes as it bathes the hepatocytes. This change in composition results in a biochemical and gaseous gradient along the cell plate. Consequently, the hepatocytes located near the portal pole of the liver cell plate will be exposed to blood with different concentrations of oxygen, carbon dioxide and many other factors from those near the central vein pole. According to the current model, this difference in the microenvironment to which hepatocytes are exposed is responsible for functional differences noted across the cell plate. One example that has been well characterized is blood oxygen level-dependent gene expression [16]. This is illustrated by erythropoietin (EPO) gene transcription in the livers of anaemic mice [17]. EPO is a hormone normally secreted by the kidneys that stimulates the production of red blood cells by the bone marrow [18]. EPO expression is dependent on oxygen tension in blood, and its mRNA levels increase when the oxygen tension is decreased [19]. In the case of anaemic animals, *in situ* hybridization identified copies of EPO mRNA in hepatocytes close to the central vein, but not in those near the portal region. This experiment demonstrates that the level of oxygen tension is not the same along the liver cell plate, and that gene expression differs in hepatocytes located near the central vein because they are subjected to lower oxygen tensions. The result described for EPO can be extrapolated to other genes with the identification of the DNA sequence called hypoxia-responsive element (HRE) [20–22]. HRE is in the promoter region of certain genes and works as an anchoring site for the hypoxia-inducible factor (HIF), a transcription factor of the helix–loop–helix family. In situations where the oxygen level is decreased, the levels of HIF increase. HIF then binds HRE and directs the synthesis of mRNA for the corresponding gene [23]. HIF mRNA is most concentrated among hepatocytes near the central vein, although there is not a zonal distribution of HIF at the protein level [24]. Other mechanisms by which differential gene expression can be attained are by changes not only in the microenvironment, but also in the intrinsic sensitivity of hepatocytes to hormones. The effects of hormones, growth factors and cytokines on cells are generally mediated by the corresponding receptors on the plasma membrane. One of the known effects of receptor stimulation is to modify the expression of other genes, allowing the cell to adapt to the demands of that specific moment. By expressing different levels of receptors, cells can respond in different ways to the microenvironment and therefore express distinct sets of genes [25,26]. Glucagon, V_{1a} vasopressin, insulin and α1 and β1 adrenergic receptors predominate in the areas surrounding the central vein, while EGF and adenosine triphosphate (ATP) receptors are more concentrated near the portal vein [14,15].

Metabolism

Metabolic considerations deal with the differential metabolism of the main categories of small molecules across the liver cell plate. These include metabolism of oxidative energy, carbohydrates, lipids, amino acids and nitrogen, bile formation and metabolism of xenobiotics.

Oxidative energy metabolism

The liver has a high metabolic activity and, therefore, its energy demands are significant. Oxygen is the final substrate oxidized in the respiratory chain, and its gradient decreases from the periportal to pericentral region, so hepatocytes located near the portal region have higher levels of oxidative metabolism. As a result, hepatocytes near the portal region not only have higher activities of succinate dehydrogenase and cytochrome oxidase, but they also contain mitochondria that are larger, rounded and have more cristae to sustain higher levels of oxidative reactions [27,28].

Carbohydrate metabolism

The most important aspect of zonation of carbohydrate metabolism in the liver is the spatial segregation of gluconeogenesis in periportal hepatocytes and glycolysis in the pericentral region. This zonation is essential for the liver to regulate the blood glucose concentration properly [29]. There is considerable evidence that enzymes involved in gluconeogenic reactions, such as glucose-6-phosphatase, fructose-1,6-biphosphatase and phosphoenolpyruvate carboxykinase (PEPCK), predominate in the periportal area. The activity of glucose-6-phosphatase is twofold higher in periportal areas, in both rats and humans [30]. Studies using perfused rat livers confirm the periportal zonation of gluconeogenesis, although the directional flow of blood has been shown to be important for the location of gluconeogenesis induced by glucagon. The zonal heterogeneity of glucose-6-phosphatase and PEPCK starts at postnatal days 5 and 1, respectively, and is fully developed by the second week of age. This is believed to be a consequence of a change to a diet rich in fat and

protein after birth, as opposed to the constant source of glucose during pregnancy. By the time of weaning, the adult pattern has been established [13].

Glycolysis is localized to the pericentral region, with enzymes such as glucokinase and pyruvate kinase showing levels of around twice that observed in the periportal areas [31,32]. In terms of glucose uptake, the glucose transporter GLUT-2 is expressed in all hepatocytes, while the GLUT-1 isoform is expressed only in the subset of the most pericentral hepatocytes [12]. Another important aspect is the zonation of glycogen synthetase and glycogen phosphorylase in periportal areas, although this distribution may play a minor role in determining glycogen deposition secondary to the availability of glucose-6-phosphate.

Lipid metabolism

Lipid metabolism can be subclassified into lipogenesis, β-oxidation, ketogenesis, cholesterol biosynthesis and lipoprotein metabolism. In contrast to carbohydrate metabolism, the zonation of lipid metabolism is much less pronounced [33].

Lipogenesis, the synthesis of lipids, requires enzymes such as ATP-dependent citrate lyase and acetyl-CoA carboxylase. These two key enzymes are expressed to a slightly greater extent in pericentral regions [34,35]. This difference is more pronounced in female animals than in males. Similarly, fatty acid synthase activity is twice as high in pericentral hepatocytes than in periportal hepatocytes in females, but not in males.

β-Oxidation of fatty acids is active throughout the cell plate, because the enzymatic activity of 3-hydroxyacyl-CoA dehydrogenase does not show a portal to central gradient [34]. However, the higher volume of mitochondria in the periportal zone suggests a slightly higher level of β-oxidation in this region [36]. Studies with the enzyme carnitine palmitoyltransferase I are inconsistent, with some showing higher periportal activity, while others do not [37,38]. There is also variability in the results depending on the experimental design. Results using bezafibrate and clofibrate, showing increased carnitine acetyltransferase in periportal compared with pericentral hepatocytes, could not be reproduced with the drug clofibrate [39]. In addition, the results showing higher periportal activity first observed in rats have not been reproduced in humans [40]. Finally, although there is a gradient in the expression levels of fatty acid binding protein (FABP), with higher levels in the periportal region, this finding may not represent increased utilization of fatty acids in the periportal area but, rather, a gradient in the concentration of fatty acids due to directional blood flow [41].

Ketogenesis is another example of a process with a poorly defined gradient. β-Hydroxybutyrate dehydrogenase, a key enzyme of ketogenesis, is preferentially expressed in the pericentral region. However, the rate of ketogenesis is almost equal in hepatocytes isolated from the pericentral and periportal regions, in the absence of glucagon [34]. In the presence of that hormone, ketogenesis is significantly higher in periportal hepatocytes [42].

Ketogenesis is important during periods of starvation or diabetes, and the study of its distribution in those conditions might provide a clearer picture, but such studies are lacking.

Cholesterol biosynthesis is a metabolic pathway controlled primarily by the activity of the enzyme HMG-CoA reductase [43]. This enzyme is distributed predominantly in periportal hepatocytes, coinciding with the periportal expression of another enzyme involved in cholesterol synthesis, HMG-CoA synthase [9,44]. Drugs such as cholestyramine and mevinolin initially induce the expression of these two enzymes in periportal hepatocytes, although regions more pericentral are eventually affected as well, until a homogeneous distribution is achieved. This probably means that, under normal circumstances, cholesterol synthesis is a periportal event, although other hepatocytes might be recruited in periods of increased demand.

Lipoprotein metabolism involves the synthesis of apoenzymes that combine with lipids to form lipoprotein particles. Lipoprotein metabolism also involves the synthesis and degradation of cholesterol esters [45]. No zonation is observed for very-low-density lipoprotein (VLDL) secretion in normal rats, while there is a twofold ratio for the lipase implicated in cholesterol transport from high-density lipoproteins to tissues when comparing periportal with pericentral hepatocytes [46]. In normally fed rats, there is no zonation in the activity of lysosomal cholesteryl ester hydrolase (CEH) and acyl-CoA:cholesterol acyltransferase (ACAT), while the activity of both cytosolic and microsomal CEH is increased in the pericentral region. However, concentrations of free and esterified cholesterol in homogenates, cytosol and microsomes of periportal and pericentral cells are similar. Treatment with cholestyramine raises the pericentral/periportal ratio of ACAT and abolishes the heterogeneity in microsomal CEH, whereas the pericentral dominance of cytosolic CEH and the homogeneous distribution of lysosomal CEH are not affected [47].

Amino acid and nitrogen metabolism

The distribution of two enzymes related to nitrogen metabolism, carbamoylphosphate synthetase, involved in the synthesis of urea, and glutamine synthetase, involved in the synthesis of glutamine, is one of the best examples of liver function zonation. Glutamine synthase is expressed in very few hepatocytes surrounding the central vein, while carbamoylphosphate synthetase is present in the remainder of the parenchyma. Treatment of liver with CCl_4 destroys the pericentral hepatocytes and abolishes glutamine synthetase activity, without evidence of compensatory expression in the remaining cells. Glutamate dehydrogenase activity forms a gradient with increased levels of expression towards the pericentral region. Glutaminase activity predominates in periportal hepatocytes [11]. Periportal predominance of urea synthesis has also been demonstrated in the perfused rat liver. Therefore, there is practically no overlap between the hepatocytes involved in the synthesis of urea and glutamine. This clear separation is accompanied by zonation

of the membrane transporters and enzymes associated with the uptake and processing of substrates in those pathways. The uptake of glutamine and glutamate displays a pronounced heterogeneity and shows a strong correlation with the metabolism of ammonia [48]. Sodium-independent transport of glutamine is two- to threefold higher in pericentral hepatocytes. There is also considerable evidence that the sodium-dependent uptake of glutamate is exclusively pericentral, showing a direct correlation with glutamine synthetase distribution. In addition, α-ketoglutarate is almost exclusively taken up by pericentral, glutamine synthetase-containing hepatocytes. Up to 60% of α-ketoglutarate taken up by pericentral hepatocytes can be converted to glutamine [49].

Bile formation and secretion

Metabolism of key components of bile, including bile acids, bilirubin and glutathione, is compartmentalized along the liver cell plate. The expression of cholesterol 7α-hydroxylase, an enzyme involved in the synthesis of bile acids, is highly zonated. The ratio of expression in the pericentral to periportal region is approximately 8:1. Treatment with cholestipol leads to induction of expression in the periportal region, with the pericentral/periportal ratio dropping to 2. The production of bile acid is more than fourfold higher in pericentral compared with periportal hepatocytes. The enzyme cholesterol 26-hydroxylase shows a pericentral/periportal ratio of around 3 before and 4 after stimulation with cholestipol. These results indicate that bile acid synthesis is predominantly pericentral [10]. Conjugation of bilirubin is a central aspect of its metabolism in terms of bile secretion. Total activity of UDP-glucuronyl transferase, the enzyme responsible for the conjugation of bilirubin to glucuronic acid, is more intense in the pericentral region [50]. Glutathione is an important factor that protects hepatocytes from oxidative injuries. It is also the main component of bile acid-independent bile flow. The intracellular glutathione concentration is significantly higher in periportal hepatocytes, although there is no difference in the activity of glutathione synthetase or glutamylcystein synthetase. Glutathione-mediated antioxidant reactions are catalysed by the enzymes glutathione-S-transferases (GST) and glutathione peroxidases. The pericentral predominance of GST has been demonstrated for several isoforms [51]. Contrasting with the GST distribution, glutathione peroxidase activity is around twofold higher in periportal hepatocytes, and a selenium-dependent isoform has been localized by immunohistochemistry to that region as well [52].

Metabolism of xenobiotics

Phase I in the biotransformation of xenobiotics is catalysed by microsomal cytochrome P-450 mono-oxygenases. Total cytochrome P-450 content shows a slight increase from the periportal to the pericentral region. Pericentral hepatocytes also have a larger area of smooth endoplasmic reticulum and a higher surface density of cytochrome P-450 [53]. In addition, pheno-barbital increases cytochrome P-450 in pericentral areas and induces the proliferation of endoplasmic reticulum. Several cytochrome P-450-dependent reactions have been localized to the pericentral region. Pericentral localization has also been shown for 7-ethoxycoumarin-*O*-demethylase, 7-ethoxyresofurin-*O*-deethylase, aniline *p*-hydrolase, benzphetamine *N*-demethylase and microsomal ethanol oxidation [54]. These and other enzymes are more prominently induced in periportal cells after phenobarbital. These findings, along with immunohisto-chemistry and *in situ* hybridization, indicate that most enzymes of the cytochrome P-450 family are predominantly expressed in pericentral hepatocytes, although each specific enzyme has its characteristic pattern of distribution that can be modified during induction with drugs. NADPH-cytochrome *c* reductase activity is also higher in pericentral hepatocytes of both rats and humans.

Signalling

Signalling is central to the understanding of the liver as a func-tional unit and involves both the response of hepatocytes to external hormonal stimuli and the internal coordination of those responses coded in the form of second messengers [55]. Hepatocytes express a wide range of plasma membrane recep-tors, many of which share common second messengers [56]. Agonists or ligands for these receptors include glucagon, vaso-pressin, ATP, insulin and growth factors such as EGF, hepato-cyte growth factor (HGF) and insulin-like growth factor (IGF). The chemical messages generated by these agonists often consist of one or more of a few main types: phosphorylation or dephos-phorylation of kinases, phosphatases and other proteins [57]; generation of inositol 1,4,5-trisphosphate and an associated increase in free cytosolic calcium [58]; stimulation or inhibition of cAMP production [59]; stimulation or inhibition of nitric oxide and cGMP production [59]; phosphorylation of phospho-lipids [60]; and changes in membrane polarity [61]. Every aspect of hepatocyte function is regulated by these messengers, includ-ing secretion, gluconeogenesis, glycogenolysis, protein syn-thesis, gene transcription, cell cycle progression and apoptosis [62–65]. There is evidence in both isolated hepatocyte couplets and triplets [66] and the intact liver [67,68] that second messen-ger signals are coordinated among hepatocytes. Calcium oscilla-tions are synchronized in isolated hepatocyte couplets, and calcium waves travel from cell to cell without delay [66]. In the intact liver, there is a similarly coordinated progression of calcium oscillations [68] and calcium waves [67] along cords of hepatocytes. Intercellular coupling via gap junctions is import-ant for coordination of second messenger signals [66] but it is not the sole determinant. The direction of calcium waves along the hepatic acinus depends upon the agonist. For example, vaso-pressin induces calcium waves that travel from the pericentral to the periportal region [67,69], whereas ATP-induced calcium signals begin at random locations within the hepatic acinus [69].

The V_{1a} vasopressin receptor is expressed most heavily among pericentral hepatocytes [67], so agonist-specific patterns of cal-cium signalling *in vivo* have been attributed to such differences in receptor distribution. The molecular mechanism by which calcium signals are coordinated and oriented along the liver cell plate has been examined in detail in isolated triplets of primary hepatocytes [70,71] and in liver cell lines [72]. Collectively, these studies suggest that three factors are necessary. First, adjacent cells must communicate directly via gap junctions. This is con-sistent with the observations that second messengers such as calcium and inositol 1,4,5-trisphosphate can cross gap junctions in hepatocytes [73]. Second, in order for signals to propagate over distances greater than one or two cells, each cell must be stimulated, so that all the cells are in an excitable state. Third, one cell or group of cells must have increased expression of hormone receptor relative to the other cells. This feature allows that particular cell to have increased sensitivity to agonist, so that it will serve as a pacemaker for the other hepatocytes [72]. As the lobular distribution of different hormone receptors varies, this final feature allows the respective agonists to generate distinct signalling patterns across the hepatic lobule, which can in turn allow agonist-specific tissue responses even though dif-ferent agonists activate the same second messengers. There are several examples illustrating how liver function depends on the coordinated response to second messengers. In the isolated perfused rat liver, hormone-induced changes in both bile flow and glucose release are altered by agents that block gap junctions [74]. However, gap junction blockers do not alter bile secretion or glucose release in livers treated with agents that increase sec-ond messengers independent of hormone receptors [74]. These results suggest that the lobular pattern of second messenger acti-vation is an important component of the liver's response to hor-monal stimulation. Only subtle changes in glucose release and bile flow occur in mice lacking connexin 32, the predominant gap junction in hepatocytes [75,76], but connexin 32 knockout mice treated with endotoxin have slightly worse hypoglycaemia and much worse cholestasis than wild-type mice treated with endotoxin [77]. Intercellular signalling may also be important for liver regeneration. It has been shown that the lobular gradi-ent of V_{1a} vasopressin receptors is accentuated after partial hepatectomy and that the organized calcium wave generated is important in promoting choleresis during the initial phase of the postoperative period [78]. Thus, intra- and intercellular signalling that is properly coordinated across the hepatic lobule shapes liver function in health as well as in disease.

Conclusion

Characterizing the effects of agonists and intracellular mes-sengers on gene expression will probably help to answer the fundamental question of how gradients of enzymes, receptors and even cell structure are generated across the liver cell plate. Comparison of regulatory sequences of genes expressed in the pericentral and periportal region and identification of transcription factors acting on those elements will probably provide additional insights. Progress has been made in characterizing the transcription factors involved in the differentiation of epithelial cells into hepatocytes [79], but those factors responsible for the phenotype variation along the liver cell plate still remain unidentified.

Acknowledgement

This work was supported by NIH grants DK57751 and DK45710.

References

1 Kmiec Z (2001) Cooperation of liver cells in health and disease. *Adv Anat Embryol Cell Biol* 161 (III–XIII), 1–151.

2 Oda M, Yokomori H, Han JY *et al.* (2003) Regulatory mechanisms of hepatic microcirculation. *Clin Hemorheol Microcirc* 29 (30–4), 167–182.

3 McCuskey RS, Reilly FD (1993) Hepatic microvasculature: dynamic structure and its regulation. *Semin Liver Dis* 13 (1), 1–12.

4 Motta PM (1977) The three-dimensional fine structure of the liver as revealed by scanning electron microscopy. *Int Rev Cytol Suppl* 6, 347–399.

5 Barbera-Guillem E, Vidal-Vanaclocha F (1988) Sinusoidal structure of the liver. *Revis Biol Celular* 16, 1–34, 54–68.

6 Papageorgopoulos C, Caldwell K, *et al.* (1999) Measuring protein synthesis by mass isotopomer distribution analysis (MIDA). *Anal Biochem* 267 (1), 1–16.

7 Gebhardt R (1992) Metabolic zonation of the liver: regulation and implications for liver function. *Pharmacol Ther* 53 (3), 275–354.

8 Brinkmann A, Katz N, Sasse D *et al.* (1978) Increase of the gluconeogenic and decrease of the glycolytic capacity of rat liver with a change of the metabolic zonation after partial hepatectomy. *Hoppe Seylers Z Physiol Chem* 359 (11), 1561–1571.

9 Singer D II, Kawka W, Kazazis DM *et al.* (1984) Hydroxymethylglutaryl-coenzyme A reductase-containing hepatocytes are distributed periportally in normal and mevinolin-treated rat livers. *Proc Natl Acad Sci USA* 81 (17), 5556–5560.

10 Ugele B, Kempen HJ, Kempen JM *et al.* (1991) Heterogeneity of rat liver parenchyma in cholesterol 7 alpha-hydroxylase and bile acid synthesis. *Biochem J* 276 (Pt 1), 73–77.

11 Moorman AF, Vermeulen JL, Charles R *et al.* (1989) Localization of ammonia-metabolizing enzymes in human liver: ontogenesis of heterogeneity. *Hepatology* 9 (3), 367–372.

12 Tal M, Kahn BB, Lodish HF *et al.* (1991) Expression of the low Km GLUT-1 glucose transporter is turned on in perivenous hepatocytes of insulin-deficient diabetic rats. *Endocrinology* 129 (4), 1933–1941.

13 Jungermann K (1986) Dynamics of zonal hepatocyte heterogeneity. Perinatal development and adaptive alterations during regeneration after partial hepatectomy, starvation and diabetes. *Acta Histochem Suppl* 32, 89–98.

14 Chabot JG, Walker P, Pelletier G (1986) Distribution of epidermal growth factor binding sites in the adult rat liver. *Am J Physiol* 250 (6 Pt 1), G760–G764.

15 Tordjmann T, Berthon B, Combettes L *et al.* (1996) The location of hepatocytes in the rat liver acinus determines their sensitivity to calcium-mobilizing hormones. *Gastroenterology* 111 (5), 1343–1352.

16 Kietzmann T, Jungermann K (1997) Modulation by oxygen of zonal gene expression in liver studied in primary rat hepatocyte cultures. *Cell Biol Toxicol* 13 (4–5), 243–255.

17 Koury ST, Bondurant MC, Koury MJ *et al.* (1991) Localization of cells producing erythropoietin in murine liver by in situ hybridization. *Blood* 77 (11), 2497–2503.

18 Koury MJ, Bondurant MC (1991) The mechanism of erythropoietin action. *Am J Kidney Dis* 18 (4 Suppl 1), 20–23.

19 Gopfert T, Gess B, Eckard KU *et al.* (1996) Hypoxia signalling in the control of erythropoietin gene expression in rat hepatocytes. *J Cell Physiol* 168 (2), 354–361.

20 Hirsch-Ernst KI, Kietzmann T, Ziemann T *et al.* (2000) Physiological oxygen tensions modulate expression of the mdr1b multidrug-resistance gene in primary rat hepatocyte cultures. *Biochem J* 350 Pt 2, 443–451.

21 Jungermann K, Kietzmann T (2000) Oxygen: modulator of metabolic zonation and disease of the liver. *Hepatology* 31 (2), 255–260.

22 Vargiu C, Belliardo S, Cravanzola C *et al.* (2000) Oxygen regulation of rat hepatocyte iNOS gene expression. *J Hepatol* 32 (4), 567–573.

23 Wang GL, Semenza GL (1996) Molecular basis of hypoxia-induced erythropoietin expression. *Curr Opin Haematol* 3 (2), 156–162.

24 Keitzmann T, Cornesse Y, Brechtel K *et al.* (2001) Perivenous expression of the mRNA of the three hypoxia-inducible factor a-subunits, HIF1a, HIF2a and HIF3a, in rat liver. *Biochem J* 354, 531–537.

25 Kietzmann T, Krones-Herzig A, Jungermann K *et al.* (2002) Signaling cross-talk between hypoxia and glucose via hypoxia-inducible factor 1 and glucose response elements. *Biochem Pharmacol* 64 (5–6), 903–911.

26 Oinonen T, Nikkola E, Lindros KO *et al.* (1993) Growth hormone mediates zone-specific gene expression in liver. *FEBS Lett* 327 (2), 237–240.

27 Sokal EM, Trivedi P, Protmann B *et al.* (1989) Developmental changes in the intra-acinar distribution of succinate dehydrogenase, glutamate dehydrogenase, glucose-6-phosphatase, and NADPH dehydrogenase in the rat liver. *J Pediatr Gastroenterol Nutr* 8 (4), 522–527.

28 Wimmer M, Pette D (1979) Microphotometric studies on intraacinar enzyme distribution in rat liver. *Histochemistry* 64 (1), 23–33.

29 Jungermann K (1985) Metabolic zonation of liver parenchyma: regulation of the glucostat of the liver. *Naturwissenschaften* 72 (2), 76–84.

30 Jungermann K (1983) Functional significance of hepatocyte heterogeneity for glycolysis and gluconeogenesis. *Pharmacol Biochem Behav* 18 (Suppl 1), 409–414.

31 Fischer W, Ick M, Katz NR (1982) Reciprocal distribution of hexokinase and glucokinase in the periportal and perivenous zone of the rat liver acinus. *Hoppe Seylers Z Physiol Chem* 363 (4), 375–380.

32 Zierz S, Katz N, Jungermann K *et al.* (1983) Distribution of pyruvate kinase type L and M2 in microdissected periportal and perivenous rat liver tissue with different dietary states. *Hoppe Seylers Z Physiol Chem* 364 (10), 1447–1453.

33 Jungermann K, Katz N (1989) Functional specialization of different hepatocyte populations. *Physiol Rev* 69 (3), 708–764.

34 Katz NR, Fischer W, Giffhorn S *et al.* (1983) Distribution of enzymes of fatty acid and ketone body metabolism in periportal and perivenous rat-liver tissue. *Eur J Biochem* 135 (1), 103–107.

35 Katz NR, Fischer W, Ick M *et al.* (1983) Heterogeneous distribution of ATP citrate lyase in rat-liver parenchyma. Microradiochemical determination in microdissected periportal and perivenous liver tissue. *Eur J Biochem* 130 (2), 297–301.

36 Loud AV (1968) A quantitative stereological description of the ultrastructure of normal rat liver parenchymal cells. *J Cell Biol* 37 (1), 27–46.

37 Guzman M, Castro J (1989) Zonation of fatty acid metabolism in rat liver. *Biochem J* 264 (1), 107–113.

38 Tosh D, Alberti KG, Aquis L *et al.* (1989) Clofibrate induces carnitine acyltransferases in periportal and perivenous zones of rat liver and does not disturb the acinar zonation of gluconeogenesis. *Biochim Biophys Acta* 992 (3), 245–50.

39 Gerondaes P, Alberti KG, Aquis L *et al.* (1988) Interactions of inhibitors of carnitine palmitoyltransferase I and fibrates in cultured hepatocytes. *Biochem J* 253 (1), 169–173.

40 Gerondaes P, Alberti KG, Aquis L *et al.* (1988) Fatty acid metabolism in hepatocytes cultured with hypolipidaemic drugs. Role of carnitine. *Biochem J* 253 (1), 161–167.

41 Iseki S, Kondo H, Hitomi M *et al.* (1990) Localization of liver fatty acid-binding protein and its mRNA in the liver and jejunum of rats: an immunohistochemical and in situ hybridization study. *Mol Cell Biochem* 98 (1–2), 27–33.

42 Tosh D, Alberti GM, Aquis L *et al.* (1988) Glucagon regulation of gluconeo-genesis and ketogenesis in periportal and perivenous rat hepatocytes. Heterogeneity of hormone action and of the mitochondrial redox state. *Biochem J* 256 (1), 197–204.

43 Singh RP, Kumar R, Kapur N *et al.* (2003) Molecular regulation of cholesterol biosynthesis: implications in carcinogenesis. *J Environ Pathol Toxicol Oncol* 22 (2), 75–92.

44 Li AC, Tanaka RD, Callaway K *et al.* (1988) Localization of 3-hydroxy-3-methylglutaryl CoA reductase and 3-hydroxy-3-methylglutaryl CoA synthase in the rat liver and intestine is affected by cholestyramine and mevinolin. *J Lipid Res* 29 (6), 781–796.

45 Kang S, Davis RA (2000) Cholesterol and hepatic lipoprotein assembly and secretion. *Biochim Biophys Acta* 1529 (1–3), 223–230.

46 Verhoeven AJ, Jansen H (1989) Secretion of liver lipase activity by periportal and perivenous hepatocytes. *Biochim Biophys Acta* 1001 (2), 239–242.

47 Romero JR, Fresnedo O, Isusi E *et al.* (1999) Hepatic zonation of the formation and hydrolysis of cholesteryl esters in periportal and perivenous parenchymal cells. *Lipids* 34 (9), 907–913.

48 Haussinger D, Lamers WH, Moorman AF *et al.* (1992) Hepatocyte heterogeneity in the metabolism of amino acids and ammonia. *Enzyme* 46 (1–3), 72–93.

49 Burger HJ, Gebhardt R, Mayer C *et al.* (1989) Different capacities for amino acid transport in periportal and perivenous hepatocytes isolated by digitonin/collagenase perfusion. *Hepatology* 9 (1), 22–28.

50 Ullrich D, Fischer G, Katz N *et al.* (1984) Intralobular distribution of UDP-glucuronosyltransferase in livers from untreated, 3-methylcholanthrene- and phenobarbital-treated rats. *Chem Biol Interact* 48 (2), 181–190.

51 Wolf CR, Moll E, Frieberg T *et al.* (1984) Characterization, localization and regulation of a novel phenobarbital-inducible form of cytochrome P450, compared with three further P450-isoenzymes, NADPH P450-reductase, glutathione transferases and microsomal epoxide hydrolase. *Carcinogenesis* 5 (8), 993–1001.

52 Kera Y, Sippel HW, Pentilla KE *et al.* (1987) Acinar distribution of glutathione-dependent detoxifying enzymes. Low glutathione peroxidase activity in perivenous hepatocytes. *Biochem Pharmacol* 36 (12), 2003–2006.

53 Kanai K, Kanamura S, Watanabe J *et al.* (1986) Peri- and postnatal development of heterogeneity in the amounts of endoplasmic reticulum in mouse hepatocytes. *Am J Anat* 175 (4), 471–480.

54 Gascon-Barre M, Benbrahim N, Tremblay C *et al.* (1989) Hepatic zonation of drug metabolizing enzymes. Studies on hepatocytes isolated from the periportal or perivenous region of the liver acinus. *Can J Physiol Pharmacol* 67 (9), 1015–1022.

55 Nathanson MH (1994) Cellular and subcellular calcium signaling in gastrointestinal epithelium. *Gastroenterology* 106 (5), 1349–1364.

56 Pierce KL, Premont RT, Lefkowitz RJ *et al.* (2002) Seven-transmembrane receptors. *Nature Rev Mol Cell Biol* 3 (9), 639–650.

57 Wong W, Scott JD (2004) AKAP signalling complexes: focal points in space and time. *Nature Rev Mol Cell Biol* 5 (12), 959–970.

58 Berridge MJ, Bootman MD, Roderick HL *et al.* (2003) Calcium signalling: dynamics, homeostasis and remodelling. *Nature Rev Mol Cell Biol* 4 (7), 517–529.

59 Beavo JA, Brunton LL (2002) Cyclic nucleotide research – still expanding after half a century. *Nature Rev Mol Cell Biol* 3 (9), 710–718.

60 Bondeva, T, Pirola L, Bugarelli-Leva G *et al.* (1998) Bifurcation of lipid and protein kinase signals of PI3Kgamma to the protein kinases PKB and MAPK. *Science* 282 (5387), 293–296.

61 Rosenmund C, Stern-Bach Y, Stevens CF *et al.* (1998) The tetrameric structure of a glutamate receptor channel. *Science* 280 (5369), 1596–1599.

62 Pusl T, Nathanson MH (2004) The role of inositol 1,4,5-trisphosphate receptors in the regulation of bile secretion in health and disease. *Biochem Biophys Res Commun* 322 (4), 1318–1325.

63 Zhou XY, Shibusawa N, Naik K *et al.* (2004) Insulin regulation of hepatic gluconeogenesis through phosphorylation of CREB-binding protein. *Nature Med* 10 (6), 633–637.

64 Fruman DA, Mauvais-Jarvis F, Pollard D *et al.* (2000) Hypoglycaemia, liver necrosis and perinatal death in mice lacking all isoforms of phosphoinositide 3-kinase p85 alpha. *Nature Genet* 26 (3), 379–382.

65 Reinehr R, Becker S, Hongen A *et al.* (2004) Involvement of the Src family kinase yes in bile salt-induced apoptosis. *Gastroenterology* 127 (5), 1540–1557.

66 Nathanson MH, Burgstahler AD (1992) Coordination of hormone-induced calcium signals in isolated rat hepatocyte couplets: demonstration with confocal microscopy. *Mol Biol Cell* 3 (1), 113–121.

67 Nathanson MH, Burgstahler AD, Mewnone A *et al.* (1995) Ca2+ waves are organized among hepatocytes in the intact organ. *Am J Physiol* 269 (1 Pt 1), G167–171.

68 Robb-Gaspers LD, Thomas AP (1995) Coordination of Ca2+ signaling by intercellular propagation of Ca2+ waves in the intact liver. *J Biol Chem* 270 (14), 8102–8107.

69 Motoyama K, Karl IE, Flye MW *et al.* (1999) Effect of Ca2+ agonists in the perfused liver: determination via laser scanning confocal microscopy. *Am J Physiol* 276 (2 Pt 2), R575–585.

70 Tordjmann T, Berthon B, Claret M *et al.* (1997) Coordinated intercellular calcium waves induced by noradrenaline in rat hepatocytes: dual control by gap junction permeability and agonist. *EMBO J* 16 (17), 5398–5407.

71 Tordjmann T, Berthon B, Jacquemin E *et al.* (1998) Receptor-oriented intercellular calcium waves evoked by vasopressin in rat hepatocytes. *EMBO J* 17 (16), 4695–4703.

72 Leite MF, Hirata K, Pusl T *et al.* (2002) Molecular basis for pacemaker cells in epithelia. *J Biol Chem* 277 (18), 16313–16323.

73 Saez JC, Connor JA, Spray DC *et al.* (1989). Hepatocyte gap junctions are permeable to the second messenger, inositol 1,4,5-trisphosphate, and to calcium ions. *Proc Natl Acad Sci USA* 86 (8), 2708–2712.

74 Nathanson MH, Rios-Velez L, Burgstahler AD *et al.* (1999) Communication via gap junctions modulates bile secretion in the isolated perfused rat liver. *Gastroenterology* 116 (5), 1176–1183.

75 Nelles E, Butzler C, Jung D *et al.* (1996) Defective propagation of signals generated by sympathetic nerve stimulation in the liver of connexin 32-deficient mice. *Proc Natl Acad Sci USA* 93 (18), 9565–9570.

76 Temme A, Stumpel F, Sohl G *et al.* (2001) Dilated bile canaliculi and attenuated decrease of nerve-dependent bile secretion in connexin 32-deficient mouse liver. *Pflugers Arch* 442 (6), 961–966.

77 Correa PR, Guerra MT, Leite MF *et al.* (2004) Endotoxin unmasks the role of gap junctions in the liver. *Biochem Biophys Res Commun* 322 (3), 718–726.

78 Nicou A, Serriere V, Prigent S *et al.* (2003) Hypothalamic vasopressin release and hepatocyte Ca2+ signaling during liver regeneration: an interplay stimulating liver growth and bile flow. *FASEB J* 17 (13), 1901–1903.

79 Parviz F, Matullo C, Garrison WD *et al.* (2003) Hepatocyte nuclear factor 4alpha controls the development of a hepatic epithelium and liver morphogenesis. *Nature Genet* 34 (3), 292–296.

2.2.2 Cell biology of the hepatocyte

Allan W. Wolkoff and Phyllis M. Novikoff

The hepatocyte has been a classical subject for cell biological study [1]. In great part, this is a result of its abundance, availability for experimental examination and diversity of function. The cell biology of the hepatocyte is a large area that could not be covered in its entirety in a single brief overview. Consequently, this chapter will focus on the biology of the hepatocyte as it relates to cell polarity, cell–cell junctions and communication, the cytoskeleton and plasma membrane function as related to receptor-mediated endocytosis.

Cell polarity

Although the hepatocyte functions as a typical polarized epithelial cell, its organization is unique (Fig. 1). Unlike most polarized epithelial cells (e.g. intestinal epithelial cell), with distinct basal and apical plasma membrane domains on opposite sides of the cell, the apical domain of the hepatocyte represents a small portion of the plasma membrane (approximately 10%) and lies between cells, set off from the basolateral plasma membrane by tight junctions (see below) and forming the bile canaliculus. The basolateral (sinusoidal) and apical (canalicular) plasma membranes have distinct lipid and protein compositions, and these help to define their differential functions (Fig. 2). In general, the basolateral plasma membrane has transporters that remove substances (e.g. bile acids, drugs) from the portal venous blood by facilitated diffusion along a concentration gradient, whereas the apical plasma membrane has transporters that pump substances against a steep concentration gradient from the cell interior into the bile canaliculus using adenosine triphosphate (ATP) hydrolysis as the source of energy. Once in the bile canaliculus, there is little return of these substances to the portal blood, because of the seal that is produced by the tight junction between cells (see below).

The factors that lead to the differential sorting of proteins to specific plasma membrane domains in the hepatocyte are not entirely understood. Although most polarized epithelial cells sort proteins directly to their final destination from the site of

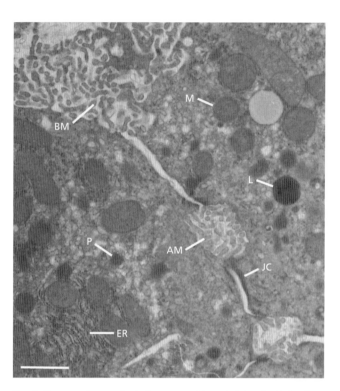

Fig. 1 Electron micrograph of a hepatocyte. The apical–basal polarity of hepatocytes is delineated by two different domains of plasma membrane, a basolateral (sinusoidal) membrane (BM) and an apical (bile canalicular) membrane (AM). Both plasma membrane domains have microvilli. Those at the BM are more numerous, longer and more slender than those at the AM. The BM microvilli project into the space of Disse where they come into direct contact with sinusoidal blood flow. The AM microvilli from adjacent hepatocytes project into a lumen to form the bile canaliculus and are exposed to bile. Junctional complexes (JC) are found adjacent to the apical membrane at the periphery of the bile canaliculus. Also labelled are endoplasmic reticulum (ER), lysosomes (L), mitochondria (M) and peroxisomes (P). Bar = 1 μm.

synthesis [2], initial evidence suggested that plasma membrane proteins trafficked to the basolateral plasma membrane after synthesis, and that those destined for the apical plasma membrane were subsequently internalized into a vesicle and delivered to the apical plasma membrane by a transcytotic process [2]. Subsequent studies revealed that a number of the apical transport pumps were delivered directly to the apical plasma membrane after synthesis [3]. Further studies suggested that apical plasma membrane proteins that had only a single transmembrane-spanning region, such as dipeptidyl peptidase IV (DPPIV), rather than the multimembrane-spanning excretory pumps, took the indirect route [4]. Interestingly, DPPIV targets directly to the apical plasma membrane in most epithelial cells other than hepatocytes [5]. The lipid compositions of basolateral and apical plasma membranes from hepatocytes are also distinct [6,7]. Cholesterol content of the apical membrane is substantially higher than that of the basolateral membrane [6], and this is reflected in reduced membrane fluidity of apical compared with basolateral membranes [7]. The mechanisms for differential sorting of lipids to these plasma membrane domains are not known.

Fig. 2 Colocalization of (a) actin and (b) the organic anion transporter OATP1A1 [55] in a section of rat liver by fluorescence confocal microscopy. A section of rat liver was aldehyde fixed, and OATP1A1 was visualized by exposure to primary antibody followed by Cy3-coupled secondary antibody. Actin filaments were subsequently visualized using fluorescein isothiocyanate (FITC) phalloidin. As seen from the arrowheads in (a), actin is especially abundant around the bile canaliculi (apical plasma membrane). As seen from the arrows in (b), OATP1A1 is present on the sinusoidal (basolateral) plasma membrane and is not present in areas identified as bile canaliculi (arrowheads). Bar = 10 μm.

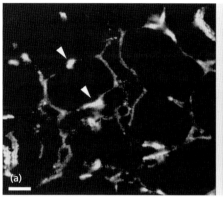
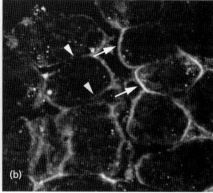

Cell–cell junctions and communication

Hepatocytes interact with each other by specific intercellular junctional complexes that serve to establish cellular polarity as well as structure the organ into well-defined plates of cells [8]. These complexes surround the bile canaliculi (apical plasma membrane) and include desmosomes as well as gap, tight and adherens junctions. Tight junctions are the most apical of these junctional complexes, establishing cell polarity and providing a barrier function that prevents solute and water flow through the paracellular space [9]. They form a continuous band around each cell and are composed of a complex of several integral membrane proteins that include occludin and claudins [9,10]. A number of peripheral membrane proteins, including ZO-1, ZO-2 and ZO-3, are found in this complex [9,10]. Interestingly, gap junctional proteins have been found to interact with occludin and ZO-1, and coordinate regulation of these complexes has been suggested [8–11]. Desmosomes are found in areas that resemble dense plaques and are localized towards the basolateral side of tight junctions. They are attached to the cytoplasmic intermediate filament network and are composed of proteins from at least three distinct gene families, namely cadherins, armadillo proteins and plakins [12]. The adherens junction is another contact structure localized towards the basolateral side of tight junctions where it serves to anchor bundles of actin filaments. These junctions also represent large complexes of proteins that include cadherins and catenins [13,14].

Gap junctions are the major subcellular structures that permit the transfer of low-molecular-weight molecules between adjacent cells [9,15,16]. These molecules include various signal transduction agents such as inositol 1,4,5-triphosphate (IP_3) and cyclic adenosine monophosphate (cAMP), as well as Ca^{2+} and electrical signals [16–18]. The gap junctions are constituted by binding of hexamers of a connexin protein that form hemichannels at the surface of each of two adjacent cells. Although over 20 connexins have been described, the major connexin in hepatocytes is connexin 32, although there is a small amount of connexin 26 as well [16]. Recent studies have indicated that mutations in the connexin 32 gene are responsible for the X-linked form of Charcot–Marie–Tooth syndrome, a neurological disorder presenting as a peripheral neuropathy [19]. Interestingly, there is no evidence for liver dysfunction in these individuals. However, when liver from connexin 32 knockout mice was stressed following endotoxin administration, a more prolonged hypoglycaemia and cholestasis were observed, when compared with wild-type animals [16]. These alterations in hepatic stress response probably result from uncoupling of intercellular signalling mechanisms and suggest that similar abnormalities may be seen in connexin 32-deficient patients under conditions of stress.

Cytoskeleton

The hepatocyte cytoskeleton is an important determinant of polarized cell function. The major components of the cytoskeleton are intermediate filaments, microtubules and microfilaments. In contrast to microfilaments and microtubules that are polymers of actin and tubulin, respectively, over 50 different intermediate filament proteins have been described, and they are expressed in a cell type-specific manner. On the basis of structural characteristics, the intermediate filament proteins have been divided into five types [20,21]. Types 1 and 2 consist of two groups of keratins, representing the largest subgroups of intermediate filament proteins. Epithelial cells express at least one type 1 (acidic) and one type 2 (neutral/basic) keratin which, in the case of hepatocytes, are keratin 8 (type 2) and keratin 18 (type 1). These proteins form a complex network residing just below the actin-based microfilaments that surround the plasma membrane and are anchored to the plasma membrane at desmosomes, which are specialized junctions between adjacent cells. Although the function of intermediate filaments in hepatocytes is not known, several transgenic mouse models have indicated that altered expression of the hepatocyte keratins is associated with increased hepatocyte mechanical fragility and susceptibility to injury [20,22–24].

Microfilaments, polymers of actin, form a thin belt around the periphery of hepatocytes [25]. Interestingly, these actin filaments are especially concentrated around the bile canalicular (apical) plasma membrane (Fig. 2) [26]. Although it has been suggested that this abundant bile canalicular distribution might be important for contraction of the canaliculus and the consequent force that initiates bile flow [27,28], there has been little recent work in this potentially important area. Within the hepatocyte, actin filaments are organized into networks and bundles, under the regulation of a number of proteins that bind to actin. Although actin structures are important determinants of cell shape and motility in many cell types, their function in the hepatocyte remains to be clarified. As these bundles of actin lie immediately below the hepatocyte plasma membrane [25], they form a barrier to entry into the cell of structures such as endocytic vesicles (see below). Myosins are molecules that can bind to actin and move on microfilaments in the presence of ATP [29]. They have the ability to bind specific vesicular cargo and facilitate its movement thorough the microfilamentous barrier [29]. Directly below and arranged perpendicular to the actin layer is a network of microtubules [25].

Microtubules are polymers of tubulin that emanate from an organizing centre. In hepatocytes, this microtubule organizing centre is near the nucleus. Owing to the biochemical characteristics of tubulin, its polymers (microtubules) have a directional polarity in which what has been termed the minus end is at the microtubule organizing centre near the cell nucleus, while the plus end is towards the cell surface [25,30]. Functionally, these polarized regions of the microtubule can be differentiated by the rate at which extension in the presence of unpolymerized tubulin occurs: the minus end grows slowly, while the plus end grows rapidly, on account of its preferential binding of tubulin. Recent studies have indicated an important role for microtubules in serving as 'railway tracks' along which intracellular vesicles and organelles can ride, powered by kinesins and dyneins, microtubule-based motors [31].

Receptor-mediated endocytosis

Receptor-mediated endocytosis is a process in which the binding of a ligand to a specific cell surface receptor initiates an intricate series of events resulting in internalization of the ligand–receptor complex into a vesicle that is processed to discrete destinations within the cell (Fig. 3). A hepatocyte-specific ligand that has been the subject of much investigation is asialoorosomucoid (ASOR). ASOR is prepared by removal of the terminal sialic acid residues on the carbohydrate chains of orosomucoid (α1-acid glycoprotein). This desialylated glycoprotein binds virtually irreversibly to a receptor on the hepatocyte surface plasma membrane that has been termed the asialoglycoprotein receptor [32]. Although the physiological function of this receptor is not known, it mediates internalization and processing of its bound ligand by a process that serves as a prototype for receptor-mediated endocytosis of other ligands, including low-density lipoproteins [33,34]. Following binding of ASOR to its cell surface receptor, the ligand–receptor complex is internalized into a vesicle that is coated with the protein clathrin [35–37]. Following uncoating, this vesicle acidifies [38], and this results in the unbinding of ligand from receptor [39]. This endocytic vesicle then undergoes a series of fissions, the consequence of which is the eventual segregation of ligand from receptor, resulting in their localization into separate daughter vesicles [33,35,36]. Following segregation, one group of daughter vesicles that contain the majority of receptor and a reduced content of ligand recycles to the cell surface. The other group of daughter vesicles that contain little receptor but most of the ligand [40] traffics through the cell to the lysosome, where ligand is degraded [33,36,39]. Lysosomes are spherical membrane-delimited organelles, first discovered in hepatocytes by biochemical procedures and then demonstrated in intact hepatocytes by microscopy [41,42]. Subsequently, these organelles were shown to be ubiquitous in virtually all cell types, where they play a major role in degradation of endocytosed and endogenous macromolecules [42,43]. This degradative function is mediated by enzymes within lysosomes that include a variety

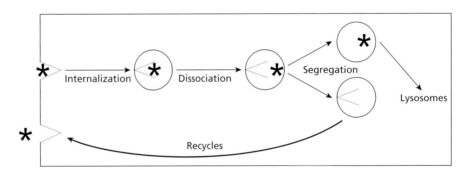

Fig. 3 Pathway of receptor-mediated endocytosis. Asialoorosomucoid (ASOR) is a hepatocyte-specific ligand that has been the subject of much investigation. ASOR (indicated by *) binds virtually irreversibly to a receptor on the hepatocyte surface plasma membrane that has been termed the asialoglycoprotein receptor. Binding to its receptor initiates internalization of the complex into an endocytic vesicle. Following acidification of this vesicle, ligand dissociates from receptor. This endocytic vesicle then undergoes a series of fissions that result in the eventual segregation of ligand from receptor and their localization into separate daughter vesicles. Following segregation, one group of daughter vesicles that contain the majority of receptor and a reduced content of ligand recycles to the cell surface. The other group of daughter vesicles that contain little receptor but most of the ligand traffics through the cell to the lysosome, where ligand is degraded [33,36,39]. Although the physiological function of the asialoglycoprotein receptor is not known, it mediates internalization and processing of its bound ligand by a process that serves as a prototype for receptor-mediated endocytosis of many other ligands.

of acid hydrolases capable of breaking down the major classes of biological macromolecules (e.g. carbohydrates, lipids, proteins, nucleic acids) into smaller components. In hepatocytes, lysosomes are distributed throughout the cytoplasm with a greater concentration near the bile canaliculus. Lysosomes exhibit a heterogeneous morphological appearance, and the different types are referred to in the literature as dense bodies, autophagic vacuoles, phagocytic vacuoles, pinocytic vacuoles, multivesicular bodies, residual bodies and tubular lysosomes. All types of lysosomes contain at least one acid hydrolase. Defects in their membrane or deficiencies in their enzyme content have resulted in the development of a number of human pathologies including a variety of lysosomal storage diseases [44].

Although little was known about the mechanism by which endocytic vesicles undergo fission and sort ligand from receptor, a number of studies suggested a role for microtubules and molecular motors in this process [25,30,33,45–52]. After internalization of ligand–receptor complexes, endocytic vesicles attach to and move along microtubules (Fig. 4). In recent studies, the process of segregation of ligand and receptor in early endocytic vesicles was reconstituted *in vitro* on microtubules using a novel fluorescence microscopy procedure in which microtubules have been attached to the surface of glass microscopy chambers (Fig. 5) [53,54]. In these studies, rat liver

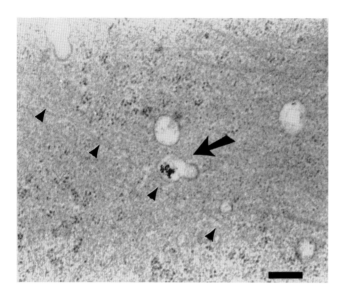

Fig. 4 Association of an endocytic vesicle with a microtubule in a hepatocyte. This is a transmission electron micrograph obtained 60 min after single-wave endocytosis of gold-conjugated ASOR by overnight cultured rat hepatocytes. An endocytic vesicle containing the gold label (arrow) is found in close proximity to a microtubule (arrowheads). In the endocytic vesicle shown in this micrograph, label is localized to one pole. Bar = 200 nm. Reprinted from ref. 30, with permission.

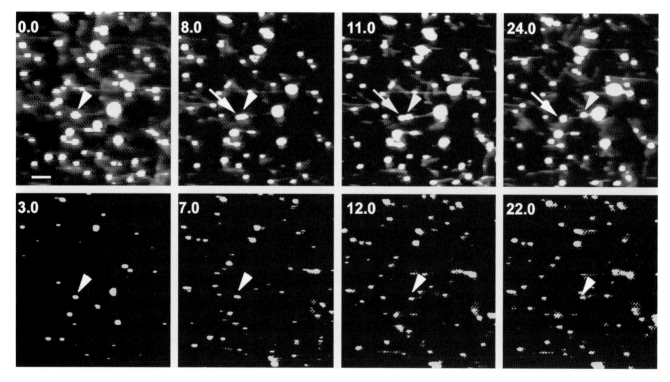

Fig. 5 Fission of a microtubule-bound endocytic vesicle *in vitro*. Texas red asialoorosomucoid (ASOR)-containing vesicles and rhodamine-labelled microtubules are in the top row. The bottom row shows the asialoglycoprotein receptor as visualized following incubation with a primary antibody and a Cy2-labelled secondary antibody. Time in seconds after addition of 50 μM ATP is shown at the upper left of each panel. Initially, the arrowhead points to a single vesicle that contains both ligand and receptor. Following the addition of ATP, this vesicle is seen to elongate and eventually to split into two daughter vesicles. Although both these daughter vesicles contain fluorescent ASOR, the one on the right contains almost all the receptor. Bar = 10 μm.

endocytic vesicles were fluorescently labelled by injection of rats with fluorescent ASOR for 5 or 15 min prior to liver harvest and vesicle purification. It was found that 5-min vesicles contained both ASOR and its receptor, indicating that they were early (presegregation) endocytic vesicles. In contrast, 15-min vesicles contained ligand but little receptor, indicating that they were late (postsegregation) endocytic vesicles. These two groups of vesicles bound to microtubules in the microscopy assay, and a substantial fraction of each group moved along the microtubules following ATP addition. However, only the early endocytic vesicles underwent fission into daughter vesicles [53,54]. Evidence suggested that this fission event was mediated by a classical kinesin motor molecule that moves towards the plus end of microtubules and a novel minus-end directed kinesin known as KifC2 [54]. The activity of KifC2 was regulated by Rab4, a small guanosine 5′-triphosphate (GTP) binding protein that is present on these early endocytic vesicles [31,54]. The late endocytic vesicles had a different complement of motor molecules and Rab proteins [31], being highly associated with dynein, a motor molecule that mediates minus end-directed movement on microtubules, Rab7, and Kif3A, a plus end-directed kinesin that was not present on the early endocytic vesicles [31,54]. These studies indicate that, over this relatively short time (10 min), acquisition and exchange of specific motor and regulatory proteins regulates the transition of early to late endocytic vesicles. The mechanism by which these important processes occur is currently under investigation.

Summary

Although simple in appearance, the hepatocyte is a complex and unique epithelial cell with subcellular structures that support important and life-sustaining biological processes. There has been much recent progress in the elucidation of these cellular components at the molecular level, and it has become apparent that there is a great deal of interaction and cross-talk between these structures within the cell. Despite this progress and novel insight into structure–function relationships within the hepatocyte, much remains to be learned regarding areas that include mechanisms to define and maintain cell polarity, cytoskeletal and motor function and interaction, and trafficking mechanisms for subcellular components. The importance of such investigation is not just theoretical, but may have major implications regarding the pathobiology and treatment of the many disorders characterized by disruption of normal hepatocyte function and homeostasis.

Acknowledgement

Supported by NIH grants CA006576, DK41918 and DK23026.

References

1 Novikoff AB, Essner E (1960) The liver cell. Some new approaches to its study. *Am J Med* 29, 102–131.

2 Ihrke G, Martin GV, Shanks MR *et al.* (1998) Apical plasma membrane proteins and endolyn-78 travel through a subapical compartment in polarized WIF-B hepatocytes. *J Cell Biol* 141, 115–133.

3 Kipp H, Arias IM (2002) Trafficking of canalicular ABC transporters in hepatocytes. *Annu Rev Physiol* 64, 595–608.

4 Bastaki M, Braiterman LT, Johns DC *et al.* (2002) Absence of direct delivery for single transmembrane apical proteins or their 'secretory' forms in polarized hepatic cells. *Mol Biol Cell* 13, 225–237.

5 Casanova JE, Mishumi Y, Ikehara Y *et al.* (1991) Direct apical sorting of rat liver dipeptidylpeptidase IV expressed in Madin–Darby canine kidney cells. *J Biol Chem* 266, 24428–24432.

6 Kremmer T, Wisher MH, Evans WH (1976) The lipid composition of plasma membrane subfractions originating from the three major functional domains of the rat hepatocyte cell surface. *Biochim Biophys Acta* 455, 655–664.

7 Storch J, Schachter D, Inoue M *et al.* (1983) Lipid fluidity of hepatocyte plasma membrane subfractions and their differential regulation by calcium. *Biochim Biophys Acta* 727, 209–212.

8 Kojima T, Yamamoto T, Murata M *et al.* (2003) Regulation of the blood–biliary barrier: interaction between gap and tight junctions in hepatocytes. *Med Electron Microsc* 36, 157–164.

9 Kojima T, Spray DC, Kokai Y *et al.* (2002) Cx32 formation and/or Cx32-mediated intercellular communication induces expression and function of tight junctions in hepatocytic cell line. *Exp Cell Res* 276, 40–51.

10 Yamamoto T, Kojima T, Murata M *et al.* (2004) IL-1beta regulates expression of Cx32, occludin, and claudin-2 of rat hepatocytes via distinct signal transduction pathways. *Exp Cell Res* 299, 427–441.

11 Kojima T, Sawada N, Chiba H *et al.* (1999) Induction of tight junctions in human connexin 32 (hCx32)-transfected mouse hepatocytes: connexin 32 interacts with occludin. *Biochem Biophys Res Commun* 266, 222–229.

12 Yin T, Green KJ (2004) Regulation of desmosome assembly and adhesion. *Semin Cell Dev Biol* 15, 665–677.

13 Tepass U (2002) Adherens junctions: new insight into assembly, modulation and function. *BioEssays* 24, 690–695.

14 Nagafuchi A (2001) Molecular architecture of adherens junctions. *Curr Opin Cell Biol* 13, 600–603.

15 Kojima T, Sawada N, Duffy HS *et al.* (2001) Gap and tight junctions in liver: composition, regulation, and function. In: Arias IM, Boyer JL, Chisari FV *et al.* (eds) *The Liver, Biology and Pathobiology*, 4th edn. Philadelphia: Lippincott Williams & Wilkins, pp. 29–46.

16 Correa PR, Guerra MT, Leite MF *et al.* (2004) Endotoxin unmasks the role of gap junctions in the liver. *Biochem Biophys Res Commun* 322, 718–726.

17 Revel JP, Karnovsky MJ (1967) Hexagonal array of subunits in intercellular junctions of the mouse heart and liver. *J Cell Biol* 33, C7–C12.

18 Spray DC (1996) Molecular physiology of gap junction channels. *Clin Exp Pharmacol Physiol* 23, 1038–1040.

19 Bergoffen J, Scherer SS, Wang S *et al.* (1993) Connexin mutations in X-linked Charcot–Marie–Tooth disease. *Science* 262, 2039–2042.

20 Omary MB, Ku NO, Toivola DM (2002) Keratins: guardians of the liver. *Hepatology* 35, 251–257.

21 Kumemura H, Harada M, Omary MB *et al.* (2004) Aggregation and loss of cytokeratin filament networks inhibit golgi organization in liver-derived epithelial cell lines. *Cell Motil Cytoskeleton* 57, 37–52.

22 Ku NO, Michie SA, Soetikno RM *et al.* (1996) Susceptibility to hepatotoxicity in transgenic mice that express a dominant-negative human keratin 18 mutant. *J Clin Invest* 98, 1034–1046.

23 Ku NO, Michie S, Oshima RG *et al.* (1995) Chronic hepatitis, hepatocyte fragility, and increased soluble phosphoglycokeratins in transgenic mice expressing a keratin 18 conserved arginine mutant. *J Cell Biol* 131, 1303–1314.

24 Zatloukal K, Stumptner C, Fuchsbichler A *et al.* (2004) The keratin cytoskeleton in liver diseases. *J Pathol* 204, 367–376.

25 Novikoff PM, Cammer M, Tao L *et al.* (1996) Three-dimensional organization of rat hepatocyte cytoskeleton: relation to the asialoglycoprotein endocytosis pathway. *J Cell Sci* 109, 21–32.

26 Bergwerk AJ, Shi X, Ford AC *et al.* (1996) Immunologic distribution of an organic anion transport protein in rat liver and kidney. *Am J Physiol* 271, G231–G238.

27 Tsukada N, Phillips MJ (1993) Bile canalicular contraction is coincident with reorganization of pericanalicular filaments and co-localization of actin and myosin-II. *J Histochem Cytochem* 41, 353–363.

28 Tsukada N, Ackerley CA, Phillips MJ (1995) The structure and organization of the bile canalicular cytoskeleton with special reference to actin and actin-binding proteins. *Hepatology* 21, 1106–1113.

29 Chan W, Calderon G, Swift AL *et al.* (2005) Myosin II regulatory light chain is required for trafficking of bile salt export protein to the apical membrane in Madin–Darby canine kidney cells. *J Biol Chem* 280, 23741–23747.

30 Goltz JS, Wolkoff AW, Novikoff PM *et al.* (1992) A role for microtubules in sorting endocytic vesicles in rat hepatocytes. *Proc Natl Acad Sci USA* 89, 7026–7030.

31 Bananis E, Nath S, Gordon K *et al.* (2004) Microtubule-dependent movement of late endocytic vesicles *in vitro*: requirements for dynein and kinesin. *Mol Biol Cell* 15, 3688–3697.

32 Stockert RJ (1995) The asialoglycoprotein receptor: relationships between structure, function, and expression. *Physiol Rev* 75, 591–609.

33 Wolkoff AW, Klausner RD, Ashwell G *et al.* (1984) Intracellular segregation of asialoglycoproteins and their receptor: a prelysosomal event subsequent to dissociation of the ligand–receptor complex. *J Cell Biol* 98, 375–381.

34 Stockert RJ, Potvin B, Tao L *et al.* (1995) Human hepatoma cell mutant defective in cell surface protein trafficking. *J Biol Chem* 270, 16107–16113.

35 Mellman I (1996) Endocytosis and molecular sorting. *Annu Rev Cell Dev Biol* 12, 575–625.

36 Mukherjee S, Ghosh RN, Maxfield FR (1997) Endocytosis. *Physiol Rev* 77, 759–803.

37 Marsh M, McMahon RT (1999) The structural era of endocytosis. *Science* 285, 215–220.

38 Forgac M (1998) Structure, function and regulation of the vacuolar (H$^+$)-ATPases. *FEBS Lett* 440, 258–263.

39 Harford J, Wolkoff AW, Ashwell G *et al.* (1983) Monensin inhibits intracellular dissociation of asialoglycoproteins from their receptor. *J Cell Biol* 96, 1824–1828.

40 Geuze HJ, Slot JW, Strous GJAM *et al.* (1984) Intracellular receptor sorting during endocytosis: comparative immunoelectron microscopy of multiple receptors in rat liver. *Cell* 37, 195–204.

41 De Duve C, Wattiaux R (1966) Functions of lysosomes. *Annu Rev Physiol* 28, 435–492.

42 Novikoff AB, Novikoff PM (1988) Lysosomes. In: Arias IM, Jakoby WB, Popper H *et al.* (eds) *The Liver: Biology and Pathobiology*, 2nd edn. New York: Raven Press, pp. 227–239.

43 Cuervo AM (2004) Autophagy: in sickness and in health. *Trends Cell Biol* 14, 70–77.

44 Vellodi A (2005) Lysosomal storage disorders. *Br J Haematol* 128, 413–431.

45 Jin M, Snider MD (1993) Role of microtubules in transferrin receptor transport from the cell surface to endosomes and the Golgi complex. *J Biol Chem* 268, 18390–18397.

46 Satir P (1994) Motor molecules of the cytoskeleton. Possible functions in the hepatocyte. In: Arias IM, Boyer JL, Fausto N *et al.* (eds) *The Liver: Biology and Pathobiology*, 3rd edn. New York: Raven Press, pp. 45–52.

47 Thatte HS, Bridges KR, Golan DE (1994) Microtubule inhibitors differentially affect translational movement, cell surface expression, and endocytosis of transferrin receptors in K562 cells. *J Cell Physiol* 160, 345–357.

48 Lafont F, Burkhardt JK, Simons K (1994) Involvement of microtubule motors in basolateral and apical transport in kidney cells. *Nature* 372, 801–803.

49 Oda H, Stockert RJ, Collins C *et al.* (1995) Interaction of the microtubule cytoskeleton with endocytic vesicles and cytoplasmic dynein in cultured rat hepatocytes. *J Biol Chem* 270, 15242–15249.

50 Hamm-Alvarez SF, Wei X, Berndt N *et al.* (1996) Protein phosphatases independently regulate vesicle movement and microtubule subpopulations in hepatocytes. *Am J Physiol* 271, C929–C943.

51 Hamm-Alvarez SF, Sheetz MP (1998) Microtubule-dependent vesicle transport: modulation of channel and transporter activity in liver and kidney. *Physiol Rev* 78, 1109–1129.

52 Murray JW, Bananis E, Wolkoff AW (2000) Reconstitution of ATP-dependent movement of endocytic vesicles along microtubules *in vitro*: an oscillatory bidirectional process. *Mol Biol Cell* 11, 419–433.

53 Bananis E, Murray JW, Stockert RJ *et al.* (2000) Microtubule and motor-dependent endocytic vesicle sorting *in vitro*. *J Cell Biol* 151, 179–186.

54 Bananis E, Murray JW, Stockert RJ *et al.* (2003) Regulation of early endocytic vesicle motility and fission in a reconstituted system. *J Cell Sci* 116, 2749–2761.

55 Wang P, Wang JJ, Xiao Y *et al.* (2005) Interaction with PDZK1 is required for expression of organic anion transporting protein 1A1 (OATP1A1) on the hepatocyte surface. *J Biol Chem* 280, 30143–30149.

2.2.3 Molecular biology of the liver cell

Sundararajah Thevananther and Saul J. Karpen

Introduction

The diversified and specialized liver functions are primarily supported by hepatocytes, which exhibit enormous capacity to respond to stressors and environmental cues effectively by activating discrete cell signalling cascades initiated at the cell surface receptors. Eventually, short-term and long-term changes occur within the cell, by modification of the activity of a broad variety of resident proteins (such as kinases, phosphatases and P-450 enzymes), modulation of the transcription of mRNA molecules

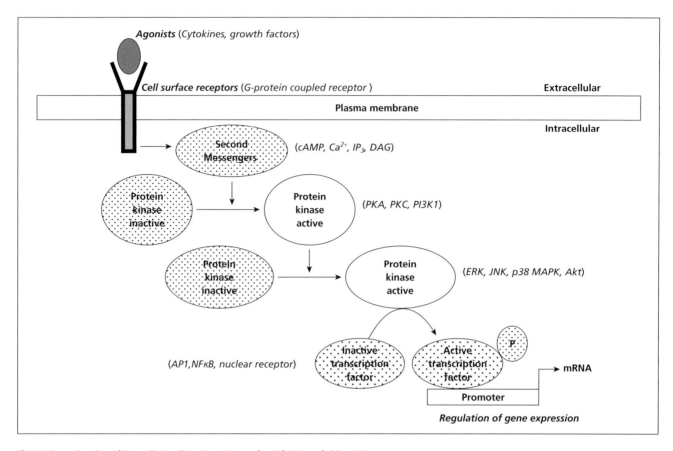

Fig. 1 General outline of liver cell signalling. See main text for definitions of abbreviations.

and synthesis of new proteins and by changes in the function or expression of nuclear transcription factors. Altogether, these processes are known as molecular adaptation, and the molecular arsenal within hepatocytes applied to cell signalling is interrelated, balanced and poised for the ultimate goal of reducing toxicity and restoring homeostasis in the most effective and expedient fashion possible. Without such an integrated, complex and balanced set of signalling responses, hepatocytes may be underdeveloped or over-reaching in their responses to stressors.

In essence, the general plan of cell signalling is to spread out the signal to as many proteins and effector molecules as possible in order to provide the maximum effective response. In some ways, it is tempting to think that the processes of cell signalling are deeply ingrained in the hepatocyte's central position at the crossroads of metabolism, which involves the production, handling and detoxification of dietary products and potential toxins from within (endobiotics) as well as from the environment (xenobiotics). The scope of this chapter will be limited to highlighting the role of signal transduction in the regulation of gene expression by its influence on the activity of transcription factors. This will include a description of key components of prototype signal transduction pathways in the liver cell with specific details regarding receptor activation, generation of second messengers, activation of kinases and phosphatases,

posttranslational modification of critical hepatic transcription factors and their role in the regulation of gene expression in the liver (Fig. 1). A detailed description of all the interrelated and competing mechanisms at play in the hepatocyte that constitute cell signalling is beyond the scope of this chapter, and the reader is referred to several recent excellent reviews [1–10].

Signal transduction

Activation of cell surface receptors and ion channels

Receptors and ion channels expressed at the cell surface 'sense' changes in the extracellular milieu of hepatocytes and modify the biological response to a multitude of physiological and pathological factors. Initiating changes in cell function and gene expression in response to environmental cues is one of the central and evolutionarily conserved ways in which the hepatocyte enacts its responses.

G protein-coupled receptors

G protein-coupled receptors are heptahelical transmembrane proteins whose activity is modulated via changes in agonist concentrations at the cell surface. Receptor–agonist interactions initiate a cascade of downstream events that is critically dependent on the subset of trimeric G proteins (α, β, γ) that interact with receptors. Receptor–G_α protein interaction leads to the activation and dissociation of G_α from $G_{\beta\gamma}$ and generation of second messengers such as cyclic adenosine monophosphate (cAMP), inositol 1,4,5-triphosphate (IP_3) and diacylglycerol (DAG). Cellular responses to fluctuations in hormones and growth factors are dependent on the types and abundance of G protein-coupled receptors expressed at the sinusoidal and canalicular surface of hepatocytes [11].

Receptor tyrosine kinases

Peptide growth factor signalling is transduced mostly via the activation of receptor tyrosine kinases (RTKs). RTKs are a class of cell surface receptors with a single transmembrane domain separating the extracellular domains, with affinity for peptide growth factors such as insulin and epidermal growth factor, from the intracellular cytoplasmic domains with tyrosine kinase activity. Autophosphorylation of RTKs activates a cascade of small GTPases such as Ras, Rac, RhoA and Cdc42 [9].

Ion channels

Ion channels play integral roles in modulating a variety of synthetic and secretary functions of hepatocytes. Hepatocytes express ligand-gated and voltage-sensitive anion and cation channels that regulate ion exchange with the extracellular milieu. Cell volume regulation is one of the most fundamental homeostatic mechanisms and essential for normal hepatocyte function [12]. Cell swelling evokes a series of signalling events resulting in the activation of K^+ and Cl^- efflux via ion channels, which plays a key role in the regulatory volume decrease and restoration of homeostasis [13]. Ion fluxes induced by the activity of ion channels influence several key events in the life cycle of hepatocytes, such as cell cycle control, proliferation, survival and apoptosis [14]. Several ion channels are linked to the cytoskeleton, and ion channel function is greatly affected by the changes in the submembranous cytoskeleton.

Generation of second messengers

Activation of cell surface receptors and ion channels results in the generation of second messengers such as cyclic nucleotides (cAMP, cGMP), lipids (IP_3, DAG), Ca^{2+}, prostaglandins and nitric oxide (NO).

cAMP

A large number of hormones, peptides and neurotransmitters interact with several G protein-coupled receptors. The αs subunit of G proteins ($G_{\alpha s}$) activates adenylate cyclase, which catalyses the generation of cAMP from adenosine triphosphate (ATP). Increase in intracellular cAMP levels leads to the activation of a cAMP-dependent kinase, protein kinase A (PKA). The effects of cAMP are primarily mediated via the activation of PKA and influence a wide range of metabolic, synthetic and secretory

functions of hepatocytes. For example, PKA phosphorylates hormone-sensitive lipase and perilipin, and results in increased lipolysis. Conversely, activation of the αi subunit of G proteins ($G_{\alpha i}$) inhibits lipolysis via the inhibition of adenylate cyclase and reductions in the intracellular cAMP levels. Phosphodiesterases participate in the termination of cAMP/PKA signalling by hydrolysing and reducing intracellular cAMP levels [4].

Lipids

IP_3 and DAG play important roles in the activation of Ca^{2+} signalling and protein kinase C (PKC). Agonists such as ATP and vasopressin binding at the $G_{\alpha q}$ protein-coupled cell surface receptors lead to the generation of IP_3 and DAG. The αq subunit of G protein interacts with the enzyme phospholipase C (PLCβ) and activates the translocation of the enzyme to the plasma membrane. In addition, the dimeric $\beta\gamma$ subunits enhance the membrane tethering of PLCβ, promote the hydrolysis of phosphatidylinositol 4,5-bisphosphate and stimulate the production of Ca^{2+}-mobilizing second messengers IP_3 and DAG. IP_3, in turn, activates the release of Ca^{2+} via the activation of IP_3 receptors (IP_3Rs) located in the endoplasmic reticulum, whereas DAGs play a role in the activation of conventional and novel PKCs.

In addition to G protein-coupled receptors, the phosphoinositide signalling pathway can be activated by the agonist-induced dimerization and tyrosine autophosphorylation of RTKs, creating high-affinity docking sites for SH2-containing PLCγ, which in turn catalyses the generation of IP_3 and DAG [15].

Ca^{2+}

Intracellular Ca^{2+} is a versatile second messenger in hepatocytes that plays a central role in regulating multiple hepatic functions and influencing varied processes such as secretion, contraction, metabolism, gene transcription and cell proliferation and apoptosis [16]. Intracellular cytosolic Ca^{2+} levels are influenced by upstream signalling events that activate the release of Ca^{2+} from intracellular stores (endoplasmic reticulum, Golgi, nucleoplasmic reticulum) as well as the Ca^{2+} influx from the extracellular milieu. The spatial and temporal patterns of calcium signals are believed to be responsible for determining the specificity and functional outcome of Ca^{2+} signalling. The subcellular distribution of the three isoforms of IP_3 receptors (types 1, 2 and 3), which differ in their affinity for IP_3 and regulation by Ca^{2+}, shape the amplitude, duration and wave patterns of Ca^{2+} transients in the cytosol. Nucleoplasmic reticulum enriched in type 2 IP_3Rs serves as a distinct reservoir of Ca^{2+} within the nuclei and is responsible for the localized generation of Ca^{2+} signals within the nucleus. The versatility of Ca^{2+} signalling within hepatocytes is underlined by their distinct ability to independently modulate Ca^{2+} signalling in the cytosolic vs. nuclear compartments [6,17,18].

Prostanoids

Prostaglandins are believed to play a role in mitogenic signal transduction in the regenerating liver and hepatocellular carcinoma. Phospholipase A_2 (PLA$_2$) activity leads to arachidonic acid release from the plasma membrane. Metabolism of arachidonic acids by the cyclo-oxygenases (COXs) leads to the generation of prostanoids, including prostaglandins and thromboxanes, in the liver. Hepatocyte growth factor receptor-mediated activation of mitogen-activated protein kinases (MAPKs) and elevations in intracellular Ca^{2+} are believed to play a role in the activation of PLA$_2$ [19,20].

Nitric oxide (NO)

The free radical NO has emerged in recent years as a small signalling molecule playing protective roles against hepatocyte apoptosis induced by tumour necrosis factor α (TNFα) and Fas ligand [21]. NO is synthesized in the cytosol and mitochondria by constitutive and inducible nitric oxide synthases (cNOS and iNOS). Under normal conditions, lower levels of NO generated act as a messenger and cytoprotective (antioxidant) factor, via direct interactions with transition metals and other free radicals. However, proinflammatory signalling leads to elevations in NO, which in turn binds and activates soluble guanylyl cyclase, leading to the conversion of guanosine triphosphate (GTP) into cyclic GMP (cGMP). Increased cGMP levels via the activation of protein kinase G (PKG) protect hepatocytes against ischaemia–reperfusion injury [22].

Activation of signalling cascades

Protein kinases influence cellular functions by catalysing the addition of a phosphate group to proteins at serine, threonine or tyrosine residues, thus serving as molecular switches discretely turning 'on' and 'off' protein function in a specific manner [23]. Hepatocellular signalling cascades often consist of multiple protein kinases acting in tandem, facilitating signal amplification and target protein modification in order to adapt and respond to the changes in the environment. Among the multiple protein kinases expressed in hepatocytes, the following are discussed below based on their functional significance for hepatocytes.

Protein kinase A

PKA is a tetrameric holoenzyme consisting of two regulatory and two catalytic subunits. cAMP binding at the regulatory subunits results in the dissociation of the PKA–protein complex. The activated catalytic subunits are released from cytoplasmic anchoring sites and phosphorylate a variety of cytoplasmic and nuclear substrates on serine sites within the canonical sequence X-Arg-Arg-X-Ser-X. Binding of MgATP at the regulatory subunit I (RI) stabilizes the holoenzyme by raising the threshold for cAMP concentrations required for activation. Autophosphorylation of the regulatory subunit II (RII) leads to the destabilization of the holoenzyme and activation of catalytic subunits. The specificity of PKA action is determined in part by anchoring PKA to subcellular sites through the association of the regulatory subunits with A-kinase anchoring proteins. PKA activity plays a key role in the polarized localization of proteins

and lipids into distinct apical and canalicular membrane domains in hepatocytes [24,25].

Protein kinase C (PKC)

PKCs are a family of serine/threonine kinases and consist of a family of at least 12 isoforms, classified into classical, novel and atypical PKCs based on their distinct mode of activation. The conventional PKC isoforms (cPKCα, βI, βII and γ) are activated by Ca^{2+} and phospholipids such as DAGs. The novel PKC isoforms (nPKCδ, ϵ, η and θ) are Ca^{2+} independent, and the atypical PKC isoforms (aPKCζ and λ) are independent of both Ca^{2+} and DAG [26].

Mitogen-activated protein kinases

MAPKs are important signal transducing enzymes connecting cell surface receptors to critical regulatory targets within hepatocytes. MAPK activity is controlled by a three-tiered cascade of MAPKs, MAPK kinases (MAPKK, MKK or MEK) and MAPKK kinase or MEK kinase (MAPKKK or MEKK). Several effector kinases such as MAPK-activated protein kinases (MAPKAPs) are activated by MAPKs, and MAPK signalling is attenuated by the action of MAPK phosphatases [5].

Hepatocytes express at least four distinct groups of MAPKs, i.e. extracellular signal-regulated kinases (ERK1/2 or p44/42 MAPK), c-jun N-terminal kinases (JNK1 and 2), p38 MAPK (p38α/α/$\gamma\delta$) and ERK5 [27–29]. Several growth factor and cytokine actions are mediated via the activation of multiple MAPK signalling pathways, influencing hepatocyte survival and proliferation. ERK1/2 activation in response to the activation of receptor tyrosine kinases by growth factors stimulates hepatocyte proliferation and survival [30]. Whereas JNK1/2 and p38 MAPK, collectively known as the stress-activated protein kinases (SAPKs), are activated by ultraviolet radiation, inflammatory cytokines and DNA damaging agents are linked to divergent liver functions such as the downregulation of gene expression during acute phase response, hepatocyte proliferation during liver regeneration and hepatocyte apoptosis [3,31–33].

Several distinct mechanisms ensure the specificity of MAPK activation. First, scaffolding proteins such as JIP1 organize JNK1/2 (MAPK), MKK7 (MAPKK) and MLK1 (MAPKKK) into a specific signalling cassette. Second, sequential physical interaction between members of a given cascade ensures the effective activation of a signalling pathway, as in the case of JNK1/2, which is bound by the N-terminal extension of MKK4 (MAPKK), which also interacts with the catalytic domain of MEKK1 (MAPKKK). Typically, the phosphoacceptor sites of MAPKs are composed of serine or threonine followed by a proline, and the neighbouring amino acids further increase the specificity of binding by the catalytic pocket of the kinase. Finally, full specificity is ensured through a docking interaction mediated by an additional site in the kinase that recognizes a distinct site other than the phosphoacceptor site in the substrate. For example, JNK recognizes and interacts with a short sequence that precedes the two principal phosphoacceptor sites, Ser63 and Ser73, outside its catalytic pocket,[2,8].

Phosphatidylinositol-3-kinases (PI3Ks)

PI3Ks are heterodimers consisting of a catalytic subunit (p110) and a regulatory subunit (p85), and they phosphorylate at the 3′-OH group of the inositol ring in inositol lipids. Upon activation of receptor tyrosine kinases, PI3Ks associate with the receptor through its SH2 domains in the regulatory subunit, leading to the activation of the catalytic subunit of the enzyme. PI3K activity is responsible for the generation of the second messenger phosphatidylinositol 3,4,5-trisphosphate (PIP_3) from phosphatidylinositol 4,5-biphosphate at the inner leaflet of the plasma membrane. PIP_3 binding at the PH domain of proteins such as Akt/protein kinase B (PKB) and activation of downstream signalling play important roles in tumorigenesis and tumour progression in hepatocellular carcinoma. The PTEN phosphatase is a natural antagonist of the PI3K/Akt signalling pathway, and hepatitis B virus X protein (HBx)-mediated activation of Akt signalling is associated with a decrease in PTEN levels [34]. In addition to their effects on hepatocyte proliferation and metastasis, PI3K/Akt pathways influence vesicular trafficking, bile formation and bile acid secretion [35,36].

Rho GTPases

Apart from the heterotrimeric G proteins, which transduce signals from the serpentine G protein-coupled receptors (GPCRs), another superfamily of small G proteins, consisting of the Rho family of GTPases (Rho, Rac, Cdc42), plays key roles in the regulation of a variety of cellular processes in hepatocytes. Activation of receptor tyrosine kinases and GPCRs leads to the activation of Rho guanine nucleotide exchange factors (GEFs) and their Rho GTPase substrates. GEFs destabilize the inactive GDP–G protein complex, inducing the release of GDP and the binding of cytosolic GTP, activating the G proteins. GTPase-activating proteins (GAPs) induce the hydrolysis of GTP bound to G proteins and inactivate them [9].

The Rho family of GTPase-mediated signalling molecules plays key roles in the organization of the cell cytoskeleton and the cell–cell and cell–matrix interactions, which influence hepatocyte polarity, gene transcription and growth regulation. Additionally, small GTPases play integral roles in the activation of JNK signalling and stimulation of DNA synthesis in primary hepatocytes in response to known agonists such as TNFα and hepatocyte growth factor [37].

Transcription factors and regulation of gene expression

In addition to alterations in the activity of cell surface receptors, second messengers and intracellular kinases, one of the major ways in which hepatocytes respond to external stimuli in a sustained fashion is to reprogramme mRNA transcription. In general, the primary mediators of gene regulation are nuclear proteins, typically referred to as transcription factors. In many ways, transcription factors can be thought of as proteins that bridge the gap between DNA regulatory sequences in genes (promoter regions) and the freely mobile proteins in the cell that execute changes initiated by cell signalling cascades [38,39]. Although, in a general sense, transcription factors can be thought of as DNA-binding proteins, they cannot effect transcription alone [40]. It is best to consider these DNA-binding proteins as anchors for the transcription factor complex, which includes co-regulators, cofactors, chromatin-modifying proteins and RNA polymerases, which together constitute a transcription initiation complex. Recent evidence even indicates that small RNA molecules are components of the transcription initiation complex [41,42]. A detailed review of the role of all members of the transcription initiation complex in regulating gene expression in hepatocytes is beyond the scope of this chapter, but highlighting a few select transcription factors, families and their interactions and responses to cell signalling processes will serve as informative examples of hepatocyte response [7,43,44]. Given their central roles as the ultimate effector molecules of cell signalling cascades, we will focus on the following target transcription factors and families: AP1, NFκB, the forkhead family and multiple members of the nuclear receptor superfamily.

AP1 and NFκB

These two transcription factor complexes have become recognized as the centrepieces of the hepatocyte's response to inflammation and infection, but they also play pivotal roles in cell survival, growth response to injury and apoptosis [3,31,45–51]. Nearly all cells in the body engage AP1 and NFκB complexes in response to stressors and injury, and their central role in hepatocyte functions ranges from acute phase response and intermediary metabolism to toxin disposal. In addition, it is important to recognize that AP1 and NFκB are both critically involved in the development of the liver, as single gene deletions in critical components of these two proteins are lethal *in utero*, and the mice do not form livers [32,52–54].

AP1 is a complex of two proteins that contains either homodimers of c-jun or heterodimers of c-jun with c-fos. These are potent regulators of gene transcription for those genes that have AP1 response elements, but they also interact with multiple different proteins in order to spread out the signal [55]. It is important to note that there are many different pathways that lead to the activation of AP1, and they generally involve phosphorylation of pre-existing components of the AP1 complex that then activates it. The one that appears to be most relevant is one of the MAPKs, in particular c-jun N-terminal kinase or JNK [33]. Once JNK is activated, it phosphorylates c-jun. AP1 target genes are numerous in the liver and are present not only in hepatocytes, but also in Kupffer cells, stellate cells, cholangiocytes and all associated inflammatory cells. In Kupffer cells and inflammatory cells, activated AP1 induces the expression of a broad variety of cytokines and other secreted inflammatory proteins. In hepatocytes, activation of both c-jun and AP1 alters the expression of several genes essential for cell survival, whereas sustained activation of JNK and AP1 can be deleterious to the cell [50].

The other primary component of the two-pronged induction of intracellular signalling associated with inflammation is NFκB. Similar in concept to AP1, activation of select kinases activates NFκB by releasing it from an inactive complex. Like AP1, NFκB is a two-part transcription factor assembly (p50 and p65) that is retained in the cytoplasm in an inactive form in complex with other proteins including an inhibitor, IκB [47,56]. In response to the activation of certain cell surface receptors (e.g. cytokine receptors), upstream kinases activate IκB kinase (IKK), which leads to the phosphorylation and degradation of inhibitory IκB and releases NFκB, which then targets to the nucleus. Once in the nucleus, NFκB can change gene expression by binding to target sequences within appropriate promoter contexts. As is the case for AP1, the NFκB protein complex has activities that extend far beyond those of binding to DNA elements in promoter regions, and also has broad interactions with a variety of proteins involved in transcription as well as basic cellular functions and cell survival. Finally, NFκB plays a critical role in cell cycle regulation and hepatocellular carcinogenesis, perhaps best understood in its role as an antiapoptotic agent [51,57]. Although we now understand a lot more about NFκB and AP1, it is quite apparent that the competing, overlapping and contradictory target gene regulations of these two potent transcription factors are still being determined. One example of NFκB activation leading to export of toxins is the rapid and profound activation of the *MDR1b* gene by NFκB [58]. This multispecific substrate transporter is responsible for the export of a broad variety of toxins and drugs from the hepatocyte.

Among the more interesting and exciting findings over the past few years is an ongoing relationship between adaptive immunity and innate immunity, which extends beyond T and B cells to incorporate hepatocytes as the central components of the immune system. This is an ancient arrangement, conserved through evolution, with homologies between the fat body in *Drosophila* and mammalian livers [59,60]. With respect to innate immunity, hepatocytes have receptors for pathogens and pathogen-specific molecules on their cell surface, generally grouped as members of the Toll-like receptor (TLR) family [10,61,62]. This makes intuitive sense, recognizing where the liver is anatomically, the constant delivery of foods, toxins, bacteria and bacterial products to the portal circulation and its role as an excretory organ. Among the more recent findings is that activation of TLR4, the cell surface receptor for lipopolysaccharide, activates a broad variety of changes in cell signalling within hepatocytes. This central player in innate immunity activates many components of the acute phase response, including activation of AP1 and NFκB. The other overlapping means of responding to inflammatory signals is generally referred to as adaptive immunity, via activation of receptors for the central

proinflammatory cytokines TNFα, interleukin (IL)-1β and IL-6, the three main cytokines involved in the liver's response to inflammation. In liver disease, complex and overlapping activations of multiple intracellular signalling pathways from the TLRs and cytokine receptors may be 'firing' simultaneously.

Forkhead (HNF3) family

The HNF3 α, β and γ isoforms identified as key regulators of the expression of serum proteins (e.g. transferrin, albumin, transthyretin) are more accurately referred to as members of the forkhead (FOXa) family of transcription factors [63,64]. These transcription factors are involved in growth, development, neoplasia, inflammation, regeneration and response to injury, and are themselves regulated by posttranslational modifications such as phosphorylation and interaction with other cellular proteins.

Nuclear receptors

Members of the nuclear receptor (NR) superfamily are intimately involved in orchestrating the transcriptional programme of a broad range of processes and functions within hepatocytes [65]. These ligand-regulated transcription factors can directly modulate the response to either excess or insufficient endobiotics, nutritional substances and inflammation, as well as engaging the protective response to exogenous substances such as drugs and toxins (xenobiotics) [7,66]. Nuclear receptors are present in all metazoans, and there are 48 members of the human nuclear receptor superfamily. The structural organization of nuclear receptors has been relatively preserved among its members, and includes activation domains, DNA-binding domains and, of particular interest, the ligand-binding domains. The nuclear receptor activity is regulatable by small molecule ligands. Many of these ligands are substances involved in liver metabolism such as fatty acids, sterols and bile acids. There is overwhelming evidence in recent years suggesting that several genes involved in diverse cellular processes in the liver, such as regulation of glucose metabolism, fatty acid synthesis and oxidation, cholesterol metabolism and bile acid homeostasis, are all regulated by NR superfamily members [38,67–71]. For example, intracellular bile acid homeostasis is primarily regulated by three nuclear receptors, CAR, PXR and FXR, of which the last two can be activated directly by primary bile acids acting as ligands. Over the past few years, it has been clear that the nuclear receptors CAR, PXR and FXR are central to the adaptive response to cholestasis, orchestrating changes in membrane transport, metabolism, conjugation and export of bile acids in states where bile acids are inappropriately retained intracellularly [66].

These three nuclear receptors cannot function alone, or as homodimers, but function as heterodimers partnering with the central nuclear receptor, RXR. It is likely that the ligand for RXR is 9 cis-retinoic acid, whereas PXR is activated by a broad variety of xenobiotics, including drugs such as rifampicin, whereas CAR activation is complex and may not involve any ligand binding [72]. These nuclear receptors are not immune to interactions with cell signalling cascades. Most nuclear receptors are phosphoproteins and, in particular, the nuclear receptor partner, RXR, is highly regulatable by a cell signalling cascade such as JNK [1,73]. Moreover, activation of cell signalling molecules such as JNK, AP1 and NFκB, can directly regulate several of these nuclear receptors either by direct interactions or by competition for binding to sites in promoter regions. Animal models of activation of inflammation with either lipopolysaccharide or cytokines generally reduce the functional activity and occasionally the mRNA expression of CAR, FXR and PXR. In the context of inflammation, activation of certain cell signalling pathways negatively affects the capacity of hepatocytes to handle bile acids, exacerbating the ongoing liver disease. Thus, there seems to be synergy, in a negative fashion, between chronic inflammatory signalling and ongoing liver disease from any initiating cause. Recent evidence suggests that there may be ways of interfering with this impaired response using a variety of nuclear receptor ligands.

In addition to direct modification of nuclear receptors by cell signalling pathways, there are known direct interactions of key signalling intermediates and nuclear receptors. Among the more relevant interactions is the NFκB binding to the DNA-binding domain of RXR, which interferes with its function [74]. Moreover, there are components of the transcription factor assembly, which not only include nuclear receptors and core regulators but also AP1 and other small molecules, that can shuttle between the cytoplasm and the nucleus and participate in transcription.

Conclusions of integration of cell signalling and transcription

In addition to rapid activation of signal transduction cascades that facilitate the hepatocyte to elicit a quick response to stressors, long-term changes and cellular adaptation appear to be best effected by changes in the transcriptional programme, by ultimately altering the function and efficacy of regulatory transcription factors. These, in turn, can alter the expression and function of cellular proteins involved in signal transduction, thereby providing an effective feedback mechanism. Some of the cellular responses are components of the acute phase response, and are generally thought to be beneficial in the short term but, if prolonged and persistent, could be detrimental. It is a delicate balancing act that the hepatocytes perform in order to safely and effectively perform their duties as the central responders to xenobiotics and stressors. Of therapeutic interest is that cell signalling cascades (kinases), as well as NR family members, are potential therapeutic targets, which may be able to augment the beneficial aspects of the integration of cell signalling and transcriptional reprogramming and minimize the negative consequences.

References

1 Rochette-Egly C (2003) Nuclear receptors: integration of multiple signalling pathways through phosphorylation. Cell Signal 15, 355–366.

2 Bogoyevitch MA, Boehm I, Oakley A et al. (2004) Targeting the JNK MAPK cascade for inhibition: basic science and therapeutic potential. Biochim Biophys Acta 1697, 89–101.

3 Brenner DA (1998) Signal transduction during liver regeneration. J Gastroenterol Hepatol 13(Suppl.), S93–95.

4 Carmen GY, Victor SM (2006) Signalling mechanisms regulating lipolysis. Cell Signal 18, 401–408.

5 Chang L, Karin M (2001) Mammalian MAP kinase signalling cascades. Nature 410, 37–40.

6 Gasper LD, Pierodon N, Thomas AP (2005) Calcium signaling. In: Dufour JF, Clavien PA (eds) Signaling Pathways in Liver Diseases. Berlin: Springer-Verlag.

7 Karpen SJ (2002) Nuclear receptor regulation of hepatic function. J Hepatol 36, 832–850.

8 Nishina H, Wada T, Katada T (2004) Physiological roles of SAPK/JNK signaling pathway. J Biochem (Tokyo) 136, 123–126.

9 Schiller MR (2006) Coupling receptor tyrosine kinases to Rho GTPases-GEFs what's the link. Cell Signal 18, 1834–1843.

10 Schwabe RF, Seki E, Brenner DA (2006) Toll-like receptor signaling in the liver. Gastroenterology 130, 1886–1900.

11 Hepler JR, Gilman AG (1992) G proteins. Trends Biochem Sci 17, 383–387.

12 Haussinger D, Reinehr R, Schliess F (2006) The hepatocyte integrin system and cell volume sensing. Acta Physiol (Oxford) 187, 249–255.

13 Lang F, Ritter M, Volkl H et al. (1993) The biological significance of cell volume. Ren Physiol Biochem 16, 48–65.

14 Stutzin A, Hoffmann EK (2006) Swelling-activated ion channels: functional regulation in cell-swelling, proliferation and apoptosis. Acta Physiol (Oxford) 187, 27–42.

15 Balla T (2006) Phosphoinositide-derived messengers in endocrine signaling. J Endocrinol 188, 135–153.

16 Nathanson MH, Schlosser SF (1996) Calcium signaling mechanisms in liver in health and disease. Prog Liver Dis 14, 1–27.

17 Echevarria W, Leite MF, Guerra MT et al. (2003) Regulation of calcium signals in the nucleus by a nucleoplasmic reticulum. Nature Cell Biol 5, 440–446.

18 Leite MF, Thrower EC, Echevarria W et al. (2003) Nuclear and cytosolic calcium are regulated independently. Proc Natl Acad Sci USA 100, 2975–2980.

19 Adachi T, Nakashima S, Saji S et al. (1995) Roles of prostaglandin production and mitogen-activated protein kinase activation in hepatocyte growth factor-mediated rat hepatocyte proliferation. Hepatology 21, 1668–1674.

20 Wu T (2006) Cyclooxygenase-2 in hepatocellular carcinoma. Cancer Treat Rev 32, 28–44.

21 Hatano E, Bennett BL, Manning AM et al. (2001) NF-kappaB stimulates inducible nitric oxide synthase to protect mouse hepatocytes from TNF-alpha-and Fas-mediated apoptosis. Gastroenterology 120, 1251–1262.

22 Kim JS, Ohshima S, Pediaditakis P et al. (2004) Nitric oxide: a signaling molecule against mitochondrial permeability transition- and pH-dependent cell death after reperfusion. Free Radic Biol Med 37, 1943–1950.

23 Hunter T (1995) Protein kinases and phosphatases: the yin and yang of protein phosphorylation and signaling. Cell 80, 225–236.

24 Mukhopadhayay S, Ananthanarayanan M, Stieger B *et al.* (1997) cAMP increases liver Na$^+$-taurocholate cotransport by translocating transporter to plasma membranes. *Am J Physiol* 273, G842–848.

25 Gatmaitan ZC, Nies AT, Arias IM (1997) Regulation and translocation of ATP-dependent apical membrane proteins in rat liver. *Am J Physiol* 272, G1041–1049.

26 Newton AC (2001) Protein kinase C: structural and spatial regulation by phosphorylation, cofactors, and macromolecular interactions. *Chem Rev* 101, 2353–2364.

27 Liang T, Xu S, Yu J *et al.* (2005) Activation pattern of mitogen-activated protein kinases in early phase of different size liver isografts in rats. *Liver Transpl* 11, 1527–1532.

28 Nishioka H, Kishioka T, Iida C *et al.* (2006) Activation of mitogen activated protein kinase (MAPK) during D-galactosamine intoxication in the rat liver. *Bioorg Med Chem Lett* 16, 3019–3022.

29 Bradham CA, Stachlewitz RF, Gao W *et al.* (1997) Reperfusion after liver transplantation in rats differentially activates the mitogen-activated protein kinases. *Hepatology* 25, 1128–1135.

30 Desbois-Mouthon C, Wendum D, Cadoret A *et al.* (2006) Hepatocyte proliferation during liver regeneration is impaired in mice with liver-specific IGF-1R knockout. *FASEB J* 20, 773–775.

31 Gunawan BK, Liu ZX, Han D *et al.* (2006) c-Jun N-terminal kinase plays a major role in murine acetaminophen hepatotoxicity. *Gastroenterology* 131, 165–178.

32 Eferl R, Sibilia M, Hilberg F *et al.* (1999) Functions of c-Jun in liver and heart development. *J Cell Biol* 145, 1049–1061.

33 Czaja MJ (2003) The future of GI and liver research: editorial perspectives. III. JNK/AP-1 regulation of hepatocyte death. *Am J Physiol Gastrointest Liver Physiol* 284, G875–879.

34 Michl P, Downward J (2005) Mechanisms of disease: PI3K/AKT signaling in gastrointestinal cancers. *Z Gastroenterol* 43, 1133–1139.

35 Webster CR, Blanch CJ, Phillips J *et al.* (2000) Cell swelling-induced translocation of rat liver Na(+)/taurocholate cotransport polypeptide is mediated via the phosphoinositide 3-kinase signaling pathway. *J Biol Chem* 275, 29754–29760.

36 Webster CR, Anwer MS (1999) Role of the PI3K/PKB signaling pathway in cAMP-mediated translocation of rat liver Ntcp. *Am J Physiol* 277, G1165–1172.

37 Auer KL, Contessa J, Brenz-Verca S *et al.* (1998) The Ras/Rac1/Cdc42/SEK/JNK/c-Jun cascade is a key pathway by which agonists stimulate DNA synthesis in primary cultures of rat hepatocytes. *Mol Biol Cell* 9, 561–573.

38 Glass CK (2006) Going nuclear in metabolic and cardiovascular disease. *J Clin Invest* 116, 556–560.

39 Smith JM, Koopman PA (2004) The ins and outs of transcriptional control: nucleocytoplasmic shuttling in development and disease. *Trends Genet* 20, 4–8.

40 Smith CL, O'Malley BW (2004) Coregulator function: a key to understanding tissue specificity of selective receptor modulators. *Endocr Rev* 25, 45–71.

41 Jeong JW, Kwak I, Lee KY *et al.* (2006) The genomic analysis of the impact of steroid receptor coactivators ablation on hepatic metabolism. *Mol Endocrinol* 20, 1138–1152.

42 Togashi M, Borngraeber S, Sandler B *et al.* (2005) Conformational adaptation of nuclear receptor ligand binding domains to agonists: potential for novel approaches to ligand design. *J Steroid Biochem Mol Biol* 93, 127–137.

43 Wagner M, Trauner M (2005) Transcriptional regulation of hepatobiliary transport systems in health and disease: implications for a rationale approach to the treatment of intrahepatic cholestasis. *Ann Hepatol* 4, 77–99.

44 Kaplowitz N (2002) Biochemical and cellular mechanisms of toxic liver injury. *Semin Liver Dis* 22, 137–144.

45 Kountouras J, Boura P, Lygidakis NJ (2001) Liver regeneration after hepatectomy. *Hepatogastroenterology* 48, 556–562.

46 Herrlich P (2001) Cross-talk between glucocorticoid receptor and AP-1. *Oncogene* 20, 2465–2475.

47 Heyninck K, Wullaert A, Beyaert R (2003) Nuclear factor-kappa B plays a central role in tumour necrosis factor-mediated liver disease. *Biochem Pharmacol* 66, 1409–1415.

48 Vanden Berghe W, De Bosscher K, Vermeulen L *et al.* (2002) Induction and repression of NF-kappa B-driven inflammatory genes. *Ernst Schering Res Found Workshop*, 233–278.

49 Morgan ET, Li-Masters T, Cheng PY (2002) Mechanisms of cytochrome P450 regulation by inflammatory mediators. *Toxicology* 181–182:207–210.

50 Sakurai T, Maeda S, Chang L *et al.* (2006) Loss of hepatic NF-kappaB activity enhances chemical hepatocarcinogenesis through sustained c-Jun N-terminal kinase 1 activation. *Proc Natl Acad Sci USA* 103, 10544–10551.

51 Liu H, Lo CR, Czaja MJ (2002) NF-kappaB inhibition sensitizes hepatocytes to TNF-induced apoptosis through a sustained activation of JNK and c-Jun. *Hepatology* 35, 772–778.

52 Karin M (2006) Nuclear factor-kappaB in cancer development and progression. *Nature* 441, 431–436.

53 Tanaka M, Fuentes ME, Yamaguchi K *et al.* (1999) Embryonic lethality, liver degeneration, and impaired NF-kappa B activation in IKK-beta-deficient mice. *Immunity* 10, 421–429.

54 Beg AA, Sha WC, Bronson RT *et al.* (1995) Embryonic lethality and liver degeneration in mice lacking the RelA component of NF-kappa B. *Nature* 376, 167–170.

55 Hess J, Angel P, Schorpp-Kistner M (2004) AP-1 subunits: quarrel and harmony among siblings. *J Cell Sci* 117, 5965–5973.

56 Baldwin AS Jr (1996) The NF-kappa B and I kappa B proteins: new discoveries and insights. *Annu Rev Immunol* 14, 649–683.

57 Dobrovolskaia MA, Kozlov SV (2005) Inflammation and cancer: when NF-kappaB amalgamates the perilous partnership. *Curr Cancer Drug Targets* 5, 325–344.

58 Cherrington NJ, Slitt AL, Li N *et al.* (2004) Lipopolysaccharide-mediated regulation of hepatic transporter mRNA levels in rats. *Drug Metab Dispos* 32, 734–741.

59 Meister M, Lemaitre B, Hoffmann JA (1997) Antimicrobial peptide defense in *Drosophila*. *Bioessays* 19, 1019–1026.

60 Sondergaard L (1993) Homology between the mammalian liver and the *Drosophila* fat body. *Trends Genet* 9, 193.

61 Liu S, Gallo DJ, Green AM *et al.* (2002) Role of toll-like receptors in changes in gene expression and NF-kappa B activation in mouse hepatocytes stimulated with lipopolysaccharide. *Infect Immun* 70, 3433–3442.

62 Vodovotz Y, Liu S, McCloskey C *et al.* (2001) The hepatocyte as a microbial product-responsive cell. *J Endotoxin Res* 7, 365–373.

63 Costa RH, Kalinichenko VV, Holterman AX *et al.* (2003) Transcription factors in liver development, differentiation, and regeneration. *Hepatology* 38, 1331–1347.

64 Clevidence DE, Overdier DG, Tao W *et al.* (1993) Identification of nine tissue-specific transcription factors of the hepatocyte nuclear factor 3/forkhead DNA-binding-domain family. *Proc Natl Acad Sci USA* 90, 3948–3952.

65 Folkertsma S, van Noort PI, Brandt RF *et al.* (2005) The nuclear receptor ligand-binding domain: a family-based structure analysis. *Curr Med Chem* 12, 1001–1016.

66 Boyer JL (2005) Nuclear receptor ligands: rational and effective therapy for chronic cholestatic liver disease? *Gastroenterology* 129, 735–740.

67 Houten SM, Watanabe M, Auwerx J (2006) Endocrine functions of bile acids. *EMBO J* 25, 1419–1425.

68 Tirona RG, Kim RB (2005) Nuclear receptors and drug disposition gene regulation. *J Pharm Sci* 94, 1169–1186.

69 Eloranta JJ, Meier PJ, Kullak-Ublick GA (2005) Coordinate transcriptional regulation of transport and metabolism. *Methods Enzymol* 400, 511–530.

70 Ory DS (2004) Nuclear receptor signaling in the control of cholesterol homeostasis: have the orphans found a home? *Circ Res* 95, 660–670.

71 Dussault I, Forman BM (2002) The nuclear receptor PXR: a master regulator of 'homeland' defense. *Crit Rev Eukaryot Gene Expr* 12, 53–64.

72 Karpen SJ (2005) Exercising the nuclear option to treat cholestasis: CAR and PXR ligands. *Hepatology* 42, 266–269.

73 Rochette-Egly C (2005) Dynamic combinatorial networks in nuclear receptor-mediated transcription. *J Biol Chem* 280, 32565–32568.

74 Fernandez-Martin JL, Kurian S, Farmer P *et al.* (1998) Tumor necrosis factor activates a nuclear inhibitor of vitamin D and retinoid-X receptors. *Mol Cell Endocrinol* 141, 65–72.

2.2.4 Hepatic transport processes

Ronald P.J. Oude Elferink

The liver takes up amino acids, sugars and nucleic acids that are absorbed in the small intestine. For each of these classes of nutrients, specific transporters are present in the sinusoidal membrane of the hepatocytes. Similarly, transporters are present that mediate the secretion of metabolites from the hepatocyte to the blood for delivery to peripheral tissues. The apical membrane of two adjacent hepatocytes forms the bile canaliculus in which primary bile is secreted. Evidently, this also involves a large set of transporters for the highly diverse spectrum of compounds that are excreted into bile.

In general, four types of transport processes across membranes can be discerned [1]:

- simple diffusion;
- facilitated diffusion;
- secondary active transport;
- primary active transport.

Simple diffusion

The plasma membrane bilayer, mainly made up of phospholipids and cholesterol, forms a tight barrier for hydrophilic compounds. Hence, all hydrophilic and amphipathic compounds need transporter proteins in order to enter cells. In principle, hydrophobic compounds are able to diffuse through plasma membrane. However, it is becoming more and more evident that most, if not all, bioactive compounds in the body are transported in and out of cells through transporter proteins. This does not exclude the possibility that hydrophobic compounds (including certain drugs) can enter cells partly or entirely through simple diffusion. An important difference between simple diffusion and protein-mediated transport is that the rate of entry into cells is linearly related to the concentration outside the cell. In contrast, protein-mediated transport of organic compounds can be saturated at sufficiently high concentrations of the transported compound.

Facilitated diffusion

This is the simplest form of transport mediated by transporter proteins and always follows the concentration gradient. Two types of transporters can be discerned in this context: channels and exchangers (Fig. 1).

Channels

Channels simply represent pores in the membrane that are made up of one or more protein subunits. Certain regions of these

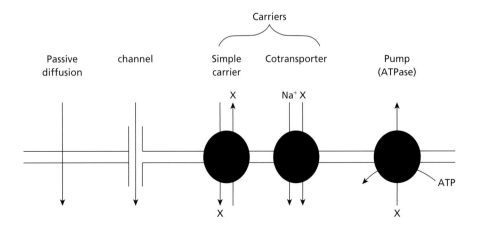

Fig. 1 Different classes of transporter proteins.

proteins form cylindrical α-helices that pass through the membrane. The simplest channels consist of six such transmembrane regions, which are arranged in such a way that they form a pore in the membrane bilayer. The pores can be in an open and a closed state. The transition between these two states is highly regulated by intracellular messengers, voltage, pH or ion concentration. In the opened state, the pore only allows passage of ions for which the channel has affinity. Typically, channels only transport electrolytes such as Na^+, K^+ and Cl^- and not organic compounds such as glucose or amino acids, which are too big to pass through a channel. Most channels are highly specific for certain ions. Thus, a chloride channel only transports Cl^- and not Na^+ or K^+. Channels do not undergo a change in conformation during the transport of a single molecule across the membrane. They simply represent a pore that is in the open or closed state. As a consequence, transport through channels is virtually insaturable. In addition, transport rates through channels are orders of magnitude faster than through carrier proteins.

An important example of a channel is the cystic fibrosis transmembrane regulator (CFTR); this is a channel specific for Cl^- ions that is regulated by intracellular cyclic adenosine monophosphate (cAMP) and by intracellular adenosine triphosphate (ATP) levels. This channel is defective in cystic fibrosis. The functioning of many cell types depends on proper channel function of CFTR and, therefore, many tissues are affected in patients with cystic fibrosis. CFTR is also expressed in cholangiocytes and contributes to bile flow generated by these cells [2].

Carrier proteins

A second form of facilitated diffusion is through carrier proteins. In contrast to channels, these proteins bind a substrate and subsequently undergo a conformational change to release the substrate at the other side of the membrane. Substrates can be either electrolytes or organic compounds. Usually, carriers can transport in either direction, although the affinity of binding on each side of the membrane may be different. Simple carriers transport substrates only down their concentration gradient. Usually, carriers are much less tightly regulated than channels. An example of a carrier is the glucose transporter GLUT2 that is present in the basolateral membrane of hepatocytes [3]. This carrier can mediate either the uptake of glucose into the hepatocyte or the release from cells depending on the prevailing concentration in the cytosol and the sinusoidal blood.

Secondary active transport

Cotransport (symporters) and countertransport (antiporters)

More complicated forms of carriers are the symporters and antiporters (Fig. 1). These transporters bind two different substrates either on the same side of the membrane (symporter) or on the opposite side of the membrane (antiporter). In this way, the transport of one substrate is coupled to that of the other. This mechanism can be used to derive energy from a concentration gradient of the first substrate and use this to drive the transport of the second substrate. Many symporters have the Na^+ ion as the driving force for transport of a second substrate. As the sodium concentration outside the cell is high whereas it is low within the cell, transport of the sodium ion down its concentration gradient (into the cell) can be used to transport a second substrate up its concentration gradient. An example of this coupled transport is the system A transporter for neutral amino acids [4]. By coupling transport of amino acids to that of sodium, the cell is capable of concentration of the amino acid in the cytosol (uphill transport).

An example of an antiporter or countertransport system is the anion exchanger AE2, which is present in the apical membrane of hepatocytes and cholangiocytes [5]. This transporter exchanges Cl^- ions for HCO_3^- ions and is important for intracellular pH homeostasis. Because the intracellular Cl^- concentration is much lower than that outside the cell, this transporter can mediate the extrusion of bicarbonate. In this way, inward chloride transport down the concentration gradient is coupled to outward and uphill bicarbonate transport.

Primary active transport

ATPases

The most complex type of transport is primary active transport, which is always mediated by transport ATPases (Fig. 1). These transporters use the energy liberated by the hydrolysis of ATP to drive transport against the concentration gradient. In this way, enormous concentration gradients (100- to 1000-fold) can be generated. Examples of such transporters are the Ca^{2+} ATPases that pump calcium ions outside the cell and inside the endoplasmic reticulum. This transport can involve more than one type of substrate. For example, the Na^+-K^+ ATPase, which is the motor of many transport processes in the cell, extrudes Na^+ ions from the cell and allows entry of K^+ ions. This causes the large concentration difference of these two ions between the cytosol and the extracellular milieu, which is used by many different secondary active transporters. Transport ATPases not only exist for electrolytes but also for organic compounds. Notably, the superfamily of ATP binding cassette (ABC) transporters mediates a host of different transport processes involving drugs, lipids, peptides and many other compounds [6].

Relevant transport systems in the hepatocyte

As described above, the main motor of transport across the plasma membrane of all cells including the hepatocyte is the Na^+-K^+ ATPase (Fig. 2). Potassium concentrated in the cell is partly lost via the potassium channel in the basolateral membrane. This creates an inside negative membrane potential,

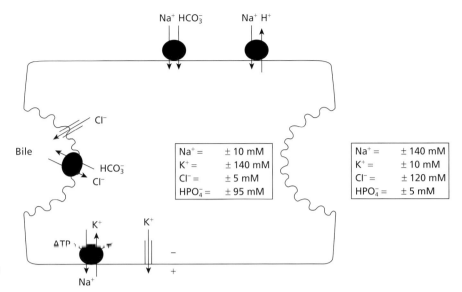

Fig. 2 The main transporters for electrolytes in hepatocytes.

which is also used by many transport processes. Maintenance of a proper intracellular pH (slightly lower than the external pH) is of crucial importance to many enzymatic reactions in the cytosol. As hepatocytes take up and extrude many acidic compounds, pH homeostasis must be quite active in hepatocytes. Intracellular acidification can be counteracted by sodium-dependent bicarbonate uptake across the basolateral membrane as well as by sodium-proton exchange (NHE1 exchanger) across this membrane, although the latter seems to be less active in hepatocytes. The canalicular membrane harbours a chloride–bicarbonate exchanger (AE2) that is capable of acidifying the

intracellular milieu. The latter transporter is activated by alkaline pH and cAMP [7].

There are two kinds of glucose carriers: one type (SGLT family) mediates active uptake by cotransport with sodium. This is important, for example, in the apical membrane of enterocytes that need to concentrate glucose from the lumen. The second type of glucose carriers are bidirectional transporters (the GLUT family), which merely transport glucose down the concentration gradient The liver is a professional glucose-producing organ and, therefore, the latter class (more specifically GLUT2) is active in this cell type (Fig. 3). There is a large family of amino

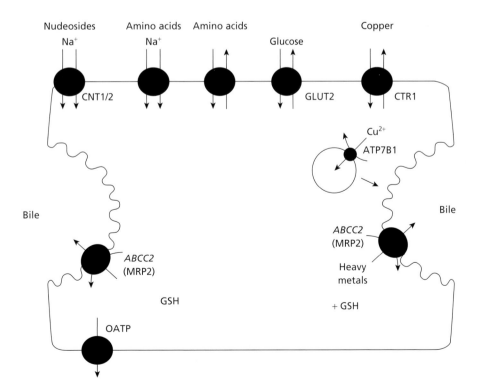

Fig. 3 Transporters for various solutes in hepatocytes. GSH, glutathione.

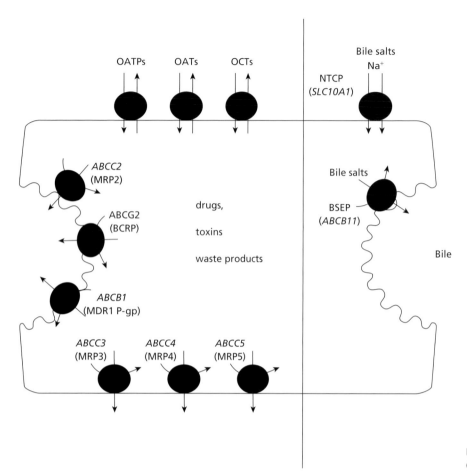

Fig. 4 Transporters in hepatocytes for drugs (left) and bile salts (right).

acid transporters (members of the solute carrier family; SLCs), some of which are mere exchangers and others which are sodium driven and therefore concentrative. The difference between these transporters mainly involves different substrate specificity [8].

The liver expresses concentrative (sodium-dependent) transporters for nucleosides from the CNT family. Concentrative uptake of nucleosides is particularly important during cell division, as illustrated by the fact that these transporters are upregulated during hepatic regeneration [9].

The liver plays an important role in homeostasis and disposition of metal ions. Copper is taken up into hepatocytes by the carrier CTR1 [10]. Heavy metals are also taken up by hepatocytes and disposed into bile. For some heavy metals, the latter process is mediated by ABCC2 (MRP2, the canalicular pump for organic compounds), which transports cadmium, zinc and copper in a glutathione-dependent mechanism [11]. Under normal conditions, however, most copper secretion into bile is mediated by a vesicular pathway in which copper is first sequestered into vesicles by the ATP-dependent copper transporter ATP7B, which is deficient in Wilson's disease (see Chapter 16.1).

The hepatocyte is also a major supplier of glutathione (GSH) to peripheral tissues. GSH is very important in all cells for detoxification of peroxides via GSH-dependent peroxidases. GSH is also important for detoxification of drugs and toxins via

conjugation with this tripeptide. To this end, the hepatocyte secretes relatively large amounts of this valuable tripeptide into the circulation. The mechanism has not been fully elucidated, but may involve the members of the OATP family, which are involved in the uptake of a major spectrum of drugs [12].

The hepatocyte fulfils a very important role in the detoxification of drugs, toxins and waste products. To this end, it is harnessed with a spectrum of transporters, both in the basolateral and in the apical membrane (Fig. 4). The transporters in the basolateral membrane involve members of the OATP, the OAT and the OCT families, which are all members of the superfamily of solute carriers (SLCs) [13]. These transporters are largely thought to be simple carriers, although they can also be secondarily active. An example of the latter case is the OATPs, which may take up drugs by simultaneous countertransport of GSH. As the intracellular GSH concentration is more than 100-fold higher than the plasma concentration, this represents a very powerful concentrative mechanism for drug uptake into the liver. These noxious compounds can be conjugated with charged moieties such as glucuronide, glutathione and sulphate, and subsequently pumped into bile across the canalicular membrane by different ABC transporters. These involve ABCC2 (MRP2), which largely transports organic anions (stimulated or not by

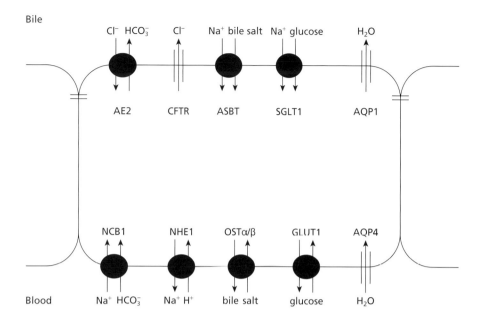

Fig. 5 Some important transport systems in cholangiocytes.

GSH), ABCG2 (breast cancer-related protein, BCRP), which transports many charged and uncharged compounds, and ABCB1 (MDR1 P-glycoprotein), which mainly transports uncharged or cationic amphilic compounds [6]. Conjugated compounds can also be transported back into the blood by pumps such as ABCC3, ABCC4 and ABCC5, resulting in urinary excretion after filtration or active excretion in the kidney.

Finally, bile salts are taken up into the hepatocyte via a sodium-dependent mechanism involving NTCP (SLC10A1). This secondary active transport ensures concentration within the hepatocyte. At the canalicular pole of the cell, the ABCB11 (or bile salt export pump, BSEP) pumps the bile salts into the canaliculus. ATP hydrolysis provides sufficient energy to reach concentration gradients of more than 100-fold. This combined secondary active transport across the basolateral membrane and primary active transport across the canalicular membrane leads to concentration gradients across the hepatocyte of more than 1000-fold (from low micromolar to high millimolar concentrations). More detailed information on the transporters involved in bile formation can be found in Chapter 2.6.

Transport in cholangiocytes

Cholangiocytes modify bile mainly by excretion of bicarbonate. Net bicarbonate excretion is thought to occur by simultaneous action of the chloride bicarbonate exchanger AE2 and the chloride channel CFTR (Fig. 5), although there are also data to suggest that CFTR is capable of excreting bicarbonate by itself. The localization of AE2 in the apical membrane of hepatocytes and cholangiocytes [5] is striking, as this transporter is localized in the basolateral membrane of various other epithelia, such as parietal cells and enterocytes [14]. Similar to the situation in hepatocytes, bicarbonate can be taken up across the basolateral membrane via sodium-dependent bicarbonate transport (NCB1).

It is postulated that water channels (aquaporins) contribute to the net water flow into bile ducts. Indeed, aquaporin 1 (AQP1, in the apical membrane) and aquaporin 4 (AQP4, in the basolateral membrane) are expressed in the cholangiocyte, but it is not clear how much these channels contribute to water flow [15].

Bile flow is stimulated by the hormone secretin, which induces intracellular production of cAMP upon binding to its receptor. It has become clear recently that cAMP induces the mobilization of various transporter proteins from intracellular stores to the plasma membrane. Insertion of CFTR, AE2 and aquaporin provides a mechanism to stimulate bicarbonate excretion by cholangiocytes and subsequent water flow [16].

Cholangiocytes are able to absorb bile salts via the sodium-dependent bile salt transporter ASBT followed by transport via the bile salt exchanger OSTα/β in the basolateral membrane [17]. It is not clear how bile salt absorption by bile ducts quantitatively compares with excretion by hepatocytes. Probably only minor amounts of bile salt are reabsorbed in the bile ducts.

Cholangiocytes also reabsorb glucose that has entered bile via the sodium-dependent glucose transporter SGLT1 in the apical membrane of these cells. The absorbed glucose is then released into the blood via the glucose carrier GLUT1 in the basolateral membrane [18].

References

1 Stein WD (1986) *Transport and Diffusion across Cell Membranes.* Orlando: Academic Press.
2 Feranchak AP, Sokol RJ (2001) Cholangiocyte biology and cystic fibrosis liver disease. *Semin Liver Dis* 21, 471–488.
3 Mueckler M (1994) Facilitative glucose transporters. *Eur J Biochem* 219, 713–725.
4 Moseley RH (1996) Hepatic amino acid transport. *Semin Liver Dis* 16, 137–145.

5 Martinez-Anso E, Castillo JE, Diez J *et al.* (1994) Immuno-histochemical detection of chloride/bicarbonate anion exchangers in human liver. *Hepatology* 19, 1400–1406.

6 Borst P, Oude Elferink RP (2002) Mammalian ABC transporters in health and disease. *Annu Rev Biochem* 71, 537–592.

7 Strazzabosco M, Boyer JL (1996) Regulation of intracellular pH in the hepatocyte. Mechanisms and physiological implications. *J Hepatol* 24, 631–644.

8 Moseley RH (1996) Hepatic amino acid transport. *Semin Liver Dis* 16, 137–145.

9 Pastor-Anglada M, Felipe A, Casado FJ *et al.* (1998) Nucleoside transporters and liver cell growth. *Biochem Cell Biol* 76, 771–777.

10 Wijmenga C, Klomp LW (2004) Molecular regulation of copper excretion in the liver. *Proc Nutr Soc* 63, 31–39.

11 Dijkstra M, Havinga R, Vonk RJ *et al.* (1996) Bile secretion of cadmium, silver, zinc and copper in the rat. Involvement of various transport systems. *Life Sci* 59, 1237–1246.

12 Ballatori N, Hammond CL, Cunningham JB *et al.* (2005) Molecular mechanisms of reduced glutathione transport: role of the MRP/CFTR/ABCC and OATP/SLC21A families of membrane proteins. *Toxicol Appl Pharmacol* 204, 238–255.

13 Hediger MA, Romero MF, Peng JB *et al.* (2004) The ABCs of solute carriers: physiological, pathological and therapeutic implications of human membrane transport proteins. Introduction. *Pflugers Arch* 447, 465–468.

14 Alper SL, Darman RB, Chernova MN *et al.* (2002) The AE gene family of Cl/HCO$_3^-$ exchangers. *J Nephrol* 15 (Suppl. 5), S41–S53.

15 Marinelli RA, Pham LD, Tietz PS *et al.* (2000) Expression of aquaporin-4 water channels in rat cholangiocytes. *Hepatology* 31, 1313–1317.

16 Tietz PS, Marinelli RA, Chen XM *et al.* (2003) Agonist-induced coordinated trafficking of functionally related transport proteins for water and ions in cholangiocytes. *J Biol Chem* 278, 20413–20419.

17 Ballatori N, Christian WV, Lee JY *et al.* (2005) OSTalpha-OSTbeta: a major basolateral bile acid and steroid transporter in human intestinal, renal, and biliary epithelia. *Hepatology* 42, 1270–1279.

18 Masyuk AI, Masyuk TV, Tietz PS *et al.* (2002) Intrahepatic bile ducts transport water in response to absorbed glucose. *Am J Physiol Cell Physiol* 283, C785–C791.

2.2.5 Modulation of liver function by hepatic nerves

Gerhard P. Püschel

Anatomical background

Hypothalamic centres

The two principal hypothalamic regions where the signals for the neural control of liver functions are generated are the ventromedial hypothalamic nucleus and the lateral hypothalamic area. The former sends signals to the liver via sympathetic autonomic nerves and, in general terms, enhances the release of fuel substrates from the liver. The latter sends parasympathetic signals to the liver which favour the replenishment of hepatic energy stores. The function of the ventromedial and lateral hypothalamic nuclei is modulated and coordinated by the periventricular region which receives nervous and humoral (e.g. leptin, insulin, glucose) signals from the periphery and other brain regions.

Afferent hepatic nerves

There are two types of afferent nerves emerging from the liver: vagal and spinal afferent nerves.

The vagal afferent neurons are located in the nodose ganglia. They project their central processes to the nucleus of the solitary tract. Their axons travel with the common hepatic branch of the vagus nerve, to which, however, they contribute only a minor portion. The vagal afferents terminate in the outer layers of the larger branches of the extrahepatic and intrahepatic bile ducts and in the adventitia of the portal vein. They transmit information about metabolite, hormone or cytokine concentration to the hypothalamus. Terminals of the vagal afferents have not been detected in the intralobular area of the liver parenchyma in rat. Because rat parenchyma is scarcely innervated in general, this might not reflect the intralobular distribution of vagal afferent nerves in other vertebrate species including man [1].

The spinal afferents stem from the dorsal root of the lower half of the thoracic medulla. Calcitonin gene-related peptide (CGRP) appears to be an accepted specific marker that has been used for immunohistochemical studies on their distribution along with retrograde labelling studies. Both techniques indicate that the intrahepatic distribution of spinal afferents is similar to that of vagal afferents. No CGRP-positive fibres were detected in the parenchyma of rodents or guinea pig and, in human liver, few fibres were detected in the portal tract [2].

Efferent hepatic nerves

Sympathetic hepatic nerves originate from the ventromedial hypothalamic nucleus. Fibres descend via the medullary reticular formation to the intermediolateral cell column in the thoracolumbar spinal cord. From here, preganglionic neurons project to a collateral ganglia, i.e. the coeliac ganglion and superior mesenteric ganglion, where the postganglionic sympathetic nerve fibres originate [3,4]. The postganglionic nerves enter the liver via an anterior and a posterior portal plexus accompanying the hepatic artery and portal vein. A few fibres also enter the liver together with the hepatic vein. In most mammals including man, aminergic nerves enter the liver lobules to a varying extent. They are found in close vicinity to stellate cells but also contact hepatocytes, sinusoidal endothelial cells and Kupffer cells. Density is highest close to the portal fields and declines along the sinusoid.

Parasympathetic hepatic efferent nerves originate in the lateral hypothalamic area, whence connections aim at the nucleus vagus/ambiguous. These vagal nuclei supply efferent parasympathetic nerves to the hepatic branch of the vagal nerve. The parasympathetic fibres form a plexus that is separate from that of the catecholaminergic nerves [4] and enter the liver at the hilus together with the sympathetic fibres. Parasympathetic nerves normally synapse on postsynaptic nerves at intramural ganglia. Few reports exist about hilar or intrahepatic parasympathetic ganglia, and their existence is still a matter of debate [4]. Functional evidence argues in favour of their existence. It has been assumed, however, that part of the parasympathetic fibres of the hepatic branch of the vagus nerve indirectly affect liver function by modulating sympathetic nerve activity in the coeliac ganglion [5]. Cholinergic fibres terminate at the terminal branches of the hepatic artery, portal vein and bile duct or in the portal area. In no vertebrate species have intralobular cholinergic nerves been detected histochemically [3].

Species differences

One has to keep in mind that the intrahepatic distribution and density of liver nerve terminals varies greatly between species. Man and guinea pig, among mammals, have the highest density of intralobular nerves, followed by dog and cat, whereas the most commonly used rodent animal models have a rather scarce intralobular innervation [6]. This holds true for a large array of neurotransmitters, i.e. catecholamines, and various neuropeptides. The density of intralobular innervation is inversely correlated with the density of gap junction between hepatocytes [4,7], indicating that a cell-to-cell signal propagation might compensate for direct innervation in animals with sparse innervation.

Regulation by hepatic nerves of liver haemodynamics

Regulation of macrovascular haemodynamics

In vivo stimulation of sympathetic splanchnic nerves in cats and dogs reduced hepatic blood flow and lowered the blood volume in intrahepatic capacitance vessels, thereby replenishing the systemic circulation [8] (Fig. 1). In isolated liver perfused with constant pressure, stimulation of sympathetic hepatic nerves reduced portal and arterial flow, whereas stimulation of sympathetic hepatic nerves in livers perfused with constant flow increased perfusion pressure. Independent of the perfusion model, a redistribution of flow was observed as a consequence of the regulation of the sinusoidal haemodynamics.

Regulation of sinusoidal haemodynamics

In vivo microscopy revealed that stimulation of the vagus dilated sinusoids and opened previously closed sinusoids in rat liver, reducing the erythrocyte flow velocity in each individual liver sinusoid without affecting the total volumetric flow in the observed microscopic field. In contrast, stimulation of sympathetic hepatic nerves in isolated perfused rat liver resulted in a redistribution of flow, apparently closing some sinusoids and leaving part of the parenchyma hypoxic [8] (Fig. 1). The regulation of the sinusoidal blood flow occurs at the level of presinusoidal sphincters [9] or by contractile cells, most probably stellate cells, along the sinusoid [10]. In addition to the intrasinusoidal haemodynamics, the fluid exchange between the sinusoid and the Disse space may be regulated by variation in the size of the fenestrae and, hence, the porosity of the sinusoidal endothelial cell in response to, for example, serotonin and nitric oxide [9]. Thus, the access of macromolecular complexes to the hepatocyte may be regulated [11]. Via these haemodynamic changes, hepatic nerve action may secondarily affect liver metabolism.

Regulation of liver metabolism by hepatic nerves

Liver metabolism is tightly regulated. It is subject to control by metabolite levels, circulating hormones and efferent hepatic nerves. These different modes of control are tightly interrelated. This makes it difficult to discern the contribution of one particular branch of this control system, i.e. the direct modulation of liver metabolism by hepatic efferent nerves (Fig. 1). In addition, haemodynamic variations in response to circulating mediators or locally released neurotransmitters may affect liver metabolism because they lead to hypo- or hyperperfusion of the parenchyma with subsequent changes in oxygen and substrate supply or metabolite washout. Different experimental approaches have been taken to eliminate these confounding factors in order to assess the direct impact of hepatic nerves on liver metabolism. Studies in whole animals with removed or clamped endocrine organs have been used as well as different models of isolated perfused liver. All these systems have their particular limitations [12]. Nevertheless, all the data taken together provide strong evidence for the possibility of a direct control by efferent nerves of hepatic metabolism.

On the other hand, afferent hepatic nerves in whole animal studies and liver perfusion systems have been shown to convey information about portal or hepatic metabolite levels to the central nervous system (CNS) or to locally integrate information about metabolite levels.

Regulation by efferent sympathetic hepatic nerves

Carbohydrate metabolism
In whole animal studies in cat, dog, pig, sheep, rabbit, rat and man, stimulation of splanchnic nerves or liver nerves increased systemic blood glucose levels or hepatic glucose output determined by microdialysis [12, and references therein]. The majority of experiments were performed under conditions that supposedly precluded indirect humoral modulation of hepatic

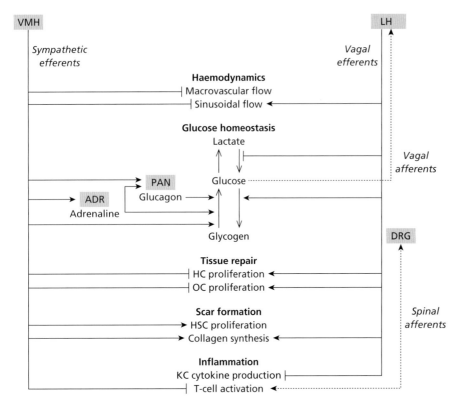

Fig. 1 Modulation by hepatic nerves of liver functions. Various functions of hepatocytes and non-parenchymal liver cells are modulated by a direct and indirect action of sympathetic and parasympathetic efferent hepatic nerves. The CNS can be informed about hepatic metabolite levels by vagal afferents. Spinal afferents can modulate immune cell function by retrograde signalling. ADR, adrenals; DRG, dorsal root ganglia; HC, hepatocyte; HSC, hepatic stellate cell; KC, Kupffer cell; LH, lateral hypothalamus; OC, oval cell; PAN, pancreas; VMH, ventromedial hypothalamus; → stimulation; —| inhibition.

glucose output, i.e. in adrenalectomized and/or pancreatectomized animals or by hormonal clamp of the pancreas. Similarly, in perfused guinea pig, mouse, rat or tree shrew, liver electrical field stimulation of nerve bundles around the liver hilus enhanced hepatic glucose output and, depending on the perfusion medium (erythrocyte-free vs. erythrocyte-containing), increased hepatic lactate output or shifted lactate uptake to output [12]. The increase in glucose output was independent of haemodynamic alterations. It was accompanied by a noradrenalin spillover and was blocked by α adrenergic receptor antagonists. Glycogenolysis was the primary source of nerve stimulation-dependent released glucose, whereas gluconeogenesis, which was inhibited by mercaptopicolinic acid, contributed only a minor fraction to nerve stimulation-dependent glucose output but accounted for almost 100% of the basal hepatic glucose output in rat livers perfused with erythrocyte-containing media.

Conflicting evidence exists concerning the physiological significance of direct neural sympathetic control of hepatic glucose output for systemic glucose supply in response to stress or activity. The activity of sympathetic hepatic nerves is suppressed by high and increased by low blood glucose levels. Direct stimulation of hepatic glucose release by sympathetic hepatic liver nerves appears to be able to blunt insulin- or activity-induced hypoglycaemia in *in vivo* animal models, in which hormonal response is impaired as a result of surgical removal or pharmacological clamping of endocrine pancreas and

adrenals. However, if the endocrine axis is intact, an activity- or hypoglycaemia-dependent increase in circulating glucagon rather than hepatic sympathetic nerve action was the main stimulus to augment hepatic glucose production [12]. With functionally intact adrenals and endocrine pancreas, the action of hepatic nerves appeared to be dispensable for stress-induced glucose release in different animal and human models.

Lipid metabolism

Much less information is available about the modulation by sympathetic hepatic nerves of hepatic lipid metabolism. In whole animal studies, liver denervation caused a reduction in hepatic carnitine palmitoyltransferase activity, fatty acid oxidation and very-low-density lipoprotein (VLDL) formation. This was taken as indirect evidence that sympathetic hepatic nerves might increase hepatic fatty acid utilization. In perfused liver, however, ketone body formation and the secretion of the VLDL apolipoprotein B was suppressed rather than increased by stimulation of sympathetic hepatic nerves or infusion of sympathetic neurotransmitters [12]. The different timeframe might account for this apparent discrepancy. Also, cholesterol production from ^{14}C acetate decreased after surgical dissection of the splanchnic nerve, indicating that an elevated sympathetic tone might augment hepatic cholesterol synthesis. No information is available concerning the relative contribution to the control of hepatic lipid metabolism of hepatic nerves compared with humoral control systems; however, as for the control of carbohydrate metabolism, direct control of lipid metabolism by hepatic nerves is presumably of minor importance.

Other metabolic functions

Independently of the accompanying haemodynamic alterations, stimulation of sympathetic hepatic nerves in perfused liver increased urate formation, reduced bile acid synthesis and bile flow and attenuated xenobiotic extraction [12]. Stimulation of sympathetic hepatic nerves led to a rapid swelling of hepatocytes and stellate cells as a result of a redistribution of electrolytes and a compensatory release of the organic osmolytes taurine and myoinositol from these cells [13]. Amino acid and ammonia metabolism were also affected by sympathetic nerve stimulation; however, the effects were largely dependent on haemodynamic alterations. Thus, urea and glutamine output as well as ammonia uptake were reduced, while glutamate and glutathione output was increased [12].

Mechanism of intrahepatic signal propagation of efferent sympathetic nerves

The apparent lack of intralobular nerve terminals, especially in rodents, was inconsistent with the observation that electrical stimulation of hepatic nerves elicited pronounced metabolic changes that were independent of haemodynamic alterations. Two models were proposed to explain the apparent discrepancy: a hepatocyte-to-hepatocyte signal propagation via gap junctions; and a signal propagation by paracrine stimulation of hepatocytes with mediators released from non-parenchymal liver cells in response to stimulation of hepatic nerves. Evidence for both models was brought forward.

Inositol trisphosphate, which is generated in hepatocytes in response to noradrenalin released from nerve terminals in the periportal region, can diffuse via gap junctions and propagate the signal from hepatocyte to hepatocyte to the perivenous region along the acinus. Pharmacological blockade of gap junctional conductivity as well as downregulation or elimination of the gap junction protein connexin 32 inhibited the nerve stimulation-dependent increase in glucose output [12].

The other model supposes that nerves ending close to non-parenchymal liver cells, specifically hepatic stellate cells, elicit the release of eicosanoids, which can act on hepatocytes further downstream in the sinusoid. In support of this hypothesis, nerve stimulation-dependent increase in glucose output from isolated perfused liver was attenuated by inhibition of phospholipase A_2 or cyclo-oxygenase in rat and in the more densely innervated guinea pig liver. Prostaglandin $F_{2\alpha}$, which was released from hepatic stellate cells in response to synaptic concentrations of noradrenalin and adenosine triphosphate (ATP) and appeared as spillover in perfused rat liver after electrical field stimulation of hepatic nerves, stimulated glucose output from perfused rat livers and glycogen phosphorylase activity in isolated rat hepatocytes via the prostaglandin $F_{2\alpha}$ (FP) receptor. In contrast to hepatic stellate cells, Kupffer cells appeared not to contribute to nerve stimulation-dependent eicosanoid formation [12].

Regulation by efferent parasympathetic hepatic nerves

Much less information is available on the contribution of parasympathetic hepatic nerves in the control of liver metabolism. Most information concerns the hepatic glucose balance (Fig. 1). The insulin-dependent glycogen deposition in isolated perfusion systems or hepatocyte cultures is surprisingly low when compared with the *in vivo* situation. A possible explanation for this enigma may be that *in vivo* parasympathetic efferent nerves act in parallel to insulin to warrant an efficient glucose clearance from the portal blood. In favour of such a model, stimulation of the parasympathetic nuclei in the lateral hypothalamus or the peripheral cut end of the hepatic branch of the vagus nerve activated glycogen synthase in rabbit, and acute hepatic vagotomy diminished the rate of glycogen deposition after a glucose load [14]. In rats that had undergone acute selective hepatic vagotomy, replenishment of glycogen stores after refeeding was severely impaired [15], and incorporation of labelled glucose into glycogen was decreased [16]. In perfused rat liver, the small insulin-dependent glucose uptake was markedly potentiated by stimulation of hepatic nerves after α and β adrenergic receptor blockade. In support of a physiological significance of these experiments, it was also found that the firing rate of the hepatic efferent branch of the vagus nerve was linearly related to blood glucose concentrations between 3 and 25 mM, the physiological range of (portal) glucose concentrations [17]. However, a simple synergism between the parasympathetic neurotransmitter acetylcholine and insulin has been excluded [18].

Parasympathetic control of hepatic glucose balance is not restricted to the increase in glucose uptake. In the postresorptive phase, liver produces glucose from gluconeogenesis by default. Part of this gluconeogenesis depends on the presence of glucagon. After pharmacological blockade of sympathetic signal transmission, electrical field stimulation of hepatic nerves inhibited the glucagon-elicited glucose release from perfused rat liver. Similarly, stimulation of hepatic nerves *in vivo* in cat decreased basal glucose output if sympathetic nerve fibres were destroyed prior to the experiment [12]. Conversely, selective hepatic vagotomy increased basal glucose output [16] or attenuated the suppression by insulin of glucagon-induced glucose output [15] from rat livers *in vivo*. Most recent evidence suggests that an impairment of this parasympathetic control of hepatic glucose production might contribute to the fatty acid-induced hepatic overproduction of glucose in type 2 diabetes [19]. It was suggested that hypothalamic sensing of elevated free fatty acids increases the vagal output to the liver, which results in a decrease in glycogenolysis to compensate for the fatty acid-dependent increase in hepatic gluconeogenesis.

Contribution of afferent nerves to metabolic regulation

Many studies show the existence of portal sensors for metabolites or hormones. These sensors modulate the discharge rate of afferents in response to portal infusions of glucose [17], amino acids [20], fatty acids and, to a lesser extent, lipids [21] as well as hormones [22,23]. Integration of these signals in the CNS affects feeding behaviour and hepatic metabolism (Fig. 1).

As an example, portal infusion of 2,5-anhydro-D-mannitol increased the discharge rate of vagal afferents, inhibited hepatic glucose release and augmented food intake. The last effects were abolished after hepatic branch vagotomy [24]. Similarly, portal infusion of fatty acid [25] or mercaptoacetate [26] augmented the discharge rate of vagal afferents and inhibited feeding. The afferents might thus be physiologically relevant for fat-induced hypophagia, and an improper function of hepatic afferents has been implicated as one possible cause contributing to aberrant feeding behaviour in diabetic animals [27]. Central registration of the abundance of hepatic glycogen stores via hepatic afferents has also been implicated in fasting-induced mobilization of free fatty acids from adipose tissue.

The existence of two types of osmo- (or sodium-) sensitive afferent fibers has been firmly established with electrophysiological methods in the hepatic branch of the vagus nerve: one increasing the discharge rate in response to hyperosmolarity, the other increasing the discharge rate in response to hypoosmolarity. Although both fibres have been implicated in the regulation of vasopressin release [28], the evidence is, however, somewhat controversial [29], and a physiological relevance might be limited to a very short-term reaction to an oral hypo- or hyperosmolar load.

Metabolite sensing in the portal area also allows the distinction between exogenous gut-derived glucose, which reaches the liver via the portal vein, and endogenous glucose, which enters the hepatic circulation via the hepatic artery. Delivery of exogenous glucose builds up a portal–arterial glucose gradient with higher glucose concentration in the portal vein that generates a portal signal. This portal signal increases the insulin-dependent hepatic glucose extraction in living dogs [30], isolated rat liver simultaneously perfused via portal vein and hepatic artery [31] and in conscious freely moving rats [32]. Conversely, increase in the glucose concentration in the hepatic artery abolishing the gradient between portal vein and hepatic artery attenuated hepatic glucose uptake in comparison with the same glucose load administered solely via the portal vein [33], despite an equally high glucose load to the liver. The size of the gradient seems to be irrelevant as long as the portal glucose concentration is about 1 mM above the arterial concentration [34]. A further increase did not result in a parallel increase in fractional glucose extraction. The increase by the portal signal in insulin-dependent glucose uptake is most probably mediated by parasympathetic fibres [35]. The portal signal is probably generated by glucose-sensitive neurons in the portal vein whose discharge rate is inversely correlated with the portal glucose concentration. Because the isolated perfused liver is disconnected from signal input from the CNS, it was assumed that the portal–arterial glucose gradient might be sensed by an intrahepatic neuronal network [35]. However, the hypothalamus cannot

be excluded as an additional arterial reference site. There is evidence that GLP-1 might be involved in the generation of the signal in response to the portal–arterial glucose gradient [36]. The portal signal was absent in mice lacking the GLP-1 receptor [37]. A recent study showed that, in humans, hepatic glucose extraction was not greater after duodenal glucose administration than after peripheral glucose administration [38]. Assuming that duodenal glucose administration, in contrast to peripheral glucose administration, will create a portal–arterial glucose gradient, this might indicate that a portal signal does increase hepatic glucose uptake in humans.

The portal signal might not only be relevant to insulin-dependent hepatic glucose disposal but also to the coordination between hepatic and peripheral glucose deposition. Two opposing observations were made in this regard. In dog, a portal–arterial glucose gradient increased hepatic but decreased peripheral (hind limb) glucose utilization [39], whereas in mice, the portal signal increased peripheral but not hepatic glucose extraction and resulted in hypoglycaemia. Sensing of the portal–arterial gradient was dependent on the Glut2 glucose transporter and GLP-1 receptor (probably in the portal sensing area). For the portal signal to increase peripheral glucose uptake, the Glut4 transporter and AMP kinase but not the insulin receptor were required in skeletal muscle [40].

Interplay between hepatic nerves and humoral control of extrahepatic metabolism

Hepatic afferent and efferent nerves may modulate the hormone-dependent regulation of extrahepatic metabolism either by altering the level of circulating hormones or by adjusting the sensitivity of peripheral tissues to circulating hormones. Evidence was provided for both routes. Thus, adrenaline release from suprarenal glands in response to insulin-induced hypoglycaemia in dogs was attenuated by hepatic denervation [41]. However, this was not observed in exercise-induced hypoglycaemia in vagotomized rats [42]. There is indirect evidence that autonomic nerve activity might influence the hepatic extraction rate of glucoregulatory hormones, however, direct evidence is lacking [12]. Although signalling by hepatic nerves appears not directly to influence insulin degradation by the liver or pancreatic insulin release after portal (prandial) glucose delivery, it might modulate insulin-dependent glucose utilization. A putative hepatic factor called hepatic insulin sensitizing substance (HISS) that was released in response to the stimulation of vagal efferents increased insulin-dependent glucose deposition in skeletal muscle in rat, cat and dog [43,44]. In an insulin sensitivity assay, the amount of glucose needed to achieve euglycaemia after injection of an insulin dose was reduced by about 50% in animals that either underwent mechanical hepatic denervation or vagotomy or received the parasympathetic antagonist atropine or the NO synthase inhibitor L-NAME (N-nitro-L-arginine methyl ester). The effect of pharmacological or mechanical denervation was reversed by

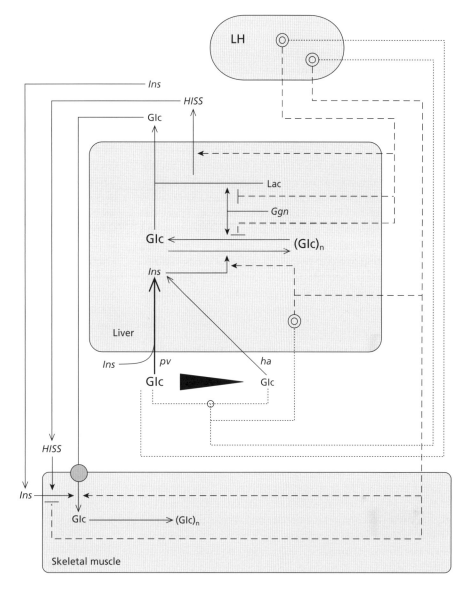

Fig. 2 Parasympathetic control of hepatic and extrahepatic glucose utilization. Glucose delivery from the gut is sensed by portal glucose sensors either as absolute glucose concentration or as a portal–arterial glucose gradient. Thereby, a portal signal is generated which is integrated either locally by a putative intrahepatic neuronal network or by the brain. Via the efferent parasympathetic nerves, this signal suppresses the glucagon-stimulated glycogenolysis and gluconeogenesis, and potentiates the insulin-dependent glycogen synthesis. Parasympathetic efferents also stimulate the release of a putative hepatic insulin sensitizing substance (HISS), which augments skeletal muscle insulin-dependent glucose uptake. The portal signal, by an ill-defined mechanism possibly involving parasympathetic efferents to the skeletal muscle, appears to inhibit insulin-dependent and to increase insulin-independent glucose uptake. Ggn, glucagon; Glc, glucose; (Glc)$_n$, glycogen; ha, hepatic artery; Ins, insulin; Lac, lactate; pv, portal vein; ...... vagal afferents; – – – – vagal efferents; → stimulation; ⊣ inhibition.

an intraportal infusion of either acetylcholine or the synthetic NO source SIN-1 (3-morpholinosydnonimine) or nitroglycerin, thus implying the sequential action of muscarinergic and nitrergic parasympathetic nerve fibres in the release of HISS [12,43]. The role of parasympathetic nerves in glucose handling is summarized in Figure 2.

Regulation by hepatic nerves of hepatic immune function and liver repair

From *in vivo* studies, it has long been evident that the hepatic nerves may impact on the severity of toxic liver injury [45]. Elevation of the sympathotonus in spontaneously hypertensive rats [46] or by electrical stimulation of the ventromedial hypothalamic area aggravated CCl$_{4-}$ or demethylnitrosamine-induced liver damage. *In vitro* studies with perfused rat liver indicate that this effect was not entirely due to elevated circulat-

ing catecholamine levels but could be attributed, at least in part, to a direct action of hepatic nerves [47]. In contrast, sympathetic hepatic nerves conferred a protection rather than a sensitization to immune cell-mediated liver injury, while peptidergic afferent nerves sensitized to immune cell-dependent liver injury [48]. Thus, depending on the noxious principle, hepatic nerve activity may be either protective or detrimental in the development of liver damage. Possible explanations for this ambiguous role of hepatic nerves are given below.

Regulation by hepatic nerves of regeneration of parenchyma and scar formation

In response to an acute toxic damage, the liver attempts to compensate for the loss of parenchyma by hepatocyte proliferation. If the hepatocyte compartment loses its capacity to divide, another progenitor cell compartment comes into play, the oval cell compartment. Recent work has demonstrated that the activation of the oval cell compartment is enhanced by decreasing the sympathetic impact on the liver [49]. Proliferation of a hepatic progenitor cell compartment was enhanced by activation of the parasympathetic input (Fig. 1). Similarly, hepatocyte proliferation, which was dependent on an intact parasympathetic supply to the liver, was observed after lesioning the sympathetic nuclei in the ventromedial hypothalamic area [50]. Liver may also react to loss of parenchyma by scar formation. The principal sources of fibrous material for this scar formation are hepatic stellate cells. Indirect evidence was provided that both parasympathetic and sympathetic hepatic nerves, which terminate in close proximity to hepatic stellate cells, might increase scar formation by stimulating hepatic stellate cell proliferation and collagen synthesis [49] (Fig. 1).

Both inhibition of parenchymal cell proliferation and stimulation of hepatic stellate cell proliferation and collagen formation might contribute to the exacerbation by sympathetic hepatic nerves of toxic liver damage observed *in vivo*.

Regulation by hepatic nerves of immune cell function

Resident macrophages (Kupffer cells) that are a rich source of cytokines during local and systemic inflammation are the major immune cell population of the liver. They are in close contact with hepatic nerve endings. Stimulation of the efferent branch of the parasympathetic nervous system attenuated the endotoxin-elicited cytokine production in non-parenchymal liver cells and thereby prevented the development of an endotoxinaemic shock [51]. Apart from Kupffer cells, T cells contribute significantly to the immune cell compartment of the liver. While their number is low under normal conditions, their number dramatically increases during inflammation due to recruitment from the circulation. Although, in contrast to Kupffer cells, they appear not to be in direct contact with hepatic nerve endings, their function may be modulated by neurotransmitters released into the tissue. Immune cell function may be modulated by sympathetic neurotransmitters and opioids, which might inhibit the cytokine release from hepatic immune cells and prevent their activation [48] (Fig. 1). Thereby, sympathetic neurotransmitters may attenuate the immune cell-dependent liver injury caused in hepatitis models such as endotoxin/galactosamine hepatitis. In contrast to the potentially beneficial effect of sympathetic efferent nerves on immune cell-mediated liver injury, peptidergic afferent nerves appear to be of crucial importance to induce and maintain galactosamine/endotoxin hepatitis in mice. Elimination of spinal afferents by capsaicin treatment of neonatal mice completely abolished the development of inflammation in this model. The deleterious effect of peptidergic afferents seems to be mediated by neurokinins [52]. In addition to stimulating immune cells, peptidergic afferent nerves may act directly on the hepatocyte to increase apoptosis. They also appear to increase hepatic fibrosis [53]. Along with the modulation of immune cell function, these last two mechanisms may contribute to the aggravation of liver injury by peptidergic afferent nerves in hepatitis models.

Impact of hepatic denervation after transplantation

During liver transplantation all hepatic nerves are transected and reinnervation of allografts is scarce. Although this apparently does not lead to a gross dysregulation of hepatic functions, some side-effects of liver transplantation might possibly be attributed to the persisting denervation [54], although unequivocal evidence is still lacking. Thus the hepatic vasoconstrictory response to hypovolemia is lacking, making patients more susceptible to hypovolemic shock. The transplanted liver appears to be insulin-resistant due to the lack of a parasympathetic input and patients who have undergone liver transplantation in comparison with kidney transplant patients are prone to weight gain as a result of an increased fat intake, which may be due to the missing portohypothalamic signalling in response to fatty acid ingestion.

References

1 Berthoud HR (2004) Anatomy and function of sensory hepatic nerves. *Anat Rec A Discov Mol Cell Evol Biol* 280, 827–835.

2 Akiyoshi H, Gonda T, Terada T (1998) A comparative histochemical and immunohistochemical study of aminergic, cholinergic and peptidergic innervation in rat, hamster, guinea pig, dog and human livers. *Liver* 18, 352–359.

3 Uyama N, Geerts A, Reynaert H (2004) Neural connections between the hypothalamus and the liver. *Anat Rec A Discov Mol Cell Evol Biol* 280, 808–820.

4 McCuskey RS (2004) Anatomy of efferent hepatic nerves. *Anat Rec A Discov Mol Cell Evol Biol* 280, 821–826.

5 Berthoud HR, Powley TL (1993) Characterization of vagal innervation to the rat celiac, suprarenal and mesenteric ganglia. *J Auton Nerv Syst* 42, 153–169.

6 Metz W, Forssmann WG (1980) Innervation of the liver in guinea pig and rat. *Anat Embryol (Berl)* 160, 239–252.

7 Reilly FD, McCuskey PA, McCuskey RS (1978) Intrahepatic distribution of nerves in the rat. *Anat Rec* 191, 55–67.

8 Gardemann A, Püschel GP, Jungermann K (1992) Nervous control of liver metabolism and hemodynamics. *Eur J Biochem* 207, 399–411.

9 Oda M, Yokomori H, Han JY (2003) Regulatory mechanisms of hepatic microcirculation. *Clin Hemorheol Microcirc* 29, 167–182.

10 Ueno T, Bioulac-Sage P, Balabaud C *et al.* (2004) Innervation of the sinusoidal wall: regulation of the sinusoidal diameter. *Anat Rec A Discov Mol Cell Evol Biol* 280, 868–873.

11 Gatmaitan Z, Varticovski L, Ling L *et al.* (1996) Studies on fenestral contraction in rat liver endothelial cells in culture. *Am J Pathol* 148, 2027–2041.

12 Püschel GP (2004) Control of hepatocyte metabolism by sympathetic and parasympathetic hepatic nerves. *Anat Rec A Discov Mol Cell Evol Biol* 280, 854–867.

13 Häussinger D (2004) Neural control of hepatic osmolytes and parenchymal cell hydration. *Anat Rec A Discov Mol Cell Evol Biol* 280, 893–900.

14 Shimazu T (1996) Innervation of the liver and glucoregulation: roles of the hypothalamus and autonomic nerves. *Nutrition* 12, 65–66.

15 Xue C, Aspelund G, Sritharan KC *et al.* (2000) Isolated hepatic cholinergic denervation impairs glucose and glycogen metabolism. *J Surg Res* 90, 19–25.

16 Matsuhisa M, Yamasaki Y, Shiba Y *et al.* (2000) Important role of the hepatic vagus nerve in glucose uptake and production by the liver. *Metabolism* 49, 11–16.

17 Niijima A (1989) Neural mechanisms in the control of blood glucose concentration. *J Nutr* 119, 833–840.

18 Akpan JO, Gardner R, Wagle SR (1974) Studies on the effects of insulin and acetylcholine on activation of glycogen synthase and on glycogenesis in hepatocytes. *Biochem Biophys Res Commun* 61, 222–229.

19 Lam TK, Pocai A, Gutierrez-Juarez R *et al.* (2005) Hypothalamic sensing of circulating fatty acids is required for glucose homeostasis. *Nature Med* 11, 320–327. Epub Feb 27 2005.

20 Torii K, Niijima A (2001) Effect of lysine on afferent activity of the hepatic branch of the vagus nerve in normal and L-lysine-deficient rats. *Physiol Behav* 72, 685–690.

21 Randich A, Spraggins DS, Cox JE *et al.* (2001) Jejunal or portal vein infusions of lipids increase hepatic vagal afferent activity. *Neuroreport* 12, 3101–3105.

22 Nishizawa M, Nakabayashi H, Kawai K *et al.* (2000) The hepatic vagal reception of intraportal GLP-1 is via receptor different from the pancreatic GLP-1 receptor. *J Auton Nerv Syst* 80, 14–21.

23 Uneyama H, Niijima A, Tanaka T *et al.* (2002) Receptor subtype specific activation of the rat gastric vagal afferent fibers to serotonin. *Life Sci* 72, 415–423.

24 Lutz TA, Niijima A, Scharrer E (1996) Intraportal infusion of 2,5-anhydro-D-mannitol increases afferent activity in the common hepatic vagus branch. *J Auton Nerv Syst* 61, 204–208.

25 Cox JE, Tyler WJ, Randich A *et al.* (2001) Celiac vagotomy reduces suppression of feeding by jejunal fatty acid infusions. *Neuroreport* 12, 1093–1096.

26 Lutz TA, Diener M, Scharrer E (1997) Intraportal mercaptoacetate infusion increases afferent activity in the common hepatic vagus branch of the rat. *Am J Physiol* 273, R442–445.

27 la Fleur SE, Ji H, Manalo SL *et al.* (2003) The hepatic vagus mediates fat-induced inhibition of diabetic hyperphagia. *Diabetes* 52, 2321–2330.

28 Adachi A, Kobashi M (1998) Role of hepatic afferent nerves in the controle of saline and water intake. In: Häussinger D, Jungermann K (eds) *Liver and the Nervous System*. Norwell, MA: Kluwer Academic Publisher.

29 Carlson SH, Wyss JM (1999) Hepatic denervation does not affect plasma vasopressin response to intragastric hypertonic saline in conscious rats. *Am J Physiol* 277, E161–E167.

30 Adkins BA, Myers SR, Hendrick GK *et al.* (1987) Importance of the route of intravenous glucose delivery to hepatic glucose balance in the conscious dog. *J Clin Invest* 79, 557–565.

31 Gardemann A, Strulik H, Jungermann K (1986) A portal-arterial glucose concentration gradient as a signal for an insulin-dependent net glucose uptake in perfused rat liver. *FEBS Lett* 202, 255–259.

32 Cardin S, Emshwiller M, Jackson PA *et al.* (1999) Portal glucose infusion increases hepatic glycogen deposition in conscious unrestrained rats. *J Appl Physiol* 87, 1470–1475.

33 Hsieh PS, Moore MC, Neal DW *et al.* (2000) Importance of the hepatic arterial glucose level in generation of the portal signal in conscious dogs. *Am J Physiol Endocrinol Metab* 279, E284–292.

34 Ogihara N, Kawamura W, Kasuga K *et al.* (2004) Characterization of the portal signal during 24-hour glucose delivery in unrestrained, conscious rats. *Am J Physiol Endocrinol Metab* 6, 6.

35 Stümpel F, Jungermann K (1997) Sensing by intrahepatic muscarinic nerves of a portal-arterial glucose concentration gradient as a signal for insulin-dependent glucose uptake in the perfused rat liver. *FEBS Lett* 406, 119–122.

36 Nishizawa M, Moore MC, Shiota M *et al.* (2003) Effect of intraportal glucagon-like peptide-1 on glucose metabolism in conscious dogs. *Am J Physiol Endocrinol Metab* 284, E1027–1036. Epub 2003 Feb 4.

37 Burcelin R, Da Costa A, Drucker D *et al.* (2001) Glucose competence of the hepatoportal vein sensor requires the presence of an activated glucagon-like peptide-1 receptor. *Diabetes* 50, 1720–1728.

38 Fery F, Tappy L, Deviere J *et al.* (2004) Comparison of intraduodenal and intravenous glucose metabolism under clamp conditions in humans. *Am J Physiol Endocrinol Metab* 286, E176–183. Epub 2003 Oct 7.

39 Moore MC, Cardin S, Edgerton DS *et al.* (2004) Unlike mice, dogs exhibit effective glucoregulation during low-dose portal and peripheral glucose infusion. *Am J Physiol Endocrinol Metab* 286, E226–233. Epub 2003 Sep 30.

40 Burcelin R, Crivelli V, Perrin C *et al.* (2003) GLUT4, AMP kinase, but not the insulin receptor, are required for hepatoportal glucose sensor-stimulated muscle glucose utilization. *J Clin Invest* 111, 1555–1562.

41 Lamarche L, Yamaguchi N, Peronnet F (1995) Hepatic denervation reduces adrenal catecholamine secretion during insulin-induced hypoglycemia. *Am J Physiol* 268, R50–57.

42 Latour MG, Cardin S, Helie R *et al.* (1995) Effect of hepatic vagotomy on plasma catecholamines during exercise-induced hypoglycemia. *J Appl Physiol* 78, 1629–1634.

43 Lautt WW (2004) A new paradigm for diabetes and obesity: the hepatic insulin sensitizing substance (HISS) hypothesis. *J Pharmacol Sci* 95, 9–17.

44 Moore MC, Satake S, Baranowski B *et al.* (2002) Effect of hepatic denervation on peripheral insulin sensitivity in conscious dogs. *Am J Physiol Endocrinol Metab* 282, E286–296.

45 Foster JH (1963) Nervous factors in toxic liver injury. *Surg Forum* 14, 74–76.

46 Hsu CT, Schichijo K, Ito M *et al.* (1993) The effect of chemical sympathectomy on acute liver injury induced by carbon tetrachloride in spontaneously hypertensive rats. *J Auton Nerv Syst* 43, 91–96.

47 Iwai M, Shimazu T (1996) Exaggeration of acute liver damage by hepatic sympathetic nerves and circulating catecholamines in perfused liver of rats treated with D-galactosamine. *Hepatology* 23, 524–529.

48 Neuhuber WL, Tiegs G (2004) Innervation of immune cells: evidence for neuroimmunomodulation in the liver. *Anat Rec A Discov Mol Cell Evol Biol* 280, 884–892.

49 Oben JA, Diehl AM (2004) Sympathetic nervous system regulation of liver repair. *Anat Rec A Discov Mol Cell Evol Biol* 280, 874–883.

50 Kiba T (2002) The role of the autonomic nervous system in liver regeneration and apoptosis – recent developments. *Digestion* 66, 79–88.

51 Borovikova LV, Ivanova S, Zhang M *et al.* (2000) Vagus nerve stimulation attenuates the systemic inflammatory response to endotoxin. *Nature* 405, 458–462.

52 Bang R, Biburger M, Neuhuber WL *et al.* (2004) Neurokinin-1 receptor antagonists protect mice from CD95- and tumor necrosis factor-alpha-mediated apoptotic liver damage. *J Pharmacol Exp Ther* 308, 1174–1180. Epub 2003 Nov 14.

53 Casini A, Lippe IT, Evangelista S *et al.* (1991) Sensory denervation with capsaicin reduces the liver collagen deposition induced by common bile duct obstruction in rats. *Adv Exp Med Biol* 298, 285–293.

54 Colle I, Van Vlierberghe H, Troisi R *et al.* (2004) Transplanted liver: consequences of denervation for liver functions. *Anat Rec A Discov Mol Cell Evol Biol* 280, 924–931.

2.2.6 *In vitro* techniques: isolated organ perfusion, slices, cells and subcellular elements

Bruno Stieger

The liver simultaneously fulfils a variety of functions. It is an important mediator of energy homeostasis, is central in the biosynthesis of plasma proteins, plays a key role in the metabolism of endogenous metabolic endproducts and xenobiotics and produces bile [1]. The liver consists of a variety of different cell types, the vast majority being hepatocytes complemented with endothelial cells, stellate cells and Kupffer cells. The elucidation of the mechanisms involved in the interplay of these various cell types, as well as understanding the physiological processes running in parallel, requires a variety of different *in vivo* and *in vitro* methods. An early successful example of the application of *in vitro* techniques was the demonstration with an isolated perfused liver setup that the liver is the predominant site of albumin synthesis in the body [2]. *In vitro* methods use systems ranging from those with great complexity such as perfused liver or primary hepatocytes to sometimes seemingly simple approaches such as membrane vesicles isolated from plasma membrane domains or intracellular organelles, as well as cloned proteins studied in heterologous expression systems.

This chapter intends to give an overview of commonly used *in vitro* methods in the delineation of the various functions of the liver. All topics covered in this chapter have been reviewed extensively. Therefore, the reader is referred to the references to retrieve in-depth information. In some cases, references will be made to individual findings. They will often relate to problems of transport research, as our laboratory has gained most of its methodological experience in this area. Owing to space limitations, a selection of references had to be made.

Perfused liver

The perfused liver permits the investigation of liver function under conditions that resemble normal physiology. There are examples in which liver function can be studied in an almost *in vivo* situation, e.g. by the *in vivo* determination of the clearance of asialorosomucoid from the circulation by the asialoglyoprotein receptor [3], in the bile fistula rat with collection of bile and testing for the clearance of cholephilic substances [4] or assessing the integrity of tight junctions using markers such as dextrans [5]. There are, however, critical limitations to these models: there is only a limited amount of blood that can be sampled and the number of data points that can be obtained in a single experiment is limited. Also, the composition of the blood cannot be controlled or altered without possibly harming the animal. Diversion of bile leads to a depletion of the bile salt pool and, consequently, to alterations in bile formation.

Perfusion of the liver is possible *in situ* or in an isolated setup [6–10]. The first setup allows the study of the liver in a condition with intact innervation in a living animal. In all setups, the essential components are a pump, an oxygenator, a system to control the temperature of the perfusate and a flow regulator. Two directions of perfusate flow are possible. In the antegrade mode, the inflow of the perfusate is via the portal vein with efflux via the hepatic vein, whereas in the retrograde mode, the direction of flow is reversed to influx via the hepatic vein and efflux via the portal vein. The perfusate may be delivered to the organ in an open (non-recirculating or single-pass perfusion) or in a recirculating manner. The recirculating setup is useful for the study of compounds which are slowly taken up by the liver or are slowly secreted. Accumulation of such compounds in the perfusate will facilitate their detection. The drawback of this setup is the accumulation of toxic metabolites in the perfusate, which will consequently impair the vitality of the perfused organ. The perfused organ is unique in that the relative contribution of various compartments of the liver to the clearance of substances from the perfusate can be studied. Such experiments are performed and analysed by the multiple indicator dilution method [11]. Furthermore, using specific inhibitors or activators, the contribution of various different cell types to whole organ physiology can be studied.

Methods have been developed to perfuse lobes or parts of human liver [12]. The human liver samples have to be of high quality and high viability for successful perfusions and good results.

Liver slices

The investigation of liver functions using the perfused liver setup is a powerful methodology, in particular with respect to the elucidation of whole organ homeostasis. However, it is limited to organ availability, which is particularly difficult for studies with human liver. Samples of high-quality human livers are limited for *in vitro* studies by ethical considerations and by the severe shortage of donor organs. An alternative approach is to use liver slices [13–15]. Liver slices are used to study hepatic drug metabolism as well as hepatotoxicity of xenobiotics [15], but they are also applied to transport research [14,16]. A particular advantage of liver slices is that they can be used to isolate intermediate metabolites of drugs or endogenous substances, as such metabolites accumulate in the culture medium during the culture period. However, this also occurs with toxic metabolites, which can become a limiting factor of the culture time.

The slices have a diameter of about 6–10 mm and a thickness of a few 100 μm. For best results, they are prepared by specialized equipment employing mechanical high-precision tissue slicers. Using a mechanical device allows the preparation of multiple slices with very similar thickness from small tissue cylinders and is important to increase the reproducibility of results. The mechanical preparation of the liver slices has the advantage that it allows the investigation of liver tissue with its different cell types in a physiological architecture. Hence, cell types different from hepatocytes can be investigated [17]. Furthermore, tissue slicing can be applied to livers of various species without modifications. This is different from enzymatic methods for cell isolation, which require adaptations to different species. Hence, liver slices are ideally suited to investigate species differences. Additionally, liver slices can also be used to assess interorgan as well as intraorgan differences in hepatic functions. The optimal thickness of the slices is determined by the following consideration, which is crucial for the viability and survival time. Slices exceeding a certain thickness will lead to damaged cells in their core as a result of limited supply of nutrients and/or oxygen with consequent ischaemia and will lead, ultimately, to necrosis. In contrast, slices below a certain thickness will have a large proportion of damaged cells in comparison with the total number of cells in one slice. The thickness of the slices also influences the access of macromolecules (e.g. proteins) to the cells in the interior of the slice.

Isolated hepatocytes and liver cell lines

The perfused liver and liver slices allow us to study liver function in a context close to an *in vivo* situation. The availability of human liver samples for *in vitro* studies is limited. However, if such material is available, the amount may exceed what is necessary for *in vitro* experiments. Owing to the large number of hepatocytes available from one perfusion, many more experimental data points can be obtained from one single liver (or experiment). Therefore, studies with isolated hepatocytes are an important tool in *in vitro* liver research.

Primary hepatocytes can be isolated from many species with collagenase perfusion. This is usually done with the two-step procedure or a modification thereof developed by Berry and Friend [18–22]. Primary hepatocytes can be used immediately after isolation to perform the investigations in suspension. This system allows experiments to be performed for only a few hours. However, primary hepatocytes can also be stored in suspension at 4°C in University of Wisconsin solution (up to 48 h for primary rat hepatocytes) [23,24]. Alternatively, primary hepatocytes can be cultured in a monolayer configuration for a few days. It is important to realize that primary cultured hepatocytes gradually lose many liver-specific functions [19,25] leading, among other problems, to downregulation of the expression of hepatocellular transport systems [26].

To improve the degree of differentiation over extended culture times, various culture methods have been used. Hepatocytes can be cultivated in a so-called sandwich configuration [20,27]. In this setup, hepatocytes are cultivated on collagen for a short time period and thereafter covered with a layer of collagen. This leads to a marked improvement in cell polarity and expression of liver-specific functions. An alternative approach is to cultivate hepatocyte couplets rather than monolayers of single hepatocytes [28]. This system has the advantage of being polar and competent for canalicular secretion. It also offers the unique potential to study intracellular processes at the light microscopic level [29]. Coculturing of hepatocytes with other cells can be used to improve the state of differentiation of primary cultured hepatocytes [30]. However, this setup has an important limitation. Investigations of hepatocyte-specific functions in such mixed culture systems require careful control experiments to demonstrate hepatocyte specificity of findings.

As in the intact liver, the lack of direct accessibility of the canalicular lumen in primary cultured hepatocytes and in cultured liver slices is basically problematic. This lack of access becomes important in experiments in which transport of metabolites or cholephilic substances across the canalicular membrane is to be investigated. In order to circumvent this problem, primary cultured hepatocytes have been cultured on gas-permeable, porous supports, and canaliculi were subsequently punctured with microneedles to collect primary bile [31]. Alternatively, the dependence of the functional integrity of tight junctions on the presence of millimolar calcium has been explored [32]. Transport experiments in the presence and absence of calcium chelators were used to determine canalicular transport in sandwich-cultured primary hepatocytes [33].

Isolation of cells from the liver is not restricted to hepatocytes. It is also possible to isolate cholangiocytes and functional bile duct units for *in vitro* experiments [34]. A combination of several methods is necessary to obtain highly purified Kupffer cells [35]. For the study of the structure and function of hepatic endothelial fenestrae, isolation and culture of endothelial cells was instrumental [36].

Experiments with primary cultured hepatocytes require a sufficient supply of fresh liver tissue of high quality for cell isolation. In the case of human hepatocytes, this is often difficult. Therefore, many different hepatoma cell lines were established. All these cell lines can be cultured and propagated easily. However, all of them show different and variable degrees of differentiation [37,38]. This variable differentiation requires selection of hepatomas expressing the functions to be studied. Bile acids in the culture medium may induce, to some degree, differentiation of hepatoma cell lines [39]. As an alternative source of hepatocyte cell lines, primary hepatocytes have been transformed by transfection with simian virus 40 large T antigen [40].

Primary cultured hepatocytes are hard to expand. Using culture conditions in the presence and absence of serum, it was possible to expand first dedifferentiated hepatocytes and to obtain, after expansion, some degree of hepatocytic differentiation by changing to a chemically defined culture medium containing growth factors [41]. Alternatively, generation of cell hybrids has been used to establish cell lines stably expressing hepatocyte-specific functions [42,43]. Among them, WIF-B cells and clones thereof have proved to be a most valuable tool in the study of hepatocytic functions and the generation of hepatocyte polarity *in vitro*.

Recently, a new avenue for obtaining a large number of hepatoctyes has opened. Adult stem cells, in particular bone marrow-derived stem cells, have demonstrated an unexpected plasticity. Evidence has been presented that subpopulations of bone marrow-derived stem cells can be differentiated *in vivo* and *in vitro* into hepatocytes [44–47]. Similar results were reported for stem cells derived from umbilical cord blood [48,49] or for monocytes [50]. However, these findings are controversially debated [51,52]. If *in vitro* differentiation of stem cells into hepatocytes can be established as a routine method, this would provide a seemingly unlimited source of hepatocytes. Hepatocytes derived from adult stem cells could potentially also be used for autologous transplantation and, hence, avoid the necessity of lifelong immunosuppression after heterologous cell (or organ) transplantation. The adult liver contains progenitor cells at different stages of differentiation [53]. Mitaka and coworkers were able to isolate so-called small hepatocytes from rat liver. In contrast to hepatocytes, small hepatocytes can be expanded into differentiated hepatocytes in culture [54]. These hepatocytes also become competent for bile secretion [55]. It seems unlikely, however, that small hepatocytes will constitute a major source of differentiated hepatocytes, as their rate of expansion is very slow and does not exceed a limited number of cell divisions. Michalopoulos and coworkers developed a method to obtain organoids in culture in a two-step procedure [56]. This procedure led to aggregates of different cell types, some of which resembled liver cell plates. This approach could be useful for studying the interaction of different cell types *in vitro*.

Isolated subcellular fractions

In order to study single cellular processes under well-defined and controlled conditions, working with subcellular fractions offers an ideal complementation to experiments with isolated cells. This is particularly important if experimental conditions are to be controlled on either side of biological membranes. There are many different methods for isolating subcellular fractions [57]. It should be kept in mind that subcellular fractions are usually heterogeneous and not free from contaminating membranes of different subcellular origin [58–60]. By combining different isolation procedures, the purity of the isolated fractions can be significantly improved, but at the expense of the yield of the subcellular fraction of interest.

Using isolated subcellular fractions allows us to perform experiments in conditions such as, for example, broad pH ranges, which are not compatible with cell vitality. Such conditions are required, for example, to investigate the energetics of transport processes or to investigate leak permeabilities of membranes. However, the latter may be introduced by the isolation method [61]. Additionally, experiments can be performed in the absence of cytosolic binding proteins [62]. This is important for the liver, which handles a large variety of poorly water-soluble, but tightly protein bound, substances. Subcellular fractions also allow us to study the sidedness of membrane-associated processes, in particular transport processes [63]. Transport experiments using subcellular fractions are performed with the rapid filtration technique [64,65]. This methodology allows us to work with very short incubation times, which are often shorter than what can be achieved in isolated organs or cells.

A prominent example of the power of isolated subcellular fractions is the dissection of hepatocellular processes involved in vectorial bile acid transport [62,66]. While work with the isolated perfused rat liver and isolated hepatocytes clearly established the uptake mechanisms for bile acids into hepatocytes, the elucidation of the secretory step across the canalicular membrane was only possible with isolated canalicular membrane vesicles. It was only possible to demonstrate with isolated vesicles that canalicular bile salt secretion is a primary active, adenosine triphosphate (ATP)-dependent process [67].

Additionally, it is also possible to identify the subcellular localization of proteins (such as, for example, the bile salt export pump) or cellular processes in the absence of antibodies [68,69]. Also, experiments with isolated plasma membrane fractions from the basolateral (sinusoidal and lateral) membrane and from the canalicular plasma membrane vesicles allow the study of domain-specific transport processes without the complication of simultaneous efflux of transported substrates, as occurs in other setups. Experiments with subcellular fractions are not restricted to experiments with plasma membrane-derived vesicles, but can also be performed with isolated organelles.

Cloned proteins

In order to characterize an individual protein functionally, it is necessary to obtain the pure protein in a sufficient amount for biochemical experiments. This requires the purification of the protein of interest. This is not feasible in many cases for membrane proteins. An attractive alternative approach is to clone membrane proteins and subsequently to study them in heterologous expression systems. A very powerful method for isolating proteins is to use functional expression cloning of the transport protein of interest in *Xenopus laevis* oocytes [70,71]. This technique is particularly well adapted to clone uptake transport systems, for example from hepatocytes [72]. This method of cloning starts by expressing total mRNA in oocytes in order to test whether the desired transport function is expressed. After enrichment of the mRNA of interest, a cDNA library is constructed and subsequently screened by *in vitro* translation of cRNA, which is expressed in oocytes. Once a single clone is obtained, the cDNA can be sequenced and cRNA used for transient expression of the cloned transport protein in oocytes for full characterization. In the case of proteins belonging to gene families or where limited sequence information is available, cloning of desired proteins is possible by homology screening of

Table 1 Comparison of K_m values of Na$^+$-dependent taurocholate transport in different experimental systems in rat liver.

Experimental system		K_m (µM)	Reference
Perfused liver		25	[86]
		61	[87]
Hepatocyte monolayers		33	[88]
		30	[89]
Hepatocyte suspensions		19	[90]
		26	[91]
		21	[92]
		12	[93]
		30	[94]
Membrane vesicles		56	[95]
		52	[96]
		46	[97]
Xenopus laevis oocytes		25	[98]
COS-7	Transient	29	[99]
HPTC	Stable	25	[100]
McArdle RH-7777	Stable	13	[101]
CHO 9–6	Stable	34	[102]
HeLa	Stable	8	[103]

libraries. Such an approach was used, for example, to clone rat organic anion transport protein 1a4 (Oatp1a4, formerly Oatp2 [73,74], or the bile salt export pump (Bsep) [75]).

For full characterization of transport proteins mediating uptake of, for example, bile acids or amino acids, transporters are heterologously expressed transiently or permanently in mammalian cells (for examples, see Table 1). It is important that the expression system does not contain an endogenous transport activity. In cases where endogenous transport systems are present, e.g. in oocytes, it may be difficult to characterize the exogenous transporter clearly. This is, for example, the case for amino acids [76]. Interestingly, oocytes show barely any uptake activity for bile acids but express an export system [77].

Many export systems in the canalicular membrane belong to the superfamily of ATP-binding cassette (ABC) transport proteins. To demonstrate the ability of Bsep to transport bile acids in an ATP-dependent manner and to characterize this transporter functionally, it was transiently expressed with the baculovirus system in the Sf9 cell line from insects [75]. As conjugated bile acids are poorly membrane permeable, isolated membrane vesicles are used to perform transport studies. Thus, there is no need to isolate specifically inside-out vesicles.

In order to demonstrate that the transport protein of interest was cloned, a full characterization with respect to kinetic parameters and driving forces is required. This necessitates complete information on the properties of the transport protein of interest in its 'natural' environment in organs, cells or membrane vesicles. As an example, the rat sodium bile acid cotransporter Ntcp, heterologously expressed in various expression systems, is compared with respect to its kinetic parameters as determined *in situ* in Table 1. Comparison of Ntcp expressed in amphibian *X.*

laevis oocytes and mammalian cell lines revealed similar transport properties for all the different expression systems. These data indicate that membrane composition may not necessarily be a critical parameter for the characterization of transport proteins in heterologous expression systems.

Heterologous expression of membrane proteins also works well for intracellular proteins such as, for example, cytochrome P-450s (e.g. a recent example in [78]). Cells transfected with individual human CYPs are the starting material for the preparation of microsomal fractions expressing individual CYPs. Such microsomes are widely used to study *in vitro* drug metabolism.

Epithelial transport is unidirectional or vectorial for many substrates. Polar expression of transport systems in polarized cell lines such as the renal Madin Darby canine kidney (MDCK) cell line or the pig kidney cell line LLCP-K$_1$ allows the reconstitution of 'secretory' units. For example, Ntcp and organic anion-transporting polypeptides are expressed in the basolateral plasma membrane of hepatocytes and are sorted to the basolateral plasma membrane domain in transfected MDCK cells [79,80]. The organic anion transporter multidrug resistance protein 2 (Mrp2) and Bsep are expressed in the canalicular membrane of hepatocytes and are sorted to the apical domains of transfected MDCK cells [80,81]. Coexpression of basolateral uptake systems with these apical transporters allows the study of vectorial transport of Mrp2 and Bsep substrates [80,81]. Such systems can be viewed as 'columnar hepatocytes' and have the advantage of direct experimental access to the apical membrane domain. Additionally, in epithelial cell lines transfected with uptake and export transport systems, transcellular flux of substrates is reconstructed. In principle, multiple transport systems can be stably transfected into heterologous expression systems, as has been demonstrated for coexpression of Oatps and Mrps [82].

Outlook

With the development of powerful methods for large-scale sequencing, for the analysis of the entire transcriptome or protein pattern of cells or for the simultaneous detection of intermediates of different metabolic pathways, additional important tools have been made available for the study of hepatic functions in health and disease [83–85]. Utilizing these new methods together with the established methods of *in vitro* techniques will undoubtedly lead to important synergies and, consequently, to a much better understanding of physiological and pathophysiological hepatocellular processes. Ultimately, these new approaches should improve both diagnostics and treatment of patients.

References

1 Arias IM, Boyer JL, Fausto N *et al.* (eds) (2001) *The Liver: Biology and Pathobiology*, 4th edn. Philadelphia, PA: Lippincott Williams & Wilkins, p. 1088.

2 Miller LL, Bly CG, Watson ML *et al.* (1951) The dominant role of the liver in plasma protein synthesis. *J Exp Med* 94, 431–453.

3 Ashwell G, Morell AG (1974) The role of surface carbohydrates in the hepatic recognition and transport of circulating glycoproteins. *Adv Enzymol Relat Areas Mol Biol* 41, 99–128.

4 Kuipers F, Havinga R, Bosschieter H *et al.* (1985) Enterohepatic circulation in the rat. *Gastroenterology* 88, 403–411.

5 Rahner C, Stieger B, Landmann L (1996) Structure–function correlation of tight junctional impairment after intrahepatic and extrahepatic cholestasis in rat liver. *Gastroenterology* 110, 1564–1578.

6 Meijer DK, Keulemans K, Mulder GJ (1981) Isolated perfused rat liver technique. *Methods Enzymol* 77, 81–94.

7 Gores GJ, Kost LJ, LaRusso NF (1986) The isolated perfused rat liver: conceptual and practical considerations. *Hepatology* 6, 511–517.

8 Wolkoff AW, Johansen KL, Goeser T (1987) The isolated perfused rat liver: preparation and application. *Anal Biochem* 167, 1–14.

9 Brouwer KL, Thurman RG (1996) Isolated perfused liver. *Pharm Biotechnol* 8, 161–192.

10 vom Dahl S, Haussinger D (1997) Experimental methods in hepatology. Guidelines of the German Association for the Study of the Liver (GASL). Liver perfusion – technique and applications. *Z Gastroenterol* 35, 221–226.

11 Tirona RG, Schwab AJ, Geng W *et al.* (1998) Hepatic clearance models: comparison of the dispersion and Goresky models in outflow profiles from multiple indicator dilution rat liver studies. *Drug Metab Dispos* 26, 465–475.

12 Melgert BN, Olinga P, Weert B *et al.* (2001) Cellular distribution and handling of liver-targeting preparations in human livers studied by a liver lobe perfusion. *Drug Metab Dispos* 29, 361–367.

13 Lerche-Langrand C, Toutain HJ (2000) Precision-cut liver slices: characteristics and use for in vitro pharmaco-toxicology. *Toxicology* 153, 221–253.

14 Olinga P, Hof IH, Merema MT *et al.* (2001) The applicability of rat and human liver slices to the study of mechanisms of hepatic drug uptake. *J Pharmacol Toxicol Methods* 45, 55–63.

15 Vickers AE, Fisher RL (2004) Organ slices for the evaluation of human drug toxicity. *Chem Biol Interact* 150, 87–96.

16 Elferink MG, Olinga P, Draaisma AL *et al.* (2004) LPS-induced downregulation of MRP2 and BSEP in human liver is due to a posttranscriptional process. *Am J Physiol Gastrointest Liver Physiol* 287, G1008–1016.

17 van de Bovenkamp M, Groothuis GM, Draaisma AL *et al.* (2005) Precision-cut liver slices as a new model to study toxicity-induced hepatic stellate cell activation in a physiologic milieu. *Toxicol Sci* 85, 632–638.

18 Berry MN, Friend DS (1969) High-yield preparation of isolated rat liver parenchymal cells: a biochemical and fine structural study. *J Cell Biol* 43, 506–520.

19 Strain AJ (1994) Isolated hepatocytes: use in experimental and clinical hepatology. *Gut* 35, 433–436.

20 LeCluyse EL, Bullock PL, Parkinson A *et al.* (1996) Cultured rat hepatocytes. *Pharm Biotechnol* 8, 121–159.

21 Berry MN, Grivell AR, Grivell MB *et al.* (1997) Isolated hepatocytes – past, present and future. *Cell Biol Toxicol* 13, 223–233.

22 Gebhardt R, Hengstler JG, Muller D *et al.* (2003) New hepatocyte in vitro systems for drug metabolism: metabolic capacity and recommendations for application in basic research and drug development, standard operation procedures. *Drug Metab Rev* 35, 145–213.

23 Sandker GW, Weert B, Merema MT *et al.* (1993) Maintenance of viability and transport function after preservation of isolated rat hepatocytes in various simplified University of Wisconsin solutions. *Biochem Pharmacol* 46, 2093–2096.

24 Mitry RR, Hughes RD, Dhawan A (2002) Progress in human hepatocytes: isolation, culture and cryopreservation. *Semin Cell Dev Biol* 13, 463–467.

25 Maher JJ (1988) Primary hepatocyte culture: is it home away from home? *Hepatology* 8, 1162–1166.

26 Rippin SJ, Hagenbuch B, Meier PJ *et al.* (2001) Cholestatic expression pattern of sinusoidal and canalicular organic anion transport systems in primary cultured rat hepatocytes. *Hepatology* 33, 776–782.

27 Berthiaume F, Moghe PV, Toner M *et al.* (1996) Effect of extracellular matrix topology on cell structure, function, and physiological responsiveness: hepatocytes cultured in a sandwich configuration. *FASEB J* 10, 1471–1484.

28 Graf J, Boyer JL (1990) The use of isolated rat hepatocyte couplets in hepatobiliary physiology. *J Hepatol* 10, 387–394.

29 Milkiewicz P, Roma MG, Elias E *et al.* (2002) Pathobiology and experimental therapeutics in hepatocellular cholestasis: lessons from the hepatocyte couplet model. *Clin Sci (Lond)* 102, 603–614.

30 Guillouzo A, Morel F, Langouet S *et al.* (1997) Use of hepatocyte cultures for the study of hepatotoxic compounds. *J Hepatol* 26 (Suppl 2), 73–80.

31 Petzinger E, Follmann W, Acker H *et al.* (1988) Primary liver cell cultures grown on gas permeable membrane as source for the collection of primary bile. *In Vitro Cell Dev Biol* 24, 491–499.

32 Harhaj NS, Antonetti DA (2004) Regulation of tight junctions and loss of barrier function in pathophysiology. *Int J Biochem Cell Biol* 36, 1206–1237.

33 Liu X, LeCluyse EL, Brouwer KR *et al.* (1999) Biliary excretion in primary rat hepatocytes cultured in a collagen-sandwich configuration. *Am J Physiol* 277, G12–21.

34 Boyer JL (1996) Bile duct epithelium: frontiers in transport physiology. *Am J Physiol* 270, G1–5.

35 Valatas V, Xidakis C, Roumpaki H *et al.* (2003) Isolation of rat Kupffer cells: a combined methodology for highly purified primary cultures. *Cell Biol Int* 27, 67–73.

36 Gatmaitan Z, Varticovski L, Ling L *et al.* (1996) Studies on fenestral contraction in rat liver endothelial cells in culture. *Am J Pathol* 148, 2027–2041.

37 Miyazaki M, Namba M (1994) Hepatocellular carcinomas. In: Hay RJ, Park J-G, Gazdar A (eds) *Atlas of Human Tumor Cell Lines*. San Diego, CA: Academic Press, pp. 185–212.

38 Ferro M, Bassi AM, Penco S *et al.* (1993) Use of established hepatoma cell lines in biotoxicology. *Cytotechnology* 11 (Suppl 1), S126–129.

39 Ng KH, Le Goascogne C, Amborade E *et al.* (2000) Reversible induction of rat hepatoma cell polarity with bile acids. *J Cell Sci* 113, 4241–4251.

40 Kobayashi N, Noguchi H, Fujiwara T *et al.* (2000) Establishment of a highly differentiated immortalized adult human hepatocyte cell line by retroviral gene transfer. *Transplant Proc* 32, 2368–2369.

41 Block GD, Locker J, Bowen WC *et al.* (1996) Population expansion, clonal growth, and specific differentiation patterns in primary cultures of hepatocytes induced by HGF/SF, EGF and TGF alpha in a chemically defined (HGM) medium. *J Cell Biol* 132, 1133–1149.

42 Blumrich M, Zeyen-Blumrich U, Pagels P *et al.* (1994) Immortalization of rat hepatocytes by fusion with hepatoma cells. II. Studies on

the transport and synthesis of bile acids in hepatocytoma (HPCT) cells. *Eur J Cell Biol* 64, 339–347.

43 Cassio D, Hamon-Benais C, Guerin M *et al.* (1991) Hybrid cell lines constitute a potential reservoir of polarized cells: isolation and study of highly differentiated hepatoma-derived hybrid cells able to form functional bile canaliculi in vitro. *J Cell Biol* 115, 1397–1408.

44 Theise ND, Nimmakayalu M, Gardner R *et al.* (2000) Liver from bone marrow in humans. *Hepatology* 32, 11–16.

45 Alison MR, Poulsom R, Jeffery R *et al.* (2000) Hepatocytes from non-hepatic adult stem cells. *Nature* 406, 257.

46 Schwartz RE, Reyes M, Koodie L *et al.* (2002) Multipotent adult progenitor cells from bone marrow differentiate into functional hepatocyte-like cells. *J Clin Invest* 109, 1291–1302.

47 Avital I, Inderbitzin D, Aoki T *et al.* (2001) Isolation, characterization, and transplantation of bone marrow-derived hepatocyte stem cells. *Biochem Biophys Res Commun* 288, 156–164.

48 Hong SH, Gang EJ, Jeong JA *et al.* (2005) In vitro differentiation of human umbilical cord blood-derived mesenchymal stem cells into hepatocyte-like cells. *Biochem Biophys Res Commun* 330, 1153–1161.

49 Wang Y, Nan X, Li Y *et al.* (2005) Induction of umbilical cord blood-derived β_2m-c-Met$^+$ cells into hepatocyte-like cells by coculture with CFSC/HGF cells. *Liver Transpl* 11, 635–643.

50 Ruhnke M, Ungefroren H, Nussler A *et al.* (2005) Differentiation of in vitro-modified human peripheral blood monocytes into hepatocyte-like and pancreatic islet-like cells. *Gastroenterology* 128, 1774–1786.

51 Menthena A, Deb N, Oertel M *et al.* (2004) Bone marrow progenitors are not the source of expanding oval cells in injured liver. *Stem Cells* 22, 1049–1061.

52 Cantz T, Sharma AD, Jochheim-Richter A *et al.* (2004) Reevaluation of bone marrow-derived cells as a source for hepatocyte regeneration. *Cell Transplant* 13, 659–666.

53 Sell S (2001) Heterogeneity and plasticity of hepatocyte lineage cells. *Hepatology* 33, 738–750.

54 Mitaka T, Sato F, Mizuguchi T *et al.* (1999) Reconstruction of hepatic organoid by rat small hepatocytes and hepatic nonparenchymal cells. *Hepatology* 29, 111–125.

55 Sidler Pfandler MA, Hochli M, Inderbitzin D *et al.* (2004) Small hepatocytes in culture develop polarized transporter expression and differentiation. *J Cell Sci* 117, 4077–4087.

56 Michalopoulos GK, Bowen WC, Zajac VF *et al.* (1999) Morphogenetic events in mixed cultures of rat hepatocytes and nonparenchymal cells maintained in biological matrices in the presence of hepatocyte growth factor and epidermal growth factor. *Hepatology* 29, 90–100.

57 Packer L, Fleischer S (eds) (1997) *Biomembranes.* San Diego, CA: Academic Press.

58 Stieger B, Murer H (1983) Heterogeneity of brush-border-membrane vesicles from rat small intestine prepared by a precipitation method using Mg/EGTA. *Eur J Biochem* 135, 95–101.

59 Murer H, Gmaj P, Stieger B *et al.* (1989) Transport studies with renal proximal tubular and small intestinal brush border and basolateral membrane vesicles: vesicle heterogeneity, coexistence of transport system. *Methods Enzymol* 172, 346–364.

60 Kast C, Stieger B, Winterhalter KH *et al.* (1994) Hepatocellular transport of bile acids. Evidence for distinct subcellular localizations of electrogenic and ATP-dependent taurocholate transport in rat hepatocytes. *J Biol Chem* 269, 5179–5186.

61 Murer H, Biber J, Gmaj P *et al.* (1984) Cellular mechanisms in epithelial transport: advantages and disadvantages of studies with vesicles. *Mol Physiol* 6, 55–82.

62 Meier PJ (1996) Hepatocellular transport systems: from carrier identification in membrane vesicles to cloned proteins. *J Hepatol* 24 (Suppl 1), 29–35.

63 Walter H (1975) Tightness and orientation of vesicles from guinea-pig kidney estimated from reactions of adenosine triphosphatase dependent on sodium and potassium ions. *Eur J Biochem* 58, 595–601.

64 Murer H, Kinne R (1980) The use of isolated membrane vesicles to study epithelial transport processes. *J Membr Biol* 55, 81–95.

65 Boyer JL, Meier PJ (1990) Characterizing mechanisms of hepatic bile acid transport utilizing isolated membrane vesicles. *Methods Enzymol* 192, 517–533.

66 Meier PJ, Boyer JL (1990) Preparation of basolateral (sinusoidal) and canalicular plasma membrane vesicles for the study of hepatic transport processes. *Methods Enzymol* 192, 534–545.

67 Keppler D, Arias IM (1997) Hepatic canalicular membrane. Introduction: transport across the hepatocyte canalicular membrane. *FASEB J* 11, 15–18.

68 Stieger B, O'Neill B, Meier PJ (1992) ATP-dependent bile-salt transport in canalicular rat liver plasma-membrane vesicles. *Biochem J* 284, 67–74.

69 Kaufmann M, Muff R, Stieger B *et al.* (1994) Apical and basolateral parathyroid hormone receptors in rat renal cortical membranes. *Endocrinology* 134, 1173–1178.

70 Sigel E (1990) Use of *Xenopus* oocytes for the functional expression of plasma membrane proteins. *J Membr Biol* 117, 201–221.

71 Romero MF, Kanai Y, Gunshin H *et al.* (1998) Expression cloning using *Xenopus laevis* oocytes. *Methods Enzymol* 296, 17–52.

72 Hagenbuch B, Jacquemin E, Meier PJ (1994) Na$^+$-dependent and Na$^+$-independent bile acid uptake systems in the liver. *Cell Physiol Biochem* 4, 198–205.

73 Hagenbuch B, Meier PJ. (2004) Organic anion transporting polypeptides of the OATP/*SLC*21 family: phylogenetic classification as OATP/*SLCO* superfamily, new nomenclature and molecular/functional properties. *Pflugers Arch* 447, 653–665.

74 Noe B, Hagenbuch B, Stieger B *et al.* (1997) Isolation of a multi-specific organic anion and cardiac glycoside transporter from rat brain. *Proc Natl Acad Sci USA* 94, 10346–10350.

75 Gerloff T, Stieger B, Hagenbuch B *et al.* (1998) The sister of P-glycoprotein represents the canalicular bile salt export pump of mammalian liver. *J Biol Chem* 273, 10046–10050.

76 Van Winkle LJ (1993) Endogenous amino acid transport systems and expression of mammalian amino acid transport proteins in *Xenopus* oocytes. *Biochim Biophys Acta* 1154, 157–172.

77 Shneider BL, Moyer MS (1993) Characterization of endogenous carrier-mediated taurocholate efflux from *Xenopus laevis* oocytes. *J Biol Chem* 268, 6985–6988.

78 Omasa T, Kim K, Hiramatsu S *et al.* (2005) Construction and evaluation of drug-metabolizing cell line for bioartificial liver support system. *Biotechnol Prog* 21, 161–167.

79 Sun AQ, Ananthanarayanan M, Soroka CJ *et al.* (1998) Sorting of rat liver and ileal sodium-dependent bile acid transporters in polarized epithelial cells. *Am J Physiol Gastrointest Liver Physiol* 275, G1045–1055.

80 Cui Y, Konig J, Keppler D (2001) Vectorial transport by double-transfected cells expressing the human uptake transporter SLC21A8 and the apical export pump ABCC2. *Mol Pharmacol* 60, 934–943.

81 Mita S, Suzuki H, Akita H *et al.* (2005) Vectorial transport of bile salts across MDCK cells expressing both rat Na$^+$-taurocholate

cotransporting polypeptide and rat bile salt export pump. *Am J Physiol Gastrointest Liver Physiol* 288, G159–167.

82 Kopplow K, Letschert K, Konig J *et al.* (2005) Human hepatobiliary transport of organic anions analyzed by quadruple-transfected cells. *Mol Pharmacol* 68, 1031–1038.

83 Shackel NA, Gorrell MD, McCaughan GW (2002) Gene array analysis and the liver. *Hepatology* 36, 1313–1325.

84 Chignard N, Beretta L (2004) Proteomics for hepatocellular carcinoma marker discovery. *Gastroenterology* 127, S120–125.

85 Griffin JL, Bollard ME (2004) Metabonomics: its potential as a tool in toxicology for safety assessment and data integration. *Curr Drug Metab* 5, 389–398.

86 Reichen J, Paumgartner G (1976) Uptake of bile acids by perfused rat liver. *Am J Physiol* 231, 734–742.

87 Dietmaier A, Gasser R, Graf J *et al.* (1976) Investigations on the sodium dependence of bile acid fluxes in the isolated perfused rat liver. *Biochim Biophys Acta* 443, 81–91.

88 Van Dyke RW, Stephens JE, Scharschmidt BF (1982) Bile acid transport in cultured rat hepatocytes. *Am J Physiol Gastrointest Liver Physiol* 243, G484–492.

89 Liang D, Hagenbuch B, Stieger B *et al.* (1993) Parallel decrease of Na(+)-taurocholate cotransport and its encoding mRNA in primary cultures of rat hepatocytes. *Hepatology* 18, 1162–1166.

90 Schwarz LR, Burr R, Schwenk M *et al.* (1975) Uptake of taurocholic acid into isolated rat-liver cells. *Eur J Biochem* 55, 617–623.

91 Anwer MS, Kroker R, Hegner D (1976) Effect of albumin on bile acid uptake by isolated rat hepatocytes. Is there a common bile acid carrier? *Biochem Biophys Res Commun* 73, 63–71.

92 Blitzer BL, Ratoosh SL, Donovan CB *et al.* (1982) Effects of inhibitors of Na^+-coupled ion transport on bile acid uptake by isolated rat hepatocytes. *Am J Physiol Gastrointest Liver Physiol* 243, G48–53.

93 Kuhn WF, Gewirtz DA (1988) Stimulation of taurocholate and glycocholate efflux from the rat hepatocyte by arginine vasopressin. *Am J Cell Physiol* 254, G732–740.

94 Follmann W, Petzinger E, Kinne RK (1990) Alterations of bile acid and bumetanide uptake during culturing of rat hepatocytes. *Am J Cell Physiol* 258, C700–712.

95 Inoue M, Kinne R, Tran T *et al.* (1982) Taurocholate transport by rat liver sinusoidal membrane vesicles: evidence of sodium cotransport. *Hepatology* 2, 572–579.

96 Duffy MC, Blitzer BL, Boyer JL (1983) Direct determination of the driving forces for taurocholate uptake into rat liver plasma membrane vesicles. *J Clin Invest* 72, 1470–1481.

97 Zimmerli B, Valantinas J, Meier PJ (1989) Multispecificity of Na^+-dependent taurocholate uptake in basolateral (sinusoidal) rat liver plasma membrane vesicles. *J Pharmacol Exp Ther* 250, 301–308.

98 Hagenbuch B, Stieger B, Foguet M *et al.* (1991) Functional expression cloning and characterization of the hepatocyte Na+/bile acid cotransport system. *Proc Natl Acad Sci USA* 88, 10629–10633.

99 Boyer JL, Ng OC, Ananthanarayanan M *et al.* (1994) Expression and characterization of a functional rat liver Na+ bile acid cotransport system in COS-7 cells. *Am J Physiol Gastrointest Liver Physiol* 266, G382–387.

100 Platte HD, Honscha W, Schuh K *et al.* (1996) Functional characterization of the hepatic sodium-dependent taurocholate transporter stably transfected into an immortalized liver-derived cell line and V79 fibroblasts. *Eur J Cell Biol* 70, 54–60.

101 Torchia EC, Shapiro RJ, Agellon LB (1996) Reconstitution of bile acid transport in the rat hepatoma McArdle RH-7777 cell line. *Hepatology* 24, 206–211.

102 Schroeder A, Eckhardt U, Stieger B *et al.* (1998) Substrate specificity of the rat liver Na(+)-bile salt cotransporter in *Xenopus laevis* oocytes and in CHO cells. *Am J Physiol Gastrointest Liver Physiol* 274, G370–375.

103 Hata S, Wang P, Eftychiou N *et al.* (2003) Substrate specificities of rat oatp1 and ntcp: implications for hepatic organic anion uptake. *Am J Physiol Gastrointest Liver Physiol* 285, G829–839.

2.3 Metabolism

2.3.1 Carbohydrates and the liver

Guenther Boden

Introduction

After a carbohydrate-containing meal, the liver maintains plasma glucose concentration within a narrow range by taking up one-quarter to one-third of the absorbed glucose, oxidizing some of it and storing the rest as glycogen or converting it into fat. In the postabsorptive state, the liver provides much needed glucose to the central nervous system and other glucose-utilizing tissues by breaking down glycogen (a process called glycogenolysis, GL) and/or by new formation of glucose from non-glucose precursors (a process called gluconeogenesis, GNG). Disturbances of any one of these processes can result in either hyperglycaemia or hypoglycaemia. This chapter focuses on glucose, the physiologically most important carbohydrate, and gives a brief overview of the pivotal role of the liver in glucose metabolism under normal and abnormal conditions.

Hepatic glucose metabolism in the postprandial state

After a meal, the liver plays a pivotal role in maintaining blood glucose homeostasis by regulating, minute by minute, hepatic glucose production and uptake.

Glucose production

After a mixed meal ($\sim$ 60% carbohydrate, $\sim$ 20% fat and $\sim$ 15% protein), endogenous glucose production (EGP; over 90% of which comes from the liver, with the remainder derived from the kidneys) falls to very low rates (0–20% of basal) (reviewed in [1]). During this period, blood sugar concentrations are predominantly maintained by absorption of meal-derived glucose, while EGP decreases to 20% or less of basal (postabsorptive

rates). As intestinal absorption of carbohydrate decreases several hours after the meal, EGP rises slowly towards basal levels.

These changes in EGP are controlled primarily by two pancreatic hormones, insulin and glucagon.

Insulin is secreted by the pancreatic β cells directly into the portal circulation. The liver extracts and degrades between 50% and 80% of the insulin entering it on first pass [2,3] and, thus, even basal insulin concentrations are approximately three times higher in the portal than in the peripheral circulation [1]. Insulin secretion is stimulated by changes in blood levels of glucose, fatty acids and amino acids (with glucose being the strongest secretagogue). Insulin secretion can be modified by an as yet unidentified portal signal (presumably mediated by the parasympathetic nervous system) [4], by several gastrointestinal hormones including glucose-dependent intestinal peptide (GIP) and glucagon-like peptide 1 (GLP1) [2,5], and by the central nervous system (cephalic phase).

Hepatic glucose production is exquisitely sensitive to changes in insulin levels. The four- to 10-fold rise in hepatic sinusoidal insulin typically seen after a carbohydrate-rich meal almost completely inhibits hepatic glucose production. There is little information on the effect of insulin on renal glucose production, but insulin presumably suppresses renal glucose production as well. Insulin suppresses EGP through direct and indirect actions. In the direct pathway, insulin lowers glucose production primarily by stimulating glycogen synthesis [6]. In the indirect pathway, by inhibiting proteolysis and lipolysis, insulin decreases the supply of gluconeogenic precursors such as amino acids and free fatty acids (FFAs) to the liver. This results in a decrease in glucose production, presumably by reducing GNG [7,8]. In addition, insulin can lower hepatic GNG and blood glucose levels by direct action on adenosine triphosphate (ATP)-sensitive K channels in the mediobasal hypothalamus [9].

Glucagon is secreted by the pancreatic α cells. Like insulin, glucagon is secreted directly into the portal circulation but, unlike insulin, the liver degrades only $\sim$ 15–25% of the glucagon entering it [10]. Glucagon secretion is stimulated by hypoglycaemia, amino acids, and sympathetic and parasympathetic nervous stimulation. Glucagon secretion is decreased by hyperglycaemia, and high FFA and somatostatin levels. Glucagon rapidly increases EGP by promoting glycogenolysis via an increase in the phosphorylase reaction [6]. After a mixed meal containing carbohydrates, protein and fat, both insulin and glucagon concentrations rise in the portal circulation, but the rise in insulin exceeds that of glucagon. The net effect is an increase in the insulin/glucagon ratio and a sharp decrease in EGP. After a protein/fat-rich meal containing little or no carbohydrates, glucagon rises much more than insulin. The low insulin/glucagon ratio results in a rise in EGP, which prevents the hypoglycaemia that would occur if the amino acid-stimulated insulin secretion was unopposed by a larger amino acid-stimulated glucagon secretion.

Glucose uptake

The liver takes up one-quarter to one-third of an ingested glucose load during the initial 4–5 h after ingestion of a mixed meal. Most of this glucose is stored as glycogen; the remainder is oxidized or converted into fat.

Postprandial glycogen synthesis is driven by portal venous hyperglycaemia and by high insulin/glucagon ratios. Hyperinsulinaemia stimulates glycogen synthase flux, while hyperglycaemia inhibits glycogen phosphorylase flux [6]. Thus, postprandial hyperglycaemia and hyperinsulinaemia together stimulate glycogen synthesis and inhibit GL, resulting in a rapid and profound decrease in EGP.

Glycogen is synthesized via two different pathways. The direct pathway (glucose to glucose-6-phosphate to glucose-1-phosphate to UDP glucose to glycogen) accounts for ~ 50% of glycogen synthesis during the postabsorptive phase and increases postprandially to 60–70% of glycogen synthesis, while the indirect pathway (three carbon glucose precursors to glucose-6-phosphate to glucose-1-phosphate to UDP glucose to glycogen) accounts for the remainder [1].

Hepatic glucose metabolism in the postabsorptive state

During the postabsorptive state, all macronutrients have ceased to enter the circulation from the digestive tract and all meal-associated changes in hormone secretion have returned to basal. For practical purposes, it is the time after an overnight fast and before breakfast. Under these conditions, the liver of a healthy person weighing ~ 70 kg produces glucose at a rate of ~ 10 g/h, of which ~ 6 g/h is taken up by the central nervous system, with the rest going to all other tissues including skeletal muscle, adipose tissue, red blood cells, renal medulla, etc. [11]. The postabsorptive blood glucose concentration of a person weighing 70 kg is ~ 90 mg/dL, and ~ 19 g of glucose, i.e. less than a 2-h supply, is present in the extracellular space (assumed to be ~ 30% of body weight).

The vital role of the liver in supplying glucose for use mainly in the central nervous system during an overnight fast is regulated by insulin and glucagon. The low postabsorptive insulin levels reduce glycogen synthesis to very low rates and allow glucagon to stimulate GL, resulting in an increase in EGP to ~ 10 g/h. Hence, it has been estimated that, after an overnight fast, basal plasma glucagon levels are responsible for 75% or more of EGP [12].

Gluconeogenesis (GNG) and glycogenolysis (GL)

EGP has two components. GNG, which is the formation of glucose from non-glucose precursors (lactate, pyruvate, glucogenic amino acids and glycerol), and GL, which is glucose derived from the breakdown of glycogen stored in the liver. Despite its physiological importance, accurate and quantitative information from human subjects on rates of GNG and GL is limited, primarily because of methodological problems. Specifically, the labelled precursors used to measure GNG are diluted to an unpredictable degree in the oxalocetic acid pool, which is shared by GNG and the tricarboxylic acid cycle [13]. Recently, however, several methods have become available that allow non-invasive measurement of *in vivo* rates of GNG and GL in humans [14–17]. Of those, the ^2H_2O method, which was developed and validated by Landau *et al.* [17] to measure GNG, is currently most widely used. This method depends on the incorporation of ^2H from ^2H_2O into carbon 5 of glucose (Fig. 1). It measures GNG from all sources, including lactate, pyruvate, glucogenic amino acids and glycerol, and avoids the problems related to precursor dilution. On the other hand, the ^2H_2O method determines only GNG-derived glucose that enters the glucose space, that is the glucose-6-phosphate to glucose flux. It does not detect GNG-derived glucose that is deposited in glycogen or cycles from glucose-6-phosphate to glycogen and back to glucose-6-phosphate and thus does not enter the blood. When GNG is determined by this method, GL can be calculated by subtracting

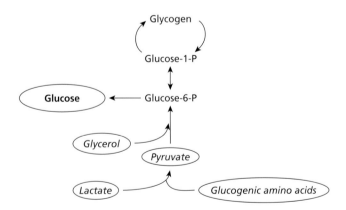

Fig. 1 Schematic representation of GNG as measured with ^2H_2O. This method determines glucose derived from pyruvate and glycerol, which enters the glucose space.

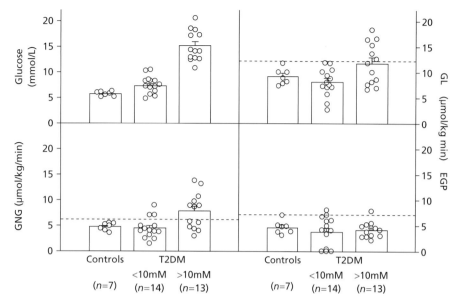

Fig. 2 Plasma glucose, GNG, GL and EGP in 14 patients with type 2 diabetes mellitus (T2DM) who had fasting plasma glucose levels of < 10 mM, in 13 patients with T2DM with fasting plasma glucose levels of > 10 mM and in seven non-diabetic control subjects. Shown are means ± SE. Broken horizontal lines represent mean ± 2 SD of control subjects. The data show that higher rates of GNG and EGP are seen mostly in patients with fasting plasma glucose levels > 10 mmol/L who have more than modest degrees of insulin deficiency [26].

GNG from EGP (GL = EGP–GNG). GL can also be obtained by directly measuring liver glycogen concentration with ^{13}C-nuclear magnetic resonance spectroscopy in combination with magnetic resonance imaging of the liver volume and isotopic measurement of EGP [14]. Use of these newer methods have shown the following:

1 In healthy people after an overnight fast, GNG and GL contribute about equally to EGP. As fasting progresses, the absolute contribution of GNG (in μmol/h) remains essentially unchanged, whereas GL decreases as glycogen stores become depleted. As a result, after more than 40 h of fasting, GNG accounts for over 90% of EGP.

2 Acutely rising serum insulin levels reduce EGP primarily by suppressing GL and, to a much lesser extent, GNG [18,19].

3 Acute elevations of plasma FFA levels raise GNG and lower GL, whereas acute lowering of FFA levels lower GNG and raise GL [20]. Because of the reciprocal changes in GNG and GL, EGP remains essentially unchanged [21]. This so-called hepatic autoregulation of EGP seems to be regulated by insulin in the following way. Rising FFA levels stimulate GNG and insulin secretion. The rise in insulin levels suppresses GL.

4 Abnormally elevated plasma FFA levels cause hepatic insulin resistance, i.e. they inhibit insulin-mediated suppression of EGP, which is due to inhibition by FFA of the normal insulin suppression of GL [19].

5 After a mixed meal, net hepatic glycogen synthesis increases by ~ 50% resulting in about 20% of the ingested glucose being deposited as glycogen in the liver [22].

Diabetes

Patients with type 2 diabetes frequently have higher rates of GNG and EGP than non-diabetic control subjects [23–26]. There is, however, a great deal of overlap in GNG and EGP between diabetic patients and non-diabetic control subjects, and absolutely higher than normal rates of GNG and EGP are usually seen only in patients with fasting plasma glucose concentrations of > 10 mmol/L [26] (Fig. 2). It needs to be recognized, however, that the 'normal' rates of GNG and EGP in patients with type 2 diabetes are abnormal in view of the fact that insulin and glucose levels are commonly elevated in these patients and that both hyperglycaemia and hyperinsulinaemia inhibit EGP in healthy subjects. In addition, patients with type 2 diabetes also seem to have dysfunctional hepatic autoregulation. For instance, when plasma FFA levels were lowered in patients with type 2 diabetes, these patients were unable to compensate for the decrease in GNG with an increase in GL; when FFA levels were raised, GNG rose but GL did not decrease appropriately [27].

In patients with type 1 diabetes mellitus, injection of insulin resulted in an acute decrease in EGP, which was due to a decrease in GL with little change in GNG (glucose concentrations were clamped at 6.5 mmol/L) [28]. In patients with type 1 diabetes during a phase of acute insulin deficiency, which developed 4–8 h after the last insulin injection, EGP rose from 9.5 to 14.3 mmol/L, which was again due to an increase in GL with little change in GNG, and glucose rose from 6.2 to 10.5 mmol/L. Thus, acute regulation of EGP in patients with type 1 diabetes is brought about primarily by changes in GL with little or no participation of GNG [28].

The reason for the increased EGP in patients with type 2 diabetes is incompletely compensated hepatic insulin resistance. Although the causes of the hepatic insulin resistance are not completely understood, there are known defects in postreceptor insulin signalling. The normally functioning direct and indirect insulin pathways (see above), which result in insulin-induced suppression of EGP, involve tyrosine phosphorylation of several intracellular proteins including insulin receptor substrates (IRS-1/2), phosphoinositide-3 kinase (PI3K), phosphoinositide-dependent kinase (PDK-1), protein kinase B (Akt) and glycogen synthase kinase-3 (GSK-3) [29]. In obesity-associated insulin resistance, the most common type of hepatic insulin resistance, instead of tyrosine phosphorylation, there is serine phosphorylation of IRS-1/2 by several serine kinases including pyruvate kinase C (PKC) and IκB kinase (IKK). Serine phosphorylation results in degradation of IRS-1/2 and thereby interrupts insulin signalling [30].

Non-alcoholic fatty liver disease (NAFLD) (see also Chapter 13)

NAFLD refers to a series of liver disorders ranging from simple steatosis to steatohepatitis, advanced fibrosis and cirrhosis in patients who do not abuse ethanol. In the United States, steatosis has been estimated to occur in more than two-thirds of the obese population and in more than 90% of morbidly obese subjects. Steatohepatitis affects ~ 20% of obese and ~ 50% of morbidly obese people. All obese diabetic patients have at least some degree of steatosis, while ~ 50% have steatohepatitis and ~ 90% have cirrhosis (reviewed in [31]).

Hepatic insulin resistance and increased generation of inflammatory cytokines are currently believed to be important for the development of steatohepatitis. In that respect, high fat feeding in rodents results in hepatic and systemic insulin resistance, as well as hepatic steatosis associated with subacute hepatic inflammation, activation of the proinflammatory NF-κB pathway and the production of several cytokines [32].

Cirrhosis

Cirrhosis of the liver is the result of many different causes, including hepatitis induced by toxins (most frequently by ethanol), NAFLD (see above), by viral infections (hepatitis A, B and C) [33] and by autoimmune inflammatory disorders (see Section 6, Cirrhosis). Thus, it is a heterogeneous disorder, which makes discussion of carbohydrate metabolism in cirrhosis difficult. In general, however, many patients with moderate liver disease, who are in a reasonably normal nutritional state, have normal or near-normal EGP rates (1.8–2.2 mg/kg/min after an overnight fast) and blood glucose levels. As most of these patients are insulin resistant [34], their normal rate of EGP and blood glucose levels are the result of compensated hepatic, as well as peripheral, insulin resistance. A significant proportion of cirrhotic patients, however, are glucose intolerant, indicating that they are unable to meet the increased insulin requirements of a carbohydrate load [35].

Several studies have reported that the contribution of GL to EGP is decreased and the contribution of GNG is increased in patients with cirrhosis. For instance, Petersen et al. [35] have determined changes in hepatic glycogen content with ^{13}C-nuclear magnetic resonance spectroscopy [14] before and after an overnight fast and found that net hepatic GL was 3.5 times lower (13% vs. 40% of EGP) in cirrhotic patients than in healthy control subjects whereas GNG was increased (87% vs. 60% of EGP). Comparable results were obtained in the same patients when GNG was measured with the ^2H_2O method [35]. Earlier, Owen et al. [36] had determined EGP and GNG by measuring arterial venous differences of glucose and GNG precursors across the liver. They found that, after an overnight fast, GNG accounted for 67% and GL for 33% of hepatic glucose production in cirrhotic patients. This was an increase in GNG and a decrease in GL compared with healthy subjects studied with the same technique by Wahren et al. [37]. The reason for the relative decrease in GL is not clear, but may be related to a decrease in glycogen content in patients with cirrhosis of the liver. Thus, it appears that many patients with cirrhosis of the liver maintain a relatively normal hepatic glucose production by increasing GNG to compensate for a decrease in GL. This may be one reason why these patients have a tendency to become protein depleted.

References

1 Cherrington AD (2001) Control of glucose production in vivo by insulin and glucagon. In: Jefferson LS, Cherrington AD (eds) *The Endocrine Pancreas and Regulation of Metabolism*. New York: Oxford University Press, pp. 759–785.

2 Ishida T, Chap Z, Chou J et al. (1983) Differential effects of oral, peripheral intravenous, and intraportal glucose on hepatic glucose uptake and insulin and glucagon extraction in conscious dogs. *J Clin Invest* 72, 590–601.

3 Duckworth WC, Bennett RG, Hamel FG (1998) Insulin degradation: progress and potential. *Endocr Rev* 19, 608–624.

4 Stumpel F, Jungermann K (1997) Sensing by intrahepatic muscarinic nerves of a portal-arterial glucose concentration gradient as a signal for insulin-dependent uptake in the perfused rat liver. *FEBS* 406, 119–122.

5 Radziuk J, Inculet R (1983) The effects of ingested and intravenous glucose and glucogenic substrate in normal man. *Diabetes* 32, 977–981.

6 Petersen KF, Laurent D, Rochman DL et al. (1998) Mechanism by which glucose and insulin net hepatic glycogenolysis in humans. *J Clin Invest* 101, 1203–1209.

7 Prager R, Wallace O, Olefsky JM (1987) Direct and indirect effects of insulin to inhibit hepatic glucose output in obese subjects. *Diabetes* 36, 607–611.

8 Ader M, Bergman RN (1990) Peripheral effects of insulin dominate suppression of fasting hyperglycemia. *Am J Physiol* 258, E1029–E1032.

9 Pocal A, Lam TKT, Gutierrez-Juarez R et al. (2005) Hypothalamic K_{ATP} channels control hepatic glucose production. *Nature* 434, 1026–1031.

10 Dobbins RL, Davis SN, Neal DW et al. (1995) Compartmental modeling of glucagon kinetics in the conscious dog. *Metabolism* 44, 452–459.

11 Cahill GF, Jr (1970) Starvation in man. *N Engl J Med* 282, 668–675.

12 Liljenquist JE, Mueller GL, Cherrington AD et al. (1977) Evidence for an important role of glucagon in the regulation of hepatic glucose production in normal man. *J Clin Invest* 59, 369–374.

13 Katz J (1985) Determination of gluconeogenesis in vivo with ^{14}C-labeled substrates. *Am J Physiol Regul Integr Comp Physiol* 248, R391–R399.

14 Rothman DL, Magnusson I, Katz LD *et al.* (1991) Quantitation of hepatic glycogenesis and gluconeogenesis in fasting humans with ^{13}C NMR. *Science* 254, 573–576.

15 Hellerstein MK, Neese RA, Linfoot P *et al.* (1997) Hepatic gluconeogenic fluxes and glycogen turnover during fasting in humans. A stable isotope study. *J Clin Invest* 100, 1305–1319.

16 Katz J, Tayek JA (1998) Gluconeogenesis and the Cori cycle in 12-, 20-, and 40-h-fasted humans. *Am J Physiol* 275, E537–E542.

17 Landau BR, Wahren J, Chandramouli V *et al.* (1996) Contributions of gluconeogenesis to glucose production in the fasted state. *J Clin Invest* 98, 378–385.

18 Gastaldelli A, Toschi E, Pettiti M *et al.* (2001) Effect of physiological hyperinsulinemia on gluconeogenesis in nondiabetic subjects and in type 2 diabetic patients. *Diabetes* 50, 1807–1812.

19 Boden G, Cheung P, Stein TP *et al.* (2002) FFA cause hepatic insulin resistance by inhibiting insulin suppression of glycogenolysis. *Am J Physiol* 283, E12–E19.

20 Chen X, Iqbal N, Boden G (1999) The effects of free fatty acids on gluconeogenesis and glycogenolysis in normal subjects. *J Clin Invest* 103, 365–372.

21 Boden G (2003) Effects of free fatty acids on gluconeogenesis and glycogenolysis. *Life Sci* 72, 977–988.

22 Taylor R, Magnussen I, Rothman DL *et al.* (1996) Direct assessment of liver glycogen storage by 13C-nuclear magnetic resonance spectroscopy and regulation of glucose homeostasis after a mixed meal in normal subjects. *J Clin Invest* 97, 126–132.

23 Ferrannini E, Barrett E, Bevilacqua S *et al.* (1983) Effect of fatty acids on glucose production and utilization in man. *J Clin Invest* 72, 1737–1747.

24 Magnusson I, Rothman DL, Katz LD *et al.* (1992) Increased rate of gluconeogenesis in type II diabetes mellitus. *J Clin Invest* 90, 1323–1327.

25 Wajngot A, Chandramouli V, Schumann WC *et al.* (2001) Quantitative contributions of gluconeogenesis to glucose production during fasting in type 2 diabetes mellitus. *Metabolism* 50, 47–52.

26 Boden G, Chen X, Stein TP (2001) Gluconeogenesis in moderately and severely hyperglycemic patients with type 2 diabetes mellitus. *Am J Physiol* 280, E23–E30.

27 Boden G, Chen X, Capulong E *et al.* (2001) Effects of free fatty acids on gluconeogenesis and autoregulation of glucose production in type 2 diabetes. *Diabetes* 50, 810–816.

28 Boden G, Cheung P, Homko C (2003) Effects of acute insulin excess and deficiency on gluconeogenesis and glycogenolysis in type 1 diabetes. *Diabetes* 52, 133–137.

29 Zick Y (2001) Insulin resistance: a phosphorylation-based uncoupling of insulin signaling. *Trends Cell Biol* 11, 437–441.

30 Samuel VT, Liu ZX, Qu X *et al.* (2004) Mechanism of hepatic insulin resistance in non-alcoholic fatty liver disease. *J Biol Chem* 279, 32345–32353.

31 Angulo P (2002) Nonalcoholic fatty liver disease. *N Engl J Med* 346, 1221–1231.

32 Cai D, Yuan M, Frantz DF *et al.* (2005) Local and system insulin resistance resulting from hepatic activation of IKK-β and NF-κB. *Nature Med* 11, 183–190.

33 Fartoux L, Poujol-Robert A, Guechot J *et al.* (2005) Insulin resistance is a cause of steatosis and fibrosis progression in chronic hepatitis C. *Gut* 54 (7), 1003–1008.

34 Stewart A, Johnston DG, Alberti KGMM (1983) Hormone and metabolic profiles in alcoholic liver disease. *Eur J Clin Invest* 13, 397–403.

35 Petersen KF, Krssak M, Navarro V *et al.* (1999) Contributions of net hepatic glycogenolysis and gluconeogenesis to glucose production in cirrhosis. *Am J Physiol* 276, E529–E535.

36 Owen OE, Reichle FA, Mozzoli MA *et al.* (1981) Hepatic, gut and renal substrate flux rates in patients with hepatic cirrhosis. *J Clin Invest* 68, 240–252.

37 Wahren J, Felig P, Cerasi E *et al.* (1972) Splanchnic and peripheral glucose and amino acid metabolism in diabetes mellitus. *J Clin Invest* 51, 1870–1878.

2.3.2 Lipoprotein metabolism

Erez F. Scapa, Keishi Kanno and David E. Cohen

Introduction

Lipoproteins are macromolecular aggregates of lipids and proteins that function to transport otherwise insoluble lipid molecules through the plasma. This chapter will discuss the structure and function of lipoproteins. Emphasis will be placed on the transport of triglycerides and cholesterol, which constitute the principal lipids carried by lipoprotein particles.

Triglycerides, which consist of three fatty acids esterified to a glycerol molecule, are insoluble in water [1]. Triglycerides are either absorbed from the diet following a meal or assembled by the liver. Lipoproteins transport triglycerides to muscles, which utilize the fatty acids as a key source of energy. Triglycerides are also transported to adipose tissue, where the fatty acids are taken up by adipocytes, reassembled and stored for later use by the body.

Cholesterol is a critical regulator of membrane structure and function. Its concentration in membranes preserves bilayer fluidity and governs the formation of microdomains. Microdomains facilitate the association of plasma membrane proteins that participate in critical cell functions, including signal transduction and receptor–ligand binding. In addition to its role in membrane biology, cholesterol is the substrate for bile salt and steroid hormone biosynthesis (see also Chapter 2.3.6) [2]. Oxidized cholesterol molecules (i.e. oxysterols) serve as ligands for nuclear hormone receptors, which regulate cellular lipid metabolism [3]. Although cholesterol is absorbed in substantial amounts by the intestine, there does not appear to be a dietary cholesterol requirement. This is because virtually all cells in the body synthesize cholesterol molecules.

An important determinant of the physical state of cholesterol is whether the hydroxyl group is esterified to a long-chain fatty acid. For cholesterol to reside in membranes, this hydroxyl group must be unesterified. Molecules of esterified cholesterol (i.e. cholesteryl esters) are too insoluble even to be accommodated within membrane bilayers in more than trace quantities.

The liver is the only organ capable of degrading cholesterol and eliminating it from the body. As a result, excess cholesterol must be transported by lipoproteins through the plasma to the liver. This process is commonly referred to as reverse cholesterol transport.

Lipoprotein structure

Overview

Although different types of lipoprotein particles circulate in the plasma, their structures are similar (Fig. 1), reflecting common physicochemical mechanisms for transporting water-insoluble lipids. Lipoproteins are assembled from polar and neutral lipids, as well as specific proteins, which are referred to as apoproteins or apolipoproteins. Apolipoproteins are amphiphilic proteins capable of interacting with both lipids and the surrounding aqueous environment of the plasma. The principal lipid components of lipoproteins include the non-polar lipids, triglycerides and cholesteryl esters, and the polar lipids, phospholipids and unesterified cholesterol [1]. The hydrophobic core of a lipoprotein particle contains non-polar lipids. The amphiphilic coat comprises polar lipids and apolipoproteins, which create a stable emulsion of the core. The phospholipids orient themselves as a monolayer surrounding the hydrophobic core, and the apoproteins align themselves at the lipid–plasma interface [4]. Because it is a polar lipid, unesterified cholesterol resides within the phospholipid monolayer of the surface coat of the lipoprotein.

The lipoproteins present in plasma are: chylomicrons (CM), very-low-density lipoproteins (VLDL), low-density lipoproteins (LDL), intermediate-density lipoproteins (IDL) and high-density lipoproteins (HDL). The characteristics of lipoproteins [4], which are categorized by density using ultracentrifugation or by electrophoretic mobility using agarose gels, are listed in Table 1. Lipoprotein size increases in proportion to the triglyceride and cholesteryl ester contents of the core, whereas the percentage of phospholipids comprising the coat decreases as a result of the corresponding decrease in surface-to-volume ratio. The density of lipoproteins is proportional to their protein contents, and inversely proportional to their lipid contents, whereas mobility on agarose gels depends upon both size and charge [4].

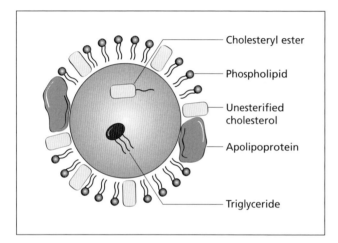

Fig. 1 Lipoprotein structure. The surface coat of lipoprotein particles comprises the polar lipids, unesterified cholesterol and phospholipids, as well as apolipoproteins. The non-polar lipids, cholesteryl esters and triglycerides, are contained in the core. Unless otherwise indicated in subsequent figures, phospholipid and whesterified cholesterol molecules are not shown for clarity.

Image labels: Cholesteryl ester, Phospholipid, Unesterified cholesterol, Apolipoprotein, Triglyceride

Apolipoproteins

Apolipoproteins are commonly identified using the abbreviation 'apo' followed by a capital letter identifying the particular protein (e.g. apoA-I). From a structural standpoint, an important common feature of these proteins is their amphiphilicity (i.e. their capacity to interact with both lipids and water). This property is primarily attributable to α-helical secondary structural elements with distinct hydrophobic and hydrophilic surfaces. These allow apolipoproteins to orient themselves at the lipid–water interface of lipoproteins and stabilize the particles. In general, apolipoproteins associate reversibly with lipids and,

Table 1 Characteristics of plasma lipoproteins.[a]

	CM	VLDL	IDL	LDL	HDL
Density (g/mL)	< 0.95	0.95–1.006	1.006–1.019	1.019–1.063	1.063–1.210
Diameter (nm)	75–1200	30–80	25–35	18–25	5–12
Total lipid (% wt)	98	90	82	75	67
Composition (% dry weight)					
Protein	2	10	18	25	33
Triglyerides	83	50	31	9	8
Unesterified cholesterol plus cholesteryl esters	8	22	29	45	30
Phospholipids (% wt lipid)	7	18	22	21	29
Electrophoretic mobility[b]	None	Pre-β	β	β	α or pre-β

[a]Adapted from ref. 4 with permission.

[b]Electrophoretic mobility of lipoprotein particles is designated relative to migration of plasma α- and β-globulins.

thereby, may exchange among lipoprotein particles in plasma. The exceptions are apoB-48 and apoB-100. Hydrophobic β-sheet elements contained in apoB-48 and apoB-100 embed within the lipid aggregate of lipoprotein particles, so that these apolipoproteins remain tightly associated with their respective lipoprotein particles and do not exchange [5].

Triglyceride delivery to muscle and adipose tissue: metabolism of apoB-containing lipoproteins

Overview

The apoB-containing lipoproteins include CM, VLDL, IDL and LDL. Their primary function is the delivery of dietary and endogenous triglycerides to muscle and fat tissue. As will be discussed later, a secondary function of apoB-containing lipoproteins is to assist with reverse cholesterol transport.

ApoB

A single apoB gene is transcribed principally in the intestine and liver. Other than its tissue-specific expression, regulation of apoB expression is largely posttranscriptional. As depicted in Figure 2, a key point in the posttranscriptional regulation of apoB metabolism occurs when mRNA transcripts from the apoB gene undergo an editing process [6]. A cytosine within the mRNA coding sequence is converted to a uracil. As a result, a codon that is normally translated into a glutamine is instead converted to a stop codon, resulting in a truncated apoB protein. The editing process is the result of tissue-specific expression of proteins collectively known as the apoB editing complex. The catalytic protein apobec-1 is responsible for deaminating cytosine [6]. In humans, apoB editing occurs in the intestine and not the liver. As a result, the edited apoB transcript in the intestine is translated into a 2152-amino-acid (aa) protein. Owing to the absence of apobec-1 expression in liver, the full-length 4536-aa protein is translated. Because intestinal apoB is 48% of the length in aa of the apoB expressed in liver, the proteins are referred to as apoB-48 and apoB-100 respectively.

Assembly and secretion of apoB-containing lipoproteins

ApoB-48 and apoB-100 undergo posttranslational modification in the endoplasmic reticulum. Disulphide bond formation appears to occur cotranslationally and requires the presence of protein disulphide isomerase (PDI), which is a luminal protein in the endoplasmic reticulum that mediates protein folding [7].

The secretion of apoB-containing lipoproteins depends critically upon the availability of triglycerides and the presence of microsomal transfer protein (MTP). MTP is a heterodimeric protein consisting of M and P subunits. The P subunit of MTP is PDI. The M subunit of MTP catalyses intermembrane transfer of triglycerides and other lipids *in vitro*. Whereas the precise role of MTP in lipoprotein assembly and secretion is incompletely understood, it appears that MTP–apoB binding and MTP lipid transfer activity are required for particle formation. Figure 3 illustrates a schematic model of how MTP participates in the assembly of apoB-containing lipoproteins, a process commonly referred to as lipidation. Consistent with its critical role in the assembly of CM and VLDL, mutations in MTP result in abetalipoproteinaemia, which is characterized by hypolipidaemia and absence in plasma of apoB-containing lipoproteins [8]. During lipoprotein assembly within the hepatocyte or enterocyte, a single apoB-100 or apoB-48 becomes embedded in a VLDL or CM particle respectively [9].

Once assembled, secretion of CM and VLDL occurs by exocytosis. CM particles first enter the lymph and subsequently the blood via the thoracic duct. In contrast, VLDL particles are secreted from the liver directly into the bloodstream. CM particles are generally larger and more variable in size than VLDL [10]. Whereas particle assembly occurs by a similar mechanism, the cellular pathways for secretion of CM and VLDL differ. Anderson's disease (also known as CM retention disease) represents a failure of exocytosis of CM from enterocytes in the setting of normal VLDL secretion [10]. Moreover, CM secretion can be inhibited pharmacologically without affecting VLDL secretion [10].

When the intracellular supply of triglyceride molecules is reduced, degradation of apoB-48 and apoB-100 occurs by both

Fig. 2 Editing of apoB mRNA. The apoB gene, with exons represented by squares and introns by lines, is transcribed in both the intestine and the liver. In the intestine, but not the liver, a protein complex containing apobec-1 modifies a single nucleotide in the apoB mRNA. As a result, the codon containing this nucleotide is converted to a premature stop codon, as indicated by the position of the 'X'. The protein that is translated in the intestine (apoB-48) is only 48% as long as the full-length protein that is translated in the liver (apoB-100).

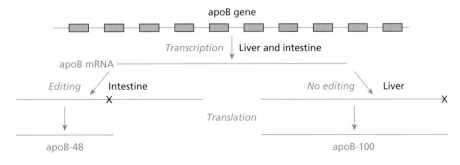

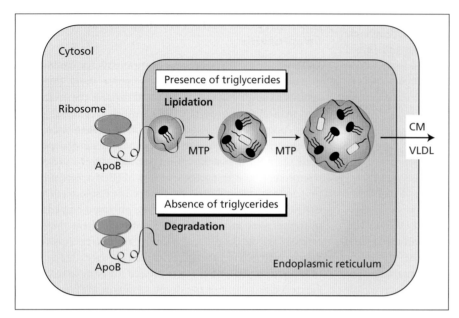

Fig. 3 Assembly and secretion of CM and VLDL particles. CM and VLDL particles are assembled and secreted by similar mechanisms in the enterocyte and hepatocyte respectively. The apoB protein (i.e. apoB-48 or apoB-100) is translated by ribosomes and enters the lumen of the endoplasmic reticulum. If triglycerides are available, the apoB protein is lipidated by the action of microsomal triglyceride transfer protein (MTP) in two distinct steps, accumulating triglyceride as well as cholesteryl ester molecules. The resulting CM or VLDL particle is secreted by exocytosis into the lymphatics by enterocytes or into the plasma by hepatocytes. In the absence of triglycerides, the apoB protein is degraded.

proteasomal and non-proteasomal pathways [11]. Similarly, the genetic absence of MTP results in rapid intracellular degradation of apoB-48 and apoB-100 [12]. In either case, lipoprotein secretion is reduced. Constitutive translation of apoB-48 allows for the prompt and highly efficient absorption of large quantities of triglycerides from the diet following a meal [10]. During fasting, apoB-48 is degraded in the intestine, whereas, in liver, continued lipidation of apoB-100 with endogenous triglycerides ensures that the metabolic demands of muscle tissue are met. When insulin levels are low, fatty acids are released from adipose tissue through the action of hormone-sensitive lipase and delivered to the liver via plasma. Among the metabolic fates of these fatty acids is incorporation into VLDL particles for delivery to muscle tissue. In the setting of insulin resistance, an inappropriately high flux of fatty acids from adipose tissue to the liver serves to increase VLDL secretion [13].

Intravascular metabolism of apoB-containing lipoproteins

As depicted in Figure 4, the delivery of triglycerides by apoB-containing lipoproteins to muscle and adipose tissue is determined to a large extent by tissue-specific expression and activity of lipoprotein lipase (LPL). LPL is abundantly expressed only on the vascular surface endothelia that line the capillary beds of cardiac, skeletal muscle and adipose tissues [14]. This enzyme hydrolyses triglycerides in the cores of CM and VLDL to form monoglycerides and fatty acids. Fatty acids that are taken up by muscle cells are consumed by oxidative metabolism as a direct source of energy. Within adipose tissue, fatty acids are re-esterified and stored as triglyceride droplets.

LPL is synthesized in parenchymal cells of muscle and adipose tissues. Within each tissue, the LPL expression level depends on

metabolic demand for fatty acids and can vary severalfold. Once translated, the protein is exocytosed and translocated across both the intercellular space and the endothelial cell. LPL is then anchored to the vascular surface of the endothelial cell by electrostatic interactions with charged sulphated proteoglycans on the plasma membrane. When infused intravascularly, heparin displaces LPL by competing for binding to these proteoglycans.

The relative expression of LPL in muscle vs. adipose tissue plays a key role in the preferential trafficking of triglycerides to muscle tissue during fasting and to adipose tissue in the postprandial state [14]. This is achieved principally by posttranscriptional mechanisms. In the fed state, insulin increases LPL mRNA levels in adipocytes, apparently by increasing mRNA stability. In the fasted state, altered glycosylation patterns of LPL in adipocytes lead to cellular retention of the enzyme and decreased expression on the endothelial surface.

Before encountering LPL, triglyceride-rich CM and VLDL particles must first acquire apoC-II (Fig. 4a), which is required for LPL activity (Fig. 4b). In contrast to apoB molecules, which remain embedded in CM and VLDL, apoC-II is an exchangeable apolipoprotein. ApoC-II molecules are acquired by CM and VLDL by exchange from HDL particles, which serve as a reservoir for exchangeable apoproteins in addition to their functions in cholesterol transport which are described below [15,16]. Within approximately 5 min following lipoprotein secretion, CM and VLDL acquire the content of apoC-II that is required for optimal LPL activity [16]. This lag period appears to be important for allowing widespread vascular distribution of apoB-containing lipoproteins to occur prior to hydrolysis [16]. Consistent with a central role in promoting lipoprotein–LPL interactions, patients with genetic defects in apoC-II manifest high plasma triglyceride concentrations [17].

Owing to the large sizes of triglyceride-rich lipoproteins, a single particle interacts with multiple LPL molecules [16]. Each LPL is bound and activated by one molecule of apoC-II (Fig. 4b). VLDL and CM also undergo a series of binding and detachment events during catabolism. Because several molecules of LPL simultaneously catabolize triglycerides from VLDL or CM, hydrolysis occurs at a rapid rate so that half the core triglycerides are consumed in approximately 10–15 min.

Whereas apoC-II promotes LPL-mediated hydrolysis of triglycerides in the cores of CM and VLDL, apoC-III functions to inhibit LPL activity [16]. ApoC-III appears to be secreted in association with CM and VLDL particles, and concentrations of apoC-III in plasma correlate directly with plasma triglyceride concentrations [15]. The function of apoC-III may be to help promote the widespread distribution of these triglyceride-rich particles throughout the body.

The activity of LPL reduces the triglyceride contents of CM and VLDL particles, which become relatively enriched in cholesteryl esters. Lipolysis of apoB-containing particles continues until about 80% of the initial triglyceride content has been removed from CM and about 50% from VLDL [16]. At this point, apoC-II is transferred to HDL, and HDL-associated apoE is acquired (Fig. 4c) [18]. The resulting CM and VLDL particles that contain apoE but lack apoC-II are referred to as 'remnants' [19].

Removal of apoB-containing lipoproteins from the circulation

ApoE plays a central role in CM and VLDL remnant uptake by receptor-mediated pathways. It is expressed in most tissues, but most prominently in liver and brain. In humans, apoE exists as three isoforms, apoE-2, apoE-3 and apoE-4 [20]. These isoforms differ in primary structure as a result of amino acid substitutions that influence the physical–chemical properties of the molecule by altering intramolecular disulphide bond formation [20]. Epidemiologically, inheritance of apoE-4 has been correlated with increased risk of developing Alzheimer's disease [21].

As illustrated in Figure 5, the liver efficiently removes CM remnants through receptor-mediated clearance [22]. Once the activity of LPL has sufficiently reduced particle size, CM remnants enter the space of Disse via endothelial fenestrations [19]. Within the space of Disse, CM remnants interact with heparan sulphate proteoglycan (HSPG) molecules. This represents the first of three steps in the process of CM uptake and is referred to as sequestration. Sequestration accounts for the rapid disappearance

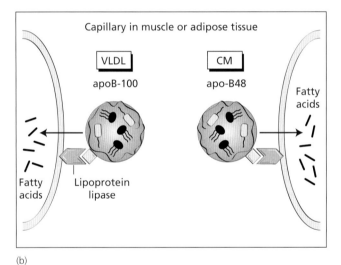

(a)

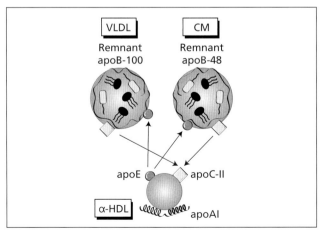

(b)

(c)

Fig. 4 (*opposite*) Metabolism of apoB-containing lipoproteins. (a) Following secretion, CM and VLDL particles are activated for lipolysis when they encounter HDL particles in the plasma and acquire the exchangeable apolipoprotein apoC-II. (b) When CM and VLDL circulate into capillaries of muscle or fat tissue, apoC-II promotes binding of the particle to lipoprotein lipase, which is bound to the surface of endothelial cells. Lipoprotein lipase mediates hydrolysis of triglycerides, but not cholesteryl esters, from the core of the lipoprotein particle. The resulting fatty acids are taken up into muscle or fat tissue. (c) Upon completion of hydrolysis, CM and VLDL lose affinity for lipoprotein lipase. When an HDL particle is encountered, apoC-II is transferred back to HDL particles in exchange for apoE. The resulting particles are CM and VLDL remnants.

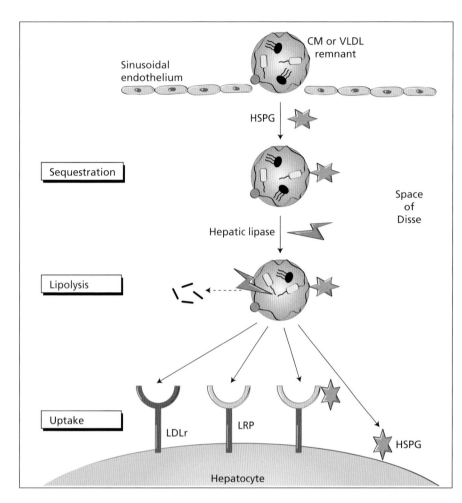

Fig. 5 Hepatic uptake of remnant particles. The activity of lipoprotein lipase results in remnant lipoprotein particles that are small enough in size to enter the space of Disse. Remnant lipoproteins are sequestered in the space of Disse by binding to high-molecular-weight heparan sulphate proteoglycan (HSPG) molecules. This is followed by binding of hepatic lipase, which promotes lipolysis of some residual triglycerides in the core of the remnant lipoproteins and the release of fatty acids (as indicated by the dashed arrow). Uptake of remnant lipoprotein particles into hepatocytes is mediated by the LDL receptor (LDLr), the LDL-related protein (LRP), a complex formed between LRP and HSPG or HSPG alone. Figure adapted from ref. 19, with permission.

of CM remnants from plasma. The second phase of CM clearance is a lipolytic processing step that occurs within the space of Disse. CM remnants bind to hepatic lipase, which is expressed by hepatocytes. It promotes CM remnant uptake by further modifying the lipid content of the particle. Finally, remnant particles are taken up into hepatocytes. The LDL receptor is a high-affinity receptor for apoE [23] that is expressed mainly in the liver, but also on a variety of cell types [22]. The LDL receptor-related protein (LRP) also plays a central role in the uptake of remnant particles through apoE-mediated interactions [19,20,24]. In addition, CM remnant uptake occurs through interactions with HSPG alone or in combination with LRP [19]. On account of these redundant mechanisms for CM remnant uptake, CM remnant particles do not tend to accumulate, even if one of the receptor pathways is disrupted [19].

About half of VLDL remnants are cleared directly by the liver, essentially as described for CM remnant particles. However, the remaining VLDL remnants are subjected to additional LPL-mediated triglyceride hydrolysis to form IDL particles, which are smaller remnant particles that may be cleared from the plasma by the same mechanisms [25]. A fraction of IDL is subject to further triglyceride hydrolysis by hepatic lipase. Presumably

because of the decrease in size that ensues, apoE dissociates from the particles, forming LDL. LDL are cholesteryl ester-rich particles that contain apoB-100, but no other apolipoproteins [16].

Plasma clearance of LDL particles occurs as the result of interactions with the LDL receptor [23]. Because the LDL receptor is the only receptor that effectively clears LDL particles from the plasma, mutations in the LDL receptor or proteins that support its function constitute the genetic basis for familial hypercholesterolaemia [23,26]. The LDL receptor is regulated in response to cellular cholesterol levels. When intracellular cholesterol levels are reduced, such as occurs during therapy with statin drugs, the LDL receptor is upregulated as a result of the proteolytic processing and activity of sterol response element binding protein 2 (SREBP-2) [27].

Reverse cholesterol transport: HDL metabolism

Overview

Whereas apoB-containing lipoproteins function primarily in

the delivery of triglycerides to muscle and adipose tissue, HDL particles are largely responsible for reverse cholesterol transport [28], whereby excess cholesterol molecules from tissues are removed and delivered to the liver for elimination via bile.

Apolipoproteins associated with HDL

ApoA-I is the major structural protein of HDL particles. It is the principal determinant of particle structure and receptor binding. ApoA-II is also a major apolipoprotein of HDL, but its precise role in the structure and metabolism of HDL is not well understood [29]. ApoA-I and apoA-II are both exchangeable apolipoproteins, and HDL particles may contain apoA-I alone or both apoA-I and apoA-II. As described above, other exchangeable apolipoproteins that are critical for apoB-containing particle metabolism variably associate with HDL particles.

Formation of HDL particles

The process of HDL formation begins when lipid-poor apoA-I secreted by the liver interacts with adenosine triphosphate (ATP) binding cassette protein A1 (ABCA1) on the plasma membrane of hepatocytes (Fig. 6) [30]. Although ABCA1 is expressed on the plasma membrane of a variety of cell types, its presence in hepatocytes regulates HDL formation [31]. In patients with Tangier disease, genetic inactivation of ABCA1 leads to a marked reduction in plasma HDL concentrations [32]. ABCA1 is required for cellular efflux of phospholipids and unesterified cholesterol in response to interactions between apoA-I in plasma and the hepatocyte plasma membrane [30,32]. The interaction of apoA-I and ABCA1 results in the formation of small pre-β-migrating HDL (pre-β-HDL) particles that are discoidal in shape [33].

Formation of pre-β-HDL is an essential step in reverse cholesterol transport, but these particles are not optimized for the removal of cholesterol from plasma membranes of extrahepatic tissues. Therefore, it is critical that pre-β-HDL undergo a maturation process to form spherical α-migrating HDL. α-HDL particles are referred to as HDL for simplicity and are highly efficient acceptors of excess cholesterol from cells. The maturation process is accomplished by the activity of lecithin–cholesterol acyltransferase (LCAT) [16]. LCAT is a circulating enzyme that is synthesized in liver. As shown in Figure 6b, it binds to HDL particles and catalyses the transfer of a fatty acid from phosphatidylcholine (also known as lecithin) to the hydroxyl group of unesterified cholesterol. The result is the formation of a cholesteryl ester and a lysophosphatidylcholine molecule [34]. The lysophosphatidylcholine is transferred to albumin in the plasma [16]. The newly formed cholesteryl ester spontaneously relocates from the surface of HDL to the core of the particle. As a result, LCAT transforms discoidal pre-β-HDL to spherical HDL particles.

HDL-mediated removal of cholesterol from cells

Efflux of unesterified cholesterol from plasma membranes to α-migrating HDL particles is the principal mechanism for cholesterol removal from cells in extrahepatic tissues (Fig. 6a and b) [35]. When the particle is in close proximity to a cell, unesterified cholesterol molecules within the plasma membrane desorb and traverse the aqueous plasma until they are incorporated into the phospholipid-rich surface coat of HDL. This is a process of passive diffusion that is controlled principally by the cholesterol concentration gradient between plasma membranes and HDL. Scavenger receptor class B type 1 (SR-BI) is expressed on a variety of cell types. *In vitro*, this receptor mediates the bidirectional flux of unesterified cholesterol between cells and HDL particles [30]. It has been proposed that HDL particles in the plasma may become tethered by SR-BI to cells [30] and, when the concentration gradient favours cellular efflux, this could promote the net movement of unesterified cholesterol to HDL [30]. Recent studies *in vitro* also suggest that ATP binding cassette proteins G1 and G4 may play significant roles in promoting cholesterol movement from cells to HDL particles [36].

Optimization of HDL-mediated cholesterol removal from cells

Ongoing cholesterol removal from cells to the surface coat of HDL requires a sustained concentration gradient [37]. This is achieved by the collective activities of three circulating plasma proteins (Fig. 6a and b). In addition to allowing HDL to mature from a discoidal to a spherical particle, LCAT activity allows unesterified cholesterol that is transferred to the surface of spherical HDL particles to be relocated to the core.

Whereas LCAT removes unesterified cholesterol from the surface of the particle, its enzymatic activity also consumes surface phosphatidylcholines, which are essential for HDL to increase in size and to accept additional cholesterol molecules from cells [16]. Phospholipid transfer protein (PLTP) is a plasma protein that replenishes the surface coat of HDL using phospholipids from remnant apoB-containing lipoprotein particles. The gradient for this transfer of phospholipids is established by the activity of LPL. As triglycerides contained within the cores of VLDL and CM are hydrolysed by LPL, their surface-to-volume ratio increases. PLTP removes excess surface phospholipids and transfers them to HDL particles [38]. This replaces phosphatidylcholine molecules that are hydrolysed by LCAT, allowing for particle growth. Based on studies in genetically engineered mice, PLTP activity constitutes the source of as much as 80% of HDL phospholipids [38].

Cholesterol ester transfer protein (CETP) promotes the transfer of cholesteryl esters from the cores of HDL particles to remnants of apoB-containing lipoproteins in exchange for triglyceride molecules from the cores of the remnant particles.

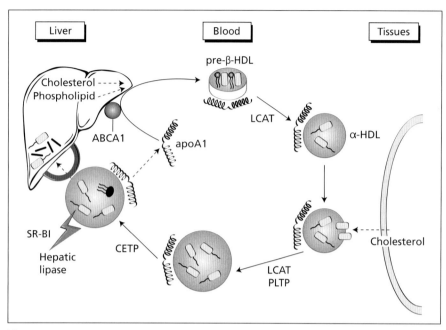

(a)

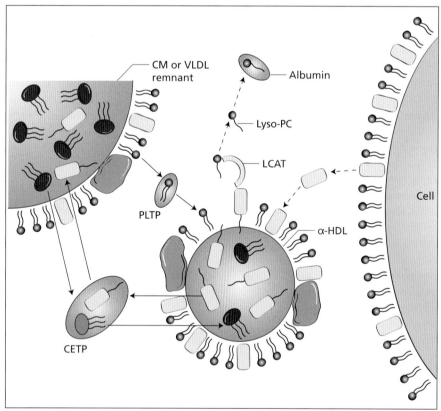

(b)

Fig. 6 Reverse cholesterol transport (a) The process of reverse cholesterol transport begins when apoA-I is secreted from the liver. ApoA-I in plasma interacts with ATP binding cassette protein AI (ABCA1), which incorporates a small amount of phospholipid and unesterified cholesterol from hepatocyte plasma membranes to form a discoidal-shaped pre-β-HDL particle. On account of the activity of lecithin–cholesterol acyltransferase (LCAT) in plasma, pre-β-HDL particles mature to form spherical α-HDL. Spherical α-migrating HDL particles function to accept excess unesterified cholesterol from the plasma membranes of cells in a wide variety of tissues. The unesterified cholesterol is transferred from the cell to nearby HDL particles by diffusion through the plasma. As explained in (b), LCAT and phospholipid transfer protein (PLTP) increase the capacity of HDL to accept unesterified cholesterol molecules from cells by allowing for expansion of the core and the surface coat of the particle. Cholesteryl ester transfer protein (CETP) exchanges some of the cholesteryl ester molecules from the core of HDL for triglycerides from the core of remnant particles. Whereas remnant particles are taken up by a variety of receptors on the liver (Fig. 5), HDL particles interact with scavenger receptor class B type I (SR-BI), which mediates selective hepatic uptake of cholesteryl esters, but not apoA-I. This process is facilitated when hepatic lipase hydrolyses triglycerides from the core of the particle. The remaining apoA-I molecules may begin the cycle of reverse cholesterol transport again. In (a), solid arrows indicate metabolic events in HDL metabolism, whereas dashed arrows denote transfer of molecules. (b) LCAT, PLTP and CETP promote the removal of excess cholesterol from the plasma membranes of cells. LCAT removes a fatty acid from a phosphatidylcholine molecule in the surface coat of α- (or pre-β-)HDL and esterifies an unesterified cholesterol molecule on the surface of the particle. The resulting lysophosphatidylcholine (lyso-PC) becomes bound to albumin in the plasma, whereas the cholesteryl ester migrates spontaneously into the core of the lipoprotein particle. The unesterified cholesterol molecules that are consumed by LCAT are replaced by unesterified cholesterol from cells. HDL phospholipids that are consumed by LCAT action are replaced with excess phospholipids from remnant particles by the activity of PLTP. As described in (a), CETP increases the efficiency of cholesterol movement to the liver by exchanging cholesteryl ester molecules from the core of α-HDL for triglycerides from the core of remnant particles. In (b), solid arrows denote protein-mediated lipid transfer, whereas dashed arrows indicate that lipids move by diffusion through the plasma.

This transfer of cholesteryl esters allows HDL to continue to accept cholesterol from tissues. Moreover, it utilizes remnant particles, which have completed their function in triglyceride delivery and are destined for hepatic clearance, for the ancillary purpose of assisting with reverse cholesterol transport. The activity of CETP also enriches HDL with triglycerides, forming the more buoyant HDL particles. As described below, this helps to increase the efficiency with which HDL delivers cholesterol to the liver [39,40]. Considering that a fraction of VLDL remnants are ultimately transformed into LDL particles, the activity of CETP also increases plasma LDL cholesterol concentrations, while decreasing the plasma concentrations of HDL cholesterol.

Hepatic uptake of HDL cholesterol from plasma

In addition to the cholesterol that is delivered to the liver by remnant particles via CETP, HDL transports cholesterol directly to the liver. As illustrated in Figure 6a, SR-BI, which is highly expressed in liver, promotes the selective uptake of lipids, but not protein, from HDL particles [41].

The process of SR-BI-mediated selective lipid uptake into hepatocytes is facilitated by the activity of hepatic lipase. Hepatic lipase promotes hydrolysis of HDL triglycerides and phospholipids, and this optimizes the SR-BI-mediated hepatic uptake of cholesteryl esters [42]. When the HDL particle decreases in size, apoA-1 molecules dissociate and interact with ABCA1 to promote the formation of new pre-β-HDL particles [33].

Summary and conclusions

This chapter has described how the structures of lipoproteins are optimally suited for their functions in the transport of insoluble triglyceride and cholesterol molecules through the plasma. The primary role of apoB-containing lipoproteins is to deliver dietary triglycerides from the intestine and endogenous triglycerides from the liver to muscle or adipose tissue depending upon metabolic needs. HDL metabolism facilitates the transport of excess cellular cholesterol from extrahepatic tissues to the liver. Owing to the activity of CETP in plasma, remnants of apoB-containing lipoproteins also assist with reverse cholesterol transport. An appreciation of these principles should provide the foundation for understanding genetic and acquired disorders of lipoprotein metabolism, as well as the molecular and cellular mechanisms of lipid-lowering therapies.

Acknowledgements

This work was supported by National Institutes of Health (grants DK56626 and DK48873), an Established Investigator Award from the American Heart Association and an International HDL research Awards Program grant to DEC. ES is the recipient of an American Liver Foundation Irwin M. Arias Postdoctoral Research Fellowship Award.

References

1 Small DM (1986) *The Physical Chemistry of Lipids: From Alkanes to Phospholipids. Handbook of Lipid Research*. New York: Plenum Press.

2 Agellon LB (2002) Metabolism and function of bile acids. In: Vance DE, Vance JE (eds) *Biochemistry of Lipids, Lipoproteins and Membranes*, 4th edn. Amsterdam: Elsevier, pp. 433–448.

3 Chawla A, Repa JJ, Evans RM *et al.* (2001) Nuclear receptors and lipid physiology: opening the X-files. *Science* 294 (5548), 1866–1870.

4 Jonas A (2002) Lipoprotein structure. In: Vance DE, Vance JE (eds) *Biochemistry of Lipids, Lipoproteins and Membranes*, 4th edn. Amsterdam: Elsevier, pp. 483–504.

5 Vance JE (2002) Assembly and secretion of lipoproteins. In: Vance DE, Vance JE (eds) *Biochemistry of Lipids, Lipoproteins and Membranes*, 4th edn. Amsterdam: Elsevier, pp. 505–526.

6 Anant S, Davidson NO (2001) Molecular mechanisms of apolipoprotein B mRNA editing. *Curr Opin Lipidol* 12 (2), 159–165.

7 Wang L, Fast DG, Attie AD (1997) The enzymatic and non-enzymatic roles of protein-disulfide isomerase in apolipoprotein B secretion. *J Biol Chem* 272 (44), 27644–27651.

8 Wetterau JR, Aggerbeck LP, Bouma ME *et al.* (1992) Absence of microsomal triglyceride transfer protein in individuals with abetalipoproteinemia. *Science* 258 (5084), 999–1001.

9 Hussain MM, Shi J, Dreizen P (2003) Microsomal triglyceride transfer protein and its role in apoB-lipoprotein assembly. *J Lipid Res* 44 (1), 22–32.

10 Hussain MM (2000) A proposed model for the assembly of chylomicrons. *Atherosclerosis* 148 (1), 1–15.

11 Pan M, Cederbaum AI, Zhang YL *et al.* (2004) Lipid peroxidation and oxidant stress regulate hepatic apolipoprotein B degradation and VLDL production. *J Clin Invest* 113 (9), 1277–1287.

12 Wang S, McLeod RS, Gordon DA *et al.* (1996) The microsomal triglyceride transfer protein facilitates assembly and secretion of apolipoprotein B-containing lipoproteins and decreases cotranslational degradation of apolipoprotein B in transfected COS 7 cells. *J Biol Chem* 271 (24), 14124–14133.

13 Ginsberg HN (2000) Insulin resistance and cardiovascular disease. *J Clin Invest* 106 (4), 453–458.

14 Mead JR, Irvine SA, Ramji, DP (2002) Lipoprotein lipase: structure, function, regulation, and role in disease. *J Mol Med* 80 (12), 753–769.

15 Shachter NS (2001) Apolipoproteins C-I and C-III as important modulators of lipoprotein metabolism. *Curr Opin Lipidol* 12 (3), 297–304.

16 Fielding PE, Fielding CJ (2002) Dynamics of lipoprotein transport in the human circulatory system. In: Vance DE, Vance JE (eds) *Biochemistry of Lipids, Lipoproteins and Membranes*, 4th edn. Amsterdam: Elsevier, pp. 527–552.

17 Jong MC, Hofker MH, Havekes LM (1999) Role of ApoCs in lipoprotein metabolism: functional differences between ApoC1, ApoC2, and ApoC3. *Arterioscler Thromb Vasc Biol* 19 (3), 472–484.

18 Cooper AD (1997) Hepatic uptake of chylomicron remnants. *J Lipid Res* 38 (11), 2173–2192.

19 Mahley RW, Ji ZS (1999) Remnant lipoprotein metabolism: key pathways involving cell-surface heparan sulfate proteoglycans and apolipoprotein E. *J Lipid Res* 40 (1), 1–16.

20 Mahley RW, Rall SC, Jr (2000) Apolipoprotein E: far more than a lipid transport protein. *Annu Rev Genomics Hum Genet* 1, 507–537.

21 Corder EH, Saunders AM, Strittmatter WJ *et al.* (1993) Gene dose of apolipoprotein E type 4 allele and the risk of Alzheimer's disease in late onset families. *Science* 261 (5123), 921–923.

22 Schneider WJ (2002) Lipoprotein receptors. In: Vance DE, Vance JE (eds) *Biochemistry of Lipids, Lipoproteins and Membranes*, 4th edn. Amsterdam: Elsevier, pp. 553–572.

23 Brown MS, Goldstein JL (1986) A receptor-mediated pathway for cholesterol homeostasis. *Science* 232 (4746), 34–47.

24 Herz J, Hamann U, Rogne S *et al.* (1988) Surface location and high affinity for calcium of a 500-kd liver membrane protein closely related to the LDL-receptor suggest a physiological role as lipoprotein receptor. *EMBO J* 7 (13), 4119–4127.

25 Packard CJ, Shepherd J (1997) Lipoprotein heterogeneity and apolipoprotein B metabolism. *Arterioscler Thromb Vasc Biol* 17 (12), 3542–3556.

26 Garcia CK, Wilund K, Arca M *et al.* (2001) Autosomal recessive hypercholesterolemia caused by mutations in a putative LDL receptor adaptor protein. *Science* 292 (5520), 1394–1398.

27 Horton JD, Goldstein JL, Brown MS (2002) SREBPs: activators of the complete program of cholesterol and fatty acid synthesis in the liver. *J Clin Invest* 109 (9), 1125–1131.

28 Silver DL, Jiang XC, Arai T *et al.* (2000) Receptors and lipid transfer proteins in HDL metabolism. *Ann NY Acad Sci* 902, 103–111; discussion 111–102.

29 Blanco-Vaca F, Escola-Gil JC, Martin-Campos JM *et al.* (2001) Role of apoA-II in lipid metabolism and atherosclerosis: advances in the study of an enigmatic protein. *J Lipid Res* 42 (11), 1727–1739.

30 Yancey PG, Bortnick AE, Kellner-Weibel G *et al.* (2003) Importance of different pathways of cellular cholesterol efflux. *Arterioscler Thromb Vasc Biol* 23 (5), 712–719.

31 Timmins JM, Lee JY, Boudyguina E *et al.* (2005) Targeted inactivation of hepatic Abca1 causes profound hypoalphalipoproteinemia and kidney hypercatabolism of apoA-I. *J Clin Invest* 115 (5), 1333–1342.

32 Lawn RM, Wade DP, Garvin MR *et al.* (1999) The Tangier disease gene product ABC1 controls the cellular apolipoprotein-mediated lipid removal pathway. *J Clin Invest* 104 (8), R25–31.

33 Rye KA, Barter PJ (2004) Formation and metabolism of prebeta-migrating, lipid-poor apolipoprotein A-I. *Arterioscler Thromb Vasc Biol* 24 (3), 421–428.

34 Jonas A (2000) Lecithin cholesterol acyltransferase. *Biochim Biophys Acta* 1529 (1–3), 245–256.

35 Rothblat GH, de la Llera-Moya M, Atger V *et al.* (1999) Cell cholesterol efflux: integration of old and new observations provides new insights. *J Lipid Res* 40 (5), 781–796.

36 Wang N, Lan D, Chen W *et al.* (2004) ATP-binding cassette transporters G1 and G4 mediate cellular cholesterol efflux to high-density lipoproteins. *Proc Natl Acad Sci USA* 101 (26), 9774–9779.

37 Ng DS (2004) Insight into the role of LCAT from mouse models. *Rev Endocr Metab Disord* 5 (4), 311–318.

38 Jiang XC, Bruce C, Mar J *et al.* (1999) Targeted mutation of plasma phospholipid transfer protein gene markedly reduces high-density lipoprotein levels. *J Clin Invest* 103 (6), 907–914.

39 Rye KA, Clay MA, Barter PJ (1999) Remodelling of high density lipoproteins by plasma factors. *Atherosclerosis* 145 (2), 227–238.

40 Barter PJ, Brewer HB, Jr, Chapman MJ *et al.* (2003) Cholesteryl ester transfer protein: a novel target for raising HDL and inhibiting atherosclerosis. *Arterioscler Thromb Vasc Biol* 23 (2), 160–167.

41 Acton S, Rigotti A, Landschulz KT *et al.* (1996) Identification of scavenger receptor SR-BI as a high density lipoprotein receptor. *Science* 271 (5248), 518–520.

42 Martinez LO, Jacquet S, Terce F *et al.* (2004) New insight on the molecular mechanisms of high-density lipoprotein cellular interactions. *Cell Mol Life Sci* 61 (18), 2343–2360.

2.3.3 Protein and amino acid metabolism

Margaret E. Brosnan and John T. Brosnan

Introduction

The liver is a major organ of amino acid metabolism. It is responsible for the disposal of much of the dietary amino acid load; it is the only organ with a complete urea cycle; it is capable of synthesizing some amino acids; and it produces glucose from muscle-derived amino acids during starvation and in diabetes. Hepatic amino acid metabolism is finely regulated. There is evidence that the liver is largely responsible for maintaining circulating amino acid homeostasis. The liver also plays a critical role in the biosynthesis of key molecules from amino acids, e.g. creatine and glutathione. It also uses amino acids and glutathione in the conjugation of xenobiotics and toxic molecules to ensure their elimination from the body. In addition, there is good evidence that amino acids play a crucial regulatory role in controlling the turnover of hepatic proteins.

Amino acid pools and amino acid transport

Rapidly frozen rat liver contains a total of 20 μmol/g, which translates into an intracellular concentration of about 40 mM [1]. This figure ignores compartmentation between and within cells, however. Nevertheless, it gives an accurate picture of the magnitude of the hepatic intracellular amino acid pool. Given that the liver cell, like plasma, experiences an osmotic pressure of about 305 mOsM, it is apparent that free amino acids account for about 13% of all intracellular osmolytes. The amino acids with the highest hepatic concentrations include taurine (7.5 mM), aspartate (6.3 mM), glutamate (2.8 mM), glutamine (10.6 mM), glycine (4.0 mM) and alanine (4.7 mM). By also measuring plasma amino acids, intracellular/extracellular concentration ratios can be calculated (Table 1). Very high ratios (> 10) were identified for taurine, aspartate, glutamate, glutamine, glycine, alanine and histidine. No amino acid displayed a ratio significantly less than 1. These ratios are largely a result of the operation of hepatic amino acid transporters.

Hepatocytes communicate with their environment via their plasma membranes, either by signal transduction or via transport. Enormous progress has been made in the field of amino acid transport as our knowledge has advanced from kinetic to molecular characterization. Different amino acid transporters are responsible for the transport of groups of structurally similar amino acids. Transport of the three classes of amino acids (zwitterionic, cationic and anionic) is effected by a number of different transporters with different (though overlapping) specificities. Energetically, we can divide these transport systems into two classes: sodium-linked transporters (an example of secondary active transport) that employ the Na^+ electrochemical

Table 1 Hepatic intracellular amino acid concentrations and intracellular/extracellular concentration ratios.

Amino acid	Hepatic concentration (mM)	Intracellular/extracellular ratio
Taurine	7.53	57
Aspartate	6.27	412
Threonine	0.46	1.8
Serine	0.53	3.0
Asparagine	0.13	3.2
Glutamate	2.83	29
Glutamine	10.63	18
Proline	1.21	6.5
Glycine	3.97	17
Alanine	4.65	11
Citrulline	0.09	1.4
Valine	0.27	1.7
Methionine	0.18	3.3
Isoleucine	0.19	2.4
Leucine	0.30	2.2
Tyrosine	0.09	0.8
Phenylalanine	0.12	2.1
Ornithine	0.31	5.2
Lysine	0.98	2.9
Histidine	1.01	20
Arginine	0.10	0.8

From ref. 1.

gradient to drive inward amino acid translocation against a concentration gradient; and sodium-independent transporters that facilitate amino acid transport in either direction, depending on the concentration gradient (an example of facilitated diffusion).

Among the most important hepatic amino acid transporters are systems A, ASC, L and N for neutral (zwitterion) amino acids, system y^+ for cationic amino acids and X_{AG}^- and X_C^- for anionic amino acids [2]. System A is a sodium-dependent transporter with preference for neutral amino acids with small side-chains (e.g. alanine and serine). System ASC is also sodium dependent and exhibits a preference for alanine, serine, cysteine and threonine, although it can also transport bulky amino acids such as leucine, valine and methionine at a lower rate. This transporter exhibits a marked trans-stimulation and is thought to exchange the extracellular and intracellular pools of a number of amino acids. System L favours amino acids with bulky side-chains (branched-chain and aromatic amino acids). It is not sodium dependent, and its active exchange properties suggest that it may mediate efflux from cells rather than influx. System N is a sodium-dependent transporter with rather narrow substrate specificity. It transports glutamine, asparagine and histidine – amino acids that contain nitrogen in their side-chains. The most active cationic transporter is system y^+, a high-affinity sodium-independent transporter that acts on lysine, histidine and arginine. Two anionic transporters are of note. System X_{AG}^- transports glutamate and aspartate, and this is accompanied by sodium cotransport and potassium countertransport. System X_C^- transports cystine into hepatocytes in exchange for glutamate

and is thought to provide the limiting substrate (cysteine) for hepatic glutathione synthesis. Much progress has recently been made in the molecular and kinetic characterization of these transporters. Nevertheless, it is apparent that the combination of a multitude of transporters with overlapping specificity and differing energetics, as well as facilitation of both uptake and exchange, makes the physiological interpretation of the roles of these transporters challenging.

These amino acid transporters are regulated with regard to both their expression and the cell types in which they are expressed. For example, system A activity is rapidly stimulated by glucagon via a mechanism that does not require protein synthesis. System A activity is also upregulated by insulin via a mechanism that requires gene transcription. Uptake of the anionic amino acids, glutamate and aspartate, is much more rapid in hepatocytes at the perivenous terminus of the hepatic acinus than in the periportal hepatocytes [3].

Metabolic disposal of dietary amino acids

Adults ingesting a typical western diet consume ~ 80–100 g of protein per day. The common textbook statement that these amino acids are oxidized in the liver cannot be true because, even if no other fuel were oxidized there, it would oblige the consumption of more oxygen than the liver actually consumes [4]. The solution to this conundrum is threefold. First, there is appreciable oxidation of a number of amino acids in the gastrointestinal tract [5]. Secondly, the branched-chain amino acids (which comprise about 20% of total dietary amino acids) largely escape splanchnic metabolism and are mostly metabolized in skeletal muscle. Thirdly, even in the fed state, the hepatic disposal of amino acids involves the conversion of their carbon skeletons to glucose and to ketone bodies, which are released, as universal fuels, for other tissues. This enables the liver to accommodate dietary amino acid disposal within the bounds of its oxygen consumption. In an adult in nitrogen balance, the daily dietary amino acid intake must be oxidized in a 24-h period. If the liver were too efficient in the clearance of absorbed amino acids, none would be available for peripheral tissues. Rather, after meals, the liver must consume only excess amino acids. An equal priority, however, is to have sufficient amino acids available for protein synthesis both in peripheral tissues and in the liver itself. In the postprandial period, the liver will metabolize amino acids released by peripheral tissues, principally muscle.

The catabolism of individual amino acids is tightly controlled, particularly the essential amino acids. This control is accomplished in a number of ways. An important role may be ascribed to glucagon, which is secreted at a higher rate upon ingestion of a high-protein meal. Glucagon activates phenylalanine hydroxylase by means of phosphorylation; it stimulates glycine and glutamine catabolism; and, together with glucorticoids, it induces the synthesis of a number of amino acid-catabolizing enzymes. Glucagon can also regulate the catabolism of a variety of amino acids, as evidenced by the generalized hypoaminoacidaemia in patients suffering from glucagonoma. A variety of mechanisms prevent the depletion of amino acids, in particular the essential amino acids. Many enzymes that initiate amino acid catabolism exhibit rather high K_ms for their amino acid substrates. However, simple Michaelis–Menten kinetics do not provide sufficient sensitivity to substrate concentrations. A number of additional mechanisms have evolved to conserve these amino acids. The hepatic isoform of S-adenosylmethionine synthase, the first enzyme of methionine catabolism, is activated by its product, S-adenosylmethionine. This regulatory feature provides the necessary sigmoidal dependence on amino acid concentrations [6]. Another regulatory stratagem is provided by the inducibility of some of the enzymes of essential amino acid catabolism. Enzymes such as tyrosine aminotransferase, ornithine aminotransferase, tryptophan dioxygenase, threonine dehydratase and histidase exhibit large-amplitude (as much as 10-fold) changes in activity. They also have short half-lives, so that they promptly return to very low activities when the stimulus is removed. The importance of these effects is clear – the induction of these enzymes permits increased catabolism of these amino acids when the supply is high, whereas the return to very low activities when the supply is low conserves these essential amino acids [7].

Covalent modification of key enzymes is also employed as a regulatory strategem. The branched-chain α-keto acid dehydrogenase (BCKDH), the controlling enzyme complex of branched-chain amino acid catabolism, is inhibited by phosphorylation; removal of the phosphate by a protein phosphatase reverses the inhibition. The BCKDH phosphatase is activated by α-ketoisocaproate. This mechanism produces a system that is particularly sensitive to α-keto acid concentration as it serves both as a substrate and as an agent that facilitates the conversion of the BCKDH to the active form. Phenylalanine hydroxylase, the flux-generating step in phenylalanine catabolism, affords another example of regulation by substrate concentration and by covalent modification. The enzyme can exist in both dimeric and tetrameric forms. Glucagon activates the enzyme by means of protein kinase A phosphorylation. In addition to its role as a substrate, phenylalanine promotes its conversion to the more active, tetrameric form. Both types of activation appear to act synergistically. Again, as in the control of BCKDH, this mechanism produces a regulatory system that is particularly sensitive to substrate (phenylalanine) concentration, much more so than could be accomplished via Michaelis–Menten kinetics alone.

Hepatic zonation of amino acid metabolism

Metabolic heterogeneity of hepatocytes along the hepatic acinus is also an important feature of hepatic amino acid metabolism. This phenomenon is well established for both glutamine and ornithine metabolism. The liver contains both glutaminase and glutamine synthetase. However, they are not expressed in the same hepatocytes. Glutaminase is found in the periportal region, for about the first third of the hepatic acinus, and can efficiently provide ammonia to carbamoylphosphate synthetase for urea synthesis. Glutamine synthetase is found in the perivenous hepatocytes where it is restricted to a layer of no more than one or two cells, which surround the terminal hepatic venule. Glutamine synthetase plays an important role in determining the low ammonia concentration of blood that leaves the liver, as it removes ammonia which has escaped the urea cycle [8]. Ornithine aminotransferase is also restricted to the same perivenous hepatocytes as glutamine synthetase; indeed, the entire pathway of arginine catabolism occurs in these hepatocytes [9]. Thus, the localization of the arginine catabolic pathway in hepatocytes that do not contain the urea cycle ensures that urea synthesis is not compromised by catabolic depletion of the cycle intermediates.

Hepatic amino acid metabolism during starvation

Gluconeogenesis from amino acids plays a crucial role during starvation in providing glucose for obligatory glucose-utilizing tissues, particularly the brain. These amino acids are primarily derived from skeletal muscle although, in the very short term, amino acids derived from hepatic proteolysis are also employed. The pattern of amino acids released by muscle is not a reflection of the amino acid composition of muscle protein. Rather, there is a considerable intramuscular amino acid metabolism that reconfigures the pattern of released amino acids. More than 50%

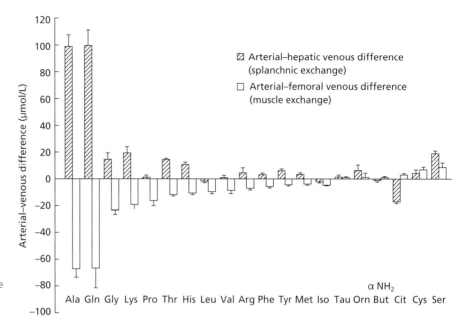

Fig. 1 Net splanchnic and peripheral exchange of amino acids in normal, postabsorptive man. Reproduced, with permission, from ref. 10.

of the released amino acids consist of alanine and glutamine. The carbon skeleton of alanine primarily arises from pyruvate of glycolytic origin. Its amino group arises, via transamination, from other amino acids, principally the branched-chain amino acids. This alanine is converted to glucose by the liver. This 'glucose–alanine cycle' plays a major role in ferrying these amino groups to the liver for detoxification, without the risk of hyperammonaemia. However, it does not really produce 'new' glucose; rather, it recycles glucose carbon, and some investigators have referred to it as 'glucopalaeogenesis' to emphasize the point that it produces 'old' glucose. The glutamine released by muscle has a variety of fates, including renal metabolism for acid–base regulation and use as a fuel by the small intestine. Alanine is an important product of intestinal glutamine metabolism and also becomes available to the liver for gluconeogenesis. Alanine is, therefore, generally acknowledged as the principal glucogenic amino acid. Yet, the role played by other amino acids should not be overlooked. Such amino acids as glycine, lysine, proline, threonine, histidine, arginine, phenylalanine and tyrosine are released by muscle and converted to glucose by the liver (Fig. 1). Although individually of less importance than alanine and glutamine, together they make a substantial contribution to hepatic gluconeogenesis [10].

Specialized functions of amino acids

Amino acids display considerable metabolic plasticity and, therefore, play a variety of roles. These include roles in one-carbon metabolism, biosyntheses, glutathione function and cell signalling. A number of these roles are highlighted below, rather than providing an exhaustive account.

Amino acids, methylation reactions and one-carbon metabolism

The folic acid, one-carbon pool provides cells with considerable flexibility in providing one-carbon groups of different oxidation states for biosynthetic and other purposes. Amino acids are the key providers of these one-carbon groups, which are generated during the catabolism of glycine, serine, histidine and tryptophan. The catabolism of serine and glycine probably supplies the bulk of the one-carbon pool by the reactions catalysed by serine hydroxymethyltransferase (reaction 1) and the glycine cleavage enzyme (reaction 2):

$$\text{Serine} + \text{THF} \leftrightarrow \text{glycine} + \text{N}^5,\text{N}^{10}\text{-methylene THF} \tag{1}$$

$$\text{Glycine} + \text{NAD}^+ + \text{THF} \rightarrow \text{CO}_2 + \text{NADH} \\ + \text{N}^5,\text{N}^{10}\text{-methylene THF} + \text{NH}_4^+ \tag{2}$$

(Tetrahydrofolate is abbreviated as THF). In addition, labile methyl groups are provided directly in the diet as methionine and choline. The one-carbon pool provides one-carbon groups for functions such as the synthesis of purine nucleotides and thymine. However, it is the abundance and variety of methylation reactions that best illustrate the importance of one-carbon metabolism.

Figure 2 provides an outline of methionine metabolism (also see Chapter 2.3.9). The key first step is the conversion of methionine to *S*-adenosylmethionine (SAM). SAM is the universal methyl donor for a remarkably large number of methylation reactions. Indeed, a recent bioinformatic analysis of a number of genomes, including human, suggests that between 0.6% and 1.6% of all genes may code for methyltransferases.

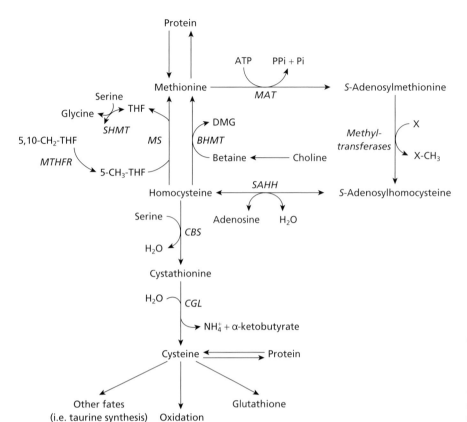

Fig. 2 Methionine metabolism in liver. MAT, methionine adenosyltransferase; SAHH, S-adenosylhomocysteine hydrolase; BHMT, betaine:homocysteine methyltransferase; SHMT, serine hydroxymethyltransferase; MTHFR, methylenetetrahydrofolate reductase; CBS, cystathionine β-synthase; CGL, cystathionine γ-lyase; MS, methionine synthase.

Methyltransferases catalyse the transfer of methyl groups from SAM to an acceptor to produce the methylated acceptor and S-adenosylhomocysteine (SAH) [11]. These methyltransferases include enzymes involved in the synthesis of small molecules (e.g. creatine, carnitine, phosphatidylcholine, epinephrine), methylation of nucleic acids (DNA methylation is a major mechanism for the regulation of gene expression, chromosome inactivation and genomic imprinting), RNA methylation (e.g. RNA capping), methylation of specific amino acid residues of proteins (e.g. protein repair, intracellular localization) and detoxification (e.g. methylation of arsenite and xenobiotic compounds).

Although methylation reactions occur in all cells of the body, they are of the greatest quantitative significance in the liver. Creatine synthesis (reaction 3) and phosphatidylcholine synthesis (reaction 4) account for about 70% of SAM utilization in the body:

$$\text{Guanidinoacetate} + \text{SAM} \rightarrow \text{creatine} + \text{SAH} \qquad (3)$$

$$\text{Phosphatidylethanolamine} + 3\,\text{SAM} \rightarrow$$
$$\text{phosphatidylcholine} + 3\,\text{SAH} \qquad (4)$$

Reaction (3) is catalysed by guanidinoacetate methyltransferase (GAMT) and reaction (4) by phosphatidylethanolamine methyltransferase (PEMT). The liver is the dominant site of both GAMT and PEMT expression.

SAH, once produced by methylation reactions, is hydrolysed to adenosine and homocysteine [11]. Some of this homocysteine is released into the plasma. We now appreciate that the liver is the principal source of plasma homocysteine because of the quantitatively dominant role played by the liver in methylation reactions. This is significant because elevated plasma homocysteine has been implicated as a risk factor for cardiovascular disease, Alzheimer's disease and fractures. Metabolism of homocysteine, rather than its release into the circulation, is the fate of most of the homocysteine that arises within the liver. Homocysteine may be metabolized in two different ways – by trans-sulphuration and by remethylation. The trans-sulphuration pathway consists of two enzymes, cystathionine β-synthase and cystathionine γ-lyase. This sequence of reactions is irreversible, which means that methionine can be converted to cysteine but cysteine cannot be converted to methionine. This, in turn, provides the biochemical basis for the well-known nutritional observation that methionine is an essential amino acid but that cysteine is not essential, provided that an adequate supply of methionine is available.

Homocysteine metabolism also occurs via remethylation to methionine [11]. In the liver, this can occur via two quite separate enzymes. Methionine synthase, one of only two vitamin B12-requiring enzymes in mammals, employs N^5-methylTHF as a methyl donor. This N^5-methylTHF arises as a result of the reduction of N^5,N^{10}-methyleneTHF by reduced nicotinamide adenine dinucleotide phosphate (NADPH), a reaction catalysed by methylenetetrahydrofolate reductase (MTHFR). Methionine synthase occurs ubiquitously throughout the body. However, a second enzyme, betaine:homocysteine methyltransferase (BHMT), which is found in the liver and kidneys of humans, can also remethylate homocysteine to methionine. In this case, the methyl group is provided by betaine, which arises during choline catabolism and is also a minor dietary constituent.

Methionine metabolism provides a fascinating example of the interplay between amino acid metabolism and vitamin status. Deficiencies of a number of B vitamins are known to cause elevated plasma homocysteine. As the two enzymes of the trans-sulphuration pathway contain pyridoxal phosphate as prosthetic groups, pyridoxal deficiency impairs this pathway and increases homocysteine levels. As methionine synthase contains methylcobalamin as its prosthetic group and employs N^5-methylTHF as a substrate, it is hardly surprising that deficiency of either vitamin B12 or folic acid results in elevated plasma homocysteine [12].

Deeper analysis reveals more sophisticated interactions. Methionine synthase can be viewed as playing two critical roles. On the one hand, homocysteine retains the carbon skeleton of methionine, and its methylation conserves this essential amino acid. Support for this function of methionine synthase is afforded by findings that a higher proportion of homocysteine is remethylated to methionine on feeding a diet low in methionine. However, methionine synthase also plays a crucial role in folate metabolism. This is best exemplified by the methyl trap hypothesis, which accounts for the fact that cobalamin deficiency often results in a functional folate deficiency [13]. This hypothesis postulates that cobalamin deficiency, which leads to decreased methionine synthase activity, will result in an accumulation of much of a cell's folate as N^5-methylTHF, with consequent depletion of the other THF coenzymes. The methyl trap is exacerbated by the fact that N^5-methylTHF is the principal folate form that is provided to cells from the circulation and must be metabolized by methionine synthase to provide the other THF coenzymes that are required by the cell. Clearly, there is a very close interrelationship between the metabolism of methionine, homocysteine and folate.

Creatine synthesis

Although the liver does not employ the creatine kinase system for its energy metabolism, it is very much involved in creatine synthesis. Creatine and creatine:phosphate break down spontaneously to creatinine, which is excreted in the urine. In young adults, some 1.5–2 g of creatinine are excreted each day, which means that a comparable quantity of creatine must be replaced. Replacement occurs by a combination of diet and synthesis in omnivores, but strict vegetarians need to synthesize all their creatine. Creatine synthesis involves a very simple metabolic pathway, but it requires no fewer than three amino acids. The first step, catalysed by the glycine:L-arginine amidinotransferase

(AGAT), involves the transfer of an amidino group from arginine to glycine to produce guanidinoacetate and ornithine (reaction 5):

$$\text{Glycine} + \text{arginine} \rightarrow \text{guanidinoacetate} + \text{ornithine} \quad (5)$$

The second reaction involves the methylation of guanidinoacetate to produce creatine (reaction 3). This reaction is predominantly found in the liver, which is the principal site of creatine synthesis. However, in humans, both liver and kidney can produce guanidinoacetate. A consideration of the quantitative aspects of creatine synthesis is revealing. After accounting for the 0.5 g of creatine that may be obtained in the diet, it is calculated that an 18- to 29-year-old man will synthesize about 1.5 g of creatine per day. This requires 2 g of arginine, which is about 40–50% of all the arginine ingested by an individual with a typical North American protein intake. In addition, as noted above, creatine synthesis consumes approximately 35% of SAM-derived methyl groups. Creatine synthesis is clearly a major pathway in amino acid metabolism.

Glutathione synthesis and function
(see also Chapter 2.3.9)

Glutathione (γ-glutamyl-cysteinyl glycine) plays important roles in many tissues but is particularly important in the liver. It exists in both reduced (GSH) and oxidized glutathione disulphide (GSSG) forms, which are interconverted by the enzyme glutathione reductase (reaction 6):

$$\text{GSSG} + \text{NADPH} + \text{H}^+ \Leftrightarrow 2\,\text{GSH} + \text{NADP}^+ \quad (6)$$

In cells, the great bulk of glutathione (~ 95%) occurs in the reduced form.

A detailed review of glutathione metabolism is found in Chapter 2.3.9.

Regulatory functions of amino acids in liver

In addition to their roles as substrates for key biosyntheses (e.g. protein, glutathione and creatine synthesis) and in intracellular metabolism (urea cycle, malate–aspartate shuttle), amino acids are important regulatory molecules that act through signalling pathways. In the liver, this is particularly apparent in the control of protein synthesis and proteolysis, as both are very active processes. Although the liver only accounts for about 2% of body weight, it is responsible for about 18% of total body protein synthesis (53 g/day in a 70-kg man) [14]. This rate of hepatic protein synthesis can increase substantially during inflammation and infections when the synthesis of acute-phase proteins is greatly increased. In healthy individuals, the liver produces about 15–20 g of albumin per day; this is very sensitive to nutritional status, in particular to protein intake. Hepatic proteolysis, which is a highly active process, is also sensitive to nutritional status, being markedly increased early in starvation. Amino acids, together with insulin, are major controllers of both hepatic protein synthesis and proteolysis.

The synthesis of individual proteins is generally regulated by rates of gene expression, which affect the abundance of individual mRNAs. In addition to this primarily transcriptional control of the synthesis of specific proteins, regulation also occurs at the translational level and can affect the synthesis of classes of proteins or even of all proteins. Amino acids and insulin increase hepatic protein synthesis through partly shared signalling networks. Leucine is the principal amino acid that promotes protein synthesis in a variety of tissues, including the liver. Its effects in liver are not as global as in muscle, although it does increase the synthesis of a number of strategically important proteins. An outline of the mechanism of this effect has become apparent through the work of Kimball and Jefferson [15], although much remains to be learned.

Provision of leucine to hepatocytes results in enhanced phosphorylation of 4E-BP1 (the binding protein for the eukaryotic initiation factor, eIF4E) and S6K1, the ribosomal protein S6 kinase. Enhanced phosphorylation of 4E-BP1 releases eIF4E, which is required for the binding of mRNA to the 43S preinitiation complex. Phosphorylation of S6K1 results in its activation and, subsequently, in the phosphorylation of ribosomal protein

(rp) S6. In turn, the phosphorylation of rpS6 results in the enhanced translation of mRNAs that contain an uninterrupted stretch of pyrimidine bases adjacent to the 5′ cap. Proteins encoded by these mRNAs include ribosomal proteins, elongation factors and polyA-binding proteins. Both 4E-BP1 and S6K1 are downstream targets of the serine/threonine protein kinase, mTOR, which is viewed as a key target of leucine's action. Amino acids that increase cell volume (*vide infra*) can also stimulate hepatic protein synthesis.

Hepatic protein turnover is mediated both by proteosome-catalysed proteolysis and by macroautophagy; the latter process is dominant in the liver and is regulated by both insulin and amino acids [16]. Macroautophagy is a complex process in which cytoplasmic material is sequestered in autophagosomes, followed by acidification of these organelles and their fusion with lysosomes. It is a non-specific process in that most constituents of the cytosol are engulfed and degraded. However, proteins constitute the great bulk of cytoplasmic material, so that macroautophagy is rightly characterized as a means of effecting protein turnover. There seem to be two parallel means whereby amino acids suppress macroautophagy. Amino acids that are transported into cells via sodium-linked, concentrative transporters tend to increase cell hydration and inhibit

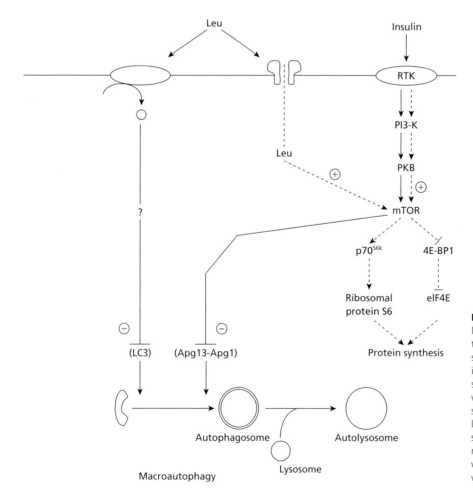

Fig. 3 Proposed signalling pathways for leucine (Leu) and regulatory amino acids in the control of macroautophagy and protein synthesis. One pathway for macroautophagy is independent of mTOR, does not affect protein synthesis and may involve leucine's interaction with a plasma membrane sensor. The other signalling pathway involves an intracellular leucine sensor, requires mTOR and both stimulates protein synthesis and suppresses macroautophagy; it shares common elements with insulin's signalling pathway. Reproduced, with permission, from ref. 18.

macroautophagy via a mitogen-activated protein (MAP) kinase-mediated mechanism. The other mechanism involves amino acids (e.g. leucine, phenylalanine and tyrosine) that are not concentrated within the liver but appear to exert their actions via an mTOR-mediated pathway.

Recent studies have clarified the mechanism by which glutamine and system A substrates affect macroautophagy. The accumulation of these amino acids within cells, together with the cotransported Na+ (which is partly exchanged for K+), is followed by a flux of water into the cell to equilibrate the osmotic pressure on both sides of the cell membrane. The resulting increase in cell volume (cell hydration) results in an immediate activation of MAP kinases, in particular ERK and p38^{MAPK}. This latter kinase brings about the inhibition of macroautophagy at the level of the formation of the autophagosome [17]. More work is needed to elucidate the complete mechanism, but the key role of cell swelling is confirmed by experiments that demonstrated a comparable degree of inhibition of proteolysis when cells were swollen in hypo-osmotic media.

Amino acids such as leucine, phenylalanine and tyrosine are agonists for another mechanism whereby amino acids inhibit macroautophagy [16,18]. The mechanism appears to involve mTOR, as rpS6, which is downstream from mTOR, becomes rapidly phosphorylated with the same kinetics as the inhibition of proteolysis. Rapamycin, an inhibitor of mTOR, could partly overcome the inhibition of autophagic proteolysis by amino acids. Again, much work remains before we will have a complete picture of the mechanism. The phosphorylation of rpS6 does not implicate this protein in the inhibition of macroautophagy; rather, it should be taken as indicating an efficient regulatory system in which mTOR activation plays a role in both the stimulation of protein synthesis and the suppression of proteolysis. There is also evidence for an mTOR-independent mechanism whereby these amino acids can suppress macroautophagy. This appears to be another example of redundant cell signalling systems. Figure 3 summarizes these mechanisms.

These new insights into amino acid-mediated cell signalling have considerable physiological significance. Amino acids signal their availability for anabolic processes, not only by being available as substrates, but also by more sophisticated mechanisms. Simultaneously, they signal the need to suppress catabolic processes. mTOR and cell hydration emerge as important 'interpreters' of amino acid availability. Recent studies also suggest that leucine may act via mTOR-independent mechanisms. It is clear that mTOR is not only an amino acid-responsive kinase but also a more general nutrient sensor; it can be antagonized by the adenosine monophosphate (AMP)-stimulated kinase which responds to the AMP/ATP ratio. The interaction and synergy of amino acid signalling with that of insulin remains to be fully elucidated. Finally, a crucial unsolved issue is the identification of the precise molecule(s) that interact(s) with regulatory amino acids such as leucine. However, it can be confidently asserted that recent work on amino acid signalling has revealed a new vista in amino acid metabolism that is likely to become even more important in the future.

References

1 Wijekoon EP, Skinner C, Brosnan ME *et al.* (2005) Amino acid metabolism in the Zucker diabetic fatty rat: effects of insulin resistance and of type 2 diabetes. *Can J Physiol Pharmacol* 82, 506–514.
2 Malandro MS, Kilberg MS (1996) Molecular biology of amino acid transporters. *Annu Rev Biochem* 65, 305–336.
3 Stoll B, McNelly S, Buscher HP *et al.* (1991) Functional hepatocyte heterogeneity in glutamate, aspartate and alpha-ketoglutarate uptake; a histoautoradiographical study. *Hepatology* 13, 247–253.
4 Jungas RL, Halperin ML, Brosnan JT (1992) Quantitative analysis of amino acid oxidation and related gluconeogenesis in humans. *Physiol Rev* 72, 419–448.
5 Stoll B, Henry J, Reeds PJ *et al.* (1998) Catabolism dominates the first-pass intestinal metabolism of dietary essential amino acids in milk protein-fed piglets. *J Nutr* 128, 606–614.
6 Martinov MV, Vitvitsky VM, Moshasov EV *et al.* (2000) A substrate switch: a new mode of regulation in the methionine metabolic pathway. *J Theor Biol* 204, 521–532.
7 Krebs HA (1972) Some aspects of the regulation of fuel supply in omnivorous animals. *Adv Eng Regul* 10, 397–420.
8 Haussinger D (1996) Hepatic glutamine transport and metabolism. *Adv Enzymol Relat Areas Mol Biol* 72, 43–86.
9 O'Sullivan D, Brosnan JT, Brosnan ME (1998) Hepatic zonation of the catabolism of arginine and ornithine in the perfused rat liver. *Biochem J* 330, 627–632.
10 Felig P (1975) Amino acid metabolism in man. *Annu Rev Biochem* 44, 933–955.
11 Finkelstein JD (1990) Methionine metabolism in mammals. *J Nutr Biochem* 1, 228–237.
12 Selhub J (1999) Homocysteine metabolism. *Annu Rev Nutr* 19, 217–246.
13 Shane B, Stokstad EL (1985) Vitamin B$_{12}$–folate interrelationships. *Annu Rev Nutr* 5, 115–141.
14 Brosnan JT, Young VR (2003) Integration of metabolism 2: protein and amino acids. In: Gibney MJ, Macdonald IA, Roche HM (eds) *Nutrition and Metabolism.* Oxford: Blackwell Science, pp. 43–73.
15 Kimball SR, Jefferson LS (2004) Molecular mechanisms through which amino acids mediate signaling through the mammalian target of rapamycin. *Curr Opin Nutr Metab Care* 7, 39–44.
16 Meijer AJ, Dubbelhuis PF (2003) Amino acid signaling and the integration of metabolism. *Biochem Biophys Res Commun* 313, 397–404.
17 Haussinger D, Graf D, Weiergraber OH (2001) Glutamine and cell signaling in liver. *J Nutr* 131, 25095–25145.
18 Kadowaki M, Kanazawa T (2003) Amino acids as regulators of proteolysis. *J Nutr* 133, 20525–20565.

2.3.4 Mitochondria and energy formation

Dominique Pessayre

Mitochondria are double-membrane organelles derived evolutionarily from bacteria. They have their own DNA and reproduce asexually, but only women transmit mitochondrial DNA. Mitochondria represent remarkable biochemical machines that are able to harness the energy produced by the oxidation of fat and other energetic substrates in a form usable by the cell.

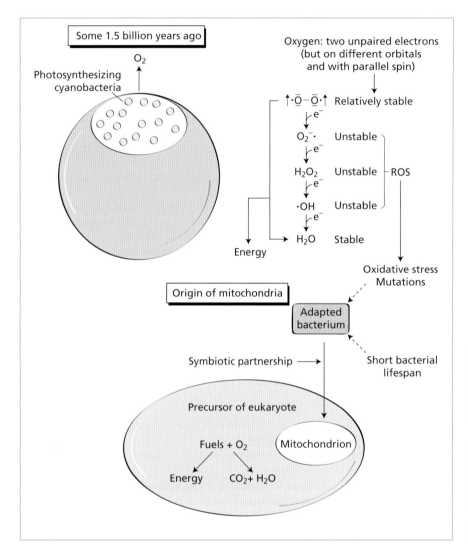

Fig. 1 Oxygen and the origin of mitochondria. Some 1.5 billion years ago, photosynthesizing cyanobacteria began releasing oxygen in the atmosphere. Although oxygen is a diradical, it is relatively stable because its two unpaired electrons are located on different orbitals and have a parallel spin. Yet, oxygen is avid for electrons. Its full reduction into water (by four successive electrons) releases considerable energy. However, its incomplete reduction by one, two or three electrons produces reactive oxygen species (ROS), which cause oxidative stress and gene mutations. The resulting high mutation rate, combined with the short lifespan and rapid turnover of bacteria, has enabled them to adapt quickly to the oxidizing environment. Thanks to a symbiotic partnership, these adapted bacteria have become our present-day mitochondria. They indirectly burn fuels with oxygen to provide considerable energy, with limited ROS formation and no immediate toxicity.

Origin and structure of mitochondria

Some 1.5 billion years ago, photosynthesizing cyanobacteria began releasing oxygen in the earth's atmosphere (Fig. 1) [1]. Oxygen is an atypical molecule (Fig. 1). Although it is a diradical, its two unpaired electrons are located on different orbitals and have a parallel spin, making oxygen a relatively stable molecule [2]. Yet, oxygen is avid for electrons. Its incomplete reduction by one, two or three successive electrons produces reactive oxygen species (ROS), which react with biological molecules to cause oxidative stress and gene mutations (Fig. 1) [1]. However, the full reduction of oxygen by four successive electrons forms a stable product (water) and releases considerable energy (Fig. 1). Therefore, the advent of oxygen evolutionarily was both a severe threat to life (due to the toxicity of ROS) and also a great opportunity (due to the energetic potential of fuel oxidation).

Thanks to their short lifespan and rapid turnover, bacteria took advantage of the high mutation rate triggered by ROS to adapt quickly to the new oxygen environment (Fig. 1). They developed biochemical machines enabling them indirectly to burn fuels with oxygen and produce usable energy, while minimizing ROS formation and toxicity. Rather than trying to emulate the biochemical perfection of bacteria, other forms of life have associated with them. Through a symbiotic partnership, these adapted bacteria have become our present-day mitochondria (Fig. 1) [3].

Like their bacterial ancestors, mitochondria have two membranes. The circular outer membrane surrounds the intermembrane space, while the folded inner membrane invaginates into cristae, which protrude into the mitochondrial matrix.

Like bacteria, mitochondria also have their own circular DNA located in the mitochondrial matrix [4].

Mitochondrial DNA (mtDNA)

Sperm cell mitochondria are ubiquitinated and are degraded in the fertilized ovum, so that mtDNA is only transmitted by women [5]. Most somatic cells, including hepatocytes, contain

Fig. 2 Transcription and replication of the mitochondrial genome. The human mitochondrial DNA (mtDNA) is a double-stranded circular DNA of 16 569 bp. Its transcription is mediated by a mitochondrial RNA polymerase and is enhanced by the binding of mitochondrial transcription factor A (mtTFA) to enhancer elements located upstream of the heavy strand promoter (HSP) and the light strand promoter (LSP). Transcription of the heavy strand starts at nucleotide 561 (within the HSP) and proceeds counterclockwise. After synthesis of the two ribosomal RNAs, transcription may be arrested by the binding of mitochondrial termination factor (mtTERM), or it may proceed to form a large polycistronic precursor RNA encoding for 12 polypeptides and 14 tRNAs. Transcription of the light strand starts at nucleotide 407 (within the LSP) and proceeds clockwise to form a single polycistronic precursor RNA, encoding one polypeptide and eight tRNAs. The replication of mtDNA is mediated by DNA polymerase γ and is asymmetrical. Only the heavy strand is replicated initially. Replication starts at the origin of replication of the heavy strand (O_H), after a short RNA primer formed by the transcriptional machinery. The need for this RNA primer explains why mtTFA also modulates the replication of mtDNA. Mitochondrial single-stranded binding protein (mtSSB) binds to the single-stranded heavy chain and also activates replication. Replication of the heavy strand proceeds clockwise. It may arrest after a few hundred basepairs (thus forming the basal 'D-loop'), probably due to the binding of regulatory factors to the termination-associated sequence (TAS). Alternatively, replication may continue to form the whole daughter heavy strand. When the displacement front has gone beyond the origin of replication of the light strand (O_L), the replication of the light strand then starts counterclockwise after a short RNA primer introduced by a DNA primase. A6 and A8, subunit 6 or 8 of ATP synthase; cyt b, cytochrome *b*; COx, subunit of cytochrome c oxidase; ND, subunit of NADH dehydrogenase; rRNA, ribosomal RNA. Grey dots represent the 22 different mitochondrial tRNAs, which also serve as punctuations.

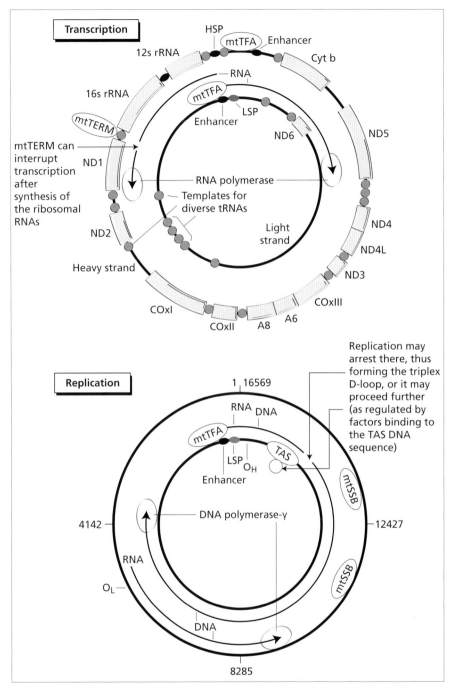

hundreds of mitochondria, and each mitochondrion usually contains a few copies of mtDNA. All mtDNA copies are identical in healthy young persons. However, in persons with inborn mitochondrial cytopathies and in elderly subjects, intact mtDNA copies coexist with mtDNA genomes with point mutations or DNA rearrangements, such as deletions or duplications.

The human mtDNA is a small (16 569 bp), circular, double-stranded DNA (Fig. 2), which is normally twisted into a super-coiled form [4]. The proportion of heavy vs. light DNA bases

differs slightly between the two mtDNA strands. Their different buoyancies on denaturing caesium chloride gradients have led to their appellation as the 'heavy strand' and the 'light strand' respectively. At the so-called 'displacement loop' (D-loop), mtDNA contains a third DNA strand. This localized triplex structure is due to the interrupted replication of the heavy strand, as discussed below.

Although most of the ancient bacterial genes have been lost, or have migrated to nuclear DNA [6], the human mtDNA still encodes for the two ribosomal mitochondrial RNAs, all 22 mitochondrial tRNAs and 13 of the polypeptides of the respiratory chain, including adenosine triphosphate (ATP) synthase [4]. Information is tightly packed on mtDNA (Fig. 2). With the exception of a few regulatory sequences, mtDNA consists mainly of coding sequences with no introns. Furthermore, the short DNA sequences encoding for mitochondrial tRNAs also serve as punctuation dots [4].

The transcription of mtDNA is mediated by a mitochondrial RNA polymerase and is enhanced by the binding of mitochondrial transcription factor A (mtTFA) to enhancer sequences located upstream of the heavy strand promoter and the light strand promoter [4]. Mitochondrial transcription factor B (mtTFB) may favour the interaction with RNA polymerase [4]. As shown in Fig. 2, the transcription of the heavy strand proceeds counterclockwise, while the transcription of the light strand runs clockwise.

DNA polymerase γ replicates mtDNA. It has proofreading activity, enabling it to remove the last added nucleotide, if mispaired [4]. The replication of mtDNA is asymmetrical (Fig. 2). Only the heavy strand is initially replicated. Replication starts at the origin of replication of the heavy strand (O_H), after a short RNA primer. This primer is formed by the transcriptional machinery and begins at the site for the initiation of transcription of the heavy strand. The need for this RNA primer explains why mtTFA enhances not only the transcription, but also the replication of mtDNA (Fig. 2). Other factors enhancing mtDNA replication are mitochondrial single-stranded binding protein (mtSSB) and the DNA helicase, twinkle. Replication of the heavy strand proceeds clockwise. It can arrest after a few hundred basepairs, thus forming the basal D-loop, or can proceed further on. The arrest or continuation of replication may be modulated by the binding of regulatory factors to the termination-associated sequence (TAS) (Fig. 2). When about two-thirds of the heavy strand has been replicated, and the displacement front has gone past the origin of replication of the light strand (O_L), the light strand begins to be replicated counterclockwise, after a short RNA primer introduced by a mitochondrial DNA primase [4].

Whereas mitochondria contain all the enzymes necessary for base excision repair, they cannot remove some bulky DNA lesions, such as pyrimidine dimers and interstrand cross-links [7,8]. However, heavily damaged mtDNA molecules can be degraded by mitochondrial nucleases, and then replaced by the synthesis of new mtDNA molecules replicated from unaltered mtDNA templates [8].

Mitochondrial protein import

With the exception of the 13 polypeptides encoded by mtDNA, the thousand or so other proteins present in mitochondria are encoded by nuclear DNA, synthesized within the cytoplasm and imported into the mitochondria, either cotranslationally or posttranslationally (Fig. 3) [9,10]. Although all imported polypeptides enter the mitochondria through the Tom40

(translocase of outer membrane 40) complex, import routes then differ with the destination of the protein (Fig. 3) [9].
• Polypeptides that are destined to form β-barrel proteins inside the outer membrane are carried by small Tim (translocase of inner membrane) proteins of the intermembrane space to the SAM (sorting and assembly machinery) complex, which inserts these proteins into the outer membrane (Fig. 3).
• Polypeptides that are destined to form multispanning proteins in the inner membrane are carried by the same small Tim proteins to the Tim22 (translocase of inner membrane 22) complex (also called the 'twin-pore translocase' because of its two pores), which inserts these proteins inside the inner membrane (Fig. 3) [9].
• Finally, polypeptides that are destined for the mitochondrial matrix are usually synthesized with an N-terminal, positively charged presequence achieving an α-helical configuration. These polypeptides cross the inner mitochondrial membrane through the Tim23 complex (also called the 'presequence translocase'). Their import is driven by the membrane potential and also by an ATP-driven pulling mechanism mediated by mitochondrial Hsp70, which is bound to Tim44. Mitochondrial processing peptidase (MPP) then removes the presequence inside the matrix (Fig. 3).

Most enzymes responsible for the tricarboxylic acid cycle, and all the proteins or enzymes involved in the replication, stability, translation and repair of mtDNA, are targeted to the mitochondrial matrix. Respiratory chain polypeptides are targeted to the inner mitochondrial membrane, except for cytochrome c, which is targeted to the intermembrane space but mostly associates with cardiolipin on the cytosolic face of the mitochondrial inner membrane. Finally, some β-oxidation enzymes are targeted to the mitochondrial inner membrane, while others are directed to the mitochondrial matrix.

Mitochondrial β-oxidation of fatty acids

Although peroxisomes contribute to the oxidation of fatty acids (particularly that of very-long-chain fatty acids), fatty acid oxidation mainly occurs within mitochondria.

Unlike medium-chain or short-chain fatty acids, long-chain fatty acids cannot directly enter the mitochondria. They must first be activated into a CoA thioester and then transported into the mitochondria by a carnitine-dependent shuttle (Fig. 4) [11]. On the cytosolic face of the outer mitochondrial membrane, acyl-CoA synthetase initially synthesizes an acyl-adenylate intermediate and then forms the acyl-CoA thioester, with the concomitant degradation of one ATP into AMP and pyrophosphate. Carnitine palmitoyl transferase I (CPT I), which is located on the cytosolic face of the outer mitochondrial membrane, next transfers the acyl group from CoA to carnitine (Fig. 4). The acyl-carnitine formed is then translocated across the inner mitochondrial membrane by carnitine acyl-carnitine translocase, in exchange for free carnitine. Finally, carnitine palmitoyl transferase II, which is located on the matrix side of the inner membrane, reforms the long-chain fatty acyl-CoA derivative inside the mitochondrial matrix (Fig. 4).

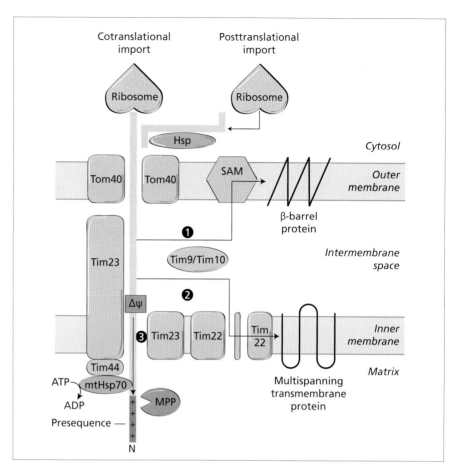

Fig. 3 Mitochondrial import of proteins. The mitochondrial proteins, which are encoded by nuclear DNA, are synthesized by cytosolic ribosomes and are imported cotranslationally or posttranslationally into the mitochondria. In the latter case, cytosolic chaperones (hsp) maintain the polypeptide in an import-competent form. All imported polypeptides cross the mitochondrial outer membrane (OM) through the translocase of outer membrane 40 (Tom40) complex. Import routes then differ with the destination of the polypeptide. (1) Polypeptides that are destined to form β-barrel proteins in the OM are brought by small Tim (translocase of the inner membrane) proteins (Tim9 and Tim10) to the sorting and assembly machinery (SAM) complex, which inserts these proteins into the OM. (2) Polypeptides that are destined to form multispanning proteins in the inner membrane (IM) are brought by the same small Tim proteins (Tim9 and Tim10) to the translocase of inner membrane 22 (Tim22) complex. Tim22, which is also called the 'twin translocase' on account of its two pores, inserts these proteins into the IM. (3) Finally, polypeptides that are destined for the mitochondrial matrix usually contain an N-terminal, positively charged presequence. They cross the inner membrane through the Tim23 complex (also called the 'presequence translocase of the inner membrane'). Their mitochondrial import is driven both by the membrane potential (Δψ) and by an ATP-driven pulling mechanism mediated by mitochondrial hsp70 (mtHsp70), which is anchored to Tim44. Mitochondrial processing peptidase (MPP) then removes the presequence in the matrix.

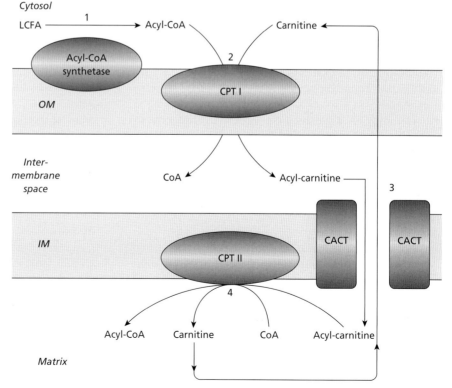

Fig. 4 Activation and mitochondrial uptake of long-chain fatty acids. (1) On the cytosolic face of the mitochondrial outer membrane (OM), the long-chain fatty acid (LCFA) is transformed by acyl-CoA synthetase into acyl-CoA. (2) Carnitine palmitoyl transferase I (CPT I), which is located on the cytosolic face of the outer membrane, transfers the acyl group from CoA to carnitine. It is unclear whether the acyl-carnitine formed is released directly into the intermembrane space by CPT I or whether it is first released outside and then crosses the outer membrane. (3) The acyl-carnitine derivative is translocated across the mitochondrial inner membrane (IM) by carnitine acyl-carnitine translocase (CACT) in exchange for free carnitine. (4) Carnitine palmitoyl transferase II (CPT II), which is located on the matrix side of the inner membrane, then reforms acyl-CoA inside the mitochondrial matrix.

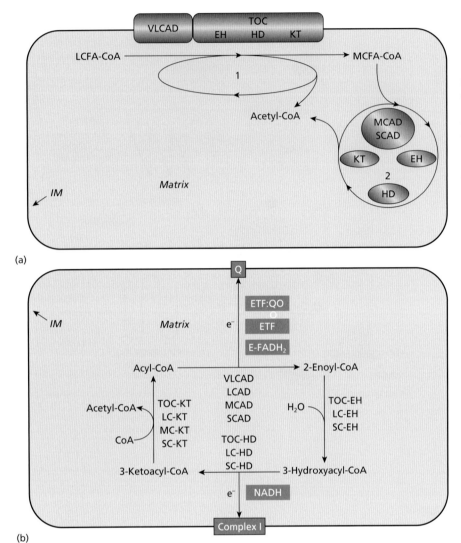

(a)

(b)

Fig. 5 Mitochondrial β-oxidation of long-chain fatty acids. (a) Successive action of membrane-bound and then soluble β-oxidation enzymes. (1) The saturated, long-chain fatty acyl-CoA (LCFA-CoA) is shortened to a medium-chain fatty acyl-CoA (MCFA-CoA) by the membrane-bound, very-long-chain acyl-CoA dehydrogenase (VLCAD) and the membrane-bound, trifunctional β-oxidation complex (TOC), which has enoyl-CoA hydratase (EH), 3-hydroxyacyl-CoA dehydrogenase (HD) and 3-ketoacyl-CoA thiolase (KT) activities. (2) The MCFA-CoA is then further split into its acetyl-CoA subunits by soluble matricial enzymes, including medium-chain and short-chain acyl-CoA dehydrogenases (MCAD and SCAD) and soluble EH, HD and KT enzymes specific for long-chain (LC), medium-chain (MC) and short-chain (SC) fatty acids. (b). β-Oxidation intermediates and fate of electrons. The β-oxidation cycle successively involves a first dehydrogenation, a hydration step, a second dehydrogenation and, finally, thiolysis, which releases acetyl-CoA. Electrons coming from acyl-CoA dehydrogenases are transferred to an enzyme-bound FAD, thus forming E-FADH$_2$, and are then shuttled by electron transfer flavoprotein (ETF) and ETF-ubiquinone oxidoreductase (ETF:QO), to the ubiquinone (Q) of the respiratory chain, thus forming ubiquinol. Electrons coming from 3-hydroxyacyl-CoA dehydrogenases are transferred to NAD$^+$, thus forming NADH, which feeds electrons into complex 1 of the respiratory chain.

Mitochondrial β-oxidation progressively shortens the acyl-CoA by two carbon units at each cycle (Fig. 5) [11]. Each β-oxidation cycle involves a first dehydrogenation leading to *trans*-2-enoyl-CoA, a hydration step forming L-3-hydroxyacyl-CoA, a second dehydrogenation leading to 3-ketoacyl-CoA and, finally, thiolytic cleavage by CoA, releasing acetyl-CoA and an acyl-CoA shortened by two carbon atoms.

First membrane-bound and then soluble enzymes successively shorten a saturated long-chain fatty acyl-CoA (Fig. 5) [12]. The membrane-bound, very-long-chain acyl-CoA dehydrogenase (VLCAD) is also very active with long-chain fatty acids and mediates the first dehydrogenation step of the β-oxidation cycle. The membrane-bound, trifunctional β-oxidation complex (TOC) then completes the β-oxidation cycle through its enoyl-CoA hydratase, 3-hydroxyacyl-CoA dehydrogenase and 3-ketoacyl-CoA thiolase activities. This membrane-bound system (VLCAD and TOC) may shorten the saturated long-chain fatty acid into a medium-chain fatty acid (Fig. 5). Further shortening is then mediated by matrix enzymes, including medium-

chain and short-chain acyl-CoA dehydrogenases (MCAD and SCAD) and soluble enoyl hydratases, 3-hydroxyacyl-CoA dehydrogenases and 3-ketoacyl-CoA thiolases specific for long-, medium- or short-chain fatty acids (Fig. 5) [11,12].

Owing to the high activity of the membrane-bound system, the soluble, long-chain acyl-CoA dehydrogenase (LCAD) is redundant for the β-oxidation of saturated long-chain fatty acids. However, LCAD is involved in the β-oxidation of unsaturated long-chain fatty acids, thus compensating for the poor activity of VLCAD for unsaturated substrates [12].

The two main steps regulating the β-oxidation flux are carnitine palmitoyl transferase I, which modulates the entry of long-chain fatty acids into the mitochondria, and acyl-CoA dehydrogenases, whose activities are relatively sluggish compared with the high activities of other β-oxidation enzymes [13].

Each β-oxidation cycle removes four electrons. The two electrons removed by acyl-CoA dehydrogenases transiently form an enzyme-bound E-FADH$_2$. These electrons are then shuttled by electron transfer flavoprotein (ETF) and ETF-ubiquinone oxidoreductase (ETF:QO) to the ubiquinone (Q) of the respiratory chain close to complex III, thus forming ubiquinol (Fig. 5). In contrast, the electrons removed by 3-hydroxyacyl-CoA dehydrogenases are transferred to NAD$^+$ to form nicotinamide adenine dinucleotide (NADH), which feeds electrons into complex I of the respiratory chain (Fig. 5). As discussed below, electrons coming from E-FADH$_2$ will produce about two ATP molecules, while those coming from NADH will form about three ATP molecules [14]. Therefore, each round of mitochondrial β-oxidation eventually leads to about five ATP molecules and one molecule of acetyl-CoA. The latter can either condense into ketone bodies, as discussed below, or may eventually undergo the tricarboxylic acid cycle to generate much more energy.

Tricarboxylic acid cycle

The final oxidation of acetyl-CoA by the tricarboxylic acid cycle (also termed the 'citric acid cycle', starts with the condensation of acetyl-CoA with oxaloacetate to form citrate (Fig. 6) [14]. This reaction is carried out by citrate synthase and involves the formation a citryl-CoA intermediate, which is then hydrolysed into CoA and citrate.

The tricarboxylic acid cycle then proceeds with the isomerization of citrate into isocitrate (mediated by aconitase), the oxidative decarboxylation of isocitrate into CO$_2$ and α-ketoglutarate (mediated by isocitrate dehydrogenase), and the CoA-supported oxidative decarboxylation of α-ketoglutarate into CO$_2$ and succinyl CoA (mediated by the α-ketoglutarate dehydrogenase complex). The cycle further proceeds with the cleavage of the thioester bond of succinyl-CoA to form succinate and one high-energy guanosine 5′-triphosphate (GTP) (mediated by the reversibly acting, succinyl-CoA synthetase). Finally, the cycle ends up with three steps resembling those involved in the β-oxidation process, with the dehydrogenation of succinate into fumarate (mediated by succinate dehydrogenase), the hydration of fumarate into malate (mediated by fumarase) and the dehydrogenation of malate into oxaloacetate (mediated by malate dehydrogenase). The overall stoichiometry of the tricarboxylic acid cycle is: acetyl-CoA + 2 H$_2$O + 3 NAD$^+$ + FAD + GDP + Pi → 2 CO$_2$ + 3 NADH + FADH$_2$ + GTP + 2 H$^+$ + CoA. As each of the three NADH molecules will eventually give about three ATP molecules and the single FADH$_2$ will form about two ATP molecules, the global energy yield of one citric acid cycle is about 11 ATP molecules, as well as one energy-rich GTP molecule, which can be used as such or can generate one more ATP molecule [14].

It is noteworthy that molecular oxygen is not immediately used in this cycle nor in the β-oxidation cycle. The oxygen

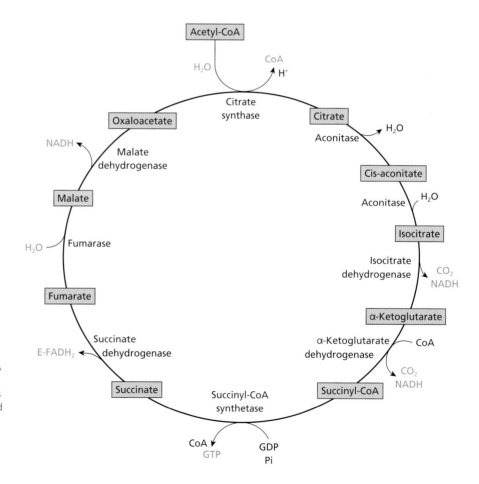

Fig. 6 Tricarboxylic acid cycle. The final oxidation of the acetate moiety of acetyl-CoA by the tricarboxylic acid cycle produces one molecule of energy-rich GTP, three molecules of NADH and one molecule of enzyme-bound FADH$_2$ within succinate dehydrogenase (E-FADH$_2$). NADH and E-FADH$_2$ then transfer their electrons to the respiratory chain to produce ATP.

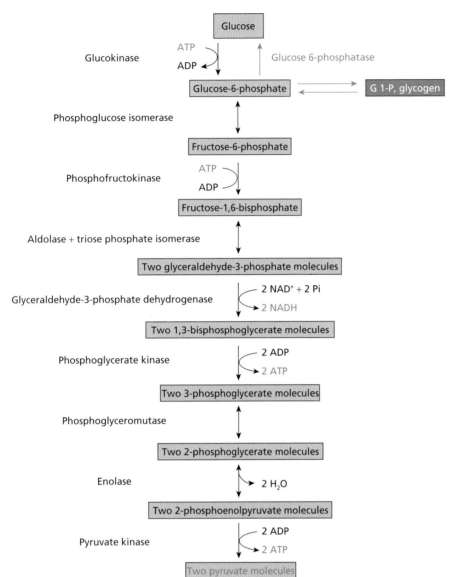

Fig. 7 Glycolysis. The glycolysis of glucose in the cytoplasm forms two molecules of pyruvate. Unless the generated NADH and pyruvate are further oxidized in mitochondria, glycolysis itself only generates two net molecules of ATP.

atoms, which end up in CO_2, come from water. However, as discussed below, the electrons, which are passed by NADH and $FADH_2$ to the respiratory chain, end up in molecular oxygen to form water. This transfer of electrons regenerates the oxidized cofactors (NAD^+ and FAD), which are necessary to sustain β-oxidation and the tricarboxylic acid cycle. Thus, even though molecular oxygen is not involved in the tricarboxylic acid cycle, oxygen is mandatory at the next step, explaining why the tricarboxylic acid cycle can only function in the presence of oxygen. In the absence of oxygen, the only metabolic pathway that can transiently provide some feeble energy is glycolysis.

Cytosolic glycolysis and the mitochondrial oxidation of pyruvate

Glycolysis is defined as the process that converts glucose into pyruvate [14]. This process, which occurs in the cytoplasm,

starts with the phosphorylation of glucose into glucose-6-phosphate. This reaction is catalysed by glucokinase in the liver and hexokinase in other organs (Fig. 7). Glucose-6-phosphate is a branching point in glucose metabolism. Its reversible isomerization to glucose-1-phosphate can lead to UDP-glucose formation and glycogen synthesis, whereas its reversible isomerization into fructose-6-phosphate can lead to glycolysis. The first committed step in glycolysis is the irreversible phosphorylation of fructose-6-phosphate into fructose-1,6-bisphosphate by phosphofructokinase. After a series of enzymatic reactions detailed in Figure 7, including the reduction of NAD^+ into NADH by glyceraldehyde-3-phosphate dehydrogenase, glycolysis ends up with the irreversible transformation of phosphoenol pyruvate into pyruvate, a reaction catalysed by pyruvate kinase (Fig. 7). Both phosphofructokinase and the liver-type pyruvate kinase are tightly regulated (through allosteric and phosphorylation events) to prevent the liver from consuming glucose when glucose is more urgently needed by brain or muscle [14]. The net stoichiometry of glycolysis is: glucose + 2 NAD$^+$ + 2 ADP + 2 Pi → 2 pyruvate + 2 NADH + 2 H$^+$ + 2 ATP + 2 H$_2$O [14].

Glycolysis cannot proceed unless the formed NADH is reoxidized into the NAD$^+$ required by glyceraldehyde-3-phosphate dehydrogenase. When there is a transient incapacity of mitochondria to reoxidize the formed NADH (for example, during strenuous muscular exercise or during tissue ischaemia), some transient relief can be obtained from the reversible reaction catalyscd by lactate dehydrogenase: NADH + H$^+$ + pyruvate → NAD$^+$ + lactate. The regeneration of NAD$^+$ allows glycolysis to continue, while the formed lactate can be oxidized at later times in the same organ (e.g. in the resting muscle) or in other organs, such as the liver. In the meantime, however, the energy yield is only two molecules of ATP for one molecule of glucose consumed, so that anaerobic glycolysis is a most wasteful way of generating energy.

However, under normal aerobic conditions, mitochondria reoxidize the NADH formed by glycolysis. Because the inner mitochondrial membrane is impermeable to NADH, its electrons rather than NADH are transferred to mitochondria. This can be achieved by two mitochondrial shuttles: the malate–aspartate or the glycerol phosphate shuttles [14]. In the cytosol, NADH regenerates NAD$^+$ by transferring its electrons to either oxaloacetate or dihydroxyacetone phosphate, which then diffuse into the mitochondria, where they release their electrons to regenerate either NADH (in the malate–aspartate shuttle) or an enzyme-bound FADH$_2$ molecule (in the glycerol phosphate shuttle) [14]. These reduced cofactors then form ATP through oxidative phosphorylation, as discussed below.

Under normal aerobic conditions, mitochondria also oxidize the pyruvate (or lactate) formed by glycolysis (Fig. 8). Mitochondrial carriers transport pyruvate or lactate into the mitochondria, where the pyruvate dehydrogenase complex catalyses the reaction: pyruvate + NAD$^+$ + CoA → acetyl-CoA + NADH. The oxidation of this acetyl-CoA in the tricarboxylic acid cycle will then generate considerable energy. Whereas the anaerobic glycolysis of glucose into pyruvate and lactate only

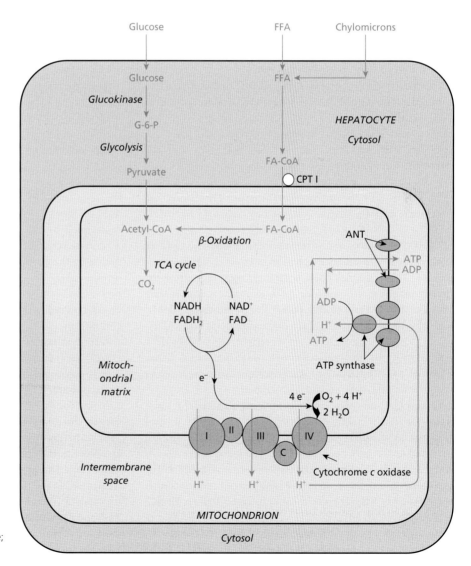

Fig. 8 Oxidative metabolism and energy production by mitochondria. The oxidation of pyruvate and free fatty acids (FFA) inside mitochondria produces NADH and FADH$_2$, which transfer their electrons to the mitochondrial respiratory chain. The flow of electrons in complexes 1, 3 and 4 is coupled with the extrusion of protons from the mitochondrial matrix into the intermembrane space. When energy is needed, these protons re-enter the matrix through ATP synthase to generate ATP from ADP. The adenine nucleotide translocator (ANT) then exchanges the formed ATP for cytosolic ADP. G-6-P, glucose 6-phosphate; LCFA-CoA, long-chain fatty acyl-CoA; CPT I, carnitine palmitoyl transferase I; TCA cycle, tricarboxylic acid cycle; c, cytochrome c.

forms two ATP molecules, the complete aerobic oxidation of glucose can provide up to 38 ATP molecules, thanks to the oxidative phosphorylation system [14].

Oxidative phosphorylation system

Oxidative phosphorylation is the process whereby the electrons stored in NADH or enzyme-bound $FADH_2$ are reacted with oxygen to form water, while part of the energy released by this exergonic reaction is harnessed to form ATP. To achieve this aim, electrons are first transferred through different respiratory chain complexes, where the electron transfer potential is converted, step by step, into an electrochemical proton gradient, which is finally converted into a phosphate transfer potential by forming energy-rich ATP molecules [14]. An analogy may be the pumping up of water behind a dam by a thermal engine, and then the opening of water valves allowing the hydrostatic flow of water into a hydroelectric turbine that generates electricity used to charge small batteries.

A total of five complexes constitute the oxidative phosphorylation system [15]. Complexes 1–4 constitute the respiratory chain, while complex 5 is ATP synthase. Depending on their original sources (NADH or enzyme-bound $FADH_2$), electrons enter the respiratory chain at different sites.
- The two electrons coming from NADH are transferred to complex 1 (also termed 'NADH-ubiquinone oxidoreductase' or 'NADH dehydrogenase'). Within this large, L-shaped complex, electrons are successively transferred to one flavin mononucleotide (FMN) and several iron–sulphur clusters to be finally donated to ubiquinone (Q), thus forming ubiquinol (QH_2). Concomitantly, four protons are pumped from the mitochondrial matrix into the intermembrane space. Therefore, the stoichiometry of the reaction catalysed by complex I is: NADH $+ 5 H_{in}^+ + Q \rightarrow NAD^+ + 4 H_{out}^+ + QH_2$ [16].
- The two electrons coming from the enzyme-bound $FADH_2$ of succinate dehydrogenase are given to complex 2. Unlike complexes 1, 3 or 4, complex 2 does not translocate protons from the mitochondrial matrix into the intermembrane space. It only transfers two electrons to ubiquinone, thus forming ubiquinol.
- Finally, the electrons coming from the enzyme-bound $FADH_2$ of acyl-CoA dehydrogenases are directly transferred by ETF and ETF:QO to ubiquinone, thus forming ubiquinol. Thus, whatever their initial site of entry (complex 1, complex 2 or ubiquinone), electrons end up in ubiquinol.

Q and QH_2 are highly mobile molecules within the inner mitochondrial membrane, allowing QH_2 to transfer its two electrons to complex 3 (also termed 'ubiquinol:cytochrome c oxidoreductase' or 'cytochrome bc_1'). The redox active sites of complex 3 include a cytochrome b with two haems (b-562 and b-566), an iron–sulphur protein (ISP) and a membrane-anchored cytochrome c_1. The 'Q cycle' theory postulates that complex 3 contains two sites for $Q/Q^-/QH_2$: an outside Q_o site located in close proximity to the intermembrane space and an inner Q_i site located in close proximity to the matrix (Fig. 9) [15]. At the

outside Q_o site, ubiquinol would produce ubiquinone by releasing its two protons into the intermembrane space and by giving one electron to the ISP (to be given next to cytochrome c_1 and then cytochrome c) and the second electron to cytochrome b [17]. Cytochrome b would then recycle this electron in the Q_i site, as explained in the legend to Figure 9. Another theory holds that ubiquinol donates its two electrons to cytochrome b, which then gives them to the ISP, en route for cytochrome c_1 and cytochrome c (Fig. 9) [18]. Whatever the path(s) of electrons, the net stoichiometry of the reaction catalysed by complex 3 is: $QH_2 + 2$ oxidized cytochrome c (Fe^{3+}) $+ 2 H_{in}^+ \rightarrow Q + 2$ reduced cytochrome c (Fe^{2+}) $+ 4 H_{out}^+$ [15].

Four reduced cytochrome c molecules finally transfer four electrons to complex 4 (cytochrome c oxidase), where the four electrons are successively, but quickly, reacted with an oxygen molecule, which is held in a tight cage so that partially reduced oxygen species are not released, but only water is safely formed [15]. The generation of water also consumes four protons, which are taken from the matrix side. Concomitantly, complex 4 transports four protons from the mitochondrial matrix into the intermembrane space. Therefore, the stoichiometry of the reaction catalysed by complex 4 is: 4 reduced cytochrome c (Fe^{2+}) $+ O_2 + 8 H_{in}^+ \rightarrow 4$ oxidized cytochrome c (Fe^{3+}) $+ 2 H_2O + 4 H_{out}^+$ [15].

Thus, the transfer of electrons through complexes 1, 3 and 4 of the respiratory chain is coupled with the extrusion of protons from the mitochondrial matrix into the mitochondrial intermembrane space. This creates a large electrochemical potential across the inner membrane, thus creating a reservoir of latent, potential energy (Fig. 8).

When energy is needed, the increase in ADP stimulates the re-entry of protons through ATP synthase (also called 'F_1F_0-ATPase', 'H^+-ATPase' or 'complex 5'), and the energy that is liberated by this re-entry is harnessed in the synthesis of ATP from ADP. The ATP formed is then extruded from mitochondria by the adenine nucleotide translocator in exchange for cytosolic ADP (Fig. 8). ATP is then used by all the cellular processes that require energy (e.g. maintenance of transmembrane ion gradients, anabolic syntheses, cell motility, muscular contraction).

ATP synthase is a wonderful biological engine (Fig. 10) [19,20]. Its transmembrane F_0 portion contains a non-rotating moiety consisting of the a subunits and a rotor made of a dozen or so c subunits (c-ring rotor). The re-entry of protons through a channel located at the junction of the a subunits and the c-ring triggers the rotation of the c-ring and the attached γ stalk. The γ stalk rotates within a cap made of three pairs of alternating α and β subunits ($\alpha_3\beta_3$ cap), which is kept immobile by the a/b_2/δ stator [20]. The rotating stalk is asymmetrical. When the stalk rotates within the $\alpha_3\beta_3$ cap, it causes rhythmic deformations of the catalytic β subunits, which may alternatively tighten around ADP and P_i, close to form ATP and fully open to release ATP. As there are three catalytic sites, one 360° rotation of the γ stalk gives rise to three ATP molecules [19].

Fig. 9 Current hypotheses for the flow of electrons within complex 3. (a) The classical 'Q cycle' theory postulates that complex 3 contains two sites for ubiquinone (Q) and its redox partners, the ubisemiquinone anion radical (Q·⁻) and ubiquinol (QH₂). The outside Q_o site would be close to the intermembrane space, and the inner Q_i site close to the matrix. Two successive ubiquinol molecules coming from other complexes may enter the outside Q_o site of complex 3, where each ubiquinol molecule would produce ubiquinone by releasing its two protons into the intermembrane space. In the process, ubiquinol would give one electron to the iron–sulphur protein (ISP), which then transfers this electron to cytochrome c_1, which in turn gives it to cytochrome c. The semiubiquinone anion radical formed from ubiquinol would then give its electron to cytochrome b (cyt b), thus forming ubiquinone, which would be returned to the region between complex 1 and complex 3. Concomitantly, cytochrome b would recycle the electrons that it receives at the Q_o site by sending them to the Q_i site. At this Q_i site, cytochrome b would first give one electron to Q, thus forming Q·⁻, and the next electron to Q·⁻, thus forming QH₂. The formed ubiquinol would then move to the Q_o site to be oxidized in exchange for ubiquinone coming from the Q_i site to be reduced. Thus, according to this scheme, for two ubiquinol molecules releasing their protons through their oxidation at the Q_o site, one molecule of ubiquinol would be regenerated at the Q_i site. (b) Another theory holds that ubiquinol instead donates its two electrons to cytochrome b, which then gives them to the iron sulphur protein (ISP), en route for cytochrome c_1, and cytochrome c.

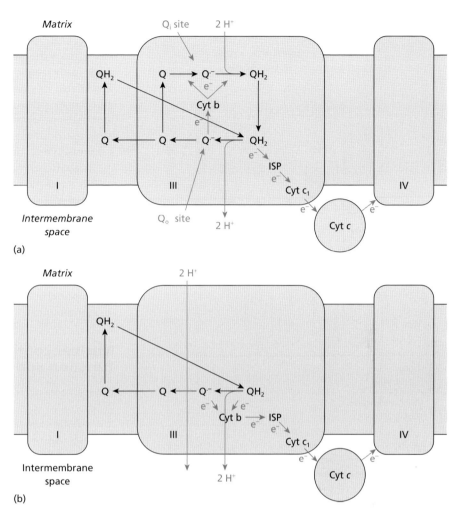

Because the driving force for ATP synthesis is the re-entry of protons, and because the flow of electrons along the respiratory chain extrudes protons at three different sites, the number of ATP molecules that can be synthesized differs with the site of electron entry into the chain. The electrons that are transferred from NADH cause the extrusion of protons at complex 1, complex 3 and complex 4 and can lead to the synthesis of about three ATP molecules for one molecule of NADH reoxidized [14]. In contrast, the electrons that are transferred by enzyme-bound FADH₂ bypass complex 1 and only permit the synthesis of about two ATP molecules for one FADH₂ reoxidized [14].

Interestingly, ATP synthase is a reversible machine. When the mitochondrial membrane potential is low, for example during ischaemia, ATP synthase functions in the reverse mode. Its ATPase activity consumes the meagre amounts of ATP formed by glycolysis to pump protons into the intermembrane space and partially to restore the mitochondrial membrane potential, which is needed to maintain mitochondrial protein import and mitochondrial viability. This ATP-depleting effect can be prevented by the binding of a matricial protein termed the inhibitor of F_1F_0-ATPase (IF₁) [21]. When the membrane potential is low (e.g. during ischaemia) and when anaerobic glycolysis causes extensive lactate formation and matrix acidification, IF₁ then binds to the F_1 moiety of ATP synthase to inhibit its ATPase activity. This attenuates the selfish use of cell ATP by deenergized mitochondria.

Except for these extreme circumstances, when mitochondria consume cell ATP for their own needs, mitochondria instead provide the cell with energy.

Regulation of fuel oxidation by energy demands

Mitochondria are thrifty organelles. They only burn fuels inasmuch as fuel oxidation is needed to satisfy the energy demands of the cell. This balance is achieved through several mechanisms, including built-in, autoregulatory mechanisms adapting fuel oxidation (and thus ATP generation) to ATP consumption.

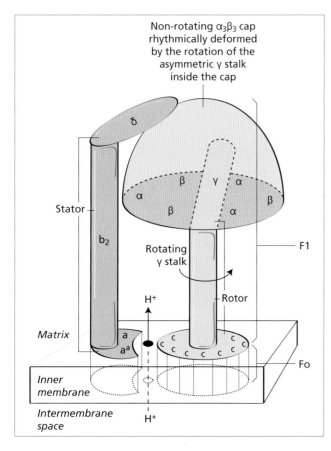

Non-rotating $\alpha_3\beta_3$ cap
rhythmically deformed
by the rotation of the
asymmetric γ stalk
inside the cap

Fig. 10 ATP synthase. The transmembrane F_0 portion of ATP synthase contains a non-rotating moiety (the a subunits) and a membrane-embedded rotor made of a dozen c subunits (the c-ring rotor). The re-entry of protons at the junction of the a subunits and the c-ring rotor triggers the rotation of the c-ring rotor and the attached γ rod, which rotates within an immobile cap made of three pairs of alternating α and β subunits ($\alpha_3\beta_3$ cap). The cap is prevented from rotating by the a/b_2/δ stator. The rotating γ stalk is asymmetrical (depicted illustratively as a bend on the figure). Its rotation within the $\alpha_3\beta_3$ cap causes rhythmic deformations of the catalytic β subunits, which may successively tighten around ADP and Pi, close to form ATP and fully open to release ATP. As there are three catalytic sites, one 360° rotation of the γ stalk produces three ATP molecules.

When energy demands are high, and ADP is high, a massive re-entry of protons into the matrix through ATP synthase decreases the mitochondrial membrane potential. This unleashes the flow of electrons in the respiratory chain, with three consequences. First, the increased flow of electrons increases the rate of proton extrusion by the respiratory chain, thus allowing the continued re-entry of protons through ATP synthase to sustain high rates of ATP generation. Second, the increased flow of electrons ends up in cytochrome c oxidase, thus increasing oxygen consumption. Finally, the increased rate of respiration is associated with an increased reoxidation of NADH and $FADH_2$ into NAD^+ and FAD, which are required to drive the oxidation of glucose, pyruvate, acyl-CoA and acetyl-CoA.

In contrast, when little energy is needed by the cell, ATP synthase is barely active and only translocates a few protons back into the matrix. The high mitochondrial membrane potential blocks the extrusion of protons into the matrix. Electrons are stuck in the respiratory chain. Oxygen consumption is low. The limited reoxidation of NADH into the NAD^+ required for mitochondrial β-oxidation and the tricarboxylic acid cycle may limit the capacity of mitochondria to oxidize fat and pyruvate. Thus, the tricarboxylic acid cycle and oxidative phosphorylation system have built-in mechanisms that automatically adapt fuel oxidation to energy consumption.

This automatic adaptation is further tuned by the regulatory effects of ATP on several critical enzymatic steps [14]. Indeed, the activities of pyruvate dehydrogenase, citrate synthase, isocitrate dehydrogenase and α-ketoglutarate dehydrogenase are modulated by ATP levels, in order to increase fuel oxidation when ATP is low and, instead, to prevent fuel oxidation when ATP is high [14].

A last level of regulation involves the effects of nuclear genes on mitochondrial function and biogenesis.

Nuclear control of mitochondrial function and biogenesis

Both mitochondrial function and mitochondrial biogenesis are controlled by nuclear genes [22]. When mitochondrial function is insufficient to sustain the cellular drain of ATP, cell ADP increases. Adenylate kinase then converts two ADP molecules into one ATP molecule and one AMP molecule [23]. The increase in AMP is sensed by AMP-activated protein kinase (AMPK), which turns off ATP-consuming pathways and switches on ATP-producing catabolic pathways [23]. In particular, AMPK phosphorylates and inactivates acetyl-CoA carboxylase, thus decreasing the synthesis of malonyl-CoA. This prevents the inhibition of CPT I by malonyl-CoA, thus allowing the translocation of long-chain fatty acyl-CoA into the mitochondria and extensive β-oxidation [23]. Finally, AMPK increases several mitochondrial oxidative enzymes, such as succinate dehydrogenase, citrate synthase and cytochrome c [24,25].

Several other factors may also modulate mitochondrial function and biogenesis in the liver, although their roles have mostly been studied in skeletal muscles, whose energy requirements vary widely with the degree of physical activity. These other factors include the Ca^{2+}/calmodulin-dependent protein kinase (CaMK), the peroxisome proliferator-activated receptor γ coactivator 1 (PGC-1) and nuclear respiratory factors 1 and 2 (NRF-1 and NRF-2). In muscles, it has been shown that CaMK induces the expression of PGC-1, which itself induces the expression of NRF-1 and NRF-2. NRF-1 and NRF-2 increase the synthesis of nuclear DNA-encoded polypeptides of the respiratory chain and also induce mtTFA [22,26]. PGC-1 binds to, and coactivates, the transcriptional function of NRF-1 on the promoter for mtTFA, which increases the transcription and replication of mtDNA [26]. Finally, PGC-1 binds to, and cooperates with, peroxisome proliferator-activated receptor-α (PPAR-α) in the transcriptional activation of nuclear genes encoding peroxisomal and mitochondrial β-oxidation enzymes, including CPT I and medium-chain acyl-CoA dehydrogenase [27]. As a consequence of these concerted actions on both nuclear genes and mtDNA genes, PGC-1 increases both the number of cardiac mitochondria and also their individual capacity to oxidize fat and to generate energy through oxidative phosphorylation [28]. Interestingly, both the AMPK- and the CaMK-mediated signals seem to act coordinately, as AMPK was required for energy deprivation-induced increases in the expression of CaMK and PGC-1 [29]. Together with the immediate regulations described in the preceding section, these nuclear changes may allow cells to increase or decrease fuel consumption depending on the energy demands of the cell.

Yet a last type of regulation concerns the different use of energetic fuels under fasted, fed or overfed conditions.

Different use of fuels by hepatic mitochondria in fasted, fed or overfed conditions (see also Chapter 13)

The handling of fuels by hepatic mitochondria is regulated in order to deliver ketone bodies and glucose to other organs when food is not available, but to store energy as glycogen and fat after meals.

In the fasting state, low insulin levels allow the massive release of free fatty acids from adipose tissue [30]. During fasting conditions, hepatic malonyl-CoA levels are low, allowing extensive mitochondrial import of long-chain free fatty acids, and thus active fatty acid β-oxidation. However, the acetyl-CoA moieties generated by hepatic mitochondrial β-oxidation are not fully oxidized in the liver, which would not be able to use this enormous amount of energy. Instead, acetyl-CoA moieties condense into ketone bodies (acetoacetate and β-hydroxybutyrate), which are secreted by the liver to be oxidized later in muscles and other peripheral tissues by the tricarboxylic acid cycle, thus sparing glucose [30]. The liver concomitantly provides other organs, such as the brain, with glucose formed from glycogen and gluconeogenesis.

In contrast, after meals, a slight increase in blood glucose increases the release of insulin by pancreatic β cells. In adipocytes, insulin inhibits hormone-sensitive lipase, thus blocking adipose tissue lipolysis. In the liver, glucose inactivates glycogen phosphorylase and activates glycogen synthetase, thus increasing glycogen stores [14]. Furthermore, both insulin and glucose trigger free fatty acid synthesis from glucose [31]. This is due to the posttranslational activation of several enzymes [14] and also to translational regulation [31]. Indeed, glucose activates carbohydrate response element binding protein (ChREBP), with two consequences. First, ChREBP stimulates liver-type pyruvate kinase, thus increasing the glycolysis of glucose into pyruvate [32]. In mitochondria, pyruvate forms acetyl-CoA, which condenses with oxaloacetate to form citrate

that translocates to the cytoplasm. Citrate lyase then catalyses the reaction: citrate + ATP + CoA + H_2O → acetyl-CoA + oxaloacetate + ADP + P_i. The acetyl-CoA, which is thus regenerated in the cytosol, is then used by acetyl-CoA carboxylase to form malonyl-CoA, which is required for the elongation of free fatty acids by fatty acid synthase. Second, ChREBP stimulates the transcription of all lipogenic genes, including acetyl-CoA carboxylase, fatty acid synthase and stearoyl-CoA desaturase, thus further increasing hepatic fatty acid and triacylglycerol synthesis [33]. Insulin cooperates with glucose in increasing fatty acid synthesis. Indeed, insulin increases the transcription of sterol regulatory element-binding protein-1c (SREBP-1c), which increases the transcriptional activation of all the enzymes required for the hepatic synthesis of fatty acids [31]. Thus, both glucose via ChREBP and insulin via SREBP-1c can increase the hepatic synthesis of free fatty acids. Furthermore, the malonyl-CoA generated by acetyl-CoA carboxylase also prevents mitochondrial β-oxidation. Malonyl-CoA inhibits CPT I, which controls the entry of long-chain fatty acids into mitochondria [30]. After a carbohydrate meal, high malonyl-CoA levels inhibit CPT I and prevent fatty acid β-oxidation [30]. Free fatty acids are not degraded, but are instead directed towards the formation of triglycerides, which are partly stored in the liver and partly secreted as very-low-density lipoproteins.

Teleologically, these various changes can be viewed as maintaining/increasing fat and glycogen stores when food is plentiful and, in contrast, using up fat and sparing glucose when food is not available. In the past, these changes have provided a satisfactory balance between energy storage and energy use, when high physical activity ensured high rates of fuel oxidation by skeletal muscle mitochondria. Nowadays, however, food intake often exceeds the limited capacity of mitochondria to burn fuels in inactive persons, causing a progressive increase in body fat stores [34].

In relatively overfed subjects, the increased hepatic synthesis of free fatty acids causes the accumulation of triglyceride droplets in the cytoplasm of hepatocytes [34]. However, the liver does not enlarge indefinitely. A new equilibrium is reached when the increased synthesis of fat is compensated by increased output pathways, including an increased mitochondrial β-oxidation of fatty acids [34]. Several adaptive changes may allow hepatic mitochondria to oxidize more fat in overfed subjects [34]. A first mechanism could be the increased hepatic concentrations of free fatty acids (FFAs) in these subjects, which may force the entry of FFAs into the mitochondria [34]. A second mechanism may involve changes in CPT I expression and its sensitivity to malonyl-CoA inhibition. CPT I is upregulated in rodent models of diabetes, and its affinity for its physiological inhibitor, malonyl-CoA, is decreased [35,36]. Loss of CPT I inhibition by malonyl-CoA could explain why β-oxidation can increase in plethoric subjects, despite high insulin and malonyl-CoA levels, which would normally block the entry of long-chain fatty acids into mitochondria [34]. An important upstream mediator of these diverse changes may be PPAR-α.

PPAR-α is activated by long-chain free fatty acids and increases the expression of enzymes involved in peroxisomal and mitochondrial β-oxidation, including CPT I [35]. PPAR-α activation also increases uncoupling protein 2 mRNA [37]. This uncoupling protein might allow the re-entry of protons from the intermembrane space into the mitochondrial matrix. This could decrease the mitochondrial membrane potential, unleash the flow of electrons in the respiratory chain, increase mitochondrial respiration and allow better reoxidation of NADH into the NAD^+ required for fatty acid oxidation.

Although these adaptive changes prevent further expansion of hepatic fat stores in overfed subjects, they do not prevent some steatosis. The unsaturated lipids of fat deposits can then be oxidized by the ROS formed by mitochondria, thus triggering lipid peroxidation and oxidative stress [34].

Formation of reactive oxygen species

The incomplete reduction of oxygen by one, two or three electrons produces ROS. The strategy devised by bacteria and mitochondria to limit ROS formation is initially to store electrons in a form (NADH or E-FADH$_2$) that is unreactive with oxygen, then to transport these electrons through a respiratory chain, which is mostly insulated from oxygen, and, finally, quickly to react four electrons with oxygen within cytochrome c oxidase to safely produce water. However, the insulation of upstream respiratory complexes from oxygen is not perfect (Fig. 11). A small fraction of the electrons that pass through complex 1 and complex 3 react with oxygen to form the superoxide anion [38]. Complex 1 releases the superoxide anion into the mitochondrial matrix, while complex 3 releases superoxide

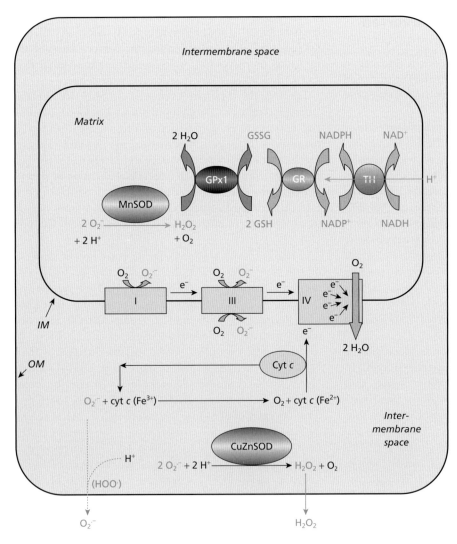

Fig. 11 Formation and inactivation of reactive oxygen species (ROS) in mitochondria. Most of the electrons that enter the respiratory chain finish in cytochrome c oxidase (complex 4), where four electrons are added quickly and in a tight cage to oxygen, so that ROS are not released, but only water is safely formed. However, upstream to complex 4, a few of the electrons donated to the respiratory chain react with oxygen to form the superoxide anion radical ($O_2 \cdot^-$). Complex 1 generates $O_2 \cdot^-$ on the matrix side. Complex 3 forms $O_2 \cdot^-$ both in the matrix and in the intermembrane space. In the matrix, manganese superoxide dismutase (MnSOD) dismutates two molecules of the superoxide anion into one oxygen molecule and one molecule of hydrogen peroxide (H_2O_2). Glutathione peroxidase 1 (GPx1) then reduces H_2O_2 into water while oxidizing two reduced glutathione (GSH) molecules into glutathione disulphide (GSSG). Glutathione reductase (GR) then regenerates GSH at the expense of NADPH. Finally, an energy-linked NAD(P)$^+$ transhydrogenase (TH) uses NADH and the mitochondrial membrane potential to regenerate NADPH from NADP$^+$. In the intermembrane space, the superoxide anion is detoxified by its reaction with oxidized (ferric) cytochrome c to form reduced (ferrous) cytochrome c, which donates its electron to complex 4 of the respiratory chain, thus regenerating oxidized cytochrome c. Although copper zinc superoxide dismutase (CuZnSOD) is mostly cytosolic, it is also imported into the intermembrane space of mitochondria, where it dismutates $O_2 \cdot^-$ into H_2O_2. Although most of the ROS formed by mitochondria are detoxified within mitochondria, some molecules of H_2O_2 can cross the outer membrane. In the acidic intermembrane space, $O_2 \cdot^-$ may be protonated to the uncharged, hydroperoxyl radical (HO$_2 \cdot$), which may also cross the outer membrane to regenerate $O_2 \cdot^-$ in the cytosol. IM, inner membrane; OM, outer membrane.

into both the mitochondrial matrix and the intermembrane space (Fig. 11) [38]. Other possible site(s) for superoxide formation may be ETF (electron transfer protein) and/or ETF:QO (ETF:quinone oxidoreductase) [38]. Superoxide generation by ETF and/or ETF:QO has been proposed as one possible explanation for the higher formation of superoxide when muscle mitochondria are energized with palmitoyl carnitine than with complex 1 substrates [38]. Overall, it is estimated that 1–2% of the oxygen consumed by mitochondria may be transformed into the superoxide anion, and that mitochondria represent the most important source of ROS in cells [39].

Being unable to completely prevent ROS formation, mitochondria have devised several systems to eliminate these ROS (Fig. 11). In particular, the superoxide radical anion is dismutated by mitochondrial manganese superoxide dismutase into hydrogen peroxide, which is detoxified into water by mitochondrial glutathione peroxidase 1 (Fig. 11) [39].

Nevertheless, residual levels of ROS can impair mitochondrial structure and function. The superoxide anion can remove one iron molecule from the cubane (4Fe–4S) cluster of mitochondrial aconitase, thus inactivating aconitase and hampering fuel oxidation in the tricarboxylic acid cycle [40]. ROS can also damage mitochondrial proteins, cardiolipin and mtDNA, thus progressively impairing mitochondrial function [41]. In some pathological conditions, a very large formation of mitochondrial ROS can trigger, or can help to trigger, mitochondrial permeability transition, which irreversibly disables mitochondria and leads to their autophagic degradation [42].

Finally, some molecules of hydrogen peroxide and possibly also of the superoxide anion (the latter probably crossing the membrane as the hydroperoxyl radical) may leak out of mitochondria [43,44] and may eventually damage extramitochondrial cell constituents, such as nuclear DNA. However, mitochondrial constituents, including mtDNA, are the main targets of mitochondrial ROS.

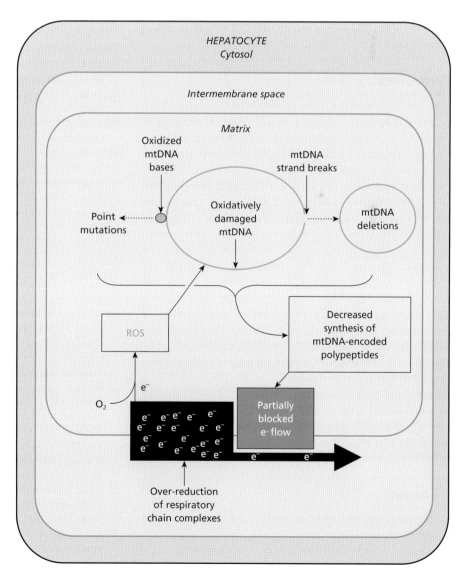

Fig. 12 Ageing of mtDNA. Reactive oxygen species (ROS) formed by the mitochondrial respiratory chain damage mtDNA. They form oxidized mtDNA bases, which may occasionally cause point mutations, and they also form mtDNA strand breaks, which may occasionally cause mtDNA deletions. Eventually, these mtDNA lesions and mutations may decrease the synthesis of mtDNA-encoded polypeptides, thus partially hampering the flow of electrons in the respiratory chain. In the overly reduced complex 1 and complex 3, the accumulated electrons may increasingly react with oxygen to form the superoxide anion radical. The increased ROS formation may further damage mtDNA. This vicious cycle, together with a decreased import of DNA repair enzymes as a consequence of the decreased membrane potential, could explain why mtDNA deletions and point mutations, which are exceptional before 40 years of age, then start to accumulate exponentially during old age.

Ageing of mitochondrial DNA

Mitochondrial ROS play an important role in the ageing process (Fig. 12). ROS oxidize mtDNA bases to form, in particular, 8-oxo-deoxyguanosine. During mtDNA replication, this modified guanine can mispair with an adenine (instead of a cytosine), and this mispairing can cause mtDNA point mutations. ROS also cause mtDNA strand breaks, which can occasionally lead to mtDNA deletions.

As these mutations accumulate over the years, they may eventually decrease the synthesis of mtDNA-encoded polypeptides, thus partially blocking the flow of electrons in the respiratory chain (Fig. 12). The over-reduction of upstream respiratory complexes may then increase mitochondrial ROS formation. Furthermore, as the mitochondrial membrane potential decreases, the membrane potential-driven import of DNA repair enzymes from the cytosol into the mitochondrial matrix may become impaired [45]. Thus, both increased mtDNA damage (due to the increased mitochondrial ROS formation) and decreased mtDNA repair (due to decreased import of repair enzymes) could explain why mtDNA deletions and point mutations increase exponentially during old age [46,47].

Overview

When photosynthesizing cyanobacteria began releasing oxygen in the atmosphere, bacteria took advantage of their quick turnover, and the high mutation rate caused by oxygen-derived ROS, to mutate and adapt to the oxygen environment. They developed truly wonderful biochemical machines, enabling them first to survive and then to thrive with energy in the new oxygen environment. Instead of trying to emulate the biochemical perfection of bacteria, other forms of life have associated with them. Assisted and controlled by nuclear genes, our mitochondrial partners oxidize or save fuels as needed, just to provide cells with the exact amount of energy they need.

However, as in all partnerships, there is some hardship. We are totally dependent on mitochondria, so that their failure is also a significant threat to health. Inborn defects, drugs or cytokines that impair mitochondrial function can cause steatosis, cell dysfunction or cell death. Furthermore, although mitochondria provide energy, they also form reactive oxygen species that contribute to ageing and death.

Death and reproduction have permitted the slow selection and adaptation of the host, providing mitochondria with an ever-adapting environment. While new species of the host have arisen and then become extinct, the mitochondrial clones have endured.

References

1 Floyd RA (1990) Role of oxygen free radicals in carcinogenesis and brain ischemia. *FASEB J* 4, 2587–2597.

2 McCord JM (2000) The evolution of free radicals and oxidative stress. *Am J Med* 108, 652–659.

3 Yang D, Oyaizu Y, Oyaizu H *et al.* (1985) Mitochondrial origins. *Proc Natl Acad Sci USA* 82, 4443–4447.

4 Taanman JW (1999) The mitochondrial genome: structure, transcription, translation and replication. *Biochim Biophys Acta* 1410, 103–123.

5 Sutovsky P, Moreno RD, Ramalho-Santos J *et al.* (1999) Ubiquitin tag for sperm mitochondria. *Nature* 402, 371–372.

6 Mourier T, Hansen AJ, Willerslev E *et al.* (2001) The human genome projects reveals a continuous transfer of large mitochondrial fragments to the nucleus. *Mol Biol Evol* 18, 1833–1837.

7 Croteau DL, Stierum RB, Bohr VA (1999) Mitochondrial DNA repair pathways. *Mutat Res* 434, 137–148.

8 LeDoux SP, Driggers WJ, Hollensworth S *et al.* (1999) Repair of alkylation and oxidative damage in mitochondrial DNA. *Mutat Res* 434, 149–159.

9 Rehling P, Brandner K, Pfanner N (2004) Mitochondrial import and the twin-pore translocase. *Nature Rev* 5, 519–530.

10 Mukhopadhyay A, Ni L, Weiner H (2004) A co-translational model to explain the in vivo import of proteins into Hela cell mitochondria. *Biochem J* 382, 385–392.

11 Bartlett K, Eaton S (2004) Mitochondrial β-oxidation. *Eur J Biochem* 271, 462–469.

12 Liang X, Le W, Zhang D *et al.* (2001) Impact of the mitochondrial enzyme organization on fatty acid oxidation. *Biochem Soc Trans* 29, 279–282.

13 Eaton S (2002) Control of mitochondrial β-oxidation flux. *Prog Lipid Res* 41, 197–239.

14 Stryer L (1988) *Biochemistry*, 3rd edn. New York: W.H. Freeman and Co.

15 Saraste M (1999) Oxidative phosphorylation at the *fin de siècle*. *Science* 283, 1488–1493.

16 Friedrich T, Bottcher B (2004) The gross structure of the respiratory complex I: a Lego System. *Biochim Biophys Acta* 1608, 1–9.

17 Trumpower BL (1990) The protonmotive Q cycle. Energy transduction by coupling of proton translocation to electron transfer by the cytochrome bc1 complex. *J Biol Chem* 265, 11409–11412.

18 Matsumo-Yagi A, Hatefi Y (2001) Ubiquinol:cytochrome *c* oxidoreductase (Complex III). Effects of inhibitors on cytochrome b reduction in submitochondrial particles and the role of ubiquinone in complex III. *J Biol Chem* 276, 19006–19011.

19 Boyer PD (1999) What makes ATP synthase spin? *Nature* 402, 247–249.

20 Capaldi RA, Aggeler R (2002) Mechanism of the F_1F_0-type ATP synthase, a biological rotary motor. *Trends Biochem Sci* 27, 154–160.

21 Cabezón E, Montgomery MG, Leslie AG *et al.* (2003) The structure of bovine F1-ATPase in complex with its regulatory protein IF1. *Nat Struct Biol* 10, 744–750.

22 Scarpulla RC (1997) Nuclear control of respiratory chain expression in mammalian cells. *J Bioenerget Biomembr* 29, 109–119.

23 Frøsig C, Jørgensen SB, Hardie DG *et al.* (2004) 5′-AMP-activated protein kinase activity and protein expression are regulated by endurance training in human skeletal muscle. *Am J Physiol Endocrinol Metab* 286, E411–417.

24 Winder WW, Holmes BF, Rubink DS *et al.* (2000) Activation of AMP-activated protein kinase increases mitochondrial enzymes in skeletal muscle. *J Appl Physiol* 88, 2219–2226.

25 Ojuka EO (2004) Role of calcium and AMP kinase in the regulation of mitochondrial biogenesis and GLUT4 levels in muscle. *Proc Nutr Soc* 63, 275–278.

26 Wu H, Kanatous SB, Thurmond FA *et al.* (2002) Regulation of mitochondrial biogenesis in skeletal muscle by CaMK. *Science* 296, 349–352.

27 Vega RB, Huss JM, Kelly DP (2000) The coactivator PGC-1 cooperates with peroxisome proliferator-activated receptor α in the transcriptional control of nuclear genes encoding mitochondrial fatty acid oxidation enzymes. *Mol Cell Biol* 20, 1868–1876.

28 Lehman JJ, Barger PM, Kovacs A *et al.* (2000) Peroxisome proliferator-activated receptor γ coactivator-1 promotes cardiac mitochondrial biogenesis. *J Clin Invest* 106, 847–856.

29 Zong H, Ren JM, Young LH *et al.* (2002) AMP kinase is required for mitochondrial biogenesis in response to chronic energy deprivation. *Proc Natl Acad Sci USA* 25, 15983–15987.

30 McGarry JD, Foster DW (1980) Regulation of hepatic fatty acid oxidation and ketone body production. *Annu Rev Biochem* 49, 395–420.

31 Browning JD, Horton JD (2004) Molecular mediators of hepatic steatosis and liver injury. *J Clin Invest* 114, 147–152.

32 Yamashita H, Takenoshita M, Sakurai M *et al.* (2001) A glucose-responsive transcription factor that regulates carbohydrate metabolism in the liver. *Proc Natl Acad Sci USA* 98, 9116–9121.

33 Lizuka K, Bruick RK, Liang G *et al.* (2004) Deficiency of carbohydrate response element binding protein (ChREBP) reduces lipogenesis as well as glycolysis. *Proc Natl Acad Sci USA* 101, 7281–7286.

34 Pessayre D, Fromenty B (2005) NASH: a mitochondrial disease. *J Hepatol* 42, 928–940.

35 Brady LJ, Brady PS, Rosmos DR (1985) Elevated hepatic mitochondrial and peroxisomal oxidative capacities in fed and starved adult obese (ob/ob) mice. *Biochem J* 231, 439–444.

36 Cook J, Gamble MSV (1987) Regulation of carnitine palmitoyl transferase by insulin results in decreased activity and decreased apparent Ki values for malonyl CoA. *J Biol Chem* 262, 2050–2055.

37 Chavin KD, Yang SQ, Lin HZ *et al.* (1999) Obesity induces expression of uncoupling protein-2 in hepatocytes and promotes liver ATP depletion. *J Biol Chem* 274, 5692–5700.

38 St-Pierre J, Buckingham JA, Roebuck SJ *et al.* (2002) Topology of superoxide production from different sites in the mitochondrial electron transport chain. *J Biol Chem* 277, 44784–44790.

39 Kowaltowski AJ, Vercesi AE (2001) Reactive oxygen generation by mitochondria. In: Lemasters JJ, Nieminen AL (eds) *Mitochondria in Pathogenesis*. New York: Kluwer Academic/Plenum Publishers, pp. 281–300.

40 Walden WE (2002) From bacteria to mitochondria: aconitase yields surprises. *Proc Natl Acad Sci USA* 99, 4138–4140.

41 Demeilliers C, Maisonneuve C, Grodet A *et al.* (2002) Impaired adaptive resynthesis and prolonged depletion of hepatic mitochondrial DNA after repeated alcohol binges in mice. *Gastroenterology* 123, 1278–1290.

42 Elmore SP, Qian T, Grissom SF *et al.* (2001) The mitochondrial permeability transition initiates autophagy in rat hepatocytes. *FASEB J* 15, 2286–2287.

43 De Grey ADNJ (2002) HO$_2$: the forgotten radical. *DNA Cell Biol* 21, 251–257.

44 Wallace MA, Liou LL, Martins J *et al.* (2004) Superoxide inhibits 4Fe-4S cluster enzymes involved in amino acid biosynthesis. Cross-compartment protection by CuZn-superoxide dismutase. *J Biol Chem* 279, 32055–32062.

45 Szczesny B, Hazra TK, Papaconstantinou J *et al.* (2003) Age-dependent deficiency in import of mitochondrial DNA glycosylases required for repair of oxidatively damaged bases. *Proc Natl Acad Sci USA* 100, 10670–10675.

46 Cortopassi GA, Shibata D, Soong NW *et al.* (1992) A pattern of accumulation of a somatic deletion of mitochondrial DNA in aging human tissues. *Proc Natl Acad Sci USA* 89, 7370–7374.

47 Wang Y, Michikawa Y, Mallidis C *et al.* (2001) Muscle-specific mutations accumulate with aging in critical human mtDNA control sites for replication. *Proc Natl Acad Sci USA* 98, 4022–4027.

2.3.5 Bilirubin metabolism

Namita Roy-Chowdhury, Yang Lu and Jayanta Roy-Chowdhury

Bilirubin in medical history

Bilirubin has attracted the attention of physicians since antiquity. Its chemistry, metabolism and disposal have been studied systematically during the last two centuries as a model for hepatic disposal of biologically important organic anions of limited aqueous solubility [1]. The discovery of several inherited disorders of bilirubin metabolism and excretion during the twentieth century has led to renewed interest in inherited diseases associated with jaundice, some of which continue to pose a therapeutic challenge, providing impetus for further research. While physicians are mainly concerned with the toxic effect of bilirubin and its importance as a liver function test, the antioxidant property of bilirubin may provide a physiological defence against oxidative injury.

Formation of bilirubin

Sources of bilirubin

Bilirubin is the breakdown product of the haem moiety of haemoglobin, other haemoproteins, such as cytochromes, catalase, peroxidase and tryptophan pyrrolase, and a small pool of free haem. In humans, 250–400 mg of bilirubin is produced daily, of which approximately 20% is produced from non-haemoglobin sources [2]. Following the injection of radio-labelled porphyrin precursors (glycine or δ-aminolaevulinic acid), an 'early-labelled peak' of bilirubin (ELP) is excreted in bile within 72 h [3]. The initial component of ELP is derived mainly from hepatic haemoproteins. This is followed by a slower component, derived from both erythroid and non-erythroid sources, which becomes prominent in conditions associated with 'ineffective erythropoiesis', e.g. congenital dyserythropoietic anaemias, megaloblastic anaemias, iron-deficiency anaemia, erythropoietic porphyria and lead poisoning [4], and in accelerated erythropoiesis [5]. The 'late-labelled peak' appears at approximately 110 days in humans and coincides with the half-life of erythrocytes.

Enzymatic mechanism of bilirubin formation

The microsomal haem oxygenase (HO) enzymes catalyse the oxidation of haem (Fig. 1). Three molecules of O_2 are consumed

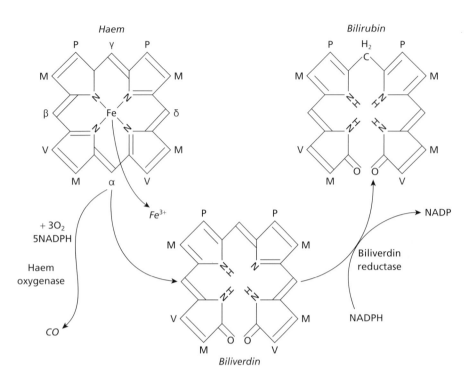

Fig. 1 Enzyme-catalysed degradation of haem. Haem degradation begins by haem oxygenase-catalysed oxidation of the α-bridge carbon of haem, which is converted to CO, leading to opening of the tetrapyrrole ring and release of the iron molecule. The resulting biliverdin molecule is subsequently reduced to bilirubin by cytosolic biliverdin reductase.

in this reaction and a reducing agent, such as nicotinamide adenine dinucleotide phosphate hydrogenase (NADPH), is needed. The α-methene bridge carbon is eliminated as CO and the iron molecule is released [6]. Of the three forms of HO, HO-1 is ubiquitous and inducible by haem [8] and stress [7]; HO-2 is a constitutive protein, expressed mainly in the brain and the testis. The catalytic activity of HO-3 is low, and this protein may function mainly as a haem binding protein. CO produced by HO activity has a vasodilatory effect and regulates the vascular tone in the liver, heart and other organs during stress. Similarly, biliverdin and its product bilirubin are potent antioxidants, which may protect tissues under oxidative stress [7,9] (see below).

Biliverdin is reduced to bilirubin by the action of cytosolic biliverdin reductases, which require NADH or NADPH for activity [10]. As discussed later, bilirubin requires energy-consuming metabolic steps for excretion in bile. Thus, the physiological advantage of its formation is not clear. The strong antioxidant activity of bilirubin may be particularly important during the neonatal period, when other antioxidants are scarce in body fluids.

Measurement of bilirubin production

Bilirubin production can be quantified from the turnover of intravenously administered radioisotopically labelled bilirubin. Plasma bilirubin clearance is proportional to the reciprocal of the area under the radiobilirubin disappearance curve [11]. Bilirubin removal is calculated as the product of plasma bilirubin concentration and clearance. At a steady state of plasma bilirubin concentration, bilirubin removal equals bilirubin production. More conveniently, bilirubin formation can be quantified from CO, which is generated in equimolar amounts with bilirubin. Following rebreathing in a closed system, CO production is calculated from the CO concentration in the rebreathing mask and/or the increment in blood carboxy-haemoglobin saturation [12]. A small fraction of the CO may be formed by intestinal bacteria, which can be a significant source of CO in intestinal bacterial overgrowth syndromes [13].

Inhibition of bilirubin production

Substances, such as tin-protoporphyrin and tin-mesoporphyrin, that bind irreversibly to HO, but are not broken down, serve as 'dead-end' inhibitors of the enzyme and reduce bilirubin production [14]. Injection of tin-mesoporphyrin lowers serum bilirubin levels by 76% in neonates [15].

Chemical characteristics of bilirubin

The tetrapyrrole structure of bilirubin IXα (1,8-dioxo-1,3,6,7-tetramethyl-2,8-divinylbiladiene-a,c-dipropionic acid [17]) was solved by Fischer and Plieninger [18]. X-ray crystallography has revealed that the propionic acid side-chains of bilirubin form hydrogen bonds with the pyrrolic and lactam sites on the opposite half of the molecule, giving rise to a distorted 'ridge tile' structure [19] (Fig. 2). Formation of hydrogen bonds requires the interpyrrolic bridges at the 5 and 15 position of bilirubin to be in *trans* or 'Z' configuration, whereby bilirubin is termed bilirubin IXα-ZZ. Engagement of all polar groups (two propionic acid carboxyls, four NH groups and two lactam oxygens) of bilirubin by the hydrogen bonds makes the molecule insoluble

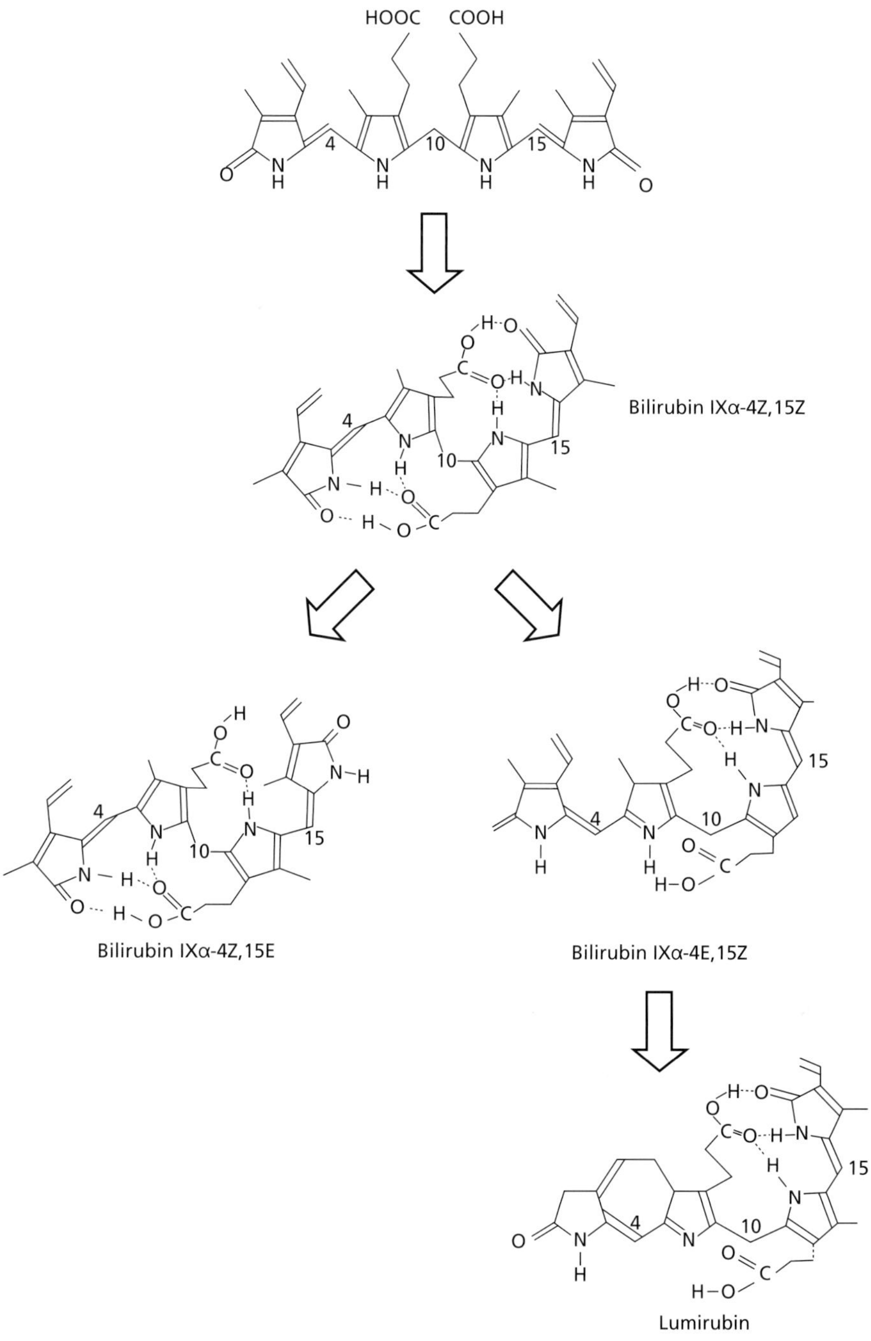

Fig. 2 Internal hydrogen bonding and photoisomerization of bilirubin. The carboxylic acid moiety of the propionic acid side-chains of bilirubin form internal hydrogen bonds with contralateral NH groups and the lactam oxygen, thereby engaging all polar groups of the molecule and making it insoluble in water. Upon exposure to light, configurational changes (Z to E) occur at the C4 and C15 interpyrrolic bridges, disrupting the hydrogen bonds. The bilirubin IXα-4E,15Z configurational isomer can be cyclized forming the so-called lumirubin. These configurational and geometric isomers are more polar than the hydrogen-bonded bilirubin IXα-4Z,15Z and are excreted in bile without requiring glucuronidation.

in water, necessitating chemical modification for excretion in bile. Disruption of the hydrogen bonds is accomplished *in vivo* by enzyme-catalysed esterification of the propionic acid carboxyl groups with a glycosyl moiety, mainly glucuronic acid (*vide infra*).

The hydrogen bonds 'bury' the central methane bridge, so that the unconjugated bilirubin reacts very slowly with diazo reagents, whereas bilirubin glucuronides, which lack hydrogen bonds, react rapidly ('direct' van den Bergh reaction). The addition of 'accelerators' such as methanol, ethanol, 6 M urea or

dimethyl sulphoxide to plasma disrupts the hydrogen bonds of bilirubin, so that both conjugated and unconjugated bilirubin react rapidly with diazo reagents ('total' van den Bergh reaction).

Bilirubin glucuronides in normal bile are 1-O-acyl conjugates linked to the propionic acid carboxyl of bilirubin in a β-D-ester linkage, which is hydrolysable by β-glucuronidase. However, during cholestasis, the migration of the 1-O-acyl bond from the C1 position to the C2, C3 or C4 position results in the generation of β-glucuronidase-resistant pigments [20], which are detectable in serum and bile by chromatographic analysis [21].

In cases of prolonged accumulation of conjugated bilirubin in plasma, as in cases of cholestasis or Dubin–Johnson syndrome, the pigment may become covalently bound to albumin [22]. This irreversibly protein-bound form, often termed delta-bilirubin, is included in the 'direct' fraction of bilirubin and is not eliminated in the bile or urine, which results in delayed clearance even after biliary obstruction or cholestasis is resolved.

Effect of light

The main absorption band of unconjugated bilirubin IXα is at 450–474 nm in most organic solvents. Upon exposure to light, the 'Z' (trans) configuration of the 5 and/or 15 carbon bridges of bilirubin switches to the 'E' (cis) configuration. The resulting configurational isomers, ZE, EZ or EE, lack internal hydrogen bonds, are more polar than bilirubin IXα-ZZ and can be excreted in bile without conjugation [23]. The non-hydrogen-bonded molecule can be stabilized slowly by cyclization of the vinyl substituent in the endovinyl half of bilirubin IXα-EZ with the methyl substituent on the internal pyrrole ring, forming the stable structural isomer, E-cyclobilirubin. Because of its stability, this molecule is quantitatively important during photo-therapy for neonatal jaundice [24]. Light and oxygen can also degrade a fraction of the bilirubin molecules into colourless fragments and biliverdin [25].

Quantification of bilirubin

Bile pigments can be quantified as native or derivatized tetrapyrroles, or after conversion to azoderivatives. Conversion to azodipyrroles by reaction with diazo reagents is the most common method of measuring serum bilirubin levels in clinical laboratories. Electrophilic attack on the central bridge splits bilirubin into two diazotized azodipyrrole molecules. As discussed above, conjugated bilirubin reacts rapidly ('direct' fraction), while total bilirubin is determined after adding an accelerator. Unconjugated bilirubin is calculated by subtracting the direct fraction from total bilirubin. As 10–15% of unconjugated bilirubin may give a 'direct' diazo reaction, this method slightly overestimates conjugated bilirubin.

Bilirubin and its conjugates in serum or bile can be quantified more accurately as intact bilirubin tetrapyrroles by high-pressure liquid chromatography [26–28]. Bilirubin mono- and diconjugates can be converted to methyl esters by alkaline methanolysis prior to separation [29] but, because the sugar groups are cleaved off, this method does not permit identification of specific conjugates.

For repeated bilirubin measurements in jaundiced infants, as an extension of clinical evaluation of jaundice, bilirubin levels can be assessed by measurement of the intensity of yellow discoloration of the skin using a special reflectance photometer [30]. Two slide tests (Ektachem) are available for determination of total bilirubin and the unconjugated, conjugated and irreversibly protein-bound fractions.

Bilirubin toxicity

Unconjugated bilirubin is toxic to many cell types, intracellular organelles and physiological processes. Bilirubin inhibits DNA synthesis [31] and ATPase activity of brain mitochondria [32], and uncouples oxidative phosphorylation. It has been reported to inhibit Ca^{2+}-activated, phospholipid-dependent protein kinase C activity and cAMP-dependent protein kinase activity [33]. Which of these toxic effects is the predominant cause of bilirubin encephalopathy remains unclear at this time. Clinically, toxic effects of bilirubin, particularly on the brain, are seen in neonates and patients with severe inherited deficiency of bilirubin conjugation. Yellow discoloration of the hippocampus, basal ganglia and nuclei of the cerebellum and brain stem, found in infants with acute bilirubin encephalopathy, is termed kernicterus. Such discoloration is not found in patients with chronic encephalopathy, in whom focal necrosis of neurons and glia is seen [34].

As all toxic effects of bilirubin are abrogated by tight binding to albumin, cerebral toxicity is usually seen when there is a molar excess of bilirubin over albumin in plasma. At serum-unconjugated bilirubin concentrations over 20 mg/dL, newborn babies are at risk of kernicterus. However, kernicterus can occur at lower concentrations in the presence of substances such as sulphonamides, radiographic contrast dyes and coumarin, which inhibit albumin–bilirubin binding by competitive or allosteric displacement [35,36]. Although immaturity of the blood–brain barrier in neonates has been implicated in the increased susceptibility of neonates to kernicterus, evidence to support this concept is insufficient. Normally, bilirubin entering the brain is cleared rapidly, but the pigment may bind to damaged and oedematous brain inhibiting its clearance, thereby increasing the susceptibility to bilirubin encephalopathy [37].

Potential beneficial effects of products of haem breakdown

Although clinicians are mainly concerned with the importance of bilirubin levels as a marker of liver disease and with the toxic effects of the pigment, biliverdin and bilirubin may exert some beneficial effects by virtue of their strong antioxidant properties. This may be relevant during the newborn period, when the level of other natural antioxidants is low. Bilirubin, which is toxic to neuronal cells at high concentrations, has been reported to have cytoprotective activity at lower concentrations. An inverse relationship between serum bilirubin levels and risk of ischaemic coronary artery disease has been observed [38], although whether such a protective effect extends to subjects with Gilbert syndrome is questionable [39]. Study of a large number of subjects in the United States has shown that the odds ratio for colorectal cancer is reduced to 0.295 in men and 0.186 in women per 1 mg/dL increment in serum bilirubin levels [40]. Similarly, a previous large study showed an inverse relationship between serum bilirubin levels and cancer mortality in a Belgian population [41]. However, such associations do not conclusively prove a causative role for bilirubin, because possible confounding variables may exist.

Bilirubin in body fluids

About 4% of bilirubin in normal plasma is conjugated, but the clinical diazo-based methods overexpress this fraction (see above). In haemolytic jaundice, there is a proportional increase in plasma-unconjugated and -conjugated bilirubin. In contrast, in inherited disorders of bilirubin conjugation, the conjugated bilirubin is absent or reduced in proportion. In biliary obstruction or hepatocellular diseases, both conjugated and unconjugated bilirubin accumulate in plasma. Bilirubin is present in exudates and other albumin-containing body fluids and binds to the elastic tissue of skin and sclera. Haem in subcutaneous haematomas is sequentially converted to biliverdin and bilirubin, resulting in a transition from green to yellow discoloration. Because of tight binding to albumin, unconjugated bilirubin is not excreted in urine in the absence of albuminuria, but conjugated bilirubin, which is less strongly bound to albumin, appears in urine. Bilirubin is present in normal human bile predominantly as diglucuronide, with bilirubin monoglucuronide and unconjugated bilirubin accounting for less than 10% and 1–4% of the pigments respectively. In the presence of reduced bilirubin glucuronidating capacity of the liver, as in Gilbert syndrome and Crigler–Najjar syndrome type 2 (see Chapter 16.6), the proportion of bilirubin monoglucuronide increases to 30% or above. In addition to the glucuronides, small amounts of glucosyl, xylosyl and mixed conjugates of bilirubin are found in human bile.

Disposition of bilirubin

Disposition of bilirubin by hepatocytes comprises several specific steps, including transport of bilirubin to hepatocytes from sites of production, uptake by and storage within hepatocytes, enzyme-catalysed conjugation with glucuronic acid, active transport into the bile canaliculus and degradation in the intestinal tract. These steps are summarized in Figure 3 and discussed briefly below.

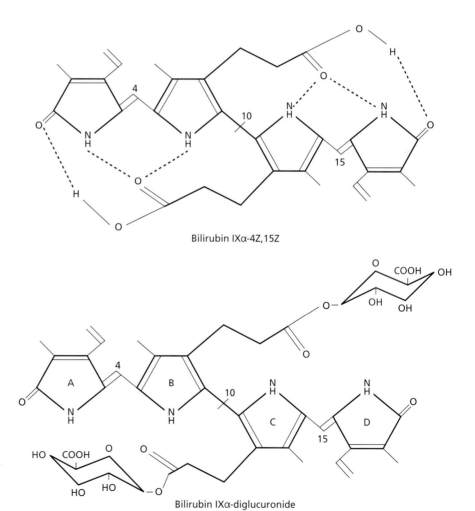

Bilirubin IXα-4Z,15Z

Bilirubin IXα-diglucuronide

Fig. 3 Glucuronidation disrupts internal hydrogen bonding of bilirubin. Glucuronidation of the propionic acid carboxyl groups results in disruption of the internal hydrogen bonds, making the molecule more polar and secretable in bile. Disruption of hydrogen bonding exposes the central CHH bridge to diazo reagents, whereby bilirubin glucuronides give the direct van den Bergh reaction.

Transport in plasma

Unconjugated bilirubin circulates in plasma bound tightly but reversibly to albumin, which prevents its excretion in urine, except during albuminuria. Albumin binding keeps bilirubin in solution and abrogates its toxic effects. Conjugated bilirubin is bound less tightly to albumin, and the unbound fraction is excreted in the urine. As mentioned above, during prolonged conjugated hyperbilirubinaemia, a fraction of conjugated bilirubin becomes irreversibly bound to albumin. This fraction, termed delta-bilirubin, is not excreted in the bile or urine and disappears slowly, reflecting the long half-life of albumin [22]. A small unbound fraction of unconjugated bilirubin is thought to be responsible for its toxicity [42]. Albumin has one high-affinity primary binding site for bilirubin. Additional sites are occupied when bilirubin is in molar excess. Normal plasma concentration of albumin (500–700 µmol/L) exceeds that of bilirubin (3–17 µmol/L). However, during exaggerated neonatal jaundice and in patients with Crigler–Najjar syndrome, the molar concentration of unconjugated bilirubin may exceed that of albumin. Hypoalbuminaemia resulting from inflammatory states, chronic malnutrition or liver disease may precipitate bilirubin toxicity. Sulphonamides, anti-inflammatory drugs, cholecystographic contrast media, fusidic acid, azapropazone, sodium caprylate and N-acetyl tryptophan displace bilirubin from albumin and increase the risk of kernicterus in jaundiced infants [43]. Binding of short-chain fatty acids to albumin causes conformational changes, decreasing bilirubin binding. Because of its pathophysiological importance, various methods have been devised to measure the unbound fraction of bilirubin and the reserve albumin binding capacity. These include ultrafiltration, ultracentrifugation, gel chromatography, affinity chromatography on albumin agarose polymers, dialysis and electrophoresis. Rapid degradation of unbound bilirubin by H_2O_2 and horseradish peroxidase has been used to distinguish it from the bound fraction.

Uptake by hepatocytes

At the sinusoidal surface of the hepatocyte (Fig. 4), bilirubin dissociates from albumin and is taken up by the hepatocyte by facilitated diffusion that requires inorganic anions, such as Cl^-. The protein(s) involved in sinusoidal bilirubin uptake have not been identified. A member of the organic anion transport protein family, termed OATP2 (also termed SLC21A6), has been proposed as the sinusoidal bilirubin transporter [44], but its importance in bilirubin transport has been questioned [45].

Storage within the liver cell

After entering the hepatocyte, bilirubin binds to the major cytosolic proteins, glutathione-S-transferases (GSTs, formerly designated ligandin or Y-protein). The GST proteins, which constitute 5% of the liver cytosol, bind various drugs, hormones, organic anions [46], a cortisol metabolite [47] and azo-dye carcinogens [48]. Bilirubin is a ligand for GSTs, but not a substrate for glutathione transfer. Binding to GSTs reduces the efflux of bilirubin from hepatocytes, thereby increasing its net uptake (Fig. 4). GST binding inhibits non-specific diffusion of bilirubin into various subcellular compartments, thereby preventing specific organellar toxicity, such as inhibition of mitochondrial respiration by bilirubin that is seen *in vitro* [49].

Conjugation of bilirubin

Conversion of unconjugated bilirubin to bilirubin diglucuronide or monoglucuronide by esterification of both or one of the propionic acid carboxyl groups is critical for efficient biliary excretion of bilirubin (Fig. 4).

Bilirubin uridine diphosphoglucuronate glucuronosyltransferase

Bilirubin is one of the many endogenous and exogenous substrates whose conjugation with glucuronic acid is mediated by one or more isoform of uridine diphosphoglucuronate glucuronosyltransferase (UGTs). UGTs are enzymes concentrated in the endoplasmic reticulum (ER) and nuclear envelope of many cell types [50]. They catalyse the transfer of the glucuronic acid moiety of UDP-glucuronic acid to the aglycone substrates, forming polar and usually less bioreactive products. Bilirubin glucuronidation is catalysed predominantly by a single UGT isoform, UGT1A1 [51]. The UGT superfamily of genes comprises two major families, UGT1 and UGT2. Nine isoforms within the UGT1A subfamily are expressed from a series of exons clustered in a unique manner on chromosome 2 at the 2q37 region [61]. Four consecutive exons (exons 2–5) located at the 3′ end of the UGT1A locus are used in nine different mRNAs. These encode the identical carboxy-terminal domains of these UGT isoforms, which contain the UDP-glucuronic acid binding site. Upstream of these four common region exons is a series of unique exons, each preceded by a separate promoter. Only one of these exons is utilized in a specific UGT mRNA. The unique exon encodes the variable N-terminal domain of the nine different UGT isoforms that impart aglycone specificity to the individual isoforms. Depending on which promoter is used, transcripts of various lengths are generated. In all cases, the unique exon, located at the 5′ end of the transcript, is spliced to exon 2, and the intervening sequence is spliced out. The genes are named according to the unique first exon. Thus, UGT1A1 utilizes the unique exon 1A1, UGT1A6 utilizes exon 1A6, etc. [53].

The presence of a separate promoter upstream from each unique region exon permits differential regulation of individual UGT isoforms during development and in response to inducing agents. UGT1A1 is expressed after birth [54] and is induced by phenobarbital and clofibrate [55]. Delayed expression of UGT1A1 is a major cause of neonatal hyperbilirubinaemia in primates. Treatment of rats with triiodothyronine markedly

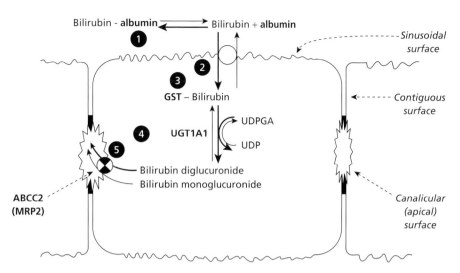

Fig. 4 Bilirubin throughput by hepatocytes. Bilirubin is transported from sites of production to hepatic sinusoids bound to albumin (1). At the sinusoidal surface of hepatocytes, bilirubin dissociates from albumin and enters hepatocytes by facilitated diffusion (2). Binding to cytosolic glutathione-*S*-transferases (GSTs) increases net uptake of bilirubin by inhibiting its efflux (3). Bilirubin is converted to mono- and diglucuronide by the action of UGT1A1, which catalyses the transfer of the glucuronic acid moiety from UDP-glucuronic acid (UDPGA) to bilirubin (4). Bilirubin glucuronides are actively transported into bile against a concentration gradient by the ATP-utilizing pump ABCC2 (also termed MRP2) (5).

reduces UGT activity towards bilirubin, whereas the activity towards 4-nitrophenol is increased [56].

In humans, the expression of UGT1A1 is limited to hepatocytes and, to a lesser extent, the proximal small intestine. UGTs are integral to ER membranes. In addition to the enzyme content, UGT1A1 activity is affected by the lipids of the ER membrane. UGT activity in native microsomal vesicles is latent [57], probably because the ER membranes pose a barrier to the polar sugar donor UDP-glucuronic acid or as a result of the constraint of the enzyme by the membranes. Based on hydrophobicity analysis, the major portion of mature UGT molecules, including the UDP-glucuronic acid and the aglycone binding sites, is thought to be located within the ER cisternae. There is a single 17-amino-acid membrane-spanning segment and a 26-amino-acid cytoplasmic tail at the carboxy-terminal end of the molecule. Full enzyme activity is manifested *in vitro* by treatment of the microsomes with membrane-permeabilizing agents, such as digitonin or alamethacin. UDP-N-acetylglucosamine (UDP-glucNac) stimulates the internalization of UDP-glucoronic acid into intact microsomal vesicles and is thought to be the natural activator of UGTs within hepatocytes. UGT1A1 forms homodimers within the ER membrane, which may be required for its full catalytic activity [58]. In addition, it may interact with other UGT isoforms, as well as other proteins of the ER.

Canalicular excretion of conjugated bilirubin

Conjugated bilirubin undergoes unidirectional transport into the bile against a concentration gradient, so that bilirubin concentration in the bile can be as high as 150-fold that in the hepatocyte. The electrochemical gradient of −35 mV, generated by the sodium pump, may help in the canalicular transport but, by itself, is too small to account for this large concentration gradient. The energy for the uphill transport of bilirubin and many other non-bile salt organic anions is derived from adenosine triphosphate (ATP) hydrolysis by the canalicular ATP-binding cassette protein, ABCC2 [also termed the MDR-related protein 2 (MRP2) or the multispecific organic anion transporter, MOAT]. ABCC2 pumps glutathione-, glucuronic acid- or sulphate-conjugated compounds across the canalicular membrane [59,60]. Canalicular transport of organic anions is unidirectional from the cytoplasm of the hepatocyte into the bile. Canalicular transport may be assisted by the membrane potential, but the contribution of membrane potential in organic anion transport has not been quantified. Mutant animals that lack ATP-dependent canalicular transport of non-bile acid organic anions retain normal activity with respect to potential-driven canalicular transport of non-bile acid organic anions, including bilirubin glucuronides [60]. The ATP-dependent canalicular organic anion transport is mediated by a canalicular membrane protein, termed canalicular multispecific organic anion transporter (cMOAT) or MRP2 [61].

Maximal bilirubin secretory capacity (Tmax) into the bile canaliculus depends on bile flow, which has bile salt-dependent and non-bile salt-dependent components. Bile acids increase the trafficking of vesicles containing MRP2 and the bile salt export pump (BSEP) from the Golgi apparatus to the apical domain of hepatocyte plasma membranes, thereby increasing the concentration of the transporters in the canalicular membrane [61].

Fate of bilirubin in the gastrointestinal tract

Although conjugated bilirubin is not substantially absorbed from the intestines, a fraction of the small amount of unconjugated bilirubin that is excreted in bile is absorbed and undergoes enterohepatic circulation. In situations in which increased amounts of unconjugated bilirubin are excreted in bile, such as e.g. during phototherapy for neonatal jaundice or Crigler–Najjar syndrome, absorption of unconjugated bilirubin from the intestine may be clinically significant [62]. In these cases, interruption of bilirubin reabsorption by ingestion of various substances, including calcium salts, can enhance the effect of phototherapy [63].

Degradation of bilirubin by intestinal bacteria generates urobilinogen and related products [64]. A major portion of the urobilinogen reabsorbed from the intestine is excreted in bile, but a small fraction is excreted in urine. Urobilinogen is colourless; its oxidation product, urobilin, contributes to the colour of normal urine and stool. During severe intrahepatic cholestasis or complete obstruction of the bile duct, urobilinogen and urobilin are absent in urine and stool, resulting in pale (so-called clay-coloured) stool. In liver disease and states of increased bilirubin production, urinary urobilinogen excretion is increased.

Alternative routes of bilirubin elimination

In the absence of bilirubin glucuronidation, a fraction of bilirubin is excreted as hydroxylated products [65], probably by the action of microsomal P450s [66] and mitochondrial bilirubin oxidase in liver [67] and other tissues.

During intrahepatic or extrahepatic cholestasis, conjugated bilirubin accumulates in plasma. In total biliary obstruction, renal excretion becomes the major pathway of bilirubin excretion [68]. Renal excretion of conjugated bilirubin depends on glomerular filtration of the non-protein-bound fraction of conjugated bilirubin.

References

1 Chen TS, Chen PS (1984) *Understanding the Liver. A History.* Westport, CT: Greenwood Press, p. 99.

2 London IM, West R, Shemin D *et al.* (1950) On the origin of bile pigment in normal man. *J Biol Chem* 184, 351–358.

3 Schwartz S, Johnson JA, Stephenson BD *et al.* (1971) Erythropoietic defects in protoporphyria: a study of factors involved in labelling of porphyrins and bile pigments from ALA-^{3}H and glycine-^{14}C. *J Lab Clin Med* 78, 411–434.

4 Robinson SH (1977) Origins of the early-labeled peak. In: Berk PD, Berlin NI (eds) *Bile Pigments: Chemistry and Physiology.* Washington, DC: US Government Printing Office, pp. 175–188.

5 Come SE, Shohet SB, Robinson SH (1974) Surface remodeling vs. whole-cell hemolysis of reticulocytes produced with erythroid stimulation or iron deficiency anemia. *Blood* 44, 817–830.

6 Tenhunen R, Marver HS, Schmid R (1969) Microsomal heme oxygenase: characterization of the enzyme. *J Biol Chem* 244, 6388–6394.

7 Elbirt KK, Bonkovsky HL (1999) Heme oxygenase: recent advances in understanding its regulation and role. *Proc Assoc Am Phys* 111, 438–447.

8 Ishizawa S, Yoshida T, Kikuchi G (1983) Induction of heme oxygenase in rat liver. *J Biol Chem* 258, 4220–4225.

9 Hayashi S, Takamiya R, Yamaguchi T *et al.* (1999) Induction of heme oxygenase-1 suppresses venular leukocyte adhesion elicited by oxidative stress: role of bilirubin generated by the enzyme. *Circ Res* 85, 663–671.

10 Tenhunen R, Ross ME, Marver HS *et al.* (1970) Reduced nicotinamide-adenine dinucleotide phosphate dependent biliverdin reductase: partial purification and characterization. *Biochemistry* 9, 298–303.

11 Jones EA, Bloomer JR, Berk PD *et al.* (1977) Quantitation of hepatic bilirubin synthesis in man. In: Berk PD, Berlin NI (eds) *Bile Pigments: Chemistry and Physiology.* Washington, DC: US Government Printing Office, pp. 189–205.

12 Berk PD, Rodkey FL, Blaschke TF *et al.* (1974) Comparison of plasma bilirubin turnover and carbon monoxide production in man. *J Lab Clin Med* 83, 29–37.

13 Westlake DW, Roxburgh JM, Talbot G (1961) Microbial production of carbon monoxide from flavinoids. *Nature* 189, 510–511.

14 Kappas A, Drummond GS, Henschke C *et al.* (1995) Direct comparison of tin-mesoporphyrin, an inhibitor of bilirubin production, and phototherapy in controlling hyperbilirubinemia in term and near-term newborns. *Pediatrics* 95 (4), 468–474.

15 Valaes T, Petmezaki S, Henschke C *et al.* (1994) Control of jaundice in preterm newborns by an inhibitor of bilirubin production: studies with tin-mesoporphyrin. *Pediatrics* 93 (1), 1–11.

16 Berk PD, Jones EA, Howe RB *et al.* (1980) Disorders of bilirubin metabolism. In: Bondy PK, Rosenberg LE (eds) *Metabolic Control and Disease*, 8th edn. Philadelphia: Saunders, p. 1009.

17 Grandchamp B, Bissel DM, Licko V *et al.* (1981) Formation and disposition of newly synthesized heme in adult rat hepatocytes in primary cultures. *J Biol Chem* 256, 11677–11683.

18 Fischer H, Plieninger H (1942) Synthese des Biliverdins (uteroverdins) und Bilirubins der Biliverdine XIII, und III, sowie der Vinulneoxanthosaure. *Hoppe Seyler Z Physiol Chem* 274, 231.

19 Bonnett R, Davis E, Hursthouse MB (1976) Structure of bilirubin. *Nature* 262 (5566), 327–328.

20 Compernolle F, Van Hees GP, Blanckaert N *et al.* (1978) Glucuronic acid conjugates of bilirubin-IXalpha in normal bile compared with post-obstructive bile. Transformation of the 1-O-acylglucuronide into 2-, 3-, and 4-O-acylglucuronides. *Biochem J* 171, 185–201.

21 Jansen PL (1981) β-Glucuronidase-resistant bilirubin glucuronides in cholestatic liver disease – determination of bilirubin metabolites in serum by means of high-pressure liquid chromatography. *Clin Chim Acta* 110, 309–317.

22 Lauff JJ, Kasper ME, Ambros RT (1983) Quantitative liquid chromatographic estimation of bilirubin species in pathological serum. *Clin Chem* 29, 800–805

23 McDonagh AF, Palma LA, Lightner DA (1982) Phototherapy for neonatal jaundice. Stereospecific and regiospecific photoisomerization of bilirubin bound to human serum albumin and NMR characterization of intramolecularly cyclized photoproducts. *J Am Chem Soc* 104, 6867.

24 Itho S, Onishi S (1985) Kinetic study of the photochemical changes of (ZZ)-bilirubin IX bound to human serum albumin. Demonstration of (EZ)-bilirubin IX as an intermediate in photochemical changes from (ZZ)-bilirubin IX to (EZ)-cyclobilirubin IX. *Biochem J* 226, 251–258.

25 McDonagh AF (1975) Thermal and photochemical reactions of bilirubin IX. *Ann NY Acad Sci* 244, 553–569.

26 Onishi S, Itho S, Kawade N *et al.* (1980) An accurate and sensitive analysis by high pressure liquid chromatography of conjugated and unconjugated bilirubin IXa and in various biological fluids. *Biochem J* 185, 281–284.

27 Spivak W, Carey MC (1985) Reverse-phase h.p.l.c. separation, quantification and preparation of bilirubin and its conjugates from native bile. *Biochem J* 225, 787–805.

28 Roy Chowdhury J, Roy Chowdhury N (1982) Quantitation of bilirubin and its conjugates by high pressure liquid chromatography. *Falk Hepatol* 11, 1649–1650.

29 Blanckaert N, Kabra PM, Farina FA *et al.* (1980) Measurement of bilirubin and its mono- and diconjugates in human serum by alkaline methanolysis and high performance liquid chromatography. *J Lab Clin Med* 96, 198–212.

30 Schumacher RE, Thornbery JM, Gutcher GR (1985) Transcutaneous bilirubinometry: a comparison of old and new methods. *Pediatrics* 76 (1), 10–14.

31 Schiff D, Chan G, Poznasky MJ (1985) Bilirubin toxicity in neural cell lines N115 and NBR10A. *Pediatr Res* 19 (9), 908–911.

32 Mustafa MG, Cowger ML, King TE (1969) Effects of bilirubin on mitochondrial reactions. *J Biol Chem* 244 (23), 6403–6414.

33 Sano K, Nakamura H, Tamotsu M (1985) Mode of inhibitory action of bilirubin on protein kinase C. *Pediatr Res* 19 (6), 587–590.

34 Vaughan VC, Allen FC, Diamond LK (1950) Erythroblastosis fetalis. IV. Further observations on kernicterus. *Pediatrics* 6, 706.

35 Gourley GR (1997) Bilirubin metabolism and kernicterus. *Adv Pediatr* 44, 173–229.

36 Odell GB (1973) Influence of binding on the toxicity of bilirubin. *Ann NY Acad Sci* 226, 225–237.

37 Lee K-S, Gartner LM (1983) Management of unconjugated hyperbilirubinemia in the newborn. *Semin Liver Dis* 3 (1), 52–64.

38 Breimer LH, Wannamethee G, Ebrahim S *et al.* (1995) Serum bilirubin and risk of ischemic heart disease in middle-aged British men. *Clin Chem* 41, 1504–1508.

39 Bosma PJ, van der Meer, IM, Bakker CT *et al.* (2003) UGT1A1*28 allele and coronary heart disease: the Rotterdam Study. *Clin Chem* 49, 1180–1181.

40 Zucker SD, Horn PS, Serman KE (2004) Serum bilirubin levels in the U.S. population: gender effect and inverse correlation with colorectal cancer. *Hepatology* 40, 827–835.

41 Temme EHM, Zhang J, Schouten EG *et al.* (2001) Serum bilirubin and 10-year mortality risk in a Belgian population. *Cancer Causes Control* 12, 887–894.

42 Bowen WR, Porter E, Waters WF (1959) The protective action of albumin in bilirubin toxicity in new born puppies. *Am J Dis Child* 98, 568–573.

43 Brodersen R (1986) Aqueous solubility, albumin binding and tissue distribution of bilirubin. In: Ostrow JD (ed.) *Bile Pigments and Jaundice*. New York: Marcel Dekker, pp. 157–181.

44 Cui Y, Konig J, Leier I *et al.* (2000) Hepatic uptake of bilirubin and its conjugates by the human organic anion-transporting polypeptide 2 (symbol SLC21A6). *J Biol Chem* 276, 9626–9630.

45 Wang P, Kim RB, Roy-Chowdhury J *et al.* (2003) Organic anion transport protein SLC21A6 (OATP2) is not sufficient for bilirubin transport. *J Biol Chem* 278 (23), 20695–20696

46 Levi AJ, Gatmaitan Z, Arias IM (1969) Two hepatic cytoplasmic protein fractions, Y and Z, and their possible role in the hepatic uptake of bilirubin, sulfobromophthalein, and other anions. *J Clin Invest* 48, 2156–2167.

47 Morey KS, Litwack G (1969) Isolation and properties of cortisol metabolite binding proteins of rat liver cytosol. *Biochemistry* 8, 4813–4821.

48 Ketterer B, Ross-Mansell P, Whitehead JK (1967) The isolation of carcinogen-binding protein from livers of rats given 4-dimethylaminoazobenzene. *Biochem J* 103, 316–324.

49 Kamisaka K, Gatmaitan Z, Moore CL *et al.* (1975) Ligandin reverses bilirubin inhibition of liver mitochondrial respiration in vitro. *Pediatr Res* 9 (12), 903–905.

50 Roy Chowdhury J, Novikoff PM, Roy Chowdhury N *et al.* (1985) Distribution of uridinediphosphoglucuronate glucuronosyl transferase in rat tissues. *Proc Natl Acad Sci USA* 82, 2990–2994.

51 Bosma PJ, Seppen J, Goldhoorn B *et al.* (1994) Bilirubin UDP-glucuronosyltransferase 1 is the only relevant bilirubin glucuronidating isoform in man. *J Biol Chem* 269 (27), 17960–17964

52 Ritter JK, Chen F, Sheen YY *et al.* (1992) A novel complex locus UGT1 encodes human bilirubin, phenol and other UDP-glucuronosyltransferase isozymes with identical carboxy termini. *J Biol Chem* 267 (5), 3257–3261.

53 Mackenzie PI, Owens IS, Burchell B *et al.* (1997) The UDP glucosyltransferase gene superfamily: recommended nomenclature update based on evolutionary divergence. *Pharmacogenetics* 7 (4), 255–269.

54 Wishart GJ (1978) Functional heterogeneity of UDP-glucuronosyl transferase as indicated by its differential development and inducibility by glucocorticoids. *Biochem J* 174 (2), 485–489.

55 Roy Chowdhury J, Roy Chowdhury N, Moscioni AD *et al.* (1983) Differential regulation by triiodothyronine of substrate-specific uridinediphosphoglucuronate glucuronyl transferases in rat liver. *Biochim Biophys Acta* 761 (1), 58–65.

56 Lilienblum W, Walli AK, Bock KW (1982) Differential induction of rat liver microsomal UDP-glucuronosyltransferase activities by various inducing agents. *Biochem Pharmacol* 31 (6), 907–913.

57 Bossuyt X, Blanckaert N (1997) Carrier-mediated transport of uridine diphosphoglucuronic acid across the endoplasmic reticulum membrane is a prerequisite for UDP-glucuronosyltransferase activity in rat liver. *Biochem J* 323, 645–648.

58 Ghosh SS, Sappal BS, Ganjam VK *et al.* (2001) Homodimerization of human bilirubin-uridine-diphosphoglucuronate glucuronosyltransferase-1 (UGT1A1) and its functional implications. *J Biol Chem* 276, 42108–42115

59 Ishikaowa T, Muller M, Klunemann C *et al.* (1990) ATP-dependent primary active transport of cysteinyl leukotrienes transport system for glutathione S-conjugates. *J Biol Chem* 265 (31), 19279–19286.

60 Nishida T, Gatmaitan Z, Roy-Chowdhury J *et al.* (1992) Two distinct mechanisms for bilirubin glucuronide transport by rat bile canalicular membrane vesicles. *J Clin Invest* 90 (5), 2130–2135.

61 Gatmaitan ZC, Nies AT, Arias IM (1997) Regulation and translocation of ATP-dependent apical membrane proteins in rat liver. *Am J Physiol* 272, G1041–G1049.

62 Brodersen R, Herman LS (1963) Intestinal reabsorption of unconjugated bilirubin. A possible contributing factor in neonatal jaundice. *Lancet* 1, 1242.

63 Van der Veere CN, Jansen PL, Sinaasappel M *et al.* (1997) Oral calcium phosphate: a new therapy for Crigler–Najjar disease? *Gastroenterology* 112, 455–462.

64 Watson CJ (1977) The urobilinoids: milestones in their history and some recent developments. In: Berk PD, Berlin NI (eds) *Bile Pigments: Chemistry and Physiology*. Washington, DC: US Government Printing Office, pp. 469–482.

65 Berry CS, Zarembo JE, Ostrow JD (1972) Evidence for conversion of bilirubin to dihydroxyl derivatives in the Gunn rat. *Biochem Biophys Res Commun* 49 (5), 1366–1375.

66 Kapitulnik J, Ostrow JD (1978) Stimulation of bilirubin catabolism in jaundiced Gunn rats by an inducer of microsomal mixed function mono oxygenases. *Proc Natl Acad Sci USA* 75 (2), 682–685.

67 Cardenas-Vazquez R, Yokosuka O *et al.* (1986) Enzymic oxidation of unconjugated bilirubin by rat liver. *Biochem J* 236 (3), 625–633.

68 Cameron JL, Filler RM, Iber FL *et al.* (1966) Metabolism and excretion of 1⁴C-labeled bilirubin in children with biliary atresia. *N Engl J Med* 274 (5), 231–236.

2.3.6 Metabolism of bile acids

Peter L.M. Jansen and Klaas Nico Faber

Introduction

Bile acids are synthesized in the liver from cholesterol; they are secreted in bile and stored in the gallbladder. After a meal, the gallbladder contracts, and stored bile is transferred to the duodenum and via the jejunum to the ileum. This movement is stimulated by intestinal propulsion. In the ileum, 90–95% of bile salts are reabsorbed and returned to the liver. The remainder is lost to the colon, where primary bile salts are transformed by bacterial metabolism into secondary bile salts. Some of the secondary bile salts are also reabsorbed, and the rest is removed with the faeces. Primary and secondary bile salts return to the liver via the portal circulation. In the liver, bile salts are taken up into hepatocytes, thereby completing the enterohepatic cycle.

Bile acids serve a number of functions: (i) they are the main solutes in bile and, as such, they are important for the generation of the so-called bile salt-dependent bile flow; (ii) bile salts are indispensable for the secretion of cholesterol and phospholipids from the liver; (iii) in bile, bile salts form mixed micelles that keep fat-soluble organic compounds in solution, including fat-soluble vitamins; (iv) in the intestine, bile salts promote the dissolution and hydrolysis of triglycerides by pancreatic enzymes; (v) bile salts act as signalling molecules in the regulation of enzymes and transporters of drug and intermediary metabolism.

The adult human liver produces about 500 mg of bile acids per day [1,2]. About three times this amount represents the total bile acid pool size that cycles through the enterohepatic circulation [2]. Bile acids complete an enterohepatic cycle about eight times per day. Enterohepatic cycling represents an efficient system for reusage of active components. Enterohepatic cycling not only serves to reclaim bile acids, but it also enables bile acids to act as messengers that carry signals from intestine to liver. Thus, they regulate their own synthesis and transport rates. Bile acids are also able to repress hepatic fatty acid and triglyceride synthesis [3,4].

Biosynthesis and metabolic defects

At least 16 different enzymes are involved in the biosynthesis of bile salts [1,5,6]. Most of these enzymes are active in the neutral (or classic) and acidic (or alternative) pathways, the two main routes for the conversion of cholesterol to the primary bile acids cholic acid (CA) and chenodeoxycholic acid (CDCA) (Fig. 1). The neutral pathway starts with the hydroxylation of the sterol nucleus of cholesterol by 7α-hydroxylase (CYP7A1) in the endoplasmic reticulum. CYP7A1 is regarded as the rate-limiting enzyme in bile acid biosynthesis, exemplified by the fact that mice deficient for Cyp7a1 have a 75% reduced bile acid pool size causing vitamin deficiencies, lipid malabsorption and liver failure [7–9]. The acidic pathway starts with the hydroxylation of the cholesterol side-chain by sterol 27-hydroxylase (CYP27). The CYP27 product, 5-cholesten-3β-27-diol, is not a substrate for CYP7A1, but is hydroxylated at the C7 position by an alternative P450 enzyme, CYP7B1. From here on, the neutral and acidic pathways largely overlap. Double hydroxylated CDCA and triple hydroxylated CA are the principal bile acids. Their ratio depends on the activity of sterol 12α-hydroxylase (CYP8B1). Bile acid synthesis is completed in hepatocyte peroxisomes, where bile acid coenzyme A:amino acid N-acyltransferase (BAAT) conjugates either taurine or glycine to CA or CDCA. At least 95% of the bile acid pool is generated through these two pathways. Extensive intracellular transport of bile acid intermediates occurs between various organelles. Transport in and out of these organelles may be mediated by transport proteins, but these have not been characterized in detail yet.

Bile acid synthesis defects (BASD) are rare genetic disorders that are the underlying cause of approximately 2% of persistent cholestasis in infants (see also Chapter 16.10, Genetic cholestatic diseases). BASDs are recognized by the absence or reduction of normal primary bile salts in serum and/or urine. Instead, non-typical bile acids and sterols are often detected in the body fluids of these patients. These can be identified by fast atom bombardment ionization–mass spectrometry (FAB-MS) and gas chromatography–mass spectrometry (GC-MS). Disease-causing mutations have been identified in 9 out of the 16 bile acid biosynthesis enzymes (Table 1). Cholestasis is a common clinical presentation of these diseases. The associated liver diseases may vary from mild to life-threatening but, in many cases, can be managed by replacement of deficient primary bile salts. This not only leads to restoration of normal bile function, but also induces feedback inhibition on the production of toxic bile acid intermediates.

Patients with CYP7A1 deficiency have a markedly reduced bile acid synthesis rate [10]. Symptoms include hyperlipidaemia, premature vascular disease and gallstones. A mutation in the *CYP7A* gene that results in truncation of the enzyme has been detected in these patients. Only one case of CYP7B1 deficiency has been reported to date [11]. This child produced no primary bile acids, and serum concentrations of the toxic 27α-hydroxy cholesterol were increased. A mutation was identified in the *CYP7B1* gene that truncates and inactivates the enzyme. In addition, it was found that expression of CYP7A, at both the mRNA and activity level, was absent. Bile acid treatment was ineffective, suggesting that the biosynthesis of toxic 27α-hydroxy cholesterol cannot be suppressed.

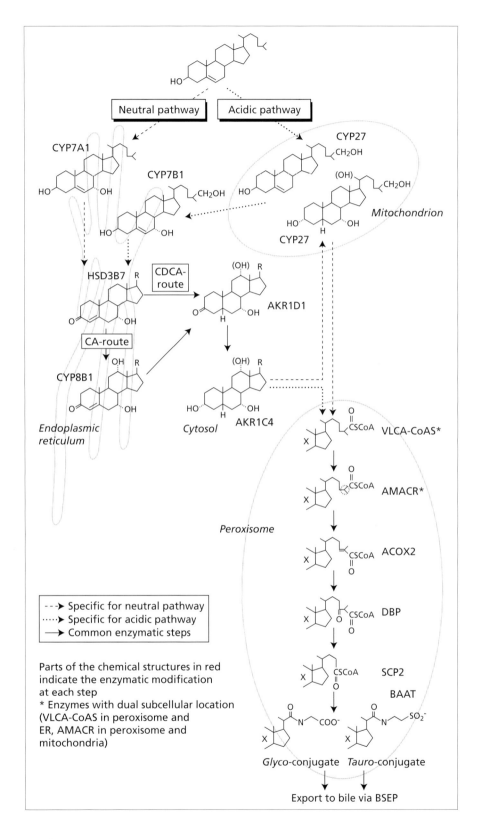

Fig. 1 Biosynthesis of bile acids in the liver. AMACR, α-methylacyl-CoA racemase; BSEP, bile salt export pump; ER, endoplasmic reticulum.

Table 1 Enzymes of the neutral and acidic pathways of bile acid synthesis.

Enzyme	Abbreviation	Mw	Tissue	Organelle	Disease symptoms	Mouse knock-out [ref.]
Cholesterol 7α-hydroxylase	CYP7A1	57 660	Liver	ER	Hypercholesterolemia, premature gallstone disease, NH	[7,8]
Sterol 27-hydroxylase	CYP27A1	56 900	Many	Mito	CTX, progressive CNS neuropathy, cholestanol and bile alcohol accumulation	[65]
Oxysterol 7α-hydroxylase	CYP7B1	58 255	Many, liver enriched	ER	Hyperoxysterolaemia, NLF	[66]
3β-hydroxy-Δ^5-C_{27} steroid oxidoreductase	HSD3B7	40 929	Many	ER	NLF, hepatotoxic bile acid intermediate accumulation	
Sterol 12α-hydroxylase	CYP8B1	58 078	Liver	ER	ND	
Δ^4-3-oxosteroid 5β-reductase	AKR1D1	37 377	Many	Cytosol	NLF, hepatotoxic bile acid intermediate accumulation	
3α-hydroxysteroid dehydrogenase	AKR1C4	37 095	Many	Cytosol	ND	
Bile acid CoA synthetase	BACS	70 312		ER/Perox	ND	
Very long-chain acyl-coenzyme A synthetase	VLCA-CoAS					
Alpha-methylacyl-CoA racemase 2-methylacyl-CoA racemase	AMACR	42 359	Liver Kidney	Perox/Mito	Adult onset sensory motor neuropathy, neonatal liver disease, pristanic acid accumulation	
Branched-chain acyl CoA oxidase	ACOX2	76 826	Many	Perox	Nd	
D-bifunctional enzyme	DBP	79 686	Many	Perox	Hypotonia, liver enlargement, developmental defects, pristanic acid/C_{27} bile acid accumulation	[67]
Thiolase 2 sterol carrier protein-2/sterol carrier protein-x	SCP2 SCPx	58 993	Liver enriched	Perox	ND	[68]
Bile acid CoA: amino acid N-acyltransferase	BAAT	46 296	Liver only	Perox	Familial hypercholanaemia, fat malabsorption, vitamin K deficiency	[69]
Enzymes of alternative routes						
Cholesterol 24-hydroxylase	CYP46A1	56 821	Brain	ER	ND	
Cholesterol 25-hydroxylase	CH25H	31 700	Many	ER	NH with fibrosis	Cited in ref. 1
Oxysterol 7α-hydroxylase	CYP39A1	54 129	Many	ER	ND	Cited in ref. 1

Mito, mitochondrion; ER, endoplasmic reticulum; Perox, peroxisome; CTX, Cerebrotendinous xanthomatosis; ND, no disease; NLF, neonatal liver failure; NH, neonatal hepatitis.

Mutations in the gene encoding 3β-hydroxy C_{27}-steroid dehydrogenase/isomerase (3βHSD) represent the most common disorders of bile acid biosynthesis [12–16]. Clinical manifestations may start at any age and include cholestasis, fat malabsorption, vitamin deficiency, pruritus and poor growth. Urine and plasma bile acid levels are high and consist of abnormal conjugates of the unoxidized precursors di- and tri-hydroxy-Δ-5-cholenic acids. These abnormal bile acids are poorly transported across the canalicular membrane and interfere with the adenosine triphosphate (ATP)-dependent transport of cholic acid. 3βHSD deficiency can be treated successfully by administration of primary bile acids. Patients with Δ^4-3-oxosteroid 5β reductase deficiency (AKR1D1) present with neonatal cholestasis [17,18]. Urine and serum levels of primary bile acids were low but Δ^4-3-oxo bile acid concentrations were elevated. Administration of primary bile acids constitutes successful therapy in these patients. Treatment by ursodeoxycholic acid is not sufficient, probably because this bile acid does not feedback to inhibit bile acid synthesis and thus does not prevent the production of hepatotoxic Δ^4-3-oxo bile acids.

Cerebrotendinous xanthomatosis (CTX) is caused by a deficiency of mitochondrial CYP27 [19,20]. CTX is a slowly progressive chronic disease characterized by early dementia and xanthomata. Bile acid synthesis is reduced, but the clinical manifestations are caused by the accumulation of cholesterol and cholestenol in the brain. This gradually disrupts the myelin sheets surrounding the neurons. If diagnosed early, CTX can be treated effectively with bile acid therapy. Deficiency of the conjugation enzyme BAAT has been reported to cause familial hypercholanaemia (FHCA). Patients present with high serum bile salt concentrations, fat malabsorption and vitamin K deficiency [21].

The final enzymatic steps of bile acid biosynthesis take place in peroxisomes. Zellweger syndrome (ZS) is a genetic disorder that affects the formation of these organelles. Mutations in over a dozen different genes have been shown to be the molecular cause of ZS or the related disorders neonatal adrenoleucodystrophy and Refsum disease [22]. These genes encode proteins that are involved in transporting newly synthesized enzymes to peroxisomes or are essential for the formation of the peroxisomal membrane. Indirectly, these mutations also affect the enzymes in peroxisomes. This may also affect bile acid synthesis. Patients present with cerebral neuronal migration disorder, craniofacial dysmorphism, psychomotor retardation and chronic liver disease. ZS is generally fatal in the first 2 years of life. Biochemically, these patients are characterized by increased levels of very-long-chain fatty acids, atypical mono-, di- and tri-C_{27} hydroxy bile acids (such as cholestanoic acid) and hyperpipecolic acidaemia.

Hepatic secretion and enterohepatic cycling of bile salts

Although bile salts can diffuse through membranes, hepatocytes and ileal mucosal cells express proteins that efficiently pump bile salts in and out of these cells. The sodium-dependent taurocholate cotransporting polypeptide (NTCP, SLC10A1) is located at the sinusoidal plasma membrane domain of hepatocytes (Fig. 2). The apical sodium-dependent bile salt transporter (ASBT, SLC10A2) is similar to NTCP, but is specifically expressed at the luminal surface of mucosa cells in the ileum [23,24]. These are high-affinity bile salt transport systems that allow the absorption of bile salts from the portal blood or the bowel lumen respectively. Both are sodium dependent with an out-to-in sodium gradient that drives this transport. In

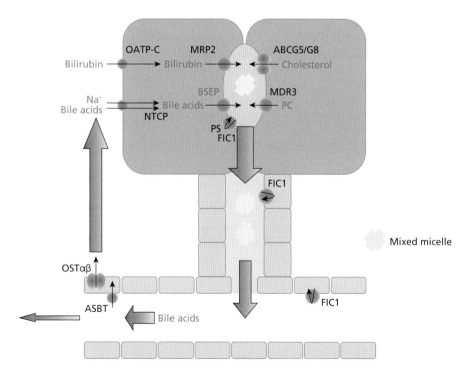

Fig. 2 Transporters involved in bile formation in liver and intestine. PC, phosphatidylcholine; PS, phosphatidylserine; GGT, gamma-glutamyltransferase.

addition, hepatocytes contain other transport proteins that may import bile salts, including the organic anion transporting polypeptide-C (OATP-C, SLC21A6), OATP-A (SLC21A3), OATP-B (SLC21A9) and OATP8 (SLC21A8) [25]. These transporters have a broad substrate specificity, they are bidirectional and do not need sodium for their transport activity. NTCP is believed to be the predominant bile salt transporter responsible for efficient hepatic uptake. Only a small fraction of portal blood bile salts spills over in the general circulation. Even the high bile salt concentrations that enter the portal circulation after a meal are efficiently dealt with by the liver.

No clinically important genetic defects of NTCP have been recognized thus far. In two children with familial hypercholanaemia, NTCP was normal [26]. In acquired forms of cholestasis, such as autoimmune, alcoholic and drug-induced hepatitis, obstructive cholestasis and primary biliary cirrhosis, NTCP levels are reduced [27–29]. This is a meaningful adaptation as it prevents the intracellular accumulation of bile salts.

How bile salts traverse the interior of the hepatocyte is not clear. In the simplest model, bile salts just dissolve in the cytosol. In this model, the cytosolic bile salt concentration is governed by the net balance between passive influx and active efflux. As bile salts are cytotoxic, influx and efflux of bile salts has to be well coordinated in order to avoid accumulation. This calls for a well-organized short-term regulation of influx and efflux transport proteins.

Bile salt secretion from hepatocytes to bile is mediated by the bile salt export pump BSEP (ABCB11). This is a bile salt-specific pump with the highest affinity for tauro- and glycochenodeoxycholic acid [30,31]. However, it also transports taurocholic acid, glycocholic acid and tauroursodeoxycholic acid and even unconjugated bile acids, albeit with lower affinity [31,32]. BSEP is a member of a large family of proteins known as the ATP-binding cassette (ABC) transporters, which have a wide range of transport functions. These proteins use ATP to pump their substrates against steep concentration gradients. This enables BSEP to build up a biliary bile salt concentration into the millimolar range, a concentration well above the critical micellar concentration. Pure bile salt micelles are extremely cytotoxic because of a detergent-like membranolytic activity. This activity has to

be neutralized, and this is accomplished by incorporation of phospholipids, cholesterol and other organic molecules.

In the canalicular lumen, bile salt micelles interact with the lumen-facing leaflet of the canalicular membranes that is enriched with phosphatidylcholine and cholesterol [33]. These are extracted into the bile salt micelle and contribute to the formation of the characteristic bile salt–phospholipid–cholesterol mixed micelle. Phospholipid transfer from the inner to the outer leaflet that faces the canalicular lumen is mediated by multidrug-resistant protein 3, MDR3 (ABCB4; in rodents mdr2, abcb4) [34]. Genetic deficiency of MDR3 causes a disease called progressive familial intrahepatic cholestasis (PFIC) type 3 [35,36] (Table 2). In this disease, phospholipid transfer through the canalicular membrane is abrogated, and this results in bile without phospholipids. Bile salt transfer is undisturbed, and the bile that is produced under these conditions is extremely cytotoxic. It damages surrounding hepatocytes and bile duct epithelial cells. Hence, liver histology of these patients shows portal inflammation, bile duct proliferation and periportal fibrosis.

BSEP gene mutations are the cause of PFIC type 2 or benign recurrent intrahepatic cholestasis (BRIC) type 2 (see also Chapter 16.10, Genetic cholestatic diseases). PFIC type 2 is characterized by neonatal hepatitis and persistent cholestasis with malabsorption, stunted growth and haemorrhagic diathesis as a result [37,38]. Patients often present with subdural haematoma in the first months of life. This can be prevented by early vitamin K supplementation. This disease provides proof for the functional importance of BSEP. Less severe defects cause a more benign type of relapsing cholestasis, BRIC type 2 [39].

PFIC type 1 and BRIC type 1 result from mutations of the *FIC1* gene affecting the FIC1 (ATP8B1) protein [40,41]. As an aminophospholipid translocator, malfunction of FIC1 affects the distribution of phosphatidylserine (PS) across the two plasma membrane leaflets. Too much PS in the outer membrane leaflet makes the outer membrane leaflet unstable. *Fic1–/–* mice have excessive outer leaflet-anchored proteins in their bile [42]. How cholestasis develops from FIC1 deficiency is not well understood.

Drug-induced cholestasis is a frequently observed, clinically relevant adverse effect of drugs. A great number of drugs and complementary medication can cause this disease. Many *BSEP*

Table 2 Transport defects.

Transport protein	Abbreviation	Membrane domain	Tissue	Disease symptoms	Mouse knock-out [ref.]
FIC1	ATP8B1	Canalicular	Liver, bile duct, intestine, pancreas	PFIC type 1, cholestasis first episodic later permanent, low GGT; BRIC type 1, episodic cholestasis; intrahepatic cholestasis of pregnancy	[70]
BSEP	ABCB11	Canalicular	Liver	PFIC type 2, permanent cholestasis, low GGT; BRIC type 2, episodic cholestasis	[71]
MDR 3	ABCB4	Canalicular	Liver	PFIC type 3, cholestasis, pruritus, high GGT; intrahepatic cholestasis of pregnancy; intrahepatic cholelithiasis	[34]

gene mutations and polymorphisms have been described [43–46]. However, a relation between these polymorphisms and drug-induced cholestasis or hepatitis remains difficult to prove and, to date, no clear connection between these and drug-induced cholestasis has been established.

The ASBT (SLC10A2) mediates the uptake of bile salts in the terminal ileum and is responsible for the preservation of bile salts in the enterohepatic circulation [24,47]. Mutations that affect the function of this protein cause bile acid-induced diarrhoea [48]. Jejunum also expresses OATP-B. However, OATP-B has a rather narrow substrate specificity and is not a good bile salt carrier [49,50]. Rat jejunum expresses Oatp3 that can serve as alternative transporter for glycine- and taurine-conjugated bile salts.

Organic solute transporter (OST) α and β act as heterodimers and mediate bile salt transport across the serosal membrane, thus allowing bile salt entry into the portal circulation [51]. They are specifically expressed in the ASBT-containing cells of the terminal ileum but also in hepatocytes. ASBT and OSTαβ are responsible for the vectorial transport of bile salts from the intestinal lumen to the portal circulation.

Bile acids as signalling molecules

It has long been known that bile acid synthesis and enterohepatic cycling are highly regulated processes. In recent years, important progress has been made in understanding the molecular mechanism involved in this process, recognizing that bile salts themselves are the crucial signalling molecules.

The nuclear hormone receptors (NHR) belong to a family of proteins that, upon binding an appropriate ligand, can activate or suppress gene expression [52] (see also Chapter 3.4, Cellular cholestasis). Promoter regions of genes contain characteristic nucleotide sequences for binding NHRs. These consist of two hexamers separated by a spacer of 0–8 nucleotides. Class II NHRs function as heterodimers in which the common retinoid X receptor RXRα complexes with a partner that can be farnesoid X receptor (FXR), constitutive androstane receptor (CAR), pregnane X receptor (PXR), the liver X receptor (LXR), the retinoic acid receptor (RAR), the peroxisomal proliferator-activated receptor (PPAR) or the vitamin D receptor (VDR) [53]. These members of the NHR family have received their names from the first ligands identified. Natural and much more potent ligands have been characterized for these NHRs, making their historic names deceptive as they do not reflect their actual function. A typical example is FXR, which is strongly activated by bile acids. NHRs reside either in the nucleus (PXR) or in the cytoplasm and move to the nucleus upon binding a ligand (CAR) [54]. Drugs, bile acids and intermediates of bile acid biosynthesis, the oxysterols, are major ligands for these NHRs. FXR binds bile salts with high affinity and thus serves as a bile acid biosensor. FXR affects a great number of target genes, with an emphasis on genes related to bile acid synthesis and transport, lipid and carbohydrate metabolism.

In the human small intestine, ASBT expression is negatively regulated by bile salts; at high bile salt concentrations, the expression of ASBT is downregulated [55,56]. This is mediated by the FXR-dependent induction of a protein called small heterodimer partner-1 (SHP-1). This protein negatively interferes with the RAR:RXR-dependent transcription of ASBT. Expression of the export proteins OSTαβ is also controlled by FXR [57]. Activation of FXR leads to an increased expression of OSTαβ. Thus, bile acids regulate their own intestinal absorption, and FXR regulation protects ileum cells from high bile salt concentrations.

After intestinal absorption, bile acids are taken up from the portal blood into the liver. Here they also bind and activate FXR, which induces SHP-1 expression. SHP-1 then interferes with LXR-dependent transcription of CYP7A1 and with RAR:RXR-dependent transcription of NTCP, thus reducing bile acid biosynthesis as well as bile acid uptake [52,58]. NTCP is downregulated during cholestasis, and this is caused by SHP-dependent and SHP-independent mechanisms. For the short-term regulation, it is relevant to note that Ntcp is a cAMP-dependent phosphoprotein. This allows the rapid regulation of Ntcp activity by phosphorylation [59].

While hepatic bile acid synthesis and uptake are negatively regulated by FXR, bile acid export is positively regulated. The BSEP gene contains a bile acid response element that provides a site for interaction with FXR:RXRα that increases transcription of this gene [60,61]. The combined downstream effects of bile acid-activated FXR results in the protection of hepatocytes against bile acid toxicity. Bile acids and drugs also serve as ligands for PXR, CAR and VDR [62]. The main function of these proteins is to provide protection against bile salt and drug toxicity. They have overlapping ligand specificity and regulate the transcription of an overlapping number of target genes, which includes many members of the cytochrome P450 family and ABC transport proteins. Induction of these proteins allows detoxification by biotransformation and secretion of harmful substances. Proof of these concepts comes from studies with PXR–/– and CAR–/– knockout mice, which are quite vulnerable to bile salt and drug toxicity [63,64].

Conclusions

Bile acids are important as emulsifiers of fat in the intestine, and an intact enterohepatic cycling of bile salts is indispensable for daily nutrition. Without bile, patients rapidly lose weight and become catabolic. Bile acids are also necessary for the intestinal uptake of fat-soluble vitamins. Therefore, infants with cholestasis often present with haemorrhagic complications due to vitamin K deficiency.

In view of the many proteins associated with bile acid metabolism, it is perhaps not surprising that there are many genetic diseases that affect bile acid biosynthesis or secretion. Cholestasis is a common phenotype in these diseases. A proper admixture of the three main components of bile – bile acids, phospholipids and cholesterol – is needed not only to prevent gallstone formation but also to avoid hepatocyte and bile duct damage. Retention of bile acids due to impaired secretion may result in hepatocyte injury. However, the liver possesses a number of adaptations that function to prevent the accumulation of bile acids. Liver injury occurs when adaptation fails.

For the treatment of cholestatic liver disease, the repertoire of drugs and interventions is limited. Primary bile salts are used for the treatment of the genetic bile acid synthesis defects. Ursodeoxycholic acid is useful for the treatment of chronic cholestatic liver diseases, in particular primary biliary cirrhosis. Also, patients with intrahepatic cholestasis of pregnancy and patients with MDR3 deficiency benefit from ursodeoxycholic acid treatment. Partial external biliary diversion is a therapeutic option for patients with PFIC types 1 and 2. For severe genetic forms of cholestasis, liver transplantation is a life-saving procedure. Gene therapy and hepatocyte transplantation remain unfulfilled promises. New insights into transcriptional regulation by NHRs offer an opportunity for drug development, and this will be likely to expand the number of drugs available for the treatment of cholestatic liver disease.

References

1 Russell DW (2003) The enzymes, regulation, and genetics of bile acid synthesis. *Annu Rev Biochem* 72, 137–174.
2 Bisschop PH, Bandsma RH, Stellaard F *et al.* (2004) Low-fat, high-carbohydrate and high-fat, low-carbohydrate diets decrease primary bile acid synthesis in humans. *Am J Clin Nutr* 79 (4), 570–576.
3 Chawla A, Repa JJ, Evans RM *et al.* (2001) Nuclear receptors and lipid physiology: opening the X-files. *Science* 294 (5548), 1866–1870.
4 Watanabe M, Houten SM, Wang L *et al.* (2004) Bile acids lower triglyceride levels via a pathway involving FXR, SHP, and SREBP-1c. *J Clin Invest* 113 (10), 1408–1418.
5 Bjorkhem I, Eggertsen G (2001) Genes involved in initial steps of bile acid synthesis. *Curr Opin Lipidol* 12 (2), 97–103.
6 Bove KE, Heubi JE, Balistreri WF *et al.* (2004) Bile acid synthetic defects and liver disease: a comprehensive review. *Pediatr Dev Pathol* 7 (4), 315–334.
7 Ishibashi S, Schwarz M, Frykman PK *et al.* (1996) Disruption of cholesterol 7alpha-hydroxylase gene in mice. I. Postnatal lethality reversed by bile acid and vitamin supplementation. *J Biol Chem* 271 (30), 18017–18023.
8 Schwarz M, Lund EG, Setchell KD *et al.* (1996) Disruption of cholesterol 7alpha-hydroxylase gene in mice. II. Bile acid deficiency is overcome by induction of oxysterol 7alpha-hydroxylase. *J Biol Chem* 271 (30), 18024–18031.
9 Arnon R, Yoshimura T, Reiss A *et al.* (1998) Cholesterol 7-hydroxylase knockout mouse: a model for monohydroxy bile acid-related neonatal cholestasis. *Gastroenterology* 115 (5), 1223–1228.
10 Pullinger CR, Eng C, Salen G *et al.* (2002) Human cholesterol 7alpha-hydroxylase (CYP7A1) deficiency has a hypercholesterolemic phenotype. *J Clin Invest* 110 (1), 109–117.
11 Setchell KD, Schwarz M, O'Connell NC *et al.* (1998) Identification of a new inborn error in bile acid synthesis: mutation of the oxysterol 7alpha-hydroxylase gene causes severe neonatal liver disease. *J Clin Invest* 102 (9), 1690–1703.
12 Clayton PT, Leonard JV, Lawson AM *et al.* (1987) Familial giant cell hepatitis associated with synthesis of 3 beta, 7 alpha-dihydroxy-and 3 beta, 7 alpha, 12 alpha-trihydroxy-5-cholenoic acids. *J Clin Invest* 79 (4), 1031–1038.
13 Ichimiya H, Nazer H, Gunasekaran T *et al.* (1990) Treatment of chronic liver disease caused by 3 beta-hydroxy-delta 5-C27-steroid dehydrogenase deficiency with chenodeoxycholic acid. *Arch Dis Child* 65 (10), 1121–1124.
14 Witzleben CL, Piccoli DA, Setchell K (1992) A new category of causes of intrahepatic cholestasis. *Pediatr Pathol* 12 (2), 269–274.
15 Horslen SP, Lawson AM, Malone M *et al.* (1992) 3 beta-hydroxy-delta 5-C27-steroid dehydrogenase deficiency; effect of chenodeoxycholic acid therapy on liver histology. *J Inherit Metab Dis* 15 (1), 38–46.
16 Jacquemin E, Setchell KD, O'Connell NC *et al.* (1994) A new cause of progressive intrahepatic cholestasis: 3 beta-hydroxy-C27-steroid dehydrogenase/isomerase deficiency. *J Pediatr* 125 (3), 379–384.
17 Setchell KD, Suchy FJ, Welsh MB *et al.* (1988) Delta 4-3-oxosteroid 5 beta-reductase deficiency described in identical twins with neonatal hepatitis. A new inborn error in bile acid synthesis. *J Clin Invest* 82 (6), 2148–2157.
18 Shneider BL, Setchell KD, Whitington PF *et al.* (1994) Delta 4-3-oxosteroid 5 beta-reductase deficiency causing neonatal liver failure and hemochromatosis. *J Pediatr* 124 (2), 234–238.
19 Cali JJ, Hsieh CL, Francke U *et al.* (1991) Mutations in the bile acid biosynthetic enzyme sterol 27-hydroxylase underlie cerebrotendinous xanthomatosis. *J Biol Chem* 266 (12), 7779–7783.
20 Sawada N, Sakaki T, Kitanaka S *et al.* (2001) Structure–function analysis of CYP27B1 and CYP27A1. Studies on mutants from patients with vitamin D-dependent rickets type I (VDDR-I) and cerebrotendinous xanthomatosis (CTX). *Eur J Biochem* 268 (24), 6607–6615.
21 Carlton VE, Harris BZ, Puffenberger EG *et al.* (2003) Complex inheritance of familial hypercholanemia with associated mutations in TJP2 and BAAT. *Nature Genet* 34 (1), 91–96.
22 Depreter M, Espeel M, Roels F (2003) Human peroxisomal disorders. *Microsc Res Tech* 61 (2), 203–223.
23 Meier PJ, Eckhardt U, Schroeder A *et al.* (1997) Substrate specificity of sinusoidal bile acid and organic anion uptake systems in rat and human liver. *Hepatology* 26 (6), 1667–1677.
24 Wong MH, Oelkers P, Craddock AL *et al.* (1994) Expression cloning and characterization of the hamster ileal sodium-dependent bile acid transporter. *J Biol Chem* 269 (2), 1340–1347.
25 Kullak-Ublick GA, Stieger B, Meier PJ (2004) Enterohepatic bile salt transporters in normal physiology and liver disease. *Gastroenterology* 126 (1), 322–342.
26 Shneider BL, Fox VL, Schwarz KB *et al.* (1997) Hepatic basolateral sodium-dependent-bile acid transporter expression in two unusual cases of hypercholanemia and in extrahepatic biliary atresia. *Hepatology* 25 (5), 1176–1183.
27 Kojima H, Nies AT, Konig J *et al.* (2003) Changes in the expression and localization of hepatocellular transporters and radixin in primary biliary cirrhosis. *J Hepatol* 39 (5), 693–702.
28 Zollner G, Fickert P, Silbert D *et al.* (2003) Adaptive changes in hepatobiliary transporter expression in primary biliary cirrhosis. *J Hepatol* 38 (6), 717–727.
29 Zollner G, Fickert P, Zenz R *et al.* (2001) Hepatobiliary transporter expression in percutaneous liver biopsies of patients with cholestatic liver diseases. *Hepatology* 33 (3), 633–646.
30 Gerloff T, Stieger B, Hagenbuch B *et al.* (1998) The sister of P-glycoprotein represents the canalicular bile salt export pump of mammalian liver. *J Biol Chem* 273 (16), 10046–10050.
31 Noe J, Stieger B, Meier PJ (2002) Functional expression of the canalicular bile salt export pump of human liver. *Gastroenterology* 123 (5), 1659–1666.
32 Mita S, Suzuki H, Akita H *et al.* (2005) Vectorial transport of bile salts across MDCK cells expressing both rat Na+-taurocholate cotransporting polypeptide and rat bile salt export pump. *Am J Physiol Gastrointest Liver Physiol* 288 (1), G159–G167.
33 Crawford AR, Smith AJ, Hatch VC *et al.* (1997) Hepatic secretion of phospholipid vesicles in the mouse critically depends on mdr2 or MDR3 P-glycoprotein expression. Visualization by electron microscopy. *J Clin Invest* 100 (10), 2562–2567.

34 Smit JJ, Schinkel AH, Oude Elferink RP *et al.* (1993) Homozygous disruption of the murine mdr2 P-glycoprotein gene leads to a complete absence of phospholipid from bile and to liver disease. *Cell* 75 (3), 451–462.

35 Deleuze JF, Jacquemin E, Dubuisson C *et al.* (1996) Defect of multidrug-resistance 3 gene expression in a subtype of progressive familial intrahepatic cholestasis. *Hepatology* 23 (4), 904–908.

36 De Vree JM, Jacquemin E, Sturm E *et al.* (1998) Mutations in the MDR3 gene cause progressive familial intrahepatic cholestasis. *Proc Natl Acad Sci USA* 95 (1), 282–287.

37 Strautnieks SS, Bull LN, Knisely AS *et al.* (1998) A gene encoding a liver-specific ABC transporter is mutated in progressive familial intrahepatic cholestasis. *Nature Genet* 20 (3), 233–238.

38 Jansen PL, Strautnieks SS, Jacquemin E *et al.* (1999) Hepatocanalicular bile salt export pump deficiency in patients with progressive familial intrahepatic cholestasis. *Gastroenterology* 117 (6), 1370–1379.

39 van Mil SW, van der Woerd WL, van der Brugge G *et al.* (2004) Benign recurrent intrahepatic cholestasis type 2 is caused by mutations in ABCB11. *Gastroenterology* 127 (2), 379–384.

40 Bull LN, Carlton VE, Stricker NL *et al.* (1997) Genetic and morphological findings in progressive familial intrahepatic cholestasis [Byler disease (PFIC-1) and Byler syndrome]: evidence for heterogeneity. *Hepatology* 26 (1), 155–164.

41 Bull LN, van Eijk MJ, Pawlikowska L *et al.* (1998) A gene encoding a P-type ATPase mutated in two forms of hereditary cholestasis. *Nature Genet* 18 (3), 219–224.

42 Paulusma CC, Groen A, Kunne C *et al.* (2006) Atp8b1 deficiency in mice reduces resistance of the canalicular membrane to hydrophilic bile salts and impairs bile salt transport. *Hepatology* 44 (1), 195–204.

43 Noe J, Kullak-Ublick GA, Jochum W *et al.* (2005) Impaired expression and function of the bile salt export pump due to three novel ABCB11 mutations in intrahepatic cholestasis. *J Hepatol* 43 (3), 536–543.

44 Pauli-Magnus C, Lang T, Meier Y *et al.* (2004) Sequence analysis of bile salt export pump (ABCB11) and multidrug resistance p-glycoprotein 3 (ABCB4, MDR3) in patients with intrahepatic cholestasis of pregnancy. *Pharmacogenetics* 14 (2), 91–102.

45 Hayashi H, Takada T, Suzuki H *et al.* (2005) Two common PFIC2 mutations are associated with the impaired membrane trafficking of BSEP/ABCB11. *Hepatology* 41 (4), 916–924.

46 Wang L, Soroka CJ, Boyer JL (2002) The role of bile salt export pump mutations in progressive familial intrahepatic cholestasis type II. *J Clin Invest* 110 (7), 965–972.

47 Craddock AL, Love MW, Daniel RW *et al.* (1998) Expression and transport properties of the human ileal and renal sodium-dependent bile acid transporter. *Am J Physiol* 274 (1 Pt 1), G157–G169.

48 Wong MH, Oelkers P, Dawson PA (1995) Identification of a mutation in the ileal sodium-dependent bile acid transporter gene that abolishes transport activity. *J Biol Chem* 270 (45), 27228–27234.

49 Kullak-Ublick GA, Ismair MG, Stieger B *et al.* (2001) Organic anion-transporting polypeptide B (OATP-B) and its functional comparison with three other OATPs of human liver. *Gastroenterology* 120 (2), 525–533.

50 Kobayashi D, Nozawa T, Imai K *et al.* (2003) Involvement of human organic anion transporting polypeptide OATP-B (SLC21A9) in pH-dependent transport across intestinal apical membrane. *J Pharmacol Exp Ther* 306 (2), 703–708.

51 Dawson PA, Hubbert M, Haywood J *et al.* (2005) The heteromeric organic solute transporter alpha-beta, Ostalpha–Ostbeta , is an ileal basolateral bile acid transporter. *J Biol Chem* 280 (8), 6960–6968.

52 Chiang JY (2004) Regulation of bile acid synthesis: pathways, nuclear receptors, and mechanisms. *J Hepatol* 40 (3), 539–551.

53 Karpen SJ (2002) Nuclear receptor regulation of hepatic function. *J Hepatol* 36 (6), 832–850.

54 Moore JT, Moore LB, Maglich JM *et al.* (2003) Functional and structural comparison of PXR and CAR. *Biochim Biophys Acta* 1619 (3), 235–238.

55 Neimark E, Chen F, Li X *et al.* (2004) Bile acid-induced negative feedback regulation of the human ileal bile acid transporter. *Hepatology* 40 (1), 149–156.

56 Li H, Chen F, Shang Q *et al.* (2005) FXR-activating ligands inhibit rabbit ASBT expression via FXR-SHP-FTF cascade. *Am J Physiol Gastrointest Liver Physiol* 288 (1), G60–G66.

57 Lee H, Zhang Y, Lee FY *et al.* (2006) FXR regulates organic solute transporter alpha and beta in the adrenal gland, kidney and intestine. *J Lipid Res* 47 (1), 1006–1011.

58 Denson LA, Sturm E, Echevarria W *et al.* (2001) The orphan nuclear receptor, shp, mediates bile acid-induced inhibition of the rat bile acid transporter, ntcp. *Gastroenterology* 121 (1), 140–147.

59 Mukhopadhyay S, Ananthanarayanan M, Stieger B *et al.* (1998) Sodium taurocholate cotransporting polypeptide is a serine, threonine phosphoprotein and is dephosphorylated by cyclic adenosine monophosphate. *Hepatology* 28 (6), 1629–1636.

60 Ananthanarayanan M, Balasubramanian N, Makishima M *et al.* (2001) Human bile salt export pump promoter is transactivated by the farnesoid X receptor/bile acid receptor. *J Biol Chem* 276 (31), 28857–28865.

61 Plass JR, Mol O, Heegsma J *et al.* (2002) Farnesoid X receptor and bile salts are involved in transcriptional regulation of the gene encoding the human bile salt export pump. *Hepatology* 35 (3), 589–596.

62 Handschin C, Meyer UA (2005) Regulatory network of lipid-sensing nuclear receptors: roles for CAR, PXR, LXR, and FXR. *Arch Biochem Biophys* 433 (2), 387–396.

63 Guo GL, Lambert G, Negishi M *et al.* (2003) Complementary roles of farnesoid X receptor, pregnane X receptor, and constitutive androstane receptor in protection against bile acid toxicity. *J Biol Chem* 278 (46), 45062–45071.

64 Stedman CA, Liddle C, Coulter SA *et al.* (2005) Nuclear receptors constitutive androstane receptor and pregnane X receptor ameliorate cholestatic liver injury. *Proc Natl Acad Sci USA* 102 (6), 2063–2068.

2.3.7 Ammonia, urea production and pH regulation

Dieter Häussinger

Ammonia plays a central role in nitrogen metabolism. It is a major byproduct of protein and nucleic acid catabolism, and its nitrogen can be incorporated into urea, amino acids, nucleic acids and many other nitrogenous compounds. Ammonia is present in body fluids as both NH_3 and NH_4^+, and these are in equilibrium according to the equation:

$$NH_3 + H^+ \leftrightarrow NH_4^+$$

The pK_a of this reaction is 9.25, so that at physiological pH there is a great excess of the ionized form. NH_3 can diffuse freely across membranes via aquaporins [1] and NH_4^+ is carried in liver by an active transport system, the RhB glycoprotein [2].

The blood ammonia concentration is normally below 35 μmol/L; this is important as ammonia is neurotoxic at higher concentrations. Excessive cerebral ammonia uptake in hyperammonaemic states leads to astrocytic glutamine accumulation and cerebral oedema, which is important in the pathogenesis of hepatic encephalopathy [3–5].

The liver is the most important site of ammonia metabolism; it removes much of the toxic ammonia presented to it by urea and glutamine synthesis. By doing so, the liver also plays a major role in the metabolic regulation of systemic pH, because hydrogen ions released from NH_4^+ during the synthesis of urea neutralize the excess bicarbonate produced by the breakdown of amino acids (see below).

Urea is electroneutral and is transported across biological membranes by facilitated diffusion. A phloretin-sensitive urea transporter is also present in liver [6], and an aquaglyceroporin, AQP9 [7], and UT-B1 [8] have also been identified as urea transporters in liver. Although urea is not further metabolized by mammalian enzymes, it interferes with the activity of K^+ channels in the plasma membrane [9] and can cause liver cell shrinkage at concentrations found in uraemia. Urea is excreted by the kidney, and is normally present in plasma and body fluids at a concentration of 3.0–6.5 mmol/L.

Sources of ammonia

Whereas urea production takes place largely within the liver, much of the ammonia used in urea synthesis is derived, directly or indirectly, from extrahepatic tissues. Ammonia is released from the intestine and the kidneys, whereas liver, resting muscle, and brain remove ammonia from the blood [10]; 25% of the nitrogen utilized in urea synthesis reaches the liver via the portal vein, from ammonia formed in the small intestine and colon (see below) [10–13]. Most of the nitrogen transported to the liver for incorporation into urea is carried not as ammonia but as amino acids, such as alanine or glutamine (see also Chapter 2.3.3).

Within the liver, glutamate and glutamine are major sources of ammonia. Glutamate is released directly from protein, but more importantly it is formed from other amino acids (except lysine and threonine) released from protein breakdown in aminotransferase reactions. Glutamate is directly formed by deamidation of glutamine, and from proline and histidine. Ammonia is released from glutamate by its oxidative deamination by glutamate dehydrogenase, a mitochondrial enzyme. Glutamate dehydrogenase is present in most tissues, but its activity is highest in the liver.

Amino acids can also be transaminated with glyoxalate to form glycine, which is deaminated by glycine oxidase to yield ammonia; this pathway is thought to be quantitatively important in mammalian ammonia production. Ammonia is generated by the deamidation of glutamine and asparagine and in the histidine lyase reaction. Ammonia is also generated from serine, threonine, cysteine, cystathione and homoserine, in pyridoxal phosphate-dependent deamination reactions, which occur mainly in the liver. Ammonia is also produced by amine oxidases, but the amounts involved are small. In addition, ammonia can be generated from the metabolism of purines and pyrimidines. Most of the ammonia produced from purine nucleotides is derived from adenosine monophosphate (AMP), in a reaction catalysed by adenylate deaminase. This pathway becomes par-

ticularly important during exercise when ammonia formation and release from muscle is increased [14].

Ammonia from the intestine

The intestine is a major site of ammonia production. Some 15–30% of the urea synthesized by the liver is degraded by bacterial ureases in the gut, with the liberation of ammonia and carbon dioxide [3,15]. Urea is hydrolysed in the mucosa or the juxtamucosal area of the colon, and to a lesser extent in the small intestine [16]. The ammonia generated in these reactions is completely absorbed and returns to the liver to be converted back to urea. The oral administration of antibiotics, such as neomycin, reduces the bacterial degradation of urea in the intestine [17].

A second source of ammonia from the gut, quantitatively of equal importance, is the intestinal mucosa itself. The small intestine produces a significant quantity of ammonia, which comes primarily from the metabolism of glutamine removed from arterial blood. The fractional glutamine extraction in the human jejunum and ileum is 24% and 9% respectively [18]. The small intestine also produces ammonia from the intraluminal amino acids, alanine, leucine and glutamine, but not from threonine, serine and glycine [19]. Most of the ammonia produced in the colon comes from bacterial degradation of urea and other nitrogenous substances; nonbacterial production accounts for only 10% of the ammonia produced in the colon; in the dog, ammonia produced by the small intestine is approximately equal to that produced in the uncleansed colon [18]. The ammonia from the intestine enters the portal circulation and the ammonia concentration in the portal vein is up to 10-fold greater than elsewhere in the circulation.

Ammonia detoxication by the liver

There are two major pathways for ammonia detoxication by the liver: urea and glutamine synthesis [10–13,20,21]. Both pathways are embedded into a sophisticated structural and functional organization in the liver acinus [10–13,20,21].

Urea production

Approximately 90% of surplus nitrogen in humans enters the urea cycle for irreversible conversion to urea, which is excreted by the kidneys. Approximately 30 g of urea is excreted daily in healthy adults. Using tracer techniques, it has been observed that calculated urea production exceeds urinary urea excretion by about 20–30% [22]. This difference is attributed to extrarenal losses, largely accounted for by the intestinal hydrolysis of urea.

The urea cycle and its enzymes
The urea cycle comprises five enzymes (Fig. 1): carbamoylphosphate synthetase I (CPS I), ornithine transcarbamylase (OTC), argininosuccinate synthetase (ASS), argininosuccinate

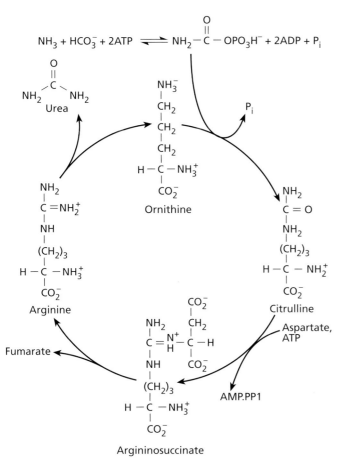

$$NH_3 + HCO_3^- + 2ATP \rightleftharpoons NH_2 - \overset{\overset{\displaystyle O}{\|}}{C} - OPO_3H^- + 2ADP + P_i$$

Fig. 1 The urea cycle.

lyase (ASL) and arginase. For efficient functioning of the pathway *in vivo*, however, further proteins are required, such as liver glutaminase [23], mitochondrial carbonic anhydrase V [24], *N*-acetylglutamate synthetase [25], the mitochondrial ornithine/citrulline antiporters ORNT1 and ORNT2 [26,27] and citrin, the mitochondrial aspartate/glutamate antiporter [28].

The liver is quantitatively the major organ involved in urea synthesis and it is doubtful whether other cell types, such as enterocytes, can produce significant amounts of urea [29]. However, at least some urea cycle enzymes are found in extra-hepatic tissues, where they are involved in providing arginine for nitric oxide (NO) synthesis (the so-called citrulline–NO cycle) [30].

The initial reaction of the urea cycle is the formation of carbamoyl phosphate from ammonia and bicarbonate (not CO_2), a reaction catalysed by CPS I, which requires *N*-acetylglutamate as an allosteric cofactor. Condensation of carbamoyl phosphate with ornithine yields citrulline (by OTC); this in turn condenses with aspartate to give argininosuccinate (by ASS), a reaction that requires the cleavage of two further high-energy phosphate bonds. Argininosuccinate is hydrolysed to fumarate and arginine (by argininosuccinase). Arginine is cleaved by arginase to give urea and ornithine. OTC, like CPS I, is also a

major mitochondrial protein [31]; the remaining enzymes are in the cytoplasm of hepatocytes. This necessitates the entry of ornithine into mitochondria and the exit of citrulline, which is brought about by the ornithine/citrulline transporters ORNT1 and 2.

This series of reactions, returning to ornithine, is known as the 'urea cycle'. It takes part not only in the removal of potentially toxic ammonia, but also in the irreversible removal of bicarbonate [32,33]. Although the arginase reaction is the major fate of arginine in liver, arginine can also be used for NO synthesis or undergo decarboxylation to form agmatine. Agmatinase converts arginine to putrescine and urea; however, the physiological role of this pathway is unclear [34].

Regulation of urea synthesis

Short-term regulation of urea synthesis occurs at the levels of substrate provision and enzyme activities, whereas long-term control is transcriptionally effected by changes in enzyme concentrations. Substrate provision for the urea cycle depends on amino acid delivery, the activity of amino acid transport systems, and amino acid metabolizing enzymes, and these factors are therefore important determinants of urea synthesis *in vivo*. The hepatic ureagenic response in humans is acutely sensitive to the plasma amino-nitrogen concentration, and urea production from an exogenous amino acid load is directly related to the plasma amino-nitrogen concentration, up to at least a concentration of 15 mmol/L [35]. Urea synthesis cannot therefore be saturated at realistic substrate concentrations.

In vitro, ASS seems to be the rate-limiting enzyme of the urea cycle at saturating ammonia concentrations. At physiologically low ammonia concentrations, however, carbamoyl phosphate synthesis is the rate-controlling step in urea synthesis [36].

Short-term regulation of urea synthesis primarily takes place at the level of ammonia and bicarbonate provision for mitochondrial CPS I, which presumably is the rate-controlling enzyme for the cycle at physiological substrate concentrations [11,12,21]. The K_m (NH_4^+) of CPS I is 1–2 mmol/L, that is, far above the portal NH_4^+ concentration of 0.2–0.3 mmol/L. Thus, the urea cycle has a low affinity for ammonia. This low affinity is in part compensated for by mitochondrial glutaminase, which is activated by its own product, ammonia, in the physiological concentration range [37]. This unique feature of liver glutaminase makes this enzyme a mitochondrial amplification system for ammonia, and glutaminase activity becomes an important determinant of urea cycle flux [12,13,21,23]. All factors known to increase urea synthesis, such as glucagon, ammonia, increased amino acid loads or alkalosis, activate glutaminase and accordingly, via amplification, ammonia provision for CPSI. Urea synthesis is also controlled at the level of mitochondrial bicarbonate supply, which is determined by pH, the CO_2 concentration and the activity of mitochondrial carbonic anhydrase V. This enzyme is required for the fast conversion of CO_2 into HCO_3^-, which is the substrate for CPS I. Its inhibition by acetazolamide blocks urea synthesis [24,38].

Short-term increases in ureagenesis are also thought to be mediated via N-acetylglutamate, a cofactor that stimulates CPS I activity [39], although its role as a short-term regulator of overall flux through the urea cycle has been disputed [40]. An intraperitoneal injection of a complete amino acid mixture causes rapid activation of ureagenesis. N-Acetylglutamate increases fivefold, causing a fivefold increase in the activity of CPS I [41]. Because the half-life of N-acetylglutamate in the liver is about 20 min, there is also a rapid response to a reduced protein intake. The concentration of ornithine may also play a role in the regulation of CPS I activity, and of flux through the urea cycle [42].

The activities of CPS I, ASS, and ASL are subject to allosteric regulation by MgATP and free Mg^{2+}. There is no feedback inhibition of the urea cycle by urea within the physiological concentration range. Only at very high urea concentrations is there some inhibition of ASL [43].

In the longer term, there are changes in urea-cycle enzyme expression following alterations in dietary protein [43–46]. Glucagon, insulin and glucocorticoids are major mediators of these responses [47]. When protein intake is increased, there is a proportional increase in the total hepatic content of all five urea-cycle enzymes, resulting in increased urea production. Long-term regulation of urea-cycle enzymes [20] primarily occurs at the level of transcription [48,49], and several proteins associated with the urea cycle such as ORNT1 [26] or glutaminase [50] are regulated in parallel. mRNA levels for CPS I and ASS also increase immediately following partial hepatectomy [51]. Glucagon, which increases during starvation, and glucocorticoids, which increase protein breakdown, are both associated with increased enzyme levels [52] and urea production. Glucagon also regulates urea synthesis by rapid mechanisms, by activation of mitochondrial glutaminase [53], amino acid transport [54], N-acetylglutamate synthesis [55], and stimulation of hepatic proteolysis [56]. Insulin probably has no direct effect on urea synthesis, but is a powerful modulator of other known hormonal regulators such as glucagon and a potent inhibitor of liver proteolysis [57], and is therefore still a major regulator of urea synthesis in vivo. Hypothyroidism is associated with increased activity of the urea-cycle enzymes in rat liver. There is no change in urea-cycle activity with hyperthyroidism [58], although urea synthesis from infused amino acids increases [59]. Growth hormone lowers urea production, possibly by reducing the supply of nitrogen to the liver [60,61]. Pregnancy and ageing are also associated with reduced urea synthesis [62,63]. Caloric restriction upregulates CPS I and glutaminase [64], whereas reduction in protein intake decreases urea synthesis [65].

Endotoxaemia [66] and interleukin-1 increase urea synthesis from amino acids in vivo [67]. In livers from endotoxaemic rats, arginase and nitric oxide synthetase can compete for arginine [68,69]. A short circuit of the urea cycle occurs under these conditions, because arginine is converted directly to citrulline and NO by inducible nitric oxide synthase; however, compared with total urea-cycle flux, this pathway of arginine metabolism is small in the hepatocyte. Flux through this citrulline–NO cycle in nonhepatic tissues is controlled by the expression of arginase and ASS and, like inducible nitric oxide synthase, is primarily regulated by cytokines [30].

Arginine protects against ammonia intoxication by stimulating N-acetylglutamate synthetase [70]. Carnitine reduces plasma ammonia and protects against acute ammonia intoxication by increasing urea synthesis [71]. Juvenile visceral steatosis mice with a defect in carnitine transport exhibit decreased expression of urea-cycle enzymes [72]. Here, probably, the accumulation of long-chain fatty acids results in an activated protein (AP)-1-dependent inhibition of the glucocorticoid activation of transcription [73]. In addition, CPS I is irreversibly inhibited by fatty acylation at physiological concentrations of palmitoyl-CoA [74]. Such phenomena provide a link between fatty acid metabolism and urea synthesis.

Drugs may influence urea synthesis. Sodium valproate increases plasma ammonia concentrations and reduces urea synthesis by 30% [75] due to a decrease of CPS I activity, but renal ammoniagenesis is also affected [76]. There is a dose-dependent inhibition of urea synthesis by acetylsalicylic acid.

Studies using isolated perfused liver preparations have shown that the pH of the perfusate influences the rate of urea production [24,77,78]. Such observations are consistent with the hypothesis that the liver plays a central role in the metabolic regulation of systemic pH (see later). Acetazolamide and loop diuretics containing a sulfonamide moiety inhibit the activity of mitochondrial carbonic anhydrase V and act as inhibitors of urea synthesis by impairing bicarbonate supply for carbamoyl phosphate synthesis [79].

Ammonia detoxication by glutamine synthesis

The other major pathway for ammonia fixation in liver is glutamine synthesis. Liver glutamine synthetase is a cytosolic enzyme and its localization in liver is restricted to a small hepatocyte subpopulation at the perivenous end of the liver acinus [23,80]. These cells are free of urea-cycle enzymes [12,21]. Thus, following the direction of sinusoidal blood flow, the two ammonia detoxication systems, urea and glutamine synthesis, are anatomically switched behind each other and present the sequence of a low- and high-affinity system for ammonia detoxication respectively [12,21]. The cells that contain glutamine synthetase have been termed perivenous scavenger cells [81], because they eliminate with high affinity the ammonia that was not used by the upstream urea-synthesizing compartment. They are of crucial importance for the maintenance of nontoxic ammonia levels in the hepatic vein: selective damage of perivenous scavenger cells does not impair upstream urea synthesis, but leads to hyperammonaemia due to a failure of scavenger function [82]. Both in vivo and in vitro, some 7 to 25% of the ammonia delivered via the portal vein escapes periportal urea synthesis and is used for glutamine synthesis [23,83]. In line with their specialization to scavenge ammonium by glutamine synthesis, the perivenous scavenger cells strongly express the NH_4^+ transporter RhB glycoprotein [2], ornithine aminotransferase [84] and the glutamate transporter GLT1 [85], and exhibit high-affinity uptake systems for α-ketoglutarate, malate and other dicarboxylates [86,87], which serve as carbon precursors for glutamine synthesis. The mechanisms underlying the strict zonal expression of glutamine synthetase are not settled [88], but may involve an intronic silencer element of the gene [89] and the Wnt/β-catenin pathway [85,90].

Small amounts of glutamine synthetase are also expressed by Kupffer cells [91]. Glutamine synthetase is strongly induced in activated hepatic stellate cells, which may significantly contribute to ammonia detoxication in fibrotic liver injury [92].

Short-term regulation of glutamine synthesis occurs at the level of substrate supply [87] and covalent modifications of the enzyme [93]. Because of the exclusive downstream localization of glutamine synthetase in the liver acinus, flux through the urea cycle in the periportal compartment will determine the amount of ammonia reaching the perivenous scavenger cells. Accordingly, all factors that regulate urea synthesis will indirectly exert control on glutamine synthesis. Also, the availability of carbon skeletons can control the rate of glutamine synthesis.

In vivo, glutamine synthetase activity is downregulated by hypophysectomy [94], endotoxaemia [93] and following portocaval anastomosis [95,96]. Glutamine and cell swelling decrease, whereas insulin and glucocorticoids increase, the levels of glutamine synthetase expression [97–99]. The age-related increase in oxidized protein in the liver and brain is accompanied by a loss of glutamine synthetase activity [100] and acetaminophen inhibits its catalytic activity [101].

The intercellular glutamine cycle and ammonia detoxication [12,13,21]

Whereas glutamine synthetase is localized in perivenous hepatocytes, glutaminase is located in periportal hepatocytes and in the mitochondria together with CPS. Here, glutaminase acts as a pH- and hormone-modulated ammonia amplifier and is an important determinant of urea-cycle flux in view of the physiologically low ammonia concentrations, which are about one order of magnitude lower than the K_m (ammonia) of CPS. Periportal glutaminase and perivenous glutamine synthetase are simultaneously active (the so-called intercellular glutamine cycle) [23]: glutamine utilized for ammonia amplification in periportal hepatocytes is resynthesized in perivenous scavenger cells from the ammonia that escaped upstream urea synthesis (Fig. 2). The regulatory properties of the intercellular glutamine cycle allow the liver to become a net producer or net consumer

Fig. 2 Structural and functional organization of hepatic ammonia and glutamine metabolism. Periportal hepatocytes contain urea-cycle enzymes and glutaminase, whereas glutamine synthetase is located in perivenous scavenger cells. Urea and glutamine synthesis are anatomically switched behind each other and represent functionally the sequence of a periportal high-capacity, but low-affinity, system and a perivenous high-affinity system for ammonia detoxication. Periportal glutaminase acts as a pH-modulated amplifier of the mitochondrial ammonia concentration and is an important determinant of urea-cycle flux. Ammonia that escapes periportal urea synthesis ('low-affinity system') is disposed of by the perivenous scavenger glutamine synthetase ('high-affinity system'). This guarantees the effective detoxication of ammonia, even when urea-cycle flux is inhibited in acidosis. At normal extracellular pH, glutaminase flux equals glutamine synthetase flux (the so-called 'intercellular glutamine cycle'): portal ammonia is completely converted into urea. In acidosis, glutaminase flux and urea synthesis decrease, whereas glutamine synthetase flux increases due to an increased ammonia delivery to perivenous hepatocytes: the liver switches ammonia detoxication from urea to net glutamine synthesis. From ref. 21.

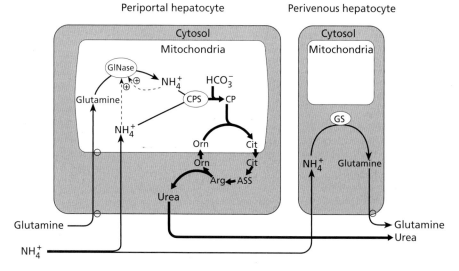

of glutamine depending on the nutritional and hormonal conditions [53,102]. Intercellular glutamine cycling also provides an effective means to shift hepatic ammonia detoxication from urea to net glutamine synthesis in acidosis.

Urea and ammonia metabolism in liver disease

Urea synthesis is reduced in severe liver disease [103] in parallel with glutamine synthesis [104], and this tends to be correlated with deterioration in other markers of hepatocellular function [105,106]. The metabolic zonation in the human hepatic lobules with respect to urea and glutamine metabolism is preserved in fibrotic lesions, but is lost in cirrhotic nodules [107].

In patients with well-compensated cirrhosis, urea production rates are similar to those of healthy controls under basal conditions, but the maximal urea production capacity in response to a protein or amino acid load is significantly reduced [35,108,109]. Reduction in the maximal capacity for urea production in patients with cirrhosis is due to a decreased activity of all five urea-cycle enzymes [110,111]. Near-normal urea production rates in cirrhosis, despite the reduced capacity of the urea cycle, are in part achieved by increased ammonia amplification due to a 4–5-fold increase in glutaminase activity [104,112,113]. Zinc supplementation speeds up the kinetics of nitrogen conversion from amino acids into urea in those with cirrhosis, but not in healthy individuals [114]. This can be explained by the zinc dependence of several urea-cycle enzymes and carbonic anhydrase V, and zinc deficiency, which is frequently found in cirrhosis.

In patients with liver disease, there is a tendency for blood ammonia levels to rise. The main reason for this is presumably the failure of the liver, because of portosystemic shunting and hepatocellular dysfunction, to remove ammonia from the portal venous blood. Liver cirrhosis is characterized by a severe scavenger cell defect [104], which also occurs after portocaval shunting [95,115]. Intestinal ammonia production is only slightly altered in liver cirrhosis [10], but may increase upon intestinal overgrowth with urease-containing bacteria [116,117]. In the presence of severe liver impairment and portosystemic shunting, skeletal muscle becomes an important organ in ammonia homeostasis [118]. In patients with chronic liver failure, muscle takes up more ammonia and releases much more glutamine than in control subjects [119,120]. The extraction of ammonia from the circulation is significantly less in patients with cirrhosis and muscle wasting [121]. Exercise causes a greater release of ammonia from muscle in patients with cirrhosis than in control subjects [122].

In patients with cirrhosis the blood ammonia, which is already high, may occasionally rise further as a result of gastrointestinal bleeding, renal failure, acid–base disturbances, diuretics and infections. Such infections inhibit perivenous glutamine synthetase, due to an inactivating tyrosine nitration of the enzyme [93].

Urea-cycle disorders [123,124]

Deficiencies in all five urea-cycle enzymes, N-acetylglutamate synthetase [125,126] and glutamine synthetase [127] have been described in humans. A genetic defect of ORNT1 leads to the hyperornithinaemia–hyperammonaemia–homocitrullinaemia syndrome [26,27], and citrin mutations can cause adult-onset type 2 citrullinaemia [29] and idiopathic neonatal hepatitis [128]. These disorders are rare and their clinical features are discussed in Chapter 22.1.

pH regulation and the liver [12,21,129,130]

The regulation of the acidity of the extracellular fluid is due primarily to the control of plasma CO_2 and HCO_3^- by the lungs, liver and kidneys. Despite its modest buffer capacity at physiological pH, the bicarbonate buffer is of special interest because the concentrations of its constituents, HCO_3^- and CO_2, can be regulated very effectively. According to the Henderson–Hasselbalch equation:

$$pH = 6.1 + \log[HCO_3^-]/[CO_2]$$

Mechanisms for the maintenance of extracellular pH must keep the $[HCO_3^-]/[CO_2]$ ratio constant. Thus, CO_2 and HCO_3^-, which are continuously generated during the oxidation of energy fuels, need to be eliminated from the body at the same velocity as they are generated metabolically. Whereas the complete oxidation of fat and carbohydrates yields CO_2 and water as the only products and the lungs fulfil the role of regulating P_{CO_2}, the hydrolysis of proteins yields bipolar amino acids, whose complete oxidation generates not only CO_2 and water, but also HCO_3^- and NH_4^+. The latter are derived from the carboxylic and amino/amido moieties of amino acids, respectively, and arise in almost equal amounts. The daily oxidation of 100 g of protein produces about 1 mol of HCO_3^- and 1 mol of NH_4^+. Thus, protein oxidation creates a strong alkali burden for the body, and the major pathway for removal of HCO_3^- is hepatic urea synthesis, which consumes 2 mol of HCO_3^- per mol of urea produced:

$$2NH_4^+ + HCO_3^- \rightleftharpoons NH_2CONH_2 + H^+ + 2H_2O$$

$$HCO_3^- + H+ \rightleftharpoons CO_2 + H_2O$$

Summary: $2NH_4^+ + 2HCO_3^- \rightarrow NH_2CONH_2 + CO_2 + 3H_2O$

In chemical terms, urea synthesis is an irreversible, energy-driven neutralization of the strong base HCO_3^- by the weak acid NH_4^+, and the average daily excretion of 30 g of urea is equivalent to the disposal of about 1 mol of HCO_3^- per day. Thus, a major function of hepatic urea synthesis is to effect this neutralization, without which the body would otherwise be confronted by a major load of alkali [32]. *In vitro* studies showed a sensitive control of hepatic urea formation by extracellular pH, which establishes a homeostatic feedback control loop between bicarbonate-consuming urea synthesis and the actual acid–base status. In this respect, it is important that the structural and functional organization of the pathways of ammonia detoxication in the liver acinus uncouples urea synthesis from the vital need to detoxify ammonia [33]. Whenever the pH and/or the HCO_3^- concentration drop in the extracellular space, the liver responds with a decrease of urea synthesis relative to the rate of protein catabolism and oxidation. Consequently, a fraction of the bicarbonate generated during protein breakdown is retained in the body and can be used to correct the underlying acidosis. The efficiency of such a mechanism is high: a 10% inhibition of ureogenesis relative to protein breakdown in acidosis will retain about 100 mmol HCO_3^- per day. In a well-balanced acid–base situation, however, the rate of bicarbonate removal (urea synthesis) from the organism must match the rate of bicarbonate production (protein catabolism) and the regulation of urea-cycle flux appears to be controlled by the rate of protein breakdown only.

pH control of urea synthesis occurs at the level of substrate provision, but not within the urea cycle itself. The mechanisms involved include pH-dependent changes in the NH_3/NH_4^+ ratio, the pH dependence of amino acid transport across the hepatocyte membrane, and the regulatory properties of mitochondrial glutaminase and carbonic anhydrase V. These enzymes adjust in a pH-dependent manner the input of the substrates ammonia and HCO_3^- into the CPS reaction, which is, *in vivo*, the rate-controlling step of urea synthesis. Lowering the extracellular pH from 7.4 to 7.3 already inhibits ammonia formation by liver glutaminase by 70% [33], mainly due to an inhibition of glutamine transport across the plasma and mitochondrial membranes [131]. Uptake across the plasma membrane is accomplished by SN1, which couples glutamine/Na^+ symport to H^+ antiport [132], and these transport characteristics may explain the inhibition of glutamine uptake by periportal cells and simultaneous augmentation of glutamine export from perivenous hepatocytes in acidosis [133]. Also, the uptake of other amino acids into the liver is inhibited in acidosis. This shifts the site of amino acid catabolism from the liver to nonhepatic tissues [134–136]. The other enzyme, mitochondrial carbonic anhydrase V, is also sensitively controlled by pH and plays an important role in providing HCO_3^- inside the mitochondria for CPS [24], because the mitochondrial membrane is impermeable to HCO_3^- but not to CO_2 [137] and the rate of spontaneous (uncatalysed) conversion of CO_2 into HCO_3^- is by far not fast enough to meet the bicarbonate requirements for intramitochondrial biosynthetic pathways [24]. In acidosis, both carbonic anhydrase and glutaminase are inhibited and, consequently, also irreversible bicarbonate consumption and urea synthesis. The regulatory properties of catalysed and uncatalysed intramitochondrial bicarbonate formation also allow discrimination of respiratory from metabolic acidosis, such that urea synthesis is inhibited much more strongly in metabolic than in respiratory acidosis. Even at a normal extracellular pH *in vitro*, the liver can respond to a decrease in buffer capacity of the extracellular

HCO_3^-/CO_2 system with an inhibition of urea synthesis and a sparing of bicarbonate.

The structural and functional organization of the pathways of nitrogen metabolism in the liver eliminates the threat of hyperammonaemia, which would otherwise result from an acidosis-induced inhibition of urea synthesis: perivenous scavenger cells maintain ammonia homeostasis by glutamine synthesis when upstream urea synthesis is switched off (Fig. 2). Acidosis shifts hepatic ammonia detoxication from bicarbonate-consuming urea synthesis to net glutamine synthesis, which is the result of both increased perivenous glutamine formation and reduced glutamine consumption at periportal glutaminase. Thus, intercellular glutamine cycling in the liver is an elegant means to adjust ammonia flux into either urea or glutamine depending on the acid–base situation. Glutamine formed by the liver and other organs during acidosis is hydrolysed in the kidney and the NH_4^+ is excreted as such into the urine. This process of so-called renal ammoniagenesis has long been known to be stimulated in acidosis and involves the action of kidney glutaminase, which is regulated by pH in an opposite way to the liver enzyme [138].

Thus, the kidneys function as a spillover for surplus NH_4^+, which cannot be disposed of by urea synthesis [130] (Fig. 3). This renal contribution is critical for the pH-stat function of the liver, because otherwise accumulation of surplus NH_4^+ in the organism, albeit in the form of glutamine, would override the acid–base control of hepatic HCO_3^- elimination by an inadaequate NH_4^+- (or glutamine-)driven stimulation of urea synthesis. With respect to ammonia and HCO_3^- homeostasis, the liver and kidney act as a team and impairment of one organ's function will give rise to acid–base disturbances. It is important to stress that it is the change of urea synthesis relative to protein breakdown that affects the bicarbonate pool in the body, whereas absolute changes of urea synthesis do not allow conclusions on bicarbonate homeostasis unless the rate of protein oxidation is assessed simultaneously. Failure to do so has led in the past to erroneous conclusions.

Clinical consequences [139–141]

Alkalosis is reportedly present in up to 70% of cirrhotic patients, whereas acidosis is found in less than 10%, which is usually a metabolic acidosis [139–141] and follows sepsis, shock and lactate accumulation. In alkalotic cirrhotic patients, the alkalosis was 13–60% metabolic, 20–50% respiratory and 10–30% mixed respiratory/metabolic [139–143]. In fulminant hepatic failure, alkalosis is present in about 75% of patients; in 30% of these cases, the alkalosis is metabolic [140]. Clearly, the acid–base status in patients with liver disease is influenced not only by the severity of liver disease itself, but also by many variables including accompanying morbidities and drugs.

Metabolic alkalosis in cirrhosis is often attributed to potassium deficiency and hyperaldosteronism, particularly as a result of diuretic therapy [144], but it may also be found without these

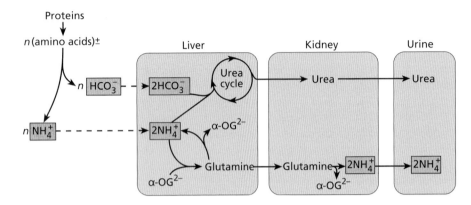

Fig. 3 Coordinated regulation of HCO_3^- and NH_4^+ homeostasis by the liver and kidneys. NH_4^+ and HCO_3^- arise in almost equimolar amounts during protein oxidation. Whereas urea synthesis irreversibly consumes HCO_3^- and NH_4^+ in a 1:1 stoichiometry, HCO_3^- is spared when urea synthesis is switched off in acidosis ('bicarbonate homeostatic response' of the liver). Under these conditions, NH_4^+ homeostasis is maintained by NH_4^+ excretion into urine ('ammonium homeostatic response' of the kidney). A feedback control loop between bicarbonate-consuming urea synthesis and the extracellular pH, $[CO_2]$ and $[HCO_3^-]$ adjusts hepatic HCO_3^- consumption to the needs of acid–base homeostasis. In metabolic acidosis, flux through the urea cycle and hepatic glutaminase is decreased, whereas flux through hepatic glutamine synthetase and renal glutaminase is increased. The coordination of these processes results in NH_4^+ disposal from the organism without concomitant HCO_3^- removal in acidosis. From ref. 79.

factors. Metabolic alkalosis in liver cirrhosis may be the result of an impaired urea synthesis [145], as suggested by an inverse relationship between plasma bicarbonate concentration in humans *in vivo* and the capacity for hepatic urea synthesis *in vitro* [104,112,146]. In view of the relationship between urea synthesis and bicarbonate homeostasis, metabolic alkalosis may not only be seen as a consequence of impaired urea synthesis, but also as representing an important driving force for residual urea synthesis in cirrhosis. This may explain why acidotic episodes can provoke hyperammonaemia in cirrhosis. In view of this, careful attention has to be paid to the acid–base status, and metabolic acidosis requires treatment [147].

The pathogenesis of respiratory alkalosis in cirrhotic patients is less clear, but elevated progesterone and oestradiol levels [148], hypoxaemia and hyperammonaemia may play a role [144,149]. It was hypothesized that hyperventilation and respiratory alkalosis represent a compensatory response of the cirrhotic patient in order to counteract the low-grade cerebral oedema that develops in response to hyperammonaemia and other precipitating factors of hepatic encephalopathy [5].

Although the liver plays a key role in lactate metabolism and lactate levels tend to be moderately elevated, overt lactic acidosis is relatively uncommon in liver disease and is usually found only when there are other factors that would increase lactate production or cause further decreases in hepatic uptake of lactate, such as shock, sepsis and bleeding [144]. In fulminant hepatitis, the development of lactic acidosis is associated with a uniformly high mortality; it has been attributed to tissue hypoxia resulting from arteriovenous shunting, as it occurred in patients with an apparently adequate systemic blood pressure, blood flow and arterial oxygen tension [150].

References

1 Jahn TP, Moller AL, Zeuthen T *et al.* (2004) Aquaporin homologues in plants and mammals transport ammonia. *FEBS Lett* 574, 31–36.

2 Weiner ID, Miller RT, Verlander JW (2003) Localization of the ammonium transporters, Rh B glycoprotein and Rh C glycoprotein, in the mouse liver. *Gastroenterology* 124, 1432–1440.

3 Hawkins RA, Jessy J, Mans AM *et al.* (1993) Effect of reducing brain glutamine synthesis on metabolic symptoms of hepatic encephalopathy. *J Neurochem* 60, 1000–1006.

4 Häussinger D, Laubenberger J, vom Dahl S *et al.* (1994) Proton magnetic resonance spectroscopy studies on human brain myo-inositol in hypo-osmolarity and hepatic encephalopathy. *Gastroenterology* 107, 1475–1480.

5 Häussinger D, Kircheis G, Fischer R *et al.* (2000) Hepatic encephalopathy in chronic liver disease, a clinical manifestation of astrocyte swelling and low-grade cerebral edema? *J Hepatol* 32, 1035–1038.

6 vom Dahl S, Häussinger D (1996) Characterization of phloretin-sensitive urea export from the perfused rat liver. *Biol Chem* 377, 25–37.

7 Carbrey JM, Gorelick-Feldman DA, Kozono D *et al.* (2003) Aquaglyceroporin AQP9, solute permeation and metabolic control of expression in liver. *Proc Natl Acad Sci USA* 100, 2945–2950.

8 Sands JM (2003) Mammalian urea transporters. *Annu Rev Physiol* 65, 543–566.

9 Hallbrucker C, von Dahl S, Ritter M (1994) Effects of urea on K^+ fluxes in perfused rat liver. *Pfluegers Arch Physiol* 428, 552–560.

10 Olde Damink S, Deutz N, Dejong C *et al.* (2002) Interorgan ammonia metabolism in liver failure. *Neurochem Int* 41, 177–188.

11 Meijer AJ, Lamers WH, Chamuleau RAFM (1990) Nitrogen metabolism and ornithine cycle function. *Physiol Rev* 70, 701–748.

12 Häussinger D, Lamers WH, Moorman AFM (1993) Metabolism of amino acids and ammonia. *Enzyme* 46, 72–93.

13 Häussinger D (1998) Hepatic glutamine transport and metabolism. *Adv Enzymol Rec Adv Mol Biol* 72, 43–86.

14 Lowenstein JM (1972) Ammonia production in muscle and other tissues, the purine nucleotide cycle. *Physiol Rev* 52, 382–414.

15 Jones EA, Smallwood RA, Craigie A *et al.* (1969) The enterohepatic circulation of urea nitrogen. *Clin Sci* 37, 825–836.

16 Wolpert E, Phillips SF, Summerskill WH (1971) Transport of urea and ammonia production in the human colon. *Lancet* 2, 1387–1390.

17 Wolpert E, Phillips SF, Summerskill WH (1970) Ammonia production in the human colon. Effects of cleansing, neomycin and acetohydroxamic acid. *N Engl J Med* 283, 159–164.

18 Weber FL, Veach G (1979) The importance of the small intestine in gut ammonium production in the fasting dog. *Gastroenterology* 77, 235–240.

19 Weber FL Jr, Friedman DW, Fresard KM (1988) *Am J Physiol* 254, G264–G268.

20 Morris SM (2002) Regulation of enzymes of the urea cycle and arginine metabolism. *Annu Rev Nutr* 22, 87–105.

21 Häussinger D (1990) Nitrogen metabolism in liver: structural and functional organization and physiological relevance. *Biochem J* 267, 281–290.

22 Walser M, Bodenlos LJ (1959) Urea metabolism in man. *J Clin Invest* 38, 1617–1626.

23 Häussinger D (1983) Hepatocyte heterogeneity in glutamine and ammonia metabolism and the role of an intercellular glutamine cycle during ureogenesis in perfused rat liver. *Eur J Biochem* 133, 269–275.

24 Häussinger D, Gerok W (1985) Hepatic urea synthesis and pH regulation. Role of CO_2, HCO_3^-, pH and the activity of carbonic anhydrase. *Eur J Biochem* 152, 381–386.

25 Beliveau-Carey G, Cheung CW, Cohen NS *et al.* (1993) Regulation of urea and citrulline synthesis under physiological conditions. *Biochem J* 292, 241–247.

26 Camacho JA, Obie C, Biery B *et al.* (1999) Hyperornithinaemia-hyperammonaemia-homocitrullinuria syndrome is caused by mutations in a gene encoding a mitochondrial ornithine transporter. *Nat Genet* 22, 151–158.

27 Camacho JA, Rioseco-Camacho N, Andrade D *et al.* (2003) Cloning and characterization of human ORNT2, a second mitochondrial ornithine transporter that can rescue a defective ORNT1 in patients with the hyperornithinemia-hyperammonemia-homocitrullinuria syndrome, a urea cycle disorder. *Mol Genet Metab* 79, 257–271.

28 Kobayashi K, Sinasac DS, Iijima M *et al.* (1999) The gene mutated in adult-onset type II citrullinaemia encodes a putative mitochondrial carrier protein. *Nat Genet* 22, 159–163.

29 Wu G (1995) Urea synthesis in enterocytes of developing pigs. *Biochem J* 312, 717–723.

30 Husson A, Brasse-Lagnel C, Fairand A *et al.* (2003) Argininosuccinate synthetase from the urea cycle to the citrulline-NO cycle. *Eur J Biochem* 270, 1887–1899.

31 Clarke S (1976) The polypeptides of rat liver mitochondria, identification of a 36, 000 dalton polypeptide as the subunit of ornithine transcarbamylase. *Biochem Biophys Res Comm* 71, 1118–1124.

32 Atkinson DE, Bourke E (1984) The role of ureagenesis in pH homeostasis. *Trends Biochem Sci* 9, 297.

33 Häussinger D, Gerok W, Sies H (1984) Hepatic role in pH regulation, role of the intercellular glutamine cycle. *Trends Biochem Sci* 9, 300–302.

34 Morris SM Jr (2004) Recent advances in arginine metabolism. *Curr Opin Clin Nutr Metab Care* 7, 45–51.

35 Vilstrup H (1980) Synthesis of urea after stimulation with amino acids, relation to liver function. *Gut* 21, 990–995.

36 Meijer AJ, Lof C, Ramos IC *et al.* (1985) Control of ureogenesis. *Eur J Biochem* 148, 189–196.

37 Häussinger D, Sies H (1979) Hepatic glutamine metabolism under the influence of the portal ammonia concentration in the perfused rat liver. *Eur J Biochem* 101, 179–184.

38 Dodgson SJ, Forster RE II (1986) Carbonic anhydrase, inhibition results in decreased urea production by hepatocytes. *J Appl Physiol* 60, 646–652.

39 Shigesada K, Aoyagi K, Tatibana M (1978) Role of acetylglutamate in ureotelism. Variations in acetylglutamate level and its possible significance in control of urea synthesis in mammalian liver. *Eur J Biochem* 85, 385–391.

40 Lund P, Wiggins D (1984) Is N-acetylglutamate a short-term regulator of urea synthesis? *Biochem J* 218, 991–994.

41 Stewart PM, Walser M (1980) Short term regulation of ureagenesis. *J Biol Chem* 255, 5270–5280.

42 Lund P, Wiggins D (1986) The ornithine requirement of urea synthesis. Formation of ornithine from glutamine in hepatocytes. *Biochem J* 239, 773–776.

43 Menyhart J, Grof J (1977) Urea as a selective inhibitor of argininosuccinate lyase. *Eur J Biochem* 75, 405–409.

44 Schimke RT (1962) Differential effects of fasting and protein-free diets on levels of urea cycle enzymes in rat liver. *J Biol Chem* 237, 1921–1924.

45 Schimke RT (1963) Studies on factors affecting the levels of urea cycle enzymes in rat liver. *J Biol Chem* 238, 1012–1018.

46 Snodgrass PJ, Lin RC (1981) Induction of urea cycle enzymes of rat liver by amino acids. *J Nutr* 111, 586–601.

47 Morris SM Jr, Moncman CL, Rand KD *et al.* (1987) Regulation of mRNA levels for five urea cycle enzymes in rat liver by diet, cyclic AMP, and glucocorticoids. *Arch Biochem Biophys* 256, 343–353.

48 Morris SM Jr (1992) Regulation of enzymes of urea and arginine synthesis. *Annu Rev Nutr* 12, 81–101.

49 Takiguchi M, Mori M (1995) Transcriptional regulation of genes for ornithine cycle enzymes. *Biochem J* 312, 649–659.

50 Dhahbi JM, Mote PL, Wingo J *et al.* (1999) Calories and aging alter gene expression for gluconeogenic, glycolytic, and nitrogen-metabolizing enzymes. *Am J Physiol* 277, E352–E360.

51 Tygstrup N, Bak S, Krog B *et al.* (1995) Gene expression of urea cycle enzymes following two-thirds partial hepatectomy in the rat. *J Hepatol* 22, 349–355.

52 Sigsgaard I, Almdal T, Hansen BA *et al.* (1988) Dexamethasone increases the capacity of urea synthesis time dependently and reduces the body weight of rats. *Liver* 8, 193–197.

53 Häussinger D, Gerok W, Sies H (1983) Regulation of flux through glutaminase and glutamine synthetase in isolated perfused rat liver. *Biochim Biophys Acta* 755, 272–278.

54 Fehlmann M, Le Cam A, Freychet P (1979) Insulin and glucagon stimulation of amino acid transport in isolated rat hepatocytes. Synthesis of a high affinity component of transport. *J Biol Chem* 254, 10431–10437.

55 Staddon JM, Bradford NM, McGivan JD (1984) Effects of glucagon *in vivo* on the N-acetylglutamate, glutamate and glutamine contents of rat liver. *Biochem J* 217, 855–857.

56 vom Dahl S, Hallbrucker C, Lang F *et al.* (1991) Regulation of liver cell volume and proteolysis by glucagon and insulin. *Biochem J* 278, 771–777.

57 Hallbrucker C, vom Dahl S, Lang F *et al.* (1991) Inhibition of hepatic proteolysis by insulin. Role of hormone-induced alterations of the cellular K+ balance. *Eur J Biochem* 199, 467–474.

58 Marti J, Portoles M, Jimenez-Nacher I *et al.* (1988) Effect of thyroid hormones on urea biosynthesis and related processes in rat liver. *Endocrinology* 123, 2167–2174.

59 Marchesini G, Fabbri A, Bianchi GP *et al.* (1989) Hepatic conversion of amino-nitrogen to urea in thyroid diseases. II. A study in hyperthyroid patients. *Metabolism* 43, 1023–1029.

60 Dahms WT, Owens RP, Kalhan SC *et al.* (1989) Urea synthesis, nitrogen balance, and glucose turnover in growth-hormone-deficient children before and after growth hormone administration. *Metabolism* 38, 197–203.

61 Wothers T, Grofte T, Jorgensen JO *et al.* (1994) Effects of growth hormone (GH) administration on functional hepatic nitrogen clearance: studies in normal subjects and GH-deficient patients *J Clin Endocrinol Metab* 78, 1220–1224.

62 Kalhan SC, Tserng KY, Gilfillan C *et al.* (1982) Metabolism of urea and glucose in normal and diabetic pregnancy. *Metabolism* 31, 824–833.

63 Fabbri A, Marchesini G, Bianchi G *et al.* (1994) Kinetics of hepatic amino-nitrogen conversion in ageing man. *Liver* 14, 288–294.

64 Dhahbi JM, Mote PL, Wingo J *et al.* (2001) Caloric restriction alters the feeding response of key metabolic enzyme genes. *Mech Ageing Dev* 122, 1033–1048.

65 Picou D, Phillips M (1972) Urea metabolism in malnourished and recovered children receiving a high or low protein diet. *Am J Clin Nutr* 25, 1261–1266.

66 Nielsen SS, Grofte T, Tygstrup N *et al.* (2005) Effect of lipopolysaccharide on in vivo and genetic regulation of rat urea synthesis. *Liver Int* 25, 177–183.

67 Heindorff H, Almdal T, Vilstrup H (1994) The in vivo effect of interleukin-1 beta on urea synthesis is mediated by glucocorticoids in rats. *Eur J Clin Invest* 24, 388–392.

68 Wettstein M, Gerok W, Häussinger D (1994) Endotoxin-induced nitric oxide synthesis in the perfused rat liver: effects of L-arginine and ammonium chloride. *Hepatology* 19, 641–647.

69 Stadler J, Barton D, Beil-Moeller H *et al.* (1995) Hepatocyte nitric oxide biosynthesis inhibits glucose output and competes with urea synthesis for L-arginine. *Am J Physiol* 268, G183–G188.

70 Kim S, Paik WK, Cohen PP (1972) Ammonia intoxication in rats: protection by N-carbamoyl-L-glutamate plus L-arginine. *Proc Natl Acad Sci USA* 69, 3530–3533.

71 Costell M, O'Connor JE, Miguez MP *et al.* (1984) Effects of L-carnitine on urea synthesis following acute ammonia intoxication in mice. *Biochem Biophys Res Commun* 120, 726–733.

72 Tomomura M, Imamura Y, Horiuchi M (1992) Abnormal expression of urea cycle enzyme genes in juvenile visceral steatosis (jvs) mice. *Biochim Biophys Acta* 1138, 167–171.

73 Tomomura M, Tomomura A, Dewan MA *et al.* (1996) Long-chain fatty acids suppress the induction of urea cycle enzyme genes by glucocorticoid action. *FEBS Lett* 399, 310–312.

74 Corvi MM, Soltys CL, Berthiaume LG (2001) Regulation of mitochondrial carbamoyl-phosphate synthetase 1 activity by active site fatty acylation. *J Biol Chem* 276, 45704–45712.

75 Hjelm M, Oberholzer V, Seakins J *et al.* (1986) Valproate-induced inhibition of urea synthesis and hyperammonaemia in healthy subjects. *Lancet* ii(8511), 859.

76 Marini AM, Zaret BS, Beckner RR (1988) Hepatic and renal contributions to valproic acid-induced hyperammonemia. *Neurology* 38, 365–371.

77 Lueck JD, Miller LL (1970) The effect of perfusate pH on glutamine metabolism in the isolated perfused rat liver. *J Biol Chem* 245, 5491–5497.

78 Häussinger D, Gerok W, Sies H (1986) The effect of urea synthesis on extracellular pH in isolated perfused rat liver. *Biochem J* 236, 261–265.

79 Häussinger D, Kaiser S, Stehle T *et al.* (1986) Liver carbonic anhydrase and urea synthesis. The effect of diuretics. *Biochem Pharmacol* 35, 3317–3322.

80 Gebhardt R, Mecke D (1983) Heterogeneous distribution of glutamine synthetase among rat liver parenchymal cells in situ and in primary culture. *EMBO J* 2, 567–570.

81 Häussinger D, Stehle T (1988) Hepatocyte heterogeneity in response to icosanoids. The perivenous scavenger cell hypothesis. *Eur J Biochem* 175, 395–403.

82 Häussinger D, Gerok W (1984) Hepatocyte heterogeneity in ammonia metabolism: impairment of glutamine synthesis in CCl$_4$ induced liver cell necrosis with no effect on urea synthesis. *Chem Biol Interact* 48, 191–194.

83 Cooper AJ, Nieves E, Coleman AE *et al.* (1987) Short-term metabolic fate of [^{13}N]ammonia in rat liver in vivo. *J Biol Chem* 262, 1073–1080.

84 Kuo FC, Hwu WL, Valle D *et al.* (1991) Colocalization in pericentral hepatocytes in adult mice and similarity in developmental expression pattern of ornithine aminotransferase and glutamine synthetase mRNA. *Proc Natl Acad Sci USA* 88, 9468–9472.

85 Cadoret A, Ovejero C, Terris B *et al.* (2002) New targets of beta-catenin signaling in the liver are involved in the glutamine metabolism. *Oncogene* 21, 8293–8301.

86 Stoll B, Hussinger D (1989) Functional hepatocyte heterogeneity. Vascular 2-oxoglutarate is almost exclusively taken up by perivenous, glutamine-synthetase-containing hepatocytes. *Eur J Biochem* 181, 709–716.

87 Stoll B, McNelly S, Buscher HP *et al.* (1991) Functional hepatocyte heterogeneity in glutamate, aspartate and alpha-ketoglutarate uptake: a histautoradiographical study. *Hepatology* 13, 247–253.

88 Lie-Venema H, Hakvoort TBM, van Hemert FJ *et al.* (1998) Regulation of the spatiotemporal pattern of expression of the glutamine synthetase gene. *Prog Nucleic Acid Res Mol Biol* 61, 243–308.

89 Gaunitz F, Deichsel D, Heise K *et al.* (2005) An intronic silencer element is responsible for specific zonal expression of glutamine synthetase in the rat liver. *Hepatology* 41, 1225–1232.

90 Ueberham E, Arendt E, Starke M *et al.* (2004) Reduction and expansion of the glutamine synthetase expressing zone in livers from tetracycline controlled TGF-beta1 transgenic mice and multiple starved mice. *J Hepatol* 41, 75–81.

91 Bode JG, Peters-Regehr T, Kubitz R *et al.* (2000) Expression of glutamine synthetase in macrophages. *J Histochem Cytochem* 48, 415–422.

92 Bode JG, Peters-Regehr T, Gressner AM *et al.* (1998) De novo expression of glutamine synthetase during transformation of hepatic stellate cells into myofibroblast-like cells. *Biochem J* 335, 697–700.

93 Görg B, Wettstein M, Metzger S *et al.* (2005) Lipopolysaccharide-induced tyrosine nitration and inactivation of hepatic glutamine synthetase in the rat. *Hepatology* 41, 1065–1073.

94 Wong BS, Chenoweth ME, Dunn A (1980) Possible growth hormone control of liver glutamine synthetase activity in rats. *Endocrinology* 106, 268–274.

95 Girard G, Butterworth RF (1992) Effect of portacaval anastomosis on glutamine synthetase activities in liver, brain, and skeletal muscle. *Dig Dis Sci* 37, 1121–1126.

96 Häussinger D, Lamers WH, Moorman AF (1993) Hepatocyte heterogeneity in the metabolism of amino acids and ammonia. *Enzyme* 46, 72–93.

97 Abcouwer SF, Bode BP, Souba WW (1995) Glucocorticoids regulate rat glutamine synthetase expression in a tissue-specific manner. *J Surg Res* 59, 59–65.

98 Warskulat U, Newsome W, Noe B *et al.* (1996) Anisoosmotic regulation of hepatic gene expression. *Biol Chem* 377, 57–65.

99 Labow BI, Souba WW, Abcouwer SF (2001) Mechanisms governing the expression of the enzymes of glutamine metabolism – glutaminase and glutamine synthetase. *J Nutr* 131, 2467S–2474S.

100 Stadtman ER, Starke-Reed PE, Oliver C *et al.* (1992) Protein modification in aging. *EXS* 62, 64–72.

101 Bulera SJ, Birge RB, Cohen SD *et al.* (1995) Identification of the mouse liver 44-kDa acetaminophen-binding protein as a subunit of glutamine synthetase. *Toxicol Appl Pharmacol* 134, 313–320.

102 Cooper AJ, Nieves E, Rosenspire KC *et al.* (1988) Short-term metabolic fate of 13N-labeled glutamate, alanine, and glutamine(amide) in rat liver. *J Biol Chem* 263, 12268–12273.

103 Rudman D, DiFulco TJ, Galambos JT *et al.* (1973) Maximal rates of excretion and synthesis of urea in normal and cirrhotic subjects. *J Clin Invest* 52, 2241–2249.

104 Kaiser S, Gerok W, Haussinger D (1988) Ammonia and glutamine metabolism in human liver slices: new aspects on the pathogenesis of hyperammonaemia in chronic liver disease. *Eur J Clin Invest* 18, 535–542.

105 Vilstrup H, Bucher D, Krog B *et al.* (1982) Elimination of infused amino acids from plasma of control subjects and of patients with cirrhosis of the liver. *Eur J Clin Invest* 12, 197–202.

106 Vilstrup H, Iversen J, Tygstrup N (1986) Glucoregulation in acute liver failure. *Eur J Clin Invest* 16, 193–197.

107 Racine-Samson L, Scoazec JY, D'Errico A *et al.* (1996) The metabolic organization of the adult human liver: a comparative study of normal, fibrotic, and cirrhotic liver tissue. *Hepatology* 24, 104–113.

108 Rypins EB, Henderson JM, Fulenwider JT *et al.* (1980) A tracer method for measuring rate of urea synthesis in normal and cirrhotic subjects. *Gastroenterology* 78, 1419–1424.

109 Rafoth RJ, Onstad GR (1975) Urea synthesis after oral protein ingestion in man. *J Clin Invest* 56, 1170–1174.

110 Khatra BS, Smith RB III, Millikan WJ (1974) Activities of Krebs-Henseleit enzymes in normal and cirrhotic human liver. *J Lab Clin Med* 84, 708–715.

111 Maier KP, Talke H, Gerok W (1979) Activities of urea-cycle enzymes in chronic liver disease. *Klin Wschr* 57, 661–665.

112 Häussinger D, Steeb R, Gerok W (1990) Ammonium and bicarbonate homeostasis in chronic liver disease. *Klin Wschr* 68, 175–182.

113 Matsuno T, Goto I (1992) Glutaminase and glutamine synthetase activities in human cirrhotic liver and hepatocellular carcinoma. *Cancer Res* 52, 1192–1194.

114 Marchesini G, Fabbri A, Bianchi G *et al.* (1996) Zinc supplementation and amino acid-nitrogen metabolism in patients with advanced cirrhosis. *Hepatology* 23, 1084–1092.

115 Häussinger D, Lamers WH, Moorman AF (1992) Hepatocyte heterogeneity in the metabolism of amino acids and ammonia. *Enzyme* 46, 72–93.

116 Hansen BA, Vilstrup H (1985) Increased intestinal hydrolysis of urea in patients with alcoholic cirrhosis. *Scand J Gastroenterol* 20, 346–350.

117 Lai D, Gorbach SL, Levitan R (1972) Intestinal microflora in patients with alcoholic cirrhosis: urea-splitting bacteria and neomycin resistance. *Gastroenterology* 62, 275–279.

118 Lockwood AH, McDonald JM, Reiman RE *et al.* (1979) The dynamics of ammonia metabolism in man. Effects of liver disease and hyperammonemia. *J Clin Invest* 63, 449–460.

119 Bessman SP, Bessman AN (1955) The cerebral and peripheral uptake of ammonia in liver disease with an hypothesis for the mechanism of hepatic coma. *J Clin Invest* 34, 622–628.

120 Fazekas JF, Ticktin HE, Shea JG (1957) Effect of 1-glutamic acid on metabolism of patients with hepatic encephalopathy. *Am J Med Sci* 234, 145–149.

121 Ganda OP, Ruderman NB (1976) Muscle nitrogen metabolism in chronic hepatic insufficiency. *Metabolism* 25, 427–430.

122 Allen SI, Conn HO (1960) Observations on the effect of exercise on blood ammonia concentration in man. *Yale J Biol Med* 33, 133–144.

123 Bachmann C (2002) Mechanisms of hyperammonemia. *Clin Chem Lab Med* 40, 653–662.

124 Brusilow SW, Horwich AL (2001) Urea cycle enzymes. In: Scriver CR, Beaudet AL, Sly WS *et al.* (eds) *The Metabolic Basis of Inherited Disease.* 8th edn. New York: McGraw Hill, pp. 1909–1963.

125 Caldovic L, Morizono H, Panglao MG *et al.* (2003) Null mutations in the N-acetylglutamate synthase gene associated with acute neonatal disease and hyperammonemia. *Hum Genet* 112, 364–368.

126 Schmidt E, Nuoffer JM, Haberle J *et al.* (2005) Identification of novel mutations of the human N-acetylglutamate synthase gene and their functional investigation by expression studies. *Biochim Biophys Acta* 1740, 54–59.

127 Häberle J, Gorg B, Rutsch F *et al.* (2005) Congenital glutamine deficiency with glutamine synthetase mutations. *N Engl J Med*, 353, 1956–33.

128 Saheki T, Kobayashi K, Iijima M *et al.* (2004) Adult-onset type II citrullinemia and idiopathic neonatal hepatitis caused by citrin deficiency: involvement of the aspartate glutamate carrier for urea synthesis and maintenance of the urea cycle. *Mol Genet Metab* 81, S20–S26.

129 Häussinger D (1988) *pH Homeostasis.* London: Academic Press.

130 Bourke E, Häussinger D (1992) pH homeostasis: the conceptual change. *Contrib Nephrol* 100, 58–88.

131 Lenzen C, Soboll S, Sies H *et al.* (1987) pH control of hepatic glutamine degradation. Role of transport. *Eur J Biochem* 16, 483–488.

132 Fei YJ, Sugawara M, Nakanishi T *et al.* (2000) Primary structure, genomic organization, and functional and electrogenic characteristics of human system N 1, a Na+- and H+-coupled glutamine transporter. *J Biol Chem* 275, 23707–23717.

133 Bode BP (2001) Recent molecular advances in mammalian glutamine transport. *J Nutr* 131, 2475S–2485S.

134 Fafournoux P, Demigne C, Remesy C *et al.* (1983) Bidirectional transport of glutamine across the cell membrane in rat liver. *Biochem J* 216, 401–408.

135 Boon L, Blommaart PJ, Meijer AJ *et al.* (1994) Acute acidosis inhibits liver amino acid transport: no primary role for the urea cycle in acid-base balance. *Am J Physiol* 267, F1015–F1020.

136 Christensen HN, Kilberg M (1995) Hepatic amino acid transport primary to the urea cycle in regulation of biologic neutrality. *Nutr Rev* 53, 74–76.

137 Balboni E, Lehninger AL (1986) Entry and exit pathways of CO_2 in rat liver mitochondria respiring in a bicarbonate buffer system. *J Biol Chem* 261, 3563–3570.

138 Curthoys NP, Watford M (1995) Regulation of glutaminase activity and glutamine metabolism. *Annu Rev Nutr* 15, 133–159.

139 Oster JR, Perez GO (1988) Acid–base homeostasis and pathophysiology in liver disease. In: Epstein M (ed.) *The Kidney in Liver Disease*, 3rd edn. Baltimore: Williams & Wilkins, pp. 119–131.

140 Record CO, Iles RA, Cohen RD *et al.* (1975) Acid–base and metabolic disturbances in fulminant hepatic failure. *Gut* 16, 144–149.

141 Dölle W (1965) *Der Säure-Basenstoffwechsel bei Leberzirrhose*. Hüthig Verlag, Heidelberg.

142 Moreau R, Hadengue A, Soupison T *et al.* (1993) Arterial and mixed venous acid-base status in patients with cirrhosis. Influence of liver failure. *Liver* 13, 20–24.

143 Bernardi M, Predieri S (2005) Disturbances of acid-base balance in cirrhosis: a neglected issue warranting further insights. *Liver Int* 25, 463–466.

144 Oster JR, Perez GO (1986) Acid-base disturbances in liver disease. *J Hepatol* 2, 299–306.

145 Guder W, Häussinger D (1987) Renal and hepatic nitrogen metabolism in systemic acid–base regulation. *J Clin Chem Clin Biochem* 25, 457–466.

146 Häussinger D (1990) Organization of hepatic nitrogen metabolism and its relation to acid-base homeostasis. *Klin Wschr* 68, 1096–1101.

147 Häussinger D, Steeb R, Gerok W (1992) Metabolic alkalosis as driving force for urea synthesis in liver disease: pathogenetic model and therapeutic implications. *Clin Investig* 70, 411–415.

148 Lustik SJ, Chhibber AK, Kolano JW *et al.* (1997) The hyperventilation of cirrhosis: progesterone and estradiol effects. *Hepatology* 25, 55–58.

149 Wichser J, Kazemi H (1974) Ammonia and ventilation: site and mechanism of action. *Respir Physiol* 20, 393–406.

150 Bihari D, Gimson AE, Lindridge J *et al.* (1985) Lactic acidosis in fulminant hepatic failure. Some aspects of pathogenesis and prognosis. *J Hepatol* 1, 405–416.

2.3.8 Protein synthesis and degradation in the liver

Armin Akhavan and Vishwanath R. Lingappa

Introduction

The proper physiological function of various organs relies on the expression of biologically active molecules such as antibodies, hormones and neurotransmitters as well as various ligands and receptors, and the signalling and other molecules by which they act. Many of these molecules are proteins, encoded in genes. Some are non-protein molecules (e.g. lipids, sugars and other small molecules such as nitric oxide gas) whose existence requires the action of proteins (e.g. enzymes that are involved in their synthesis). The DNA of the genes encoding these

proteins must be transcribed and processed into mRNAs and exported out of the nucleus into the cytoplasm, as a prerequisite for gene expression. This occurs by complex mechanisms that are outside the scope of this review. Once in the cytoplasm, mRNAs can be either quiescent, as a result of binding proteins that prevent their translation into proteins, or actively engaged in making their encoded polypeptides.

One important function of the liver is the synthesis and secretion of a wide range of proteins into the bloodstream, including blood clotting factors and transporter proteins such as lipoproteins and albumin. Another important function is the synthesis and correct localization of integral membrane proteins of the plasma membrane and other compartments. A common feature of these classes of proteins is that their fates are determined very early during translation of the mRNAs in which they are encoded. The nascent chains of these proteins are targeted to the membrane of the endoplasmic reticulum (ER), a specialized intracellular compartment that initiates their journey by subsequent vesicle fission and fusion through the secretory pathway (Fig. 1). Regulatory steps along the way ultimately determine the amount, function and/or localization of these proteins. Some of these steps, such as the initial event of translocation across (for a secretory protein) or integration into (for a membrane protein) the membrane of the ER, are, in their simplest manifestation, irreversible events. However, under certain conditions, these irreversible steps are overcome by cellular machineries that degrade undesired proteins, and thereby end their action. In this chapter, we describe first the fundamentals of early events in mRNA translation and degradation of newly synthesized secretory and membrane proteins. Subsequently, we discuss regulatory mechanisms of protein synthesis and degradation with emphasis on examples relevant to liver function and pathophysiology.

Principles of posttranscriptional gene expression

Translation of mRNA to protein

Translation of mRNA into protein starts by (i) binding of methionyl-tRNA ($tRNA_{Met}$) to the small ribosomal subunit (40S), (ii) recruitment of the complex to mRNA at the first AUG codon and (iii) joining of the large ribosomal subunit (60S) to the mRNA–40S complex. The eukaryotic initiation factors (eIF) are involved in all three steps of translation initiation [1]. Shortly before the start of translation, the eIF2 (composed of α, β and γ subunits) forms a complex with GTP and $tRNA_{Met}$ to facilitate binding to the small ribosomal subunit. The binding of this preinitiation complex, known as the 43S complex, to mRNA is assisted both in *cis* and in *trans*. The *cis* element referred to is the 'cap', a modified guanine nucleotide at the 5′ end of mRNA, which in many cases is critical for the recruitment of 43S by the eIF4 complex [2]. The eIF4 complex is composed of several proteins including: eIF4E, which physically binds the

Fig. 1 Synthesis, maturation and degradation of a membrane glycoprotein. A schematic diagram of a hepatocyte is shown indicating numbered key compartments relevant to protein synthesis and degradation. Let us consider the pathway involved in integral membrane protein biogenesis and illustrate the roles of each compartment. First, the mRNA is transcribed, processed and exported from the nucleus (1) via the nuclear pores (see arrow). Translation is initiated in the cytoplasm on free ribosomes (2) in the cytosol. Secretory and integral membrane protein nascent chains are targeted to the ER (3) via the signal recognition particle (SRP), which binds the signal sequence and is released upon interaction with the SRP receptor at the cytoplasmic face of the ER membrane (4). This results in opening of the translocon in the ER membrane and translocation/integration of the nascent polypeptide into the ER membrane. Concurrently, the nascent chain interacts with luminal proteins (such as molecular chaperones) and undergoes posttranslational modifications (such as glycosylation and signal sequence cleavage). The maturation of polypeptides continues as they exit the ER and transit the Golgi complex, composed of *cis* (6), medial (7) and *trans* (8) stacks, by vesicle fission and fusion. Vesicles (9) leaving the trans-Golgi network can take a number of different paths depending on various determinants of trafficking pathways. Thus, the mature protein is transported to its final destination at the lysosome (10) or apical (11) or basolateral (12) plasma membrane. All these events involve vesicle fusion (13). Vesicles also form by internalization from the plasma membrane (14), leading to various endosome-related compartments (15) including the lysosome (10). Before exit from the ER, membrane proteins are scrutinized by proteins termed molecular chaperones for abnormal structural features and/or covalent modifications. If recognized as misfolded or unassembled, the protein is bound by the molecular chaperone, transported out of the ER through the translocon 'in reverse' and sent for degradation by the 26S proteasome (5). There are multiple forms of the proteasome in multiple locations within the cytoplasm. Also shown are the endothelial cells (16) and red blood cells (17) on the basolateral side of the hepatocyte. Note that the apical plasma membrane comprises the bile canaliculus in the hepatocyte and represents a very small surface area compared with the much larger basolateral surface on the bloodstream side.

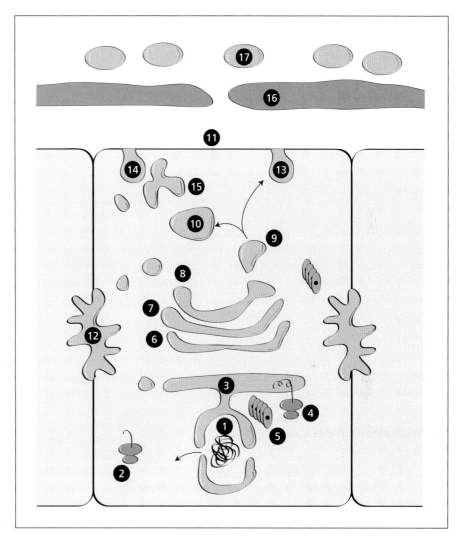

cap structure; eIF4A, which unwinds the secondary structures in the 5′ untranslated region (UTR); and eIF4G, which plays a scaffolding role by interacting with other eIFs. Subsequent to the formation of the ribosome–mRNA complex, the ribosome starts translation at the AUG codon corresponding to the first methio-nine. According to one proposal, the ribosome scans the mRNA molecule at the 5′ UTR until it reaches the first AUG codon in a favourable context (known as the Kozak sequence) [3]. An alternative mechanism for translation initiation has also been proposed (described below).

Targeting to the secretory pathway

While the basic aspects of translation initiation and elongation of secretory and membrane proteins are identical to those of the cytoplasmic proteins, the biogenesis of these different classes of proteins diverges shortly after the start of translation. Sorting and targeting of membrane and secretory proteins to the ER starts when the signal sequence emerges from the ribosome. Despite very little sequence homology between them, signal sequences can be best characterized as an extension of 20–50 amino acids containing a stretch of hydrophobic residues (the H-domain) sandwiched between a charged (N-domain) and a polar (C-domain) region, typically predicted to have a beta bend in secondary structure [4]. Extensive biochemical analyses in cell-free systems have established that the H-domain of the signal sequence is recognized by a cytoplasmic *trans*-acting factor termed the signal recognition particle (SRP). Mammalian SRP is a ribonucleoprotein consisting of six polypeptides (SRP9, SRP14, SRP19, SRP54, SRP68 and SRP72, where the numbers correspond to their molecular weight) and an RNA (SRP-RNA) [5]. Signal sequence recognition and SRP-RNA binding is attained through SRP54, a GTPase that mediates ER targeting of the ribosome–nascent chain complex when bound to GTP. During targeting, GTP hydrolysis is inhibited by both the ribosome and the signal sequence. Thus, translation is transiently arrested until targeting is completed. Following targeting, the interaction between the SRP and SRP receptor (SR) stimulates GTP hydrolysis, SRP release and the resumption of protein synthesis. SR is also composed of two GTPase subunits. The α subunit (SRα) is closely related to the GTPase domain of SRP54. SRα interacts with SRβ, which is an integral membrane protein with a GTPase domain related to Sar1 and the ARF family.

Translocation across the ER

Following ER targeting, translation resumes, with the chain entering the aqueous environment of the translocation channel, also termed the translocon. During translocation of the polypeptide chain, the ribosome is classically viewed as forming a tight seal with the translocon. This seal shields the nascent chain from the cytosolic environment [6]. At this point, many irreversible decisions are taken, and the nascent chain is folded, covalently modified and assembled into a functional unit through a dynamic network of protein–protein interactions [7]. Signal peptidase and oligosaccharyl transferase (OST) are responsible for cleavage of the signal sequence at the C-domain and addition of sugar residues to the consensus N-linked glycosylation sites respectively. The folding and assembly of the nascent chain is assisted by ER resident proteins such as calnexin, immunoglobulin heavy chain binding protein (BiP), protein disulphide isomerase (PDI) and others. In addition, in the course of translocation, whereas secretory proteins completely cross the ER membrane to enter the lumen, individual segments of topologically distinct membrane proteins are parti-

tioned between the cytosol, the lumen and the ER membrane. In order to accommodate these modifications and cope with the complexity of the topology of membrane proteins, the translocon must provide a dynamic environment for the growing polypeptide [8]. In eukaryotes, the translocon is formed from heteromeric membrane proteins referred to as the Sec61 complex (with α, β and γ subunits) [9]. This complex is necessary and, in some cases, sufficient for translocation. The translocation of the majority of proteins is facilitated by the translocating chain-associating membrane (TRAM), a multispanning glycoprotein that aids the formation of a tight ribosome–membrane junction through a signal sequence-dependent process [10]. In addition, the translocon complex interacts with the ribosome, the signal peptidase complex and the OST, as well as the translocon-associated protein (TRAP), in a manner that accommodates the enormous diversity of proteins that transit the secretory pathway. Therefore, the profile of secretory and membrane protein synthesis is dependent not only on signals encoded by the primary amino acid sequence (such as the signal sequence) but also on a dynamic interplay between cellular factors whose interactions with the nascent chain during translocation ultimately determine protein topology and folding. Mutations in the genes that encode components of the ER translocation and processing machinery have been identified in patients with autosomal-dominant polycystic liver disease [11]. The precise mechanism of integration into the ER membrane remains unclear. The simple-minded notion that hydrophobic domains are stabilized in the bilayer as they emerge from the ribosome seems untenable in the light of evidence that the translocation channel is aqueous [12,13], that multiple transmembrane loops are positioned in some cases before integration occurs [14,15] and the occurrence of discrete charged, extracytoplasmic sequences (termed stop transfer effector sequences) that are necessary for integration at subsequent hydrophobic domains, at least in some cases [16,17]. However, a specific integration receptor has yet to be identified for transmembrane protein biogenesis. Of particular interest is evidence of *trans*-acting factors that can alter the fate of a nascent chain, taking a polypeptide that would be destined to be an integral membrane protein and, instead, directing it to a different translocation/folding pathway by which it is secreted [18,19].

Beyond the ER

During and subsequent to translation and translocation, the newly synthesized proteins are either degraded (described in the next section) or further processed and matured in order to contribute to the protein's physiological function. Maturation involves non-covalent folding and covalent, post- and cotranslational modifications, as well as trafficking through the secretory pathway to the correct final destination. These events may be interconnected, for example some posttranslational modifications occur in specialized compartments (e.g. sialylation of proteins in the *trans*-Golgi network). In other cases, a posttranslational modification is a requisite for a particular compartmental trafficking event (e.g. the role of mannose residue phosphorylation in directing lysosomal enzymes out of the secretory pathway and to those organelles; see [20]).

Proteins destined for posttranslational maturation leave the ER either by a signal-mediated event (i.e. receptor–ligand interaction) or by bulk flow through budding and fusion of vesicles with consecutive organelles [21]. Budding of ER vesicles is driven by polymerization of a protein called coat protein II (COPII) from specialized ER exit sites. These vesicles lose their coat and fuse to the so-called vesicular tubular clusters (VTCs), also known as the ER–Golgi intermediate compartment. The cargo is then taken from VTCs in vesicles to the Golgi complex. ER resident proteins, however, recycle back to the ER in vesicles coated with a different protein, termed COPI.

The processing and sorting of proteins continues at the Golgi complex by sequential progress through the cis-, medial- and trans-Golgi cisternae. Transport of the cargo from trans-Golgi to the plasma membrane, lysosome or to other endomembranes takes place by clathrin-coated vesicles. In addition to COP coatomers and clathrin, various adapter proteins are involved in the transport of cargo between secretory compartments. The lectin ERGIC-53, for example, is involved in the transport of various glycoprotein cargo including clotting factors V and VIII [22]. Mutations in ERGIC-53 or an associated protein (MCFD2) cause a bleeding disorder, probably by disrupting the secretion of blood clotting factors by the liver [23].

An important dimension of postsynthetic sorting that is particularly prominent in the liver, but will not be discussed in detail here, involves directing proteins to the apical vs. the basolateral aspects of the plasma membrane [24] (see Chapter 2.2.2). In the liver, the apical plasma membrane is limited to the bile canalicular membrane, while the much larger basolateral aspect is in contact with the bloodstream via the sinusoidal space (discussed in Chapter 2.2.2). The exocyst is a cytoplasmic particle comprising multiple proteins that is involved in the trafficking of vesicles during apical vs. basolateral sorting [24]. Recent evidence suggests a regulatory connection between protein synthesis and trafficking, by which, perhaps, cells are able to 'keep count' of proteins synthesized and targeted to one membrane face vs. another [25–27]. Thus, Sec61β, a component of the translocon complex, has been associated with binding components of the exocyst, although the molecular mechanism of this interaction and the regulatory feedback loops involved remain unclear.

Degradation

Among a large number of proteases involved in protein degradation, the best understood are the lysosomal and the 26S proteasomal degradation pathways. The former takes place in lysosomes, a membrane-enclosed acidic environment filled with hydrolytic enzymes. The lysosomal degradation pathway is critical for bulk proteolysis by visceral tissues such as the liver and for clearance of unwanted proteins recycled from the plasma

membrane [28]. The proteasomal degradation pathway, on the other hand, is largely involved in processes that require fine control of protein degradation. The 26S proteasome consists of a central hollow cylinder (the 20S proteasome) and two caps on each end (the 19S caps). The 20S proteasome is composed of distinct proteases arranged with their active sites facing the inner chamber. The 19S cap includes protein subunits with ATPase activity, which unfold proteins and move them to the interior chamber. Perhaps the best understood function of proteasomes is in ER-associated degradation (ERAD) [29]. It is generally believed that the ER is equipped with machinery for the selection of misfolded or unassembled proteins that are recognized through exposure of structural tags (such as disulphide bonds) or posttranslational modifications (such as signal sequence cleavage and glycosylation) [7]. These proteins are generally believed to be misfolded forms recognized by the ER molecular chaperones that exercise a 'quality control' function over protein products before they enter the later stages of the secretory pathway. The journey of such misfolded molecules through the secretory pathway is blocked at the level of ER where they are, instead, targeted for return to the cytoplasm and destruction by the 26S proteasome complex. For example, the majority of mutations in the low-density lipoprotein receptor, which cause familial hypercholesterolaemia, result in its intracellular retention and, hence, the inability of the liver to maintain lipoprotein metabolism [30]. Other liver disorders that are caused by defective trafficking of secretory and membrane proteins include α-1-antitrypsin deficiency [31] and Laron syndrome (as a consequence of mutations in growth hormone receptor) [32].

The details of the ERAD machinery are best understood in the case of glycoproteins (Fig. 1) [33]. The lectin chaperones calnexin and calreticulin identify aberrant sugar residues on glycoproteins and retain these proteins in the ER through successive cycles of removal and readdition of glucose residues to the core sugars initially added during translocation across the ER membrane. These cycles offer the misfolded protein an opportunity to refold in a productive manner. If successful, the correctly refolded molecule is deglycosylated, released and exported to the vesicles destined for the Golgi apparatus. If refolding is unsuccessful, the consequence can be degradation by the 26S proteasome. Before degradation by the proteasome, however, these polypeptides must recross the ER membrane through a process referred to as retrotranslocation or dislocation [34]. Numerous genetic and biochemical studies have suggested that Sec61, in addition to its well-established role in translocation, is also critical for the disposal of unwanted proteins from the ER into the cytosol. Recently, two parallel reports identified Derline-1 as an ER membrane protein responsible for retrotranslocation of certain substrates [35,36]. In all cases, the driving force for extracting the polypeptide from the ER membrane is likely to be provided by the p97 ATPase complex [34]. During extraction from the ER membrane, unwanted proteins are covalently modified by the addition of a chain of small molecules referred to as ubiquitin (Ub). The polyubiquitylated proteins are targeted to the 26S proteasome, which ultimately cleaves them into small peptides but spares the Ub moiety. In order to facilitate proteasomal degradation, N-glycans are removed prior to proteolysis by a ubiquitous cytosolic N-glycanase [37].

In some cases, unwanted proteins are selected for degradation at sites other than the ER, such as in the nucleus. A recent study has identified that the characteristics of nuclear degradation machinery resemble those of ERAD [38].

Translational control of gene expression

In order to cope with the environmental and physiological challenges constantly encountered by organs and cells, the production of proteins is subject to regulation at all levels of synthesis. Since protein synthesis requires both amino acids and metabolic energy, in some instances, such as in starvation, regulation of translation initiation is an important survival factor. Regulation of protein synthesis is also important in cases where variations of protein levels are essential for the progress of cells through specific stages, such as the steps of the cell cycle and development.

Regulation of translation initiation in *cis* and in *trans*

Control of translation initiation is widespread, relying on both the structural features of individual mRNAs (*cis*-regulatory factors) and the molecules involved in the translation initiation process (*trans*-regulatory factors). Alternative models for the recruitment of ribosomes to mRNA have been proposed that are independent of the cap, such as use of an internal RNA structure known as the internal ribosomal entry site (IRES) [39]. These structures were first found in picornavirus mRNA [40] and later in hepatitis C virus and related pestiviruses [41]. These viruses manipulate cellular eIFs, either by phosphorylation or through degradation, in a manner that blocks the cap-dependent translation without compromising IRES-mediated translation [42]. By doing so, the essential eIFs, which are normally engaged by the cap-dependent translation of host mRNA, are now hijacked for the translation of viral mRNA through IRES-dependent initiation. IRES-dependent translation initiation has also been described for a number of cellular mRNAs including BiP, fibroblast growth factor 2, vascular endothelial growth factor and so on [2]. Some cellular mRNAs contain a 5' cap-dependent initiation site in addition to an IRES element located in their coding region [43]. This enables proteins of distinct functions to be generated by alternative translation initiation of a single mRNA molecule. In an extreme case, the translation of the fibroblast growth factor 2 can generate five different products through four IRES sites in addition to cap-dependent translation.

In eukaryotes, IRES-dependent translation initiation is mainly involved in the expression of a selective number of genes under conditions in which cap-dependent protein synthesis is blocked, such as during stress, some stages of the cell cycle and apoptosis

[42]. At least four kinases have been identified that are activated in response to viral infection, low levels of haem in red blood cells, amino acid starvation and during the ER stress response. These kinases typically inhibit translation initiation through phosphorylation of eIF2α. In addition, degradation of eIF4G, which prevents cap-dependent translation, has been reported in cells undergoing apoptosis or infected with certain viruses [43]. Thus, the rate and the level of translation, as well as the site of translation initiation, are governed by structural elements of mRNA and modification of eIFs.

Regulation of protein degradation

Examples of cellular processes regulated by degradation include apoptosis, development, cell cycle, antigen processing and lipid metabolism by the liver [44]. In addition, the half-life of normally short-lived proteins is thought to be determined by degradation through recognition of signals inherent in their amino acid sequence. Among these signals, the best characterized is the N-degron of the N-end rule pathway, in which the half-life of a protein is determined by the identity of its N-terminal amino acid [45].

Lipid metabolism by the liver is a prime example of regulated degradation [46]. The liver enzyme 3-hydroxy-3-methylglutaryl coenzyme A reductase (HMGR) is an integral membrane protein of the ER, and it functions as a rate-limiting enzyme for the synthesis of cholesterol. HMGR degradation is accelerated in the presence of sterol precursors of cholesterol when production is unnecessary. This process, which is similar to ERAD, is inhibited when the flux through the sterol pathway is low and HMGR activity is essential for cholesterol production. In addition to HMGR, sterol regulation by the liver is subject to regulated degradation at other levels. For example, apolipoprotein 100 (ApoB) is also degraded by the ERAD if not assembled into very-low-density lipoprotein particles in the liver secretory pathway [47,48]. Therefore, proteolysis directs many cellular processes, primarily by controlling the levels of intracellular proteins, a function that was originally solely assigned to transcription and translational control.

Future prospects: regulation of translocation and targeting

Relative to translation initiation and degradation, regulatory events at the level of targeting and translocation have primarily been limited to examples involving proofreading (accuracy) functions. However, because many important and irreversible events govern targeting and translocation steps, regulation at this stage may influence key features of proteins including localization, structure and function. In the following section, we will discuss the stages of translocation and targeting that could be points of regulation. We will also present a new view, in which these regulatory stages could control protein conformation, a concept that may provide a rationale for many phenomenological observations of protein function that cannot be explained by conventional views [49].

The opportunity to regulate targeting begins as soon as the signal sequence emerges from the ribosome. Recognition of the signal sequence by the SRP results in a transient arrest in translation [50]. At this point, the time window of translation arrest and, hence, the rate of synthesis could be regulated by signalling events. The strength of interaction between SRP and the signal sequence could also be modified in a manner preferable for some signal sequences over the others. In extreme cases, dissociation of SRP from the signal sequence may prevent targeting and generate a cytoplasmic protein that serves a different function, the same function at a distinct cellular location or that may be rapidly degraded. The last possibility has been described recently for PrP as a result of the inefficiency of signal sequence function, which generates proteasomally degraded cytosolic protein [51]. Alternatively, in the absence of bound SRP, polypeptide chains may be synthesized in the cytoplasm and, hence, available for signalling molecules and posttranslational modifications that would otherwise be inaccessible during cotranslational translocation. These modified molecules may than be translocated across the ER through posttranslational translocation [52]. Posttranslational modifications will not necessarily provide steric hindrance for translocation across the Sec61 channel, as N-linked glycosylation moieties are well tolerated for retrotranslocation through the same channel.

The next opportunity for regulation comes after targeting when the nascent chain–ribosome complex is docked at the translocon. According to the dogma, the growing chain is protected from cytosolic factors by virtue of a tight seal formed between the ribosome and the ER membrane. However, it has been shown recently that the length of the polypeptide chain accessible to cytosolic proteases varies depending on the heterogenous signal sequence [53]. Although a physiological significance for this phenomenon remains to be demonstrated, it can promote the exposure of an otherwise shielded mature domain to cytosolic factors. Indeed, pause transfer sequences have been identified in ApoB that mediate sufficient temporal and spatial opening of the ribosome membrane junction to allow for interaction with cytoplasmically applied macromolecules [54].

Each step in protein biogenesis represents a unique opportunity for regulation. Translation initiation, for example, is the last step at which a cell can decide whether to express a particular gene or not. Degradation, on the other hand, is the only way to diminish the amounts of an already existing protein. What could the regulatory process at the level of translocation accomplish that is unique and inaccessible during translation initiation or degradation? During translocation, a nascent polypeptide must acquire its proper structure through an array of interactions and modifications by ER resident proteins and cytosolically accessible molecules, as well as the ribosome. At this stage, a nascent chain is directed to multiple folded states, some of which are thermodynamically unfavourable. With reference to most developing processes, plasticity is conceivable for early translocational events that shape the structure of a protein. For instance, trans-acting factors (such as TRAM) could influence the energetics of protein folding by changing the environment of the translocon in favour of one structure over the others [55,18]. By doing so, for any unique amino acid sequence, multiple structures and, hence, functions could be assigned. Functionally and conformationally distinct proteins could be selected either by signalling molecules that impinge on trans-acting factors during translocation or by selective degradation during or after synthesis. There is precedence for both these mechanisms. First, in the case of PrP, at least three conformationally distinct forms have been identified arising from a single amino acid sequence. Two of these forms span the membrane once in the opposite direction, and the third form is fully translocated across the membrane [56]. An ER membrane protein (TRAP alpha) has been identified that favours the expression of secretory PrP over the membrane forms [18,19]. Consistent with the existence of different structures, multiple functions have been identified for PrP as both a proapoptotic and an antiapoptotic factor [57]. Second, degradation is another way in which functionally desired proteins can be selected. Cotranslational degradation is commonly observed for a large fraction of newly synthesized proteins [58,59]. In the case of the cystic fibrosis transmembrane conductance regulatory (CFTR) gene, less than 30% of newly synthesized molecules transit to post-ER compartments, with the majority of the wild-type molecules retained in the ER [60]. Whereas the ER-retained fraction degrades rapidly (half-life = 20–40 min), the post-ER fraction is remarkably stable with a half-life of hours. This quantitative heterogeneity persists even after inhibiting ER-to-Golgi traffic, indicating that differential stability is not a mere consequence of distinct localization. Instead, differential stability reflects different structural states, each with a unique folding thermodynamic. Although in the case of CFTR, the energetically unfavourable structural variant is retained in the ER, energetically unfavourable mutant proteins have been identified that exit the ER with an efficiency similar to wild type in a tissue-specific manner [61]. Together, these findings imply that the commonly observed cotranslational degradation is not merely a way to rid the cell of non-functional molecules that are structurally unstable. ERAD and other degradative machinery may serve to prune gene expression and eliminate *functional* protein conformations that are not desired at that precise time or by certain cell types. More studies are needed to see whether this and other alternative notions of regulated gene expression are generally valid or represent unusual variations observed for a small number of specialized proteins.

References

1 Gbauer F, Hentze MW (2004) Molecular mechanisms of translational control. *Nature Rev Mol Cell Biol* 5, 827–835.
2 Gingras AC, Raught B, Sonenberg N (1999) eIF4 initiation factors: effectors of mRNA recruitment to ribosomes and regulators of translation. *Annu Rev Biochem* 68, 913–963.

3 Kozak M (1986) Point mutations define a sequence flanking the AUG initiator codon that modulates translation by eukaryotic ribosomes. *Cell* 44, 283–292.

4 Martoglio B, Dobberstein B (1998) Signal sequences: more than just greasy peptides. *Trends Cell Biol* 10, 410–415.

5 Keenan RJ, Fremann DM, Stroud RM *et al.* (2001) The signal recognition particle. *Annu Rev Biochem* 70, 755–775.

6 Jungnickel B, Rapoport TA (1995) A posttargeting signal sequence recognition event in the endoplasmic reticulum membrane. *Cell* 82, 261–270.

7 Ellgaard L, Molinari M, Helenius A (1999) Setting the standards: quality control in the secretory pathway. *Science* 286, 1882–1888.

8 Hegde RS, Lingappa VR (1997) Membrane protein biogenesis: regulated complexity at the endoplasmic reticulum. *Cell* 91, 575–582.

9 Johnson AE, Waes MA (1999) The translocon: a dynamic gateway at the ER membrane. *Annu Rev Cell Dev Biol* 15, 799–842.

10 Voigt S, Jungnickel B, Hartmann E *et al.* (1996) Signal sequence-dependent function of the TRAM protein during early phases of protein transport across the endoplasmic reticulum. *J Cell Biol* 134, 25–35.

11 Drenth JPH, Martina JA, van de Kerkhof R *et al.* (2004) Polycystic liver disease is a disorder of cotranslational protein processing. *Trends Mol Med* 11, 37–42.

12 Gilmore R, Blobel G (1985) Translocation of secretory proteins across the microsomal membrane occurs through an environment accessible to aqueous perturbants. *Cell* 42, 497–505.

13 Simon SM, Blobel G (1991) A protein-conducting channel in the endoplasmic reticulum. *Cell* 65, 371–380.

14 Borel AC, Simon SM (1996) Biogenesis of polytopic membrane proteins: membrane segments assemble within translocation channels prior to membrane integration. *Cell* 85, 379–389.

15 Skach WR, Lingappa VR (1993) Amino-terminal assembly of human P-glycoprotein at the endoplasmic reticulum is directed by cooperative actions of two internal sequences. *J Biol Chem* 268, 23552–23561.

16 Yost CS, Lopez CD, Prusiner SB *et al.* (1990) Non-hydrophobic extracytoplasmic determinant of stop transfer in the prion protein. *Nature* 343, 669–672.

17 Falcone D, Do H, Johnson AE *et al.* (1999) Negatively charged residues in the IgM stop-transfer effector sequence regulate transmembrane polypeptide integration. *J Biol Chem* 274, 33661–33670.

18 Hegde RS, Voigt S, Lingappa VR (1998) Regulation of protein topology by trans-acting factors at the endoplasmic reticulum. *Mol Cell* 2, 85–91.

19 Fons RD, Bogert BA, Hegde RS (2003) Substrate-specific function of the translocon-associated protein complex during translocation across the ER membrane. *J Cell Biol* 160, 529–539.

20 Dell'Angelica EC, Payne GS (2001) Intracellular cycling of lysosomal enzyme receptors: cytoplasmic tails' tales. *Cell* 106, 395–398.

21 Lee MCS, Miller EA, Goldberg J *et al.* (2004) Bi-directional protein transport between the ER and Golgi. *Annu Rev Cell Dev Biol* 20, 87–123.

22 Appenzeller C, Anderson H, Kappeler F *et al.* (1999) The lectin ERGIC-53 is a cargo transport receptor for glycoproteins. *Nature Cell Biol* 6, 330–334.

23 Zhang B, Cunningham MA, Nichols WC *et al.* (2003) Bleeding due to disruption of a cargo-specific ER-to-Golgi transport complex. *Nature Genet* 34, 220–225.

24 Zegers MM, Hoekstra D (1998) Mechanisms and functional features of polarized membrane traffic in epithelial and hepatic cells. *Biochem J* 336, 257–269.

25 Guo W, Novick P (2004) The exocyst meets the translocon: a regulatory circuit for secretion and protein synthesis? *Trends Cell Biol* 14, 61–63.

26 Lipschutz JH, Lingappa VR, Mostov KE (2003) The exocyst affects protein synthesis by acting on the translocation machinery of the endoplasmic reticulum. *J Biol Chem* 278, 20954–20960.

27 Toikkanen JH, Miller KJ, Soderlund H *et al.* (2003) Beta subunit of the Sec61p endoplasmic reticulum translocon interacts with the exocyst complex in *Saccharomyces cerevisiae*. *J Biol Chem* 278, 20946–20953.

28 Dunn WA (1994) Autophagy and related mechanisms of lysosome-mediated protein degradation. *Trends Cell Biol* 4, 139–143.

29 Trombetta ES, Parodi AJ (2003) Quality control and protein folding in the secretory pathway. *Annu Rev Cell Dev Biol* 19, 649–676.

30 Hobbs HH, Russell DW, Brown MS *et al.* (1990) The LDL receptor locus in familial hypercholesterolemia: mutational analysis of a membrane protein. *Annu Rev Genet* 24, 133–170.

31 Stoller JK, Aboussouan LS (2005) Alpha1-antitrypsin deficiency. *Lancet* 365, 2225–2236.

32 Laron Z (1993) Disorders of growth hormone resistance in childhood. *Curr Opin Pediatr* 5, 474–480.

33 Helenius A, Abi M (2004) Roles of N-linked glycans in the endoplasmic reticulum. *Annu Rev Biochem* 73, 1019–1049.

34 Tsai B, Ye Y, Rapoport TA (2002) Retro-translocation of proteins from the endoplasmic reticulum into the cytosol. *Nature Rev Mol Cell Biol* 3, 246–255.

35 Lilley BN, Ploegh H (2004) A membrane protein required for dislocation of misfolded proteins from the ER. *Nature* 429, 834–840.

36 Ye Y, Shibata Y, Ron D *et al.* (2004) A membrane protein complex mediates retro-translocation from the ER lumen into the cytosol. *Nature* 429, 841–847.

37 Suzuki T, Park H, Lennarz WJ (2002) Cytoplasmic peptide: N-glycanase (PNGase) in eukaryotic cells: occurrence, primary structure, and potential functions. *FASEB J* 16, 635–641.

38 Gardner RG, Nelson ZW, Gottschling DE (2005) Degradation-mediated protein quality control in the nucleus. *Cell* 120, 803–815.

39 Vagner S, Galy B, Pyronnet S *et al.* (2001) Attracting the translation machinery to internal ribosome entry sites. *EMBO Rep* 2, 893–898.

40 Pelletier J, Sonenberg N (1988) Internal initiation of translation of eukaryotic mRNA directed by a sequence derived from poliovirus RNA. *Nature* 334, 320–325.

41 Tsukiyama-Kohara K, Iizuka N, Kohara M *et al.* (1992) Internal ribosomal entry site within hepatitis C viruses. *J Virol* 66, 1476–1483.

42 Komar AA, Hatzoglous M (2005) Internal ribosome entry sites in cellular mRNAs: mystery of their existence. *J Biol Chem* 280, 23425–23428.

43 Dever TE (2002) Gene-specific regulation by general translation factors. *Cell* 108, 545–556.

44 Varshavsky A (2005) Regulated protein degradation. *Trends Biochem Sci* 30, 283–286.

45 Varshavsky A (1996) The N-end rule: functions, mysteries, uses. *Proc Natl Acad Sci USA* 93, 12142–12149.

46 Hampton RY (2002) Proteolysis and sterol regulation. *Annu Rev Cell Dev Biol* 18, 345–378.

47 Fisher EA, Zhou M, Mitchell DM *et al.* (1997) The degradation of apolipoprotein B100 is mediated by the ubiquitin-proteasome pathway and involves heat shock protein 70. *J Biol Chem* 272, 20427–20434.

48 Ginsberg HN (1997) Role of lipid synthesis, chaperone proteins and proteasomes in the assembly and secretion of apoprotein B-containing

lipoproteins from cultured liver cells. *Clin Exp Pharmacol Physiol* 24, A29–A32.

49 Lingappa VR, Rutkowski DT, Hegde RS *et al.* (2002) Conformational control through translocational regulation: a new view of secretory and membrane protein folding. *BioEssays* 24, 741–748.

50 Wolin SL, Walter P (1989) Signal recognition particle mediates a transient elongation arrest of preprolactin in reticulocyte lysate. *J Cell Biol* 109, 2617–2622.

51 Rane NS, Yokovich JL, Hegde RS (2004) Protection from cytosolic prion protein toxicity by modulation of protein translocation. *EMBO J* 23, 4550–4559.

52 Hansen W, Garcia PD, Walter P (1986) In vitro protein translocation across the yeast endoplasmic reticulum: ATP-dependent posttranslational translocation of the prepro-alpha-factor. *Cell* 45, 397–406.

53 Rutkowski DT, Lingappa VR, Hegde RS (2001) Substrate-specific regulation of the ribosome-translocon junction by N-terminal signal sequences. *Proc Natl Acad Sci USA* 98, 7823–7828.

54 Hegde RS, Lingappa VR (1996) Sequence-specific alteration of the ribosome-membrane junction exposes secretory proteins to the cytosol. *Cell* 85, 217–228.

55 Hegde RS, Voigt S, Rapoport TA *et al.* (1998) TRAM regulates the exposure of the nascent secretory proteins to the cytosol during translocation into the endoplasmic reticulum. *Cell* 92, 621–631.

56 Hegde RS, Mastrianni JA, Scott MR *et al.* (1998) A transmembrane form of the prion protein in neurodegenerative disease. *Science* 279, 827–834.

57 Saghafi S, Spilman P, Tan Z *et al.* (2006) Cellular prion protein topology determines pro- and anti-apoptotic functions (submitted).

58 Schubert U, Anton LC, Gibbs J *et al.* (2000) Rapid degradation of a large fraction of newly synthesized proteins by proteasomes. *Nature* 404, 770–774.

59 Turner GC, Varshavsky A (2000) Detecting and measuring cotranslational protein degradation in vivo. *Science* 289, 2117–2120.

60 Kopito RR (1999) Biosynthesis and degradation of CFTR. *Physiol Rev* 79, S167–S173.

61 Sekijima Y, Wiseman RL, Matteson J *et al.* (2005) The biological and chemical basis for tissue-selective amyloid disease. *Cell* 121, 73–85.

2.3.9 Glutathione

José C. Fernández-Checa and Carmen García-Ruiz

Introduction

The tripeptide glutathione (GSH) is one of the most intensively studied intracellular non-protein thiols on account of the critical role that it plays in cell biochemistry and physiology. GSH is a tripeptide found in high concentrations in all cells. It is synthesized from glutamate, cysteine and glycine in the cytosol in two steps, each requiring adenosine triphosphate (ATP) hydrolysis. GSH has certain structural features responsible for its stability and biological functions. For instance, the peptide bond linking the amino-terminal glutamate and the cysteine residue of GSH is through the γ-carboxyl group of glutamate rather than

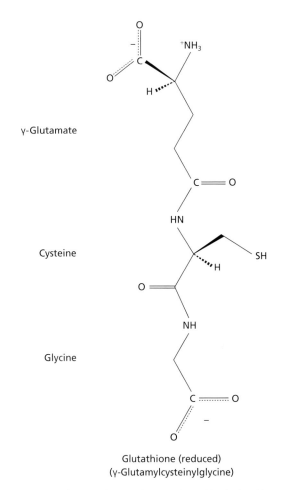

Fig. 1 Structure of GSH and its constituent amino acids. The bond between glutamate and cysteine determines the stability and resistance of GSH to hydrolysis, while its functions are mainly determined by the SH group of cysteine in its reduced form.

the conventional α-carboxyl group (Fig. 1). This unusual arrangement resists degradation by intracellular peptidases and is subject to hydrolysis by only one known enzyme, γ-glutamyltranspeptidase (GGT). Furthermore, the carboxyl-terminal glycine moiety of GSH protects the molecule against cleavage by intracellular γ-glutamylcyclotransferase. As a consequence, GSH is only metabolized extracellularly by GGT, which acts on the external face of certain cell types. Moreover, the sulphydryl group of cysteine is required for GSH's functions, in particular the regulation of disulphide bonds of proteins and the disposal of electrophiles and oxidants.

Despite its exclusive synthesis in the cytosol, GSH is distributed in intracellular organelles, including endoplasmic reticulum (ER) and mitochondria. GSH is found predominantly in its reduced form except in the ER, where it exists mainly as oxidized glutathione (GSSG) to provide the adequate environment necessary for protein metabolism. A tight connection between ER and cytosol is necessary to ensure an appropriate secretory function of the ER, as GSH in the cytosol reduces protein disulphide isomerase and restores normal disulphide formation and secretory rates. In mitochondria, however, GSH is mainly found in reduced form and represents a minor fraction of the total GSH pool (10–15%). Considering the volume of the mitochondrial matrix, the concentration of mitochondrial GSH (mGSH) may be similar to that of cytosol (10–14 mM). Owing to the widespread roles of GSH in cell physiology, changes in GSH homeostasis have been implicated in the aetiology and progression of a number of human diseases. In this chapter, we review its regulation and functions and its role in oxidative stress, hepatocyte death and liver diseases.

GSH homeostasis

GSH biosynthesis

GSH exists in high concentrations in all types of cells and is synthesized from precursor amino acids in the cytosol in two steps. The regulation of GSH biosynthesis is dependent mainly on cysteine availability and enzymatic activity [1,2]. The liver has unique features regarding GSH regulation, as hepatocytes are able to convert methionine to cysteine through the trans-sulphuration pathway. In addition, the rate of GSH biosynthesis in the hepatocyte is balanced by its rate of export, mainly into plasma and bile. The synthesis of GSH from its constituent amino acids, L-glutamate, L-cysteine and L-glycine, involves two ATP-requiring enzymatic steps (Fig. 2). The first step in GSH biosynthesis is rate limiting and catalysed by γ-glutamylcysteine synthetase (GCS), which exhibits an absolute requirement for either Mg^{2+} or Mn^{2+}. GCS is composed of a heavy (GCS-HS) and a light (GCS-LS) subunit, and each is encoded by different genes in both rat and human. The heavy subunit exhibits all the catalytic activity of the isolated enzyme and feedback inhibition by GSH. The light subunit, on the other hand, plays an important regulatory role in the overall function of the enzyme and allows the holoenzyme to be catalytically more efficient and less subject to inhibition by GSH than the heavy subunit alone.

GCS is regulated physiologically by two important factors: GSH inhibition and cysteine availability. Thus, inhibition by GSH is non-allosteric and involves binding of GSH to the glutamate site of the enzyme. A second binding site for GSH has been described and involves interaction with the thiol moiety of GSH. On the other hand, the availability of its precursor, L-cysteine, also regulates GCS. The apparent K_m values of GCS for glutamate and cysteine are 1.8 and 0.1–0.3 mM respectively. The intracellular glutamate concentration is severalfold higher than the K_m value of GCS for glutamate, but the intracellular cysteine concentration approximates the apparent K_m value of GCS for cysteine. Hence, both the availability of intracellular cysteine and the activity of GCS greatly influence the rate of GSH synthesis.

The second step in the synthesis of GSH is catalysed by GSH synthetase (GS) (Fig. 2). This enzyme has not been studied as extensively as GCS. However, GS is not subject to feedback inhibition by GSH. Overexpression of GS fails to increase GSH levels as opposed to overexpression of GCS, which increases GSH. However, GS deficiency in humans can result in dramatic metabolic consequences because the accumulated γ-glutamylcysteine is converted to 5-oxoproline, which can cause severe metabolic acidosis [3].

Because the availability of cysteine is a critical determinant of GSH synthesis, factors that regulate intracellular cysteine levels ultimately contribute to GSH biosynthesis and, hence, cellular GSH levels. Among these, the transport of cysteine or cystine (and its subsequent reduction to cysteine intracellularly) or methionine transport modulate the intracellular levels of GSH. The transport of methionine is effective in regulating GSH biosynthesis through the subsequent conversion of methionine into cysteine by the trans-sulphuration pathway (Fig. 3), which operates only in hepatocytes. In addition to the intracellular cysteine availability, the regulation of GCS is a critical step in GSH homeostasis. The activity of GCS is regulated at both the transcriptional and the posttranscriptional levels, and hormones may modulate hepatic GSH biosynthesis through GCS regulation [4].

GSH degradation

In contrast to GSH synthesis, GSH degradation occurs exclusively in the extracellular space and only in cells that express the enzyme GGT. GGT, which is abundant on the apical surface of most transporting epithelia, including liver canalicular and bile ductular membranes, is the only enzyme that can initiate catabolism of GSH, glutathione-S-conjugates and glutathione complexes under physiological conditions. Because GGT is a plasma membrane-bound enzyme with its active site on the extracellular surface of the membrane, export of GSH and its adducts into the extracellular space is the initial, and presumably regulated, step in their turnover in all mammalian cells. GGT removes the glutamyl moiety from GSH and GSH-containing compounds to yield cysteinylglycine or cysteinylglycine-S-

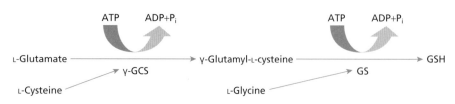

Fig. 2 GSH synthesis. The biosynthesis of GSH needs glutamate, cysteine and glycine, which are bound in two steps catalysed by γ-GCS and GS, which adds glycine to γ-glutamylcysteine. Both enzymes require ATP hydrolysis and, hence, the synthesis of GSH is energy consuming. In addition to γ-GCS, which is the rate-limiting enzyme, the availability of cysteine regulates GSH synthesis.

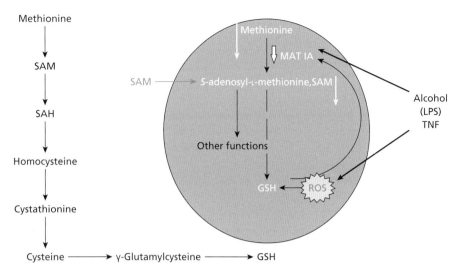

Fig. 3 The trans-sulphuration pathway and role of S-adenosyl-L-methionine (SAM) in alcohol-induced GSH regulation. In addition to the limited availability of cysteine in the biosynthesis of GSH, methionine meets the need for cysteine. It is channelled for GSH biosynthesis through the trans-sulphuration pathway, in which the sulphur of methionine is converted into cysteine. A key component of this process is SAM, which acts as a GSH precursor in hepatocytes and, hence, prevents GSH depletion induced by agents such as alcohol. LPS, lipopolysaccharide; ROS, reactive oxygen species; TNF, tumour necrosis factor.

conjugates. These compounds are substrates for dipeptidases, which hydrolyse the peptide bond between cysteine and glycine. Dipeptidases are also ectoproteins; thus, these reactions also occur in the extracellular space. The hepatic transport of GSH into plasma and bile thus contributes to its extrahepatic metabolism, which has been reviewed elsewhere [5].

Biological functions

Detoxification of Michael electrophiles and metals

Detoxification of xenobiotics or their metabolites is one of the major functions of GSH. GSH, being a nucleophile, targets electrophiles with αβ unsaturated carbonyl moieties or Michael electrophiles. These compounds form conjugates with GSH either spontaneously or enzymatically in reactions catalysed by GSH S-transferases [1]. This reaction results not only in the removal of the electrophile via its subsequent metabolism or transport out of the cell, but also in the potential depletion of GSH, particularly if GSH biosynthesis does not match the rate of electrophile elimination. The metabolism of GSH conjugates begins with cleavage of the γ-glutamyl moiety by GGT, leaving a cysteinyl–glycine conjugate. The cysteinyl–glycine bond is cleaved by dipeptidase, resulting in a cysteinyl conjugate. This is followed by N-acetylation of the cysteine conjugate, forming a mercapturic acid. The metabolism of GSH conjugates to mercapturic acid begins in the biliary tree, intestine or kidney, but the formation of the N-acetylcysteine conjugate usually occurs in the kidney.

In addition to exogenous compounds, many endogenously formed compounds also follow similar metabolic pathways. Some examples include estradiol-17-β, leukotrienes and prostaglandins [4,6]. GSH also forms metal complexes via non-enzymatic reactions. GSH is one of the most versatile and pervasive metal-binding ligands and plays an important role in metal transport, storage and metabolism. GSH functions in the mobilization and delivery of metals between ligands, in the transport of metals across cell membranes, as a source of cysteine for metal binding and as a reductant or cofactor in redox reactions involving metals. The sulphydryl group of the cysteine moiety of GSH has a high affinity for metals, forming thermodynamically stable but kinetically labile mercaptides with a number of metals, including mercury, silver, cadmium, arsenic, lead, gold, zinc and copper.

Maintenance of thiol status

As the dominant non-protein thiol in mammalian cells, GSH is essential in maintaining the intracellular redox balance and the essential thiol status of proteins [1,4,6]. To achieve this, GSH undergoes thiol–disulphide exchange in a reaction catalysed by thiol-transferase, as follows:

$$\text{Protein–SSG} + \text{GSH} \rightarrow \text{protein–SH} + \text{GSSG}$$

As this reaction is reversible, the equilibrium is determined by the redox state of the cell, which depends on the concentrations of GSH and GSSG [proportional to the log of $(GSH)^2/(GSSG)$]. Normally, cellular GSSG is kept very low (< 1% of the total GSH pool) so that protein mixed disulphide formation is limited. The thiol–disulphide equilibrium within the cell is known to regulate a diverse number of metabolic processes, including enzyme activity, transport activity and gene expression, via alteration of redox-sensitive *trans*-activating factors.

Antioxidant function

As a consequence of aerobic metabolism, all aerobic organisms are subject to a certain level of physiological oxidative stress. Mitochondrial respiration of xenobiotic transformation through cytochrome P450s yields reactive oxygen species (ROS) such as superoxide ($O_2^-\cdot$) and hydrogen peroxide, and can lead to the further production of toxic oxygen radicals that can cause lipid peroxidation and cell injury. The endogenously produced hydrogen peroxide is reduced by GSH in the presence of selenium-dependent GSH peroxidase. As a result, GSH is oxidized to GSSG, which in turn is reduced back to GSH by GSSG reductase at the expense of nictoinamide adenine dinucleotide phosphate hydrogenase (NADPH), forming a redox cycle. Either GSH peroxidase or GSH S-transferase can reduce organic peroxides. Hydrogen peroxide can also be reduced by catalase, which is present only in the peroxisome. In the mitochondria, GSH is particularly important because there is no catalase and, therefore, GSH is responsible for maintaining a functionally competent organelle [7,8]. Because mitochondria are essential for cell function, mitochondrial GSH is a vital antioxidant that regulates cell death pathways and, hence, is of significance in disease progression. In addition, GSH also works as a coenzyme for several other antioxidant enzymes such as glutaredoxins and thioredoxins.

Cysteine storage and the γ-glutamyl cycle

One of the most important functions of GSH is to store cysteine. Cysteine is extremely unstable in the extracellular space and rapidly auto-oxidizes to cystine, in a process producing potentially toxic ROS. The γ-glutamyl cycle, first described by Meister in the early 1970s, allows GSH to serve as a continuous source of cysteine [6]. In this cycle, GSH is released from the cell by carrier-mediated transporter(s), and the ectoenzyme GGT then transfers the γ-glutamyl moiety of GSH to an amino acid (the best acceptor being cystine), forming γ-glutamyl amino acid and cysteinylglycine. The γ-glutamyl amino acid can then be transported back into the cell to complete the cycle. Once inside the cell, the γ-glutamyl amino acid can be metabolized further to release the amino acid and 5-oxoproline, which can be converted to glutamate and used for resynthesis of GSH. Cysteinylglycine is broken down by dipeptidase to generate cysteine and glycine, and cysteine is then taken up and converted back to GSH, a process that occurs in most types of cells. Once inside the cell, the majority of cysteine is incorporated into GSH; some is incorporated into protein, depending on the need of the cell, and some is degraded into sulphate and taurine. For most cells, this mechanism provides a continuous source of cysteine. Thus, the γ-glutamyl cycle allows the efficient utilization of GSH as cysteine storage.

GSH compartmentation: mitochondrial GSH

GSH is synthesized exclusively in the cytosol of cells; however, it is distributed intracellularly, including in the ER and mitochondria. While GSH in the ER is important for the assembly and secretory pathway for proteins, GSH in mitochondria (mGSH) plays an essential role in the maintenance of a functionally competent organelle and has been recognized more recently to regulate cell death/survival pathways [8]. Mitochondria are the main consumers of molecular oxygen in the cell, and this process functions as a transducing device to provide the energy required for ATP synthesis in oxidative phosphorylation. Most of the oxygen consumed during oxidative phosphorylation is fully reduced to water; however, a minor percentage of oxygen is partially reduced by a single electron, generating superoxide anion that acts on the matrix side of mitochondria and from which other ROS and oxidants (e.g. hydrogen peroxide) arise as byproducts of aerobic respiration. Although mitochondria are exposed to the constant generation of oxidant species, the organelle remains functional because of the existence of an antioxidant defence system, starting with transformation of superoxide anion into hydrogen peroxide by manganese superoxide dismutase (MnSOD). If the accumulation of hydrogen peroxide is not limited, it may either oxidize mitochondrial components (proteins, lipids, DNA) or participate in a chain of reactions (Haber–Weiss–Fenton) that generate more reactive free radicals, e.g. hydroxyl radical.

The task of controlling endogenous ROS in mitochondria is mainly accomplished by GSH, because mitochondria lack catalase, and because GSH is an integral component of the redox cycle with the participation of the GSH peroxidase and NADPH-dependent GSSG reductase. Moreover, a balance between the activity of MnSOD and the GSH redox cycle must exist to ensure the efficient disposal of hydrogen peroxide [7]. As mGSH concentration is high, moderate depletion of mGSH would not be expected to have a negative impact on the disposal of hydrogen peroxide by GSH peroxidase or on mitochondrial function. However, the depletion of mGSH below a critical level would compromise the adequate reduction of hydrogen peroxide, particularly in conditions of stimulated ROS generation from the mitochondrial electron transport chain. Thus, under complex 3 inhibition by antimycin A, stimulated hydrogen peroxide generation is only observed when GSH is depleted to 2–3 nmol/mg protein [9], which corresponds to the range of the K_m of GSH peroxidase for GSH (3 mM). Furthermore, because of the existence of GSH S-transferases (GST) in mitochondria, GSH also ensures the reduction of organic hydroperoxides, including products of lipid peroxidation [7].

Thus, as inferred from its versatility in reducing oxidants and in conjugating electrophiles, mGSH plays an essential role in maintaining mitochondria in a healthy state, and its depletion may be a key event in disease pathogenesis and sensitization of cells to oxidant and drug-induced cell injury. In addition, by regulating the redox environment, mGSH influences the mitochondrial cell death pathway through mitochondrial membrane permeabilization (MMP), which is recognized to play a role in pathophysiology.

mGSH transport

The concentration of mGSH is in the range of cytosolic GSH. However, unlike cytosol, mitochondria do not contain the enzymatic machinery to synthesize GSH from its constituent amino acids. Therefore, mGSH arises from the cytosol by carrier-mediated transport located in the inner membrane that overcomes the unfavourable entry against an electrochemical gradient [10]. The earlier characterization of the transport of GSH into rat liver mitochondria indicated an active, energy-dependent process stimulated by ATP and inhibited by glutamate and upon collapse of the protonmotive force with protonophores [7,10].

Although hepatic mGSH transport has been functionally expressed in *Xenopus laevis* oocytes, the identification of the carrier(s) responsible had remained elusive until recently [11]. Indeed, the functional expression of the hepatic 2-oxoglutarate carrier in mitochondria from *Xenopus laevis*, demonstrating the transport of reduced GSH in a phenylsuccinatesensitive manner, further confirmed the suggestion that the 2-oxoglutarate carrier contributes to the transport of GSH in liver mitochondria [11]. The initial rate of 2-oxoglutarate transport in rat liver mitochondria was reduced following depletion of mGSH, suggesting a 2-oxoglutarate/GSH exchange. In contrast to the transport of GSH in kidney mitochondria, which occurs with a single kinetic component, the kinetics of GSH in rat liver mitochondria display a high-affinity and a low-affinity component. Moreover, the kinetics of 2-oxoglutarate transport in rat liver mitochondria exhibited a single Michaelis–Menten component with sensitivity to phenylsuccinate and GSH. Interestingly, the transport of 2-oxoglutarate was dependent on mitochondrial membrane fluidity, a characteristic feature of the hepatic mitochondrial transport of GSH (see below).

Thus, these studies suggest that the 2-oxoglutarate carrier may be responsible for the low-affinity transport of GSH in rat liver mitochondria in exchange for matrix 2-oxoglutarate. However, the identification of alternative carriers that account for the high-affinity transport of GSH in liver mitochondria remains to be established. In this regard, uncoupling protein 2 (UCP2) has been suggested to favour the mitochondrial transport of GSH. Although it may be conceivable that the transport of protons back into the matrix by UCP2 may favour the movement of GSH, the role of UCP2 in the transport of GSH into mitochondria remains speculative.

Regulation of mGSH transport

Recent cumulative evidence in hepatocytes and isolated mitochondria indicates that the transport of mGSH is highly dependent on appropriate membrane physical properties [8]. The function of membrane proteins including carriers can be modulated by the microenvironment of the membrane in which they are inserted, and lipid composition determines the dynamic properties of biological membranes. Both the cholesterol/phospholipid molar ratio and the (un)saturation of fatty acyl groups in phospholipids contribute to the membrane fluidity changes that correspond to the transition of membranes from gel to a liquid crystalline state. Cholesterol enrichment of cellular membranes or large multilamellar liposomes have been shown to decrease membrane fluidity monitored by fluorescence polarization of specific probes without an effect on the lifetime of the excited state of the probe. On the other hand, highly unsaturated fatty acyl chains (e.g. 20:4 and 22:6) in phospholipids are unlikely to associate with cholesterol and may thus create fluid membrane domains.

As the function of the electron transport chain can be affected by the lipid composition of the mitochondrial inner membrane, the regulation of mitochondrial GSH transport by membrane fluidity has been examined in isolated rat liver mitochondria enriched in cholesterol (reviewed in [8]). Cholesterol incorporated into mitochondria by incubation with a cholesterol–bovine serum albumin (BSA) mixture results in increased cholesterol content (two- to threefold). Although the bulk of cholesterol (70–80%) is found in the outer membrane after exposure to the cholesterol–BSA complex, the cholesterol incorporated in the inner membrane is twice as great as that present in control mitoplasts. The measurement of fluorescence polarization of fluorescent probes indicates decreased membrane fluidity in the cholesterol-enriched mitochondria. Cholesterol-enriched mitochondria display impaired initial rates of GSH uptake at different GSH concentrations, whereas the uptake of adenosine diphosphate (ADP) through the adenine nucleotide translocator remains unaffected. Moreover, the fluidization of cholesterol-enriched mitochondria by A_2C restored the mitochondrial transport of GSH despite increased cholesterol content. Thus, in addition to its regulation by the protonmotive force, ATP hydrolysis and glutamate, the mitochondrial transport of GSH is dependent on appropriate membrane fluidity.

GSH and cell death regulation

Through the maintenance of protein sulphydryls in the appropriate redox state, GSH can regulate important death/survival pathways, which modulate the fate of cells in response to apoptotic stimuli. A number of studies have shown that intracellular GSH loss, such as that induced by stimulated efflux out of the cell or its consumption, sensitizes different cell types to a variety of apoptotic stimuli (reviewed in [12]). For instance, epithelial HeLa cells expressing mutated cystic fibrosis transmembrane conductance regulator (CFTR) display resistance to hydrogen peroxide-mediated apoptosis accompanied by higher intracellular GSH stores and lower mitochondrial Bax levels. Recent studies in mouse hepatocytes in which the GSH levels were depleted by diethylmaleate or paracetamol indicated a sensitization to tumour necrosis factor (TNF)-induced apoptosis. In examining the activation of stress kinases and NF-κB-dependent survival genes, GSH depletion in the cytosol/nuclei resulted in sustained activation of Jun N-terminal kinase (JNK) by TNF. Intriguingly, while GSH depletion did not impair the nuclear DNA binding of NF-κB induced by TNF, it did prevent the induction of NF-κB-dependent survival genes such as inducible nitric oxide synthase (iNOS). These data show a differential dependence on GSH levels between the NF-κB DNA-binding activity and its transactivation, with the latter showing a requirement for critical GSH

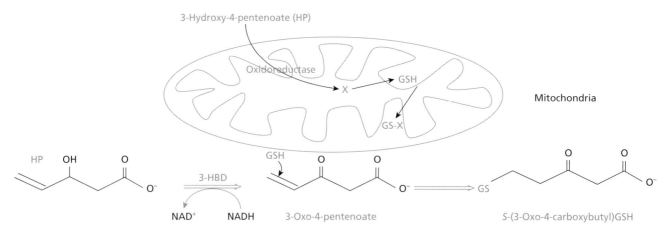

Fig. 4 Depletion of mitochondrial GSH. The biotransformation of HP into a Michael electrophile, 3-oxo-4-pentenoate, occurs selectively in the mitochondrial matrix thanks to the 3-HBD. This αβ unsaturated carbonyl is then conjugated with GSH yielding S-(3-oxo-4-carboxybutyl)GSH, resulting in the depletion of mitochondrial GSH. This pharmacological approach has been useful to learn specifically about the relevance of mitochondrial GSH in cell death regulation.

levels. Although the DNA binding of NF-κB can be modulated by the redox environment, recent findings indicate a novel pathway for the redox regulation of NF-κB based on mass spectrometry and molecular modelling of the S-glutathionylation of cysteine 62 of the p50 subunit of NF-κB. Thus, depending on the extent and mechanism of GSH depletion (efflux from cytosol of cells vs. decreased GSH/GSSG ratio), a limited storage of cell GSH can promote cell death through sustained JNK activation and/or suppression of NF-κB-dependent survival pathways.

In addition to the redox regulation of these death-promoting components, the engagement of the death-inducing signalling complex (DISC) and caspase-8 activated by ligation of death receptors relies on the appropriate redox environment for proper function. Through this mechanism, adequate GSH levels are required to ensure active DISC and caspase-8 activity after Fas stimulation in CEM and H9 cells. However, this dependence has not been observed in HepG2 or Hepa1–6 cells, indicating that the requirement of GSH for active DISC is cell-type specific. In hepatocytes, for instance, the role of GSH in sensitization to Fas or TNF is controversial. The length (prolonged vs. acute) and extent of GSH depletion (cytosolic vs. mitochondrial) may determine the fate of hepatocytes after Fas or TNF challenge. Thus, the existence of additional factors, e.g. the presence of redox-active thioredoxin in different cell types, may determine the outcome of the delicate balance between physiological antioxidants (GSH) and endogenously produced oxidants (ROS and nitric oxide) in the progression of apoptosis signalling.

Role of mGSH and susceptibility to cell death

Recently, pharmacological approaches have been used selectively to deplete mGSH in order to examine its role in the susceptibility of primary hepatocytes to death stimuli. By exploiting the selective biotransformation of (R,S)-3-hydroxy-4-pentenoate (HP) into a Michael acceptor within mitochondria by the (R)-3-hydroxybutanoate NAD+ oxidoreductase (3-HBD) (Fig. 4),

it has been possible selectively to deplete the mGSH pool in intact hepatocytes while sparing cytosolic GSH, underscoring the specific role of mGSH in apoptosis induced by TNF [13]. Preincubation of primary cultured rat hepatocytes with HP results in sensitization to TNF-mediated cell death in the absence of any other sensitization approach such as blocking protein or total RNA synthesis or NF-κB activation. mGSH-depleted hepatocytes exposed to TNF exhibit a significant and early generation of peroxides that precedes the loss of mitochondrial membrane potential, release of cytochrome c and apoptotic and necrotic demise. Similar findings have been observed when the depletion of mGSH is induced by chronic ethanol intake, which are reversed upon repletion of mGSH. On the other hand, overexpression of a mitochondrial GSH transporter, the dicarboxylate carrier, which results in substantially higher mGSH levels, protects NKK-52E cells from oxidant-induced apoptosis. In addition, mGSH depletion by triterpenoid derivatives in pancreatic cancer cells enhances apoptosis by a redox-dependent mechanism, thus further validating the crucial role of mGSH in controlling cell survival [14]. Moreover, mGSH depletion by HP has been shown to sensitize cultured hepatocytes to hypoxia-induced cell death [15]. Thus, mitochondria are both a source and a target of ROS. Through the maintenance of superoxide anion-induced hydrogen peroxide generated on the matrix side of the mitochondrial inner membrane, the pool of mGSH serves as a critical line of defence that controls the fate of cells in response to apoptosis stimuli.

In addition to ensuring the appropriate redox state of critical mitochondrial proteins (e.g. components of the mitochondrial permeability transition pore complex), GSH in mitochondria may also be vital in guarding the integrity of lipids. A recent study demonstrated the critical role of cardiolipin, in collaboration with proapoptotic Bcl-2 family members, in the formation of supramolecular openings in the outer mitochondrial membrane [16]. In addition to its fundamental role as a housekeeping lipid in the organization of individual complexes into functional units of the respiratory chain, cardiolipin has a defined distribution pattern within mitochondria and may serve as a functional link in the action of BH1–3 multidomain proteins, e.g. Bax, or BH3-only Bid, to elicit the release of cytochrome *c*. Cytochrome *c* is bound to the inner membrane by cardiolipin. Recent studies in rat liver mitochondria have characterized a two-step process in the release of cytochrome *c*, consisting of the detachment of this protein from its membrane-anchoring lipid, cardiolipin, followed by permeabilization of the outer membrane allowing the release of cytochrome *c* into the extramitochondrial environment. As the peroxidation of cardiolipin contributes to the transition from tight to loose conformation of cytochrome *c*, an additional aspect of the protective role of mGSH might involve protection of cardiolipin from ROS attack. In this regard, hepatocellular mGSH depletion by HP leads to intact cardiolipin loss and subsequent accumulation of peroxidized cardiolipin in mitochondrial membranes. Whether this step is essential for mitochondrial membrane permeabilization (MMP) and, hence, apoptosome assembly by TNF is currently being investigated in liposomes reconstituted with intact vs. peroxidized cardiolipin. Thus, either through the maintenance of vital mitochondrial proteins and/or cardiolipin, mGSH depletion associated with disease states (such as hypoxia–reperfusion injury, toxic bile acid-induced damage and chronic alcohol intake) will favour conditions for cell damage.

GSH depletion in liver diseases

Because GSH is a critical antioxidant, and ROS are recognized in the pathophysiology of liver diseases, GSH depletion is associated with, and contributes to, the progression of liver diseases. In this capacity, GSH depletion may contribute to bile acid-induced liver damage, ischaemia–reperfusion liver injury and hepatitis B and C-induced liver damage [17,18].

Alcohol-induced liver damage is among the best characterized of diseases associated with GSH depletion (see also Section 12, Alcoholic liver disease). Hepatic mitochondria are recognized targets of ethanol metabolism in the liver. Studies in animal models of chronic ethanol feeding demonstrate functional alterations in oxidative phosphorylation, while patients with alcoholic hepatitis display mitochondria with morphological aberrations. Therefore, we examined the regulation of mGSH status and transport in experimental models of chronic alcohol feeding (reviewed in [19]). Our earlier observations more than a decade ago indicated that chronic ethanol intake selectively reduced the levels of mGSH in hepatocytes. Furthermore, similar findings have been observed in rats fed ethanol intragastrically, reproducing some of the pathological findings seen in patients ranging from steatosis to inflammation and fibrosis. These studies demonstrate a progressive depletion of mGSH with ethanol intake that precedes signs of liver injury in the ethanol-fed mice. Moreover, intragastric alcohol-fed mice also exhibit mGSH depletion that is prevented by MnSOD overexpression, indicating that mGSH levels are regulated by oxidative stress. The depletion of mGSH caused by chronic alcohol feeding is seen preferentially in perivenous hepatocytes and results from a defective transport of GSH from cytosol into mitochondria, as demonstrated in *in vitro* and *in vivo* tracer kinetic studies. Consistent with the observations that mGSH depletion caused by alcohol intake is secondary to impaired transport of GSH, we have documented decreased membrane fluidity in alcohol-fed livers [19]. Furthermore, acetaldehyde stimulates *de novo* synthesis of cholesterol in HepG2 cells, which then traffics to the mitochondrial inner membrane resulting in increased order parameter and impaired transport of GSH into mitochondria [20]. The fluidization of mitochondria from alcohol-fed livers or from acetaldehyde-treated HepG2 cells with A_2C restores the ability of mitochondria to transport GSH. In agreement with the impairment of mitochondrial GSH transport by alcohol intake, raising cytosolic GSH levels with N-acetylcysteine, a GSH precursor, does not increase the mGSH level in hepatocytes from alcohol-fed livers. However, S-adenosyl-L-methionine (SAM), which, in addition to its role in promoting GSH synthesis, can prevent alterations of membrane lipid composition including cholesterol/phospholipid increase, prevents alcohol-induced membrane fluidity loss in alcohol-fed rats and normalizes the mGSH levels. Exogenous SAM prevents TNF-induced MAT1A downregulation [21], which can also contribute to the depletion of SAM and subsequent GSH levels (Fig. 3). Interestingly, treatment of alcohol-fed rats with tauroursodeoxycholic acid replenishes mGSH levels through restoration of mitochondrial membrane fluidity.

Thus, alcohol-stimulated cholesterol increase and subsequent deposition in mitochondrial membranes accounts for the impairment of GSH transport in mitochondria, leading to depleted mGSH levels. In addition to the observations in hepatocytes, the depletion of mGSH has also been observed in alveolar type 2 cells from alcohol-fed rats resulting from impaired transport of GSH into mitochondria.

In cirrhosis, which is also associated with mitochondrial dysfunction, similar findings of mGSH dysregulation may occur. For instance, secondary biliary cirrhosis in rats induced by bile duct ligation will deplete mGSH, which occurs earlier than the observed decrease in GSH levels in liver homogenates. Although the mechanism is not entirely clear, mitochondria from bile duct-ligated rats exhibit altered lipid composition, with a two- to threefold increase in the cholesterol/phospholipid ratio in the mitochondrial inner membrane, thus raising the possibility of impaired transport of GSH into mitochondria.

Thus, as cholesterol influences the mitochondrial transport of GSH via the modulation of membrane physical properties, the transport of cholesterol to mitochondria may be significant in pathological states such as alcohol-induced liver disease (ALD). Most of the cholesterol in membranes is located in the plasma membrane, representing 65–80% of the total cellular cholesterol. Mitochondria, however, are cholesterol-poor organelles, with the outer mitochondrial membrane containing more cholesterol than the inner membrane.

Although the transport to and function of cholesterol in mitochondria is best understood in steroidogenic cells, the transport of cholesterol to hepatic mitochondria may be important in the bile acid synthesis pathway through its conversion into 27-hydroxycholesterol by the sterol 27-hydroxylase (Cyp27). In addition to its function as a precursor for bile acid synthesis, 27-hydroxycholesterol regulates liver steatosis by acting as a ligand of the liver X receptor (LXR) transcription factor via induction of sterol regulatory element-binding protein (SREBP)-1c. While steroidogenic acute regulatory protein (StAR) is key for the transport of cholesterol in steroidogenic cells, a recently purified protein from rat liver mitochondria has been shown to transport cholesterol to the mitochondrial inner membrane [22]. An intermembrane protein of 57.5 kDa, which transports cholesterol between mitochondrial membranes, has been purified by cholesterol affinity chromatography. In addition, a recent study has reported the detection of StAR in human liver cells, correlating its presence with the 27-hydroxylation of cholesterol, a process that occurs in the mitochondria and is considered the rate-limiting step in bile acid synthesis via the CYP27A1-initiated 'acidic' pathway [23]. A better understanding of this process and its regulation may identify novel therapeutic targets to maintain mitochondrial function and improve mGSH transport in liver diseases.

There is also a novel mechanism for cholesterol enrichment of mitochondrial inner membrane. Acetaldehyde can stimulate *de novo* cholesterol synthesis in HepG2 cells through ER stress [20], a process characterized by the accumulation of unfolded or misfolded proteins in the ER, which signals the induction of responsive genes [24]. Acetaldehyde increases the levels of GADD153 and the ER-associated transcription factor SREBP, which regulates cholesterol synthesis by activation of the rate-limiting enzyme hydroxymethylglutaryl-CoA reductase (HMGCoAR). The acetaldehyde-stimulated mitochondrial cholesterol content in HepG2 is preceded by increased levels of GADD153 and SREBP1, mimicked by the ER stress-inducing agents tunicamycin and homocysteine and prevented by the HMGCoAR inhibitor lovastatin. In addition, homocysteine, a toxic non-protein sulphur-containing amino acid formed exclusively upon demethylation of the essential amino acid methionine, contributes to alcohol-induced liver injury through ER stress [25]. Indeed, feeding mice betaine to promote methylation of homocysteine into methionine ameliorates alcohol-induced ER stress in mouse livers, indicating that homocysteine-induced ER stress contributes to alcohol-induced liver injury. Hence, alcohol intake leads to hyperhomocysteinaemia, which in turn may elicit ER stress, thereby promoting alcohol-induced liver injury.

GSH and hepatotoxicity (see also Section 14, Toxic liver injury)

mGSH is of critical relevance in hepatotoxicity because of its role in downregulating ROS and oxidants generated in the mitochondrial electron transport chain and maintaining overall mitochondrial function. For instance, patients taking LipoKinetix, a dietary supplement marketed as a weight loss agent, developed acute hepatotoxicity, which improved spontaneously after its use was discontinued. Usnic acid, a metabolite found in lichen, is a key constituent of LipoKinetix; usnic acid induces hepatocyte necrosis associated with disruption of mitochondrial respiration and energy metabolism, leading to ATP depletion and GSH depletion [26]. Furthermore, usnic acid increases hydrogen peroxide production in mitochondria, indicating that the depletion of mGSH is necessary for the sensitization of hepatocytes to usnic acid cytotoxicity. These findings suggest that usnic acid may be responsible, at least in part, for hepatotoxicity and liver failure seen in patients taking LipoKinetix.

Paracetamol (*N*-acetyl-*p*-aminophenol, APAP) is a widely used analgesic that is considered safe when taken at therapeutic doses. However, hepatocellular necrosis occurs at higher doses or under conditions that enhance the susceptibility to APAP. APAP hepatotoxicity is mediated by its metabolite *N*-acetyl-*p*-benzoquinone imine (NAPQI), which is generated by liver cytochrome P450, particularly cytochrome P450 2E1 (CYP2E1), and is detoxified by conjugation with GSH. NAPQI initiates its toxicity by first attacking mitochondria, followed by mGSH depletion. Although APAP can decrease GSH in both cytosol and mitochondria, the kinetics of GSH depletion in hepatocytes exposed to APAP indicate that the depletion of mGSH precedes that of cytosolic GSH, establishing the relevance of this GSH pool in the hepatotoxicity of APAP [27]. Interestingly, *N*-acetyl-*m*-aminophenol (AMAP), a non-hepatotoxic regioisomer of APAP, depletes cytosolic GSH but not mGSH. Like many other drugs, APAP cytotoxicity in hepatocytes is mediated through MMP, and agents that block it, such as ciclosporin A, protect hepatocytes against APAP-induced cell death. The synergism between alcohol intake and susceptibility to APAP further illustrates the sensitization to APAP hepatocellular toxicity by mGSH depletion. Selective depletion of mGSH caused by chronic ethanol feeding contributes to the enhanced susceptibility to APAP toxicity. Furthermore, ethanol induces CYP2E1, and the enhanced APAP toxicity induced by chronic ethanol is closely associated with the magnitude of both CYP2E1 induction and mGSH depletion, as the APAP toxicity disappears when CYP2E1 and the mGSH pool return to control levels after alcohol withdrawal [28]. Thus, these observations not only explain the likely mechanisms by which ethanol potentiates the toxicity of APAP, but also help to explain the low frequency with which the interaction is observed given the high incidence of concomitant use of alcohol and APAP.

References

1 DeLeve L, Kaplowitz N (1991) Glutathione metabolism and its role in hepatotoxicity. *Pharmacol Ther* 52, 287–305.
2 Hammond CL, Lee TK, Ballatori N (2001) Novel roles for glutathione

in gene expression, cell death, and membrane transport of organic solutes. *J Hepatol* 34, 946–954.

3 Huang CS, He W, Meister A *et al.* (1995) Amino acid sequence of rat kidney glutathione synthetase. *Proc Natl Acad Sci USA* 92, 1232–1236.

4 Fernández-Checa J, Lu SC, Ookhtens *et al.* (1992) The regulation of hepatic glutathione. In: Tavoloni N, Berk PD (eds) *Hepatic Anion Transport and Bile Secretion: Physiology and Pathophysiology*. New York: Marcel Dekker, pp. 363–395.

5 Ballatori N, Hammond CL, Cunningham JB *et al.* (2005) Molecular mechanisms of reduced glutathione transport: role of the MRP/CFTR/ABCC and OATP/SLC21A families of membrane proteins. *Toxicol Appl Pharmacol* 204, 238–255.

6 Meister A (1988) Glutathione. In: Aria IM, Jakoby WB, Popper H *et al.* (eds) *The Liver: Biology and Pathobiology*, 2nd edn. New York: Raven Press, pp. 401–417.

7 Fernández-Checa JC, Kaplowitz N, Garcia-Ruiz C *et al.* (1997) GSH transport in mitochondria: defense against TNF-induced oxidative stress and alcohol-induced defect. *Am J Physiol* 273, G7–17.

8 Fernandez-Checa JC, Kaplowitz N (2005) Hepatic mitochondrial glutathione: transport and role in disease and toxicity. *Toxicol Appl Pharmacol* 204, 263–273.

9 Garcia-Ruiz C, Colell A, Morales A *et al.* (1995) Role of oxidative stress generated from the mitochondrial electron transport chain and mitochondrial glutathione status in loss of mitochondrial function and activation of transcription factor nuclear factor-kappa B: studies with isolated mitochondria and rat hepatocytes. *Mol Pharmacol* 825–834.

10 Martensson J, Lai JC, Meister A (1990) High-affinity transport of glutathione is part of a multicomponent system essential for mitochondrial function. *Proc Natl Acad Sci USA* 87, 7185–7189.

11 Coll O, Colell A, Garcia-Ruiz C *et al.* (2003) Sensitivity of the 2-oxoglutarate carrier to alcohol intake contributes to mitochondrial glutathione depletion. *Hepatology* 38, 692–702.

12 Fernandez-Checa JC (2003) Redox regulation and signaling lipids in mitochondrial apoptosis. *Biochem Biophys Res Commun* 304, 471–479.

13 Garcia-Ruiz C, Colell A, Mari M *et al.* (2003) Defective TNF-α-mediated hepatocellular apoptosis and liver damage in acidic sphingomyelinase knockout mice. *J Clin Invest* 111, 197–208.

14 Samudio I, Konopleva M, Hail N *et al.* (2005) 2-cyano, 3, 12-dioxooleana, 1, 9, diene, 28-imidazolide (CDDO-IM) directly targets mitochondrial glutathione to induce apoptosis in pancreatic cancer. *J Biol Chem* 280, 36273–36282.

15 Lluis JM, Morales A, Blasco C *et al.* (2005) Critical role of mitochondrial glutathione in the survival of hepatocytes during hypoxia. *J Biol Chem* 280, 3224–3232.

16 Kuwana T, Mackey MR, Perkins G *et al.* (2002) Bid, Bax and lipids cooperate to form supramolecular openings in the outer mitochondrial membrane. *Cell* 111, 331–342.

17 Gumpricht E, Dahl R, Yerushalmi B *et al.* (2002) Nitric oxide ameliorates hydrophobic bile acid-induced apoptosis in isolated rat hepatocytes by non-mitochondrial pathways. *J Biol Chem* 277, 25823–25830.

18 Otani K, Korenaga M, Beard MR *et al.* (2005) Hepatitis C virus core protein, cytochrome P450 2E1, and alcohol produce combined mitochondrial injury and cytotoxicity in hepatoma cells. *Gastroenterology* 128, 96–107.

19 Fernandez-Checa JC, Colell A, Garcia-Ruiz C (2002) S-Adenosyl-L-methionine and mitochondrial reduced glutathione depletion in alcoholic liver disease. *Alcohol* 27, 179–183.

20 Lluis JM, Colell A, Garcia-Ruiz C *et al.* (2003) Acetaldehyde impairs mitochondrial glutathione transport in HepG2 cells through endoplasmic reticulum stress. *Gastroenterology* 124, 708–724

21 Mari M, Colell A, Morales A *et al.* (2004) Acidic sphingomyelinase downregulates the liver-specific methionine adenosyltransferase 1A, contributing to tumor necrosis factor-induced lethal hepatitis. *J Clin Invest* 113, 895–904.

22 Soccio RE, Breslow JL (2004) Intracellular cholesterol transport. *Arterioscler Thromb Vasc Biol* 24, 1150–1160.

23 Hall EA, Ren S, Hylemon PB *et al.* (2005) Detection of the steroidogenic acute regulatory protein, StAR, in human liver cells. *Biochim Biophys Acta* 1733, 111–119.

24 Kaufman RJ (1999) Stress signaling from the lumen of the endoplasmic reticulum: coordination of gene transcriptional and translational controls. *Genes Dev* 13, 1211–1233.

25 Ji C, Kaplowitz N (2003) Betaine decreases hyperhomocysteinemia, endoplasmic reticulum stress, and liver injury in alcohol-fed mice. *Gastroenterology* 124, 1488–1499.

26 Han D, Canali R, Rettori D *et al.* (2003) Effect of glutathione depletion on sites and topology of superoxide and hydrogen peroxide production in mitochondria. *Mol Pharmacol* 64, 1136–1144.

27 Vendemiale G, Grattagliano I, Altomare E *et al.* (1996) Effect of acetaminophen administration on hepatic glutathione compartmentation and mitochondrial energy metabolism in the rat. *Biochem Pharmacol* 52, 1147–1154.

28 Zhao P, Slattery JT (2002) Effects of ethanol dose and ethanol withdrawal on rat liver mitochondrial glutathione: implication of potentiated acetaminophen toxicity in alcoholics. *Drug Metab Dispos* 30, 1413–1417.

2.3.10 Haem biosynthesis and excretion of porphyrins

Hervé Puy and Jean-Charles Deybach

Introduction

Synthesis of porphyrins occurs in nearly all living cells: in animals for haem production and in plants for chlorophyll production. Porphobilinogen (PBG) and δ-aminolaevulinic acid (ALA) are linear porphyrin precursors, whereas porphyrins are molecules that are cyclic precursors of haem. In mammalian cells, haem synthesis occurs mostly in liver and erythropoietic tissues. Eight enzymes are involved in haem synthesis from succinyl CoA and glycine; the biosynthetic pathway starts in the mitochondrion and, after passing through three cytoplasmic stages, re-enters the mitochondrion for the final steps of haem formation. Therefore, the first and last three enzymes are found in mitochondria and the others in the cytosol (Fig. 1). All these enzymes are encoded by nuclear genes, and their full-length human cDNA and genomic sequences have been isolated and characterized [1]. Haemoproteins, including haemoglobin or myoglobin, mitochondrial or microsomal cytochromes, catalase, peroxidase, nitric oxide synthase, prostaglandin endoperoxide

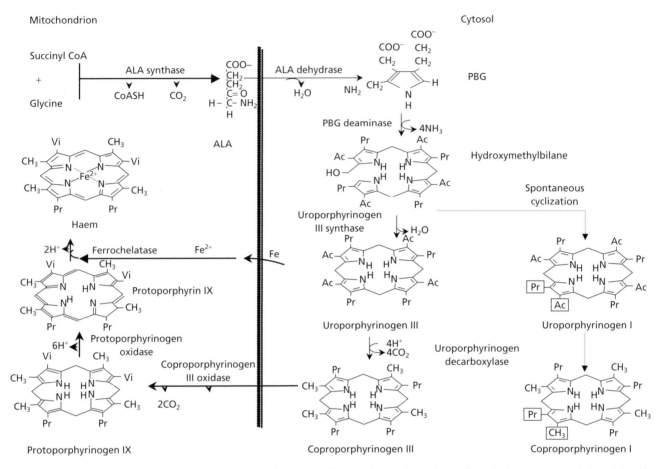

Fig. 1 The haem biosynthetic pathway. Subcellular distribution of enzymes and intermediates in the synthesis of haem is shown. ALA, δ-aminolaevulinic acid; PBG, porphobilinogen; Ac, acetyl (CH₂-COOH); CoASH, coenzyme A; Pr, propionyl (CH₂-CH₂-COOH); Vi, vinyl (CH=CH₂).

synthase, guanylate cyclase or tryptophan pyrrolase, play very important roles in electron and oxygen transport, in the activation of oxygen or hydrogen peroxide and, finally, in hydrogen peroxide decomposition.

Haem biosynthesis

Structure of porphyrins

Porphyrins are cyclic tetrapyrroles in which the pyrrole rings, conventionally designated as A, B, C and D, are linked through their carbon atoms by methene (–CH=) bridges (Fig. 1). All the cyclic tetrapyrrole intermediates of the biosynthetic pathway, with the exception of protoporphyrin IX, the last intermediate, are porphyrinogens, which are reduced forms that are rapidly oxidized to porphyrins when exposed to air with the loss of six protons. Porphyrins emit intense red fluorescence when exposed to light at around 400 nm. Thus, spectrofluorometric methods provide very sensitive detection and quantification of porphyrins (Soret band).

The naturally occurring porphyrins all have side-chains on the carbon atoms of the pyrrole rings. The porphyrin isomers differ in the arrangement of the side-chain substituents (e.g. acetyl and propionyl in uroporphyrins; methyl and propionyl in coproporphyrins). Water solubility of porphyrins is favoured by the presence of carboxylic acid side-chains. Uroporphyrin, the most water-soluble of the porphyrins, is excreted predominantly in urine, coproporphyrin mostly in urine and partly in bile, whereas protoporphyrin, the least soluble, is excreted only in the bile. There are four isomers of each of these porphyrins; only the I and III isomers occur in nature. In isomer I, the side-chains are arranged symmetrically around the ring; in isomer III, the substituents on ring D are reversed [2]. In animals, the complex between ferrous iron and protoporphyrins is usually called haem.

Biosynthesis

The two types of cells in the body that are responsible for synthesizing most of the haem are the erythropoietic cells (80%)

and the liver parenchymal cells (20%). The steps in the pathway are outlined in Figure 1.

Synthesis of porphyrin precursors: δ-aminolaevulinic acid and porphobilinogen

ALA synthase (EC 2.3.1.37), the first enzyme in the pathway, is a mitochondrial protein that requires pyridoxal phosphate as a cofactor. Two different isoenzymes, erythroid-specific or housekeeping, are encoded by two separate genes on different chromosomes (see below). It catalyses the condensation of glycine and succinyl-CoA, which is produced by the tricarboxylic acid cycle, to form ALA, which is exclusively committed to the synthesis of haem. ALA dehydrase (EC 4.2.1.24) then catalyses the condensation of two molecules of ALA to form monopyrrole PBG. The ALA dehydrase gene, situated on chromosome 9, has two codominant alleles, 1 and 2 [3]. The isoenzymes produced in the liver and erythroid tissue through tissue-specific alternative splicing are identical, with the form of splicing determined by activation of an untranslated region. The ALA dehydrase-2 isoenzyme is more electronegatively charged than ALA dehydrase-1, and its affinity for lead, which inhibits its activity by competing with the zinc atoms needed for catalytic action, is therefore higher. As a consequence, individuals with the ALA dehydrase-2 genotype are more vulnerable to lead exposure.

Synthesis of coproporphyrinogen III

Two cytoplasmic enzymes, PBG deaminase (EC 4.3.1.8) and uroporphyrinogen III cosynthetase (cosynthetase; EC 4.2.1.75), convert four molecules of PBG to uroporphyrinogen III (with liberation of four molecules of ammonia). PBG deaminase catalyses the polymerization of four molecules of PBG, yielding a linear tetrapyrrole intermediate, hydroxymethylbilane (Fig. 1). In this reaction, four units of PBG are assembled head-to-tail by the deaminase, starting with ring A and building round to ring D, to form the unrearranged bilane. The deaminase furnishes a straight-chain tetrapyrrole, hydroxymethylbilane, but it is not an enzyme for ring closure. The PBG deaminase contains, at its catalytic site, a dipyrrolomethane cofactor. The function of the dipyrrolomethane cofactor appears to be that of anchoring the substrate molecules at the catalytic site and directing the condensation of PBG to form the tetrapyrrole. Uroporphyrinogen III cosynthase then rapidly converts the intermediate into uroporphyrinogen III, a cyclic tetrapyrrole with eight carboxyl side-chains. In the absence of this ring-closing and side-chain-rearranging enzyme, an abortive I isomeric uroporphyrin is formed spontaneously, and, after partial decarboxylation to I isomeric coproporphyrinogen, is excreted via the hepatobiliary route as well as in urine. Uroporphyrinogen decarboxylase (EC 4.1.1.37), encoded on the short arm of chromosome 1, catalyses the stepwise decarboxylation of uroporphyrinogen III and converts the four acetic acid side-chains to methyl groups to form coproporphyrinogen III. The reactions, passing through 7-, 6- and 5-carboxylic states of the porphyrin molecule, take place at a single catalytic site. Only isomer III can be used in the remaining steps [3].

Synthesis of haem

Coproporphyrinogen oxidase (EC 1.3.3.3), encoded by a gene on chromosome 9, selectively converts two propionic acid chains to vinyl groups on the III isomeric form of coproporphyrinogen and then catalyses the stepwise decarboxylation to produce protoporphyrinogen IX. This mitochondrial enzyme, which requires copper for its action, is not membrane bound and was shown to be present in the intermembrane space. This localization implies that protoporphyrinogen oxidase (EC 1.3.3.4) must cross the inner membrane because haem is formed within the inner membrane (Fig. 2). Protoporphyrinogen

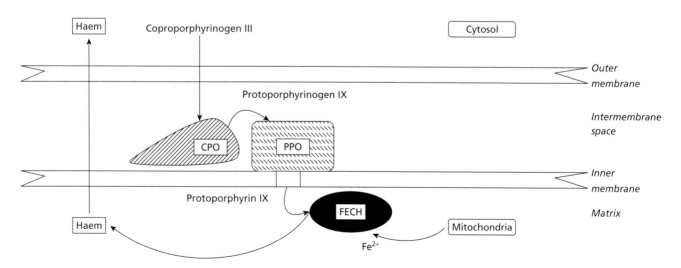

Fig. 2 Haem biosynthetic pathway. Association of the three terminal enzymes (coproporphyrinogen oxidase CPO, protoporphyrinogen oxidase PPOX, ferrochelatase FECH) with the inner mitochondrial membrane.

oxidase, encoded by a gene on chromosome 1, catalyses the oxidation of protoporphyrinogen IX to protoporphyrin IX: six hydrogen atoms are removed (four from methylene bridges and two from pyrrole rings). Only oxidized molecules (porphyrins) are brightly coloured, whereas reduced porphyrins (porphyrinogens) are colourless. The final enzymatic step in haem synthesis is the insertion of iron by the enzyme ferrochelatase (EC 4.99.1.1), which is encoded by a gene on chromosome 18 and is localized to the inner membrane of mitochondria. Unlike the three preceding enzymes in the haem biosynthetic pathway, which use porphyrinogens as substrates, ferrochelatase uses protoporphyrin IX; other dicarboxyl porphyrins, such as deutero- and mesoporphyrin IX, serve as good substrates for this enzyme *in vitro*. Only the reduced form of iron (Fe^{2+}), and not Fe^{3+}, is incorporated into protoporphyrin IX by the enzyme. Co^{2+} and Zn^{2+} are more efficient substrates for the enzyme than Fe^{2+}. Therefore, various rates of ferrochelatase activity can be obtained *in vitro*, depending upon which metal and porphyrin substrates are used. Moreover, in humans, ferrochelatase deficiency leads to free protoporphyrin accumulation, whereas iron deficiency leads to zinc protoporphyrin accumulation. The biosynthesis of haem requires 8 mol of glycine and 8 mol of succinic acid [3]. Each of the enzymes and their respective deficiency diseases are described in Chapter 16.5, Human hereditary porphyrias.

Haem catabolism

All cells are able to handle haem left over from the breakdown of haem proteins, thus preventing toxic accumulation of the compound. Haem oxygenase 1 (HO-1, EC 1.14.99.3), situated in the endoplasmic reticulum, is considered as a heat shock protein that is ubiquitously expressed, but is present in especially large amounts in liver and spleen, where the main degradation of haemoglobin takes place. Combined with nicotinamide adenine dinucleotide phosphate hydrogenase (NADPH) cytochrome 450 reductase, it cleaves one of the methene bridges of the porphyrin ring and generates carbon monoxide. The linear tetrapyrrol, biliverdin, is oxidized to bilirubin and excreted via the liver–bile route, whereas the liberated iron is reutilized. HO-1 activity is induced by a variety of stimuli, including haem itself, heavy metals, organic chemicals, endotoxins, hyperthermia, hypoglycaemia, burns and oxidative stress. Stimuli that increase HO-1 gene expression could accelerate the flux of metabolites through the haem biosynthetic pathway, and may thereby trigger clinical symptoms in some forms of hepatic porphyria by overload of the deficient enzyme [4]. The isoenzyme haem oxygenase 2 (HO-2), encoded by another gene, is not induced by the same agents that increase the transcription of the ubiquitous gene. This HO-2 gene is strongly expressed in brain, where it may serve to supply the tissue with carbon monoxide, a neuronal messenger that binds to the haem prosthetic group of guanylate cyclase generating cyclic GMP.

Regulation of haem synthesis

The mechanisms applied in the control of haem biosynthesis differ between liver and bone marrow, the two tissues that make haem in the largest amounts. Both erythroid-specific and non-erythroid or 'housekeeping' transcripts have been identified for each of the first four enzymes in the pathway. ALA is the first intermediate in the haem biosynthetic pathway exclusively committed to haem synthesis, and the rate of ALA synthesis is an important controlling step for haem formation. Erythroid-specific and housekeeping transcripts for the first step enzyme ALA synthase are encoded by two separate genes on different chromosomes: the erythroid-specific gene, expressed only in fetal liver and adult bone marrow (ALA synthase-2 on chromosome X), and the housekeeping gene, expressed in all cells (ALA synthase-1 on chromosome 3). For ALA dehydrase, porphobilinogen deaminase and uroporphyrinogen synthase, each transcript is activated from the same gene [5].

In the liver

In the liver, the haemoprotein enzymes formed, including cytochrome P450s, are rapidly turned over in response to current metabolic needs. ALA synthase-1 has many features of a rate-limiting enzyme in the production of haem. The rate of this enzyme turnover is very rapid; the half-life of mitochondrial ALA synthase-1 is among the shortest of all mitochondrial proteins. The ALA synthase-1 activity in normal liver is the lowest among all enzymes in the haem biosynthetic pathway. The free intracellular haem pool inhibits ALA synthase-1 activity via a negative feedback regulation (Fig. 3). Four potential targets for regulating the formation of the enzyme by haem have been identified: regulation of the production of ALA synthase at either (i) the transcriptional level or (ii) the translational level with a destabilization of ALA synthase mRNA by haem; (iii) modulation of the rate of entry of the enzyme into the mitochondria; or (iv) direct inhibition (Fig. 4). Basal or uninduced hepatic ALA synthase-1 provides sufficient ALA and haem to maintain normal levels of liver haemoproteins but, when the synthesis of the cytochrome P450 enzymes is induced and more haem synthesis is required, ALA synthase-1 is induced. The activity of PBG deaminase, the third enzyme in the pathway, is close to that of ALA synthase-1. Increased hepatic ALA synthase activity has been described during acute attacks in patients with acute porphyrias. ALA synthase induction is a secondary phenomenon; it is the result of exposure to several factors (such as drugs, hormones) that act on an enzyme more or less derepressed by haem deficiency. Under these conditions of ALA synthase-1 induction and increased ALA production, such as in an acute attack of an acute hepatic porphyria, PBG deaminase can become a rate-limiting metabolic step. This would account for the especially marked increases in ALA and PBG that are produced and excreted in acute intermittent porphyria (see Chapter 16.5). The activity of HO, the rate-limiting enzyme for

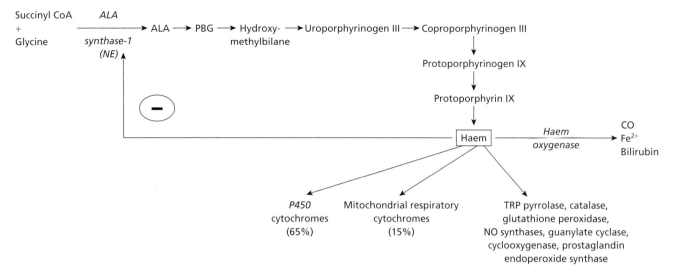

Fig. 3 Regulation of haem biosynthesis in the liver. ALA synthase-1 is rate limiting and feedback regulated by the intracellular concentration of haem. NE, non-erythroid form; TRP, tryptophan; NO, nitric oxide.

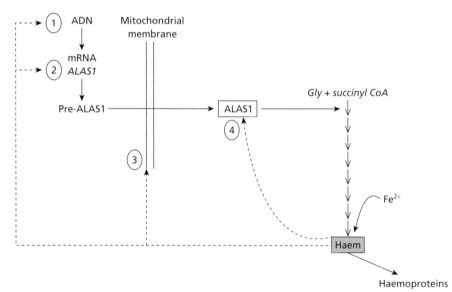

Fig. 4 Retroinhibition of hepatic ALA synthase-1 (ALAS1) activity via a negative feedback regulation mediated by the free intracellular haem pool. Four potential targets for regulating the formation of the enzyme by haem are identified: (1) the transcriptional level (*trans*-regulating factor haem responsive element: HRE), (2) the translational level with a destabilization of ALA synthase mRNA by haem, (3) modulation of the rate of entry of the enzyme into the mitochondria (mediated by a haem regulatory motif: HRM), (4) direct inhibition of the enzyme activity.

haem degradation to CO, iron and bile pigment, can also influence the level of regulatory free haem in hepatocytes. Starvation leads to increased HO activity, which may contribute to precipitating a crisis in acute hepatic porphyrias by depleting haem [6]. Conversely, attacks of these disorders can be prevented by a high carbohydrate diet. Thus, mechanisms for both haem synthesis and degradation can regulate haem formation.

In erythroid cells

In the erythroid cell, the synthesis of the enzymes participating in the formation of haem is under the control of iron and erythropoietin, formed under hypoxic conditions. Indeed,

regulatory influences in the erythrocyte act during cell differentiation and, in contrast to the liver, the erythrocyte also responds to stimuli for haem synthesis by increasing its cell numbers to meet changing requirements for haemoglobin. The haemoglobinization of the erythroid cell is controlled by the ALA synthase-2 isoenzyme, which exhibits a 75% identity in the C-terminal part with ALA synthase-1. This enzyme, produced by a gene on the X chromosome, is not inducible by the drugs that induce ALA synthase-1 in the liver and is not repressed by exogenous haem treatment. ALA synthase-2 activity is induced only during the period of active haem synthesis of the red cell, and its rate of formation, and thus its activity in the cell, is in the end regulated by the amount of free iron present. The erythroid ALA synthase-

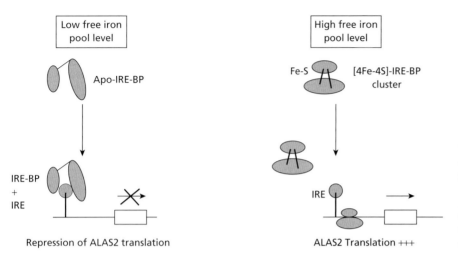

Fig. 5 Regulation of ALA synthase-2 translation by free iron/IRE/IRE-BP. In iron deficiency, the mRNA of erythroid ALA synthase-2 is blocked by attachment to an iron responsive element (IRE) of an IRE-binding protein (IRE-BP), and translation of this key enzyme is inhibited. In the presence of an excess of iron, the lack of attachment leads to an increase in the translation of the enzyme.

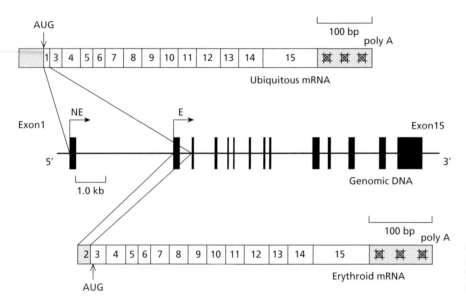

Fig. 6 Gene structure of the human porphobilinogen deaminase gene and its two transcripts produced by alternative splicing. NE, non-erythroid promoter; E, erythroid promoter.

2 gene encodes an iron-responsive element (IRE), which is a stable stem–loop structure on the mRNA with affinity for a specific cytosolic protein, the IRE-binding protein (IRE-BP). If there is enough free iron present in the erythroid cell, the IRE-BP is modified by the formation of sulphur/iron clusters; it then loses its ability to bind the IRE sequence. ALA synthase-2 translation is increased as a result, and the rate of formation of haem, and thus of globin chains as well, is activated. In iron deficiency, the unmodified IRE-BP blocks ALA synthase-2 translation by associating with its mRNA, and haem synthesis is consequently inhibited by lack of ALA synthase activity (Fig. 5). ALA dehydrase and PBG deaminase are other sites of regulation mediated by alternative splicing. The single PBG deaminase gene is located at chromosome 11q24.1–24.2 and contains 15 exons. It encodes erythroid-specific and ubiquitous isoforms of PBG deaminase that are generated by the use of separate promoters and alternative splicing of the two primary transcripts. The isoforms differ only at their NH$_2$ ends where the ubiquitous isoform extends for

an additional 17 residues, making a polypeptide of 361 amino acids (Fig. 6).

The upstream promoter is active in all tissues, and thus the enzyme encoded by the larger transcript was termed the 'housekeeping PBG deaminase'. The other promoter, located 3 kb downstream, is active only in erythroid cells. It displays some structural homology with the β-globin gene promoter, suggesting that some common *trans*-acting factors may coregulate the transcription of these genes during erythroid development. The expression of ALA synthase-2, ALA dehydrase and PBG deaminase erythroid isogenes is determined by *trans*-activation of nuclear factor GATA-1, CACC box and NF-E2 binding sites in the promoter areas [7]. Ferrochelatase, the final enzyme in haem biosynthesis, may also play a significant role in controlling the rate of haem formation in erythroid cells. Ferrochelatase deficiency in human protoporphyria results in the accumulation of protoporphyrin almost exclusively in erythroid tissue, even though ferrochelatase is deficient in all other tissues in these patients. This finding suggests that ferrochelatase activity can become rate limiting in erythroid cells, but not in other tissues, when the enzyme itself or its substrate, iron, is partially deficient. Although protoporphyrin is excreted only in the bile and accumulates in the liver in some patients, it presumably originates in the bone marrow.

Excretion of porphyrins and of porphyrin precursors

Porphyrins and porphyrin precursors are excreted in urine and/or bile (Table 1). In relation to the total rate of haem synthesis, excretion of porphyrins is very small; in other words, few porphyrins (and porphyrin precursors, ALA, PBG) 'escape' during haem formation and therefore are not transformed into bilirubin. Each day, bone marrow and liver synthesize about 375 mg of haem. In humans, the mean level of ALA excreted in urine is ~ 3 mg/day; this means that less than 0.5% of ALA synthesized each day has not been used for haem synthesis [8].

Urine

Porphyrin precursors

ALA and PBG are excreted only in the urine. After injection of labelled precursors, a large fraction of labelled ALA is excreted unaltered in urine; a small fraction is much more efficiently incorporated into hepatic haem than into haemoglobin in erythropoietic cells, probably because of the relative impermeability of the erythropoietic cell membrane to ALA. Injection-labelled PBG cannot be demonstrated in the liver, probably because it also does not pass the liver cell membrane; the impermeability of the cell membrane is only relative as, in instances

where the amount of endogenous PBG is considerably increased (for instance acute porphyrias), huge amounts of PBG are found in urine. Moderately increased excretion of precursors is also observed in patients with hepatic diseases [8].

Porphyrins

Coproporphyrin is the predominant porphyrin in normal human urine (Table 1). However, urine contains only 30–35% of the total coproporphyrin; the remainder is found in bile. This urinary and faecal distribution is combined with a differential excretion of coproporphyrin isomers. The type 3 isomer predominates (70%) over the type 1 in urine, whereas the reverse is found in bile. It is now widely accepted that the unequal excretion rates of the isomers can be attributed to a hepatic carrier that favours the excretion of the I isomer [9]. In several human liver diseases with impaired hepatic excretory mechanisms, there is an increase in the total isomer ratio towards a predominance of the type 1 compound [2]. Other porphyrins present in normal human urine include uroporphyrin and traces of porphyrins with seven, six and five carboxyl groups. The intermediates (porphyrinogens) are unstable and rapidly oxidize to their corresponding porphyrins, and a large fraction of the porphyrins present in urine are excreted in this form of reduced colourless precursors. Freshly voided urine from patients with acute porphyria may have little if any increase in concentrations of preformed porphyrin; this probably explains why urine is frequently normal in colour when freshly passed, but darkens gradually on exposure to light and air. PBG can also be converted non-enzymatically to porphyrins (mostly uroporphyrin type 1): it is therefore very important to protect urine from light and to store it between 4 and 10°C if measurement of precursors has to be carried out.

Table 1 Normal values of haem pathway metabolites in humans: data from the Centre Français des Porphyries.

	Urine (per mmol creatinine)		Faeces (per g dry weight)		Red blood cell (per L)		Plasma (per L)	
	Normal value	Method	Normal value	Method	Normal value	Method	Normal value	Method
δ-Aminolaevulinic acid (µmol)	0–3	Ion-exchange chromatography	–	–	–	–	–	
Porphobilinogen (µmol)	0–1		–	–	–	–	–	
Total porphyrin (nmol)	–	–	10–200	Quantitative spectrophotometry	500–1900	Quantitative fluorimetric scanning	10–20	Quantitative fluorimetric scanning
Uroporphyrin (nmol)	0–10	Quantitative spectrophotometry	0–2	HPLC	0–6	HPLC		Lack of fluorescence emission spectroscopy (620–630 nm)
Coproporphyrin (nmol)	0–20		0–60	HPLC	50–180	HPLC		
Protoporphyrin (nmol)	–	–	0–150	HPLC	300–1800	HPLC		

HPLC, high-pressure liquid chromatography.

Faeces

Significant amounts of porphyrins are excreted in faeces (mostly all of the protoporphyrin and 70% of coproporphyrin; Table 1). They may represent pigments that have reached the intestinal tract with the bile, except dicarboxylic porphyrins, which are mainly of dietary origin and may be derived from haem proteins of ingested food or intestinal haemorrhages; they may also be formed by intestinal microorganisms. Because of this, faecal porphyrins should be measured only if the patient's food has been devoid of bleeding or ingestion of meat in the past 3 days.

The mechanism by which protoporphyrin is excreted into bile has been studied mostly after description(s) of fatal liver disease in erythropoietic protoporphyria (see Chapter 16.5). Among haem-forming tissues, the bone marrow is the major source of protoporphyrin, a very poorly water-soluble compound: in the plasma, over 90% of protoporphyrin is bound to albumin with some bound to haemopexin. Hepatic uptake may occur through a process similar to that for other organic anions (such as bilirubin) that are bound to albumin. In the isolated, *in situ*-perfused rat liver, the overall disappearance of protoporphyrin follows first-order kinetics. Within the hepatocyte, protoporphyrin is associated with several proteins, among them one of the Z class of liver cytosolic proteins [10]. The rate-limiting step for the overall transport of protoporphyrin from plasma to bile appeared to be canalicular secretion, as less than 5% of the protoporphyrin extracted by liver was secreted into bile. This secretion should be mediated by the ABCG2/BCRP transporter, a member of the ATP-binding cassette (ABC) family [11]. The basal rate of bile secretion of porphyrins has been studied in healthy humans [12]: the flow of protoporphyrin is slightly higher than the flow of coproporphyrin; the flow of uroporphyrin is the lowest. Hepatic conjugation with glucuronic acid does not occur for protoporphyrin and coproporphyrin. Approximately 85% of hepatic protoporhyrin remains metabolically unaltered before being eliminated by bile secretion; 15% of protoporphyrin extracted by the liver may be converted to bilirubin, with non-haemoglobin haem species as intermediaries, and is also excreted in bile.

Hepatic infusion of micelle-forming bile acids facilitates canalicular protoporphyrin secretion [13]: the micelle-forming taurocholate increased biliary protoporphyrin concentration (by more than six times) and secretion (by more than 12 times) considerably more than dehydrocholate (a non-micelle-forming bile acid). Some bile acids (taurocholate and glycocholate) increase protoporphyrin metabolism 1.7- to 2.7-fold over control values. There are a number of direct and indirect ways in which bile acids might alter the metabolism of protoporphyrin, including either the stimulation of the activity of enzymes such as ferrochelatase and HO or the solubilization of protoporphyrin [14]. Before its final faecal excretion, a significant proportion of protoporphyrin is reabsorbed in the intestine and may circulate through the enterohepatic system [13]. However, it is not yet known how much intestinal microorganisms or food contribute to the total fecal porphyrin excretion.

References

1 Anderson KE, Sassa S, Bishop DF *et al.* (2001) The porphyrias. In: Scriver CR, Beaudet AL, Sly WS *et al.* (eds) *The Metabolic Basis of Inherited Disease*, 8th edn, Vol. 1. New York: McGraw-Hill Publications, pp. 2991–3062.
2 Mauzerall DC (1998) Evolution of porphyrins. *Clin Dermatol* 16, 195–201.
3 Dailey HA (1997) Enzymes of heme biosynthesis. *J Biol Inorg Chem* 2, 411–417.
4 Ponka P (1999) Cell biology of heme. *Am J Med Sci* 318, 241–256.
5 May BK, Dogra SC, Sadlon TJ *et al.* (1995) Molecular regulation of heme biosynthesis in higher vertebrates. *Prog Nucleic Acid Res Mol Biol* 51, 1–51.
6 Deybach JC, Puy H (2003) Acute intermittent porphyria from clinical to molecular aspects. In: Kadish KM, Smith KM, Guilard R (eds) *Porphyrin Handbook*. San Diego, CA: Academic Press Publications, pp. 319–338.
7 Thunell S, Harper P, Brock A *et al.* (2000) Porphyrins, porphyrin metabolism and porphyrias. *Scand J Clin Lab Invest* 60, 541–560.
8 Doss MO, Sassa S (1994) The porphyrias. In: Noe DA, Rock RC (eds) *Laboratory Medicine. The Selection and Interpretation of Clinical Laboratory Studies*. Baltimore, MD: Williams & Wilkins Publications, pp. 535–553.
9 Kaplowitz N, Javitt N, Kappas A (1972) Coproporphyrin I and 3 excretion in bile and urine. *J Clin Invest* 51, 2895–2891.
10 Vincent SH, Muller-Eberhard U (1985) A protein of the Z class of liver cytosolic proteins in the rat that preferentially blins heme. *J Biol Chem* 260, 14521–14528.
11 Zhou S, Zong Y, Ney PA *et al.* (2005) Increased expression of the Abcg2 transporter during erythroid maturation plays a role in decreasing cellular protoporphyrin IX levels. *Blood* 105, 2571–2576.
12 McCormack LR, Liem HH, Strum WB *et al.* (1982) Effects of haem infusion on biliary secretion of porphyrins, haem and bilirubin in man. *Eur J Clin Invest* 12, 257–262.
13 Ibrahim GW, Watson CJ (1968) Enterohepatic circulation and conversion of protoporphyrin to bile pigment in man. *Proc Soc Exp Biol Med* 127, 890–895.
14 Berenson MM, Marin JJ, Larsen R *et al.* (1987) Effect of bile acids on hepatic protoporphyrin metabolism in perfused rat liver. *Gastroenterology* 93, 1086–1093.

2.3.11 Vitamins and the liver (A and D)

Masataka Okuno, Rie Matsushima-Nishiwaki and Soichi Kojima

Summary

The metabolism, pathological relevance and therapeutic applications of retinoids (vitamin A and its derivatives) and vitamin D are reviewed in human hepatic disorders. Both vitamins have profound effects on cell activities, including cell growth, differentiation and apoptosis. Retinoids consist of several molecular species, including retinoic acid (RA), retinol and retinylesters. Dietary retinoids are packed in nascent chylomicrons that are taken up by the liver, in which hepatic stellate cells (HSC) store the majority of body retinoids as retinylesters. The liver supplies retinoids as retinol to meet the requirements of peripheral tissues through binding to its specific binding protein, retinol-binding protein. RA is biosynthesized from retinol in target cells and exerts its biological functions through two distinct nuclear receptors, RA receptor (RAR) and retinoid X receptor (RXR). An isomer of RA, 9,13-di-cis-RA, is involved in the development of liver fibrosis. Retinoids are prime candidates for cancer chemoprevention by reversing the carcinogenic processes through regulating cell proliferation and differentiation. Acyclic retinoid, a synthetic retinoid, successfully suppresses the development of hepatocellular carcinoma (HCC) in cirrhotic patients. Eradication of malignant clones by inducing apoptosis ('clonal deletion') is suggested as a mechanism of the chemopreventive effect. Photolysis of provitamin D3 to previtamin D3 and its thermal isomerization to vitamin D3 take place in the skin. Vitamin D3 is metabolized in the liver to 25-hydroxyvitamin D3, and then in the kidney to its biologically active form, 1,25-dihydroxyvitamin D3 [$1,25(OH)_2$D3]. As the liver plays a major role in the formation of $1,25(OH)_2$D3, osteodystrophy often occurs in patients with chronic liver diseases. $1,25(OH)_2$D3 binds to its nuclear receptor, vitamin D receptor (VDR), which forms a heterodimer with RXR and regulates downstream genes mainly related to calcium metabolism. VDR is expressed in non-parenchymal liver cells but not in hepatocytes. Vitamin D also has immunomodulatory effects, and polymorphisms of VDR are implicated in some autoimmune diseases, including autoimmune hepatitis and primary biliary cirrhosis. Use of vitamin D for the treatment of HCC is also suggested.

Metabolism and function of retinoids

Vitamin A and its analogues, collectively termed retinoids, have profound effects on cell activities, including cell growth, differentiation, apoptosis, reproduction and morphogenesis [1]. Natural retinoids consist of retinoic acid (RA, an active metabolite that binds to its nuclear receptors), retinol (a transport form in the plasma) and retinylesters (storage forms in the tissues) (Fig. 1) [2]. All natural retinoids originate in the diet as either retinylesters or provitamin A carotenoids. Dietary retinylesters and carotenoids are subjected to a series of metabolic conversions to form retinol in the intestinal mucosa. Retinol is absorbed with other dietary lipids, esterified to retinylesters and packed in nascent chylomicrons. The chylomicrons are secreted into the lymphatic system and then enter into the circulation. Most chylomicron retinylesters are taken up by the liver, the major storage site of body retinoids. The liver stores retinoids in the form of retinylesters and supplies retinoids as retinol after hydrolysis of the esters to meet the requirements of peripheral tissues.

There are specific binding proteins for retinol in the plasma and cells, retinol-binding protein (RBP) and cellular retinol-binding protein (CRBP) respectively [3]. RBP is synthesized in hepatic parenchymal cells (hepatocytes) and secreted into the plasma after binding to retinol. Although RBP has a small molecular weight of 21 kDa, as RBP usually binds to transthyretin (TTR) and forms a RBP–retinol–TTR complex, it can avoid renal glomerular filtration. After delivery of retinol to target tissues, apo-RBP loses the binding to TTR, is rapidly secreted through the glomerulus and is reabsorbed by the renal proximal tubules where RBP is degraded to its constituent amino acids. Because RBP has a short half-life of approximately 12 h, it can be used as a sensitive diagnostic tool, particularly in diseases of the liver and kidney and in malnutrition. Plasma levels of RBP as well as retinol and TTR decrease in patients with acute and chronic liver diseases. RBP and TTR levels are found to correlate highly with the reduction of traditional markers such as prothrombin and albumin, which indicate the severity of liver damage. Two types of hepatic cells are known to participate in retinoid storage and metabolism, hepatocytes and HSCs [4]. HSCs play central roles in the storage of retinoids in the liver (more than 75% of hepatic retinoid), although HSCs account for only around 5% of the total liver population. Hepatocytes take up retinoids from chylomicrons and secrete them as retinol after binding to RBP, which is also synthesized by hepatocytes. The mechanism by which retinoids are transferred between hepatocytes and HSCs remains unsolved, although some pathways are postulated. It is believed that HSCs take up retinol from a retinol–RBP complex in the intercellular space that is secreted by hepatocytes. However, some suggest that intracellular retinol bound to CRBP is transferred directly between hepatocytes and HSCs by means of membrane contacts, including desmosomes and other direct intercellular channels. HSCs esterify retinol into retinylesters (mostly retinyl palmitate) and store the esters in the cytoplasm.

A small portion of dietary retinoids is converted to RA, a bioactive hormone, absorbed through the portal vein and present in the plasma bound to albumin. The majority of RA is biosynthesized in the cells of peripheral tissues and modulates the expression of various target genes [2]. Biosynthesis of RA is mediated by alcohol dehydrogenase and aldehyde dehydrogenase, which convert retinol to retinal and retinal to RA respectively. CRBP transfers retinol to these enzymes and helps in the formation of RA. Excess RA binds to cellular RA-binding protein (CRABP) in the cytoplasm and is further oxidized to an inactive metabolite by cytochrome P450 (CYP). For example, CYPRA1 is a novel P450 that inactivates RA by hydroxylation. CRABP acts as a buffering system to control the intracellular concentration of RA, thereby provoking or inhibiting RA actions. Some enzymes and proteins that modulate biosynthesis or degradation of RA are under the control of RA itself. For example, the expression of alcohol dehydrogenase, CRBP and CRABP is upregulated by RA. Thus, the intracellular concentration of RA is under the positive and negative feedback control of RA itself. These regulatory systems can impose a type of check-and-balance mechanism on RA biosynthesis and thus its function.

Retinoid receptors

RAs exert their biological functions through two distinct nuclear receptors, RAR and RXR [5] (Fig. 2a). Both RAR and RXR

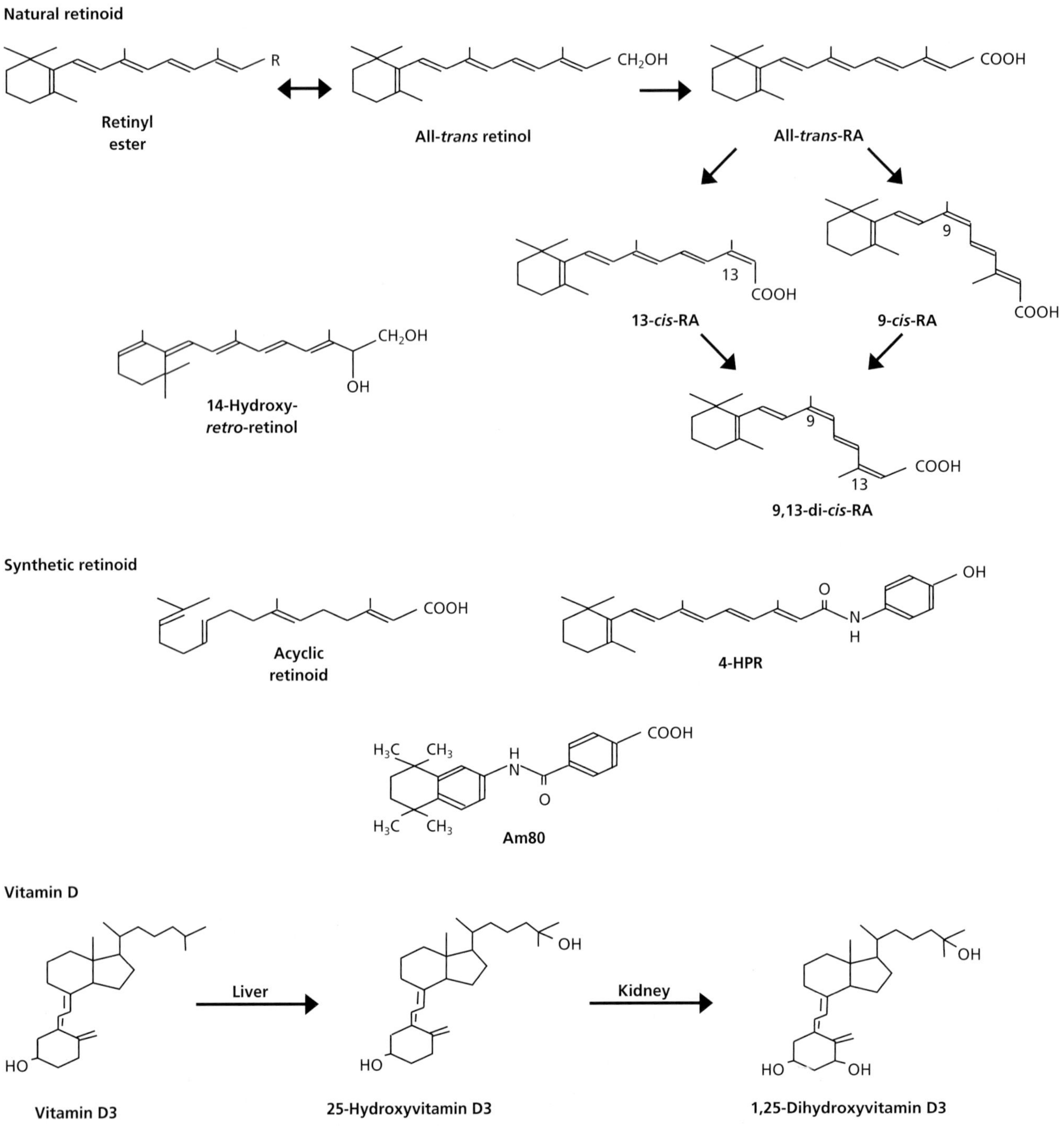

Natural retinoid

Synthetic retinoid

Vitamin D

Fig. 1 Chemical structures of retinoids and vitamin D. Retinylesters (R: fatty acid) stored in the liver are hydrolysed to all-*trans*-retinol that is then transported to target cells after binding to RBP in the circulation. RA, a bioactive hormone, is biosynthesized from retinol by alcohol dehydrogenase and aldehyde dehydrogenase in the target cells. This RA-generating process is irreversible (one-way reaction). Two isomers of RA, all-*trans*-RA and 9-*cis*-RA, activate retinoid nuclear receptor, RAR, whereas only 9-*cis* RA activates the other retinoid receptor, RXR. Another isomer of RA, 13-*cis*-RA, is used clinically for the prevention of head and neck cancers, and 9,13-di-*cis*-RA has pathological significance in liver fibrosis. 14-Hydroxy-*retro*-retinol enhances lymphocyte proliferation independently of known retinoid receptors. A number of synthetic retinoids have been developed for pharmacological applications including cancer chemotherapy and chemoprevention. Acyclic retinoid and 4-HPR successfully prevent the development of HCC and breast cancer, respectively, in clinical trials. Am80 is a promising retinoid aiming to induce second remission in relapsed acute promyelocytic leukaemia (APL) patients who have become resistant to RA therapy. Exposure to solar ultraviolet light converts a derivative of cholesterol (7-dehydrocholesterol) to previtamin D3 in the skin, which is rapidly subjected to thermal isomerization to vitamin D3. Vitamin D3 is metabolized in the liver to 25-hydroxyvitamin D3, and then in the kidney to its biologically active form, 1,25-dihydroxyvitamin D3 [1,25(OH)$_2$D3].

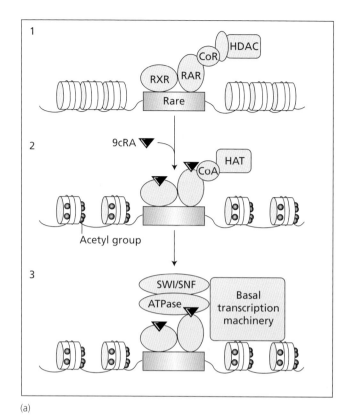
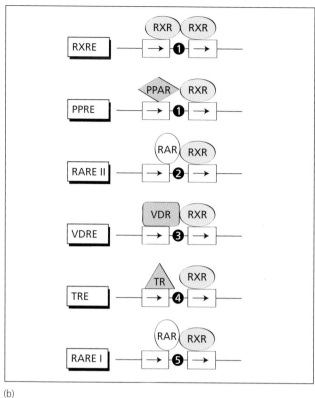

(a)   (b)

Fig. 2 (a) Transcriptional repression and activation of RAR–RXR heterodimer. In the absence of ligands (RA), RAR–RXR heterodimer is linked to corepressor complexes (CoR) and associated with histone deacetylases (HDACs). HDACs remove acetyl groups from histones, induce chromatin compaction and silence the promoter region of the target genes (repression). Binding of RA to the receptor induces its conformational alteration, which destabilizes the interaction with CoR and, instead, allows a connection to coactivators (CoAs) (derepression). CoAs mediate the association between the heterodimer and histone acetyltransferase (HAT) complexes, which induces acetylation of histones and thus leads to chromatin decondensation. Subsequently, activation of transcription takes place by contact with the basal transcription machinery, ATPase and other related factors (transactivation). (b) Direct repeats serve as hormone-response elements for RAR, RXR, VDR, thyroid receptor (TR) and peroxisome proliferator activator receptor (PPAR). The elements consist of direct repeats of core sequence AGGTCA (arrows in boxes) separated by defined numbers of nucleotides (the nucleotide number is shown between the two boxes). RXR functions as a master regulator, forming homo- and heterodimers with RXR, PPAR, RAR, VDR and TR.

consist of three subtypes, α, β and γ, characterized by a modular domain structure. The RA molecule contains four coupled double bonds and thus has several stereoisomers, including all-*trans*-RA (atRA) and 9-*cis*-RA (9cRA), 13-*cis*-RA (13cRA) and 9,13-di-*cis*-RA (dcRA) (Fig. 1). RAR interacts with both atRA and 9cRA, whereas RXR binds only to 9cRA. 13cRA and dcRA are relatively weak ligands for RAR and do not bind to RXR. AtRA and 13cRA are used for the treatment and prevention of cancer, as discussed later. DcRA is involved in the development of liver fibrosis by inducing tissue plasminogen activator in HSCs and subsequently activating transforming growth factor-β, the most potent fibrogenic cytokine [6]. Both RAR and RXR have a DNA-binding domain called C-domain and a ligand-binding domain (E-domain). RXR forms a homodimer as well as heterodimers with RAR and several other nuclear receptors. These dimers bind to their respective response elements and subsequently activate or inhibit the expression of target genes. RAR and RXR bind to an RA response element (RARE) and an

RXR response element (RXRE) respectively. These elements consist of direct repeats of the core sequence AGGTCA separated by a defined number of nucleotides. RARE has direct repeat spacers of two or five nucleotides (DR-2 and DR-5 respectively), and RXRE has a spacer of one nucleotide (DR-1) (Fig. 2b). The tissue-specific expression patterns of the receptors suggest that distinct functions of each subtype and functional redundancy make the retinoid signalling highly complex. The detailed mechanism of transactivation via RAR–RXR heterodimers has been revealed recently [7] (Fig. 2a). In the absence of RA, the RAR–RXR heterodimer binds to corepressor complexes that link between the heterodimer and histone deacetylases (HDACs). HDACs induce chromatin condensation and gene silencing by removing acetyl groups from nucleosomal histones. The binding of RA to ligand-binding domains of RAR and RXR induces the conformational changes in the domain, which allows the interaction between RAR/RXR and coactivators. Coactivators recruit histone acetyltransferases (HATs) such as

CREB-binding proteins or p300 that induce the acetylation of histone amino-terminal tails, resulting in nucleosomal repulsion and chromatin decondensation. On the other hand, a novel retinol (but not RA) metabolite, 14-hydroxy-*retro*-retinol (Fig. 1), induces lymphocyte proliferation, the activity of which cannot be substituted by any isomers of RA, implying the presence of other orphan receptors and/or other retinoid signalling pathways independent of nuclear receptors.

In HCC, both local deficiency of retinoids in the tumour tissues and unresponsiveness of the cancer cells to retinoids lead to loss of retinoid signalling and normal cell function, which seems to be linked to the development of cancer (see also Chapter 18.2, Malignant tumours) [8,9]. Alcohol consumption accelerates retinoid depletion in the cirrhotic liver associated with hepatitis virus infection, which may be related to its enhanced carcinogenic state [10]. RXRα is phosphorylated in HCC cells by extracellular signal-regulated kinase (Erk) 1/2 (also called mitogen-activated protein kinase), loses its function and is accumulated in the cancer cells [11,12], leading to their enhanced proliferation. In addition, RARβ is suggested to be a tumour suppressor gene in some tumours such as head and neck cancer [7,13]. As the RARβ–RXR heterodimer is more activated by retinoids than the RARα–RXR heterodimer, expression of RARβ as well as RXRα may be advantageous in suppressing tumour cell growth. Cells with normal retinoid signalling would be deleted and, as a result, only the remaining cells with impaired response might survive during the carcinogenic process.

Chemoprevention of HCC (see also Chapter 18.2)

Retinoids inhibit carcinogenesis at several steps (i.e. initiation, promotion and progression) and are thus prime candidates for cancer chemoprevention [14]. Recent advances in understanding the molecular mechanisms of carcinogenesis and the parallel progress in molecular targeting have stimulated the development of novel synthetic retinoids for cancer chemotherapy and chemoprevention. Some retinoids work as agonists that enhance the transactivation via RARE or RXRE, whereas others function as antagonists that inhibit the transcription induced by natural RA. In addition, novel mechanisms of retinoid receptor-independent induction of apoptosis have been reported recently with some synthetic retinoids such as 4-hydroxyphenyl retinamide (4-HPR, fenretinide) [7] (Fig. 1). In clinical studies, striking successes have been achieved in the therapy of acute promyelocytic leukaemia (APL) as well as the prevention of several malignancies, including cancers of the oral cavity, head and neck, breast, skin and liver [7,13,15]. Now, differentiation induction therapy with RA and a synthetic RAR ligand, Am80 (Fig. 1), has become standard in the treatment of APL. 13cRA is used clinically for the prevention of cancers in the oral cavity, head and neck region and the skin [7,13].

HCC, one of the most frequent cancers in the world, is an important target of cancer prevention by retinoid. HCC is closely linked to hepatitis viral infection and commonly arises in livers with chronic inflammation. The annual incidence of HCC reaches approximately as high as 3–7% in hepatitis virus-infected cirrhotic patients [16]. Moreover, the annual incidence rises to approximately 20–25% after the curative removal of the primary HCC [17,18]. Such a high carcinogenic state of the cirrhotic liver is a major cause of the limited 5-year survival rate (approximately 40%) even after the curative treatment [19]. Therefore, a new strategy to prevent post-therapeutic recurrence of HCC is required to improve further the therapeutic outcome of HCC. A number of clinical studies have attempted different strategies to suppress the development of HCC. For example, interferon (IFN) suppresses hepatic necroinflammation and thus serves to reduce the incidence of HCC [20,21]. IFN may belong to a category of biopreventive (or immunopreventive) agents, functioning as a biological response modifier. On the other hand, retinoids are chemopreventive agents, as the retinoid seems to act directly on (pre)malignant cells without modulating hepatic necroinflammation. We have developed a synthetic acyclic retinoid (all-*trans*-3,7,11,15-tetramethyl-2,4,6,10,14-hexadecapentanoic acid or polyprenoic acid), aiming for the chemoprevention of HCC (Fig. 1). A double-blind and placebo-controlled clinical study [22,23] has shown that oral administration of acyclic retinoid for 12 months significantly reduced the incidence of post-therapeutic recurrence and subsequently improved survival. In that clinical trial, serum lectin-reactive α-fetoprotein (AFP-L3), which indicates the presence of unrecognizable cancer cells in the remnant liver, disappeared in the acyclic retinoid group after administration [24]. These findings await validation in independent studies. This observation suggests a new concept in cancer chemoprevention, 'clonal deletion', the removal of latent malignant (or premalignant) cells that are invisible by diagnostic images from the organ with a hypercarcinogenic state such as cirrhosis–HCC sequence [25,26]. This concept may explain the reason why only a short-term administration (12 months) of acyclic retinoid has brought about a long-term suppressive effect on the development of HCC for several years. Once (pre)malignant clones are deleted, it would take at least several years for the development of *de novo* cancer in the cirrhotic liver. Acyclic retinoid not only functions as a RXRα ligand but also suppresses phosphorylation of RXRα by inactivating the Ras/Erk system, and thereby restores the function of RXRα [27]. Restoration of the function of RXRα leads to apoptosis induction of the cancer cells, which is a mechanism of clonal deletion. The detailed underlying molecular mechanisms of retinoid-induced apoptosis are discussed elsewhere [26]. Acyclic retinoid is now being tested in a clinical trial in Japan, aimed at chemoprevention of HCC.

Metabolism and function of vitamin D

Vitamin D is known as a 'sunshine vitamin' [28] because of its dependency on sunlight for conversion to an active metabolite. There are six vitamin D compounds, vitamin D2–D7, sharing a common basal structure with different side-chains. Among these, vitamin D2 (ergocalciferol) and vitamin D3 (cholecalciferol) exert high biological activities. In particular, vitamin D3 is the major vitamin D species in man. The first step in vitamin D3 production normally takes place in the skin. Exposure to solar ultraviolet light converts a derivative of cholesterol, 7-dehydro-cholesterol (provitamin D3), to previtamin D3 in the skin via a photolysis reaction. Previtamin D3 is then rapidly subjected to thermal isomerization to vitamin D3 in the skin. Vitamin D3 originating from either the skin or the diet is transported to the liver microsome via the circulation, where it is converted by vitamin D 25-hydroxylase to 25-hydroxyvitamin D3 [25(OH)D3], the major circulating form of vitamin D3 (Fig. 1). The 25-hydroxylation reaction is the prerequisite step for the subsequent 1α-hydroxylation and 24-hydroxylation reactions in the kidney. Namely, 25(OH)D3 enters the circulation again and, in the renal mitochondria, it is converted to 1α,25-dihydroxyvitamin D3 [1,25(OH)$_2$D3], the active form of vitamin D3, by 25(OH)D3 1α-hydroxylase, whereas the 24-hydroxylation reaction leads to inactivation and disposal of vitamin D3. Both reactions are strictly controlled by serum phosphorus as well as by parathyroid hormone, calcium and 1,25(OH)$_2$D3.

Presently, six cytochrome P450s (CYP2C11, 27A1, 2D25, 2R1, 3A4 and 2J3) are found to exhibit vitamin D 25-hydroxylation activities, and CYP27B1 and CYP24 have been established as 1α-hydroxylase and 24-hydroxylase respectively [29]. CYP24 metabolizes vitamin D and 1,25(OH)$_2$D3 to their excretion products [30]. As 24-hydroxylase is induced by 1,25(OH)$_2$D3 itself, the vitamin has a negative feedback system. Thus, vitamin D, like retinoids, is really more of a hormone than a vitamin.

Vitamin D plays a central role in calcium and phosphate homeostasis and is essential for the proper development and maintenance of bone, thus acting on the major target organs, bone and intestine, through a vitamin D receptor (VDR), which belongs to the class II steroid hormone superfamily and is closely related to RAR and RXR [30] (Fig. 2b). VDR forms a heterodimer with RXR and regulates the downstream genes via vitamin D-responsive element (VDRE), consisting of a direct repeat of consensus AGGTCA separated by three nucleotides (DR-3) (Fig. 2b). Among such genes, as described above, CYP24 (24-hydroxylase) is the most inducible gene, and participates in the degradation of vitamin D. When VDR interacts with 1,25(OH)$_2$D3, VDR moves away from the corepressor and acquires the ability to recruit coactivators after forming a heterodimer with RXR at VDRE, which is similar to the regulation of RAR/RXR (Fig. 1a). VDR is expressed not only in the well-known target cells such as osteoblasts and renal tubule cells, but also in a variety of cells including colon cells, lymphocytes and promyelocytes, suggesting novel functions for the hormone beyond osseous tissues [30]. Indeed, 1,25(OH)$_2$D3 is a potent regulator of cell growth and differentiation, with recent evidence showing inhibition of tumour invasion, angiogenesis and tumour cell death [31]. For example, 1,25(OH)$_2$D3 has been shown to induce terminal differentiation of promyelocytes to monocytes [32].

The liver is generally considered to be negative for VDR, although it is obviously a direct target organ of 1,25(OH)$_2$D3 [33]. This may be explained by the low expression of VDR in hepatic parenchymal cells but significant expression in non-parenchymal cells including sinusoidal endothelial, Kupffer, stellate and biliary epithelial cells [34]. VDR expression is also positive in HCC, and thus experimental and clinical trials to use 1,25(OH)$_2$D3 for the treatment of HCC have been suggested [31,35].

Osteodystrophy (osteomalacia and osteoporosis) is often seen in patients with advanced chronic liver diseases [36]. Serum 25(OH)D3 concentrations of < 80 nmol/L are associated with reduced calcium absorption, osteoporosis and increased fracture risk [37]. However, although serum levels of 1,25(OH)$_2$D3 are low in cirrhotic patients, this does not correlate with the bone formation rates [38]. Thus, the pathogenesis of the bone disease is multifactorial, including not only altered vitamin D metabolism, but also other factors such as impaired vitamin K activity, malnutrition and hypogonadism.

A potential link between vitamin D and the immune system has emerged as an interesting area of investigation [39]. Vitamin D interacts with helper T lymphocytes and thereby suppresses the inflammatory responses. For example, inflammatory bowel diseases (IBDs), including ulcerative colitis and Crohn's disease, are closely related to vitamin D deficiency [40]. In addition, VDR deficiency has been shown to exacerbate IBD in experimental animals. Vitamin D-deficient mice on low-calcium diets developed severe IBD, and 1,25(OH)$_2$D3 treatment of mice improved IBD symptoms [39]. Thus, the idea of using vitamin D for the suppression of IBD has been proposed. The link between VDR polymorphisms and two autoimmune-related liver diseases, autoimmune hepatitis and primary biliary cirrhosis, has also been suggested, although the underlying mechanism has not yet been clarified [41,42].

Because both retinoids and vitamin D are fat-soluble vitamins and can thus accumulate when intake is excessive, less toxic synthetic analogues have been developed for use as clinical therapeutics (for detailed descriptions of their toxic effects, see Chapter 14.2, Toxic liver injury, and Chapter 14.4, Hepatic toxicity induced by herbal medicines).

Acknowledgements

This study was supported partly by Grants-in-Aid from the Ministry of Education, Culture, Sports, Science and Technology of Japan (16290215 to SK). We are grateful to Drs T. Sano, S. Adachi, Y. Takano, A. Obora, I. Yasuda, Y. Shiratori, H. Moriwaki and Y. Muto (Gifu University, Japan).

References

1 Hansen LA, Sigman CC, Andreola F *et al.* (2000) Retinoids in chemoprevention and differentiation therapy. *Carcinogenesis* 21, 1271–1279.

2 Blaner WS, Olson JA (1994) Retinol and retinoic acid metabolism. In: Sporn MB, Roberts AB, Goodman DS (eds) *The Retinoids: Biology, Chemistry, and Medicine*, 2nd edn. New York: Raven Press, pp. 229–255.

3 Soprano DR, Blaner WS (1994) Plasma retinol-binding protein. In: Sporn MB, Roberts AB, Goodman DS (eds) *The Retinoids: Biology, Chemistry, and Medicine*, 2nd edn. New York: Raven Press, pp. 257–281.

4 Blomhoff R, Wake K (1991) Perisinusoidal stellate cells of the liver: important roles in retinol metabolism and fibrosis. *FASEB J* 5, 271–277.

5 Mangelsdorf DJ, Umesono K, Evans RM (1994) The retinoid receptors. In: Sporn MB, Roberts AB, Goodman DS (eds) *The Retinoids: Biology, Chemistry, and Medicine*, 2nd edn. New York: Raven Press, pp. 319–349.

6 Okuno M, Sato T, Kitamoto T *et al.* (1999) Increased 9,13-di-*cis* retinoic acid in rat hepatic fibrosis: implication for a potential link between retinoid loss and TGF-β mediated fibrogenesis *in vivo*. *J Hepatol* 30, 1073–1080.

7 Altucci L, Gronemeyer H (2001) The promise of retinoids to fight against cancer. *Nature Rev Cancer* 1, 181–193.

8 Kojima S, Okuno M, Matsushima-Nishiwaki R *et al.* (2004) Acyclic retinoid in the chemoprevention of hepatocellular carcinoma. *Int J Oncol* 24, 797–805.

9 Okuno M, Kojima S, Matsushima-Nishiwaki R *et al.* (2004) Retinoids in cancer chemoprevention. *Curr Cancer Drug Targ* 4, 285–298.

10 Adachi S, Moriwaki H, Muto Y *et al.* (1991) Reduced retinoid content in hepatocellular carcinoma with special reference to alcohol consumption. *Hepatology* 14, 776–780.

11 Matsushima-Nishiwaki R, Okuno M, Adachi S *et al.* (2001) Phosphorylation of retinoid X receptor a at serine 260 impairs its metabolism and function in human hepatocellular carcinoma. *Cancer Res* 61, 7675–7682.

12 Adachi S, Okuno M, Matsushima-Nishiwaki R *et al.* (2002) Phosphorylation of retinoid X receptor suppresses its ubiquitination in human hepatocellular carcinoma. *Hepatology* 35, 332–340.

13 Hong WK, Itri LM (1994) Retinoids and human cancer. In: Sporn MB, Roberts AB, Goodman DS (eds) *The Retinoids: Biology, Chemistry, and Medicine*, 2nd edn. New York: Raven Press, pp. 597–630.

14 Moon RC, Metha RG, Rao KVN (1994) Retinoids and cancer in experimental animals. In: Sporn MB, Roberts AB, Goodman DS (eds) *The Retinoids: Biology, Chemistry, and Medicine*, 2nd edn. New York: Raven Press, pp. 573–595.

15 Chen ZX, Xue YQ, Zhang R *et al.* (1991) A clinical and experimental study on all-trans retinoic acid-treated acute promyelocytic leukemia patients. *Blood* 78, 1413–1419.

16 Shiratori Y, Yoshida H, Omata M (2001) Different clinicopathological features of hepatocellular carcinoma in relation to causative agents. *J Gastroenterol* 36, 73–78.

17 Kumada T, Nakano S, Takeda I *et al.* (1997) Patterns of recurrence after initial treatment in patients with small hepatocellular carcinoma. *Hepatology* 25, 87–92.

18 Koda M, Murawaki Y, Mitsuda A *et al.* (2000) Predictive factors for intrahepatic recurrence after percutaneous ethanol injection therapy for small hepatocellular carcinoma. *Cancer* 88, 529–537.

19 Kakumu S (2002) Trends in liver cancer researched by the liver cancer study group of Japan. *Hepatol Res* 24, S21–S27.

20 Nishiguchi S, Kuroki T, Nakatani S *et al.* (1995) Randomized trial of effects of interferon-alpha on the incidence of hepatocellular carcinoma in chronic active hepatitis C with cirrhosis. *Lancet* 346, 1051–1055.

21 Yoshida H, Shiratori Y, Moriyama M *et al.* (1999) Interferon therapy reduces the risk for hepatocellular carcinoma: National surveillance program of cirrhotic and noncirrhotic patients with chronic hepatitis C in Japan. *Ann Intern Med* 131, 174–181.

22 Muto Y, Moriwaki H, Ninomiya M *et al.* (1996) Prevention of second primary tumors by an acyclic retinoid, polyprenoic acid, in patients with hepatocellular carcinoma. *N Engl J Med* 334, 1561–1567.

23 Muto Y, Moriwaki H, Saito A (1999) Prevention of second primary tumors by an acyclic retinoid in patients with hepatocellular carcinoma. *N Engl J Med* 340, 1046–1047.

24 Moriwaki H, Yasuda I, Shiratori Y *et al.* (1997) Deletion of serum lectin-reactive a-fetoprotein by acyclic retinoid: a potent biomarker in the chemoprevention of second primary hepatoma. *Clin Cancer Res* 3, 727–731.

25 Moriwaki H, Okuno M, Shiratori Y *et al.* (2000) Clonal deletion, a novel strategy of cancer control that falls between cancer chemoprevention and cancer chemotherapy: a clinical experience in liver cancer. In: Okita K (ed.) *Frontiers in Hepatology: Progress in Hepatocellular Carcinoma Treatment*. Tokyo: Springer-Verlag, pp. 97–103.

26 Okuno M, Sano T, Matsushima-Nishiwaki R *et al.* (2001) Apoptosis induction by acyclic retinoid: a molecular basis of 'clonal deletion' therapy for hepatocellular carcinoma. *Jpn J Clin Oncol* 31, 359–362.

27 Matsushima-Nishiwaki R, Okuno M, Takano Y *et al.* (2003) Molecular mechanism for growth suppression of human hepatocellular carcinoma cells by acyclic retinoid. *Carcinogenesis* 24, 1353–1359.

28 DeLuca HF (2004) Overview of general physiologic features and functions of vitamin D. *Am J Clin Nutr* 80, 1689S–1696S.

29 Ohyama Y, Yamasaki T (2004) Eight cytochrome P450s catalyze vitamin D metabolism. *Front Biosci* 9, 3007–3018.

30 Jones G, Strugnell SA, DeLuca HF (1998) Current understanding of the molecular actions of vitamin D. *Physiol Rev* 78, 1193–1231.

31 Pourgholami MH, Morris DL (2004) 1,25-Dihydroxyvitamin D3 in lipiodol for the treatment of hepatocellular carcinoma: cellular, animal and clinical studies. *J Steroid Biochem Mol Biol* 89–90, 513–518.

32 Suda T, Ueno Y, Fujii K *et al.* (2002) Vitamin D and bone. *J Cell Biochem* 88, 259–266.

33 Sandgren ME, Bronnegard M, DeLuca HF (1991) Tissue distribution of the 1,25-dihydroxyvitamin D3 receptor in the male rat. *Biochem Biophys Res Commun* 181, 611–616.

34 Gascon-Barre M, Demers C, Mirshahi A *et al.* (2003) The normal liver harbors the vitamin D nuclear receptor in nonparenchymal and biliary epithelial cells. *Hepatology* 37, 1034–1042.

35 Dalhoff K, Dancey J, Astrup L *et al.* (2003) A phase II study of the vitamin D analogue Seocalcitol in patients with inoperable hepatocellular carcinoma. *Br J Cancer* 89, 252–257.

36 Crosbie OM, Freaney R, McKenna MJ *et al.* (1999) Bone density, vitamin D status, and disordered bone remodeling in end-stage chronic liver disease. *Calcif Tissue Int* 64, 295–300.

37 Heaney RP (2004) Functional indices of vitamin D status and ramifications of vitamin D deficiency. *Am J Clin Nutr* 80, 1706S–1709S.

38 Diamond T, Stiel D, Mason R *et al.* (1989) Serum vitamin D metabolites are not responsible for low turnover osteoporosis in chronic liver disease. *J Clin Endocrinol Metab* 69, 1234–1239.

39 Cantorna MT, Zhu Y, Froicu M *et al.* (2004) Vitamin D status, 1,25-dihydroxyvitamin D3, and the immune system. *Am J Clin Nutr* 80, 1717S–1720S.

40 Andreassen H, Rungby J, Dahlerup JF *et al.* (1997) Inflammatory bowel disease and osteoporosis. *Scand J Gastroenterol* 32, 1247–1255.

41 Vogel A, Strassburg CP, Manns MP (2002) Genetic association of vitamin D receptor polymorphisms with primary biliary cirrhosis and autoimmune hepatitis. *Hepatology* 35, 126–131.

42 Fan L, Tu X, Zhu Y *et al.* (2005) Genetic association of vitamin D receptor polymorphisms with autoimmune hepatitis and primary biliary cirrhosis in the Chinese. *J Gastroenterol Hepatol* 20, 249–255.

2.3.12 Normal iron metabolism

Kyle E. Brown

Introduction

Iron is an essential nutrient, but one with considerable potential for toxicity. It is therefore understandable that the uptake and disposition of iron are controlled by elaborate physiological mechanisms. Although the highly regulated nature of iron metabolism has been recognized for decades, the mechanisms governing its regulation have only recently been elucidated. This has been made possible by the discovery of a variety of proteins involved in iron transport, as well as the iron-regulatory hormone, hepcidin. The aim of this chapter is to provide an overview of iron metabolism with an emphasis on these new discoveries, particularly as they relate to the liver.

Overview of iron metabolism

Before describing these discoveries, a brief review of iron metabolism is necessary. Iron metabolism is a highly conservative process characterized by recycling. The body of the average adult male contains approximately 5 g of iron, of which the single largest component is the haemoglobin contained in the erythrocytes. At the end of their relatively short lifespan, these cells are destroyed, their haemoglobin catabolized and the resulting iron made available for reuse in the synthesis of haemoglobin, myoglobin or any of a number of iron-requiring enzymes, including the cytochrome P450 system, ribonucleotide reductase and the prolyl hydroxylases. In an iron-replete individual, some iron is stored, primarily in the liver, spleen and bone marrow. Hence, once absorbed, iron is conserved. This observation is underscored by the fact that there is no regulated pathway for the excretion of iron, and daily iron loss is negligible, resulting mostly from desquamation of cells.

Given the lack of a regulated means of excreting iron, the control of iron uptake is clearly of paramount importance. The duodenum and proximal jejunum are the main sites of absorption of dietary iron. Haem iron is absorbed more efficiently than non-haem iron, apparently by endocytosis of the intact iron–protoporphyrin complex at the enterocyte brush border.

Iron is then liberated from the haem moiety by the action of haem oxygenase and enters the intracellular iron pool from which it can be transferred across the basolateral membrane, bind to transferrin and enter the circulation. In contrast, the absorption of non-haem iron is more limited, in part as a result of its more complex uptake. As detailed below, absorption of non-haem iron requires reduction of ferric iron at the brush border membrane, followed by internalization by a proton-coupled transporter. Presumably, once iron derived from non-haem sources enters the intracellular iron pool within the enterocyte, its fate is similar to that of haem-derived iron. It is worth noting that, although a great deal has been learned about the mechanisms controlling iron absorption, iron stores exert a major influence on this process under physiological conditions but the means by which iron stores are sensed remains unclear.

Iron transport and uptake mechanisms

Because of the ability of iron to catalyse the production of reactive intermediates, its uptake and transit through the body require mechanisms to diminish its reactivity and thus prevent free radical generation. One of the means by which this is accomplished is by the binding of iron to proteins for transportation and storage. Thus, iron is transported in the blood bound to transferrin. Each molecule of transferrin can bind two atoms of ferric iron. Transferrin-bound iron is taken up at the cell membrane by the interaction of transferrin with the extracellular ligand-binding domain of the transferrin receptor 1 (TfR1). Upon binding of transferrin to TfR1, the entire complex is internalized by receptor-mediated endocytosis. Iron dissociates from transferrin in the acidic milieu of the endosome and then enters the intracellular iron pool, from which it is incorporated into iron-containing proteins, while apotransferrin and TfR1 are recycled to the cell membrane.

The abundance of TfR1 is regulated by cellular iron status, while the identical mechanism controls expression of the iron-storage protein ferritin in an inverse manner. Cellular iron content determines the composition of a cytosolic protein termed the iron regulatory protein 1 (IRP1). Under iron-replete conditions, IRP1 contains a 4Fe–4S cluster that is unable to bind to iron-responsive elements (IRE) in the mRNAs of TfR1 and ferritin. When cellular iron content is low, the iron–sulphur cluster is disassembled, liberating an apo-IRP that binds to specific stem–loop structures in the 3′ or 5′ untranslated regions (UTRs) of the mRNAs encoding these proteins. In the case of TfR1, the IREs are located in the 3′ UTR, and binding of IRP1 increases the stability of the message and enhances the synthesis of TfR1. Conversely, binding of IRP1 to the IREs in the 5′ UTR of ferritin mRNA mediates translation repression. Thus, under iron-replete conditions, there is more rapid turnover of TfR1 mRNA, leading to diminished translation and cell-surface expression of TfR1, reduced uptake of transferrin-bound iron and an expanded capacity for iron storage through increased synthesis of ferritin. Cellular iron deficiency, on the other hand, reverses these phenomena by promoting TfR1 expression and uptake of transferrin-bound iron while diminishing synthesis of ferritin.

In contrast to TfR1, the recently described transferrin receptor 2 (TfR2) has a rather restricted tissue distribution, with the liver the predominant site of expression, and lower levels reported in erythroid precursors and enterocytes [1]. Interestingly, both the 3′ and the 5′ UTRs of TfR2 mRNA lack IREs, indicating that its regulation differs from that of TfR1. Consistent with this observation, hepatic TfR2 expression is not downregulated by iron overload [2]. Given that the liver is a major site for iron storage, the high level of expression of TfR2 and its lack of responsiveness to iron status might be viewed as a protective mechanism, selectively diverting iron to hepatocytes under conditions in which circulating levels of transferrin-bound iron are high and peripheral iron stores are replete. However, the notion that TfR2 merely serves as a reserve is contradicted by the finding that subjects with mutations affecting TfR2 develop a form of non-*HFE* haemochromatosis (type 3) [3]. These observations indicate that TfR2 must serve additional functions, perhaps playing a role in modulating intestinal iron uptake and/or sensing of body iron stores.

In normal individuals, nearly all cellular acquisition of iron from blood occurs via transferrin receptor-mediated uptake, as virtually all the iron in the circulation is bound to transferrin. In circumstances in which the binding capacity of transferrin becomes saturated, as for example in iron loading disorders, iron forms low-molecular-weight complexes, the most abundant of which is iron citrate. It has been known for years that hepatic clearance of this non-transferrin-bound iron (NTBI) is rapid and highly efficient. Furthermore, studies in isolated perfused rat livers and cultured hepatocytes indicated that hepatic uptake of NTBI involves a membrane carrier protein whose iron transport function is subject to competition by other divalent metal ions. Based on these characteristics, it appears that the recently discovered divalent metal transporter 1 (DMT1; also known as DCT1 and Nramp-2) is the major transporter accounting for hepatic uptake of NTBI.

Using a cDNA library prepared from iron-deficient rat intestine, the DMT1 transcript was identified by its ability to increase iron uptake in *Xenopus* oocytes [4]. DMT1 has subsequently been shown to transport various divalent metal ions in a manner that is coupled to the transport of protons. Although DMT1 mRNA is broadly expressed in mammalian tissues including liver, its highest level of expression is found in the proximal intestine, consistent with its role in the absorption of dietary non-haem iron. Two isoforms of DMT1 have been described. The form of DMT1 that predominates in the intestine has an IRE in its 3′ UTR, indicating that the stability of this transcript is regulated by cellular iron status in a manner similar to that of TfR1. Reciprocal changes in duodenal DMT1 expression *vis-à-vis* iron status have been demonstrated in iron-deficient rats and in humans with iron deficiency and iron overload [5]. Collectively, these data provide evidence for a negative feedback

loop in which iron status regulates intestinal DMT1 expression, which in turn controls iron uptake.

Less is known about the regulation and function of DMT1 in the liver. Data concerning the regulation of DMT1 expression by iron status in the liver are inconsistent, with some studies reporting that iron deficiency increases DMT1 mRNA in a manner similar to that of the intestine, while others find no change with altered iron status. Rather surprisingly, livers of rats fed an iron-deficient diet are reported to lack DMT1 immunoreactivity, while those from animals fed an iron-enriched diet demonstrate a pattern of DMT1 reactivity similar to that in the livers of animals fed a control diet, only much more intense [6]. This finding may reflect induction of the non-IRE-regulated form of DMT1, which contains metal responsive elements in its 5′ regulatory region. Nonetheless, it is unclear why the IRE-regulated form of DMT1 (which is also present in liver) is repressed in liver under conditions of iron deficiency. It is evident that the regulation of DMT1 expression in the liver requires further study.

Questions also remain regarding the cellular localization of DMT1 in the liver. While *in situ* hybridization of DMT1 mRNA demonstrated diffuse, low-level expression confined to hepatocytes, results of quantitative polymerase chain reaction (PCR) studies on carefully isolated liver cell populations indicate that DMT1 transcripts are present in hepatocytes, sinusoidal endothelial cells, Kupffer cells and hepatic stellate cells, with the highest levels of expression observed in the last two cell types [7]. These results are particularly interesting in view of the finding that DMT1 immunoreactivity in normal rat liver is observed along the sinusoids, consistent with expression of the transporter on the microvilli of hepatocytes, where it can take up NTBI (or other divalent metals) from the subendothelial space. However, based on the PCR results and the immunostaining, one or more types of sinusoidal lining cells may also acquire iron from sinusoidal blood via DMT1. Further studies are needed to determine the sources and significance of non-parenchymal cell DMT1 expression.

Another issue relevant to DMT1 in liver is the mechanism by which iron is reduced prior to uptake by the transporter. Under physiological conditions, iron exists predominantly in the ferric (+3) state. Uptake by cellular transport systems requires that iron undergoes reduction to the ferrous (+2) state. Recent studies have identified a ferric reductase that is highly expressed in the proximal intestine, termed duodenal cytochrome *b* (Dcytb) [8]. A haem protein, Dcytb, is upregulated by conditions that stimulate iron absorption, including iron deficiency, chronic anaemia and hypoxia. The mechanism by which its expression is upregulated in these conditions is unclear, as there are no obvious IREs in the mRNA of Dcytb. Nevertheless, the localization of Dcytb on the brush border of duodenal enterocytes closely mirrors that of DMT1, supporting the concept that Dcytb supplies ferrous iron to DMT1. Presumably, hepatocellular uptake of NTBI via DMT1 has a similar requirement for ferrous iron. However, whether the reductase that serves this

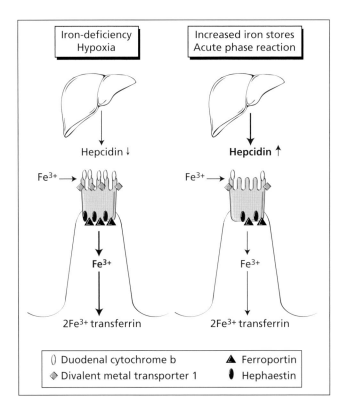

Fig. 1 Schematic representation of effects of various stimuli on hepcidin and its effects on iron transporters in the enterocyte. Dcytb, duodenal cytochrome *b*; DMT1, divalent metal transporter 1; Fpn, ferroportin; Heph, hephaestin.

function on hepatocytes (and other liver cells that express DMT1) is identical to Dcytb is currently unknown.

Iron mobilization and export (see Fig. 1)

Given that the liver is a site of iron storage under physiological conditions, it is apparent that there must be mechanisms by which iron stored in the liver can be mobilized and exported to extrahepatic tissues. Under normal physiological circumstances, Kupffer cells play a prominent role in interorgan iron trafficking. One of the primary sites of erythrocyte turnover, Kupffer cells, along with the reticuloendothelial cells of the spleen and bone marrow, ingest senescent or damaged red blood cells, catabolize the haemoglobin and release the iron. Collectively, the quantity of iron that is recycled from erythrocytes through the macrophage compartment on a daily basis is severalfold greater than that taken up through the intestine. Hence, the contribution of Kupffer cells to total body iron economy is both qualitatively and quantitatively important. It is therefore not surprising that Kupffer cells are the major type of liver cell that express a recently described iron exporter, ferroportin (Fpn; also known as Ireg1 and MTP1) [9–11].

In the intestine, Fpn expression is upregulated by iron deficiency and anaemia. Although this makes sense from a

physiological perspective, it is somewhat surprising in view of the presence of IREs in the 5′ UTR of Fpn mRNA, rather than in the 3′ UTR as would be expected, given the similarity of its regulation to that of DMT1 and TfR1. As illustrated by the example of ferritin, binding of IRPs to IREs in the 5′ region generally results in translational repression. It has been proposed that the IRE in the 5′ UTR may be non-functional in the intestine. If so, this suggests that Fpn expression may be regulated by different mechanisms in different tissues and/or cell types, as the intensity of Fpn staining of Kupffer cells in murine livers is reported to increase with iron loading [11].

Consistent with its role in iron absorption, Fpn is expressed at high levels along the basolateral membrane in mature enterocytes of the duodenal villi. In addition, Fpn transcripts are also detected in liver, spleen, kidney and placenta. In murine liver, hepatocytes as well as Kupffer cells show immunoreactivity for Fpn, albeit less intense. The quantitative PCR study on isolated cells from rat livers discussed above reported similar levels of Fpn transcripts in hepatocytes, Kupffer cells and stellate cells, and lower levels in sinusoidal endothelial cells [7]; however, Fpn protein has not been demonstrated in the last two cell types. Interestingly, the subcellular localization of Fpn appears to differ between hepatocytes and Kupffer cells, being localized to the plasma membrane along the sinusoidal border in the former and cytoplasmic in the latter [11]. It has been proposed that the intracellular localization of Fpn in Kupffer cells (which is also observed in RAW267.4 cells, a murine macrophage cell line) indicates that Fpn does not directly export iron across the plasma membrane in these cells but, rather, that it may participate in intracellular trafficking of iron, perhaps through the secretory pathway. Further studies are needed to determine whether Fpn is involved in multiple pathways of iron export.

Like cellular uptake of iron, efflux of iron from cells requires ferroxidase activity. It has been known for some time that ceruloplasmin, a copper-containing plasma ferroxidase synthesized by hepatocytes, plays an important role in iron homeostasis. Aceruloplasminaemia results in a form of iron overload that is recapitulated in mice with a targeted disruption of the ceruloplasmin gene [12]. Interestingly, although the ceruloplasmin knockout mice accumulate iron in both hepatocytes and Kupffer cells, intestinal iron absorption is unaffected by ceruloplasmin deficiency.

The recent discovery of a homologue of ceruloplasmin that is expressed at high levels in intestinal villi, termed hephaestin, probably accounts for this observation [13]. Despite their similarities, the function of hephaestin is distinct from that of ceruloplasmin, as mutations in hephaestin lead to iron deficiency rather than iron overload. This is illustrated by the sex-linked anaemia (*sla*) mouse, in which a mutation in hephaestin impairs the transfer of iron out of the enterocyte, resulting in microcytic, hypochromic anaemia. The divergent phenotypes of the ceruloplasmin knockout and the *sla* mouse appear to indicate that one ferroxidase has little if any ability to substitute functionally for the other. As hephaestin is membrane bound, this may indicate a requirement for close physical proximity of the ferroxidase to Fpn for efficient iron export, at least in the enterocyte. In this context, it is interesting to contrast hepatocytes, which have low levels of Fpn protein and lack detectable hephaestin transcripts, with Kupffer cells, which have more robust levels of Fpn and express hephaestin transcripts, albeit at levels that are considerably lower than the intestine [7]. Taken together, these observations suggest either that the ferroxidase activity of ceruloplasmin can indeed substitute for hephaestin in Fpn-expressing cells in the liver (but not in the intestine), or that hepatocytes and possibly Kupffer cells as well may employ additional means to promote iron export, such as upregulation of hephaestin in response to iron loading and/or the expression of alternative exporters or ferroxidases.

Another gene involved in iron metabolism that is highly expressed in the liver as well as the intestine is HFE (see also Chapter 16.2, Haemochromatosis). Originally identified on the basis of a high frequency of HFE mutations in patients with genetic haemochromatosis, wild-type HFE protein forms a complex at the plasma membrane with TfR1 and β2-microglobulin. Studies in transfected cells indicate that the stoichiometry of these components influences the rate of recycling of TfR1, thus modulating iron uptake [14]. Nonetheless, the precise mechanism whereby HFE mutations lead to iron loading remains speculative. While immunohistochemistry for HFE demonstrates a distinctive pattern of intracellular perinuclear staining in the epithelial cells of the small intestine [15], immunoreactivity for HFE in liver has been variously ascribed to bile ducts, sinusoidal lining cells, Kupffer cells and endothelial cells. Furthermore, these studies are at variance with results of PCR and Western blot analysis of isolated liver cells demonstrating that hepatocytes are the major source of HFE in rat liver, with a minor contribution from Kupffer cells [7]. Additional studies are needed to resolve this discrepancy and provide further insight into the function of HFE.

In contrast to the genes encoding HFE and proteins involved in iron transport, haemojuvelin mRNA is not abundantly expressed in the intestine. Rather, the highest levels of expression are seen in skeletal muscle, with lower levels in cardiac muscle and liver, where haemojuvelin transcripts are localized to periportal hepatocytes. Haemojuvelin was discovered by positional cloning of the locus associated with juvenile haemochromatosis [16]. Subsequently, two groups have reported that targeted deletion of haemojuvelin in mice results in iron overload [17,18]. While the function of haemojuvelin is unknown, it has been proposed that haemojuvelin is 'upstream' of hepcidin in the pathways controlling iron metabolism, as both patients with iron overload resulting from haemojuvelin mutations and haemojuvelin knockout mice fail to respond to their iron burden with an appropriate increase in hepcidin. A direct interaction between these two proteins seems unlikely, however, given that hepatic expression of haemojuvelin is not altered in mice treated with parenteral iron, while the same livers show a robust increase in hepcidin mRNA. Thus, the available data demonstrate lack of responsiveness of haemojuvelin to iron as well as divergent regulation of haemojuvelin and hepcidin in normal animals treated with iron.

A major advance in the understanding of iron metabolism was the discovery of the iron regulatory hormone hepcidin. Hepcidin was originally identified as an antimicrobial peptide isolated from human urine [19]. The liver is the predominant source of hepcidin, where the 84-amino-acid prepropeptide is synthesized and cleaved to yield 20- and 25-amino-acid peptides that are released into the circulation and filtered by the kidney. Consistent with release into the blood from hepatocytes, hepcidin immunoreactivity is observed along the sinusoidal borders of hepatocyte membranes, with accentuated staining of periportal (zone 1) hepatocytes [20].

The initial finding linking hepcidin to iron metabolism came about through the use of subtractive hybridization to identify genes upregulated by iron overload in murine livers [21]. Later studies demonstrated that hepcidin knockout mice develop a form of iron overload reminiscent of hereditary haemochromatosis [22], while mice with overexpression of hepcidin have severe iron-deficiency anaemia [23]. These data led to the conclusion that hepcidin is a negative regulator of intestinal iron absorption, an inference that has since been confirmed by administration of synthetic hepcidin to rodents.

In addition to iron status, hepcidin expression is modulated by hypoxia and inflammation [24]. In the latter case, hepcidin is an acute-phase reactant, and its induction in response to inflammatory mediators accounts for several phenomena associated with anaemia of chronic disease [25,26]. Although the responsiveness of hepcidin to interleukin-1, interleukin-6 and tumour necrosis factor-α is established, the mechanism by which these mediators influence hepcidin expression is not known. Evidence to date indicates that hepcidin expression is regulated primarily at the transcriptional level. CCAAT enhancer binding protein α, a transcription factor involved in the control of many hepatocyte-specific genes, is a major positive regulator of hepcidin gene expression in the basal state [27]. However, the mechanisms involved in the induction or suppression of hepcidin expression in response to various stimuli have not been delineated, including the means by which iron status modulates hepcidin. There are no apparent IREs in the hepcidin transcript. Furthermore, isolated hepatocytes do not respond to exogenous iron in cell culture [21], suggesting that, *in vivo*, some other cell type senses iron levels and communicates that information to hepatocytes. Although Kupffer cells are likely candidates for this function, recent studies in rodents have shown an appropriate hepcidin response to iron following elimination of Kupffer cells [28,29]. Hence, this aspect of hepcidin biology remains poorly understood.

Subsequent studies have provided insight into the mechanisms by which hepcidin modulates iron absorption. Within a week of being placed on a low-iron diet, rats show a twofold increase in intestinal iron absorption that is temporally associated with a significant drop in hepatic hepcidin expression, and increases in duodenal mRNAs for Dcytb, DMT1 and Fpn [30] (see Fig. 1). Although the increase in Fpn mRNA under these circumstances is of relatively small magnitude, the increase in Fpn protein is more substantial. A similar pattern is seen in the intestine of hepcidin knockout mice, providing additional evidence that hepcidin suppresses the expression of these iron transporters. While the role of hepcidin in the regulation of Dcytb and DMT1 has not been characterized, several reports have established that Fpn is a major target of hepcidin's action. As suggested by the observations discussed above, hepcidin appears to regulate Fpn expression by two distinct mechanisms. The first is at the level of Fpn transcripts, which are decreased following stimulation of endogenous hepcidin production or administration of recombinant hepcidin [31]. The second involves binding of hepcidin to Fpn at the cell membrane, causing internalization and degradation of Fpn, thus diminishing iron transfer [32]. These mechanisms are clearly not mutually exclusive and, while either or both probably contribute to the decrease in intestinal iron absorption in response to hepcidin, it is unclear at present whether Fpn expression in liver cells is regulated in the same manner. In mice treated with iron, intestinal Fpn expression is low, consistent with the known effects of hepcidin. In the liver, however, Fpn is increased, particularly in Kupffer cells [11]. This may result from enhanced translation due to the presence of the IRE in the 5′ UTR of Fpn mRNA. If so, this effect must predominate over the hepcidin-induced increase in Fpn turnover. Alternatively, the distinctive intracellular pattern of Fpn in Kupffer cells implies that Fpn may not physically interact with hepcidin in macrophages, again raising the possibility of differential regulation of Fpn in liver vs. intestine. Further characterization of the effect of hepcidin on the regulation of iron transporters in the liver and its physiological consequences will help to clarify these issues.

The development of iron overload in hepcidin knockout mice [22] and humans with mutations in the hepcidin gene [33] is clearly explicable by the effects of hepcidin on intestinal iron absorption. Since the discovery of hepcidin, several authors have reported that hepcidin expression fails to increase in response to increased iron stores in other disease states characterized by iron loading. For example, hepcidin expression is inappropriately low in iron-loaded subjects with hereditary haemochromatosis [34] and haemojuvelin mutations [16]. Similar findings are reported in a variety of iron-loading anaemias [35]. These observations have led to the concept that 'upstream' iron-related proteins such as HFE and haemojuvelin must in some way control hepcidin expression such that, when these proteins are mutated, dysregulation of hepcidin results. It is clear that the response of hepcidin is defective in all these disorders, as 'appropriate' levels of hepcidin would prevent the progressive accumulation of iron. Nonetheless, it is unclear whether there are direct interactions between hepcidin and other 'upstream' iron regulatory proteins, or whether endogenous iron loading (secondary to HFE or haemojuvelin mutations, for example, as opposed to administration of dietary or parenteral iron) leads to aberrant sensing of iron stores, thus accounting for the dysregulation of hepcidin expression, which then becomes the final common pathway of iron overload. Efforts to elucidate this question are limited by the current lack of knowledge regarding the mechanism by which iron status regulates hepcidin expression.

References

1 Kawabata H, Yang R, Hirama T *et al.* (1999) Molecular cloning of transferrin receptor 2. *J Biol Chem* 274, 20826–20832.

2 Fleming RE, Migas MC, Holden CC *et al.* (2000) Transferrin receptor 2: continued expression in mouse liver in the face of iron overload and in hereditary hemochromatosis. *Proc Natl Acad Sci USA* 97, 2214–2219.

3 Roetto A, Totaro A, Piperno A *et al.* (2001) New mutations inactivating transferrin receptor 2 in hemochromatosis type 3. *Blood* 97, 2555–2560.

4 Gunshin H, Mackenzie B, Berger UV *et al.* (1997) Cloning and characterization of a mammalian proton-coupled metal-ion transporter. *Nature* 388, 482–488.

5 Zoller H, Koch RO, Theurl I *et al.* (2001) Expression of duodenal iron transporters divalent-metal iron transporter 1 and ferroportin 1 in iron deficiency and iron overload. *Gastroenterology* 120, 1412–1419.

6 Trinder D, Oates PS, Thomas C *et al.* (2000) Localisation of divalent metal transporter 1 (DMT1) to the microvillus membrane of rat duodenal enterocytes in iron deficiency, but to hepatocytes in iron overload. *Gut* 46, 270–276.

7 Zhang A-S, Xiong S, Tsukamoto H *et al.* (2004) Localization of iron metabolism-related mRNAs in rat liver indicate that HFE is expressed predominantly in hepatocytes. *Blood* 103, 1509–1514.

8 McKie AT, Barrow D, Latunde-Dada GO *et al.* (2001) An iron-regulated ferric reductase associated with the absorption of dietary iron. *Science* 291, 1755–1758.

9 Donovan A, Brownlie A, Zhou Y *et al.* (2000) Positional cloning of zebrafish *ferroportin*1 identifies a conserved vertebrate iron exporter. *Nature* 403, 776–781.

10 McKie AT, Marciani P, Rolfs A *et al.* (2000) A novel duodenal iron-regulated transporter, IREG1, implicated in the basolateral transfer of iron to the circulation. *Mol Cell* 5, 299–309.

11 Abboud S, Haile DJ (2000) A novel mammalian iron-regulated protein involved in intracellular iron metabolism. *J Biol Chem* 275, 19906–19912.

12 Harris ZL, Durley AP, Man TK *et al.* (1999) Targeted gene disruption reveals an essential role for ceruloplasmin in cellular iron efflux. *Proc Natl Acad Sci USA* 96, 10812–10817.

13 Vulpe CD, Kuo Y-M, Murphy TL *et al.* (1999) Hephaestin, a ceruloplasmin homologue implicated in intestinal iron transport, is defective in the *sla* mouse. *Nature Genet* 21, 195–199.

14 Waheed A, Grubb JH, Zhou XY *et al.* (2002) Regulation of transferrin-mediated iron uptake by HFE, the protein defective in hereditary hemochromatosis. *Proc Natl Acad Sci USA* 99, 3117–3122.

15 Parkkila S, Waheed A, Britton RS *et al.* (1997) Immunohistochemistry of HLA-H, the protein defective in patients with hereditary hemochromatosis, reveals unique pattern of expression in gastrointestinal tract. *Proc Natl Acad Sci USA* 94, 2534–2539.

16 Papanikolaou G, Samuels ME, Ludwig EH *et al.* (2004) Mutations in *HFE*2 cause iron overload in chromosome 1q-linked juvenile hemochromatosis. *Nature Genet* 36, 77–82.

17 Huang FW, Pinkus JL, Pinkus GS *et al.* (2005) A mouse model of juvenile hemochromatosis. *J Clin Invest* 115, 2187–2191.

18 Niederkofler V, Salie R, Arber S (2005) Hemojuvelin is essential for dietary iron sensing, and its mutation leads to severe iron overload. *J Clin Invest* 115, 2180–2186.

19 Park CH, Valore EV, Waring AJ *et al.* (2001) Hepcidin, a urinary antimicrobial peptide synthesized in the liver. *J Biol Chem* 276, 7806–7810.

20 Kulaksiz H, Gehrke SG, Janetzko A *et al.* (2004) Pro-hepcidin: expression and cell specific localisation in the liver and its regulation in hereditary haemochromatosis, chronic renal insufficiency, and renal anaemia. *Gut* 53, 735–743.

21 Pigeon C, Ilyin G, Courselaud B *et al.* (2001) A new mouse liver-specific gene, encoding a protein homologous to human antimicrobial peptide hepcidin, is overexpressed during iron overload. *J Biol Chem* 276, 7811–7819.

22 Nicolas G, Bennoun M, Devaux I *et al.* (2001) Lack of hepcidin gene expression and severe tissue iron overload in upstream stimulatory factor 2 (USF2) knockout mice. *Proc Natl Acad Sci USA* 98, 8780–8785.

23 Nicolas G, Bennoun M, Porteu A *et al.* (2002) Severe iron deficiency anemia in transgenic mice expressing liver hepcidin. *Proc Natl Acad Sci USA* 99, 4596–4601.

24 Nicolas G, Chauvet C, Viatte L *et al.* (2002) The gene encoding the iron regulatory peptide hepcidin is regulated by anemia, hypoxia, and inflammation. *J Clin Invest* 110, 1037–1044.

25 Nemeth E, Rivera S, Gabayan V *et al.* (2004) IL-6 mediates hypo-ferremia of inflammation by inducing the synthesis of the iron regulatory hormone hepcidin. *J Clin Invest* 113, 1271–1276.

26 Lee P, Peng H, Gelbart T *et al.* (2005) Regulation of hepcidin transcription by interleukin-1 and interleukin-6. *Proc Natl Acad Sci USA* 102, 1906–1910.

27 Courselaud B, Pigeon C, Inoue Y *et al.* (2002) C/EBPα regulates hepatic transcription of hepcidin, an antimicrobial peptide and regulator of iron metabolism. *J Biol Chem* 277, 41163–41170.

28 Montosi G, Corradini E, Garuti C *et al.* (2005) Kupffer cells and macrophages are not required for hepatic hepcidin activation during iron overload. *Hepatology* 41, 545–552.

29 Lou D-Q, Lesbordes J-C, Nicolas G *et al.* (2005) Iron- and inflammation-induced hepcidin gene expression in mice is not mediated by Kupffer cells *in vivo*. *Hepatology* 41, 1056–1064.

30 Frazer DM, Wilkins SJ, Becker EM *et al.* (2002) Hepcidin expression inversely correlates with the expression of duodenal iron transporters and iron absorption in rats. *Gastroenterology* 123, 835–844.

31 Yeh K-Y, Yeh M, Glass J (2004) Hepcidin regulation of ferroportin 1 expression in the liver and intestine of the rat. *Am J Physiol* 286, G385–G394.

32 Nemeth E, Tuttle MS, Powelson J *et al.* (2004) Hepcidin regulates cellular iron efflux by binding to ferroportin and inducing its internalization. *Science* 306, 2090–2093.

33 Roetto A, Papanikolaou G, Politou M *et al.* (2003) Mutant antimicrobial peptide hepcidin is associated with severe juvenile hemochromatosis. *Nature Genet* 33, 21–22.

34 Bridle KR, Frazer DM, Wilkins SJ *et al.* (2003) Disrupted hepcidin regulation in *HFE*-associated haemochromatosis and the liver as a regulator of body iron homeostasis. *Lancet* 361, 669–673.

35 Papanikolaou G, Tzilianos M, Christakis JI *et al.* (2005) Hepcidin in iron overload disorders. *Blood* 105, 4103–4105.

2.3.13 Normal copper metabolism and lowering copper to subnormal levels for therapeutic purposes

George J. Brewer, Edward D. Harris and Fred K. Askari

Introduction

In this chapter, we will first provide a review of current knowledge about copper metabolism. Copper is an essential trace element, and the normal diet contains an average of about 1.0 mg. This is about 25% more than is required, and most of the excess is normally excreted by the liver into the bile for loss in the stool. Hence, the liver is important in regulating copper balance and other aspects of metabolism. Excellent progress has been made in understanding copper metabolism in the body, thanks in part to discoveries of the genes that cause two copper-related diseases, ATP7A for Menkes' disease and ATP7B for Wilson's disease (see Chapter 16.1). Progress has also been helped by the elucidation of the roles of copper chaperones, evolutionarily conserved genes whose protein products facilitate transfer of copper to target proteins or vesicles. In the second part of the chapter, a new area involving copper will be reviewed, that of the therapeutic use of lowering copper to subnormal levels to treat cancer and diseases of inflammation and fibrosis.

Copper metabolism and its role in health and disease

Introduction

The essentiality of copper in human health has been recognized for more than 70 years. Severe copper deficiency, whether genetic or acquired, can produce devastating disease and death. The toxic properties of copper were brought to the forefront of scientific attention when a disease described by Wilson in the early 1900s called 'hepatolenticular degeneration' was later discovered to be due to copper accumulation and toxicity [1]. The liver plays a prominent role in copper distribution to organs and regulates overall system homeostasis. Bile, not urine, for eventual loss in the stool, is the major excretory route for copper. Normal urine copper loss is 20–50 µg/day, whereas stool copper loss is in the order of 1.0 mg/day. Transport through the blood to the absorption surfaces of cells has yet to be clarified with certainty. Transport through the membrane and into cytosolic proteins, however, is becoming better understood [2]. The discovery of two structurally related membrane-bound Cu-ATPases, ATP7A and ATP7B, defective in Menkes' and Wilson's diseases, respectively, has provided insight into intracellular copper movement and control of its excretion from the cell. These discoveries have also provided unprecedented biochemical insights into diseases of copper metabolism and have formed the basis upon which much of the current theories of cellular copper movement and homeostasis rest.

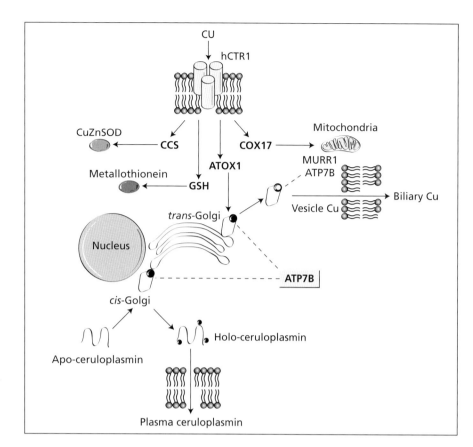

Fig. 1 Overview of liver copper metabolism. Shown are protein chaperones (ATOX1, CCS, COX17) that move intracellular Cu to target proteins. Major excretory routes are the bile and via incorporation into ceruloplasmin. ATP7B, the only Cu-ATPase expressed in liver, performs dual functions in secreting copper from the liver. CuZnSOD, copper/zinc superoxide dismutase; GSH, glutathione; hCTR1, copper transporter.

Chemical properties and copper toxicity

Because copper is a redox metal, unfettered copper is a potential oxidant (or reductant) of cellular proteins, lipids and nucleic acids. This property mandates copper to be in a bound form and not a free ion in blood, extracellular fluids or cytosol. Of its two major valencies, Cu(I) and Cu(II), Cu(I) behaves as a progenitor of free radicals. As a $3d^{10}$ metal ion, Cu(I) also has the potential to antagonize Zn(II). Protein-bound forms of copper are generally responsible for targeted transport to functional biomolecules. The metallothioneins, a family of sulphydryl-rich metal-binding proteins, limit the buildup of mobile copper in cells and work with excretory systems to maintain a steady-state level in the cytosol. Metallothionein synthesis *de novo* is prompted by sudden influxes of copper and other metals into the cell, which clearly demonstrates a genetic-level response system to prevent buildup of copper and other toxic metals in cells and tissues [3]. The protective effects of metallothionein are overwhelmed over time, however, when systems designed to transport copper into bile or release copper from the cell fail to function because of genetic mutations.

The role of the liver in copper homeostasis

The prevailing understanding is that copper absorption occurs mostly at the intestinal mucosa, and copper utilization culminates with the incorporation of Cu(I) and Cu(II) ions into cellular enzymes or storage proteins. The liver intervenes as a major hub for copper distribution to peripheral organs or excretion in the bile (Fig. 1). Dietary copper entering the liver from the portal circulation passes into the liver parenchymal cells after being handed off from binding sites primarily on serum albumin. Transport through the membranes will be discussed below. Upon entering the hepatocytes, copper is met by glutathione (GSH) and sequestered. Another series of proteins, the copper chaperones (Table 1), direct copper to intracellular enzymes or organelles. When bound to chaperones, copper is then positioned to be incorporated directly into either enzymes such as copper/zinc superoxide dismutase [4] or vesicles that represent intracellular compartments along the secretory pathway [5]. The intracellular compartments represent staging areas for incorporating copper into ceruloplasmin or into biliary canaliculi. For example, ATP7B, a Cu-ATPase that is defective in Wilson's disease, is positioned strategically to receive copper from ATOX1 (formerly HAH1), a copper chaperone, and excrete copper from liver via the biliary canaliculi [6]. Precisely how ATP7B governs the movement of copper into the bile is unknown but, clearly, an impairment in that step shifts copper homeostasis towards a failure of biliary excretion and the amassing over time of large amounts of copper in the liver and the rest of the body. Thus, a fault in both copies of the ATP7B gene prevents biliary copper excretion and holo-ceruloplasmin biosynthesis, which are the hallmarks of Wilson's disease.

Table 1 Copper chaperones and transporters.

	Organism	Target or function	Reference
Chaperone			
ATX1	Yeast	CCC_2 protein	[30]
ATOX1	Human orthologue of ATX1 (formerly HAH1)	ATP7A, ATP7B	[6]
CCS	Yeast, human (formerly Lys7 in yeast)	Apo-superoxide dismutase	[12]
COX17	Yeast, mouse, human	Mitochondria	[13]
Transporters			
Ctr1p	Yeast	Membrane copper transport	[7]
hCTR1	Human orthologue of Ctr1p	Membrane copper transport	[7]

Transmembrane movement and the copper chaperones

Gaining access to a cell requires movement across the membrane. hCTR1, a membrane copper transporter in humans (Table 1), has a counterpart in the yeast, Ctr1p, and it is through studies of the yeast protein that many of the properties of copper transporters in humans have become known [7]. Based on these studies, one can surmise that hCtr1 is selective only for Cu(I). This observation necessitates a copper reductase enzyme that changes Cu(II) to Cu(I) to coordinate with transmembrane movement. Precisely how the Cu(I) ions move through the hCTR1 portal is unknown, but recent data suggest that a mechanism involving endocytosis of the carrier is an option [8,9].

Once inside the cell, the metabolic fate of copper relies on copper chaperones, as introduced in the previous section. Chaperones are copper-binding proteins that perform two important functions: (i) sequestering copper to prevent free metal-catalysed oxidations; and (ii) recognizing and conducting copper transfer to intracellular proteins or vesicles. Ions generally rely on the mass action principle to drive the movement of freely diffusible forms. Because free copper concentration is negligible in a cell, it cannot drive reactions and, because of the demand of the many different proteins that require copper for function, intracellular movement relies on copper-binding transport proteins to target specific proteins [10]. A chaperone-bound copper in transit is able to exchange with a target protein, such as enzymes or other proteins, or a membrane-bound Cu-ATPase. Copper chaperones emulate the copper sites on the target protein, thus facilitating the transprotein transfer of copper from chaperone to target [11]. At the present time, several such chaperones are known (Table 1). CCS (copper chaperone for superoxide dismutase) delivers copper to a major antioxidant enzyme in the cell [12]. COX17 is required to move copper into the mitochondria for the binding and assembly of cytochrome *c* oxidase [13] and is essential in embryonic development [14]. ATOX1 mediates the entrance of copper into the secretory pathway through ATP7A and ATP7B, which drive an energy-dependent relocation of copper into vesicles [15].

Cu-ATPases in absorption and cellular homeostasis

There are two phases to intracellular copper transport and movement; these are soluble and vesicle associated. The soluble phase includes components that provide copper to cytosolic enzymes; the vesicle phase is believed to be part of the *trans*-Golgi network for excreting copper from cells. As noted above, two different but functionally similar Cu-ATPases, ATP7A and ATP7B (Table 2), provide the entrance. Wilson's and Menkes' diseases have roots in genetic impairments in ATP7B and ATP7A respectively. ATP7A is found in practically every cell tested, with the exception of adult hepatocytes [16]. ATP7B is prominent in liver, kidney and brain and plays less of a role in other organs [17]. Vesicles laden with ATP7A or ATP7B are mobile and transverse the space between the Golgi and cell surfaces to release copper as part of intestinal absorption or into the biliary canaliculi at the apical surface of hepatocytes. Vesicles that contain ATP7A provide copper to enzymes such as tyrosinase (pigmentation) [18], lysyl oxidase (connective tissue integrity) [19], dopamine-β-monooxygenase (neurotransmitter biosynthesis) [20] or peptidylglycine α-amidating monooxygenase (PAM, neuropeptide hormone biosynthesis; Table 3) [21]. Enhancing the concentration of extracellular copper instigates movement of vesicles towards the plasma membrane [22]. Movement and direction are a function of residues in the N-terminal, copper-binding domain of ATP7A. An exposed dileucine signal at the C-terminal is believe to control

Table 2 Copper regulatory proteins.

Regulatory proteins	Defect	Reference
ATP7A	Causes Menkes' disease	[16]
ATP7B	Causes Wilson's disease	[17]
Murr1	Causes canine copper toxicosis in Bedlington terriers	[25]
XIAP	None known – interacts with Murr1	[29]

Table 3 Neuropeptide hormones that depend on peptidylglycine α-amidating monooxygenase for activity.

Hormone	Biological function	Adverse effects with ageing
Gastrin	Gastric acid secretion	Gastric cancer
Adrenomedullin	Prostate cell growth	Prostrate hypertrophy, cancer
Oleamide	Sleep, lipid synthesis	Sleep disorders, depression
Pancreastatin	Insulin control	Type 2 diabetes
Oxytocin	Water homeostasis	General hydration, skin laxity
Vasopressin	Water homeostasis	General hydration, skin laxity
Substance P	Emotions	Depression
Substance K	Neural transmission	Brain function
Galanin	Neuron modulator	Perception of pain, food intake, memory
Neuropeptide Y	Appetite	Obesity
Cholecystokinin	Satiation	Hyperphagia
Calcitonin	Bone metabolism	Osteoporosis
Releasing hormones		
Corticotrophin	Corticosteroid levels	Immunocompetence, infection
Thyrotrophin	Thyroid hormone levels	Metabolic pace
Melanocyte	Pigmentation, energy	Skin colour, obesity
Gonadotrophin	Sexual hormones	Sexual development, drive

localization of vesicles to the *trans*-Golgi network [23]. Connecting ATP7A and ATP7B, two functionally similar proteins, with two dissimilar diseases has given invaluable insight into pathways of copper movement and homeostasis. Identifying ATP7B with Wilson's disease is a clear indication that ATP7B (i) incorporates copper into ceruloplasmin for excretion into the plasma and (ii) delivers copper to the apical environment of the liver cell. Identifying ATP7A with Menkes' disease tags this Cu-ATPase as an indispensable factor in the absorption of copper across the intestine as well as movement across the blood–brain barrier [24] and into other cells such as the kidney. Moreover, connecting ATP7A-laden vesicles with copper incorporation into apo-tyrosinase, apo-lysyl oxidase and apo-PAM gives a molecular understanding of the phenotypes that are seen in experimental copper deficiencies and inborn genetic diseases, such as Menkes' disease, and age-related impairments in copper metabolism.

Future directions

Several recent discoveries could have an important impact on our understanding of copper metabolism and disease. Murr1 (Table 2) is the name given to a factor that is defective in canines that amass liver copper [25]. The discovery of Murr1 has resolved a mystery as to why Bedlington terriers and some other canine breeds have a Wilson-like copper toxicosis yet, unlike Wilson's disease, have a perfectly functional ATP7B. In humans, the *MURR1* gene maps to chromosome 2. Stuehler *et al.* [26] reported that 19 (30%) of 63 patients with Wilson's disease had mutations in the *MURR1* gene. As to its mechanism, recent studies have shown that Murr1 binds to ATP7B, possibly to direct the movement of that protein to the apical surface of hepatocytes, which is essential to release copper into the bile [27]. Murr1, however, is detected in all tissues and cell types, which

suggests that its role in copper homeostasis extends beyond ATP7B binding and movement [28]. A unique interaction between Murr1 and an apoptosis-suppressing protein, XIAP (Table 2), leads to a reduced level of copper in the cell [29]. XIAP, which is known to inhibit certain caspases, interacts with Murr1 to hasten its destruction through a ubiquitin-dependent proteolysis. Cells from *XIAP* knockout mice have reduced copper levels, whereas cells in which Murr1 is suppressed have the expected elevation in cellular copper. The data, therefore, suggest that XIAP indirectly controls cellular copper homeostasis by regulating the turnover of Murr1.

A second discovery relates ATOX1 to the immunophillin protein FKBP52 [30]. The latter is required to render immunosuppressive factors functional. Precisely why ATOX1 binds strongly to the protein is unclear at this time, but the data suggest other factors, regulatory or structural, are involved in the pathway of copper movement in cells. Finally, recognizing that ATP7A is required to incorporate copper into PAM in the brain [21] has linked copper with the biosynthesis of at least 15 neuropeptide hormones, all requiring this structural modification to become functional (Table 3). By being a critical factor in the activation of neuropeptide hormones, copper is elevated to the point of being one of the most important biominerals in cognitive development in early life and, in the later stages, in senescence, diabetes, osteoporosis, cancer and other disorders that occur with ageing.

Lowering copper to subnormal levels for therapeutic purposes

Introduction

In the past, lowering copper levels for therapeutic purposes was used primarily for the treatment of Wilson's disease, a disease of copper accumulation and copper toxicity. Wilson's disease is covered in Chapter 16.1, and here therefore, we are not referring to Wilson's disease, but to a series of disease conditions that now appear to be potentially treatable by lowering copper levels. Copper levels are essentially normal in these diseases to begin with, but are lowered by therapy to a midrange, not so low as to cause clinical copper deficiency, but low enough to inhibit certain processes involved in specific diseases (for reviews see [31–33]). These processes are angiogenesis, fibrosis and inflammation, and the diseases are cancer, diseases of excessive fibrosis and diseases of excessive inflammation.

Copper and angiogenesis

It is now well established that angiogenesis is required for cancer growth and progression [34,35], and that antiangiogenic therapies are a valid approach to cancer treatment [36]. The essential role of copper in angiogenesis is not so well known, but nonetheless the research in this area dates back two decades [37,38]. It was shown that mild copper deficiency in rabbits, produced by penicillamine and a low copper diet, reduced the angiogenic response in the cornea to known angiogenic stimulants [38]. Tumours explanted to brains of rats and rabbits made copper deficient by this same approach grew more slowly and failed to show vascular invasion of normal tissue, compared with tumours explanted into control rabbits [39,40].

Most of the antiangiogenic, anticancer work that has been done using the lowered copper level approach, subsequent to the work mentioned above, has been done using the anticopper drug, tetrathiomolybdate (TM), originally introduced for the treatment of Wilson's disease [41]. This drug has also been used for the antifibrotic and anti-inflammatory studies discussed later in the chapter. The only significant toxicity of copper-lowering therapy with TM in these diseases is overtreatment. The mild copper deficiency produced from overtreatment causes mild bone marrow suppression with anaemia and/or leucopenia, easily corrected by decreasing the dose of TM.

Lowering copper levels with TM for cancer therapy

Preclinical studies

Numerous preclinical studies have established the efficacy of TM in preventing the growth of various cancers in mice. One study used transgenic mice (Her-2/*neu*) genetically programmed to develop mammary cancer during the first year of life [42]. TM given daily by oral gavage beginning on day 100 completely prevented the development of visible mammary tumours, while most of the controls had developed gross tumours by day 270 ($P < 0.01$). The study was stopped, and a few TM-treated mice were autopsied. Histological sections of the breasts in these mice revealed small, avascular clusters of tumour cells. A few TM-treated mice were followed after stopping TM, and they all developed gross mammary tumours.

Another study used xenografts of SUM149 inflammatory breast cancer cells in mice, and TM markedly inhibited tumour growth and caused reduced microvessel density compared with controls [42]. In another study, Dunning prostate cancer cells were injected into nude mice [43]. TM treatment retarded tumour growth. Combination therapy with TM and the PHSCN peptide sequence, a competitive inhibitor of a fibronectin sequence, improved survival and the number of metastatic lesions.

In a lung cancer model study in mice, Lewis lung high metastatic cancer cells were injected into the upper leg [44]. Radiation therapy significantly slowed tumour growth, TM therapy also significantly slowed tumour growth, and the combination was additive in slowing tumour growth. The effect of TM in squamous cell carcinoma cells was evaluated in another mouse study and showed dramatic inhibition of tumour growth [45]. A combination study with doxorubicin against the SUM149 inflammatory breast cancer cells injected into nude mice was reported [46]. TM or doxorubicin alone significantly inhibited tumour growth, while the combination completely prevented tumour growth. Apoptosis of tumour cells was enhanced in all treatment groups, but especially in the combination therapy group.

A study of TM therapy was carried out in dogs affected with a variety of advanced and metastatic cancers [47]. Nine dogs in this 13-dog study were evaluable. Three of the nine had relatively prolonged periods of disease stabilization, and a fourth dog, with metastatic osteosarcoma, had a relatively prolonged partial remission.

Clinical studies

A phase I/II study of 42 patients with advanced and metastatic cancer was carried out [48]. Eighteen patients were evaluable. Freedom from progression averaged 11 months, much longer than the 1–2 months expected in this type of patient if they were on no treatment. Quality of life was stabilized after steady deterioration in the period prior to treatment. Particularly positive results were seen in a few patients. One patient, with metastatic chondrosarcoma, has survived 5 years with what appears to be a complete remission. Using a blood flow-sensitive ultrasound technique, it was possible to show drastic blood flow reduction in a metastasis as a result of TM therapy in a patient with metastatic renal cancer.

Nine phase II trials of TM therapy in specific advanced cancers have been initiated. One, on renal cancer, has been completed and published [49]. Four out of nine evaluable patients had at least 6 months of disease stabilization, but results overall were not strongly positive. Preliminary results in other trials, such as mesothelioma and hepatocellular cancer, are more encouraging.

Mechanism of action

The anticancer mechanism of action almost certainly involves reducing copper availability. This conclusion is based in part on *in vitro* studies in which TM inhibition of endothelial cell tube formation, under the influence of fibroblastic growth factor, was abrogated by copper supplementation [42]. Second, anticancer effects have been obtained with two different anticopper drugs, TM as reviewed above and penicillamine as studied by Brem *et al.* [39,40]. These two drugs both lower copper availability, but through completely different mechanisms of action.

A further conclusion is that the anticancer mechanism of action of lowering copper levels is almost certainly due to anti-angiogenic effects. *In vitro* studies of TM action have shown inhibition of numerous angiogenic cytokines [vascular endothelial growth factor, fibroblastic growth factor, interleukin-6, nuclear factor kappa B (NF-κB), and interleukin-8] [42]. *In vivo* studies during TM therapy have also shown inhibition of angiogenic cytokines, including NF-κB [50]. Both clinical and preclinical studies have shown inhibition of blood flow or decreased microvessel density as a result of TM therapy [48]. Numerous angiogenic cytokines have been shown to bind copper or to be copper dependent [33].

Lowering copper levels with TM for antifibrotic therapy

The pathway for fibrosis involves activation of transforming growth factor beta (TGF-β), a cytokine that activates connective tissue growth factor (CTGF), which in turn activates numerous genes involved in fibrosis (see Section 6, Cirrhosis). Excessive activation of this pathway is believed to cause fibrotic disease, such as pulmonary fibrosis, cirrhosis of various types, interstitial renal fibrosis (the endstage of many types of kidney disease) and scleroderma, to name but a few [51]. It has been hypothesized that this pathway is copper dependent, based upon one of the activators of TGF-β being SPARC (secreted protein acidic and rich in cysteine), known to be copper dependent, and the high cysteine content of CTGF, often an indicator of copper binding [33].

The copper dependence of fibrosis was tested in the bleomycin mouse model of pulmonary fibrosis. TM therapy almost completely prevented the pulmonary fibrosis from bleomycin [52]. TGF-β protein levels were elevated in the lungs of bleomycin-treated animals, and this elevation was almost completely prevented by TM [53]. Protection by TM against fibrotic disease was also tested in the carbon tetrachloride mouse model of cirrhosis [54]. After 12 weeks of carbon tetrachloride injections, untreated mice developed severe fibrosis. Fibrosis from carbon tetrachloride injections was prevented by TM therapy. Serum TGF-β levels were elevated by carbon tetrachloride, and this elevation was almost completely prevented by TM. The protection of TM against excessive fibrosis seems to be independent of any effect of TM on preventing inflammation [52–54].

Lowering copper levels with TM for anti-inflammatory therapy

It was noted in the bleomycin studies that TM therapy inhibited tumour necrosis factor (TNF)α messenger levels in the lungs of bleomycin-treated animals at 7 days compared with bleomycin-treated controls [53]. This led to a series of four studies evaluating TM therapy in inflammation models. In all four cases, TM therapy strongly inhibited the inflammatory responses [54,55]. These models are concanavalin A-induced hepatitis, paracetamol (acetaminophen)-induced hepatitis, adriamycin-induced cardiac inflammation and injury, and lupus adenopathy in the *lpr* mouse model. In most of these models, concomitant with suppression by TM of markers of inflammation and injury, inhibition of serum TNFα and/or another inflammatory cytokine, interleukin-1-beta (IL-1β), was shown when toxin- or disease-challenged animals were compared with the same animals receiving TM therapy. Inhibition of these cytokines seems to reduce inflammation, as shown by the efficacy of TNFα antibodies in various inflammatory diseases [56–59]. The mechanism by which TM inhibits these cytokines is not known. One possibility is that suppression of IL-2 release by activated T lymphocytes, which has been shown to result from TM therapy, results in less activation of inflammatory cells and therefore less release of TNFα and IL-1β by these cells.

Comment on prospects for antifibrotic and anti-inflammatory therapy with TM

Only clinical trials will determine whether copper-lowering therapy with TM will have clinical efficacy in fibrotic and inflammatory diseases is clinical trials. This approach is further advanced with fibrotic than with inflammatory diseases. Clinical trials are either under way, or under active planning, for idiopathic pulmonary fibrosis, primary biliary cirrhosis and scleroderma. There is essentially no effective treatment for fibrotic diseases such as these. Regarding inflammatory diseases, much of modern medicine deals with the discomfort and additional injury produced by inflammation in a large variety of diseases, many of them autoimmune. Therapeutic agents, such as steroids, non-steroidal anti-inflammatory drugs (NSAIDs), chemotherapeutic drugs and antibodies against specific inflammatory proteins (such as TNFα), have some efficacy. However, efficacy is only partial, and myriads of patients have continuing discomfort and tissue injury in spite of the best treatment. Time will tell whether copper-lowering therapy with TM can be of value against these diseases.

Summary

In this chapter we have first reviewed and summarized the exciting progress in understanding normal copper metabolism. The discovery that genetic defects in ATP7A and ATP7B cause Menkes' and Wilson's diseases, respectively, has not only provided a molecular basis for these diseases, but has also allowed an increasingly detailed understanding of copper transport and utilization in the body. The discoveries of numerous chaperones for moving copper between specific molecules has not only provided insight into mechanisms of copper movement, but also

Table 4 Published therapeutic uses of lowering copper to subnormal levels.

Mechanism	Diseases	Reference to work so far
Angiogenesis	Cancer	[39,40,42–50]
	Retinopathy	[60]
Antifibrosis	Pulmonary fibrosis	[52,53]
	Cirrhosis	[54]
Anti-inflammatory	Concanavalin A	[54]
	Paracetamol liver injury	[55]

underscores two principles about copper. One is that free copper is very toxic and simple diffusion and molecular uptake is not permissible. The second is the extreme evolutionary conservatism of copper-handling molecules, which go back in evolution at least as far as yeast.

Second, we have reviewed a new area for the use of anticopper drugs (summarized in Table 4). For a very long time, anticopper drugs have had one primary clinical use, the treatment of copper toxicity from excessive accumulation of copper such as in Wilson disease, canine copper toxicosis or copper-poisoned sheep. Here, we introduce the concept that lowering copper availability to a midrange can have therapeutic efficacy in a wide array of diseases.

References

1 Wilson SA (1912) Progressive lenticular degeneration: a familial nervous disease associated with cirrhosis of the liver. *Brain* 34, 295–507.

2 Harris ED (2003) Basic and clinical aspects of copper. *Crit Rev Clin Lab Sci* 40 (5), 547–586.

3 Sone T, Yamaoka K, Minami Y *et al.* (1987) Induction of metallothionein synthesis in Menkes' and normal lymphoblastoid cells is controlled by the level of intracellular copper. *J Biol Chem* 262 (12), 5878–5885.

4 Bartnikas TB, Gitlin JD (2003) Mechanisms of biosynthesis of mammalian copper/zinc superoxide dismutase. *J Biol Chem* 278 (35), 33602–33608.

5 Harrison MD, Jones CE, Dameron CT (1999) Copper chaperones: function, structure and copper-binding properties. *J Biol Inorg Chem* 4 (2), 145–153.

6 Hamza I, Schaefer M, Klomp LW *et al.* (1999) Interaction of the copper chaperone HAH1 with the Wilson disease protein is essential for copper homeostasis. *Proc Natl Acad Sci USA* 96 (23), 13363–13368.

7 Sharp PA (2003) Ctr1 and its role in body copper homeostasis. *Int J Biochem Cell Biol* 35 (3), 288–291.

8 Klomp AE, Tops BB, Van Denberg IE *et al.* (2002) Biochemical characterization and subcellular localization of human copper transporter 1 (hCTR1). *Biochem J* 364 (Pt 2), 497–505.

9 Petris MJ, Smith K, Lee J *et al.* (2003) Copper-stimulated endocytosis and degradation of the human copper transporter, hCtr1. *J Biol Chem* 278 (11), 9639–9646.

10 Markossian KA, Kurganov BI (2003) Copper chaperones, intracellular copper trafficking proteins. Function, structure, and mechanism of action. *Biochemistry (Mosc)* 68 (8), 827–837.

11 Huffman DL, O'Halloran TV (2001) Function, structure, and mechanism of intracellular copper trafficking proteins. *Annu Rev Biochem* 70, 677–701.

12 Culotta VC, Klomp LW, Strain J *et al.* (1997) The copper chaperone for superoxide dismutase. *J Biol Chem* 272 (38), 23469–23472.

13 Beers J, Glerum DM, Tzagoloff A (1997) Purification, characterization, and localization of yeast Cox17p, a mitochondrial copper shuttle. *J Biol Chem* 272 (52), 33191–33196.

14 Takahashi Y, Kako K, Kashiwabara S *et al.* (2002) Mammalian copper chaperone Cox17p has an essential role in activation of cytochrome C oxidase and embryonic development. *Mol Cell Biol* 22 (21), 7614–7621.

15 Prohaska JR, Gybina AA (2004) Intracellular copper transport in mammals. *J Nutr* 134 (5), 1003–1006.

16 Mercer JF, Livingston J, Hall B *et al.* (1993) Isolation of a partial candidate gene for Menkes disease by positional cloning. *Nature Genet* 3 (1), 20–25.

17 Lutsenko S, Efremov RG, Tsivkovskii R *et al.* (2002) Human copper-transporting ATPase ATP7B (the Wilson's disease protein): biochemical properties and regulation. *J Bioenerg Biomembr* 34 (5), 351–362.

18 Petris MJ, Strausak D, Mercer JF (2000) The Menkes copper transporter is required for the activation of tyrosinase. *Hum Mol Genet* 9 (19), 2845–2851.

19 Tchaparian EH, Uriu-Adams JY, Keen CL *et al.*(2000) Lysyl oxidase and P-ATPase-7A expression during embryonic development in the rat. *Arch Biochem Biophys* 379 (1), 71–77.

20 Barnes N, Tsivkovskii R, Tsivkovskaia N *et al.* (2005) The copper-transporting ATPases, Menkes and Wilson disease proteins, have distinct roles in adult and developing cerebellum. *J Biol Chem* 280 (10), 9640–9645.

21 Steveson TC, Ciccotosto GD, Ma XM *et al.* (2003) Menkes protein contributes to the function of peptidylglycine alpha-amidating monooxygenase. *Endocrinology* 144 (1), 188–200.

22 Petris MJ, Mercer JF, Culvenor JG *et al.* (1996) Ligand-regulated transport of the Menkes copper P-type ATPase efflux pump from the Golgi apparatus to the plasma membrane: a novel mechanism of regulated trafficking. *EMBO J* 15 (22), 6084–6095.

23 Petris MJ, Camakaris J, Greenough M *et al.* (1998) A C-terminal di-leucine is required for localization of the Menkes protein in the trans-Golgi network. *Hum Mol Genet* 7 (13), 2063–2071.

24 Qian Y, Tiffany-Castiglioni E, Welsh J *et al.* (1998) Copper efflux from murine microvascular cells requires expression of the Menkes disease Cu-ATPase. *J Nutr* 128 (8), 1276–1282.

25 van De SB, Rothuizen J, Pearson PL *et al.* (2002) Identification of a new copper metabolism gene by positional cloning in a purebred dog population. *Hum Mol Genet* 11 (2), 165–173.

26 Stuehler B, Reichert J, Stremmel W *et al.* (2004) Analysis of the human homologue of the canine copper toxicosis gene MURR1 in Wilson disease patients. *J Mol Med* 82 (9), 629–634.

27 Tao TY, Liu F, Klomp L *et al.* (2003) The copper toxicosis gene product Murr1 directly interacts with the Wilson disease protein. *J Biol Chem* 278 (43), 41593–41596.

28 Wijmenga C, Klomp LW (2004) Molecular regulation of copper excretion in the liver. *Proc Nutr Soc* 63 (1), 31–39.

29 Burstein E, Ganesh L, Dick RD *et al.* (2004) A novel role for XIAP in copper homeostasis through regulation of MURR1. *EMBO J* 23 (1), 244–254.

30 Portnoy ME, Rosenzweig AC, Rae T *et al.* (1999) Structure-function analyses of the ATX1 metallochaperone. *J Biol Chem* 274 (21), 15041–15045.

31 Brewer GJ (2001) Copper control as an antiangiogenic anticancer therapy: lessons from treating Wilson's disease. *Exp Biol Med* 226 (7), 665–673.

32 Brewer GJ, Merajver SD (2002) Cancer therapy with tetrathiomolybdate: antiangiogenesis by lowering body copper – a review. *Integr Cancer Ther* 1 (4), 327–337.

33 Brewer GJ (2003) Tetrathiomolybdate anticopper therapy for Wilson's disease inhibits angiogenesis, fibrosis and inflammation. *J Cell Mol Med* 7 (1), 11–20.

34 Folkman J (1971) Tumor angiogenesis: therapeutic implications. *N Engl J Med* 285 (21), 1182–1186.

35 Folkman J (1995) Angiogenesis in cancer, vascular, rheumatoid and other disease. *Nature Med* 1 (1), 27–31.

36 Brem S (1999) Angiogenesis and cancer control: from concept to therapeutic trial. *Cancer Control* 6 (5), 436–458.

37 Raju KS, Alessandri G, Ziche M *et al.* (1982) Ceruloplasmin, copper ions, and angiogenesis. *J Natl Cancer Inst* 69 (5), 1183–1188.

38 Ziche M, Jones J, Gullino PM (1982) Role of prostaglandin E1 and copper in angiogenesis. *J Natl Cancer Inst* 69 (2), 475–482.

39 Brem SS, Tsanaclis AM, Zagzag D (1990) Anticopper treatment inhibits pseudopodial protrusion and the invasive spread of 9L gliosarcoma cells in the rat brain. *Neurosurgery* 26 (3), 391–396.

40 Brem SS, Zagzag D, Tsanaclis AM *et al.* (1990) Inhibition of angiogenesis and tumor growth in the brain. Suppression of endothelial cell turnover by penicillamine and the depletion of copper, an angiogenic cofactor. *Am J Pathol* 137 (5), 1121–1142.

41 Brewer GJ, Hedera P, Kluin KJ *et al.* (2003) Treatment of Wilson disease with ammonium tetrathiomolybdate: III. Initial therapy in a total of 55 neurologically affected patients and follow-up with zinc therapy. *Arch Neurol* 60 (3), 379–385.

42 Pan Q, Kleer CG, van Golen KL *et al.* (2002) Copper deficiency induced by tetrathiomolybdate suppresses tumor growth and angiogenesis. *Cancer Res* 62 (17), 4854–4859.

43 van Golen KL, Bao L, Brewer GJ *et al.* (2002) Suppression of tumor recurrence and metastasis by a combination of the PHSCN sequence and the antiangiogenic compound tetrathiomolybdate in prostate carcinoma. *Neoplasia* 4 (5), 373–379.

44 Khan MK, Miller MW, Taylor J *et al.* (2002) Radiotherapy and antiangiogenic TM in lung cancer. *Neoplasia* 4 (2), 164–170.

45 Cox C, Merajver SD, Yoo S *et al.* (2003) Inhibition of the growth of squamous cell carcinoma by tetrathiomolybdate-induced copper suppression in a murine model. *Arch Otolaryngol Head Neck Surg* 129 (7), 781–785.

46 Pan Q, Bao LW, Kleer CG *et al.* (2003) Antiangiogenic tetrathiomolybdate enhances the efficacy of doxorubicin against breast carcinoma. *Mol Cancer Ther* 2 (7), 617–622.

47 Kent MS, Madewell BR, Dank G *et al.* (2004) An anticopper antiangiogenic approach for advanced cancer in spontaneously occurring tumors, using tetrathiomolybdate: a pilot study in a canine animal mode. *J Trace Elem Exp Med* 17 (1), 9–20.

48 Brewer GJ, Dick RD, Grover DK *et al.* (2000) Treatment of metastatic cancer with tetrathiomolybdate, an anticopper, antiangiogenic agent: Phase I study. *Clin Cancer Res* 6 (1), 1–10.

49 Redman BG, Esper P, Pan Q *et al.* (2003) Phase II trial of tetrathiomolybdate in patients with advanced kidney cancer. *Clin Cancer Res* 9 (5), 1666–1672.

50 Pan Q, Bao LW, Merajver SD (2003) Tetrathiomolybdate inhibits angiogenesis and metastasis through suppression of the NFkappaB signaling cascade. *Mol Cancer Res* 1 (10), 701–706.

51 Border WA, Noble NA (1994) Transforming growth factor beta in tissue fibrosis. *N Engl J Med* 331 (19), 1286–1292.

52 Brewer GJ, Ullenbruch MR, Dick RB *et al.* (2003) Tetrathiomolybdate therapy protects against bleomycin-induced pulmonary fibrosis in mice. *J Lab Clin Med* 141 (3), 210–216.

53 Brewer GJ, Dick R, Ullenbruch MR *et al.* (2004) Inhibition of key cytokines by tetrathiomolybdate in the bleomycin model of pulmonary fibrosis. *J Inorg Biochem* 98 (12), 2160–2167.

54 Askari FK, Dick RB, Mao M *et al.* (2004) Tetrathiomolybdate therapy protects against concanavalin A and carbon tetrachloride hepatic damage in mice. *Exp Biol Med* 229 (8), 857–863.

55 Ma S, Hou G, Dick RD *et al.* (2004) Tetrathiomolybdate protects against liver injury from acetaminophen in mice. *J Appl Res Clin Exp Ther* 4 (3), 419–426.

56 Elliott MJ, Maini RN, Feldmann M *et al.* (1993) Treatment of rheumatoid arthritis with chimeric monoclonal antibodies to tumor necrosis factor alpha. *Arthritis Rheum* 36 (12), 1681–1690.

57 Shanahan JC, St Clair W (2002) Tumor necrosis factor-alpha blockade: a novel therapy for rheumatic disease. *Clin Immunol* 103 (3 Pt 1), 231–242.

58 D'Haens G, Van Deventer S, Van Hogezand R *et al.* (1999) Endoscopic and histological healing with infliximab anti-tumor necrosis factor antibodies in Crohn's disease: a European multicenter trial. *Gastroenterology* 116 (5), 1029–1034.

59 Mease PJ, Goffe BS, Metz J *et al.* (2000) Etanercept in the treatment of psoriatic arthritis and psoriasis: a randomised trial. *Lancet* 356 (9227), 385–390.

60 Elner SG, Elner VM, Yoshida A *et al.* (2005) Effects of tetrathiomolybdate in a mouse model of retinal neovascularization. *Invest Ophthalmol Vis Sci* 46 (1), 299–303.

2.3.14 Trace elements and the liver

Brent A. Neuschwander-Tetri

Life would not be possible without a large number of 'trace' elements, each serving critical roles in metabolism and function (Table 1). This chapter reviews the function and relevant biology of trace elements with respect to the liver. Because copper has a special role as a trace element with respect to normal liver function and liver disease, it is covered in more detail in Chapter 2.3.13 and is not discussed further here.

Trace elements are necessary for normal function and are therefore associated with morbid deficiency states. They are also commonly toxic when present in excess, and this chapter will touch briefly on toxicity as it relates to the essential trace elements. Actual values for liver, plasma and total body content of the trace elements that are used to assess deficiency states and toxicity are catalogued in other resources and are not reviewed here [1–4]. Although such values are important in forensic medicine and epidemiological studies, they are rarely relevant to the routine practice of clinical medicine [5]. Accurate

Table 1 Physiological trace elements in the body.[a]

Element	Function(s)	Causes of deficiency	Deficiency: hepatic consequences	Deficiency: non-hepatic consequences	Changes in liver disease
Arsenic	Uncertain[b]				
Cobalt	Cobalamin (vitamin B12)	Multiple	Fatty liver disease	Multiple	Impaired elimination of vitamin B12 degradation products
Chromium	Improves insulin signalling	Defined diet without supplementation	Impaired glucose tolerance	Impaired glucose tolerance	Hepatic accumulation in chronic liver disease
Fluorine	Uncertain[b]				
Iodine	Thyroid hormone				
Lead	Uncertain[b]				
Manganese	Cofactor for multiple enzymes (e.g. MnSOD, pyruvate carboxylase, phosphoenolpyruvate carboxykinase, arginase, prolidase)	Defined diet without supplementation	Impaired glucose tolerance, elevated ammonia levels, impaired cholesterol synthesis, impaired clotting factor synthesis	Impaired glucose tolerance, dermatitis	Decreased urinary excretion and increased liver concentration in alcoholic cirrhotics [58] Increased levels in globus pallidus in cirrhotics, may cause extrapyramidal symptoms [53]
Molybdenum	Xanthine oxidase Aldehyde oxidase Sulphite oxidase	Defined diet without supplementation	Altered sulphur amino acid metabolism	Not established	
Nickel	Nickel[b] known to have a catalytic role in six bacterial enzymes (including urease), but no eukaryotic enzymes				
Selenium	See Table 2	Dietary protein deficiency Dietary protein solely from Se-deficient areas	Oxidant stress	See text	Low serum levels in chronic liver disease [26]
Silicon	Uncertain[b]				
Tin	Uncertain[b]				
Vanadium	Uncertain[b]				
Zinc	Cofactor for multiple enzymes and transcription factors	Increased urinary loss in cirrhosis Alcoholism Malabsorption (e.g. coeliac disease, inflammatory bowel disease)	Altered ammonia metabolism	Encephalopathy in cirrhotics	Low serum levels in chronic liver disease [26] Low liver levels in alcoholic cirrhosis [58]

[a]Copper is discussed in Chapter 2.3.13.
[b]Certain elements may have physiological roles based on animal studies of specific dietary deficiencies, but requirements and specific functions in humans are not known [5,7].

assessment of trace element levels in organs such as the liver continues to be refined as technologies such as scanning transmission electron microscopic analysis are developed. Nonetheless, the necessity and function of certain elements such as boron, nickel, tin and vanadium continues to be debated (Table 1) because dietary deficiency models in animals sometimes suggest that they are essential, yet their specific functions at the molecular level have not been established [5,6]. Described below are the functions of major trace elements relevant to the liver with special emphasis on selenium, an element now recognized to play a unique role in human biology. The importance of many trace elements in nutrition and disease was reviewed extensively by an expert panel [7], and the summary below includes many of their key findings.

Selenium

Selenium has a special role in the normal function of the liver and tissues throughout the body. Found directly below sulphur on the periodic table, selenium thus shares many of the chemical properties of sulphur [8]. In fact, most selenium in the body is found in selenoproteins, which contain the amino acid seleno-cysteine (Sec), a modification in which selenium is found in place of the sulphur atom of cysteine. Failure to produce seleno-proteins in the liver causes liver necrosis in mice, attesting to the importance of selenium in normal liver function [9]. Selenium is also incorporated into proteins as selenomethionine from ingested selenomethionine. In contrast to the specific incorpo-ration of Sec in proteins, selenomethionine (Se-met) replaces methionine arbitrarily during translation depending on the relative abundance of Se-met [10]. Although Se-met may exert different local steric effects from methionine, it has not been found to have specific biological functions [11].

The story of how Sec becomes incorporated into selenopro-teins is one that has challenged the accepted dogma of protein synthesis pathways as it has unfolded over the past three decades. While one possible mechanism of selenium incorpora-tion could be replacement of the sulphur atom in cysteine by selenium through posttranslational peptide modification, the surprising reality is that Sec is preformed as a unique amino acid and incorporated during translation. The conceptual difficulty this raised is that it contradicted the decades-old paradigm that the 64 possible ribonucleotide triplets of mRNA encode either insertion of 20 specific amino acids or translational termination. Understanding how Sec, now considered to be the 21st amino acid, could be synthesized and incorporated during translation required a revision of this paradigm.

Through a number of elegant experiments conducted over the past two decades, Sec is now recognized to be translationally inserted into nascent peptide chains by a unique transfer RNA, t-RNA[Ser]Sec, which recognizes the UGA codon, a codon canon-ically identified as a termination signal (Fig. 1). In the context of several proteins acting *in trans* and a specific *cis*-acting hairpin sequence in the 3′ untranslated regions of selenoprotein mRNA transcripts, the UGA codon is recognized as the signal for Sec insertion into nascent peptides [12–15]. Genetic deletion of t-RNA[Ser]Sec in mice is embryonically lethal, attesting to the importance of this pathway [9]. Adding to this complexity was the finding that t-RNA[Ser]Sec directly participates in the enzy-matic formation of Sec. The t-RNA is first charged with serine, but the bound serine is subsequently converted to Sec while still

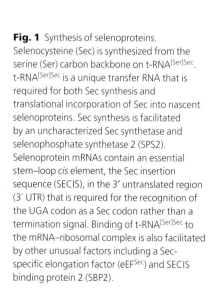

Fig. 1 Synthesis of selenoproteins. Selenocysteine (Sec) is synthesized from the serine (Ser) carbon backbone on t-RNA[Ser]Sec. t-RNA[Ser]Sec is a unique transfer RNA that is required for both Sec synthesis and translational incorporation of Sec into nascent selenoproteins. Sec synthesis is facilitated by an uncharacterized Sec synthetase and selenophosphate synthetase 2 (SPS2). Selenoprotein mRNAs contain an essential stem–loop *cis* element, the Sec insertion sequence (SECIS), in the 3′ untranslated region (3′ UTR) that is required for the recognition of the UGA codon as a Sec codon rather than a termination signal. Binding of t-RNA[Ser]Sec to the mRNA–ribosomal complex is also facilitated by other unusual factors including a Sec-specific elongation factor (eEF[Sec]) and SECIS binding protein 2 (SBP2).

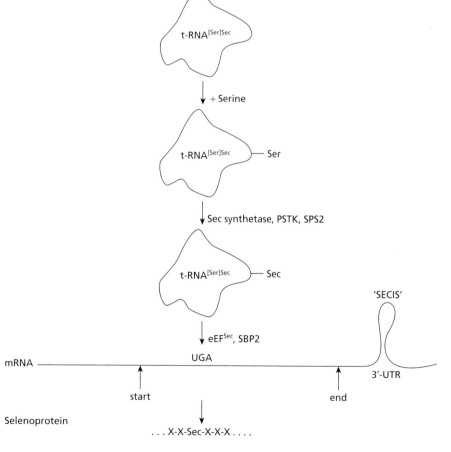

attached to t-RNA[Ser]Sec [16]. In no other case is a t-RNA known to participate catalytically in the modification of a bound amino acid. The unique enzymes needed for these steps were first elucidated in bacteria and then defined in eukaryotes, although many details remain to be clarified [12,17]. An interesting recent observation with respect to liver disease is that the antigenic epitope for antisoluble liver antigen (anti-SLA), an antibody associated with autoimmune hepatitis, appears to be t-RNA[Ser]Sec [18].

Biological functions of selenium

The biological functions of selenium are mediated primarily by Sec in selenoproteins. Early tracer studies with ^{75}Se identified several major selenoproteins that included glutathione peroxidase (GPx) and selenoprotein P (SelP). Until recently, computer algorithms used to identify open reading frames in genes could not accurately identify UGA codons that encode Sec instead of translational termination. However, the recognition of an obligate and unique 3' *cis* element in selenoprotein transcripts led to new computational approaches that subsequently identified a total of 25 putative selenoproteins, now identified as the 'selenoproteome' of the mammalian genome (Table 2) [19]. Reconciling the selenoproteome with previously identified selenoproteins has been complicated by the existence of multiple alternative splice forms of many of the transcripts.

The enzymatic function of selenoproteins typically depends on the presence of a negatively charged deprotonated selenium and, for this reason, the Sec is usually located within the active site. The pK$_a$ of the selenol group of Sec is substantially higher than the analogous sulphydryl of cysteine and, as such, is mostly deprotonated (R-Se$^-$) at physiological pH. By comparison, the pK$_a$ of cysteine is lower, and it is mostly protonated (R-SH) at physiological pH. Thus, Sec is a much more facile nucleophile than cysteine at reactive sites of selenoprotein enzymes. Three examples of selenoproteins are described below.

The first selenoprotein to be characterized was glutathione peroxidase 1 (GPx1), an enzyme that catalytically eliminates hydrogen peroxide and lipid hydroperoxides in the cytosol and mitochondria using glutathione as an electron donor. The highest cellular concentrations of GPx1 are found in the liver. Catalase, a non-selenium-dependent enzyme, also eliminates hydrogen peroxide but is confined to peroxisomes and does not participate in the general intracellular defence against oxidant stress. Moreover, catalase does not eliminate lipid hydroperoxides. Although oxidant stress impairs normal cellular functions, overexpression of GPxs may adversely influence normal redox-mediated cellular signalling [20]. For example, mice that overexpress GPx1 in the liver develop features of insulin resistance, suggesting that too much antioxidant defence could have a negative impact on normal insulin signalling [21].

Another selenoprotein, thioredoxin reductase (TrxR), plays an important role in most organs in maintaining normal redox status. TrxR-1 is localized to the cytoplasm where, in addition to its role in thiol redox regulation, it is essential for deoxynucleotide synthesis. Another form, TrxR-2, is located within mitochondria and prevents oxidant injury caused by the constitutive release of superoxide from the mitochondrial electron transport chain. Deletion of TrxR (but not GPx1 or SelP) induces a cellular stress response [22], and human tumour cells treated with tumour necrosis factor (TNF)α undergo increased apoptosis when they lack Sec in TrxR. In addition, non-physiological trace elements such as gold and platinum actively inhibit TrxR [23].

All Sec-containing selenoproteins except SelP contain only one Sec, whereas SelP, thought to serve as a transport protein for selenium, has 10 Sec. Although many tissues express SelP, impaired liver synthesis of SelP reduces serum levels by 75% in mice, indicating that the liver serves a primary role in the synthesis and secretion of this selenium transport protein [9,24]. Evidence that liver-synthesized and secreted SelP is required by other organs is provided by a liver-specific knockout of SelP in mice that demonstrates impaired renal synthesis of selenoproteins [25].

Deficiency states

Profound liver-specific deficiency of selenoproteins causes liver necrosis and death in genetically modified mice that cannot synthesize selenoproteins in the liver [9]. Dietary selenium deficiency in humans is unlikely to mimic this extreme phenotype, and such overt liver manifestations of selenium deficiency have not been described clinically. However, low selenium levels have been found in patients with chronic liver disease [26–28], and selenium-deficient rodents have higher serum liver enzymes and markers of oxidant stress [29,30]. Studies in cultured cells have shown that selenium deficiency in hepatocytes leads to cell death by oxidative stress, but many malignant hepatocellular carcinoma cell lines survive in culture despite selenium deficiency, possibly indicating the resistance of liver cancer to normal oxidant-mediated mechanisms of cell death.

A diverse diet usually contains sufficient selenium to meet the recommended daily allowance of 55–70 μg per day and prevent a deficiency state. However, with the new recognition of multiple Sec-containing proteins, this assertion is being revisited to determine whether some of the previously unknown proteins may be impaired by inadequate selenium status despite a diet containing the currently recommended amount [31,32]. Dietary protein is an important source of selenium. Rats fed a protein-deficient diet had low GPx levels and exhibited increased sensitivity to liver injury induced by carbon tetrachloride [33], abnormalities that could be ameliorated by selenium supplements [34]. Acute alcohol feeding has also been shown to decrease hepatic selenium levels in animal studies, whereas deficiency states in people are usually associated with consuming food produced in a limited geographical region (e.g. certain regions in New Zealand and China) and are associated with growth retardation, defective spermatogenesis, cataracts and cardiomyopathy.

Table 2 Selenoprotein functions.

Selenoprotein	Function	Comments
GPx1[a]	Eliminates cytosolic hydrogen peroxide and lipid hydroperoxides; most abundant in the liver	First selenoprotein characterized; also called cystosolic GPx
GPx2	Gastrointestinal mucosal antioxidant, inhibits absorption of lipid hydroperoxides [36]	Originally described in gut mucosa but also found in liver
GPx3	Plasma antioxidant	Secreted glycoprotein, kidneys may be the major source; 'plasma GPx'
GPx4	Eliminates diverse hydroperoxides [59]	May regulate intracellular signalling [60]; 'phospholipid hydroperoxide GPx'
GPx6	Unknown function	Identified by genomic analysis [19]
H	Hypothetical protein	
I	Selenocysteine synthesis	
J	Hypothetical protein	
K	Putative membrane protein	
M	Unknown function [61]	Abundant in brain
N, SEPN1	Possible antioxidant in muscle	Possible role in muscular dystrophy; requires prenylation for function, HMG-CoA reductase inhibitors may interfere and cause myopathy [62]
O	Hypothetical protein	
P, SelP	Selenium storage and transport [24]	10 selenocysteines per molecule, widely expressed in different organs; liver may be the major source of circulating SelP
R, MsrB1	Methionine sulfoxide reductase [63]	
S	Putative membrane protein	
SPS2	Essential for tRNA[Ser]Sec synthesis	Possible selenium donor
T	Hypothetical protein	
Trx1	Catalyses flavin-mediated reduction of oxidized thioredoxin	Localized to cytosol
Trx2	Thioredoxin reduction	Localized to mitochondria
Trx3	Thioredoxin reduction	Localized to testis
V	Hypothetical protein	
W	Probable antioxidant function	Most abundant in cardiac and skeletal muscle
X	Hypothetical protein	mRNA abundant in liver, leukocytes
Z	Hypothetical protein	mRNA abundant in liver, kidney
DI-1[b]	Catalyses the monodeiodination of thyroxine (T4) to the active thyroid hormone (T3) or inactive form (rT3)	Found in liver, may play a role in liver-specific effects of thyroid hormone
DI-2	Conversion of T4 to T3 and rT3	Not localized to liver
DI-3	Conversion of T4 to rT3	Primarily localized to the CNS
Sep15, 15 kDa protein	Possible role in endoplasmic reticulum protein folding	High expression in liver; localized to the endoplasmic reticulum [35,64]

[a]GPx, glutathione peroxidase (note, GPx5 is not a selenoprotein).
[b]DI, iodothyronine diodinase [65].
CNS, central nervous system; HMG-CoA, hydroxymethylglutaryl-CoA.
Adapted from refs 19, 12 and 10.

As is true of many other trace elements and vitamins, suboptimal health attributed to mild and clinically undetected deficiency states has been proposed and is the basis for selenium supplementation as an antioxidant in many multivitamins and other supplements. Disease states that have been attributed to moderately low selenium levels include cancer, susceptibility to viral infections, progression of AIDS, defective spermatogenesis, arthritis, vascular disease, asthma and immune system dysregulation [12,35]. Mice lacking both GPx1 and GPx2 have been found to develop ulcerative colitis and colon cancers, attesting to the potential importance of selenium enzymes in preventing inflammation and neoplasia [36,37]. On the other hand, the selenium-dependent thioredoxin pathway is antiapoptotic and may favour the survival of malignant cells.

Selenium provided in dietary supplements is typically in forms such as sodium selenite or selenate, although the primary dietary source may be selenomethionine in plant proteins [11,38]. Other organic forms of selenium have been found to be a potentially useful source as well [39] and, despite major differences between selenite supplements and selenate supplements

[40], the best approach to dietary selenium supplementation has not been established.

Toxicity of selenium

In general, excess selenium intake is rare in humans but is a significant environmental issue for animals. Liver selenium levels are increased in elderly people from the Faeroe Islands where whales are a dietary mainstay, and also in Inuits of the Arctic North American continent [41]. Environmentally, selenium accumulates in the groundwater in specific geographical regions having poor drainage, and wetland birds that dwell in such regions develop selenium toxicity. Cattle and sheep grazing in such regions also develop colourfully named syndromes such as 'blind staggers' and 'alkali disease' attributed to selenium toxicity, although hepatic manifestations of selenium toxicity have not been described.

Routes of selenium excretion have not been fully identified. The liver converts Se-met to Sec, and Sec is converted to serine and selenide, possibly involving an enzyme that specifically removes selenium from Sec [42]. Selenide is di- or trimethylated and then exhaled or excreted [11]. Additionally, a water-soluble carbohydrate conjugate, Se-methyl-N-acetylselenohexosamine, has been identified as a major urinary selenium metabolite in one study [43]. Whether secretory mechanisms can compensate for excessive intake is unknown, although selenium levels do reach a steady-state level during nutritional supplementation with Se-met [11]. The specific role of the liver in these metabolic pathways has not been established.

Zinc

The liver plays a central role in zinc homeostasis, removing it from albumin in the blood and distributing it to the body as needed. Hormonal stimuli such as glucocorticoids and epinephrine upregulate hepatic zinc uptake by upregulating hepatic metallothionein levels [44]. Zinc serves as an essential cofactor for over 100 enzymes and zinc finger transcription factors that are necessary for intermediary metabolism in the liver and other organs. It serves a major antioxidant function as a cofactor for copper–zinc superoxide dismutase, the first line of defence against cytosolic reactive oxygen intermediates generated in the liver. The specific effects of zinc deficiency on these metabolic steps have not been fully elucidated.

Excretion of zinc is mostly in the stool; biliary secretion is minimal, and most zinc lost in the stool originates from gut mucosa and pancreatic secretions. Cirrhotics have increased urinary zinc loss and can become zinc deficient. Zinc supplements, typically zinc sulphate, 220 mg three times daily in cirrhotics, may be effective in treating portosystemic encephalopathy and muscle cramps [26,45–47], although these data have been disputed [48]. Zinc supplements increase metallothionein expression, which can impair normal copper uptake. This is the desired effect when zinc is used to treat Wilson's disease, but the importance of impaired copper uptake in cirrhotics taking zinc supplements requires further investigation.

Chromium

Chromium in its various forms is both an industrial toxin and a commonly used dietary supplement. The toxicity of chromium depends on its redox state. Whereas Cr VI (i.e. chromate) is a known industrial toxin and carcinogen, Cr III is hypothesized to improve insulin sensitivity by enhancing postreceptor insulin signalling [49]. Cr VI is a strong oxidizing agent but is rapidly reduced to Cr III when ingested. The effect of Cr III on insulin signalling is the rationale for its promotion in forms such as chromium picolinate as a dietary supplement to prevent or improve diabetes. It has also been promoted as an aid in weight reduction and as a stimulant for increasing muscle mass, although controlled clinical trials have not confirmed these claims. The uptake of chromium by hepatocytes is facilitated by an anion channel, probably the same channel that mediates the uptake of other anions such as phosphate.

Chromium has the potential to accumulate in the liver of patients with chronic liver disease, and excess dietary supplements should be avoided in this group [7]. One case of severe hepatotoxicity attributed to chromium picolinate use has been reported [50]. It is not secreted into the bile and, thus, cholestasis is not a cause of chromium accumulation. Accumulation in the liver may develop in long-term peritoneal dialysis patients, although the significance of this is uncertain [51].

Manganese

Manganese is a cofactor for a number of enzymes important for intermediary metabolism, including the hepatic urea cycle enzyme arginase. However, deficiency syndromes and how they affect normal metabolism in the liver are not well described [52]. A provocative finding with respect to fatty liver disease was that manganese-deficient animals developed insulin resistance and glucose intolerance, but clinical studies of supplements have not been found to improve insulin sensitivity or diabetes. As a cofactor for prolinase, an enzyme needed for proline synthesis, and glucosyltransferases, enzymes needed for glycosaminoglycan synthesis, manganese also plays a role in extracellular matrix production and maturation.

Manganese absorbed from food is avidly taken up by the liver and distributed to tissues bound to transferrin and albumin. The mechanisms of absorption appear to be regulated in parallel with iron absorption such that iron deficiency increases manganese absorption from the gastrointestinal tract and iron excess reduces manganese absorption. Excess manganese is secreted into the bile, and some authorities recommend that supplements should be avoided in patients with chronic liver disease to avoid hepatic accumulation [7]. Manganese has been shown to accumulate in the globus pallidus of the brain in patients with cirrhosis [53].

Cobalt

Cobalt is best known as the catalytic centre of the corrin ring in cobalamin, the active core of vitamin B12. Vitamin B12 is synthesized by gut bacteria and is thus not directly affected by altered hepatic metabolism. However, the liver plays a central role in enterohepatic circulation of vitamin B12 and the disposal of corrinoid metabolites of vitamin B12 through biliary secretion of degradation products. Alterations in vitamin B12 function leading to manifestations of a deficiency state have thus been attributed to altered hepatic metabolism of B12 [54].

Molybdenum

Molybdenum is an essential cofactor for three enzymes: sulphite oxidase, xanthine oxidase and aldehyde oxidase. Sulphite oxidase is essential for the hepatic metabolism of sulphur-containing molecules such as cysteine and the formation of taurine. Whether molybdenum deficiency impairs the production of the bile acid taurocholic acid or alters the function of bile is not known. The second molybdenum enzyme, xanthine oxidase, metabolizes purines and is required for the elimination of degraded nucleotides. It has also been proposed to be a significant source of superoxide generation during ischaemia–reperfusion injury. Lastly, aldehyde oxidase requires molybdenum as a cofactor. It is known for its role in the hepatic metabolism of ingested ethanol from toxic acetaldehyde to acetate, but it also plays a key role in eliminating other more toxic aldehydes such as the lipid peroxidation product 4-hydroxynonenal.

Despite these known metabolic roles of molybdenum, there are no recognized hepatic effects of molybdenum deficiency or excess. This metal does undergo enterohepatic circulation and crosses cell membranes through an anion channel. It interacts with copper to form thiomolybdate complexes that increase copper elimination and cause copper deficiency. This interaction is the rationale for its use to promote copper excretion in patients with Wilson's disease.

Toxicity and elimination of trace elements

The liver has a central role in the uptake and disposition of many trace elements, especially the heavy metals [55]. Metallothionein, a cytosolic metal-binding protein composed of 25–30% cysteines, binds heavy metals, prevents their toxic interaction with other cellular components and facilitates their elimination. Metallothionein is especially important in the uptake and detoxification of cadmium [56]. Stress markedly upregulates hepatic metallothionein expression, but the reason for this is uncertain [57]. The liver also has the highest glutathione levels of any organ, and glutathione plays an important role in the biliary secretion of heavy metals, especially copper, cadmium, mercury, lead and zinc [55]. Although cholestasis is commonly associated with hepatic copper accumulation, the impact of impaired biliary secretion on the disposal of other heavy metals is less certain.

Summary

Trace elements serve essential metabolic functions in the liver, and the liver plays a central role in the disposition of most trace elements. Much work is needed to identify optimal measures of trace element adequacy and the functional consequences of deficiency states.

References

1 Versieck J (1985) Trace elements in human body fluids and tissues. *Crit Rev Clin Lab Sci* 22, 97–184.
2 Aalbers TG, Houtman JP, Makkink B (1987) Trace-element concentrations in human autopsy tissue. *Clin Chem* 33, 2057–2064.
3 Iyengar V, Woittiez J (1988) Trace elements in human clinical specimens: evaluation of literature data to identify reference values. *Clin Chem* 34, 474–481.
4 Rahil-Khazen R, Bolann BJ, Myking A *et al.* (2002) Multi-element analysis of trace element levels in human autopsy tissues by using inductively coupled atomic emission spectrometry technique (ICP-AES). *J Trace Elem Med Biol* 16, 15–25.
5 Linder MC (1984) Other trace elements and the liver. *Semin Liver Dis* 4, 264–276.
6 Nielsen FH (1985) The importance of diet composition in ultratrace element research. *J Nutr* 115, 1239–1247.
7 Institute of Medicine Food and Nutrition Board (2001) *Dietary Reference Intakes for Vitamin A, Vitamin K, Boron, Chromium, Copper, Iodine, Iron, Manganese, Molybdenum, Nickel, Silicon, Vanadium, and Zinc. A Report of the Panel on Micronutrients, Subcommittees on Upper Reference Levels of Nutrients and of Interpretation and Uses of Dietary Reference Intakes, and the Standing Committee on the Scientific Evaluation of Dietary Reference Intakes.* Washington, DC: National Academy Press.
8 Jacob C, Giles GI, Giles NM *et al.* (2003) Sulfur and selenium: the role of oxidation state in protein structure and function. *Angewandte Chem Int Edn in English* 42, 4742–4758.
9 Carlson BA, Novoselov SV, Kumaraswamy E *et al.* (2004) Specific excision of the selenocysteine tRNA[Ser]Sec (*Trsp*) gene in mouse liver demonstrates an essential role of selenoproteins in liver function. *J Biol Chem* 279, 8011–8017.
10 Behne D, Kyriakopoulos A (2001) Mammalian selenium-containing proteins. *Annu Rev Nutr* 21, 453–473.
11 Schrauzer GN (2000) Selenomethionine: a review of its nutritional significance, metabolism and toxicity. *J Nutr* 130, 1653–1656.
12 Driscoll DM, Copeland PR (2003) Mechanism and regulation of selenoprotein synthesis. *Annu Rev Nutr* 23, 17–40.
13 Ramos A, Lane AN, Hollingworth D *et al.* (2004) Secondary structure and stability of the selenocysteine insertion sequences (SECIS) for human thioredoxin reductase and glutathione peroxidase. *Nucleic Acids Res* 32, 1746–1755.
14 Diamond AM (2004) On the road to selenocysteine. *Proc Natl Acad Sci USA* 101, 13395–13396.
15 Howard MT, Aggarwal G, Anderson CB *et al.* (2005) Recoding

elements located adjacent to a subset of eukaryal selenocysteine-specifying UGA codons. *EMBO J* 24, 1596–1607.

16 Carlson BA, Xu X-M, Kryukov GV *et al.* (2004) Identification and characterization of phosphoseryl-tRNA[Ser]Sec kinase. *Proc Natl Acad Sci USA* 101, 12848–12853.

17 Mehta A, Rebsch CM, Kinzy SA *et al.* (2004) Efficiency of mammalian selenocysteine incorporation. *J Biol Chem* 279, 37852–37859.

18 Torres-Collado AX, Czaja AJ, Gelpi C (2005) Anti-tRNP[ser]sec/SLA/LP autoantibodies. Comparative study using in-house ELISA with a recombinant 48.8 kDa protein, immunoblot, and analysis of immuno-precipitated RNAs. *Liver Int* 25, 410–419.

19 Kryukov GV, Castellano S, Novoselov SV *et al.* (2003) Charac-terization of mammalian selenoproteomes. *Science* 300, 1439–1443.

20 Arthur JR (2000) The glutathione peroxidases. *Cell Mol Life Sci* 57, 1825–1835.

21 McClung JP, Roneker CA, Mu W *et al.* (2004) Development of insulin resistance and obesity in mice overexpressing cellular glutathione peroxidase. *Proc Natl Acad Sci USA* 101, 8852–8857.

22 Mostert V, Hill KE, Burk RF (2003) Loss of activity of the selenoen-zyme thioredoxin reductase causes induction of hepatic heme oxyge-nase-1. *FEBS Lett* 541, 85–88.

23 Nordberg J, Arnér ESJ (2001) Reactive oxygen species, antioxidants, and the mammalian thioredoxin system. *Free Radic Biol Med* 31, 1287–1312.

24 Hill KE, Zhou J, McMahan WJ *et al.* (2003) Deletion of selenoprotein P alters distribution of selenium in the mouse. *J Biol Chem* 278, 13640–13646.

25 Schweizer U, Streckfuss F, Pelt P *et al.* (2005) Hepatically derived selenoprotein P is a key factor for kidney but not for brain selenium supply. *Biochem J* 386, 221–226.

26 Loguercio C, De Girolamo V, Federico A *et al.* (2001) Relationship of blood trace elements to liver damage, nutritional status, and oxidative stress in chronic nonalcoholic liver disease. *Biol Trace Elem Res* 81, 245–254.

27 Jain SK, Pemberton PW, Smith A *et al.* (2002) Oxidative stress in chronic hepatitis C: not just a feature of late stage disease. *J Hepatol* 36, 805–811.

28 Aboutwerat A, Pemberton PW, Smith A *et al.* (2003) Oxidant stress is a significant feature of primary biliary cirrhosis. *Biochim Biophys Acta* 1637, 142–150.

29 Matsumoto K-I, Ui I, Satoh K *et al.* (2002) Evaluation of oxidative damage in the liver of selenium-deficient rats. *Redox Rep* 7, 351–354.

30 Moskovitz J, Stadtman ER (2003) Selenium-deficient diet enhances protein oxidation and affects methionine sulfoxide reductase (MsrB) protein level in certain mouse tissues. *Proc Natl Acad Sci USA* 100, 7486–7490.

31 Brown KM, Arthur JR (2001) Selenium, selenoproteins and human health: a review. *Public Health Nutr* 4, 593–599.

32 Pagmantidis V, Bermano G, Villette S *et al.* (2005) Effects of Se-depletion on glutathione peroxidase and selenoprotein W gene expression in the colon. *FEBS Lett* 579, 792–796.

33 Gonzalez-Reimers E, Lopez-Lirola A, Olivera RM *et al.* (2003) Effects of protein deficiency on liver trace elements and antioxidant activity in carbon tetrachloride-induced liver cirrhosis. *Biol Trace Elem Res* 93, 127–140.

34 He Y-T, Liu D-W, Ding L-Y *et al.* (2004) Therapeutic effects and molecular mechanisms of anti-fibrosis herbs and selenium on rats with hepatic fibrosis. *World J Gastroenterol* 10, 703–706.

35 Diwadkar-Navsariwala V, Diamond AM (2004) The link between selenium and chemoprevention: a case for selenoproteins. *J Nutr* 134, 2899–2902.

36 Esworthy RS, Aranda R, Martín MG *et al.* (2001) Mice with combined disruption of Gpx1 and Gpx2 genes have colitis. *Am J Physiol Gastroint Liver Physiol* 281, G848–G855.

37 Chu FF, Esworthy RS, Chu PG *et al.* (2004) Bacteria-induced intestinal cancer in mice with disrupted Gpx1 and Gpx2 genes. *Cancer Res* 64, 962–968.

38 Schrauzer GN (2001) Nutritional selenium supplements: product types, quality, and safety. *J Am Coll Nutr* 20, 1–4.

39 Li L, Xie Y, El-Sayed WM *et al.* (2004) Characteristics of selenazolidine prodrugs of selenocysteine: toxicity, selenium levels, and glutathione peroxidase induction in A/J mice. *Life Sci* 75, 447–459.

40 Mueller AS, Pallauf J, Rafael J (2003) The chemical form of selenium affects insulinomimetic properties of the trace element: investigations in type II diabetic dbdb mice. *J Nutr Biochem* 14, 637–647.

41 Milman N, Laursen J, Byg K-E *et al.* (2004) Elements in autopsy liver tissue samples from Greenlandic Inuit and Danes. V. Selenium meas-ured by X-ray fluorescence spectrometry. *J Trace Elem Med Biol* 17, 301–306.

42 Mihara H, Kurihara T, Watanabe T *et al.* (2000) cDNA cloning, purification, and characterization of mouse liver selenocysteine lyase. Candidate for selenium delivery protein in selenoprotein synthesis. *J Biol Chem* 275, 6195–6200.

43 Kobayashi Y, Ogra Y, Ishiwata K *et al.* (2002) Selenosugars are key and urinary metabolites for selenium excretion within the required to low-toxic range. *Proc Natl Acad Sci USA* 99, 15932–15936.

44 Cousins RJ (1986) Toward a molecular understanding of zinc metabolism. *Clin Physiol Biochem* 4, 20–30.

45 Reding P, Duchateau J, Bataille C (1984) Oral zinc supplementation improves hepatic encephalopathy. Results of a randomised controlled trial. *Lancet* 2, 493–495.

46 Marchesini G, Fabbri A, Bianchi G *et al.* (1996) Zinc supplementation and amino acid-nitrogen metabolism in patients with advanced cirrhosis. *Hepatology* 23, 1084–1092.

47 Kugelmas M (2000) Preliminary observation: oral zinc sulfate replace-ment is effective in treating muscle cramps in cirrhotic patients. *J Am Coll Nutr* 19, 13–15.

48 Baskol M, Ozbakir O, Coskun R *et al.* (2004) The role of serum zinc and other factors on the prevalence of muscle cramps in non-alcoholic cirrhotic patients. *J Clin Gastroenterol* 38, 524–529.

49 Vincent JB (2000) Quest for the molecular mechanism of chromium action and its relationship to diabetes. *Nutr Rev* 58, 67–72.

50 Cerulli J, Grabe D, Gauthier I *et al.* (1998) Chromium picolinate toxic-ity. *Ann Pharmacother* 32, 428–431.

51 Borguet F, Wallaeys B, Cornelis R *et al.* (1996) Transperitoneal absorption and kinetics of chromium in the continuous ambulatory peritoneal dialysis patient – an experimental and mathematical analysis. *Nephron* 72, 163–170.

52 Keen CL, Ensunsa JL, Watson MH *et al.* (1999) Nutritional aspects of manganese from experimental studies. *Neurotoxicology* 20, 213–223.

53 Spahr L, Butterworth RF, Fontaine S *et al.* (1996) Increased blood manganese in cirrhotic patients: relationship to pallidal magnetic resonance signal hyperintensity and neurological symptoms. *Hepatology* 24, 1116–1120.

54 Lambert D, Benhayoun S, Adjalla C *et al.* (1997) Alcoholic cirrhosis and cobalamin metabolism. *Digestion* 58, 64–71.

55 Ballatori N (1991) Mechanisms of metal transport across liver cell plasma membranes. *Drug Metab Rev* 23, 83–132.

56 Klaassen CD, Liu J (1998) Metallothionein transgenic and knock-out mouse models in the study of cadmium toxicity. *J Toxicol Sci* 23 (Suppl 2), 97–102.

57 Jacob ST, Ghoshal K, Sheridan JF (1999) Induction of metallothionein by stress and its molecular mechanisms. *Gene Expr* 7, 301–310.

58 Rodriguez-Moreno F, Gonzalez-Reimers E, Santolaria-Fernandez F *et al.* (1997) Zinc, copper, manganese, and iron in chronic alcoholic liver disease. *Alcohol* 14, 39–44.

59 Ran Q, Liang H, Gu M *et al.* (2004) Transgenic mice overexpressing glutathione peroxidase 4 are protected against oxidative stress-induced apoptosis. *J Biol Chem* 279, 55137–55146.

60 Imai H, Nakagawa Y (2003) Biological significance of phospholipid hydroperoxide glutathione peroxidase (PHGPx, GPx4) in mammalian cells. *Free Radic Biol Med* 34, 145–169.

61 Korotkov KV, Novoselov SV, Hatfield DL *et al.* (2002) Mammalian selenoprotein in which selenocysteine (Sec) incorporation is supported by a new form of Sec insertion sequence element. *Mol Cell Biol* 22, 1402–1411.

62 Baker SK (2005) Molecular clues into the pathogenesis of statin-mediated muscle toxicity. *Muscle Nerve* 31, 572–580.

63 Kim H-Y, Gladyshev VN (2004) Methionine sulfoxide reduction in mammals: characterization of methionine-R-sulfoxide reductases. *Mol Biol Cell* 15, 1055–1064.

64 Korotkov KV, Kumaraswamy E, Zhou Y *et al.* (2001) Association between the 15-kDa selenoprotein and UDP-glucose:glycoprotein glucosyltransferase in the endoplasmic reticulum of mammalian cells. *J Biol Chem* 276, 15330–15336.

65 Beckett GJ, Arthur JR (2005) Selenium and endocrine systems. *J Endocrinol* 184, 455–465.

2.3.15 Hepatic metabolism of drugs

Chris Liddle and Catherine A.M. Stedman

General concepts

Drug metabolism is the process by which drug molecules are chemically altered, usually to more polar metabolites that exhibit increased water solubility to allow elimination in urine or bile and/or increased access to excretory transporters. The liver is quantitatively and qualitatively the most important site of drug metabolism, although extrahepatic metabolism of drugs is also well recognised, both in the gastrointestinal mucosa and by circulating enzymes such as esterases. Drug metabolism is likely to be a byproduct of metabolic pathways that metabolize endogenously synthesized compounds (endobiotics) such as steroids, sterols, bile acids and eicosanoids. This is supported by the observation that hepatic enzymes involved in drug metabolism often have these endobiotic compounds as substrates, and that some hepatocellular transporters that handle bile acids also transport drugs [1,2].

One of the most surprising features of hepatic drug-metabolizing pathways is their ability to cope with a seemingly endless array of drug substrates. Thus, many of the newer fully synthetic drugs that have no close structural counterparts in nature are successfully metabolized by the liver and irreversibly removed or 'cleared' from the body. This broad substrate recognition is achieved by the presence of multiple drug-metabolizing enzymes in the hepatocyte, and many can metabolize multiple substrates. For example, the calcium channel blocker nifedipine is almost entirely metabolized by the cytochrome P450 (P450) CYP3A4, an enzyme with very broad substrate recognition that is responsible for the metabolism of some 50% of all therapeutic drugs. In contrast, the benzodiazepine diazepam is metabolized by P450s belonging to the CYP2C, 2D and 3A subfamilies to several primary metabolites, some retaining pharmacological activity. Thus, individual drugs may be metabolized in very different ways, and variation in the expression of individual enzymes and transporters for genetic or other reasons may have complex effects, which may sometimes be difficult to model and predict in advance.

Central role of the liver in drug metabolism

In terms of both gross anatomy and microstructure, the liver is ideally designed as a drug clearance organ (Fig. 1). Most foreign chemical compounds (xenobiotics), including therapeutic drugs, enter the body by absorption from the gastrointestinal tract. As covered in Chapter 2.1.1 of this book, venous drainage from most of the gastrointestinal tract is via the portal vein to the liver. Along with drug-metabolizing enzymes and drug transporters expressed in the intestinal mucosa, the liver provides an effective barrier that prevents xenobiotics from entering the systemic circulation. The fraction of an absorbed drug metabolized on this initial postabsorptive pass through the liver is termed 'first-pass clearance' and, factored together with the fraction of the drug absorbed from the gastrointestinal tract, determines the 'bioavailability' or the fraction of an orally administered drug that reaches the systemic circulation as intact drug [3]. For some drugs, the extent of first-pass clearance can be so great that oral administration is largely ineffective; for example, glyceryl trinitrate and lidocaine (lignocaine).

Within the hepatic lobular architecture, drug metabolism is not evenly distributed. Some important drug-metabolizing P450s such as CYP3A4 are predominantly expressed in pericentral (zone 3) hepatocytes [4]. One reason for this functional specialization may be that metabolism can give rise to highly toxic electrophilic intermediates, which may lead to cell death. With metabolic segregation, only pericentral necrosis occurs, rather than massive necrosis if highly reactive molecules cannot be successfully detoxified.

Drug-metabolizing enzymes

Phase I metabolism refers to a basic structural alteration of a drug molecule, whereas in phase II metabolism, a water-soluble

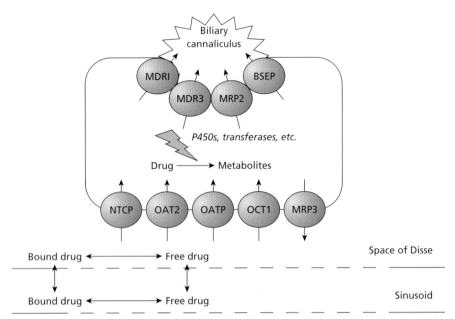

Fig. 1 Organization of drug metabolism at the level of the hepatocyte. Portal blood enters hepatic sinusoids where free drug molecules are transported into hepatocytes. Within hepatocytes, enzyme-mediated metabolism occurs prior to excretion of drug and drug metabolites by transport into bile or back into the circulation. BSEP, bile salt export pump; MDR, multidrug resistance protein; MRP, multidrug resistance-associated protein; OAT, organic anion transporter; OCT, organic cation transporter; NTCP, Na$^+$-taurocholate cotransporting polypeptide.

Table 1 Major human drug-metabolizing cytochrome P450s and receptors responsible for inductive regulation.

Cytochrome P450 family	Member	Regulating receptor
CYP1	CYP1A1	AhR
	CYP1A2	AhR
CYP2	CYP2A6	CAR
	CYP2A13	
	CYP2B6	CAR, PXR
	CYP2C8	PXR
	CYP2C9	CAR, PXR
	CYP2C18	
	CYP2C19	PXR, CAR
	CYP2D6	
	CYP2E1	
	CYP2F1	
	CYP2J2	
CYP3	CYP3A4	PXR, CAR
	CYP3A5	PXR, CAR
	CYP3A7[a]	PXR

AhR, aryl hydrocarbon receptor; CAR, constitutive androstane receptor; PXR, pregnane X receptor.
[a]Expressed in fetal liver and uterine endometrium.

moiety is attached or 'conjugated' to the drug. P450 enzymes are the predominant catalysts of phase I metabolism in the liver. P450s comprise a gene superfamily with 57 members in the human genome. A subset of approximately 15 P450 enzymes belonging to the CYP1, 2 and 3 gene families mediates 70–80% of all phase I-dependent metabolism of therapeutic drugs (Table 1) and participates in the metabolism of countless other xenobiotic chemicals. P450s from other families subserve a vari-

ety of specialized functions, particularly cholesterol and steroid synthesis and fatty acid metabolism [1,5].

P450 enzymes function as mono-oxygenases that insert one atom of oxygen into the substrate molecule. They have been alternatively referred to as 'mixed function oxidases' on account of their wide substrate specificities. Within hepatocytes, drug-metabolizing P450s are located in the smooth endoplasmic reticulum, in contrast to some synthetic P450s that are localized to the mitochondrial inner membrane. Drug-metabolizing P450 enzymes accomplish a wide variety of metabolic reactions including aliphatic and aromatic hydroxylation, *O*-, *S*- and *N*-dealkylation, oxidative and reductive dehalogenation, *N*-oxidation and *N*-hydroxylation, demethylation and deamination [6]. For example, CYP2D6 catalyses the *O*-demethylation of codeine to form morphine (Fig. 2), where the metabolite possesses greater pharmacological activity than the parent drug. Phase I-generated metabolites may be sufficiently water soluble for immediate elimination or may form substrates for phase II enzymes.

Phase II metabolism involves the conjugation of a hydrophilic chemical moiety to a drug molecule. Enzymes that accomplish this task are collectively known as 'transferases', as they catalyse the transfer of a moiety from a donor molecule to the drug recipient. For example, the UDP-glucuronosyltransferases (UGT) catalyse the transfer of the sugar α-glucuronic acid from the donor molecule uridine-α-glucuronide to a substrate molecule, as exemplified by morphine (Fig. 2). Most transferases also belong to gene families with individual members catalysing the conjugation of a distinct but often overlapping range of substrates. A list of enzymes commonly involved in phase II human drug metabolism is presented in Table 2. An important function of phase II enzymes is the detoxification of reactive molecules that may be generated by phase I drug metabolism [7].

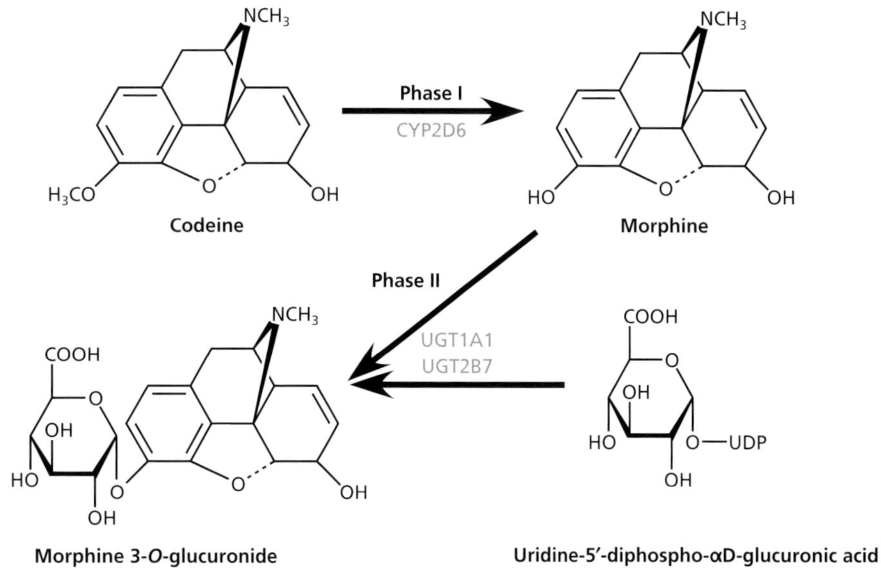

Fig. 2 Phases of hepatic drug metabolism as exemplified by codeine. Codeine is converted to morphine by CYP2D6-mediated *O*-demethylation, a phase I reaction. Morphine is subsequently conjugated by phase II enzymes UDP-glucuronosyltransferases (UGT) to form both 3-*O*- and 6-*O*-glucuronide metabolites, the pharmacologically inactive 3-*O* metabolite being shown in this figure.

Table 2 Some major human phase II drug-metabolizing enzymes and receptors implicated in regulation.

Superfamily	Function	Substrate examples	Gene families[a]	Receptors implicated in regulation[b]	
Glutathione *S*-transferases (GST)	Catalyse nucleophilic attack by GSH on non-polar compounds	Adriamycin, BCNU, busulfan, carmustine, chlorambucil, cyclophosphamide, DDT, inorganic arsenic, pesticides	GSTA[c] GSTM GSTP GSTS GSTT1 GSTZ GSTO	GSTA2	CAR, PXR AhR
Sulphotransferases (SULT)	Sulphation	Steroid hormones, bile acids, isoflavones, paracetamol, minoxidil	SULT1[d] SULT2 SULT4	SULT1A1 SULT2A1	CAR VDR
N-acetyltransferases (NAT)	*N*-acetylation, *O*-acetylation	Arylamines *N*-hydroxylated heterocyclic amines	NAT1 NAT2		
UDP-glucuronosyltransferases (UGT)	Glucuronidation	Bilirubin, paracetamol, morphine, zidovudine, NSAIDs	UGT1A UGT2B	UGT1A1 UGT1A6 UGT2B4 UGT2B7	PXR, CAR, HNF1α AhR, SHP FXR, ?PPAR HNF1α

BCNU, carmustine; GSH, reduced glutathione; NSAID, non-steroidal anti-inflammatory drug.
[a]Only significant human families are listed.
[b]Only nuclear receptors implicated in the regulation of human enzymes are listed.
[c]Cytosolic GSTs are shown; mitochondrial and microsomal GSTs are not shown.
[d]Only cytosolic SULTs are included in the nomenclature.

Drug transporters

Cloning and characterization of plasma membrane-bound hepatocyte transporters has revealed that many drugs enter and exit hepatocytes by energy-dependent transporters rather than by simple diffusion (Fig. 1, Table 3) [8]. The predominant transporters involved in drug uptake are members of the solute carrier (SLC) transporter superfamily, which are located on the sinusoidal (basolateral) plasma membrane. In contrast, transporters responsible for the excretion of drugs and drug metabolites from hepatocytes belong to the ATP-binding cassette (ABC) transporter superfamily and are located on

Table 3 Major hepatic drug transporters: nomenclature, function and nuclear receptor regulation.

Trivial symbol (gene symbol)	Name	Nuclear receptor	Function and substrates
Basolateral membrane of hepatocyte			
OATP1B1 (SLCO1B1)[a]	Organic anion-transporting	FXR, HNF1α,	Hepatic uptake of organic anions and cations
OATP1B3 (SLCO1B3)[b]	proteins	?PXR	e.g. enalapril, digoxin, HMG-CoA reductase inhibitors, BA, bilirubin
OCT1 (SLC22A1)	Organic cation transporter		Hepatic uptake of hydrophilic organic cations
			e.g. cimetidine, choline, dopamine, acyclovir, zidovudine
OAT2 (SLC22A7)	Organic anion transporter		Hepatic uptake of organic anions and drugs
			e.g. salicylate, methotrexate, non-steroidal anti-inflammatory drugs
NTCP (SLC10A1)	Na$^+$-taurocholate cotransporting polypeptide	SHP/FXR	Na$^+$-dependent uptake of conjugated BA from portal blood
MRP1 (ABCC1)	Multidrug resistance-	PXR	Drug export from hepatocytes, e.g. VP16, colchicine, etoposide
MRP3 (ABCC3)	associated proteins	PXR, FTF ?CAR	Organic solute transporter: extrudes BA conjugates, methotrexate, etoposide
MRP4 (ABCC4)			Mediates glutathione efflux from hepatocytes into blood by cotransport with BA; also exports purine and nucleoside analogues
Canalicular membrane of hepatocyte			
MDR1 (ABCB1)	Multidrug resistance-1	PXR	Excretion of organic cations, xenobiotics and cytotoxins to bile e.g. colchicine, doxirubicin, adriamycin, vinblastine, paclitaxel, vincristine
MDR3 (ABCB4)	Multidrug resistance-3	FXR, PPARα	Phospholipid export pump: translocates phosphatidylcholine from inner to outer leaflet of membrane bilayer
MRP2 (ABCC2)	Multidrug resistance-associated protein-2	PXR,CAR ?FXR	Mediates multispecific organic anion transport into bile, e.g. bilirubin diglucuronide, sulphates, glutathione conjugates, vinblastine, sulphinpyrazone
BSEP (ABCB11)	Canalicular bile salt export pump	FXR	ATP-dependent transport of monovalent bile salts and ?paclitaxel into bile
FIC1 (ATP8B1)	Familial intrahepatic cholestasis-1		Potential aminophospholipid-translocating ATPase
AE2 (SLC4A2)	Chloride–bicarbonate anion exchanger isoform-2		Facilitates bicarbonate secretion into bile, stimulates BA-independent bile flow
ABCG5/ABCG8	'Half ABC transporters'	FXR, PXR LXR	Transport sterols into bile. May partially mediate biliary cholesterol secretion
BCRP (ABCG2)	'Half ABC transporters'		Mediates cellular extrusion of sulphated conjugates, ?estramustine

BA, bile acids; CAR, constitutive androstane receptor; FTF, fetal transcription factor (also called liver receptor homologue 1, LRH1); FXR, farnesoid X receptor; LXR, liver X receptor; MDR1 protein is also known as P-glycoprotein; PPAR, peroxisome proliferator-activated receptor; PXR, pregnane X receptor; SHP, short heterodimer partner; HNF, hepatocyte nuclear factor.
[a]OATP1B1 is also known as OATP-C, OATP2, LST-1.
[b]OATP1B3 is also known as OATP8, LST-2.

the biliary canalicular (apical) plasma membrane, where they mediate the excretion of drugs into bile, or on the sinusoidal membrane, where they mediate efflux back into the circulation. Hepatocyte transporters and their functions are covered in more detail in Chapter 2.2.4.

Interindividual differences in drug metabolism

Clinicians are well aware that individual dose requirements of drugs for patients can very widely, even in the absence of obvious confounding factors such as drug–drug interactions [9]. For many drugs, a significant component of this inter-individual difference can be attributed to variability in drug

metabolism [10]. Importantly, metabolism cannot be reliably predicted by simple anthropomorphic characteristics such as body mass, body surface area, gender, age or race. While some variability can now be attributed to allelic variation within drug-metabolizing genes (Table 4), hepatic and intestinal expression of the most important and abundant human P450 enzyme CYP3A4 exhibits a unimodal distribution that cannot be explained by genetic polymorphism [5]. As CYP3A4 is intimately involved in the metabolism of many endogenously synthesized compounds, such as bile acids and ecosinoids in addition to therapeutic drugs, it now seems likely that variation in CYP3A4 may be the result of homeostatic regulatory mechanisms. In this respect, nuclear receptors that have endogenous ligands, such as the farnesoid X receptor (FXR) and the

Table 4 Genetic polymorphisms of some major human drug-metabolizing enzymes and transporters.

Gene	Major allelic variants	Prevalence of PM phenotype (%)		Examples of drugs affected by PM status
		Caucasian	Asian	
CYP1A2	CYP1A2*1K	–	–	Phenytoin, caffeine
CYP2A6	CYP2A6*4, CYP2A6*9	~ 0	2–4	Nicotine
CYP2B6	CYP2B6*6	–	–	Cyclophosphamide
CYP2C9	CYP2C9*2, CYP2C9*3	1–2	0.04	Phenytoin, glipizide, tolbutamide, warfarin, irbesartan
CYP2C19	CYP2C19*2, CYP2C19*3	2–5	10–25[a]	Diazepam, omeprazole, lansoprazole, imipramine, fluoxetine, sertraline, nelfinavir
CYP2D6	CYP2D6*4, CYP2D6*5, CYP2D6*10, CYP2D6*17, CYP2D6*41, CYP2D6*2xn[b]	5–10	1–2	Codeine, metoprolol, tricyclic antidepressants, venlafaxine, ondansetron, tropisetron, perhexiline
DPD	DPYD*2A	3	?	5-Fluorouracil
NAT	NAT2*5B, NAT2*6A[c]	50	< 40	Isoniazid, procainamide, hydralazine, sulphonamides
TPMT	TPMT*2, TPMT*3A, TPMT*3C	0.3	< 0.3	Azathioprine, 6-mercaptopurine
UGT1A1	UGT1A1*28, UGT1A1*6, UGT1A1*27	0.5–10	~ 3	Irinotecan, lamotrigine
MDR1	C3435T, G2677T	–	–	Digoxin, ciclosporin, tacrolimus, protease inhibitors
OATP1B1	OATP-C*5, OATP-C*1b	< 2%	–	Pravastatin

DPD, dihydropyrimidine dehydrogenase; PM, poor metabolizer; TPMT, thiopurine S-methyltransferase.
[a]The CYP2C19 PM phenotype is more common throughout Polynesia and Micronesia, with an incidence between 38% and 79%.
[b]CYP2D6 gene duplication results in increased CYP2D6 activity, the ultrarapid metabolizer (UM) phenotype. At least 75 CYP2D6 alleles have been identified.
[c]Phenotypes include slow, intermediate or fast acetylators. NAT1*, wide heterogeneity; NAT2*, at least 13 point mutations described [36].

pregnane X receptor (PXR), as well as other transcription factors important in the expression of liver-predominant genes such as hepatocyte nuclear factor 4α (HNF4α) and CCAAT/enhancer-binding protein β (C/EBPβ), have all been shown to be important regulators of CYP3A4 gene transcription [11–14].

Regulation of drug-metabolizing pathways

In an evolutionary sense, the ability to respond to a potentially toxic chemical challenge through the upregulation of endobiotic and xenobiotic metabolizing and transporting genes would be expected to confer a survival advantage. It is therefore not surprising that many drug disposition pathways are inherently variable and are capable of responding to a wide range of chemical stimuli. Recent work has shown that several drug-metabolizing and -transporting genes are subject to adaptive regulation, predominantly by nuclear receptors [15]. Members of the nuclear receptor superfamily function as ligand-activated transcription factors and have critical roles in diverse cellular processes. A subset of nuclear receptors that heterodimerize with the receptor for 9-cis retinoic acid-α (RXR) recognises a range of small lipophilic molecules that includes xenobiotic compounds, including a range of therapeutic drugs. The two receptors identified to date that have this role are PXR and the constitutive androstane receptor (CAR) [16]. PXR and CAR are capable of transcriptional induction of an array of drug-metabolizing and -transporting genes that cover all phases of hepatic drug disposition (Tables 1–3). In addition, nuclear receptors that appear to have exclusively endobiotic ligands such as the farnesoid X receptor (FXR) and the vitamin D receptor (VDR) have also been implicated in the regulation of drug-metabolizing pathways. Interestingly, PXR, FXR and VDR are all capable of binding and responding to bile acids, reinforcing the concept that drug metabolism is interrelated with cholesterol and bile acid homeostasis [17]. CAR appears to subserve additional roles in bilirubin and energy homeostasis [18], although its precise roles as an endogenous regulator remain enigmatic.

Role of genetic variation (pharmacogenetics)

The term 'pharmacogenetics' can be defined as the study of genetically determined variation in drug response. Pharmacogenomics is the use of genetic information to individualize drug therapy, a science that is still in its infancy. We now recognize that many genes involved in drug metabolism and transport are subject to genetic polymorphism, which may result in changes in drug disposition and, hence, both drug efficacy and drug toxicity [9,10]. All phases of drug disposition are now recognized to be affected by genetic variability, and some clinically relevant examples are listed in Table 4.

To date, genetic variation in cytochrome P450-mediated metabolism has been most intensively studied, and polymorphic forms of P450s are responsible for the development of a significant number of adverse drug reactions (ADRs) [19].

High-throughput analysis of P450 polymorphisms is already commercially available, but its impact on drug prescribing is not yet clear. All genes encoding P450 enzymes in families 1–3 are polymorphic to some degree. However, the functional importance of the variant alleles differs, and the frequencies of their distribution in different ethnic groups also vary. In general, four phenotypes can be identified: poor metabolizers (PMs), who lack the functional enzyme; intermediary metabolizers (IMs), who are heterozygous for one deficient allele or carry two alleles that cause reduced activity; extensive metabolizers (EMs), who have two normal alleles; and ultrarapid metabolizers (UMs), who have multiple gene copies, a trait that is dominantly inherited. The consequences of PM status have been well characterized for some genotypes (e.g. CYP2D6), and this results in slow drug metabolism, high drug concentrations at ordinary dosage, a higher risk of ADRs and, in some cases, no response to some prodrugs (e.g. codeine). In contrast, UM status results in nonresponse to drugs that are substrates for the enzyme, particularly well demonstrated with tricyclic antidepressants. For nortriptyline, the optimum dose varies from as low as 20 mg/day in PMs to 500 mg/day in UMs [19]. While genotyping CYP2D6 mutations could prove clinically useful, over 70 allelic variants of this gene have been described, which makes this approach technically difficult and expensive.

An alternative approach to assessing variation in hepatic metabolism is to phenotype through the use of pharmacokinetic studies in which the patient is given a marker drug for a particular metabolic pathway and serum or urinary drug levels are used to estimate the rate of clearance. While technically feasible, this approach has not been widely adopted largely because of the inconvenience and cost involved, with clinicians usually opting for a pragmatic approach, adjusting drug dose based on signs of efficacy or toxicity. At present, the only pharmacogenetic test in routine clinical use is the genotyping or phenotyping of thiopurine S-methyltransferase (TPMT), an enzyme that is crucial for the detoxification of the immunosuppressant 6-mercaptopurine, particularly in bone marrow where alternative metabolism through xanthine oxidase is not present [20].

More recently, it has been appreciated that genetic polymorphism has important effects on phase II enzymes as well as drug transporters such as MDR1 and OATP2. There is still controversy as to whether, and to what extent, the pharmacokinetics and pharmacodynamics of drugs are modified by the various genotypes of *MDR1*. In contrast to the P450 polymorphisms, no loss-of-function mutations have been described for *MDR1* in humans, and the differences between genotypes with respect to protein expression are moderate when compared, for example, with CYP2D6 [21].

Factors determining the rate of hepatic drug clearance

Several factors determine the rate at which the liver clears a drug from the body [22]. The most important of these are: (i) hepatic blood flow, which determines the rate at which drugs

are delivered to the liver; (ii) binding to plasma proteins, as only unbound drug can be taken up by hepatocytes; (iii) affinity for hepatocyte uptake transporters; and (iv) the intrinsic affinity of hepatic enzymes for the drug as a substrate. The relative importance of these factors varies greatly for individual drugs, with hepatic blood flow being the main determinant of the rate of metabolism for very high metabolic clearance drugs and the other factors assuming more importance for drugs with low metabolic clearance. This has significant implications for patients with liver disease (see below).

Metabolic drug–drug interactions

At the level of hepatic drug metabolism, the two mechanisms of drug–drug interactions are induction and inhibition of drug-metabolizing enzymes. Examples of both are listed in Table 5. Inductive drug–drug interactions occur when an inducing drug causes an increase in the metabolism of coadministered drugs with a resultant diminution in their therapeutic effect. The most important enzyme affected by this form of interaction is CYP3A4 because of the potential magnitude of its induction and the vast array of drugs metabolized by this P450 enzyme [23]. Only relatively recently have the mechanisms of CYP3A4 induction by inducing drugs such as rifampicin, phenytoin, carbamazepine and the herbal remedy St John's Wort been elucidated. Most, if not all, CYP3A4-inducing drugs are now recognized to be ligands for PXR, a nuclear receptor that is highly expressed in hepatocytes and intestinal epithelial cells. PXR/RXR heterodimers bind to response elements in the regulatory upstream region of the CYP3A4 gene, resulting in transcriptional activation [12]. Several other drug-metabolizing genes and drug transporters are also induced by ligand-activated PXR, while a lesser number are activated by other receptors, including CAR and the aryl hydrocarbon receptor (AhR) [24,25].

Inhibition of metabolism by coadministered drugs is also a common cause of drug–drug interactions and occurs by two basic mechanisms. The most common mechanism of inhibition is simple competition between drugs for access to the catalytic pocket of the relevant drug-metabolizing enzyme. Some drugs are highly effective competitors for P450 enzymes, including cimetidine, ketoconazole and indinavir. The second way in which drugs inhibit P450s, often referred to as 'mechanism-based P450 inhibition', involves the formation of a catalytically inactive, covalently bound complex between a metabolite of the substrate drug and the P450 enzyme [26]. Macrolide antibiotics such as erythromycin and clarithromycin as well as tamoxifen, fluoxitine and the anti-HIV agents ritonavir and delavirdine are examples of drugs that interact in this way.

Role of metabolism in drug activation and drug toxicity

Drug metabolism usually results in metabolites with less pharmacological activity and less toxicity, but this is not always the

Table 5 Drug substrates, inhibitors and inducers of some cytochrome P450 enzymes.

P450 enzyme	Common drug substrates	Inhibitors	Inducers
CYP1A2	Clozapine, clomipramine, estrogen, fluvoxamine, haloperidol, tacrine, theophylline	Amiodarone, cimetidine, fluoroquinolones, ticlopidine	Polycyclic aromatic hydrocarbons omeprazole, ritonavir, phenobarbital
CYP2C9	Phenytoin, warfarin, tolbutamide, glipizide	Amiodarone, fluconazole, miconazole, phenylbutazone, sulphinpyrazone	Carbamazepine, phenobarbital, rifampin, St John's Wort
CYP2D6	Alprenolol, bufuralol, carvedilol, metoprolol, propranolol, timolol, amitriptyline, clomipramine, desipramine, imipramine, nortriptyline, flecainide, mexiletine, propafenone, fluoxetine, haloperidol, paroxetine, perphenazine, venlafaxine, codeine, dextromethorphan	Clomipramine, quinidine, fluoxetine, haloperidol, paroxetine	Not inducible
CYP2E1	Paracetamol, benzene, ethanol, isoflurane, theophylline	Disulfiram, diethyl-dithiocarbamate	Ethanol, isoniazid
CYP3A	Diltiazem, felodipine, nifedipine, verapamil, ciclosporin, tacrolimus, alprazolam, midazolam, triazolam, atorvastatin, lovastatin, clarithromycin, erythromycin, indinavir, nelfinavir, ritonavir, saquinavir, losartan, sildenafil	Diltiazem, verapamil, itraconazole, ketoconazole, clarithromycin, erythromycin, troleandomycin, delavirdine, indinavir, ritonavir, saquinavir, grapefruit juice, mifepristone, nefazodone	Rifabutin, rifampin, rifapentine, carbamazepine, phenobarbital, phenytoin, topiramate, efavirenz, nevirapine, St John's Wort

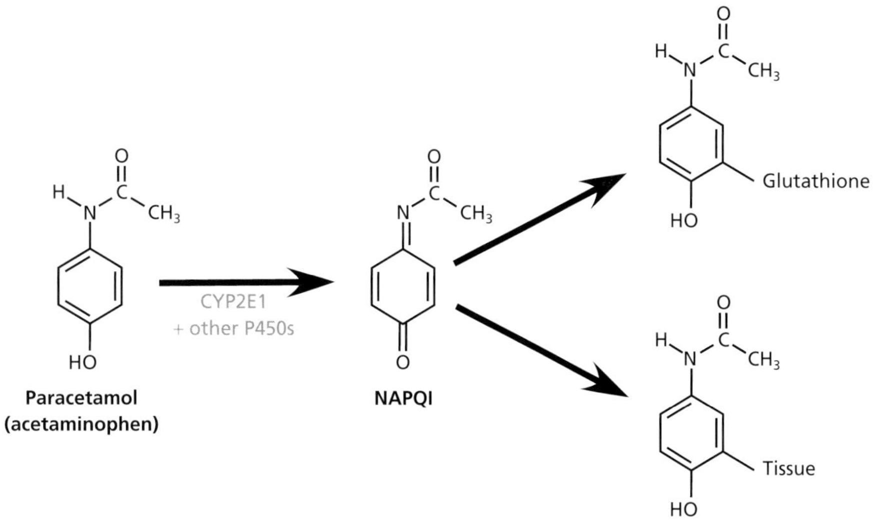

Fig. 3 Metabolic activation of paracetamol (acetaminophen) to a hepatotoxic metabolite. Phase I metabolism, predominantly mediated by CYP2E1, involves N-hydroxylation of paracetamol to form the electrophilic intermediate N-acetyl-p-benzoquinone imine (NAPQI). NAPQI is in turn detoxified by a spontaneous reaction with hepatic glutathione. Non-detoxified NAPQI can bind covalently to macromolecules within hepatocytes causing hepatic necrosis, as occurs in paracetamol overdose.

case. For example, irinotecan, a drug used for the chemotherapy of colorectal cancer, is a prodrug that requires metabolic activation by CYP3A4 to a compound named SN-38, which is the active pharmacological agent. SN-38 is subsequently detoxified by conjugation with α-glucuronic acid catalysed by UGT1A1. Individuals with the common genetic hyperbilirubinaemia Gilbert's syndrome are partially deficient in UGT1A1 and experience excessive toxicity when administered standard doses of irinotecan [27]. Metabolic activation applies not only to therapeutic drugs. Of concern is that some procarcinogens, such as heterocyclic amines, can be activated by P450 enzymes to carcinogenic metabolites [28].

Drug metabolism also contributes to both dose-related and idiosyncratic drug-induced hepatotoxicity. Paracetamol is a classic example of dose-related toxicity. The P450-mediated phase I metabolism of paracetamol (acetaminophen) gives rise to the reactive intermediate N-acetyl-p-benzoquinone imine (NAPQI), which is detoxified by a spontaneous reaction with hepatic glutathione (Fig. 3), a cysteine-containing triamino acid peptide. In the setting of paracetamol overdose, the rate of formation of NAPQI exhausts hepatic-reduced glutathione stores, and hepatocellular toxicity ensues [7]. While reactive metabolites have been identified for many drugs exhibiting idiosyncratic toxicity, the mechanisms by which tissue damage occurs and propagates remain poorly understood. It is thought that some idiosyncratic hepatic reactions to drugs are the result of drug metabolites being covalently bound to cellular proteins, either causing altered protein function or engendering an immunological response with subsequent recruitment of inflammatory cells, production of proinflammatory cytokines and Fas- or porin-mediated induction of apoptosis [7] (see also Chapters 3.1 and 14.1). In the past, it has been difficult to estimate the likelihood of a drug causing idiosyncratic hepatotoxicity, but recent advances in proteomics and metabolomics may begin to allow prediction of the proclivity of a drug to cause this form of toxicity, before human studies are undertaken [29].

Drug metabolism in liver disease, portal hypertension and systemic disease states

Liver disease and portal hypertension

In advanced liver disease, drug metabolism mediated by some P450 enzymes or enzyme subfamilies, particularly CYP1A, 2C19 and 3A, appears to be impaired to an extent that cannot be explained by simple hepatocellular loss, and suggests specific downregulation of these genes [30]. This loss of metabolism varies with the cause of liver disease; for example, in patients with a predominant cholestatic aetiology, CYP3A activity is relatively preserved [31], possibly because of positive regulation by retained bile acids acting though PXR and FXR. There is a strong relationship between quantitative measures of hepatic drug metabolism such as the aminopyrine breath test and the Child–Pugh score [30], although such metabolic measurements may not be better predictors of the severity of liver disease than clinical assessment in combination with more readily available and less expensive biochemical tests.

In the presence of portal hypertension, hepatic blood flow may be reduced in combination with increased portal–systemic shunting through collateral blood vessels. This can dramatically increase the bioavailability of high clearance drugs, for example propranolol, a drug that is commonly used in cirrhotic patients to lower portal vascular pressure. Such patients often require a relatively low dose of this drug to achieve a therapeutic effect and avoid side-effects such as excessive bradycardia. At the other end of the spectrum, the rate of metabolism of low clearance drugs is particularly sensitive to any factor that affects the availability of drug-metabolizing enzymes, as occurs with loss of hepatocellular mass in liver disease. A good example is diazepam, which exhibits a 50% reduction in clearance in advanced liver disease [32]. An additional factor that alters drug disposition in advanced liver disease is decreased plasma protein binding due to decreased hepatic protein synthesis. This results in increased action of drugs that usually circulate in a highly bound state. Issues relating to prescribing drugs in patients with liver diseases are covered in Chapter 23.3.

Drug metabolism in inflammatory states

In the early 1980s, it was recognized that theophylline toxicity occurred in children with influenza, despite being on a nontoxic dose of the drug prior to falling ill [33]. It was subsequently shown that several inflammatory states were associated with decreased expression of some hepatic P450 enzymes and that interleukin-1, interleukin-6, interferons and bacterial lipopolysaccharide were capable of mediating this phenomenon, predominantly operating through transcriptional repression [34]. More recently, it has been proposed that some patients with advanced cancer may experience excessive toxicity from chemotherapy because of diminished hepatic metabolism of anticancer drugs, even when the malignant process does not directly involve the liver. In this situation, it appears that the cancer is modulating drug-metabolizing enzymes through either the direct or the indirect release of proinflammatory cytokines [35].

References

1 Nebert DW, Russell DW (2002) Clinical importance of the cytochromes P450. *Lancet* 360 (9340), 1155–1162.

2 Handschin C, Meyer UA (2005) Regulatory network of lipid-sensing nuclear receptors: roles for CAR, PXR, LXR, and FXR. *Arch Biochem Biophys* 433 (2), 387–396.

3 Shen DD, Kunze KL, Thummel KE (1997) Enzyme-catalyzed processes of first-pass hepatic and intestinal drug extraction. *Adv Drug Deliv Rev* 27 (2–3), 99–127.

4 Yokose T, Doy M, Taniguchi T *et al.* (1999) Immunohistochemical study of cytochrome P450 2C and 3A in human non-neoplastic and neoplastic tissues. *Virchows Arch* 434 (5), 401–411.

5 Wilkinson GR (2005) Drug metabolism and variability among patients in drug response. *N Engl J Med* 352 (21), 2211–2221.

6 Ortiz de Montellano PR (ed.) (1995) *Cytochrome P-450: Structure, Mechanism and Biochemistry*, 2nd edn. New York: Plenum Press.

7 Park BK, Kitteringham NR, Maggs JL *et al.* (2005) The role of metabolic activation in drug-induced hepatotoxicity. *Annu Rev Pharmacol Toxicol* 45, 177–202.

8 Mizuno N, Niwa T, Yotsumoto Y *et al.* (2003) Impact of drug transporter studies on drug discovery and development. *Pharmacol Rev* 55 (3), 425–461.

9 Weinshilboum R (2003) Inheritance and drug response. *N Engl J Med* 348 (6), 529–537.

10 Meyer UA (2004) Pharmacogenetics – five decades of therapeutic lessons from genetic diversity. *Nature Rev Genet* 5 (9), 669–676.

11 Gnerre C, Blattler S, Kaufmann MR *et al.* (2004) Regulation of CYP3A4 by the bile acid receptor FXR: evidence for functional binding sites in the CYP3A4 gene. *Pharmacogenetics* 14 (10), 635–645.

12 Goodwin B, Hodgson E, Liddle C (1999) The orphan human pregnane X receptor mediates the transcriptional activation of CYP3A4 by rifampicin through a distal enhancer module. *Mol Pharmacol* 56 (6), 1329–1339.

13 Tirona RG, Lee W, Leake BF *et al.* (2003) The orphan nuclear receptor HNF4α determines PXR- and CAR-mediated xenobiotic induction of CYP3A4. *Nature Med* 9 (2), 220–224.

14 Martinez-Jimenez CP, Gomez-Lechon MJ, Castell JV *et al.* (2005) Transcriptional regulation of the human hepatic CYP3A4:

identification of a new distal enhancer region responsive to CCAAT/enhancer-binding protein β isoforms (liver activating protein and liver inhibitory protein). *Mol Pharmacol* 67 (6), 2088–2101.

15 Tirona RG, Kim RB (2005) Nuclear receptors and drug disposition gene regulation. *J Pharm Sci* 94 (6), 1169–1186.

16 Liddle C, Goodwin B (2002) Regulation of hepatic drug metabolism: role of the nuclear receptors PXR and CAR. *Semin Liver Dis* 22 (2), 115–122.

17 Eloranta JJ, Kullak-Ublick GA (2005) Coordinate transcriptional regulation of bile acid homeostasis and drug metabolism. *Arch Biochem Biophys* 433 (2), 397–412.

18 Goodwin B, Moore JT (2004) CAR: detailing new models. *Trends Pharmacol Sci* 25 (8), 437–441.

19 Ingelman-Sundberg M (2004) Pharmacogenetics of cytochrome P450 and its applications in drug therapy: the past, present and future. *Trends Pharmacol Sci* 25 (4), 193–200.

20 Givens RC, Watkins PB (2003) Pharmacogenetics and clinical gastroenterology. *Gastroenterology* 125 (1), 240–248.

21 Eichelbaum M, Fromm MF, Schwab M (2004) Clinical aspects of the MDR1 (ABCB1) gene polymorphism. *Ther Drug Monit* 26 (2), 180–185.

22 Birkett DJ (2002) *Pharmacokinetics Made Easy*, 2nd edn. Roseville, NSW: McGraw-Hill.

23 Liddle C, Robertson GR (2003) Predicting inductive drug-drug interactions. *Pharmacogenomics* 4 (2), 141–152.

24 Maglich JM, Stoltz CM, Goodwin B *et al.* (2002) Nuclear pregnane x receptor and constitutive androstane receptor regulate overlapping but distinct sets of genes involved in xenobiotic detoxification. *Mol Pharmacol* 62 (3), 638–646.

25 Whitlock JP, Jr (1999) Induction of cytochrome P4501A1. *Annu Rev Pharmacol Toxicol* 39, 103–125.

26 Zhou S, Yung Chan S, Cher Goh B *et al.* (2005) Mechanism-based inhibition of cytochrome P450 3A4 by therapeutic drugs. *Clin Pharmacokinet* 44 (3), 279–304.

27 Innocenti F, Iyer L, Ratain MJ (2001) Pharmacogenetics of anticancer agents: lessons from amonafide and irinotecan. *Drug Metab Dispos* 29 (4 Pt 2), 596–600.

28 Wogan GN, Hecht SS, Felton JS *et al.* (2004) Environmental and chemical carcinogenesis. *Semin Cancer Biol* 14 (6), 473–486.

29 Liebler DC, Guengerich FP (2005) Elucidating mechanisms of drug-induced toxicity. *Nature Rev Drug Discov* 4 (5), 410–420.

30 Villeneuve JP, Pichette V (2004) Cytochrome P450 and liver diseases. *Curr Drug Metab* 5 (3), 273–282.

31 George J, Murray M, Byth K *et al.* (1995) Differential alterations of cytochrome P450 proteins in livers from patients with severe chronic liver disease. *Hepatology* 21 (1), 120–128.

32 Hebert MF. Guide to drug doses in hepatic disease. In: Speight TM, Holford NHG (eds) *Avery's Drug Treatment*, 4th edn. Auckland: Adis International Ltd.

33 Kraemer MJ, Furukawa CT, Koup JR *et al.* (1982) Altered theophylline clearance during an influenza B outbreak. *Pediatrics* 69 (4), 476–480.

34 Morgan ET (2001) Regulation of cytochrome P450 by inflammatory mediators: why and how? *Drug Metab Dispos* 29 (3), 207–212.

35 Slaviero KA, Clarke SJ, Rivory LP (2003) Inflammatory response: an unrecognised source of variability in the pharmacokinetics and pharmacodynamics of cancer chemotherapy. *Lancet Oncol* 4 (4), 224–232.

2.4 Synthetic function

2.4.1 Albumin and other carrier proteins

Richard A. Weisiger

Soluble proteins make up 6.4–8.3% of plasma by weight [1], a value comparable to their concentration in cell water [2]. Many plasma proteins are synthesized by the liver. Their concentrations may decrease in the setting of liver disease, malnutrition or protein-losing states such as nephrotic syndrome, severe burns, bowel inflammation, intestinal lymphangiectasia or major bleeding episodes. The most abundant plasma proteins have little or no enzymatic activity. Instead, their function is typically binding to other molecules, generically referred to as *ligands*. Some plasma binding proteins that have been characterized are listed in Table 1. Most of these proteins bind to only one (or a few related) molecules with high affinity. For example, haemopexin binds haem, retinol-binding protein binds retinol, and transferrin binds iron. In contrast, other binding proteins such as albumin and alpha-fetoprotein are far less selective.

Albumin is the most important serum binding protein in terms of concentration (about 4.2%) [1,3] and number of different ligands bound. The latter include fatty acids [4], unconjugated bilirubin [5], many divalent cations such as copper [6,7], hydrophobic bile acids [6] and a variety of drugs and toxins [6,8–11] (Table 2). Albumin's broad specificity reflects not only

Table 1 Soluble binding proteins found in plasma.

Binding protein	Ligand	References
Afamin	Vitamin E, probably others	[18,65,36]
Albumin	See Table 2	
Alpha-fetoprotein	Long-chain fatty acids, bilirubin, many others	[66]
Avidins	Biotin	[67]
Ceruloplasmin	Copper	[68]
Cholesterol ester transfer protein	Cholesterol	[33]
Corticosteroid-binding globulin	Steroid hormones	[69]
Folate-binding protein	Folic acid	[6]
Haptoglobin	Haemoglobin	[6]
Haemopexin	Haem	[6]
Lipocalins	Retinoids, arachidonic acid, steroids, pheromones	[70]
Lipoproteins	Triglycerides, cholesterol, bile acids, vitamin E	[6]
Phospholipid transfer protein	Phospholipids	[71,72]
Retinol-binding protein	Retinols	[73,74]
Sex hormone-binding globulin	Testosterone, dihydrotestosterone, estradiol	[75]
Thyroxine-binding globulin	Thyroxine	[76]
Transcobalamins	Vitamin B12	[77,78]
Transcortin	Corticoids	[79]
Transferrin	Iron	[6]
Transthyretin	Thyroxine	[73]
Vitamin D-binding protein	Vitamin D	[6]

Table 2 Some molecules bound by plasma albumin.

Amino acids (tryptophan, cysteine)	[17,80]
Bilirubin	[5,6,29]
Cationic metal ions (Ag, Ca, Cd, Co, Cu, Hg, Mg, Mn, Ni, Zn)	[3,6,7,81–83]
Chloride	[6]
Many drugs (e.g. coumadin, digitalis, ibuprofen, diazepam, lidocaine, furosemide, valproic acid, phenytoin)	[6,8]
Medium- and long-chain fatty acids	[6,84]
Certain bile acids (e.g. lithocholate, chenodeoxycholate)	[6,85]
Certain steroid hormones (cortisone, estradiol, progesterone, aldosterone)	[6]
Thyroxine	[6, 86]
Certain toxins (e.g. aflatoxin, digitoxin, 'organic anions')	[9–11]

the presence of several discrete binding sites [6], but also its ability to adapt its three-dimensional conformation in response to binding [12,13], thus creating a better fit between the binding site and the ligand. This ability is termed *conformational adaptability* [14]. Even when no ligands are bound, albumin is constantly sampling from a large library of conformations in a process known as *conformational breathing* [14]. This variability helps to explain why it took so long to crystallize albumin in a form suitable for determining its detailed three-dimensional structure [6,15,16].

Human serum albumin consists of a single polypeptide chain of 585 amino acids with a molecular weight of 66 700 Da [9,17]. It contains six homologous subdomains that individually retain binding capacity when separated by proteolysis [15]. It is part of a multigene family that also includes alpha-fetoprotein, afamin and vitamin D-binding protein [15,18]. Synthesis of albumin is restricted to the liver, and albumin levels typically decline as the severity of liver disease worsens. The serum albumin concentration is an important part of the Child–Pugh score for assessing the severity of liver disease [19], but is not used in the MELD score for determining liver transplantation priority, in part because such critically ill patients often have other conditions (such as gastrointestinal bleeding) that may lower the albumin level [20,21]. Hyperalbuminaemia, when seen, is nearly always due to dehydration rather than increased synthesis.

Functions of albumin and other plasma binding proteins

Convection

The primary function of blood is to transport molecules to and from tissues by convection (flow). Without this function, important metabolites such as glucose and oxygen would become depleted, and products of metabolism such as carbon dioxide and lactate would accumulate to toxic levels. The most dramatic example of failure of convective transport is cardiac

arrest, which causes rapid and severe damage to most tissues. However, selective failure of convective transport can occur even with normal cardiac output if binding protein concentrations are low. For example, a very low haemoglobin level selectively blocks convective transport of oxygen, causing ischaemia. Congenital absence of transcobalamin blocks vitamin B12 transport, causing brain damage [22,23]. Congenital retinol-binding deficiency blocks the transport of retinol, causing atrophy of the retina [24]. Congenital haptoglobin deficiency is associated with seizures caused by the accumulation of haemoglobin and its degradation products in the brain [25]. Interestingly, congenital lack of serum albumin causes few manifestations in otherwise healthy persons, probably because other plasma proteins with overlapping binding specificities compensate for its absence [26]. Nevertheless, critically ill patients with hypoalbuminaemia have greatly decreased survival rates even with normal nutrition, and replacing albumin seems to improve their survival [27].

The rate at which a molecule is transported by the bloodstream is proportional to its concentration. For lipophilic and amphipathic molecules, this concentration is very low unless binding proteins are present, reflecting their limited solubility in water and their strong tendency to bind to tissues. Plasma binding proteins may increase the rate of convective transport of their ligands by many orders of magnitude. They are often called *carrier proteins* in recognition of this important role.

It may seem counterintuitive that protein binding can make a ligand more available to tissues. Indeed, bilirubin is cleared by liver much more efficiently in the absence of albumin than in its presence [28], suggesting that the opposite should be true. However, the maximum possible concentration of unbound bilirubin in plasma is so tiny, about 7 nM [29], that normal blood flow cannot deliver nearly enough bilirubin to the liver to keep up with the rate of production, even if the efficiency of removal is 100%. On the other hand, the concentration of albumin-bound bilirubin in plasma is large enough that only a small fraction needs to be removed to keep up with bilirubin production. In summary, protein binding makes ligands more available to sites of metabolism and excretion within the body by increasing their rates of convection from one tissue to another.

By a similar mechanism, binding proteins are also important in hormone signalling. Thyroid and steroid hormones are relatively hydrophobic and tend to bind strongly to tissues [30,31]. In the absence of binding proteins, these hormones bind to the first cells they encounter [30,31], thus preventing rapid signalling to other cells. By competing with cellular binding sites for these hormones, plasma binding proteins for thyroid [32], steroid [6,33] and other lipophilic hormones maintain a uniform circulating pool that bathes all cells with similar hormone concentrations, allowing changes in hormone levels to propagate rapidly and uniformly throughout the body [30]. In general, the activity of a hormone is proportional to the unbound ('free') hormone concentration [34]. Plasma hormone binding proteins buffer this concentration against rapid changes while promoting a uniform distribution throughout the body.

Diffusion

Convection alone cannot deliver dissolved molecules to the cell surface. No matter how vigorously the extracellular fluid is 'stirred' (e.g. by flow or turbulence), a very thin layer of unstirred plasma always remains just above the plasma membrane [35]. The only way for soluble molecules to cross this layer is by diffusion. The thickness of this layer varies among tissues. It is relatively small in the liver, where fenestrations in the endothelial cells allow plasma proteins direct access to the subendothelial (Disse) space [36]. Erythrocytes passing through the liver sinusoids may 'massage' the endothelium, thus both increasing the rate of exchange of plasma with the subendothelial space [36] and reducing the thickness of the unstirred layer. In contrast, cells in less metabolically active tissues may be located one or more cell diameters from the nearest capillary, requiring metabolites to diffuse much greater distances to reach them.

Diffusion is the random motion of dissolved molecules across a concentration gradient. Although the unstirred plasma layer is typically very small, it can greatly limit the rate at which small molecules move into and out of cells [35,37]. According to Fick's law, the steady diffusional flux (J) is proportional to the concentration difference of the diffusing molecule (ΔC) and its diffusion constant (D) (a measure of its rate of random motion) and inversely related to the square of the thickness of the layer (x) (Eq. 1).

$$J = \Delta C \, D / x^2 \qquad (1)$$

Because of their low solubility in water [29,38], many hydrophobic molecules such as fatty acids and bilirubin cannot even approach a sufficient concentration in plasma to drive observed rates of uptake across this layer in the liver and other metabolically active tissues [37]. In much the same way that they increase convection, binding proteins also increase the diffusional flux of their ligands by increasing the amount of dissolved ligand available for diffusion [37]. While it is true that binding to the protein lowers the ligand's diffusion constant by a factor of about 10, this is more than compensated for by the increase in the soluble concentration (often by many orders of magnitude). These higher concentrations allow for larger values of ΔC, resulting in a net increase in the diffusion rate [37].

Interactions with cell membranes

Cellular uptake of protein-bound ligands may occur by several possible mechanisms. Some binding proteins randomly release their ligands in the general vicinity of the target cell membrane, while others deliver them carefully to specific sites on the cell surface or even within the cell. Many cells have receptors for binding proteins on their surface (e.g. transferrin [6]). Binding to these receptors is typically followed by receptor-mediated endocytosis of the entire protein–ligand complex, dissociation of the ligand from the binding protein in the acid lysosomal compartment and return of the binding protein to the plasma

[6]. In other cases, however, the complex may serve a signalling function. Sex steroid-binding protein allows certain sex hormones to activate adenyl cyclase without ever entering the cell by reversibly binding to a specific G protein-linked receptor on the cell surface [39]. Only certain sex hormones are able to activate the receptor when bound to the binding protein [39].

Cellular uptake may also draw on a pool of unbound ligand at the cell surface that is rapidly replenished by dissociation from the binding protein. Dissociation may either be spontaneous or catalysed by an interaction of the binding protein with the cell surface. If sufficiently slow, the rate of dissociation may limit the rate of cellular uptake by allowing the unbound ligand concentration to become depleted at the cell surface. Dissociation-limited uptake has been demonstrated for avidly bound molecules such as bilirubin and fatty acids [37,40]. Indeed, the affinity of albumin for bilirubin and long-chain fatty acids may represent a compromise between the need to limit the toxicity of these molecules (which favours more avid binding) and the need for rapid dissociation of the ligand from albumin prior to uptake (which favours less avid binding). Under physiological conditions, the hepatic uptake rate of fatty acids and bilirubin is influenced by many processes (including the rates of plasma flow into the liver, diffusion across the unstirred plasma layer, transport across the plasma membrane, diffusion through the cell cytoplasm and metabolism or excretion), each of which has a roughly comparable rate [41]. The detailed process by which binding proteins facilitate diffusion of their ligands across extracellular water layers was first defined by Bass and Pond [42] and has since been validated in a variety of physiological settings [43–45].

Limiting toxicity

Many molecules that bind to plasma proteins are potentially toxic. This includes endogenous molecules such as bilirubin and long-chain fatty acids, heavy metal ions such as iron and copper, and exogenous drugs and toxins such as digitalis, aminoglycosides and warfarin. These molecules cause little or no toxicity while bound to plasma proteins, but interfere with critical cell functions when present at sufficient concentrations within tissues. Binding to plasma proteins provides a relatively safe place to store these molecules while they await cellular metabolism or elimination.

For example, children with congenital absence of hepatic bilirubin uridine diphosphate (UDP)-glucuronal transferase may develop brain damage (kernicterus) from the accumulation of high levels of unconjugated bilirubin in neural tissues [46]. Bilirubin inhibits important cellular functions such as the Na^+/K^+-ATPase and peptide phosphorylation in the brain [47,48]. However, brain damage does not occur until the storage capacity of plasma albumin is exceeded [6,46]. Likewise, long-chain fatty acids can cause damage to cell membranes and inhibit some enzymes when present at high concentrations [49–51]. However, high plasma concentrations are needed to support maximum cardiac and skeletal muscle output. Binding of more than 99.99% of the plasma fatty acids to albumin greatly reduces this potential toxicity while keeping the fatty acids in a form that is rapidly available for metabolism. Finally, in patients with haemochromatosis, liver and other tissues do not become loaded with iron until after transferrin is saturated [52], allowing the formation of small iron complexes that are rapidly cleared by the liver [53,54]. Without binding proteins such as transferrin, iron ions release toxic free radicals as they repeatedly cycle between the ferrous and ferric states [55].

Plasma binding proteins also influence drug effectiveness and toxicity. Warfarin causes toxicity by blocking the formation of clotting factors in the liver, an effect that is used therapeutically by the drug coumadin. However, the full effect of a daily dose of coumadin does not become manifest until after the plasma binding sites on albumin have been loaded. Persons with hypoalbuminaemia are more susceptible to warfarin toxicity [56,57]. Hypoalbuminaemia is also a risk factor for aminoglycoside toxicity [58]. In a similar way, plasma binding increases the amount of a dietary toxin that must be ingested to produce toxicity. The important role of plasma binding in modulating tissue concentrations of drugs is underscored by the fact that measurement of unbound drug concentrations is increasingly used to monitor therapy [59]. Monitoring unbound concentrations is particularly important in patients with disturbed plasma binding due to hypoalbuminaemia or the presence of competitive inhibitors of binding such as uraemic toxins or certain drugs [59].

Targeting ligands to specific tissues

Binding proteins may help to direct their ligands to specific tissues that express receptors for the protein. This mechanism makes optimum use of ligands that are in limited supply or may cause toxicity if delivered to the wrong tissues. For example, transcobalamins target vitamin B12 to cells expressing the transcobalamin receptor [60], and transferrin targets iron to cells expressing the transferrin receptor [6]. When expressed, the receptor for sex steroid-binding globulin renders cells sensitive to the hormonal effects of certain steroid hormones [39].

Oncotic functions

Albumin provides approximately 80% of the colloid osmotic pressure in normal blood, reflecting its high concentration and relatively low molecular weight. Significant decreases in serum albumin levels due to liver failure, bleeding, nephrotic syndrome or protein-losing enteropathy are associated with the accumulation of fluid in extracellular compartments (e.g. oedema, ascites) [61]. Cerebral oedema may be life threatening and reflects not only low albumin levels, but also increased permeability of the cerebral vessels [62]. Administration of albumin reduces the reaccumulation of ascites after paracentesis [63] and has been used to treat cerebral oedema as well [64].

References

1 Bennet JC, Plum F (eds) (1996) *Cecil Textbook of Medicine*, 20th edn. Philadelphia, PA: W.B. Saunders Co.

2 Luby-Phelps K, Lanni F, Taylor DL (1988) The submicroscopic properties of cytoplasm as a determinant of cellular function. *Annu Rev Biophys Biophys Chem* 17, 369–396.

3 Peters T, Reed RG (1978) Serum albumin as a transport protein. In: Sund H (ed.) *Transport by Proteins*. Berlin: Walter de Gruyter, pp. 57–73.

4 Ashbrook JD, Spector AA, Santos EC *et al.* (1975) Long chain fatty acid binding to human plasma albumin. *J Biol Chem* 250, 2333–2338.

5 Brodersen R (1979) Binding of bilirubin to albumin. *CRC Crit Rev Clin Lab Sci* 11, 305–399.

6 Carter DC, Ho JX (1994) Structure of serum albumin. *Adv Protein Chem* 45, 153–203.

7 Masuoka J, Saltman P (1994) Zinc(II) and copper(II) binding to serum albumin. A comparative study of dog, bovine, and human albumin. *J Biol Chem* 269, 25557–25561.

8 Meijer DK, van der Sluijs P (1989) Covalent and noncovalent protein binding of drugs: implications for hepatic clearance, storage, and cell-specific drug delivery. *Pharm Res* 6, 105–118.

9 Kragh-Hansen U (1990) Structure and ligand binding properties of human serum albumin. *Dan Med Bull* 37, 57–84.

10 Dirr HW, Schabort JC (1987) Characterization of the aflatoxin B1-binding site of rat albumin. *Biochim Biophys Acta* 913, 300–307.

11 Doucet J, Fresel J, Hue G *et al.* (1993) Protein binding of digitoxin, valproate and phenytoin in sera from diabetics. *Eur J Clin Pharmacol* 45, 577–579.

12 Hvidt AA, Wallevik K (1972) Conformational changes in human serum albumin as revealed by hydrogen-deuterium exchange studies. *J Biol Chem* 247, 1530–1535.

13 Wilting J, Kremer JM, Ijzerman AP *et al.* (1982) The kinetics of the binding of warfarin to human serum albumin as studied by stopped-flow spectrophotometry. *Biochim Biophys Acta* 706, 96–104.

14 Scheider W (1977) Real-time measurement of dielectric relaxation of biomolecules: kinetics of a protein-ligand binding reaction. *Ann NY Acad Sci* 303, 47–58.

15 Geisow MJ (1992) Human serum albumin structure – solved. *Trends Biotechnol* 10, 335–337.

16 Petitpas I, Grune T, Bhattacharya AA *et al.* (2001) Crystal structures of human serum albumin complexed with monounsaturated and polyunsaturated fatty acids. *J Mol Biol* 314, 955–960.

17 Peters T, Jr (1985) Serum albumin. *Adv Protein Chem* 37, 161–245.

18 Lichenstein HS, Lyons DE, Wurfe, MM *et al.* (1994) Afamin is a new member of the albumin, alpha-fetoprotein, and vitamin D-binding protein gene family. *J Biol Chem* 269, 18149–18154.

19 Schneider PD (2004) Preoperative assessment of liver function. *Surg Clin North Am* 84, 355–373.

20 Srikureja W, Kyulo NL, Runyon BA *et al.* (2005) MELD score is a better prognostic model than Child–Turcotte–Pugh score or discriminant function score in patients with alcoholic hepatitis. *J Hepatol* 42, 700–706.

21 Freeman RB, Jr, Wiesner RH, Roberts JP *et al.* (2004) Improving liver allocation: MELD and PELD. *Am J Transplant* 4 (Suppl 9), 114–131.

22 Qian L, Quadros EV, Regec A *et al.* (2002) Congenital transcobalamin II deficiency due to errors in RNA editing. *Blood Cells Mol Dis* 28, 134–142; discussion 143–135.

23 Kaikov Y, Wadsworth LD, Hall CA *et al.* (1991) Transcobalamin II deficiency: case report and review of the literature. *Eur J Pediatr* 150, 841–843.

24 Seeliger MW, Biesalski HK, Wissinger B *et al.* (1999) Phenotype in retinol deficiency due to a hereditary defect in retinol binding protein synthesis. *Invest Ophthalmol Vis Sci* 40, 3–11.

25 Manoharan A (1997) Congenital haptoglobin deficiency. *Blood* 90, 1709a.

26 Russi E, Weigand K (1983) Analbuminemia. *Klin Wochenschr* 61, 541–545.

27 Vincent JL, Dubois MJ, Navickis RJ *et al.* (2003) Hypoalbuminemia in acute illness: is there a rationale for intervention? A meta-analysis of cohort studies and controlled trials. *Ann Surg* 237, 319–334.

28 Stollman YR, Gartner U, Theilmann L *et al.* (1983) Hepatic bilirubin uptake in the isolated perfused rat liver is not facilitated by albumin binding. *J Clin Invest* 72, 718–723.

29 Brodersen R (1979) Bilirubin. Solubility and interaction with albumin and phospholipid. *J Biol Chem* 254, 2364–2369.

30 Mendel CM, Weisiger RA, Jones AL *et al.* (1987) Thyroid hormone-binding proteins in plasma facilitate uniform distribution of thyroxine within tissues: a perfused rat liver study. *Endocrinology* 120, 1742–1749.

31 Mendel CM, Kuhn RW, Weisiger RA (1991) Uptake of corticosterone by the perfused rat liver. *Endocrinology* 129, 27–32.

32 Ekins R, Edwards P, Newman B (1982) The role of binding-proteins in hormone delivery. In: Ekins RP (ed.) *Free Hormones in Blood*. New York: Elsevier Press, pp. 3–43.

33 Ruggeri RB (2005) Cholesteryl ester transfer protein: pharmacological inhibition for the modulation of plasma cholesterol levels and promising target for the prevention of atherosclerosis. *Curr Topics Med Chem* 5, 257–264.

34 Mendel CM, Cavalieri RR, Köhrle J (1992) Thyroxine (T_4) transport and distribution in rats treated with EMD 21388, a synthetic flavonoid that displaces T_4 from transthyretin. *Endocrinology* 130, 1525–1532.

35 Barry PH, Diamond JM (1984) Effects of unstirred layers on membrane phenomena. *Physiol Rev* 64, 763–872.

36 Wisse E, De Zanger RB, Charrels K *et al.* (1985) The liver sieve: considerations concerning the structure and function of endothelial fenestrae, the sinusoidal wall and the space of Disse. *Hepatology* 5, 683–692.

37 Weisiger RA (1998) Impact of extracellular and intracellular diffusion barriers on hepatic uptake kinetics. In: Linehan JH (ed.) *Whole Organ Approaches to Cellular Metabolism*. New York: Springer-Verlag, pp. 389–423.

38 Vorum H, Brodersen R, Kragh-Hansen U *et al.* (1992) Solubility of long-chain fatty acids in phosphate buffer at pH 7.4. *Biochim Biophys Acta Lipids Lipid Metab* 1126, 135–142.

39 Rosner W, Hryb DJ, Khan MS *et al.* (1999) Sex hormone-binding globulin mediates steroid hormone signal transduction at the plasma membrane. *J Steroid Biochem Mol Biol* 69, 481–485.

40 Weisiger RA (1985) Dissociation from albumin: a potentially rate-limiting step in the clearance of substances by the liver. *Proc Natl Acad Sci USA* 82, 1563–1567.

41 Luxon BA, Holly DC, Milliano MC, Weisiger RA (1998) Sex differences in multiple steps in the hepatic transport of palmitate support a balanced uptake mechanism. *Am J Physiol* 274, G52–G61.

42 Bass L, Pond SM (1988) The puzzle of rates of cellular uptake of protein-bound ligands. In: Rescigno A (ed.) *Pharmacokinetics: Mathematical and Statistical Approaches to Metabolism and Distribution of Chemicals and Drugs*. London: Plenum Press, pp. 241–265.

43 Weisiger RA, Pond SM, Bass L (1989) Albumin enhances unidirectional fluxes of fatty acid across a lipid-water interface: theory and experiments. *Am J Physiol* 257, G904–G916.

44 Weisiger RA, Pond SM, Bass L (1991) Hepatic uptake of protein-bound ligands: extended sinusoidal perfusion model. *Am J Physiol* 261, G872–G884.

45 Pond SM, Davis CKC, Bogoyevitch MA *et al.* (1992) Uptake of palmitate by hepatocyte suspensions: facilitation by albumin? *Am J Physiol* 262, G883–G894.

46 Ahlfors CE, Wennberg RP (2004) Bilirubin–albumin binding and neonatal jaundice. *Semin Perinatol* 28, 334–339.

47 Hansen TW (2001) Bilirubin brain toxicity. *J Perinatol* 21 (Suppl 1), S48–51; discussion S59–62.

48 Kawai K, Cowger ML (1981) Effect of bilirubin on ATPase activity of human erythrocyte membranes. *Res Commun Chem Pathol Pharmacol* 32, 123–135.

49 Rhoads DE, Ockner RK, Peterson NA *et al.* (1983) Modulation of membrane transport by free fatty acids: inhibition of synaptosomal sodium-dependent amino acid uptake. *Biochemistry* 22, 1965–1970.

50 Khan WA, Blobe GC, Hannun YA (1992) Activation of protein kinase C by oleic acid. *J Biol Chem* 267, 3605–3612.

51 Gordon GB (1977) Saturated free fatty acid toxicity. II. Lipid accumulation, ultrastructural alterations, and toxicity in mammalian cells in culture. *Exp Mol Pathol* 27, 262–276.

52 Franchini M, Veneri D (2005) Recent advances in hereditary hemochromatosis. *Ann Haematol* 84, 347–352.

53 Brissot P, Wright TL, Ma WL *et al.* (1985) Efficient clearance of non-transferrin-bound iron by rat liver Implications for hepatic iron loading in iron overload states. *J Clin Invest* 76, 1463–1470.

54 Wright TL, Brissot P, Ma WL *et al.* (1986) Characterization of non-transferrin-bound iron clearance by rat liver. *J Biol Chem* 261, 10909–10914.

55 Herbert V, Shaw S, Jayatilleke E *et al.* (1994) Most free-radical injury is iron-related: it is promoted by iron, hemin, holoferritin and vitamin C, and inhibited by desferoxamine and apoferritin. *Stem Cells* 12, 289–303.

56 Tincani E, Mazzali F, Morini L (2002) Hypoalbuminemia as a risk factor for over-anticoagulation. *Am J Med* 112, 247–248.

57 Piroli RJ, Passananti GT, Shively CA *et al.* (1981) Antipyrine and warfarin disposition in a patient with idiopathic hypoalbuminemia. *Clin Pharmacol Ther* 30, 810–816.

58 Gamba G, Contreras AM, Cortes J *et al.* (1990) Hypoalbuminemia as a risk factor for amikacin nephrotoxicity. *Rev Invest Clin* 42, 204–209.

59 Dasgupta A (2002) Clinical utility of free drug monitoring. *Clin Chem Lab Med* 40, 986–993.

60 Sennett C, Rosenberg LE, Mellman IS (1981) Transmembrane transport of cobalamin in prokaryotic and eukaryotic cells. *Annu Rev Biochem* 50, 1053–1086.

61 Halvorsen L, Holcroft JW (1988) Albumin: mechanisms of edema formation. *Nutr Clin Pract* 3, 222–225.

62 Blei AT, Larsen FS (1999) Pathophysiology of cerebral edema in fulminant hepatic failure. *J Hepatol* 31, 771–776.

63 Arroyo V (2002) Pathophysiology, diagnosis and treatment of ascites in cirrhosis. *Ann Hepatol* 1, 72–79.

64 Gurkan F, Haspolat K, Yaramis A *et al.* (2001) Beneficial effect of human albumin on neonatal cerebral edema. *Am J Ther* 8, 253–254.

65 Voegele AF, Jerkovic L, Wellenzohn B *et al.* (2002) Characterization of the vitamin E-binding properties of human plasma afamin. *Biochemistry* 41, 14532–14538.

66 Aoyagi Y, Ikenaka T, Ichida F (1979) Alpha-fetoprotein as a carrier protein in plasma and its bilirubin-binding ability. *Cancer Res* 39, 3571–3574.

67 Korpela J (1984) Avidin, a high affinity biotin-binding protein, as a tool and subject of biological research. *Med Biol* 62, 5–26.

68 Giurgea N, Constantinescu MI, Stanciu R *et al.* (2005) Ceruloplasmin – acute-phase reactant or endogenous antioxidant? The case of cardiovascular disease. *Med Sci Monit* 11, RA48–51.

69 Breuner CW, Orchinik M (2002) Plasma binding proteins as mediators of corticosteroid action in vertebrates. *J Endocrinol* 175, 99–112.

70 Flower DR (1996) The lipocalin protein family: structure and function. *Biochem J* 318 (Pt 1), 1–14.

71 Stein O, Stein Y (2005) Lipid transfer proteins (LTP) and atherosclerosis. *Atherosclerosis* 178, 217–230.

72 van Tol A (2002) Phospholipid transfer protein. *Curr Opin Lipidol* 13, 135–139.

73 Raghu P, Sivakumar B (2004) Interactions amongst plasma retinol-binding protein, transthyretin and their ligands: implications in vitamin A homeostasis and transthyretin amyloidosis. *Biochim Biophys Acta* 1703, 1–9.

74 Zanotti G, Berni R (2004) Plasma retinol-binding protein: structure and interactions with retinol, retinoids, and transthyretin. *Vitam Horm* 69, 271–295.

75 Rosner W, Hryb DJ, Khan MS *et al.* (1991) Sex hormone-binding globulin: anatomy and physiology of a new regulatory system. *J Steroid Biochem Mol Biol* 40, 813–820.

76 Palha JA (2002) Transthyretin as a thyroid hormone carrier: function revisited. *Clin Chem Lab Med* 40, 1292–1300.

77 Fernandes-Costa F, Metz J (1982) Vitamin B12 binders (transcobalamins) in serum. *Crit Rev Clin Lab Sci* 18, 1–30.

78 von Castel-Dunwoody KM, Kauwell GP, Shelnutt KP *et al.* (2005) Transcobalamin 776C→G polymorphism negatively affects vitamin B-12 metabolism. *Am J Clin Nutr* 81, 1436–1441.

79 Yamamoto M, Ariyoshi Y, Matsui N (1982) The serum concentrations of unbound, transcortin bound and albumin bound cortisol in patients with dysproteinemia. *Endocrinol Jpn* 29, 639–646.

80 Bowmer CJ, Lindup WE (1978) Binding of phenytoin, L-tryptophan and O-methyl red to albumin. Unexpected effect of albumin concentration on the binding of phenytoin and L-tryptophan. *Biochem Pharmacol* 27, 937–942.

81 Zucker SD, Goessling W, Zeidel ML *et al.* (1994) Membrane lipid composition and vesicle size modulate bilirubin intermembrane transfer. Evidence for membrane-directed trafficking of bilirubin in the hepatocyte. *J Biol Chem* 269, 19262–19270.

82 Kragh-Hansen U, Vorum H (1993) Quantitative analyses of the interaction between calcium ions and human serum albumin. *Clin Chem* 39, 202–208.

83 Lovstad RA (2004) A kinetic study on the distribution of Cu(II)-ions between albumin and transferrin. *Biometals* 17, 111–113.

84 Spector AA (1975) Fatty acid binding to plasma albumin. *J Lipid Res* 16, 165–179.

85 Takikawa H, Sugiyama Y, Hanano M *et al.* (1987) A novel binding site for bile acids on human serum albumin. *Biochim Biophys Acta* 926, 145–153.

86 Hoshikawa S, Mori K, Kaise N *et al.* (2004) Artifactually elevated serum-free thyroxine levels measured by equilibrium dialysis in a pregnant woman with familial dysalbuminemic hyperthyroxinemia. *Thyroid* 14, 155–160.

2.4.2 The liver and coagulation

Maria T. DeSancho and Stephen M. Pastores

Introduction

The liver plays a major role in haemostasis, as most of the coagulation factors, anticoagulant proteins and components of the fibrinolytic system are synthesized by hepatic parenchymal cells. Additionally, the reticuloendothelial system of the liver helps to regulate coagulation and fibrinolysis by clearing these coagulation factors from the circulation. Finally, because the liver is a highly vascularized organ with vital venous systems draining through the parenchyma, liver diseases can affect abdominal blood flow and predispose patients to significant bleeding problems.

The aetiology of impaired haemostasis resulting from abnormal liver function is often multifactorial and may include impaired coagulation factor synthesis, synthesis of dysfunctional coagulation factors, increased consumption of coagulation factors, altered clearance of activated coagulation factors and quantitative and qualitative platelet disorders. In this chapter, we will review the normal physiology of haemostasis, describe the role of the liver in the haemostatic system and discuss the coagulation abnormalities that may occur in patients with liver disease and during liver transplantation.

Physiology of haemostasis

Normal haemostatic balance is dependent on a complex interplay between procoagulant, anticoagulant and fibrinolytic proteins. Initiation of coagulation begins when tissue factor (TF) is exposed after an injury to the vessel wall (Fig. 1). TF forms a

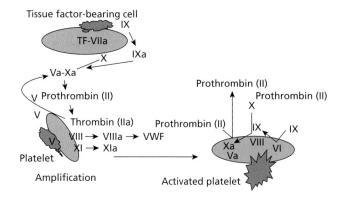

Fig. 1 Tissue factor (TF) is the major initiator of coagulation. Tissue factor-bearing cells include stimulated monocytes, endothelial cells and vascular smooth muscle cells. Exposure of TF to blood is rapidly followed by the formation of a complex between TF and factor VIIa that activates both factor IX and X, leading to generation of thrombin. Thrombin also activates factor V, VIII, XI and platelets.

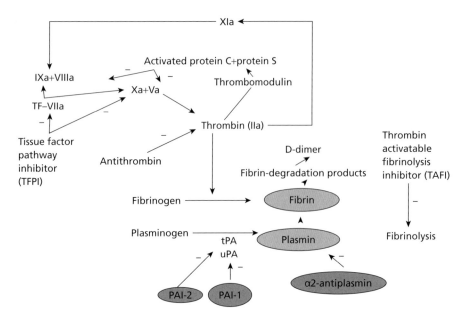

Fig. 2 The fibrinolytic and natural anticoagulant pathways.

complex with activated factor VII (factor VIIa) present in the plasma. The TF/factor VIIa complex converts factor X to factor Xa, which, in turn, along with a cofactor, factor Va, converts pro-thrombin (factor II) to thrombin (factor IIa) [1]. Although this process generates a small amount of thrombin, this thrombin serves to prime the coagulation cascade by increasing the enzymatic activity of factor VIIa, making it 100-fold more active. In addition, thrombin activates factor V, VIII, XI and platelets, which form the infrastructure to amplify the enzymatic reactions of the coagulation cascade. Ultimately, thrombin is formed directly by the TF/VIIa complex activating factor X to Xa or indirectly by converting factor IX to factor IXa, which in turn complexes with its cofactor, factor VIIIa, to convert factor X to factor Xa. The large amount of thrombin that is generated cleaves fibrinogen to fibrin monomers, which in turn spontaneously polymerize and are cross-linked by factor XIIIa (which itself is activated by thrombin) to produce a stable clot. At this time, thrombin-activatable fibrinolysis inhibitor (TAFI) becomes fully active and serves to diminish the incorporation and activation of plasminogen, leading to delayed clot lysis (Fig. 2).

TF-dependent generation of thrombin is rapidly inhibited by TF pathway inhibitor (TFPI), which binds TF/VIIa/Xa forming the quaternary complex TFPI/Xa/TF/VIIa, which is internalized by the TF-bearing cell. The main endogenous anticoagulant system is the protein C-dependent system. Protein C and its cofactor protein S are both vitamin K-dependent factors synthesized by the liver. Protein C binds to an endothelial cell protein C receptor (ECPR) and is activated by thrombin bound to thrombomodulin, another endothelial cell membrane-based protein [2]. The activated protein C complex inactivates factors VIIIa and Va (Fig. 2). Another important endogenous anticoagulant system involves antithrombin (AT), also primarily produced in the liver, which inactivates thrombin (IIa), factors Xa,

IXa, XIa and XIIa. The anticoagulant activity of AT can be increased by up to 1000-fold in the presence of heparin. Another vitamin K-dependent anticoagulant is protein Z, whose structure is similar to coagulation factors VII, IX, X, protein C and protein S. However, in contrast to these other vitamin K-dependent factors, protein Z is not a serine protease and plays an important role in inhibiting coagulation by serving as a cofactor for the inactivation of factor Xa by forming a complex with the plasma protein Z-dependent protease inhibitor. The role of alterations in the protein Z levels has been evaluated in different disease states, with conflicting findings [3]. Finally, to prevent excess clotting, fibrin is digested by the fibrinolytic system, the major components of which are plasminogen and tissue-type plasminogen activator (tPA) (Fig. 2). Both these proteins are incorporated into polymerizing fibrin, where they interact to generate plasmin, which in turn acts on fibrin to dissolve the preformed clot. Plasminogen binds to fibrin at specific lysine binding sites and to tPA. The binding of plasminogen to tPA converts the proenzyme plasminogen to active proteolytic plasmin. Plasmin cleaves polymerized fibrin strands at multiple sites and releases fibrin degradation products (FDPs) [3].

The fibrinolytic system is regulated by three serine proteinase inhibitors: alpha2-antiplasmin (α_2-PI), plasminogen activator inhibitor-1 (PAI-1) and plasminogen activator inhibitor-2 (PAI-2) (Fig. 2). α_2-PI is secreted by the liver, is present within platelets and serves to immediately inactivate free plasmin, whereas PAI-1 is the most important and most rapidly acting physiological inhibitor of both tPA and urokinase-type plasminogen activator (uPA). PAI-2, originally purified from human placenta, inhibits both two-chain tPA and two-chain uPA with comparable efficiency, but it is less effective towards single-chain tPA [4].

Role of the liver in the haemostatic system

The liver is the primary site of synthesis of most of the clotting factors and the proteins involved in the fibrinolytic system. These include all the vitamin K-dependent coagulation proteins (factors II, VII, IX, X, protein C, protein S and protein Z), as well as factor V, XIII, fibrinogen, antithrombin, α_2-PI and plasminogen. The notable exceptions are von Willebrand factor (VWF), tPA, thrombomodulin, TPFI and uPA. The VWF, tPA, thrombomodulin and TFPI are synthesized in endothelial cells, while uPA is expressed by endothelial cells, macrophages, renal epithelial cells and some tumour cells [4].

Vitamin K, a fat-soluble vitamin, is required to achieve proper levels of procoagulant factors (II, VII, IX and X) and anticoagulant factors (proteins C, S and Z). These factors require vitamin K as a cofactor for post-ribosomal modification to render them physiologically active. All the vitamin K-dependent factors have in their amino-terminal several glutamic acid residues that must be converted to gamma-carboxyglutamic acid residues. This process is crucial to allow these proteins to bind calcium ions to form bridges to phospholipid surfaces, which are essential for the formation of activation complexes [5]. Finally, the liver plays a vital role in the regulation of anticoagulation. Removal of activated clotting and fibrinolytic factors, especially tPA, is mediated through the hepatic reticuloendothelial system [6].

Haemostatic abnormalities in liver disease

Various haemostatic abnormalities can occur in patients with liver disease and, in general, the severity of these abnormalities is dependent on the degree of hepatic dysfunction (Table 1).

Coagulation defects in acute liver disease

Liver disease can cause both quantitative and qualitative abnormalities in coagulation factors. Commonly, the vitamin K-dependent factors decrease first, starting with factor VII and protein C owing to their short half-life (6 h), followed by reductions in factor II and X levels. Factor V levels are decreased in both acute and chronic liver disease [7]. Factor IX levels are usually only modestly reduced until advanced stages of liver disease. In contrast, VWF (synthesized by the endothelial cells) and factor VIII levels may be normal even in the presence of advanced liver disease because there is an increased production of factor VIII by the sinusoidal endothelial cells when the liver is damaged, combined with decreased clearance of the VWF/factor VIII complex.

Fibrinogen levels are rarely decreased and may even be elevated because of abnormal non-functional fibrinogen (dysfibrinogenaemia) related to defective polymerization. A decrease in fibrinogen levels may indicate the presence of

Table 1 Hemostatic changes in patients with liver disease.

Haemostatic abnormality	Mechanism
Hypocoagulability	Decreased synthesis of coagulation factors (except VIII and VWF)
	Hypofibrinogenaemia (endstage liver failure)
	Vitamin K deficiency (II, VII, IX, X)
	Decreased clearance of degraded coagulation factors
Hypercoagulability	Decreased synthesis of natural anticoagulant proteins antithrombin (AT), proteins C, S and Z
	Decreased clearance of activated coagulation factors
Dysfibrinogenaemia	Synthesis of abnormal fibrinogen
Hyperfibrinolysis	Increased levels of circulating tPA activity due to impaired hepatic clearance
	Decreased synthesis of fibrinolytic inhibitors (PAI-1 and α2-antiplasmin)
	Decreased thrombin-activatable fibrinolytic inhibitor (TAFI)
Quantitative and qualitative platelet defects:	Decreased bone marrow production (due to decreased thrombopoietin)
	Splenic sequestration
Thrombocytopenia	Immune-mediated platelet destruction
	Folate and vitamin B12 deficiencies
Thrombocytopathies	Direct effect of ethanol
	Non-specific platelet aggregation abnormalities

disseminated intravascular coagulation (DIC) or progression to fulminant hepatitis with hepatic failure.

In a study of patients with significant liver injury and associated coagulopathy, factors II, V, VII and X were reduced to a similar degree and were significantly lower than factors IX and XI [8]. Factor VIII, however, was increased as well as interleukin 6 (IL-6), tumour necrosis factor-alpha (TNFα), thrombin–antithrombin (TAT) and soluble TF levels [9]. Of note, all the decreased factor levels were directly activated by TF. In patients with acute fulminant hepatic failure, the haemostatic alterations are attributed to quantitative and qualitative platelet defects, impaired synthesis and clearance of the coagulation factors and related inhibitory proteins and enhanced fibrinolysis. DIC may also play a role; however, DIC is difficult to distinguish from changes resulting from impaired hepatic synthesis and clearance alone [10]. In a study of 42 patients with acute fulminant hepatic failure, the activities of plasminogen and its inhibitor α_2-PI were reduced while tPA activity was normal. PAI-1, however, was greatly increased, indicating a shift towards inhibition of fibrinolysis in these patients. TAT complex levels and D-dimer, a fragment of cross-linked fibrin in plasma, were also significantly increased, indicating activation of coagulation and fibrinolysis respectively. Thus, gross abnormalities of the fibrinolytic system occur in fulminant liver failure but, because inhibitory activity appears to be present in adequate quantities, this limits the incidence of bleeding due to fibrinolysis [11].

Coagulation defects in chronic liver disease

In patients with liver cirrhosis, most coagulation factors and inhibitors of the coagulation and fibrinolytic systems are markedly reduced because of impaired protein synthesis, except for factor VIII and fibrinogen levels, which may be normal or increased. Possible explanations for the increased factor VIII levels are the increased hepatic biosynthesis of VWF and decreased expression of low-density lipoprotein receptor-related protein, both of which modulate the level of factor VIII in plasma, rather than increase factor VIII synthesis [12]. Because fibrinogen is an acute-phase reactant, its synthesis tends to be preserved in patients with stable cirrhosis.

The deficiencies in vitamin K-dependent factors in cirrhosis may occur by several mechanisms, including reduced hepatic synthesis and reduced absorption of bile salts required for absorption of vitamin K-dependent factors, which may occur in the setting of cholestatic liver disease. Other contributing factors include poor oral intake and treatment with antibiotics that destroy the intestinal bacteria that synthesize vitamin K. As with acute liver disease, the reductions in coagulation factors parallel the degree of progression of liver disease.

In addition to impaired synthesis of clotting factors, excessive fibrinolysis, DIC, thrombocytopenia and platelet dysfunction account for the diverse spectrum of haemostatic defects in chronic or endstage liver disease [13] (Table 1).

The abnormalities of the fibrinolytic system are complex and result from impaired synthesis and altered clearance of the fibrinolytic factors. One of the most striking mechanisms is an imbalance between tPA and its specific inhibitor (PAI-1), which results in an increase in free tPA in the plasma and a reduction in α_2-PI. TAFI plays an important regulatory role in fibrinolysis. TAFI is a procarboxypeptidase synthesized by the liver and, upon activation by thrombin or plasmin, TAFI is converted into TAFIa. TAFIa inhibits fibrinolysis by removing C-terminal lysines from partially degraded fibrin, causing a decrease in the cofactor function of fibrin in the plasminogen activation catalysed by tPA, resulting in decreased plasmin generation [14,15]. Thrombin is the most likely activator of TAFI and, when thrombin is complexed to thrombomodulin, TAFI activation is increased by more than 1000-fold [16]. The levels of TAFI are markedly reduced in cirrhotic patients and correlate with the severity of disease [16,17].

In addition to the reduced hepatic synthesis of clotting factors, cirrhotic patients also have a significant deficit of natural anticoagulants, particularly protein C and antithrombin [18]. Activated protein C (APC), is the main anticoagulant that, in combination with its cofactor protein S, downregulates thrombin generation *in vivo* by inhibiting the action of the cofactors factors Va and VIIIa. AT complexed to endothelial heparin-like substances inhibits thrombin (factor IIa) directly through the formation of an equimolar complex and indirectly through the inhibition of the serine proteases (factors IX, X, XI and XII). Thrombin formation is also downregulated by the TFPI, which specifically inhibits the complex of TF and VIIa [1].

Recent studies have indicated that standard coagulation tests such as prothrombin time (PT) and activated partial thromboplastin time (aPTT) may not reflect the true coagulation status of patients with liver cirrhosis. This is because these tests do not take into account the activation of the primary endogenous anticoagulant protein C, levels of which are considerably reduced in cirrhosis. Tripodi *et al.* [19] reported impairment of thrombin generation measured without thrombomodulin, consistent with the reduced levels of procoagulant factors typically seen in cirrhosis. However, when the test was modified by adding thrombomodulin, patients generated as much thrombin as control subjects. The authors concluded that thrombin generation is normal in cirrhosis and that the reduction in procoagulant factors in these patients is compensated for by the reduction in anticoagulant factors, thus leaving the coagulation balance unaltered. Furthermore, their findings suggest that measurement of thrombin generation in the presence of thrombomodulin may be more suitable for the evaluation of bleeding risk [19].

Thrombocytopenia

Patients with liver disease may develop quantitative (thrombocytopenia) and/or qualitative platelet abnormalities (thrombocytopathies) such as impaired platelet adhesion and aggregation. The aetiology of thrombocytopenia in these patients is often attributed to splenic sequestration (hypersplenism), but may also occur as a result of platelet destruction mediated by platelet-associated immunoglobulins (PAIgG) [20] and impaired hepatic synthesis and/or increased degradation of thrombopoietin (TPO) by platelets sequestered in the congested spleen [21].

Mild to moderate thrombocytopenia occurs in 16–52% of patients with acute hepatitis with or without cirrhosis. Severe thrombocytopenia can occur as a consequence of aplastic anaemia, a rare complication of acute hepatitis [22]. Idiopathic immune thrombocytopenia (ITP) has also been reported in patients with hepatitis C [23]. Cocaine may cause thrombotic thrombocytopenic purpura associated with toxic acute hepatitis [24]. Ethanol directly suppresses platelet formation and decreases the lifespan of platelets, both of which contribute to thrombocytopenia commonly seen with alcohol-related liver disease [25]. Other aetiologies including medications, folate and vitamin B12 deficiencies, severe infections and DIC should also be considered in evaluating thrombocytopenia in patients with liver disease within the appropriate clinical setting.

Thrombocytopenia is a more common feature of chronic liver disease and has been reported in 49–64% of cirrhotic patients [26]. The primary mechanism for thrombocytopenia is thought to be due to hypersplenism secondary to portal hypertension, which results in increased platelet sequestration and destruction. There is also increased destruction of platelets by immunological mechanisms that result from increased PAIgG. Increased levels of PAIgG have been reported in 55–88% of patients with chronic liver disease [20,27]. The elevated levels of PAIgG correlate inversely with the platelet count in some [20,28], but not all studies [27]. Recently, diminished protein synthesis in the liver has been reported to cause inadequate synthesis of TPO [29]. TPO is a glycoprotein produced primarily in the liver that acts to increase the basal production rate of megakaryocytes and platelets. TPO levels are significantly lower in cirrhotic patients with thrombocytopenia than in those with normal platelet counts. Serum TPO levels correlate inversely with the severity of liver disease [30,31]. Finally, platelet counts post liver transplantation also correlate with TPO levels, regardless of splenic size [32].

Intravascular activation and increased consumption of platelets in the diseased liver as a result of low-grade DIC is also a possible but controversial mechanism of thrombocytopenia. In patients with alcohol-induced cirrhosis, the thrombocytopenia may result from folate deficiency, direct toxic effects of ethanol on megakaryocytopoiesis [33,34] and increased platelet activation [35].

Platelet function abnormalities

In patients with chronic liver disease, impaired platelet aggregation with different agonists including adenosine diphosphate (ADP), thrombin, epinephrine and ristocetin has been described [36]. The abnormal platelet aggregation is thought to be caused by circulating platelet inhibitors (fibrin degradation products and D-dimers), plasmin degradation of platelet receptors, dysfibrinogenaemia and excess nitric oxide synthesis [13,37]. Conversely, hyper-responsiveness rather than a defective platelet/VWF interaction is observed in cirrhosis, which may compensate for other haemostatic problems; this appears to be mediated primarily by increased VWF levels [38]. The platelet function defects may account for the prolongation of the bleeding time in 40% of patients with cirrhosis and correlates with disease severity [39,40]. Erythropoietin is the primary stimulus to erythrocyte production and also induces megakaryocyte formation. Treatment with erythropoietin significantly increases platelet counts and platelet function in patients with alcoholic liver cirrhosis [41].

Disseminated intravascular coagulation

Low-grade DIC is commonly found in patients with endstage liver disease (ESLD). This syndrome is typically characterized by thrombocytopenia, prolongation of the PT and aPTT, decreased fibrinogen and elevated levels of fibrin degradation products (FDPs). Additionally, elevated levels of prothrombin activation

fragment F1 + 2, fibrinopeptide A, D-dimer and TAT complexes are also observed in varying degrees [42–44]. The frequency and severity of DIC tends to correlate with the stage of liver disease [13,42,44,45].

The aetiology of DIC in chronic liver disease is multifactorial and includes release of procoagulants from injured hepatocytes, impaired clearance of activated clotting factors, decreased synthesis of coagulation inhibitors and endotoxin entry into the portal circulation [13].

The diagnosis of DIC in patients with chronic or endstage liver disease is often difficult and challenging, as the coagulation defects in both disorders are quite similar. Typically, an elevated D-dimer is more specific for DIC as it indicates activation of both coagulation and fibrinolysis, whereas high levels of fibrinogen degradation products (FDP) or dysfunctional fibrinogen are more common in ESLD [46]. Importantly, decreasing levels of factor VIII and fibrinogen with an increased D-dimer level on serial testing is more characteristic of DIC.

Clinically significant DIC is uncommon in patients with liver disease, usually complicates severe bacterial infections or severe sepsis and can also develop in patients with peritoneovenous shunts [47].

Haemostatic changes in liver transplant

Complex coagulation disorders may occur during liver transplantation including preoperative coagulation abnormalities due to the underlying liver disease and haemostatic changes related to the transplantation, all of which may contribute to severe bleeding. Prior to the anhepatic phase, there are usually no serious haemostatic alterations. Bleeding during transplantation is greatly influenced by the activation of the fibrinolytic system, which occurs during the anhepatic and reperfusion phases. The hyperfibrinolysis is mediated by an intense release of tPA and a lack of hepatic clearance during the neohepatic period. A second fibrinolytic burst results from release of tPA by the endothelial cells of the revascularized graft [48]. Conversely, PAI-1 decreases during the anhepatic period and increases during the neohepatic period [49]. A preserved capacity to generate thrombin and less fibrinolytic activation during the anhepatic phase occurs in primary biliary cirrhosis compared with other types of cirrhosis [50].

Factors that influence the risk of bleeding during liver surgery also include the presence of cirrhosis, portal hypertension, high levels of central venous pressure, renal dysfunction and the length of graft preservation [49]. A hypercoagulable state has occasionally been reported in some patients with neoplasm or Budd–Chiari syndrome [45,51]. Platelet count decreases during liver transplantation with a nadir at the time of reperfusion, and may worsen in the case of a damaged organ graft. It has been suggested that the transplanted liver has a major role in the thrombocytopenia with intrahepatic platelet sequestration, local thrombin generation on the damaged graft endothelium,

Laboratory abnormality	Haemostatic defect
Prolonged PT and normal aPTT	PT corrects with mixing studies → factor VII deficiency
Prolonged PT and aPTT	PT and aPTT correct with mixing studies → factors I, II, V, X deficiencies
Prolonged thrombin time (TT) and reptilase time (RT)	Dysfibrinogenaemia
Shortened euglobulin lysis time	Decreased PAI-1, decreased α_2-PI, increased tPA (during liver transplant)
Thrombocytopenia (verified by manual interpretation of the peripheral blood smear)	Platelet sequestration Immune-mediated thrombocytopenia Decreased synthesis of thrombopoietin
Prolonged bleeding time/abnormal platelet aggregation studies	Thrombocytopathies
Marked increase in D-dimer, low fibrinogen and normal factor VIII	Possible DIC (in the proper clinical setting)

Table 2 Laboratory features of coagulopathy of liver disease.

platelet extravasation and increased phagocytosis by the Kupffer cells as potential mechanisms. Platelet function abnormalities have also been described after revascularization, whereby hypothermia enhances splanchnic platelet dysfunction and prolongs coagulation reaction time by reducing enzymatic activity [52]. Release of exogenous heparin from the harvested graft after donor heparinization or endogenous heparin-like substances from the damaged ischaemic graft endothelium may also play a role in the coagulopathy at reperfusion [53]. Haemodilution secondary to fluid replacement and the preservation solution from the donor liver can additionally reduce plasma levels of coagulation factors at reperfusion [54].

Laboratory testing for coagulation defects in liver disease

Initial standard screening tests in patients with liver disease should include a PT, aPTT, complete blood count with examination of the peripheral blood smear and a fibrinogen level. In selected patients, additional testing should include a D-dimer test, thrombin time (TT), reptilase time (RT), euglobulin clot lysis time and a bleeding time (Table 2).

Often, the clotting tests remain normal until clotting factor levels fall to less than 30–40% of normal. In mild liver disease, the PT is prolonged, but the aPTT is usually normal. As the liver disease progresses, both PT and aPTT levels are prolonged, although in compensated cirrhosis, the high factor VIII level may blunt the prolongation of the aPTT. It is important to note, however, that international normalized ratio (INR) values may not be accurately reflective of the coagulopathy in patients with ESLD [55].

Fibrinogen levels are either normal or increased in patients with stable chronic liver disease.

In decompensated cirrhosis or DIC, severe hypofibrino-

genaemia (< 100 mg/dL) is present, resulting in marked prolongation of the PT, aPTT and TT. Functional abnormalities of fibrinogen or dysfibrinogenaemias are diagnosed by a prolongation of the TT and RT.

Therapy for haemostatic abnormalities in liver disease

The management of haemostatic abnormalities in patients with liver disease is often difficult and challenging. Therapy is directed at correction of haemostatic defects in patients who are actively bleeding or who require surgery or other invasive procedures. Additionally, therapy should be targeted to the type of procedure and site and severity of bleeding. The bleeding risk appears to be higher in patients with multiple haemostatic defects, renal failure or a previous history of bleeding.

Vitamin K

Vitamin K deficiency in patients with severe acute liver disease may be treated with one dose of 10 mg of vitamin K administered intravenously (i.v.) [56]. In patients whose prolonged PT does not completely correct with vitamin K therapy, impaired hepatic synthesis of coagulation factors from parenchymal liver disease must be suspected as the cause of the coagulopathy. Other patient subgroups in whom vitamin K may be useful include patients with primary biliary cirrhosis and those with chronic liver disease who are receiving broad-spectrum antibiotics and have poor nutritional intake [57].

Plasma

Fresh frozen plasma (FFP) is prepared from units of whole blood and from plasmapheresis. Plasma contains all the coagulation factors. Transfusion of FFP is the main therapy for patients with liver disease and coagulopathy who are actively bleeding [58]. However, the response to FFP is unpredictable. The use of FFP for the correction of moderate to severe coagulopathy prior to invasive procedures, e.g. percutaneous liver biopsy, is controversial and more studies are needed [59]. In general, it is recommended that, if the PT is prolonged by < 4 seconds, percutaneous biopsy can be undertaken safely. If the PT is prolonged by 4–6 seconds, FFP transfusion may allow the PT to decrease to the desired range. However, if the PT is prolonged by > 6 seconds, other biopsy techniques may need to be considered [60]. The recommended dose of FFP is 10–15 mL/kg. In the majority of patients with chronic liver disease, repeated transfusions of FFP every 12 h may be required for complete correction of the PT. There is currently no consensus on the volume of FFP or type of infusion regimens required to prevent or treat bleeding [13,59]. If FFP is given, repeat coagulation tests should be performed as soon as the infusion is completed to guide further management [59]. Potential adverse effects of FFP include volume overload, transmission of bloodborne infections, transfusion-related acute lung injury (TRALI) and allergic, febrile or haemolytic reactions.

Cryoprecipitate

Cryoprecipitate is prepared from FFP and is rich in fibrinogen, factor VIII, VWF, factor XIII and fibronectin. Each bag of cryoprecipitate contains 80–100 IU/mL factor VIII and at least 140 mg of fibrinogen [59]. Cryoprecipitate is indicated in patients with severe coagulopathy and hypofibrinogenaemia (< 100 mg/dL) or dysfibrinogenaemia.

DDAVP

Deamino-8-D-arginine vasopressin (desmopressin acetate or DDAVP) is a synthetic analogue of antidiuretic hormone, which raises the plasma levels of factor VIII and VWF and enhances platelet adhesion to the vessel wall. The agent is usually administered at a dose of 0.3 µg/kg by i.v. infusion over 20–30 min. In patients with liver cirrhosis, DDAVP may be used to shorten or normalize the prolonged bleeding time in those who need invasive procedures [61]. However, in two randomized trials, DDAVP did not reduce intraoperative blood loss and transfusion requirements in patients undergoing hepatectomy or control bleeding in cirrhotic patients with acute variceal bleeding [62,63].

Platelets

Platelet transfusions are indicated in patients with liver disease who are actively bleeding and have a platelet count below 50 000/µL or known history of platelet dysfunction. Prophylactic platelet transfusions may be necessary before invasive procedures (e.g. percutaneous liver biopsy) in patients with platelet counts < 50 000/µL [64]. A 1-h post-transfusion platelet count is commonly used to determine the efficacy of platelet transfusion and to guide subsequent therapy. Patients with marked splenomegaly, however, may not respond with an increase in platelet count after transfusion because of increased sequestration of the transfused platelets. Failure to increase the platelet count after transfusion may also be observed in patients with DIC, severe infection and alloimmunization due to platelet-specific and/or human leukocyte antigen (HLA) antibodies [13].

Antifibrinolytic agents

Epsilon aminocaproic acid, tranexamic acid and aprotinin are antifibrinolytic agents that inhibit plasmin generation and have been demonstrated to decrease bleeding associated with fibrinolysis in chronic liver disease [65] and intraoperative blood loss and transfusion requirements during liver transplantation [66–68]. These agents are contraindicated in patients with DIC and must only be used in selected patients with bleeding caused by excessive fibrinolysis.

Recombinant factor VIIa (rFVIIa)

Recombinant activated factor VII (rFVIIa) is a genetically engineered concentrate of human coagulation factor VIIa, which is structurally similar to native human plasma-derived factor VIIa. By enhancing thrombin generation on activated platelets, rFVIIa promotes the formation of a stable fibrin clot that is resistant to premature lysis [69]. This agent is Food and Drug Administration (FDA) approved for the treatment of haemophilia A and B patients with inhibitors against factors VIII and IX. Limited studies have shown correction of coagulopathy and decreased bleeding with the use of rFVIIa in patients with acute and chronic hepatic failure [70]. In these studies, rFVIIa was administered at doses ranging from 5 to 80 mg/kg i.v. for at least two doses [71–73]. Further studies are needed to identify the optimal dosing and confirm the safety, efficacy and cost–benefit of rFVIIa in patients with liver disease. Similarly, rFVIIa has been used to control bleeding associated with coagulopathy in patients undergoing orthotopic liver transplantation, including Jehovah's Witness patients [74]. Caution should be undertaken in administering rFVIIa to patients with DIC, coronary artery disease and severe sepsis because of their higher risk of thrombosis [75,76].

Thrombopoietin

TPO is a relatively lineage-specific cytokine that stimulates megakaryocyte growth and maturation *in vitro* and is a potent *in vivo* thrombopoietic growth factor. This cytokine may be potentially useful for reducing bleeding in patients with thrombocytopenia due to liver disease or preparing these patients for liver transplantation [77], although it is not FDA approved to date.

Conclusions

The liver plays a crucial role in haemostasis as it is responsible for the synthesis of most of the clotting and fibrinolytic proteins and the clearance of these coagulation factors from the circulation. Acute and chronic liver diseases are associated with a spectrum of haemostatic defects, and their severity tends to parallel the degree of hepatic injury. The aetiology of impaired haemostasis due to liver disease is multifactorial and includes impaired synthesis of coagulation factors, vitamin K deficiency, altered clearance of activated coagulation factors, excessive fibrinolysis, DIC and quantitative and qualitative platelet disorders. Standard laboratory testing should be supplemented with more specific tests of activation of the coagulation and fibrinolytic systems. The management of symptomatic haemostatic changes in patients with liver disease requires a multidisciplinary approach directed at correction of the haemostatic defects in patients who are actively bleeding or who require surgery or other invasive procedures.

References

1 Rosenberg RD, Aird WC (1999) Vascular-bed-specific hemostasis and hypercoagulable states. *N Engl J Med* 340(20), 1555–1564.

2 Esmon CT (2003) The protein C pathway. *Chest* 124(3 Suppl), 26S–32S.

3 Sofi F, Cesari F, Fedi S *et al.* (2004) Protein Z: 'light and shade' of a new thrombotic factor. *Clin Lab* 50(11–12), 647–652.

4 Cesarman-Maus G, Hajjar KA (2005) Molecular mechanisms of fibrinolysis. *Br J Haematol* 129(3), 307–321.

5 Borowski M, Furie BC, Bauminger S *et al.* (1986) Prothrombin requires two sequential metal-dependent conformational transitions to bind phospholipid. conformation-specific antibodies directed against the phospholipid-binding site on prothrombin. *J Biol Chem* 261(32), 14969–14975.

6 Greenberg DL, Davie EW (2001) Blood coagulation factors: their complimentary DNA, genes and expression. In: Coluan RW, Hirsh J, Marder VJ, Clower AW, George JN (eds) *Hemostasis and Thrombosis: Basic Principles and Clinical Practice*. Philadelphia, PA: Lippincott Williams and Wilkins, pp. 21–57.

7 Mammen EF (1994) Coagulation defects in liver disease. *Med Clin North Am* 78(3), 545–554.

8 Kerr R (2003) New insights into haemostasis in liver failure. *Blood Coagul Fibrinolysis* 14(Suppl 1), S43–45.

9 Kerr R, Newsome P, Germain L *et al.* (2003) Effects of acute liver injury on blood coagulation. *J Thromb Haemost* 1(4), 754–759.

10 Pereira SP, Langley PG, Williams R (1996) The management of abnormalities of hemostasis in acute liver failure. *Semin Liver Dis* 16(4), 403–414.

11 Pernambuco JR, Langley PG, Hughes RD *et al.* (1993) Activation of the fibrinolytic system in patients with fulminant liver failure. *Hepatology* 18(6), 1350–1356.

12 Hollestelle MJ, Geertzen HG, Straatsburg IH *et al.* (2004) Factor VIII expression in liver disease. *Thromb Haemost* 91(2), 267–275.

13 Kujovich JL (2005) Hemostatic defects in end stage liver disease. *Crit Care Clin* 21(3), 563–587.

14 Wang W, Boffa MB, Bajzar L *et al.* (1998) A study of the mechanism of inhibition of fibrinolysis by activated thrombin-activatable fibrinolysis inhibitor. *J Biol Chem* 273(42), 27176–27181.

15 Nesheim M, Bajzar L (2005) The discovery of TAFI. *J Thromb Haemost* 3(10), 2139–2146.

16 Colucci M, Binetti BM, Branca MG *et al.* (2003) Deficiency of thrombin activatable fibrinolysis inhibitor in cirrhosis is associated with increased plasma fibrinolysis. *Hepatology* 38(1), 230–237.

17 Van Thiel DH, George M, Fareed J (2001) Low levels of thrombin activatable fibrinolysis inhibitor (TAFI) in patients with chronic liver disease. *Thromb Haemost* 85(4), 667–670.

18 Castelino DJ, Salem HH (1997) Natural anticoagulants and the liver. *J Gastroenterol Hepatol* 12(1), 77–83.

19 Tripodi A, Salerno F, Chantarangkul V *et al.* (2005) Evidence of normal thrombin generation in cirrhosis despite abnormal conventional coagulation tests. *Hepatology* 41(3), 553–558.

20 Sanjo A, Satoi J, Ohnishi A *et al.* (2003) Role of elevated platelet-associated immunoglobulin G and hypersplenism in thrombocytopenia of chronic liver diseases. *J Gastroenterol Hepatol* 18(6), 638–644.

21 Rios R, Sangro B, Herrero I *et al.* (2005) The role of thrombopoietin in the thrombocytopenia of patients with liver cirrhosis. *Am J Gastroenterol* 100(6), 1311–1316.

22 Zeldis JB, Dienstag JL, Gale RP (1983) Aplastic anemia and non-A, non-B hepatitis. *Am J Med* 74(1), 64–68.

23 Narita R, Asaumi H, Abe S *et al.* (2003) Idiopathic thrombocytopenic purpura with acute hepatitis C viral infection. *J Gastroenterol Hepatol* 18(4), 462–463.

24 Balaguer F, Fernandez J, Lozano M *et al.* (2005) Cocaine-induced acute hepatitis and thrombotic microangiopathy. *JAMA* 293(7), 797–798.

25 Scharf RE, Aul C (1988) Alcohol-induced disorders of the hematopoietic system. *Z Gastroenterol* 26 (Suppl 3), 75–83.

26 Bashour FN, Teran JC, Mullen KD (2000) Prevalence of peripheral blood cytopenias (hypersplenism) in patients with nonalcoholic chronic liver disease. *Am J Gastroenterol* 95(10), 2936–2939.

27 Pereira J, Accatino L, Alfaro J *et al.* (1995) Platelet autoantibodies in patients with chronic liver disease. *Am J Hematol* 50(3), 173–178.

28 Nagamine T, Ohtuka T, Takehara K *et al.* (1996) Thrombocytopenia associated with hepatitis C viral infection. *J Hepatol* 24(2), 135–140.

29 Panasiuk A, Prokopowicz D, Zak J *et al.* (2004) Reticulated platelets as a marker of megakaryopoiesis in liver cirrhosis; relation to thrombopoietin and hepatocyte growth factor serum concentration. *Hepatogastroenterology* 51(58), 1124–1128.

30 Ishikawa T, Ichida T, Sugahara S *et al.* (2002) Thrombopoietin receptor (c-mpl) is constitutively expressed on platelets of patients with liver cirrhosis, and correlates with its disease progression. *Hepatol Res* 23(2), 115–121.

31 Giannini E, Botta F, Borro P *et al.* (2003) Relationship between thrombopoietin serum levels and liver function in patients with chronic liver disease related to hepatitis C virus infection. *Am J Gastroenterol* 98(11), 2516–2520.

32 Goulis J, Chau TN, Jordan S *et al.* (1999) Thrombopoietin concentrations are low in patients with cirrhosis and thrombocytopenia and are restored after orthotopic liver transplantation. *Gut* 44(5), 754–758.

33 Peltz S (1991) Severe thrombocytopenia secondary to alcohol use. *Postgrad Med* 89(6), 75–76, 85.

34 Levine RF, Spivak JL, Meagher RC *et al.* (1986) Effect of ethanol on thrombopoiesis. *Br J Haematol* 62(2), 345–354.

35 Ogasawara F, Fusegawa H, Haruki Y *et al.* (2005) Platelet activation in patients with alcoholic liver disease. *Tokai J Exp Clin Med* 30(1), 41–48.

36 Thomas DP, Ream VJ, Stuart RK (1967) Platelet aggregation in

patients with Laennec's cirrhosis of the liver. *N Engl J Med* 276(24), 1344–1348.

37 Albornoz L, Bandi JC, Otaso JC *et al.* (1999) Prolonged bleeding time in experimental cirrhosis: role of nitric oxide. *J Hepatol* 30(3), 456–460.

38 Beer JH, Clerici N, Baillod P *et al.* (1995) Quantitative and qualitative analysis of platelet GPIb and von Willebrand factor in liver cirrhosis. *Thromb Haemost* 73(4), 601–609.

39 Blake JC, Sprengers D, Grech P *et al.* (1990) Bleeding time in patients with hepatic cirrhosis. *Br Med J* 301(6742), 12–15.

40 Hsu WC, Lee FY, Lee SD *et al.* (1994) Prolonged bleeding time in cirrhotic patients: relationship to peripheral vasodilation and severity of cirrhosis. *J Gastroenterol Hepatol* 9(5), 437–441.

41 Homoncik M, Jilma-Stohlawetz P, Schmid M *et al.* (2004) Erythropoietin increases platelet reactivity and platelet counts in patients with alcoholic liver cirrhosis: a randomized, double-blind, placebo-controlled study. *Aliment Pharmacol Ther* 20(4), 437–443.

42 Vukovich T, Teufelsbauer H, Fritzer M *et al.* (1995) Hemostasis activation in patients with liver cirrhosis. *Thromb Res* 77(3), 271–278.

43 Bakker CM, Knot EA, Stibbe J *et al.* (1992) Disseminated intravascular coagulation in liver cirrhosis. *J Hepatol* 15(3), 330–335.

44 Violi F, Ferro D, Basili S *et al.* (1995) Prognostic value of clotting and fibrinolytic systems in a follow-up of 165 liver cirrhotic patients. CALC group. *Hepatology* 22(1), 96–100.

45 Kemkes-Matthes B, Bleyl H, Matthes KJ (1991) Coagulation activation in liver diseases. *Thromb Res* 64(2), 253–261.

46 Carr JM (1989) Disseminated intravascular coagulation in cirrhosis. *Hepatology* 10(1), 103–110.

47 Harmon DC, Demirjian Z, Ellman L *et al.* (1979) Disseminated intravascular coagulation with the peritoneovenous shunt. *Ann Intern Med* 90(5), 774–776.

48 Porte RJ, Knot EA, Bontempo FA (1989) Hemostasis in liver transplantation. *Gastroenterology* 97(2), 488–501.

49 Ozier Y, Steib A, Ickx B *et al.* (2001) Haemostatic disorders during liver transplantation. *Eur J Anaesthesiol* 18(4), 208–218.

50 Segal H, Cottam S, Potter D *et al.* (1997) Coagulation and fibrinolysis in primary biliary cirrhosis compared with other liver disease and during orthotopic liver transplantation. *Hepatology* 25(3), 683–688.

51 Lewis JH, Bontempo FA, Awad SA *et al.* (1989) Liver transplantation: intraoperative changes in coagulation factors in 100 first transplants. *Hepatology* 9(5), 710–714.

52 Himmelreich G, Hundt K, Neuhaus P *et al.* (1992) Decreased platelet aggregation after reperfusion in orthotopic liver transplantation. *Transplantation* 53(3), 582–586.

53 Bayly PJ, Thick M (1994) Reversal of post-reperfusion coagulopathy by protamine sulphate in orthotopic liver transplantation. *Br J Anaesth* 73(6), 840–842.

54 Rohrer MJ, Natale AM (1992) Effect of hypothermia on the coagulation cascade. *Crit Care Med* 20(10), 1402–1405.

55 Robert A, Chazouilleres O (1996) Prothrombin time in liver failure: time, ratio, activity percentage, or international normalized ratio? *Hepatology* 24(6), 1392–1394.

56 Pereira SP, Rowbotham D, Fitt S *et al.* (2005) Pharmacokinetics and efficacy of oral versus intravenous mixed-micellar phylloquinone (vitamin K1) in severe acute liver disease. *J Hepatol* 42(3), 365–370.

57 Sallah S, Bobzien W (1999) Bleeding problems in patients with liver disease. Ways to manage the many hepatic effects on coagulation. *Postgrad Med* 106(4), 187–190, 193–195.

58 Kaul VV, Munoz SJ (2000) Coagulopathy of liver disease. *Curr Treat Options Gastroenterol* 3(6), 433–438.

59 O'Shaughnessy DF, Atterbury C, Bolton Maggs P *et al.* (2004) Guidelines for the use of fresh-frozen plasma, cryoprecipitate and cryosupernatant. *Br J Haematol* 126(1), 11–28.

60 Grant A, Neuberger J (1999) Guidelines on the use of liver biopsy in clinical practice. British Society of Gastroenterology. *Gut* 45(Suppl 4), IV1–IV11.

61 Mannucci PM (2000) Desmopressin (DDAVP) in the treatment of bleeding disorders: the first twenty years. *Haemophilia* 6(Suppl 1), 60–67.

62 de Franchis R, Arcidiacono PG, Carpinelli L *et al.* (1993) Randomized controlled trial of desmopressin plus terlipressin vs. terlipressin alone for the treatment of acute variceal hemorrhage in cirrhotic patients: a multicenter, double-blind study, new Italian endoscopic club. *Hepatology* 18(5), 1102–1107.

63 Wong AY, Irwin MG, Hui TW *et al.* (2003) Desmopressin does not decrease blood loss and transfusion requirements in patients undergoing hepatectomy. *Can J Anaesth* 50(1), 14–20.

64 Sue M, Caldwell SH, Dickson RC *et al.* (1996) Variation between centers in technique and guidelines for liver biopsy. *Liver* 16(4), 267–270.

65 Hu KQ, Yu AS, Tiyyagura L *et al.* (2001) Hyperfibrinolytic activity in hospitalized cirrhotic patients in a referral liver unit. *Am J Gastroenterol* 96(5), 1581–1586.

66 Kahl BS, Schwartz BS, Mosher DF (2003) Profound imbalance of pro-fibrinolytic and anti-fibrinolytic factors (tissue plasminogen activator and plasminogen activator inhibitor type 1) and severe bleeding diathesis in a patient with cirrhosis: correction by liver transplantation. *Blood Coagul Fibrinolysis* 14(8), 741–744.

67 Boylan JF, Klinck JR, Sandler AN *et al.* (1996) Tranexamic acid reduces blood loss, transfusion requirements, and coagulation factor use in primary orthotopic liver transplantation. *Anesthesiology* 85(5), 1043–1048; discussion 30A–31A.

68 Neuhaus P, Bechstein WO, Lefebre B *et al.* (1989) Effect of aprotinin on intraoperative bleeding and fibrinolysis in liver transplantation. *Lancet* 2(8668), 924–925.

69 Hedner U (2004) Dosing with recombinant factor VIIa based on current evidence. *Semin Hematol* 41(1 Suppl 1), 35–39.

70 Ejlersen E, Melsen T, Ingerslev J *et al.* (2001) Recombinant activated factor VII (rFVIIa) acutely normalizes prothrombin time in patients with cirrhosis during bleeding from oesophageal varices. *Scand J Gastroenterol* 36(10), 1081–1085.

71 Shami VM, Caldwell SH, Hespenheide EE *et al.* (2003) Recombinant activated factor VII for coagulopathy in fulminant hepatic failure compared with conventional therapy. *Liver Transpl* 9(2), 138–143.

72 Pavese P, Bonadona A, Beaubien J *et al.* (2005) FVIIa corrects the coagulopathy of fulminant hepatic failure but may be associated with thrombosis: a report of four cases. *Can J Anaesth* 52(1), 26–29.

73 Bosch J, Thabut D, Bendtsen F *et al.* (2004) Recombinant factor VIIa for upper gastrointestinal bleeding in patients with cirrhosis: a randomized, double-blind trial. *Gastroenterology* 127(4), 1123–1130.

74 Jabbour N, Gagandeep S, Peilin AC *et al.* (2005) Recombinant human coagulation factor VIIa in Jehovah's Witness patients undergoing liver transplantation. *Am Surg* 71(2), 175–179.

75 O'Connell KA, Wood JJ, Wise RP *et al.* (2006) Thromboembolic adverse events after use of recombinant human coagulation factor VIIa. *JAMA* 295(3), 293–298.

76 Ramsey G (2006) Treating coagulopathy in liver disease with plasma transfusions or recombinant factor VIIa: an evidence-based review. *Best Pract Res Clin Haematol* 19(1), 113–126.

77 Kuter DJ, Begley CG (2002) Recombinant human thrombopoietin: basic biology and evaluation of clinical studies. *Blood* 100(10), 3457–3469.

2.4.3 Function and metabolism of collagen and other extracellular matrix proteins

Rebecca G. Wells

Introduction

The extracellular matrix (ECM) occupies a small percentage of the volume of the normal liver, yet plays a disproportionately important role in liver function in health and disease. ECM proteins are both signalling molecules and architectural elements of the liver and are responsible for maintaining the differentiated state of normal hepatocytes and non-parenchymal cells. In liver fibrosis and cirrhosis, there are changes in the distribution, quantity and relative proportions of collagens and other ECM proteins (Fig. 1); these result in altered cell phenotypes, architectural distortion with abnormal blood flow, impaired diffusion and altered cell signalling.

ECM proteins in the normal liver

The normal liver encompasses physically separate regions with different matrix and cellular compositions. The matrix in the capsule and surrounding the bile ducts and central venous region is similar to that in other epithelial organs, with an organized basement membrane of collagen IV, laminin, entactin and perlecan. The interstitium of the portal space contains the fibrillar collagens I, III and V as well as collagen VI and fibronectin [1].

The space of Disse, which lies in between sinusoidal endothelial cells (SEC) and hepatocytes, has a matrix unique in the liver and the body. This narrow space, less than 1 μM wide, lacks the continuous laminin, perlecan and entactin that are found in most basement membranes [2]. Although collagen IV is present, it is in discrete discontinuous deposits not associated with laminin or perlecan. Fibronectin is abundant, applied closely to the microvilli of hepatocytes. Collagens III and VI are also found in the space of Disse, collagen III in discontinuous deposits and collagen VI arranged relatively homogeneously, increasing from the portal to the central region [3]. Structure is provided by

a continuous network of thick collagen I cables, which extend into the lobular areas from the adjacent portal tracts [1]. This unusual matrix is essential for maintaining the differentiation of hepatocytes and SEC as well as other non-parenchymal cells [4]. Gradients of matrix material are found in the sinusoids and may have functional relevance, resulting in phenotypical differences between cells in the periportal vs. central regions [1,5].

ECM proteins in the fibrotic liver

Fibrosis results in a nearly 10-fold increase in the expression of matrix proteins in the liver. The most impressive change is the capillarization of the sinusoids, in which the sparse, atypical matrix of the space of Disse is replaced by a complete and continuous basement membrane, with accompanying loss of fenestration of the sinusoidal endothelium. This process begins with an increase in cellular isoforms of fibronectin in the space of Disse, followed by increases in collagens I, III and IV and the appearance of laminin. As fibrosis progresses, portal to central gradients are lost, and the new matrix becomes continuous [6] (see also Chapters 4.1 and 6.1). This results in loss of the differentiated phenotype of the resident cells of the space of Disse, in particular SEC, hepatocytes and hepatic stellate cells (HSC). Additionally, the increased ECM impairs the normal exchange of soluble proteins and fluids between sinusoidal blood and adjacent liver cells.

When fibrosis advances to cirrhosis, the normal architecture of the liver is lost with the formation of increasingly dense fibrous septae of fibronectin and collagens I, III, V and VI. These bands of matrix may become progressively stabilized (for example through collagen cross-linking) and protease resistant, impeding remodelling and the resolution of cirrhosis.

Structure and key features of specific ECM proteins

The ECM and its individual components are multifunctional. They have architectural and barrier functions, regulate growth factors and are themselves signalling molecules (Table 1). There are multiple complex interactions between different matrix components, making it difficult to understand the function of individual proteins. A variety of related mesenchymal cells in the liver synthesize normal and pathological matrix, suggesting that fibrosis is best understood as a generalized process rather than one limited to specific ECM molecules or specific fibrogenic cells such as HSC (see also Chapters 6.1 and 6.2).

Fig. 1 (*opposite*) Distribution of major matrix components in normal and fibrotic liver. A liver acinus is shown graphically to demonstrate changes in extracellular matrix (ECM) distribution in normal and diseased liver. Note that continuity between portal, parenchymal and central structures is not shown due to controversy regarding their relative anatomy. The size of the space of Disse compared with the sinusoidal space is greatly exaggerated, particularly in the normal liver. The interrelationship between different ECM components is not well understood and is shown only schematically. The organized basement membrane shown contains collagens VIII, XIX, XV, XIV and XVIII in addition to collagen IV, laminin, perlecan, and entactin. Proteoglycans other than perlecan are not shown. PV, portal vein; CV, central vein; HA, hepatic artery; SC, hepatic stellate cell; EC, sinusoidal endothelial cell; PF, portal fibroblast; SD, space of Disse; BD, bile duct; H, hepatocyte; TS, thick, organized septa; S, sinusoid; P, portal tract.

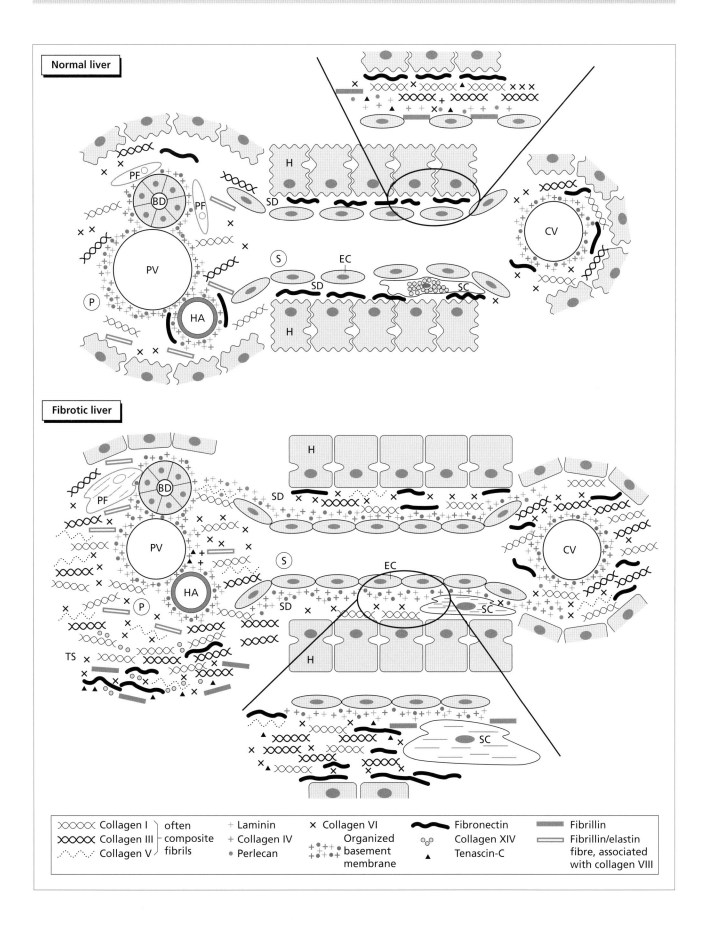

Normal liver

Fibrotic liver

⨯⨯⨯⨯⨯ Collagen I	often	+ Laminin	⨯ Collagen VI	▬▬ Fibronectin
⨯⨯⨯⨯⨯ Collagen III	composite fibrils	+ Collagen IV	Organized basement membrane	₀°₀ Collagen XIV
∿∿∿∿ Collagen V		• Perlecan		▲ Tenascin-C

Fibrillin

Fibrillin/elastin fibre, associated with collagen VIII

Table 1 Functions of ECM proteins in the liver.

Mechanical and architectural
    Tensile strength
    Resilience
    Scaffolds for supramolecular assemblies
    Anchors and connectors for blood vessels, nerves, other cells and other
    matrix components
    Filtration barrier
    Migration substrates and barriers
Signalling
    Ligands for integrins and other signalling receptors
    Signalling receptors and coreceptors
    Sources of biologically active fragments (regulation of growth and
    apoptosis)
    Sequestration and targeting of growth factors
    Damage sensors

Collagens

Collagen structure and synthesis

The major structural proteins in both normal and fibrotic liver are collagens, ECM proteins with sizeable domains of Gly-Xaa-Yaa repeats, where X and Y are often proline and hydroxyproline respectively. This basic structure, with a central glycine and a rotation-limiting proline, allows the formation of a rigid triple helix (Fig. 2). Variations in chain composition among collagen family members are important for function, allowing differences in structural characteristics and network formation as well as different interactions with proteoglycans, receptors, growth factors and other ECM proteins in supramolecular assemblies (Table 2).

The fibrillar collagens (see below) are the most abundant collagens in the liver, and their synthesis is potentially regulated at multiple steps. Although the topic is beyond the scope of this

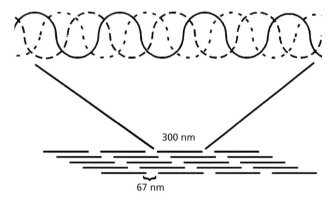

Fig. 2 Fibril arrangement of the fibrillar collagens. Collagen chains made up of repeating Gly-Xaa-Yaa motifs form right-handed triple helices 300 nm long (top). The hydrogen atom side-chains of the glycine residues pack into the centre of the triple helix; the rigid helical geometry is maintained by the proline and hydroxyproline residues, which usually occupy the second and third positions of the repeat. Fibrils of collagens I, III and V are formed by the staggered, parallel packing of many triple helices with a periodicity of 67 nm (bottom).

chapter, the fibrillar collagens are subject to significant transcriptional and posttranscriptional regulation; transcription of the collagen $\alpha 1(I)$ chain in particular is regulated by complex interactions involving both 5' stem–loop and 3' untranslated region (UTR) binding proteins [7]. The fibrillar collagens are synthesized with N- and C-terminal propeptide sequences, the latter playing an important role in protein folding. Nascent chains undergo several kinds of posttranslational modification: vitamin C-dependent proline hydroxylation by prolyl-4-hydroxylase on the polypeptides, which is essential for the stability of the triple helix, hydroxylation on lysine residues by lysyl hydroxlase, which is important for fibril packing, and N- and O-linked glycosylation. After secretion into the extracellular space, collagen chains are cleaved by N- and C-propeptidases and form fibrils. Fibril formation is also modulated at multiple levels including retention of the N-terminal propeptides of collagens III and V, which can regulate lateral fibril growth, and association with the FACIT collagens or decorin (see below), which can regulate fibril thickness [4].

Collagen cross-linking enzymes

Mature collagen fibrils undergo interchain cross-linking, which is essential for mechanical stability. There are three major families of enzymes important in collagen cross-linking; these enzymes also participate in cross-linking of other matrix molecules including elastin and fibronectin. Tissue transglutaminase is a multifunctional protein which mediates the formation of ϵ-(γ-glutamyl lysine) cross-links in collagens and other ECM molecules, rendering them resistant to proteolysis [8]. It is increased in transdifferentiating HSC in culture and is found in myofibroblasts in the fibrotic liver [9–11]. Cross-links typical of tissue transglutaminase action have been demonstrated in the residual fibrous septae of rats with partially resolved fibrosis, suggesting that cross-linking modulates matrix degradation and fibrosis resolution [12] (see also Chapter 6.1).

The lysyl oxidases (LOX) catalyse the oxidative deamination of lysine and hydroxylysine in collagen and of lysine in elastin, leading to the formation of aldehydes, which then condense with neighbouring groups to form covalent cross-links. Although present in the normal liver, LOX family members increase dramatically in fibrosis, including very early after injury and before fibrogenic myofibroblasts appear [13,14]. LOX-mediated cross-links render collagens resistant to degradation and may also play a causal role in the initiation of fibrosis [13,15].

Lysyl hydroxylases catalyse the conversion of lysine into hydroxylysine and thereby determine the route of collagen cross-linking by LOX. The hydroxylysine route appears to be particularly important in diminishing the susceptibility of collagen to proteolysis and is the major pathway for cross-link formation in human cirrhosis [7,16,17].

Collagens in the liver

Ten collagens have been identified in the adult liver. These are divided into two groups based on structure, the fibrillar and the

Table 2 Collagens of the liver.

Type	Composition	Structure
Fibrillar		
I	$[\alpha1(I)]_2[\alpha2(I)]$	300-nm rigid fibrils, 67-nm periodicity
		Uninterrupted triple helices
		Forms composite structures with collagens III and V
		Non-collagenous N- and C-terminal propeptides cleaved before fibril assembly
III	$[\alpha1(III)]_3$	Same as for collagen I
V	$[\alpha1(V)]_2[\alpha2(V)])$	Same as for collagen I
Non-fibrillar		
Network forming		
IV	$[\alpha1(IV)]_2[\alpha2(IV)]$	400-nm-long chains
		Triple helix with multiple interruptions
		Forms filamentous network via N- and C-terminal and lateral associations
VI	$[\alpha1(VI)][\alpha2(VI)][\alpha3(VI)]$	105-nm triple helix
		Large N- and C-terminal globular domains with von Willebrand factor (VWF) A and fibronectin (Fn) type 3 repeats
		Forms antiparallel dimers, then tetramers and networks
VIII	$[\alpha1(VIII)]_2[\alpha2(VIII)]$	130-nm-long chains
		Interrupted triple helices
		Large C-terminal and small N-terminal globular domains
		Forms hexagonal lattices in some tissues
FACITS (fibril associated with interrupted triple helices)		
XIV	$[\alpha1(XIV)]_3$	Two short collagenous domains with three non-collagenous domains
		Glycosaminoglycan (GAG) modified
		N-terminal domain with Fn type 3 repeats and VWF A domains
		Associates with surface of collagen fibrils
XIX	$[\alpha1(XIX)]_3$	Five short collagenous and six non-collagenous domains
		Associates with surface of collagen fibrils
Multiplexins (multiple triple-helical domains and interruptions)		
XV	$[\alpha1(XV)]_3$	Interrupted triple helix
		Large N- and C-terminal globular domains
		Chondroitin sulphate GAGs
		Highly homologous to collagen XVIII
XVIII	$[\alpha1(XVIII)]_3$	Interrupted triple helix
		Large N- and C-terminal globular domains
		Heparan sulphate GAGs
		Cleavage of C-terminal domain NC1 generates endostatin

non-fibrillar collagens (see Table 1). Although the fibrillar collagens, particularly collagens I and III, are generally regarded as the most important in fibrosis on the basis of their quantity as well as mechanical characteristics, it is now understood that other collagens also contribute to fibrosis in important ways.

Fibrillar collagens (I, III and V)

The fibrillar collagens I, III and V all increase significantly in fibrosis; together with collagen IV, they are the most abundant ECM proteins in the liver. They are mechanically important, contributing tensile strength. The fibrillar collagens do not form separate structures but, rather, may be incorporated into composite fibrils, with the relative contribution of each collagen determining the diameter and mechanical properties of the fibril as well as the sensitivity of the fibril to different proteases [4,18,19].

Collagen I has few interruptions in the Gly-Xaa-Yaa structure, enabling it to form rigid triple-helical fibrils, with three amino acids per turn. Many other matrix molecules (including collagens III, V, VI, fibronectin and proteoglycans) are found on the surface of collagen I. Collagen III is structurally similar. It is the first collagen to increase in chronic liver disease; although later replaced in part by collagen I, it remains highly expressed [20]. Collagen V is an abundant collagen that acts as a connector to other collagen types and may be important in initiating the growth of other collagen fibrils [21,22].

Non-fibrillar collagens

The collagens in this group do not form fibrils but, instead, contain combinations of collagenous and non-collagenous domains that enable them to form a variety of different three-dimensional structures. The non-fibrillar collagens in the liver can be divided into three groups based on structure: the network-forming collagens, the FACITS (fibril-associated with interrupted triple helices) and the multiplexins (multiple triple-helical domains and interruptions).

Network-forming collagens (IV, VI, and VIII) The network-forming collagens have many interruptions in their triple-helical chains, which give them flexibility. This flexibility enables them to make linear, axial and lateral associations and so form networks, not fibres [23]; it also allows them to interact with multiple other proteins and macromolecules.

Collagen IV, the main component of most basement membranes, has many variants, although in liver it occurs almost exclusively in the form $[\alpha 1(IV)]_2[\alpha 2(IV)]$. The ends of this collagen cross-link to enable the formation of a three-dimensional network, which anchors and stabilizes other basement membrane components, including perlecan and laminin. Collagen IV is synthesized primarily by endothelial cells, suggesting an active role for these cells in the capillarization of the sinusoids [24].

Collagen VI is a heterotrimeric collagen that forms branching filamentous networks and binds to many additional matrix proteins [4,23,25]. It surrounds the fibres of loosely packed collagens I and III and may anchor structures such as nerves, blood vessels and other cells into place, in part by interconnections with collagen IV in endothelial cell basement membranes [25,26]. Collagen VI is increased up to 10-fold in liver fibrosis. Soluble collagen VI is increased in the circulation of patients with chronic liver disease, which can promote mesenchymal cell (and potentially HSC) proliferation, and is also a potent inhibitor of apoptosis. For these reasons, collagen VI has been proposed as a sensor for tissue damage, with the release of the soluble form stimulating proliferation of surrounding cells and wound healing [4,27,28].

Collagen VIII forms tetrahedral assemblies and, in some cases, hexagonal lattices [23]. It appears to be associated with the basement membrane as well as the elastic fibres of the portal triad, and may serve as a bridge between other matrix molecules. It is especially important in the vasculature, playing a role in angiogenesis [29–31]. Although collagen VIII has been minimally studied in the liver, in other injury models it stimulates smooth muscle cell migration and matrix metalloproteinase (MMP) synthesis and thus may be involved in differentiation and remodelling in wound healing [29,32].

FACIT collagens (XIV, XIX) The FACITs consist of alternating short triple-helical domains and non-triple-helical domains

and, as a result, are highly flexible. Rather than forming fibrils themselves, they associate with pre-existing fibrils of other collagens.

Collagen XIV (also known as undulin) is widely expressed in liver, particularly on the surface of mature, dense fibrils of collagens I and III; it is not seen in the disorganized tissue of actively fibrogenic regions [33,34]. Interestingly, the procollagen I N-proteinase (which cleaves the N-propeptide of collagen I) is bound to collagen XIV, raising the possibility that collagen XIV provides spatial control in regulating the growth of the fibrillar collagens [35]. In the liver, collagen XIV is absent from the sinusoidal space, but is abundant in the portal tract. It increases in fibrosis and can suppress proliferation of HSC and fibroblasts; these effects, as well as its association with dense collagen fibres, suggest a role in established rather than ongoing fibrosis [4]. The other FACIT collagen in the liver, collagen XIX, is primarily found in basement membranes and, to a small extent, in the sinusoids [36]. It has a significant vascular association and may be involved in angiogenesis.

Multiplexin collagens (XV, XVIII) The multiplexin collagens XVIII and XV are structurally homologous proteoglycans with central triple-helical domains and multiple non-collagenous regions which give them flexibility. Collagen XVIII derived from tissues is heparan sulphate linked, whereas collagen XV has chondroitin sulphate modifications [37–39]. Both are found in basement membranes, where they may organize the basement membrane and link it to the underlying matrix.

Collagen XVIII is unusual in that it is increased only twofold in diseased liver compared with normal liver. It is synthesized primarily by hepatocytes and biliary epithelial cells in both states, and is localized in a continuous distribution in both basement membranes and the perisinusoidal space [36,40,41]. Most of the increase in collagen XVIII in disease is along sinusoids that have undergone capillarization, suggesting that it may contribute to this process. Collagen XVIII is also found in the diseased liver in the basement membrane surrounding ductular hepatocytes, proliferating bile ductules and cirrhotic nodules; this distribution implies a potential role in ECM breakdown and remodelling, as well as the ductular reaction and angiogenesis [40,41]. Intact collagen XVIII supports endothelial cell survival, migration and proliferation, and also has the potential to sequester heparan sulphate and heparan sulphate-binding growth factors [31]. The C-terminal globular domain of collagen XVIII can be cleaved by a variety of proteases including MMPs and elastases to generate endostatin, a heparin-binding protein that inhibits angiogenesis and mediates apoptosis [39].

Non-collagenous proteins of the ECM

Fibronectin

Fibronectin is an abundant and widely distributed ECM glycoprotein with multiple domains, including a heparin-binding N-terminus, a collagen-binding domain and an Arg-Gly-Asp

(RGD) motif-containing cell-binding domain with multiple repeated sequences termed type 3 repeats. Unlike many other matrix components, assembly of fibronectin is driven by interaction with its integrins (via the cell-binding domain), suggesting that it plays a particularly important role in the interaction between cells and the surrounding ECM. In the normal liver, fibronectin is found in the portal region around basement membranes and also in a perisinusoidal, speckled pattern; it is the most abundant ECM protein in the normal space of Disse, coating hepatocytes as well as normal collagen fibrils [2]. With its multiple domains, fibronectin probably functions to connect the surfaces of both endothelial cells and hepatocytes to collagen bundles. Fibronectin is one of the first matrix proteins to increase in fibrosis, with significantly increased deposition in the space of Disse, the portal region and fibrotic bands; as a result, it has been called a fibrotic 'pacemaker' [2,42,43].

There are multiple splice variants of fibronectin. Variant EIIIA is expressed primarily during repair of liver injury. It stimulates the activation of fibroblasts and HSC to myofibroblasts in culture [44]. Transforming growth factor (TGF)-β induces production of EIIIA by endothelial cells, suggesting one mechanism among many whereby TGF-β induces fibrosis [45].

Tenascin-C

The tenascins are oligomeric glycoproteins with complex, multidomain structures including fibronectin type 3 repeats. Although the tenascins are highly conserved across vertebrate species and are tightly regulated, their functions are not well understood. Tenascin-C is the best characterized member of the family and the only one known to be expressed in the liver. It antagonizes cell attachment to fibronectin and appears to block fibronectin-mediated signalling at the level of focal adhesion kinase and Rho-mediated pathways; it stimulates growth pathways, including Wnt pathways [46–48]. Tenascin-C also binds multiple additional proteins including integrins, a variety of proteoglycans, adhesion molecules and collagens [49].

Tenascin-C is upregulated in liver fibrosis. In the normal liver, it is found as discontinuous deposits in the sinusoids, but is absent from portal tracts [50–52]. In rat models of fibrosis, tenascin-C is expressed transiently and is found in early septae (at the interface between the parenchyma and the scar) but not in organized areas of fibrosis, suggesting that it has a role in early deposition of ECM. Tenascin-C in the fibrotic liver is synthesized and secreted by HSC [13,50–53].

Laminins

The laminins are a family of large heterotrimeric (α, β, γ chains) glycoproteins typically found in basement membranes associated with collagen IV, perlecan and a variety of other molecules including the glycoprotein nidogen (entactin). They self-assemble into a mesh-like structure and play an important role in the architecture of the basement membrane. Laminins interact with cell surface receptors to regulate additional functions including development and differentiation [54].

Several laminin chains are found in the liver, although their distributions vary [55,56]. In the normal liver, laminins are found in the basement membrane structures of the portal region, with small, focal deposits in the sinusoidal space [1,2]. In the cirrhotic liver, there is a marked increase in laminin deposition, which is found surrounding single or small groups of hepatocytes. Laminin is heavily deposited in the space of Disse in the fibrotic liver along with collagen IV and perlecan, eventually forming a continuous basement membrane [2]. HSC are important laminin-producing cells [56].

Elastin and fibrillin

Elastin and the fibrillins are the major components of elastic fibres in the body and are responsible for many of the mechanical properties of tissues, in particular resilience. Elastic fibres are formed from fibrillin microfibrils with or without a core of elastin. Assembly begins with fibrillin arrays forming transglutaminase cross-linked beaded microfibrils. Elastin binds to these microfibrils, undergoes ordered self-assembly and is then stabilized by LOX-mediated cross-links, which render it highly protease resistant [57]. The function of the different elastic fibres in the liver is not well understood. Both fibrillin and elastin bind to multiple other ECM components including collagens and proteoglycans. Fibrillin can mediate signalling by binding to integrin $\alpha_V\beta_3$; it also binds to TGF-β and may regulate TGF-β targeting [57]. Fibrillin may be cleaved into antiadhesive fragments by proteases, potentially modulating cell/matrix interactions and enhancing cell migration [58].

Fibrillin-1, the only family member studied in the liver, is found associated with elastin in vessel walls and portal tract connective tissue. Unlike elastin, fibrillin-1 is also found adjacent to the limiting plate and lining the sinusoids, forming a continuous network in the space of Disse, where it may have a mechanical role in sinusoidal wall adaptation to variations in blood flow [59]. Fibrillin-1 expression increases in fibrosis where it is found in areas of newly developing matrix (surrounding myofibroblasts invading the parenchyma), around the ductular basement membrane and in the dense septae of organized matrix [58, 59]. Elastin, unlike fibrillin, is not found around invading myofibroblasts or in the space of Disse [58,60,61]. Fibrillin is thought to be produced by both quiescent and activated HSC and portal fibroblasts; elastin, in contrast, appears be produced only by portal fibroblasts and myofibroblasts [58,59].

Proteoglycans and hyaluronic acid

Proteoglycans are proteins with glycosaminoglycan (GAG) modifications. They have multiple functions including maintaining the structural integrity of the ECM, forming a highly charged barrier to the passage of other molecules and regulating growth factor signalling by binding to and sequestering many growth factors including fibroblast growth factor (FGF)-2. Some proteoglycans, in particular the syndecans, heparan sulphate proteoglycans that increase dramatically in fibrosis, are now recognized as signalling receptors [62–65]. Additionally, certain proteases copurify with proteoglycans; this is increased in cirrhosis. There is a fivefold increase in proteoglycan expression in fibrosis. Given the many functions of proteoglycans, they are likely to play a significant role in regulating liver function [66].

Heparan, dermatan and chondroitin sulphate proteoglycans are found in the normal liver, with heparan sulphate proteoglycans comprising approximately 60% of the total [66]. In the cirrhotic liver, chondroitin and dermatan sulphate proteoglycans are disproportionally increased; there are also subtle changes in the side-chain composition of individual proteoglycans, which may affect their function [62,66]. Heparan sulphate proteoglycans are primarily synthesized by hepatocytes in the normal and diseased liver while, in contrast, increases in chondroitin and dermatan sulphate proteoglycans in disease are mediated largely by HSC [66].

The basement membrane proteoglycans include perlecan and collagens XVIII and XV (see above). Perlecan is a large, modular heparan sulphate proteoglycan that interacts with a variety of other proteins including other basement membrane proteins (laminin, collagen IV), heparan sulphate-binding growth factors and fibrillin-1. Perlecan serves as an architectural component of the basement membrane as well as a reservoir for growth factors and a filter for soluble proteins [67]. In the normal liver, perlecan is present in the portal and central venous basement membranes as well as the sinusoids. In fibrosis, it is increased up to eightfold and is modified with the addition of chondroitin sulphate as well as heparan sulphate. Perlecan is increased around reactive bile ductules and markedly increased in sinusoids and the space of Disse, where it is incorporated into the basement membrane, reflecting the capillarization of the sinusoids [62–64,68]. SEC are a major source of perlecan *in vivo* [43].

Decorin, a small chondroitin sulphate proteoglycan, is also increased in cirrhosis. Decorin binds to collagen VI, fibronectin and thrombospondin and appears to be required for the assembly of collagen XIV to the surface of collagen I [4]. Normally located in the space of Disse and portal region, decorin is found prominently in the fibrotic septae of the diseased liver [68,69].

Hyaluronic acid (HA) is a pure carbohydrate polymer composed of repeating disaccharide units present in the extracellular matrix. HA has a high rate of turnover for an ECM molecule, and liver SEC are responsible for a significant amount of its catabolism [70]. It is a minor component of the liver ECM, although significantly increased in fibrotic livers [71,72]; HA and one of its receptors, CD44, increase in parallel in liver fibrosis [73]. An ECM rich in HA is highly hydrated, promotes migration and is specifically important in the migration of HSC in liver disease [74].

Other matrix proteins

A variety of other matrix proteins are present in the liver and upregulated during fibrogenesis including, although not limited to, entactin, thrombospondin, vitronectin, secreted protein acidic and rich in cysteine (SPARC; osteonectin), the *GPI*-linked protein glypican and the proteoglycans aggrecan and betaglycan.

Receptors for ECM proteins

Many of the functions of ECM molecules are mediated by their signalling receptors, heterodimeric (α, β) membrane proteins termed integrins. Matrix-bound integrins initiate cell signalling through a variety of pathways and thereby regulate cell growth, differentiation and migration; in the liver, they are important regulators of fibrosis and tissue remodelling. Integrin expression by the different cells of the liver reflects the specific composition of the underlying matrix, such that hepatocytes and SEC express a unique panel of integrins while biliary epithelial cells express integrins typical of most epithelial cells. In fibrosis, hepatocyte and SEC integrin expression changes to a more epithelial-like pattern and may contribute to the development of fibrosis [75,76]. Integrins may play a role in initiating and maintaining the activation of HSC; they also potentially regulate contractility, proliferation and apoptosis in activated cells [77].

A newly identified class of membrane proteins, the discoidin domain receptors (DDRs), are non-integrin tyrosine kinase receptors for fibrillar collagens. In HSC, these receptors may mediate collagen-induced MMP upregulation and proliferation, although their role in liver fibrosis is not known [78].

Matrix homeostasis and degradation in the liver

Matrix deposition in the normal liver is a dynamic process reflecting ongoing synthesis and degradation. Because the collagens and other matrix proteins of the fibrotic liver are highly cross-linked (see above) and relatively resistant to proteolysis, their degradation requires a specialized group of more than 25 proteases, the MMPs. The MMPs are divided into five families, although they show significant functional overlap [79] (see also Chapter 6.1).

Several MMPs deserve note. The interstitial collagenases (MMPs -1, -8, -13 and possibly -2 and -14) are the only MMPs able to cleave native collagens I and III in their triple-helical domains, and they play a key role in fibrosis and its resolution. The gelatinases (MMPs -2 and -9), however, are also important as they degrade collagen IV, elastin, fibronectin and laminin in addition to denatured fibrillar collagens that have been partially unfolded by interstitial collagenases. MMP-2 (gelatinase A) demonstrates increased activity in parallel with the development of fibrosis, particularly at intermediate stages; it degrades the normal perisinusoidal matrix as part of the parenchymal remodelling involved in progression of disease, enabling HSC migration [80–83].

Regulation of matrix degradation is important in both normal and diseased tissue. In the normal liver, avoiding excess degradation is critical for avoiding tissue injury. In fibrosis, there are changes in both deposition and degradation of matrix components. Resolution of fibrosis requires remodelling of the abnormal matrix; mice expressing a collagenase-resistant collagen I have decreased resolution of fibrosis even after removal of the original profibrogenic insult [84]. The expression and proteolytic activation of the MMPs are subject to complex regulation by growth factors, other proteases including other MMPs, and the matrix itself via integrin-mediated signalling. An important level of regulation is derived from a family of inhibitors, the tissue inhibitors of metalloproteinases (TIMPs), which bind in a non-covalent and reversible manner to the active sites of the MMPs. TIMP-1 and -2 have both been shown to be highly upregulated in fibrosis [81,85,86]. Their importance is illustrated by the demonstration that matrix deposition is enhanced in a CCl_4 model of fibrosis in mice overexpressing TIMP-1 in the liver [87]. HSCs are a key cellular source of the MMPs, their activators and the TIMPs [83].

Conclusion

The ECM is now recognized to be a complex and dynamic rather than a static component of the liver. Although the fibrillar collagens and fibronectin are justifiably the subject of much attention, there is increasing appreciation for the role of other collagens, proteoglycans and additional minor components of the ECM in regulating liver function. Liver cells and the ECM have a bidirectional relationship: almost all liver cells produce some matrix, and most are in turn phenotypically regulated by the ECM. Recent research has focused on the role of fibrogenic cells in addition to HSC and will probably yield important insights in the future. A further area of intense research will be on new functions of the matrix including mechanisms of ECM-mediated regulation of cell phenotype.

References

1 Martinez-Hernandez A, Amenta PS (1993) The hepatic extracellular matrix. I. Components and distribution in normal liver. *Virchows Arch A Pathol Anat Histopathol* 423 (1), 1–11.

2 Hahn E, Wick G, Pencev D *et al.* (1980) Distribution of basement membrane proteins in normal and fibrotic human liver: collagen type IV, laminin, and fibronectin. *Gut* 21 (1), 63–71.

3 Loreal O, Clement B, Schuppan D *et al.* (1992) Distribution and cellular origin of collagen VI during development and in cirrhosis. *Gastroenterology* 102 (3), 980–987.

4 Schuppan D, Ruehl M, Somasundaram R *et al.* (2001) Matrix as a modulator of hepatic fibrogenesis. *Semin Liver Dis* 21 (3), 351–372.

5 Reid LM, Fiorino AS, Sigal SH *et al.* (1992) Extracellular matrix gradients in the space of Disse: relevance to liver biology. *Hepatology* 15 (6), 1198–1203.

6 Martinez-Hernandez A, Amenta PS (1993) The hepatic extracellular matrix. II. Ontogenesis, regeneration and cirrhosis. *Virchows Arch A Pathol Anat Histopathol* 423 (2), 77–84.

7 Brenner DA, Waterboer T, Choi SK *et al.* (2000) New aspects of hepatic fibrosis. *J Hepatol* 32(1 Suppl), 32–38.

8 Mehta K, Fok JY, Mangala LS (2006) Tissue transglutaminase: from biological glue to cell survival cues. *Front Biosci* 11, 173–185.

9 Grenard P, Bresson-Hadni S, El Alaoui S *et al.* (2001) Transglutaminase-mediated cross-linking is involved in the stabilization of extracellular matrix in human liver fibrosis. *J Hepatol* 35 (3), 367–375.

10 Mirza A, Liu SL, Frizell E *et al.* (1997) A role for tissue transglutaminase in hepatic injury and fibrogenesis, and its regulation by NF-kappaB. *Am J Physiol* 272 (2 Pt 1), G281–288.

11 Schnabel C, Sawitza I, Tag CG *et al.* (2004) Expression of cytosolic and membrane associated tissue transglutaminase in rat hepatic stellate cells and its upregulation during transdifferentiation to myofibroblasts in culture. *Hepatol Res* 28 (3), 140–145.

12 Issa R, Zhou X, Constandinou CM *et al.* (2004) Spontaneous recovery from micronodular cirrhosis: evidence for incomplete resolution associated with matrix cross-linking. *Gastroenterology* 126 (7), 1795–1808.

13 Desmouliere A, Darby I, Costa AM *et al.* (1997) Extracellular matrix deposition, lysyl oxidase expression, and myofibroblastic differentiation during the initial stages of cholestatic fibrosis in the rat. *Lab Invest* 76 (6), 765–778.

14 Kim Y, Peyrol S, So CK *et al.* (1999) Coexpression of the lysyl oxidase-like gene (LOXL) and the gene encoding type III procollagen in induced liver fibrosis. *J Cell Biochem* 72 (2), 181–188.

15 Vater CA, Harris ED, Jr, Siegel RC (1979) Native cross-links in collagen fibrils induce resistance to human synovial collagenase. *Biochem J* 181 (3), 639–645.

16 Ricard-Blum S, Bresson-Hadni S, Vuitton DA *et al.* (1992) Hydroxypyridinium collagen cross-links in human liver fibrosis: study of alveolar echinococcosis. *Hepatology* 15 (4), 599–602.

17 van der Slot AJ, Zuurmond AM, van den Bogaerdt AJ *et al.* (2004) Increased formation of pyridinoline cross-links due to higher telopeptide lysyl hydroxylase levels is a general fibrotic phenomenon. *Matrix Biol* 23 (4), 251–257.

18 Geerts A, Schuppan D, Lazeroms S *et al.* (1990) Collagen type I and III occur together in hybrid fibrils in the space of Disse of normal rat liver. *Hepatology* 12 (2), 233–241.

19 Romanic AM, Adachi E, Kadler KE *et al.* (1991) Copolymerization of pNcollagen III and collagen I. pNcollagen III decreases the rate of incorporation of collagen I into fibrils, the amount of collagen I incorporated, and the diameter of the fibrils formed. *J Biol Chem* 266 (19), 12703–12709.

20 Ramadori G, Knittel T, Saile B (1998) Fibrosis and altered matrix synthesis. *Digestion* 59 (4), 372–375.

21 Birk DE, Fitch JM, Babiarz JP *et al.* (1988) Collagen type I and type V are present in the same fibril in the avian corneal stroma. *J Cell Biol* 106 (3), 999–1008.

22 Becker J, Schuppan D, Rabanus JP *et al.* (1991) Immunoelectron microscopic localization of collagens type I, V, VI and of procollagen type III in human periodontal ligament and cementum. *J Histochem Cytochem* 39 (1), 103–110.

23 Knupp C, Squire JM (2005) Molecular packing in network-forming collagens. *Adv Protein Chem* 70, 375–403.

24 Herbst H, Frey A, Heinrichs O *et al.* (1997) Heterogeneity of liver cells expressing procollagen types I and IV in vivo. *Histochem Cell Biol* 107 (5), 399–409.

25 Griffiths MR, Shepherd M, Ferrier R *et al.* (1992) Light microscopic and ultrastructural distribution of type VI collagen in human liver: alterations in chronic biliary disease. *Histopathology* 21 (4), 335–344.

26 Keene DR, Engvall E, Glanville RW (1988) Ultrastructure of type VI collagen in human skin and cartilage suggests an anchoring function for this filamentous network. *J Cell Biol* 107 (5), 1995–2006.

27 Ruhl M, Sahin E, Johannsen M *et al.* (1999) Soluble collagen VI drives serum-starved fibroblasts through S phase and prevents apoptosis via down-regulation of Bax. *J Biol Chem* 274 (48), 34361–34368.

28 Atkinson JC, Ruhl M, Becker J *et al.* (1996) Collagen VI regulates normal and transformed mesenchymal cell proliferation in vitro. *Exp Cell Res* 228 (2), 283–291.

29 Shuttleworth CA (1997) Type VIII collagen. *Int J Biochem Cell Biol* 29 (10), 1145–1148.

30 Sawada H, Konomi H (1991) The alpha 1 chain of type VIII collagen is associated with many but not all microfibrils of elastic fiber system. *Cell Struct Funct* 16 (6), 455–466.

31 Ricard-Blum S, Dublet B, van der Rest M (2000) *Unconventional Collagens. Type VI, VII, VIII, IX, X, XII, XIV, XVI, and XIX.* Oxford: Oxford University Press.

32 Hou G, Mulholland D, Gronska MA *et al.* (2000) Type VIII collagen stimulates smooth muscle cell migration and matrix metalloproteinase synthesis after arterial injury. *Am J Pathol* 156 (2), 467–476.

33 Schuppan D, Cantaluppi MC, Becker J *et al.* (1990) Undulin, an extracellular matrix glycoprotein associated with collagen fibrils. *J Biol Chem* 265 (15), 8823–8832.

34 Milani S, Grappone C, Pellegrini G *et al.* (1994) Undulin RNA and protein expression in normal and fibrotic human liver. *Hepatology* 20 (4 Pt 1), 908–916.

35 Colige A, Beschin A, Samyn B *et al.* (1995) Characterization and partial amino acid sequencing of a 107-kDa procollagen I N-proteinase purified by affinity chromatography on immobilized type XIV collagen. *J Biol Chem* 270 (28), 16724–16730.

36 Myers JC, Li D, Bageris A *et al.* (1997) Biochemical and immunohistochemical characterization of human type XIX defines a novel class of basement membrane zone collagens. *Am J Pathol* 151 (6), 1729–1740.

37 Halfter W, Dong S, Schurer B *et al.* (1998) Collagen XVIII is a basement membrane heparan sulfate proteoglycan. *J Biol Chem* 273 (39), 25404–25412.

38 Li D, Clark CC, Myers JC (2000) Basement membrane zone type XV collagen is a disulfide-bonded chondroitin sulfate proteoglycan in human tissues and cultured cells. *J Biol Chem* 275 (29), 22339–22347.

39 Iozzo RV (2005) Basement membrane proteoglycans: from cellar to ceiling. *Nature Rev Mol Cell Biol* 6 (8), 646–656.

40 Jia JD, Bauer M, Sedlaczek N *et al.* (2001) Modulation of collagen XVIII/endostatin expression in lobular and biliary rat liver fibrogenesis. *J Hepatol* 35 (3), 386–391.

41 Musso O, Rehn M, Saarela J *et al.* (1998) Collagen XVIII is localized in sinusoids and basement membrane zones and expressed by hepatocytes and activated stellate cells in fibrotic human liver. *Hepatology* 28 (1), 98–107.

42 Odenthal M, Neubauer K, Meyer zum Buschenfelde KH *et al.* (1993) Localization and mRNA steady-state level of cellular fibronectin in rat liver undergoing a CCl4-induced acute damage or fibrosis. *Biochim Biophys Acta* 1181 (3), 266–272.

43 Rescan PY, Loreal O, Hassell JR *et al.* (1993) Distribution and origin of the basement membrane component perlecan in rat liver and primary hepatocyte culture. *Am J Pathol* 142 (1), 199–208.

44 Tomasek JJ, Gabbiani G, Hinz B *et al.* (2002) Myofibroblasts and mechano-regulation of connective tissue remodelling. *Nature Rev Mol Cell Biol* 3 (5), 349–363.

45 George J, Wang SS, Sevcsik AM *et al.* (2000) Transforming growth factor-beta initiates wound repair in rat liver through induction of the EIIIA-fibronectin splice isoform. *Am J Pathol* 156 (1), 115–124.

46 Wenk MB, Midwood KS, Schwarzbauer JE (2000) Tenascin-C suppresses Rho activation. *J Cell Biol* 150 (4), 913–920.

47 Midwood KS, Schwarzbauer JE (2002) Tenascin-C modulates matrix contraction via focal adhesion kinase- and Rho-mediated signaling pathways. *Mol Biol Cell* 13 (10), 3601–3613.

48 Ruiz C, Huang W, Hegi ME *et al.* (2004) Growth promoting signaling by tenascin-C (corrected). *Cancer Res* 64 (20), 7377–7385.

49 Hsia HC, Schwarzbauer JE (2005) Meet the tenascins: multifunctional and mysterious. *J Biol Chem* 280 (29), 26641–26644.

50 Van Eyken P, Geerts A, De Bleser P *et al.* (1992) Localization and cellular source of the extracellular matrix protein tenascin in normal and fibrotic rat liver. *Hepatology* 15 (5), 909–916.

51 Yamada S, Ichida T, Matsuda Y *et al.* (1992) Tenascin expression in human chronic liver disease and in hepatocellular carcinoma. *Liver* 12 (1), 10–16.

52 Van Eyken P, Sciot R, Desmet VJ (1990) Expression of the novel extracellular matrix component tenascin in normal and diseased human liver. An immunohistochemical study. *J Hepatol* 11 (1), 43–52.

53 Miyazaki H, Van Eyken P, Roskams T *et al.* (1993) Transient expression of tenascin in experimentally induced cholestatic fibrosis in rat liver: an immunohistochemical study. *J Hepatol* 19 (3), 353–366.

54 Colognato H, Yurchenco PD (2000) Form and function: the laminin family of heterotrimers. *Dev Dyn* 218 (2), 213–234.

55 Sasaki T, Giltay R, Talts U *et al.* (2002) Expression and distribution of laminin alpha1 and alpha2 chains in embryonic and adult mouse tissues: an immunochemical approach. *Exp Cell Res* 275 (2), 185–199.

56 Kikkawa Y, Mochizuki Y, Miner JH *et al.* (2005) Transient expression of laminin alpha1 chain in regenerating murine liver: restricted localization of laminin chains and nidogen-1. *Exp Cell Res* 305 (1), 99–109.

57 Kielty CM, Sherratt MJ, Shuttleworth CA (2002) Elastic fibres. *J Cell Sci* 115 (Pt 14), 2817–2828.

58 Lorena D, Darby IA, Reinhardt DP *et al.* (2004) Fibrillin-1 expression in normal and fibrotic rat liver and in cultured hepatic fibroblastic cells: modulation by mechanical stress and role in cell adhesion. *Lab Invest* 84 (2), 203–212.

59 Dubuisson L, Lepreux S, Bioulac-Sage P *et al.* (2001) Expression and cellular localization of fibrillin-1 in normal and pathological human liver. *J Hepatol* 34 (4), 514–522.

60 Porto LC, Chevallier M, Peyrol S *et al.* (1990) Elastin in human, baboon, and mouse liver: an immunohistochemical and immunoelectron microscopic study. *Anat Rec* 228 (4), 392–404.

61 Velebny V, Kasafirek E, Kanta J (1983) Desmosine and isodesmosine contents and elastase activity in normal and cirrhotic rat liver. *Biochem J* 214 (3), 1023–1025.

62 Kovalszky II, Nagy JO, Gallai M *et al.* (1997) Altered proteoglycan gene expression in human biliary cirrhosis. *Pathol Oncol Res* 3 (1), 51–58.

63 Roskams T, Moshage H, De Vos R *et al.* (1995) Heparan sulfate proteoglycan expression in normal human liver. *Hepatology* 21 (4), 950–958.

64 Roskams T, Rosenbaum J, De Vos R *et al.* (1996) Heparan sulfate proteoglycan expression in chronic cholestatic human liver diseases. *Hepatology* 24 (3), 524–532.

65 Tkachenko E, Rhodes JM, Simons M (2005) Syndecans: new kids on the signaling block. *Circ Res* 96 (5), 488–500.

66 Gressner AM (1994) Activation of proteoglycan synthesis in injured liver – a brief review of molecular and cellular aspects. *Eur J Clin Chem Clin Biochem* 32 (4), 225–237.

67 Levavasseur F, Loreal O, Lietard J *et al.* (1995) Basement membrane gene expression in the liver. *J Hepatol* 22 (2 Suppl), 10–19.

68 Gallai M, Kovalszky I, Knittel T *et al.* (1996) Expression of extracellular matrix proteoglycans perlecan and decorin in carbon-tetrachloride-injured rat liver and in isolated liver cells. *Am J Pathol* 148 (5), 1463–1471.

69 Hogemann B, Edel G, Schwarz K *et al.* (1997) Expression of biglycan, decorin and proteoglycan-100/CSF-1 in normal and fibrotic human liver. *Pathol Res Pract* 193 (11–12), 747–751.

70 McCourt PA (1999) How does the hyaluronan scrap-yard operate? *Matrix Biol* 18 (5), 427–432.

71 Scott JE, Bosworth TR, Cribb AM *et al.* (1994) The chemical morphology of extracellular matrix in experimental rat liver fibrosis resembles that of normal developing connective tissue. *Virchows Arch* 424 (1), 89–98.

72 Murata K, Ochiai Y, Akashio K (1985) Polydispersity of acidic glycosaminoglycan components in human liver and the changes at different stages in liver cirrhosis. *Gastroenterology* 89 (6), 1248–1257.

73 Satoh T, Ichida T, Matsuda Y *et al.* (2000) Interaction between hyaluronan and CD44 in the development of dimethylnitrosamine-induced liver cirrhosis. *J Gastroenterol Hepatol* 15 (4), 402–411.

74 Kikuchi S, Griffin CT, Wang SS *et al.* (2005) Role of CD44 in epithelial wound repair: migration of rat hepatic stellate cells utilizes hyaluronic acid and CD44v6. *J Biol Chem* 280 (15), 15398–15404.

75 Scoazec JY (1995) Expression of cell–matrix adhesion molecules in the liver and their modulation during fibrosis. *J Hepatol* 22 (2 Suppl), 20–27.

76 Languino LR, Wells RG (2001) Integrins. In: Arias IM (ed.) *The Liver: Biology and Pathobiology*, 4th edn. Philadelphia: Lippincott Williams & Wilkins, pp. 475–482.

77 Zhou X, Murphy FR, Gehdu N *et al.* (2004) Engagement of alphav-beta3 integrin regulates proliferation and apoptosis of hepatic stellate cells. *J Biol Chem* 279 (23), 23996–24006.

78 Olaso E, Ikeda K, Eng FJ *et al.* (2001) DDR2 receptor promotes MMP-2-mediated proliferation and invasion by hepatic stellate cells. *J Clin Invest* 108 (9), 1369–1378.

79 Benyon RC, Arthur MJ (2001) Extracellular matrix degradation and the role of hepatic stellate cells. *Semin Liver Dis* 21 (3), 373–384.

80 Takahara T, Furui K, Funaki J *et al.* (1995) Increased expression of matrix metalloproteinase-II in experimental liver fibrosis in rats. *Hepatology* 21 (3), 787–795.

81 Benyon RC, Iredale JP, Goddard S *et al.* (1996) Expression of tissue inhibitor of metalloproteinases 1 and 2 is increased in fibrotic human liver. *Gastroenterology* 110 (3), 821–831.

82 Takahara T, Furui K, Yata Y *et al.* (1997) Dual expression of matrix metalloproteinase-2 and membrane-type 1-matrix metalloproteinase in fibrotic human livers. *Hepatology* 26 (6), 1521–1529.

83 Bedossa P, Paradis V (2003) Liver extracellular matrix in health and disease. *J Pathol* 200 (4), 504–515.

84 Issa R, Zhou X, Trim N *et al.* (2003) Mutation in collagen-1 that confers resistance to the action of collagenase results in failure of recovery from CCl4-induced liver fibrosis, persistence of activated hepatic stellate cells, and diminished hepatocyte regeneration. *FASEB J* 17 (1), 47–49.

85 Iredale JP, Benyon RC, Arthur MJ *et al.* (1996) Tissue inhibitor of metalloproteinase-1 messenger RNA expression is enhanced relative to interstitial collagenase messenger RNA in experimental liver injury and fibrosis. *Hepatology* 24 (1), 176–184.

86 Herbst H, Wege T, Milani S *et al.* (1997) Tissue inhibitor of metalloproteinase-1 and -2 RNA expression in rat and human liver fibrosis. *Am J Pathol* 150 (5), 1647–1659.

87 Yoshiji H, Kuriyama S, Miyamoto Y *et al.* (2000) Tissue inhibitor of metalloproteinases-1 promotes liver fibrosis development in a transgenic mouse model. *Hepatology* 32 (6), 1248–1254.

2.5 Regulation of the liver cell mass

2.5.1 Control of liver cell proliferation

Nisar P. Malek and K. Lenhard Rudolph

Control of liver cell cycle entry and progression

The liver is a quiescent organ that has enormous capacity to regenerate in response to injury [1]. This capacity is regulated through the ordered activation and inactivation of regulatory proteins which govern the entry and exit of liver cells from the cell cycle [2]. Our understanding of the molecular basis of these processes is mainly derived from studies in cultured primary hepatocytes, established liver cancer cell lines and also from the analysis of mouse strains with defined defects in genes that are involved in cell cycle regulation. Given the enormous amount of data that have been published on the regulation of hepatocyte proliferation, we will focus only on the role of key cell cycle regulatory proteins in liver cell cycle control in this chapter. Special emphasis will be given to studies that have used mouse model systems to explore liver cell regeneration *in vivo*.

The two-third hepatectomy model in mice and rats has been used extensively to explore the basic molecular mechanism of liver cell proliferation [3]. During the process of liver regeneration, hepatocytes proceed through different stages, which have previously been organized into a so-called initiation or priming phase during which the quiescent hepatocytes are rendered replication competent, the division phase in which the hepatocytes proceed through different phases of the cell cycle and finally divide into two cells, and a termination phase which leads to the termination of liver cell proliferation when organ mass is restored [4].

Under physiological conditions, i.e. in the absence of organ damage or loss, quiescent liver cells are arrested in the G0 state of the cell cycle. A central mediator of cellular quiescence is the retinoblastoma (Rb) protein [5]. Depending on its phosphorylation status, Rb can either repress or activate the expression of a multitude of critical target genes, which control the entry into the division phase of the hepatocyte cell cycle. Hypophosphorylated Rb binds to proteins of the E2F family of transcription factors and blocks their transactivation capacity [6]. Upon phosphorylation, Rb releases E2F, which leads to the expression of E2F target genes and progression into the cell cycle. Using inducible Rb knockout mice, it was shown that acute loss of Rb function in hepatocytes results in unscheduled induction of cell proliferation even in the absence of sufficient mitogenic stimulation [7].

In addition to Rb, a proteolytic system maintains quiescence of hepatocytes by limiting the expression of cyclins to restricted phases of the cell cycle. This system consists of the anaphase-promoting complex (APC) and the skp/cullin/F-box (SCF) multiprotein complex [8]. These degradation systems regulate the ubiquitylation and subsequent proteasomal turnover of cyclins and other important cell cycle regulators. Ablation of the APC2 subunit of APC in mouse liver leads to the accumulation of cyclin A, which induces an unscheduled entry of mouse hepatocytes into the cell cycle [9]. Together, these studies show that the proliferative quiescence of hepatocytes is an actively maintained state, which requires the activity of several proteins and multiprotein complexes.

Upon liver cell damage or loss of organ mass, liver cells exit G0 and enter the G1 phase. An important mediator of this process is the cyclin D protein which, after binding to cdk4 (cyclin-dependent kinase 4 or 6), can phosphorylate the Rb protein, thus allowing the activation of the E2F-dependent transcriptional programme. Cyclin D1 is a highly unstable protein with a half-life of ~ 15 min [10]. Therefore, induction and maintenance of cyclin D1 expression is primarily dependent on continuous transcription of the cyclin D1 gene. Several signalling cascades activate the cyclin D1 promoter in response to mitogenic stimulation, thereby connecting extracellular mitogenic signalling cascades with the core cell cycle machinery, namely phosphorylation of the Rb protein [2]. Conversely, overexpression of cyclin D1 in mouse hepatocytes leads to cell cycle entry without further mitogenic stimulation. Nevertheless, even short-term expression of cyclin D1 in liver cells leads to severe genetic alterations, including centrosome abnormalities and chromosomal aberrations, reinforcing the notion that central regulators of cell proliferation are frequently involved in cellular transformation processes [11,12]. The expression of cyclin D/cdk4 kinase complexes during the G1 phase leads to the induction of cyclin E/cdk2 activity through E2F-dependent transcription of the cyclin E gene. Importantly, the loss of the cyclin D1 gene in the mouse can be fully rescued through the expression of the cyclin E cDNA in the cyclin D genomic locus. Therefore, the only essential downstream function of cyclin D is to allow cyclin E expression during the G1 phase of the cell cycle [13]. Cyclin E expression also promotes proliferation of mouse hepatocytes *in vivo*; however, this function requires the coexpression of the skp2 protein, a member of the F-box protein family, which plays a crucial role in the destruction of the cyclin kinase inhibitor p27kip1 [14,15]. Cyclin kinase inhibitors (cki) fall into two classes: the ink4 group (p15, p16, p18, p19) and the cip/kip group (p21, p27, p57). The main function of ckis is to regulate the activity of cyclin/cdk complexes throughout the cell division cycle by directly binding and inhibiting the active kinase complex [16]. However, this dogma has recently been challenged through the generation of mouse models with deletions in the cyclin E1/E2 and cdk2 genes [17,18]. Surprisingly, the phenotype of cdk2 knockout mice is restricted to a defect in meiotic cell division, while cell proliferation in cyclin E1/E2 double knockout mice was only impaired when cells were released from quiescence. Moreover, p27 and p21 still inhibited the cell division after overexpression in cdk2 knockout cells, indicating that cdk2 cannot stand as the essential target of these ckis [19]. Nevertheless, loss or overexpression of these proteins in hepatocytes leads to severe phenotypes in the corresponding mouse models. For instance, liver-specific overexpression of p21 in transgenic mice leads to a dramatic impairment in liver cell proliferation, runted liver and body growth and a significant increase in polyploid cells [20]. Stabilization of the p27 protein through loss of skp2 also blocks hepatocyte proliferation in G1 but, at the same time, leads to cellular growth and an increase in cell size of the affected hepatocytes [21]. In these experiments, cellular growth was accompanied by multiple rounds of endoreduplication [21]. Conversely, serial transplantation experiments using p27 knockout hepatocytes showed that loss of this protein greatly increases the proliferative abilities of liver cells [22]. Together, these findings demonstrate that p27 turnover is critical for the control of hepatocyte proliferation by regulating a molecular switch, which controls proliferation or cellular growth of hepatocytes.

Polyploidization might also serve a physiological role as it is frequently accompanied by cellular growth. In fact, an increase in DNA content without a concurrent mitotic division but followed by an enlargement in cell mass might offer an alternative to mitosis in certain cell types including liver cells. Recently, an elegant study using isolated rat hepatocytes and live cell videomicroscopy characterized the mechanism of liver cell polyploidization at the cellular level. It was shown that the generation of 4n hepatocytes is a result of impaired cytokinesis in a fraction of 2n mononuclear liver cells, which results in the generation of binucleated 2n hepatocytes. These cells then underwent normal mitosis which, however, required the clustering of two centrosomes at each pole of the cells and ultimately resulted in the formation of a bipolar spindle and 4n hepatocytes [23]. The molecular mechanisms that control these processes are unknown at this point.

Another important regulator of liver cell proliferation is the Foxm1b protein, a member of the Forkhead Box (Fox) family of transcription factors. Foxm1b expression controls the expression of several cell cycle regulatory proteins including the cdc25B phosphate, cyclin D1 and cyclin B1. Overexpression of Foxm1b accelerates the onset of hepatocyte DNA replication, while loss of the protein leads to a failure to enter mitosis and polyploidization, demonstrating the protein's central role in the process of liver regeneration [24]. Importantly, loss of Foxm1b also leads to an almost complete inhibition of liver cancer formation after treatment of Foxm1b knockout (Foxm1b–/–) mice with the DNA-damaging agent diethylnitrosamine (DEN). While Foxm1b–/– mice still developed altered enzyme foci, which represent the earliest detectable lesions in this model system, they did not show hepatocellular adenomas or carcinomas. Interestingly, all tumours in Foxm1b–/– mice showed strong nuclear p27kip1 expression, suggesting that this cki prevented cellular division in response to DEN treatment [25].

An important role in the development of liver cancer (see Chapter 18.2.1) was also demonstrated for the transcription factor c-jun. C-jun mediates several cellular processes, including proliferation and survival. Using inducible c-jun knockout mice to study its role in liver cancer development, it was demonstrated that inactivation of this transcription factor significantly reduced the number and size of hepatic tumours. The impaired tumour development coincided with the induction of the tumour suppressor protein p53, which led to the induction of noxa, a proapoptotic gene, and subsequent death of the transformed cells. These studies pointed to an antiapoptotic role of c-jun through the suppression of the p53 gene, thus promoting the early stages of hepatocellular carcinoma (HCC) development [26,27].

Telomere shortening, senescence and telomerase

Despite the ability of liver cells to re-enter the cell cycle during organ regeneration, it has long been observed that liver regeneration is impaired at the endstage of chronic liver diseases and during cirrhosis formation (see Chapters 6.1–6.3 and 2.5.2), indicating that the regenerative capacity of human liver cells is limited. A potential explanation for this phenomenon might come from telomere biology. Telomeres consist of simple tandem nucleotide repeats [(TTAGGG)n in humans] that are located at each end of chromosomes [27]. Telomeres are heterochromatic and do not encode any gene product, but have an essential function for cell viability, which is to cap and protect the chromosomal ends. As the chromosomal end is in principle similar to a double-strand break, chromosomal capping is necessary to avoid activation of DNA damage responses, chromosomal fusions and chromosomal instability (CIN). Beside the length of telomere repeats, the higher order structure [28,29] of the telomeres formed by the binding of specific proteins to the telomere [30] is important for the telomere capping function. Owing to the end-replication problem of DNA polymerase and processing of the telomere termini during the cell cycle, telomeres shorten during each round of cell division by 50–100 bp in human cells [31]. The ongoing telomere shortening is compensated for by the enzyme 'telomerase', which can synthesize telomeres de novo [32,33]. Telomerase consists of two essential components: telomerase reverse transcriptase (TERT), which is the catalytic subunit of the enzyme; and telomerase RNA component (TERC), which is the functional RNA and serves as a template for telomere sequence synthesis. In humans, telomerase is active during embryogenesis but is repressed postnatally in most somatic tissues and remains active only in immature germ cells and certain stem and progenitor cells [34].

On account of the repression of telomerase, telomeres of human cells shorten during each cell division (see above), and the replicative lifespan of human cells is limited by this mechanism to 50–70 cell divisions [35]. However, overexpression of telomerase can elongate the lifespan of primary human cells including hepatocytes [36,37]. Telomere shortening limits the lifespan of primary human cells by inducing senescence, which is characterized by a permanent cell cycle arrest. Senescence is induced when telomeres reach a critical short length and lose their capping function. It has been shown that the dysfunctional telomeres provoke a DNA damage response including the activation of ATM/ATR/p53/Chk2/p21/p16 pathways [38,39]. When cells lose p53 or Chk2 function, they can bypass the senescence checkpoint and continue to proliferate despite the presence of telomere dysfunction [40,41]. As a consequence, chromosomal fusions and breakage of fused chromosomes induce CIN (see below and [42]), and cells will eventually reach a second checkpoint called crisis, which is characterized by massive CIN and apoptosis [43].

In humans, telomeres shorten during ageing in a variety of tissues and organs [44]. There is some correlation between age-related telomere shortening and cell turnover of different organs, and the rate of telomere shortening is increased during chronic diseases that increase the rate of cell turnover [44]. There is growing evidence that telomere shortening and senescence impair the regenerative capacity of organs and tissues during human ageing and chronic disease [44].

Telomere shortening, senescence and telomerase in ageing liver and chronic liver diseases

Normal healthy liver does not show significant levels of telomerase activity [45]. The liver is a quiescent organ with a very low rate of cell division, yet the liver shows significant telomere shortening during ageing [46]. During chronic liver disease, low levels of telomerase reactivation have been detected by some investigators. However, it remains a subject of debate to what extent this really reflects telomerase activation of regenerating hepatocytes or whether it is induced by infiltration of telomerase-positive lymphocytes. It has been shown in a variety of studies that there is accelerated telomere shortening during chronic liver disease and at the cirrhosis stage [46], clearly indicating that the level of telomerase is not sufficient to compensate for telomere shortening during chronic liver disease. Telomere shortening in chronic liver disease and cirrhosis predominantly affects hepatocytes, and there is an accumulation of SA-βGal (senescence marker)-positive hepatocytes during cirrhosis development [46]. In agreement with these data, an activation of senescence checkpoint signalling has been detected at the cirrhosis stage.

Direct experimental evidence for a role of telomere shortening in cirrhosis formation came from studies in telomerase knockout mice. Telomere shortening in mTERC–/– mice led to impaired liver regeneration and premature development of fibrosis and steatosis in response to chronic liver damage [47]. Impaired liver regeneration correlated with the induction of senescence in hepatocytes with critically short telomeres. Thus, telomere shortening led to a reduction in the pool of proliferative cells that have the capacity to re-enter the cell cycle and to regenerate the organ in response to damage [48]. In addition, the studies in mTERC–/– mice support the concept that telomerase gene therapy can improve the regenerative capacity of organs with critically short telomeres in vivo [47].

These concepts derived from mouse models and the telomere length analysis from human diseased liver (see above) indicate that telomere shortening and senescence contribute to a decrease in hepatocyte proliferation that is recognized during cirrhosis development in humans [49,50]. Together, these studies have led to a new model of cirrhosis formation [51]; according to this model, telomere shortening and senescence limit the regenerative capacity of hepatocytes during chronic liver disease. When the regenerative reserve of the liver falls beneath a critical threshold, stellate cells become activated and form fibrotic scar tissue (Fig. 1). The data from mouse models indicate that telomerase activation could be used for the treatment of liver cirrhosis. However, a detailed understanding of telomere shortening and telomerase reactivation during cancer formation is necessary to predict the potential cancer risk of such therapies.

Telomere shortening, senescence and telomerase in liver cancer

Telomere shortening and senescence are regarded as potent tumour suppressor mechanisms inhibiting immortal growth of transformed cells in the human body. In line with this hypothesis, over 90% of human tumours show a reactivation of telomerase, indicating that telomere stabilization is essential

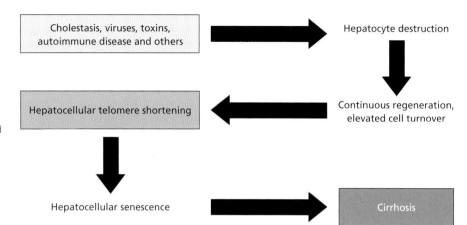

Fig. 1 The telomere hypothesis of cirrhosis formation (reprinted with permission from [46]). Chronic liver diseases lead to an elevated rate of hepatocyte cell turnover, which accelerates telomere shortening, finally culminating in hepatocyte senescence and cessation of regeneration. Continuous liver damage at this point provokes an activation of stellate cells and fibrotic scarring (see Chapters 1.6, 6.1 and 6.2).

for tumour survival and progression [52]. However, in the vast majority of human cancers including HCC, telomeres are very short, much shorter than in the non-transformed surrounding tissue. These data point to an apparent paradox: on the one hand, telomere shortening and senescence are supposed to function as a tumour suppressor mechanism but, on the other hand, telomere shortening is associated with tumour development, indicating that it might represent a tumour risk factor. Indeed, the risk of HCC development increases sharply at the cirrhosis stage (see Chapters 6.3 and 18.2.1), which is characterized by telomere shortening (see above), and the majority of HCC show significant telomere shortening compared with non-transformed surrounding tissue or regenerative nodules [52]. In addition, a strong increase in cancer incidence has been observed in other tissues during ageing and at the endstage of chronic diseases, indicating that senescence as a tumour suppressor mechanism functions well in young age and in tissues with long telomeres but loses effectiveness in tissues with shortened telomeres.

A possible explanation came from studies in mTERC–/– mice revealing a dual role for telomere shortening during cancer initiation and progression. In line with the classical view that telomere shortening acts as a tumour suppressor mechanism, tumour progression was impaired in mTERC–/– mice [53,54]. Impaired tumour progression correlated with activation of senescence signalling pathways (upregulation of p53) in tumour cells of mTERC–/– compared with mTERC+/+ mice. Upregulation of p53 in tumour cells of mTERC–/– mice correlated with increased rates of apoptosis and impaired proliferation of tumour cells *in vivo* [55]. In contrast to the suppression of macroscopic tumours, telomere shortening in mTERC–/– mice was associated with an increase in tumour initiation [55,56]. Increased tumour initiation induced by telomere shortening was linked to chromosomal instability, which is a major mechanism driving tumorigenesis in aged humans and at the endstage of chronic disease. When telomeres lose the capping function, CIN evolves because chromosomes will fuse, and breakage of the chromosomes occurs during anaphase of the cell cycle. As a morphological correlate, chromatin bridges of stretched and

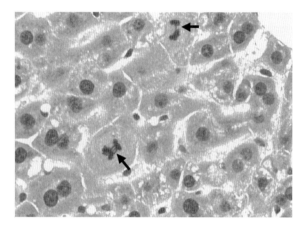

Fig. 2 Telomere shortening induces chromosomal instability (CIN). Loss of telomere capping function results in chromosomal fusions. When cells containing fused chromosomes enter the cell cycle, the chromosomal fusions will break during anaphase. As a morphological correlate, chromatin bridges are seen in anaphase (anaphase bridges, black arrows). The breakage of fused chromosomes results in chromosomal gains and losses in the daughter cells and newly generates telomere free ends at the breakpoints, which will again fuse and break during the next round of cell division. These repeated 'fusion–bridge–breakage cycles' generate CIN of cells with dysfunctional telomeres.

breaking chromosomes appear during anaphase (Fig. 2). A sharp increase in anaphase bridges was observed during liver regeneration and in early tumours of mTERC–/– mice, pointing to a mechanism of tumour initiation in response to telomere shortening [44,52]. Together, these data suggest that telomere shortening has a dual role in cancer formation. On the one hand, telomere shortening induces CIN and tumour initiation. On the other hand, telomere shortening suppresses progression of tumours, which instead need to stabilize telomere ends to avoid an overload of instability and cancer cell death (Fig. 3). This suggests that telomere shortening during ageing and chronic (liver) disease could contribute to the increased rate of tumour initiation observed in this clinical setting (see

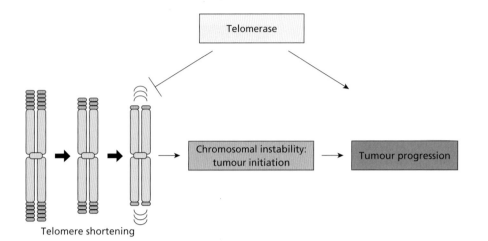

Fig. 3 Telomere shortening has a dual role in cancer. Telomere shortening causes chromosomal fusions and fusion–bridge–breakage cycles (Fig. 2) resulting in CIN and tumour initiation. However, tumour progression requires stabilization of telomere ends to limit ongoing CIN. The telomere hypothesis of HCC development indicates that telomeres shorten during chronic liver diseases and cirrhosis formation. This results in telomere dysfunction, CIN and HCC initiation. At this stage, massive CIN selects for reactivation of telomerase necessary for the stabilization of chromosomes.

Chapters 6.3 and 18.2.1). However, the tumours that evolve in response to telomere shortening apparently need to reactivate telomerase to stabilize telomeres and to prevent ongoing CIN to allow tumour progression. This model could explain the coexistence of critically short telomeres, CIN and high levels of telomerase activity prevalent in most human epithelial cancer cells including HCC [52]. In support of the hypothesis that telomere shortening leads to CIN and cancer initiation in human HCC, a strong correlation between telomere shortening and increase in copy number of chromosome 8 – a hallmark cytogenetic alteration in human HCC – was observed [57]. As tumour suppression in response to telomere shortening was linked to an activation of senescence signalling involving p53 (see above), it appeared a logical consequence that loss of p53 amplified the development of CIN and epithelial cancer initiation induced by telomere shortening in mTERC–/– mice [58]. Heterozygous deletion of p53 alleviated suppression of hepatocarcinogenesis in mice with short telomeres [59]. In humans, the p53 signalling pathway is defective in over 70% of HCC [60], indicating that there could be a cooperation between telomere shortening and loss of p53 function. The role of telomerase reactivation in tumours arising from cells with dysfunctional telomeres and mutant p53 has now to be investigated. Recent data in mouse models have revealed experimental evidence that massive telomere dysfunction induced apoptosis independent of p53 gene status [61], indicating that telomerase activation and telomere stabilization might be essential for tumour progression even in the absence of p53. In agreement with this assumption, it was found that oligonucleotide telomerase inhibitors impaired the growth of p53 mutant human hepatoma in a xenotransplant model [62].

Regarding the use of telomerase activators for improvement of hepatocyte regeneration at the cirrhosis stage (see above), it will be important to elucidate which of the mechanisms induced by telomere dysfunction – impaired regeneration, increased tumour initiation, impaired tumour progression – is dominantly affecting organismal survival. One mouse study has revealed that, in the setting of chronic liver damage, the negative impact of telomere shortening on liver regeneration outweighs the tumour suppressor effects of telomere shortening on hepatocarcinogenesis in terms of overall survival [63].

Outlook

Research work over the last decades has improved our understanding of the control of liver cell proliferation during regeneration, cirrhosis formation and hepatocarcinogenesis. In cancer, promising molecular therapies are now emerging. Similarly, it appears possible that the mechanisms of cell cycle control, telomere length control and senescence will translate into the development of new therapies to improve endogenous regeneration and cell transplantation therapies. Additional areas of interest are: (i) the development of biological ageing markers to improve individual therapies and the assessment of individual risk of disease progression; and (ii) the identification of markers indicating the risk of tumour development, thus allowing the optimization of tumour prevention and screening.

References

1 Fausto N (2004) Liver regeneration and repair: hepatocytes, progenitor cells, and stem cells. *Hepatology* 39 (6), 1477–1487.
2 Sherr CJ, Roberts JM (2004) Living with or without cyclins and cyclin-dependent kinases. *Genes Dev* 18 (22), 2699–2711.
3 Michalopoulos GK, DeFrances M (2005) Liver regeneration. *Adv Biochem Eng Biotechnol* 93, 101–134.
4 Zimmermann A (2004) Regulation of liver regeneration. *Nephrol Dial Transplant* 19 (Suppl 4), 6–10.
5 Liu H, Dibling B, Spike B *et al.* (2004) New roles for the RB tumor suppressor protein. *Curr Opin Genet Dev* 14 (1), 55–64.
6 Attwooll C, Denchi EL, Helin K (2004) The E2F family: specific functions and overlapping interests. *EMBO J* 23 (24), 4709–4716.
7 Mayhew CN, Bosco EE, Fox SR *et al.* (2005) Liver-specific pRB loss results in ectopic cell cycle entry and aberrant ploidy. *Cancer Res* 65 (11), 4568–4577.
8 Vodermaier HC (2004) APC/C and SCF: controlling each other and the cell cycle. *Curr Biol* 14 (18), R787–796.

9 Wirth KG, Ricci R, Gimenez-Abian JF *et al.* (2004) Loss of the anaphase-promoting complex in quiescent cells causes unscheduled hepatocyte proliferation. *Genes Dev* 18 (1), 88–98.

10 Diehl JA, Cheng M, Roussel MF *et al.* (1998) Glycogen synthase kinase-3beta regulates cyclin D1 proteolysis and subcellular localization. *Genes Dev* 12 (22), 3499–3511.

11 Nelsen CJ, Kuriyama R, Hirsch B *et al.* (2005) Short term cyclin D1 overexpression induces centrosome amplification, mitotic spindle abnormalities, and aneuploidy. *J Biol Chem* 280 (1), 768–776.

12 Nelsen CJ, Rickheim DG, Timchenko NA *et al.* (2001) Transient expression of cyclin D1 is sufficient to promote hepatocyte replication and liver growth in vivo. *Cancer Res* 61 (23), 8564–8568.

13 Geng Y, Whoriskey W, Park MY *et al.* (1999) Rescue of cyclin D1 deficiency by knockin cyclin E. *Cell* 97 (6), 767–777.

14 Nelsen CJ, Hansen LK, Rickheim DG *et al.* (2001) Induction of hepatocyte proliferation and liver hyperplasia by the targeted expression of cyclin E and skp2. *Oncogene* 20 (15), 1825–1831.

15 Carrano AC, Eytan E, Hershko A *et al.* (1999) SKP2 is required for ubiquitin-mediated degradation of the CDK inhibitor p27. *Nature Cell Biol* 1 (4), 193–199.

16 Sherr CJ, Roberts JM (1999) CDK inhibitors: positive and negative regulators of G1-phase progression. *Genes Dev* 13 (12), 1501–1512.

17 Geng Y, Yu Q, Sicinska E *et al.* (2003) Cyclin E ablation in the mouse. *Cell* 114 (4), 431–443.

18 Ortega S, Prieto I, Odajima J *et al.* (2003) Cyclin-dependent kinase 2 is essential for meiosis but not for mitotic cell division in mice. *Nature Genet* 35 (1), 25–31.

19 Martin A, Odajima J, Hunt SL *et al.* (2005) Cdk2 is dispensable for cell cycle inhibition and tumor suppression mediated by p27(Kip1) and p21(Cip1). *Cancer Cell* 7 (6), 591–598.

20 Wu H, Wade M, Krall L *et al.* (1996) Targeted in vivo expression of the cyclin-dependent kinase inhibitor p21 halts hepatocyte cell-cycle progression, postnatal liver development and regeneration. *Genes Dev* 10 (3), 245–260.

21 Kossatz U, Dietrich N, Zender L *et al.* (2004) Skp2-dependent degradation of p27kip1 is essential for cell cycle progression. *Genes Dev* 18 (21), 2602–2607.

22 Karnezis AN, Dorokhov M, Grompe M *et al.* (2001) Loss of p27(Kip1) enhances the transplantation efficiency of hepatocytes transferred into diseased livers. *J Clin Invest* 108 (3), 383–390.

23 Guidotti JE, Bregerie O, Robert A *et al.* (2003) Liver cell polyploidization: a pivotal role for binuclear hepatocytes. *J Biol Chem* 278 (21), 19095–19101.

24 Wang X, Kiyokawa H, Dennewitz MB *et al.* (2002) The Forkhead Box m1b transcription factor is essential for hepatocyte DNA replication and mitosis during mouse liver regeneration. *Proc Natl Acad Sci USA* 99 (26), 16881–16886.

25 Kalinichenko VV, Major ML, Wang X *et al.* (2004) Foxm1b transcription factor is essential for development of hepatocellular carcinomas and is negatively regulated by the p19ARF tumor suppressor. *Genes Dev* 18 (7), 830–850.

26 Eferl R, Ricci R, Kenner L *et al.* (2003) Liver tumor development. c-Jun antagonizes the proapoptotic activity of p53. *Cell* 112 (2), 181–192.

27 Behrens A, Sibilia M, David JP *et al.* (2002) Impaired postnatal hepatocyte proliferation and liver regeneration in mice lacking c-jun in the liver. *EMBO J* 21 (7), 1782–1790.

28 Blackburn EH (1991) Structure and function of telomeres. *Nature* 350 (6319), 569–573.

29 Griffith JD, Comeau L, Rosenfield S *et al.* Mammalian telomeres end in a large duplex loop. *Cell* (1999) 97 (4), 503–514.

30 Phan AT, Mergny JL (2002) Human telomeric DNA: G-quadruplex, i-motif and Watson–Crick double helix. *Nucleic Acids Res* 30 (21), 4618–4625.

31 Smogorzewska A, De Lange T (2004) Regulation of telomerase by telomeric proteins. *Annu Rev Biochem* 73, 177–208.

32 Allsopp RC, Chang E, Kashefi-Aazam M *et al.* (1995) Telomere shortening is associated with cell division in vitro and in vivo. *Exp Cell Res* 220 (1), 194–200.

33 Meyerson M, Counter CM, Eaton EN *et al.* (1997) hEST2, the putative human telomerase catalytic subunit gene, is up-regulated in tumor cells and during immortalization. *Cell* 90 (4), 785–795.

34 Nakayama J, Tahara H, Tahara E *et al.* (1998) Telomerase activation by hTRT in human normal fibroblasts and hepatocellular carcinomas. *Nature Genet* 18 (1), 65–68.

35 Allsopp RC, Harley CB (1995) Evidence for a critical telomere length in senescent human fibroblasts. *Exp Cell Res* 219 (1), 130–136.

36 Bodnar AG, Ouellette M, Frolkis M *et al.* (1998) Extension of life-span by introduction of telomerase into normal human cells. *Science* 279 (5349), 349–352.

37 Wege H, Le HT, Chui MS *et al.* (2003) Telomerase reconstitution immortalizes human fetal hepatocytes without disrupting their differentiation potential. *Gastroenterology* 124 (2), 432–444.

38 d'Adda di Fagagna F, Reaper PM, Clay-Farrace L *et al.* (2003) A DNA damage checkpoint response in telomere-initiated senescence. *Nature* 426 (6963), 194–198.

39 Satyanarayana A, Greenberg RA, Schaetzlein S *et al.* (2004) Mitogen stimulation cooperates with telomere shortening to activate DNA damage responses and senescence signaling. *Mol Cell Biol* 24 (12), 5459–5474.

40 Gire V, Roux P, Wynford-Thomas D *et al.* (2004) DNA damage checkpoint kinase Chk2 triggers replicative senescence. *EMBO J* 23 (13), 2554–2563.

41 Chin L, Artandi SE, Shen Q *et al.* (1999) p53 deficiency rescues the adverse effects of telomere loss and cooperates with telomere dysfunction to accelerate carcinogenesis. *Cell* 97 (4), 527–538.

42 Kirk KE, Harmon BP, Reichardt IK *et al.* (1997) Block in anaphase chromosome separation caused by a telomerase template mutation. *Science* 275 (5305), 1478–1481.

43 Wright WE, Shay JW (1992) The two-stage mechanism controlling cellular senescence and immortalization. *Exp Gerontol* 27 (4), 383–389.

44 Djojosubroto MW, Choi YS, Lee HW *et al.* (2003) Telomeres and telomerase in aging, regeneration and cancer. *Mol Cells* 15 (2), 164–175.

45 Lechel A, Manns MP, Rudolph KL (2004) Telomeres and telomerase: new targets for the treatment of liver cirrhosis and hepatocellular carcinoma. *J Hepatol* 41, 491–497.

46 Wiemann SU, Satyanarayana A, Tsahuridu M *et al.* (2002) Hepatocyte telomere shortening and senescence are general markers of human liver cirrhosis. *FASEB J* 16 (9), 935–942.

47 Rudolph KL, Chang S, Millard M *et al.* (2000) Inhibition of experimental liver cirrhosis in mice by telomerase gene delivery. *Science* 287 (5456), 1253–1258.

48 Satyanarayana A, Wiemann SU, Buer J *et al.* (2003) Telomere shortening impairs organ regeneration by inhibiting cell cycle re-entry of a subpopulation of cells. *EMBO J* 22 (15), 4003–4013.

49 Delhaye M, Louis H, Degraef C *et al.* (1999) Hepatocyte proliferative activity in human liver cirrhosis. *J Hepatol* 30 (3), 461–471.

50 Delhaye M, Louis H, Degraef C *et al.* (1996) Relationship between hepatocyte proliferative activity and liver functional reserve in human cirrhosis. *Hepatology* 23 (5), 1003–1011.

51 Tillmann HL, Manns MP, Rudolph KL (2005) Merging models of hepatitis C virus pathogenesis. *Semin Liver Dis* 25 (1), 84–92.

52 Satyanarayana A, Manns M, Rudolph K (2004) Telomeres and telomerase: a dual role in hepatocarcinogenesis. *Hepatology* 40 (2), 276–283.

53 Greenberg RA, Chin L, Femino A *et al.* (1999) Short dysfunctional telomeres impair tumorigenesis in the INK4a(delta2/3) cancer-prone mouse. *Cell* 97 (4), 515–525.

54 Gonzalez-Suarez E, Samper E, Flores JM *et al.* (2000) Telomerase-deficient mice with short telomeres are resistant to skin tumorigenesis. *Nature Genet* 26 (1), 114–117.

55 Rudolph KL, Millard M, Bosenberg MW *et al.* (2001) Telomere dysfunction and evolution of intestinal carcinoma in mice and humans. *Nature Genet* 28 (2), 155–159.

56 Farazi PA, Glickman J, Jiang S *et al.* (2003) Differential impact of telomere dysfunction on initiation and progression of hepatocellular carcinoma. *Cancer Res* 63 (16), 5021–5027.

57 Plentz R, Gebel M, Mann M *et al.* (2005) Telomere shortening correlates with increasing aneuploidy of chromosome 8 on a cellular level in primary human hepatocellularcarcinoma, *Hepatology* 42, 522–526.

58 Artandi SE, Chang S, Lee SL *et al.* (2000) Telomere dysfunction promotes non-reciprocal translocations and epithelial cancers in mice. *Nature* 406 (6796), 641–645.

59 Farazi PA, Glickmann J, Horner J *et al.* (2006) Cooperative interactions of p53 mutation, telomere dysfunction, and chronic liver damage in hepatocellular carcinoma. *Cancer Res* 66 (9), 4766–4773.

60 Tannapfel A, Busse C, Weinans L *et al.* (2001) INK4a-ARF alterations and p53 mutations in hepatocellular carcinomas. *Oncogene* 20 (48), 7104–7109.

61 Lechel A, Satyanarayana A, Ju Z *et al.* (2005) The cellular level of telomere dysfunction determines induction of senescence or apoptosis in vivo. *EMBO Rep* 6 (3), 275–281.

62 Djojosubroto MW, Chin AC, Go N *et al.* (2005) Telomerase antagonists GRN163 and GRN163L inhibit tumor growth and increase chemosensitivity of human hepatoma. *Hepatology* 42 (5), 1127–1136 .

63 Wiemann SU, Satyanarayana A, Buer J *et al.* (2004) Contrasting effects of telomere shortening on organ homeostasis, tumor suppression, and survival during chronic liver damage. *Oncogene* 24 (9), 1501–1509.

2.5.2 Regeneration of chronically injured liver

Anna Mae Diehl

As in other organs, maintenance of tissue integrity in the liver requires a balance between cell death and regeneration so that cells undergoing natural age-related apoptosis are replaced by healthy cells that maintain vital tissue-specific functions. Liver injury amplifies the rate and magnitude of cell death. Consequently, recovery from liver damage necessitates accentuated regenerative responses to restore liver architecture and function to the premorbid state.

The adult liver has tremendous regenerative capacity, as evidenced by complete reconstitution of functional liver mass within weeks of partial hepatectomy (PH) [1]. The regenerative response evoked by acute liver damage has been studied for decades. That work identified several factors that promote the proliferation of mature hepatocytes and delineated pathways that modulate hepatocyte cell cycle progression and viability (reviewed in [2,3]). Because regeneration of bile ducts and hepatic blood vessels following acute liver injury has been less well studied (reviewed in [4,5]), how replacement of those structures is coordinated with recovery of the hepatocyte mass is less certain. Nevertheless, because hepatic regeneration following acute injury has been the subject of numerous recent reviews, it will not be discussed extensively in this chapter. Rather, we will focus on mechanisms that mediate the regeneration of chronically injured livers.

Chronic liver damage results from insufficient regeneration

Chronic liver injury poses a significant health threat. Chronic liver damage is among the leading causes of premature death in adults [6,7]. Given that the liver typically regenerates completely following massive acute injury, it is curious that repetitive, seemingly milder, insults are often not completely repaired, leading to persistent (and sometimes progressive) liver damage. This observation raises the intriguing possibility that chronic liver damage is more attributable to subpar repair than to unusually severe injury.

That insufficient liver regeneration may play a key role in the pathogenesis of chronic liver damage of various aetiologies merits consideration. At first glance, this concept appears to contradict liver biopsy evidence of increased hepatocyte DNA synthesis in chronically damaged livers [8]. Although the latter finding suggests that a regenerative response is attempting to repair the injured tissue, it must not match the substantially increased rate of liver cell death because hepatocyte 'dropout', 'piecemeal necrosis', apoptosis and 'ballooning' (indicative of ongoing necrosis) generally predominate [9]. In addition, chronic liver injury itself sometimes results in replacement of hepatocytes and bile ducts with fibrous tissue. Thus, persistent liver injury appears gradually to deplete regenerative capacity, resulting in sustained loss of normal liver architecture and function.

Why liver regeneration falters during chronic injury is unclear. It is not known whether certain injuries also inhibit regeneration, or if some individuals are simply unable to mount a normal regenerative response to injury that is efficiently repaired by most others. Similarly, it is poorly understood how age, gender, diet, comorbid conditions and their treatments affect any given individual's hepatic regenerative capacity, thus changing the degree of liver damage that ensues during chronic exposure to a constant level of injury. All these questions have obvious clinical relevance. Thus, it is imperative that we learn more about the mechanisms that regulate the regeneration of chronically injured livers.

Unfortunately, research in this area is sparse. In contrast to acute liver regeneration studies that typically focus on proliferative responses of mature hepatocytes, most investigations of repair in chronically injured livers focus on fibrogenesis. Consequently, it is poorly understood how dying hepatocytes or cholangiocytes are replaced during chronic liver injury. Also unknown is how efforts to compensate for increased rates of hepatic epithelial cell death relate to fibrotic responses, including increased proliferation of hepatic stellate cells (HSC) and their activation to a more myofibroblastic phenotype. The remainder of this chapter will summarize information about mechanisms that mediate the replacement of various liver cell populations in chronically injured livers, highlighting differences between acute and chronic repair.

Mechanisms for hepatocyte replacement during liver injury

Proliferation of mature hepatocytes

Healthy livers

Mature hepatocytes rarely replicate in healthy adult livers. The low proliferative index matches the low prevalence of hepatocyte apoptosis. In health, there is a gradient of hepatocyte DNA synthesis across the liver lobule, with most proliferation occurring in periportal hepatocytes and least in hepatocytes near terminal hepatic venules [3]. This gradient may be driven by the progressive decline in proliferative activity in ageing progeny from resident, periportal progenitor cells [10]. Alternatively, the portal-to-central gradient of soluble, gut-derived hepatotrophic factors may be responsible for the fall off in proliferative activity [11,12]. Portal blood might also carry in precursor cells from the marrow-like environment of the spleen, which may provide a reservoir for exogenous liver progenitors [13]. The potential importance of portal venous factors (soluble or cellular) as regulators of basal levels of hepatocyte proliferation is supported by evidence that otherwise healthy livers atrophy when deprived of portal blood [12]. Also, hepatocyte proliferation normally fluctuates over the course of the day and is highest postprandially, when portal venous blood flow to the liver increases [14].

Acutely injured livers

Acute loss of liver mass generally elicits a robust proliferative response in residual healthy hepatocytes, as evidenced by dramatically increased rates of DNA synthesis and mitoses in mature-appearing (i.e. differentiated) adult hepatocytes after 70% PH or acute exposure to hepatotoxins [3]. However, the ultimate proliferative capacity of any given mature hepatocyte has been difficult to assess. In uninjured livers, most mature hepatocytes have exited proliferative phases of the cell cycle and live in a growth-arrested (G0) state. The extent to which some or all of these cells can re-enter the cell cycle and replicate after liver injury remains uncertain, despite decades of research.

When cultured in the presence of growth factors, primary adult hepatocytes proliferate poorly on most matrices, despite robustly upregulating prereplicative genes and DNA synthesis. Sparse proliferation may merely be an artefact of arduous isolation protocols or suboptimal culture conditions [3]. Indeed, hepatocyte transplantation experiments have generated support for the concept that mature hepatocytes generally retain considerable capacity for proliferation *in vivo*. In one study, labelled hepatocytes isolated from adult rat donor livers were transplanted directly into one lobe of a recipient rat's liver after ligating portal vein branches to the other lobes [15]. Deprived of portal blood flow, those segments involuted. Eventually, the entire liver mass was reconstituted by donor hepatocytes. Based on the number of hepatocytes that were transplanted, the authors concluded that a single hepatocyte can divide at least 34 times, giving rise to 1.7×10^{10} daughter cells. This implies that a single rat hepatocyte has the clonogenic potential to generate 50 adult rat livers. However, it is difficult to exclude the possibility that the donor liver cells used in these studies might have included progenitor cells.

Another widely cited argument for the high proliferative capability of mature hepatocytes is the adult liver's ability to regenerate completely after PH [1]. Indeed, the ancient Greek myth about Prometheus revolves around the liver's ability to regenerate after pieces of liver have been removed. To monitor the kinetics of DNA synthesis following PH, rats were partially hepatectomized and killed at various times during the first day and 1, 2, 3, 7 and 14 days after PH. One hour before killing, each rat was injected intraperitoneally with tritiated thymidine or bromodeoxyuridine to label newly synthesized DNA, and autoradiography or immunohistochemistry was done to calculate the hepatocyte labelling index during the previous hour [16,17]. These studies demonstrate that DNA synthesis (S phase) in mature hepatocytes begins at around 24 h, and the labelling index reaches its peak value of 3–4% on day 3 after PH. This represents a 26-fold (2600%) increase in the hepatocyte labelling index over basal, pre-PH values. During the same time, hepatocytes double their ploidy, suggesting that half the observed labelling index increase is due to DNA accumulation and half to cell division. If this interpretation is valid, then the hepatocyte production rate increases 13-fold during the initial 72 h after PH. However, the morphometry of regenerating livers suggests that hepatocyte proliferation may not be this robust because the hepatic acini increase in size by only about 15% during this time period. This is not sufficient to accommodate the number of hepatocytes that would be generated by an acute 1300% increase in proliferative activity [16]. This finding suggests that much of the acute post-PH increase in hepatocyte labelling index occurs because damaged hepatocyte DNA is being repaired. Nevertheless, some mature hepatocytes do proliferate after PH [3].

Traditionally, the PH model is considered to be a 'pure' model of regeneration because the remnant liver lobes are not directly manipulated (i.e. injured) at the time of PH [1]. However, serum aminotransferase levels usually increase after PH. Also, careful inspection of liver sections typically reveals increased apoptotic bodies, as well as scattered foci of swollen hepatocytes, that are variably associated with haemorrhage and small cell infiltrates [18–20]. Thus, in many ways, PH resembles acute exposure to hepatotoxic drugs because both insults result in liver injury and abrupt loss of functioning hepatocytes. Subpopulations of surviving mature hepatocytes subsequently proliferate and the liver regenerates its mass within 10–14 days [21].

Chronically injured livers

In contrast to hepatocytes in healthy livers, mature hepatocytes in chronically injured livers exhibit markedly reduced and delayed proliferative responses to PH [22,23]. The replication defect appears to be intrinsic to the hepatocytes themselves, as primary hepatocytes isolated from chronically injured livers respond poorly to mitogens in cell culture [24]. The mechanisms for inhibited proliferative capacity are being elucidated, and seem to be related to chronic injury-related stress. Even very mild forms of chronic liver injury, such as steatosis, elicit such stress. Hepatocytes in fatty livers are chronically exposed to increased levels of inflammatory mediators, including tumour necrosis factor (TNF)α and interleukin (IL)-6, cytokines that promote hepatocyte replication in healthy livers. Chronic exposure to TNFα increases reactive oxygen species production and can also induce cellular apoptosis. Hepatocytes typically survive these threats by upregulating various antiapoptotic and antioxidant defences [25,26]. However, these survival mechanisms are apparently insufficient for complete protection because rates of hepatocyte apoptosis are increased in both experimental animals and patients with fatty livers [27,28], and surviving hepatocytes exhibit evidence of oxidative damage to nuclear and mitochondrial DNA [27].

Viable but damaged cells in chronically injured livers elicit various adaptive mechanisms, including the induction of stress-related kinases that activate cyclin-dependent kinase inhibitors to restrict cell cycle progression [23]. The resultant replicative senescence prevents the duplication of sublethally damaged hepatocytes, while preserving liver-specific functions. Although this is generally beneficial, it compromises the efficiency of liver regeneration by removing mature hepatocytes from the regenerative response. Hence, recovery from a superimposed injury (such as PH) is prolonged in fatty livers, and the liver remains damaged for longer.

Stress-related replicative senescence in mature hepatocytes is not a phenomenon that is restricted to chronic fatty liver diseases. Mature hepatocytes of mice that are genetically deficient in PARP, an important DNA repair enzyme, also exhibit replicative senescence [24]. Although the livers of young PARP-deficient mice appear grossly normal, closer inspection demonstrates accumulation of hepatocytes with damaged DNA. Following PH, induction of DNA synthesis in mature, PARP-deficient hepatocytes is significantly inhibited. Moreover, the rate of entry into S phase is markedly reduced when primary hepatocytes from PARP-deficient mice are cultured with mitogens. Given that cellular DNA damage triggers growth arrest, the findings in PARP-deficient mice are not surprising. Together with the results from mice with fatty livers [23], and patients with chronic viral hepatitis [9], these data demonstrate that most viable hepatocytes in chronically injured livers have sustained damage and become senescent. Consequently, mechanisms other than mature hepatocyte replication must be evoked to replace dying hepatocytes.

Hepatocyte hypertrophy and polyploidy

Hepatocytes enlarge (i.e. hypertrophy) in many chronic liver diseases. A report from Thorgeirsson's group [29] suggests that hepatic hypertrophy is a compensatory mechanism to restore normal liver mass when hepatocyte proliferation is inhibited. Rats that underwent PH after being treated with 5-fluorouracil to inhibit hepatocyte proliferation were able to recover liver mass without inducing hepatic DNA synthesis. The initial, acute restoration of liver mass was accomplished by enlargement (hypertrophy) of the periportal hepatocytes. However, the hypertrophied state was not stable because, once the DNA synthesis inhibitor was withdrawn, the enlarged hepatocytes entered the cell cycle, and normal liver structure and DNA content were re-established [29]. Therefore, hypertrophy of residual surviving hepatocytes appears to be a temporizing response that transiently boosts liver mass following a bout of hepatocyte death.

DNA replication without cell division (i.e. polyploidy) contributes to cellular hypertrophy. Polyploidy occurs whenever DNA damage outstrips base excision repair mechanisms [30]. This occurs following exposure to 5-fluorouracil and other DNA-damaging agents. Hepatocytes with non-lethal damage become arrested in G2 so that they can be repaired, while those that acquired irreparable DNA damage after exiting the G1 checkpoint are deleted. Even in healthy animals, acute liver injury evoked by PH increases the number of polyploid hepatocytes [31]. Sustained exposure to oxidative stress amplifies this response. Thus, hepatocyte polyploidy is increased in chronically injured livers, indicating that the proportion of mature hepatocytes that are capable of replication is reduced.

Differentiation of hepatic progenitors

Although replication of mature hepatocytes is severely crippled during chronic liver injury, atrophy is a relatively rare, late response to chronic injury. Hence, there must be other mechanisms to replace dead hepatocytes. Studies of liver biopsies from patients and animals with various aetiologies of chronic liver injury indicate that expansion and differentiation of hepatic progenitors are the predominant forces that maintain hepatocyte mass in chronically injured livers.

Even healthy adult livers contain progenitors [32]. These progenitor populations are heterogeneous [33]. Some are bipotential (i.e. capable of generating either cholangiocytes or hepatocytes), but whether any are more pluripotent is debated [34–37]. Thus, it is uncertain whether resident hepatic progenitors can generate other types of liver cells (e.g. endothelial cells, stellate cells, resident hepatic immune cells) or non-hepatic epithelia (e.g. pancreas, intestine, kidney, lung). Liver progenitor subpopulations might be replenished from extrahepatic sources, such as bone marrow, but the extent to which this occurs is also debated, as is the process involved (i.e. fusion or transdifferentiation) [38–42]. Whether or not any of these progenitors are true stem cells, capable of infinite self-renewal while generating progeny that differentiate into adult liver cells, is obscure.

Resident hepatic progenitors (oval cells)

Phenotype

To date, the best characterized hepatic progenitors are small cells with scant cytoplasm and an oval-shaped nucleus that reside along the canals of Hering. These cells have been dubbed 'oval cells', 'ductular cells' or 'neocholangiolar cells' based on their morphology and localization along structures that comprise the proximal portion of the intrahepatic biliary system [32,34,43,44]. Expansion of oval cells commonly occurs in various types of chronic liver injury, and is typically described by hepatic pathologists as 'ductular reaction' or 'neocholangiolar proliferation' [9,45–48]. Oval cells variably express poorly characterized cytokeratin antigens, such as OV-1 and OV-6, isoforms of pyruvate kinase (muscle pyruvate kinase; mpk) and γ-glutamyltransferase (γ-GT) that distinguish them from mature hepatocytes and cholangiocytes [49–51]. Some also express surface markers, including c-kit, Sca-1 and CD34, and chemokine receptors (CXCR-4) that are expressed by other types of progenitors [35,52–54]. That oval cells are capable of differentiating into cholangiocytes or hepatocytes is demonstrated by their ability to generate progeny that express biliary cytokeratins, such as CK19, or hepatocyte proteins, such as HNF-4α, α-fetoprotein and albumin [55,56].

Regulatory factors

Immunohistochemistry demonstrates that oval cells accumulate in the livers of patients with chronic viral hepatitis, autoimmune and congenital liver diseases and alcoholic and non-alcoholic fatty liver disease [9,45–48]. Similar cells accumulate in rodents with chronic liver disease [23]. Oval cell accumulation parallels fibrosis stage. Hence, the greatest expansion of oval cells occurs in cirrhotic livers, where oval cells typically localize near activated HSC [23,48]. This association may be driven by paracrine signalling, because HSC produce stem cell-derived factor (SDF)-1, the ligand for CXCR-4 that is expressed by oval cells [54]. Both cell types produce hedgehog (Hh) family ligands (unpublished data). Hh proteins are potent morphogens that promote the viability of various types of progenitor cells [37], including the endodermal progenitors that generate the embryonic liver bud [57]. Similar to other epithelial progenitors [37], some mouse oval cells and stellate cells from mice, rats and humans also express Patched, the cell surface receptor for Hh (unpublished data). Thus, oval cells and HSC may provide each other with important viability signals that permit each cell population to expand during chronic liver injury.

Origin and fate

Other than fairly circumstantial evidence that biliary damage induces oval cells to differentiate into cholangiocytes, and hepatocyte death provokes differentiation along the hepatocyte lineage [32], little is known about factors that determine oval cell fate. It is not known whether some oval cells are true stem cells, capable of infinite self-renewal, or if oval cells are merely progeny of a more stem cell-like progenitor that resides in the liver or some other tissue(s). Experiments with mice that have been rendered genetically deficient in telomerase suggest that stem-like cells do play a role in maintaining adult liver mass.

Because infinite self-renewal is a unique characteristic of stem cells, they require telomerase to repair chromosomal deletions that occur during DNA replication [58]. Consequently, telomerase activity is generally high in fetal tissues and falls with age [59]. However, there are significant tissue-related differences in this ageing response [60]. Adult rat, mice and human livers retain considerable telomerase activity [61]. In healthy adult livers, telomerase mRNA is detected in occasional sinusoidal cells and rare hepatocytes (but not in most mature hepatocytes and cholangiocytes). Injured livers have many more telomerase-positive cells, with frequent expression noted in sinusoidal cells and infiltrating mononuclear cells, and occasional expression in proliferative, ductular cells and hepatocytes [62,63].

Given these findings (and contrary to some studies cited earlier), it is unlikely that most mature hepatocytes can replicate indefinitely, and not surprising that widespread telomere shortening occurs in regenerating livers following the acute injury of PH [64]. Cells with critically shortened telomeres are senescent and never re-enter the cell cycle. Thus, following an acute injury, regeneration is accomplished by subpopulations of non-senescent cells with sufficient telomere reserves to support replication.

These non-senescent cells may encompass a spectrum of the more differentiated progeny of rare liver stem-like cells that persist into adulthood. If true, the latter are the 'seeds' that generate replacement hepatocytes to continuously replenish liver cells that are consumed during day-to-day hepatocyte turnover. The requirement for stem-like cells in adult livers was unmasked by provoking sudden massive hepatocyte loss in telomerase-deficient mice that cannot maintain their stem cell populations. Unlike normal mice, such mice become cirrhotic after experiencing a single insult that abruptly deletes a large number of hepatocytes (e.g. PH) [65]. In retrospect, similarly dismal outcomes were reported in older studies that subjected adult rats to hepatic irradiation (another type of stem cell-depleting insult) prior to PH [66]. Inherited stem cell depletion that results from dysfunctional telomere maintenance also promotes cirrhosis in humans [67].

Together, these findings demonstrate that adult liver mass is maintained by progenitors that continuously differentiate to replace dying mature hepatocytes. This process is taxed when liver injury increases the death rate of more mature liver cells. Whether oval cells are the telomerase-expressing progenitors that fuel regeneration is unknown. It is also conceivable that liver progenitors may simply require factors produced by some other type of telomerase-positive stem cell.

Potential extrahepatic sources of hepatic progenitors

Bone marrow and umbilical cord blood harbour multipotent stem-like cells. Several laboratories have shown that transplantation of bone marrow- or cord blood-derived progenitors can rescue mice from various types of fatal, acute liver damage. Repopulation of recipient liver parenchyma with donor-derived hepatocytes has been demonstrated repeatedly [39,40,42,68–74]. However, the extent and duration of repopulation has varied widely among different reports. Few studies have examined whether reconstitution of the hepatocyte compartment is preceded by the appearance of donor-derived oval cells, and those that have looked report discrepant results.

Grompe and collaborators have presented compelling evidence that donor cells simply fuse with recipient hepatocytes to regenerate livers in their FAH-deficient mouse model of tyrosinaemia and liver failure [75,76]. However, the general relevance of these findings is uncertain because FAH deficiency damages progenitor cells [77]. Further confounding data interpretation in these experiments, donor bone marrow cells were obtained from animals with Fanconi's anaemia, another progenitor cell defect [78]. Thus, it is difficult to know whether fusion of progenitors and residual mature hepatocytes occurs predominantly when progenitors are defective or is a more typical response.

Studies of mice with other types of acute and chronic liver injury suggest that fusion is probably not a common phenomenon during liver regeneration [40,72,79,80]. These studies also demonstrate that differentiation of donor-derived cells into hepatocytes can definitely occur in living animals. These findings complement abundant data from cell culture experiments showing that bone marrow- and cord blood-derived progenitors can differentiate into functional hepatocytes [41,74]. Less certain is whether this generation of hepatocytes from extrahepatic progenitors evolves through oval cell-like intermediaries, and how often this mechanism is evoked during repair of acute or chronic liver injury. Thus, it remains conceivable that circulating stem-like cells mainly provide factors that optimize the differentiation and proliferation of resident liver progenitors, including oval cells.

Mechanisms that regulate cholangiocyte replacement

Proliferation of mature cholangiocytes

Evidence for DNA synthesis in bile duct cells (i.e. large cholangiocytes) after PH or carbon tetrachloride-induced liver injury demonstrates that, like mature hepatocytes, mature cholangiocytes can also proliferate under certain circumstances [81,82]. During post-PH liver regeneration, bile duct DNA synthesis is coincident with that of liver sinusoidal cells, following peak hepatocyte DNA synthesis by about a day. Studies in cultured cholangiocytes, as well as in experimental animals demonstrate that cholangiocyte proliferation is induced by some of the same factors that promote hepatocyte proliferation, including insulin, insulin-like growth factor, hepatocyte growth factor (HGF), IL-6 and epidermal growth factor (EGF). Also, like hepatocyte proliferation, cholangiocyte proliferation is inhibited by transforming growth factor (TGF)-β [83,84]. In addition to these factors, various neurohumoral factors regulate cholangiocyte proliferation. Vagotomy has potent antiproliferative effects on cholangiocytes, despite exacerbating cholangiocyte apoptosis induced by bile duct ligation [83]. Serotonin also inhibits cholangiocyte proliferation. In contrast, cholangiocytes proliferate in response to nerve growth factor (NGF), which increases spontaneously following bile duct ligation [84]. Estrogens also promote cholangiocyte proliferation, while estrogen antagonists, such as tamoxifen, inhibit it [85].

Cholangiocytes produce several growth-regulatory peptides, including HGF, IL-6 and NGF, and use these to autoregulate their proliferation [4,84]. Net proliferative activity appears to be governed by modulation of protein kinase A (PKA) and protein kinase C (PKC) signalling, with the former stimulating p42/p44 and p38 mitogen-activated protein kinases (MAPK) and cellular proliferation, while the latter inhibits these events. In addition to directly promoting proliferation, some trophic factors, such as taurocholate, also activate AKT and phosphatidyl-inositol-3 (PI3) kinase. The upregulation of these survival pathways enhances the actions of cholangiocyte mitogens.

HSC produce some of the neurohumoral factors and cytokines that regulate cholangiocyte growth. This is intriguing, particularly as the phenotype of stellate cells themselves is also modulated by these factors. Thus, it is likely that cross-talk between stellate cells and adjacent cholangiocytes regulates the response to bile duct injury.

Expansion and differentiation of cholangiocyte progenitors

Many types of acute and chronic liver injury (not merely injury that is restricted to bile ducts) are followed by proliferation of immature bile ductular cells. Some of these cells are bipotential hepatic progenitors (oval cells), and others are their immediate progeny (small cholangiocytes). It has even been suggested that hepatocytes might transdifferentiate into hepatocytes during some types of bile duct injury [86]. Proliferation of immature ductular cells is most evident along the edges of portal triads, at the portal–parenchymal interface, where small ductular-like structures (i.e. neocholangioles) accumulate. As recovery proceeds, these structures disappear, presumably because the ductular cells that are differentiating along the cholangiocyte lineage migrate into bile ducts to replace dying mature cholangiocytes.

Chronic bile duct damage: cell death exceeds replacement

Given that mature cholangiocytes can proliferate, and adult livers normally contain progenitors for cholangiocytes, it is uncertain why ductopenia and bile duct strictures are consequences of certain types of chronic liver injury. Bile ducts are particularly vulnerable to damage from chronic immune attack, ischaemia and obstruction [4]. The relative contributions of increased cholangiocyte death rates and inhibited cholangiocyte replacement to eventual bile duct destruction remain largely unexamined. However, studies of liver biopsies from patients with primary biliary cirrhosis suggest that loss of cholangiocyte progenitors (i.e. defective repair) is important [87]. Such livers exhibit reduced numbers of canals of Hering, the most proximal portion of the bile drainage pathway with a cholangiocyte lining. Oval cells localize to canals of Hering. Thus, reduced numbers of these structures may signify a depletion of progenitor pools that are available to replace dying bile duct cells, leading to eventual ductopenia.

Mechanisms that regulate hepatic endothelial replacement

The hepatic endothelium is targeted for destruction during acute and chronic liver injury induced by ischaemia–reperfusion and hepatotoxins, including chemotherapeutic agents and ethanol. Endothelial damage also occurs in more obscure hepatic vasculopathies, such as Budd–Chiari syndrome, and during hepatic allograft rejection. Thus, endothelial cells must be replaced during repair of various types of liver injury. The mechanisms for this are poorly understood.

The endothelia of large blood vessels and many capillary beds are replenished by circulating endothelial progenitors, some of which are derived from bone marrow progenitors [88,89]. There has been relatively little research about the role of bone marrow-derived endothelial progenitors in maintaining (or restoring) hepatic vascular integrity. *In situ* analysis of donor and recipient cells following liver and bone marrow transplantation suggests that this may occur. However, whether or not circulating endothelial progenitors contribute significantly to endothelial repair in other settings has been debated [90,91].

Certain resident liver cells produce matrix molecules and soluble factors that regulate angiogenesis [5]. For example, HSC are rich local sources of leptin and vascular endothelial growth factor. Thus, it is conceivable that increased release of these factors by activated stellate cells in the subendothelial spaces of injured livers may stimulate the proliferation of residual mature endothelial cells and/or differentiation of nearby endothelial progenitors. Conversely, endothelial cells themselves express adhesion molecules and chemotactic molecules that recruit other types of cells, including bone marrow-derived endothelial progenitors, into the liver [92]. The hepatic sinusoidal endothelia might also elaborate signals that influence the phenotype of resident stellate cells. Pertinent to these points, Wanless and colleagues have suggested that endothelial dysfunction may contribute to the genesis of cirrhosis during chronic liver injury [93,94].

Mechanisms that regulate hepatic stellate cell replacement

Healthy livers

Virtually nothing is known about the mechanisms that maintain HSC populations in healthy livers. Even in uninjured livers, mesenchymal populations are composed of heterogeneous cell types [95–98]. The prototypical 'quiescent' HSC is retinoid rich and expresses several neural markers, such as glial fibrillary acidic protein and nestin, as well as desmin, a mesenchymal marker [99,100]. In uninjured livers, histological assessment of retinoid-rich sinusoidal cells suggests that the ratio of HSC to hepatocytes is relatively constant [100,101]. Long-term coculture studies of mature hepatocytes and HSC demonstrate that HSC processes can form tight junctions with hepatocytes, suggesting that cell-to-cell communication between hepatocytes and HSC may regulate the phenotypes of both cell types [102]. However, because standard isolation protocols do not yield perfectly pure populations of quiescent HSC [99], and standard culture conditions quickly activate HSC to a myofibroblastic phenotype that expresses α-smooth muscle actin (Asma) and type 1 collagen [95], characterization of the gene expression profile of truly quiescent HSC has proved difficult. Recently, Tsukamoto and colleagues reported culture conditions that appear to revert activated HSC to a more quiescent phenotype. Under such conditions, HSC resemble mature adipocytes, expressing transcription factors, such as PPARγ and C/EBP family members, that induce genes that promote lipid accumulation and inhibit the production of inflammatory mediators, type 1 collagen and smooth muscle cell markers, such as Asma [103].

Acute liver injury

During both acute and chronic liver injury, the liver accumulates HSC [98,104]. Following acute liver injury evoked by PH, HSC in the residual liver become activated to a myofibroblastic phenotype and proliferate [105–107]. In the rat, the onset of HSC proliferation lags behind that of the hepatocyte compartment by ~ 24 h. Attempts to isolate HSC during the first few days following PH have demonstrated that acute liver injury dramatically accentuates the physical association that exists between hepatocytes and HSC. Thus, most HSC (and hepatocyte) preparations from post-PH livers are significantly contaminated with the other cell type [108]. This has confounded efforts to analyse the effect of acute liver injury on HSC gene expression.

Brenner and colleagues have used another strategy to address this question. Recently, they generated double transgenic mice that express genes that encode two different fluorescent markers (EGFP and RGFP) under the respective control of two promoters that transduce distinct genes that are induced during HSC activation (Asma and type 1 collagen) [98]. Consequently, EGFP and RGFP mark cells that have turned on gene expression of Asma and/or collagen in these double transgenic mice. Initial studies of the double transgenic mice have yielded somewhat unanticipated results. Namely, unlike cultures of primary HSC that coordinately upregulate Asma and collagen gene expression during spontaneous *in vitro* activation, transgenic mice respond to liver injury by accumulating cells that express Asma alone (without collagen induction), collagen alone (without Asma) and cells that co-induce both Asma and collagen. Only the last subpopulation matches the culture-activated HSC that have formed the basis of our current understanding of activated HSC. Much remains to be learned about the two other subpopulations and, at this point, it remains uncertain which subpopulation contains the prototypical 'quiescent' HSC that have acquired an activated phenotype. This is a critical issue because cells that are (+) for Asma or collagen I alone might also contribute to the repair of injured livers.

Chronic liver injury

A major difference between the HSC response to acute and chronic liver injury appears to be the duration of HSC activation [98]. Following circumscribed (acute) liver injury, proliferation of activated, myofibroblastic HSC occurs transiently because activated HSC ultimately undergo apoptosis [109]. Hence, apoptosis of injury-activated myofibroblastic HSC plays a major role in reducing the liver burden of these cells back to basal levels [110].

The fact that activated HSC survive at all, let alone proliferate transiently, is intriguing because the microenvironment of injured livers contains numerous noxious factors, including proapoptotic cytokines such as TGF-β. Activated HSC are not impervious to TGF-β because they express receptors for this cytokine and activate TGF-β-regulated signalling cascades to induce collagen gene expression [111]. However, unlike neighbouring hepatocytes, myofibroblastic HSC do not undergo growth arrest or apoptosis when confronted with TGF-β.

In endodermally derived tissues, such as the kidney and liver, cells that are resistant to TGF-β-mediated apoptosis are known to be involved in mesenchymal–epithelial transitions [112]. In fact, in the kidney, it is TGF-β-resistant cells with an epithelial lineage that are driven to acquire a fibroblastic phenotype when exposed to TGF-β (so-called 'epithelial-to-mesenchymal transition' or EMT). Removal of TGF-β or exposure to HGF promotes reversion of the fibroblastic-appearing cells to their more typical, epithelial phenotype ('mesenchymal-to-epithelial transition' or MET) [113]. At present, it is unproven whether similar events occur in the liver. However, the kidney data are certainly provocative given evidence that TGF-β promotes cirrhosis (i.e. accumulation of myofibroblastic cells at the expense of mature hepatocytes) [95,98], while HGF limits the accumulation of activated HSC [110] and promotes the reconstitution of the hepatic parenchyma after liver injury [114]. In this regard, it is important to recall the close physical association between activated, myofibroblastic HSC and oval cells (putative liver epithelial progenitors) in chronically injured livers. Might cirrhosis result from events that drive oval cells (or their progenitors) along a fibroblastic, as opposed to an epithelial, lineage (i.e. EMT)? Conversely, do treatments that promote 'reversal' of cirrhosis simply induce the opposite response (i.e. MET)? Research is needed to delineate the mechanisms that direct repair towards one, as opposed to the other, response.

Summary

This review has summarized evidence that liver remodelling (repair) is a daily event in healthy adults. 'Healthy' remodelling/repair involves both proliferation of mature liver cells and differentiation of their progenitors. Chronic liver injury stresses these responses, unmasking inefficiencies and deficiencies in mechanisms that are designed to balance the reconstitution of different liver cell populations, thereby preserving normal liver architecture and function. Chronic liver damage manifests when healthy remodelling/repair responses are broken. Chronic hepatitis, cirrhosis and hepatocellular carcinoma are extreme manifestations of dysfunctional repair.

References

1 Higgins GM, Andersen RM (1931) Experimental pathology of liver: restoration of liver of the white rat following partial surgical removal. *Arch Pathol* 12, 186–202.

2 Fausto N, Riehle KJ (2005) Mechanisms of liver regeneration and their clinical implications. *J Hepatobiliary Pancreat Surg* 12, 181–189.

3 Michalopoulos GK, DeFrances M (2005) Liver regeneration. *Adv Biochem Eng Biotechnol* 93, 101–134.

4 Strazzabosco M, Fabris L, Spirli C (2005) Pathophysiology of cholangiopathies. *J Clin Gastroenterol* 39, S90–S102.

5 Medina J, Arroyo AG, Sanchez-Madrid F *et al.* (2004) Angiogenesis in chronic inflammatory liver disease. *Hepatology* 39, 1185–1195.

6 Vong S, Bell BP (2004) Chronic liver disease mortality in the United States, 1990–1998. *Hepatology* 39, 476–483.

7 Adams LA, Lymp JF, St Sauver J *et al.* (2005) The natural history of nonalcoholic fatty liver disease: a population-based cohort study. *Gastroenterology* 129, 113–121.

8 Vemuru RP, Aragona E, Gupta S (1992) Analysis of hepatocellular proliferation: study of archival liver tissue is facilitated by an endogenous marker of DNA replication. *Hepatology* 16, 968–973.

9 Clouston AD, Powell EE, Walsh MJ *et al.* (2005) Fibrosis correlates with a ductular reaction in hepatitis C: roles of impaired replication, progenitor cells and steatosis. *Hepatology* 41, 809–818.

10 Zajicek G, Oren R, Weinreb MJ (1985) The streaming liver. *Liver* 5, 293–300.

11 Kennedy S, Rettinger S, Flye MW *et al.* (1995) Experiments in transgenic mice show that hepatocytes are the source for postnatal liver growth and do not stream. *Hepatology* 22, 160–168.

12 Schweizer W, Duda P, Tanner S *et al.* (1995) Experimental atrophy/hypertrophy complex (AHC) of the liver portal vein, but not bile duct obstruction, is the main driving forces for the development of AHC in the rat. *J Hepatol* 23, 71–78.

13 Fernandez-Salguero P, Pineau T, Hilbert DM *et al.* (1995) Immune system impairment and hepatic fibrosis in mice lacking the dioxin-binding Ah receptor. *Science* 268, 638–639.

14 Souto M, Llanos JM (1985) The circadian optimal time for hepatectomy in the study of liver regeneration. *Chronobiol Int* 2, 169–175.

15 Ilan Y, Roy-Chowdhury N, Prakash R *et al.* (1997) Massive repopulation of rat liver by transplantation of hepatocytes into specific lobes of the liver and ligation of portal vein branches to other lobes. *Transplantation* 64, 8–13.

16 Zajicek G, Arber N, Schwartz-Arad D (1991) Streaming liver. VIII: Cell production rates following partial hepatectomy. *Liver* 11, 347–351.

17 Werlich T, Stiller KJ, Machnik G (1998) Experimental studies on the stem cell concept of liver regeneration. *Exp Toxicol Pathol* 50, 73–77.

18 Kanashima R, Nagasue N, Kobayashi M *et al.* (1980) A comparative study of lysomal enzyme contents in blood and liver of rats following partial hepatectomy. *Hepatogastroenterology* 27, 448–456.

19 Colletti LM, Kunkel SL, Green M *et al.* (1996) Hepatic inflammation following 70% hepatectomy may be related to up-regulation of epithelial neutrophil activating protein-78. *Shock* 6, 397–402.

20 Greco M, Moro L, Pellecchia G *et al.* (1998) Release of matrix proteins from mitochondria to cytosol during prereplicative phase of liver regeneration. *FEBS Lett* 427, 179–182.

21 Chung H, Hong DP, Jung JY *et al.* (2005) Comprehensive analysis of differential gene expression profiles on carbon tetrachloride-induced rat liver injury and regeneration. *Toxicol Appl Pharmacol* 206, 27–42.

22 Yang SQ, Lin HZ, Mandal AK *et al.* (2001) Disrupted signaling and inhibition of liver regeneration in obese mice with fatty livers: implications for nonalcoholic fatty liver disease pathogenesis. *Hepatology* 34, 694–706.

23 Roskams T, Yang SQ, Koteish A *et al.* (2003) Oxidative stress and oval cell accumulation in mice and humans with alcoholic and non-alcoholic fatty liver disease. *Am J Pathol* 163, 1301–1311.

24 Yang S, Koteish A, Lin H *et al.* (2004) Oval cells compensate for damage and replicative senescence of mature hepatocytes in mice with fatty liver disease. *Hepatology* 39, 403–411.

25 Rashid A, Wu T-C, Huang CC *et al.* (1999) Mitochondrial proteins that regulate apoptosis and necrosis are induced in mouse fatty liver. *Hepatology* 29, 1131–1138.

26 Yang SQ, Zhu H, Li Y *et al.* (2000) Mitochondrial adaptations to obesity-related oxidant stress. *Arch Biochem Biophys* 378, 259–268.

27 Gao D, Wei C, Chen L *et al.* (2004) Oxidative DNA damage and DNA repair enzyme expression are inversely related in murine models of fatty liver disease. *Am J Physiol Gastrointest Liver Physiol* 287, G1070–1077.

28 Feldstein AE, Gores GJ (2005) Apoptosis in alcoholic and non-alcoholic steatohepatitis. *Front Biosci* 10, 3093–3099.

29 Nagy P, Teramoto T, Factor VM *et al.* (2001) Reconstitution of liver mass via cellular hypertrophy in the rat. *Hepatology* 33, 339–345.

30 Strathdee G, Sansom OJ, Sim A *et al.* (2001) A role for mismatch repair in control of DNA ploidy following damage. *Oncogene* 20, 1923–1927.

31 Zajicik G, Schwartz-Arad D, Bartfeld E (1989) The streaming liver. V: Time and age-dependent changes of hepatocyte DNA content, following partial hepatectomy. *Liver* 9, 164–171.

32 Fausto N (2004) Liver regeneration and repair: hepatocytes, progenitor cells, and stem cells. *Hepatology* 39, 1477–1487.

33 Thorgeirsson SS, Grisham JW (2003) Overview of recent experimental studies on liver stem cells. *Semin Liver Dis* 23, 303–312.

34 Novikoff PM, Yam A (1998) Stem cells and rat liver carcinogenesis: contributions of confocal and electron microscopy. *J Histochem Cytochem* 46, 613–626.

35 Jensen CH, Jauho EI, Santoni-Rugiu E *et al.* (2004) Transit-amplifying ductular (oval) cells and their hepatocytic progeny are characterized by a novel and distinctive expression of delta-like protein/preadipocyte factor 1/fetal antigen 1. *Am J Pathol* 164, 1347–1359.

36 Liu C, Schreiter T, Dirsch O *et al.* (2004) Presence of markers for liver progenitor cells in human-derived intrahepatic biliary epithelial cells. *Liver Int* 24, 669–678.

37 Jones PH (1997) Epithelial stem cells. *Bioessays* 19, 683–690.

38 Austin TW, Lagasse E (2003) Hepatic regeneration from hematopoietic stem cells. *Mech Dev* 120, 131–135.

39 Grompe M (2003) The role of bone marrow stem cells in liver regeneration. *Semin Liver Dis* 23, 363–372.

40 Grove JE, Bruscia E, Krause DS (2004) Plasticity of bone marrow-derived stem cells. *Stem Cells* 22, 487–500.

41 Jang YY, Collector MI, Baylin SB *et al.* (2004) Hematopoietic stem cells convert into liver cells within days without fusion. *Nature Cell Biol* 6, 532–539.

42 Dalakas E, Newsome PN, Harrison DJ *et al.* (2005) Hematopoietic stem cell trafficking in liver injury. *FASEB J* 19, 1225–1231.

43 Oh SH, Hatch HM, Petersen BE (2002) Hepatic oval 'stem' cell in liver regeneration. *Semin Cell Dev Biol* 13, 405–409.

44 Saxena R, Theise N (2004) Canals of Hering: recent insights and current knowledge. *Semin Liver Dis* 24, 43–48.

45 Roskams T, Desmet V (1998) Ductular reaction and its diagnostic significance. *Semin Diagn Pathol* 15, 259–269.

46 Mandache E, Vidulescu C, Gherghiceanu M *et al.* (2002) Neoductular progenitor cells regenerate hepatocytes in severely damaged liver: a comparative ultrastructural study. *J Cell Mol Med* 6, 59–73.

47 Falkowski O, An HJ, Ianus IA *et al.* (2003) Regeneration of hepatocyte 'buds' in cirrhosis from intrabiliary stem cells. *J Hepatol* 39, 357–364.

48 Eleazar JA, Memeo L, Jhang JS *et al.* (2004) Progenitor cell expansion: an important source of hepatocyte regeneration in chronic hepatitis. *J Hepatol* 41, 983–991.

49 Tian YW, Smith PG, Yeoh GC (1997) The oval-shaped cell as a candidate for a liver stem cell in embryonic, neonatal and precancerous liver: identification based on morphology and immunohistochemical staining for albumin and pyruvate kinase isoenzyme expression. *Histochem Cell Biol* 107, 243–250.

50 Roskams T, De Vos R, Van Eyken P et al. (1998) Hepatic OV-6 expression in human liver disease and rat experiments: evidence for hepatic progenitor cells in man. J Hepatol 29, 455–463.

51 Libbrecht L, Desmet V, Van Damme B et al. (2000) The immunohistochemical phenotype of dysplastic foci in human liver: correlation with putative progenitor cells. J Hepatol 33, 76–84.

52 Crosby HA, Nijjar SS, de Goyet J de V et al. (2002) Progenitor cells of the biliary epithelial cell lineage. Semin Cell Dev Biol 13, 397–403.

53 Hatch HM, Zheng D, Jorgensen ML et al. (2002) SDF-1alpha/CXCR4: a mechanism for hepatic oval cell activation and bone marrow stem cell recruitment to the injured liver of rats. Cloning Stem Cells 4, 339–351.

54 Kollet O, Shivtiel S, Chen YQ et al. (2003) HGF, SDF-1, and MMP-9 are involved in stress-induced human CD34+ stemcell recruitment to the liver. J Clin Invest 112, 160–169.

55 Malhi H, Irani AN, Gagandeep S et al. (2002) Isolation of human progenitor liver epithelial cells with extensive replication capacity and differentiation into mature hepatocytes. J Cell Sci 115, 2679–2688.

56 Wang X, Foster M, Al-Dhalimy M et al. (2003) The origin and liver repopulating capacity of murine oval cells. Proc Natl Acad Sci USA 100(Suppl. 1), 11881–11888.

57 Deutsch G, Jung J, Zheng M et al. (2001) A bipotential precursor population for pancreas and liver with embryonic endoderm. Development 128, 871–881.

58 Henson NL, Heaton ML, Holland BH et al. (2005) Karyotypic analysis of adult pluripotent stem cells. Histol Histopathol 20, 769–784.

59 von Zglinicki T, Martin-Ruiz CM (2005) Telomeres as biomarkers for ageing and age-related diseases. Curr Mol Med 5, 197–203.

60 Prowse KR, Creider CW (1995) Developmental and tissue-specific regulation of mouse telomerase and telomere length. Proc Natl Acad Sci USA 92, 4818–4822.

61 Yamaguchi Y, Nozawa K, Savoysky EH et al. (1998) Change in telomerase activity of rat organs during growth and aging. Exp Cell Res 242, 120–127.

62 Ogami M, Ikura Y, Nishiguchi S et al. (1999) Quantitative analysis and in situ localization of human telomerase RNA in chronic liver disease and hepatocellular carcinoma. Lab Invest 79, 15–26.

63 Kotoula V, Hytiroglou P, Pyrpasopoulou A et al. (2002) Expression of human telomerase reverse transcriptases in regenerative and precancerous lesions of cirrhotic livers. Liver 22, 57–69.

64 Satyanarayana A, Wiemann SU, Buer J et al. (2003) Telomere shortening impairs organ regeneration by inhibiting cell cycle re-entry of a subpopulation of cells. EMBO J 22, 4003–4013.

65 Rudolph KL, Chang S, Millard M et al. (2000) Inhibition of experimental liver cirrhosis in mice by telomerase gene delivery. Science 287, 1185–1187.

66 Geraci JP, Jackson KL, Mariano MS et al. (1985) Hepatic injury after whole-liver irradiation in the rat. Radiat Res 101, 508–518.

67 Mason PJ, Wilson DB, Bessler M (2005) Dyskeratosis congenita – a disease of dysfunctional telomere maintenance. Curr Mol Med 5, 159–170.

68 Petersen BE, Bowen WC, Patrene KD et al. (1999) Bone marrow as a potential source of hepatic oval cells. Science 284, 1168–1170.

69 Theise ND, Badve S, Saxena R et al. (2000) Derivation of hepatocytes from bone marrow cells in mice after radiation-induced myeloablation. Hepatology 31, 235–240.

70 Avital I, Inderbitzin D, Aoki T et al. (2001) Isolation, characterization, and transplantation of bone marrow-derived hepatocyte stem cells. Biochem Biophys Res Commun 288, 156–164.

71 Gao J, Denni JE, Muzic RF et al. (2001) The dynamic in vivo distribution of bone marrow-derived mesenchymal stem cells after infusion. Cells Tissues Organs 169, 12–20.

72 Herzog EL, Chai L, Krause DS (2003) Plasticity of marrow-derived stem cells. Blood 102, 3483–3493.

73 Kucia M, Ratajczak J, Ratajczak MZ (2005) Bone marrow as a source of circulating CXCR4+ tissue-committed stem cells. Biol Cell 97, 133–146.

74 Laurson J, Selden C, Hodgson HJ (2005) Hepatocyte progenitors in man and in rodents – multiple pathways, multiple candidates. Int J Exp Pathol 86, 1–18.

75 Wang X, Willenbring H, Akkari Y et al. (2003) Cell fusion is the principal source of bone-marrow-derived hepatocytes. Nature 422, 897–901.

76 Vassilopoulos G, Wang PR, Russell DW (2003) Transplanted bone marrow regenerates liver by cell fusion. Nature 422, 901–904.

77 Zebrini C, Weinberg DS, Hollister KA (1992) DNA ploidy abnormalities in the liver of children with hereditary tyrosinemia type I. Correlation with histopathologic features. Am J Pathol 140, 1111–1115.

78 Li X, Leteurtre F, Rocha V et al. (2003) Abnormal telomere metabolism in Fanconi's anaemia correlates with genomic instability and the probability of developing severe aplastic anaemia. Br J Haematol 120, 836–845.

79 Theise ND, Krause DS (2002) Bone marrow to liver: the blood of Prometheus. Semin Cell Dev Biol 13, 411–417.

80 Jang YY, Sharkis SJ (2004) Metamorphosis from bone marrow derived primitive stem cells to functional liver cells. Cell Cycle 3, 980–982.

81 Tracy TF, Jr, Bailey PV, Goerke ME et al. (1991) Cholestasis without cirrhosis alters regulatory liver gene expression and inhibits hepatic regeneration. Surgery 110, 176–182; discussion 182–173.

82 LeSage GD, Glaser SS, Marucci L et al. (1999) Acute carbon tetrachloride feeding induces damage of large but not small cholangiocytes from BDL rat liver. Am J Physiol 276, G1289–1301.

83 de Groen PC, Vroman B, Laakso K et al. (1998) Characterization and growth regulation of rat intrahepatic bile duct epithelial cell line under hormonally derived serum-free conditions. In Vitro Cell Dev Biol Anim 34, 704–710.

84 LeSage GD, Glaser SS, Alpini G (2001) Regulation of cholangiocyte proliferation. Liver 21, 73–80.

85 Alvaro D, Alpini G, Onori P et al. (2002) Alfa and beta estrogen receptors and the biliary tree. Mol Cell Endocrinol 193, 105–108.

86 Michalopoulos GK, Barua L, Bowen WC (2005) Transdifferentiation of rat hepatocytes into biliary cells after bile duct ligation and toxic biliary injury. Hepatology 41, 535–544.

87 Saxena R, Hytiroglou P, Thung SN et al. (2002) Destruction of canals of Hering in primary biliary cirrhosis. Hum Pathol 33, 983–988.

88 Asahara T, Kawamoto A (2004) Endothelial progenitor cells for postnatal vasculogenesis. Am J Physiol Cell Physiol 287, C572–579.

89 Tavian M, Zheng B, Oberlin E et al. (2005) The vascular wall as a source of stem cells. Ann NY Acad Sci 1044, 41–50.

90 Fujii H, Hirose T, Oe S et al. (2002) Contribution of bone marrow cells to liver regeneration after partial hepatectomy in mice. J Hepatol 36, 653–659.

91 Stadtfeld M, Graf T (2005) Assessing the role of hematopoietic plasticity for endothelial and hepatocyte development by non-invasive lineage tracing. Development 132, 203–213.

92 Theuerkauf I, Zhou H, Fischer HP (2001) Immunohistochemical patterns of human liver sinusoids under different conditions of pathologic perfusion. Virchows Arch 438, 498–504.

93 Wanless IR, Shiota K (2004) The pathogenesis of nonalcoholic steatohepatitis and other fatty liver diseases: a four-step model including the role of lipid release and hepatic venular obstruction in the progression to cirrhosis. *Semin Liver Dis* 24, 99–106.

94 Ward NL, Haninec AL, Van Slyke P *et al.* (2004) Angiopoietin-1 causes reversible degradation of the portal microcirculation in mice: implications for treatment of liver disease. *Am J Pathol* 165, 889–899.

95 Friedman SL (2004) Stellate cells: a moving target in hepatic fibrogenesis. *Hepatology* 40, 1041–1043.

96 Pinzani M, Rombouts K (2004) Liver fibrosis: from the bench to clinical targets. *Dig Liver Dis* 36, 231–242.

97 Ramadori G, Saile B (2004) Portal tract fibrogenesis in the liver. *Lab Invest* 84, 153–159.

98 Bataller R, Brenner DA (2005) Liver fibrosis. *J Clin Invest* 115, 209–218.

99 Geerts A, Niki T, Hellemans K *et al.* (1998) Purification of rat hepatic stellate cells by side scatter-activated cell sorting. *Hepatology* 27, 590–598.

100 Senoo H (2004) Structure and function of hepatic stellate cells. *Med Electron Microsc* 37, 3–15.

101 Enzan H, Himeno H, Hiroi M *et al.* (1997) Development of hepatic sinusoidal structure with special reference to Ito cells. *Microsc Res Tech* 39, 336–349.

102 Riccalton-Banks L, Liew C, Bhandari R *et al.* (2003) Long-term culture of functional liver tissue: three-dimensional coculture of primary hepatocytes and stellate cells. *Tissue Eng* 9, 401–410.

103 She H, Xiong S, Hazra S *et al.* (2005) Adipogenic transcriptional regulation of hepatic stellate cells. *J Biol Chem* 280, 4959–4967.

104 Jin YL, Enzan H, Kuroda N *et al.* (2003) Tissue remodeling following submassive hemorrhagic necrosis in rat livers induced by an intraperitoneal injection of dimethylnitrosamine. *Virchows Arch* 442, 39–47.

105 Ramalho LN, Zucoloto S, Ramalho FS *et al.* (2003) Effect of antihypertensive agents on stellate cells during liver regeneration in rats. *Arq Gastroenterol* 40, 40–44.

106 Balabaud C, Bioulac-Sage P, Desmouliere A (2004) The role of hepatic stellate cells in liver regeneration. *J Hepatol* 40, 1023–1026.

107 Higashi N, Sato M, Kojima N *et al.* (2005) Vitamin A storage in hepatic stellate cells in the regenerating rat liver: with special reference to zonal heterogeneity. *Anat Rec A Discov Mol Cell Evol Biol* 286, 899–907.

108 Mabuchi A, Mullaney I, Sheard P *et al.* (2004) Role of hepatic stellate cells in the early phase of liver regeneration in rat: formation of tight adhesion to parenchymal cells. *Comp Hepatol* 3 (Suppl. 1), S29.

109 Rippe RA (1998) Life or death: the fate of the hepatic stellate cell following hepatic injury. *Hepatology* 27, 1447–1448.

110 Kim WH, Matsumoto K, Bessho K *et al.* (2005) Growth inhibition and apoptosis in liver myofibroblasts promoted by hepatocyte growth factor leads to resolution from liver cirrhosis. *Am J Pathol* 166, 1017–1028.

111 Date M, Matsuzaki K, Matsushita M *et al.* (2000) Modulation of transforming growth factor beta function in hepatocytes and hepatic stellate cells in rat liver injury. *Gut* 46, 719–724.

112 Valdes F, Alvarez AM, Locascio A *et al.* (2002) The epithelial mesenchymal transition confers resistance to the apoptotic effects of transforming growth factor Beta in fetal rat hepatocytes. *Mol Cancer Res* 1, 68–78.

113 Li Y, Yang J, Dai C *et al.* (2003) Role for integrin-linked kinase in mediating tubular epithelial to mesenchymal transition and renal interstitial fibrogenesis. *J Clin Invest* 112, 503–516.

114 Shiota G, Kunisada T, Oyama K *et al.* (2000) In vivo transfer of hepatocyte growth factor gene accelerates proliferation of hepatic oval cells in a 2-acetylaminofluorene/partial hepatectomy model in rats. *FEBS Lett* 470, 325–330.

2.6 Excretion

2.6.1 Physiology of bile formation

Martin Wagner and Michael Trauner

Physiological functions of bile

Bile secretion represents the exocrine function of the liver, which is accomplished by both hepatocytes and bile duct epithelial cells (cholangiocytes). Bile has several important physiological functions: it is critical for lipid digestion and absorption; it represents an important route of elimination for various endo- and xenobiotics; and it also has important trophic and immunological properties (Table 1).

Bile composition

Bile is a complex aqueous solution consisting of organic and inorganic solutes, the latter comprising mainly electrolytes found in similar concentrations as in plasma. Organic constituents include bile acids, bile pigments such as bilirubin, cholesterol, phospholipids and proteins such as albumin and immunoglobins (Ig) (Fig. 1, Table 2). Bile acids are synthesized from cholesterol in pericentral hepatocytes and – together with bile acids returning to the liver via the enterohepatic circulation

Table 1 Physiological functions of bile.

Lipid digestion and absorption	Bile acids promote dietary lipid absorption in the small intestine by solubilizing lipids and their digestion products as micelles
Excretion of endobiotics	Elimination of excess cholesterol, conjugated bilirubin, aged proteins and metals
Excretion of xenobiotics	Elimination of lipophilic, highly protein-bound drugs, toxins and carcinogens after hepatic conversion into amphipathic metabolites
Mucosal defence	Achieved by antibacterial properties of bile acids and secretion of secretory IgA
Signalling properties	Bile acids regulate their own synthesis, biliary excretion and intestinal uptake, cholangiocyte proliferation and gallbladder secretory activity

– are actively secreted into bile [1]. In bile, they form mixed micelles with phospholipids and cholesterol, thereby promoting their biliary elimination. Formation of mixed micelles also lowers the detergent activity of monomeric bile acids in the bile

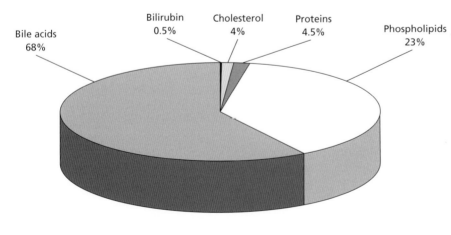

Bile acids
68%

Bilirubin
0.5%

Cholesterol
4%

Proteins
4.5%

Phospholipids
23%

Fig. 1 Bile composition. Typical bile composition in healthy humans. Values are derived from Moseley RH (1996) Bile secretion and cholestasis. In: Kaplowitz N (ed.) *Liver and Biliary Disease*, 2nd edn. Baltimore: William & Wilkins, pp. 185–204.

Table 2 Bile composition.

Water
Organic anions
    Bile acids, bilirubin, glutathione
Lipids
    Cholesterol, phosphatidylcholine
Proteins, peptides, amino acids
    Plasma proteins (e.g. albumin, IgA), hepatocellular enzymes (e.g. alkaline
    phosphatase)
Electrolytes
    Na^+, K^+, Cl^-, HCO_3^-, Ca^{2+}, Mg^{2+}, SO_4^{2-}, PO_4^{2-}
Nucleotides
    Adenosine triphosphate (ATP), diphosphate (ADP), monophosphate
    (AMP)
Heavy metals
    Cu^{2+}, Mn^{2+}, Fe^{2+}, Zn^{2+}

duct lumen and prevents toxicity of high biliary bile acid concentrations (mM) to cholangiocytes [2]. The major bile pigment is bilirubin, the endproduct of haem metabolism. Unconjugated bilirubin is rapidly taken up by hepatocytes and converted into more hydrophilic glucuronides, which are then excreted and give bile its typical colour [3].

Lipid digestion and absorption

Bile acids promote dietary lipid absorption by solubilizing lipids as micelles in the small intestine. These absorptive micelles contain solubilized fatty acids and monoglycerides formed by the action of pancreatic enzymes on dietary triglycerides. Fat-soluble vitamins are also poorly absorbed without bile acids [1,4]. There are two reasons for the high intestinal concentrations of bile acids above their critical micellar concentrations required for solubilization of biliary lipids: bile acids are concentrated in the gallbladder; and cell membranes and paracellular junctions within the biliary systems are impermeable to ionized bile acids [1,4].

Excretory function

Bile is not only an important route of elimination for xenobiotics including drugs and their metabolites, environmental toxins and carcinogens, but also for endogenous compounds (termed endobiotics) such as cholesterol, bilirubin, sex steroids and metals including copper and iron. As the liver is equipped with phase I (hydroxylation) and phase II (conjugation) enzymes (e.g. P-450 cytochromes, sulphatases, glucuronidases), these compounds can be either detoxified (e.g. unconjugated bilirubin converted into bilirubin diglucuronide) or otherwise metabolized (e.g. cholesterol converted into bile acids) before

being excreted into bile. As such, cholesterol excretion into bile is one of the most important routes for cholesterol elimination from the body. Per day, roughly 1.1 g of cholesterol is eliminated via faeces, of which one-third is converted to bile acids and two-thirds are excreted as neutral steroids [5].

Signalling

Bile components such as bile acids not only serve as detergents for the digestion and absorption of dietary lipids and vitamins, but also have a broad spectrum of signalling properties within the liver and following their excretion into the biliary tract and the intestine. As such, bile acids modulate the expression of genes involved in bile formation (e.g. induction of the bile salt export pump, BSEP) and bile acid metabolism (e.g. suppression of the rate-limiting enzyme of bile acid synthesis, cholesterol 7α-hydroxylase, CYP7A1) by binding and activating nuclear receptors such as the classical bile acid receptor farnesoid X receptor, FXR [5,6]. Moreover, bile acids can activate second messenger systems such as cyclic adenosine monophosphate (cAMP) and kinases such as protein kinase A (PKA), protein kinase C (PKC), phosphatidylinositol 3-kinase (PI3K) and mitogen-activated protein kinases (MAPK) (see below) [6,7]. This enables bile acids to regulate their own synthesis and excretion in hepatocytes, and to modulate cholangiocyte and intestinal functions such as cellular proliferation and enterohepatic circulation [5,8,9]. Bile acids can induce the production of intestinal factors that send signals to the liver: an important example is the fibroblast growth factor 15 (FGF15). It is produced in the intestine, reaches the liver via the portal circulation and binds to a hepatic FGF receptor (FGFR4). This cascade ultimately contributes to the negative feedback inhibition of bile acid synthesis [10].

Mucosal defence

Bile also plays a critical role in mucosal immunity of the intestine through biliary excretion of Ig and the antibacterial properties of bile acids. Secretory IgA aggregates bacteria, inhibits their motility and prevents their adherence to the epithelial cells [11]. Growth of anaerobes is readily suppressed by the unconjugated (but not conjugated) cholic acid (CA), chenodeoxycholic acid (CDCA) and ursodeoxycholic acid (UDCA) in the intestinal flora, while growth of aerobes is less affected. *In vitro* studies suggest that unconjugated dihydroxy bile acids [e.g. deoxycholic acid (DCA)] also have antibacterial activity against *Helicobacter pylori* [12]. Moreover, in addition to their detergent bacteriostatic activities, bile acids may limit intestinal bacterial overgrowth and translocation by transcriptional modulation of an inflammatory response via stimulation of the bile acid receptor FXR in the intestine [13]. Bile also contains significant amounts of the antioxidant tocopherol, which may prevent oxidative injury to the bile duct epithelium and intestine.

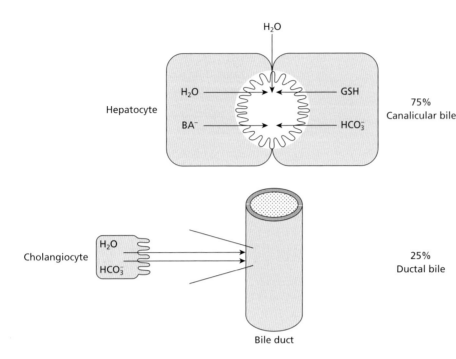

Fig. 2 Origin of bile. Seventy per cent of total bile production originates from hepatocytes. The majority of canalicular bile is formed by active excretion of bile acids (BA; bile acid-dependent fraction). Hepatocellular bicarbonate (HCO_3^-) and glutathione (GSH) secretion are the major constituents of the bile acid-independent fraction. Depending on species, up to 30% of bile comes from bile ducts, with HCO_3^- accounting for the most relevant proportion. Water (H_2O) passively follows the osmotic gradients generated by the actively excreted biliary compounds at the level of hepatocytes and cholangiocytes.

General principles of bile secretion

Anatomical considerations

Bile is secreted into bile canaliculi, which are minute channels arranged as a network of tubuli between adjacent hepatocytes. The hepatocyte is a polygonal polarized cell with three functionally distinct membrane domains: the basal (sinusoidal) membrane comprising approximately 35% of the cell surface; the lateral (intercellular) membrane comprising 50%; and the apical (canalicular) membrane constituting about 15% of the cell surface. As the endothelial cells of hepatic sinusoids are fenestrated, the sinusoidal membrane is in direct contact with plasma via the space of Disse. The sinusoidal membrane contains uptake systems for membrane-impermeable organic solutes that utilize sodium and pH gradients across the membrane. The canalicular membrane contains adenosine triphosphate (ATP)-dependent transporters that excrete organic solutes such as bile acids and glutathione into the canalicular lumen. Tight junctions seal off the bile canaliculi and separate the canalicular from the basolateral domain. The lipid composition of the canalicular membrane differs from that of the basolateral membrane, which explains its relative resistance to the detergent action of high concentrations of bile acids (mM) in bile. The canaliculi empty bile into small terminal bile ductules, termed canals of Hering and lined in part by cholangiocytes and hepatocytes; these are followed by intralobular ducts that are fully lined with cholangiocytes. After entering the portal tract, the interlobular ducts finally acquire a basal membrane and are supplied by a peribiliary vascular plexus. The interlobular ducts are followed by septal ducts, area ducts, segmental ducts and the hepatic right and left duct. Finally, bile is stored in the gallbladder (if present)

and reaches the intestine via the common bile duct. Functionally, bile ducts can be divided into small (< 15-µm diameter) and large (> 15-µm diameter) ducts [8].

Osmotic principle of bile formation

Bile secretion is an osmotic process driven by active excretion of organic solutes (i.e. mainly bile acids, bicarbonate, glutathione), which is coupled to passive para- and transcellular inflow of water and filterable solutes (e.g. electrolytes, glucose, amino acids) until an osmotic equilibrium is achieved (Fig. 2). As tight junctions between the hepatocytes are negatively charged, cations can passively follow the actively excreted anions into bile canaliculi, while the negative charges of the tight junctions prevent backdiffusion of the excreted anions. In contrast to renal excretion, hydrostatic filtration (as occurs in glomeruli) does not play a role in bile formation [14]. Up to 95% of bile consists of water, which can cross the plasma membrane through the lipid portion of the bilayer by diffusion or through aquaporin water channels (AQPs) in response to the osmotic gradients generated by the active transport of solutes. In contrast to previous assumptions, the transcellular route for water accounts for most of the water flux with only a minimal paracellular contribution via the tight junctions. Transcellular water movement across cholangiocytes can be 10 times higher than in hepatocytes [15].

Canalicular and ductal bile formation

Normal bile production in man accounts for approximately 600 mL/day. Bile is primarily secreted at the level of bile canaliculi of hepatocytes (canalicular bile), followed by modifications through the bile duct epithelium (ductal bile) (Fig. 2). This canalicular fraction accounts for ~ 75% of daily bile production in man and is further modified by secretory and absorptive processes as it passes along the bile ductules and ducts. The quantity of ductal bile varies significantly by species and in response to hormonal stimuli, ranging from as little as 5% in rats to as much as 25–40% of bile secretion in man [16]. Canalicular bile acid excretion is a saturable ATP-dependent process mediated by ATP-binding cassette (ABC) transporters for bile acids and non-bile acid organic anions, and represents the rate-limiting step in bile formation. Ductal modifications in bile composition only take place in ductules > 15 μm in diameter that express transport systems such as the cystic fibrosis transmembrane conductance regulator (CFTR) and hormone (e.g. secretin, vasoactive intestinal peptide) receptors [8,17,18]. Secretin is released after vagal stimulation and contact of acidic gastric content with the duodenal mucosa, resulting in induction of a bicarbonate-rich bile secretion from bile ducts and alkalinization of the biliary pH. The effects of secretin on ductal bile secretion are counteracted by other hormones such as gastrin and somatostatin [8,18].

Bile acid-dependent and -independent bile flow

Canalicular excretion of conjugated bile acids – the most abundant biliary organic solutes – represents the major driving force for the 'bile acid-dependent' fraction of bile flow (Fig. 3). Bile acids are highly concentrated up to 1000-fold in bile via active transport mechanisms from sinusoidal blood into bile, the major concentration step being from the cytoplasm into the bile canaliculus (~ 100-fold). In addition to their osmotic activity, bile acids promote canalicular phospholipid and cholesterol secretion and form mixed biliary micelles with them. Bile acids that do not form micelles and/or have a high critical micellar

concentration (e.g. C23- or C22-nor-bile acids) have greater choleretic effects as they are osmotically more active. Hypercholeresis induced by nor-bile acids is mainly accompanied by ductal bicarbonate (HCO_3^-) secretion resulting from exchange to non-ionic diffusion of unconjugated bile acids across the bile duct epithelium (so-called 'cholehepatic shunting') [1,4].

Canalicular excretion of reduced glutathione (GSH) and HCO_3^- accounts for the major components of the 'bile acid-independent' fraction of bile flow [16] (Fig. 3). However, HCO_3^- secretion occurs mainly at the level of bile duct epithelial cells (cholangiocytes), in response to stimulation by hormones and neuropeptides such as secretin, vasoactive intestinal peptide and bombesin.

Enterohepatic circulation of bile acids and other biliary constituents

Many biliary compounds such as bile acids, bilirubin, estrogens or drugs undergo an intensive enterohepatic circulation, i.e. are reabsorbed in the intestine, taken up again by the liver and resecreted into bile (Fig. 4); some compounds repeat this cycle several times before being eliminated in the faeces. As a result of the high degree of intestinal bile acid conservation, only 0.5 g of bile acids are lost through faecal excretion and must be replaced by *de novo* bile acid synthesis, accounting for only 3–5% of the bile acids excreted into bile [1,4,5,19]. Unconjugated bile acids, which are reabsorbed after bacterial deconjugation in the intestine, are almost completely reamidated with glycine and taurine. The human bile acid pool circulates from 6 to 10 times a day, resulting in a daily bile salt excretion of 20–40 g. The human pool size accounts for approximately 50–60 μmol/kg body weight, averaging 3–4 g of bile acids in total. Bile acid concentrations in the bile canaliculus and ductules/ducts are in the range of 20–50 mmol/L and reach concentrations as high as 300 mmol/L in the gallbladder, whereas they are diluted to 1–10 mmol/L in

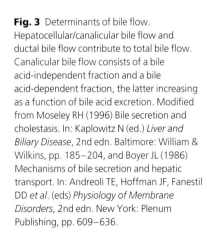

Fig. 3 Determinants of bile flow. Hepatocellular/canalicular bile flow and ductal bile flow contribute to total bile flow. Canalicular bile flow consists of a bile acid-independent fraction and a bile acid-dependent fraction, the latter increasing as a function of bile acid excretion. Modified from Moseley RH (1996) Bile secretion and cholestasis. In: Kaplowitz N (ed.) *Liver and Biliary Disease*, 2nd edn. Baltimore: William & Wilkins, pp. 185–204, and Boyer JL (1986) Mechanisms of bile secretion and hepatic transport. In: Andreoli TE, Hoffman JF, Fanestil DD *et al.* (eds) *Physiology of Membrane Disorders*, 2nd edn. New York: Plenum Publishing, pp. 609–636.

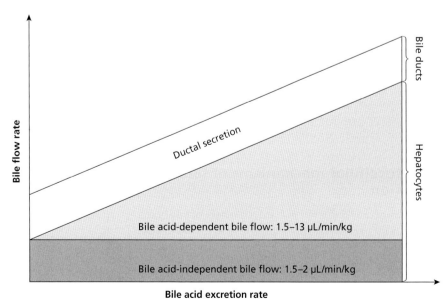

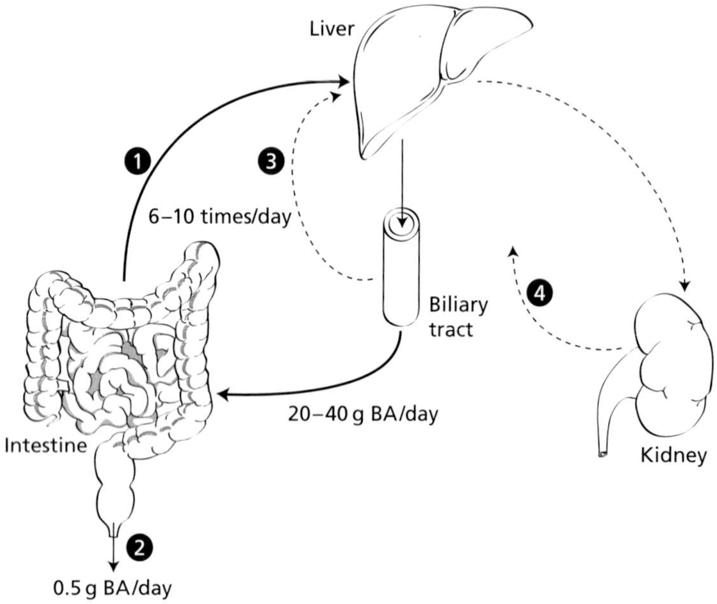

Fig. 4 Enterohepatic circulation of bile acids (BA). Bile acids circulate from 6 to 10 times a day between liver and intestine. The liver excretes 20–40 g of bile acids per day into the biliary tract, which are reabsorbed in the terminal ileum and taken up again by the liver (1). Only 0.5 g are lost via faeces (2) and must be replaced by *de novo* synthesis in the liver. (3) Cholehepatic shunting from cholangiocytes via the peribiliary plexus is quantitatively negligible under physiological conditions, but may become an important escape route for bile acids under cholestatic conditions. (4) Nephrohepatic shunting minimizes renal loss of glomerularly filterable bile acids that have escaped the first-pass clearance of the liver.

the gastrointestinal tract and – following their intestinal reabsorption – are as low as 20–50 µmol/L in the portal vein and only 5 µmol/L after efficient first-pass extraction in the systemic venous plasma [4].

Bile acids that escape the first-pass clearance by the liver are filtered at the glomerulus and excreted into urine, where they are reabsorbed by transporters in the brush border of the proximal convoluted tubule ('nephrohepatic' cycle between kidney and liver [4,20] (Fig. 4). Under normal conditions, urinary bile acid losses are minimal as a result of this renal bile acid conservation. However, some metabolic liver products are preferentially excreted into plasma and, subsequently, urine rather than bile, even under normal conditions. Under pathological, cholestatic conditions with disruption of the enterohepatic circulation, these pathways may be 'alternatively' used by biliary compounds not normally excreted into urine [21]. Bile acids may also undergo 'cholehepatic shunting' from the bile duct lumen, via cholangiocytes and the periductular capillary plexus, back to hepatocytes [20] (Fig. 4). Although this pathway plays a minor role for conjugated bile acids under normal physiological conditions, it may also become an important escape route under cholestatic conditions with bile stasis in obstructed ducts [20].

Hepatocellular mechanisms of bile secretion

Formation of canalicular bile includes: (i) uptake of biliary constituents at the basolateral/sinusoidal membrane; (ii) transcellular/intracellular transport; followed by (iii) canalicular excretion (Fig. 5). Bile formation normally depends not only on the proper function of hepatobiliary transport systems, but also on an intact cytoskeleton, as required for the movement of vesicles and

bile canalicular contractions, cell junctions that seal off the bile canaliculi and maintain cell polarity, and signal transduction cascades that regulate and coordinate these processes [22] (Fig. 6).

Hepatocellular uptake of biliary compounds

Bile acids encounter the basolateral (sinusoidal) membrane of hepatocytes mostly in their albumin-bound form. While dihydroxy bile acids are almost completely albumin bound, protein binding decreases with the degree of bile acid hydroxylation [4]. Bile acid–albumin complexes pass the fenestrae of the sinusoidal epithelium into the space of Disse, where bile acids dissociate from albumin [23,24]. Bile acids are then efficiently removed from portal plasma by high-affinity, low K_m-transporting polypeptides in the basolateral sinusoidal membrane. Hepatic first-pass clearance of conjugated bile acids ranges from 75% to 90% depending on their biochemical structure [23]. Unconjugated bile acids enter the hepatocyte mainly by passive diffusion or via Na^+-independent mechanisms, while conjugated bile acids are taken up largely by Na^+-dependent mechanisms. Under normal conditions, bile acid uptake occurs mainly in periportal hepatocytes of zone 1. Under cholestatic or postprandial conditions with higher bile acid concentrations, hepatocytes are also recruited in zone 3. Hepatocytes in zone 1 are also more efficiently involved in the canalicular excretion of bile acids than those in zone 3. This indicates that, under physiological conditions, bile acid-dependent bile flow appears to be predominantly a function of zone 1 [23,25].

High-affinity Na^+-dependent bile salt uptake into hepatocytes is mediated by a Na^+/taurocholate cotransporter (NTCP/ *SLC10A1*) whereas a family of multispecific organic anion transporters (OATPs/*SLC21A*) facilitate Na^+-independent bile

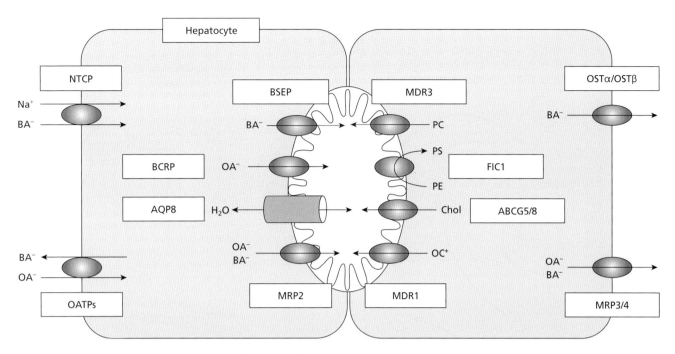

Fig. 5 Hepatocellular transport proteins. Bile acids (BA⁻) and non-bile acid organic anions (OA⁻) are taken up by the liver via the Na+/taurocholate cotransporter (NTCP) and organic anion transport proteins (OATPs) located at the basolateral membrane. On the canalicular pole, the bile salt export pump (BSEP) actively transports bile acids into the lumen and is the main determinant of the bile acid-dependent bile flow. The multidrug resistance-associated protein (MRP)2 actively excretes bilirubin, glutathione (GSH) and also certain divalent (e.g. glucuronidated and sulphated) bile acids. Water passively follows along an osmotic gradient mainly via water channels, termed aquaporins (AQP). Excretion of lipids is mediated by the multidrug resistance (MDR) protein MDR3, which flips phosphatidylcholine (PC) from the inner to the outer leaflet of the canalicular membrane, and by the two-half transporter ABC G5/8, which transports cholesterol (Chol). The definitive function of FIC1 is still unclear, but it may represent a flippase for aminophospholipids [phosphatidylserine (PS), phosphatidylethanolamine (PE)] from the outer to the inner lipid layer. Organic cations (OC+) and many drugs are effluxed via another member of the MDR family, MDR1. BCRP, breast cancer-related protein. Basolateral excretion of bile acids is mediated via the ABC transporters MRP3 and MRP4 and via the organic solute transporter OSTα/OSTβ.

acid uptake and mostly amphipathic organic compounds including conjugated and unconjugated bile acids [26] (Fig. 5). Na⁺-independent bile acid uptake is quantitatively less important than Na⁺-dependent uptake and is mediated by exchange with intracellular anions (e.g. GSH, HCO₃⁻). In contrast to NTCP, OATPs are not restricted exclusively to hepatocytes, but are also expressed in multiple tissues including kidney, neuronal structures and intestine. Apart from conjugated and unconjugated bile acids, OATPs also have broader substrate preferences, including bilirubin, neutral steroids, eicosanoids, numerous xenobiotics and many more [27]. Additional basolateral uptake systems include organic anion transporters (OATs) and organic cation transporters (OCTs) [28].

In addition to these uptake systems, the basolateral membrane also contains efflux pumps. Members of the multidrug resistance-related proteins (MRPs) MRP3/*ABCC3* and MRP4/*ABCC4* are normally expressed at very low levels in hepatocytes (Fig. 5), but can be upregulated in cholestasis, which may explain the shift towards renal excretion of bile acids in patients with chronic, longstanding cholestasis [5]. Members of the OATP family also remain candidates for bile acid efflux at the basolateral membrane, as they may be able to operate as bidirectional exchangers. The heteromeric organic solute transporter

alpha-beta, OSTα/OSTβ, represents another basolateral bile acid export system [29].

Intracellular transport of biliary compounds

The mechanisms of intracellular bile acid transport from the basolateral to the canalicular hepatocyte membrane are poorly understood. Two possible transfer mechanisms have been proposed: carrier-mediated diffusion and vesicular transport. For a given bile acid, the intracellular transport mechanism largely depends on its intracellular concentration, hydrophobicity and the affinity for intracellular binding proteins. Significant amounts of bile acids cannot exist in free (unbound) form in the cytoplasm, as their detergent properties would be toxic [23]. Under physiological conditions, the majority of amidated bile acids bind to intracellular bile acid-binding proteins and diffuse to the canalicular membrane along the prevailing basolateral → canalicular bile acid concentration gradient [26]. Bile acid-binding proteins also frequently have other (predominant) physiological functions. As such, 3α-hydroxysteroid dehydrogenase (3α-HSD), glutathione *S*-transferases (GST) and the liver fatty acid-binding proteins (L-FABP) have been implicated

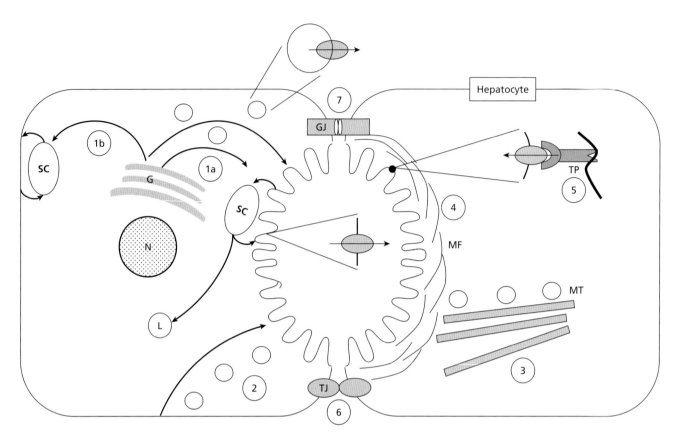

Fig. 6 Role of vesicular targeting, cytoskeleton and cell junctions for bile secretion. (1a) Vesicles containing canalicular transport proteins are either directly targeted from the Golgi apparatus (G) to the canalicular membrane or intermediately stored in a subapical compartment (SC) from which a rapid insertion into the canalicular membrane is possible. The other way around, there is retrieval from the canalicular membrane into the subapical compartment, possibly followed by lysosomal (L) and proteosomal degradation of the transport protein. (1b) Vesicular trafficking also occurs at the basolateral membrane. Similarly, transporter cycling between a submembranous compartment and the basolateral membrane can occur. (2) A microtubule-dependent transcytotic vesicular pathway mediates the transfer of solutes and proteins into bile. (3) Microtubules (MT) are also responsible for the transport of transporter-containing vesicles from the Golgi apparatus to the plasma membrane or a submembranous compartment. (4) The pericanalicular microfilament sheath (MF) consisting of an actin–myosin network mediates canalicular contractions, which in turn facilitate bile flow from pericentral to periportal regions. (5) Tethering proteins (TP) cross-link transport proteins with actin filaments. (6) Tight junctions (TJ) seal off the canalicular space and prevent regurgitation of biliary constituents while (7) gap junctions (GJ) facilitate intercellular communication. N, nucleus.

as hepatocellular bile acid-binding proteins for their intracellular transfer [30].

The more hydrophobic bile acids are, the more they tend to depend on vesicular trafficking for their transcellular transport. [31]. Thus, under high bile acid loads, hydrophobic bile acids (e.g. lithocholic acid) may accumulate within membrane-bound compartments and may be transported by vesicle-mediated mechanisms. As the evidence for vesicular transport has mostly been obtained indirectly from (microtubule) inhibition studies, the results could also reflect impaired targeting of transporters rather than 'true' direct vesicular transport of biliary constituents [7,32].

Canalicular mechanisms of bile secretion

Canalicular bile secretion represents the rate-limiting step in bile formation. Most canalicular transporters belong to the class

of ATP-binding cassette (ABC) transporters (see Chapter 2.2.4) such as the multidrug resistance (MDR) P-glycoproteins (ABCB subfamily) or the MRP (ABCC subfamily) [5] (Fig. 5). As such, the canalicular membrane contains a bile salt export pump (BSEP/*ABCB11*) for monovalent bile acids, a conjugate export pump (MRP2/*ABCC2*) for divalent bile acids and various other amphipathic conjugates, including bilirubin diglucuronide and GSH (a major determinant of bile acid-independent canalicular bile flow), and a multidrug export pump (MDR1/*ABCB1*) for bulky amphipathic organic cations (e.g. various drugs) (Fig. 5) [5,9]. Another transport system is the breast cancer-related protein (BCRP/*ABCG2*) for sulphated conjugates, including dehydroepiandrosteronesulphate and estrone-3 sulphate. After secretion, biliary bile acids drive the secretion of phosphatidyl-choline and cholesterol from the outer leaflet of the canalicular membrane. The continuous transport of phospholipids from the inner to the outer leaflet is mediated by the murine phospholipid flippase Mdr2/*Abcb4* or its human orthologue MDR3/*ABCB4* [2,33]. Biliary cholesterol transport was long thought to be passive, but recent studies suggest a role for the sterol half-transporters ABCG5/8, which also mediate efflux of plant sterols such as sitosterol [34]. The relevance of these transporters is exemplified by the development of severe cholestasis as a result of hereditary defects in the various transport systems [35].

Under physiological conditions, bile acid and lipid excretion are tightly coupled. Bile acids solubilize phospholipids and cholesterol from the canalicular membrane. With increasing bile acid output and as a function of bile acid hydrophobicity, biliary phospholipid excretion increases [2]. Biliary phospholipids consist almost exclusively of phosphatidylcholine, while the canalicular membrane also contains sphingomyelin, phosphatidylserine and -etholamine, which are critical determinants of membrane polarity and fluidity [2]. Mdr2/MDR3 is a specific flippase for phosphatidylcholine but not sphingomyelin and phosphatidylserine and -etholamine. A common hypothesis for coupled bile acid–phospholipid excretion suggests that the translocation of phospholipids to the outer canalicular leaflet results in phospholipid-rich, less rigid microdomains. Simultaneously, ongoing bile acid excretion via BSEP leads to high supramicellar concentrations of bile acids that further destabilize these microdomains. Phospholipid translocation then leads to the formation of vesicles that pinch off as vesicular structures [2,36]. The high biliary concentrations of phospholipids and cholesterol also protect cholangiocytes from the detergent effects of bile acids via the formation of mixed micelles. This is supported by findings in Mdr2 gene knockout mice (Mdr2–/–) [33], which develop sclerosing cholangitis attributed to the misbalance in the biliary bile acid/phospholipid ratio, resulting in a toxic bile that damages the bile duct epithelium [37].

Additional canalicular transporters include the putative aminophospholipid flippase FIC1/*ATP8B1*, mutations in which are responsible for familial intrahepatic cholestasis type 1 [5] and aquaporins (i.e. AQP8 on the canalicular membrane), water channels that mediate transcellular water transport (see above). The most relevant ATP-independent transporter at the canalicular membrane is a Cl^-/HCO_3^- exchanger (AE2/*SLC4A2*), which, together with MRP2, accounts for the largest part of the bile acid-independent canalicular bile fraction [5,9]. Taken together, AE2 and MRP2 are the major driving forces for bile acid-independent bile flow, while BSEP drives bile acid-dependent flow (Fig. 5).

Vesicular trafficking and bile formation

Movement of vesicles within hepatocytes (vesicular trafficking) serves: (i) to regulate the number of transporters within the cell membrane by targeting of transport and other membrane proteins to and from the cell surface; and (ii) to transport compounds contained within the vesicular lumen (transcytosis), for example, immunoglobulins, hydrophobic bile acids or

hormones (Fig. 6). Rapid insertion and retrieval of canalicular transporters such as MRP2, Mdr2 (MDR3 in humans) and BSEP to and from the canalicular membrane are necessary to rapidly meet the varying demands of normal bile secretion. Canalicular ABC transporters reside within submembranous endosomal pools that can be mobilized in response to several stimuli such as bile acids themselves, hypo-osmolarity (resulting in cell swelling), pH changes (alkalinization), cAMP, activation of PKC, PI3K and MAPK [32]. Additive effects of bile acids and cAMP further suggest the existence of different intrahepatic pools for the recruitment of ABC transporters to the canalicular membrane, one mobilized by taurocholate, the other by cAMP. While Mdr1 and Mdr2 are directly targeted from the Golgi apparatus to the canalicular membrane, Bsep follows an indirect route via subapical intracellular pools before entering the canalicular membrane [32] (Fig. 6). Pulse–chase experiments have revealed that Bsep undergoes rapid cycling between the canalicular membrane and a subapical endocytotic compartment [38,39].

In addition to targeting and insertion, retrieval of transporters from the canalicular membrane is also a tightly regulated process [7]. Hyperosmolarity and other pathological stimuli such as endotoxin (lipopolysaccharide, LPS), cytokines, biliary obstruction, phalloidin and oxidative stress result in retrieval of membrane transporters with a reduction in the number of functional transporters in the canalicular membrane. The retrieved membrane transporters may initially undergo reinsertion from a subapical vesicular compartment, but are later degraded by the lysosomal or ubiquitin–proteasome pathway [5,7] (Fig. 6).

Recent evidence suggests that not only canalicular but also basolateral membrane transporters (e.g. Ntcp) are regulated by insertion and retrieval in a similar fashion. As such, Ntcp may recycle between the basolateral membrane and a submembranous pool [6,40]. Phosphorylation of specific tyrosine residues on the cytoplasmic tail of rat Ntcp appears to be involved in targeting of this basolateral transporter to this specific plasma membrane domain [5,40].

Role of cytoskeleton in bile formation

The importance of an intact cytoskeleton for bile formation (Fig. 6) is emphasized by findings in cholestasis, where cytoskeletal changes result in the loss of apical microvilli, diminished contractility of the canalicular membrane and impaired vesicle movement, and may contribute to the leakiness of tight junctions [22].

Microtubules (MTs)

Targeting of membrane components, transcytosis and canalicular exocytosis/endocytosis of vesicles ('vesicular trafficking') depend on intact MTs. Canalicular ABC transporters (e.g. Bsep, Mrp2, Mdr2) are targeted in tubulovesicular compartments that move along MTs [6,7,39,41]. Vesicle transport along MTs is driven by the motor proteins dynein and kinesin [41]. Bile acids can interfere with the function of these motor proteins [42]. Stimulation of bile acid and other organic anion excretion can be abrogated by MT inhibitors such as colchicine and vinblastin [43], consistent with the notion that mobilization of additional transporters via vesicular trafficking depends on MTs.

Intermediate filaments (IFs)

These are expressed in hepatocytes as cytokeratin (CK) 8 and 18, which mechanically support the bile canaliculus as pericanalicular sheaths. The CK–IF network has long been considered a rather static structure for mechanical stability of hepatocytes; however, studies in gene knockout mice have revealed their importance for non-mechanical functions as well, such as modulation of toxic stress and apoptosis [44]. IF networks also provide a flexible intracellular scaffolding for actin and microtubules [45–47] and thus may be critical for normal bile formation.

Microfilaments

These are enriched in the pericanalicular area and form a contractile web around the canaliculus. Actin microfilaments provide contractile activity of the bile canaliculi and, therefore, play an important role in intrahepatic propulsion of bile. Disruption of microfilaments (e.g. by actin inhibitors such as cytochalasins B and D) results in dilatation of the bile canaliculi and cholestasis [45]. Under normal conditions, actin filaments are also intimately associated with tight junctions. Cholestasis interferes with this association, resulting in disturbed tight junction morphology and function [22]. Moreover, microfilaments are also involved in the regulation of hepatic bile acid uptake via translocation of the bile acid importer Ntcp from a submembranous endosomal compartment into the basolateral membrane [48]. Thus, targeting of Ntcp to the plasma membrane consists of two steps: (i) delivery of Ntcp to the region of the plasma membrane via MTs; and (ii) insertion of Ntcp into the plasma membrane, in a microfilament- and cAMP-sensitive fashion [48]. Impaired actin polymerization also inhibits cycling of Bsep from the canaliculus to its intracellular compartments [39].

Tethering proteins

These cross-link actin microfilaments and integral membrane proteins. The dominant protein of the ezrin–radixin–moesin family, radixin, interacts with the cytoplasmatic domain of the canalicular bilirubin export pump MRP2. Mice lacking radixin have lower canalicular Mrp2 and develop conjugated hyperbilirubinaemia, as radixin may be required for proper canalicular localization of Mrp2 [49]. However, radixin may also be essential for maintenance of the canalicular localization of other ABC transporters including Bsep, and plays a critical role in the general ultrastructure of the canalicular membrane. In addition, recent studies using yeast two-hybrid screens have identified HAX-1 – a cytoskeleton-associated, cortactin-interacting protein – as a binding partner of Bsep, Mdr1 and Mdr2; these studies suggest a role for HAX-1 in the internalization of BSEP,

and possibly other ABC transporters, from the canalicular membrane [50]. With a similar approach, myosin II regulatory light chain was identified as playing a role in Bsep trafficking to the apical membrane [51]. This suggests that (at least for Bsep) different tethering proteins may be involved in insertion and retrieval. At the cholangiocyte level, binding of CFTR and Na^+/H^+ exchanger (NHE)3 to the actin cytoskeleton via the ezrin/EBP50 complex is essential for the reciprocal regulation of CFTR and NHE3 activities by PKA [52].

Cell junctions and bile formation

Cell junctions play a critical role in bile formation by maintaining cell polarization and osmotic gradients, as well as by participating in cell communication required for coordination of bile secretion (Fig. 6).

Tight junctions

Throughout the gastrointestinal tract, tight junctions create the paracellular barrier required to separate tissue spaces and maintain electrochemical gradients used for transport. In the liver, tight junctions form a 'blood–bile barrier', separating sinusoidal blood from the canalicular content. Tight junctions between the hepatocytes have a negative charge and are thus cation selective, preventing backdiffusion of the actively secreted anions. Localization and expression of major tight junction proteins [i.e. zonula occludens-1 (ZO-1) and occludin] are altered in cholestasis, resulting in increased paracellular permeability, regurgitation of biliary constituents into plasma and collapse of the osmotic gradient in the bile canaliculi [22,53].

Gap junctions

These are hexameric hemichannels that consist of connexin 26 and 32 in hepatocytes and allow cell-to-cell movement of solutes, ions, water and second messengers, providing an intercellular communication pathway. Cell-to-cell signalling via gap junctions thus provides a mechanism for coordinating the response of hepatocytes to external stimuli (e.g. hormones). This can be achieved via synchronized spread of hormone-induced Ca^{2+} waves [54]. Thus, gap junctions enable coordinated contractions of bile canaliculi from centrizonal to periportal hepatocytes through intercellular communication. Impaired gap junction communication and disturbed Ca^{2+} signalling may contribute to cholestasis [22].

Mechanisms of ductal bile formation

Bile ductules and ducts not only represent the collecting system for bile, but are also capable of modifying canalicular bile by secretory and reabsorbtive processes during passage through the intrahepatic biliary tree. Experiments in rats suggest that only larger bile ducts (> 15 μm diameter) contribute to ductal bile secretion, while small bile ducts remain 'passive' [8,55]. Bile duct epithelial cells (cholangiocytes) are equipped with

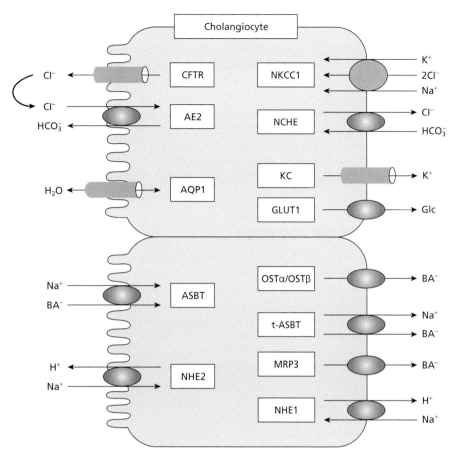

Fig. 7 Cholangiocellular transport proteins. The chloride/bicarbonate (Cl^-/HCO_3^-) anion exchanger (AE2) mediates ductular HCO_3^- excretion in exchange for Cl^-, which is extruded by the cystic fibrosis transmembrane conductance regulator (CFTR). Efflux of Cl^- generates a lumen-negative potential, which favours movement of Na^+ into the bile duct lumen through a paracellular pathway followed by water along the osmotic gradients via aquaporins (AQP). Ductal bile acid (BA^-) reabsorption is mediated via the apical sodium-dependent bile acid cotransporter ASBT; basolateral bile acid export is mediated by a truncated form of ASBT (t-ASBT), the multidrug resistance-associated protein (MRP)3 or organic solute transporter $OST\alpha$/$OST\beta$. HCO_3^- uptake is mediated via the basolateral Cl^-/HCO_3^- exchanger (NCHE). A Na^+-K^+-ATPase and K^+ channel (KC) maintain the Na^+ gradient and membrane potential difference. A Na^+/K^+/$2Cl^-$ cotransporter (NKCC1) actively imports Cl^- ions and is a major determinant of the consecutive apical fluid secretion. Reabsorption of glucose (Glc) is mediated via a basolateral glucose transporter (GLUT1). NHE, Na^+/H^+ exchanger.

transporters and hormone receptors required for their secretory and absorptive functions (Fig. 7). The majority of biliary bile acids is conjugated and absorbed in a Na^+-dependent manner via the apical bile acid transporter Asbt [56] (Fig. 7). Monomeric unconjugated bile acids and dihydroxy bile acids and C23 nor-dihydroxy bile acids can passively enter cholangiocytes in exchange for HCO_3^-, thus inducing a bicarbonate-rich hypercholeresis, a mechanism termed 'cholehepatic shunting' [21,23]. Conjugated bile acids can efflux to the plasma of the periductal capillary plexus [4] (Fig. 7). However, bile acid uptake into cholangiocytes may serve trophic and signalling functions of bile acids in cholangiocytes, rather than contributing to a cholehepatic shunting of conjugated bile acids under physiological conditions [57]. Still, cholehepatic shunting may play a role under cholestatic conditions to limit bile acid stasis in obstructed bile ducts [20].

The CFTR/*ABCC7* Cl^- channel and the Cl^-/HCO_3^- anion exchanger (AE2/*SLC4A2*) provide the molecular basis for ductal bile (bicarbonate) secretion and are expressed only in large bile ducts (Fig. 7). Apical Cl^- efflux is mediated by CFTR, a cAMP-dependent Cl^- channel that is encoded by *ABCC7* and activated by secretin via the second messenger cAMP [8,18]. In addition to cAMP-dependent CFTR, there are Ca^{2+}-dependent

Cl^- channels that may represent important therapeutic targets in cystic fibrosis. Opening of Cl^- channels in the apical membrane leads to efflux of Cl^- and the generation of a lumen-negative potential, which favours movement of Na^+ into the bile duct lumen through a paracellular pathway and water via aquaporins. Moreover, the change in the apical Cl^- gradient facilitates HCO_3^- extrusion via AE2. Thus, bile undergoes increasing dilution and alkalinization as it traverses the bile duct system. In addition, the cholangiocyte contains several exchange systems mediating the movement of ions required for ductal bile secretions (Fig. 7). Cholangiocytes also reabsorb glucose and amino acids [8]. As in hepatocytes, vesicular trafficking and regulated insertion of transporters into the apical membrane play a critical role in bile formation [58]. For example, secretin induces exocytosis of preformed vesicles containing AQP1 and CFTR in cholangiocytes [18].

Modification of bile by gallbladder epithelium

In species that possess a gallbladder, most of the bile acid pool during the fasting state is stored in that organ, where bile acids are present in concentrations up to 300 mM [4]. Such high concentrations are achieved by removal of water and electrolytes by the gallbladder epithelium via a Na^+/H^+ exchanger, which also results in acidification of bile. As the gallbladder epithelium is exposed to a much more aggressive biliary milieu for longer periods of time than the bile duct epithelium, mucins are required as an additional protective factor. Unconjugated bile acids can traverse the gallbladder epithelium by simple diffusion, while conjugated bile acids require active transport systems. As such, the human gallbladder epithelium contains bile acid and organic anion uptake systems such as ASBT and OATP-A, and exporters such as MRP2 and MRP3 [59,60]. Cholesterol secretion into the gallbladder lumen is mediated via ABCG5/8 [61].

Regulation of bile secretion

To meet physiological demands and daily variations, transcriptional and posttranscriptional mechanisms regulate hepatobiliary transport processes and bile formation. Rapid changes in bile secretory function are usually mediated by posttranscriptional events [e.g. insertion/retrieval of transporters, direct transporter modifications by phosphorylation (P) and phosphoinositide (PI)-3-kinase products (PI-P_{1-3})], while transcriptional changes have more delayed but long-term effects [7].

Transcriptional regulation

Ligand-activated nuclear (orphan) receptors (NRs) and liver-enriched transcription factors play a key role in the transcriptional regulation of hepatobiliary transport (Table 3) (also see Chapter 2.2.3). NRs are activated by biliary constituents (e.g. bile acids, bilirubin), lipid products (e.g. oxysterols) and xenobiotics and facilitate the positive feedforward and negative feedback regulation of hepatic transport and phase I/II metabolism of these compounds [62]. So far, three nuclear receptors have been shown to be activated by bile acids: the farnesoid X receptor FXR (NR1H4) by classic bile acids such as chenodeoxycholic acid, deoxycholic acid, lithocholic acid and cholic acid; the pregnane X receptor PXR (NR1I2) by lithocholic acid and potentially ursodeoxycholic acid; and the vitamin D receptor VDR (NR1I1) by hydrophobic bile acids such as lithocholic acid [62–64]. The constitutive androstane receptor CAR (NR1I3) is activated by bilirubin [20,63], but a role for bile acid sensing has been postulated. These are class II nuclear receptors, which heterodimerize with the retinoid X receptor alpha RXRα (NR2B1) before binding to distinct DNA response elements of target gene promoters. In addition to these ligand-activated nuclear receptors, other factors such as the hepatocyte nuclear factor (HNF) family of transcription factors, CCAAT/enhancer binding protein (C/EBP), sterol-responsive element binding protein (SREBP), signal transducers and activators of transcription (STAT) and nuclear factor kappa B (NFκB) also play an important role in the regulation of hepatobiliary transporter expression (Table 3). These transcription factors are activated by hormones, cytokines and their signalling cascades [5].

Posttranscriptional mechanisms

In addition to transcriptional regulation of transport systems, posttranscriptional and posttranslational changes such as targeting and sorting, transporter redistribution, transporter protein degradation (e.g. via lysosomal or the ubiquitin–proteasome pathway), direct protein modifications [e.g. (de-) phosphorylation, (de-) glycosylation], changes in membrane fluidity or cis-/trans-inhibition of transport systems by cholestatic agents (e.g. drugs) can also play an important role in the regulation of hepatobiliary transport [5–7,32].

Second messenger systems and bile secretion

Bile secretion by hepatocytes and cholangiocytes is rapidly regulated by the integration of signals from prosecretory/choleretic and antisecretory/cholestatic hormones (Table 4). Signals from these hormones are translated into activation of second messenger systems such as cAMP, cGMP and changes in cytosolic Ca^{2+} (for details see Chapter 2.2.3) [6,16]. Downstream kinases (e.g. PKA, PKC, MAPK, PI3K) in turn then further transduce these signals and alter target protein (i.e. transporter) function via phosphorylation/dephosphorylation. Some hormones (e.g. secretin, bombesin) act exclusively at the level of cholangiocytes because their receptors are only present on those cells and not on hepatocytes. In contrast, the glucagon and vasopressin receptors are selectively expressed on hepatocytes. In addition to hormones, gases (NO, CO) and bile acids themselves are capable of activating some of these signalling cascades (Table 4). NO stimulates bile flow by activation of guanylyl cyclase, resulting in the formation of cGMP, which in turn stimulates GSH and HCO_3^- excretion [65,66]. Higher concentrations may be cholestatic by impairing bile canalicular contraction [67], increasing tight junction permeability [68] and impairing ductular bile secretion [69]. Inhibition of CO, which accumulates during haem metabolism, increases bile acid-dependent bile flow and bile acid secretion [70].

cAMP–protein kinase A (PKA)

cAMP stimulates sinusoidal bile acid uptake, transcytotic vesicle trafficking and canalicular excretion of bile acids, other organic anions and HCO_3^- in hepatocytes [6]. In contrast to cAMP, cGMP does not stimulate bile acid excretion but only bile acid-independent bile flow by promoting biliary HCO_3^- and GSH excretion [65]. cAMP increases Ntcp content in sinusoidal membranes and Mrp2, Mdr2 and Bsep in canalicular membranes in a microtubule-dependent fashion [6]. The cAMP effects are thought to be mediated via PKA, a cAMP-dependent kinase, which in turn results in activation of the PI3K pathway and increases in cytosolic Ca^{2+} (see below), ultimately leading to vesicle movement and transporter translocation. Moreover, Ntcp is a serine/threonine phosphatide which, on addition of cAMP, is dephosphorylated, leading to increased retention of Ntcp in the plasma membrane [6]. In addition to Ntcp, Oatp1

Table 3 Transcriptional regulation of bile secretion: role of nuclear receptors, ligands/activators, target genes and physiological effects.

Nuclear receptor	Ligands/activators	Target genes (examples)	Effects
FXR (*NR1H4*)	Bile acids: chenodeoxycholic acid > deoxycholic acid = lithocholic acid > cholic acid	Basolateral uptake systems in liver (e.g. NTCP, OATP2, OATP8), canalicular export pumps (BSEP, MRP2, MDR3), bile acid synthesis enzymes (e.g. CYP7A1, CYP8B1)	Stimulation of bile acid-dependent and -independent bile flow (glutathione excretion). Reduction in hepatocellular bile acid uptake and bile acid synthesis (indirectly via induction of transcriptional repressor SHP)
PXR (*NR1I2*)	Rifampicin, dexamethasone, bile acids (lithocholic acid, potentially ursodeoxycholic acid), phenobarbital, statins, St John's Wort, xenobiotics	Hepatobiliary transporters (MRP2, MRP3, MDR1, rodent Oatp2), phase I and II detoxifying enzymes, bile acid synthesis (CYP7A1)	Stimulation of alternative basolateral bile acid efflux, stimulation of bilirubin glucuronidation and excretion, stimulation of phase I and II detoxification reactions in liver
CAR (*NR1I3*)	Bilirubin, phenobarbital, several xenobiotics	Hepatobiliary transporters (MRP2, MRP3, MRP4, MDR1), phase I and II detoxifying enzymes	Stimulation of alternative basolateral bile acid efflux, stimulation of bilirubin glucuronidation and excretion, stimulation of phase I and II detoxification reactions
PPARα (*NR1C1*)	Fatty acids, fibrates, statins, eicasanoids, leukotrienes, NSAIDs	Hepatobiliary transporters (ASBT, rodent Mdr2)	Stimulation of biliary phospholipid excretion (via Mdr2), stimulation of bile acid uptake in terminal ileum (via ASBT)
VDR (*NR1I1*)	Lithocholic acid, vitamin D	Bile acid detoxifying cytochromes and enzymes (CYP3A4, SULT2A1) in intestine and liver, hepatobiliary transporters (MRP3, ASBT)	Stimulation of intestinal bile acid detoxification, physiological effect on bile formation still unclear
GR (*NR3C1*)	Glucocorticoids, potentially ursodeoxycholic acid	Bile acid uptake systems (ASBT, NTCP)	Stimulation of bile acid uptake and canalicular excretion, beneficial effects in cholestatic jaundice ('steroid whitewash') may be mediated by direct transporter effects (induction of bilirubin export pump MRP2) in addition to anti-inflammatory effects
STAT5	Prolactin, placental lactogen, growth hormone	Hepatobiliary transporters (NTCP)	Stimulation of hepatic bile acid uptake
HNF1α (*TCF1*)	–	Hepatobiliary transporters (OATP2, OATP8, rodent Ntcp, Oatp1, Oatp2, Oatp4, OATP1B1, OATP1A3, Asbt)	Master transcription factor for the regulation of uptake transport systems on the basolateral membrane
HNF4α (*NR2A1*)	–	Hepatobiliary transporters (OATP2, rodent Ntcp, Oatp1), bile acid synthesis enzymes (CYP7A1, CYP8B1)	Mainly indirect effects via HNF1α in the regulation of uptake transport systems on the basolateral membrane

NSAIDs, non-steroidal anti-inflammatory drugs.

transport activity has also been shown to be regulated by serine phosphorylation [71,72].

Ca²⁺–protein kinase C (PKC)

The effects of intracellular Ca^{2+} on bile secretion are complex, given the multiple levels of actions and the multitude of possible effects, including increases in tight junction permeability, reduction in basolateral bile acid uptake, stimulation of bile canalicular contractions and canalicular excretion of bile acids and non-bile acid organic anions [6]. Some of these Ca^{2+} effects are mediated by PKC. Tauroursodeoxycholic acid (TUDCA) stimulates hepatocyte exocytosis by increasing cytosolic Ca^{2+} and translocation of the Ca^{2+}-sensitive PKCα to the hepatocellular membrane [73,74]. This may stimulate the insertion of canalicular transporters into the canalicular membrane. In contrast, the cholestatic taurolithocholic acid (TLCA) translocates Ca^{2+}-independent PKCε to the canalicular membrane, reduces binding of PKCα and impairs hepatobiliary exocytosis [73,74].

Phosphatidylinositol 3-kinase (PI3K)

Several different bile acids have been shown to activate PI3K [6]. PI3K is required for vesicular trafficking of ABC transporters

Table 4 Hormones and other mediators, their second messengers and effects on bile formation.

Hormone/mediator	Second messenger	Target cells/effect
Secretin	cAMP ↑, PKA	Cholangiocytes: stimulation of a bicarbonate-rich flow
Somatostatin	cAMP ↓	Cholangiocytes: inhibition of basal and secretin-induced bile flow
Gastrin	IP_3, Ca^{2+}, PKC ↑	Cholangiocytes: no effect on basal bile flow and bicarbonate excretion, but inhibition of secretin-induced choleresis
Bombesin	Unknown (independent of cAMP, cGMP and Ca^{2+})	Cholangiocytes: induction of a bicarbonate-rich bile flow
VIP	Unknown (cAMP independent, yet unidentified pathways)	Cholangiocytes: induction of a bicarbonate-rich bile flow Hepatocytes: mild stimulation of bile acid-dependent bile flow in rodents
Glucagon	cAMP ↑, Ca^{2+}	Hepatocytes: stimulation of bile acid-independent bile flow
Vasopressin	IP_3, Ca^{2+}, PKC	Hepatocytes: reduction in bile acid-independent bile flow
Insulin	↓ Secretin-induced cAMP in cholangiocytes	Cholangiocytes: inhibition of secretin-induced ductal bile secretion Hepatocytes: stimulation of bile acid-independent canalicular bile fraction
Acetylcholine	IP_3, Ca^{2+}	Cholangiocytes: induction of a bicarbonate-rich bile flow
Endothelin	IP_3, Ca^{2+}, ↓ secretin-induced cAMP	Hepatocytes: inhibition of bile flow, endothelin antagonists increase bile acid-independent bile flow (glutathione and bicarbonate excretion) Cholangiocytes: inhibition of secretin-induced choleresis
NO	cGMP ↑	Hepatocytes: stimulation of bile acid-independent bile flow (bicarbonate and glutathione excretion)
Bile acids		
Ursodeoxycholic acid	Ca^{2+}, PKCα ↑, MAPK	Hepatocytes: stimulation of vesicular exocytosis, canalicular insertion of canalicular transporters (Mrp2 and Bsep); stimulation of bile acid-dependent and -independent bile flow Cholangiocytes: stimulation of Cl^- excretion and Cl^-/HCO_3^- exchange
Lithocholic acid	PKCε ↑, PKCα ↓	Hepatocytes: inhibits PKCα-dependent Bsep phosphorylation and activation, reduction in bile acid-dependent bile flow

VIP, vasoactive intestinal polypeptide.

from intracellular pools to the bile canaliculus in response to bile acids and cell swelling. Inhibition of PI3K with wortmannin inhibits taurocholate-induced bile flow by about 50%, underlining the importance of the PI3K pathway. In addition, PI3K is also required for maximal transport activity of Mrp2, Mdr2 and Bsep [32,75,76]. Moreover, PI3K is involved in cell swelling- and cAMP-induced Ntcp translocation at the basolateral membrane [6].

Mitogen-activated protein kinases (MAPK)
MAPK signalling pathways (ERK1/2 and p38) mediate, at least in part, stimulation of bile flow and Bsep translocation to the canalicular membrane induced by changes in cell volume (swelling) and TUDCA [6,7].

Biliary compounds regulating bile secretion
In addition to classic hormonal signals, secretory functions of the biliary epithelium are also paracrinally regulated by molecules secreted into bile (e.g. bile acids, GSH, purinergic mediators). As such, ATP is released into bile in mM concentrations and binds

to purinergic receptors on cholangiocytes where this process stimulates ductal bicarbonate secretion [77].

Acknowledgements

This work was supported by grants P15502 and P18613-B05 from the Austrian Science Fund, grant 10266 from the Jubilee Funds of the Austrian National Bank and a GEN-AU grant from the Austrian Ministry for Science (to MT).

References

1 Hofmann AF (1999) Bile acids: the good, the bad, and the ugly. *News Physiol Sci* 14, 24–29.
2 Oude Elferink RP, Groen AK (2000) Mechanisms of biliary lipid secretion and their role in lipid homeostasis. *Semin Liver Dis* 20(3), 293–305.
3 Jansen PL, Bosma PJ, Chowdhury JR (1995) Molecular biology of bilirubin metabolism. *Prog Liver Dis* 13, 125–150.
4 Hofmann AF (1999) The continuing importance of bile acids in liver and intestinal disease. *Arch Intern Med* 159(22), 2647–2658.

5 Trauner M, Boyer JL (2003) Bile salt transporters: molecular characterization, function, and regulation. *Physiol Rev* 83(2), 633–671.

6 Anwer MS (2004) Cellular regulation of hepatic bile acid transport in health and cholestasis. *Hepatology* 39(3), 581–590.

7 Haussinger D, Schmitt M, Weiergraber O *et al.* (2000) Short-term regulation of canalicular transport. *Semin Liver Dis* 20(3), 307–321.

8 Marzioni M, Glaser SS, Francis H *et al.* (2002) Functional heterogeneity of cholangiocytes. *Semin Liver Dis* 22(3), 227–240.

9 Kullak-Ublick GA, Stieger B, Meier PJ (2004) Enterohepatic bile salt transporters in normal physiology and liver disease. *Gastroenterology* 126(1), 322–342.

10 Inagaki T, Choi M, Moschetta A *et al.* (2005) Fibroblast growth factor 15 functions as an enterohepatic signal to regulate bile acid homeostasis. *Cell Metab* 2(4), 217–225.

11 Reynoso-Paz S, Coppel RL, Mackay IR *et al.* (1999) The immunobiology of bile and biliary epithelium. *Hepatology* 30(2), 351–357.

12 Itoh M, Wada K, Tan S *et al.* (1999) Antibacterial action of bile acids against *Helicobacter pylori* and changes in its ultrastructural morphology: effect of unconjugated dihydroxy bile acid. *J Gastroenterol* 34(5), 571–576.

13 Inagaki T, Moschetta A, Lee YK *et al.* (2006) Regulation of antibacterial defense in the small intestine by the nuclear bile acid receptor. *Proc Natl Acad Sci USA* 103(10), 3920–3925.

14 Sperber I (1959) Secretion of organic anions in the formation of urine and bile. *Pharmacol Rev* 11, 109–134.

15 Marinelli RA, Gradilone SA, Carreras FI *et al.* (2004) Liver aquaporins: significance in canalicular and ductal bile formation. *Ann Hepatol* 3(4), 130–136.

16 Nathanson MH, Boyer JL (1991) Mechanisms and regulation of bile secretion. *Hepatology* 14, 551–566.

17 Alpini G, Roberts S, Kuntz SM *et al.* (1996) Morphological, molecular, and functional heterogeneity of cholangiocytes from normal rat liver. *Gastroenterology* 110(5), 1636–1643.

18 Baiocchi L, LeSage G, Glaser S *et al.* (1999) Regulation of cholangiocyte bile secretion. *J Hepatol* 31(1), 179–191.

19 Kullak-Ublick GA (2000) Hepatic transport of bile salts. *Semin Liver Dis* 20, 273–292.

20 Trauner M, Wagner M, Fickert P *et al.* (2005) Molecular regulation of hepatobiliary transport systems: clinical implications for understanding and treating cholestasis. *J Clin Gastroenterol* 39(4), S111–S124.

21 Hofmann AF (1993) The cholehepatic circulation of unconjugated bile acids: an update. In: Paumgartner G, Stiehl A, Gerok W (eds) *Bile Acids and the Hepatobiliary System*. Boston: Kluwer, pp. 143–160.

22 Trauner M, Meier PJ, Boyer JL (1998) Molecular pathogenesis of cholestasis. *N Engl J Med* 339(17), 1217–1227.

23 Meier PJ (1995) Molecular mechanisms of hepatic bile salt transport from sinusoidal blood into bile. *Am J Physiol* 269(6 Pt 1), G801–G812.

24 Arias IM (1990) The biology of hepatic endothelial cell fenestrae. *Prog Liver Dis* 9, 11–26.

25 Kullak-Ublick G-A, Stieger B, Hagenbuch B *et al.* (2000) Hepatic transport of bile salts. *Semin Liver Dis* 20, 273–292.

26 Meier PJ, Stieger B (2002) Bile salt transporters. *Annu Rev Physiol* 64, 635–661.

27 Hagenbuch B, Meier PJ (2003) The superfamily of organic anion transporting polypeptides. *Biochim Biophys Acta* 1609(1), 1–18.

28 Faber KN, Muller M, Jansen PL (2003) Drug transport proteins in the liver. *Adv Drug Deliv Rev* 55(1), 107–124.

29 Dawson PA, Hubbert M, Haywood J *et al.* (2005) The heteromeric organic solute transporter {alpha}–{beta}, Ost{alpha}–Ost{beta}, is an ileal basolateral bile acid transporter. *J Biol Chem* 280(8), 6960–6968.

30 Agellon LB, Torchia EC (2000) Intracellular transport of bile acids. *Biochim Biophys Acta* 1486(1), 198–209.

31 Crawford JM, Strahs DC, Crawford AR *et al.* (1994) Role of bile salt hydrophobicity in hepatic microtubule-dependent bile salt secretion. *J Lipid Res* 35(10), 1738–1748.

32 Kipp H, Arias IM (2000) Intracellular trafficking and regulation of canalicular ATP-binding cassette transporters. *Semin Liver Dis* 20(3), 339–351.

33 Smit JJ, Schinkel AH, Oude Elferink RP *et al.* (1993) Homozygous disruption of the murine mdr2 P-glycoprotein gene leads to a complete absence of phospholipid from bile and to liver disease. *Cell* 75(3), 451–462.

34 Yu L, Hammer RE, Li-Hawkins J *et al.* (2002) Disruption of Abcg5 and Abcg8 in mice reveals their crucial role in biliary cholesterol secretion. *Proc Natl Acad Sci USA* 99(25), 16237–16242.

35 Jansen PL, Sturm E (2003) Genetic cholestasis, causes and consequences for hepatobiliary transport. *Liver Int* 23(5), 315–322.

36 Crawford AR, Smith AJ, Hatch VC *et al.* (1997) Hepatic secretion of phospholipid vesicles in the mouse critically depends on mdr2 or MDR3 P-glycoprotein expression. Visualization by electron microscopy. *J Clin Invest* 100(10), 2562–2567.

37 Fickert P, Fuchsbichler A, Wagner M *et al.* (2004) Regurgitation of bile acids from leaky bile ducts causes sclerosing cholangitis in Mdr2 (Abcb4) knockout mice. *Gastroenterology* 127(1), 261–274.

38 Kipp H, Pichetshote N, Arias IM (2001) Transporters on demand: intrahepatic pools of canalicular ATP binding cassette transporters in rat liver. *J Biol Chem* 276(10), 7218–7224.

39 Wakabayashi Y, Lippincott-Schwartz J, Arias IM (2004) Intracellular trafficking of bile salt export pump (ABCB11) in polarized hepatic cells: constitutive cycling between the canalicular membrane and rab11-positive endosomes. *Mol Biol Cell* 15(7), 3485–3496.

40 Anwer MS, Gillin H, Mukhopadhyay S *et al.* (2005) Dephosphorylation of Ser-226 facilitates plasma membrane retention of Ntcp. *J Biol Chem* 280(39), 33687–33692.

41 Hamm-Alvarez SF, Sheetz MP (1998) Microtubule-dependent vesicle transport: modulation of channel and transporter activity in liver and kidney. *Physiol Rev* 78(4), 1109–1129.

42 Marks DL, LaRusso NF, McNiven MA (1995) Isolation of the microtubule-vesicle motor kinesin from rat liver: selective inhibition by cholestatic bile acids. *Gastroenterology* 108(3), 824–833.

43 Crawford JM, Berken CA, Gollan JL (1988) Role of the hepatocyte microtubular system in the excretion of bile salts and biliary lipid: implications for intracellular vesicular transport. *J Lipid Res* 29(2), 144–156.

44 Zatloukal K, Stumptner C, Fuchsbichler A *et al.* (2004) The keratin cytoskeleton in liver diseases. *J Pathol* 204(4), 367–376.

45 Tsukada N, Ackerley CA, Phillips MJ (1995) The structure and organization of the bile canalicular cytoskeleton with special reference to actin and actin-binding proteins. *Hepatology* 21(4), 1106–1113.

46 Omary MB, Coulombe PA, McLean WH (2004) Intermediate filament proteins and their associated diseases. *N Engl J Med* 351(20), 2087–2100.

47 Omary MB, Ku NO, Toivola DM (2002) Keratins: guardians of the liver. *Hepatology* 35(2), 251–257.

48 Dranoff JA, McClure M, Burgstahler AD *et al.* (1999) Short-term regulation of bile acid uptake by microfilament-dependent translocation of rat ntcp to the plasma membrane. *Hepatology* 30(1), 223–229.

49 Kikuchi S, Hata M, Fukumoto K *et al.* (2002) Radixin deficiency causes conjugated hyperbilirubinemia with loss of Mrp2 from bile canalicular membranes. *Nature Genet* 31(3), 320–325.

50 Ortiz DF, Moseley J, Calderon G *et al.* (2004) Identification of HAX-1 as a protein that binds bile salt export protein and regulates its abundance in the apical membrane of Madin–Darby canine kidney cells. *J Biol Chem* 279(31), 32761–32770.

51 Chan W, Calderon G, Swift AL *et al.* (2005) Myosin II regulatory light chain is required for trafficking of bile salt export protein to the apical membrane in Madin-Darby canine kidney cells. *J Biol Chem* 280(25), 23741–23747.

52 Fouassier L, Duan CY, Feranchak AP *et al.* (2001) Ezrin–radixin–moesin-binding phosphoprotein 50 is expressed at the apical membrane of rat liver epithelia. *Hepatology* 33(1), 166–176.

53 Mitic LL, Van Itallie CM, Anderson JM (2000) Molecular physiology and pathophysiology of tight junctions I. Tight junction structure and function: lessons from mutant animals and proteins. *Am J Physiol Gastrointest Liver Physiol* 279(2), G250–G254.

54 Echevarria W, Arias IM (2004) Gap junctions in the liver. In: Trauner M, Jansen PLM (eds) *Molecular Pathogenesis of Cholestasis.* New York, NY: Landes Bioscience, Kluwer Academic/Plenum Publishers, pp. 36–47.

55 Kanno N, Lesage G, Glaser S *et al.* (2000) Functional heterogeneity of the intrahepatic biliary epithelium. *Hepatology* 31(3), 555–561.

56 Lazaridis KN, Pham L, Tietz P *et al.* (1997) Rat cholangiocytes absorb bile acids at their apical domain via the ileal sodium-dependent bile acid transporter. *J Clin Invest* 100(11), 2714–2721.

57 Lesage G, Glaser S, Alpini G (2001) Regulation of cholangiocyte proliferation. *Liver* 21(2), 73–80.

58 Tietz PS, Marinelli RA, Chen XM *et al.* (2003) Agonist-induced coordinated trafficking of functionally related transport proteins for water and ions in cholangiocytes. *J Biol Chem* 278(22), 20413–20419.

59 Rost D, Konig J, Weiss G *et al.* (2001) Expression and localization of the multidrug resistance proteins MRP2 and MRP3 in human gallbladder epithelia. *Gastroenterology* 121(5), 1203–1208.

60 Chignard N, Mergey M, Veissiere D *et al.* (2001) Bile acid transport and regulating functions in the human biliary epithelium. *Hepatology* 33(3), 496–503.

61 Plosch T, Bloks VW, Terasawa Y *et al.* (2004) Sitosterolemia in ABC-transporter G5-deficient mice is aggravated on activation of the liver-X receptor. *Gastroenterology* 126(1), 290–300.

62 Karpen SJ (2002) Nuclear receptor regulation of hepatic function. *J Hepatol* 36(6), 832–850.

63 Eloranta JJ, Kullak-Ublick GA (2005) Coordinate transcriptional regulation of bile acid homeostasis and drug metabolism. *Arch Biochem Biophys* 433(2), 397–412.

64 Chiang JY (2004) Regulation of bile acid synthesis: pathways, nuclear receptors, and mechanisms. *J Hepatol* 40(3), 539–551.

65 Trauner M, Nathanson MH, Rydberg StA *et al.* (1997) Endotoxin impairs biliary glutathione and HCO_3^- excretion and blocks the choleretic effect of nitric oxide in rat liver. *Hepatology* 25, 1184–1191.

66 Myers NC, Grune S, Jameson HL *et al.* (1996) cGMP stimulates bile acid-independent bile formation and biliary bicarbonate excretion. *Am J Physiol* 270(3 Pt 1), G418–G424.

67 Dufour JF, Turner TJ, Arias IM (1995) Nitric oxide blocks bile canalicular contraction by inhibiting inositol trisphosphate-dependent calcium mobilization. *Gastroenterology* 108(3), 841–849.

68 Burgstahler AD, Nathanson MH (1995) NO modulates the apicolateral cytoskeleton of isolated hepatocytes by a PKC-dependent, cGMP-independent mechanism. *Am J Physiol* 269(5 Pt 1), G789–G799.

69 Spirli C, Fabris L, Duner E *et al.* (2003) Cytokine-stimulated nitric oxide production inhibits adenylyl cyclase and cAMP-dependent secretion in cholangiocytes. *Gastroenterology* 124(3), 737–753.

70 Sano T, Shiomi M, Wakabayashi Y *et al.* (1997) Endogenous carbon monoxide suppression stimulates bile acid-dependent biliary transport in perfused rat liver. *Am J Physiol* 272(5 Pt 1), G1268–G1275.

71 Glavy JS, Wu SM, Wang PJ *et al.* (2000) Down-regulation by extracellular ATP of rat hepatocyte organic anion transport is mediated by serine phosphorylation of oatp1. *J Biol Chem* 275(2), 1479–1484.

72 Guo GL, Klaassen CD (2001) Protein kinase C suppresses rat organic anion transporting polypeptide 1- and 2-mediated uptake. *J Pharmacol Exp Ther* 299(2), 551–557.

73 Paumgartner G, Beuers U (2002) Ursodeoxycholic acid in cholestatic liver disease: mechanisms of action and therapeutic use revisited. *Hepatology* 36(3), 525–531.

74 Paumgartner G, Beuers U (2004) Mechanisms of action and therapeutic efficacy of ursodeoxycholic acid in cholestatic liver disease. *Clin Liver Dis* 8(1), 67–81, vi.

75 Misra S, Ujhazy P, Varticovski L *et al.* (1999) Phosphoinositide 3-kinase lipid products regulate ATP-dependent transport by sister of P-glycoprotein and multidrug resistance associated protein 2 in bile canalicular membrane vesicles. *Proc Natl Acad Sci USA* 96(10), 5814–5819.

76 Misra S, Varticovski L, Arias IM (2003) Mechanisms by which cAMP increases bile acid secretion in rat liver and canalicular membrane vesicles. *Am J Physiol Gastrointest Liver Physiol* 285(2), G316–G324.

77 Strazzabosco M, Fabris L, Spirli C (2005) Pathophysiology of cholangiopathies. *J Clin Gastroenterol* 39(4 Suppl. 2), S90–S102.

2.6.2 Motility of the biliary tree

Mayank Bhandari and James Toouli

Introduction

The presence of the gallbladder and biliary tract was described in some of the earliest recorded observations of man [1], but their role in digestion was not appreciated. In the sixteenth century, a membrane near the distal end of the common bile duct, thought to impede reflux of duodenal contents into the bile duct, was described but it was not until 1887 that this structure was described as a sphincter and named after Rugero Oddi, who published a detailed description of its anatomy [2]. Following the discovery of the hormone cholecystokinin (CCK), it was shown to contract the gallbladder and reduce sphincter of Oddi resistance. These and subsequent studies firmly established that an intimate relationship existed between gallbladder contraction, sphincter of Oddi function and the flow of bile into the duodenum.

Anatomy

Embryology

The gallbladder and bile ducts arise from the caudal portion of a diverticular anlage that originates from the ventral floor of the foregut. The pancreas develops from two foregut buds in the region of the future duodenum. Anatomical studies showed that the distal muscularis propria of the bile duct and pancreatic duct are independent from duodenal musculature. In studies of the human fetus, Boyden showed that the sphincter of Oddi, appearing approximately 5 weeks after the intestinal musculature, arises *de novo* from mesenchyme.

Morphology

The biliary tract comprises the bile ducts, gallbladder, cystic duct and the sphincter of Oddi. Bile flows from the hepatocytes into canaliculi, which communicate with numerous interlobular ducts. These in turn drain into two main hepatic ducts. The main right and left hepatic ducts fuse at the porta hepatis to form the common hepatic duct. The cystic duct joins the common hepatic duct at a variable distance caudal to the porta hepatis to form the common bile duct.

The human gallbladder is a pear-shaped muscular sac with a resting volume of 35–50 mL. It lies in the fossa on the right inferior surface of the liver. The gallbladder is divided anatomically into the blunt-ended fundus, the body and the neck, which leads to the cystic duct. A sacculation at the neck of the gallbladder is known as Hartman's pouch. The cystic duct is of variable length, usually joining the common hepatic duct at an acute angle to form the common bile duct.

The common bile duct passes dorsal to the first part of the duodenum lying in a groove either within or posterior to the head of the pancreas and enters the second part of the duodenum through the major duodenal papilla in association with the pancreatic duct of Wirsung. The junction of the terminal common bile duct, pancreatic duct and duodenum at the papilla assumes one of three configurations that may be likened to a Y, V or U. In approximately 70% of subjects, the ducts open into a common channel and thus have a Y configuration. This common channel drains into the duodenum through a single orifice on the duodenal papilla of Vater. In approximately 20% of subjects, the common channel is almost non-existent, and the two ducts have a common V shape opening on the papilla. In 10% of subjects, the common bile duct and pancreatic duct have separate openings on the tip of the papilla; these openings lie adjacent to each other and give a U-shaped configuration. The terminal parts of the common bile duct and pancreatic duct, the common channel and major duodenal papilla of Vater are invested by varying thickness of smooth muscle and together form the sphincter of Oddi segment.

The major part of the human sphincter of Oddi lies within the duodenal wall and is anatomically and functionally independent of the duodenal muscle.

Distinct sphincters lie at the terminal end of the common bile duct (sphincter choledochus), the terminal end of the pancreatic duct (sphincter pancreaticus) and the common channel (sphincter ampullae) [3]. However, more recently, Hand [4], using a combination of radiological, duct cast techniques and histological sectioning methods, did not distinguish separate sphincters and concluded from his human autopsy studies that the common bile duct and pancreatic duct become fused in a common connective tissue sheath outside the duodenal wall and pass together through a slit in the duodenal muscle known as the 'choledochal window'. The lumina, however, do not join at this level but are separated by a thick muscular septum. In most subjects, fusion of the two lumina occurs in the submucosal layer of the duodenum to form a common channel varying in length between 2 and 17 mm. Before entering the duodenum, each duct becomes completely surrounded by circular muscle, some of which forms a figure of eight pattern around the two ducts. The point at which the smooth muscle starts on each duct is readily identified radiologically as a notch. Distal to the notch, each lumen becomes narrow as it traverses the duodenal wall, this narrowing being associated with a thickening of the duct wall due to smooth muscle, connective tissue and mucous glands. As the ducts pass through the duodenal wall, longitudinal muscle fibres interdigitate between the circular ductular muscle fibres and the duodenal muscle. The ducts emerge from the duodenal muscle layers to have a course of variable length through the duodenal submucosa before opening on to the papilla of Vater; throughout this submucosal course, the ducts are ensheathed by circularly orientated smooth muscle. Manometric studies in man support Hand's description of the sphincter of Oddi in that separate sphincteric zones have not been identified [5].

The mucosa of the human sphincter of Oddi segment is lined by columnar epithelium and contains numerous mucus-secreting glands. The mucosa is thrown into longitudinal folds likened to mucosal valvules [6]. These folds are least marked proximally and increase distally, becoming maximal in the common channel. The mucosal folds may occasionally be seen projecting through the orifice of the duodenal papilla.

Innervation

The extrahepatic biliary tract is innervated by dense networks of extrinsic and intrinsic nerves that regulate smooth muscle tone and epithelial cell function of the extrahepatic biliary tree. The coeliac ganglia contribute both motor and sensory nerves made up of sympathetic fibres, which originate in the T7–T10 spinal segments. Hepatic plexus is formed by nerve fibres from both the vagi, which supply parasympathetic motor nerves to the extrahepatic biliary system [7].

The wall of the biliary tract is composed of three layers, namely serosal, muscularis and mucosal layers. Ganglionated nerve plexuses are located in the subserosal and the subepithelial layers. Histochemical studies have shown that the gallbladder is richly supplied with both adrenergic and cholinergic ganglia. In addition, studies [8] have shown the presence of immuno-reactive peptidergic nerves that can be labelled to detect vasoactive intestinal polypeptide (VIP). The sphincter of Oddi has a rich ganglionic plexus. It has a predominance of cholinergic ganglia and a smaller number of adrenergic ganglia.

Immunohistochemical studies from our laboratory have demonstrated the presence of a wide range of peptidergic neurones in the sphincter region. These include galanin, substance P and somatostatin-containing nerves. In addition, the inhibitory transmitter nitric oxide has been demonstrated in nerves to the sphincter and is thought to have an important function in modulating sphincter relaxation. It has been shown that the nerves in the sphincter region communicate with the proximal biliary tract, the gallbladder and the duodenum [9,10].

Physiology

Gallbladder

Fluid transport and its regulation

The gallbladder concentrates hepatic bile by selective reabsorption of bile constituents. In addition, studies have shown that, under both physiological and pathological conditions, reversal of fluid transport across the gallbladder mucosa occurs, and net secretion into the gallbladder lumen results. Sodium and chloride ions are absorbed from the gallbladder lumen by both active and passive transport mechanisms. Water absorption is thought to be passive and secondary to active solute movement resulting from osmotic equilibration of transported solute within the epithelium. The secretion of water and electrolytes by the gallbladder mucosa is an active process that can take place against hydrostatic and osmotic gradients [11]. Animal *in vitro* and *in vivo* studies have demonstrated that a number of gastrointestinal peptides affect gallbladder fluid transport. Cyclic adenosine monophosphate (cAMP) acts as a second messenger for the effects of several mediators and has been implicated in sodium and chloride transport in rabbit and necturus gallbladder. Vasoactive intestinal polypeptide (VIP) and secretin have been shown to modify gallbladder fluid transport at concentrations that suggest a physiological role. However, other peptides, such as glucagon, cholecystokinin, neurotensin, bombesin, motilin and somatostatin, which have been shown to enhance absorption *in vitro*, may act to potentiate or inhibit the effects of the major peptides [12].

Application of prostaglandins of the E and F series to *in vitro* animal gallbladder preparations have demonstrated inhibition of fluid absorption by arachidonic acid [13]. In animal studies, bile salts, female sex hormones and autonomic nerve stimulation have also been shown to influence fluid transport.

During fasting, the normal gallbladder absorbs fluid at a rate corresponding to one-third of the fasting gallbladder volume. After feeding, there is reversal of the direction of gallbladder transport from a net absorption to a net secretion into the gallbladder lumen. The net water transport across the gallbladder wall may be influenced by both humoral factors and autonomic nerves. During inflammation of the gallbladder, often associated with cystic duct obstruction, the absorptive capacity of the gallbladder mucosa is lost, and net secretion into the lumen results, producing a hydrops. This pathological effect appears to be mediated by prostaglandin release due to the formation of lysolecithin by hydrolysis of phospholipid in the gallbladder. This process can be reversed by indomethacin, supporting the belief that at least part of the change in fluid transport may result from endogenous prostaglandin formation.

Gallbladder motility

Gallbladder filling depends on the rate of bile secretion from the liver and the resistance to flow through the sphincter of Oddi. Only 50% of secreted hepatic bile enters the gallbladder during fasting; the remaining bile passes into the duodenum without concentration by the gallbladder. Release of CCK after ingestion of food causes the gallbladder to have a slow steady contraction which delivers bile into the duodenum for 20 min or longer while generating an intraluminal gallbladder pressure that is generally only a little elevated above that in the common bile duct. About 75% of gallbladder volume is ejected during CCK stimulation. The slow emptying of the gallbladder is typical of a graded tonic smooth muscle contraction such as that which occurs in the fundus of the stomach during gastric emptying of liquids. The hormones that affect gallbladder motility are shown in Table 1.

Estimations of human fasting gallbladder volume by ultrasound techniques have shown a mean volume of approximately 17 mL in normal subjects. In the past, it was thought that the gallbladder volume gradually increased during fasting until the mean maximal volume was reached and only emptied after a food stimulus. However, studies in dogs [14] and opossums have shown that the gallbladder contracts by up to 40% of maximal contractile capacity during the interdigestive period, and that these gallbladder contractions occur during phase II of the migrating motor complex (MMC). The periodic gallbladder contractions during fasting empty concentrated viscous bile and enable gallbladder refilling with dilute hepatic bile. Studies in man using ultrasound estimation of gallbladder volume confirm that a similar cyclical pattern of gallbladder volume changes occur, in association with phase III of the MMC [15]. The controlling mechanism that produces gallbladder volume changes during fasting is unknown. A potential candidate is motilin, a hormone produced by the mucosa of the proximal small intestine. Serum motilin levels show cyclic changes during MMC cycles with the peak values preceding phase III MMC

Table 1 Hormones affecting gallbladder motility.

Prokinetic agents	Inhibitors
CCK	VIP
Secretin (with CCK)	Somatostatin
Motilin	Neurotensin
Substance P	Pancreatic polypeptide
Gastrin releasing peptide	Peptide YY
Neuropeptide Y	Histamine (H2 receptors)
Histamine (H1 receptors)	

activity. In animal studies, motilin has been shown to produce gallbladder contraction [14].

The ability of a fatty meal to elicit gallbladder contraction has been well documented in man and a number of animal species. Proteins entering the duodenum also produce gallbladder contraction, but carbohydrates have only a minimal effect. Endogenous CCK is released from the mucosa of the proximal small intestine, and studies that measure serum CCK levels by radioimmunoassay have shown that gallbladder contraction induced by intraduodenal infusion of fat correlates directly with the level of circulating CCK [16].

The role of autonomic nerves in regulating gallbladder volume is not clear. The innervation of the gallbladder mainly plays a facilitatory role to that of gastrointestinal hormones and peptides, which are the prime regulators of gallbladder motility. In one study, increased fasting volume of the human gallbladder was demonstrated after vagotomy [17]. A number of studies have investigated the effect of vagal stimulation and vagotomy on gallbladder contractility [18], but the results have generally been inconclusive. Similarly, studies of sympathetic innervation have produced inconstant and variable findings, and the role of the sympathetic autonomic nervous system in gallbladder motility requires further study [19].

Cystic duct

Accumulating evidence suggests that the cystic duct is not merely a passive conduit between the gallbladder and the common bile duct, but may play an active role in the flow of bile into and out of the gallbladder. Histologically, an anatomically prominent sphincter, as described by Lutken, does not appear to be present; however, a thin layer of smooth muscle is evident in the wall of the duct and, along with the prominent mucosal folds that make up the valves of Heister, the cystic duct may act as a variable resistor to flow.

Flow studies in dogs have demonstrated resistance to flow across the cystic duct, the resistance being equal whether perfusion was carried either into or out of the gallbladder [20]. Significant reductions in flow were induced following systemic intravenous or local intra-arterial injection of morphine, adrenalin or CCK, suggesting that the cystic duct performs like a sphincter in modulating flow through its lumen. Studies in the prairie dog gallstone model have shown that cystic duct resistance to flow increases prior to gallstone formation in these animals [21]. These studies suggest that abnormalities in cyst duct formation may be implicated in the pathophysiology of gallstone formation.

Common bile duct

The role of the common bile duct in the control of bile flow has been confused because of anatomical differences in the species studied. As in the cystic duct, histological studies in man have demonstrated only thin longitudinally orientated layers of smooth muscle within the walls of the common bile duct [22]. The major tissue component appears to be elastic fibres. However, in other species such as sheep, the common bile duct is invested with circularly orientated smooth muscle which exhibits peristaltic activity.

The weight of evidence suggests that the human common bile duct does not have a primary propulsile function. However, the elastic fibres and the longitudinally orientated smooth muscle provide a tonic pressure that may help to overcome the tonic resistance of the sphincter of Oddi. The diameter of the human common bile duct before and after cholecystectomy has been the subject of controversy. Part of the controversy has resulted from methodology used in determining duct size. It has become quite obvious that duct size as determined by ultrasonography and magnetic resonance cholangiography (MRC) cannot be equated to duct size determined by endoscopic retrograde cholangiography (ERCP) or intraoperative extraluminal measurements. Ultrasound and MRC measurement records the non-distended lumen, whereas at ERCP, contrast produces distension. Intraoperative measurements include wall thickness. In general, the normal diameter of the common bile duct as determined by ultrasound is less than 6 mm, by retrograde cholangiography less than 10 mm, and by intraoperative extraluminal measurements less than 12 mm. What has become clear is that the common bile duct does not increase in diameter significantly following cholecystectomy [23,24]. The major cause of dilated common bile duct is increased intraluminal pressure, which is generally produced by either primary or secondary obstruction at the sphincter of Oddi.

Motility of the sphincter of Oddi

The primary function of the sphincter of Oddi is to control the delivery of bile and pancreatic juice into the duodenum. This is possible because of low pressure within the bile duct. Approximately 800–1500 mL of bile flows through the human sphincter of Oddi. Various studies in animals and man have tried to evaluate the mechanism by which the sphincter of Oddi controls the flow of bile and pancreatic secretions. These studies have shown that there is anatomical variability between species and also that the sphincter of Oddi motility differs from one species to another. Thus, while many commonalities exist, one has to be circumspect in translating animal data directly into the motility and function of the human sphincter of Oddi.

Sphincter of Oddi motility studies in animals

In vivo studies in dogs, cats, rabbits, monkeys and opossums have demonstrated that the sphincter of Oddi exhibits muscle contractions that are independent of duodenal activity. The results from the dog studies suggested that the sphincter of Oddi has a milking effect on bile, thus propelling small volumes of fluid from the common bile duct into the duodenum [25]. Manometric and electromyographic studies of the opossum sphincter of Oddi demonstrated phasic contractions that propagate along the entire length from the cephalic to the caudal end [26]. The common bile duct and pancreatic duct proximal to the sphincter do not demonstrate spontaneous motor activity.

Analysis of simultaneous cineradiography, trans-sphincteric flow and electromyographic recordings from the opossum sphincter of Oddi has demonstrated the effect of the phasic contractions on the flow of bile into the duodenum. The predominant mechanism of common bile duct emptying in the opossum is the antegrade sphincter of Oddi phasic contraction. A wave of contraction begins at the junction of the common bile duct and sphincter of Oddi stripping the contents of the sphincter of Oddi segment into the duodenum. During the period of sphincter of Oddi contraction, flow into the common bile duct ceases, and there is no flow from the common bile duct into the sphincter of Oddi segment. Next, the sphincter of Oddi relaxes, and passive flow of bile occurs from the common bile duct into the sphincter of Oddi segment. After filling of the sphincter of Oddi segment, a wave of contraction begins again at the junction of the common bile duct and sphincter segment, and the cycle repeats itself. The overall effect of the phasic contractions is to promote flow from the common bile duct into the duodenum. During sphincter contraction, or systole, flow from the common bile duct into the sphincter of Oddi segment stops, and flow into the sphincter segment occurs only during sphincter relaxation or diastole. Increasing the frequency of sphincter contractions by administering the sphincter agonists phenylephrine (50 µg/kg i.v.) and bethanechol (30 µg/kg i.v.) decreased the diastolic interval between contractions and decreased the time available for passive flow of fluid from the common bile duct into the sphincter segment. Initially, an increase in the frequency of sphincter phasic contractions produced an increase in flow across the sphincter. However, as the frequency of contractions increases further, flow decreases because of the decrease in the diastolic interval. When the frequency of contractions exceeds eight per minute, the diastolic interval is abolished, and there is no flow across the sphincter of Oddi segment in the opossum. Recent studies have shown that the sphincter may act as a pump or a resistor and that the bile duct pressure influences it [27]. This intrinsic activity is controlled by interstitial nerves of Cajal and is modulated by hormones [28], peptides such as adenosine triphosphate (ATP) and adenosine [29] and nitric oxide [30].

In cats, an intravenous bolus of CCK inhibited the phasic contractions and produced a fall in sphincter tone. Following administration of the neurotoxin tetrodotoxin, CCK administration no longer produced inhibition, but instead caused contraction in the sphincter of Oddi. The investigators concluded that CCK produces its effect by stimulation of non-adrenergic non-cholinergic inhibitory neurones, with this effect overriding a lesser, direct smooth muscle stimulatory action of the hormone [28]. Neurohistochemical studies have demonstrated both adrenergic and cholinergic neurons within the sphincter of Oddi, and experiments in animals have determined the pharmacological effects of histamine, cholinergic and adrenergic stimulation on the sphincter muscle [26]. However, the physiological significance of these drug actions on the sphincter of Oddi requires further investigation.

The function of the vagus nerve in sphincter of Oddi physiology remains obscure. Sphincter of Oddi neurons probably receive vagal input, and their activity is modulated by release of neuropeptides from sensory fibres, a significant source of excitatory synaptic input to these cells arising from the duodenum. This duodenum–sphincter of Oddi circuit is likely to play an important role in the coordination of sphincter of Oddi tone with gallbladder motility in the process of gallbladder emptying [31]. Studies in dogs suggested that, following vagal transaction, the resistance to flow across the sphincter of Oddi is decreased [32]. However, in the prairie dog, increased resistance to flow through the sphincter of Oddi occurs after truncal vagotomy. Results from vagal stimulation studies have failed to define clearly the role of the vagus in biliary dynamics.

Studies carried out in opossums with chronically implanted electrodes positioned in the sphincter of Oddi and the small intestine have demonstrated that the phasic activity of the sphincter of Oddi is omnipresent [33]. However, the frequency of the phasic contractions varies periodically during fasting. Four phases that are analogous to the phases of the intestinal interdigestive MMC have been described for the sphincter of Oddi. Food ingestion and the intravenous infusion of CCK and pentagastrin abolish the periodic nature of the interdigestive sphincter of Oddi contractions and, in this species, ingested food produced an increase in contractile frequency, which increased the flow of bile into the duodenum. The physiological function of the periodic sphincter of Oddi contractions during fasting might be similar to that proposed for intestinal MMC, which is to act as a housekeeper to eliminate any debris that may accumulate at the lower end of the bile duct. In addition, this activity of the sphincter may modulate the volume of bile passing into either the duodenum or the gallbladder during fasting.

The Australian opossum sphincter of Oddi demonstrates an activity that is similar to that of the human sphincter. In this species, inhibition of sphincter phasic contractions promotes the flow of bile. It has been shown that this inhibition is mediated by neural release of nitric oxide [28]. There is evidence that nitric oxide mediates the caerulein and CCK octapeptide-mediated relaxation of the canine sphincter of Oddi [34]. Table 2 illustrates the effects of various bioactive agents on the sphincter of Oddi.

Sphincter of Oddi motility in man

Cineradiographic studies of the human sphincter of Oddi exhibit rhythmic contractions that propel contrast into the duodenum [35]. Sphincter of Oddi pressure studies conducted at the time of biliary tract surgery demonstrated variations in pressure thought to be the manometric equivalent of the cineradiographic contractions [36]. Resistance to outflow of fluid from the common bile duct into the duodenum was also demonstrated by the intraoperative studies. This resistance was

Table 2 Effects of various bioactive agents on the sphincter of Oddi.

Stimulator	Inhibitor
Morphine met-encephalin	Tramadol
Galanin	Glucagon
Substance P	CGRP
CCK	CCK
Neuropeptide Y	Peptide YY
Nitric oxide	Somatostatin

CGRP, calcitonin gene-related peptide.

reduced after administration of CCK octapeptide or smooth muscle relaxants such as amylnitrite [37].

Manometric recordings from within the sphincter of Oddi segment [38] have been made via a pressure-sensitive catheter introduced into the sphincter of Oddi via a duodenoscope (Fig. 1). They have demonstrated that the human sphincter of Oddi is characterized by prominent phasic contractions superimposed on a basal sphincter of Oddi pressure 3 mmHg above the pressure in the common bile duct and pancreatic duct (Fig. 2). The amplitude of the phasic contractions is approximately 130 mmHg, and the mean frequency is four per min.

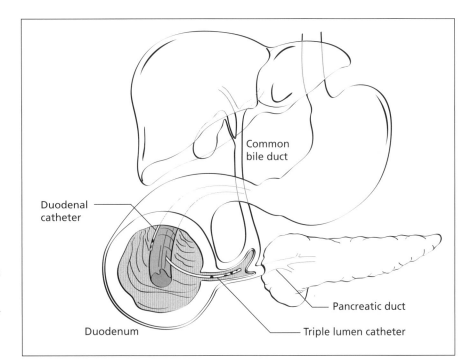

Fig. 1 Sphincer of Oddi manometry using a triple lumen perfused catheter. The catheter is introduced into the bile duct via the biopsy channel of a duodenoscope. The recording ports of the catheter are positioned to register pressure changes from the sphincter. A separate catheter attached to the endoscope records duodenal pressure.

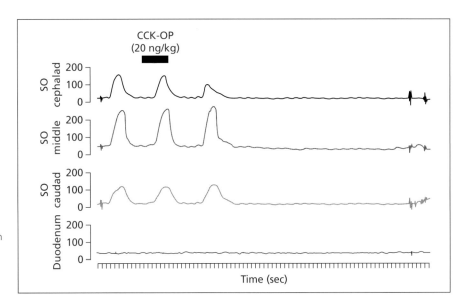

Fig. 2 Recording from the Sphincter of Oddi and a separate duodenal catheter. The sphincter contractions are characterized by phasic contractions which are superimposed on a basal pressure. Administration of the octapeptide of cholecystokinin produces inhibition of the phasic contractions and a fall in basal pressure.

Table 3 Pressures recorded from the sphincters of Oddi of normal subjects.

	Normal		Abnormal
	Median	Range	
Basal pressure (mmHg)	15	3–35	>40
Amplitude (mmHg)	135	95–195	>300
Frequency (n/min)	4	2–6	>7
Sequences (%)			
Antegrade	80	12–100	
Simultaneous	13	0–50	
Retrograde	9	0–50	

Analysis of the direction of propagation of the phasic contractions during a continuous 3-min period demonstrated that the majority of contractions (60%) are orientated in an antegrade direction from the common bile duct towards the duodenum. A smaller number of contractions occurred either simultaneously (24%) or had a retrograde orientation (15%). Intravenous bolus injection of CCK octapeptide (20 ng/kg) normally produces inhibition of the phasic contractions and a fall in the basal sphincter of Oddi pressure. Table 3 shows the pressures recorded from the sphincter of Oddi of normal subjects. Studies from patients with T-tubes inserted in the common bile duct following bile duct exploration [39] have shown that the frequency of sphincter of Oddi phasic contractions during fasting exhibits a periodicity in relation to duodenal MMC, similar to that demonstrated in the opossum.

Following the ingestion of a meal, bile flow across the sphincter of Oddi is promoted by inhibition or reduction in the amplitude of the phasic contractions and a fall in the sphincter of Oddi basal pressure. This effect on the human sphincter of Oddi is similar to that following intravenous injection of the CCK octapeptide. Consequently, in man, unlike the American opossum, bile flow occurs mainly between sphincter of Oddi phasic contractions during the period of diastole. The phasic contractions do propel small volumes of bile into the duodenum, but this is not the major means by which bile flow occurs. The phasic contractions in man may function to prevent reflux of duodenal contents into either the bile or the pancreatic ducts, and to maintain the ducts free from small debris. In order to promote flow across the human sphincter of Oddi, inhibition or reduction in the phasic contractions and a fall in basal pressure is necessary.

References

1 Glenn F, Grafe WR, Jr (1966) Historical events in biliary tract surgery. *Arch Surg* 93, 848–852.

2 Oddi R (1887) D'une disposition a sphincter speciale de l'ouverture du canal cholidoque. *Arch Ital Biol* 8, 371–322.

3 Boyden EA (1937) The sphincter of Oddi in man and certain representative mammals. *Surgery* 1, 24–37.

4 Hand BH (1963) An anatomical study of the choledochoduodenal area. *Br J Surg* 50, 486–494.

5 Toouli J, Geenen JE, Hogan WJ et al. (1982) Sphincter of Oddi motor activity: a comparison between patients with common bile duct stones and controls. *Gastroenterology* 82, 111–117.

6 Tansy MF, Salkin L, Innes DL et al. (1975) The mucosal lining of the intramural common bile duct as a determinant of ductal opening pressure. *Am J Dig Dis* 20, 613–625.

7 Burnett W, Gairns FW, Bacsich J (1964) Some observations on the innervation of the extrahepatic biliary system in man. *Ann Surg* 159, 8–26.

8 Sundler F, Alumets J, Hakanson R et al. (1977) VIP innervation of the gallbladder. *Gastroenterology* 72, 1375–1377.

9 Wen-Qin Cai, Gabella G (1983) Innervation of the gallbladder and biliary pathways in the guinea pig. *J Anat* 136, 97–109.

10 Padbury RTA, Furness JB, Baker RA et al. (1993) Projection of nerve cells from the duodenum to the sphincter of Oddi and gallbladder of the Australian possum. *Gastroenterology* 104, 130–136.

11 Saccone GTP, Harvey JR, Baker RA et al. (1994) Intramural neural pathways between the duodenum and sphincter of Oddi in the Australian brush-tailed possum *in vivo*. *J Physiol* 481(2), 447–456.

12 Wood JR, Svanvik J (1983) Gallbladder water and electrolyte transport and its regulation. *Gut* 24, 579–593.

13 Wood JR, Brennan LJ, Hombrey JM et al. (1982) Effects of regulatory peptides on gallbladder function. *Scand J Gastroenterol* 17(Suppl.), 78.

14 Thornell E, Jansson R, Kral JG et al. (1979) Inhibition of prostaglandin synthesis as a treatment of biliary pain. *Lancet* 1, 584.

15 Takahashi I, Suzuki T, Aizawa et al. (1982) Comparison of gallbladder contractions induced by motilin and cholecystokinin in dogs. *Gastroenterology* 82, 419–424.

16 Toouli J, Bushell M, Stevenson G et al. (1986) Gallbladder emptying in man related to fasting duodenal migrating motor contractions. *Aust NZ J Surg* 56, 147–151.

17 Weiner I, Kazutomo I, Fagan CJ et al. (1981) Release of cholecystokinin in man, correlation of blood levels with gallbladder contraction. *Ann Surg* 194, 321–327.

18 Johnson FE, Boyden EA (1952) The effect of double vagotomy on the motor activity of the human gallbladder. *Surgery* 32, 591–601.

19 Benevantano TC, Rosen RG (1969) The physiological effect of acute vagal section of canine biliary dynamics. *J Surg Res* 9, 331–334.

20 Persson CGA (1972) Adrenoreceptors in the gall bladder *Acta Pharmacol* 32, 177–185.

21 Scott GW, Otto WJ (1979) Resistance and sphincter-like properties of the cystic duct. *Surg Gynaecol Obstet* 149, 177–182.

22 Pitt HA, Roslyn JJ, Kuchenbocker SL et al. (1981) The role of cystic duct resistance in the pathogenesis of cholesterol gallstones. *J Surg Res* 30, 508–514.

23 Toouli J, Watts J McK (1971) In vitro motility studies on the canine and human extrahepatic biliary tracts. *Aust NZ J Surg* 40, 380–387.

24 Le Quesne LP, Wihtsid CG, Hand BT (1959) The common bile duct after cholecystectomy. *Br Med J* 1, 329–332.

25 Hunt DR, Scott AJ (1989) Changes in bile duct diameter after cholecystectomy: 5 year perioperative study. *Gastroenterology* 97, 1485–1488.

26 Watts J McK, Dunphy JE (1966) The role of the common bile duct in biliary dynamics. *Surg Gynaecol Obstet* 122, 1207–1281.

27 Toouli J, Dods WJ, Honda R et al (1983) Motor function of the opossum sphincter of Oddi. *J Clin Invest* 71, 208–220.

28 Grivell MB, Woods CM, Grivell AR *et al.* (2004) The possum sphincter of Oddi pumps or resists flow depending on common bile duct pressure: a multilumen manometry study. *J Physiol* 558(Pt 2), 611–622.

29 Behar J, Biancani P (1980) Effect of cholecystokinin and the octapeptide of cholecystokinin on the feline sphincter of Oddi and gallbladder. Mechanisms of action. *J Clin Invest* 66, 1231–1239.

30 Woods CM, Toouli J, Saccone GT (2003) A2A and A3 receptors mediate the adenosine-induced relaxation in spontaneously active possum duodenum *in vitro*. *Br J Pharmacol* 138(7), 1333–1339.

31 Baker RA, Saccone GTP, Toouli J (1993) Nitric oxide mediates nonadrenergic, noncholinergic neural relaxation of the sphincter of Oddi of the Australian brush tailed possum. *Gastroenterology* 105, 1746–1753.

32 Onesmo B, Balemba MJ, Salter GM (2004) Innervation of the extrahepatic biliary tract. *Anat Rec A Discov Mol Cell Evol Biol* 280(1), 836–847.

33 Pitt HA, Doty JE, Roslyn JJ *et al.* (1981) The role of altered extrahepatic biliary function in the pathogenesis of gallstones after vagotomy. *Surgery* 90, 418–425.

34 Honda R, Toouli J, Dodds WJ *et al.* (1982) Relationship of sphincter of Oddi spike bursts to gastro-intestinal myoelectric activity in conscious opossums. *J Clin Invest* 69, 770–778.

35 Woods CM, Mawe GM, Toouli J *et al.* (2005) Sphincter of Oddi: understanding its control and function. *Neurogastroenterol Motility* 17, 31–40.

36 Hess W (1979) Physiology of the sphincter of Oddi. In: Classen M, Geenen J, Kawai K (eds) *The Papilla Vateri and its Diseases.* Proceedings of the International Workshop of the World Congress of Gastroenterology held in Madrid, 1978. Köln: Verlag Gerhard Witzstock, pp. 14–21.

37 Cushieri A, Hughes JH, Cohen M (1972) Biliary pressure studies during cholecystectomy. *Br J Surg* 59, 267–273.

38 Butsch WL, McGowan JM, Waslters W (1936) Clinical studies on the influence of certain drugs in relation to biliary pain and to the variations in intrabiliary pressure. *Surg Gynaecol Obstet* 63, 451–456.

39 Geenen JE, Hogan WJ, Dodds WJ *et al.* (1980) Intraluminal pressure recording from the human sphincter of Oddi. *Gastroenterology* 78, 371–324.

2.7 Immunology of the liver

2.7.1 Cytokines in liver physiology and pathology

Tom Luedde and Christian Trautwein

Cellular communication by cytokines

It is of fundamental importance that cells are able to communicate with each other. This is achieved by the interaction of cellular receptors, which signal internally to the nucleus, and external factors, which are able to bind these receptors. Cytokines are small-molecular-weight messengers secreted by one cell to alter the behaviour of either itself (autocrine messenger), a closely related cell (paracrine messenger) or cells in different organs (endocrine messenger). Whereas most cytokines are soluble, some may be membrane bound, e.g. Fas ligand (FasL). They are produced by virtually all cell types and have a broad variety of functions. Cytokines produced by leukocytes with effects mainly on other white blood cells are named interleukins (ILs). Cytokines with a chemoattractant activity are called chemokines. Cytokines that interfere with viral replication are called interferons, and those causing differentiation and proliferation of stem cells are called colony-stimulating factors [1].

Basic principles of cytokine action in the liver

The liver is an exceptional organ in terms of its metabolic, synthetic and detoxifying functions. In addition, it has the unique potential to regenerate after tissue loss and, for example, plays an important role in the regulation process that keeps blood glucose stable. All these and many other functions represent the organ's ability to execute the proper reaction towards the body's demands and keep it in homeostasis. Therefore, the liver appears to be a preferred source for and target of cytokine signalling, and the regulation of the network connecting cytokines, receptors and signalling pathways in the liver is tremendously complex.

Initially, knowledge about the function of cytokines in the liver was mainly based on studies in cell culture systems using immortalized hepatoma cell lines. This enabled the elucidation of signalling networks downstream of cytokine receptors, but these experimental systems did not allow analysis of intercellular communication in a physiological milieu. Subsequently, the use of transgenic animals and the gene knockout technology facilitated the analysis of cytokine effects in an intact organism, but again these studies were limited by the embryonic lethality of mice with germline deletion(s) of crucial genes. Currently, conditional gene targeting based on the cre/loxP system has emerged as a powerful new tool for the study of gene functions *in vivo* in the adult mouse. This technique allows a specific gene to be deleted only in a particular tissue, leaving its expression elsewhere in the body intact.

Cytokine pathways evolved very early in evolution. For example, the nuclear factor (NF)κB signalling pathway – a key mediator of the action of tumour necrosis factor (TNF) in higher organisms – is already found in *Drosophila* and molluscs [2], where its function is to combat infection. This physiological function has mainly been preserved in higher organisms, but the same pathway is also integrated into many other organs' functions, e.g. during development, growth control or the control of cell death. NFκB signalling withholds several 'control elements' that keep this pathway and its components in a stable balance to avoid organ damage under normal conditions. In fact, increasingly, studies now underscore the fact that the deregulation of cytokine-related pathways in the liver may amplify or mediate liver damage in response to various pathogenic agents.

Cytokines are key modulators of liver function

Hepatocytes express a variety of receptors for cytokines, which can be divided into different families (Table 1). Among these, death receptor ligands from the TNF family of cytokines are involved in almost all critical processes in liver physiology and pathology. This family comprises several ligands, e.g. TNF, FasL

Table 1 Cytokines in the liver.

TNF family	IL-6 family	IL-1 family	Growth factors	Interferons	Chemokines
TNF	IL-6	IL-1α	HGF	IFNγ	IL-8
FasL	LIF	IL-1β	EGF		ENA-78
TRAIL	OSM		TGFα		IP-10
	Cardiotropin 1		TGFβ		MIP-2
	CNF		IGF-I		
	IL-11		IGF-II		
			PDGF		
			FGF-1 and FGF-2		
			Activin A		

TNF, tumour necrosis factor; FasL, Fas ligand; TRAIL, tumour necrosis factor-related apoptosis-inducing ligand; IL-6, interleukin 6; LIF, leukaemia inhibitory factor; OSM, oncostatin M; CNF, ciliary neurotropic factor; IL-11, interleukin 11; IL-1α/β, interleukin 1α/β; HGF, hepatocyte growth factor; EGF, epidermal growth factor; TGFα/β, transforming growth factor α/β; IGF-I/II, insulin-like growth factor I/II; PDGF, platelet-derived growth factor; FGF-1/2, fibroblast growth factor 1/2; IFNγ, interferon γ; IL-8, interleukin 8; ENA-78, epithelial neutrophil-activating peptide 78; IP-10, interferon-inducible protein 10; MIP-2, macrophage inflammatory protein 2.

and tumour necrosis factor-related apoptosis-inducing ligand (TRAIL), which exist in a soluble or cell bound form and activate structurally related receptor proteins known as the TNF receptor superfamily, including TNF receptor 1 (TNF-R1), TNF-R2, Fas and death receptor 3 (DR3), DR4 and DR5 [3]. The IL-6 family of cytokines has several members which, by interacting with adaptor molecules, complex with a signal transducing molecule named gp130, thereby activating downstream pathways and signal molecules such as the signal transducers and activators of transcription (STAT) (mainly STAT-3) [4]. IL-1 members activate similar downstream targets as TNF, e.g. NFκB. Moreover, receptors for growth factors, such as epidermal growth factor (EGF), transforming growth factors (TGF)α and TGFβ, hepatocyte growth factor (HGF), insulin-like growth factor (IGF)-1 and IGF-2, may control proliferation of hepatocytes during embryogenesis or liver regeneration [5].

Non-parenchymal cells (NPCs) of the liver, function both as recipients of cytokine-driven messages, and also synthesize cytokines. Kupffer cells (KCs), resident tissue macrophages, synthesize pro-inflammatory cytokines such as IL-1, IL-6 and TNF upon activation as a result of phagocytosis or binding of endotoxin [6]. These released cytokines stimulate hepatocytes and other non-parenchymal liver cells in a paracrine manner. Activation of KCs may also be induced by cytokines such as interferon gamma (IFNγ), the receptors of which are expressed on KCs. Chemokines released by KCs and hepatic stellate cells (HSCs) mediate migration of neutrophils and blood monocytes. Moreover, sinusoidal endothelial cells are targets for pro-inflammatory cytokines to express cell adhesion molecules and may also produce cytokines [7]. Cytokines are also critical regulators of hepatic fibrosis and injury (see Chapter 6.2, Cellular and molecular pathobiology, pharmacological intervention and biochemical assessment of liver fibrosis).

Due to the complexity of the cytokine network, it is not the intention of this chapter to describe in detail the action of all these cytokines in the liver. For a brief overview, Table 2 summarizes the functions of some key cytokines in models of liver physiology and pathology. In contrast, we will focus mainly on the action of one cytokine as an example of how cytokines and cytokine-dependent signalling pathways are involved in the physiological function of the liver and how their alteration can lead to the development and progression of liver disease. Recent studies have revealed that alterations of TNF and TNF-dependent signalling pathways have an enormous impact in different liver disease models and thus might be an attractive target for pharmaceutical intervention, as has become the case for inflammatory bowel disease or rheumatoid arthritis [8].

Death receptor ligands modulate cell death in the liver

Excessive hepatocyte apoptosis and necrosis have been implicated in a number of acute and chronic liver diseases, e.g. viral and autoimmune hepatitis, cholestatic disease, alcoholic or drug-/toxin-induced liver injury and transplantation-associated liver damage, including graft rejection [9]. Studies in patients and animal models have strongly implicated death receptor ligands such as TNF in the induction of apoptosis and in triggering destruction of the liver [10].

TNF was originally identified by its capacity to induce haemorrhagic necrosis in mouse tumours [11], but severe side-effects led to a failure of its use as a systemic anticancer chemotherapeutic agent [12,13]. A very prominent effect was the direct cytotoxic role of TNF for human hepatocytes, resulting in increased levels of serum aminotransferases and bilirubin. Since then, many clinical studies have underscored the crucial role of TNF in fulminant hepatic failure (FHF) and other liver diseases. TNF participates in many forms of hepatic pathology, including ischaemia–reperfusion injury, alcoholic and viral hepatitis and injury from hepatotoxins [14–17]. Exogenous TNF induces

Table 2 Cytokine function in different models of liver physiology and pathology.

Biological model and reference	Cytokines involved	Cytokine function
Liver development [6]	FGF-1 and FGF-2	Differentiation of hepatic endoderm
	HGF	Growth of hepatoblasts
	OSM	Differentiation of hepatocytes
	TGFβ	Induction of Vg1
Liver regeneration [5,65]	TNF	Induction of IL-6 production in KCs
	TNF, IL-6	Priming of hepatocytes ($G_0 \rightarrow G_1$)
	HGF, EGF, TGFα	Growth factors, cell cycle progression (G1→S)
	TGF-β, Activin A	Inhibition of liver regeneration
	IFNγ	Inhibition of liver regeneration
	ENA-78, MIP-2 and other CXC chemokines	Stimulation of hepatocyte proliferation
Acute phase response [6,53]	IL-1α/β, TNF	Stimulation of synthesis of type 1 acute-phase proteins (APPs) (C-reactive protein, serum amyloid-A)
	IL-6, CNF, OSM, LIF	Stimulation of synthesis of type 2 APPs (fibrinogen, haptoglobin)
Liver fibrosis [6]	TNF, IL-1, IL-6, IL-8	Damage factors
	TGFβ, PDGF, TNF, IGF-1, IL-1	Activating factors
	TGFβ, PDGF, TNF	Surviving factors
Acute and chronic liver failure [9]	TNF, FasL, TGFβ	Hepatocyte apoptosis, necrosis
	IL-6	Survival signal
Liver cancer [6,66]	HGF, IGF-2, TGFα, TGFβ	Hepatic mitogens
	TNF, IL-1, HGF, EGF	Metastasis
	TNF	Possibly pro- and anti-tumorogenic effects, pro-proliferative vs. pro-apoptotic

FGF-1/2, fibroblast growth factor 1/2; HGF, hepatocyte growth factor; OSM, oncostatin M; TGFβ, transforming growth factor β; TNF, tumour necrosis factor α; IL-6, interleukin 6; EGF, epidermal growth factor; TGFα, transforming growth factor α; IFNγ, interferon γ; ENA-78, epithelial neutrophil-activating peptide 78; MIP-2, macrophage inflammatory protein 2; CXC, IL-1α/β, interleukin 1α/β, CNF, ciliary neurotropic factor; LIF, leukaemia inhibitory factor; IL-8, interleukin 8; PDGF, platelet-derived growth factor; IGF-I, insulin-like growth factor I; FasL, Fas ligand; IGF-2, insulin-like growth factor 2; TGFα, transforming growth factor α.

FHF and hepatocyte apoptosis in combination with other toxins [17]. In patients with FHF, serum levels of TNF, TNF-R1 and TNF-R2 are markedly increased and these changes correlate directly with disease activity. In explanted livers of patients with FHF, infiltrating mononuclear cells expressed high amounts of TNF and hepatocytes overexpressed TNF-R1 [18]. Thus, it is very likely that the TNF system is involved in the pathogenesis of hepatic failure in humans, and its significance has also been shown clearly in several animal models of hepatic failure, e.g. the endotoxin/ᴅ-galactosamine (GalN) and the concanavalin A (ConA) models [19,20].

TNF activates pro- and antiapoptotic signalling cascades
(see also Chapter 3.1)

Activation of the caspase cascade

Fas and TNF facilitate programmed cell death in a similar manner by activation of caspases. The most important target of both pathways orchestrating cellular death is the aspartate-specific cysteine protease or caspase cascade, consisting of initiator caspases such as caspases-8 and -9 and executioner caspases, e.g. caspase-3, -6 and -7. As proteolytic cleavage generates the mature caspases, one way in which these enzymes are activated is via the action of proteases, including other caspases [21]. TNF signals through two distinct cell surface receptors, TNF-R1 and TNF-R2, of which TNF-R1 initiates the majority of TNF's biological activities. Binding of TNF to its receptor leads to the release of the inhibitory protein silencer of death domains (SODD) from TNF-R1's intracellular domain. This leads to the recognition of the intracellular TNF-R1 domain by the adapter protein TNF receptor-associated death domain (TRADD), which in turn recruits Fas-associated death domain (FADD). FADD recruits caspase-8 to the TNF-R1 complex, where it becomes activated and initiates the protease cascade, leading to activation of executioner caspases and apoptosis (Fig. 1). In contrast to TNF-dependent signalling, Fas can interact directly with the death domain of FADD without recruiting TRADD [22,23]. In several studies, involvement of mitochondria and the release of

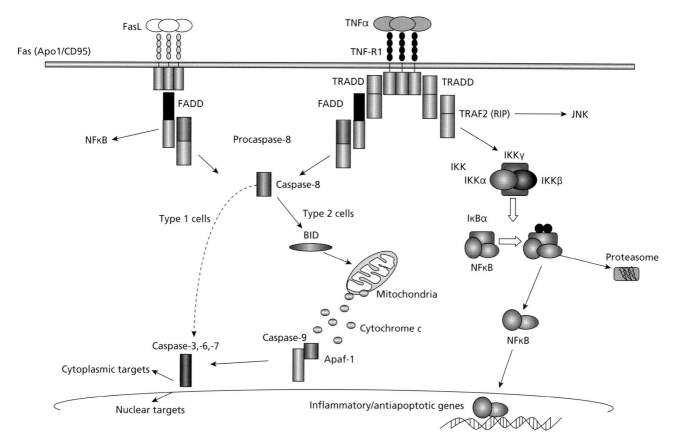

Fig. 1 FasL- and TNFα-dependent signalling in the liver.

cytochrome *c* in the apoptotic process has been demonstrated, and this was also shown for Fas- and TNF-mediated apoptosis in the liver [24,25].

Activation of the NFκB pathway

In addition to activation of caspases, ligand binding of TNF to its receptor also leads to the activation of alternative pathways, e.g. the nuclear factor (NF)κB pathway. Activation of the NFκB pathway is mediated by interaction of both TNF receptors with the receptor-associated factors 1 and 2 (TRAF-1 and TRAF-2). NFκB is a transcription factor consisting of a dimer of different subunits (e.g. p50 and p65), which is normally retained in the cytoplasm through interaction with its inhibitor IκB. TNF-induced activation of NFκB relies on phosphorylation of two conserved serines (Ser32 and Ser36 in human IκBα) in the *N*-terminal regulatory domain of IκBs. After phosphorylation, the IκBs undergo a second posttranslational modification: polyubiquitination followed by the degradation of IκB proteins by the proteasome, thus releasing NFκB from its inhibitory IκB binding partner, so that it can translocate to the nucleus and activate transcription of NFκB-dependent target genes [26]. A high-molecular-weight complex that mediates the phosphorylation of IκB has been purified and characterized. This complex consists of three tightly associated IκB kinase (IKK) polypep-

tides: IKK1 (also called IKKα) and IKK2 (IKKβ) are the catalytic subunits of the kinase complex [27–29]. Moreover, it contains a regulatory subunit called NEMO (NFκB essential modulator), IKKγ or IKKAP-1 [30–32]. In the context of TNF-mediated apoptosis, NFκB appears to provide a prosurvival signal. Evidence that NFκB governs critical antiapoptotic proteins comes from well-described animal models. Injection of TNF into mice and addition of TNF to hepatic cells resulted in activation of nuclear translocation and of DNA binding of NFκB [33].

In contrast to Fas-mediated apoptosis, hepatocytes are resistant to apoptosis induced by TNF or lipopolysaccharide (LPS), a potent inducer of endogenous TNF in the liver, unless they are treated with inhibitors of transcription (e.g. cycloheximide or actinomycin D), which block the expression of (antiapoptotic) proteins [17,34,35]. Specific blockade of NFκB activation by adenoviral-directed overexpression of the NFκB superrepressor IκB (which retains the dimeric NFκB in the cytoplasm as it contains mutations at the phosphorylation sites) significantly enhanced TNF-mediated apoptosis of hepatocytes [36]. A similar result was obtained by treatment of hepatocytes with the proteasome inhibitor lactacystin, which prevents degradation of IκBs, and an antibody against p65 protein [37].

Further evidence for the central role of the NFκB pathway in preventing apoptosis in hepatocytes comes from genetic experiments. Knockout mice lacking the p65 subunit of NFκB die between embryonic (E) days 15 and 16 as a result of fetal hepatocyte apoptosis [38]. This is caused by increased sensitivity towards TNF, as TNF/p65 double-deficient mice are rescued from embryonic lethality [39]. It is presumed to involve the transcriptional induction of various apoptotic suppressors. Among these genes are the cellular inhibitors of apoptosis (c-IAPs), e.g. c-IAP1 and c-IAP2, which bind directly and inhibit effector caspases, such as caspase-3 and caspase-7, and prevent activation of procaspase-6 and procaspase-9 [40].

TNF in experimental disease models of the liver

TNF/NF-κB in liver regeneration
(see also Chapter 2.5.2)

In mammals, the liver is distinguished by its capacity to regenerate lost parenchymal mass in response to, for example, surgical resection, viral injury or toxic exposure [5]. Therefore, it has been a major challenge to evaluate the extra- and intracellular events that orchestrate this highly complex process driving quiescent, fully differentiated hepatocytes through distinct stages including priming of hepatocytes, cell cycle progression, proliferation and cessation of regeneration [41]. A well-established model for studying liver regeneration is that of partial (two-thirds) hepatectomy (PH) in rodents.

Several growth factors can interact with receptors on the cell membrane activating intracellular signalling pathways involved in target gene activation in hepatocytes. The growth factors have been characterized according to their mitogenic capacity. Therefore, at present, hepatocyte growth factor (HGF), epidermal growth factor (EGF) and transforming growth factor (TGF)α can be classified as mitogens, while insulin and epinephrine are classified as comitogens. These factors activate intracellular signalling cascades such as the Ras/MAPkinase pathway, which couple the extracellular signals to the major regulating molecules of the cell cycle machinery, such as the cyclin-dependent kinases (CDK) [41].

Besides the direct role of growth factors, cytokines such as TNF and IL-6 are also involved in priming hepatocytes towards cell cycle progression. Initially, it was found that there is cascade of events leading, first, to elevated TNF and, consecutively, to increased IL-6 serum levels. Additionally, experiments indicated that anti-TNF antibodies inhibit proliferation of hepatocytes, again indicating that the molecule might be involved in controlling cell cycle progression of hepatocytes. The importance of TNF and NFκB signalling was further confirmed by the fact that liver regeneration is defective in TNFR-1 knockout mice, which do not show hepatic NFκB activation after PH [42]. However, it remains uncertain whether NFκB is able directly to promote hepatocyte proliferation in this model. NFκB can directly stimulate the transcription of genes that encode G1 cyclins, and a κB site is present within the cyclin D1 promoter [43,44].

However, recent results questioned a direct involvement in hepatocytes and highlighted its role in non-parenchymal cells (NPC) such as KCs. Chaisson et al. [45] used transgenic mice that expressed the non-degradable IκBα superrepressor specifically in hepatocytes, and these mice showed normal hepatocyte proliferation after PH. Moreover, mice lacking the IKKβ (IKK2) subunit in hepatocytes showed normal liver regeneration [46]. TNF-induced NFκB activation in NPCs leads to the production of another important cytokine, IL-6. IL-6 is not absolutely necessary for liver regeneration, but has a protective, antiapoptotic function in this process [47], underscoring the fact that, instead of a direct proliferative effect, TNF-dependent NFκB activation in NPC is part of an IL-6 production pathway that protects hepatocytes from apoptosis during liver regeneration.

TNF/NF-κB in liver cancer (see also Chapter 18.2.1)

According to Hanahan and Weinberg [48], tumorigenesis requires six essential alterations to normal cell physiology: self-sufficiency in growth signals; insensitivity to growth inhibition; evasion of apoptosis; immortalization; sustained angiogenesis; and tissue invasion and metastasis. As outlined in this chapter, TNF and NFκB are able to induce several of these cellular alterations. A recent study demonstrated constitutive activation of NFκB in hepatocellular carcinoma (HCC) [49]. Moreover, two important animal studies using transgenic and conditional knockout mice that alter expression of specific members of the TNF/NFκB axis have highlighted the essential function of this pathway in the initiation and promotion of carcinogenesis in the liver:

In one study, the function of TNF/NFκB has been studied in an inflammatory liver carcinogenesis model by using the mdr-2 knockout mouse that develops a chronic cholangitis and subsequently hepatocellular carcinomas (HCC) [50]. The authors demonstrated that early neoplastic events in this model are related to the biliary system and occur independently of cytokine effects on hepatocytes. In contrast, during later steps of tumour promotion, TNF is expressed mainly by endothelial and inflammatory cells, subsequently leading to activation of NFκB in the surrounding hepatocytes. Interestingly, when this activation of NFκB is blocked by transgenic overexpression of a non-degradable IκB form, no effect on early events of carcinogenesis are detected, whereas during later stages of tumorigenesis the number and size of tumours was markedly decreased in these mice compared with mice that could activate NFκB, which was accompanied by stronger apoptosis of hepatocytes. A similar effect could be shown by treatment with anti-TNF-antibodies. Thus, the authors concluded that acquisition of oncogenic mutations renders hepatocytes specifically sensitive towards apoptosis, which has to be blocked by NFκB activated by TNF in order for promotion of HCC.

In another study, the different outcomes of NFκB function in hepatocytes were compared with those in non-parenchymal liver cells including KCs in a chemical liver carcinogenesis model [51]. After exposure of young mice to the carcinogenic drug diethylnitrosamine (DEN), hepatocytes undergo apoptosis, which is enhanced in mice with a conditional IKK2 knockout that cannot activate NFκB specifically in hepatocytes. This increased apoptosis then leads to the release of cytokines including TNF and IL-6 from hepatic KCs, which in turn stimulates hepatocellular proliferation leading to increased size and number of liver tumours, compared with wildtype mice. The central role of cytokines released by the non-parenchymal liver cells in this model is underscored by the fact that mice also lacking IKK2 in hepatocytes and KCs and which have a defect in NFκB activation in both cell types secrete less of the cytokines such as TNF and IL-6 and therefore develop less rather than more HCCs.

Taken together, these and similar studies have highlighted the new therapeutic options of cytokine targeting in the liver. Instead of treating the primary cause of inflammation, which is often not possible in chronic hepatitis, treatment of the secondary events that lead to tumours, (e.g. anti-TNF-dependent strategies), might be a more realistic aim in cancer treatment.

TNF/NF-κB in local and systemic insulin-resistance (see also Chapter 2.3.1)

Recent studies have revealed that local inflammation and cytokines produced by liver cells also have a strong impact on systemic functions. For example, feeding of mice with a high-fat diet that leads to systemic insulin resistance is accompanied by hepatic NFκB activation and increased secretion of the cytokines TNF, IL-6 and IL-1β [52]. Furthermore, by constitutively activating NFκB in the liver using the hepatocyte-specific overexpression of a dominant active IKK2 form, an increased local and systemic insulin resistance is observed in these mice, even when fed a normal diet. This effect was mediated by an increased release of NFκB-dependent cytokines from the liver and was accompanied by a reduced insulin receptor-dependent signalling. Complementing this finding, the inhibition of hepatic NFκB signalling leads to diminished cytokine release and decreased insulin resistance in mice fed with a high-fat diet [53], thus underscoring the therapeutic potential of cytokine modulation in the development of diabetes mellitus.

IL-6: a protective cytokine in liver failure?

IL-6 belongs to a family of cytokines comprising IL-6, IL-11, leukaemia inhibitory factor (LIF), oncostatin M, ciliary neurotropic factor, novel neurotrophin 1/B cell stimulating factor 3 and cardiotropin 1 [4]. IL-6 binds to hepatocytes by interacting with an 80-kd membrane glycoprotein (gp80) that complexes with a signal transducing molecule, gp130 (Fig. 2a). Binding of gp130 leads to dimerization of the intracellular domains of two gp130 molecules, which promotes association

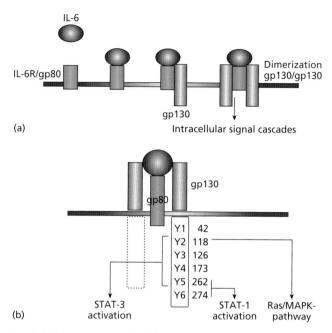

Fig. 2 IL-6 dependent signalling. (a) IL-6 binding and receptor dimerization. (b) Signal transduction through gp130.

with receptor-associated Janus kinases (JAKs: JAK1, JAK2, and TYK). The JAKs become activated and phosphorylate different tyrosine residues on the gp130 molecule. Depending on the location of the phosphorylated tyrosines, signal transducers and activators of transcription (STAT) proteins (mainly STAT-3) and also the Ras/mitogen-activated protein (MAP) kinase pathway become activated and trigger numerous downstream effects mediated by the signalling of IL-6 and related cytokines (Fig. 2b) [4].

As outlined above, IL-6 is one of the key regulators of the initial steps of liver regeneration. An important role of IL-6-dependent signalling in the liver is also attributed to the induction of the acute phase response [54,55]. STAT-3 participates in transcriptional activation. gp130 may also promote anti-apoptotic effects in different cell types. For example, activation of STAT-3 in B cells and human myeloma cells activates anti-apoptotic genes such as *BCL2* and *BCLXL*, protecting them from Fas-dependent apoptosis [56]; similar results occur in T cells: STAT-3-deficient T cells are severely impaired in IL-6-induced proliferation – due to the profound defect in IL-6-mediated prevention of apoptosis. In hepatocytes, IL-6 protects from transforming growth factor (TGF)β-induced apoptosis by blocking TGFβ-induced activation of caspase-3 via rapid tyrosine phosphorylation of phosphatidylinositol 3 kinase (PI 3 kinase), which constitutively activates the protein kinase Akt [57].

In humans, there is strong evidence that IL-6 is directly involved in the pathogenesis of different diseases, including multiple myeloma and congestive heart disease [58,59]. Recently, we analysed the potential role of IL-6 in the development of acute and chronic liver injury in humans and examined its pathophysiological basis in animal models. We found a direct correlation of IL-6 expression in serum and liver tissue with disease progression in patients with FHF. Additionally, there was an abolished acute-phase response and an increased susceptibility to LPS-induced liver injury in mice deficient for functional gp130 in hepatocytes [60,61], allowing us to define genes that are protective during T cell-mediated liver injury [62].

Cytokines and cytokine-dependent pathways as a therapeutic target

As outlined above, a growing number of studies have implicated cytokines and cytokine-dependent pathways in the development of liver failure, chronic liver disease, hepatic inflammation and liver carcinogenesis. Numerous chemical compounds, monoclonal antibodies and viral vectors that inhibit or modulate cytokines (e.g., TNF or the NFκB pathway) are under development [63]. For example, pharmacological inhibitors of caspases, including the caspase-8 inhibitor IETD-CHO and the caspase-3 inhibitor DEVD-CHO, have shown beneficial effects in experimental *in vivo* models of TNFα- and Fas-induced liver failure [64,65]. However, the examples given in this chapter also emphasize the complexity of functions that these pathways regulate depending on the disease model or cell type. Therefore, the pharmacological inhibition of a specific molecule or pathway in a certain clinical setting might result in unpredictable and fatal consequences in the same or other tissues and organs. Currently, there is no pharmacological method that allows the specific targeting of molecules in a certain tissue. Hence, at present, animal models that allow gene targeting in a specific cell type will prove to be valuable tools to define more clearly the effects of the modulation of cytokines, cytokine receptors or cytokine-dependent pathways. Alternatively, future research efforts might highlight the role of more downstream effectors of cytokine pathways, the function of which can be attributed specifically to a certain role in pathogenesis such as carcinogenesis, which could then be targeted by a systemic drug therapy.

One of the most difficult problems in clinical hepatology is the progression of chronic inflammation, including chronic hepatitis or primary sclerosing cholangitis (PSC) towards hepatocellular or cholangiocellular carcinoma, respectively. Although huge diagnostic efforts are taken in the surveillance of these patients, cancer is still not always diagnosed in time for a curative treatment. With a more thorough understanding of the function of cytokines in the liver, gained from animal disease models, it might be possible to improve diagnostic tools as well as to develop drugs that inhibit or slow down the sequence from inflammation to cancer.

References

1 Parkin J, Cohen B (2001) An overview of the immune system. *Lancet* 357, 1777–1789.

2 Montagnani C, Kappler C, Reichhart JM *et al.* (2004) Cg-Rel, the first Rel/NF-kappaB homolog characterized in a mollusk, the Pacific oyster *Crassostrea gigas. FEBS Lett* 561, 75–82.

3 Schulze-Osthoff K, Ferrari D, Los M *et al.* (1998) Apoptosis signaling by death receptors. *Eur J Biochem* 254, 439–459.

4 Streetz KL, Luedde T, Manns MP *et al.* (2000) Interleukin 6 and liver regeneration. *Gut* 47, 309–312.

5 Michalopoulos GK, DeFrances MC (1997) Liver regeneration. *Science* 276, 60–66.

6 Decker K (1990) Biologically active products of stimulated liver macrophages (Kuppfer cells). *Eur J Biochem* 192, 245–261.

7 Ramadori G, Armbrust T (2001) Cytokines in the liver. *Eur J Gastroenterol Hepatol* 13, 777–784.

8 Siddiqui MA, Scott LJ (2005) Infliximab: a review of its use in Crohn's disease and rheumatoid arthritis. *Drugs* 65, 2179–2208.

9 Neuman MG (2001) Apoptosis in diseases of the liver. *Crit Rev Clin Lab Sci* 38, 109–166.

10 Luedde T, Liedtke C, Manns MP *et al.* (2002) Losing balance: cytokine signaling and cell death in the context of hepatocyte injury and hepatic failure. *Eur Cytokine Netw* 13, 377–383.

11 Carswell EA, Old LJ, Kassel RL *et al.* (1975) An endotoxin-induced serum factor that causes necrosis of tumors. *Proc Natl Acad Sci USA* 72, 3666–3670.

12 Feinberg B, Kurzrock R, Talpaz M *et al.* (1988) A phase I trial of intravenously-administered recombinant tumor necrosis factor-alpha in cancer patients. *J Clin Oncol* 6, 1328–1334.

13 Kimura K, Taguchi T, Urushizaki I *et al.* (1987) Phase I study of recombinant human tumor necrosis factor. *Cancer Chemother Pharmacol* 20, 223–229.

14 Colletti LM, Remick DG, Burtch GD *et al.* (1990) Role of tumor necrosis factor-alpha in the pathophysiologic alterations after hepatic ischemia/reperfusion injury in the rat. *J Clin Invest* 85, 1936–1943.

15 Felver ME, Mezey E, McGuire M *et al.* (1990) Plasma tumor necrosis factor alpha predicts decreased long-term survival in severe alcoholic hepatitis. *Alcohol Clin Exp Res* 14, 255–259.

16 Gonzalez-Amaro R, Garcia-Monzon C, Garcia-Buey L *et al.* (1994) Induction of tumor necrosis factor alpha production by human hepatocytes in chronic viral hepatitis. *J Exp Med* 179, 841–848.

17 Leist M, Gantner F, Naumann H *et al.* (1997) Tumor necrosis factor-induced apoptosis during the poisoning of mice with hepatotoxins. *Gastroenterology* 112, 923–934.

18 Streetz K, Leifeld L, Grundmann D *et al.* (2000) Tumor necrosis factor alpha in the pathogenesis of human and murine fulminant hepatic failure. *Gastroenterology* 119, 446–460.

19 Gantner F, Leist M, Lohse AW *et al.* (1995) Concanavalin A-induced T-cell-mediated hepatic injury in mice: the role of tumor necrosis factor. *Hepatology* 21, 190–198.

20 Pfeffer K, Matsuyama T, Kundig TM *et al.* (1993) Mice deficient for the 55 kd tumor necrosis factor receptor are resistant to endotoxic shock, yet succumb to *L. monocytogenes* infection. *Cell* 73, 457–467.

21 Martin SJ, Green DR (1995) Protease activation during apoptosis: death by a thousand cuts? *Cell* 82, 349–352.

22 Ashkenazi A, Dixit VM (1998) Death receptors: signaling and modulation. *Science* 281, 1305–1308.

23 Chen G, Goeddel DV (2002) TNF-R1 signaling: a beautiful pathway. *Science* 296, 1634–1635.

24 Bradham CA, Qian T, Streetz K *et al.* (1998) The mitochondrial permeability transition is required for tumor necrosis factor alpha-

mediated apoptosis and cytochrome c release. *Mol Cell Biol* 18, 6353–6364.

25 Yin XM, Wang K, Gross A *et al.* (1999) Bid-deficient mice are resistant to Fas-induced hepatocellular apoptosis. *Nature* 400, 886–891.

26 Yamamoto Y, Gaynor RB (2004) IkappaB kinases: key regulators of the NF-kappaB pathway. *Trends Biochem Sci* 29, 72–79.

27 DiDonato JA, Hayakawa M, Rothwarf DM *et al.* (1997) A cytokine-responsive IkappaB kinase that activates the transcription factor NF-kappaB. *Nature* 388, 548–554.

28 Mercurio F, Zhu H, Murray BW *et al.* (1997) IKK-1 and IKK-2: cytokine-activated IkappaB kinases essential for NF-kappaB activation. *Science* 278, 860–866.

29 Regnier CH, Song HY, Gao X *et al.* (1997) Identification and characterization of an IkappaB kinase. *Cell* 90, 373–383.

30 Mercurio F, Murray BW, Shevchenko A *et al.* (1999) IkappaB kinase (IKK)-associated protein 1, a common component of the heterogeneous IKK complex. *Mol Cell Biol* 19, 1526–1538.

31 Rothwarf DM, Zandi E, Natoli G *et al.* (1998) IKK-gamma is an essential regulatory subunit of the IkappaB kinase complex. *Nature* 395, 297–300.

32 Yamaoka S, Courtois G, Bessia C *et al.* (1998) Complementation cloning of NEMO, a component of the IkappaB kinase complex essential for NF-kappaB activation. *Cell* 93, 1231–1240.

33 FitzGerald MJ, Webber EM, Donovan JR *et al.* (1995) Rapid DNA binding by nuclear factor kappa B in hepatocytes at the start of liver regeneration. *Cell Growth Differ* 6, 417–427.

34 Lehmann V, Freudenberg MA, Galanos C (1987) Lethal toxicity of lipopolysaccharide and tumor necrosis factor in normal and D-galactosamine-treated mice. *J Exp Med* 165, 657–663.

35 Leist M, Gantner F, Bohlinger I *et al.* (1994) Murine hepatocyte apoptosis induced in vitro and in vivo by TNF-alpha requires transcriptional arrest. *J Immunol* 153, 1778–1788.

36 Nagaki M, Naiki T, Brenner DA *et al.* (2000) Tumor necrosis factor alpha prevents tumor necrosis factor receptor-mediated mouse hepatocyte apoptosis, but not fas-mediated apoptosis: role of nuclear factor-kappaB. *Hepatology* 32, 1272–1279.

37 Bellas RE, FitzGerald MJ, Fausto N *et al.* (1997) Inhibition of NF-kappa B activity induces apoptosis in murine hepatocytes. *Am J Pathol* 151, 891–896.

38 Beg AA, Baltimore D (1996) An essential role for NF-kappaB in preventing TNF-alpha-induced cell death. *Science* 274, 782–784.

39 Doi TS, Marino MW, Takahashi T *et al.* (1999) Absence of tumor necrosis factor rescues RelA-deficient mice from embryonic lethality. *Proc Natl Acad Sci USA* 96, 2994–2999.

40 Deveraux QL, Roy N, Stennicke HR *et al.* (1998) IAPs block apoptotic events induced by caspase-8 and cytochrome *c* by direct inhibition of distinct caspases. *EMBO J* 17, 2215–2223.

41 Fausto N (2000) Liver regeneration. *J Hepatol* 32, 19–31.

42 Yamada Y, Kirillova I, Peschon JJ *et al.* (1997) Initiation of liver growth by tumor necrosis factor: deficient liver regeneration in mice lacking type I tumor necrosis factor receptor. *Proc Natl Acad Sci USA* 94, 1441–1446.

43 Guttridge DC, Albanese C, Reuther JY *et al.* (1999) NF-kappaB controls cell growth and differentiation through transcriptional regulation of cyclin D1. *Mol Cell Biol* 19, 5785–5799.

44 Hinz M, Krappmann D, Eichten A *et al.* (1999) NF-kappaB function in growth control: regulation of cyclin D1 expression and G0/G1-to-S-phase transition. *Mol Cell Biol* 19, 2690–2698.

45 Chaisson ML, Brooling JT, Ladiges W *et al.* (2002) Hepatocyte-specific

inhibition of NF-kappaB leads to apoptosis after TNF treatment, but not after partial hepatectomy. *J Clin Invest* 110, 193–202.

46 Maeda S, Chang L, Li ZW *et al.* (2003) IKKbeta is required for prevention of apoptosis mediated by cell-bound but not by circulating TNFalpha. *Immunity* 19, 725–737.

47 Wuestefeld T, Klein C, Streetz KL *et al.* (2003) Interleukin-6/glycoprotein 130-dependent pathways are protective during liver regeneration. *J Biol Chem* 278, 11281–11288.

48 Hanahan D, Weinberg RA (2000) The hallmarks of cancer. *Cell* 100, 57–70.

49 Tai DI, Tsai SL, Chang YH *et al.* (2000) Constitutive activation of nuclear factor kappaB in hepatocellular carcinoma. *Cancer* 89, 2274–2281.

50 Pikarsky E, Porat RM, Stein I *et al.* (2004) NF-kappaB functions as a tumour promoter in inflammation-associated cancer. *Nature* 431(7007): 461–6.

51 Maeda S, Kamata H, Luo JL *et al.* (2005) IKKbeta couples hepatocyte death to cytokine-driven compensatory proliferation that promotes chemical hepatocarcinogenesis. *Cell* 121, 977–990.

52 Cai D, Yuan M, Frantz DF *et al.* (2005) Local and systemic insulin resistance resulting from hepatic activation of IKK-beta and NF-kappaB. *Nature Med* 11, 183–190.

53 Arkan MC, Hevener AL, Greten FR *et al.* (2005) IKK-beta links inflammation to obesity-induced insulin resistance. *Nature Med* 11, 191–198.

54 Trautwein C, Boker K, Manns MP (1994) Hepatocyte and immune system: acute phase reaction as a contribution to early defence mechanisms. *Gut* 35, 1163–1166.

55 Zhang D, Sun M, Samols D *et al.* (1996) STAT3 participates in transcriptional activation of the C-reactive protein gene by interleukin-6. *J Biol Chem* 271, 9503–9509.

56 Catlett-Falcone R, Landowski TH, Oshiro MM *et al.* (1999) Constitutive activation of Stat3 signaling confers resistance to apoptosis in human U266 myeloma cells. *Immunity* 10, 105–115.

57 Chen RH, Chang MC, Su YH *et al.* (1999) Interleukin-6 inhibits transforming growth factor-beta-induced apoptosis through the phosphatidylinositol 3-kinase/Akt and signal transducers and activators of transcription 3 pathways. *J Biol Chem* 274, 23013–23019.

58 Ludwig H, Nachbaur DM, Fritz E *et al.* (1991) Interleukin-6 is a prognostic factor in multiple myeloma. *Blood* 77, 2794–2795.

59 Tsutamoto T, Hisanaga T, Wada A *et al.* (1998) Interleukin-6 spillover in the peripheral circulation increases with the severity of heart failure, and the high plasma level of interleukin-6 is an important prognostic predictor in patients with congestive heart failure. *J Am Coll Cardiol* 31, 391–398.

60 Streetz KL, Tacke F, Leifeld L *et al.* (2003) Interleukin 6/gp130-dependent pathways are protective during chronic liver diseases. *Hepatology* 38, 218–229.

61 Streetz KL, Wustefeld T, Klein C *et al.* (2003) Lack of gp130 expression in hepatocytes promotes liver injury. *Gastroenterology* 125, 532–543.

62 Klein C, Wustefeld T, Assmus U *et al.* (2005) The IL-6-gp130-STAT3 pathway in hepatocytes triggers liver protection in T cell-mediated liver injury. *J Clin Invest* 115, 860–9.

63 Karin M, Cao Y, Greten FR *et al.* (2002) NF-kappaB in cancer: from innocent bystander to major culprit. *Nature Rev Cancer* 2, 301–310.

64 Bajt ML, Lawson JA, Vonderfecht SL *et al.* (2000) Protection against Fas receptor-mediated apoptosis in hepatocytes and nonparenchymal cells by a caspase-8 inhibitor in vivo: evidence for a postmitochondrial processing of caspase-8. *Toxicol Sci* 58, 109–117.

65 Bajt ML, Vonderfecht SL, Jaeschke H (2001) Differential protection with inhibitors of caspase-8 and caspase-3 in murine models of tumor necrosis factor and Fas receptor-mediated hepatocellular apoptosis. *Toxicol Appl Pharmacol* 175, 243–252.

2.7.2 Intrahepatic lymphocytes

Wajahat Z. Mehal

Introduction

The immune system is central to liver injury in a variety of diseases including autoimmunity, viral hepatitides and many drug reactions. Such immune-mediated pathology will be discussed in detail in the sections focusing on individual diseases. This section will discuss the unique lymphocyte populations and immune properties of the healthy liver. The anatomical location of the liver constantly exposes it to large amounts of foreign antigens, and the most common immunological response to these is the development of antigen-specific immunological tolerance. This is much more complex than the immune system simply not responding to the antigen. Foreign antigens in the liver result in a range of dynamic immune responses that ultimately result in physical removal of lymphocytes, decreased ability of lymphocytes to become activated and the development of regulatory lymphocytes.

Understanding the molecular and cellular mechanisms underlying immune responses to hepatic antigens is directly relevant to viral hepatitis because antigens of hepatitis B virus (HBV) and hepatitis C virus (HCV) and alloantigens after transplantation induce varying degrees of immune tolerance. In many pathological situations, there is, however, a robust immune response to foreign and even self-antigens. An understanding of the factors that regulate the balance between induction of tolerance and the mounting of an immune response is necessary to design disease-specific therapies. In addition to conventional immune responses, novel roles in regulating liver fibrosis have also been identified for liver lymphocytes.

Localization and function

The healthy liver contains a very large and diverse population of lymphocytes [1]. Intrahepatic lymphocytes are defined as lymphocytes that are firmly attached to the liver and are not simply in the intrahepatic blood. The size of the intrahepatic population in the healthy liver is easily underestimated on microscopy but, on digestion, 1 g of healthy human and murine liver tissues yields approximately 10 million lymphocytes [2,3]. Taking the size of the liver into account, this is approximately 30% as many lymphocytes as in the spleen. The unexpected abundance of lymphocytes in the healthy liver is matched by their variety.

Table 1 Lymphocyte populations in the liver and spleen.

	Normal liver (%)	Spleen (%)
TCR-αβ	25	60
TCR-γδ	10	2–3
Natural killer T (NK-T) cells	30	1–2
Natural killer (NK) cells	25	5
B cells	5	25
Dendritic cells (DC)	5	2–3
c-kit+ cells	<1	<1
	Most in cell cycle	Most in G0
	Most with activation markers	Few with activation markers

Table 1 displays the types and percentages of intrahepatic lymphocytes and contrasts these features with those of the spleen.

Natural killer (NK) and NK-T cells

The liver contains a large population of NK and NK-T cells. NK cells were initially identified as Pit cells and large granular lymphocytes. They express inhibitory and excitatory receptors that predominantly use the presence of major histocompatibility complex (MHC) class I antigens on other cells to establish self and non-self [4]. The best known function of NK cells is cytotoxicity, and they possess a number of proapoptotic mediators such as CD95 ligand and perforin/granzyme, as well as secretion of interferon (IFN)-γ and tumour necrosis factor (TNF)α [5]. Unlike other lymphocytes, NK cells demonstrate spontaneous cytotoxicity, which can be further enhanced by IFN-α/β, interleukin (IL)-2, IL-12, IL-15 and IL-18 [6]. The cytotoxic activity of NK cells has been demonstrated in a range of *in vivo* model systems to provide protection against tumours, viruses and other intracellular pathogens such as malarial parasites. Activation of NK cells also serves as a bridge to activation of the adaptive immune response. This is predominantly through secretion of IFN-γ, resulting in an upregulation of adhesion and co-stimulatory molecules, activation of dendritic cells and recruitment of more NK cells from the bone marrow [7].

NK-T cells share many of the features of NK cells (expression of NK1.1 and IL-2Rβ) but, in addition, have features of classic T cells [expression of an αβ T-cell receptor (TCR), CD3, CD69 and CD62L] [8,9]. As such, NK-T cells are positioned between the innate and adaptive immune systems. This is further reflected by the limited diversity of their TCRs. In mice, NK-T cells express TCR with an invariant Vα14–Jα281alpha chain paired with a Vβ8 beta chain. The TCRs of NK-T cells undergo selection and activation on the class I-like molecule CD1, which is expressed on hepatocytes, and also on dendritic cells, B cells, T cells and macrophages [10]. As suggested by their phenotype, NK-T cells have functions that overlap with NK cells, particularly a robust cytotoxic response. Unlike NK cells, NK-T cells require a stimulatory signal for the development of cytotoxicity. This is typically activation by the TCR, but may be as little as the presence of IL-2 or IL-18 [6]. The identity of the natural antigens recognized by the NK-T cell receptor on the CD1 molecule has been an area of great interest. The three-dimensional structure of the CD1 molecule predicts that it accommodates hydrophobic ligands, and this has been confirmed experimentally [11,12]. It is important to note that CD1 (unlike class I MHC molecules) is relatively invariant. There is, however, much more structural promiscuity, with one CD1 molecule able to bind a wide range of lipid antigens [13]. In addition, humans have five isoforms of CD1, providing further flexibility in lipid antigen presentation. This allows NK-T cells to monitor CD1-expressing cells for the presence of a wide variety of microbial lipid molecules, as well as abnormal lipid molecules on neoplastic cells.

In addition to delivering a cytotoxic signal to cells expressing unusual lipid molecules presented on CD1, activation of NK-T cells results in activation of NK cells and other cell types including CD8+ T cells and B cells via cross-talk. Kupffer cells are an important intermediary for the activation of NK cells by NK-T cells [14]. NK-T cells may have additional novel functions, such as limiting fibrosis by inducing apoptosis of hepatic stellate cells, which are currently being explored.

Collectively, NK and NK-T cells provide the liver with a large population of lymphocytes with cytotoxic function. This cytotoxic function is important in the removal of tumour cells with loss of class I molecules or expression of abnormal lipid molecules, and also removal of cells that express non-self lipids from pathogens.

Dendritic cells and presentation of hepatic antigens to the immune system

The best characterized functions of dendritic cells (DC) are the phagocytosis of antigens from peripheral tissues, migration to lymph nodes and maturation into efficient antigen presentation cells resulting in activation of T cells [15]. While these are certainly important, it has become clear that DC can also regulate the immune response and induce tolerance to self- and foreign antigens [16]. Dendritic cells collectively express many cell surface markers, including CD11c, CD8, CD11b, CD40, CD80, CD83, CD86, B220, CD45, MHC class I and II. There has been much controversy on the classification of subsets of DC based on selective expression of these markers. The reciprocal expression of CD8 and CD11b has been used to divide DC into CD8+CD11b– (lymphoid DC) and CD8–CD11b+ (myeloid DC) [17]. Lymphoid DC are present in the thymus and in the liver at a much lower percentage. In the thymus, they are responsible for deleting developing T cells with autoreactive potential, and thus may be specialized for maintaining tolerance [18]. For example, infusion of donor lymphoid DC prior to cardiac transplantation prolongs graft survival. Plasmacytoid DC form another well-defined population, which is identified in mice by the presence of B220 expression and, in humans, by CD123 [19]. In both species, plasmacytoid DC produce large amounts of type 1 interferons upon stimulation by pathogens via pattern recognition receptors, or activated T cells via CD40. In addition, maturation of DC is associated with upregulation of MHC class II, CD80, CD86 and enhanced ability to prime T cells.

Hepatic DC reside mostly around the portal triads and have an immature phenotype based on lack of expression of co-stimulatory molecules, but they do express MHC class I and II. Consistent with this phenotype, they are able to internalize antigen by phagocytosis and have poor ability to activate T cells. It has been shown recently that the liver is a major site for the translocation of immature DC from the blood to the lymphatic compartment [20,21]. Immature DC will phagocytose carbon-laden particles, enter the liver, translocate across the sinusoidal endothelium and drain to the coeliac nodes. This process is relatively fast, with carbon-laden DC appearing in coeliac nodes within 2 h of injection into the venous circulation. During their passage through the liver, there is frequent contact with Kupffer cells and some upregulation of MHC class II, suggesting DC maturation. Antigen presentation by murine hepatic DC results in poor allostimulation of T cells *in vitro* and, *in vivo*, results in secretion of IL-10 in secondary lymphoid tissue. This is in contrast to the production of IFN-γ and IL-12 by mature bone marrow-derived DC [22]. Most features of hepatic DC suggest that they have a weak ability to induce T-cell activation and are biased to tolerization. The unique anatomy of the liver allows naive T cells in the blood to come into contact with hepatic DC, further augmenting liver DC-induced tolerance.

Unlike other organs, there is a significant amount of evidence that non-DC liver cell populations can present hepatic antigens to naive T cells [23–26]. As efficient antigen presentation requires the coordinated presentation of MHC–peptide complexes, co-stimulatory molecules and the presence of appropriate cytokines, it was predicted that antigen presentation by such non-professional antigen-presenting cells will result in weak T-cell priming. This was confirmed by *in vitro* antigen presentation experiments using hepatocytes, sinusoidal endothelium and Kupffer cells [24–26]. The best *in vivo* evidence for antigen presentation is for sinusoidal endothelium [27]. This unique population expresses molecules that promote antigen uptake, including the mannose and scavenger receptors. In addition, they express a number of co-stimulatory molecules including CD40, CD80 and CD86. Antigen presentation by sinusoidal endothelial cells results in passive apoptosis of CD8+ T cells and development of CD4+ T cells towards a regulatory phenotype [23]. From studies in transgenic mice, it is also clear that antigen expression limited to hepatocytes results in T-cell tolerance with low levels of antigen, and deletion of T cells with high levels of antigen. As antigen originally limited to a single cell population can be taken up by other cell populations and subsequently presented (cross-presentation), the conclusions from transgenic expression of antigen on hepatocytes are not definitive.

Table 2 Phenotype and known functions of intrahepatic lymphocytes.

TCRαβ	These make up the majority of T cells. Posses either CD4 or CD8 as coreceptors and have a polyclonal TCR. They are activated by engagement of the TCR by appropriate MHC–peptide complex. CD8+ T cells typically become cytotoxic T cells on activation. CD4+ T cells can differentiate into Th1 (inflammatory; cytokines IFN-γ, LT-α) or Th2 (helper; cytokines IL-4, IL-5, IL-10) cells or have features of both
TCR low CD4–CD8–	An unusual cell type found in the liver with low levels of TCR, lacking CD4 and CD8 coreceptors, but possessing B220. They also possess activation markers, are undergoing cell cycle, and a proportion are also undergoing apoptosis. Most probably mature T cells that have undergone activation and are now undergoing apoptosis. May contain generated extrathymic T cells
TCR-γδ	T cells with a distinctive TCR able to recognize antigen independent of MHC molecules. They recognize antigens that are poorly recognized by conventional T cells and have cytotoxic function as well as cytokine secretion biased towards a Th2 profile
Natural killer NK-T	TCR receptor of limited diversity and additional inhibitory receptors. Low numbers in most organs except for bone marrow and liver. Activated via the TCR and have high cytotoxicity potential with production of IFN-γ, TNFα, IL-2 and IL-4
Natural killer (NK)	Many of the features of NK-T cells but no TCR. Similar to NK-T cells, present in high percentage in bone marrow and liver. Demonstrate spontaneous cytotoxicity, especially if target does not express MHC class I molecules
B	Undergo development in bone marrow and possess a polyclonal immunoglobulin receptor. On activation via cell surface IgM, produce immunoglobulin which can cause complement-mediated lysis and recruit other cells and molecules
Dendritic (DC)	Naïve cells phagocytose and acquire specialized antigen-presenting function on activation The liver is a major site for the activation and translocation of DC from blood to the lymphatic compartment

TCR-γδ T cells

T cells with the γδ TCR constitute a small but distinct lymphoid population in the blood and other organs of most mammals [28–30]. The γδ TCR is composed of a relatively small number of germline gene segments, with non-diverse canonical γδ TCRs predominating in different anatomical sites. The crystal structure of the γδ TCR reveals similarities with the immunoglobulin molecule, predicting that the γδ TCR can bind antigens directly rather than as an antigen–MHC complex [31]. This is borne out by functional experiments, and γδ T cells can clearly recognize heat shock proteins directly, but some γδ TCRs can also recognize antigen bound to class II and class Ib molecules [32]. Major classes of γδ TCR ligands are microbe-derived alkyl amines and metabolites of the isoprenoid biosynthesis pathway. Upon activation, γδ T cells possess a range of effector functions, including granule and CD95L-dependent cytotoxicity, production of a range of cytokines including IFN-γ, TNFα, IL-10, transforming growth factor (TGF)-β and IL-4 [33]. γδ T cells also produce cytokines which are relatively unique to them, including fibroblast growth factor-7 and connective tissue growth factor, suggesting a role in maintaining epithelial integrity and wound repair [34]. These properties suggest that γδ T cells fulfil a role in initiating an immune response against pathogenic antigens such as phosphoantigens that are not well recognized by conventional T cells and, as they can recognize antigen directly without the need for antigen processing, they can respond earlier than conventional αβ T cells.

The above features of γδ T cells apply to hepatic γδ T cells. In addition to this, in mice, the liver is an organ shown to be uniquely enriched in a Thy-1-positive γδ T-cell population, which makes up about 50% of hepatic γδ T cells. The Thy-1-positive γδ T-cell population has a limited γ and δ TCR repertoire and is known to secrete greater amounts of IL-4 than other

γδ T cells and relatively large amounts of IFN-γ [35]. Some of these properties are analogous to NK-T cells, suggesting a similar differentiation programme in the liver for these two different cell types.

TCR-αβ T cells (see Table 2)

These are the most familiar T cells that make up the majority of T cells in the secondary lymphoid organs (spleen and lymph nodes) [15]. A number of differences between the liver and the secondary lymphoid organs are present. The vast majority of αβ T cells in lymph nodes and spleen are naïve and do not express activation markers, whereas in the liver, the majority express activation markers such as CD69 or CD44 high. A significant percentage of liver αβ T cells also express an unusual molecule, B220, which is typically associated with B cells, but is also found on T cells undergoing activation-induced apoptosis [36]. Cell cycle analysis shows that, consistent with the presence of activation markers, the majority of αβ T cells in the liver are undergoing cell cycle, and approximately 15% at any time have evidence of apoptosis. Thus, in contrast to the naïve population of T cells in lymph nodes, αβ T cells in the normal liver are activated, undergoing cell cycle and also undergoing cell death.

Two related sets of experimental observations provided important clues to the origin of this large and peculiar liver αβ T-cell population. First, when large numbers of T cells in mice are activated near simultaneously, there is mobilization of αβ T cells from lymph nodes and spleen, followed over 1–2 days by a massive accumulation of αβ T cells in the liver [37]. Secondly, direct infusion of activated T cells into the portal vein results in retention of the vast majority in the liver [38]. These and other data have established that the normal liver has the unusual capacity to retain activated T cells, which contrasts with other organs in which retention occurs in the presence of inflammation. The healthy liver has a unique set of features responsible for retention of activated T cells. Hepatic sinusoids have an interconnected set of channels with relatively low blood flow and a diameter of approximately 6.5 μM. This approximates the diameter of naive T cells, but is less than that of activated T cells. The sinusoids are also populated with a very mobile population of Kupffer cells, which traverse sinusoids, blocking and frequently reversing blood flow [39]. This low flow, interrupted flow pattern maximizes the contact of activated T cells entering the liver with the sinusoidal endothelium and other cells in the sinusoidal lumen. One prediction from this is that selectins, which are important in initiating rolling of fast-moving lymphocytes, will have a minimal role in hepatic retention of lymphocytes and this is the case from studies on selectin-deficient mice. The integrins that are responsible for firm adhesion of lymphocytes are important in hepatic retention of T cells, with intercellular adhesion molecule (ICAM)-1 and vascular cell adhesion molecule (VCAM)-1 having the major role [38,40]. Normal hepatic vascular and sinusoidal endothelium also express vascular adhesion protein (VAP)-1, which enhances lymphocyte retention by its enzymatic activity as an amine oxidase [41].

After retention in the liver, activated T cells can undergo cell division, effector function with release of IFN-γ, perforin/granzyme-induced cytotoxicity and apoptosis. Certain features promote intrahepatic apoptosis of intrahepatic T cells, including the presence of large quantifies of high-affinity antigen, particularly on Kupffer cells, and a large population of responding T cells. These features are most closely met with soluble food antigens entering the liver in large quantities. This results in apoptosis of activated T cells entering the liver with specificity for food antigens, ensuring that food antigens do not promote significant T-cell responses. An important molecular signal which induces apoptosis in hepatic CD8+ T cells is the alternative co-stimulatory molecule B7-H1 [42]. In its absence, an immune response results in less intrahepatic T cell apoptosis and greater liver injury [43]. Even in the absence of intrahepatic antigen, there is hepatic retention and eventual T-cell apoptosis, but also significant effector function. For example, most of the antiviral T-cell response against hepatitis B antigens is non-cytolytic [44]. This is followed by a more limited cytolytic response against hepatocytes with remaining viral antigen [45]. Such regulation of the two effector responses is presumed to clear viral infections with the induction of minimum hepatocyte apoptosis.

Regulation of the hepatic T-cell response

The hepatic immune response encompasses extremes, with hyporesponsiveness and tolerance on most exposures to foreign antigens, but a florid response with fulminant liver failure in others. A central question in liver immunology is understanding how the immune components reviewed above are regulated. There are a number of candidate processes, many or all of which may be important. T-cell apoptosis in response to high-affinity

antigen has already been noted above. Hepatocyte injury is an important stimulus to an effective hepatic immune response in experimental models. This may overcome hepatic hyporesponsiveness by the generation of danger signals that were hypothesized over a decade ago and have recently been identified as metabolites of nucleotide degradation along the uric acid pathway [46]. Production of type 1 interferons (IFN-α/β) triggered by viral infection of hepatocytes is another candidate, resulting in recruitment of T cells and stimulation of IL-15, which promotes CD8+ T-cell survival [47,48]. In addition, type 1 interferons may provide a vital maturation signal to hepatic DC. Type 1 interferons may therefore provide an important switch between tolerance and an adaptive T-cell response. Finally, regulatory T cells in the liver may induce immunosuppression above the baseline in conditions such as hepatocellular cancer (HCC) and chronic viral hepatitis [49,50]. The concept of regulator T cells has been investigated for over 30 years, but better tools in the last 10 years have allowed this field to develop [51]. In principle, these are functionally hyporesponsive cells with very little or no production of IL-12, but production of IL-10, TGF-β and CTLA-4. The best characterized T-cell type with regulator function is the thymic-derived CD4+ T cells also expressing the CD25 marker [52]. However, NK-T and γδ T cells can also have similar functional properties. There is direct evidence for increased CD4+CD25+ T cells within tumour tissue of patients with HCC [49]. In patients with chronic HBV, the frequency of circulating regulatory T cells was significantly higher than in non-infected individuals [50]. These studies are preliminary but suggest a significant role for regulatory T cells in shaping the hepatic immune response.

Lymphocytes and liver fibrosis

The majority of liver pathology resulting in fibrosis has a significant inflammatory component. This is certainly true for chronic viral infections, but also for alcoholic liver diseases and non-alcoholic steatohepatitis. This observation raises questions about the influence of the inflammatory response, distinct from hepatocyte injury, in the progression of fibrosis. It also raises questions about the ability of stellate cells to proliferate and function in the setting of a florid T-cell response such as in chronic HBV infection.

A comparable amount of liver injury has been shown to result in greater fibrosis in the setting of a T helper (Th)2 immune response than a Th1 immune response [53]. The presence of IFN-γ in the Th1 response is central to minimizing liver fibrosis. Hepatic CD8+ T cells from fibrotic livers are able to induce fibrosis when transferred into mice with no liver injury, demonstrating the profibrogenic ability of such CD8+ T cells independent of liver injury [54]. Finally, experiments in mice lacking the co-stimulatory molecule B7-H1 demonstrate that B7-H1 expressed on hepatic stellate cells protects them from T cell-mediated cytotoxicity by inducing apoptosis of activated T cells [55].

References

1 Park S, Murray D, John B *et al.* (2002) Biology and significance of T-cell apoptosis in the liver. *Immunol Cell Biol* 80 (1), 74–83.

2 Crispe IN (2003) Hepatic T cells and liver tolerance. *Nature Rev Immunol* 3 (1), 51–62.

3 Mehal WZ, Azzaroli F, Crispe IN (2001) Immunology of the healthy liver: old questions and new insights. *Gastroenterology* 120 (1), 250–260.

4 Kane KP, Lavender KJ, Ma BJ (2004) Ly-49 receptors and their functions. *Crit Rev Immunol* 24 (5), 321–348.

5 Smyth MJ, Cretney E, Kelly JM *et al.* (2005) Activation of NK cell cytotoxicity. *Mol Immunol* 42 (4), 501–510.

6 Dao T, Mehal WZ, Crispe IN (1998) IL-18 augments perforin-dependent cytotoxicity of liver NK-T cells. *J Immunol* 161 (5), 2217–2222.

7 Wiltrout RH (2000) Regulation and antimetastatic functions of liver-associated natural killer cells. *Immunol Rev* 174, 63–76.

8 Moretta L, Bottino C, Pende D *et al.* (2002) Human natural killer cells: their origin, receptors and function. *Eur J Immunol* 32 (5), 1205–1211.

9 Elewaut D, Kronenberg M (2000) Molecular biology of NK T cell specificity and development. *Semin Immunol* 12 (6), 561–568.

10 Mandal M, Chen XR, Alegre ML *et al.* (1998) Tissue distribution, regulation and intracellular localization of murine CD1 molecules. *Mol Immunol* 35 (9), 525–536.

11 Seki S, Habu Y, Kawamura T *et al.* (2000) The liver as a crucial organ in the first line of host defense: the roles of Kupffer cells, natural killer (NK) cells and NK1.1 Ag+ T cells in T helper 1 immune responses. *Immunol Rev* 174, 35–46.

12 Schmieg J, Gonzalez-Aseguinolaza G, Tsuji M (2003) The role of natural killer T cells and other T cell subsets against infection by the pre-erythrocytic stages of malaria parasites. *Microbes Infect* 5 (6), 499–506.

13 Bendelac A, Rivera MN, Park SH *et al.* (1997) Mouse CD1-specific NK1 T cells: development, specificity, and function. *Annu Rev Immunol* 15, 535–562.

14 Wesley JD, Robbins SH, Sidobre S *et al.* (2005) Cutting edge: IFN-gamma signaling to macrophages is required for optimal Valpha14i NK T/NK cell cross-talk. *J Immunol* 174 (7), 3864–3868.

15 Janeway C, Travers P, Capra D *et al.* (2005) *Immunobiology: the Immune System in Health and Disease*, 6th edn. London: Current Biology; Garland Publications.

16 Mellor AL, Munn DH (2004) IDO expression by dendritic cells: tolerance and tryptophan catabolism. *Nature Rev Immunol* 4 (10), 762–774.

17 Lau AH, Thomson AW (2003) Dendritic cells and immune regulation in the liver. *Gut* 52 (2), 307–314.

18 McLellan AD, Kampgen E (2000) Functions of myeloid and lymphoid dendritic cells. *Immunol Lett* 72 (2), 101–105.

19 Colonna M, Trinchieri G, Liu YJ (2004) Plasmacytoid dendritic cells in immunity. *Nature Immunol* 5 (12), 1219–1226.

20 Kudo S, Matsuno K, Ezaki T *et al.* (1997) A novel migration pathway for rat dendritic cells from the blood: hepatic sinusoids-lymph translocation. *J Exp Med* 185 (4), 777–784.

21 Matsuno K, Ezaki T, Kudo S *et al.* (1996) A life stage of particle-laden rat dendritic cells in vivo: their terminal division, active phagocytosis, and translocation from the liver to the draining lymph. *J Exp Med* 183 (4), 1865–1878.

22 Thomson AW, Drakes ML, Zahorchak AF *et al.* (1999) Hepatic dendritic cells: immunobiology and role in liver transplantation. *J Leuk Biol* 66 (2), 322–330.

23 Crispe IN (2003) Hepatic T cells and liver tolerance. *Nature Rev Immunol* 3 (1), 51–62.

24 Bertolino P, Heath WR, Hardy CL *et al.* (1995) Peripheral deletion of autoreactive CD8+ T cells in transgenic mice expressing H-2Kb in the liver. *Eur J Immunol* 25 (7), 1932–1942.

25 Knolle PA, Uhrig A, Hegenbarth S *et al.* (1998) IL-10 down-regulates T cell activation by antigen-presenting liver sinusoidal endothelial cells through decreased antigen uptake via the mannose receptor and lowered surface expression of accessory molecules. *Clin Exp Immunol* 114 (3), 427–433.

26 Roland CR, Walp L, Stack RM *et al.* (1994) Outcome of Kupffer cell antigen presentation to a cloned murine Th1 lymphocyte depends on the inducibility of nitric oxide synthase by IFN-gamma. *J Immunol* 153 (12), 5453–5464.

27 Limmer A, Ohl J, Kurts C *et al.* (2000) Efficient presentation of exogenous antigen by liver endothelial cells to CD8+ T cells results in antigen-specific T-cell tolerance. *Nature Med* 6 (12), 1348–1354.

28 Pennington DJ, Silva-Santos B, Hayday AC (2005) Gammadelta T cell development – having the strength to get there. *Curr Opin Immunol* 17 (2), 108–115.

29 Kabelitz D, Wesch D (2003) Features and functions of gamma delta T lymphocytes: focus on chemokines and their receptors. *Crit Rev Immunol* 23 (5–6), 339–370.

30 Hayday AC (2000) [gamma][delta] cells: a right time and a right place for a conserved third way of protection. *Annu Rev Immunol* 18, 975–1026.

31 Allison TJ, Winter CC, Fournie JJ *et al.* (2001) Structure of a human gammadelta T-cell antigen receptor. *Nature* 411 (6839), 820–824.

32 Allison TJ, Garboczi DN (2002) Structure of gammadelta T cell receptors and their recognition of non-peptide antigens. *Mol Immunol* 38 (14), 1051–1061.

33 Tsukaguchi K, de Lange B, Boom WH (1999) Differential regulation of IFN-gamma, TNF-alpha, and IL-10 production by CD4(+) alphabetaTCR+ T cells and vdelta2(+) gammadelta T cells in response to monocytes infected with *Mycobacterium tuberculosis*-H37Ra. *Cell Immunol* 194 (1), 12–20.

34 Girardi M, Lewis J, Glusac E *et al.* (2002) Resident skin-specific gammadelta T cells provide local, nonredundant regulation of cutaneous inflammation. *J Exp Med* 195 (7), 855–867.

35 Gerber DJ, Azuara V, Levraud JP *et al.* (1999) IL-4-producing gamma delta T cells that express a very restricted TCR repertoire are preferentially localized in liver and spleen. *J Immunol* 163 (6), 3076–3082.

36 Mehal WZ, Crispe IN (1998) TCR ligation on CD8+ T cells creates double-negative cells in vivo. *J Immunol* 161 (4), 1686–1693.

37 Huang L, Soldevila G, Leeker M *et al.* (1994) The liver eliminates T cells undergoing antigen-triggered apoptosis in vivo. *Immunity* 1 (9), 741–749.

38 Mehal WZ, Juedes AE, Crispe IN (1999) Selective retention of activated CD8+ T cells by the normal liver. *J Immunol* 163 (6), 3202–3210.

39 MacPhee PJ, Schmidt EE, Groom AC (1995) Intermittence of blood flow in liver sinusoids, studied by high resolution in vivo microscopy. *Am J Physiol* 269, G692.

40 Lalor PF, Shields P, Grant A *et al.* (2002) Recruitment of lymphocytes to the human liver. *Immunol Cell Biol* 80 (1), 52–64.

41 Lor PF, Edwards S, McNab G *et al.* (2002) Vascular adhesion protein-1 mediates adhesion and transmigration of lymphocytes on human hepatic endothelial cells. *J Immunol* 169 (2), 983–992.

42 Zha Y, Blank C, Gajewski TF (2004) Negative regulation of T-cell function by PD-1. *Crit Rev Immunol* 24 (4), 229–237.

43 Dong H, Zhu G, Tamada K *et al.* (2004) B7-H1 determines accumulation and deletion of intrahepatic CD8(+) T lymphocytes. *Immunity* 20 (3), 327–336.

44 Guidotti LG, Chisari FV (2001) Noncytolytic control of viral infections by the innate and adaptive immune response. *Annu Rev Immunol* 19, 65–91.

45 Anon (2005) Oscillating CD8+ T cell effector functions after antigen recognition in the liver. *Immunity* 23 (1), 53–63.

46 Shi Y, Evans JE, Rock KL (2003) Molecular identification of a danger signal that alerts the immune system to dying cells. *Nature* 425 (6957), 516–521.

47 Salazar-Mather TP, Orange JS, Biron CA (1998) Early murine cytomegalovirus (MCMV) infection induces liver natural killer (NK) cell inflammation and protection through macrophage inflammatory protein 1alpha (MIP-1alpha)-dependent pathways. *J Exp Med* 187 (1), 1–14.

48 Mattei F, Schiavoni G, Belardelli F *et al.* (2001) IL-15 is expressed by dendritic cells in response to type I IFN, double-stranded RNA, or lipopolysaccharide and promotes dendritic cell activation. *J Immunol* 167 (3), 1179–1187.

49 Unitt E, Rushbrook SM, Marshall A *et al.* (2005) Compromised lymphocytes infiltrate hepatocellular carcinoma: the role of T-regulatory cells. *Hepatology* 41 (4), 722–730.

50 Franzese O, Kennedy PT, Gehring AJ *et al.* (2005) Modulation of the CD8+-T-cell response by CD4+ CD25+ regulatory T cells in patients with hepatitis B virus infection. *J Virol* 79 (6), 3322–3328.

51 Chang KM (2005) Regulatory T cells and the liver: a new piece of the puzzle. *Hepatology* 41 (4), 700–702.

52 Shevach EM (2002) CD4+ CD25+ suppressor T cells: more questions than answers. *Nature Rev Immunol* 2 (6), 389–400.

53 Shi Z, Wakil AE, Rockey DC (1997) Strain-specific differences in mouse hepatic wound healing are mediated by divergent T helper cytokine responses. *Proc Natl Acad Sci USA* 94 (20), 10663–10668.

54 Safadi R, Ohta M, Alvarez CE *et al.* (2004) Immune stimulation of hepatic fibrogenesis by CD8 cells and attenuation by transgenic interleukin-10 from hepatocytes. *Gastroenterology* 127 (3), 870–882.

55 Yu MC, Chen CH, Liang X *et al.* (2004) Inhibition of T-cell responses by hepatic stellate cells via B7-H1-mediated T-cell apoptosis in mice. *Hepatology* 40 (6), 1312–1321.

2.7.3 Antibody production and transport in the liver

Alvin B. Imaeda and Wajahat Z. Mehal

Introduction and description of B-cell differentiation

The liver is uniquely positioned between the external and internal immune environments and needs to function in a dual role of surveillance against dangerous pathogens and tolerance of benign food antigens. The previous two chapters have focused on the roles of cytokines and T cells in the liver and immune function, and Chapter 1.5 has reviewed Kupffer cells. This chapter will focus on immunoglobulin (Ig) and B cells, particularly IgA, as it is the most thoroughly studied immunoglobulin in the liver. IgA plays an important role in the immunity of the gut and liver, and also helps to prevent unnecessary inflammatory responses against benign or easily cleared antigens.

B cells initially develop in the bone marrow where they undergo a series of developmental steps that result in secretion of immunoglobulin with little affinity for self-antigens, but high affinity for a large but finite repertoire of foreign antigens. Within the bone marrow, an irreversible random process of gene segment rearrangement occurs, bringing several gene segments together to form the variable region of an immunoglobulin receptor. If a successful rearrangement occurs, further rearrangement on the other chromosome is halted, allowing expression of a receptor of a single specificity. B cells expressing receptors with high affinity for self-antigens undergo programmed cellular death, minimizing the production of autoantibodies. The developing cells home to different tissues including spleen, peripheral lymph nodes and gut-associated lymphoid tissue (GALT). There, they express cell surface IgM and IgD receptors, and require ligation of these receptors by specific antigen in order to undergo further maturation. Maturation can occur through both T cell-dependent and T cell-independent mechanisms. T cell-independent B-cell activation results primarily in IgM-producing plasma cells, whereas T cell-dependent activation allows gene rearrangement resulting in a γ, α or ε constant region to produce IgG, IgA or IgE respectively. A process called somatic hypermutation introduces many point mutations throughout the variable region of the gene, and B cells with appropriate affinity for antigen are selected to divide and mature [1]. Adhesion molecules and chemokines control homing of the B cells to specific tissues where they mature into plasma cells or memory cells. Immunoglobulin class switching from IgM to IgG, IgA or IgE is controlled, at least in part, by locally produced cytokines. For example, B cells primed with antigen in the lamina propria preferentially become IgA-producing B cells as a result of transforming growth factor (TGF)-β, interleukin (IL)-6 and IL-10 produced by the stromal cells in this tissue [2].

The liver plays an important role in the biology and function of the mucosal humoral immune system. It plays a key role in the transport, function and clearance of IgA. The cell biology of IgA was delineated in animal liver and bile models in the 1980s. Limited confirmatory studies were carried out with human systems with some interesting differences found in the physiology among different species. The normal patterns of IgA metabolism are altered in disease states such as cirrhosis, and especially in all stages of alcoholic liver disease.

IgA synthesis

IgA is produced by the body in larger quantities than any other antibody isotype. Its serum half-life is 5–6 days compared with

Table 1 IgA subtypes and their characteristics.

	Serum	Secretory tissues
IgA form	Monomeric	Dimeric/polymeric
	IgA1 80–90%	IgA1 40–70%
	IgA2 10–20%	IgA2 30–60%
J chain and secretory chain	Nearly absent	Present
Origin	Bone marrow	Local mucosal tissue
Function	Unknown, possibly	Neutralization and clearance,
	opsonization and ADCC	no significant opsonization or ADCC
Catabolism	ASGP-R on hepatocytes?	ASGP-R on hepatocytes?
		Through secretions after transcytosis
Alcohol effects	Increased IgA2	IgA1 deposits in hepatic sinusoids
		and renal mesangium

ADCC, antibody-dependent, cell-mediated cytotoxicity; ASGP-R, asialoglycoprotein receptor.

20–23 days for IgG, and most of the IgA is present in external secretions. Consequently, blood levels for IgA are much lower than those of IgG [3,4]. Humans have two different isotypes of IgA, IgA1 and IgA2 (Table 1). Bone marrow, spleen and serum have approximately 80–90% IgA1 and 10–20% IgA2, whereas mucosal tissues have a higher percentage, approximately 30–60%, of IgA2 [5,6]. The majority of IgA is monomeric or dimeric, with very small amounts of tetrameric forms. The predominant form in human serum is monomeric (mIgA), whereas at mucosal surfaces, secretory IgA is dimeric or polymeric (pIgA) [7–9]. Each monomer consists of two alpha heavy chains and two kappa or lambda light chains, linked by disulphide bonds. Two additional chains are covalently bound to human secretory IgA. In the dimeric form, a small glycoprotein called the J chain links the two immunoglobulin molecules together by the Fc portion of the alpha chains [10]. Additionally, a secretory chain component (SC) from the polymeric immunoglobulin receptor is attached to the Fc portion as the immunoglobulin is secreted into the luminal compartment as described below [11] (see Fig. 1a).

IgA is synthesized by antigen-primed plasma cells in the GALT, which includes Peyer's patches, isolated lymphoid follicles and the lamina propria just beneath the basement membrane of gut surface epithelia. Therefore, IgA must be transported back to its primary site of action on the luminal aspect of the epithelium. Secretory component (SC) is an approximately 550-amino-acid polypeptide with five Ig-like domains and is expressed preferentially on the basolateral membrane (submucosal side) of intestine, lung, breast and other secreting organs. Polymeric, but not monomeric, forms of IgA bind to SC on the basolateral surface of cells [12]. The complex is internalized into endocytic vesicles and, through a SC-directed process called transcytosis, it is specifically routed to the apical (luminal) surface of the epithelial cell. There, the complex is cleaved and released into the external environment [12,13] (see Fig. 1b). A component of SC remains attached to the IgA complex and may serve to protect the molecule from environmental proteases [14].

IgA secretion in the hepatobiliary system: rats vs. human

The discovery of IgA as the major protein component of bile in rats led to the study of IgA in the hepatobiliary system and the eventual understanding of the synthesis and secretion of IgA as described above [15]. Hepatobiliary transport of IgA results in IgA secretion into bile. This results in transport of IgA into the gut with localization of its effector function in surveillance of the bile and gut mucosa and eventual excretion.

Significant species differences in the transport of IgA are present. The rat, rabbit and chicken are efficient at hepatic transport of plasma IgA into bile, whereas man, dog and guinea pig are inefficient at this transport [16]. This correlates with expression of SC, as the efficient transporters express SC on hepatocytes, whereas man and the other inefficient transporters express SC on intra- and extrahepatic biliary epithelium but not hepatocytes [12,17,18]. These species differences result in widely different quantities of biliary excretion of pIgA, about 35 mg/kg/day for rats and rabbits and only about 1 mg/kg/day for man, dog and guinea pig [16]. Therefore, widely different amounts of pIgA are available in these different species to survey the biliary compartment. This suggests that different quantities of pIgA are available to protect the luminal gut compartment in different species. However, Jonard et al. [7] have shown that, in contrast to rat, the primary source of pIgA to enter the intestinal lumen in humans is from the bowel mucosa, not from bile. Similarly, the primary source of human biliary pIgA, although far less concentrated than in rats, is from the biliary ductal epithelium and perhaps the gallbladder mucosa and not hepatocytes as in rats [17–19]. Although no specific evidence exists to explain this dichotomy, the two systems seem to employ different strategies. In rats, IgA originates from plasma cells primed in the gut, traverses the mesenteric lymph system or portal venous blood and is then secreted by hepatocytes into the bile and drained back into the gut. A system with high pIgA concentration, but probably lower specificity, is present in the rat. In man, a more

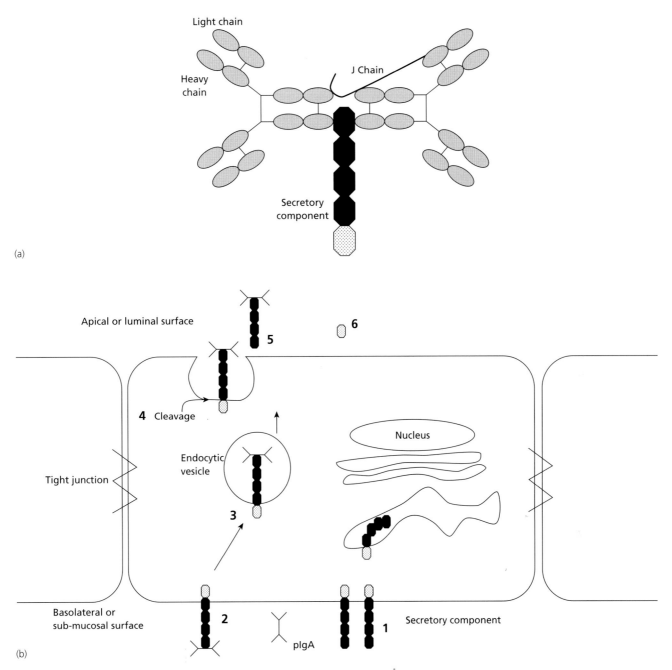

Fig. 1 (a) Topographical representation of interaction between two monomeric IgA molecules, J chain and secretory component. Each ellipse represents an immunoglobulin domain. (b) Diagrammatic representation of transcytosis of IgA. (1) Expression of secretory component on the basolateral membrane. (2) Binding of pIgA to secretory component [note: this includes J chain; see (a)]. (3) Endocytosis of the pIgA–secretory component complex. (4) Cleavage of secretory component and exocytosis. (5) Secretory IgA (sIgA). (6) Cytoplasmic tail of secretory component.

localized priming in the lamina propria to supply gut IgA or in peribiliary lymph nodes to supply biliary IgA provides smaller quantities of probably highly specific antibodies. It is important to note that IgM also binds to SC, and small amounts of IgM as well as IgG are found in human bile [8].

Multiple other factors probably influence secretion of IgA into bile. This has been examined to a limited extent in animal models and cell culture models. As might be expected, bile flow decreases the concentration of IgA secreted into bile [20]. Other factors regulate expression of SC in some model systems, and thus may also influence secretion of pIgA into bile and other compartments. For example, androgen increases free SC in rat tears, and estradiol stimulates secretion of SC into the uterine cavity [21,22]. In cultured rat hepatocytes, dexamethasone and cortisol increase secretion of SC. This is inhibited by an inhibitor of protein synthesis and, interestingly, is also inhibited by estradiol [23]. Finally, interferon gamma and tumour necrosis factor (TNF)α upregulate expression of SC on a human colonic carcinoma cell line [18,24]. The role of these mediators of IgA secretion in humans is not known.

Immunoglobulin catabolism

Studies in mice and primates aimed at identifying sites of IgA catabolism have shown that the greatest uptake of radiolabelled mIgA and pIgA occurs in the liver. Parenchymal cells are more active than non-parenchymal cells in the uptake. Competitive inhibition studies with asialofeutin suggest that the receptor responsible for this uptake is the asialoglycoprotein receptor (ASGP-R) [25]. The ASGP-R is expressed on hepatocytes of many species, including humans. It binds to terminal galactose residues on desialylated glycoproteins and directs them to vesicles that fuse to lysosomes, leading to degradation of the proteins. Only about 0.5–8% of ligands that bind the ASGP-R escape the degradative pathway and are then secreted into bile [26]. This suggests that the primary function of binding of IgA to ASGP-R is for clearance of IgA. This is more important for serum IgA, the predominant subtype of which is IgA1, as mucosal IgA2 can be excreted through stool and other secretions. Studies looking at ASGP-R binding and catabolism of IgA1 vs. IgA2, using in vitro or a somewhat artificial in vivo system, have shown contradictory results [18,27,28].

The transferrin receptor can bind IgA1 when expressed on renal mesangial cells and possibly when expressed on dividing lymphocytes. The functional significance of this interaction is unclear, but transferrin receptor has been implicated in IgA nephropathy [29,30]. A possible role for transferrin receptor in the binding and clearance of IgA in the liver has not been determined.

IgG and IgM are also cleared by the liver, but by different mechanisms and cell types than IgA. Studies in rats show that IgG is catabolized in tissues throughout the body including skin, muscle, liver, kidney, bone marrow and spleen. On a weight basis, liver and spleen are the most active, and non-parenchymal cells are much more active in catabolism than hepatocytes [31]. The Fc receptor Brambell (FcRB) is a saturable receptor that binds and protects IgG from lysosomal catabolism and is likely to be responsible for its longer half-life than other immunoglobulins [32]. In studies of IgM catabolism, 60–80% of IgM is degraded in the liver. Again, in contrast to IgA, non-parenchymal cells are more active than parenchymal cells in degradation of IgM [33].

The function of IgA in the hepatobiliary system

IgA is the predominant form of immunoglobulin that affects the mucosal surfaces. This includes the intestinal, respiratory and reproductive tracts, the lactating breast and the salivary and tear glands. Mucosal IgA is not an effective opsonin for phagocytosis,

and it does not effectively fix complement. Additionally, it acts primarily in the environment in which complement and phagocytes are not normally present. Its inability to induce inflammation may be important in order to maintain both the physical epithelial barrier and tolerance against benign antigens [29]. IgA thus serves as the first line of defence in preventing agents from penetrating the epithelial barrier. IgA may also allow clearance of pathogens in secretions, bile and stool through transcytosis of bacteria that have penetrated the epithelium or by interception of intracellular virus or bacteria during transcytosis. IgA is involved in neutralization of bacterial toxins, bacteria, viruses, food antigens and other toxins. In fact, IgA antibodies against multiple organisms or toxins have been demonstrated in bile, either occurring naturally or after infection or inoculation with agents including cholera toxin (rat) [34, 35], *Vibrio cholerae* (rat, monkey) [18,36], *Escherichia coli* (man) [37] and *Giardia lamblia* (rat) [38]. Finally, CD89, the FcαRI, is a relatively newly described Fc receptor for IgA. It is expressed on phagocytes, including Kupffer cells. Binding of IgA-opsonized organisms by CD89 is expected to result in phagocytosis and clearance of bloodborne pathogens, as well as antibody-dependent, cell-mediated cytoxicity (ADCC) [29]. Interestingly, mucosal type IgA (sIgA) does not bind this receptor, only serum pIgA and IgA immune complexes. IgA–antigen complexes are not cleared through hepatocytes into bile in man; however, alternative pathways to clear IgA complexes in the liver are present. These include the FcαRI on Kupffer cells and the ASGP-R on hepatocytes that primarily direct their ligands to lysosomes [39]. Secretion of IgA into bile in man may primarily serve to provide an immune surveillance mechanism for the biliary tree, rather than a major source of IgA for the intestinal lumen. However, IgA-deficient individuals are not particularly prone to severe biliary tract infections, and IgM may provide additional protection [40].

Immunoglobulins and liver disease

Liver disease has interesting effects on IgA, particularly alcoholic liver disease. Severe liver damage or cirrhosis of any aetiology can lead to an elevation in serum IgA [41,42]. Interestingly, however, alcohol use even with only mild changes in liver histology leads to elevations in serum IgA [43,44]. This has been called an IgA-associated disorder linking it to such diseases as Berger's disease (primary IgA nephropathy), Henoch–Schonlein purpura and IgA-producing myeloma.

The mechanism of increased serum IgA and deposits in the liver sinusoids is unclear. A simple explanation is that alcohol affects hepatic IgA catabolism, perhaps by decreasing uptake via ASGP-R [28]. This probably accounts for some of these findings; however, evidence suggests that the situation is more complex with an increase in IgA synthesis. There is some evidence that IgA-producing B cells are spontaneously active in alcoholic liver disease, although T-cell function is depressed [45,46]. Multiple studies have shown an increase in IgA antibodies against bacteria or bacterial products, as well as dietary components in alcoholic liver disease [47–49]. The specific reasons for this increase in response to microbial and food antigens are unclear but may include disease-specific, disease-non-specific and severity-related mechanisms. Alcohol may influence immune function by decreasing Kupffer cell phagocytic activity or by decreasing gut epithelial barrier function leading to increased antigen availability [50,51]. Severe liver damage of any aetiology may additionally lead to decreased clearance of antigens, leading to increased stimulation of the mucosal immune system. Interestingly, hepatic sinusoidal IgA is primarily mIgA, whereas serum shows an increase in the proportion of pIgA2 [41,42,52]. The reasons for the increased proportion of IgA2 in serum, and the IgA1 in hepatic sinusoidal deposits in alcoholic liver disease, remain to be fully investigated. Limited evidence suggests that sinusoidal IgA deposits may be found in non-alcoholic steatohepatitis (NASH) that are indistinguishable from those seen with alcoholic liver disease [53].

Of additional interest is the finding that patients with alcoholic liver disease have increased titres of IgA and IgG antibodies that recognize acetaldehyde-modified protein condensates [54]. This suggests a direct link between alcohol metabolites and antigen stimulation of IgA-producing plasma cells, implying a role for these antibodies in alcohol-related liver disease. However, no liver-related pathogenicity of the increased titres of IgA has been shown, and these antibodies may decrease hepatic inflammation [55].

In addition to alcohol-related liver disease, serum IgA is elevated in primary biliary cirrhosis (PBC) [42,56]. Reports of elevation of IgA in extrahepatic biliary obstruction have not been confirmed, but serum SC is elevated in both extrahepatic biliary obstruction and PBC [42]. Elevations in serum and mucosal IgA in PBC may be mechanistically related to pathogenesis of the disease, rather than being a result of the liver injury. Specifically, IgA antibodies against pyruvate dehydrogenase complex are proposed to bind to this complex during transcytosis in salivary, lachrymal and biliary epithelial cells [57]. This complex is part of the antimitochondrial antibody–antigen complex implicated as self-antigen in PBC. This binding could potentially contribute to the pathogenesis, but this has not been proven (see Chapter 11.1).

In the healthy liver, B cells make up only about 5% of lymphocytes. In disease states such as autoimmune hepatitis, PBC, chronic hepatitis B and chronic hepatitis C, collections of lymphocytes termed intrahepatic lymphoid follicles (ILFs) have been seen. In chronic hepatitis C, these have been shown to include well-formed germinal centres similar to those in spleen that allow differentiation, clonal selection and affinity maturation of B cells [58]. As discussed for antibodies above, the functional significance of B-cell collections in the liver has not been defined in any of these diseases. In hepatitis B and hepatitis C, the T-cell response is the main determinant in clearing infection, and the role of antibodies in clearance, control or even persistence is not known (please see Chapter 9.1 for a full discussion of hepatitis B and hepatitis C).

IgA nephropathy associated with liver disease

Liver disease is a common cause of IgA nephropathy; in fact, it is the most common form of secondary IgA nephropathy [59]. The majority of the data for IgA nephropathy associated with liver disease are from patients with alcoholic liver disease; however, this form of nephropathy is seen in some patients with liver disease of other aetiologies as well [52]. The incidence of glomerular abnormalities seen in patients with liver disease ranges from 50% to 100% of those with cirrhosis. The glomerular deposits are usually mesangial IgA deposits [60]. Small amounts of IgG, IgM and complement may also be present. Like the deposits in the hepatic sinusoids and in primary IgA nephropathy, the mesangial deposits in hepatic IgA nephropathy are primarily IgA1 [59]. This may be a consequence of the increased production and decreased clearance of IgA or, alternatively, antigen(s) or immune complexes may drive this deposition. Recent studies investigating the role of the FcαRI in IgA nephropathy and alcoholic nephropathy have suggested that increases in IgA stimulate shedding of the FcαRI. It is proposed that complexes of the receptor and IgA may contribute to the pathogenesis [29,61]. Additionally, increased renal mesangial expression of the transferrin receptor which binds IgA has been implicated in the pathogenesis of this disease [30]. Regardless, only a small percentage of patients have clinically apparent disease. One series found 9.6% of all cirrhotic patients with nephritis and 1.6% with nephrotic syndrome [62]. Most patients are asymptomatic and may have only microscopic haematuria and mild proteinuria [59]. Treatment options for alcoholic IgA nephropathy have not been defined, and overall prognosis is directly related to the degree of underlying liver disease.

References

1 Janeway C, Travers P, Capra D *et al.* (2005) *Immunobiology: the Immune System in Health and Disease*, 6th edn. London: Garland Publications.

2 Fagarasan S *et al.* (2001) In situ class switching and differentiation to IgA-producing cells in the gut lamina propria. *Nature* 413, 639–643.

3 Conley ME, Delacroix DL (1987) Intravascular and mucosal immunoglobulin A: two separate but related systems of immune defense? *Ann Intern Med* 106, 892.

4 Mestecky J *et al.* (1986) The human IgA system: a reassessment. *Clin Immunol Immunopathol* 40, 105.

5 Crago SS *et al.* (1984) Distribution of IgA1-, IgA2- and J chain-containing cells in human tissues. *J Immunol* 132, 16.

6 Kett K *et al.* (1986) Different subclass distribution of IgA-producing cells in human lymphoid organs and various secretory tissues. *J Immunol* 136, 3631.

7 Jonard PP *et al.* (1984) Secretion of immunoglobulins and plasma proteins from the jejunal mucosa: transport rate and origin of polymeric immunoglobulin A. *J Clin Invest* 74, 525–535.

8 Delacroix DL *et al.* (1982) Selective transport of polymeric immunoglobulin A in bile: quantitative relationships of monomeric and polymeric immunoglobulin A, immunoglobulin M and other proteins in serum, bile and saliva. *J Clin Invest* 70, 230–241.

9 Newkirk MM *et al.* (1983) Estimation of polymeric IgA in human serum: an assay based on binding of radiolabeled human secretory component with applications in the study of IgA nephropathy, IgA monoclonal gammopathy, and liver diseases. *J Immunol* 130, 1176.

10 Mestecky J *et al.* (1974) Site of J chain attachment to human polymeric IgA. *Proc Natl Acad Sci USA* 71, 544.

11 Kuhn LC, Kraehenbuhl JP (1981) The membrane receptor for polymeric immunoglobulin is structurally related to secretory component from rabbit liver and mammary gland. *J Biol Chem* 256, 12490–12495.

12 Takahashi I, Nakane PK, Brown WR (1982) Ultrastructural events in the translocation of polymeric IgA by rat hepatocytes. *J Immunol* 128, 1181–1187.

13 Breitfeld PP *et al.* (1990) Deletions in the cytoplasmic domain of the polymeric immunoglobulin receptor differentially affect endocytotic rate and postendocytotic traffic. *J Biol Chem* 265, 13750–13757.

14 Brown WR, Newcomb RW, Ishizaka K (1970) Proteolytic degradation of exocrine and serum immunoglobulins. *J Clin Invest* 49, 1374–1380.

15 Lemaitre-Coelho I, Jackson GDF, Vaerman JP (1977) Rat bile as a convenient source of secretory IgA and free secretory component. *Eur J Immunol* 7, 588–590.

16 Brown WR, Kloppel TM (1989) The liver and IgA: immunological, cell biological and clinical implications. *Hepatology* 9 (5), 763–784.

17 Nagura H *et al.* (1981) IgA in human bile and liver. *J Immunol* 126, 587–595.

18 Tomana M, Kulhavy R, Mestecky J (1988) Receptor-mediated binding and uptake of immunoglobulin A by human liver. *Gastroenterology* 94, 762–770.

19 Green FHY, Fox H (1972) An immunofluorescent study of the distribution of immunoglobulin-containing cells in the normal and inflamed human gall bladder. *Gut* 13, 379–384.

20 Kloppel TM *et al.* (1987) Uncoupling of the biliary secretory pathways for IgA and its receptor, secretory component, by brief periods of cholestasis. *Am J Physiol* 253 (2), G232–G240.

21 Sullivan DA, Wira CR (1981) Estradiol regulation of secretory component in the female reproductive tract. *J Steroid Biochem* 15, 439–444.

22 Sullivan DA, Bolch KJ, Allansmith MR (1984) Hormonal influence on the secretory immune system of the eye: androgen regulation of secretory component levels in rat tears. *J Immunol* 132, 1130–1135.

23 Wira CR, Colby E (1985) Regulation of secretory component by glucocorticoids in primary cultures of rat hepatocytes. *J Immunol* 134, 1744–1748.

24 Kvale D *et al.* (1988) Tumor necrosis factor-alpha up-regulates expression of secretory component, the epithelial receptor for polymeric Ig. *J Immunol* 140, 3086–3089.

25 Moldoveanu Z *et al.* (1990) Site of catabolism of autologous and heterologous IgA in non-human primates. *Scand J Immunol* 32, 577–583.

26 Schif JM, Fisher MM, Underdown BJ (1984) Receptor-mediated biliary transport of immunoglobulin A and asialoglycoprotein: sorting and missorting of ligands revealed by two radiolabeling methods. *J Cell Biol* 98, 79–89.

27 Hopf U *et al.* (1978) In vivo and in vitro binding of IgA to plasma membranes of hepatocytes. *Scand J Immunol* 8, 543–549.

28 Rifai A *et al.* (2000) The N-glycans determine the differential blood clearance and hepatic uptake of human immunoglobulin (Ig)A1 and IgA2 isotypes. *J Exp Med* 191 (12), 2171–2181.

29 Monteiro RC, van de Winkel JGJ (2003) IgA Fc receptors. *Annu Rev Immunol* 21, 177–204.

30 Moura IC *et al.* (2001) Identification of the transferrin receptor as a novel immunoglobulin (Ig)A1 receptor and its enhanced expression on mesangial cells in IgA nephropathy. *J Exp Med* 194, 417–425.

31 Henderson LA, Baynes JW, Thorpe SR (1982) Identification of sites of IgG catabolism in the rat. *Arch Biochem Biophys* 215 (1), 1–11.

32 Junghans RP, Anderson CL (1996) The protection receptor for IgG catabolism is the B2-microglobulin-containing neonatal intestinal transport receptor. *Proc Natl Acad Sci USA* 93, 5512–5516.

33 Chroneos ZC, Baynes JW, Thorpe SR (1995) Identification of liver endothelial cells as the primary site of IgM catabolism in the rat. *Arch Biochem Biophys* 319 (1), 63–73.

34 Vaerman JP *et al.* (1985) Neutralization of cholera toxin by rat bile secretory IgA antibodies. *Immunology* 54, 601–603.

35 Tamaru T, Brown WR (1985) IgA antibodies in rat bile inhibit cholera toxin-induced secretion in ileal loops in situ. *Immunology* 55, 579–583.

36 Cooper GN *et al.* (1984) Intestinal antibodies in rats following exposure to live *Vibrio cholerae*. *Aust J Exp Biol Med Sci* 62, 465–477.

37 Dahlgren UIH, Svanvik J, Eden CS (1986) Antibodies to *Escherichia coli* and anti-adhesive activity in paired serum, hepatic and gall bladder bile samples. *Scand J Immunol* 24, 251–260.

38 Loftness TJ *et al.* (1984) Occurrence of specific secretory immunoglobulin A in bile after inoculation of Giardia lamblia trophozoites into rat duodenum. *Gastroenterology* 87, 1022–1029.

39 Schiff JM, Huling SL, Jones AL (1986) Receptor-mediated uptake of asialoglycoprotein by the primate liver initiates both lysosomal and transcellular pathways. *Hepatology* 6, 837–847.

40 Cunningham-Rundles C (2001) Physiology of IgA and IgA deficiency. *J Clin Immunol* 21 (5), 303–309.

41 Van De Wiel A *et al.* (1987) Characteristics of serum IgA and liver IgA deposits in alcoholic liver disease. *Hepatology* 7 (1), 95–99.

42 Delacroix DL *et al.* (1983) Changes in size, subclass, and metabolic properties of serum immunoglobulin A in liver diseases and in other diseases with high serum immunoglobulin A. *J Clin Invest* 71, 358–367.

43 Seilles E *et al.* (1995) Serum secretory IgA and secretory component in patients with non-cirrhotic alcoholic liver diseases. *J Hepatol* 22, 278–285.

44 Goldin RD, Cattle S, Boylston TW (1986) IgA deposition in alcoholic liver disease. *J Clin Pathol* 39, 1181–1185.

45 Van De Wiel A *et al.* (1987) Spontaneous IgA synthesis by blood mononuclear cells in alcoholic liver disease. *Scand J Immunol* 25, 181–187.

46 Nouri-Aria KT *et al.* (1986) T and B cell function in alcoholic liver disease. *J Hepatol* 2, 195–207.

47 Nolan JP *et al.* (1986) IgA antibody to lipid A in alcoholic liver disease. *Lancet* 1, 176–179.

48 Staun-Olsen P *et al.* (1983) *Escherichia coli* antibodies in alcoholic liver disease. *Scand J Gastroenterol* 18, 889–896.

49 Bjorneboe M, Prytz H, Orskov F (1972) Antibodies to intestinal microbes in serum of patients with cirrhosis of the liver. *Lancet* 1, 58–60.

50 Lahnborg G, Friman L, Bergman L (1981) Reticuloendothelial function in patients with alcoholic cirrhosis. *Scand J Gastroenterol* 16, 481–489.

51 Van De Wiel A, Schuurman H, Kater L (1987) Alcoholic liver disease: an IgA-associated disorder. *Scand J Gastroenterol* 22, 1025–1030.

52 Van De Wiel A *et al.* (1986) Characteristics of IgA deposits in liver and skin of patients with liver disease. *Am J Clin Pathol* 86, 724–730.

53 Nagore N, Scheuer PJ (1988) Does a linear pattern of sinusoidal IgA deposition distinguish between alcoholic an diabetic liver disease? *Liver* 8 (5), 281–286.

54 Viitala K *et al.* (1997) Serum IgA, IgG, and IgM antibodies directed against acetaldehyde-derived epitopes: relationship to liver disease severity and alcohol consumption. *Hepatology* 25 (6), 1418–1424.

55 Parlesak A, Schafer C, Bode C (2002) IgA against gut-derived endotoxins: does it contribute to suppression of hepatic inflammation in alcohol-induced liver disease? *Dig Dis Sci* 47 (4), 760–766.

56 Fukuda Y, Imoto M, Hayakawa T (1985) Serum levels of secretory immunoglobulin A in liver disease. *Am J Gastroenterol* 80, 237–241.

57 Palmer JM *et al.* (2000) Secretory autoantibodies in primary biliary cirrhosis (PBC). *Clin Exp Immunol* 122 (3), 423–428.

58 Murakami J *et al.* (1999) Functional B-cell response in intrahepatic lymphoid follicles in chronic hepatitis C. *Hepatology* 30 (1), 143–150.

59 Pouria S, Feehally J (1999) Glomerular IgA deposition in liver disease. *Nephrol Dialysis Transplant* 14, 2279–2282.

60 Newell G (1987) Cirrhotic glomerulonephritis: incidence, morphology, clinical features, and pathogenesis. *Am J Kidney Dis* 9 (3), 183–190.

61 Launay P *et al.* (2000) Fcá receptor (CD89) mediates the development of immunoglobulin A (IgA) nephropathy (Berger's disease). Evidence for pathogenic soluble receptor-IgA complexes in patients and CD89 transgenic mice. *J Exp Med* 191, 1999–2009.

62 Nakamoto Y *et al.* (1981) Characteristics of hepatic IgA glomerulonephritis as the major part. *Virchows Arch A* 392, 45–54.

3 Basic concepts in pathobiology

3.1 Hepatocyte apoptosis and necrosis

Henning Schulze-Bergkamen, Marcus Schuchmann and Peter R. Galle

Introduction

The balance between cell division and cell death is a basic feature of the development and maintenance of liver homeostasis. There is increasing evidence that inappropriately controlled cell death is associated with several liver diseases. Liver failure and liver cancer are prototypical settings with uncontrolled massive cell death, on the one hand, or resistance to apoptosis, which is considered to be a hallmark of cancer cells, on the other hand. From the point of view of a metazoan organism, a single cell has many ways to die or survive at the wrong time: one separates an impairment of the intrinsic active cell death programme, apoptosis, from death due to (oncotic) necrosis, autophagy or mitotic catastrophe.

This chapter will mainly focus on the molecular mechanisms involved in the apoptotic cell death programme. Possible interactions between non-apoptotic and apoptotic cell death pathways are delineated, and new targets for the design of therapeutics that are aimed at modulating the death of liver cells are discussed.

The phenomenon of apoptosis and its morphology

Apoptosis is a common property of multicellular organisms in order to eliminate unwanted and potentially harmful cells. Apoptosis is actively controlled and occurs in a programmed fashion; thus, it is also referred to as programmed cell death (PCD).

Morphological observations, which today are recognized as distinct apoptotic morphological changes, were first described by Carl Vogt in 1842. The phenomenon of PCD was first called apoptosis (Greek, meaning 'falling off') in 1972, occurring in the liver after portal vein ligation [1]. However, it took about two decades before the importance of active cell death became generally accepted as a mechanism of controlling tissue and organ cellularity in concert with its functional counterpart, mitosis. Apoptosis is now known to play a fundamental role in physiological processes such as mammalian development and immune reactions [2]. During embryonic growth, apoptosis is the main mechanism for the removal of unnecessary tissue. In the adult organism, apoptosis regulates the balance between cell proliferation and death. When cells are no longer needed, infected, aged or have become seriously damaged, they are cleared by apoptosis [3]. In the immune system, potentially autoreactive and useless immune cells are mainly eliminated by apoptosis.

Morphological features in the pathobiology of liver diseases, now recognized as part of the apoptotic process, have been described in earlier chapters. Terms such as 'shrinking necrosis', 'acidophil bodies' and 'Councilman bodies' were used to describe apoptotic hepatocytes before the term 'apoptosis' was coined [4]. Along with the distinct morphological alterations, apoptosis is accompanied by various biochemical changes. As these changes are not specific for hepatocyte apoptosis, morphological assessment still presents the 'gold standard' for the identification of apoptotic cell death.

During the process of apoptosis, cells shrink and lose their contact with neighbouring cells [5]. Chromatin condenses at the nuclear membrane and the nucleolus dissociates. At the same time, the cytoplasm shows condensation and the formation of cytoplasmic blebs ('zeiosis'). Fragmentation of the cytoplasm and the nucleus results in membrane-bound, subcellular fragments, referred to as apoptotic bodies, which still contain intact organelles.

An inherent part of the apoptotic programme is the rapid phagocytosis of apoptotic bodies. Apoptotic hepatocytes are mainly phagocytosed by Kupffer cells. This process requires the recognition of membrane markers that are expressed on the outer surface of apoptotic cells [6]. An important signal for removal is the outside exposure of phosphatidylserine, which is normally localized exclusively to the inner leaflet of the plasma membrane. However, in liver cells, the asialoglycoprotein receptor may mainly mediate the clearance of apoptotic cells [7].

Phagocytosis of apoptotic cells is typically not accompanied by profound inflammatory reactions. Apoptotic bodies maintain their membrane integrity, thus avoiding the liberation of potentially toxic intracellular contents. In addition, the clearance by Kupffer cells is a rapid process, which prevents triggering of the immune response that may follow spontaneous lysis of apoptotic bodies. However, in pathological conditions, hepatocellular apoptosis may cause inflammatory reactions such as infiltration of neutrophils [8]. The same applies for necrosis, in which membrane integrity is lost, and the resulting cytolysis elicits an inflammatory response [9].

Presumably, the most remarkable feature of apoptosis is its highly regulated nature. The molecular pathways leading to apoptosis are tightly controlled by a complex network of proteins and their endogenous inhibitors. Various checkpoints in apoptosis pathways allow the cell to prevent the engagement of the death machinery under physiological conditions or to start or continue the death programme in pathological conditions.

Biochemistry of apoptosis

As a result of the activation of intracellular proteases and endonucleases, profound biochemical changes such as DNA fragmentation and degradation of cellular proteins accompany apoptosis.

Transglutaminases

Transglutaminases are a family of thiol- and Ca^{2+}-dependent acyltransferases, which catalyse cross-links between glutamine and lysine residues. Transglutaminase 2 is known to be induced during the *in vivo* apoptotic programme and appears to be required for the formation of the rigid structure of the tightly scaled apoptotic bodies that contain extensively cross-linked proteins. Recently, it has been shown that the clearance of apoptotic hepatocytes is defective in the absence of transglutaminase 2, resulting in the accumulation of apoptotic cells and inflammatory reactions [10].

Proteases

Apoptosis is accompanied by the proteolytic breakdown of structural proteins and proteins involved in signalling [11]. The activation of cysteinyl aspartate-specific proteases, caspases, is central to most apoptotic pathways and occurs in a programmed fashion. Originally, caspases were identified in the nematode *Caenorhabditis elegans* [12]. The human genome encodes 13 distinct caspases. Caspases are synthesized as inactive precursors. Upon specific cleavage at defined aspartate residues, they are activated. The so-called 'initiator caspases', including caspase-2, -8, -9 and -10, are recruited to large protein complexes such as the death-inducing signalling complex (DISC) or the apoptosome (see below). These caspases cleave and activate 'executioner' caspases, mainly caspase-3, -6, and -7, which subsequently cleave other proteins, e.g. poly-(ADP-ribose) polymerase or histone H1. Caspase activation has been viewed as being synonymous with apoptotic cell death. However, caspases also contribute to processes that do not culminate in cell death [13]. For

example, caspases-1, -4 and -5 are involved in inflammatory cytokine production and may not propagate cell death signals.

Apart from caspases, other proteases such as cathepsins have been implicated in hepatocyte apoptosis. Cathepsins are among the most abundant lysosomal enzymes. Activation of death receptors as well as different stress stimuli can trigger permeabilization of lysosomes, resulting in a translocation of cathepsins into the cytoplasm. Cathepsin activity can result in apoptotic features, dependent on and independent of caspase activity [14]. Cathepsin B actively participates in hepatocyte apoptosis, e.g. after exposure of hepatocytes to tumour necrosis factor (TNF) [15]. In cathepsin B knockout mice, hepatocytes are resistant to TNF-mediated apoptosis [16]. Inhibition of cathepsin B attenuates hepatic injury after bile duct ligation [17].

Calpains have also been implicated in apoptotic cell death in the liver after ischaemic injury [18]. Calpains are a group of calcium-dependent, non-lysosomal cysteine proteases contributing to cell injury by proteolysis of a plethora of substrates.

Endonucleases

Endonuclease activity results in a characteristic fragmentation of genomic DNA into oligonucleosomes ('DNA laddering'). First, DNA is cleaved into 300- and 50-kb fragments [19]. Second, DNA is cleaved into 180- to 200-bp fragments, resulting from multiple single-stranded nicks in the internucleosomal linker region.

Methods for the investigation of apoptosis

There is general agreement that the only universal features of apoptosis are the distinct morphological changes, such as chromatin condensation and nuclear fragmentation [20]. Widely used methods include the identification of the characteristic internucleosomal DNA fragmentation by DNA laddering after gel electrophoresis [5] or an *in situ* demonstration using the terminal deoxynucleotidyl transferase-mediated deoxyuridine triphosphate nick end labelling (TUNEL) assay [21]. DNA laddering or positive TUNEL staining, however, are not an unequivocal proof of apoptosis, as they may not distinguish internucleosomal DNA cleavage of apoptosis from the pattern of DNA cleavage in necrosis, e.g. in the model of bile duct ligation-associated liver injury [22]. An evaluation of the cellular morphology by electron microscopy may additionally be performed.

Some routine flow cytometry methods are based on the fact that DNA fragmentation is associated with a decrease in the DNA binding of dyes such as propidium iodide, which can be readily detected by flow cytometry [23].

Detection of proteins involved in the apoptotic process is an additional possibility for assessing apoptosis, although most candidate proteins are not absolutely specific for apoptosis. Another marker for apoptosis is phosphatidylserine, which is externalized at the cell membrane in the early phase of apoptosis and can be detected by annexin V labelling in flow cytometry [24].

An additional approach to investigate apoptosis pathways is to monitor the activity of caspases. A number of assays have been developed that measure caspase activity through the use of specific fluorogenic substrates [25]. In addition, cleaved caspase substrates such as cytokeratin 18 can be detected by enzyme-linked immunosorbent assay (ELISA) or by immunoblotting, e.g. in the sera of patients undergoing liver injury. It is important to note, however, that caspase activity does not automatically reflect apoptosis cascades (see below).

Activation of mitochondria is a central event in apoptosis, but also occurs in other modes of cell death. It is reflected by a mitochondrial outer membrane permeabilization (MOMP), which can be measured by flow cytometry or by detection of proteins released from the mitochondrial space (e.g. cytochrome *c*).

In conclusion, no specific assay or parameter, except the morphological changes *in vivo*, allows a clear distinction between apoptosis and other cell death patterns.

Mechanisms of apoptosis

Although apoptosis of hepatocytes can be triggered by several different stimuli, apoptotic signalling is mainly transduced by two major molecular pathways, an extrinsic pathway mediated by death receptors on the cell surface and an intrinsic pathway, which is triggered at the mitochondrial level (Fig. 1). Both pathways culminate in the activation of caspases and endonucleases, which ultimately degrade the cellular constituents.

Extrinsic death pathway

The extrinsic death pathway is initiated by binding of death receptor ligands to specific death receptors on the cell surface (Fig. 2). Death receptors belong to the TNF superfamily, which is characterized by a sequence of two to five cysteine-rich extracellular repeats. The death receptors share a homologous intracellular death domain (DD), which is essential for the transduction of the apoptotic signal [26]. The most widely expressed death receptors on hepatocytes are CD95 (Fas/APO-1) and TNF receptor 1 (CD120a).

CD95 (Fas/APO-1)/CD95L

Among the death receptors, CD95 has been characterized most extensively [27]. It is a widely expressed glycosylated transmembrane protein that is expressed in most tissues. Hepatocytes constitutively express CD95 on their surface, rendering the liver highly sensitive towards CD95-mediated apoptosis [28]. Thus, mice injected with agonistic CD95 antibodies rapidly die of liver failure. Correspondingly, human hepatocytes are highly sensitive to CD95 triggering *in vitro* [28,29]. The ligand of CD95, CD95L, is a transmembrane protein mainly expressed on activated T and B cells, as well as in immune-privileged sites such as the testis and eyes. Under pathological conditions, CD95L is also found in the liver, e.g. on activated T cells and on hepatocytes. In addition to a membrane-bound form, a soluble form of CD95L exists, which is generated by extracellular metalloproteinase activity [30].

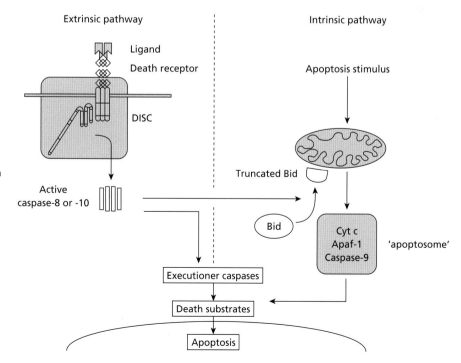

Fig. 1 The two main pathways for the initiation of apoptosis. Apoptosis can be triggered by two alternative pathways. The extrinsic pathway is initiated by binding of ligands to specific death receptors on the cell surface. The intrinsic pathway is initiated at the mitochondria by various stimuli. Initiator caspases such as caspase-8, -9 and -10 activate executioner caspases such as caspase-3, -6 and -7. Executioner caspases cleave death substrates and, finally, apoptosis occurs. Apaf-1, apoptotic protease activating factor-1; cyt c, cytochrome c; DISC, death-inducing signalling complex.

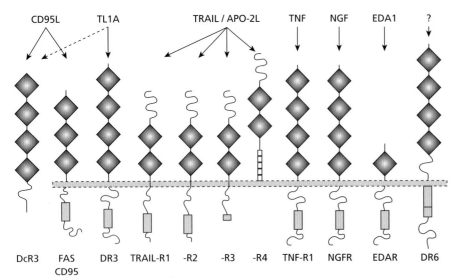

Fig. 2 Death receptors and their ligands. So far, eight members of the death receptor family have been characterized: TNFR1 (tumour necrosis factor receptor 1), CD95 (also known as APO-1 or Fas), DR3, TRAIL-R1 and TRAIL-R2 (TNF-related apoptosis-inducing ligand receptor 1 and 2), DR6, ectodysplasin A receptor (EDAR) and nerve growth factor receptor (NGFR). Death receptors are distinguished by a cytoplasmic region termed the death domain. After triggering by their corresponding ligands, a number of molecules are recruited to the death domains. Death ligands also interact with decoy receptors (DcRs) that do not possess death domains [TRAIL-R3, TRAIL-R4, DcR3 and osteoprotegrin (not shown)]. Receptors are given below the scheme, ligands at the top. The question mark indicates the unknown ligand for DR6. TL1A, endothelial cell-derived TNF-like factor.

The crucial determinant of death receptor signalling is the formation of a multimeric complex of proteins triggered by receptor cross-linking with their natural ligands. The structure formed is called the death-inducing signalling complex (DISC) [31]. The DISC of CD95 consists of trimerized CD95, the adapter Fas-associated death domain protein (FADD/Mort1), caspase-8 and caspase-10 [32]. FADD is recruited to the DISC after trimerization of CD95 and is capable of binding caspase-8 and -10, resulting in activation of the caspase cascade.

Depending on the cell type, either of two different pathways is activated downstream of CD95 after DISC formation. In type I cells, the death signal is propagated by a cascade that is initiated by the activation of large amounts of caspase-8 at the DISC and subsequent activation of downstream caspases. In type II cells, propagation of the apoptotic signal depends on its amplification via mitochondria [33]. *In vivo* studies with Bid-deficient mice indicate that hepatocytes are CD95 type II cells [34].

TNF

TNFR1 can signal a diverse range of activities including apoptosis, proliferation and inflammation. Its ligand, TNF, is produced by many cell types, including lymphoid cells and macrophages, and also activates TNFR2. At least one of these two TNF receptors is present in almost every cell [35]. Although most of the biological activities of TNF appear to be transduced by TNFR1, many can also be mediated by TNFR2. Exposure to TNF results in activation of transcription factors, such as AP-1 and NFκB. Following ligand-induced trimerization, TNFR1 recruits a multivalent adapter molecule, termed TNFR1-associated death domain protein, which binds to a number of signalling molecules such as TRAF2, FADD and RIP. TNF-induced apoptosis is most likely to be mediated via FADD-induced caspase-8 recruitment, while TRAF2 and RIP recruitment results in activation of the protein kinase JNK, AP-1 and NFκB. NFκB and

AP-1 mediate important immunoregulatory functions. NFκB activation can also protect cells against apoptosis.

TNF-related apoptosis-inducing ligand (TRAIL)

The death receptor ligand TRAIL is a type II transmembrane protein that interacts with at least five members of the TNF receptor superfamily [36]. TRAIL rapidly induces apoptosis in a wide variety of transformed cell lines. TRAIL-R1 and -R2 contain a cytoplasmic death domain and are capable of transducing an apoptotic signal upon ligation of TRAIL [37]. TRAIL-R1 and -R2 are also present on hepatocytes. However, it is debatable whether the TRAIL receptor is expressed on hepatocytes and whether these cells are sensitive to the specific ligand TRAIL [38].

Transforming growth factor (TGF)-beta

TGF-β1 can induce growth arrest and apoptosis in many cell types including hepatocytes [39]. The specific high-affinity receptors of TGF-β1 are present on essentially all cells, and TGF-β1 is expressed in most tissues. TGF-β1 is released, e.g. from activated hepatic stellate cells (HSC), and acts as a pro-fibrogenic master cytokine by the following mechanisms:
· It stimulates the transdifferentiation of HSC into myofibroblasts.
· It stimulates matrix synthesis in myofibroblasts.
· It inhibits matrix degradation.
· It induces apoptosis of hepatocytes.

Intrinsic death pathway

The intrinsic pathway is initiated at the mitochondrial level. Mitochondria act as integrating sensors of various death stimuli. A range of BH3-only members of the Bcl-2 family (see below) trigger the mitochondrial signalling cascade by acting as sentinels for cell stress, damage or infection [40]. Upon activation, they are mobilized to initiate mitochondrial outer membrane permeabilizatiion (MOMP) through post-translational modification, resulting in the release of effector molecules such as cytochrome *c*, Smac/DIABLO (second mitochondrial-derived activator of caspase/directed IAP binding protein with low pI) and apoptosis-inducing factor (AIF) from the intermembranous space of mitochondria. Once cytochrome *c* is released into the cytosol, the apoptosome is assembled, which is a multiprotein complex in which Apaf-1 serves as an oligomerization platform for assembly and autoproteolytic activation of caspase-9. Subsequently, caspase-9 activates further downstream caspases. Smac/DIABLO facilitates caspase activation by sequestering caspase inhibitors. AIF is thought to induce apoptotic changes in a caspase-independent manner.

Molecules involved in the regulation of hepatocyte apoptosis

A variety of molecules influence the apoptotic sensitivity of hepatocytes in physiological and pathological conditions. Key molecules that are thought to play a major role in hepatic apoptosis pathways are discussed below.

p53

Mutations in the *TPp53* gene (the gene that encodes human p53) are the most common genetic alteration observed in human cancer [41]. p53, as a guardian of the genome, transduces the diversity of signals arising from stress and damage into tumour-suppressive apoptotic and growth-arresting responses. p53 can be activated by kinases such as the DNA-dependent protein kinase and ATM (ataxia telangiectasia, mutated). ATM phosphorylates p53, which leads to the abrogation of p53 binding to the ubiquitin ligase Mdm-2 and activation of p53. Subsequently, p53 regulates the expression of several pro- and antiapoptotic genes at transcriptional and posttranscriptional levels. For example, in the context of DNA damage, p53 can result in the transcriptional activation of the BH3-only proteins Puma and Noxa, which can promote MOMP. In addition, p53 can transcriptionally activate death receptors as well as death ligands. A transcription-independent proapoptotic effect involves direct interactions of p53 and MOMP inducers at the mitochondrial level.

Bcl-2 family

The Bcl-2 family is a well-established family of proteins playing a pivotal role in preserving mitochondrial integrity. Common to all Bcl-2 family members are the Bcl-2 homology regions (BH1–4). These proteins are predominantly localized to the outer mitochondrial membrane (OMM), but also to other cellular membranes. The family is split into multidomain antiapoptotic proteins (e.g. Bcl-2, Bcl-x$_L$ and Mcl-1), multidomain proapoptotic proteins containing three BH domains (e.g. Bax and Bak) and the proapoptotic BH3-only proteins containing only one BH region (e.g. Bid, Bim, Noxa, Puma). Multidomain proapoptotic Bcl-2 proteins are thought to catalyse MOMP by triggering oligomerization of BH3-only proteins (Fig. 3). BH3-only proteins most probably initiate MOMP by inducing

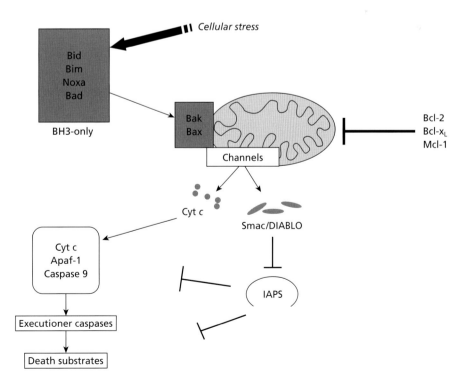

Fig. 3 Regulation of mitochondrial activation. Various stimuli can initiate mitochondrial activation. A subfamily of proapoptotic Bcl-2 proteins, the 'BH3-only proteins', act as sentinels for cell stress and damage and can be mobilized to initiate mitochondrial outer membrane permeabilization (MOMP) by triggering oligomerization of Bax and/or Bak in the outer mitochondrial membrane. Oligomerization results in the formation of channels that permit the escape of several molecules into the cytoplasm.

oligomerization of Bax and Bak in the OMM [42]. Bax and Bak can form channels in the OMM through which many proteins escape from the mitochondrial intermembranous space. BH3-only proteins fall into two subfamilies: those that can directly trigger opening of the Bax–Bak channel to precipitate MOMP (such as Bid and Bim) and those that sensitize the opening of the channel by neutralizing members of the antiapoptotic Bcl-2 family (such as Puma and Noxa). The antiapoptotic members, Bcl-2 representing the paradigm, mainly reside in the OMM and counter the effect of proapoptotic members.

Inhibitor of apoptosis (IAP) family

In humans, eight members of the IAP family have been identified so far, including XIAP, c-IAP1/2 and survivin. IAPs are endogenous inhibitors of caspases and therefore counteract apoptosis. They may also function as ubiquitin ligases, promoting the degradation of caspases. Some of the proteins that are released from mitochondria, e.g. Smac/DIABLO, can bind to IAPs and thereby relieve their caspase inhibition.

NFκB

NFκB was originally discovered as a result of its role in regulating gene expression in immune and inflammatory responses. However, activation of NFκB can protect liver cells from the apoptotic cascade induced by TNF and other stimuli, mainly by its effect on the transcription of antiapoptotic genes, e.g. c-FLIP, cellular IAPs and Bcl-x_L [43].

FLIP

FLIPs [FADD-like interleukin-1β-converting enzyme-like protease (FLICE/caspase-8)-inhibitory proteins] interfere directly at the level of death receptors. In human cells, two splice variants, a long form (FLIP$_L$) and a short form (FLIP$_S$), have been identified, both sharing structural homology with procaspase-8 but lacking catalytic activity. The structural homology allows FLIP molecules to bind to the DISC and thereby prevent the activation of caspase-8 [2].

Regulation of apoptosis under physiological conditions

Apoptosis under physiological conditions allows the removal of damaged or unwanted cells with virtually no proinflammatory response in the surrounding tissue. In rodents, only about one to five apoptotic cells per 10 000 hepatocytes are found [44], preferentially located in zone 3 around the hepatic venules [45]. It has been proposed that hepatocytes originate from the portal area and progress towards the perivenular region, where they are eliminated via apoptosis.

On increased functional demand, e.g. in overfeeding, in pregnancy, during severe protein loss or after treatment with a wide range of drugs (such as phenobarbital), rodent liver enlarges as a result of hypertrophy and hyperplasia. Once the stimulus is removed, the liver returns to its normal size by removing excessive hepatocytes via apoptosis.

Regulation of apoptosis under pathological conditions

Balance between cell division and cell death is a basic feature in the development and maintenance of liver homeostasis. Disturbances in this balance can cause liver diseases: too much cell death can cause liver injury, too little cell death is a prerequisite for the development of hepatocellular carcinoma. Thus, a tight control of the equilibrium between life and death in the liver is necessary.

During liver injury, hepatocytes, endothelial cells and cholangiocytes are driven to die by apoptosis due to the accumulation of cytokines such as TNF, IL-1β and interferon (IFN)-γ, as well as toxic metabolites, reactive oxygen species (ROS), bile acids and other substances.

Deregulation of the apoptosis programme is pathophysiologically involved in acute as well as chronic liver diseases, including cholestasis [46], hepatitis C [47] and alcoholic and non-alcoholic steatohepatitis (NASH) [48,49]. The most dramatic liver disease, fulminant hepatic failure (FHF), is characterized by uncontrolled massive death of hepatocytes [28], e.g. in patients with acute Wilson disease [50].

In both humans and rodents, apoptosis of hepatocytes in acute and chronic liver diseases is generally mediated by death receptors, in particular CD95. Increased CD95 expression has been observed in several liver diseases [28]. High CD95 expression makes hepatocytes quite sensitive to cytotoxic T cells expressing CD95L. In addition, the specific ligand of CD95, CD95L, can be detected in sera of patients with liver diseases. For example, CD95L derived from the placenta can enter the liver via the fetomaternal circulation causing liver damage in patients with haemolysis, elevated liver enzymes and low platelets (HELLP) syndrome [51]. In contrast, enhanced expression of CD95L on hepatocellular carcinoma cells might result in active destruction of lymphocytes, thus contributing to an immune evasion of cancer cells [52].

Caspases play an important role in liver injury. Their activity reflects the extent of liver injury. For example, increased caspase activation can be found not only in liver biopsies, but also in sera from patients with hepatitis C [53]. In addition, serum caspase activity correlates with the extent of steatosis and the progression of fibrosis [54]. Other proteases, such as cathepsin D, can induce cell death independently of caspase activity via triggering of AIF release from mitochondria [55].

Toxic and metabolic liver injury

Several drugs and toxins or their metabolites can cause liver injury by both necrosis and/or apoptosis. For many hepatotoxic substances, evidence for induction of apoptosis has been obtained, e.g. for ethanol [28], paracetamol [56] and cytostatic drugs [57]. In alcoholic hepatitis, hepatocyte apoptosis is frequently observed and correlates with disease severity. Apoptosis is partly induced by CYP2E1-dependent formation of ROS and lipid peroxides, which can cause mitochondrial activation. In addition, the CD95 as well as the TNF death receptor system contribute to liver injury.

In NASH, apoptosis is also involved in disease progression [49]. As in alcoholic hepatitis, expression of the death receptors CD95 and TNFR1 is significantly enhanced on hepatocytes [48]. In addition, the lysosomal enzyme cathepsin B is thought to play an important role in apoptosis induction in NASH, as its inhibition profoundly inhibits liver injury.

Viral hepatitis and immune-mediated liver diseases

Viral infections of the liver can cause apoptosis. Councilman bodies, a characteristic pathological feature of viral hepatitis, closely resemble apoptotic cells. Apoptosis can be induced either as a direct cytopathic effect of viruses or as a result of the host immune response. In hepatitis B or C, activated cytotoxic T cells expressing CD95L may kill infected hepatocytes expressing CD95 [28]. Other pathways, including the TNF system, have also been implicated in hepatocyte apoptosis during viral infection. Elimination of virus-infected cells by apoptosis may be counteracted by viral-encoded proteins, which abrogate apoptotic pathways, e.g. CrmA. In hepatitis C, multiple virus-derived proteins counteract apoptosis induction as a possible mechanism to maintain persistent infection [8].

In autoimmune hepatitis, lymphocytic infiltration also causes hepatocyte apoptosis. In host-vs.-graft reaction in allograft rejection, upregulation of apoptosis-associated factors, such as TGF-β1, is observed.

Cholestatic liver disease

Bile acids have been shown to trigger hepatocyte apoptosis by activation of death receptors, in particular CD95 [46]. Interestingly, CD95-dependent apoptosis has been described as being activated in the absence of ligand interaction. TRAIL-R2 is also transcriptionally induced in persistent cholestasis and is thought to contribute to liver injury [58].

Hepatic fibrosis

In contrast to physiological conditions, increased hepatocyte apoptosis under pathological conditions is associated with an inflammatory response. Upon persistent inflammation, fibrogenesis can occur, mainly as a consequence of the activation of hepatic stellate cells (HSC) following their transdifferentiation into myofibroblasts [59]. Kupffer cells, the major phagocytes of apoptotic bodies in the liver, can express death ligands and

proinflammatory cytokines, thereby accelerating hepatocyte apoptosis and inflammatory reactions. Importantly, HSC also engulf apoptotic bodies in the liver, a process that is associated with activation of quiescent HSC and with production of TGF-β, a potent profibrogenic cytokine.

Hepatocarcinogenesis

The development of hepatocellular carcinoma (HCC) has been associated with defective apoptosis and increased cell proliferation. HCC cells often show alterations in the expression of tumour suppressor genes, DNA repair genes, genes involved in the cell cycle and genes involved in apoptosis. Mutations in the tumour suppressor gene p53 are among the most common alterations observed in HCC [60]. The p53 protein is activated as a result of DNA damage. Dysfunctional p53 allows the tumour cell to escape apoptosis induction (see section on Molecules involved in the regulation of hepatocyte apoptosis). Other alterations leading to apoptosis resistance are downregulation of death receptors, such as CD95, or enhanced expression of anti-apoptotic proteins, such as Bcl-x$_L$. In addition, expression of CD95L enables HCC cells to actively kill immune cells [52].

Hepatocyte necrosis

Contrary to the controlled cellular death programme in apoptosis, necrosis (or recently renamed oncosis or oncotic necrosis) is a more chaotic mechanism of cell death. It results from metabolic disruption with energy depletion and loss of adenosine triphosphate (ATP), ion dysregulation and enhanced degradative hydrolase activity. In the presence of oxygen, toxic oxygen species may be generated followed by lipid peroxidation. Loss of ATP leads to cellular oedema, rounding and swelling of mitochondria, dilation of the endoplasmic reticulum, lysosomal disruption and the formation of plasma membrane protrusions called blebs [61]. Bleb formation, which is caused by disrupted cellular volume control and cytoskeletal disturbances, is reversible, e.g. after reoxygenation. If injury continues, necrotic cell death occurs by failure of the plasma membrane permeability barrier, leading to bleb rupture and the release of cellular components. The release of cellular contents triggers an inflammatory response in the surrounding tissue [1].

Similar to the intrinsic death pathway in apoptosis, damage to mitochondria appears to be a key event in early progression of necrosis [9]. In addition, proteases are involved in the induction of necrotic cell death. Calpains, for example, have been implicated as an intracellular mediator leading to necrosis. Upon activation, they dissociate from the membrane and exert proteolytic activity on a plethora of substrates, such as cytoskeletal and membrane proteins, resulting in an alteration of the mitochondrial membrane potential [62]. Interestingly, necrosis can also be regulated and may involve caspase activation [63].

Cell death by necrosis can frequently be observed in ischaemic injury in the liver, e.g. during shock, liver surgery or transplantation. A typical stimulus for necrosis in the liver is cold hepatic ischaemia followed by reperfusion, which leads to necrosis within minutes [64].

Recent studies report a major role of necrotic cell death in chronic liver injury as well. In the model of experimental bile duct ligation in rats, liver injury is almost exclusively caused by necrosis [22]. However, CD95-mediated apoptosis has also been discussed as contributing to liver injury in cholestasis [46].

Other forms of cell death in liver injury

During the last decade, most research activities in hepatology dealing with liver injury focused on the evaluation of apoptosis pathways. In the past, the terms 'programmed cell death (PCD)' and 'apoptosis' have frequently been used as synonyms, and PCD as well as apoptosis has been equated with caspase activation. However, there is accumulating evidence that hepatocytes can die via PCD without typical features of apoptosis or necrosis and independently of caspase activation. Caspase-independent cell death is an important protective mechanism for an organism to eliminate harmful cells in case of a failure of caspase activation [13]. Thus far, various forms of caspase-independent PCD have been described, depicted as autophagy, paraptosis, mitotic catastrophe, anoikis and others (Fig. 4). In autophagy, cells die by chewing themselves up [65]. Unlike apoptosis, cells are degraded with little or no help from phagocytes and use their own lysosomal system for degradation. Autophagy helps to eliminate longlived proteins and plays an important role in cellular remodelling. Hepatocytes of liver grafts show autophagic vacuoles after reperfusion, suggesting that warm reperfusion acts as a stress stimulus triggering autophagic degeneration [66]. The role of autophagy in the pathogenesis of other liver diseases continues to be explored. In carcinogenesis of HCC, breakdown of autophagy might play an important role [67].

The differentiation between autophagy and another form of cell death, called paraptosis, is not clear so far. Paraptosis is characterized by swelling of mitochondria and the endoplasmic reticulum (ER), leading to cytoplasmic vacuolation [68]. Its role in liver injury has not yet been defined. The same applies for another type of cell death depicted as mitotic catastrophe. It results from abnormal mitosis due to defective cell cycle checkpoints and leads to the formation of interphase cells with multiple micronuclei [69]. Anoikis occurs if hepatocytes lose their contact with the extracellular matrix. Indicators of apoptosis do not appear until the cell has become non-adherent, because the loss of adhesion is the cause and not the result of cell death. For hepatocyte survival, β1 integrin-mediated attachment to hepatic extracellular matrix is a prerequisite to avoid anoikis [70].

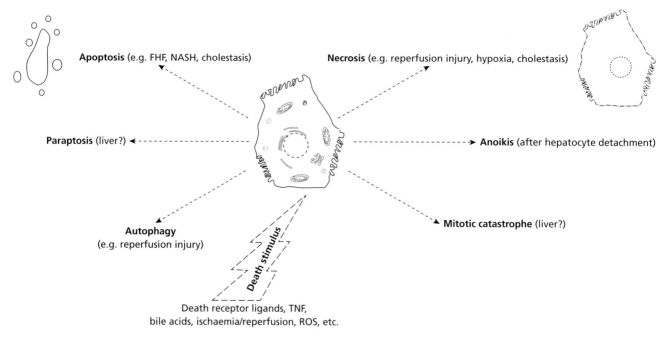

Fig. 4 Modes of cell death in the liver. Hepatocytes can die from different modes of cell death. Apoptosis occurs in physiological as well as pathological conditions and represents a highly organized and genetically controlled type of cell death leading to shrinkage of the cell and disintegration into small apoptotic bodies. Paraptosis involves cytoplasmic vacuolation independent of caspase activity and in the absence of typical nuclear changes. Its role in liver diseases is not yet defined. Necrosis (or oncosis/oncotic necrosis) leads to cellular oedema and disruption of the cell membrane, e.g. in reperfusion liver injury. In autophagy, the cell's own lysosomal system leads to degradation of organelles and cell death. Breakdown of autophagy has been hypothesized to contribute to the development of hepatocellular carcinoma. Anoikis occurs if hepatocytes lose their contact with the extracellular matrix. Mitotic catastrophe occurs after mitotic failure, but has not been described as contributing to liver injury so far. FHF, fulminant hepatic failure; NASH, non-alcoholic steatohepatitis; ROS, reactive oxygen species; TNF, tumour necrosis factor.

Mixed patterns of cell death in liver injury

Hepatocyte apoptosis and necrosis as well as other forms of cell death may occur in parallel in pathological conditions. The contribution of certain specific death modes to liver injury is often elusive for the following reasons:

1 Morphological and molecular overlaps. Although many biochemical and immunological assays have been developed to characterize apoptosis, none of the changes monitored in these assays is unique to apoptosis (see the section on Methods for the investigation of apoptosis).

2 Certain death stimuli may lead to different modes of cell death. In various liver diseases, critical death stimuli have been identified. However, death stimuli such as cytokines, bile acids or ROS can trigger different modes of cell death in parallel. For example, if detoxification of ROS is impaired in the liver, oxidative stress occurs, e.g. in obstructive cholestasis [71]. A decision between necrotic and apoptotic cell death upon oxidative stress may depend on the intracellular ATP level. A marked depletion in ATP facilitates necrotic cell death, whereas high levels of ATP favour the development of apoptosis.

3 Molecular switches between different modes of cell death. Apoptosis induction may be followed by secondary necrosis, when ATP is eventually depleted during apoptosis [72]. Ineffective elimination of apoptotic bodies may also result in a switch from apoptosis to necrosis caused by an inflammatory response. In contrast, if the necrosis pathway is inhibited, death stimuli may eventually force the cell into apoptosis [64]. Several mediators, such as nitric oxide (NO), have been described to function as potent modulators of death programmes by ATP depletion or inactivation of caspases.

4 Activation of proteases may result in different death modes. Lysosomal proteases, such as cathepsins, may trigger different death modes in liver injury. Low release of lysosomal proteases triggers apoptosis, whereas massive release leads to necrosis [73]. Calpains have been implicated as an intracellular mediator leading to apoptosis as well as necrosis [74,75].

5 Cross-talk between different proteolytic systems. Cross-talk between caspases, cathepsins, calpains and other proteases influences the mode of cell death in liver injury and further complicates the differentiation between specific death programmes.

6 Underestimation of apoptotic cell death. The extent of apoptotic cell death is frequently underestimated because: (i) apoptosis is a rapid event with an estimated duration of 2–3 h; and (ii) only scattered single cells may be affected, and apoptotic bodies, which are readily eliminated, are small.

Targeting cell death in liver diseases

Liver injury is caused by a complex picture of cell death patterns. As the apoptosis programme is deranged in a series of liver diseases, many therapeutic approaches target the apoptotic cascade (Fig. 5). A series of publications describe successful rescue of animals from FHF, for example by blocking caspase activity [76], expression of antiapoptotic Bcl-2 family members [77] and expression of dominant negative FADD/MORT1 [78,79]. The discovery of RNA interference opens up new opportunities to specifically target apoptosis pathways, e.g. through down-regulating genes encoding CD95 or caspase-8 [80,81]. Other approaches target death receptor ligands. For example, FLINT (LY498919) has been shown to effectively bind CD95L and LIGHT, another TNF receptor family ligand, and may have therapeutic benefits in liver diseases in which the pathogenesis is believed to be related to inappropriate apoptosis [82].

Caspases are an attractive target not only for antiapoptotic interventions in acute, but also in chronic hepatitis [83]. Caspase inhibitors have already entered clinical trials in patients with liver diseases, e.g. in patients with hepatitis C [84]. However, inhibition of caspases might not be effective in

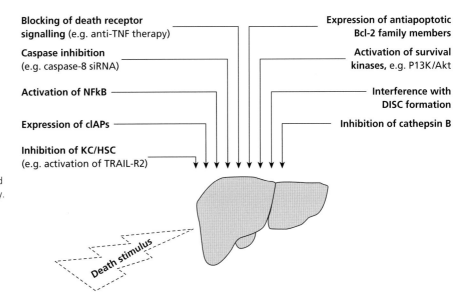

Fig. 5 Prosurvival strategies for the treatment of liver diseases. Much effort has been devoted to the search for strategies to inhibit liver injury. Most of these efforts target apoptosis pathways, such as inhibition of caspases and death receptor signalling. KC, Kupffer cells; HSC, hepatic stellate cells; cIAP, cellular inhibitor of apoptosis; DISC, death-inducing signalling complex; siRNA, small interfering RNA.

certain complex pathophysiological conditions for the following reasons:

• Interference with caspase activity may not alter the extent of death, but rather the shape of the demise [85].

• Caspase inhibitors can prevent the appearance of certain, but not all features of apoptosis [86].

• Deletion of single caspases may have only localized and partial effects on cell death, whereas broad-range caspase inhibitors may inhibit unrelated proteases, whose activity may be necessary for survival.

• Several forms of cell death, including apoptosis-like death, can occur in a caspase-independent manner or are even accelerated by caspase inhibitors.

Other approaches to reducing cell death in liver injury include inhibition of calpains and cathepsins. Calpain inhibition reduces the number of apoptotic sinusoidal endothelial cells (SEC). This may be of special interest for the prevention of reperfusion injuries in clinical transplantation, as apoptosis of SEC is a key feature in this scenario [87]. Inhibition of cathepsin B is of therapeutic interest, e.g. for the attenuation of hepatic injury in cholestasis [88] or reperfusion injury [89].

Targeting of TGF-β may also inhibit hepatocyte apoptosis. Experimental therapeutic strategies are focused on inactivation of TGF-β by overexpression of soluble TGF-β receptors as scavengers, by intracellular overexpression of mediators inhibiting TGF-β signalling or by inhibition of TGF-β synthesis.

Other approaches include inhibition of MOMP by expression of antiapoptotic members of the Bcl-2 family as well as pharmacological inhibition of the permeability transition pore of mitochondrion-specific ion channels.

Growth factors such as hepatocyte growth factor have been shown to inhibit CD95-mediated apoptosis of human hepatocytes and might be applied in liver diseases in which the CD95 system is involved [90].

The design of antiapoptotic therapeutic strategies should consider the overlapping death programmes in hepatocytes. Inhibition of apoptosis may have little effect on the survival of liver cells if a decrease in apoptosis is compensated for by an increase in the fractions of cells that undergo permanent growth arrest with features of cell senescence or die through the process of mitotic catastrophe. Considering the fact that switches between different cell death modes can occur that are dependent on the mediators and tissue conditions, targeting of individual death pathways may not be sufficient to ameliorate liver injury effectively. In addition, blocking of cell death in the liver may not only promote survival of hepatocytes, but also that of potentially harmful cells, including hepatic NKT cells. NKT cells are abundant in the normal liver and are thought to contribute to the pathophysiology of FHF and other forms of liver injury [91]. An antiapoptotic therapy regimen may also trigger liver fibrosis by preventing cell death of HSC [92]. Finally, promotion of cell survival in liver injury may favour carcinogenesis of HCC, as death of abnormal cells in the liver is an important process in preventing clonal expansion and tumour formation (Fig. 6).

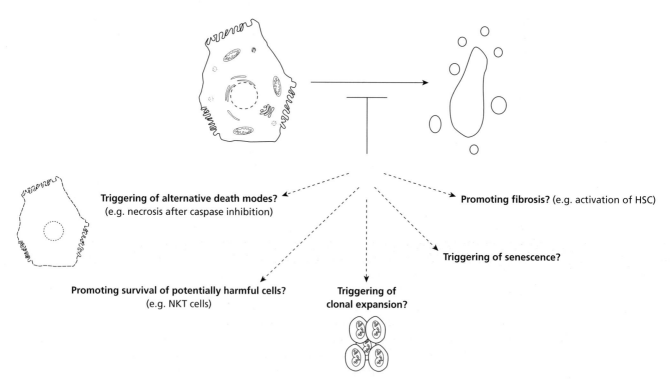

Fig. 6 Pitfalls of antiapoptotic therapy strategies for liver diseases. Targeting death pathways in the liver is a powerful tool for the treatment of liver diseases. However, possible side-effects should be considered. Senescence: a signal transduction programme leading to irreversible cell cycle arrest. HSC, hepatic stellate cells; NKT cells, natural killer T cells.

Despite possible limitations, the investigation of novel approaches for the inhibition of liver cell death will probably lead to new treatment options in clinical hepatology.

Conclusion

Death programmes in the liver enable the elimination of damaged and unwanted cells *in vivo*. In acute and chronic liver injury, the balance between death and survival is disturbed. Enhanced liver cell death through apoptosis and necrosis is a key pathogenic feature of liver diseases. However, under pathological conditions, various cell death patterns in hepatocytes cannot be classified as either necrosis or apoptosis, e.g. various forms of programmed cell death independent of caspase activity. In addition, overlaps between the signalling pathways of different death programmes make exclusive definitions artificial. It still remains elusive which factors determine the type of death. Research currently being conducted in this exciting field is likely to be beneficial for the future treatment of liver diseases.

References

1 Kerr JF, Wyllie AH, Currie AR (1972) Apoptosis: a basic biological phenomenon with wide-ranging implications in tissue kinetics. *Br J Cancer* 26 (4), 239–257.

2 Krammer PH (2000) CD95's deadly mission in the immune system. *Nature* 407 (6805), 789–795.

3 Jacobson MD, Weil M, Raff MC (1997) Programmed cell death in animal development. *Cell* 88 (3), 347–354.

4 Alison MR, Sarraf CE (1994) Liver cell death: patterns and mechanisms. *Gut* 35 (5), 577–581.

5 Wyllie AH, Kerr JF, Currie AR (1980) Cell death: the significance of apoptosis. *Int Rev Cytol* 68:251–306.

6 Savill J, Fadok V, Henson P *et al.* (1993) Phagocyte recognition of cells undergoing apoptosis. *Immunol Today* 14 (3), 131–136.

7 Dini L, Falasca L, Lentini A *et al.* (1993) Galactose-specific receptor modulation related to the onset of apoptosis in rat liver. *Eur J Cell Biol* 61 (2), 329–337.

8 Guicciardi ME, Gores GJ (2005) Apoptosis: a mechanism of acute and chronic liver injury. *Gut* 54 (7), 1024–1033.

9 Rosser BG, Gores GJ (1995) Liver cell necrosis: cellular mechanisms and clinical implications. *Gastroenterology* 108 (1), 252–275.

10 Szondy Z, Sarang Z, Molnar P *et al.* (2003) Transglutaminase 2–/– mice reveal a phagocytosis-associated crosstalk between macrophages and apoptotic cells. *Proc Natl Acad Sci USA* 100 (13), 7812–7817.

11 Patel T, Gores GJ, Kaufmann SH (1996) The role of proteases during apoptosis. *FASEB J* 10 (5), 587–597.

12 Miura M, Zhu H, Rotello R *et al.* (1993) Induction of apoptosis in fibroblasts by IL-1 beta-converting enzyme, a mammalian homolog of the C. elegans cell death gene ced-3. *Cell* 75 (4), 653–660.

13 Kroemer G, Martin SJ (2005) Caspase-independent cell death. *Nature Med* 11 (7), 725–730.

14 Jaattela M (2004) Multiple cell death pathways as regulators of tumour initiation and progression. *Oncogene* 23 (16), 2746–2756.

15 Werneburg NW, Guicciardi ME, Bronk SF *et al.* (2002) Tumor necrosis factor-alpha-associated lysosomal permeabilization is cathepsin B dependent. *Am J Physiol Gastrointest Liver Physiol* 283 (4), G947–956.

16 Guicciardi ME, Miyoshi H, Bronk SF *et al.* (2001) Cathepsin B knock-out mice are resistant to tumor necrosis factor-alpha-mediated hepatocyte apoptosis and liver injury: implications for therapeutic applications. *Am J Pathol* 159 (6), 2045–2054.

17 Canbay A, Guicciardi ME, Higuchi H *et al.* (2003) Cathepsin B inactivation attenuates hepatic injury and fibrosis during cholestasis. *J Clin Invest* 112 (2), 152–159.

18 Kohli V, Madden JF, Bentley RC *et al.* (1999) Calpain mediates ischemic injury of the liver through modulation of apoptosis and necrosis. *Gastroenterology* 116 (1), 168–178.

19 Oberhammer F, Wilson JW, Dive C *et al.* (1993) Apoptotic death in epithelial cells: cleavage of DNA to 300 and/or 50 kb fragments prior to or in the absence of internucleosomal fragmentation. *EMBO J* 12 (9), 3679–3684.

20 Cotter TG, al-Rubeai M (1995) Cell death (apoptosis) in cell culture systems. *Trends Biotechnol* 13 (4), 150–155.

21 Gavrieli Y, Sherman Y, Ben-Sasson SA (1992) Identification of programmed cell death in situ via specific labeling of nuclear DNA fragmentation. *J Cell Biol* 119 (3), 493–501.

22 Gujral JS, Liu J, Farhood A *et al.* (2004) Functional importance of ICAM-1 in the mechanism of neutrophil-induced liver injury in bile duct-ligated mice. *Am J Physiol Gastrointest Liver Physiol* 286 (3), G499–507.

23 Nicoletti I, Migliorati G, Pagliacci MC *et al.* (1991) A rapid and simple method for measuring thymocyte apoptosis by propidium iodide staining and flow cytometry. *J Immunol Methods* 139 (2), 271–279.

24 Homburg CH, de Haas M, von dem Borne AE *et al.* (1995) Human neutrophils lose their surface Fc gamma RIII and acquire annexin V binding sites during apoptosis in vitro. *Blood* 85 (2), 532–540.

25 Stennicke HR, Salvesen GS (1997) Biochemical characteristics of caspases-3, -6, -7, and -8. *J Biol Chem* 272 (41), 25719–25723.

26 Tartaglia LA, Ayres TM, Wong GH *et al.* (1993) A novel domain within the 55 kd TNF receptor signals cell death. *Cell* 74 (5), 845–853.

27 Schmitz I, Kirchhoff S, Krammer PH (2000) Regulation of death receptor-mediated apoptosis pathways. *Int J Biochem Cell Biol* 32 (11–12), 1123–1136.

28 Galle PR, Hofmann WJ, Walczak H *et al.* (1995) Involvement of the CD95 (APO-1/Fas) receptor and ligand in liver damage. *J Exp Med* 182 (5), 1223–1230.

29 Schulze-Bergkamen H, Untergasser A, Dax A *et al.* (2003) Primary human hepatocytes – a valuable tool for investigation of apoptosis and hepatitis B virus infection. *J Hepatol* 38 (6), 736–744.

30 Suda T, Hashimoto H, Tanaka M *et al.* (1997) Membrane Fas ligand kills human peripheral blood T lymphocytes, and soluble Fas ligand blocks the killing. *J Exp Med* 186 (12), 2045–2050.

31 Kischkel FC, Hellbardt S, Behrmann I *et al.* (1995) Cytotoxicity-dependent APO-1 (Fas/CD95)-associated proteins form a death-inducing signaling complex (DISC) with the receptor. *EMBO J* 14 (22), 5579–5588.

32 Lavrik I, Golks A, Krammer PH (2005) Death receptor signaling. *J Cell Sci* 118 (Pt 2), 265–267.

33 Scaffidi C, Fulda S, Srinivasan A *et al.* (1998) Two CD95 (APO-1/Fas) signaling pathways. *EMBO J* 17 (6), 1675–1687.

34 Li S, Zhao Y, He X *et al.* (2002) Relief of extrinsic pathway inhibition by the Bid-dependent mitochondrial release of Smac in Fas-mediated hepatocyte apoptosis. *J Biol Chem* 277 (30), 26912–26920.

35 Tartaglia LA, Goeddel DV (1992) Two TNF receptors. *Immunol Today* 13 (5), 151–153.

36 Wiley SR, Schooley K, Smolak PJ *et al.* (1995) Identification and characterization of a new member of the TNF family that induces apoptosis. *Immunity* 3 (6), 673–682.

37 Walczak H, Degli-Esposti MA, Johnson RS *et al.* (1997) TRAIL-R2: a novel apoptosis-mediating receptor for TRAIL. *EMBO J* 16 (17), 5386–5397.

38 Mori E, Thomas M, Motoki K *et al.* (2004) Human normal hepatocytes are susceptible to apoptosis signal mediated by both TRAIL-R1 and TRAIL-R2. *Cell Death Differ* 11 (2), 203–207.

39 Oberhammer FA, Pavelka M, Sharma S *et al.* (1992) Induction of apoptosis in cultured hepatocytes and in regressing liver by transforming growth factor beta 1. *Proc Natl Acad Sci USA* 89 (12), 5408–5412.

40 Huang DC, Strasser A (2000) BH3-only proteins – essential initiators of apoptotic cell death. *Cell* 103 (6), 839–842.

41 Levine AJ (1997) p53, the cellular gatekeeper for growth and division. *Cell* 88 (3), 323–331.

42 Danial NN, Korsmeyer SJ (2004) Cell death: critical control points. *Cell* 116 (2), 205–219.

43 Schuchmann M, Galle PR (2002) Dead or alive – NF-kappaB, the guardian which tips the balance. *J Hepatol* 36 (6), 827–828.

44 Bursch W, Taper HS, Lauer B *et al.* (1985) Quantitative histological and histochemical studies on the occurrence and stages of controlled cell death (apoptosis) during regression of rat liver hyperplasia. *Virchows Arch B Cell Pathol Incl Mol Pathol* 50 (2), 153–266.

45 Benedetti A, Jezequel AM, Orlandi F (1988) Preferential distribution of apoptotic bodies in acinar zone 3 of normal human and rat liver. *J Hepatol* 7 (3), 319–324.

46 Miyoshi H, Rust C, Roberts PJ *et al.* (1999) Hepatocyte apoptosis after bile duct ligation in the mouse involves Fas. *Gastroenterology* 117 (3), 669–677.

47 Patel T, Roberts LR, Jones BA *et al.* (1998) Dysregulation of apoptosis as a mechanism of liver disease: an overview. *Semin Liver Dis* 18 (2), 105–114.

48 Ribeiro PS, Cortez-Pinto H, Sola S *et al.* (2004) Hepatocyte apoptosis, expression of death receptors, and activation of NF-kappaB in the liver of nonalcoholic and alcoholic steatohepatitis patients. *Am J Gastroenterol* 99 (9), 1708–1717.

49 Feldstein AE, Canbay A, Angulo P *et al.* (2003) Hepatocyte apoptosis and fas expression are prominent features of human nonalcoholic steatohepatitis. *Gastroenterology* 125 (2), 437–443.

50 Strand S, Hofmann WJ, Grambihler A *et al.* (1998) Hepatic failure and liver cell damage in acute Wilson's disease involve CD95 (APO-1/Fas) mediated apoptosis. *Nature Med* 4 (5), 588–593.

51 Strand S, Strand D, Seufert R *et al.* (2004) Placenta-derived CD95 ligand causes liver damage in hemolysis, elevated liver enzymes, and low platelet count syndrome. *Gastroenterology* 126 (3), 849–858.

52 Strand S, Hofmann WJ, Hug H *et al.* (1996) Lymphocyte apoptosis induced by CD95 (APO-1/Fas) ligand-expressing tumor cells – a mechanism of immune evasion? *Nature Med* 2 (12), 1361–1366.

53 Bantel H, Lugering A, Poremba C *et al.* (2001) Caspase activation correlates with the degree of inflammatory liver injury in chronic hepatitis C virus infection. *Hepatology* 34 (4 Pt 1), 758–767.

54 Seidel N, Volkmann X, Langer F *et al.* (2005) The extent of liver steatosis in chronic hepatitis C virus infection is mirrored by caspase activity in serum. *Hepatology* 42 (1), 113–120.

55 Bidere N, Lorenzo HK, Carmona S *et al.* (2003) Cathepsin D triggers Bax activation, resulting in selective apoptosis-inducing factor (AIF) relocation in T lymphocytes entering the early commitment phase to apoptosis. *J Biol Chem* 278 (33), 31401–31411.

56 Tsukidate K, Yamamoto K, Snyder JW *et al.* (1993) Microtubule antagonists activate programmed cell death (apoptosis) in cultured rat hepatocytes. *Am J Pathol* 143 (3), 918–925.

57 Muller M, Strand S, Hug H *et al.* (1997) Drug-induced apoptosis in hepatoma cells is mediated by the CD95 (APO-1/Fas) receptor/ligand system and involves activation of wild-type p53. *J Clin Invest* 99 (3), 403–413.

58 Higuchi H, Grambihler A, Canbay A *et al.* (2004) Bile acids up-regulate death receptor 5/TRAIL-receptor 2 expression via a c-Jun N-terminal kinase-dependent pathway involving Sp1. *J Biol Chem* 279 (1), 51–60.

59 Canbay A, Friedman S, Gores GJ (2004) Apoptosis: the nexus of liver injury and fibrosis. *Hepatology* 39 (2), 273–278.

60 Staib F, Hussain SP, Hofseth LJ *et al.* (2003) TP53 and liver carcinogenesis. *Hum Mutat* 21 (3), 201–216.

61 Lemasters JJ, DiGuiseppi J, Nieminen AL *et al.* (1987) Blebbing, free Ca2+ and mitochondrial membrane potential preceding cell death in hepatocytes. *Nature* 325 (6099), 78–81.

62 Aguilar HI, Botla R, Arora AS *et al.* (1996) Induction of the mitochondrial permeability transition by protease activity in rats: a mechanism of hepatocyte necrosis. *Gastroenterology* 110 (2), 558–566.

63 Schwab BL, Guerini D, Didszun C *et al.* (2002) Cleavage of plasma membrane calcium pumps by caspases: a link between apoptosis and necrosis. *Cell Death Differ* 9 (8), 818–831.

64 Jaeschke H, Lemasters JJ (2003) Apoptosis versus oncotic necrosis in hepatic ischemia/reperfusion injury. *Gastroenterology* 125 (4), 1246–1257.

65 Gozuacik D, Kimchi A (2004) Autophagy as a cell death and tumor suppressor mechanism. *Oncogene* 23 (16), 2891–2906.

66 Lu Z, Dono K, Gotoh K *et al.* (2005) Participation of autophagy in the degeneration process of rat hepatocytes after transplantation following prolonged cold preservation. *Arch Histol Cytol* 68 (1), 71–80.

67 Shintani T, Klionsky DJ (2004) Autophagy in health and disease: a double-edged sword. *Science* 306 (5698), 990–995.

68 Sperandio S, de Belle I, Bredesen DE (2000) An alternative, nonapoptotic form of programmed cell death. *Proc Natl Acad Sci USA* 97 (26), 14376–14381.

69 Castedo M, Perfettini JL, Roumier T *et al.* (2004) Cell death by mitotic catastrophe: a molecular definition. *Oncogene* 23 (16), 2825–2837.

70 Pinkse GG, Voorhoeve MP, Noteborn M *et al.* (2004) Hepatocyte survival depends on beta1-integrin-mediated attachment of hepatocytes to hepatic extracellular matrix. *Liver Int* 24 (3), 218–226.

71 Gujral JS, Farhood A, Bajt ML *et al.* (2003) Neutrophils aggravate acute liver injury during obstructive cholestasis in bile duct-ligated mice. *Hepatology* 38 (2), 355–363.

72 Lemasters JJ, Nieminen AL, Qian T *et al.* (1998) The mitochondrial permeability transition in cell death: a common mechanism in necrosis, apoptosis and autophagy. *Biochim Biophys Acta* 1366 (1–2), 177–196.

73 Bursch W (2001) The autophagosomal–lysosomal compartment in programmed cell death. *Cell Death Differ* 8 (6), 569–581.

74 Squier MK, Miller AC, Malkinson AM *et al.* (1994) Calpain activation in apoptosis. *J Cell Physiol* 159 (2), 229–237.

75 Arora AS, de Groen P, Emori Y *et al.* (1996) A cascade of degradative hydrolase activity contributes to hepatocyte necrosis during anoxia. *Am J Physiol* 270 (2 Pt 1), G238–245.

76 Rodriguez I, Matsuura K, Ody C *et al.* (1996) Systemic injection of a tripeptide inhibits the intracellular activation of CPP32-like proteases in vivo and fully protects mice against Fas-mediated fulminant liver destruction and death. *J Exp Med* 184 (5), 2067–2072.

77 Lacronique V, Mignon A, Fabre M *et al.* (1996) Bcl-2 protects from lethal hepatic apoptosis induced by an anti-Fas antibody in mice. *Nature Med* 2 (1), 80–86.

78 Streetz K, Leifeld L, Grundmann D *et al.* (2000) Tumor necrosis factor alpha in the pathogenesis of human and murine fulminant hepatic failure. *Gastroenterology* 119 (2), 446–460.

79 Schuchmann M, Varfolomeev EE, Hermann F *et al.* (2003) Dominant negative MORT1/FADD rescues mice from CD95 and TNF-induced liver failure. *Hepatology* 37 (1), 129–135.

80 Zender L, Hutker S, Liedtke C *et al.* (2003) Caspase 8 small interfering RNA prevents acute liver failure in mice. *Proc Natl Acad Sci USA* 100 (13), 7797–7802.

81 Song E, Lee SK, Wang J *et al.* (2003) RNA interference targeting Fas protects mice from fulminant hepatitis. *Nature Med* 9 (3), 347–351.

82 Wroblewski VJ, McCloud C, Davis K *et al.* (2003) Pharmacokinetics, metabolic stability, and subcutaneous bioavailability of a genetically engineered analog of DcR3, FLINT [DcR3(R218Q)], in cynomolgus monkeys and mice. *Drug Metab Dispos* 31 (4), 502–507.

83 Bajt ML, Vonderfecht SL, Jaeschke H (2001) Differential protection with inhibitors of caspase-8 and caspase-3 in murine models of tumor necrosis factor and Fas receptor-mediated hepatocellular apoptosis. *Toxicol Appl Pharmacol* 175 (3), 243–252.

84 Valentino KL, Gutierrez M, Sanchez R *et al.* (2003) First clinical trial of a novel caspase inhibitor: anti-apoptotic caspase inhibitor, IDN-6556, improves liver enzymes. *Int J Clin Pharmacol Ther* 41 (10), 441–449.

85 Leist M, Single B, Castoldi AF *et al.* (1997) Intracellular adenosine triphosphate (ATP) concentration: a switch in the decision between apoptosis and necrosis. *J Exp Med* 185 (8), 1481–1486.

86 McCarthy NJ, Whyte MK, Gilbert CS *et al.* (1997) Inhibition of Ced-3/ICE-related proteases does not prevent cell death induced by oncogenes, DNA damage, or the Bcl-2 homologue Bak. *J Cell Biol* 136 (1), 215–227.

87 Natori S, Selzner M, Valentino KL *et al.* (1999) Apoptosis of sinusoidal endothelial cells occurs during liver preservation injury by a caspase-dependent mechanism. *Transplantation* 68 (1), 89–96.

88 Guicciardi ME, Gores GJ (2004) Cheating death in the liver. *Nature Med* 10 (6), 587–588.

89 Baskin-Bey ES, Canbay A, Bronk SF *et al.* (2005) Cathepsin B inactivation attenuates hepatocyte apoptosis and liver damage in steatotic livers after cold ischemia–warm reperfusion injury. *Am J Physiol Gastrointest Liver Physiol* 288 (2), G396–402.

90 Schulze-Bergkamen H, Brenner D, Krueger A *et al.* (2004) Hepatocyte growth factor induces Mcl-1 in primary human hepatocytes and inhibits CD95-mediated apoptosis via Akt. *Hepatology* 39 (3), 645–654.

91 Ajuebor MN, Aspinall AI, Zhou F *et al.* (2005) Lack of chemokine receptor CCR5 promotes murine fulminant liver failure by preventing the apoptosis of activated CD1d-restricted NKT cells. *J Immunol* 174 (12), 8027–8037.

92 Wright MC, Issa R, Smart DE *et al.* (2001) Gliotoxin stimulates the apoptosis of human and rat hepatic stellate cells and enhances the resolution of liver fibrosis in rats. *Gastroenterology* 121 (3), 685–698.

3.2 Ischaemia–reperfusion injury to the liver

Nazia Selzner and Pierre A. Clavien

Ischaemic injury of the liver can be divided into three types: (i) cold (or hypothermic); (ii) warm (or normothermic); and (iii) rewarming [1,2]. Cold ischaemia occurs almost exclusively in the transplant setting where it is applied intentionally to reduce the metabolic activities of the graft while the organ awaits implantation. Warm ischaemia occurs during liver surgery, trauma, shock and transplantation, when hepatic inflow occlusion (Pringle manoeuvre) or inflow and outflow (total vascular exclusion) are induced to minimize blood loss while dividing liver parenchyma. Rewarming ischaemia occurs during manipulation of the graft (for example, *ex situ* split liver preparation) or during the period of implantation of the graft when the cold liver is subjected to room or body temperature. Of note, injury to the liver cells after any type of ischaemia is apparent mainly after reperfusion when oxygen supply and blood elements are restored to the liver. While the main mechanisms of injury appear to share common pathways, recent evidence suggests important differences between cold and warm ischaemic injury. Therefore, the two forms of ischaemia and the protective strategies for each form will be discussed separately in this chapter.

Warm (normothermic) ischaemia

Warm ischaemic injury is common during liver surgery, various forms of shock, trauma and transplantation. For example, ischaemia is intentionally applied to the liver by occluding hepatic inflow (Pringle manoeuvre) during the time of transection of the liver parenchyma to prevent bleeding. Ischaemia is tolerated only for a period of about 1 h in normal and about 30 min in cirrhotic livers, and the duration of ischaemia correlates with the degree of reperfusion injury [3].

Warm ischaemia leads rapidly to the death of hepatocytes [4,5]. The severe injury of hepatocytes is preceded by massive death of endothelial cells [6]. Kupffer cells, the resident hepatic macrophages, play a major role in the mechanism of warm ischaemic injury. Upon reperfusion, Kupffer cells are activated [7]. This is evidenced by structural changes, formation of oxygen free radicals, increased phagocytosis and release of various cytokines including tumour necrosis factor alpha (TNFα)

(Fig. 1) [8–10]. After reperfusion, leukocytes adhere to the denuded sinusoids and contribute significantly to the injury [11,12]. Both TNFα and interleukin 1 (IL-1), released by activated Kupffer cells, can upregulate CD11b expression on leukocytes and recruit these cells into the sinusoids [13]. The mechanism of injury involves the release of reactive oxygen intermediates. Other potential substances released by neutrophils include various proteases and hypochloric acid [14]. There is a growing body of evidence suggesting that host T cells also participate in hepatic ischaemic injury. TNFα and IL-1 can recruit and activate CD4+ T lymphocytes in the liver during the early phase of reperfusion [15], which autoamplify Kupffer cell activation and neutrophil recruitment into the liver [16].

Leukocyte recruitment into sinusoids during the early phase of reperfusion is also mediated through activation of the complement cascade. The complement chains rapidly activated by cellular proteins released during reperfusion engage complement receptors on neutrophils and their recruitment into sinusoids [17].

Further binding of the various components mentioned above (cytokines, oxygen free radicals, etc.) to their respective receptors during the early stages of reperfusion initiates the complex machinery leading to the death of hepatocytes.

Different forms of cell death

Two distinct forms of cell death are recognized: necrosis, a passive mechanism of cell death due to overwhelming injury; and a more tightly regulated process called programmed cell death or apoptosis (see Chapter 3.1). They can be distinguished by morphological and biochemical criteria as well as by their sensitivity to pharmacological or genetic manipulation.

The main features of necrosis are early cell and organelle swelling, ion dysregulation, adenosine triphosphate (ATP) depletion and activation of degradative enzymes. These processes culminate in the rupture of the cell membrane with release of intracellular proteins, metabolites and ions. The cell debris represents a strong stimulus for inflammatory processes, which typically accompany necrosis.

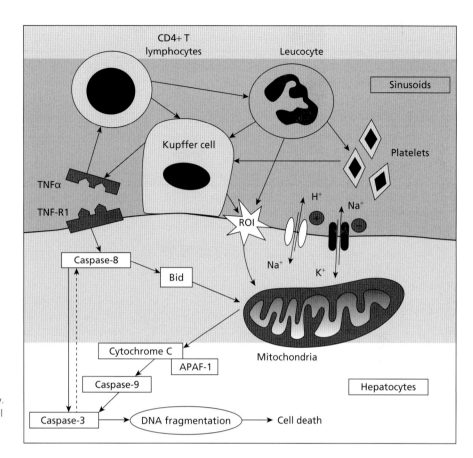

Fig. 1 Mechanisms of warm ischaemic injury. Major pathways including TNFα-mediated cell death and generation of reactive oxygen intermediates (ROI) are indicated.

Apoptosis was originally described in lymphoid cells and appears to be the primary process by which normal cell death occurs during development or by which cell numbers are maintained in tissues with rapid cell turnover such as intestinal epithelium or skin. Under physiological conditions, apoptosis occurs as a continuous and serial event affecting selective cells with rapid and silent removal of the dead cells though macrophages. Studies with cytosolic extracts of cells, which have been induced to undergo apoptosis in a synchronous manner, have shown that apoptosis can be divided into biochemically and morphologically distinct phases. In the first phase, the 'initiation phase', a tightly regulated molecular machinery involving various proteases is activated. In the second 'committed or effector phase', the molecular machinery becomes fully activated, as shown by the ability of the cytosolic extracts of committed cells to induce apoptotic changes in nuclei. Only after this, in the third phase, or 'degradation phase', do the hallmarks of apoptosis become evident. These include morphological changes including DNA fragmentation and the formation of apoptotic bodies.

Necrosis and apoptosis have long been viewed as fundamentally different processes. Although necrosis was thought to be the predominant form of death triggered by severe cellular injury or extreme environmental perturbation, cell death with features of apoptosis can occur after major stress to the cells. Whether necrosis or apoptosis predominates and eventually accounts for a given cell's demise may depend on both intrinsic (e.g. cell type, developmental state of the cell, ATP or fat content) [18] and extrinsic factors (e.g. the nature and severity of the insult, pharmacological interventions). Further complicating the task of distinguishing necrosis from apoptosis, these death cascades may share some common mediators. Lemasters [19] introduced the theory of 'necrapoptosis' for such mixed forms of cell death. It postulates that a process begins with a common death signal or toxic stress that culminates in either cell lysis (necrotic cell death) or programmed cellular resorption (apoptosis), depending on other modifying factors such as the decline in cellular ATP levels or fat content (steatosis) (Fig. 2).

In the context of hepatic ischaemia and reperfusion injury, a controversy has emerged in recent years over whether necrotic or apoptotic cell death accounts for the severe parenchymal injury [4,20]. Some investigators reported that the overwhelming majority of parenchymal injury observed is caused by massive necrotic alterations [4]. In contrast, others showed that specific inhibition of apoptosis significantly prevented parenchymal injury and improved animal survival after prolonged periods of ischaemia [21–24]. For example, we have demonstrated that apoptotic cell death is initiated by binding of TNFα to the specific receptor TNF-R1 on the cell membrane of hepatocytes in a mouse model of normothermic ischaemic injury [9] (Fig. 1). The apoptotic signal is then transferred into the cell where

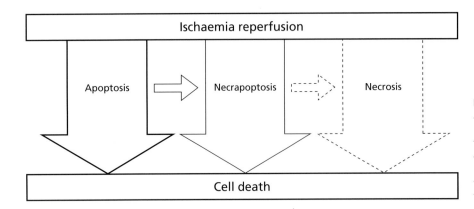

Fig. 2 Mixed forms of cell death with apoptotic and necrotic features have been proposed and have led to the creation of the term 'necrapoptosis'. Death pathways with early features of apoptosis followed by some necrotic changes are possible, depending on the nature and the severity of the insult and on the condition of the affected cell.

different caspases are activated. This process leads to DNA fragmentation and cell death. In this process, the mitochondria act as amplifiers of the signal, allowing even weak signals to have deleterious effects [25]. Blocking early mechanisms of apoptosis (the first and second phases from above) can prevent parenchymal injury. Several protective strategies based on specific blockage of the pathways of injury have been developed over the past decades. These strategies can be divided into surgical interventions and the use of pharmacological agents.

Protective strategies

Surgical strategies

While many strategies to protect against warm ischaemic injury have been proposed in various animal models, only two have finally made the transition into clinical practice, namely intermittent clamping [3] and ischaemic preconditioning [26].

Ischaemic preconditioning consists of a brief period of ischaemia followed by a short interval of reperfusion before the actual surgical procedure, with a prolonged ischaemic stress [27]. During the surgery, hepatic inflow is occluded by placing a vascular clamp or a loop around the portal triad (i.e. portal vein, hepatic artery and bile duct), rendering the whole organ ischaemic. After an ischaemic interval of 10–15 min, the clamp is removed and the liver is reperfused for 10–15 min before the prolonged ischaemic insult (Fig. 3). Our current understanding of the underlying biological principle is that cells primed by various kinds of subinjurious stress trigger defence mechanisms against subsequent lethal injury of the same or a different type [28–30]. The phenomenon was initially discovered in the myocardium by Murry *et al.* [31] in 1986. Subsequently, beneficial effects were shown in various tissues including skeletal muscle [32], kidney [33], lung [34], intestine [35] and liver [26,36–38]. Although the benefit of ischaemic preconditioning in the liver has already been suggested in a clinical pilot study [26] and a large randomized study [38], knowledge of the molecular mechanisms remains vague. Several mediators have been proposed to play a critical role in the protective pathways including adenosine [27], nitric oxide [36], oxidative stress [39],

some heat shock proteins (Hsps; e.g. Hsp72 and haem oxygenase 1/Hsp32) [40] and TNFα [9,41,42].

In addition to the extracellular mediators, studies in heart and liver indicate that the ischaemic preconditioning process involves the activation of intracellular messengers such as protein kinase C, adenosine monophosphate-activated protein kinase, p38 mitogen-activated protein kinase, Ik kinase and signal transducers and activators of transcription [43–45]. The downstream consequences of these pathways could be cytoprotective by abrogation of cell death pathways (such as activation of vacuolar ATP, inhibition of intracellular sodium accumulation and cell swelling), stimulation of antioxidant and other cellular protective mechanisms, and by initiation of entry into the cell cycle.

Intermittent clamping consists of multiple cycles of short intervals of ischaemia (10–30 min) and reperfusion (5–15 min) [46] (Fig. 3). Although the protective mechanisms of this concept still remain elusive, intermittent clamping is currently used in practice by many centres. In a prospective randomized study, Belghiti *et al.* [3] showed that cycles of short intervals of ischaemia (15 min) and reperfusion (5 min) provided protection in patients undergoing major liver resection. We have compared this protocol with ischaemic preconditioning [22] in a mouse model and found that both strategies provide comparable protection for ischaemic intervals of up to 75 min. For longer ischaemic intervals, only intermittent clamping conferred significant protection. We therefore concluded that ischaemic preconditioning is preferable for most liver resections because each period of reperfusion in the intermittent clamping strategy may cause significant bleeding.

Pharmacological strategies

Many pharmacological agents have been shown to confer protection against ischaemic injury in the liver. However, none of these strategies has found its way into routine clinical practice.

Caspase inhibition

Caspases belong to the family of cysteine proteinases. Specific isoforms are involved in the initiation and execution phase of

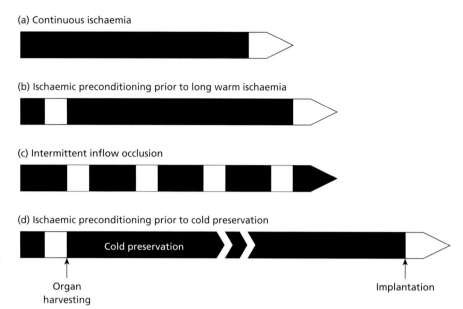

Fig. 3 Several surgical strategies exist to overcome the negative effects of prolonged ischaemia ■ (solid box) and reperfusion □ (open box) (a). To prevent warm ischaemic injuries, the options include ischaemic preconditioning (b) and intermittent inflow occlusion (c). Experimental studies suggest that normothermic ischaemic preconditioning prior to hypothermic preservation also protects against cold ischaemic injuries (d).

apoptosis. Among these isoforms, caspase-8 is activated during the early phases, and caspase-3 is activated during the late phase of apoptosis [25]. Suppression of their activation, or inhibition of their activity, reduces or completely abolishes apoptosis in cell culture models. In a rat model of warm ischaemia, Cursio *et al.* [23,47] demonstrated maximal caspase activation 3 h after reperfusion. Pretreatment of the animals with a specific caspase inhibitor 2 min prior to ischaemia resulted in significant improvement in lethal injury that normally occurred 24–48 h after ischaemia. The protective effect of caspase inhibition has also been confirmed by other groups in different models of cold and warm ischaemia [21,48].

Other proteases, such as calpain, have been reported as mediators of preservation–reperfusion injury [49–51]. Calpains are a group of non-lysosomal, cytoplasmic, calcium-dependent cysteine proteases involved in proteolysis of several cytoskeletal and membrane proteins [52]. Several group have reported the protective effects of calpain inhibition in cold [53,54] and warm ischaemic injury [5].

TNFα as initiator of the apoptotic cascade

In 1990, Colletti *et al.* [10] provided the first evidence suggesting that prolonged ischaemic intervals lead to a burst of various cytokines including TNFα. Other groups subsequently confirmed this finding [9,42,55]. Various approaches to block the TNFα signalling pathway upon reperfusion have been used, including TNFα antibody [10,41,55], pretreatment with the methylxanthine derivate, pentoxifylline (inhibitor of TNFα synthesis and release in Kupffer cells) [9] or the use of TNF-R1 knockout mice [9]. Each of these approaches was found to confer protection against reperfusion injury and animal death after prolonged ischaemic insult to the liver. The finding that TNFα acts at an early stage before any evidence of morphological features suggests that this cytokine represents an appealing

target for preventive strategies. However, so far, no clinical studies have been presented that would show a beneficial effect of pentoxifylline on ischaemic liver injury.

The role of Kupffer cells and antioxidants

There is growing evidence that the activation of resident macrophages (Kupffer cells) of the liver contributes to ischaemic injury in the liver [55–57]. Activated Kupffer cells release a variety of potentially harmful mediators, including TNFα [9,10,41] and reactive oxygen species [56,58,59], during the reperfusion period.

The most damaging form of reactive oxygen species generated in mitochondria of the Kupffer cells is the hydroxyl radical (OH˙). One of the major and most sensitive targets of OH˙ is the mitochondrial DNA [57–60]. OH˙ attacks deoxyribose and causes the release of nucleic acids of mitochondrial DNA, resulting in strand breaks. OH˙ can also directly attack bases, leading to modifications with a loss of DNA integrity and, hence, impaired transcription. Although the role of reactive oxygen species in a number of liver diseases is generally accepted, the detailed mechanisms of reactive oxygen involvement are under debate. The most convincing hypothesis of reactive oxygen-induced cell injury is the destruction of cellular membranes through peroxidation of lipids. In addition, all mitochondrial constituents, proteins, lipids and mitochondrial DNA [61], are potential targets for reactive oxygen species-mediated damage. Through such damage, a gradual impairment of defences in mitochondria will enhance the effect of further oxidative stress. In the liver, the involvement of reactive oxygen has been suggested in apoptotic cell death of hepatocytes and endothelial cells [62]. One possible explanation is that oxidative stress can induce the mitochondrial membrane permeability transition, a central event preceding cell death [63]. Another potential target of reactive oxygen species could be the caspases [64]. Caspases can be activated by low concentrations of hydrogen peroxide, while higher levels inhibit enzymatic activity, presumably due to oxidation of critical sulphydryl groups.

Owing to the central role of oxidative stress in the setting of ischaemia–reperfusion, a large number of studies have attempted to identify methods to either prevent or neutralize oxidative stress [65–68]. It has also been demonstrated that strategies aiming at overexpressing antioxidant proteins (e.g. superoxide dismutase [69,70]) may confer protection against extended ischaemic injury. However, none of these strategies has found its way into routine clinical practice, with the exception of some antioxidant ingredients that were introduced into preservation solutions.

Cold (hypothermic) ischaemia

Liver transplantation has experienced dramatic success over the past 15 years and has become the treatment of choice for many patients with endstage liver disease. While major progress has been made in several areas of transplantation, such as selection of recipients and immunosuppression, ischaemic injury remains an important limiting factor for the full success of the procedure. During the various phases of transplantation, the liver graft is exposed to different types of ischaemic stress, including normothermic ischaemia before or during harvesting of the organ from the donor, cold ischaemia during the period of preservation and rewarming during graft implantation.

Hypothermia, while necessary to slow metabolism during the period of preservation, causes morphological changes in some sinusoidal endothelial cells [21,71–73]. They become rounded, detached and slough into the sinusoidal lumen; however, most cells remain alive until reperfusion as assessed by Trypan blue [74] and in situ terminal deoxynucleotidyl transferase-mediated dUTP nick end labelling (TUNEL) assay studies [73]. Adhesion of the platelets to the sinusoid lining induces sinusoidal endothelial cell (SEC) apoptosis upon reperfusion of the cold ischaemic liver [75]. Finally, leukocytes and platelets synergistically exacerbate SEC injury by the induction of apoptosis [76].

The injuries due to low-temperature preservation are different from warm ischaemic injury in many aspects. The main feature of the warm ischaemia type of injury is massive and early (3–6 h) apoptosis of hepatocytes after reperfusion. In contrast, cold storage is associated with diffuse SEC damage within 30–60 min of reperfusion while hepatocytes remain morphologically normal [77]. The degree of endothelial cell detachment has been shown to correlate with the duration of cold ischaemia [1,78–79]. Several recent reports have pointed out that activation of matrix metalloproteinases is a critical feature of SEC detachment during cold hepatic preservation prior to reperfusion [80]. Matrix metalloproteinases are also important contributors to angiogenesis.

Upon reperfusion of the cold preserved graft, SEC undergo apoptosis with subsequent DNA fragmentation and cell death

[73]. The strong correlation between the degree of apoptosis and graft viability suggests that SEC apoptosis is a critical process in cold ischaemic injury. While a number of intracellular mediators of apoptosis are known, the data regarding the initiating extracellular processes are scarce. Disruption of the endothelial wall leads to leukocyte [11,56,76,81] and platelet adhesion [75,82], which induces microcirculatory disturbances.

Protective strategies

Cooling of the organ and preservation solutions

Reduction of metabolic activity by cooling of the organ to 1–4°C was among the first strategies designed to protect against ischaemic injury [83]. This strategy may safely preserve the liver for transplantation for up to 8 h, whereas livers kept at room temperature tolerate only about 1 h of ischaemia. Cooling requires the application of a perfusion/preservation solution. Thus, efforts were directed at designing an effective solution that would extend the period for safe preservation. The development of University of Wisconsin (UW) cold preservation solution in the mid-1980s [83] provided a breakthrough in liver transplantation allowing organ sharing across large distances. The solution was developed empirically and was supposed to act on the known and speculated negative effects of hypothermia. These negative effects include: (i) cell swelling caused by inhibition of the membrane pump Na^+/K^+ ATPase regulating cell volume; (ii) intracellular acidosis caused by anaerobic metabolism and lactate accumulation [84]; (iii) disturbances in the homeostasis of cytosolic Ca [85]; and (iv) free-radical generation [86]. The solution contains a cocktail of substances such as lactobionate, raffinose, phosphate buffer, glutathione, colloids (hydroxyethylstarch) and various ions. Despite the lack of understanding as to how the ingredients confer protection, the UW solution still remains the most widely used preservation solution. Other solutions such as Eurocollins (with high glucose content and very high osmolarity) or Celsior (with mannitol, glutamate and histidine buffer) are less effective and have been abandoned in clinical practice. Finally, Bretschneider's histidine–tryptophan–ketoglutarate (HTK) was designed for cardiac preservation and was formulated to retard acidosis (histidine), to prevent membrane injury (tryptophan) and to provide a substrate for energy metabolism (ketoglutarate). This solution was also tested by several groups in liver transplantation and has been shown to be equally as effective as the UW solution during the usual periods of cold preservation used in human transplantation [87,88].

Ischaemic preconditioning

As in the warm ischaemic liver, ischaemic preconditioning is potentially an effective approach to preventing preservation injury [89] (Fig. 3). Our group has recently demonstrated that ischaemic preconditioning is protective during the period of cold storage of the liver prior to reperfusion, by reducing endothelial cell detachment and matrix metalloproteinase activity [89]. The protective effect is mediated by a short sublethal burst of oxygen free radicals. Indeed, a mild burst of oxidative stress generated during the process of ischaemic preconditioning induces natural defence mechanisms against subsequent lethal injury, as also demonstrated in a model of warm ischaemia [39]. However, the clinical benefit and applicability of ischaemic preconditioning in liver transplantation remains to be established.

Conclusion

Ischaemia and reperfusion injuries remain important in liver surgery, transplantation and various forms of shock. Hepatic ischaemia can be divided into two types, normothermic (warm) and cold (organ preservation) ischaemia. While some injurious mechanisms are common for these two types, such as initial apoptosis of SEC followed by hepatocyte injury, critical differences exist, such as resistance of hepatocytes to cold ischaemic injury. Apoptosis appears to be involved in both types of injury as various antiapoptotic strategies have been shown by several groups to confer a high degree of protection, including improved survival following long ischaemic insult. The future lies in a better understanding of the underlying mechanisms of injury, and a closer look at protective strategies such as ischaemic preconditioning may lead to the identification of effective molecules enhancing tolerance to ischaemic injury.

References

1 Clavien PA, Harvey PR, Strasberg SM (1992) Preservation and reperfusion injuries in liver allografts. An overview and synthesis of current studies. *Transplantation* 53 (5), 957–978.

2 Selzner N, Rudiger H, Graf R *et al.* (2003) Protective strategies against ischemic injury of the liver. *Gastroenterology* 125 (3), 917–936.

3 Belghiti J, Noun R, Malafosse R *et al.* (1999) Continuous versus intermittent portal triad clamping for liver resection: a controlled study. *Ann Surg* 229 (3), 369–375.

4 Gujral JS, Bucci TJ, Farhood A *et al.* (2001) Mechanism of cell death during warm hepatic ischemia–reperfusion in rats: apoptosis or necrosis? *Hepatology* 33 (2), 397–405.

5 Kohli V, Madden JF, Bentley RC *et al.* (1999) Calpain mediates ischemic injury of the liver through modulation of apoptosis and necrosis. *Gastroenterology* 116 (1), 168–178.

6 Kohli V, Selzner M, Madden JF *et al.* (1999) Endothelial cell and hepatocyte deaths occur by apoptosis after ischemia–reperfusion injury in the rat liver. *Transplantation* 67 (8), 1099–1105.

7 Caldwell-Kenkel JC, Currin RT, Tanaka Y *et al.* (1991) Kupffer cell activation and endothelial cell damage after storage of rat livers: effects of reperfusion. *Hepatology* 13 (1), 83–95.

8 Jaeschke H (1999) Kupffer cell-induced oxidant stress during hepatic ischemia–reperfusion: does the controversy continue? *Hepatology* 30 (6), 1527–1528.

9 Rudiger HA, Clavien PA (2002) Tumor necrosis factor alpha, but not Fas, mediates hepatocellular apoptosis in the murine ischemic liver. *Gastroenterology* 122 (1), 202–210.

10 Colletti LM, Remick DG, Burtch GD *et al.* (1990) Role of tumor necrosis factor-alpha in the pathophysiologic alterations after hepatic ischemia/reperfusion injury in the rat. *J Clin Invest* 85 (6), 1936–1943.

11 Clavien PA, Harvey PR, Sanabria JR *et al.* (1993) Lymphocyte adherence in the reperfused rat liver: mechanisms and effects. *Hepatology* 17 (1), 131–142.

12 Jaeschke H, Smith CW (1997) Mechanisms of neutrophil-induced parenchymal cell injury. *J Leukoc Biol* 61 (6), 647–653.

13 Bajt ML, Farhood A, Jaeschke H (2001) Effects of CXC chemokines on neutrophil activation and sequestration in hepatic vasculature. *Am J Physiol Gastrointest Liver Physiol* 281 (5), G1188–1195.

14 Weiss SJ. (1989) Tissue destruction by neutrophils. *N Engl J Med* 320 (6), 365–376.

15 Zwacka RM, Zhang Y, Halldorson J *et al.* (1997) CD4(+) T-lymphocytes mediate ischemia/reperfusion-induced inflammatory responses in mouse liver. *J Clin Invest* 100 (2), 279–289.

16 Le Moine O, Louis H, Demols A *et al.* (2000) Cold liver ischemia–reperfusion injury critically depends on liver T cells and is improved by donor pretreatment with interleukin 10 in mice. *Hepatology* 31 (6), 1266–1274.

17 Jaeschke H, Farhood A, Bautista AP *et al.* (1993) Complement activates Kupffer cells and neutrophils during reperfusion after hepatic ischemia. *Am J Physiol* 264 (4 Pt 1), G801–809.

18 Selzner M, Rudiger HA, Sindram D *et al.* (2000) Mechanisms of ischemic injury are different in the steatotic and normal rat liver. *Hepatology* 32 (6), 1280–1288.

19 Lemasters JJ. (1999) Necrapoptosis and the mitochondrial permeability transition: shared pathways to necrosis and apoptosis. *Am J Physiol* 276 (1 Pt 1), G1–6.

20 Clavien PA, Rudiger HA, Selzner M (2001) Mechanism of hepatocyte death after ischemia: apoptosis versus necrosis. *Hepatology* 33 (6), 1555–1557.

21 Natori S, Selzner M, Valentino KL *et al.* (1999) Apoptosis of sinusoidal endothelial cells occurs during liver preservation injury by a caspase-dependent mechanism. *Transplantation* 68 (1), 89–96.

22 Rudiger HA, Kang KJ, Sindram D *et al.* (2002) Comparison of ischemic preconditioning and intermittent and continuous inflow occlusion in the murine liver. *Ann Surg* 235 (3), 400–407.

23 Cursio R, Gugenheim J, Ricci JE *et al.* (1999) A caspase inhibitor fully protects rats against lethal normothermic liver ischemia by inhibition of liver apoptosis. *FASEB J* 13 (2), 253–261.

24 Bilbao G, Contreras JL, Eckhoff DE *et al.* (1999) Reduction of ischemia–reperfusion injury of the liver by *in vivo* adenovirus-mediated gene transfer of the antiapoptotic Bcl-2 gene. *Ann Surg* 230 (2), 185–193.

25 Scaffidi C, Fulda S, Srinivasan A *et al.* (1998) Two CD95 (APO-1/Fas) signaling pathways. *EMBO J* 17 (6), 1675–1687.

26 Clavien PA, Yadav S, Sindram D *et al.* (2000) Protective effects of ischemic preconditioning for liver resection performed under inflow occlusion in humans. *Ann Surg* 232 (2), 155–162.

27 Peralta C, Hotter G, Closa D *et al.* (1997) Protective effect of preconditioning on the injury associated to hepatic ischemia-reperfusion in the rat: role of nitric oxide and adenosine. *Hepatology* 25 (4), 934–937.

28 Jaeschke H (2003) Molecular mechanisms of hepatic ischemia-reperfusion injury and preconditioning. *Am J Physiol Gastrointest Liver Physiol* 284 (1), G15–26.

29 Cavalieri B, Perrelli MG, Aragno M *et al.* (2002) Ischemic preconditioning attenuates the oxidant-dependent mechanisms of reperfusion cell damage and death in rat liver. *Liver Transpl* 8 (11), 990–999.

30 Schauer RJ, Gerbes AL, Vonier D *et al.* (2003) Induction of cellular resistance against Kupffer cell-derived oxidant stress: a novel concept

of hepatoprotection by ischemic preconditioning. *Hepatology* 37 (2), 286–295.

31 Murry CE, Jennings RB, Reimer KA (1986) Preconditioning with ischemia: a delay of lethal cell injury in ischemic myocardium. *Circulation* 74 (5), 1124–1136.

32 Pang CY, Forrest CR (1995) Acute pharmacologic preconditioning as a new concept and alternative approach for prevention of skeletal muscle ischemic necrosis. *Biochem Pharmacol* 49 (8), 1023–1034.

33 Turman MA, Bates CM (1997) Susceptibility of human proximal tubular cells to hypoxia: effect of hypoxic preconditioning and comparison to glomerular cells. *Ren Fail* 19 (1), 47–60.

34 Du ZY, Hicks M, Winlaw D *et al.* (1996) Ischemic preconditioning enhances donor lung preservation in the rat. *J Heart Lung Transplant* 15 (12), 1258–1267.

35 Hotter G, Closa D, Prados M *et al.* (1996) Intestinal preconditioning is mediated by a transient increase in nitric oxide. *Biochem Biophys Res Commun* 222 (1), 27–32.

36 Peralta C, Closa D, Hotter G *et al.* (1996) Liver ischemic preconditioning is mediated by the inhibitory action of nitric oxide on endothelin. *Biochem Biophys Res Commun* 229 (1), 264–270.

37 Yadav SS, Sindram D, Perry DK *et al.* (1999) Ischemic preconditioning protects the mouse liver by inhibition of apoptosis through a caspase-dependent pathway. *Hepatology* 30 (5), 1223–1231.

38 Clavien PA, Selzner M, Rudiger HA *et al.* (2003) A prospective randomized study in 100 consecutive patients undergoing major liver resection with versus without ischemic preconditioning. *Ann Surg* 238 (6), 843–850; discussion 851–852.

39 Rudiger HA, Graf R, Clavien PA (2003) Sub-lethal oxidative stress triggers the protective effects of ischemic preconditioning in the mouse liver. *J Hepatol* 39 (6), 972–977.

40 Redaelli CA, Tian YH, Kubulus D *et al.* (2002) Hyperthermia preconditioning induces renal heat shock protein expression, improves cold ischemia tolerance, kidney graft function and survival in rats. *Nephron* 90 (4), 489–497.

41 Colletti LM, Kunkel SL, Walz A *et al.* (1996) The role of cytokine networks in the local liver injury following hepatic ischemia/reperfusion in the rat. *Hepatology* 23 (3), 506–514.

42 Peralta C, Fernandez L, Panes J *et al.* (2001) Preconditioning protects against systemic disorders associated with hepatic ischemia–reperfusion through blockade of tumor necrosis factor-induced P-selectin up-regulation in the rat. *Hepatology* 33 (1), 100–113.

43 Carini R, De Cesaris MG, Splendore R *et al.* (2000) Ischemic preconditioning reduces Na(+) accumulation and cell killing in isolated rat hepatocytes exposed to hypoxia. *Hepatology* 31 (1), 166–172.

44 Carini R, De Cesaris MG, Splendore R *et al.* (2001) Signal pathway involved in the development of hypoxic preconditioning in rat hepatocytes. *Hepatology* 33 (1), 131–139.

45 Teoh N, Dela Pena A, Farrell G (2002) Hepatic ischemic preconditioning in mice is associated with activation of NF-kappaB, p38 kinase, and cell cycle entry. *Hepatology* 36 (1), 94–102.

46 Makuuchi M, Mori T, Gunven P *et al.* (1987) Safety of hemihepatic vascular occlusion during resection of the liver. *Surg Gynecol Obstet* 164 (2), 155–158.

47 Cursio R, Gugenheim J, Panaia-Ferrari P *et al.* (1998) Improvement of normothermic rat liver ischemia/reperfusion by muramyl dipeptide. *J Surg Res* 80 (2), 339–344.

48 Kobayashi A, Imamura H, Isobe M *et al.* (2001) Mac-1 (CD11b/CD18) and intercellular adhesion molecule-1 in ischemia–reperfusion injury of rat liver. *Am J Physiol Gastrointest Liver Physiol* 281 (2), G577–585.

49 Wang M, Sakon M, Umeshita K *et al.* (2001) Prednisolone suppresses ischemia–reperfusion injury of the rat liver by reducing cytokine production and calpain mu activation. *J Hepatol* 34 (2), 278–283.

50 Squier MK, Miller AC, Malkinson AM *et al.* (1994) Calpain activation in apoptosis. *J Cell Physiol* 159 (2), 229–237.

51 Arora AS, de Groen P, Emori Y *et al.* (1996) A cascade of degradative hydrolase activity contributes to hepatocyte necrosis during anoxia. *Am J Physiol* 270 (2 Pt 1), G238–245.

52 Croall DE, DeMartino GN (1991) Calcium-activated neutral protease (calpain) system: structure, function, and regulation. *Physiol Rev* 71 (3), 813–847.

53 Kohli V, Gao W, Camargo CA, Jr *et al.* (1997) Calpain is a mediator of preservation-reperfusion injury in rat liver transplantation. *Proc Natl Acad Sci USA* 94 (17), 9354–9359.

54 Upadhya GA, Topp SA, Hotchkiss RS *et al.* (2003) Effect of cold preservation on intracellular calcium concentration and calpain activity in rat sinusoidal endothelial cells. *Hepatology* 37 (2), 313–323.

55 Wanner GA, Muller PE, Ertel W *et al.* (1999) Differential effect of anti-TNF-alpha antibody on proinflammatory cytokine release by Kupffer cells following liver ischemia and reperfusion. *Shock* 11 (6), 391–395.

56 Jaeschke H, Farhood A (1991) Neutrophil and Kupffer cell-induced oxidant stress and ischemia–reperfusion injury in rat liver. *Am J Physiol* 260 (3 Pt 1), G355–362.

57 Mochida S, Arai M, Ohno A *et al.* (1994) Oxidative stress in hepatocytes and stimulatory state of Kupffer cells after reperfusion differ between warm and cold ischemia in rats. *Liver* 14 (5), 234–240.

58 Rymsa B, Wang JF, de Groot H (1991) O_2^- release by activated Kupffer cells upon hypoxia–reoxygenation. *Am J Physiol* 261 (4 Pt 1), G602–607.

59 Jaeschke H (1998) Mechanisms of reperfusion injury after warm ischemia of the liver. *J Hepatobiliary Pancreat Surg* 5 (4), 402–408.

60 Coito AJ, Buelow R, Shen XD *et al.* (2002) Heme oxygenase-1 gene transfer inhibits inducible nitric oxide synthase expression and protects genetically fat Zucker rat livers from ischemia-reperfusion injury. *Transplantation* 74 (1), 96–102.

61 Boveris A, Chance B (1973) The mitochondrial generation of hydrogen peroxide. General properties and effect of hyperbaric oxygen. *Biochem J* 134 (3), 707–716.

62 Adachi S, Zeisig M, Moller L (1995) Improvements in the analytical method for 8-hydroxydeoxyguanosine in nuclear DNA. *Carcinogenesis* 16 (2), 253–258.

63 Richter C, Gogvadze V, Laffranchi R *et al.* (1995) Oxidants in mitochondria: from physiology to diseases. *Biochim Biophys Acta* 1271 (1), 67–74.

64 Omar R, Nomikos I, Piccorelli G *et al.* (1989) Prevention of postischaemic lipid peroxidation and liver cell injury by iron chelation. *Gut* 30 (4), 510–514.

65 Karwinski W, Soreide O (1997) Allopurinol improves scavenging ability of the liver after ischemia/reperfusion injury. *Liver* 17 (3), 139–143.

66 Ozaki M, Nakamura M, Teraoka S *et al.* (1997) A novel anti-oxidant compound, protects the rat liver from ischemia–reperfusion injury. *Transpl Int* 10 (2), 96–102.

67 Zhong Z, Froh M, Connor HD *et al.* (2002) Prevention of hepatic ischemia-reperfusion injury by green tea extract. *Am J Physiol Gastrointest Liver Physiol* 283 (4), G957–964.

68 Sewerynek E, Reiter RJ, Melchiorri D *et al.* (1996) Oxidative damage in the liver induced by ischemia–reperfusion: protection by melatonin. *Hepatogastroenterology* 43 (10), 898–905.

69 Rauen U, Polzar B, Stephan H *et al.* (1999) Cold-induced apoptosis in cultured hepatocytes and liver endothelial cells: mediation by reactive oxygen species. *FASEB J* 13 (1), 155–168.

70 Czaja MJ (2002) Induction and regulation of hepatocyte apoptosis by oxidative stress. *Antioxid Redox Signal* 4 (5), 759–767.

71 Otto G, Wolff H, David H (1984) Preservation damage in liver transplantation: electron-microscopic findings. *Transplant Proc* 16 (5), 1247–1248.

72 McKeown CM, Edwards V, Phillips MJ *et al.* (1988) Sinusoidal lining cell damage: the critical injury in cold preservation of liver allografts in the rat. *Transplantation* 46 (2), 178–191.

73 Gao W, Bentley RC, Madden JF *et al.* (1998) Apoptosis of sinusoidal endothelial cells is a critical mechanism of preservation injury in rat liver transplantation. *Hepatology* 27 (6), 1652–1660.

74 Holloway CM, Harvey PR, Strasberg SM (1990) Viability of sinusoidal lining cells in cold-preserved rat liver allografts. *Transplantation* 49 (1), 225–229.

75 Sindram D, Porte RJ, Hoffman MR *et al.* (2000) Platelets induce sinusoidal endothelial cell apoptosis upon reperfusion of the cold ischemic rat liver. *Gastroenterology* 118 (1), 183–191.

76 Sindram D, Porte RJ, Hoffman MR *et al.* (2001) Synergism between platelets and leukocytes in inducing endothelial cell apoptosis in the cold ischemic rat liver: a Kupffer cell-mediated injury. *FASEB J* 15 (7), 1230–1232.

77 Clavien PA (1998) Sinusoidal endothelial cell injury during hepatic preservation and reperfusion. *Hepatology* 28 (2), 281–285.

78 Momii S, Koga A (1990) Time-related morphological changes in cold-stored rat livers. A comparison of Euro-Collins solution with UW solution. *Transplantation* 50 (5), 745–750.

79 Gao W, Washington MK, Bentley RC *et al.* (1997) Antiangiogenic agents protect liver sinusoidal lining cells from cold preservation injury in rat liver transplantation. *Gastroenterology* 113 (5), 1692–1700.

80 Upadhya GA, Strasberg SM (1999) Evidence that actin disassembly is a requirement for matrix metalloproteinase secretion by sinusoidal endothelial cells during cold preservation in the rat. *Hepatology* 30 (1), 169–176.

81 Takei Y, Marzi I, Gao WS *et al.* (1991) Leukocyte adhesion and cell death following orthotopic liver transplantation in the rat. *Transplantation* 51 (5), 959–965.

82 Cywes R, Packham MA, Tietze L *et al.* (1993) Role of platelets in hepatic allograft preservation injury in the rat. *Hepatology* 18 (3), 635–647.

83 Belzer FO, Southard JH (1988) Principles of solid-organ preservation by cold storage. *Transplantation* 45 (4), 673–676.

84 Woods HF, Krebs HA (1971) Lactate production in the perfused rat liver. *Biochem J* 125 (1), 129–139.

85 Marsh DC, Belzer FO, Southard JH (1990) Hypothermic preservation of hepatocytes. II. Importance of Ca2 and amino acids. *Cryobiology* 27 (1), 1–8.

86 Brass CA, Narciso J, Gollan JL (1991) Enhanced activity of the free radical producing enzyme xanthine oxidase in hypoxic rat liver. Regulation and pathophysiologic significance. *J Clin Invest* 87 (2), 424–431.

87 Hatano E, Kiuchi T, Tanaka A *et al.* (1997) Hepatic preservation with histidine-tryptophan-ketoglutarate solution in living-related and cadaveric liver transplantation. *Clin Sci (Lond)* 93 (1), 81–88.

88 Erhard J, Lange R, Scherer R *et al.* (1994) Comparison of histidine-tryptophan-ketoglutarate (HTK) solution versus University of Wisconsin (UW) solution for organ preservation in human liver transplantation. A prospective, randomized study. *Transpl Int* 7 (3), 177–181.

89 Sindram D, Rudiger HA, Upadhya AG *et al.* (2002) Ischemic preconditioning protects against cold ischemic injury through an oxidative stress dependent mechanism. *J Hepatol* 36 (1), 78–84.

3.3 Genetics and liver diseases

3.3.1 Genetic polymorphisms in liver disease

Hongjin Huang and Ramsey Cheung

Polymorphisms associated with liver diseases

Similar to other complex diseases, the clinical manifestations of liver diseases are the outcome of the interactions between host genetic determinants and environmental factors. In recent years, there have been an increasing number of studies to identify genetic variations that are associated with different phenotypes of liver diseases. A single nucleotide polymorphism (SNP), the most common type of genetic variation, is a stable single base substitution distributed throughout the human genome. The frequency of a given SNP in individuals has been estimated to be 1 in 1000 base pairs. In the following discussion, we only include associations between SNPs and disease susceptibilities, and focus our discussion on the 'validated markers', which are defined as SNPs that have a positive association with similar clinical endpoints in two or more independent studies (Table 1).

Non-alcoholic fatty liver diseases (NAFLD): MTP (see also Chapter 13.1)

According to the Third National Health and Nutrition Examination Survey, NAFLD may account for 5.5% of the population with unexplained aminotransferase levels [1], making this the most common cause of liver disease. In fact, 'burned-out' non-alcoholic steatohepatitis (NASH) is likely to be the major cause of 'cryptogenic' cirrhosis [2]. The clinical presentation of NAFLD and NASH are similar, but predictors of progressive liver disease include an aspartate aminotransferase (AST)/alanine aminotransferase (ALT) ratio > 1, older age, presence of type 2 diabetes mellitus or obesity or presence of metabolic syndrome [3–5]. However, despite the fact that a majority of individuals with obesity and insulin resistance will have steatosis, only 9–26% and 25% of those groups, respectively, will ever develop NASH [6,7], suggesting that other environmental and genetic factors also play a determining role. One family study reported the presence of NASH in seven out of eight studied kindreds, while another study found that 18% of 90 patients with NASH had an affected first-degree relative, supporting the role of genetic risk factors [8,9]. So far, the only validated genetic association with NASH is in the microsomal triglyceride transfer protein (*MTP*) gene. The G allele of the promoter SNP −493G/T in *MTP* leads to decreased transcription of *MTP*, resulting in a reduced export of triglyceride from hepatocytes and increased intracellular accumulation of triglyceride [10]. Bernard *et al.* [10] reported the association of −493G/T with biological surrogates of NASH, such as ALT, sex and body mass index (BMI) in 271 type 2 diabetic patients. Namikawa *et al.* [11] reported its direct association with NASH in 63 patients with biopsy-proven NASH in comparison with 150 healthy control subjects. We have confirmed this association in a study of 127 NAFLD patients (50 of whom had biopsy-proven NASH) and 60 normal subjects with matched BMI. In our study, 128T [in complete linkage disequilibrium (LD) with − 493G/T] was associated with a decreased risk of NASH relative to both the 'normal' group (OR = 0.2, $P = 0.0001$) and the 'steatosis only' group [odds ratio (OR) = 0.4, $P = 0.05$] [12]. The various approaches to determine the role of genes in NAFLD have been reviewed recently by Day [13].

Alcoholic liver disease: ADH, ALDH2 and CYP2E1 (see also Section 12)

Although excessive alcohol intake is the major risk factor for alcoholic liver disease, and fatty change of the liver is almost universal in subjects with excessive alcohol use, only a minority of these subjects develop alcoholic hepatitis, and 4–20% develop cirrhosis [14,15]. Factors associated with the development of alcoholic liver disease other than the level of alcohol consumption typically include gender, nutrition and coexisting

Table 1 Genetic markers validated in two or more studies in liver diseases.

Gene	Polymorphism	Country	Patients	Controls	P	Endpoint	Year	Authors	Ref.
Nonalcoholic fatty liver disease (NAFLD)									
MTP	−493G/T	Japan	63	150	0.001	NASH[a] vs. normal[b]	2004	Namikawa et al.	[11]
		US	127	60	0.0001	NASH[a] vs. normal[b]	2005	Huang et al.	[12]
Alcoholic liver disease (ALD)									
ADH2	ADH2*1	Japan	80	60[b]	0.029	ALC[c] vs. ALNC[d]	1995	Yamauchi et al.	[19]
		China	75	235[b]	<0.05	ALC[c] vs. normal[b]	1997	Chao et al.	[20]
		Australia	114	200[b]	<0.05	ALC[c] vs. normal[b]	2002	Frenzer et al.	[21]
		China	165	65[b]	<0.05	ALD[e] vs. AD[f]	2002	Yu et al.	[22]
		Korean	22	100[b]	<0.05	ALC[c] vs. normal[b]	2004	Kim et al.	[23]
ALDH2	ALDH2*1	China	75	235[b]	<0.05	ALC[c] vs. normal[b]	1997	Chao et al.	[20]
		China	165	65[b]	<0.05	ALD[e] vs. AD[f]	2002	Yu et al.	[22]
		Korean	22	100[b]	<0.05	ALC[c] vs. normal[b]	2004	Kim et al.	[23]
CYP2E1	CYP2E1*c2	Japan	80	60[b]	0.013	ALC[c] vs. ALNC[d]	1995	Yamauchi et al.	[19]
		Japan	68		0.019	ALD[e] vs. heavy drinkers	1997	Tanaka et al.	[24]
		Korean	22	100[b]	<0.05	ALC[c] vs. normal[b]	2004	Kim et al.	[23]
Primary biliary cirrhosis (PBC)									
CTLA1	49A/G	England	200	200	0.000063	PBC[g] vs. normal[b]	2000	Agarwal et al.	[29]
		China	77	160	0.0046	PBC[g] vs. normal[b]	2004	Fan et al.	[30]
VDR	BsmII	Germany	74	214	0.009	PBC[g] vs. normal[b]	2002	Vogel et al.	[31]
		Hungary	33	160	<0.03	PBC[g] vs. normal[b]	2002	Lakatos et al.	[32]
		Hungary	31	51	0.01	PBC[g] vs. normal[b]	2000	Halmos et al.	[33]
		China	58	160	0.01	PBC[g] vs. normal[b]	2005	Fan et al.	[34]
IFN response in chronic hepatitis C									
IL10	−592A/C, −819C	Australia	43		<0.05	SVR[h] vs. NR[i]	1999	Edwards-Smith et al.	[39]
		UK	303		<0.05	SVR[h] vs. NR[i]	2003	Knapp et al.	[40]
MxA	−88G/T	Japan	115		0.0018	SVR[h] vs. NR[i]	2000	Hijikata et al.	[42]
		Japan	159		<0.05	SVR[h] vs. NR[i]	2001	Hijikata et al.	[43]
		Japan	235		<0.05	SVR[h] vs. NR[i]	2004	Suzuki et al.	[44]
CCR5	59029G/A	US	171		0.05	SVR[h] vs. NR[i]	2003	Promrat et al.	[46]
		Japan	105		0.03	SVR[h] vs. NR[i]	2004	Konishi et al.	[47]
Fibrosis risk in chronic hepatitis C									
DDX5	S480A	US	1051		<0.05	F3-4 vs. F0-2	2004	Huang et al.	[53]
CPT1A	A275T	US	1133		<0.05	F3-4 vs. F0-2	2005	Huang et al.	[54]
HFE	C282Y	US	119		0.01	Mean fibrosis stage	2002	Bonkovsky et al.	[57]
		Germany	246	200[b]	<0.05	F2-4 vs. F0-1	2003	Gehrke et al.	[58]
		Germany	166		0.026	F2-4 vs. F0-1	2004	Geier et al.	[59]
TGFB1	L10P, R25P	Germany	46		0.024	Mean fibrosis stage	2002	Gewaltig et al.	[62]
		Germany	210	50[b]	<0.05	F3-4 vs. F0-2	2005	Wang et al.	[63]
TNF	−308G/A	US	144		0.03	F4 vs. F0-3	2000	Yee et al.	[65]
		India	52		0.04	F3-4 vs. F0-2	2004	Goyal et al.	[66]

For each disease or trait, we only included the 'validated markers', defined as SNPs that have a positive association, with the same or similar clinical endpoints, in two or more independent studies.

[a] Non-alcoholic steatohepatitis.
[b] Normal healthy population.
[c] Alcoholic liver cirrhosis.
[d] Alcoholic liver non-cirrhosis.
[e] Alcoholic liver diseases.
[f] Alcohol dependent.
[g] Primary biliary cirrhosis.
[h] Sustained virological responders.
[i] Non-responders.

viral hepatitis [14]. A study of 15 924 male twin pairs found high concordance for alcoholism and related cirrhosis among monozygotic twins, suggesting that genetics may play a major role [16]. Most research has focused on the candidate genes of enzymes involved in alcohol metabolism. Alcohol dehydrogenase (ADH), cytochrome P-4502E1 (*CYP2E1*) and aldehyde dehydrogenase-2 (ALDH2) are the three key enzymes responsible for hepatic metabolism of ethanol and its metabolite, acetaldehyde. ADH consists of three genes, *ADH1*, *ADH2* and *ADH3*, forming a gene cluster on chromosome 4q21–23 [17]. The *ADH2*1* polymorphism results in a less active beta 2 subunit. Similarly, the c2 allele at the 5′ flanking region of *CYP2E1* causes a lower basal *CYP2E1* activity and, in the *ALDH2*2* polymorphism, a G/A mutation at codon 487 produces an inactive ALDH2 [18]. To a certain extent, these genotypes have accounted for the individual differences in alcohol and acetaldehyde blood concentrations after drinking [18]. Multiple studies, with sample sizes varying from 80 to 328, have confirmed the association of these polymorphisms with alcohol-induced liver fibrosis, alcoholic cirrhosis and hepatocellular carcinoma (Table 1) [19–24].

Primary biliary cirrhosis (PBC): CTLA-4 and VDR
(see Chapter 11.1)

PBC is a chronic autoimmune disease with destruction of the intrahepatic bile ducts. Over 90% of patients have detectable antimitochrondrial antibody, directed at the pyruvate dehydrogenase E2 complex. The disease predominantly affects women with a female to male ratio of 9:1, and a peak incidence in the fifth decade of life. It is more common in northern Europe [25]. Genetic factors clearly play an important role, with a concordance rate of PBC in monozygous twins of up to 63%, the second highest rate among autoimmune diseases [26]. In addition, 4–6% of the first-degree relatives of patients with PBC also develop the disease. However, different from most autoimmune conditions, PBC has only weak association with human leucocyte antigen (HLA) alleles (the usual genetic elements for autoimmunity) [27], suggesting that other genetic factors may play an important role, in addition to environmental factors. Cytotoxic T-lymphocyte antigen-4 (CTLA-4) is expressed by activated T cells, and negatively regulates the activation of T cells [28]. The SNP 49A/G leads to the change of Thr to Ala in the protein leader peptide, reducing the inhibitory function of CTLA-4 [28]. The 49A/G polymorphism was first associated with the predisposition to PBC in a large study of 200 Caucasian patients [29], and the results were confirmed recently in 77 Chinese PBC patients [30]. Another gene, vitamin D receptor (*VDR*), codes for the receptor of an immunomodulator, 1,25-dihydroxyvitamin D3. Polymorphisms in *VDR* have been associated with various other autoimmune diseases [27]. The *Bsm*II polymorphism in *VDR* has been significantly associated with PBC in German, Hungarian and Chinese patients [31–34].

Treatment response in patients with chronic hepatitis C: IL-10, MxA, CCR5

Several viral and host factors, such as pretreatment viral load, hepatitis C virus (HCV) genotype, rapid or early virological response, absence of cirrhosis, younger age, sex and race, have been identified as predictors of response to interferon (IFN)-based antiviral therapy [35,36]. Nevertheless, genetic markers could complement and improve the current predictive value in making treatment decisions. SNPs within the promoter region of the gene for the cytokine interleukin 10 (IL-10) have been studied extensively. IL-10, an immune suppressor, inhibits the secretion of proinflammatory and antiviral cytokines, as well as the development and activation of CD4+ T-helper lymphocytes with a Th1 phenotype [37]. Three well-defined promoter SNPs, −1082, −819 and −592, (with the last two in complete LD), influence the level of IL-10 secretion [38]. Edwards-Smith *et al.* [39] found that, in 43 HCV patients, those with genotypes or haplotypes of these three SNPs resulted in higher expression of the IL-10 gene and had a poor response to IFNα therapy. This association was confirmed in a larger study with 303 HCV patients treated with IFN [40]. The second SNP related to IFN response has been identified in gene *MxA*, which is induced by IFN and involved in clearance of HCV in IFN-treated patients [41]. Hijikata *et al.* [42] first reported the significant association of −88G/T with sustained virological response to IFN therapy in a cohort of 115 HCV patients, and confirmed the results when more patients (*n* = 159) were enrolled [43]. The association was validated in another independent cohort of 235 patients [44]. However, all these studies were conducted in a Japanese population, and the association in non-Japanese populations has not been established. The third SNP has been reported in the CC chemokine receptor 5 (CCR5) gene, which codes for a receptor for cell entry of human immunodeficiency virus-1 (HIV-1). Its promoter, SNP 59029, has been associated with HIV disease progression [45]. This marker was marginally associated with a sustained response to IFN therapy in 171 patients with mixed races [46], and the association was confirmed in 105 Japanese patients [47].

Fibrosis progression in patients with chronic hepatitis C: DDX5, CPT1A, HFE, TGF-β1 and TNF
(see also Section 6)

The fibrosis progression rate is highly variable among subjects with chronic hepatitis C infection. Overall, it is estimated that only about 20% of chronically infected subjects progressed to cirrhosis after 20 years [48]. Previously identified clinical risk factors for fibrosis progression included male gender, excessive alcohol use, older age at time of infection and the presence of steatosis on liver biopsy [49–51]. However, many patients with these characteristics have mild disease, while other patients without these factors have cirrhosis [52]. Therefore, host genetic factors are important in determining fibrosis risk in HCV patients.

In a multicentre study of over 1000 chronic hepatitis C patients from four US academic centres, we have identified two novel genetic polymorphisms that were associated with fibrosis risk [53,54]. DDX5, a RNA helicase also known as p68, has previously been shown to interact with the HCV RNA-dependent RNA polymerase in the NS5B region [55]. This suggests that DDX5 is a human cellular factor involved in HCV RNA replication. The second one is CPT1A, a key enzyme in the carnitine-dependent transport across the mitochondrial inner membrane. Deficiency of CPT1A causes a decreased rate of fatty acid beta-oxidation, resulting in fatty liver diseases [56]. Our results indicate that DDX5 and CPT1A SNPs are associated with the risk of developing bridging fibrosis/cirrhosis in multiple cohorts [53,54].

At least three studies have also identified polymorphisms of the *HFE* (haemochromatosis) gene as contributing to fibrosis risk. C282Y and H63D are the two common missense mutations in *HFE*, contributing to hepatic iron overload. Bonkovsky *et al.* [57] first reported in a study of 119 HCV patients that patients with the C282Y mutation had a higher mean fibrosis score (stage 2.6 vs. 1.8) compared with those without the mutation. In a similar study, C282Y was associated with advanced fibrosis (F2–4 vs. F0–1) in 246 HCV patients [58]. A third analysis of 166 patients further confirmed the positive association of C282Y with advanced fibrosis (F2–4) [59]. Another well-studied gene is the gene coding for transforming growth factor β1 (TGF-β1), a profibrogenic cytokine that stimulates the synthesis and inhibits the degradation of a large number of extracellular matrix proteins [60]. Two coding SNPs, L10P and R25P, could potentially change the secretion levels of TGF-β1 [61]. These two SNPs have been correlated with higher stages of fibrosis in a study of 46 patients [62], and were associated with bridging fibrosis/cirrhosis (F3–F4) in 210 Caucasian patients [63]. The other validated SNP for fibrosis risk is the promoter SNP –308A in the gene for tumour necrosis factor (TNF). As a major inflammatory mediator, TNFα could affect liver fibrogenesis by stimulating hepatic stellate cells [64]. The –308A promoter SNP was significantly associated with cirrhosis in 144 patients with chronic hepatitis C [65], and with bridging fibrosis/cirrhosis in 52 patients [66].

Identification of disease-associated polymorphisms: candidate gene vs. genome-wide study

Genetic studies to identify disease associations can be broadly divided into candidate gene studies, which use resequencing or association approaches, and genome-wide studies, which use genome-wide linkage mapping or genome-wide association approaches. So far, most published genetic studies in liver diseases have focused on the candidate gene approach, in which polymorphisms in a few candidate genes with known biological functions have been studied (Tables 1 and 2). While this approach does identify interesting markers, it limits the findings

to known biological pathways. However, genome-wide association study is becoming feasible as a result of the completion of the human genome sequence, the deposition of millions of SNPs into public databases, the rapid improvements in SNP genotyping technology and the International HapMap Project.

Genome-wide association studies, in which a dense set of SNPs across the genome are typed to survey the disease association, have at least two advantages. First, in comparison with the candidate gene approach, a genome-wide study offers an unbiased, yet fairly comprehensive, option for all genes and diseases independent of any known pathophysiology. Second, for most complex diseases caused by common variants with modest effects, the association approach is much more powerful than the linkage approach [67–69].

Markers in a genome-wide scan can be selected based on LD or potential functions, or the combination of both. LD is the non-random association of alleles at two or more loci on a chromosome. The rationale for LD-based markers is that most of the common SNPs in the genome can be divided into groups (haplotype blocks), in which the genotype of one SNP accurately predicts those of the correlated neighbouring ones. On the basis of current data, it is estimated that a few hundred thousand well-chosen SNPs should be adequate to cover most of the genome [67–69]. Obviously, this approach is dependent on the clear understanding of the LD pattern, and efficient statistical methods to select the tagging SNPs, both of which are still in progress. On the other hand, based on the fact that most mutations causing Mendelian disorders are missense mutations, Botstein and Risch [70] proposed that genome-wide association should focus on missense mutations. As there are only one or two missense SNPs per gene, this strategy requires only 30 000–60 000 SNPs [67]. In the genome-wide study we performed on patients with chronic hepatitis C, 68.3% of SNPs are coding functional SNPs (missense, nonsense, acceptor and donor splice sites); the remainder are non-coding, putative regulatory SNPs that may affect the level of gene expression, i.e. SNPs located at putative transcription factor binding sites, or 5'/3' untranslated regions [53,54].

Study design and data analysis

Despite the increasing interest in finding genetic markers associated with different liver diseases, very few markers have been validated in multiple studies (Tables 1 and 2). This is a common problem observed in other disease association studies and precludes these markers from being usefully incorporated into clinical practice [71]. In a comprehensive review by Hirschhorn *et al.* [71] of > 600 positive disease associations that have been reported, 166 (27.7%) have been studied three or more times, but only six (1%) have been consistently replicated. Similarly, we found that, of the > 115 associations in different liver diseases that have been reported, 28 SNPs (24%) have been studied in two or more sample sets, but only 14 SNPs (12%) have been

Table 2 Polymorphisms reported in liver disease.

Diseases	SNPs/genes reported[a]	SNPs/genes reported in more than two studies[b]	SNPs/genes validated in more than two studies[c]
Non-alcoholic fatty liver disease (NAFLD)	ADRB2, ADRB3, AGT, ALDH2, CD14, HFE, IL10, IL1B, MTP, PEMT, PPARA, PPARG, TGFB1, TNF	MTP, PPARA	MTP
Alcohol-induced liver disease (ALD)	ADH1, ADH2, ADH3, ALDH2, CD14, CTLA4, CYP2E1, IL10, IL1RN, SOD2	ADH1, ADH2, ADH3, ALDH2, CYP2E1, IL-1RN	ADH2, ALDH2, CYP2E1
Primary biliary cirrhosis (PBC)	ABCB1, CD14, CD14 ligand, CTLA4, CYP2D6, CYP2E1, FAS, HLA, IL10, IL1B, L1RN, IL-2, IL6, MBL2, MDR1, NOS3, NR1I2, NRAMP1, PXR, SPP1, TNF, VDR	CTLA4, IL-10, TNF, VDR	CTLA4, VDR
IFN response in chronic hepatitis C	CCR2, CCR5, CTLA4, NB3, HFE, HLA-B, HLA-DRB1, IFNG, IL10, IL1B, IRF1, LMP2, LMP7, MBL, MxA, OPN, RANTES, TAP1, TAP2, TGFB1, TNFA	CCR2, CCR5, IL-10, LMP7, MxA, RANTES, TNFA	CCR5, IL-10, MxA
Fibrosis risk in chronic hepatitis C	ACE, AGT, AGTR1, ApoE, C5, CR2, CCR3, CCR5, COMT, CPT1A, CX3CR1, CYP17, CYP2C19, DDX5, EPHX1, F2, F5, FAS, HFE, HLA, HO1, IFNG, IL10, IL1A, IL1B, IL1RA, IL4, IL6, LDLR, LTA, MBL, MCP1, MCP2, MMP1, MMP3, MMP9, MPO, MTHFR, P53, RANTES, SRD5A2, TAP2, TFR1, TGFB1, TNF	CPT1A, DDX5, HFE, IL1B, TFR1, TGB1, TNF, MPO, HLA	CPT1A, DX5, HFE, TGB1, TNF

For each disease or trait, we included: a, all reported associations; b, associations reported in two or more studies; and c, validated associations. The 'validated markers' are described in detail in the text and Table 1.

validated with positive associations (Table 2). The number of validated makers would be even less (2–3, ~ 1%) if the criteria of Hirschhorn *et al.* [71] were applied.

Here, we discuss the main issues encountered in the association studies and possible solutions. Some of these problems have been reviewed in detail recently [68,72–74].

Sample size

The power to detect an association is determined by the effect size of a disease locus, the frequency of the disease allele(s), the frequency of the tested marker allele(s), the extent of LD between the tested marker and the disease locus and the sample size [75]. While the first four factors are intrinsic properties of the disease and genetic allele, sample size is the only controllable variable that will determine the statistical power of a study. If, in an ideal association study scenario, we assume an OR of 2 as effect size, a 10% frequency of the disease allele and a 100% LD between the tested marker and the disease allele, the required sample size is close to 300 cases and control subjects for detecting such an association, with a statistical power of 80% at a significance level of $P < 0.05$. Obviously, most of the studies listed in Table 2 are undersized even for such an optimal scenario, which is the main source of false positives (type 1 error) and non-replicable results. For the study of complex diseases including liver diseases, sample size should ideally be calculated based on more practical or suboptimal conditions, such as weak effects, rare alleles and partial LD [75]; therefore, the required sample size would be even larger.

Control population

The selection of control subjects is critical as any systematic difference between cases and control subjects can appear as a disease association. One solution is the matched case–control design. Depending on the specific liver disease, the general demographics and related risk factors, such as age, sex, alcohol consumption, viral subtype, etc., should be similar between cases and control subjects. More importantly, the most serious confounder from the genetics perspective is ethnicity, also known as population stratification [76]. This occurs when the cases and control subjects are unintentionally drawn from two or more ethnic groups or subgroups. Stratification will occur if one of these subgroups has higher disease prevalence, or the frequency of some markers varies substantially between ethnic groups. Therefore, cases that contain a predominant ethnic group must be matched to appropriate control subjects of the same ethnicity. If possible, a few sets of control populations can be selected based on various substructures that might exist in the case population. Another solution is to use family-based studies such as the transmission disequilibrium test (TDT). This method is immune to false-positive results from ethnic admixture because ethnicity is controlled internally. The disadvantages are that it requires the affected offspring and their parents to be accessible, and 50% more genotyping than in case–control studies to achieve similar power [73,74,76]. This approach is also not feasible for diseases such as alcoholic cirrhosis or chronic hepatitis C, where it would be hard to find a family with multiple members with alcoholic cirrhosis or infected with HCV.

Clinical endpoints

To identify replicable genetic markers, it is important to have well-defined, commonly acceptable and clinically relevant phenotypes with minimal sampling error. For example, in studying fibrosis risk in patients with chronic hepatitis C, we chose fibrosis stage as the clinical endpoint. We have defined 'cases' as patients with bridging fibrosis or cirrhosis (stage 3–4), while 'control subjects' are those with no or mild fibrosis (stage 0–2). By grouping patients in this manner, we maximized our chances of identifying SNPs associated with fibrosis progression if such SNPs really existed. We intentionally did not group patients according to fibrosis progression rate, which is a value calculated from fibrosis stage on liver biopsy and estimated duration of infection. There were at least three potential sources of error in using fibrosis rate as the clinical endpoint: sampling variation from liver biopsy, uncertainty in determining the duration of HCV infection by recall of risk factor(s), and linearity of fibrosis progression rate. Numerous studies have demonstrated that the accuracy of staging fibrosis in a liver biopsy specimen is affected by the liver biopsy size, quality and experience of the examining pathologist [77–80]. However, such variation is nearly always limited to a single stage [77–80]. Fibrosis staging from liver biopsy is more accurate at the extremes, especially for cirrhosis [80,81], or when fibrosis is stratified into mild (metavir F0–1) vs. advanced (metavir F2–4).

Follow-up genotyping

It is important to realize that, in most cases, the original positive marker may be in LD with the true disease loci or with another marker of better allele frequency or effect size. To explore this possibility, positive associations should be followed up by testing adjacent markers and constructing the haplotype structure in the region.

Interaction with other genetic or environmental factors

If the association is dependent on gene–gene and gene–environment interactions, the association is only replicable in populations with appropriate genetic and environment characteristics [67,71]. In PBC, for example, there is a geographical pattern and the genetic association is often limited to certain geographical areas [26].

Suggested work flow for a genetic epidemiological study

Based on the above discussions, we propose a work flow for future association studies in liver disease as shown in Figure 1.

An ideal case–control association study should comprise a minimum of two large sample sets, namely discovery and

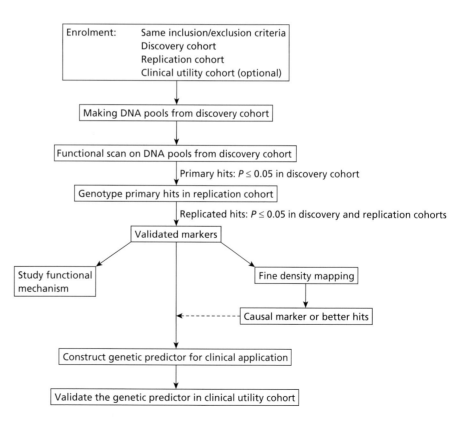

Fig. 1 Proposed study design for association studies between genetic markers and disease phenotypes.

replication cohorts, with a minimum of 250 cases and 250 control subjects in each cohort. All subjects should be enrolled under the same inclusion and exclusion criteria, using well-defined clinical endpoint(s) of interest. DNAs from the discovery cohort are pooled based on the studied clinical endpoints, major risk factors and demographics. Genome-wide scan is performed on pools of the discovery cohort, and significant markers from discovery can be genotyped in the replication cohort. 'Validated markers' are defined as those markers with significant association in both the discovery and the replication cohorts, with the same risk allele and ORs of similar magnitude. Validated markers are individually genotyped in all samples from the discovery and replication cohorts to confirm the association. For all confirmed markers, additional SNPs in the same LD block should be genotyped to identify causal mutations or markers with better ORs and/or allele frequencies. Simultaneously, functional mechanisms of these markers and their genes should be studied in relation to specific liver disease. Furthermore, using combined discovery and replication samples as training sets, statistical methods can be employed to construct the genetic signature selected from all validated hits. The predictive model will then be verified in the clinical utility cohort.

Summary

Association studies have identified interesting genetic polymorphisms influencing disease manifestations and treatment responses in patients with liver diseases. However, most genetic studies in liver diseases have utilized candidate gene approaches, which limit findings to the few genes with known biological function. In addition, small sample size and lack of replication sample sets further hinder the identification of 'true' disease-associated markers. At present, over 10 million SNPs have been identified in over 26 000 genes in the human genome, a small fraction (< 1%) of which, so-called 'functional SNPs' that alter the functions of the gene products, are likely to be potential disease-causing SNPs. A functional genomic scan, performed on a large scale, with well-designed sample sets enables investigators to identify reliable genetic markers that can be integrated into clinical practice.

References

1 Clark JM, Brancati FL, Diehl AM (2003) The prevalence and etiology of elevated aminotransferase levels in the United States. *Am J Gastroenterol* 98(5), 960–967.

2 Ong J, Younossi ZM, Reddy V *et al.* (2001) Cryptogenic cirrhosis and posttransplantation nonalcoholic fatty liver disease. *Liver Transpl* 7(9), 797–801.

3 Angulo P, Keach JC, Batts KP *et al.* (1999) Independent predictors of liver fibrosis in patients with nonalcoholic steatohepatitis. *Hepatology* 30(6), 1356–1362.

4 Neuschwander-Tetri BA, Caldwell SH (2003) Nonalcoholic steatohepatitis: summary of an AASLD Single Topic Conference. *Hepatology* 37(5), 1202–1219.

5 Marchesini G, Bugianesi E, Forlani G *et al.* (2003) Nonalcoholic fatty liver, steatohepatitis, and the metabolic syndrome. *Hepatology* 37(4), 917–923.

6 Wanless IR, Lentz JS (1990) Fatty liver hepatitis (steatohepatitis) and obesity: an autopsy study with analysis of risk factors. *Hepatology* 12(5), 1106–1110.

7 Erbey JR, Silberman C, Lydick E (2000) Prevalence of abnormal serum alanine aminotransferase levels in obese patients and patients with type 2 diabetes. *Am J Med* 109(7), 588–590.

8 Struben VM, Hespenheide EE, Caldwell SH (2000) Nonalcoholic steatohepatitis and cryptogenic cirrhosis within kindreds. *Am J Med* 108(1), 9–13.

9 Willner IR, Waters B, Patil SR *et al.* (2001) Ninety patients with non-alcoholic steatohepatitis: insulin resistance, familial tendency, and severity of disease. *Am J Gastroenterol* 96(10), 2957–2961.

10 Bernard S, Touzet S, Personne I *et al.* (2000) Association between microsomal triglyceride transfer protein gene polymorphism and the biological features of liver steatosis in patients with type II diabetes. *Diabetologia* 43(8), 995–999.

11 Namikawa C, Shu-Ping Z, Vyselaar JR *et al.* (2004) Polymorphisms of microsomal triglyceride transfer protein gene and manganese superoxide dismutase gene in non-alcoholic steatohepatitis. *J Hepatol* 40(5), 781–786.

12 Huang H, Merriman RB, Chokkalingam AP *et al.* (2005) Novel genetic markers associated with risk of non-alcoholic steatohepatitis in patients with non-alcoholic fatty liver diseases. *Gastroenterology* 128(4, Suppl. 2), A694–695.

13 Day CP (2004) The potential role of genes in nonalcoholic fatty liver disease. *Clin Liver Dis* 8(3), 673–691.

14 Diehl AM (2002) Liver disease in alcohol abusers: clinical perspective. *Alcohol* 27(1), 7–11.

15 Maddrey WC (2000) Alcohol-induced liver disease. *Clin Liver Dis* 4(1), 115–131.

16 Hrubec Z, Omenn GS (1981) Evidence of genetic predisposition to alcoholic cirrhosis and psychosis: twin concordances for alcoholism and its biological end points by zygosity among male veterans. *Alcohol Clin Exp Res* 5(2), 207–215.

17 Yoshida A, Hsu LC, Yasunami M (1991) Genetics of human alcohol-metabolizing enzymes. *Prog Nucleic Acid Res Mol Biol* 40, 255–287.

18 Higuchi S, Matsushita S, Masaki T *et al.* (2004) Influence of genetic variations of ethanol-metabolizing enzymes on phenotypes of alcohol-related disorders. *Ann NY Acad Sci* 1025, 472–480.

19 Yamauchi M, Maezawa Y, Mizuhara Y *et al.* (1995) Polymorphisms in alcohol metabolizing enzyme genes and alcoholic cirrhosis in Japanese patients: a multivariate analysis. *Hepatology* 22(4 Pt 1), 1136–1142.

20 Chao YC, Young TH, Tang HS *et al.* (1997) Alcoholism and alcoholic organ damage and genetic polymorphisms of alcohol metabolizing enzymes in Chinese patients. *Hepatology* 25(1), 112–117.

21 Frenzer A, Butler WJ, Norton ID *et al.* (2002) Polymorphism in alcohol-metabolizing enzymes, glutathione S-transferases and apolipoprotein E and susceptibility to alcohol-induced cirrhosis and chronic pancreatitis. *J Gastroenterol Hepatol* 17(2), 177–182.

22 Yu C, Li Y, Chen W *et al.* (2002) Genotype of ethanol metabolizing enzyme genes by oligonucleotide microarray in alcoholic liver disease in Chinese people. *Chin Med J (Engl)* 115(7), 1085–1087.

23 Kim MS, Lee DH, Kang HS *et al.* (2004) [Genetic polymorphisms of alcohol-metabolizing enzymes and cytokines in patients with alcohol induced pancreatitis and alcoholic liver cirrhosis.] *Korean J Gastroenterol* 43(6), 355–363.

24 Tanaka F, Shiratori Y, Yokosuka O *et al.* (1997) Polymorphism of alcohol-metabolizing genes affects drinking behavior and alcoholic liver disease in Japanese men. *Alcohol Clin Exp Res* 21(4), 596–601.

25 Kaplan MM, Gershwin ME (2005) Primary biliary cirrhosis. *N Engl J Med* 353(12), 1261–1273.

26 Selmi C, Invernizzi P, Zuin M *et al.* (2005) Genetics and geoepidemiology of primary biliary cirrhosis: following the footprints to disease etiology. *Semin Liver Dis* 25(3), 265–280.

27 Invernizzi P, Selmi C, Mackay IR *et al.* (2005) From bases to basis: linking genetics to causation in primary biliary cirrhosis. *Clin Gastroenterol Hepatol* 3(5), 401–410.

28 Tivol EA, Schweitzer AN, Sharpe AH (1996) Costimulation and autoimmunity. *Curr Opin Immunol* 8(6), 822–830.

29 Agarwal K, Jones DE, Daly AK *et al.* (2000) CTLA-4 gene polymorphism confers susceptibility to primary biliary cirrhosis. *J Hepatol* 32(4), 538–541.

30 Fan LY, Tu XQ, Cheng QB *et al.* (2004) Cytotoxic T lymphocyte associated antigen-4 gene polymorphisms confer susceptibility to primary biliary cirrhosis and autoimmune hepatitis in Chinese population. *World J Gastroenterol* 10(20), 3056–3059.

31 Vogel A, Strassburg CP, Manns MP (2002) Genetic association of vitamin D receptor polymorphisms with primary biliary cirrhosis and autoimmune hepatitis. *Hepatology* 35(1), 126–131.

32 Lakatos LP, Bajnok E, Hegedus D *et al.* (2002) Vitamin D receptor, oestrogen receptor-alpha gene and interleukin-1 receptor antagonist gene polymorphisms in Hungarian patients with primary biliary cirrhosis. *Eur J Gastroenterol Hepatol* 14(7), 733–740.

33 Halmos B, Szalay F, Cserniczky T *et al.* (2000) Association of primary biliary cirrhosis with vitamin D receptor BsmI genotype polymorphism in a Hungarian population. *Dig Dis Sci* 45(6), 1091–1095.

34 Fan L, Tu X, Zhu Y *et al.* (2005) Genetic association of vitamin D receptor polymorphisms with autoimmune hepatitis and primary biliary cirrhosis in the Chinese. *J Gastroenterol Hepatol* 20(2), 249–255.

35 Lindsay KL (2002) Introduction to therapy of hepatitis C. *Hepatology* 36 (5S1), S114–120.

36 Ferenci P (2004) Predictors of response to therapy for chronic hepatitis C. *Semin Liver Dis* 24(S2), 25–31.

37 Moore KW, O'Garra A, de Waal Malefyt R *et al.* (1993) Interleukin-10. *Annu Rev Immunol* 11, 165–190.

38 Eskdale J, Keijsers V, Huizinga T *et al.* (1999) Microsatellite alleles and single nucleotide polymorphisms (SNP) combine to form four major haplotype families at the human interleukin-10 (IL-10) locus. *Genes Immun* 1(2), 151–155.

39 Edwards-Smith CJ, Jonsson JR, Purdie DM *et al.* (1999) Interleukin-10 promoter polymorphism predicts initial response of chronic hepatitis C to interferon alfa. *Hepatology* 30(2), 526–530.

40 Knapp S, Hennig BJ, Frodsham AJ *et al.* (2003) Interleukin-10 promoter polymorphisms and the outcome of hepatitis C virus infection. *Immunogenetics* 55(6), 362–369.

41 Giannelli G, Guadagnino G, Dentico P *et al.* (2004) MxA and PKR expression in chronic hepatitis C. *J Interferon Cytokine Res* 24(11), 659–663.

42 Hijikata M, Ohta Y, Mishiro S (2000) Identification of a single nucleotide polymorphism in the MxA gene promoter (G/T at nt −88) correlated with the response of hepatitis C patients to interferon. *Intervirology* 43(2), 124–127.

43 Hijikata M, Mishiro S, Miyamoto C *et al.* (2001) Genetic polymorphism of the MxA gene promoter and interferon responsiveness of hepatitis C patients: revisited by analyzing two SNP sites (−123 and −88) *in vivo* and *in vitro. Intervirology* 44(6), 379–382.

44 Suzuki F, Arase Y, Suzuki Y *et al.* (2004) Single nucleotide polymorphism of the MxA gene promoter influences the response to interferon monotherapy in patients with hepatitis C viral infection. *J Viral Hepat* 11(3), 271–276.

45 Kostrikis LG, Huang Y, Moore JP *et al.* (1998) A chemokine receptor CCR2 allele delays HIV-1 disease progression and is associated with a CCR5 promoter mutation. *Nature Med* 4(3), 350–353.

46 Promrat K, McDermott DH, Gonzalez CM *et al.* (2003) Associations of chemokine system polymorphisms with clinical outcomes and treatment responses of chronic hepatitis C. *Gastroenterology* 124(2), 352–360. Erratum in: *Gastroenterology* (2003) 124(4), 1168.

47 Konishi I, Horiike N, Hiasa Y *et al.* (2004) CCR5 promoter polymorphism influences the interferon response of patients with chronic hepatitis C in Japan. *Intervirology* 47(2), 114–120.

48 Thomas DL, Seeff LB (2005) Natural history of hepatitis C. *Clin Liver Dis* 9(3), 383–498.

49 Poynard T, Bedossa P, Opolon P (1997) Natural history of liver fibrosis progression in patients with chronic hepatitis C. The OBSVIRC, METAVIR, CLINIVIR, and DOSVIRC groups. *Lancet* 349, 825–832.

50 Wright M, Goldin R, Fabre A *et al.* (2003) Measurement and determinants of the natural history of liver fibrosis in hepatitis C virus infection: a cross sectional and longitudinal study. *Gut* 52, 574–579.

51 Ramesh S, Sanyal AJ (2004) Hepatitis C and nonalcoholic fatty liver disease. *Semin Liver Dis* 24, 399–413.

52 Marcellin P, Asselah T, Boyer N (2002) Fibrosis and disease progression in hepatitis C. *Hepatology* 36, S47–56.

53 Huang H, Shiffman ML, Cheung RC *et al.* (2006) Identification of two gene variants associated with risk of advanced fibrosis in patients with chronic hepatitis C. *Gastroenterology* 130, 1679–1687.

54 Huang H, Wright TL, Tuason O *et al.* (2005) Association of fibrosis risk in HCV patients with a missense single nucleotide polymorphism in a gene encoding carnitine palmitoyltransferase 1A (CPT1A). *J Hepatol* 42(Suppl. 2), 22.

55 Goh PY, Tan YJ, Lim SP *et al.* (2004) Cellular RNA helicase p68 relocalization and interaction with the hepatitis C virus (HCV) NS5B protein and the potential role of p68 in HCV RNA replication. *J Virol* 78(10), 5288–5298.

56 Bonnefont JP, Djouadi F, Prip-Buus C *et al.* (2004) Carnitine palmitoyltransferases 1 and 2: biochemical, molecular and medical aspects. *Mol Aspects Med* 25, 495–520.

57 Bonkovsky HL, Troy N, McNeal K *et al.* (2002) Iron and HFE or TfR1 mutations as comorbid factors for development and progression of chronic hepatitis C. *J Hepatol* 37(6), 848–854.

58 Gehrke SG, Stremmel W, Mathes I *et al.* (2003) Hemochromatosis and transferrin receptor gene polymorphisms in chronic hepatitis C: impact on iron status, liver injury and HCV genotype. *J Mol Med* 81(12), 780–787.

59 Geier A, Reugels M, Weiskirchen R *et al.* (2004) Common heterozygous hemochromatosis gene mutations are risk factors for inflammation and fibrosis in chronic hepatitis C. *Liver Int* 24(4), 285–294.

60 Border WA, Noble NA (1994) Transforming growth factor beta in tissue fibrosis. *N Engl J Med* 331(19), 1286–1292.

61 He B, Xu C, Yang B *et al.* (1998) Linkage and association analysis of genes encoding cytokines and myelin proteins in multiple sclerosis. *J Neuroimmunol* 86(1), 13–19.

62 Gewaltig J, Mangasser-Stephan K, Gartung C *et al.* (2002) Association

of polymorphisms of the transforming growth factor-beta1 gene with the rate of progression of HCV-induced liver fibrosis. *Clin Chim Acta* 316(1–2), 83–94.

63 Wang H, Mengsteab S, Tag CG *et al.* (2005) Transforming growth factor-beta1 gene polymorphisms are associated with progression of liver fibrosis in Caucasians with chronic hepatitis C infection. *World J Gastroenterol* 11(13), 1929–1936.

64 Friedman SL (1997) Molecular mechanisms of hepatic fibrosis and principles of therapy. *J Gastroenterol* 32(3), 424–430.

65 Yee LJ, Tang J, Herrera J *et al.* (2000) Tumor necrosis factor gene polymorphisms in patients with cirrhosis from chronic hepatitis C virus infection. *Genes Immun* 1(6), 386–390.

66 Goyal A, Kazim SN, Sakhuja P *et al.* (2004) Association of TNF-beta polymorphism with disease severity among patients infected with hepatitis C virus. *J Med Virol* 72(1), 60–65.

67 Hirschhorn JN, Daly MJ (2005) Genome-wide association studies for common diseases and complex traits. *Nature Rev Genet* 6(2), 95–108.

68 Wang WY, Barratt BJ, Clayton DG *et al.* (2005) Genome-wide association studies: theoretical and practical concerns. *Nature Rev Genet* 6(2), 109–118.

69 Goldstein DB, Ahmadi KR, Weale ME *et al.* (2003) Genome scans and candidate gene approaches in the study of common diseases and variable drug responses. *Trends Genet* 19(11), 615–622.

70 Botstein D, Risch N (2003) Discovering genotypes underlying human phenotypes: past successes for mendelian disease, future approaches for complex disease. *Nature Genet* 33(Suppl.), 228–237.

71 Hirschhorn JN, Lohmueller K, Byrne E *et al.* (2002) A comprehensive review of genetic association studies. *Genet Med* 4, 45–61.

72 Colhoun HM, McKeigue PM, Davey Smith G (2003) Problems of reporting genetic associations with complex outcomes. *Lancet* 361, 865–972.

73 Cardon LR, Bell JI (2001) Association study designs for complex diseases. *Nature Rev Genet* 2(2), 91–99.

74 Risch NJ (2000) Searching for genetic determinants in the new millennium. *Nature* 405(6788), 847–856.

75 Zondervan KT, Cardon LR (2004) The complex interplay among factors that influence allelic association. *Nature Rev Genet* 5(2), 89–100.

76 Cardon LR, Palmer LJ (2003) Population stratification and spurious allelic association. *Lancet* 361(9357), 598–604.

77 Regev A, Berho M, Jeffers LJ *et al.* (2002) Sampling error and intraobserver variation in liver biopsy in patients with chronic HCV infection. *Am J Gastroenterol* 97, 2614–2618.

78 Bedossa P, Dargere D, Paradis V (2003) Sampling variability of liver fibrosis in chronic hepatitis C. *Hepatology* 38, 1449–1457.

79 Afdal NH, Nunes D (2004) Evaluation of liver fibrosis: a concise review. *Am J Gastroenterol* 99, 1160–1174.

80 Rousselet MC, Michalak S, Dupre F *et al.* (2005) Sources of variability in histological scoring of chronic viral hepatitis. *Hepatology* 41, 257–264.

81 Poynard T, Mathurin P, Lai CL *et al.*; PANFIBROSIS Group (2003) A comparison of fibrosis progression in chronic liver diseases. *J Hepatol* 38(3), 257–265.

3.3.2 Immunogenetics of liver disease

Peter T. Donaldson

Immunogenetics is now recognized as a major subspeciality within the field of complex disease genetics. Understanding the genetic basis of complex disease has been heralded as one of the major challenges of the postgenome era. There are three major goals: (i) to use the new genetics in disease diagnosis; (ii) to use the new genetics in patient management and care (including development of individualized therapies – although this is more suited to pharmacogenetics); and (iii) to use the new genetics to advance our understanding of disease pathology. Of these three promises, the last is perhaps the most realistic for immunogenetics.

Immunogenetics grew out of an early interest in the immune recognition of tumours and blossomed with the advent of transplantation in a clinical setting. Consequently, a major focus for this subspeciality has been (and still is) the human major histocompatibility complex (MHC). More recently, the genome project has revealed a vast array of inherited variation in immune regulatory proteins, and it now seems that almost all 'immune response (IR) genes' are polymorphic. As the immune response is a central process in most, if not all, human diseases, it is of no surprise to find that IR genes play a very significant role in the development and progression of non-Mendelian (complex) liver disease.

The first immunogenetic studies in liver disease were conducted in the early 1970s [1]. These investigations broke most of the rules for genetic association studies that we know today, but nevertheless described key genetic associations upon which much later work has been based. Not all those early studies have withstood the test of time (Table 1). Those that do survive scrutiny have evolved. This evolution reflects a growing knowledge of the human genome, a better understanding of linkage disequilibrium and a better understanding of the role played by haplotypes.

Today, immunogenetics is split into two broad categories concerning either MHC or non-MHC genes. The strongest and most reproducible genetic associations in liver disease are with MHC alleles and haplotypes. However, there is an increasing body of evidence to suggest involvement of non-MHC IR genes. In this section, I will consider the state of knowledge for both MHC and non-MHC IR genes in liver disease, discuss some of the current theories to explain these associations and try to illustrate the way forward for immunogenetic studies.

Human MHC

The human MHC maps to 7.6 Mb of chromosome 6p21.3. The full map of the human MHC was published recently and is more complex than previously envisaged [2]. The extended MHC (xMHC) encodes 421 gene loci, of which 252 are

Table 1 Summary of early studies of HLA in autoimmune and viral liver disease.

Disease	Association	Author and year
PSC	A1 and **B8**	Schrumpf et al. (1982)
	B12 (44) (later B44)	Chapman et al. (1983)
	DR3	Chapman et al. (1983)
	DR13	Farrant et al. (1992)
Type 1 AIH	**A1 and B8**	Mackay & Morris (1972)
	Dw3 (later DR3)	Opelz et al. (1977)
	DR3	Donaldson et al. (1991)
	DRw4 (later DR4)	Williams et al. (1978)
	DR4	Donaldson et al. (1991)
PBC	A1 and B8	Eddleston et al. (1974)
	DR2	Miyamori et al. (1983)
	DR3	Ercilla et al. (1979)
	DR4	Johnston et al. (1987)
	DR8	Gores et al. (1987)
	DR11	Gores et al. (1987)
HBV	DR2	Almarri and Batchelor (1994)*
	DR6	van Hattum et al. (1987)
	DR7	Almarri and Batchelor (1994)*
HCV	**DR5-DQ3**	Peano et al. (1994)
	DR5-DQ3	Zavaglia et al. (1996)

AIH, autoimmune hepatitis; HBV, hepatitis B virus; HCV, hepatitis C virus; PBC, primary biliary cirrhosis; PSC, primary sclerosing cholangitis. All the above studies are described as 'early' either on grounds of the year of the original publication or on the basis of the technology used for HLA typing. With one exception (*) all were based on serological typing, which is based on restriction fragment length polymorphism (RFLP) analysis. Associations which have been widely replicated are highlighted. Note that nomenclature has changed and technology has evolved permitting higher resolution genotyping and subdivision of some allelic families. For example, the DR6 family can be divided into approximately 63 *DRB1*13* and 48 *DRB1*14* alleles.

expressed genes, 30 are classified as transcripts and 139 are pseudogenes. The xMHC is characterized by extreme linkage disequilibrium and a very high degree of polymorphism (56 of the 252 expressed xMHC genes are known to be polymorphic). This polymorphism includes single nucleotide polymorphism (SNPs), deletion/insertion polymorphism (DIPs) and two large regions of duplication.

Within the xMHC, it is possible to recognize clusters and superclusters that appear to have arisen from both small- and large-scale segmental duplications. Currently, six clusters and six superclusters are recognized. Among these are three that are of immediate interest: the human leucocyte antigen (HLA) class I supercluster, the tumour necrosis factor (TNF) cluster and the HLA class II cluster.

The HLA class I supercluster comprises: the classical HLA *A*, *B* and *Cw* loci; the non-classical HLA *E*, *F* and more distant *HFE* locus; the class I-like genes *MICA* and *MICB*; and 12 pseudogenes. Both classical and non-classical HLA class I gene products

are involved in the natural killer (NK) cell-mediated immune responses through presentation of antigens to CD8+ T cells and recognition of the leukocyte receptor complex or natural killer complex. The expression profile of the class I-like *MICA* and *MICB* indicates a possible role in mucosal immunity. HFE, on the other hand, although resembling a classical HLA class I protein (including the interaction with β2-microglobulin), is involved in iron metabolism, rather than in antigen processing and presentation. Although early studies described genetic linkage between the HLA *A* locus and idiopathic haemochromatosis (IH), this was later found to be a result of linkage disequilibrium with the *HFE* locus 4 Mb telomeric of HLA *A*.

The TNF gene cluster comprises the genes encoding TNFα, lymphotoxin-α and lymphotoxin-β. All three are cytokines involved in the inflammatory immune response.

The HLA class II cluster comprises the classical HLA *DP*, *DQ* and *DR* genes and the non-classical HLA *DM* and *DO* genes. The products of these genes form heterodimers involved in antigen presentation to CD4+ T cells (*DP*, *DQ*, *DR*) and peptide exchange and loading into class II molecules (*DM*, *DO*).

Interestingly, although there are many class I-like genes in the genome, there are (as yet) no class II-like genes outside the xMHC.

Genes of the human MHC in clinical liver disease

Despite the apparent complexity of the xMHC, studies in liver disease have concentrated on relatively few of the genes encoded therein. The areas of interest include members of the HLA class I supercluster (HLA *A*, *B* and, to a lesser extent, *Cw* and *MICA*), the class II cluster (HLA *DR*, *DQ* and, to a lesser extent, *DP*) and a single member of the TNF cluster (*TNFA*). In addition, a few studies have looked at the MHC-encoded complement genes *C4A* and *C4B*. A map of the xMHC can be found at www.nature.com/nrg/journal/v5/n12/poster/MHCmap; data on individual genes can found at www.ncbi.nih.gov/MHC; and up-to-date HLA nomenclature can be found at www.anthonynolan.org.uk/research.

Much has been written about how we should study genetically complex diseases. However, very little of this advice has (until recently) had any impact on the strategies applied to the study of genetically complex liver diseases. The basic data that would indicate to a classical geneticist that the diseases listed below have a significant heritable component are simply not available. Most of these diseases are rare in families, and most are diseases of adulthood presenting in later life, ruling out the possibilities of genetic studies based on linkage analysis of families or affected sib pairs. Consequently, studies of these diseases have been almost entirely restricted to case–control association analyses. Yet despite this, there have been some very promising findings in this area of research, in particular in the study of autoimmune and, more recently, viral liver diseases.

Table 2 Summary of HLA haplotypes in autoimmune liver disease.

Disease	Population	Haplotype	Risk ratio
PBC	Japan	**DRB1***0803-DQ3-DPB1*0501*	NA
	NEC-Europe and NEC-USA	**DRB1*0801**-DQA1*0401-DQB1*0402*	8.16
PSC	NEC-Europe	[a]B8-**MICA*008**-TNFA*2-DRB3*0101-**DRB1*0301**-DQB1*0201*	2.69
		DRB3*0101-DRB1*1301-DQA1*0103-**DQB1*0603**	3.8
		MICA*008-DRB5*0101-DRB1*1501-DQA1*0102-**DQB1*0602**	1.52
		DRB4*0103-DRB4*0401-DQA1*03-**DQB1*0302**	0.26
		DRB4*0103-DRB1*0701-DQA1*0201-**DQB1*0303**	0.15
		MICA*002	0.15
AIH	NEC-Europe and NEC-USA	[a]A1-B8-MICA*008-TNFA*2-DRB3*0101-**DRB1*0301**-DQB1*0201*	4.6–5.51
		DRB4*0103-**DRB1*0401**-DQA1*0301-DQB1*0301*	3.3–3.7
		DRB5*0101-**DRB1*1501**-DQA1*0102-DQB1*0602*	0.32–0.4
	Japan	Bw54-DRB4*-**DRB1*0405**-DQA1*0301-DQB1*0401*	
	Argentina and Brazil	Adults: DRB4*0101-**DRB1*0405**	10.4
		Children: DRB3*0101-**DRB1*1301**-DQA1*0103-DQB1*0603*	16.3
		Children: DRB3*0101-**DRB1*0301**-DQA1*0501-DQB1*0201*	3.0

NEC, northern European Caucasoid. All studies are based on adult cases unless otherwise marked. Protective haplotypes are underlined and have risk values < 1. The current allele(s) of interest (i.e. candidate primary susceptibility/resistance allele shown) are in bold on each haplotype.
[a]HLA 8.1 haplotype.

The MHC and autoimmune liver disease

The strongest associations have been reported in the autoimmune liver diseases, primary sclerosing cholangitis (PSC) and type 1 autoimmune hepatitis (AIH) (Table 2) [3]. At first glance, there are striking similarities between the two. Both PSC and AIH are associated with an increased frequency of the HLA 8.1 haplotype. However, closer scrutiny reveals that susceptibility and resistance for these diseases may map to different gene loci within the MHC. Thus, in PSC, MHC-encoded susceptibility appears to involve either a combination of *DRB–DQB* and the *MICA* alleles or perhaps *MICA* alone [3], whereas in type 1 AIH, MHC-encoded susceptibility appears to be related very closely to specific *DRB1* alleles that carry lysine or arginine at position 71 [4].

Primary sclerosing cholangitis

In PSC, studies have consistently reported an increased risk of disease associated with the HLA 8.1 haplotype and with the HLA *DRB3*0101-DRB1*1301-DQA1*0103-DQB1*0603* haplotype [3]. The association with the HLA *DRB5*0101-DRB1*1501-DQA1*0102-DQB1*0602* haplotype is more controversial [5]. Interestingly, other than B8, there have been no reproducible associations with classical HLA class I alleles in PSC [5], indicating that susceptibility and resistance to PSC do not map to these gene loci. However, data on *MICA* allele frequencies in PSC indicate a five- to sixfold increased risk of PSC associated with homozygosity for *MICA*008* and a 14-fold reduced risk associated with one or more copies of the *MICA*002* allele (Table 2)

[3,5]. This provides strong evidence to suggest a significant role for *MICA* in MHC-encoded susceptibility/resistance to PSC. Yet, *MICA* alone cannot account for all the observed MHC associations as the HLA *DRB3*0101-DRB1*1301-DQA1*0103-DQB1*0603* haplotype does not carry *MICA*008*, and neither of the other two HLA haplotypes associated with disease resistance carry *MICA*002*.

These observations have important implications for our understanding of the pathogenesis of PSC. In PSC, the potential involvement of the *MICA* genes indicates a more prominent role for the innate immune response. MICα molecules are expressed on gastrointestinal and thymic epithelia and are also seen in non-diseased liver. MICα molecules may be induced by stress including heat shock. These molecules are ligands for T cells expressing the NKG2D activatory receptor, which activates γδ T cells and NK cells. The 'normal' liver has a large resident population of γδ T cells, NK and natural (N)T cells, and increased numbers of γδ T cells and NK cells have also been documented in PSC livers [6].

There is evidence that *MICA*008* homozygosity may be associated with a loss of MICα function. All *MICA* alleles carry a variable number of short tandem repeat (STR) sequences. The STR encoded on all *MICA*008* haplotypes, the 5.1STR, encodes a MICα molecule with a short, perhaps even, unstable cytoplasmic segment. If PSC arises as a result of infection, heat shock induction of MICα on biliary epithelium would be a crucial step in the activation of intrahepatic γδ T cells and NK cells, leading to cytokine secretion and cytolytic effector functions. In individuals homozygous for *MICA*008*, unstable expression of MICα may cause failed immune activation, with the consequence of persistent infection. Persistent infection carries with it an ever-increasing risk of recognition of self (auto)antigens through collateral damage and/or exposure of cryptic epitopes.

There is particular interest in innate immunity in inflammatory bowel disease (IBD) at present, and it is tempting, given the observation that two-thirds of all PSC patients may develop ulcerative colitis (UC) at some stage in their illness, to consider the potential for genetic overlap, in which case a common link with innate immunity would perhaps be fitting. Indeed, studies of the MHC suggest that PSC patients with concurrent IBD are less likely to have the *DR4* or *DR7* haplotypes than those without [7], and more recent studies indicate that the *CARD4* polymorphism associated with increased risk of IBD and UC may be a risk factor for PSC/UC overlap [8].

Autoimmune hepatitis type 1

In Europe and North America, there are very clear strong associations between increased risk for type 1 AIH and both the HLA 8.1 and *DRB4*0101-DRB1*0401-DQA1*0301-DQB1*0301* haplotypes (Table 2) [4]. The latter association is secondary to the former and is more pronounced in patients with late-onset disease. There no are significant associations with HLA *A*, *B* or *Cw* on the second haplotype, no significant associations (independent of HLA 8.1) with either *TNFA* or *MICA* and no single shared *DQA*, *DQB* or *DPB* allele or sequence carried on both these haplotypes. These observations led to the development of the 'lysine/arginine DRβ-71 hypothesis' in type 1 AIH [4].

According to this hypothesis, MHC-encoded susceptibility and resistance depends primarily on the amino acid residue encoded at position 71 of the DRβ polypeptide. Both *DRB1*0301* and *DRB1*0401* encode lysine at position 71, and susceptibility alleles in other populations (including *DRB1*0404* and *DRB1*0405*) have arginine 71 (Table 3). These are both basic, highly charged, polar amino acids and are positioned over the P4 and P7 binding pockets of the expressed HLA-DR molecule. The allele *DRB1*1501*, which is associated with a reduced risk of type 1 AIH, encodes alanine 71, a small non-charged residue. Substitution of lysine/arginine for alanine would have a profound effect on the peptide-binding properties of the expressed DR molecule, and it this idea upon which the 'lysine/arginine DRβ-71 hypothesis' is based.

Type 1 AIH is a classical autoimmune disease. The genetic association with HLA *DRB1* points to the MHC class II antigen presenting pathway and events in T-cell activation as the key to understanding disease initiation. This fits well with the characteristics of type 1 AIH as a predominantly T cell-mediated disease. However, the lysine/arginine 71 model does not tell us much about the autoantigen in type 1 AIH and is not universal. A number of alternative models have been proposed, but none of them fits the European/North American data [4]. Different models for each population (if they are valid) may suggest that different genetic associations have arisen in different populations, depending on the prevailing environmental risk factors:

for example, in South America, where hepatitis A virus is endemic, persistent infection is associated with carriage of the HLA *DRB1*1301* [9] allele, the same allele carried by the majority of children who develop type 1 AIH in that population. Thus, these HLA associations may provide the 'molecular footprint' of the prevailing environmental trigger(s) that precipitate the disease in different populations.

A further level of complexity exists whereby European and North American patients with *DRB1*0301* have quite different clinical characteristics from those with the *DRB1*0401* haplotype, although both haplotypes carry lysine 71 [4], indicating that, although lysine/arginine 71 may be the primary determinant of disease susceptibility (at least in European and North America) to type 1 AIH, other genes within the MHC (or closely linked genes) may modify the clinical phenotype.

Primary biliary cirrhosis (PBC)

Studies of PBC [3,10], the most common of the three autoimmune liver diseases, consistently report weak but significant associations with alleles of the HLA DR8 family (*DRB1*0801* in Europeans and *DRB1*0803* in Japan). The risk of disease for those with these alleles is approximately two to three times greater than for those without (Table 2). However, in Europeans, this association accounts for only 15–25% of patients. This may indicate that the true association lies elsewhere along the chromosome with *DRB1*0801* acting as a linkage marker.

In the case of PBC, these findings are not in keeping with the picture of a T cell-mediated autoimmune disease, suggesting that some thought should be given to the role of non-classical MHC and other immunogenes in PBC.

The MHC and viral hepatitis

The relationship between the host MHC IR genes and viral hepatitis has been quite widely explored (see Table 4), with particular emphasis being placed on HLA [3,11]. In most cases, the risk of infection is not itself genetically determined, but host HLA genes do play a role in determining the outcome following exposure to the virus. Not all the immunogenetic studies in viral hepatitis have been replicated but, among the more reproducible and interesting findings are the following observations: individuals who have the *DRB1*1301* [12] allele are more prone to persistent hepatitis A virus (HAV) infection; individuals with *DRB1*1302* [13] are more prone to persistent hepatitis B virus (HBV) infection; and individuals with *DQB1*0301* haplotypes [14,15] are more likely to have self-limiting hepatitis C virus (HCV) infection (Table 4).

Most studies on the immunogenetics of viral liver disease are based on the European population where the major concern has been HCV. Although there have been a few studies of HAV and HBV, with the exception of the two studies above [12,13], most of these have been based on small numbers, and the findings from these studies have not been widely replicated. In contrast,

Table 3 *DRB1* alleles and amino acids associated with type 1 AIH.

Allele	Amino acid (single letter code) and position				
	13	26	67–72	74	86
*DRB1*0301*	S	Y	LLEQKR	R	V
*DRB1*0401*	H	F	LLEQKR	A	G
*DR1*0404*	H	F	LLEQRR	A	G
*DRB1*0405*	H	F	LLEQRR	A	G
*DRB1*1301*	**S**	**F**	**ILEDER**	**A**	**V**
*DRB1*1501*	R	F	ILEQAR	A	V

Bold type illustrates the major susceptibility alleles for type 1 AIH. Underlining denotes association in paediatric cases of type 1 AIH from Argentina. Normal type shows protective haplotype. Sequences for second expressed DRB gene on each haplotype are not shown. Analysis of pooled data for the King's and Mayo published series (205 patients) indicates tyrosine (Y) at DRβ-26 has odds ratio (OR) of 3.52 and arginine (R) at DRβ-74 has an OR of 3.74; whereas lysine (K) at DRβ-71 has an OR of 8.78 and all three possibilities are highly significant ($P < 0.00000001$).

there is a considerable volume of work on HCV, much of which has been replicated.

At first glance, the current literature on HLA and HCV appears to be contradictory [3,8,11,12]. There are a number of reasons for this. Many of the early studies focused on the potential relationship between HLA and the risk of infection with HCV. Early studies were based on poor-quality HLA serotyping and were often based on small numbers [16]. More recently, investigators have used DNA-based techniques focusing on the role of HLA in determining outcome following viral infection. Even so, many studies remain small (with low numbers in informative subgroups), and most studies fail to correct for confounding variables such as viral genotype, viral load, route of infection, gender, age and alcohol intake.

Currently, one major finding stands out from the rest. Alric *et al.* [14] found a higher frequency of the *DRB1*11-DQB1*0301* haplotype in French patients with untreated self-limiting (acute) infection compared with those with persistent (chronic) infection. This is particularly pertinent because the majority (estimated at 50–80%) of those infected with HCV become chronic carriers. Cramp *et al.* [15] later suggested that a different haplotype, *DRB*04-DQB1*0301*, was responsible for this effect. In each case, the authors found increased frequencies of the predominant *DQB1*0301* haplotype in their particular population, thus suggesting that the *DQB1*0301* allele is responsible for this effect, rather than a particular *DRB1* allele.

Based on these observations [14,15], we may expect that individuals with *DQB1*0301* would have a more vigorous immune response to HCV peptides, and indeed they do [17]. In addition, studies have shown that these patients have a greater response to a range of HCV peptides and are more likely to have a multispecific IR as opposed to a monospecific response when

challenged with different HCV-derived peptides *in vitro* (M. Cramp, unpublished observations). A multispecific IR may be essential to combat mechanisms by which the virus evades immune-mediated destruction.

Although the data on *DQB1*0301* are very exciting, there are dissenting voices. Studies in the Irish population have been particularly informative in describing associations with the HLA 8.1 haplotype rather than with either of the common *DQB1*0301* haplotypes above [3,18]. The Irish study population [18] is unique in being composed of a single cohort of women who contracted HCV following immunization with a single batch of infected rhesus antibody. Thus, in this series, the confounding variables of gender, viral genotype, viral load and route of infection are all neutral. However, the findings reported in this cohort have not been replicated in the population at large.

Overlap between MHC associations in autoimmune and viral liver disease

It is interesting to note that the key HLA haplotypes in viral infection (Table 4) are also implicated in type 1 AIH and PSC (Table 2). Although there is no absolute correlation between haplotypes that promote viral persistence and those which promote autoimmune disease, there are significant areas of overlap. For example, *DRB1*0301* and *DRB1*1301* promote viral persistence and autoimmunity, whereas *DRB1*1501* and *DRB1*0701*, which protect from type 1 AIH and PSC, respectively, may both promote HCV persistence. This may all be coincidence, reflecting the fact that the HLA alleles above are all common alleles. However, there are many other common *DRB1* alleles that do not appear in these lists, and it is interesting to speculate about the potential biological basis of this overlap.

Non-MHC immune response genes in clinical liver disease

In the last decade, there has been a plethora of studies investigating non-MHC IR genes. This has been fuelled by the genome project and the knowledge that nearly all human genes are polymorphic. Thus, any gene that encodes an immune-active protein may be targeted for study. This has created a vast, mostly negative, literature populated with failed genetic association studies. Investigators have simply thrown caution to the wind and selected candidates of convenience rather biologically plausible candidates. Early success with the MHC has also fuelled a false expectation that all studies will reveal relatively strong genetic effects (odds ratios > 3). With hindsight, we now know this is not likely in the majority of cases and, therefore, we need to plan our studies so that we can detect relatively weak effects (odds ratios as low as 1.2).

If we consider the key processes in the immune response, we can break our list of candidates into subsections dealing with:

early antigen presentation (so-called signal 1), involving HLA, the T-cell receptor (TCR) and immunoglobulin genes; late antigen presentation (so-called signal 2), involving, among other genes, those encoding the cytotoxic T-lymphocyte antigen-4 (CTLA-4) molecule and related accessory molecules (CD28, as well as B7.1 and B7.2, also known as CD80 and CD81); inflammation, especially the cytokine networks; termination, restoration and repair, especially cytokines involved with wound healing and apoptosis.

In addition, there are a number of genes involved in the innate immune response that do not fall easily into this simple division, for example the killer cell immunoglobulin-like receptor (KIR) genes.

Genes involved in early antigen presentation in clinical liver disease

Other than HLA, very little is known about the role of the other genes involved in early antigen presentation in either auto-immune or viral liver disease. Although there are some early data on both Ig and TCR genes in type 1 AIH, investigators have avoided studying these gene complexes because most of their variation arises from somatic mutation and recombination.

Genes involved in late antigen presentation in clinical liver disease

One of the critical processes in the immune response is governed by the balance between rival accessory molecules CTLA-4 and CD28. In the immediate aftermath of MHC–peptide–TCR interaction, a second signal is required to determine the course of events. Initially, CD4+ T cells expressing CD28 interact with the antigen-presenting cells (APC) through the CD80/CD81 ligand to provide this signal. However, it appears that switching from immune activation to immune memory occurs through the upregulation of CTLA-4 on CD4+, CD25+ T cells. These cells compete with the CD28+ T cells, effectively downregulating the immune response. There are numerous SNPs in the *CTLA4* gene on chromosome 2q33; two of these, commonly referred to as A+49G and CT60 [7], have received particular attention [3,19]. Preliminary studies of the A+49G SNP identified associations with both PBC and type 1 AIH, although these have not been replicated in all populations studied [3]. This may reflect both closer linkage with the functional SNP CT60 (which has not yet been investigated in either disease) or the relatively weak effect of this polymorphism, which may demand large-scale studies for reproducible results.

As T-cell immune responses predominate in immunity to both HBV and HCV, we may also expect *CTLA4* to have a potential role in determining the outcome following viral infection. However, data to support this have not been forthcoming, although there is an isolated (and unconfirmed) report of an association with response to interferon/ribavirin in HCV [20].

Genes involved in inflammation in clinical liver disease

The inflammatory immune response is orchestrated by the cytokine network. Cytokines are also important in wound healing and repair and in the downregulation (termination) of the immune response.

Early studies in liver disease focused on the MHC-encoded proinflammatory cytokine tumour necrosis factor α gene (*TNFA*). Although mostly negative, this stimulated interest in investigating other (non-MHC-encoded) cytokine genes in liver disease, starting with the proinflammatory cytokines, interleukin (IL)-1 and IL-6, interferon-γ, then spreading to the immunoregulatory cytokines IL-4 and IL-10. For the most part, these studies examined preselected single SNPs or, occasionally, multiple SNPs in the target gene. With a few possible exceptions (including preliminary data on *IL1* genes in PBC [10], and on the *IL*10 promoter polymorphisms in alcoholic liver disease [21] and HCV [22]), these studies have been blank or remain controversial.

Overall, the lack of success in the majority of these studies can be attributed to the complexity of the cytokine network (especially the degree of redundancy in the system), the limited scope of many of these studies and the small numbers available for study. We must also question the non-hypothesis-constrained approach of many investigators, which, although valid under some circumstances, will always have a much larger failure rate than a hypothesis-based approach.

Genes involved in termination of the immune response, restoration of immune homeostasis and tissue repair in clinical liver disease

Termination of the immune response is an important process that is often overlooked by immunologists in their search to understand disease pathology. Key within this process is apoptosis and, recently, there has been some interest in the potential role of polymorphism in the FAS gene (correct gene name TNF receptor superfamily 6 or *TNFRSF*6) in both autoimmune and viral liver disease, although studies so far have failed to identify any significant relationships.

Termination of the immune response is also linked with restoration of immune homeostasis and tissue repair. The latter process is particular important in liver disease where abnormalities in the tissue repair mechanisms may lead to fibrosis and cirrhosis. Key components in tissue repair are the family of matrix metalloproteinases (MMPs) and their tissue inhibitors (tissue inhibitors of matrix metalloproteinases or TIMPs). These genes encode a complex network of interacting proteins that regulate collagen metabolism. These proteins have immune regulatory properties and interact with various cytokines including IL-1 and transforming cell growth factor beta (TCGF-β). Studies of *MMP*1, *MMP*3 and *MMP*9 as well as *TGFB*1 and various *IL*1

Virus	Population	Haplotype/allele
HAV	Argentina	Children: *DRB3*0101-**DRB1*1301**-DQA1*0103-DQB1*0603*
HBV	Gambia acute infection	*DRB3*0301-**DRB1*1302**-DQA1*0102-DQB1*0501*
		*DRB3*0301-**DRB1*1302**-DQA1*0102-DQB1*0604*
		[a]*DRB3*0301-**DRB1*1301**-DQA1*0103-DQB1*0603*
HCV	NEC-Europe acute infection	*DRB3*0101-DRB1*1101-DQA1*0501-**DQB1*0301***
		*DRB3*0101-DRB1*1104-DQA1*0501-**DQB1*0301***
		*DRB4*0103-DRB1*0401-DQA1*03-**DQB1*0301***
		[b]***DRB1*0101**-DQA1*0101-DQB1*0501*
HCV	NEC-USA	***DRB1*0101**-DQA1*0101-DQB1*0501*
	Black-USA	*DRB1*0101-DQA1*0101-DQB1*0501*
HCV	NEC-Europe chronic infection	[c]*DRB5*0101-DRB1*1501-DQA1*0102-DQB1*0602*
		*DRB3*0101-**DRB1*0301**-DQA1*0501-DQB1*0201*
		[c]*DRB4*0103-DRB1*0701-DQA1*0201-DQB1*0201*

Table 4 Summary of key HLA haplotypes associated with acute (self-limiting) vs. protracted (chronic) infection in viral hepatitis.

NEC, northern European Caucasoid. Summary represents key selected studies only. All studies based on adult cases unless marked otherwise.
[a]This association was neither confirmed nor refuted by Thursz *et al.* [13].
[b]This association applies to the Irish rhesus patient study group only.
[c]These two haplotypes are consistently found at higher frequencies in patients with chronic HCV infection but are rarely statistically significant. However, the effect of the haplotype may be weak and most studies are underpowered to detect such weak effects.

family member genes have been conducted in PSC. Associations have been described with both *MMP*3 [23] and *MMP*1 [24], although there is no consensus on the former observation, and the latter report has yet to be confirmed in an independent series.

Non-MHC genes involved in the innate immune response in clinical liver disease

Innate and adaptive immunity overlap and interact. In clinical liver disease, studies of the MHC have considered the complement genes *C2*, *C4A*, *C4B*, as well as *MICA* and *TNFA*, all of which have roles in innate immunity. Although there are strong reported associations with specific *C4* alleles in AIH [4] and PBC [10], these may be secondary to linkage disequilibrium with genes of the MHC class II cluster.

More recently, investigators have started to look at the KIR genes. The KIR genes map to chromosome 19q13.4 within the leukocyte receptor complex cluster (LRC). KIRs form receptor–ligand pairs with particular groups of HLA class I *B* and *Cw* alleles and are involved in regulation of NK cell activation. Because the KIR and HLA genes are located on different chromosomes, some individuals lack appropriate pairings and may be more susceptible to failure of NK regulation. The KIR region shows variation in gene content, number and type as well as allelic polymorphism and is particularly complex. The *KIR2DL3* haplotype has been associated with resolving HCV infection, suggesting a role for NK cells in HCV clearance [25]. However, this association is dependent upon possession of a particular HLA class I family group, and the full meaning of this association is not yet clear.

Directions for future studies

Much can be learned about potential disease genes by looking at studies of other (similar) diseases. Investigations in IBD provide an excellent example.

IBD is a complex clinical syndrome, made up mostly of Crohn's disease and ulcerative colitis. Genetic studies reveal a polygenic picture with a number of gene loci suspected, and recent studies have identified several of the major players in susceptibility to both Crohn's disease and ulcerative colitis. The identification of *CARD15* as a major gene for Crohn's disease has changed the perception of the disease pathology, highlighting likely mechanisms of disease genesis and informing the debate on which genes to investigate in related disorders. The recent identification of the gene *CARD4*, which encodes the human NOD1 homologue (located on chromosome 7 – a linkage region for IBD), may have implications for PSC, as it has been shown to be particularly common in IBD patients with ulcerative colitis and PSC.

Overall, studies of the MHC in autoimmune and viral liver disease have been more fruitful than those of non-MHC genes. HLA polymorphisms are mostly functional and are biologically relevant; HLA genes are inherited in tightly conserved haplotypes with several other IR genes, each encoding key components in both the innate as well as the acquired immunity. Thus, HLA haplotypes may each carry several disease-promoting alleles, possibly acting as multihit disease cassettes. This multihit model may explain the relative strength of MHC associations compared with those for non-MHC genes. However, we should not be complacent. So far, studies have considered only 12 of the 56 polymorphic genes of the human MHC, and there is much work still to be done unravelling the role of MHC genes in liver disease.

In contrast, non-MHC genes may have relatively weak effects (although not exclusively, for example *CARD15*), and few of the studies conducted so far in liver disease have been designed to detect such small risk values. To be successful, future studies of liver disease will need to be inclusive and based on large collections of well-characterized patients. They will need to employ high-throughput genotyping and will have to explore whole pathways and networks, rather than single preselected SNPs and genes as most current studies have done.

References

1 Tiwari JL, Terasaki PI (1985) Gastroenterology. In: Tiwari JL, Terasaki PI (eds) *HLA and Disease Associations*, 1st edn. New York: Springer-Verlag, pp. 232–263.

2 Horton R, Wilming L, Rand V *et al.* (2004) Gene map of the extended human MHC. *Nature Rev Genet* 5, 889–899.

3 Donaldson PT (2004) Recent advances in clinical practice: genetics of liver disease: immunogenetics and disease pathogenesis. *Gut* 53, 599–608.

4 Donaldson PT (2002) Genetics in autoimmune hepatitis. *Semin Liver Dis* 22, 353–363.

5 Donaldson PT, Norris S (2001) Immunogenetics in PSC. *Balliere's Best Pract Res Clin Gastroenterol* 15, 611–627.

6 Doherty DG, O'Farrelly C (2003) Lymphoid repertoires in healthy liver. In: Gershwin ME, Vierling JM, Manns MP (eds) *Liver Immunology*, 1st edn. Philadelphia: Hanley Belfus, pp. 31–46.

7 Donaldson PT, Norris S (2002) Evaluation of the role of MHC class II alleles, haplotypes and selected amino acid sequences in primary sclerosing cholangitis. *Autoimmunity* 35, 555–564.

8 McGovern DPB, Hysi P, Ahmed T *et al.* (2005) Association between a complex insertion/deletion polymorphism in NOD1 (CARD4) and susceptibility to inflammatory bowel disease. *Hum Mol Genet* 14, 1245–1250.

9 Pando M, Larriba J, Fernandez GC *et al.* (1999) Paediatric and adult forms of type 1 autoimmune hepatitis in Argentina: evidence for differential genetic predisposition. *Hepatology* 30, 1374–1380.

10 Jones DEJ, Donaldson PT (2003) Genetic factors in the pathogenesis of primary biliary cirrhosis. *Clin Liver Dis* 7, 841–864.

11 Thio CL, Thomas DL, Carrington M *et al.* (2000) Chronic viral hepatitis and the human genome. *Hepatology* 31, 819–827.

12 Fainboim L, Velasco MCC, Marcos CY *et al.* (2001) Protracted, but not acute, hepatitis A virus infection is strongly associated with HLA-DRB1*1301, a marker for paediatric autoimmune hepatitis. *Hepatology* 33, 1512–1517.

13 Thursz MR, Kwiatkowski D, Allsopp COM *et al.* (1995) Association between an MHV class II allele and clearance of hepatitis B virus in the Gambia. *N Engl J Med* 332, 1065–1069.

14 Alric L, Fort M, Izopet J *et al.* (2000) Study of host- and virus-related factors associated with spontaneous hepatitis C virus clearance. *Tissue Antigens* 56, 154–158.

15 Cramp M, Carucci P, Underhill J *et al.* (1998) Association between HLA class II genotype and spontaneous clearance of hepatitis C viremia. *J Hepatol* 29, 207–213.

16 Donaldson PT (1999) HLA and susceptibility to hepatitis C virus – commentary. *Eur J Clin Invest* 29, 280–283.

17 Harcourt G, Hellier S, Bunce M *et al.* (2001) Effect of HLA class II genotype on T helper lymphocyte responses and viral control in hepatitis C virus infection. *J Viral Hepatol* 8, 174–179.

18 McKiernan SM, Hagan R, Curry M *et al.* (2000) The MHC is a major determinant of viral status, but not fibrotic stage, in individuals infected with hepatitis C. *Gastroenterology* 118, 1124–1130.

19 Ueda H, Howson JM, Esposito L *et al.* (2003) Association of the T-cell regulatory gene CTLA4 with susceptibility to autoimmune disease. *Nature* 423, 506–511.

20 Yee LJ, Perez KA, Tang J *et al.* (2003) Association of CTLA4 polymorphisms with sustained response to interferon and ribavirin therapy for chronic hepatitis C virus infection. *J Infect Dis* 187, 1264–1271.

21 Grove J, Daly AK, Bassendine MF *et al.* (2000) Interleukin-10 promoter region polymorphism and susceptibility to advanced alcoholic liver disease. *Gut* 46, 540–545.

22 Yee LJ, Tang J, Gibson AW *et al.* (2001) Interleukin-10 polymorphisms as predictors of sustained response in antiviral therapy for chronic hepatitis C infection. *Hepatology* 33, 708–712.

23 Satsangi J, Chapman RWG, Haldar N *et al.* (2001) A functional polymorphism of the stromelysin gene (MMP-3) influences susceptibility to primary sclerosing cholangitis. *Gastroenterology* 121, 124–130.

24 Wienke K, Louka AS, Spurkland A *et al.* (2004) Association of matrix metalloproteinase-1 and -3 promoter polymorphisms with clinical subsets of Norwegian primary sclerosing cholangitis patients. *J Hepatol* 41, 209–214.

25 Khakoo SI, Thio CL, Martin MP *et al.* (2004) HLA and NK cell inhibitory receptor genes in resolving hepatitis C virus infection. *Science* 305, 872–874.

3.3.3 Genetic determinants of complex liver diseases: mouse models and quantitative trait locus analysis

Frank Lammert

Introduction

Many common liver diseases are the result of complex interactions between environmental factors and multiple genes. It is assumed that a large number of liver-specific disease genes determine the clinical outcomes of patients following exposure to acute or chronic liver injury, and that individuals who carry certain combinations of these genes are most susceptible. In the past decade, techniques and resources for genome analysis, in particular quantitative trait locus (QTL) analysis, have been established to identify and localize the genes that contribute to polygenic (complex) diseases in rodent models under defined environmental conditions. QTL analysis is based on experimental crosses of genetically distinct inbred mouse strains. This chapter describes the impact of these genomic approaches in mouse models on our understanding of the complex genetics of chronic liver diseases. Complex liver diseases such as liver fibrosis and hepatocellular carcinoma demonstrate how mouse models represent an invaluable tool to identify unknown pathomechanisms, to investigate how systems of genes work together in health and disease processes and to define new therapeutic targets.

Monogenic and polygenic (complex) liver diseases

Even in the early 1900s, the wide variability in the severity of liver diseases led clinicians to suggest that there are hereditary factors affecting the traits. However, simple (monogenic) diseases (also known as Mendelian traits) represent only a small portion of the total number of human liver disorders, with Wilson's disease [1] and classic haemochromatosis [2] as prominent examples. In contrast, many common liver diseases are determined by the interaction of multiple genes (epistasis) and the interactions of these genes with different environmental factors (polygenic or multifactorial diseases). The risk alleles are not sufficient to cause the disease, but they confer susceptibility to manifestation and/or progression of the disease. Examples of such complex liver diseases include liver cirrhosis and hepatocellular carcinoma.

The approaches to identifying the genetic determinants of complex liver diseases can be separated into different categories: candidate gene methods that test genetic variants of a potential susceptibility gene for association with a liver disease; and positional cloning approaches (forward genetics), which use genetic markers to perform an unbiased scan of the whole genome. Candidate gene association studies are often based on unrelated cases and control subjects and offer the advantages of speed, relatively low cost and the possibility of identifying genes with small allele effects [3]. However, prior knowledge of the pathophysiology is a requirement for the candidate gene approach, and therefore limits its utility.

In addition to human genetics, mouse models can be used for gene discovery in complex diseases (Fig. 1), as recently highlighted by the Complex Trait Consortium [4]. Whereas genetic studies in humans are often hindered by difficulty in ascertaining sufficient numbers of affected individuals and the fact that environmental factors are difficult to control, mouse genetics offers more accessible and lower cost tools for gene identification. Compared with humans, genetic analysis in mice is facilitated by: (i) inbreeding of mouse strains, i.e. mating of siblings through at least 20 generations, to reduce allelic diversity; (ii) rapid and systematic generation of progeny; (iii) the ability to control environmental influences; and (iv) powerful experimental systems unique to mice [5].

To date, case–control (association-based) studies for the detection of QTLs have dominated studies of complex diseases in humans, whereas in mouse genetics, linkage (segregation-based) studies prevail. Linkage studies observe the co-inheritance of genetic markers and target loci in a segregating population. In contrast, large samples of unrelated human individuals are traditionally analysed using association-based approaches, which compare the frequency of specific genotypes between cases and control subjects.

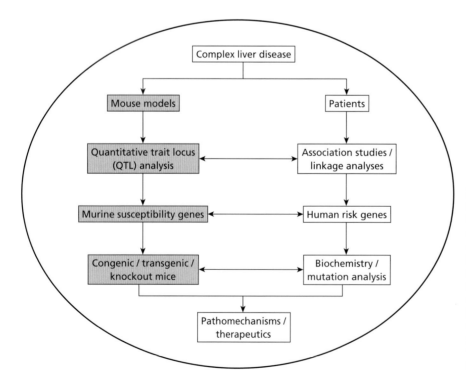

Fig. 1 Complementary genetic analysis of complex liver diseases in mice and humans. Human risk genes can be identified in association (case–control) studies or linkage analyses in families. Mouse models allow the identification of susceptibility genes using quantitative trait locus (QTL) analysis and congenic mice. The pathophysiological consequences of biochemical alterations and mutations in humans can be studied in transgenic and knockout mice. It should be noted that the experimental findings can be transferred between mice and humans at each step in the analysis.

Table 1 Experimental design of a QTL analysis in inbred mice.

Experimental step	Items
1 Inbred strain survey	Selection of strains, finding a phenotypical difference among inbred strains
2 Characterization of parental strains and F1 progeny	Inheritance pattern, differences in expression for gender and age, subphenotypes
3 Experimental cross	F2 or backcross, size of cross
4 Genome analysis	Selection of genetic markers, selective genotyping, phenotypical pooling
5 Data analysis	QTL mapping software, thresholds for statistical significance
6 Functional testing of candidate genes	Congenics, transgenics and knockout mice

Quantitative trait locus (QTL) analysis in inbred mice

A QTL is a genetic locus whose alleles affect the phenotypical variation of a disease [4]. For locus identification, a segregating experimental cross of inbred mouse strains is phenotyped and then genotyped for markers that differ between the parental strains and are distributed evenly throughout the entire genome. In general, QTLs are mapped by statistically locating the genomic regions in which the degree of genotypical similarity correlates maximally with the degree of phenotypical similarity among the progeny [6–8]. Table 1 lists the experimental stages of QTL analysis.

The first step in QTL analysis is an inbred strain survey. By definition, inbred mice are the result of at least 20 brother × sister matings, resulting in mice that are homozygous for all alleles and thus genetically identical. For a strain survey, a quantitative phenotype is determined in multiple inbred strains in response to an environmental challenge such as a high-fat diet or exposure to hepatotoxins. To increase the likelihood of resolving the genetic complexity, the phenotype of interest should be very narrowly defined, or a subset of the overall disease phenotype should be chosen for the genetic analysis. The strains are then ordered along the phenotypical spectrum to identify genetically susceptible and resistant strains. Figure 2 illustrates an example, the strain survey for CCl_4-induced liver fibrosis [9], showing hepatic hydroxyproline concentrations, which reflect collagen contents in liver, as a quantitative trait in seven inbred mouse strains [10].

Once the strain spectrum is determined, the genetic variability that gives rise to the phenotypical differences can be explored by *in silico* and/or experimental QTL analysis. Experimental crossing of inbred mouse strains can be regarded as the central procedure in QTL analysis (Table 1). Two inbred strains that differ phenotypically are bred to obtain intercross or backcross progeny (Fig. 3). An intercross (F2) tests genotype–phenotype associations in a cross of F1 progeny. Whereas F1 mice are heterozygous at every locus and genetically identical to each other, a recombination of the parental genetic material is possible during meiosis of the F1 mice and becomes genotypically and phenotypically visible in the F2 generation. A continuously distributed quantitative trait in an F2 design suggests that multiple genes contribute to the phenotype, as expected for a polygenic trait (Fig. 4). Similarly, a backcross tests marker–trait association in progeny obtained by backcrossing F1 mice to one of the parental lines (Fig. 3).

Microsatellites (simple sequence length polymorphisms, SSLPs) have been widely used as genetic markers in QTL analysis. These markers are short repetitive DNA sequences [e.g. $(CA)_n$] with known chromosomal locations throughout the mouse genome. Because microsatellites are abundant, vary in size across inbred mouse strains and are easily determined by polymerase chain reaction (PCR)-based assays, they are convenient for use as genetic markers in QTL studies. More recently, single nucleotide polymorphisms (SNPs) have been identified and genotyped in large panels of inbred mice [11,12]. A SNP can be considered to be a form of point mutation that has been evolutionarily successful enough to recur in a significant proportion of a species'

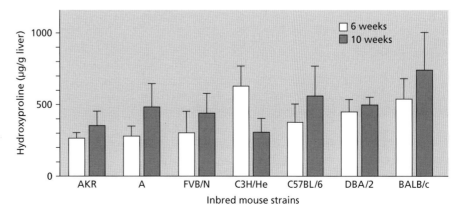

Fig. 2 Inbred strain survey for liver fibrosis. Hepatic hydroxyproline levels (representing hepatic collagen contents) in inbred mouse strains before and after treatment with CCl_4. Hydroxyproline levels (µg/g liver) at 6 and 10 weeks are represented by white and grey bars respectively. Strains AKR, A and FVB/N were significantly more resistant towards hepatic fibrosis, whereas C57BL/6, DBA/2 and BALB/c mice were more susceptible. From ref. 10, with permission.

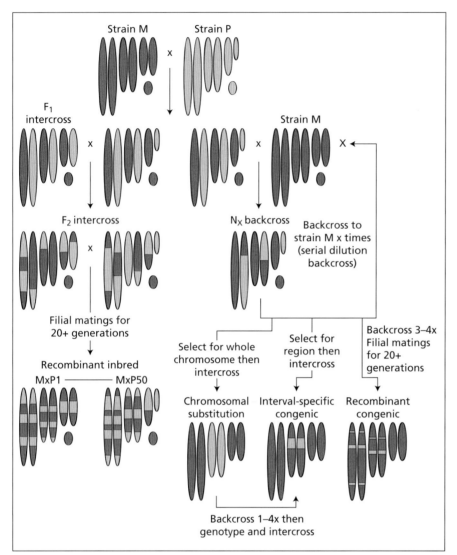

Fig. 3 Experimental mouse crosses for QTL analysis (see text for details). M, maternal; P, paternal.

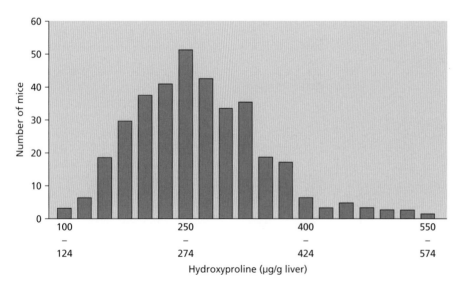

Fig. 4 Polygenic inheritance of liver fibrosis. Distribution of hepatic hydroxyproline levels in intercross (F2) progeny of fibrosis-susceptible BALB/c and resistant A/J mice [(A/J × BALB/c)F1 × (A/J × BALB/c)F1] after treatment with CCl_4 for 6 weeks. According to hydroxyproline levels (μg/g liver), mice were divided into phenotypical classes, as indicated on the abscissa. The intercross shows a normal (Gaussian) distribution of hydroxyproline levels, consistent with polygenic (non-Mendelian) inheritance of fibrosis susceptibility. From ref. 10, with permission.

Table 2 QTL analysis of complex liver diseases in inbred mice.

Liver disease	QTLs	References
Cholesterol cholelithiasis	Lith1 (lithogenic gene 1) – Lith23	[32,34–40,75,76]
Haemochromatosis	Hfe-modifier 1 – Hfe-modifier 4	[26]
Liver fibrosis	Hfib1 (hepatic fibrogenic gene 1) – Hfib2	[10,53]
Non-alcoholic fatty liver disease	Lcho1 (liver cholesterol accumulation 1) – Lcho4	[77,78]
Porphyria cutanea tarda	Hcbip1 (hexachlorobenzene-induced porphyria 1) – Hcbip2	[79,80]
Schistosomiasis	Rsm1 (resistance to *Schistosoma mansoni* 1)	[81]

population. The two SNP alleles can be reliably determined (e.g. using TaqMan assays), but genetic diversity and thus information content across different strains is lower compared with microsatellites (see Chapter 3.6 for more information about molecular techniques).

For the final QTL analysis, all intercross or backcross progeny are phenotyped and genotyped for microsatellites or SNPs that differ between the parental strains and densely cover the whole genome (Table 1). The rationale behind QTL identification is the fact that parental alleles are distributed randomly to offspring. Therefore, for any loci not contributing to a disease phenotype, parental alleles are randomly represented between sufficiently large pools of susceptible and resistant mice. However, strain-specific alleles for loci that determine susceptibility are over-represented in the affected progeny. Linkage analysis of phenotypes and genotypes is performed using genetic mapping software such as MapManager QTX [13] or R/qtl [14], which allow user-friendly identification (e.g. by regression analysis or interval mapping) [15] and statistical validation of linkage. The logarithm of the odds ratio (LOD) score, the traditional statistics for genetic linkage, is a measure of the strength of evidence for the presence of a QTL. The LOD score is the odds ratio comparing the hypothesis of a QTL at a particular location vs. that of no QTL. LOD scores ≥ 3 are generally considered to indicate significant results, albeit theoretical thresholds have been calculated for specific cross designs [16] and, alternatively, empirical thresholds, which correct for multiple testing, can be calculated by permutation tests [17].

Table 2 lists complex liver diseases that have been studied in QTL analyses and are discussed in the following sections.

Liver fibrosis

Fibrosis or scarring of the liver is a common consequence of all chronic liver diseases irrespective of aetiology (see also Section 6). It represents the generalized response of the liver to chronic injury and is characterized by excessive deposition of extracellular matrix by activated hepatic stellate cells [18–20]. The molecular basis of this process is complex and involves the interplay of many factors, of which growth factors, cytokines and chemoattractants are prominent. The marked variability in progression of fibrosis has been attributed to age, gender and environmental factors [21], but host genetic factors are also

likely to contribute to the variable course of fibrosis in response to chronic injury [22]. Shi *et al.* [9] were first to show that the fibrotic response differs among inbred mouse strains. Liver injury induced with CCl_4 resulted in severe fibrosis in BALB/c mice, whereas C57BL/6 mice developed comparatively less fibrosis. Of note, fibrogenic BALB/c mice exhibited a T-helper 2 (Th2) response, whereas C57BL/6 mice displayed a Th1 response, consistent with the common paradigm that Th1/Th2 cytokine subsets modulate the fibrotic response of the liver [23].

Subsequently, Hillebrandt *et al.* [10] performed a systematic inbred strain survey (Fig. 2) to identify unknown susceptibility loci for liver fibrosis. For QTL analysis, F1 hybrids of susceptible BALB/c and resistant A/J inbred strains were intercrossed to obtain 358 F2 progeny. Linkage analysis of phenotypes and genotypes identified QTLs on chromosomes 2 and 15 that significantly affect the histological stage of fibrosis and hepatic collagen content [10].

Haemochromatosis

QTL analysis can also be used to identify gene loci that determine the severity and progression of a monogenic disease, and not manifestation of the disease *per se*. Hereditary haemochromatosis is a common disorder of iron homeostasis characterized by increased dietary iron absorption and progressive iron accumulation, mainly in the liver (see also Chapter 16.2). Most patients are homozygous for the C282Y mutation in the *HFE* gene encoding an atypical human leucocyte antigen (HLA) class I protein that interacts with the transferrin receptor 1 and regulates the iron regulator hepcidin [24]. However, not all individuals carrying the haemochromatosis-predisposing genotype in the general population become iron loaded [25]. Genetic modifiers have been shown to influence disease penetrance, but their number and chromosomal locations remain unknown, and their identification is hampered by complex interactions with environmental factors. To circumvent these difficulties, Bensaid *et al.* [26] bred congenic inbred mouse strains for the *Hfe* gene that differ strongly in their propensity to develop hepatic iron loading. Strains are denoted as congenic (Fig. 3) if a chromosomal region has been transferred from one strain to another by recurrent backcrossing (≥ 10) of a founder individual to a recipient strain [27]. Marker-assisted breeding of congenic mouse strains (speed congenics) is possible over five generations

[28]. To localize the loci controlling hepatic iron loading, 1028 progeny from an F2 intercross between the C57BL/6 and DBA/2 Hfe-deficient strains were selectively genotyped and phenotyped for iron overload. The QTL analysis, which is denoted 'modifier scan' in this setting, identified four loci on chromosomes 7, 8, 11 and 12 that modify the haemochromatosis phenotype. The LOD scores of all three loci were > 6, indicating significant linkage, and the QTL regions contained several genes recently shown to exert important roles in the regulation of iron metabolism [26].

A similar QTL analysis employed mice deficient in the product of the β_2-microglobulin class I light chain gene, which fail to express HFE and other major histocompatibility complex (MHC) class I family proteins and manifest many characteristics of the haemochromatosis phenotype [29]. Analysis of the iron-loading phenotype in β_2-microglobulin congenic strains showed that the genetic background is a major determinant in iron loading. Resistance and susceptibility to iron overload segregated as complex traits in backcross progeny. Both studies [26,29] demonstrate the polygenic pattern of hepatic iron loading in Hfe-deficient mice and indicate that multiple modifier genes influence the severity of iron overloading and haemochromatosis, which was originally considered to represent a classic monogenic liver disease [2]. Examination of candidate genes residing at the modifier loci and genetic analysis of the syntenic chromosomal regions in humans will provide important insights into the heterogeneous disease presentation observed among HFE C282Y homozygotes [25].

Cholelithiasis (see also Chapter 19.3)

Familial clustering and an increased concordance of the trait in monozygotic twins compared with dizygotic twins [30] indicate that gallstone disease has a strong genetic component. However, the identification of human lithogenic genes is hampered by the multifactorial pathogenesis of gallstones. Gallstones are likely to result from the complex interaction of susceptibility genes, female gender, advanced age and environmental factors such as high-carbohydrate, high-fat and low-fibre diets and low physical activity [31]. The mouse is a suitable model to study the pathogenesis of cholesterol gallstone formation, as inbred mouse strains challenged with a lithogenic diet (containing 15% fat, 1% cholesterol and 0.5% cholic acid) show different prevalence rates of cholesterol gallstones [5,32]. As a tool for genetic mapping, Khanuja et al. [32] used recombinant inbred (RI) strains derived from strains representing the extremes of a strain survey. RI strains [33] are derived by successive (≥ 20) crosses between siblings from an initial cross between two parental strains (Fig. 3). These RI strains are homozygous for one of the parental alleles at every locus, but differ in the representation of these strains across the genome. RI strains can accelerate mapping by circumventing the costly and time-consuming experimental crosses. Recently, the genotypes of RI lines have been determined for very dense sets of SNPs [12]. Thus, a method for rapid identification of QTLs is to perform a phenotype survey across an RI panel whose parental strains represent phenotypical extremes of the inbred strain survey, and to identify the QTLs underlying the RI strain phenotype data.

With respect to cholecystolithiasis, QTL mapping in experimental crosses of several inbred mouse strains was successfully employed to localize the whole ensemble of lithogenic (Lith) loci that determine the gallstone phenotypes in inbred mouse lines. The results of several QTL analyses have been summarized in a 'gallstone map' [5] (Fig. 5). As illustrated, the formation of gallstones and mucin, which is considered to be a precursor to stone formation, is a polygenic trait determined by several loci on different chromosomes [5]. The Lith1 locus on chromosome 2 was identified in a genomewide scan of backcross progeny from the gallstone-susceptible strain C57L/J and the resistant strain AKR/J [32]. Since then, more than 20 murine Lith loci and several candidate genes (ABC transporters for biliary lipids, nuclear receptors, mucins) have been identified (Table 2) [34–40]. Lith1 and other loci have been confirmed and fine-mapped in congenic strains generated by introgressing the susceptible Lith alleles into resistant background strains, which induces hypersecretion of biliary cholesterol and other gallstone-related phenotypes [41].

Genomic toolbox for narrowing susceptibility loci: from QTL to gene

A QTL can be large and usually contains hundreds of genes, but identifying the causal gene remains difficult. Because the resolution of QTL mapping is low, any linked region(s) identified probably span(s) many megabases (Mb). The identification of recombinant progeny within the critical region can narrow the candidate region, or SNP association studies can be performed across the region. If strain sequence data are available, one can proceed to direct sequence comparison to identify polymorphisms. The literature is revisited once linkage has been established to query the locus as a region for any known risk factors, and also to determine whether candidate genes from any relevant microarray studies reside within the region [42]. It is important to generate a gene list for the linked region, and to examine the genes that could have a pathobiological function related to the liver disease. Afterwards, selective breeding strategies can be pursued in mice to harness in vivo genetic recombination to narrow the candidate region and therefore reduce the number of candidate genes. Examples of selective breeding include interval-specific congenic strains and recombinant congenic strains (Fig. 3). The comparison between different congenic strains possessing overlapping chromosomal interval regions helps to define the region that harbours the QTL gene more precisely [7]. Recombinant congenic strains are formed by crossing two inbred strains, followed by a few backcrosses to one of the parental strains and subsequent inbreeding without selection [43]. Such inbred strains consist of randomly fixed chromosomal segments of the donor strain on the background of the recipient strain to which it was backcrossed. Alternatively,

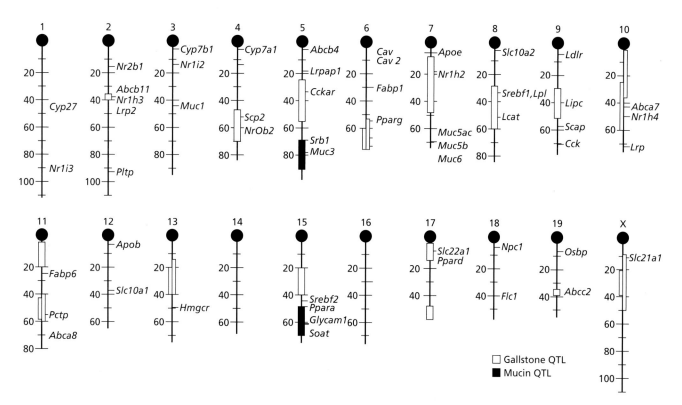

Fig. 5 Murine 'gallstone map'. Composite map of candidate genes and quantitative trait loci (QTLs) for cholesterol gallstone formation. A vertical line represents each mouse chromosome, with the centromere at the top; genetic distances from the centromere (horizontal black lines) are indicated to the left of the chromosomes in centiMorgans (cM). Gallstone QTLs (Lith genes) are represented by white rectangles, and QTLs for mucin formation, a common precursor of stones, by black rectangles. Candidate genes are indicated by horizontal lines with the gene symbols to the right. Updated from ref. 5, new version available from http://pga.jax.org/qtl/index.

Table 3 Summary of bioinformatics tools for dissection of mouse QTLs [45].

Bioinformatics tool	Methodology	Resolution
Comparative genomics	Identifies regions of chromosomal synteny in QTLs that are concordant across species	10–20 Mb
Combined cross analysis	Recodes genotype information from multiple crosses detecting a shared QTL into one susceptible and one resistant genotype to combine the crosses in a single QTL analysis	10–20 Mb
Genomewide haplotype analysis	Associates conserved haplotype patterns across the genome with a phenotype in inbred strains	< 5 Mb
Interval-specific haplotype analysis	Detects regions identical by descent within QTLs shared in multiple crosses	< 5 Mb
Sequence comparison	Searches strain-specific sequence databases for regulatory or coding polymorphisms within the QTL interval	10–20 genes
Expression comparison	Searches microarray databases to identify genes expressed in an organ of interest or genes exhibiting differential expression between the strains of interest	10–20 genes

consomic mice (also known as chromosome substitution strains) may be used (Fig. 3), which are panels of inbred strains bred to differ by a single chromosome [44]. By comparing the phenotypes of these mice, one can determine which chromosome confers a specific phenotype [42].

Recently developed bioinformatics methods, including comparative genomics, combined cross analysis, genomewide and interval-specific haplotype analysis, followed by sequence and expression analysis, each facilitated by public databases, provide new tools for narrowing mouse QTLs (Table 3; see Plate 3.3.3.1,

facing p. 72) [45,46] (see Chapter 3.6). Comparative genomics is based on the structural conservation among all mammalian genomes. The gene content and linear organization of genes along chromosomal segments in mice correspond to that found in humans, with ~ 340 syntenic segments conserved between the two species [47]. Experimental evidence suggests that causal genes underlying rodent QTLs are often conserved as disease genes in humans. Therefore, cross-species conservation (synteny) can be used to compare linked regions across human and animal models and to determine whether candidate loci across a number of model organisms are likely to harbour orthologous genes. However, as chromosomal segments conserved between rodents and humans are often large, comparative genomic analysis only modestly narrows a QTL interval in most cases (Table 3).

Combined cross analysis and haplotype analysis are based on the unusual nature of the inbred mouse genome, which is a mixture of DNA from different subspecies [48]. Combined cross analysis is a statistical method of integrating data from existing QTL crosses to narrow the QTL interval provided that the same causal gene underlies the QTL in each cross [49]. QTLs are often found at the same chromosomal location in multiple crosses, and all strains carrying the susceptibility allele at a QTL share the same ancestral allele of the causal gene. Thus, combined cross analysis provides increased power to detect QTLs with small effects [49].

An alternative way to narrow QTL intervals based on the structure of the genome is haplotype analysis [50]. Genomewide and interval-specific haplotype analysis can be used to narrow experimentally derived QTLs (Table 3). The innovative idea of a computer algorithm to link phenotypes to genotypes in inbred mouse strains [51] stimulated the development of genomewide haplotype analysis, which predicts the location of QTLs affecting a trait without a priori knowledge of the loci. It should be noted that these methods have also been called 'association mapping', as they are based on genetic association, whereas experimental QTL analysis (Table 1) employs genetic linkage. There are now several newly developed computational methods that input phenotype values across inbred strains of mice to rapidly predict genetic susceptibility loci without the need to derive experimental crosses of inbred strains. Each of these methods uses a database of strain-specific genetic markers. The methods also use strain data on characteristic combinations of SNP alleles on

single chromosomes that are inherited together (haplotypes). Inbred mice share haplotypes across 30–60% of the mouse genome [11]. Pletcher et al. [52] grouped inbred strains based on inferred haplotypes (determined by three consecutive SNPs) and tested for phenotypical differences between the groups. They sequentially applied sliding three-SNP windows across the genome to identify QTLs in which the different haplotype groups showed distinct phenotypes. This type of analysis was applied for a phenotype that scored the formation of gallstones in 25 strains of male mice [52]. Eleven regions were produced that exceeded the threshold for statistical significance at a genomewide level ($P = 0.0004$), and seven of these regions fell within the range of experimentally identified QTLs for gallstone formation or mucin accumulation (Table 4, Fig. 5).

In interval-specific haplotype analysis, genetic markers covering a critical QTL interval are grouped into the strains that carry the high allele and those that possess the low allele. Any region with genotypes that are shared between the high-allele strains but differ from the low-allele strains is considered a haplotype region likely to contain the QTL gene [45]. To refine a QTL for liver fibrosis on mouse chromosome 2, which was detected previously in an experimental intercross between fibrosis-susceptible BALB/c and the resistant A/J inbred strains, we [53] used interval-specific haplotype analysis with a dense SNP map and hepatic collagen concentrations from seven inbred mouse strains (Fig. 2) as input quantitative data. We inferred haplotypes from three-SNP windows with an average size of 900 kb and calculated the strength of the genetic association at each haplotype on the basis of the genotype–phenotype pairings. The refined QTL separated into two long-range haplotypes, which carry the complement factor 5 (C5) as QTL gene at the distal end [53]. Haplotype association mapping is still a developing method, and issues that need to be addressed include the required number of

Table 4 Comparison of in silico and experimental QTLs for cholecystolithiasis (modified from [52]).

In silico QTL			Experimental QTL		Reference
Chromosome	QTL position (Mb)	P value	Cross	QTL position (Mb, 95% CI)[a]	
2	173–175	0.000078	(129S1 × CAST)F2	176 (159–182)	[38]
3	84–87	0.000418	–	–	
4	28–29	0.000388	(A × AKR) × AKR	4 (0–29)	[34]
5	99–102	0.000135	(SM × NZB)F2	106 (60–115)	[52]
6	10–13	0.000127	(DBA/2 × CAST)F2	2 (0–15)	[37]
10	79–82	0.000225	–	–	
11	95–97	0.000349	(SWR × AKR) × AKR[b]	122 (95–129)	[35]
12	40–46	0.000279	–	–	
14	59–63	0.000190	–	–	
15	82–95	0.000088	(A × AKR) × AKR	102 (89–telomere)	[34]
16	69–71	0.000173	(129S1 × CAST)F2	70 (49–95)	[38]

[a]QTL regions were defined as experimentally determined 95% confidence intervals (CI) or as ± 10-cM intervals around the peak position with the highest logarithm of the odds ratio score.
[b]QTL for gallbladder mucin, an early step in gallstone formation.

inbred strains and the minimum SNP density to detect small haplotypes [45].

The molecular bases for QTLs are DNA polymorphisms affecting the expression or the function of a gene product. Genome sequence databases enable *in silico* sequence comparisons of whole QTL intervals to detect sequence variants. Sequence comparison of susceptible and resistant strains can reveal strain-specific polymorphisms underlying QTLs. If genomic sequence data for strains of interest are not available, individual candidate genes within the QTL are resequenced in those strains to find genetic changes that could be responsible for a phenotype. These include alterations in the coding sequence that change an amino acid sequence or the stop codon, sequence alterations in a splice junction that may affect processing of the mRNA transcript, and sequence alterations in other non-coding regulatory regions. DNA regions can also be compared across species to highlight regions of conservation. Specific software tools [54,55] assess the degree of conservation and are useful in detecting which non-coding regions are likely to be functionally important. A complementary strategy to searching sequence databases is investigating gene expression databases to identify genes that are differentially expressed between strains for many tissues. Such expression differences can be mapped to chromosomal intervals with QTL mapping methods such as WebQTL [56,57]. WebQTL is a website (http://www.genenetwork.org/) that contains genotype and expression data from many RI strain sets. The WebQTL databases comprise several biological traits and microarray-based gene expression data (including liver) from the RI lines. A search function detects correlations between RNA expression and biological traits, and mapping functions identify QTLs for a selected trait.

Functional genomics

Gene arrays (transcriptomics) and proteomics are increasingly used to phenotypically characterize the expression profiles of liver tissue or serum from patients with liver diseases (see Chapter 3.6). Expression data provide much insight into the pathobiology of a process, but do not necessarily reveal underlying disease genes, as the causal gene residing in a QTL may not be differentially expressed in the disease state. However, gene arrays can also be incorporated into functional genomics of complex liver diseases, as illustrated by the examples below.

Liver metabolism

Fine mapping of QTLs and validation of positional candidates are time-consuming and not always successful. Therefore Schadt and his group [58] developed a hybrid procedure to map loci involved in complex traits that leverages the strengths of forward and reverse genetic approaches (see Plate 3.3.3.2, facing p. 72). By integrating genotypes and hepatic microarray data in RI strains and experimental crosses, they showed that clinical QTLs controlling cholesterol and leptin levels and other metabolic traits are enriched for clusters of QTLs that determine the hepatic expression levels of genes associated with these metabolic traits (eQTLs). By matching patterns of gene expression in segregating mouse populations (forward genetics) with expression responses induced in knockout mice (reverse genetics), genes controlling clusters of eQTLs and clinical QTLs could be mapped (see Plate 3.3.3.2, facing p. 72). The utility of this approach was demonstrated by identifying 5-lipoxygenase as the gene underlying a QTL with pleiotropic effects on lipid metabolism in an F2 cross between strains C57BL/6 and DBA/2 [58].

Hepatocellular carcinoma

The majority of cDNA microarray-based gene expression profiling studies on human hepatocellular carcinoma (HCC) have focused on identifying genes associated with clinical features of HCC patients (see Chapters 3.5 and 18.2.1). Although notable success has been achieved, this approach still faces significant challenges on account of the heterogeneous nature of HCC (and other cancers) as well as the many confounding factors embedded in gene expression profile data. The underlying molecular basis for HCC heterogeneity, which hampers both treatment and prognostic predictions, is still largely unknown. Genetically modified mice have been used extensively for analysing the molecular mechanisms that occur during tumour development. However, in many cases, it is uncertain to what extent the mouse models reproduce features observed in the corresponding human conditions [59]. This is due largely to lack of precise methods for direct and comprehensive comparison at the molecular level of the mouse and human tumours. These limitations can be overcome by cross-species comparison of multiple gene expression data sets from human tumours and mouse models, which allow the identification of critical regulatory modules in the expression profiles. The success of this new experimental approach, comparative functional genomics, suggests that gene expression signatures reflecting similar HCC phenotypes are conserved across species and that integration of independent data sets enhances the ability to identify key regulatory elements in tumour development [60].

For most microarray studies, the challenge resides in deriving biological meaning from an overwhelming amount of data. Although the ability to measure large numbers of genes affords new insight by identifying genes that would not have been imagined to participate in a process, it is difficult to derive meaning from even a small experiment without analysis tools that identify biological themes present in expression data [GenMAPP, MAPPFinder (http://www.genmapp.org/), EASE (http://david.abcc.hcifcrf.gov/)]. These tools visualize gene expression data on maps representing biological pathways and groupings of genes, and identify over-represented functional gene categories with respect to all assayed genes using a number of categorization systems, including gene ontology, biological pathways, chromosomal localizations and protein domains.

Recently, microarray analysis was used to determine global gene expression patterns of HCCs from seven different mouse models and human HCCs from predefined subclasses to obtain direct comparison of the molecular features of mouse and human HCCs [59]. Gene expression patterns in HCCs from Myc, E2f1 and Myc/E2f1 transgenic mice were most similar to those of the better survival group of human HCCs, whereas the expression patterns in HCCs from Myc/TGFα transgenic mice and in diethylnitrosamine-induced mouse HCCs were most similar to those of the poorer survival group of human HCCs (see Plate 3.3.3.3, facing p. 72). These results suggest that these two classes of mouse models recapitulate the molecular characteristics of subclasses of human HCCs. In contrast, gene expression patterns of HCCs from Acox1 knockout and ciprofibrate-treated mice were least similar to those observed in either subclass of human HCCs [59]. As hepatocarcinogenesis is driven by peroxisome proliferation in these two models, the findings are in line with previous studies suggesting that humans are insensitive to the hepatotoxic effects of peroxisome proliferation [61]. The similarity of gene expression profiles between human and mouse models is in good agreement with the phenotypical HCC characteristics. Human HCCs with increased proliferation, decreased apoptosis and higher genomic instability can be paired with mouse models with the same characteristics. Thus, this approach can effectively identify appropriate mouse models to study human HCCs. Furthermore, cross-species similarity of gene expression patterns allows prioritization of genes obtained from human gene expression profiling studies and focus on genes whose expression is altered during hepatocarcinogenesis in both species (see Plate 3.3.3.3, facing p. 72).

Functional testing of QTL genes in genetically engineered mice

Although the unequivocal identification of the gene underlying a QTL is technically demanding [7,62], recently, genes for several QTLs including liver fibrosis, cholelithiasis, diabetes, obesity, atherosclerosis and modifiers of colorectal cancer have been identified successfully [63]. The tracking of a particular genetic variant with disease in susceptible strains of mice, and the nature of the sequence alteration, with attention towards the predicted impact on protein function, are important considerations in making the case for the involvement of a particular gene. However, in order to verify that a particular allele is pathogenic, additional functional testing has to be performed. Formal proof of gene discovery requires demonstration that replacement with a gene variant produces the phenotypical variant of interest [4].

Gene targeting followed by transgenic complementation, e.g. with recombined bacterial artificial chromosomes [64,65] or knockin technology [66] in mice, are *in vivo* approaches that are appropriate for functional validation. For liver fibrosis, interval-specific congenic mice (Fig. 3) and transgenesis with recombined bacterial artificial chromosomes demonstrated that

the gene encoding complement factor C5 [67] underlies a QTL on mouse chromosome 5 [53]. Genetically engineered mice for candidate genes may also be available from several sources, which should be queried before generating a mouse model *de novo* [42]. For example, Bay Genomics PGA (http://baygenomics.ucsf.edu/) and the German Gene Trap Consortium (http://tikus.gsf.de/) have generated libraries from insertional mutations in mouse embryonic stem (ES) cells available to the scientific community for the purpose of generating knockout mice. 'Gene trap' vectors carrying reporter genes for localizing expression and other multipurpose alleles amenable to a wide range of postinsertional modifications were used in ES cells to randomly inactivate genes, and thousands of genes have been trapped [68,69]. Short interfering (si) RNA technology for posttranscriptional gene silencing is an emerging technology for both *in vitro* and *in vivo* functional testing that may also be applied to functional validation of candidate genes in liver diseases [42]. Alternatively, pharmacological interventions using antibodies or small molecules can be used. For example, small molecule inhibitors of the C5 receptor displayed antifibrotic effects *in vivo*, further supporting the identity of C5 and the fibrogenic QTL on chromosome 12 [53].

Suggested workflow for gene discovery in mouse models of complex liver diseases and future perspectives for clinical practice

Based on the above discussions, Figure 6 proposes a workflow for studies to discover genes for complex liver diseases in mouse models. Once a susceptibility locus has been identified in the mouse and the QTL has been narrowed by the above approaches and proven to be pathophysiologcially relevant in mice, these results should be investigated in humans. The final proof of a causal QTL gene can be produced by demonstrating the phenotype in genetically engineered mice and confirming the association of the gene with the disease in human populations, as recently reported for Tnfsf4 in atherosclerosis [70] and C5 in liver fibrosis [53]. Previous studies have focused on nucleotide polymorphisms as genetic variants, but variation in gene copy number might be yet another source of interindividual differences. Recently, copy number variation of the *Fcgr3* gene encoding a receptor for Fc fragments of immunoglobulins was identified as a determinant of susceptibility to immunologically mediated glomerulonephritis in rats and humans [71]. The finding that gene copy number polymorphism predisposes to an immunologically mediated disease in two mammalian species provides evidence for the importance of genome plasticity in the evolution of complex diseases. It is to be expected that these mechanisms also apply to liver diseases, albeit experimental proof has yet to be provided.

The mouse studies demonstrate how QTL analysis leads to the identification of new gene loci affecting complex liver diseases.

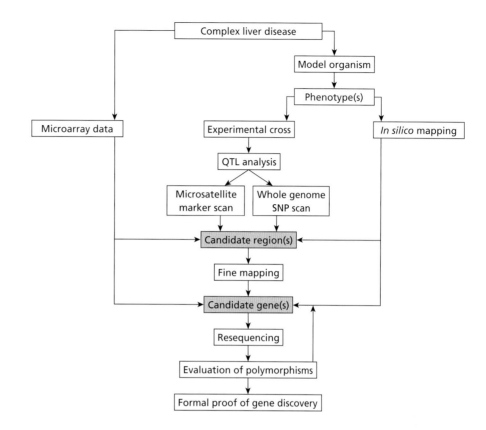

Fig. 6 Flow diagram of the gene discovery process in complex liver diseases. Modified from [42].

Moreover, the findings indicate that similar sets of genes regulate complex liver diseases in mouse models and humans and that variations in evolutionarily conserved genes alter the same pathobiological pathways across species [72]. In the future, the whole ensemble of susceptibility genes in mouse models of liver diseases will be studied in association and family studies in humans. As pointed out, multiple genes contribute to complex liver diseases, but most genetic studies in humans have focused on single genes. Recently, a study from Australia [73] detected associations between polymorphisms in six genes (*APOE, CCR5, CTLA4, HFE, MTP, SOD2*) and progressive liver fibrosis in chronic hepatitis C, with individual odds ratios ranging from 2.1 to 4.5. The odds ratios between rapidly progressing fibrosis and the possession of at least three, four or five at-risk alleles increased to 9.1, 15.5 and 24.1 respectively [73]. Using logistic regression analysis, a predictive equation could be developed and tested using a second cohort of patients with advanced fibrosis. Future combined analyses of human genes will be facilitated by the recent completion of the International HapMap Project [74], which catalogues the common patterns of DNA sequence variation of all human genes in different populations worldwide. It is anticipated that haplotype-based studies in large, well-characterized cohorts with chronic liver diseases will allow the determination of genetic risk profiles that promote rapid disease progression and help to select the most beneficial and personalized therapies (see Plate 3.3.3.4, facing p. 72).

References

1 Roberts EA, Schilsky ML (2003) A practice guideline on Wilson disease. *Hepatology* 37, 1475–1492.

2 Bacon BR (1989) Joseph H. Sheldon and hereditary hemochromatosis: historical highlights. *J Lab Clin Med* 113, 761–762.

3 Risch N, Merikangas K (1996) The future of genetic studies of complex human diseases. *Science* 273, 1516–1517.

4 The Complex Trait Consortium (2003) The nature and identification of quantitative trait loci: a community's view. *Nature Rev Genet* 4, 911–916.

5 Lammert F, Carey MC, Paigen B (2001) Chromosomal organization of candidate genes involved in cholesterol gallstone formation: a murine gallstone map. *Gastroenterology* 120, 221–238.

6 Lander ES, Schork NJ (1994) Genetic dissection of complex traits. *Science* 265, 2037–2048.

7 Darvasi A (1998) Experimental strategies for the genetic dissection of complex traits in animal models. *Nature Genet* 18, 19–24.

8 Doerge RW (2002) Mapping and analysis of quantitative trait loci in experimental populations. *Nature Rev Genet* 3, 43–52.

9 Shi Z, Wakil AE, Rockey DC (1997) Strain-specific differences in mouse hepatic wound healing are mediated by divergent T helper cytokine responses. *Proc Natl Acad Sci USA* 94, 10663–10668.

10 Hillebrandt S, Goos C, Matern S *et al.* (2002) Genome-wide analysis of hepatic fibrosis in inbred mice identifies the susceptibility locus Hfib1 on chromosome 15. *Gastroenterology* 123, 2041–2051.

11 Wiltshire T, Pletcher MT, Batalov S *et al.* (2003) Genome-wide single-nucleotide polymorphism analysis defines haplotype patterns in mouse. *Proc Natl Acad Sci USA* 100, 3380–3385.

12 Yalcin B, Fullerton J, Miller S et al. (2004) Unexpected complexity in the haplotypes of commonly used inbred strains of laboratory mice. *Proc Natl Acad Sci USA* 101, 9734–9739.

13 Manly KF, Cudmore RH, Meer JM (2001) Map Manager QTX, cross-platform software for genetic mapping. *Mamm Genome* 12, 930–932.

14 Broman KW, Wu H, Sen S et al. (2003) R/qtl: QTL mapping in experimental crosses. *Bioinformatics* 19, 889–890.

15 Lander ES, Botstein D (1989) Mapping mendelian factors underlying quantitative traits using RFLP linkage maps. *Genetics* 121, 185–199.

16 Lander E, Kruglyak L (1995) Genetic dissection of complex traits: guidelines for interpreting and reporting linkage results. *Nature Genet* 11, 241–247.

17 Churchill GA, Doerge RW (1994) Empirical threshold values for quantitative trait mapping. *Genetics* 138, 963–971.

18 Gressner AM (1998) The cell biology of liver fibrogenesis – an imbalance of proliferation, growth arrest and apoptosis of myofibroblasts. *Cell Tissue Res* 292, 447–452.

19 Friedman SL (2004) Mechanisms of disease: mechanisms of hepatic fibrosis and therapeutic implications. *Nature Clin Pract Gastroenterol Hepatol* 1, 98–105.

20 Bataller R, Brenner DA (2005) Liver fibrosis. *J Clin Invest* 115, 209–218.

21 Poynard T, Bedossa P, Opolon P (1997) Natural history of liver fibrosis progression in patients with chronic hepatitis C. *Lancet* 349, 825–832.

22 Bataller R, North KE, Brenner DA (2003) Genetic polymorphisms and the progression of liver fibrosis: a critical appraisal. *Hepatology* 37, 493–503.

23 Wynn TA (2004) Fibrotic disease and the T_H1/T_H2 paradigm. *Nature Rev Immunol* 4, 583–594.

24 Feder JN, Gnirke A, Thomas W et al. (1996) A novel MHC class I-like gene is mutated in patients with hereditary haemochromatosis. *Nature Genet* 13, 399–408.

25 Adams PC, Reboussin DM, Barton JC et al. (2005) Hemochromatosis and iron-overload screening in a racially diverse population. *N Engl J Med* 352, 1769–1778.

26 Bensaid M, Fruchon S, Mazeres C et al. (2004) Multigenic control of hepatic iron loading in a murine model of hemochromatosis. *Gastroenterology* 126, 1400–1408.

27 Snell GD (1978) Congenic resistant strains of mice. In: Morse HC (ed.) *Origins of Inbred Mice.* New York, NY: Academic Press, pp. 119–155.

28 Markel P, Shu P, Ebeling C et al. (1997) Theoretical and empirical issues for marker-assisted breeding of congenic mouse strains. *Nature Genet* 17, 280–284.

29 Sproule TJ, Jazwinska EC, Britton RS et al. (2001) Naturally variant autosomal and sex-linked loci determine the severity of iron overload in beta 2-microglobulin-deficient mice. *Proc Natl Acad Sci USA* 98, 5170–5174.

30 Katsika D, Grjibovski A, Einarsson C et al. (2005) Genetic and environmental influences on symptomatic gallstone disease: a Swedish study of 43 141 twin pairs. *Hepatology* 41, 1138–1143.

31 Lammert F, Sauerbruch T (2005) Mechanisms of disease: the genetic epidemiology of gallbladder stones. *Nature Clin Pract Gastroenterol Hepatol* 2, 423–433.

32 Khanuja B, Cheah YC, Hunt M et al. (1995) Lith1, a major gene affecting cholesterol gallstone formation among inbred strains of mice. *Proc Natl Acad Sci USA* 92, 7729–7733.

33 Bailey DW (1971) Recombinant-inbred strains. An aid to finding identity, linkage, and function of histocompatibility and other genes. *Transplantation* 11, 325–327.

34 Lammert F, Wang DQ, Wittenburg H et al. (2002) Lith genes control mucin accumulation, cholesterol crystallization, and gallstone formation in A/J and AKR/J inbred mice. *Hepatology* 36, 1145–1154.

35 Wittenburg H, Lammert F, Wang DQ et al. (2002) Interacting QTLs for cholesterol gallstones and gallbladder mucin in AKR and SWR strains of mice. *Physiol Genomics* 8, 67–77.

36 Wittenburg H, Lyons MA, Li R et al. (2003) FXR and ABCG5/ABCG8 as determinants of cholesterol gallstone formation from quantitative trait locus mapping in mice. *Gastroenterology* 125, 868–881.

37 Lyons MA, Wittenburg H, Li R et al. (2003) Lith6: a new QTL for cholesterol gallstones from an intercross of CAST/Ei and DBA/2J inbred mouse strains. *J Lipid Res* 44, 1763–1771.

38 Lyons MA, Wittenburg H, Li R et al. (2003) New quantitative trait loci that contribute to cholesterol gallstone formation detected in an intercross of CAST/Ei and 129S1/SvImJ inbred mice. *Physiol Genomics* 14, 225–239.

39 Lyons MA, Korstanje R, Li R et al. (2005) Single and interacting QTLs for cholesterol gallstones revealed in an intercross between mouse strains NZB and SM. *Mamm Genome* 16, 152–163.

40 Wittenburg H, Lyons MA, Li R et al. (2005) Association of a lithogenic Abcg5/Abcg8 allele on chromosome 17 (Lith9) with cholesterol gallstone formation in PERA/EiJ mice. *Mamm Genome* 16, 495–504.

41 Paigen B, Schork NJ, Svenson KL et al. (2000) Quantitative trait loci mapping for cholesterol gallstones in AKR/J and C57L/J strains of mice. *Physiol Genomics* 4, 59–65.

42 Burch LH, Schwartz DA (2005) Finding fibrosis genes: the lung. In: Varga J, Brenner DA, Phan SH (eds) *Fibrosis Research: Methods and Protocols.* Totowa, NJ: Humana Press, pp. 293–313.

43 Demant P, Hart AA (1986) Recombinant congenic strains – a new tool for analyzing genetic traits determined by more than one gene. *Immunogenetics* 24, 416–422.

44 Nadeau JH, Singer JB, Matin A et al. (2000) Analysing complex genetic traits with chromosome substitution strains. *Nature Genet* 24, 221–225.

45 DiPetrillo K, Wang X, Stylianou IM et al. (2005) Bioinformatics toolbox for narrowing rodent quantitative trait loci. *Trends Genet* 21, 683–692.

46 Flint J, Valdar W, Shifman S et al. (2005) Strategies for mapping and cloning quantitative trait genes in rodents. *Nature Rev Genet* 6, 271–286.

47 Pennacchio LA, Baroukh N, Rubin EM (2003) Human–mouse comparative genomics: successes and failures to reveal functional regions of the human genome. *Cold Spring Harb Symp Quant Biol* 68, 303–309.

48 Wade CM, Kulbokas EJ, Kirby AW et al. (2002) The mosaic structure of variation in the laboratory mouse genome. *Nature* 420, 574–578.

49 Li R, Lyons MA, Wittenburg H et al. (2005) Combining data from multiple inbred line crosses improves the power and resolution of quantitative trait loci mapping. *Genetics* 169, 1699–1709.

50 Cuppen E (2005) Haplotype-based genetics in mice and rats. *Trends Genet* 21, 318–322.

51 Grupe A, Germer S, Usuka J et al. (2001) In silico mapping of complex disease-related traits in mice. *Science* 292, 1915–1918.

52 Pletcher MT, McClurg P, Batalov S et al. (2004) Use of a dense single nucleotide polymorphism map for in silico mapping in the mouse. *PLoS Biol* 2, e393.

53 Hillebrandt S, Wasmuth HE, Weiskirchen R et al. (2005) Complement factor 5 is a quantitative trait gene that modifies liver fibrogenesis in mice and humans. *Nature Genet* 37, 835–843.

54 Dubchak I, Brudno M, Loots GG et al. (2000) Active conservation of noncoding sequences revealed by three-way species comparisons. *Genome Res* 10, 1304–1306.

55 Mayor C, Brudno M, Schwartz JR *et al.* (2000) VISTA: visualizing global DNA sequence alignments of arbitrary length. *Bioinformatics* 16, 1046–1047.

56 Chesler EJ, Lu L, Wang J *et al.* (2004) WebQTL: rapid exploratory analysis of gene expression and genetic networks for brain and behavior. *Nature Neurosci* 7, 485–486.

57 Chesler EJ, Lu L, Shou S *et al.* (2005) Complex trait analysis of gene expression uncovers polygenic and pleiotropic networks that modulate nervous system function. *Nature Genet* 37, 233–242.

58 Mehrabian M, Allayee H, Stockton J *et al.* (2005) Integrating genotypic and expression data in a segregating mouse population to identify 5-lipoxygenase as a susceptibility gene for obesity and bone traits. *Nature Genet* 37, 1224–1233.

59 Lee JS, Chu IS, Mikaelyan A *et al.* (2004) Application of comparative functional genomics to identify best-fit mouse models to study human cancer. *Nature Genet* 36, 1306–1311.

60 Thorgeirsson SS, Lee JS, Grisham JW (2006) Functional genomics of hepatocellular carcinoma. *Hepatology* 43, S145–S150.

61 Lee JS, Thorgeirsson SS (2005) Genetic profiling of human hepatocellular carcinoma. *Semin Liver Dis* 25, 125–132.

62 Moore KJ, Nagle DL (2000) Complex trait analysis in the mouse: the strengths, the limitations and the promise yet to come. *Annu Rev Genet* 34, 653–686.

63 Korstanje R, Paigen B (2002) From QTL to gene: the harvest begins. *Nature Genet* 31, 235–236.

64 Zhang Y, Buchholz F, Muyrers JP *et al.* (1998) A new logic for DNA engineering using recombination in *Escherichia coli*. *Nature Genet* 20, 123–128.

65 Glaser S, Anastassiadis K, Stewart AF (2005) Current issues in mouse genome engineering. *Nature Genet* 37, 1187–1193.

66 Nebert DW, Dalton TP, Stuart GW *et al.* (2000) 'Gene-swap knock-in' cassette in mice to study allelic differences in human genes. *Ann NY Acad Sci* 919, 148–170.

67 Guo RF, Ward PA (2005) Role of C5a in inflammatory responses. *Annu Rev Immunol* 23, 821–852.

68 Stryke D, Kawamoto M, Huang CC *et al.* (2003) BayGenomics: a resource of insertional mutations in mouse embryonic stem cells. *Nucleic Acids Res* 31, 278–281.

69 Schnutgen F, De-Zolt S, van Sloun P *et al.* (2005) Genomewide production of multipurpose alleles for the functional analysis of the mouse genome. *Proc Natl Acad Sci USA* 102, 7221–7226.

70 Wang X, Ria M, Kelmenson PM *et al.* (2005) Positional identification of TNFSF4, encoding OX40 ligand, as a gene that influences atherosclerosis susceptibility. *Nature Genet* 37, 365–372.

71 Aitman TJ, Dong R, Vyse TJ *et al.* (2006) Copy number polymorphism in Fcgr3 predisposes to glomerulonephritis in rats and humans. *Nature* 439, 851–855.

72 Paigen K (1995) A miracle enough: the power of mice. *Nature Med* 1, 215–220.

73 Richardson MM, Powell EE, Barrie HD *et al.* (2005) A combination of genetic polymorphisms increases the risk of progressive disease in chronic hepatitis C. *J Med Genet* 42, e45.

74 Altshuler D, Brooks LD, Chakravarti A *et al.* (2005) A haplotype map of the human genome. *Nature* 437, 1299–1320.

75 Machleder D, Ivandic B, Welch C *et al.* (1997) Complex genetic control of HDL levels in mice in response to an atherogenic diet. Coordinate regulation of HDL levels and bile acid metabolism. *J Clin Invest* 99, 1406–1419.

76 Paigen B, Schork NJ, Svenson KL *et al.* (2000) Quantitative trait loci mapping for cholesterol gallstones in AKR/J and C57L/J strains of mice. *Physiol Genomics* 4, 59–65.

77 Schwarz M, Davis DL, Vick BR *et al.* (2001) Genetic analysis of cholesterol accumulation in inbred mice. *J Lipid Res* 42, 1812–1819.

78 Rangnekar AS, Lammert F, Igolnikov A *et al.* (2006) Quantitative trait loci analysis of mice administered the methionine-choline deficient dietary model of experimental steatohepatitis. *Liver Int* 26, 1000–1005.

79 Akhtar RA, Smith AG (1998) Chromosomal linkage analysis of porphyria in mice induced by hexachlorobenzene-iron synergism: a model of sporadic porphyria cutanea tarda. *Pharmacogenetics* 8, 485–494.

80 Robinson SW, Clothier B, Akhtar RA *et al.* (2002) Non-ahr gene susceptibility loci for porphyria and liver injury induced by the interaction of 'dioxin' with iron overload in mice. *Mol Pharmacol* 61, 674–681.

81 Correa-Oliveira R, James SL, McCall D *et al.* (1986) Identification of a genetic locus, Rsm-1, controlling protective immunity against *Schistosoma mansoni*. *J Immunol* 137, 2014–2019.

3.4 Cellular cholestasis

Stefano Fiorucci

Cholestasis is defined as the impairment of normal bile flow resulting either from a functional defect at the level of the hepatocyte or from obstruction at the bile duct level [1]. Non-obstructive cholestasis can result from infections, the use of certain drugs and autoimmune, metabolic or genetic disorders. In recent years, a number of transport proteins involved in bile formation have been identified (see Chapter 16.10, Genetic cholestatic diseases). The recognition that specific gene mutations lead to progressive familial intrahepatic cholestasis has provided compelling evidence of the importance of these hepatic transporters in bile formation. Full details on inherited cholestatic disorders are described elsewhere (see Chapter 16.10). This chapter is focused on changes in hepatocellular transporter expression observed in experimental and human cholestatic conditions.

Accumulation of bile acid and bilirubin is the hallmark of cholestasis. The hepatic clearance of bile acids and bilirubin can be divided into four phases that include the following: phase 0, hepatic uptake; phase I, metabolism (e.g. hydroxylation); phase II, detoxification (e.g. conjugation); and phase III, excretion. These processes are regulated by a number of nuclear receptors (NRs) and their ligands that are the major determinants of the functional expression of genes that determine these pathways, together with enzymes that control bile acid synthesis (Tables 1 and 2).

Molecular basis of hepatobiliary transport

The main membrane transporters that primarily determine hepatic bile production are now largely characterized at the molecular level. Most of them have been cloned from both human and rodent tissues [2]. Information on the localization, nomenclature and function of hepatobiliary transporters is listed elsewhere in this book (see Chapter 2.3.6).

Table 1 The nuclear receptor superfamily.

Class I: Homodimers; steroid receptors	Class II: RXR heterodimers	Class III: Orphan homodimers	Class IV: Orphan monomers	Class V: Ligand-binding domain less
GR Glucocorticoid receptor	CAR Constitutive androstane receptor	RXR Retinoid X receptor	LRH-1 Liver receptor homologue 1	SHP Small heterodimer partner
AR Androgen receptor	FXR Farnesoid X receptor	COUP-TF Chicken ovalbumin upstream promoter transcription factor		
ER Estrogen receptor	LXR Liver X receptor	HNF4 Hepatocyte nuclear factor 4		
MR Mineralocorticoid receptor	PPAR Peroxisomal proliferator receptor			
PR Progesterone receptor	PXR Pregnane X receptor			
	RAR Retinoic acid receptor			
	TR Thyroid receptor			
	VDR Vitamin D receptor			

Table 2 Nuclear receptors involved in the regulation of bile acid synthesis and secretion.

Nuclear receptor	Ligands	Target genes
RXRα	9-*cis* retinoic acid	Heterodimeric partner of other class II receptors[a]
RAR	All-*trans* retinoic acid	*NTCP, MRP2*
FXR	Bile acids	*BSEP, SHP, UGTs, SULTs, MRP2, MDR3*
PXR	Xenobiotics, ursodeoxycholic acid, rifampicin C	*CYP3A, OATP, MRP2, MRP4, GST*
CAR	Xenobiotics, phenobarbital	*CYP3A, OATP-C, MRP2, MRP4, UGT, SULTs, GSTs*
LXR	Oxysterols	*CYP7A, CYP8B, ABCG5/8*
SHP	None	Inhibits *CYP7A, CYP8B, NTCP*
FTF	Bile acids	*CYP7A, CYP7A, 8B1, MRP3*
VDR	Vitamin D	*CYP3A, SULTs*
HNF1	None	*NTCP, CYP7A*

[a]See Table 1.

Sinusoidal uptake of biliary solutes

The sinusoidal membrane of hepatocytes contains several carrier proteins that facilitate entry into the liver of bile acids and other lipid-soluble organic substances, including physiological substrates (i.e. bilirubin), as well as drugs and xenobiotics. Bile salt uptake (phase 0) is mediated by Na^+-dependent and -independent mechanisms. The Na^+ taurocholate co-transporting polypeptide (NTCP) and a growing family of multispecific organic anion transporters are the major proteins involved in this step of bile formation. NTCP is exclusively expressed in the liver, strictly localized on the basolateral membrane of hepatocytes and is the predominant Na^+-dependent bile acid transporter of the hepatocyte. The NTCP transports mainly conjugated bile salts, taking advantage of the membrane-inward direction of the Na^+ gradient, which is maintained by the Na^+/K^+-ATPase of the hepatocytes [1,2].

The sinusoidal Na^+-independent transport of bile acids and organic anions is mediated by the growing family of organic anion-transporting polypeptides (OATPs). The OATPs are a family of polyspecific transporters with overlapping substrate affinity that are involved in the uptake of unconjugated bile acids. In addition, OATPs mediate the uptake of bilirubin conjugates, thyroid hormones, neutral steroids, reduced glutathione, bicarbonate and xenobiotics [2–4]. In contrast to NTCP, OATPs are expressed in extrahepatic tissues, particularly the small intestine, kidney and brain, underscoring their role in the overall disposition of amphipathic compounds. In addition, some OATPs work as bidirectional transporters at high intracellular substrate concentrations, allowing the extrusion of potentially dangerous compounds. Other transport proteins, such as the liver homologues of the kidney organic anion transporters (OATs) and polyspecific organic cation transporters (OCTs), have also been identified recently at the sinusoidal domain of hepatocytes [3].

Canalicular transport of biliary solutes

After intracellular transport, which might involve binding, sequestration, biotransformation or conjugation, endo- and xenobiotics are secreted across the canalicular membrane of the hepatocyte. This process (which provides the primary driving force for the generation of bile flow, phase III) is mediated by transporters of the ATP-binding cassette (ABC) superfamily [5]. ABC transporters present in the canalicular membrane are: (i) the bile export pump (BSEP), which mediates secretion of bile acids into the canaliculus; (ii) the multidrug-resistant associated protein 2 (MRP2), which transports anionic conjugates of many lipophilic substances and reduced glutathione; (iii) the multidrug-resistant 1 (*MDR1*) gene product, which acts as a transporter of bulky cationic compounds and steroids; and (iv) the *MDR3* gene product, which acts as a phospholipid flippase. Three additional 'half ABC transporters', which contain only six of the 12 transmembrane domains typical of ABC transporters, have been identified recently in the canalicular membrane: ABCG5 and ABCG8, which regulate cholesterol secretion, and ABCG2, which preferentially transports sulphate conjugates. The canalicular membrane also contains an anion exchanger that excretes bicarbonate into bile, and a P-type ATPase (familial intrahepatic cholestasis 1; FIC1) thought to participate in the transport of aminophospholipids from the outer to the inner leaflet of liver or biliary cell membranes.

Basolateral transport

Sinusoidal bile acids efflux (phase III) is mediated by OATPs or ABC transporters located at the basolateral membrane of hepatocytes. MRP3 and MRP4 transport, among other physiological substrates, non-sulphated and sulphated bile salts [6,7]. Although MRP3 is minimally expressed in normal livers, it is inducible. MRP4 is expressed in the liver to a greater degree and functions as an ATP-dependent co-transporter of reduced glutathione, together with monoanionic bile acids. Given the vectorial nature of hepatobiliary transport, the export to the portal blood of compounds normally excreted into bile might serve as an alternative pathway for elimination of biliary constituents, limiting the accumulation of toxic endo- and xenobiotics when the canalicular secretory pathway is disrupted.

Hepatocellular changes in cholestatic diseases

With the exception of paediatric cholestasis or familial progressive cholestasis, where specific mutations have been identified, in cholestatic diseases, alterations in transporter expression are thought to represent a compensatory (anticholestatic) response that aims to limit hepatocellular accumulation of potentially toxic biliary constituents and provide alternative excretory routes for bile access in cholestasis [8]. Thus, cholestatic injury in rodents results in a marked reduction in mRNA and protein levels of Ntcp and other organic anion-transporting proteins (i.e. Oatp1 and Mrp2) and, to a lesser extent, of Bsep. Thus, Bsep is more stably expressed than the other transporters (Ntcp, Oatp1 and Mrp2) and might continue to excrete bile salts even under cholestatic conditions [9–14]. In contrast, expression of Mdr1 at the canalicular membrane and isoforms of Mrp (Mrp1, Mrp3 and Mrp4) at the basolateral membrane increases following cholestatic injury. In addition, Oatp isoforms, Oatp2 and Oatp4, are relatively well preserved under cholestatic conditions. The maintained expression of Oatp2 and Oatp4 might facilitate efflux of bile salts by virtue of their function as anion exchangers. Similarly, the observed upregulation of Mrp3 and Mrp4 might contribute to the secretion of sulphated bile salts, which are increased in cholestasis. Upregulation of basolateral Mrp3 might also explain the appearance of conjugated bilirubin in plasma and urine during cholestasis. Finally, under cholestatic conditions, adaptive changes in organic anion transporters also occur in the kidney, favouring the renal excretion of bile acids and other biliary constituents [14]. Expression of NTCP and OATP2, as well as BSEP and MRP2, is reduced in patients with acute inflammation-induced cholestasis, highlighting a role for proinflammatory mediators in regulating transporter expression [15]. In primary biliary cirrhosis (PBC), changes in transporter expression evolve in a stage-dependent manner. In early PBC stages, no change in bile acid or organic anion transporters is seen. With disease progression, OATP2 and NTCP are partially downregulated, whereas MRP3 and MDR1 expression is upregulated. The expression of canalicular BSEP and MRP2 is essentially unchanged [16–19].

Molecular mechanisms of regulation of hepatic transporters in cholestasis

One of the more intriguing, and increasingly appreciated, means of hepatic self-regulation in bile acid synthesis and endo-/xenobiotic transport is provided by members of the NR superfamily [20–22]. NRs are ligand-inducible transcription factors that specifically regulate the expression of target genes involved in metabolism, development and reproduction. NRs can be divided into at least five classes [23–26] (Table 1).

1 Class I ('classical' or 'steroid') receptors include those for progesterone, estrogens, androgens, glucocorticoids and mineral corticoids. Type 1 receptors are sequestered in non-productive associations with heat shock proteins and, in this state, do not influence the rate of transcription of their cognate promoters. These receptors bind to palindromic repeats in a homodimeric head-to-head arrangement only in the presence of ligand.

2 Class II includes receptors for thyroid hormone, all-*trans* retinoic acid (RAR) and vitamin D3. Unlike type 1 receptors, these receptors bind constitutively to response elements that contain direct or inverted repeats and exhibit promiscuous dimerization patterns, many involving heterodimerization with retinoid X receptor (RXR). This class could be further divided into permissive heterodimers, in which RXR ligand is able to activate transcription (e.g. peroxisome proliferator-activating receptor), and non-permissive heterodimers that require the ligand of the RXR partner receptor to activate the transcription (Table 1).

3 A third subclass contains 9-*cis* retinoic acid, orphan receptors and other receptors that form a functional unit as homodimers.

4 This class contains a nuclear orphan receptor LRH-1 (liver receptor homologue 1).

5 This class includes receptors such as SHP (small heterodimer partner), the product of a FXR–RXR responsive gene that retains the typical receptor structure but lacks the DNA-binding domain.

Several ligand-activated transcription factors and members of the NR superfamily are involved in the regulation of expression/activity of key steps in bile acid synthesis and transmembrane transport (Table 2); among these, the farnesoid X receptor (FXR), the constitutive androstane receptor (CAR) and pregnane X receptor (PXR) are the best characterized (Table 1; Fig. 1). FXR is a cellular sensor of bile acids [20,21,23,27–31]. The hydrophobic bile acid chenodeoxycholic acid (CDCA) is the most potent physiological agonist of FXR. FXR is expressed in the liver, intestine, adrenal glands and kidney, and regulates various critical steps in the enterohepatic circulation of bile acids. Upon ligation by CDCA and/or other synthetic and non-synthetic ligands, FXR complexes with RXR to increase the expression of BSEP, MDR3 and MRP2 in the liver and IBAPB (the ileal bile acid-binding protein) in the small intestine [32]. FXR also activates the transcription of the short or small heterodimeric partner (*SHP*), which in turn inhibits transcription of *CYP7A* and *CYP8B* [22,29,30,33] (Fig. 1), thereby providing feedback inhibition of bile acid synthesis. These adaptive changes mediated by FXR protect the liver from the injurious effects of the hepatic accumulation of bile acids during cholestasis. Thus, there has been considerable interest in the development of synthetic FXR agonists for the treatment of cholestatic liver disease, and several compounds have been shown to be

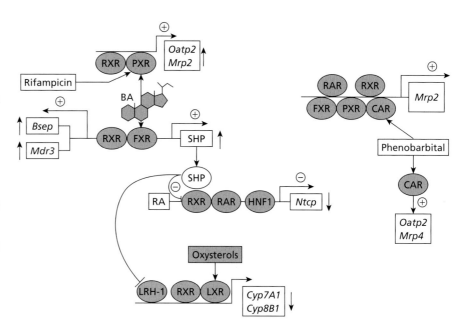

Fig. 1 Molecular mechanisms mediating the regulation of hepatocellular transporters by nuclear receptors (NRs). Left. FXR is a bile acid sensor. In the presence of increased concentrations of bile acids in hepatocytes, FXR complexes with RXR and, in its heterodimeric form, induces the expression of the SHP. In its turn, SHP inhibits the expression of Ntcp. In addition, SHP displaces LRH-1 from its binding site in the promoter of Cyp7A1 and Cyp8B1, causing a suppression of the conversion of cholesterol into bile acids. In addition, FXR activation causes a direct induction of Bsep and Mdr3. These changes lead to reduced bile acid uptake and synthesis and increased excretion through Bsep and Mdr3. Bile acids are also PXR ligands. Activation of PXR upregulates the expression of Oatp2 and Mrp2. Rifampicin is a PXR ligand. Right. Activation of Car by phenobarbital leads to upregulation of Mrp2 expression and induction of Oatp2 and Mrp4.

hepatoprotective in rat and mouse models of cholestasis [34,35]. Synthetic FXR ligands protect rats from ethinylestradiol-induced cholestasis by increasing the expression of Shp, Bsep and Mrp2 and reducing the synthesis of Cyp7a1 and Cyp8b1 as well as the expression of Ntcp [36,37]. Further emphasizing the essential role of *Fxr* in cholestasis, mice harbouring a mutated *Fxr* gene appear to be unable to upregulate Bsep and other *Fxr*-regulated events in response to feeding with cholic acid. *Fxr* null mice also develop cholesterol gallstones because of deficiency in the excretion of bile acids and phospholipids [33].

CAR, the constitutive androstane receptor, is another important nuclear receptor involved in adaptive responses to cholestasis and hyperbilirubinaemia [38]. CAR plays an important role in the detoxification of bile acids by stimulating bile acid sulphation through the activation of steroid sulphotransferases (SULT2A9). CAR also mediates the response of the liver to phenobarbital and has been shown to be an important determinant of the expression of pathways involved in bilirubin clearance including hepatic uptake by Oatp2, binding to the intracellular proteins gluthathione-*S*-transferases (A1 and 2), conjugation with glucuronide by the microsomal bilirubin uridine 5′ diphosphate-glucuronosyltransferase (UGT1A1), and excretion of bilirubin diglucuronide into bile by Mrp2. Activation of CAR in mice is necessary and sufficient to mediate resistance to the hepatotoxicity of lithocholic acid. CAR also coordinately upregulates both Sult2a1, which sulphates hydroxy-bile acids, and Mrp4. In humans, the CAR agonist phenobarbital reduces jaundice in neonates and both serum bilirubin and bile acid levels in patients with PBC [38–43].

PXR (NR112) is closely related to CAR, and both nuclear receptors coordinately regulate a similar group of genes that determine hepatic oxidative metabolism, conjugation reactions and transmembrane transport [44–46]. Examples of these genes include many of the cytochrome P-450s, the glutathione-

S-transferases, the uridine 5′ diphosphate-glucuronosyltransferases, the sulphotransferases (*SULTs*), the *MRPs* and the *OATPs*, all of which are important in the elimination of xenobiotics and the hepatic clearance of endogenous compounds such as bile acids and bilirubin. Pxr stimulates expression of Oatp2, which is involved in bile acid and organic anion or cation transport, and Cyp3a, which is involved in bile acid hydroxylation and detoxification. Finally, another transcription factor, hepatocyte nuclear factor 1α (HNF1α), appears to play a role in mediating bile acid-induced suppression of *OATP2* [47]. Thus, changes in transporter expression during cholestasis appear to be mediated by biliary constituents, mainly bile acids acting on a set of NRs including FXR, PXR and CAR, as well as HNF1α.

Therapeutic perspectives

Ursodeoxycholic acid (UDCA) is a weak, if any, ligand for FXR but a better ligand for PXR [48]. The anticholestatic effect of UDCA is, at least in part, mediated by stimulation of transporter expression or function. UDCA stimulates vesicular exocytosis and insertion of transporters in the canalicular membrane, and increases Bsep, Mrp2, Mrp3 and Mrp4 protein levels in experimental animals and BSEP, MDR3 and MRP4 on the canalicular membrane in humans [49,50]. More recently, UDCA has also been shown to increase Cyp3a4 expression, a relevant detoxification pathway for bile acids. Other studies have found no effects of UDCA on CYP3A metabolic activity in patients with PBC [51,52]. UDCA therapy also increases the hydrophobicity of the bile acid pool and has antiapoptotic and anti-inflammatory effects that could be affecting the clinical outcome. Thus, it is not clear to what extent UDCA's beneficial effect in cholestasis relates to its properties as a NR ligand.

Rifampicin is an effective treatment for severe pruritus in the cholestatic patient and has been associated with increased

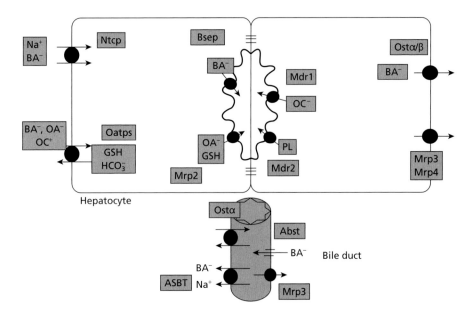

Fig. 2 Adaptive changes in hepatic transporters in rodent models of cholestasis. Animal models of obstructive cholestasis associate with changes in the expression/activity of several hepatocellular transporters. These changes represent an adaptation rather than a causative factor, but might contribute to maintain the functional disturbance observed in cholestatic disorders. Adaptive changes include reduction in expression of Ntcp and Oatp and increased expression/activity of Mrp1, Mrp3 and Mdr1. Bsep remains largely unchanged as well as Mdr2. Administration of an FXR ligand increases Bsep, Mrp2, Mrp3 and Mrp4 expression [36].

urinary excretion of bile acid glucuronides [53,54]. Rifampicin is a potent PXR ligand and increases the expression of CYP3A4, UGT1A1, MRP2, MRP3 and CYP3A metabolism in patients with PBC [44,45]. Long-term treatment of patients with PBC with rifampicin tends to decrease serum bilirubin levels and induces remission in some patients with benign recurrent intrahepatic cholestasis. The beneficial effects on pruritus have been postulated to be mediated by phase I hydroxylation reactions of the hydrophobic bile acids lithocholic and deoxycholic acid via CYP3A4 followed by glucuronidation or sulphation. Owing to complementary action, an interesting therapeutic approach would be the combination of rifampicin plus UDCA in the treatment of cholestatic disorders [50]. The ability of these two drugs to increase the expression of CYP3A4, UGT1A1 and MRP2 (rifampicin) and BSEP, MDR3 and MRP4 (UDCA) suggests that the two drugs might have additive effects [55].

In addition to FXR, CAR and PXR, other receptors such as the retinoic acid receptor, the vitamin D receptor and the glucocorticoid receptor are involved in regulating some of these pathways. Corticosteroids have been shown to stimulate expression of Bsep and Mrp2 [56] in hepatocytes and cholangiocellular transporters in cholangiocytes [57]. These effects account for the beneficial effects of corticosteroids in the treatment of cholestatic jaundice ('steroid whitewash') [57].

Gene transcriptional regulation is enormously complex, and multiple or redundant nuclear factors are almost always involved. This suggests that combinations of specific nuclear receptor ligands may be useful in maximizing the induction of gene expression. In addition, other cofactors, activators, repressors, histone acetylators and methylation reactions also influence gene transcription and may become appropriate targets in the future for therapeutic intervention with small molecules as their specific actions are defined [58].

Note

By convention, the names of human hepatobiliary transporter genes are capitalized, whereas rodent genes and their products are written in lower case with capitalization of the first letter. In addition, transporter genes are set in italics, whereas gene products are set in roman.

Another FXR-regulated bile acid transporter the organic solute transporter (OST)α/β has been identified in hepatocytes, cholangiocytes and intestinal and renal cells. Activation of this transporter increases excretion of bile acids for hepatocytes [59].

References

1 Trauner M, Boyer JL (2003) Bile salt transporters: molecular characterization, function, and regulation. *Physiol Rev* 83, 633–671.

2 Meier PJ, Stieger B (2002) Bile salt transporters. *Annu Rev Physiol* 64, 635–661.

3 Pellicciari R, Constantino C, Fiorucci S (2005) Farnesoid X receptor: from structure to potential clinical applications. *J Med Chem* 48, 5383–5403.

4 Li L, Meier PJ, Ballatori N (2000) Oatp2 mediates bidirectional organic solute transport: a role for intracellular glutathione. *Mol Pharmacol* 58, 335–340.

5 Borst P, Elferink RO (2002) Mammalian ABC transporters in health and disease. *Annu Rev Biochem* 71, 537–592.

6 König J, Rost D, Cui Y *et al.* (1999) Characterization of the human multidrug resistance protein isoform MRP3 localized to the basolateral hepatocyte membrane. *Hepatology* 29, 1156–1163.

7 Rius M, Nies AT, Hummel-Eisenbeiss *et al.* (2003) Cotransport of reduced glutathione with bile salts by MRP4 (ABCC4) localized to the basolateral hepatocyte membrane. *Hepatology* 38, 374–384.

8 Trauner M, Meier PJ, Boyer JL (1998) Molecular pathogenesis of cholestasis. *N Engl J Med* 339, 1217–1227.

9 Lee JM, Trauner M, Soroka CJ et al. (2000) Expression of the bile salt export pump is maintained after chronic cholestasis in the rat. Gastroenterology 118, 163–172.

10 Schrenk D, Gant TW, Preisegger KH et al. (1993) Induction of multidrug resistance gene expression during cholestasis in rats and nonhuman primates. Hepatology 17, 854–860.

11 Soroka CJ, Lee JM, Azzaroli F et al. (2001) Cellular localization and up-regulation of multidrug resistance-associated protein 3 in hepatocytes and cholangiocytes during obstructive cholestasis in rat liver. Hepatology 33, 783–791.

12 Pei QL, Kobayashi Y, Tanaka Y et al. (2002) Increased expression of multidrug resistance-associated protein 1 (mrp1) in hepatocyte basolateral membrane and renal tubular epithelia after bile duct ligation in rats. Hepatol Res 22, 58–64.

13 Wagner M, Fichert P, Zollner G et al. (2003) Role of farnesoid X receptor in determining hepatic ABC transporter expression and liver injury in bile duct-ligated mice. Gastroenterology 125, 825–838.

14 Lee J, Azzaroli F, Wang L et al. (2001) Adaptive regulation of bile salt transporters in kidney and liver in obstructive cholestasis in the rat. Gastroenterology 121, 1473–1484.

15 Zollner G, Fickert P, Zeng R et al. (2001) Hepatobiliary transporter expression in percutaneous liver biopsies of patients with cholestatic liver diseases. Hepatology 33, 633–646.

16 Zollner G, Fickert P, Silbert D et al. (2003) Adaptive changes in hepatobiliary transporter expression in primary biliary cirrhosis. J Hepatol 38, 717–727.

17 Wagnar M, Fickert P, Zollner G (2003) Role of farnesoid X receptor in determining hepatic ABC transporter expression and liver injury in bile duct-ligated mice. Gastroenterology 125, 825–838.

18 Oswald M, Kullak-Ublick GA, Paumgartner G et al. (2001) Expression of hepatic transporters OATP-C and MRP2 in primary sclerosing cholangitis. Liver 21, 247–253.

19 Kullak-Ublick GA, Beuers U, Fahney C et al. (1997) Identification and functional characterization of the promoter region of the human organic anion transporting polypeptide gene. Hepatology 26, 991–997.

20 Pellicciari R, Costantino G, Fiorucci S (2005) Farnesoid x receptor: from structure to potential clinical applications. J Med Chem 48, 5383–5403.

21 Parks DJ, Blanchard SG, Bledsoe RK et al. (1999) Bile acids: natural ligands for an orphan nuclear receptor. Science (Wash DC) 284, 1365–1368.

22 Seol W, Choi HS, Moore DD (1996) An orphan nuclear hormone receptor that lacks a DNA binding domain and heterodimerizes with other receptors. Science (Wash DC) 272, 1336–1339.

23 Kliewer SA, Lehmann JM, Willson TM (1999) Orphan nuclear receptors: shifting endocrinology into reverse. Science 284, 757–760.

24 Maglich JM, Sluder A, Guan X et al. (2001) Comparison of complete nuclear receptor sets from the human, Caenorhabditis elegans and Drosophila genomes. Genome Biol 2, 0029.1–0029.7.

25 Aranda A, Pascual A (2001) Nuclear hormone receptors and gene expression. Pharm Rev 83(1), 1269–1299.

26 Kliewer SA, Umesono K, Mangelsdorf DJ et al. (1992) Retinoid X receptor interacts with nuclear receptors in retinoic acid, thyroid hormone and vitamin D3 signalling. Nature 355, 446–449.

27 Chawla A, Repa JJ, Evans RM et al. (2001) Nuclear receptors and lipid physiology: opening the X-files. Science 294, 1866–1870.

28 Wang H, Chen J, Hollister K et al. (1999) Endogenous bile acids are ligands for the nuclear receptor FXR/BAR. Mol Cell 3, 543–553.

29 Goodwin B, Jones SA, Price RR et al. (2000) A regulatory cascade of the nuclear receptors FXR, SHP-1 and LRH-1 represses bile acid biosynthesis. Mol Cell 6, 517–526.

30 Lu TT, Makishima M, Repa JJ et al. (2000) Molecular basis for feedback regulation of bile acid synthesis by nuclear receptors. Mol Cell 6, 507–515.

31 Forman BM, Goode E, Chen J et al. (1995) Identification of a nuclear receptor that is activated by farnesol metabolites. Cell 81, 687–693.

32 Sinal CJ, Tohkin M, Miyata M et al. (2000) Targeted disruption of the nuclear receptor FXR/BAR impairs bile acid and lipid homeostasis. Cell 102, 731–744.

33 Denson LA, Sturm E, Echevarria W et al. (2001) The orphan nuclear receptor, shp, mediates bile acid-induced inhibition of the rat bile acid transporter, NTCP. Gastroenterology 121, 140–147.

34 Maloney PR, Parks DJ, Haffner CD et al. (2000) Identification of a chemical tool for the orphan nuclear receptor FXR. J Med Chem 43, 2971–2974.

35 Pellicciari R, Fiorucci S, Camaioni E et al. (2002) 6alpha-ethyl-chenodeoxycholic acid (6-ECDCA), a potent and selective FXR agonist endowed with anticholestatic activity. J Med Chem 45, 3569–3572.

36 Fiorucci S, Clerici C, Antonelli E et al. (2005) Protective effects of 6-ethyl chenodeoxycholic acid, a farnesoid X receptor (FXR) ligand, in estrogen induced cholestasis. J Pharmacol Exp Ther 313, 604–612.

37 Lu Y, Binz J, Numerick MJ et al. (2003) Hepatoprotection by the farnesoid X receptor agonist GW4064 in rat models of intra- and extrahepatic cholestasis. J Clin Invest 112, 1678–1687.

38 Kast HR, Goodwin B, Tarr PT et al. (2002) Regulation of multidrug resistance-associated protein 2 (ABCC2) by the nuclear receptors pregnane X receptor, farnesoid X-activated receptor, and constitutive androstane receptor. J Biol Chem 277, 2908–2915.

39 Saini SP, Sonoda J, Xu L et al. (2004) A novel constitutive androstane receptor-mediated and CYP3A-independent pathway of bile acid detoxification. Mol Pharmacol 65, 292–300.

40 Assem M, Schuetz EG, Leggas M et al. (2004) Interactions between hepatic Mrp4 and Sult2a as revealed by the constitutive androstane receptor and Mrp4 knockout mice. J Biol Chem 279, 22250–22257.

41 Huang W, Zhang J, Moore DD (2004) A traditional herbal medicine enhances bilirubin clearance by activating the nuclear receptor CAR. J Clin Invest 113, 137–143.

42 Bloomer JR, Boyer JL (1975) Phenobarbital effects in cholestatic liver disease. Ann Intern Med 82, 310–317.

43 Zhang J, Huang W, Qatanani M et al. (2004) The constitutive androstane receptor and pregnane X receptor function coordinately to prevent bile acid-induced hepatotoxicity. J Biol Chem 279, 49517–49522.

44 Xie W, Radominska-Pandya A, Shi Y et al. (2001) An essential role for nuclear receptors SXR/PXR in detoxification of cholestatic bile acids. Proc Natl Acad Sci USA 98, 3375–3380.

45 Staudinger L, Goodwin B, Jones SA et al. (2001) The nuclear receptor PXR is a lithocholic acid sensor that protects against liver toxicity. Proc Natl Acad Sci USA 98, 3369–3374.

46 Beigneux AP, Moser AH, Shigenaga JK et al. (2002) Reduction in cytochrome P-450 enzyme expression is associated with repression of CAR (constitutive androstane receptor) and PXR (pregnane X receptor) in mouse liver during the acute phase response. Biochem Biophys Res Commun 293, 145–149.

47 Jung D, Kullak-Ublick GA (2003) Hepatocyte nuclear factor 1 α: a key mediator of the effect of bile acids on gene expression. Hepatology 37, 622–631.

48 Paumgartner G, Beuers U (2002) Ursodeoxycholic acid in cholestatic liver disease: mechanisms of action and therapeutic use revisited. *Hepatology* 36, 525–531.

49 Fickert P, Zollner G, Fuchsbichler A *et al.* (2001) Effects of ursodeoxycholic and cholic acid feeding on hepatocellular transporter expression in mouse liver. *Gastroenterology* 121, 170–183.

50 Marshall HU, Wagner M, Zollner G *et al.* (2005) Complementary stimulation of hepatobiliary transport and detoxification systems by rifampicin and ursodeoxycholic acid in humans. *Gastroenterology* 129, 476–485.

51 Zollner G, Fickert P, Fuchsbichler A *et al.* (2003) Role of nuclear bile acid receptor, FXR, in adaptive ABC transporter regulation by cholic and ursodeoxycholic acid in mouse liver and kidney. *J Hepatol* 39, 628–630.

52 Dilger K, Denk A, Heeg MH *et al.* (2005) No relevant effect of ursodeoxycholic acid on cytochrome P450 3A metabolism in primary biliary cirrhosis. *Hepatology* 41, 595–602.

53 Ghent CN, Carruthers SG (1988) Treatment of pruritus in primary biliary cirrhosis with rifampin. Results of a double-blind, crossover, randomized trial. *Gastroenterology* 94, 488–493.

54 Wietholtz H, Marschall HU, Sjovall J *et al.* (1996) Stimulation of bile acid 6 alpha-hydroxylation by rifampicin. *J Hepatol* 24, 713–718.

55 Boyer JL (2005) Nuclear receptor ligands: rational and effective therapy for chronic cholestatic liver disease? *Gastroenterology* 129, 735–740.

56 Kubitz R *et al.* (1999) Regulation of the multidrug resistance protein 2 in the rat liver by lipopolysaccharide and dexamethasone. *Gastroenterology* 116, 401–410.

57 Alvaro D *et al.* (2002) Corticosteroids modulate the secretory processes of the rat intrahepatic biliary epithelium. *Gastroenterology* 122, 1058–1069.

58 Rizzo G, Renga B, Antonelli E *et al.* (2005) The methyl transferase PRMT1 functions as co-activator of farnesoid X receptor (FXR)/9-cis retinoid X receptor and regulates transcription of FXR responsive genes. *Mol Pharmacol* 68, 551–558.

59 Boyer JL, Trauner M, Mennone A *et al.* (2006) Upregulation of a basolateral FXR-dependent bile acid efflux transporter OSTalpha-OSTbeta in cholestasis in humans and rodents. *Am J Physiol Gastrointest Liver Physiol* 290: G1124–G1130.

3.5 Oncogenes and tumour suppressor genes

Dipankar Chattopadhyay and Helen Reeves

Introduction

Hepatocytes are highly differentiated cells with multiple metabolic and synthetic functions. In a normal adult, the life expectancy of a hepatocyte is more than 1 year, with little basal proliferation and only 0.01% of hepatocytes in the 'S phase' of the cell cycle at any one time [1,2]. The liver, however, is the major detoxifying organ of the body and is the first in line to be injured by ingested toxins. Accordingly, the liver has unusual properties of regeneration. Partial (70%) hepatectomy studies in rodents, in which the original liver mass can be restored within 7 days, highlight the dramatic nature of this regenerative capacity (see also Chapter 2.5). This response is complex and involves many growth factors and cytokines as well as the hormones insulin and glucagon. Neither the precise triggers of the early events nor the signals turning off the growth response are clearly understood. What is appreciated, however, is that persistent abuse of this tightly regulated proliferative response can result in failures in the control of these processes, which in turn can contribute to the development and progression of hepatocellular cancer (HCC). HCC most often occurs on a background of chronic liver injury associated with an ongoing healing response, of which perpetual hepatocyte proliferation is a key part. This, in association with the disorganized architecture that characterizes cirrhosis, provides an environment in which DNA damage is (i) most likely to occur and (ii) remain unrepaired (see also Chapter 18.2).

The architecture of the cirrhotic liver is disrupted by bands of fibrous scarring and regenerating nodules of hepatocytes. These nodules of hepatocytes lose the network of communicating venules, arterioles and bile ducts that are in close contact with the hepatic sinusoids in normal liver. As injury continues, the replication potential of hepatocytes gradually diminishes. The relative contribution of other cell types, such as hepatic progenitor cells or even bone marrow stem cells, to the restoration of liver mass increases [3]. Furthermore, cells with a growth advantage, whatever their origin, may flourish rather than be destroyed. The process of hepatocarcinogenesis is a progressive multistep one, perhaps originating from one aberrant mono-clonal population of hepatocytes within a regenerative nodule, but in which a series of successive events brings about hyperplasia, followed by dysplasia, eventually followed by malignant transformation into an early and then advanced HCC [4]. Significant 'events' are the molecular changes that occur in the DNA of key growth regulatory genes that are responsible for the liver's appropriate response to injury (see Fig. 1). These genes are often called oncogenes (growth-promoting genes) or tumour suppressor genes (growth-suppressive genes). Damage to these genes can disrupt proliferative control at a number of levels, including at the cell surface receptor level (IGFR, TGFBRII), the level of cytosolic signalling cascades (Ras, Raf, β-catenin) and also within the nucleus of the cell (TP53, p16). Each of these examples is an established oncogene or a tumour suppressor gene, the dysfunction of which can contribute to the development of HCC.

Genetic instability

Cancers are characterized by disorganized and accelerated growth of immortalized abnormal cells. The key features of malignant cells, as defined by Hanahan and Weinburg in 2000 [5], include the loss of normal contact inhibition, independence towards growth and antigrowth signals, resistance to apoptosis and the development of angiogenic and metastatic capabilities. These features are acquired as a result of the progressive accumulation of genetic and epigenetic events disrupting key regulatory pathways. A 'genetic' event implies that the genomic DNA is damaged in some way – perhaps by mutation, deletion or amplification of a key gene sequence. An 'epigenetic' event is one that indirectly affects the level of expression of a gene without changing its genetic sequence, an example of this being promoter hypermethylation masking transcription factor binding sites and resulting in reduced expression. Why tumours are 'genetically unstable' is unclear. In the case of HCC, it may be that numerous genetic abnormalities occur as a result of chronic liver injury associated with oxidative stress and depleted antioxidant defences. Damage to the DNA of a single cell may escape notice as a result of overstretched repair mechanisms. If the DNA damage inactivates a proapoptotic gene or activates a

Table 1 Oncogenes involved in the development and progression of HCC.

Oncogene	Method(s) of deregulation	Consequences
Ras isoforms	Activating mutation Hypomethylation and overexpression	Sustained activation of the Ras/Raf/MAP kinase pathway resulting in inappropriate mitogenic stimulation
Cyclin D1	Activating mutation ↑ wild-type levels	Cell cycle deregulation, accelerated G1/S transition
β-catenin	Mutation resistant to degradation	Sustained activation of LEF/TCF4 mitogenic signalling
c-myc	Allelic gain Hypomethylation resulting in ↑ expression	Inappropriate mitogenic stimulation
Gankyrin	Increased expression	Blocking the activity of p53 and Rb

proliferative gene, the cell may survive inappropriately or grow more rapidly, particularly in an environment encouraging hepatocyte regeneration. This growing clone of hyperproliferative or apoptosis-resistant cells may be more prone to further DNA damage.

There is some evidence, however, that tumours may be 'genetically unstable' and prone to DNA damage at the outset [6]. The commonest type of genetic instability in HCC is chromosomal instability, or CIN. DNA mutation is generally common in genetic instability, but CIN is particularly characterized by aneuploidy/variation in chromosome number and multiple areas of allelic imbalance as a result of deletions or gains of parts of chromosomes. Regions gained in cancers may contain additional copies of oncogenes, while those deleted may contain tumour suppressor genes. Extensive demethylation in centromeric sequences is common in human cancers and may have a role in the development of aneuploidy [7], while the progressive shortening of chromosome telomeres during cell division may also contribute [8,9].

Oncogenes

Oncogenes are DNA sequences that were first discovered in transforming retroviruses. Subsequent works revealed that not only were these DNA sequences capable of inducing neoplastic transformation in mammalian cells but, moreover, they were present in human neoplastic tissues. Thus, these viral oncogenes, or 'genes that cause cancer', were initially thought to be disseminated by retroviruses. Instead, they are now known to be present in all eukaryotes. Oncogenes and their gene products show close species homology and have remained almost unchanged through evolution. Genes homologous to these retroviral genes are present in normal cells and are often termed proto-oncogenes. Proto-oncogenes play pivotal roles in regulating normal cellular growth, differentiation and development. Mechanisms for activation of proto-oncogenes to oncogenes include point mutations, gross DNA rearrangements, gene amplification and promoter insertion. A number of proto-oncogenes have been found to be inappropriately active or

overexpressed in both preneoplastic and neoplastic hepatocellular lesions, as summarized in Table 1. They include genes enhancing the activity of key proliferative signalling cascades, such as the Ras/Raf/MAP kinase cascade and the Wnt pathway, as well as some downstream cell cycle regulators.

When in its active guanosine 5′-triphosphate (GTP)-bound state, the Ras protein is responsible for recruiting Raf kinase to the cell membrane and initiating the MAP kinase cascade, a key regulator of cellular proliferation. Increased activity occurs at each of level of the Ras/Raf/MAP kinase cascade in HCC. Activating mutations rendering Ras permanently in its GTP-bound state occasionally occur in HCC, while overexpression of wild-type Ras is very common [10]. Furthermore, the Ras partner, c-Raf kinase, is reportedly elevated in up to 100% of HCC and 91.2% of cirrhotic livers. The level of c-Raf overexpression is usually higher in HCC relative to cirrhotic tissues in the same individual [11]. In human HCC, increased expression of MAP kinase is also common [12]. Activated MAP kinases translocate to the nucleus and phosphorylate transcription factors, promoting the expression of proliferative genes. Overexpression of MAP kinase correlates with the increased expression of c-fos and cyclin D1, the latter promoting acceleration through the G1 checkpoint of the mammalian cell cycle. RhoB is another member of the *Ras* gene family that is overexpressed in HCC [13]. It is more associated with transformation and motility than proliferation and possibly plays a role in intrahepatic metastases of human HCC [13].

The hallmark of Wnt signalling is the stabilization of cytoplasmic β-catenin, followed by its nuclear translocation and association with LEF/TCF transcription factors. In the absence of a Wnt signal, β-catenin is phosphorylated by functional interactions with glycogen synthase kinase 3β (GSK3β), axin and the adenomatous polyposis coli (APC) protein. It is subsequently ubiquitinated and degraded via the proteosome. Inappropriate stabilization of cellular β-catenin may result in transcriptional activation of the target genes of Wnt signalling, e.g. *c-myc*, *cyclin D1* and *PPARα*, thereby mediating cellular proliferation and tumour progression. Activating mutations of β-catenin are reportedly present in 18–41% of HCC [14,15]. Mutations in

AXIN1, also necessary for efficient β-catenin degradation, are present in some HCCs and lead to β-catenin accumulation without any mutation in the β-catenin gene itself [16].

The c-myc protein is a multifunctional nuclear phosphoprotein that plays a role in cell cycle progression, apoptosis and cellular transformation. It functions as a transcription factor and is a downstream product of proliferative signalling cascades such as Wnt. The c-*myc* gene may be hypomethylated, amplified or rearranged in human HCC. It is commonly overexpressed in this cancer and has been shown to produce increased hepatocyte proliferation in an animal transgenic mouse model when coexpressed with transforming growth factor (TGF)-α [17]. Additional animal model data confirming increased expression of c-myc in diethylnitrosamine-induced murine preneoplastic foci of altered hepatocytes (FAH) suggests that its overexpression may be an early event in chemical hepatocarcinogenesis [18].

Gankyrin is a novel protein that has oncogenic properties and is overexpressed in HCC [19]. Its effects are predominantly related to its inactivation of key tumour suppressor proteins such as Rb, P16 and TP53, and it is described in more detail later in this chapter.

The mechanisms described above relate to specific genes altered by rearrangement, amplification, mutation or promoter hypomethylation. However, viral proteins disrupting proto-oncogene function also have a major role to play in HCCs arising in association with hepatitis B virus (HBV) and, to some extent, hepatitis C virus (HCV) infection. In HCC related to HBV, random integration of viral DNA into human chromosomal DNA occurs. Occasionally, this integration can interrupt the expression or function of growth-suppressive genes. Often, however, this integration enables the production of a viral protein termed HBx. The HBx protein serves the virus by promoting hepatocellular proliferation, but similarly contributes to the process of hepatocarcinogenesis. HBx activates cell signalling cascades including the MAP kinase and Janus family tyrosine kinases (JAK)/signal transducer and activators of transcription (STAT) pathways [20]. It acts as a cotranscription factor for oncogenic proteins such as c-myc, c-jun and c-fos or Ras [21]. The HBx protein may also promote cell survival by interaction with the Wnt pathway. It suppresses GSK3β activity, thereby inhibiting both β-catenin phosphorylation and its subsequent degradation. Furthermore, HBx influences the activity of Src kinase [22], a tyrosine kinase that also contributes to β-catenin localization and activity [23]. In cancers relating to HCV infection, the HCV core protein may contribute to cancer development. It promotes apoptosis resistance by interacting with several intracellular pathways, including indirect enhancement of NFκB activity [24] and inhibition of tumour necrosis factor (TNF)-induced and *Fas*-mediated apoptosis [25].

Tumour suppressor genes

The normal function of a tumour suppressor gene (TSG) is to inhibit cellular proliferation. Unlike oncogenes, they are 'recessive', as loss of function of both alleles is considered necessary to generate a mutant phenotype. The most extensively studied TSG is *TP53*, one allele of which is already mutated in the germline in the inherited Li–Fraumeni syndrome associated with the development of multiple cancers. HCC, like the majority of cancers, is most often sporadic in nature, therefore requiring both alleles to 'acquire' rather than inherit a means of inactivation. Methods of TSG inactivation/silencing include allelic loss, mutation, promoter hypermethylation and aberrant alternative splicing. While much is known about *TP53* in HCC, other TSGs include the retinoblastoma gene (*Rb*) and the cell cycle inhibitors *p16*, *p21* and *p27*. These and others have been reviewed recently [10] and are summarized in Table 2.

TP53 is located on chromosome 17p13 and encodes a nuclear protein that is involved in several cellular functions including the regulation of G1 to S transition in the cell cycle, DNA repair and apoptotic cell death. In a normal cell, the half-life of TP53 is short. However, in the presence of DNA damage caused by a carcinogen or UV light, for example, it is produced in increased amounts, becomes more stable as a result of inhibition of degradation and induces either a growth arrest or apoptosis depending on the extent of DNA damage. TP53 is therefore regarded as a gatekeeper for cellular proofreading in response to many stress signals, including DNA damage. As the DNA repair network plays a key role in faithful maintenance of the genome, abrogation of TP53 function is detrimental and potentiates increased genome instability, cancer development and progression. A reduction in wild-type TP53 function in HCC can occur as a result of an inactivating point mutation, reduced expression as a result of promoter hypermethylation or loss of an allele of *TP53*, and also as a result of interference from other cellular or viral proteins.

Although mutation of *TP53* is common in HCC, both the incidence and the specific nucleotide base changes vary with different geographical regions. The presence of a unique mutational spectrum of *TP53* has provided a strong molecular link between carcinogen exposure and HCC development. In South Africa and the Qidong area of China, a significant number of HCCs have a *TP53* R249S mutation [26,27]. This 'hotspot' mutation is associated with the high intake of aflatoxin 1 in food and may have contributed to the high incidence of HCC in theses areas [28]. In other regions where aflatoxin levels in food are low or undetectable, no such mutational specificity of the *TP53* gene has been detected.

Both host and non-host proteins can contribute to TP53 inactivation in HCC. MDM2 is a cellular protein transcriptionally activated by TP53, which in turn inhibits TP53 activity as part of a negative autoregulatory feedback loop. MDM2 inhibits the nuclear localization of TP53, inhibits the transactivation function of TP53, but also promotes its degradation. MDM2 is a ligase that promotes the ubiquitination and subsequent proteosomal destruction of TP53. Although numbers of studies on MDM2 in HCC are small, there is accumulating evidence indicating overexpression of MDM2 in this cancer, providing yet

Table 2 Tumour suppressor genes (TSG) involved in the development and progression of HCC.

TSG	Method(s) of deregulation	Consequences
P53 growth-suppressive transcription factor	Mutation and accumulation of inactive protein (28–67%) Allelic loss of 17p13 and loss of expression (17–70%)	Loss of induction of key growth-suppressive genes (*p21*, *GADD45*), apoptosis resistance secondary to disrupted targets (Bax, PIDD, NOXA, PERP, reactive oxygen species), loss of prevention of new blood vessel formation (TSP1, BAI1, Maspin, GD-AIF)
IGFR2 growth-inhibitory tyrosine kinase receptor	Inactivating mutation (25%) Allelic loss of 6q26 (23–36%)	Associated with ↑ IGF2 (hepatocyte mitogen) and ↓ TGF-β (growth inhibitor) signalling (early event)
Rb retinoblastoma protein	Inactivating mutation (15%) Allelic loss of 13q14 (18–70%)	E2F release and stimulation of G1/S cell cycle progression (early event)
PTEN	Inactivating mutation (4%) Allelic loss of 10q23 (17–27%)	Disrupts PI3 kinase/MTOR pathway. Associated with ↓ IGF secretion and ↓ VEGF expression (possibly a late event)
AXIN	Inactivating mutation (6%) Allelic loss of 16p13 (22–40%)	β-catenin accumulation, therefore loss of suppression of β-catenin-stimulated LEF/TCF4 mitogenic signalling
p16 CKI inhibitor	Allelic loss of 9p21 (20–30%) Promoter of hypermethylation	Loss of cyclin-dependent kinase inhibitor function, accelerated cell cycle progression; defective response to DNA damage
E-cadherin	Allelic loss of 16q22 (26–54%) Promoter of hypermethylation	Decreased degradation of β-catenin
RASSF1 ras association domain family protein	Allelic loss of 3p21 (62%) Promoter of hypermethylation	Loss of Ras-regulated proapoptosis, loss of inhibition of cyclin D1 accumulation
BRCA2	Allelic loss of 13q12 (18–19%) Promoter of hypermethylation Occasional germline mutation	Defect in DNA repair of double-strand breaks leading to impaired genomic integrity and cell cycle control
RIZ1 Rb interacting zinc finger protein transcription factor	Allelic loss of 1p36 (26–46%)	Loss results in inhibition of G2/M and accelerated cell cycle progression; loss of induction of apoptosis
KLF6	Allelic loss of 10p15 (40%) Inactivating mutation (0–10%)	Loss promotes proliferation, possibly as a result of lack of upregulation of cell cycle inhibitor p21

IGF, insulin-like growth factor; MTOR, mammalian target of rapamycin; VEGF, vascular endothelial growth factor.

more means of inactivating TP53 in circumstances when it is both wild type and its expression retained [29,30].

In HCC secondary to HBV infection, the presence of the HBx protein can interfere with tumour suppressor functions. The HBx protein can inhibit *TP53* sequence-specific transcriptional activation [31], TP53-mediated apoptosis [32], as well as TP53 binding to transcription-nucleotide excision repair (NER) factors, such as XPB [33]. HCV proteins may also contribute. HCV is an RNA virus, and its genome contains an open reading frame encoding a large polyprotein precursor that is then processed by a combination of cellular and viral proteases into three or four structural and at least six non-structural proteins. HCV NS5A is a non-structural protein that possibly plays a role in the development of chronic liver disease and HCC [34]. It reportedly forms complexes with TP53, repressing TP53 transactivation function by disrupting its normal DNA binding. The HCV core protein may also repress the transcriptional activity of the *TP53* promoter and is a further possible mechanism of abrogating the activity of TP53 in HCV-induced HCC [35].

The retinoblastoma susceptibility (*Rb*) gene is another TSG whose dysfunction is known to contribute to hepatocarcinogenesis. The Rb protein is a core element governing cell cycle progression. Essentially, Rb controls the cell cycle at the G1/S boundary, restricting release of the E2F transcription factor [36] by virtue of its own cyclical phosphorylation. The activity or phosphostatus of Rb depends on the activity of the cyclin-dependent kinase, CDK4, which in turn depends on interactions with agonists such as cyclin D1 and inhibitors such as P16INK4. Overall, the Rb pathway is inactivated in a number of human HCC cell lines [37] and in the majority of HCCs [38]. Cyclin D1/CDK4 phosphorylates and inactivates Rb, and mechanisms contributing to Rb inactivation in HCC include cyclin D1 over-expression [39] as well as overactivity of CDK4 as a result of reduced expression of the Cdk4 inhibitor p16INK4 [40]. Viral proteins may also alter Rb activity. HCV core protein reportedly decreases the expression of Rb, thus allowing E2F to be constitutively active, possibly promoting rapid cell proliferation [41].

Gankyrin, as mentioned previously, has been cloned by cDNA subtractive hybridization in HCC [19] and can be identified by

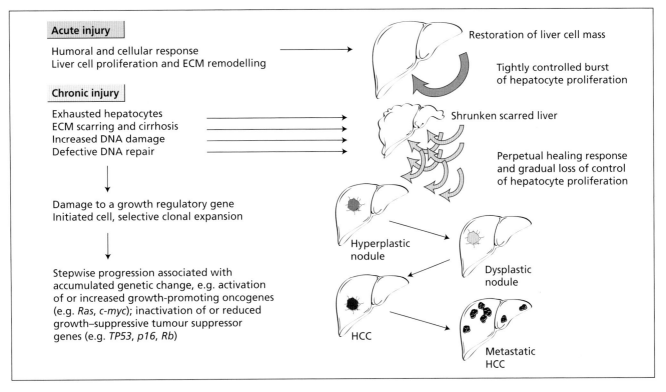

Fig. 1 The development and progression of HCC is associated with accumulated genetic change. The closely regulated burst of hepatocyte proliferation that occurs in response to acute liver injury is represented, as are the events that occur in response to persistent injury. The wound healing myofibroblast response creates a scarred distorted liver within which hepatocytes continue to regenerate, creating nodules of cells that lack the structural organization of normal liver plates and sinusoids. Within this abnormal environment, a combination of depleted defences against DNA damage, failing DNA repair mechanisms and exhausted hepatocyte replication potential permits cells that gain a proliferative advantage to survive and expand. The stepwise progression of phenotypically abnormal hepatocytes, from hyperplastic to dysplastic to early and, finally, advanced HCCs, is associated with accumulated genetic or molecular events. In particular, these events include DNA damage enhancing the activities of growth-promoting oncogenes and inactivating the growth-suppressive effects of tumour suppressor genes. The result of accumulated damage is accelerated growth of increasingly abnormal cells and the progression of HCC. ECM, extracellular matrix.

in situ examination as a highly expressed oncoprotein in HCC [42]. During hepatic carcinogenesis, gankyrin promotes the release of E2F activity as a result of binding Rb directly and bringing about its phosphorylation and inactivation [42]. Gankyrin also promotes CDK4 phosphorylation of Rb by competing with the tumour suppressor P16INK4 in its binding and inhibition of CDK4 [43]. In addition, gankyrin suppresses the activity of TP53. It interacts with MDM2, the key TP53 ubiquitin ligase, promoting the proteosomal degradation of TP53 [44]. Thus, gankyrin overexpression is common and highly disruptive in HCC. Devising a means of destroying it may prove valuable therapeutically in the years to come.

DLC1 (deleted in liver cancer 1) is a putative TSG first reported by Yuan *et al.* in 1998 [45]. A recent *in vitro* study has confirmed DLC1 as a Rho GTPase activating protein (Rho GAP) [46]. In mammalian cells, Rho GAPs are important regulators in the switching between active GTP-bound and inactive guanosine 5′-diphosphate (GDP)-bound Rho proteins. They stimulate the intrinsic GTPase activity of Rho proteins and catalyse their conversion into the inactive GDP state. This attenuates the signal-transducing activities of Rho proteins, and Rho GAPs

therefore act as negative regulators. The loss of activity of such a negative modulator may therefore confer a proliferative advantage to a cell. Deletion of the *DLC1* gene is present in a subset of hepatoma cell lines and primary HCCs [47], and it is likely that epigenetic alterations also contribute to its inactivation in primary HCC [46]. Restoration of DLC1 expression can inhibit the proliferation of hepatoma cells [47], promote caspase-3-mediated apoptosis and inhibit invasiveness *in vitro*, as well as contribute to a reduction in the ability of the cells to form tumours in athymic nude mice [48].

A number of other candidate tumour suppressor genes have been proposed in HCC, one of the most recent of which is Kruppel-like factor 6 (*KLF6*). KLF6, a ubiquitously expressed transcription factor, has been identified as a TSG inactivated by allelic loss and mutation in a number of cancers, including HCC [49]. While work to characterize the biology of this and other candidate TSGs and oncogenes continues, we recognize that there are likely to be many more unknown genetic or biological events taking place. However, there is hope that, with continued effort, we will eventually understand enough about these processes to start to make a difference to the way in which we manage this common, dismal malignancy. Presently, although we know that HCC most often occurs in individuals with cirrhotic liver disease, we have neither the accurate safe methods nor the means to identify individuals with cirrhosis within our population, let alone identify those with HCC. Understanding the molecular pathogenesis of these conditions will help us to identify both the biomarkers of the future, for use as more sensitive and less invasive diagnostic and prognostic tests, as well as, hopefully, the means to restore the control of regulated hepatocyte growth. In this way, we would hope not only to detect early malignant disease in at-risk individuals and treat it more effectively, but possibly even to prevent its development and/or progression.

References

1 Diehl AM, Rai R (1996) Review: regulation of liver regeneration by pro-inflammatory cytokines. *J Gastroenterol Hepatol* 11 (5), 466–470.

2 Michalopoulos GK, DeFrances MC (1997) Liver regeneration. *Science* 276 (5309), 60–66.

3 Forbes F, Alison M (2005) Liver stem cells in persistent viral infection, liver regeneration and cancer. In: Thomas H, Lemon S, Zuckerman A (eds) *Viral Hepatitis*, 3rd edn. Oxford: Blackwell Publishing.

4 Coleman WB (2003) Mechanisms of human hepatocarcinogenesis. *Curr Mol Med* 3 (6), 573–588.

5 Hanahan D, Weinberg RA (2000) The hallmarks of cancer. *Cell* 100 (1), 57–70.

6 Cahill DP, Kinzler KW, Vogelstein B *et al.* (1999) Genetic instability and Darwinian selection in tumours. *Trends Cell Biol* 9 (12), M57–60.

7 Esteller M (2003) Cancer epigenetics: DNA methylation and chromatin alterations in human cancer. *Adv Exp Med Biol* 532, 39–49.

8 Plentz RR, Schlegelberger B, Flemming P *et al.* (2005) Telomere shortening correlates with increasing aneuploidy of chromosome 8 in human hepatocellular carcinoma. *Hepatology* 42 (3), 522–526.

9 Satyanarayana A, Manns MP, Rudolph KL (2004) Telomeres and telomerase: a dual role in hepatocarcinogenesis. *Hepatology* 40 (2), 276–283.

10 Kremer-Tal S, Day CP, Reeves HL (2005) The genetic basis of hepatocellular cancer. In: Ali S, Mann DM, Friedman SL (eds) *Liver Diseases: Biochemical Mechanisms and New Therapeutic Insights.* Enfield, NH: Science Publishers.

11 Hwang YH, Choi JY, Kim S *et al.* (2004) Over-expression of c-raf-1 proto-oncogene in liver cirrhosis and hepatocellular carcinoma. *Hepatol Res* 29 (2), 113–121.

12 Huynh H, Nguyen TT, Chow KH *et al.* (2003) Over-expression of the mitogen-activated protein kinase (MAPK) kinase (MEK)-MAPK in hepatocellular carcinoma: its role in tumor progression and apoptosis. *BMC Gastroenterol* 3 (1), 19.

13 Genda T, Sakamoto M, Ichida T *et al.* (1999) Cell motility mediated by rho and Rho-associated protein kinase plays a critical role in intrahepatic metastasis of human hepatocellular carcinoma. *Hepatology* 30 (4), 1027–1036.

14 de La Coste A, Romagnolo B, Billuart P *et al.* (1998) Somatic mutations of the beta-catenin gene are frequent in mouse and human hepatocellular carcinomas. *Proc Natl Acad Sci USA* 95 (15), 8847–8851.

15 Miyoshi Y, Iwao K, Nagasawa Y *et al.* (1998) Activation of the beta-catenin gene in primary hepatocellular carcinomas by somatic alterations involving exon 3. *Cancer Res* 58 (12), 2524–2527.

16 Satoh S, Daigo Y, Furukawa Y *et al.* (2000) AXIN1 mutations in hepatocellular carcinomas, and growth suppression in cancer cells by virus-mediated transfer of AXIN1. *Nature Genet* 24 (3), 245–250.

17 Murakami H, Sanderson ND, Nagy P *et al.* (1993) Transgenic mouse model for synergistic effects of nuclear oncogenes and growth factors in tumorigenesis: interaction of c-myc and transforming growth factor alpha in hepatic oncogenesis. *Cancer Res* 53 (8), 1719–1723.

18 Alexandre K, Jacobovitz D, Galand P (1990) Immunohistochemical detection of c-myc and c-erbA products in diethylnitrosamine-induced preneoplastic and neoplastic liver lesions in rats. *Carcinogenesis* 11 (7), 1189–1194.

19 Higashitsuji H, Itoh K, Nagao T *et al.* (2000) Reduced stability of retinoblastoma protein by gankyrin, an oncogenic ankyrin-repeat protein overexpressed in hepatomas. *Nature Med* 6 (1), 96–99.

20 Arbuthnot P, Capovilla A, Kew M (2000) Putative role of hepatitis B virus X protein in hepatocarcinogenesis: effects on apoptosis, DNA repair, mitogen-activated protein kinase and JAK/STAT pathways. *J Gastroenterol Hepatol* 15 (4), 357–368.

21 Natoli G, Avantaggiati ML, Chirillo P *et al.* (1994) Induction of the DNA-binding activity of c-jun/c-fos heterodimers by the hepatitis B virus transactivator pX. *Mol Cell Biol* 14 (2), 989–998.

22 Bouchard MJ, Wang LH, Schneider RJ (2001) Calcium signaling by HBx protein in hepatitis B virus DNA replication. *Science* 294 (5550), 2376–2378.

23 Muller T, Choidas A, Reichmann E *et al.* (1999) Phosphorylation and free pool of beta-catenin are regulated by tyrosine kinases and tyrosine phosphatases during epithelial cell migration. *J Biol Chem* 274 (15), 10173–10183.

24 You LR, Chen CM, Lee YH (1999) Hepatitis C virus core protein enhances NF-kappaB signal pathway triggering by lymphotoxin-beta receptor ligand and tumor necrosis factor alpha. *J Virol* 73 (2), 1672–1681.

25 Marusawa H, Hijikata M, Chiba T *et al.* (1999) Hepatitis C virus core protein inhibits Fas- and tumor necrosis factor alpha-mediated apoptosis via NF-kappaB activation. *J Virol* 73 (6), 4713–4720.

26 Bressac B, Kew M, Wands J *et al.* (1991) Selective G to T mutations of p53 gene in hepatocellular carcinoma from southern Africa. *Nature* 350 (6317), 429–431.

27 Aguilar F, Hussain SP, Cerutti P (1993) Aflatoxin B1 induces the transversion of G→T in codon 249 of the p53 tumor suppressor gene in human hepatocytes. *Proc Natl Acad Sci USA* 90 (18), 8586–8590.

28 Hsu IC, Metcalf RA, Sun T *et al.* (1991) Mutational hotspot in the p53 gene in human hepatocellular carcinomas. *Nature* 350 (6317), 427–428.

29 Jablkowski M, Bocian A, Bialkowska J *et al.* (2005) A comparative study of P53/MDM2 genes alterations and P53/MDM2 proteins immunoreactivity in liver cirrhosis and hepatocellular carcinoma. *J Exp Clin Cancer Res* 24 (1), 117–125.

30 Luo YL, Cheng RX, Feng DY (2001) [Role of functional inactivation of p53 from MDM2 overexpression in hepatocarcinogenesis]. *Hunan Yi Ke Da Xue Xue Bao* 26 (1), 13–16.

31 Wang XW, Forrester K, Yeh H *et al.* (1994) Hepatitis B virus X protein inhibits p53 sequence-specific DNA binding, transcriptional activity, and association with transcription factor ERCC3. *Proc Natl Acad Sci USA* 91 (6), 2230–2234.

32 Wang XW, Gibson MK, Vermeulen W *et al.* (1995) Abrogation of p53-induced apoptosis by the hepatitis B virus X gene. *Cancer Res* 55 (24), 6012–6016.

33 Jia L, Wang XW, Harris CC (1999) Hepatitis B virus X protein inhibits nucleotide excision repair. *Int J Cancer* 80 (6), 875–879.

34 Gong GZ, Jiang YF, He Y *et al.* (2004) HCV NS5A abrogates p53 protein function by interfering with p53-DNA binding. *World J Gastroenterol* 10 (15), 2223–2227.

35 Ray RB, Steele R, Meyer K *et al.* (1997) Transcriptional repression of p53 promoter by hepatitis C virus core protein. *J Biol Chem* 272 (17), 10983–10986.

36 Muller H, Helin K (2000) The E2F transcription factors: key regulators of cell proliferation. *Biochim Biophys Acta* 1470 (1), M1–12.

37 Suh SI, Pyun HY, Cho JW *et al.* (2000) 5-Aza-2′-deoxycytidine leads to down-regulation of aberrant p16INK4A RNA transcripts and restores the functional retinoblastoma protein pathway in hepatocellular carcinoma cell lines. *Cancer Lett* 160 (1), 81–88.

38 Azechi H, Nishida N, Fukuda Y *et al.* (2001) Disruption of the p16/cyclin D1/retinoblastoma protein pathway in the majority of human hepatocellular carcinomas. *Oncology* 60 (4), 346–354.

39 Joo M, Kang YK, Kim MR *et al.* (2001) Cyclin D1 overexpression in hepatocellular carcinoma. *Liver* 21 (2), 89–95.

40 Hui AM, Sakamoto M, Kanai Y *et al.* (1996) Inactivation of p16INK4 in hepatocellular carcinoma. *Hepatology* 24 (3), 575–579.

41 Cho JW, Baek WK, Suh SI *et al.* (2001) Hepatitis C virus core protein promotes cell proliferation through the upregulation of cyclin E expression levels. *Liver* 21 (2), 137–142.

42 Tan L, Fu XY, Liu SQ *et al.* (2005) Expression of p28GANK and its correlation with RB in human hepatocellular carcinoma. *Liver Int* 25 (3), 667–676.

43 Lozano G, Zambetti GP (2005) Gankyrin: an intriguing name for a novel regulator of p53 and RB. *Cancer Cell* 8 (1), 3–4.

44 Higashitsuji H, Itoh K, Sakurai T *et al.* (2005) The oncoprotein gankyrin binds to MDM2/HDM2, enhancing ubiquitylation and degradation of p53. *Cancer Cell* 8 (1), 75–87.

45 Yuan BZ, Miller MJ, Keck CL *et al.* (1998) Cloning, characterization, and chromosomal localization of a gene frequently deleted in human liver cancer (DLC-1) homologous to rat RhoGAP. *Cancer Res* 58 (10), 2196–2199.

46 Wong CM, Lee JM, Ching YP *et al.* (2003) Genetic and epigenetic alterations of DLC-1 gene in hepatocellular carcinoma. *Cancer Res* 63 (22), 7646–7651.

47 Ng IO, Liang ZD, Cao L *et al.* (2000) DLC-1 is deleted in primary hepatocellular carcinoma and exerts inhibitory effects on the proliferation of hepatoma cell lines with deleted DLC-1. *Cancer Res* 60 (23), 6581–6584.

48 Zhou X, Thorgeirsson SS, Popescu NC (2004) Restoration of DLC-1 gene expression induces apoptosis and inhibits both cell growth and tumorigenicity in human hepatocellular carcinoma cells. *Oncogene* 23 (6), 1308–1313.

49 Kremer-Tal S, Reeves HL, Narla G *et al.* (2004) Frequent inactivation of the tumor suppressor Kruppel-like factor 6 (KLF6) in hepatocellular carcinoma. *Hepatology* 40 (5), 1047–1052.

3.6 Genomics, gene arrays and proteomics in the study of liver disease

Geoffrey W. McCaughan, Nicholas A. Shackel, Rohan Williams, Devanshi Seth,
Paul S. Haber and Mark D. Gorrell

The completed sequencing of the human genome in the year 2000 revealed that it encoded approximately 30 000 genes [1]. The functions of approximately 50% of these genes have been defined or proposed, leaving at least half the human genome with unrecognized functions. It has been estimated that these 30 000 genes encode approximately 100 000 proteins (produced predominantly by alternative splicing) [2]. Consequently, the human proteome consists of approximately 100 000 proteins/polypeptides. This enormous wealth of information has led to an explosion of studies that have characterized disease or pathophysiological states based on sampling of the human genome or proteome. This chapter reviews the emerging data from such studies related to the examination of liver diseases and liver pathobiology.

Terminology

Functional genomics

Functional genomics is the study of gene function through the utilization of high-throughput technologies, in addition to the information obtained by gene sequencing and mutation analysis (Fig. 1). Since these technologies have become available in the last 10 years, an insurmountable volume of data has been generated. It is a challenge to sift through these data and to extract meaningful information. It has been aptly put by Duyk that 'we must guard against committing the mortal sin of genomics by confusing throughput with output, which too often blurs the distinction between data and knowledge. Instead, we must

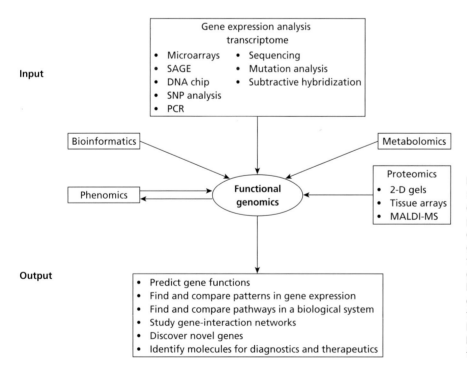

Fig. 1 Overview of functional genomics methodologies. This figure depicts a number of approaches and techniques that generate a plethora of information within a cell or organism with which to study functional genomics. A comprehensive understanding of this information with respect to functioning of genes, transcripts and proteins is essential to build functional maps of their interactions and discover novel diagnostic and therapeutic targets. The rapid development of such high-throughput technologies is no doubt building an unprecedented understanding of functional genomics in all organisms.

Fig. 2 Gene array examples showing two examples of the common types of gene array. (a) One-probe gene array, in this case using a radionucleotide probe hybridized to a nylon membrane spotted with cDNAs. Affymetrix GeneChip™ is another example of a single-probe experiment but uses a completely different high-density array and a fluorophore labelled probe. (b) Comparative hybridization (multiplexing) using two probes labelled with Cy3 and Cy5 fluorophores on a glass slide microarray.

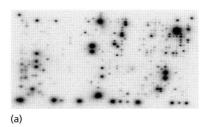
(a)

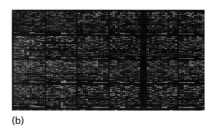
(b)

maintain the necessary focus to achieve an ever-more operational understanding of all the molecular components and the interactions that define a cell or an organism' [3].

Gene arrays

Gene arrays are tools used to simultaneously display expression profiles of thousands of genes with the aim of comparing the patterns of gene expression (profiles) of whole organisms, disease states or other aspects of pathophysiology. The technology involves high-density spotting of gene-specific DNA sequences arrayed in predetermined coordinates on a solid matrix, followed by probing with labelled RNA/DNA samples to interrogate the expression of the arrayed genes in these samples (Fig. 2). Currently, there are in excess of 235 companies that are actively involved in developing microarray technology. A recent report in *Nature* presents a list of companies and technologies that encompasses a wide range of gene array platforms including single nucleotide polymorphisms (SNP), whole genome genotyping, microRNA chips and specialized bioinformatics software in addition to platforms for expression profiling (http://www.nature.com.opac.library.usyd.edu.au/nature/journal/v435/n7044/pdf/435995a.pdf).

The gene expression profile defined by gene arrays has been called a 'transcriptome'. The liver transcriptome from adult humans has been studied using cDNA arrays in recent years [4]. A comprehensive summary of the liver transcriptome defined by different gene array technologies was reviewed recently [5]. Gene arrays are discussed in detail in later sections.

Proteomics

Proteomics is the global analysis of protein expression in a cell, tissue or body fluid to determine the function, interaction and importance in different environments and conditions, such as health and disease. Various techniques, for example two-dimensional electrophoresis, mass spectrophotometry (MS), matrix assisted laser desorption/ionization (MALDI), electrospray ionization (ESI), tissue arrays and antibody arrays, have progressed rapidly in proteomics in recent years. Proteomics is discussed in detail in later sections.

Bioinformatics

Bioinformatics refers to the use of mathematical, statistical and computational techniques to collect, analyse and store large quantities of data from biological systems. Bioinformatics includes programmes that allow normalization of data, calculate statistical significance of gene/protein expression levels and allocate gene function through data mining. Bioinformatics can handle large data sets by means of specially derived algorithms for various functions, including identification of differential gene expression, molecular pathways and gene/protein networks. Several open source and commercial bioinformatics software packages are available for high-throughput data analysis. For more information on bioinformatics tools, see later sections.

Methodologies

Gene arrays

There are a variety of gene arrays available as 'off-the-shelf' products. These include arrays covering the whole genome and specialized arrays that sample select gene expression. The basic principle involved in each is to immobilize small fragments of DNA for hundreds to thousands of genes in a grid format. Regardless of the chemistry involved in preparing the microarrays, the multiple steps involved remain similar (Fig. 3).

Microarray reproducibility within and between laboratories and across platforms has been a major issue in dealing with generated data [6]. As with other molecular biology techniques, variability is introduced at each step. This includes the variability introduced at the time of printing and the lack of standardized approaches in handling array platforms across laboratories. Variability introduced at each step is compounded, and successive sources of experimental errors are amplified, as the experiment proceeds (Figs 3 and 4).

New methodologies can minimize experimental variability at the time of performing microarray experiments. Variability can be dealt with at the time of normalization and analysis using statistical packages designed specifically to address such issues. To reduce disparities and to reproduce microarray data across laboratories, 'minimal information about a microarray

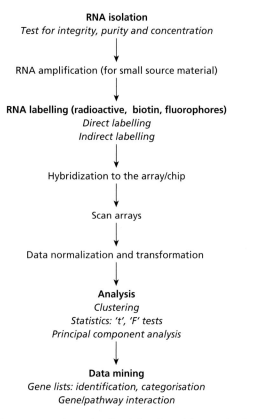

RNA isolation
Test for integrity, purity and concentration

↓

RNA amplification (for small source material)

↓

RNA labelling (radioactive, biotin, fluorophores)
Direct labelling
Indirect labelling

↓

Hybridization to the array/chip

↓

Scan arrays

↓

Data normalization and transformation

↓

Analysis
Clustering
Statistics: 't', 'F' tests
Principal component analysis

↓

Data mining
Gene lists: identification, categorisation
Gene/pathway interaction

Fig. 3 Microarray experimental outline. A flowchart of the steps involved in a microarray experiment. The importance of proper RNA isolation and ensuring good quality RNA is used is critical.

experiment' (MIAME) guidelines set standards to facilitate the publication of microarray data. Conforming to MIAME-compliant protocols (http://www.mged.org/Workgroups/MIAME/miame.html) should ensure the quality and reproducibility of the data. Recent articles [7,8] suggest that robust and reproducible microarray results can be obtained across platforms as well as laboratories, provided the experimental and analytical methods are standardized.

Experimental design

Experimental design is clearly an important step in microarray analysis (Fig. 5). Underlying every successful microarray experi-

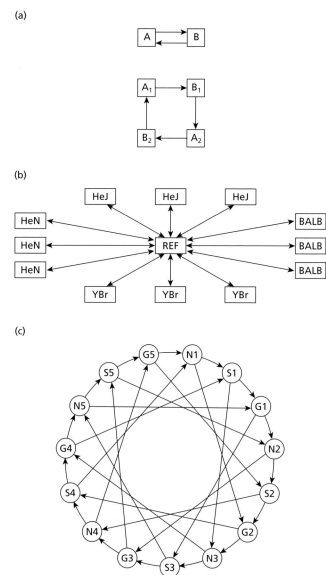

Fig. 5 Microarray experimental design. Experimental design in microarray experiments is a fundamental and often overlooked aspect. The experimental design can take many forms: (a) simple pairwise comparisons on two samples or sequential pairwise comparisons of multiple samples; (b) comparison of multiple samples to a common reference; or (c) cross comparison of all samples to each other in an experiment.

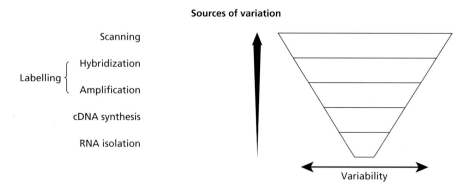

Fig. 4 Gene array experimental variation. A graphical depiction of the increasing variation in gene array experiments. Variability can be biological or technical. Importantly, technical error can be amplified at each step leading to uninterpretable or widely varying results. Minimizing methodological variation is a principal goal of gene array analysis to enable discrimination between individual and disease phenotype differences.

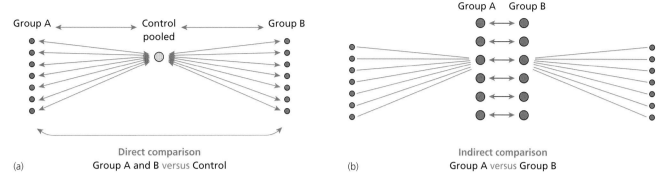

Fig. 6 Replicates in microarray experiments. The use of replicates is a critical aspect of microarray experiments. Replicates can be of two forms including (a) biological replicates in which multiple different individual samples are compared to a common control (direct comparison) or (b) technical replicates in which multiple replicates of the same samples are compared (indirect comparison). The preferred method is now the use of multiple biological replicates as this often overcomes many of the problems addressed by technical replicates when a large number of samples are analysed.

ment, the first and foremost task is to ensure that the design of the experiment is chosen to answer the specific biological question being asked. The experimental design is particularly important if the researcher chooses to use comparative two-fluorophore cohybridization. In this case, one is limited to comparing only those two samples that have been cohybridized. Choice of experimental design can vary from a simple experiment with only a simple two-group comparison to extremely complex experiments in which several groups/individual samples are compared with each other within and between groups [9] (Fig. 5).

Currently, microarray data have a resolution limit. Actual real small-fold differences in gene expression can be impossible to resolve from background variability or 'noise'. Gene array experimental 'noise' can be defined in multiple ways, including biological noise (individual phenotype variation, sex, age, diurnal changes, etc.) and technical noise (sample preparation, labelling, hybridisation efficiency, etc.). There are typically two complementary approaches used to address the problem of 'noise' in microarray experiments, downstream validation and the use of replicates. Validation of microarray results commonly uses more sensitive, independent and quantitative analysis tools such as quantitative polymerase chain reaction (qPCR) and downstream protein studies [10]. The frequent use of a small number of samples in microarray experiments has meant that statistical analysis is often unable to provide meaningful results. Therefore, the use of replicates is an important consideration in experimental design (Fig. 6). There are two kinds of replicates.

Biological replicates

Hybridizations of multiple independent samples belonging to one group are compared with samples from another group or with a reference, for example tissue from multiple test samples independently treated with drug 1 (group A) and drug 2 (group B) hybridized individually to a common reference pool and analysed statistically for direct and indirect comparisons.

Technical replicates

Repeat hybridization of the same two samples to multiple slides, for example samples from groups A and B treated with drugs 1 and 2, respectively, pooled (or individual) within the respective treatments and hybridized with each other on multiple arrays. To be able to compare samples and identify differential expression with confidence, it is necessary to include as many replicates as possible in the study. Replication facilitates estimation of experimental variability such that appropriate statistical measures (ANOVA, t-statistics, B-statistics) provide increased precision in the identification of differential expression.

Pooling of samples

Pooling samples before hybridization has been a subject of considerable debate in gene array experiments [11,12]. It is generally accepted that pooling affects the data quality and inference of results, but the exact nature of the effects is unknown. Therefore, the loss of specific information about individual samples on pooling means that this approach is generally discouraged. However, in a situation in which individual biological variability is to be reduced (e.g. for finding biomarkers or expression patterns of a group), there is an advantage in pooling together samples of a certain type. Pooling minimizes the individual differences within a group while highlighting the differences between groups. The high cost of performing microarrays is also a major factor encouraging researchers to pool samples. To overcome the shortcomings of pooling vs. non-pooling, samples with enough RNA should be hybridized individually during experimentation and, if required, data can be pooled at the time of analysis. If the amount of RNA is limited, samples can be pooled for microarrays and used singly for downstream qPCR to confirm gene array expression [10]. Conditions under which pooling is advisable and the number of arrays and samples needed for pooling have been defined [11,12].

Source of RNA

Isolation of RNA from samples is the initial and one of the most important aspects of a gene array experiment. RNA can be obtained from whole organisms, different organs or specific cell types within an organ. Techniques for isolating RNA from archival preserved tissues, either frozen or in formalin, are now available. Cell lines and primary cell cultures are yet another source of RNA. Laser capture microdissection and flow cytometry enable the isolation of specific cell populations from tissues (tumours, epithelial, stellate and inflammatory cells). Reagents and commercial kits are also available for isolating RNA from as few as 10 cells.

Commercially available standardized kits are readily available from various sources (Ambion, Invitrogen, Clontech and Qiagen). These kits help the researcher to isolate RNA with their specific requirements from a diverse range of biomaterials including prokaryotic cells and all types of animal tissues. Regardless of the source of RNA, integrity (purity and quality) is the single most important factor for successful microarray hybridization. Contaminating genomic DNA and organic solvents and salts from the RNA extraction process can severely interfere with the downstream processing of microarray experiments and produce undesirable results. There are several ways of assessing the quality and integrity of RNA. A visual analysis of total RNA is performed using electrophoresis with sharp bands for 28S and 18S rRNA and a > 1.7:1 ratio for 28S:18S rRNA being considered the benchmark for intact RNA (Fig. 7). For determining quantity and integrity, spectrophotometric measurement of absorbance at A230 nm, A260 nm and A280 nm wavelengths is recommended. A ratio of 1.7–2.0 for A260:A280 and ≥ 1.5 for A260:A230 is generally considered to be a measure of quality RNA, but impurities such as phenol, surfactants and DNA that absorb strongly in the 220- to 280-nm region can lead to misleading spectrophotometer readings. RNA can be purified by repeat extractions or using column-based methods to remove contaminating phenol. The RNA isolation method is a major consideration in experimental design, especially as some methods are incompatible with downstream labelling or hybridization. Further, the use of two different RNA isolation methods in the same microarray experiment is often not valid, given the variability and unique characteristics of the many available methods.

A comprehensive standardized system that has become a popular method of choice and is included as a standard protocol in MIAME is the use of the Agilent bioanalyser (Palo Alto, CA, USA) (Fig. 7) [13]. The bioanalyser can assess RNA degradation, DNA contamination and estimate amounts of RNA from picogram amounts of starting material. Importantly, the RNA quality within and across laboratories can be standardized using Agilent's software to calculate the RNA integrity number (RIN). The RIN ranges from 1 (totally degraded RNA) to 10 (completely intact RNA), and this is useful in comparing array data from various sources and across laboratories.

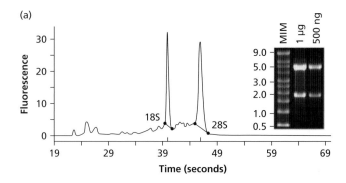

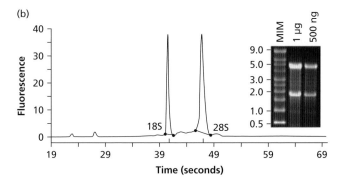

Fig. 7 Agilent Bioanalyzer assessment of RNA quality. RNA quality is one of the most important aspects of gene array analysis. RNA quality can be assessed in a number of ways including the use of an Agilent Bioanaylzer as shown here. Good-quality RNA does not have genomic DNA contamination and has a 28S to 18S ratio of intensity of > 1.7:1. (a) Human heart total RNA; (b) HeLa S3 total RNA. Reproduced with kind permission of Agilent Technologies.

RNA amplification

Microarray experiments require RNA in microgram quantities (5–100 μg) for hybridization. It becomes necessary to use amplification of RNA in cases in which obtaining the starting material is a limitation, for example microdissected biopsies, fine-needle aspirates, sorted cells and embryonic tissue. In the process of generating amplified RNA, the sensitivity of detection for low-abundance transcripts improves. However, amplification is generally avoided if possible because of uncertainty regarding the relative representation of genes within the gene pool following amplification. This is because the amplification efficiency between transcripts and batches of enzymes may not be equal. With optimized protocols, routine RNA amplification actually improves the quality of microarray results by providing more array-to-array consistency [14]. There are two major methods of RNA amplification: linear and exponential.

• Linear amplification was first described by Eberwine [15] and uses a T7 promoter and T7 RNA polymerase-dependent system that amplifies transcripts in proportion to their original abundance relative to each other. Using this method, mRNA amplifications of > 1000-fold can be achieved while still retaining the original relative transcript profile. Many of the commercially available amplification systems use this principle. Over the last decade, the T7 polymerase-based system has been refined to the extent that RNA can be amplified from as little as 1 ng of starting material and purified and labelled with fluorophores using a single kit.

- Exponential amplification utilizes PCR-based techniques with a mix of DNA polymerases and patented technology for modified oligonucleotides that amplify full-length transcripts with fidelity. The PCR is terminated in the exponential phase to avoid saturation during the reaction plateau, therefore maintaining the original relative transcript representation profile. SMART kits from Clontech Laboratories, Palo Alto, CA, USA, have been used to amplify cDNAs from RNA and used for microarrays [16–18].

Sample labelling

Radioactive, fluorescent and biotin labels are incorporated into the sample material used to interrogate the DNA targets on the arrays. Radioactive labels (^{32}P and ^{33}P) were commonly used before fluorophores were made available. Biotin is a popular label for single-colour assays, such as the Affymetrix system. Fluorophores [generally cyanine (Cy) dyes] are available to detect more than a single colour simultaneously and assist in the screening of more than one sample on the same array. Multiplexing two (or more) colour fluorophores saves samples, time and costs and, as a result, is widely used in a research-based setting. The principal advantage of using more than one fluorophore is the incorporation of a common standard across all experiments. Statistical methods for the analysis of two-colour arrays are well defined but, as yet, there is no consensus for a single probe method. However, there are other issues, such as the unequal efficiencies of incorporation of fluorophores during transcription, that confound interpretation of multiplexed experiments.

Array platforms

There are three types of platforms on which DNA is immobilized using combinatorial chemistries:

- filter or membrane arrays: nylon and plastic;
- glass slides;
- glass beads with microfibres.

The source of gene probes fixed on the above platforms can consist of genome-wide or specific information using:

- cDNA libraries;
- short oligonucleotide clone sets and expressed sequence tags (ESTs);
- long oligonucleotide clone sets and ESTs;
- focused DNA sets for specialized research/diagnostic areas.

Since the inception of DNA microarrays almost a decade ago, a number of array designs and platforms have been developed. The initial design used hundreds to thousands of cDNA or oligonucleotide probes immobilized in a grid format on nylon or plastic platforms. The next generation of array platforms were on glass slides with combinatorial chemistries to covalently bind DNA to the treated slide surface. cDNAs and oligonucleotides are printed on these slides using robotic arrayers. With recent advances in this technology, more than 30 000 DNA spots can be accommodated on a single glass array. The extent of coverage of the genome depends on the source of cDNA and oligonucleotide libraries. Affymetrix uses a different technology to synthesize the DNA target on the surface of the array. The feature density of this approach is now 5 μm and falling, enabling millions of DNA targets to be arrayed on a single GeneChip™. This enables each gene to be represented by multiple probes along the length of the transcript, and each sequence is also arrayed as a single base mismatch control of specificity. An alternative approach uses sequentially arranged glass beads in a capillary fibre, which can be rapidly probed in minutes while being highly sensitive [19–21]. In addition to complete transcriptome expression profiling, custom-made specialized arrays can also be manufactured. Such specialized arrays are generally low-density arrays and consist of specific sets of genes, for example cytokines, cancer genes and toxicology-related genes, for specialized research and/or diagnostic purposes.

Proteomics

Introduction

An organism's proteome is the complex effector of gene expression and the ultimate molecular mediator of biology and disease. However, the relationship between protein and mRNA transcript expression is not always obvious, and many proteins are regulated by posttranslational modifications (PTM) such as phosphorylation [22]. Therefore, while proteomic methods are complementary to transcriptome studies, they offer unique insights into normal physiology and pathobiology [23–25]. In contrast to transcriptome analysis, in which the expression of tens of thousands of mRNAs can be examined in a single experiment, the high-throughput analysis of the proteome is limited to hundreds or a few thousand proteins at best [24,26]. Further, the complexity of the proteome, relative abundance, sample preparation and methods of analysis all greatly influence the protein expression data obtained in these experiments. Current proteomic methods are limited by sample preparation, with prefractionation being the norm to obtain meaningful protein expression data.

Proteomic methodologies: general

Proteomic methods can be divided into those in which known peptides are assayed (closed systems) and those in which novel peptides can be analysed and/or identified (open systems). Antibody and peptide arrays are examples of closed systems, whereas MS analysis can identify potentially novel peptides [27,28]. MS methods can be further divided into those techniques that can identify proteins (based on sequence data or weight-matching protein digests) or methods that identify unique MS profiles without identifying individual proteins [for example surface-enhanced laser desorption/ionization (SELDI) profiling] [26,29,30]. Most proteomic methods involve the same basic sequential sample processing: (i) sample preparation;

(ii) sample prefractionation; (iii) sample separation; and (iv) protein identification [26,29–33]. The array variation in this approach differs by attaching protein or antibody to a substrate instead of sample separation.

An alternative classification of proteomic methods is 'top-down' or 'bottom-up' [34]. 'Top-down' proteomics studies whole proteins using methods such as two-dimensional gel electrophoresis. In contrast, 'bottom-up' proteomics uses an approach in which complex protein solutions are subject to proteolysis prior to separation (typically by chromatographic methods).

Sample preparation

Proteins, in contrast to nucleic acids, have a highly variable chemistry that frequently impedes the analysis of complete proteomes [25,35,36]. Protein interactions with lipids and nucleotides as well as other proteins need to be disrupted. Typically, a combination of detergents, reducing agents and chaotropic denaturing salts are used. To avoid non-experimental protein modification, protease, kinase and phosphatase inhibitors are included in sample buffers. Sample preparation is often biased towards the downstream methods of analysis and frequently represents the first stage in fractionating a sample for efficient analysis [37,38]. The complexity of a protein sample and the charge are primary determinants of the efficiency of MS ionization, a critical determinant of MS analysis accuracy [25,35,36]. Therefore, sample preparation and prefractionation are frequently combined before sample separation.

Sample prefractionation

Proteome complexity in virtually all organs or cells is so great that no current separation method is capable of resolving even a significant minor fraction of the proteins contained in a sample. Therefore, most biological samples are pre/subfractionated before protein separation [31,39]. Sample prefractionation can take many forms, including charge separation, affinity capture and chemical modification. Alternatively, prefractionation can be combined with cellular subfractionation to obtain membrane, nuclei and other intracellular organelles [40–42]. Laser capture microdissection can be used selectively to isolate cell subpopulations for analysis, although this approach is at the limit of sensitivity in current proteomic research [43,44]. One of the major limitations of current proteomics techniques is the inability to resolve low-abundance proteins from the few highly expressed proteins such as intracellular actin and serum albumin that account for more than 90% of the protein mass [25,35] (haemoglobin, transferrin, immunoglobulin, haptoglobin, complement and antitrypsin are other highly abundant serum proteins). This is critically important, as many proteins mediating signalling or useful as biomarkers are expressed in nanomolar or lower concentrations [25,45–47]. Therefore, an additional aim of prefractionation is to concentrate the samples following removal of these interfering high-abundance proteins. However, these approaches are not without flaws as more than 97% of the low-molecular-weight proteins are bound to larger carrier proteins [48]. Therefore, prefractionation may remove proteins of interest from the subsequent analysis. Most investigators now use panels of prefractionation methods prior to protein separation. One of the most intriguing and promising prefractionation methods uses chemical modification, such as the use of enzyme suicide substrates followed by biotin avidin affinity [49,50]. This approach has the advantage of selectively targeting a known protein subfraction. An alternative approach to selectively identifying protein subfractions uses activity-based protein profiling (ABPP), a strategy in which fluorophore-labelled (typically rhodamine), active site-directed probes are used to tag a protein [51].

Sample separation

The ability to separate and resolve individual proteins within a sample has typically been performed by two-dimensional gel electrophoresis [35,36] (Fig. 8). The first dimension, referred to as isoelectric focusing, resolves proteins based on charge using immobilized pH gradients. The second dimension resolves

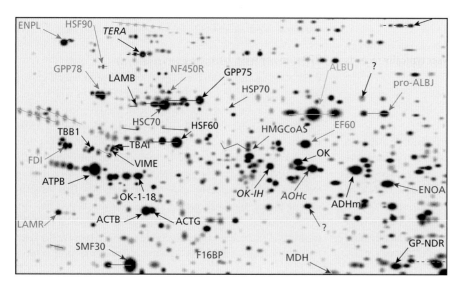

Fig. 8 Two-dimensional gel electrophoresis of F344 rat liver. Protein map of F344 rat liver analysed using 2-D gel electrophoresis. Comparison of such protein maps from two different conditions reveals differentially expressed proteins as a result of the treatment. Courtesy of Large Scale Biology Corp.

proteins based on size using sodium dodecyl sulphate-polyacrylamide gel electrophoresis (SDS-PAGE) gels. Individual proteins are visualized by Coomassie, silver or fluorophore staining (such as SYPRO ruby) [35,36,52]. A typical two-dimensional gel will resolve 1500–3000 protein spots. If the pH gradient is spread across several gels (zoom gels), 5000–10 000 proteins can be resolved. An interesting variation of the classical two-dimensional gel is DiGE (differential gel electrophoresis), in which protein samples to be compared are labelled with fluorescent dyes, mixed and then resolved on a two-dimensional gel [52,53]. In a manner similar to microarray analysis, the relative abundance is determined by resultant fluorescence. This approach has the advantage of avoiding ambiguities in spot match across gels and uses multiple common internal standards.

There are multiple limitations to two-dimensional gels including under-representation of basic and hydrophobic membrane proteins and the propensity of certain proteins to precipitate at their isoelectric point in the first dimension [54]. Additionally, two-dimensional gels are difficult to automate as well as being labour and time intensive [54]. Therefore, chromatographic techniques are now being widely adopted and frequently preferred to two-dimensional gel analysis in proteomic research [54]. There are a number of chromatographic techniques including affinity, ion-exchange, size-exclusion and reverse-phase liquid chromatography [54]. Additionally, chromatographic methods can be used to perform isoelectric focusing, chromatofocusing, free flow electrophoresis and capillary electrophoresis [54]. Combining a chromatographic first dimension followed by a second dimension separation by capillary electrophoresis or reverse-phase liquid chromatography can achieve greater resolution and sensitivity than a classical two-dimensional gel approach [54]. Over 12 000 unique proteins can be identified in a single sample using a two-dimensional chromatography approach [54]. Further, chromatography methods are readily automated, can be multiplexed and allow online MS characterization as well as protein recovery.

Protein identification

Protein identification relies on a number of MS techniques with two basic components: an ionization module and a mass analyser. The ionization module adds charge to the protein (typically by addition of a proton), and the mass analyser typically records time of flight (TOF) of a protein across an electric field (proportional to the mass) [36,54,55]. The most common proteomics technique to date is MALDI-TOF, in which an isolated sample is applied to a surface with an analyte (i.e. 2,5-dihydroxybenzoic acid), ionized and subjected to TOF. Although MS is capable of extremely accurate mass determination, the accuracy rapidly declines with proteins greater than 5 kDa [36,54,55]. Therefore, protein fragments, typically following trypsin digest, are best analysed by MS. This method is known as peptide mass fingerprinting (PMF). However, as the ionization efficiency of protein fragments is variable, MS analysis is not quantitative. Sequence information can be deduced by controlled fragmentation of peptides with MS to give peptide fragments that differ by the mass of a particular amino acid. This method is known as 'MS/MS' or 'tandem MS analysis'. Correct identification of a protein is dependent on the MS accuracy in determining molecular weight. Therefore, as many forms of posttranslational modification (PTM) change the mass of the protein, MS analysis is an ideal method of determining whether a protein has been modified in this manner [36,54,55]. However, many PTMs may be missed as MS sequence coverage of a protein is rarely complete.

The above discussion of MS analysis shows how proteins can be identified. However, MS analysis can be used to give characteristic MS profiles without identifying constituent proteins. This is done with SELDI using a ProteinChip Array (Cipehergen Biosystems) [56,57]. In this approach, prefractionation is performed using chemical (i.e. anion exchange) or biochemical (i.e. antibody) techniques. The immobilized protein subfraction on the chip is then treated with laser desorption/ionization (LDI) and subject to TOF (SELDI-TOF). This is essentially a modification of the MALDI technique in which all proteins are captured. MALDI-TOF requires sample separation before MS as each spot on the MALDI plate corresponds to a single protein; in contrast, SELDI-TOF relies on subfractionation of the chip and identification of individual proteins based on mass (not a protein fragment). However, although MALDI-TOF and SELDI-TOF can predict peptide mass up to ~ 300 kDa, the accuracy for large peptides (> 30 kDa) is poor [35,36,56,57]. Therefore, SELDI-TOF does not always accurately identify proteins, but is capable of generating MS profiles that may or may not be unique in a comparative analysis of closely related samples.

Proteomic array platforms

Array platforms in proteomic research fall into two groups. First, individual antibodies are arrayed on a surface and probed with protein samples [55,58]. Detection relies on prior protein sample labelling with a fluorophore or using a fluorescent second antibody. This is also known as forward-phase arrays (FPA). The second method arrays a protein sample, which is then probed with labelled antibody. This second technique is known as reverse-phase arrays (RPA). FPAs are plagued by low sensitivity and high variability. Current FPA platforms of many hundreds of antibodies are being used with limited success. RPAs, in contrast, have the necessary reproducibility and sensitivity for the analysis of clinical specimens. However, RPAs have to be custom made for each sample and are expensive.

Conclusions: proteomic methods

It is clear that proteomic analysis has the potential to offer unique and critically important insights into normal human biology and disease. In contrast to transcriptome analysis, proteomics is hampered by multiple technical difficulties that make it more demanding than gene array analysis. Presently, proteomic methods sample rather than profile the proteome. Additionally, sample preparation and prefractionation are critical aspects of successful proteome analysis. However, the promise of proteomic techniques in biodiscovery, biomarker

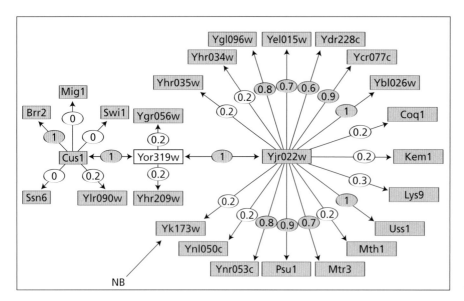

Fig. 9 Protein interaction map. Protein interaction map of *Saccharomyces cerevisiae*, including predicted biological scores. Courtesy of Hybrigenics SA.

identification and prediction of toxic responses will ensure that this is an area of functional genomics research that will continue to attract intense attention.

Bioinformatics

The explosion of high-throughput techniques since the advent of the genome sequencing projects has led to the need for innovative statistical analysis of data. Although strong quantitative traditions exist in other domains of biology and biomedical research, the adoption of quantitative approaches (as opposed to semi-quantitative or qualitative approaches) is relatively new in cell and molecular biology. There is now an established and fruitful interface between the disciplines of biology, statistics and computer science to aid these problems. In this section, we will discuss a selection of issues relevant to the interpretation of data from high-throughput experimental platforms. While the emphasis is on expression microarrays, much of the discussion is, or will be, relevant to other postgenomic measurement systems.

It is now well understood that microarray data are subject to a bewildering variety of systematic biases related to experimental and data acquisition processes [59,60]. The data processing and statistical procedures required to correct these effects collectively fall under the term 'normalization'. These include intensity-dependent biases [61–63], spatial-dependent biases and, in the case of printed glass arrays, biases related to the printing order of spotted clones or oligonucleotides [59,60].

The requirements of data analysis following these basic preprocessing and normalization steps are dependent on the overall aim of the investigation. For laboratory-scale studies, where the aim of the experiment is typically to obtain new information regarding the action of genes and pathways in the biological system under study, the emphasis should be placed on exploratory analysis. The notion of 'exploratory analysis' should not be confused with lack of statistical rigour. Methods developed in multivariate statistics over the last century may also be applied in the exploratory analysis of microarray data, for example unsupervised learning methods ('clustering' or 'pattern discovery') such as hierarchical clustering or the self-organizing map (SOM) can be used to identify groups of genes (Fig. 9) whose expression levels are related across a set of experimental conditions [4,64].

For larger scale studies, the same techniques can of course be applied but, if the aim of the study relates to the identification of genes that are predictive for a given disease or condition, then the well-established methodology of supervised learning is required [65]. Supervised learning techniques are readily available in many microarray data analysis packages and in all the generic statistical computing packages (SPSS, SAS, R/S-Plus).

The identification of differentially expressed genes is the first step, albeit a challenging one, in the overall data interpretation process. Taking a set of dozens or hundreds of genes and constructing a biologically plausible hypothesis remains an immensely difficult and time-consuming task. A vast conglomeration of data relating to gene product function exist in a variety of forms, including as free text in abstracts and papers, in 'comments fields' of biological databases (such as NCBI or Ensemble) and in more specialized, curated databases (e.g. Mouse Genome Informatics). While much of this information is readily available via web servers, such devices are optimal when used for obtaining information about a single transcript or gene product. The integration of this information from large sets of genes still results in a problem of manual data collation; thus, there is a great need for the development of methods for large-scale analysis of functional data.

Several recent developments have significant implications in relation to this goal. First, the work of the Gene Ontology Consortium has a standardized format that has largely become a default for the presentation of information about the function of gene products covering the entire spectrum of cell and molecular biology. Gene Ontology is not a database *per se* but a controlled vocabulary of terms (an 'ontology'). It should not be confused with metabolic or signalling pathway databases, such as KEGG or Reactome [66]. Several interesting analyses have been made using comparative functional genomics by analysing microarray data across many distantly related species to identify conserved 'modules' of genes whose gene products have consistent functions [67]. Such modules could be used as a basis for comparing cellular function across different conditions. In terms of annotation *per se*, there is an increasing amount of work being undertaken on literature extraction and analysis techniques, based on natural language processing, to automatically define annotational data of interest (for example to extract protein–protein interactions from publications). Although most of this work is currently in the area of methodological development, several interesting applications of text mining concepts have been published that point to the potential that these techniques might have in the future for the interpretation of high-throughput experiments [68].

Gene array data in liver disease

The liver transcriptome

As noted above, there are estimated to be in excess of 32 000 protein-encoding genes in the human genome. Furthermore, there are an unknown number of functionally significant alternatively spliced transcripts arising from these genes that may exceed 100 000. How many of these transcripts are expressed in the liver is unknown. Resources for identifying and comparing organ transcriptomes are rare. One method of inferring complexity is to examine GenBank human UniGene clusters of non-redundant gene sets [69]. These UniGene clusters are compiled from mRNA and ESTs and, as a group, represent a species' transcriptome [69]. Currently, the human UniGene assembly of clusters (Build 180) has over 5 million sequences representing 52 888 non-redundant transcripts. Parsing keyword searches [parsing string used ('liver' or 'hepatic') and 'human' for UniGene Build 180] identified approximately 26% of transcripts (representing 13 627 clusters) in liver tissue; this compares with brain (46%), lung (40%), kidney (35%), colon (32%) and heart (23%). Coulouarn *et al.* [70] used a similar approach and identified 12 638 non-redundant clusters from liver tissue (UniGene Build 129). Further, serial analysis of gene expression (SAGE) libraries can also provide some insight into the complexity of the liver transcriptome [71,72]. Two SAGE libraries from normal human liver identified 15 496 and 18 081 unique transcripts from a total number of 66 308 and 125 700 tags respectively [71,72]. In a SAGE comparison of multiple organs,

32 131 unique tags were identified (from a total of 455 325 tags); of these, 56% were expressed in the liver compared with brain (75%), breast (81%) and colon (91%) [73]. Therefore, it is clear that the normal liver has a complex transcriptome expressing many thousands of transcripts. Interestingly, the SAGE comparison of gene transcripts from various tissues has identified organ-related chromosomal domains such as 6p12.1 associated with hepatic xenobiotic metabolism [73].

Microarray analysis of normal human liver by Yano *et al.* [4] highlights many of the problems in examining the non-diseased liver transcriptome. A total of 2418 genes were examined in five normal patients with only 50% of these transcripts being detected in four out of five patients. Furthermore, only 27% of genes had coordinate expression in these normal patients. Therefore, in addition to the liver having a complex transcriptome, there appears to be significant individual variability in transcript expression. This is further highlighted by the observation of Enard *et al.* [74], who found that duplicate liver samples from the same individual differed by 12% (technical variation) but that intraspecies variation was as pronounced as interspecies variation in hepatic mRNA transcript expression comparing chimpanzees and humans. Focused specialized arrays such as the Liverpool nylon array targeting the liver transcriptome have now been synthesized and include in excess of 10 000 target genes [70]. However, such approaches fail to detect differential gene expression for transcripts not expressed in normal liver that are expressed in disease.

Gene arrays in human liver disease

Presently there are in excess of 200 published gene array studies of human liver disease or studies that utilize human liver tissue (Table 1). This represents roughly 40% of the greater than 500 published papers utilizing gene arrays to study human pathobiology. Most of these studies attempt to understand pathobiology by examining mRNA transcript expression. There are few publications in human liver disease where gene expression is correlated with clinical outcome.

Hepatitis C virus (HCV) infection (see also Section 9)
Acute HCV infection has been examined in experimental infection in the chimpanzee. Bigger *et al.* [75] used DNA array technology to study acute HCV infection in a single animal that cleared the virus. They described the strong early induction of interferon (IFN)γ-induced genes such as *ISG15* and *ISG16* with the later induction of Th1-associated transcripts such as *MIG* (CXCL9) and *IP10* (CXCL10). These genes were upregulated > 40-fold at the time of viral clearance. Also, induction of apoptosis genes (*FAS* and *TNFR*), cellular proliferation genes (*PCNA* and cyclin) and transcripts related to lipid metabolism (apidophilin) were detected.

Su *et al.* [76] used similar methods to compare chimpanzees that cleared acute HCV infection with an animal that had virus persistence. They observed upregulation of many transcripts.

Table 1 Summary of processes observed in genomics and proteomics studies of human liver disease.

Pathology	Processes observed	Reference
Normal liver	Variability of non-diseased liver transcript expression	[4,70,71]
	Acute phase response transcript expression	[70]
Hepatitis C (HCV)	Chronic infection induction of Th1 immune response, fibrosis, apoptosis and proliferation-associated genes	[75,76, 79,88,192,193]
	Acute infection induction of IFN and T cell-associated genes with viral clearance	[75,76]
	In vitro hepatocyte disruption of RIG-1 signalling in response to NS3/4A	[77]
	In vitro hepatocyte induction of NFκB response to NS5A	[194]
	IFN-associated gene induction in response to IFN and ribavirin treatment in chronic infection	[78]
	Tumour-associated gene expression including biomarker identification in HCV-associated HCC	[83,158,159[a],195–197]
	IFN- and TRAIL-associated gene expression in HCV recurrence post liver transplantation	[84,85]
Hepatitis B (HBV)	Chronic HBV infection induction of IFN, fibrosis and proliferation-associated genes	[79,88]
	HBV fibrosis (marker study)	[154[a]]
	HBV inflammation (marker study)	[161[a]]
Autoimmune hepatitis (AIH)	Chronic AIH cirrhosis induction of apoptosis inhibitors and Th1/Th2 gene expression	[80,82]
Alcohol-associated liver disease (ALD)	Annexin- and stellate cell-associated gene induction in chronic alcoholic liver disease	[89,163[a]]
Non-alcoholic fatty liver disease (NAFLD)	Steatotic liver disease	[92,93[b],94]
	Decreased expression of mitochondrial-associated gene expression in non-alcoholic steatohepatitis (NASH)	[92]
Biliary liver disease	Chronic primary biliary cirrhosis (PBC)s, Wnt pathway gene expression	[82,91]
	Chronic primary sclerosing cholangitis (PSC) cirrhosis, epithelial- and endothelial-associated gene expression	[91]
	Mac-2Bp expression in PSC-associated cholangiocarcinoma (marker study)	[162[a]]
	Imprinting gene expression in embryonic compared with perinatal biliary atresia	[95]
Hepatocellular carcinoma (HCC)	HCC differentiation- and progression-associated gene expression (marker studies)	[81,99,154[a],165,166,197[a]]
	Molecular signature in viral hepatitis-associated HCC	[100,102,103, 154[a],199]
	Metastatic HCC development-associated gene expression including osteopontin expression	[106,200]
	Prognosis/recurrence of HCC including association with RhoC expression	[107,108]
Cholangiocarcinoma	PSF2 upregulation in intrahepatic cholangiocarcinoma	[109,201]
	Mac-2Bp expression in cholangiocarcinoma (marker study)	[162[a]]

[a]Proteomic analysis.
[b]Combination of transcriptome and proteome analysis.

Those genes associated with the early response (which correlated with viral load) included many IFNα-induced genes including *STAT1*, 2′-5′ oligoadenylate synthetase, *Mx1*, *ISP15* and *p27*. Furthermore, there was induction of lipid pathway genes such as fatty acid synthetase and sterol response element binding protein (SREBP). These lipid pathway genes were associated with viral replication, and blockade of these two pathways using *in vitro* replicon experiments led to a decrease in viral replication. Additionally, there was downregulation of peroxisome proliferator-activated receptor (PPAR)α as well as hepatic lipase C and flotillin 2. The reduction in PPARα would be expected to be associated with insulin resistance, a feature of chronic HCV but, prior to this, it was not an expected aspect of acute HCV infection. Whether HCV replication *per se* results in insulin resistance clearly warrants further study. Clearance of HCV was associated with the late induction of T helper 1 (Th1) transcripts such as *CXCL9* and *CXCL10*, MHC expression and T-cell molecules such as CD8 and granzyme A. Of interest was the induction of IFNα-induced genes early in infection, as observed by Bigger *et al.* [75], but the timing did not correlate with clearance as high levels of these transcripts continued in the animal with viral persistence. This has also been seen in human studies.

Functional studies in HCV replicon systems has shown that NS3/4A was able to inhibit IFNα antiviral effector function by blocking the phosphorylation of IRF-3, a key protein in the antiviral response [77]. Thus, chronic HCV infection induces a persistent intrahepatic IFNα antiviral response, but the virus itself escapes the response via an inhibition of the effector arm. However, the intrahepatic IFNα-induced gene response is variable among individual patients. This response has been identified, by microarrays, to be higher in patients not responding to pegylated IFN and ribavirin therapy, suggesting an increased resistance to the effector arm that cannot be amplified by exogenous therapy [78]. In contrast, patients who had a sustained viral response (SVR) to pegylated IFN therapy had a lower expression of IFN genes that, by inference, can be amplified by exogenous therapy resulting in viral clearance.

Chronic HCV infection has been studied in a number of ways using array analysis. The study by Honda et al. [79] profiled gene expression using microarrays in individuals with chronic hepatitis B (HBV) and chronic HCV, comparing them with a single non-diseased control subject. The study examined liver biopsy material. Honda et al. [79] concluded that chronic HCV infection was associated with a predominant anti-inflammatory, proproliferative, antiapoptotic intrahepatic gene profile. However, an analysis of the data in these experiments indicated widespread upregulation of proinflammatory genes such as interleukin (IL)-2 receptor, CD69, CD44, IFNγ-inducible protein, major histocompatibility complex (MHC) class 1 genes and monokine induced by IFNγ. Similar findings were made in HCV cirrhosis in which proinflammatory Th1-associated transcript expression predominated [80]. HCV-associated cirrhosis has also been shown to display upregulation of a wide variety of fibrotic genes such as platelet-derived growth factor (PDGF) and transforming growth factor (TGF)-β3. These studies have also identified potential novel mediators of HCV-associated injury such as frizzled-related proteins, discoidin domain-related protein 1 (DDR1), EMMPRIN and SARP-3 [80]. These results have been expanded and analysed more rigorously by a comparison of gene profiles in patients with HCV cirrhosis, HCV and hepatocellular carcinoma (HCC) and normal liver [81]. Importantly, this analysis aimed to exclude genes expressed in normal liver, other forms of cirrhosis or HCC. This study identified 87 upregulated and 45 downregulated genes that appear to be markers of HCV liver injury [81]. Genes such as ILxR (IL-13 receptor a2), CCR4 and cartilage glycoprotein 39 (GP-39) were identified [81]. The last transcript was also identified in chronic HCV infection by a totally different genomics approach, namely suppressive subtractive hybridization [82].

The premalignant behaviour of intrahepatic HCV infection has been studied by our group by comparing HCV cirrhosis with and without HCC [83]. This approach identified upregulation of many oncogenes (i.e. TEL oncogene), immune genes (IFNγ associated) and fibrosis genes (integrins) as well as cell signalling (G-coupled receptor kinase) and proliferation-associated genes (cyclin K) in cirrhosis complicated by HCC. This indicates that there might be a premalignant cirrhotic response in HCV infection. The data suggest that there is more cellular proliferation, immune activation and fibrosis in the liver of patients with HCC than in those with cirrhosis alone. A key area of future research will be to ascertain whether such a profile can be recognized before HCC actually develops. If so, it may be used to identify and screen high-risk patients.

Gene array analysis of HCV recurrence in transplant allografts has shed new light on the molecular mechanisms of viral recurrence [84,85]. HCV recurrence in the graft is associated with expression of IFNγ-associated genes such as CXCL10 (IP-10), CXCL9 (HuMIG) and RANTES [85,86]. Further, antiviral IFNγ-associated gene expression is seen in chronic HCV recurrence and during acute rejection associated with HCV recurrence [85]. Additionally, upregulation of the NF-kappa beta (NFκB) pathway during acute rejection in association with HCV recurrence appears to alter cellular apoptosis via changes in the expression of TRIAL-associated genes [85]. Importantly, chronic HCV recurrence in grafts is associated with Th1-associated gene expression similar to that seen in chronically HCV-infected individuals who have not been transplanted [85]. In contrast, cholestatic HCV recurrence, which follows an aggressive course, is associated with a Th2 cytokine profile [85]. This suggests that the Th1 immune response suppresses viral replication while being profibrogenic [85,86]. In cholestatic HCV recurrence, the unchecked viral replication is directly fibrogenic [85,86].

HBV infection (see also Section 9)
Acute HBV infection has been analysed in the chimpanzee [87]. This study revealed several findings. First, that there was no differential gene expression during the initial phase of HBV infection and the first phase of HBV replication. This is in direct contrast to HCV infection and suggests that HBV infection acts in the initial phase as a 'stealth virus', failing to induce a significant innate immune response [87,88]. Intrahepatic gene induction is first seen during the phase of viral clearance. Gene expression during the early phase of infection was associated with T-cell receptor and antigen presentation. Following this, T-cell effector function (granzymes), T-cell recruitment (chemokines) and monocyte activation-associated gene expression was observed. A later phase of clearance was associated with the expression of B cell-related genes. At the time of writing, there are no published studies of acute or chronic HBV infection in the human. We have studied HBV cirrhotic explants and have found less differential gene expression compared with normal liver than in HCV-associated cirrhosis. This state of chronic HBV infection is characterized by upregulation of stress point, cell cycle and immune system genes. Similar findings have been reported by others (personal communications).

Alcoholic liver disease (ALD) (see also Chapter 12)
Intrahepatic gene profiling using microarrays in ethanol-fed baboons has identified increased expression of 14 different

annexin genes (including *A1* and *A2*) that were not previously implicated in the progression of fibrosis in ALD [89]. Furthermore, the intrahepatic transcriptome profile in alcoholism shares some similarity with lipopolysaccharide (LPS) administration but, in general, is significantly different from other forms of liver disease [89,90]. Cluster analysis has allowed differentiation of alcoholic hepatitis from alcoholic steatosis. Genes known to be involved in alcohol injury, such as alcohol dehydrogenases, acetaldehyde dehydrogenases, IL-8, *S*-adenosyl methionine synthetase, phosphatidylethanolamine N-transferase and several solute carriers, have been shown to be differentially expressed in alcoholic hepatitis vs. alcoholic steatosis. Many novel differentially expressed genes were identified, including claudins, osteopontin, *CD209*, selenoprotein and genes related to bile duct proliferation [89]. The most prominent categories of differentially expressed genes involved cell adhesion/extracellular matrix (ECM) proteins, oxidative stress and coagulation that were also common to endstage ALD. Overexpression of annexin A2 was also seen in alcoholic hepatitis. Genes associated with fibrosis/cell adhesion/ECM were the most prominent category in human advanced ALD, consistent with the fibrotic nature of ALD. However, these were not specific to alcohol and have been reported in primary biliary cirrhosis (PBC) and other forms of liver cirrhosis [80,91].

Non-alcoholic fatty liver disease (NAFLD)
(see also Section 13)

Non-alcoholic steatohepatitis (NASH) is the clinicopathological syndrome in NAFLD that has been most widely studied using gene array analysis of transcript expression. Studies have identified differentially expressed genes in endstage NASH cirrhosis compared with other disease states [92–94]. Decreased expression of genes associated with mitochondrial function and increased expression of genes associated with the acute-phase response were observed [92]. The latter increases were speculated as being associated with insulin resistance, a feature of NAFLD [92]. Further differential expression of genes involved in lipid metabolism, ECM remodelling, regeneration, apoptosis and detoxification have all been observed in NASH following microarray analysis [93].

Primary biliary cirrhosis (see also Chapter 11.1)

One of the major findings in an array examination of PBC endstage liver disease was the identification of a subset of genes associated with the Wnt pathway [91]. In particular, Wnt13, Wnt5A and Wnt12 were shown to be differentially expressed. Other genes particularly upregulated in PBC included transcription initiation factor 250 kDa subunit (TAFII 250), PAX3/forkhead transcription factor and patched homologue (PTC). A consistent feature of the gene array analysis of PBC was the repeated identification of *Drosophila* gene homologues that were differentially expressed (Wnt genes, hedgehog pathway, notch pathway) [91].

Autoimmune hepatitis (AIH) (see also Chapter 11.2)

The only available data on AIH is a comparison between HCV- and AIH-associated cirrhosis [80]. One of the key findings in this study was the observation that three inhibitors of apoptosis (IAP) genes were selectively differentially expressed in AIH. This is an intriguing finding. If this gene expression was identified as being in the intrahepatic lymphocyte population, then lack of apoptosis of such cells may be an important pathogenic pathway in the perpetuation of AIH. In this comparison with HCV, AIH was associated with an inflammatory gene pathway that consisted of a mix of Th1- and Th2-associated genes. Also, there was a marked upregulation of a large number of transcription factors in AIH vs. other forms of cirrhosis [80].

Primary sclerosing cholangitis (PSC) (see also Chapter 11.3)

The only available data on PSC comes in a comparison with PBC [91]. There were a far greater number of genes showing differential expression in PSC vs. non-diseased liver compared with PBC and non-diseased liver. These include genes associated with epithelial biology (amphiregulin, bullous pemphigoid antigen), inflammation (T-cell secreted protein P I-309, CTLA4), apoptosis (Bcl-2 interacting killer, Bcl-x, death-associated protein 3) and intracellular kinases such as CDK7 and JAK1.

Biliary atresia (BA) (see Chapter 22.1)

A study comparing gene expression in embryonic vs. perinatal BA has been published [95]. Gene profiling clearly separated these two conditions. The most remarkable difference was in the expression of so-called regulatory genes. In embryonic BA, 45% of differentially expressed genes were in this category vs. 15% in the perinatal form. Included in these genes were imprinting genes, and genes associated with RNA processing and cell cycle regulation that were not present in the perinatal form of BA.

Cystic fibrosis (CF) (see also Chapter 16.4)

Gene array analysis of CF-related liver injury is yet to be published. Extrahepatic sites affected by this disease (lung, pancreas and intestine) have been studied [96–98]. Importantly, gene arrays using tiling oligonucleotides with corresponding sequence mismatches offer the promise of accurate screening of over 1200 known cystic fibrosis transmembrane conductance regulator (CFTR) gene mutations in a single experiment. The promise of gene array analysis in CF-related organ disease (especially lung, liver and intestine) is immense given the inexorable nature of the disease. It is envisaged that specialized gene arrays will be used selectively in many aspects of CF research.

Hepatocellular carcinoma (see also Chapter 18.2.1)

Neoplastic proliferation in HCV-associated HCC has been studied by array analysis. A plethora of potential novel tumour markers have been identified. These include the serine/threonine kinase 15 (STK15) and phospholipase A2 (PLA2G13 and PLA2G7) that were increased in over half the tumours identified [81]. However, different studies identify different gene groups in HCV-associated HCC such as cytoplasmic dynein light chain, hepatoma-derived growth factor, ribosomal protein L6, TR3 orphan receptor and c-myc [99]. The clustering analysis in this study showed that the expression of 22 genes in HCC related to differentiation of the malignancy, with over half these genes being transcription factors or related to cell development or differentiation [99]. Although many of these genes can be implicated in HCC development, they are often identified in large gene sets in endstage disease. Therefore, whether these genes represent cause or effect is unknown. HBV-associated HCC has been studied by several groups [100–103]. Genes associated with cell proliferation, cell cycle, apoptosis and angiogenesis were deregulated in HCC tissues. Increased expression of cyclin-dependent kinases was seen, while several cell cycle negative regulators were decreased. Metastatic development has also been studied using gene arrays [104–107]. Genes identified with metastatic development included osteopontin [105]. The authors then demonstrated that neutralizing antibodies to osteopontin blocked tumour invasion *in vivo*. A study of unsupervised gene profiling of patients with HCC revealed a set of genes associated with decreased survival including RhoC [108]. These genes include a subset of proproliferative, antiapoptotic genes as well as genes involved in ubiquitination and histone modification. Gene profiles in HCC have also identified patterns of gene expression associated with tumour differentiation, vascular invasion as well as recurrence post surgery [107].

Cholangiocarcinoma (see also Chapter 19.9)

Obama *et al.* [109] used laser microdissection to compare gene expression in intrahepatic cholangiocarcinoma with noncancerous biliary epithelial cells. Over 50 upregulated genes were identified. These included forkhead and homeobox transcription factors, cadherin and survivin genes. Surprisingly, 421 genes were downregulated but not characterized in this study. Additionally, a group of 30 genes was identified as being associated with lymph node metastases. This study revealed some common findings with another studied aimed at identifying gene expression in a variety of biliary tract cancers [110].

Gene arrays in animal models

Animal models studied have included acute liver regeneration, drug toxicity, liver fibrosis, fatty liver, biliary obstruction, liver transplantation and carcinogenesis. Drug toxicity studies are numerous and include effects induced by clofibrate, PPARα agonists, carbon tetrachloride, amiodarone, arsenic and methotrexate [111–121]. In one study, a novel cDNA library highly enriched for genes expressed under a variety of hepatotoxic conditions was created and used to develop a custom oligonucleotide library [122].

An expression signature for rat liver fibrosis was identified using a cDNA 14 814 gene microarray [123]. The 'genetic fibrosis index' identified consisted of 95 genes (87 upregulated, 8 downregulated). These included genes associated with cytoskeletal proteins, cell proliferation and protein synthesis. Bile obstruction in the mouse identified three sequential main biological processes. At day 1, enzymes involved in steroid metabolism were overexpressed. This was followed by an increase in cell cycle/proliferation-associated genes at day 7, occurring at a time of maximum cholangiocyte proliferation. From days 14 to 21, genes associated with the inflammatory response and matrix remodelling were identified. Similar temporal gene expression was identified in the model of acute liver regeneration. Steroid and lipid metabolism genes were downregulated as early as 2 h post hepatectomy, whereas genes associated with cytoskeletal assembly and DNA synthesis became upregulated by 16 h and remained elevated at the 40-h time point at the peak of S phase.

Carcinogenic foci in experimental animals have been isolated and studied using gene array technology [124]. Approximately 8% of 2000 transcripts were differentially expressed in one study. These included genes with roles in signal transduction, detoxification and cytoskeletal assembly. Over 30 genes were identified as being dysregulated in these foci as well as in neonatal liver. Small-for-size liver allografts in rats showed upregulation of adhesion molecule, inflammatory mediators and apoptosis-associated genes together with downregulation of energy-metabolizing genes.

Alcoholic liver disease has been studied in the chronic enterogastric ethanol infusion model in a mouse; a total of 12 422 genes were analysed [90]. Several cytochrome P-450 genes were shown to be upregulated, while several genes involved in fatty acid metabolism (stearoyl CoA desaturase 3-hydroxyacetyl CoA dehydrogenase) and fatty acid synthetase were downregulated. In contrast, genes associated with glutathione *S*-transferase were markedly upregulated. Interestingly, a novel molecule intestinal factor was 50-fold downregulated. It was postulated that alcohol might be affecting the healthy intestinal epithelium, and downregulation of this gene might be associated with permeability changes in the intestine associated with chronic alcohol ingestion.

Proteomic data and liver disease

The liver proteome

The human proteome is complex and differs significantly depending on the organ or cell population being studied. Proteins can be subject to in excess of 100 different types of posttranslational modifications [22]. Therefore, the estimated 40 000 genes in the human genome may give rise to more than a million distinct proteins [33,54]. Utilizing an approach of parsing GenBank with keywords, we can gain insight into human organ proteome complexity. [In June 2005, the GenBank protein entries were parsed with the keyword 'human' and one of the following: 'brain', 'liver', 'lung', 'kidney', 'bowel or colon', 'heart', 'kidney' and 'serum'. A total of 91 261 protein entries were identified across all these organs. The percentage for each organ was then calculated to give an estimate of relative protein abundance. The number of individual GenBank protein entries in each organ was: brain (35 834), liver (13 195), lung (12 770), kidney (11 997), bowel/colon (6045), heart (6011) and serum (5409).] Proteomes from human brain, liver, lung, kidney, bowel/colon, heart, kidney and serum express 39%, 14%, 14%, 13%, 7%, 7% and 6%, respectively, of the proteins found in all these organs. This highlights the complexity of the brain proteome. Furthermore, the liver has a complex organ proteome. In contrast, a prototype human cell such as a lymphoblast, with a mass of 670 pg, contains 67 pg of protein from a total of 10^9 polypeptide molecules from ~ 4000 different proteins [125,126]. Within a cell, approximately 90% of the cellular protein mass results from the 100 most abundant proteins, and a further 1200 proteins account for another 7% of the protein mass that is detectable by typical proteomic analysis (from a lysate of 10^6 cells) [125,126]. However, the remaining 3% of the protein mass includes 2800 proteins (over 50% of the different protein species) and is frequently below the detection limit of most proteomic methods [125,126]. Therefore, it is important to consider the frequency of protein expression within a homogeneous cellular sample (i.e. cell lines) compared with a heterogeneous cellular sample (i.e. organs). This is an especially important consideration for hepatologists using biopsy specimens in which the non-parenchymal cell subpopulation abundance is low and subject to sampling error [127,128].

Frequently, the underlying assumption of transcriptome analysis is that changes in mRNA expression reflect changes in protein expression. There are many examples in which protein expression or function is not controlled by mRNA expression. In the intact non-diseased liver tissue, approximately 25% of the changes in mRNA transcript expression are not accompanied by changes in the expression of the corresponding protein [129]. Studies comparing mRNA and protein expression in liver are few. Anderson and Seilhamer [129] showed a poor correlation between the liver tissue abundance of 19 proteins and corresponding mRNA transcripts (correlation coefficient of only 0.48). Furthermore, they isolated 50 abundant mRNA transcripts, of which 29 encoded secreted proteins [129]. However, of the 50 most abundant proteins they isolated, none was secreted [129]. There is a bias in mRNA pools, when compared with protein expression, towards an over-representation of both secreted protein transcripts and high-abundance mRNA transcripts such as *G3PDH* [129–133]. Ultimately, the protein expression in every cell is controlled by the transcriptome, although the relationship between individual gene transcripts and the corresponding protein expression may not be clear at first.

Proteomic studies of liver disease – general comments

Proteomic studies of liver disease have fallen into the following four groups: (i) discovery of previously unrecognized proteins in a cell population or disease state [134–136]; (ii) biomarker discovery [56,137]; (iii) hepatic toxicological prediction/profiling [138–147]; and (iv) studies of known proteins or classes of proteins [49,50] (see Tables 1 and 2). Proteomics has been used successfully in biodiscovery of proteins in hepatocytes, hepatic stellate cells [134–136], hepatocellular carcinoma [137] and viral hepatitis [148–153]. In these studies, tens to hundreds of proteins were identified. However, they are limited as they sample, rather than profile, the proteome. Further observed changes in protein expression may reflect weak associations rather than a direct role in the development of pathobiology. The biodiscovery approach has been used successfully in toxicological models and used to develop characteristic profiles of protein expression that may predict intrahepatic toxicology responses [138–147]. This is an area of intense focus for pharmaceutical companies as they strive to reduce development costs and aim to predict drug toxicity earlier in the drug development cycle. Biomarker discovery is another area receiving intense focus using proteomic methods. However, for years, there has not been a new Food and Drugs Administration (FDA)-approved serum marker as this is an immense challenge. Biological sample protein concentrations vary by 12–15 orders of magnitude. Furthermore, specific serum markers are likely to be expressed at nanomolar or lower concentrations. One approach to overcome these limitations is to use a combination of potential markers that are easier to detect but with each protein marker alone having a lower specificity but high sensitivity. This is an approach currently used in serum tests of hepatic fibrosis, and proteomic methods are being used to try and identify new serum markers of hepatic fibrogenesis [53,154,155]. One of the most promising approaches is the use of accurate mass tags (AMT) or suicide substrates that selectively and reproducibly target a subproteome [49,50,156,157]. This has the added advantage of aiding prefractionation and increasing the resolution of proteins as the tag can be captured on an affinity surface [49,50].

Proteomics in human liver disease

Hepatitis C virus infection (see also Section 9)
Proteomic methodologies have been applied to a number of aspects of HCV-related liver injury. These include the study of HCV-related HCC development in which overexpression of α-enolase was identified and correlated with poorly differentiated HCC [158,159]. The response of hepatocyte cell lines to IFNγ treatment has uncovered over 54 IFN-response genes including many novel targets, an approach that may pave the way for novel therapies. Examination of protein extracts that bind to the HCV internal ribosome entry site (IRES) has identified a number of novel protein targets such as Ewing sarcoma breakpoint 1 region

protein EWS and TRAF-3. The final aspect of HCV liver injury receiving attention is the study of potential biomarkers such as heat shock protein HSP-70 associated with HCV infection progression to HCC [160].

Hepatitis B virus infection (see also Section 9)

In contrast to gene array experiments, there are a number of studies that use proteomics on sera to examine different stages of chronic HBV infection. In one study, altered proteomic profiles were identified for haptoglobin β and α2 chain apolipoprotein (Apo)A-1 and A-1V, α-1 antitrypsin, transthyretin and DNA topisomerase 11β [161]. Some of these proteins are among the most abundant serum proteins secreted by the liver and are generally associated with acute-phase inflammatory responses. What was apparent in this study was that different isoforms of some of these proteins showed distinct changes in HBV infection itself and differed at times between patients with low inflammatory scores vs. high inflammatory scores. Some examples include a decrease in cleaved haptoglobin β peptides and ApoA-1 fragments in patients with higher inflammatory scores. In comparison, some α-1-antitrypsin fragments were increased in patients with higher inflammatory scores. In an attempt to simplify such studies, deglycosylation of serum was undertaken before analysis. An alternative approach studied serum protein profiles and correlated this with disease severity using a SELDI protein chip analysis and artificial neural network models [154]. They found six fragments with a positive and 24 with a negative prediction of fibrosis stage and subsequently developed a fibrosis index with excellent precise values for significant fibrosis and cirrhosis based on the Ishak fibrosis score. The inclusion of clinical biochemical parameters such as alanine aminotransferase (ALT), bilirubin, total protein, haemoglobin and international normalized ratio (INR) strengthened the study accuracy.

AIH-, PBC- and PSC-associated liver disease
(see Section 11)

As far as we are aware, there are no published proteomic studies addressing the pathophysiology of these diseases. Cholangiocarcinoma that is associated with PSC has been studied using proteomics techniques [162]. Using tandem mass spectroscopy, Koopman et al. [162] identified Mac-2 binding protein (Mac-2BP) as a diagnostic marker in biliary carcinoma. The diagnostic accuracy of serum Mac-2BP expression in biliary carcinoma was superior to that of the established marker CA19-9. This study highlights the progression of proteomic research in liver disease: a focus initially on malignancy and biomarker discovery followed by studies of pathophysiology.

Alcoholic liver disease (ALD) and non-alcoholic fatty liver disease (NAFLD) (see Section 12 and Chapter 13)

Proteomic studies of alcoholism have, like the gene array studies, been an eclectic mix of research examining HCC development associated with alcohol, studies of hepatocyte alcohol-related

biology and neural aspects of alcohol addiction. Studies of the intrahepatic toxic effects using proteomics have helped to outline toxicology profiles that can be used for screening as well as for trying to understand the alcohol-associated liver injury. Mitochondrial ethanol hepatotoxicity is thought to involve modification of protein thiol redox state. Using two-dimensional gel proteomic studies, Venkatraman et al. [163] were able to demonstrate a decrease in the reduced thiols on aldehyde dehydrogenase and glucose-regulated protein 78. The change in aldehyde dehydrogenase reduced thiols was accompanied by a reduction in the specific activity of the enzyme. The term 'alcoholomics' has been coined to refer to the study of those proteins (i.e. the subproteome) that are directly or indirectly affected by alcohol.

There is to date only a single proteomic study of NAFLD [93]. In this study, SELDI-TOF was used to profile serum samples from 91 patients with NAFLD compared with seven obese control subjects. Twelve unique protein peaks were identified that associated with NAFLD (four associated with steatosis, four with steatosis with non-specific inflammation and four with NASH). Unfortunately, although the peak mass is shown, SELDI-TOF lacks the accuracy required to give mass determination enabling unequivocal protein identification.

Hepatocellular carcinoma (HCC) (see Chapter 18.2.1)

To date, biomarker profiling has been applied predominantly to studies of malignant tissue [164–166]. In one study, HCC development in chronic HBV infection was characterized by a significant decrease in a fragment of complement-3 and an isoform of ApoA-1 [167]. In tissue studies, expression of variants of aldehyde dehydrogenase and tissue ferritin light chain have been identified in HCC, but not in surrounding tissues. Similar studies have also identified fructose-bisphosphatase arginosuccinate synthetase and cathepsin B preprotein as downregulated in HCC tissues. In an extensive study using laser capture microscopy, Li et al. [168] identified 261 proteins differentially expressed between HCC and non-HCC hepatocytes. Kinases in the Eph family were identified along with the Ras-like family of Rho proteins. In addition, a DED box polypeptide was downregulated while three members of the spliceosome and heterogeneous nuclear ribonucleoprotein K were upregulated. SELDI-TOF MS has also been used to examine the sera of 82 patients with cirrhosis (38 without and 44 with HCC). An algorithm including the six highest scoring peaks allowed the prediction of HCC in over 90% of cases [169]. The highest discriminating peak was a C-terminal peptide of vitronectin.

Proteomic analysis of blood as a marker of liver disease: 'next generation' liver function tests?

Several studies have evaluated proteomic analysis of serum protein as a diagnostic test to assess the severity of liver disease and, in particular, for non-invasive assessment of liver fibrosis. These studies are in their infancy, with basic methodologies still unresolved. However, the early studies show that the technique has promise. In a pilot study of 46 patients with chronic hepatitis B, an artificial neural network (ANN) model was derived from the proteomic fingerprint and used to derive a fibrosis index [154]. The ANN fibrosis index correlated strongly with Ishak scores and stages of fibrosis. The areas under the receiver operating characteristic (ROC) curve for significant fibrosis (Ishak score > 2) and cirrhosis (Ishak score > 4) were both > 0.90. Inclusion of INR, total protein, bilirubin, ALT and haemoglobin in the ANN model improved the predictive power, giving accuracies > 90% for the prediction of fibrosis and cirrhosis. Another study found that pretreatment of serum proteins to remove N-glycosylation enhanced the resolution of serum polypeptide profiles [148]. This technique has the potential to improve diagnostic serum proteomics.

Chen and colleagues [170] developed a method of glycoproteomic analysis in an attempt to discover serum markers that can assist in the early detection of HBV-induced liver cancer. The authors showed that woodchucks diagnosed with HCC have dramatically higher levels of serum-associated core α-1, 6-linked fucose. One glycoprotein, Golgi protein 73 (GP73), was found to be elevated and hyperfucosylated in the serum of animals and humans with a diagnosis of HCC. Serum profiling was used to distinguish HCC from the earlier stages of HCV-related liver disease [56]. The proteomic model distinguished chronic HCV from HCV–HCC with moderate sensitivity and specificity. Inclusion of known serum markers α-fetoprotein, des-γ carboxyprothrombin and GP73 again improved the diagnostic accuracy significantly.

Proteomics in other liver disease

The metalloproteome is defined as the set of proteins that have metal binding capacity by being metalloproteins or having metal binding sites. The Cu and Zn metalloproteomes were defined in human hepatoma lines [171]. Although the gene for Wilson's disease has been identified, the mechanisms by which excess copper leads to oxidative stress and acute liver failure are not fully understood. Using an *in vitro* model of copper loading, novel copper binding proteins were isolated using proteomic techniques [140].

Although there has been limited proteomic analysis of liver tissue in models of disease, liver-associated pathobiological processes have been examined. In one study of the liver ageing process, 85 differentially expressed proteins were identified comprising antioxidation, glucose/amino acid metabolism, signal transduction and cell cycle systems [172]. In ageing, the antioxidation system showed a large increase in glutathione peroxidase and a decrease in glutathione S-transferase. Similarly, levels of glycolytic enzymes were decreased in the ageing animal. Furthermore, levels of proteins associated with signal transduction/apoptosis, for example cathepsin B, were decreased in the ageing process.

Proteomics has also been used to identify genes associated with LPS-induced liver injury. Proteins such as TRAIL receptor 2 were downregulated in the liver of LPS-treated mice whereas TNFAIP1 was significantly upregulated. Three different proteins were novel in the fatty liver proteome (aconitase succinate dehydrogenase, propanol CoA carboxylase α chain and 3-hydroxyanthrilate 3-4-dioxygenase).

Future studies

The future of 'omics' methodologies (genomics, proteomics and metabolomics) will address a number of technical and biological limitations of current techniques. Gene array analysis of mRNA transcript expression is the most developed functional genomics technique and has now been extended to the analysis of homogeneous cell populations from liver [173]. The last decade has seen this technique develop dramatically with the number of gene targets being included on arrays now enabling true transcriptome profiling as opposed to simply sampling the transcriptome. Additionally, the variability of the various gene array techniques is now better understood, with both technical and biological variability being addressed by the use of sample pooling, and technical and biological replicates. The adoption of MIAME standards for the presentation of results from gene array experiments promises better standardization, reproducibility and the ability to compare results [13,174]. The future will see the widespread development of specialized targeted gene arrays (such as fibrosis, cancer and iron metabolism arrays) as well as the use of gene arrays in clinical care. Gene array experiments that currently discriminate dissimilar cancer specimens will be able to discern much more closely related phenotypical stages in non-malignant disease progression. Additionally, the use of gene arrays covering multiple exons of an mRNA transcript will be able to detect alternative splicing, and the use of sequence mismatched oligonucleotides will detect multiple known and novel SNPs [175]. The bioinformatics analysis of gene expression data is now focused on outcome/phenotype prediction as well as uncovering biological pathway interactions, chromosomal loci identification and functional characterization in dynamic systems. These newer techniques are likely to become widely adopted research and then potentially clinically applicable methodologies.

Proteomic methods have lagged behind transcriptome analysis, and the immediate future heralds an increase in throughput, an increase in dynamic range/sensitivity and improved resolution of proteins within biological samples [35,36]. Sample preparation and prefractionation appear to be the key to improved resolution in the short term, with the use of proteomic methods to profile whole proteomes in a single specimen being a long-term distant research goal. Proteomic methods with future promise include the use of protein adjuncts to enable techniques such as DiGE and targeting of particular protein subclasses such as proteases. One particularly promising future technique is the use of imaging MS to perform a spatial profile of proteins in a tissue section (in a manner similar to SELDI-TOF but the laser actually rasters a tissue section) [176–178]. Another area of great promise in proteomic research is its use in biomarker discovery. However, these techniques are still in their infancy as a result of differences in biological protein expression. The magnitude of the problems to be solved can be gauged by recent serum protein profiling that identified 3020 serum proteins by two or more tags but required 18 laboratories and failed to detect many of the low-abundance proteins (these are potential biomarkers) (www.hupo.org). Importantly, in this analysis, those laboratories that used very accurate MS analysis and prefractionation combined with multiple chromatographic separation methods were most successful. Additional improvements include the use of protein arrays on which antibodies or antigens are fixed to a membrane [179–183]. The initial experimental use of protein arrays is likely to involve studies of the immune system, given the number of antibodies available in this discipline. Studies such as the immunotyping of leukaemias with antibody arrays have demonstrated that the technology is available in a working format [184]. The study by Haab *et al.* [185] showed that a protein microarray could be produced allowing the detection of cognate ligands at an absolute concentration below 1 ng/mL. Unfortunately, only 20% of the arrayed antibodies and 50% of the arrayed antigen provided specific and accurate measurements of their cognate ligands at or below 1.6 μg/mL and 0.34 μg/mL respectively [185]. There are many commercial antibody and protein array sources that, along with academia, are developing these methodologies. Related technologies include the ability to capture proteins or antigens using technologies such as SELDI and BIAcore (biomolecular interaction analysis), both of which are available in chip formats. A newly emerging technology that promises to increase the initial 'downstream' characterization of differentially expressed genes is tissue arrays. Tissue arrays have been produced with over 600 individual tissue samples on a single glass slide; these are then analysed by immunohistochemistry, fluorescence *in situ* hybridization (FISH) and RNA/RNA *in situ* hybridization [186–191].

Finally, multiplexing is likely to be a key 'buzzword' in the future. The ability to conserve and process a sample in multiple ways, so that it can be subjected to many analytical methods, is an approach presently receiving a lot of attention [176–178]. The use of gene array platforms to profile transcriptomes, SNPs and promoter elements is readily possible on a single sample. Further protein analysis using chromatographic techniques with in-line parallel chromatographic sample treatments and separation is being adopted and can be readily automated. The adoption of cross-platform technologies is presently cost prohibitive for many institutions but likely to become more widespread with the adoption of core facilities in commercial and academic institutions and the focus on collaborations to use the inevitable deluge of data. This leaves us with new bioinformatic challenges. The future path for functional genomics/proteomics techniques appears to be bright and paved with almost endless data. Our ultimate challenge may be to make biological sense of these data!

References

1 Venter JC, Adams MD, Myers EW *et al.* (2001) The sequence of the human genome. *Science* 291 (5507), 1304–1351.

2 Kornblihtt AR (2005) Promoter usage and alternative splicing. *Curr Opin Cell Biol* 17 (3), 262–268.

3 Duyk GM (2002) Sharper tools and simpler methods. *Nature Genet* 32 (Suppl), 465–468.

4 Yano N, Habib NA, Fadden KJ *et al.* (2001) Profiling the adult human liver transcriptome: analysis by cDNA array hybridization. *J Hepatol* 35 (2), 178–186.

5 Shackel NA, Gorrell MD, McCaughan GW (2002) Gene array analysis and the liver. *Hepatology* 36 (6), 1313–1325.

6 Lee ML, Kuo FC, Whitmore GA *et al.* (2000) Importance of replication in microarray gene expression studies: statistical methods and evidence from repetitive cDNA hybridizations. *Proc Natl Acad Sci USA* 97 (18), 9834–9839.

7 Larkin JE, Frank BC, Gavras H *et al.* (2005) Independence and reproducibility across microarray platforms. *Nature Methods* 2 (5), 337–344.

8 Irizarry RA, Warren D, Spencer F *et al.* (2005) Multiple-laboratory comparison of microarray platforms. *Nature Methods* 2 (5), 345–350.

9 Churchill GA (2002) Fundamentals of experimental design for cDNA microarrays. *Nature Genet* 32 (Suppl) 490–495.

10 Yin JL, Shackel NA, Zekry A *et al.* (2001) Real-time reverse transcriptase-polymerase chain reaction (RT-PCR) for measurement of cytokine and growth factor mRNA expression with fluorogenic probes or SYBR Green I. *Immunol Cell Biol* 79 (3), 213–221.

11 Kendziorski C, Irizarry RA, Chen KS *et al.* (2005) On the utility of pooling biological samples in microarray experiments. *Proc Natl Acad Sci USA* 102 (12), 4252–4257.

12 Kendziorski CM, Zhang Y, Lan H *et al.* (2003) The efficiency of pooling mRNA in microarray experiments. *Biostatistics* 4 (3), 465–477.

13 Brazma A, Hingamp P, Quackenbush J *et al.* (2001) Minimum information about a microarray experiment (MIAME) – toward standards for microarray data. *Nature Genet* 29 (4), 365–371.

14 Feldman AL, Costouros NG, Wang E *et al.* (2002) Advantages of mRNA amplification for microarray analysis. *Biotechniques* 33 (4), 906–912, 914.

15 Eberwine J (1996) Amplification of mRNA populations using aRNA generated from immobilized oligo(dT)-T7 primed cDNA. *Biotechniques* 20 (4), 584–591.

16 Vernon SD, Unger ER, Rajeevan M *et al.* (2000) Reproducibility of alternative probe synthesis approaches for gene expression profiling with arrays. *J Mol Diagn* 2 (3), 124–127.

17 Zhu YY, Machleder EM, Chenchik A *et al.* (2001) Reverse transcriptase template switching: a SMART approach for full-length cDNA library construction. *Biotechniques* 30 (4), 892–897.

18 Seth D, Gorrell MD, McGuinness PH *et al.* (2003) SMART amplification maintains representation of relative gene expression: quantitative validation by real time PCR and application to studies of alcoholic liver disease in primates. *J Biochem Biophys Methods* 55 (1), 53–66.

19 Kohara Y, Noda H, Okano K *et al.* (2001) DNA hybridization using 'bead-array': probe-attached beads arrayed in a capillary in a predetermined order. *Nucleic Acids Res* 29 (Suppl. 1), 83–84.

20 Kohara Y, Noda H, Okano K *et al.* (2002) DNA probes on beads arrayed in a capillary, 'Bead-array', exhibited high hybridization performance. *Nucleic Acids Res* 30 (16), e87.

21 Noda H, Kohara Y, Okano K *et al.* (2003) Automated bead alignment apparatus using a single bead capturing technique for fabrication of a miniaturized bead-based DNA probe array. *Anal Chem* 75 (13), 3250–3255.

22 Cantin GT, Yates JR, 3rd (2004) Strategies for shotgun identification of post-translational modifications by mass spectrometry. *J Chromatogr A* 1053 (1–2), 7–14.

23 Resing KA, Ahn NG (2005) Proteomics strategies for protein identification. *FEBS Lett* 579 (4), 885–889.

24 Parent R, Beretta L (2005) Proteomics in the study of liver pathology. *J Hepatol* 43 (1), 177–183.

25 Colantonio DA, Chan DW (2005) The clinical application of proteomics. *Clin Chim Acta* 357, 151–158.

26 Lane CS (2005) Mass spectrometry-based proteomics in the life sciences. *Cell Mol Life Sci* 62 (7–8), 848–869.

27 Albala JS (2001) Array-based proteomics: the latest chip challenge. *Expert Rev Mol Diagn* 1 (2), 145–152.

28 Hanash S (2003) The emerging field of protein microarrays. *Proteomics* 3 (11), 2075.

29 Lauber WM, Carroll JA, Dufield DR *et al.* (2001) Mass spectrometry compatibility of two-dimensional gel protein stains. *Electrophoresis* 22 (5), 906–918.

30 Rodland KD (2004) Proteomics and cancer diagnosis: the potential of mass spectrometry. *Clin Biochem* 37 (7), 579–583.

31 Fountoulakis M, Juranville JF, Tsangaris G *et al.* (2004) Fractionation of liver proteins by preparative electrophoresis. *Amino Acids* 26 (1), 27–36.

32 Righetti PG, Castagna A, Herbert B *et al.* (2003) Prefractionation techniques in proteome analysis. *Proteomics* 3 (8), 1397–1407.

33 Righetti PG, Castagna A, Antonioli P *et al.* (2005) Prefractionation techniques in proteome analysis: the mining tools of the third millennium. *Electrophoresis* 26 (2), 297–319.

34 Kettman JR, Frey JR, Lefkovits I (2001) Proteome, transcriptome and genome: top down or bottom up analysis? *Biomol Eng* 18 (5), 207–212.

35 Kolch W, Mischak H, Chalmers MJ *et al.* (2004) Clinical proteomics: a question of technology. *Rapid Commun Mass Spectrom* 18 (19), 2365–2366.

36 Kolch W, Mischak H, Pitt AR (2005) The molecular make-up of a tumour: proteomics in cancer research. *Clin Sci (Lond)* 108 (5), 369–383.

37 Chernokalskaya E, Gutierrez S, Pitt AM *et al.* (2004) Ultrafiltration for proteomic sample preparation. *Electrophoresis* 25 (15), 2461–2468.

38 Nabi G, N'Dow J, Hasan TS *et al.* (2005) Proteomic analysis of urine in patients with intestinal segments transposed into the urinary tract. *Proteomics* 5 (6), 1729–1733.

39 Stasyk T, Huber LA (2004) Zooming in: fractionation strategies in proteomics. *Proteomics* 4 (12), 3704–3716.

40 Schirmer EC, Florens L, Guan T *et al.* (2003) Nuclear membrane proteins with potential disease links found by subtractive proteomics. *Science* 301 (5638), 1380–1382.

41 Murayama K, Fujimura T, Morita M *et al.* (2001) One-step subcellular fractionation of rat liver tissue using a Nycodenz density gradient prepared by freezing-thawing and two-dimensional sodium dodecyl sulfate electrophoresis profiles of the main fraction of organelles. *Electrophoresis* 22 (14), 2872–2880.

42 Lopez MF, Kristal BS, Chernokalskaya E *et al.* (2000) High-throughput profiling of the mitochondrial proteome using affinity fractionation and automation. *Electrophoresis* 21 (16), 3427–3440.

43 Zang L, Palmer Toy D, Hancock WS *et al.* (2004) Proteomic analysis of ductal carcinoma of the breast using laser capture microdissection, LC-MS, and 16O/18O isotopic labeling. *J Proteome Res* 3 (3), 604–612.

44 Tadros Y, Ruiz-Deya G, Crawford BE *et al.* (2003) In vivo proteomic analysis of cytokine expression in laser capture-microdissected urothelial cells of obstructed ureteropelvic junction procured by laparoscopic dismembered pyeloplasty. *J Endourol* 17 (5), 333–336.

45 Chignard N, Beretta L (2004) Proteomics for hepatocellular carcinoma marker discovery. *Gastroenterology* 127 (5 Suppl 1), S120–125.

46 Ahmed N, Barker G, Oliva KT *et al.* (2004) Proteomic-based identification of haptoglobin-1 precursor as a novel circulating biomarker of ovarian cancer. *Br J Cancer* 91 (1), 129–140.

47 Hanash S (2003) Disease proteomics. *Nature* 422 (6928), 226–232.

48 Mehta AI, Ross S, Lowenthal MS *et al.* (2003) Biomarker amplification by serum carrier protein binding. *Dis Markers* 19 (1), 1–10.

49 Greenbaum D, Baruch A, Hayrapetian L *et al.* (2002) Chemical approaches for functionally probing the proteome. *Mol Cell Proteomics* 1 (1), 60–68.

50 Joyce JA, Baruch A, Chehade K *et al.* (2004) Cathepsin cysteine proteases are effectors of invasive growth and angiogenesis during multistage tumorigenesis. *Cancer Cell* 5 (5), 443–453.

51 Barglow KT, Cravatt BF (2004) Discovering disease-associated enzymes by proteome reactivity profiling. *Chem Biol* 11 (11), 1523–1531.

52 Patton WF (2002) Detection technologies in proteome analysis. *J Chromatogr B Anal Technol Biomed Life Sci* 771 (1–2), 3–31.

53 Henkel C, Roderfeld M, Weiskirchen R *et al.* (2005) Identification of fibrosis-relevant proteins using DIGE (difference in gel electrophoresis) in different models of hepatic fibrosis. *Z Gastroenterol* 43 (1), 23–9.

54 Neverova I, Van Eyk JE (2005) Role of chromatographic techniques in proteomic analysis. *J Chromatogr B Anal Technol Biomed Life Sci* 815 (1–2), 51–63.

55 Steel LF, Haab BB, Hanash SM (2005) Methods of comparative proteomic profiling for disease diagnostics. *J Chromatogr B Anal Technol Biomed Life Sci* 815 (1–2), 275–284.

56 Schwegler EE, Cazares L, Steel LF *et al.* (2005) SELDI-TOF MS profiling of serum for detection of the progression of chronic hepatitis C to hepatocellular carcinoma. *Hepatology* 41 (3), 634–642.

57 Cordingley HC, Roberts SL, Tooke P *et al.* (2003) Multifactorial screening design and analysis of SELDI-TOF ProteinChip array optimization experiments. *Biotechniques* 34 (2), 364–365, 368–373.

58 Utz PJ (2005) Protein arrays for studying blood cells and their secreted products. *Immunol Rev* 204, 264–282.

59 Smyth GK, Yang YH, Speed T (2003) Statistical issues in cDNA microarray data analysis. *Methods Mol Biol* 224, 111–136.

60 Smyth GK, Speed T (2003) Normalization of cDNA microarray data. *Methods* 31 (4), 265–273.

61 Yang YH, Dudoit S, Luu P *et al.* (2002) Normalization for cDNA microarray data: a robust composite method addressing single and multiple slide systematic variation. *Nucleic Acids Res* 30 (4), e15.

62 Yang YH, Buckley MJ, Speed TP (2001) Analysis of cDNA microarray images. *Brief Bioinform* 2 (4), 341–349.

63 Yang MC, Ruan QG, Yang JJ *et al.* (2001) A statistical method for flagging weak spots improves normalization and ratio estimates in microarrays. *Physiol Genomics* 7 (1), 45–53.

64 Wu LF, Hughes TR, Davierwala AP *et al.* (2002) Large-scale prediction of *Saccharomyces cerevisiae* gene function using overlapping transcriptional clusters. *Nature Genet* 31 (3), 255–265.

65 Jain KK (2000) Applications of proteomics in oncology. *Pharmacogenomics* 1 (4), 385–393.

66 Hekkelman ML, Vriend G (2005) MRS: a fast and compact retrieval system for biological data. *Nucleic Acids Res* 33 (Web Server issue), W766–769.

67 Stuart JM, Segal E, Koller D *et al.* (2003) A gene-coexpression network for global discovery of conserved genetic modules. *Science* 302 (5643), 249–255.

68 Chaussabel D, Sher A (2002) Mining microarray expression data by literature profiling. *Genome Biol* 3 (10), RESEARCH0055.

69 Yuan J, Liu Y, Wang Y *et al.* (2001) Genome analysis with gene-indexing databases. *Pharmacol Ther* 91 (2), 115–132.

70 Coulouarn C, Lefebvre G, Derambure C *et al.* (2004) Altered gene expression in acute systemic inflammation detected by complete coverage of the human liver transcriptome. *Hepatology* 39 (2), 353–364.

71 Yamashita T, Hashimoto S, Kaneko S *et al.* (2000) Comprehensive gene expression profile of a normal human liver. *Biochem Biophys Res Commun* 269 (1), 110–116.

72 Yamashita T, Honda M, Takatori H *et al.* (2004) Genome-wide transcriptome mapping analysis identifies organ-specific gene expression patterns along human chromosomes. *Genomics* 84 (5), 867–875.

73 Yamashita Y, Shimada M, Harimoto N *et al.* (2004) cDNA microarray analysis in hepatocyte differentiation in Huh 7 cells. *Cell Transplant* 13 (7–8), 793–797.

74 Enard W, Khaitovich P, Klose J *et al.* (2002) Intra- and interspecific variation in primate gene expression patterns. *Science* 296 (5566), 340–343.

75 Bigger CB, Brasky KM, Lanford RE (2001) DNA microarray analysis of chimpanzee liver during acute resolving hepatitis C virus infection. *J Virol* 75 (15), 7059–7066.

76 Su AI, Pezacki JP, Wodicka L *et al.* (2002) Genomic analysis of the host response to hepatitis C virus infection. *Proc Natl Acad Sci USA* 99 (24), 15669–15674.

77 Karayiannis P (2005) The hepatitis C virus NS3/4A protease complex interferes with pathways of the innate immune response. *J Hepatol* 43 (4), 743–745.

78 Chen L, Borozan I, Feld J *et al.* (2005) Hepatic gene expression discriminates responders and nonresponders in treatment of chronic hepatitis C viral infection. *Gastroenterology* 128 (5), 1437–1444.

79 Honda M, Kaneko S, Kawai H *et al.* (2001) Differential gene expression between chronic hepatitis B and C hepatic lesions. *Gastroenterology* 120 (4), 955–966.

80 Shackel NA, McGuinness PH, Abbott CA *et al.* (2002) Insights into the pathobiology of hepatitis C virus-associated cirrhosis: analysis of intrahepatic differential gene expression. *Am J Pathol* 160 (2), 641–654.

81 Smith MW, Yue ZN, Korth MJ *et al.* (2003) Hepatitis C virus and liver disease: global transcriptional profiling and identification of potential markers. *Hepatology* 38 (6), 1458–1467.

82 Shackel NA, McGuinness PH, Abbott CA *et al.* (2003) Novel differential gene expression in human cirrhosis detected by suppression subtractive hybridization. *Hepatology* 38 (3), 577–588.

83 McCaughan GW, Xiao XH, Zekry A *et al.* (2003) The intrahepatic response to HCV infection. In: Jilbert AR, Grgacic EVL, Vickery K *et al.* (eds) *Proceedings of the 11th International Symposium on Viral Hepatitis and Liver Disease.* Sydney: Australian Centre for Hepatitis Virology, pp. 100–106.

84 Mansfield ES, Sarwal MM (2004) Arraying the orchestration of allograft pathology. *Am J Transplant* 4 (6), 853–862.

85 McCaughan GW, Zekry A (2004) Mechanisms of HCV reinfection and allograft damage after liver transplantation. *J Hepatol* 40 (3), 368–374.

86 McCaughan GW, Zekry A (2002) Pathogenesis of hepatitis C virus recurrence in the liver allograft. *Liver Transpl* 8 (10 Suppl 1), S7–S13.

87 Wieland S, Thimme R, Purcell RH *et al.* (2004) Genomic analysis of the host response to hepatitis B virus infection. *Proc Natl Acad Sci USA* 101 (17), 6669–6674.

88 Wieland SF, Chisari FV (2005) Stealth and cunning: hepatitis B and hepatitis C viruses. *J Virol* 79 (15), 9369–9380.

89 Seth D, Leo MA, McGuinness PH *et al.* (2003) Gene expression profiling of alcoholic liver disease in the baboon (*Papio hamadryas*) and human liver. *Am J Pathol* 163 (6), 2303–2317.

90 Deaciuc IV, Doherty DE, Burikhanov R *et al.* (2004) Large-scale gene profiling of the liver in a mouse model of chronic, intragastric ethanol infusion. *J Hepatol* 40 (2), 219–227.

91 Shackel NA, McGuinness PH, Abbott CA *et al.* (2001) Identification of novel molecules and pathogenic pathways in primary biliary cirrhosis: cDNA array analysis of intrahepatic differential gene expression. *Gut* 49 (4), 565–576.

92 Sreekumar R, Rosado B, Rasmussen D *et al.* (2003) Hepatic gene expression in histologically progressive nonalcoholic steatohepatitis. *Hepatology* 38 (1), 244–251.

93 Younossi ZM, Baranova A, Ziegler K *et al.* (2005) A genomic and proteomic study of the spectrum of nonalcoholic fatty liver disease. *Hepatology* 42 (3), 665–674.

94 Younossi ZM, Gorreta F, Ong JP *et al.* (2005) Hepatic gene expression in patients with obesity-related non-alcoholic steatohepatitis. *Liver Int* 25 (4), 760–771.

95 Zhang DY, Sabla G, Shivakumar P *et al.* (2004) Coordinate expression of regulatory genes differentiates embryonic and perinatal forms of biliary atresia. *Hepatology* 39 (4), 954–962.

96 Galvin P, Clarke LA, Harvey S *et al.* (2004) Microarray analysis in cystic fibrosis. *J Cyst Fibros* 3 (Suppl 2), 29–33.

97 Norkina O, Kaur S, Ziemer D *et al.* (2004) Inflammation of the cystic fibrosis mouse small intestine. *Am J Physiol Gastrointest Liver Physiol* 286 (6), G1032–1041.

98 Srivastava M, Eidelman O, Pollard HB (1999) Pharmacogenomics of the cystic fibrosis transmembrane conductance regulator (CFTR) and the cystic fibrosis drug CPX using genome microarray analysis. *Mol Med* 5 (11), 753–767.

99 Shirota Y, Kaneko S, Honda M *et al.* (2001) Identification of differentially expressed genes in hepatocellular carcinoma with cDNA microarrays. *Hepatology* 33 (4), 832–840.

100 Kim JW, Ye Q, Forgues M *et al.* (2004) Cancer-associated molecular signature in the tissue samples of patients with cirrhosis. *Hepatology* 39 (2), 518–527.

101 Kim BY, Lee JG, Park S *et al.* (2004) Feature genes of hepatitis B virus-positive hepatocellular carcinoma, established by its molecular discrimination approach using prediction analysis of microarray. *Biochim Biophys Acta* 1739 (1), 50–61.

102 Iizuka N, Oka M, Yamada-Okabe H *et al.* (2004) Molecular signature in three types of hepatocellular carcinoma with different viral origin by oligonucleotide microarray. *Int J Oncol* 24 (3), 565–574.

103 Iizuka N, Oka M, Yamada-Okabe H *et al.* (2002) Comparison of gene expression profiles between hepatitis B virus- and hepatitis C virus-infected hepatocellular carcinoma by oligonucleotide microarray data on the basis of a supervised learning method. *Cancer Res* 62 (14), 3939–3944.

104 Qin LX, Tang ZY (2004) Recent progress in predictive biomarkers for metastatic recurrence of human hepatocellular carcinoma: a review of the literature. *J Cancer Res Clin Oncol* 130 (9), 497–513.

105 Ye QH, Qin LX, Forgues M *et al.* (2003) Predicting hepatitis B virus-positive metastatic hepatocellular carcinomas using gene expression profiling and supervised machine learning. *Nature Med* 9 (4), 416–423.

106 Pan HW, Ou YH, Peng SY *et al.* (2003) Overexpression of osteopontin is associated with intrahepatic metastasis, early recurrence, and poorer prognosis of surgically resected hepatocellular carcinoma. *Cancer* 98 (1), 119–127.

107 Tang ZY, Ye SL, Liu YK *et al.* (2004) A decade's studies on metastasis of hepatocellular carcinoma. *J Cancer Res Clin Oncol* 130 (4), 187–196.

108 Wang W, Yang LY, Huang GW *et al.* (2004) Genomic analysis reveals RhoC as a potential marker in hepatocellular carcinoma with poor prognosis. *Br J Cancer* 90 (12), 2349–2355.

109 Obama K, Ura K, Li M *et al.* (2005) Genome-wide analysis of gene expression in human intrahepatic cholangiocarcinoma. *Hepatology* 41 (6), 1339–1348.

110 Hansel DE, Rahman A, Hidalgo M *et al.* (2003) Identification of novel cellular targets in biliary tract cancers using global gene expression technology. *Am J Pathol* 163 (1), 217–229.

111 Bulera SJ, Eddy SM, Ferguson E *et al.* (2001) RNA expression in the early characterization of hepatotoxicants in Wistar rats by high-density DNA microarrays. *Hepatology* 33 (5), 1239–1258.

112 Cunningham MJ, Liang S, Fuhrman S *et al.* (2000) Gene expression microarray data analysis for toxicology profiling. *Ann NY Acad Sci* 9 (19), 52–67.

113 Huang Q, Jin X, Gaillard ET *et al.* (2004) Gene expression profiling reveals multiple toxicity endpoints induced by hepatotoxicants. *Mutat Res* 549 (1–2), 147–167.

114 Jiang Y, Liu J, Waalkes M *et al.* (2004) Changes in the gene expression associated with carbon tetrachloride-induced liver fibrosis persist after cessation of dosing in mice. *Toxicol Sci* 79 (2), 404–410.

115 Jolly RA, Goldstein KM, Wei T *et al.* (2005) Pooling samples within microarray studies: a comparative analysis of rat liver transcription response to prototypical toxicants. *Physiol Genomics* 22 (3), 346–355.

116 Jung JW, Park JS, Hwang JW *et al.* (2004) Gene expression analysis of peroxisome proliferators- and phenytoin-induced hepatotoxicity using cDNA microarray. *J Vet Med Sci* 66 (11), 1329–1333.

117 Minami K, Saito T, Narahara M *et al.* (2005) Relationship between hepatic gene expression profiles and hepatotoxicity in five typical hepatotoxicant-administered rats. *Toxicol Sci* 87 (1), 296–305.

118 Shankar K, Vaidya VS, Corton JC *et al.* (2003) Activation of PPAR-alpha in streptozotocin-induced diabetes is essential for resistance against acetaminophen toxicity. *FASEB J* 17 (12), 1748–1750.

119 Ulrich RG, Rockett JC, Gibson GG *et al.* (2004) Overview of an interlaboratory collaboration on evaluating the effects of model hepatotoxicants on hepatic gene expression. *Environ Health Perspect* 112 (4), 423–427.

120 Waring JF, Ciurlionis R, Jolly RA *et al.* (2001) Microarray analysis of hepatotoxins *in vitro* reveals a correlation between gene expression profiles and mechanisms of toxicity. *Toxicol Lett* 120 (1–3), 359–368.

121 Waring JF, Jolly RA, Ciurlionis R *et al.* (2001) Clustering of hepatotoxins based on mechanism of toxicity using gene expression profiles. *Toxicol Appl Pharmacol* 175 (1), 28–42.

122 Waring JF, Cavet G, Jolly RA *et al.* (2003) Development of a DNA microarray for toxicology based on hepatotoxin-regulated sequences. *EHP Toxicogenomics* 111 (1T), 53–60.

123 Utsunomiya T, Okamoto M, Hashimoto M *et al.* (2004) A gene-expression signature can quantify the degree of hepatic fibrosis in the rat. *J Hepatol* 41 (3), 399–406.

124 Iida M, Anna CH, Hartis J *et al.* (2003) Changes in global gene and protein expression during early mouse liver carcinogenesis induced by non-genotoxic model carcinogens oxazepam and Wyeth-14,643. *Carcinogenesis* 24 (4), 757–770.

125 Lefkovits I, Kettman JR, Frey JR (2001) Proteomic analysis of rare molecular species of translated polypeptides from a mouse fetal thymus cDNA library. *Proteomics* 1 (4), 560–573.

126 Lefkovits I, Kettman JR, Frey JR (2000) Global analysis of gene expression in cells of the immune system I. Analytical limitations in obtaining sequence information on polypeptides in two-dimensional gel spots. *Electrophoresis* 21 (13), 2688–2693.

127 Ratziu V, Charlotte F, Heurtier A *et al.* (2005) Sampling variability of liver biopsy in nonalcoholic fatty liver disease. *Gastroenterology* 128 (7), 1898–1906.

128 Regev A, Berho M, Jeffers LJ *et al.* (2002) Sampling error and intraobserver variation in liver biopsy in patients with chronic HCV infection. *Am J Gastroenterol* 97 (10), 2614–2618.

129 Anderson L, Seilhamer J (1997) A comparison of selected mRNA and protein abundances in human liver. *Electrophoresis* 18 (3–4), 533–537.

130 ter Kuile BH, Westerhoff HV (2001) Transcriptome meets metabolome: hierarchical and metabolic regulation of the glycolytic pathway. *FEBS Lett* 500 (3), 169–171.

131 Miklos GL, Maleszka R (2001) Integrating molecular medicine with functional proteomics: realities and expectations. *Proteomics* 1 (1), 30–41.

132 Miklos GL, Maleszka R (2001) Protein functions and biological contexts. *Proteomics* 1 (2), 169–178.

133 Jansen R, Gerstein M (2000) Analysis of the yeast transcriptome with structural and functional categories: characterizing highly expressed proteins. *Nucleic Acids Res* 28 (6), 1481–1488.

134 Kristensen DB, Kawada N, Imamura K *et al.* (2000) Proteome analysis of rat hepatic stellate cells. *Hepatology* 32 (2), 268–277.

135 Kawada N, Kristensen DB, Asahina K *et al.* (2001) Characterization of a stellate cell activation-associated protein (STAP) with peroxidase activity found in rat hepatic stellate cells. *J Biol Chem* 276 (27), 25318–25323.

136 Eng FJ, Friedman SL (2000) Fibrogenesis I. New insights into hepatic stellate cell activation: the simple becomes complex. *Am J Physiol Gastrointest Liver Physiol* 279 (1), G7–G11.

137 Seow TK, Liang RC, Leow CK *et al.* (2001) Hepatocellular carcinoma: from bedside to proteomics. *Proteomics* 1 (10), 1249–1263.

138 Kaplowitz N (2004) Drug-induced liver injury. *Clin Infect Dis* 38 (Suppl 2), S44–48.

139 Fella K, Gluckmann M, Hellmann J *et al.* (2005) Use of two-dimensional gel electrophoresis in predictive toxicology: identification of potential early protein biomarkers in chemically induced hepatocarcinogenesis. *Proteomics* 5 (7), 1914–1927.

140 Roelofsen H, Balgobind R, Vonk RJ (2004) Proteomic analyzes of copper metabolism in an *in vitro* model of Wilson disease using surface enhanced laser desorption/ionization-time of flight-mass spectrometry. *J Cell Biochem* 93 (4), 732–740.

141 Low TY, Leow CK, Salto-Tellez M *et al.* (2004) A proteomic analysis of thioacetamide-induced hepatotoxicity and cirrhosis in rat livers. *Proteomics* 4 (12), 3960–3974.

142 Nordvarg H, Flensburg J, Ronn O *et al.* (2004) A proteomics approach to the study of absorption, distribution, metabolism, excretion, and toxicity. *J Biomol Tech* 15 (4), 265–275.

143 Merrick BA, Bruno ME (2004) Genomic and proteomic profiling for biomarkers and signature profiles of toxicity. *Curr Opin Mol Ther* 6 (6), 600–607.

144 Guzey C, Spigset O (2002) Genotyping of drug targets: a method to predict adverse drug reactions? *Drug Safety* 25 (8), 553–560.

145 Meneses-Lorente G, Guest PC, Lawrence J *et al.* (2004) A proteomic investigation of drug-induced steatosis in rat liver. *Chem Res Toxicol* 17 (5), 605–612.

146 Gao J, Ann Garulacan L, Storm SM *et al.* (2004) Identification of *in vitro* protein biomarkers of idiosyncratic liver toxicity. *Toxicol In Vitro* 18 (4), 533–541.

147 Fountoulakis M, Suter L (2002) Proteomic analysis of the rat liver. *J Chromatogr B Anal Technol Biomed Life Sci* 782 (1–2), 197–218.

148 Comunale MA, Mattu TS, Lowman MA *et al.* (2004) Comparative proteomic analysis of de-N-glycosylated serum from hepatitis B carriers reveals polypeptides that correlate with disease status. *Proteomics* 4 (3), 826–838.

149 Garry RF, Dash S (2003) Proteomics computational analyses suggest that hepatitis C virus E1 and pestivirus E2 envelope glycoproteins are truncated class II fusion proteins. *Virology* 307 (2), 255–265.

150 Kim W, Oe Lim S, Kim JS *et al.* (2003) Comparison of proteome between hepatitis B virus- and hepatitis C virus-associated hepatocellular carcinoma. *Clin Cancer Res* 9 (15), 5493–5500.

151 Lu H, Li W, Noble WS *et al.* (2004) Riboproteomics of the hepatitis C virus internal ribosomal entry site. *J Proteome Res* 3 (5), 949–957.

152 Rosenberg S (2001) Recent advances in the molecular biology of hepatitis C virus. *J Mol Biol* 313 (3), 451–464.

153 Scholle F, Li K, Bodola F *et al.* (2004) Virus–host cell interactions during hepatitis C virus RNA replication: impact of polyprotein expression on the cellular transcriptome and cell cycle association with viral RNA synthesis. *J Virol* 78 (3), 1513–1524.

154 Poon TC, Hui AY, Chan HL *et al.* (2005) Prediction of liver fibrosis and cirrhosis in chronic hepatitis B infection by serum proteomic fingerprinting: a pilot study. *Clin Chem* 51 (2), 328–335.

155 Xu C, Chang C, Yuan J *et al.* (2004) Identification and characterization of 177 unreported genes associated with liver regeneration. *Genomics Proteomics Bioinformatics* 2 (2), 109–118.

156 Pasa-Tolic L, Masselon C, Barry RC *et al.* (2004) Proteomic analyses using an accurate mass and time tag strategy. *Biotechniques* 37 (4), 621–624, 626–633, 636 passim.

157 Bogdanov B, Smith RD (2005) Proteomics by FTICR mass spectrometry: top down and bottom up. *Mass Spectrom Rev* 24 (2), 168–200.

158 Takashima M, Kuramitsu Y, Yokoyama Y *et al.* (2005) Overexpression of alpha enolase in hepatitis C virus-related hepatocellular carcinoma: association with tumor progression as determined by proteomic analysis. *Proteomics* 5 (6), 1686–1692.

159 Kuramitsu Y, Nakamura K (2005) Current progress in proteomic study of hepatitis C virus-related human hepatocellular carcinoma. *Expert Rev Proteomics* 2 (4), 589–601.

160 Takashima M, Kuramitsu Y, Yokoyama Y *et al.* (2003) Proteomic profiling of heat shock protein 70 family members as biomarkers for hepatitis C virus-related hepatocellular carcinoma. *Proteomics* 3 (12), 2487–2493.

161 He QY, Lau GK, Zhou Y *et al.* (2003) Serum biomarkers of hepatitis B virus infected liver inflammation: a proteomic study. *Proteomics* 3 (5), 666–674.

162 Koopmann J, Thuluvath PJ, Zahurak ML *et al.* (2004) Mac-2-binding protein is a diagnostic marker for biliary tract carcinoma. *Cancer* 101 (7), 1609–1615.

163 Venkatraman A, Landar A, Davis AJ *et al.* (2004) Oxidative modification of hepatic mitochondria protein thiols: effect of chronic alcohol consumption. *Am J Physiol Gastrointest Liver Physiol* 286 (4), G521–527.

164 Liu AY, Zhang H, Sorensen CM *et al.* (2005) Analysis of prostate cancer by proteomics using tissue specimens. *J Urol* 173 (1), 73–78.

165 Wong YF, Cheung TH, Lo KW *et al.* (2004) Protein profiling of cervical cancer by protein-biochips: proteomic scoring to discriminate cervical cancer from normal cervix. *Cancer Lett* 211 (2), 227–234.

166 Wiesner A (2004) Detection of tumor markers with ProteinChip technology. *Curr Pharm Biotechnol* 5 (1), 45–67.

167 Steel LF, Shumpert D, Trotter M *et al.* (2003) A strategy for the comparative analysis of serum proteomes for the discovery of biomarkers for hepatocellular carcinoma. *Proteomics* 3 (5), 601–609.

168 Li C, Hong Y, Tan YX *et al.* (2004) Accurate qualitative and quantitative proteomic analysis of clinical hepatocellular carcinoma using laser capture microdissection coupled with isotope-coded affinity tag and two-dimensional liquid chromatography mass spectrometry. *Mol Cell Proteomics* 3 (4), 399–409.

169 Paradis V, Degos F, Dargere D *et al.* (2005) Identification of a new marker of hepatocellular carcinoma by serum protein profiling of patients with chronic liver diseases. *Hepatology* 41 (1), 40–47.

170 Chen J, Kahne T, Rocken C *et al.* (2004) Proteome analysis of gastric cancer metastasis by two-dimensional gel electrophoresis and matrix assisted laser desorption/ionization-mass spectrometry for identification of metastasis-related proteins. *J Proteome Res* 3 (5), 1009–1016.

171 She YM, Narindrasorasak S, Yang S *et al.* (2003) Identification of metal-binding proteins in human hepatoma lines by immobilized metal affinity chromatography and mass spectrometry. *Mol Cell Proteomics* 2 (12), 1306–1318.

172 Cho YM, Bae SH, Choi BK *et al.* (2003) Differential expression of the liver proteome in senescence accelerated mice. *Proteomics* 3 (10), 1883–1894.

173 Schnabl B, Purbeck CA, Choi YH *et al.* (2003) Replicative senescence of activated human hepatic stellate cells is accompanied by a pronounced inflammatory but less fibrogenic phenotype. *Hepatology* 37, 653–664.

174 Killion PJ, Sherlock G, Iyer VR (2003) The Longhorn Array Database (LAD): an open-source, MIAME compliant implementation of the Stanford Microarray Database (SMD). *BMC Bioinformatics* 4 (1), 32.

175 Mockler TC, Ecker JR (2005) Applications of DNA tiling arrays for whole-genome analysis. *Genomics* 85 (1), 1–15.

176 Rohner TC, Staab D, Stoeckli M (2005) MALDI mass spectrometric imaging of biological tissue sections. *Mech Ageing Dev* 126 (1), 177–185.

177 Maddalo G, Petrucci F, Iezzi M *et al.* (2005) Analytical assessment of MALDI-TOF imaging mass spectrometry on thin histological samples. An insight in proteome investigation. *Clin Chim Acta* 357, 210–218.

178 McDonnell LA, Piersma SR, MaartenAltelaar AF *et al.* (2005) Subcellular imaging mass spectrometry of brain tissue. *J Mass Spectrom* 40 (2), 160–168.

179 Borrebaeck CA, Ekstrom S, Hager AC *et al.* (2001) Protein chips based on recombinant antibody fragments: a highly sensitive approach

as detected by mass spectrometry. *Biotechniques* 30 (5), 1126–1130, 1132.

180 Kodadek T (2001) Protein microarrays: prospects and problems. *Chem Biol* 8 (2), 105–115.

181 Zhu H, Snyder M (2001) Protein arrays and microarrays. *Curr Opin Chem Biol* 5 (1), 40–45.

182 Walter G, Bussow K, Cahill D *et al.* (2000) Protein arrays for gene expression and molecular interaction screening. *Curr Opin Microbiol* 3 (3), 298–302.

183 Nagayama K (1997) Protein arrays: concepts and subjects. *Adv Biophys* 34, 3–23.

184 Belov L, de la Vega O, dos Remedios CG *et al.* (2001) Immunophenotyping of leukemias using a cluster of differentiation antibody microarray. *Cancer Res* 61 (11), 4483–4489.

185 Haab BB, Dunham MJ, Brown PO (2001) Protein microarrays for highly parallel detection and quantitation of specific proteins and antibodies in complex solutions. *Genome Biol* 2 (2), RESEARCH0004.

186 Hoos A, Urist MJ, Stojadinovic A *et al.* (2001) Validation of tissue microarrays for immunohistochemical profiling of cancer specimens using the example of human fibroblastic tumors. *Am J Pathol* 158 (4), 1245–1251.

187 Gillett CE, Springall RJ, Barnes DM *et al.* (2000) Multiple tissue core arrays in histopathology research: a validation study. *J Pathol* 192 (4), 549–553.

188 Ibarrola N, Pandey A (2001) Integrating DNA and tissue microarrays for cancer profiling. *Trends Biochem Sci* 26 (10), 589.

189 Andersen CL, Hostetter G, Grigoryan A *et al.* (2001) Improved procedure for fluorescence in situ hybridization on tissue microarrays. *Cytometry* 45 (2), 83–86.

190 Dhanasekaran SM, Barrette TR, Ghosh D *et al.* (2001) Delineation of prognostic biomarkers in prostate cancer. *Nature* 412 (6849), 822–826.

191 Moch H, Kononen T, Kallioniemi OP *et al.* (2001) Tissue micro-

arrays: what will they bring to molecular and anatomic pathology? *Adv Anat Pathol* 8 (1), 14–20.

192 Bigger CB, Guerra B, Brasky KM *et al.* (2004) Intrahepatic gene expression during chronic hepatitis C virus infection in chimpanzees. *J Virol* 78 (24), 13779–137792.

193 Shackel NA, McGuinness PH, Abbott CA *et al.* (2002) Insights into the pathobiology of hepatitis C virus associated cirrhosis: analysis of intrahepatic differential gene expression. *Am J Pathol* 160 (2), 641–654.

194 Girard S, Vossman E, Misek DE *et al.* (2004) Hepatitis C virus NS5A-regulated gene expression and signaling revealed via microarray and comparative promoter analyses. *Hepatology* 40 (3), 708–718.

195 Smith MW, Yue ZN, Geiss GK *et al.* (2003) Identification of novel tumor markers in hepatitis C virus-associated hepatocellular carcinoma. *Cancer Res* 63 (4), 859–864.

196 Kondoh N, Wakatsuki T, Ryo A *et al.* (1999) Identification and characterization of genes associated with human hepatocellular carcinogenesis. *Cancer Res* 59 (19), 4990–4996.

197 Yamashita T, Kaneko S, Hashimoto S *et al.* (2001) Serial analysis of gene expression in chronic hepatitis C and hepatocellular carcinoma. *Biochem Biophys Res Commun* 282 (2), 647–654.

198 Liu K, Lei XZ, Zhao LS *et al.* (2005) Tissue microarray for high-throughput analysis of gene expression profiles in hepatocellular carcinoma. *World J Gastroenterol* 11 (9), 1369–1372.

199 Kang YK, Hong SW, Lee H *et al.* (2004) Overexpression of clusterin in human hepatocellular carcinoma. *Hum Pathol* 35 (11), 1340–1346.

200 Tackels-Horne D, Goodman MD, Williams AJ *et al.* (2001) Identification of differentially expressed genes in hepatocellular carcinoma and metastatic liver tumors by oligonucleotide expression profiling. *Cancer* 92 (2), 395–405.

201 Obama K, Ura K, Satoh S *et al.* (2005) Up-regulation of PSF2, a member of the GINS multiprotein complex, in intrahepatic cholangiocarcinoma. *Oncol Rep* 14 (3), 701–706.

4 Pathology

4.1 Histological features

Valeer J. Desmet, Tania Roskams and Miguel Bruguera

Hepatocellular changes

The ground-glass hepatocyte [1] displays a more homogeneous, paler eosinophilic staining than the normal hepatocyte in all or part of its cytoplasm (see Plates 4.1.1 and 4.1.29, facing p. 72). It is most typically observed in carriers of hepatitis B virus (HBV), in whom its appearance is due to hypertrophy of the endoplasmic reticulum, loaded with HBsAg.

A more or less similar appearance of hepatocytes may be observed in drug induction, in myoclonal epilepsy (Lafora's disease), in alcoholics treated with aversion drugs (cyanamide) [2], in glycogenosis type 4 (Andersen's disease), in fibrinogen storage disease [3] and in immunosuppressed transplanted patients [4,5]. In HBV-infected patients, HBsAg can be demonstrated in ground-glass hepatocytes by special stains (Shikata's orcein stain, Victoria blue), immunohistochemical techniques, and regular and immunoelectron microscopy [6–8].

Acidophil condensation refers to a hepatocyte of reduced size, with increased density and eosinophilia of its cytoplasm, and usually pyknosis of the nucleus. The cell may assume a rhomboid outline [6,9].

Ballooning or hydropic swelling describes hepatocytes characterized by an increased volume with pale, 'empty' appearance of most of their cytoplasm; the remaining cytoplasm appears condensed in the perinuclear region (see Plates 4.1.2 and 4.1.8, facing p. 72). This lesion is thought to represent a precursor stage of lytic necrosis. It is observed in viral, toxic and ischaemic liver damage, predominantly in acinar zone 3 [6,9].

Alcoholic clear cells ('hépatite alcoolique à cellules claires' [10]) are enlarged and rounded hepatocytes with pale, rarefied cytoplasm; nuclei may be enlarged with prominent nucleoli. The cell borders are usually distinct, accentuated by pericellular fibrosis. Mallory bodies often occur in 'alcoholic clear cells' [7].

Feathery degeneration of hepatocytes is seen in cholestasis, mostly of longer duration. This lesion resembles 'hydropic swelling' with, in addition, bilirubin impregnation of the visible threads of cytoplasm. Ultrastructurally, such cells display whorls of membranous material, thought to result from intracellular membrane damage due to the detergent action of retained bile acids [11,12].

Alcoholic hyaline or Mallory body refers to an intracellular inclusion in hepatocytes, which are often pale and swollen (alcoholic clear cells). In its typical form, the Mallory body is an irregular, intensely eosinophilic mass (see Plate 4.1.3, facing p. 72). The lesion corresponds to clumps of aggregated cytokeratin filaments. Small Mallory bodies are better identified by immunostaining for cytokeratins.

The term alcoholic hyaline may be misleading because the lesion occurs in numerous other diseases besides alcoholic liver damage, especially in chronic cholestasis [13] and in non-alcoholic steatohepatitis.

In alcoholic liver disease, Mallory body-containing hepatocytes may be encircled by polymorphonuclear and/or mononuclear inflammatory cells; this lesion is known as satellitosis [7].

Megamitochondria (giant mitochondria) appear as round or cigar-shaped, intensely eosinophilic inclusions of variable size, up to the size of a nucleus (see Plate 4.1.3, facing p. 72); they are negative on periodic acid–Schiff (PAS)–diastase stained sections, in contrast to α_1-antitrypsin inclusions and phagolysosomes, with which they might be confused [7]. Their presence suggests a heavy alcohol consumption [14].

Mitochondriosis (oxyphil or oncocytic change) [15] corresponds to an increase in the number of mitochondria in hepatocytes, rendering the latter more granular and strongly eosinophilic than normal parenchymal cells. Oncocytic hepatocytes are often found in clusters.

Sanded nuclei [16] are hepatocellular nuclei stuffed with hepatitis B core particles causing peripheral margination of the chromatin. In light microscopy, the central part of the nucleus appears to be occupied by faintly eosinophilic, finely granular ('sand') material. They may be found in small numbers during the viral replicative phase of chronic viral hepatitis B. Sanded nuclei should not be confused with nuclear vacuolation [6,7].

Cytomegalovirus (CMV) inclusions may be found in all types of cells in the liver, most often in hepatocytes and bile duct cells. These are characterized by cytomegaly and the development of intranuclear basophilic inclusions, surrounded by a clear halo. The cytoplasm may be strongly basophilic. Appropriate immunostaining reveals CMV antigens [17].

Herpes simplex viral inclusions occur as two types. The more common type renders the nucleus homogeneously basophilic, with effacement of the nucleolus and most of the chromatin granules. The second type corresponds to the classic Cowdry type A inclusion: an eosinophilic, rounded or irregular inclusion surrounded by a clear halo with margination of the chromatin. Viral antigens can be identified by appropriate immunostaining [7,18].

Nuclear vacuolation corresponds to hepatocellular nuclei that appear empty on light microscopy. The vacuolation may be due to glycogen (e.g. in diabetics) or to invagination of cytoplasm or accumulation of lipid into the nucleus. This change is not very helpful in diagnosis [7,9,18].

Atrophy of hepatocytes is reflected in reduced size and increased cytoplasmic density and lipofuscin content of hepatocytes (see Plate 4.1.19, facing p. 72).

Hypoxic vacuoles are formed in anoxic conditions by invagination of the cell membrane of hepatocytes with engulfment of plasma proteins. They occur in acinar zone 3 and appear as pale-staining smaller or larger vacuoles. Appropriate immunostaining reveals the presence of albumin, fibrinogen and other plasma proteins. Electron microscopy shows that the membrane surrounding the vacuoles is not part of the endoplasmic reticulum, which differentiates the lesion from 'endoplasmic reticulum storage disorders' such as α_1-antitrypsin or fibrinogen storage [19].

Necrosis and inflammation

Acidophil body (single cell acidophil necrosis; coagulation necrosis) refers to a rounded clump of intensely eosinophilic cytoplasm, with or without a pyknotic nucleus, corresponding to necrosis of a single hepatocyte. The acidophil body is disconnected from the liver cell plate and becomes phagocytosed by Kupffer cells. The lesion is often incorrectly referred to as a Councilman (-like) body [6,9,18].

Apoptosis represents a physiological, preprogrammed mode of cell death, characterized by budding and fragmentation of a liver cell into smaller and larger 'acidophil bodies' (see Plates 4.1.2 and 4.1.4, facing p. 72). Apoptosis is an essential and vital component in liver development and growth, in physiology and in the most diverse pathological conditions. It is the way in which senescent cells are eliminated in normal liver; it plays a role in embryonic development of intrahepatic bile ducts, in regression of ductular reaction and in vanishing bile duct diseases. Apoptosis is part and parcel of focal necrosis and piecemeal necrosis in chronic hepatitis; it is a common feature in acute and fulminant hepatitis and in liver allograft rejection. Furthermore, apoptosis is a key phenomenon in several forms of toxic liver injury, in carcinogenesis and in the cell kinetics of hepatocellular carcinoma [20].

Coagulative necrosis is a form of cell death in which hepatocytes lose cohesion from surrounding cells and have a deeply eosinophilic cytoplasm. This change is typical of anoxic injury.

Lytic necrosis represents a mode of liver cell death followed by rapid disappearance of the dead cells; it is histologically recognized by lack of cells [21,22].

Confluent (lytic) necrosis refers to the disappearance of groups of contiguous hepatocytes, resulting in denudation of the reticulin framework. According to the extent of confluent necrosis, it is graded as focal or zonal, the latter occupying an entire acinar zone, usually zone 3, occasionally zone 1 (for example in severe viral hepatitis A).

Bridging hepatic necrosis represents more extensive degrees of confluent necrosis, leading to necrotic 'bridges' between adjacent vascular structures.

Central–central bridging necrosis links adjacent central veins; it corresponds to confluent necrosis in the microcirculatory periphery of a complex acinus [23].

Portal–central bridging necrosis links portal tracts and central veins; it corresponds to confluent necrosis in the microcirculatory periphery of the simple acinus.

Still higher degrees of confluent necrosis are described as panlobular, multilobular, submassive and massive necrosis [21,22].

Surgical necrosis [24] is observed in liver specimens taken during abdominal surgical interventions. It appears as acidophil necrosis of hepatocytes surrounded by neutrophil polymorphs (see Plate 4.1.5, facing p. 72). It is usually observed in acinar zone 3; the extent of the lesion increases with the duration of the operation and the degree of manipulation of the liver. This lesion is often observed after revascularization of the donor liver in liver transplantation.

Piecemeal necrosis occurs at the interface between mesenchyme (portal tracts or septa) and parenchyma (interface hepatitis). Mononuclear lymphoid cells infiltrate the mesenchyme and extend into the adjacent parenchyma, associated with progressive apoptotic cell death and disappearance of hepatocytes, thus leading to an unsharp mesenchymal–parenchymal border and gradual expansion of the mesenchymal area (see Plate 4.1.6, facing p. 72) [22].

Lymphocytic piecemeal necrosis represents the 'classic' lesion and is characterized by a predominance of lymphocytes and plasma cells (see Plate 4.1.6) [7,25].

Biliary piecemeal necrosis occurs in periportal (zone 1) locations in chronic biliary disease; it is characterized by cholate stasis of zone 1 hepatocytes, periportal ductular reaction and infiltration by inflammatory cells, including neutrophils. This lesion also creates an unsharp mesenchymal–parenchymal interphase, and thus resembles classic piecemeal necrosis architecturally, but not cytologically [7,9,25].

Fibrous piecemeal necrosis apparently represents a late stage of (biliary) piecemeal necrosis, in which connective tissue strands surround entrapped groups of hepatocytes with little cellular inflammation. Around portal tracts, it leads to the formation of new limiting plates that border seemingly enlarged portal tracts [25].

Ductular piecemeal necrosis describes a lesion that is close to biliary piecemeal necrosis, with less emphasis on periportal or paraseptal cholate stasis [25].

Liver cell rosettes [26] correspond to small groups of hepatocytes in lymphocytic or fibrous piecemeal necrosis; the cells appear hydropic and are often arranged around a central lumen [27] (see Plate 4.1.7, facing p. 72).

Focal necrosis describes cell death (usually apoptotic in nature) of a small group of hepatocytes, associated with local accumulation of mononuclear cells (lymphocytes, histiocytes); apoptotic liver cell fragments are not always identifiable between the infiltrating cells [9,28].

Spotty necrosis is virtually synonymous with focal necrosis, referring to involvement of single or very small groups of parenchymal cells (see Plate 4.1.4, facing p. 72) [9].

Emperipolesis refers to the intracellular location of a cell (usually a lymphocyte) inside a hepatocyte (see Plate 4.1.8, facing p. 72). The lymphocyte is often surrounded by a narrow clear halo. Peripolesis describes the close association between a lymphocyte and a hepatocyte; the former may be located in an indentation of the latter [7].

Biliary and cholestatic lesions

Parenchymal changes

In its histological meaning, the term cholestasis used to refer to a microscopically visible deposition of bilirubin in the liver tissue. In a strict sense, it corresponds to bilirubinostasis. As cholate stasis (see below) is another important parenchymal feature in chronic cholestatic conditions, it is more appropriate to replace the histological term cholestasis with the more precise term bilirubinostasis [7,29].

Hepatocellular bilirubinostasis corresponds to intracellular accumulation of bilirubin-stained granules in the parenchymal cells, especially in toxic cholestasis (e.g. resulting from drugs and endotoxinaemia) (see Plates 4.1.9 and 4.1.14, facing p. 72) [6,11].

Canalicular bilirubinostasis is recognized as inspissated bile plugs in more or less dilated intercellular bile canaliculi. It first occurs in acinar zone 3, but may extend up to acinar zone 1 in cholestasis of long duration (see Plate 4.1.9) [12].

Kupffer cell bilirubinostasis is represented by smaller and coarser bilirubin-stained inclusions in hypertrophic Kupffer cells. It is only observed in cholestasis of several days' duration (see Plate 4.1.9) [12].

Ductular bilirubinostasis corresponds to inspissated, bilirubin-stained concrements in more or less dilated bile ductules. It is occasionally seen in longstanding extrahepatic bile duct obstruction, especially in extrahepatic bile duct atresia in the neonate. It also occurs in severely necrotizing hepatitis [30]. In septicaemia, large bile concrements are formed in unusually dilated periportal ductules [31] (see Plate 4.1.10, facing p. 72).

Cholate stasis is a lesion of zone 1 hepatocytes in longlasting cholestasis [7,9,29]. The parenchymal cells are pale, swollen and coarsely granular. Some of the granules correspond to copper accumulation and stain with rhodamine (copper) and orcein or Victoria blue (copper-binding protein or metallothionein). Later on, bilirubin granules may also accumulate, and Mallory bodies may develop. The term cholate stasis refers to the presumed intracellular accumulation of bile salts as the suspected mechanism for this lesion.

The appearance of *cholestatic liver cell rosettes* [27] is a sign of longlasting cholestasis. It may be particularly pronounced in contraceptive steroid-induced cholestasis. Scattered through the parenchyma, groups of liver cells are arranged in a tubular fashion around a smaller or larger lumen, which may appear empty or filled with eosinophilic or bilirubin-stained material (see Plate 4.1.11, facing p. 72). The composing hepatocytes express bile duct-type cytokeratins, indicating an intermediate differentiation of these hepatocytes [29].

Xanthomatous cells (*foam cells*) occur as single cells or in clusters, in the parenchyma or portal tracts or both, in the case of longlasting cholestasis. They correspond to lipid-laden histiocytes, related to hyperlipidaemia and hypercholesterolaemia [32].

Bile infarct (*Charcot–Gombault infarct*) represents an area of paraportal necrosis of liver parenchyma; the central part of the necrotic zone, in particular, is impregnated with bilirubin (which has affinity for necrotic tissue) (see Plate 4.1.12, facing p. 72). With time, the necrotic mass becomes organized in a fibrous scar. This lesion is mainly (but not exclusively) observed in longstanding extrahepatic bile duct obstruction [32].

Bile lake refers to a large mass (larger than the usual extracellular bile plug of canalicular bilirubinostasis) in the parenchyma of a cholestatic liver [26,32].

Portal and periportal changes

Bile extravasates are mainly seen in the late stages of large duct obstruction; they represent inspissated bile concrements in ducts associated with erosion and necrosis of the epithelial lining of the duct. The bile mass in contact with portal connective tissue may incite a foreign body giant cell reaction.

Lymphocytic cholangitis [25] describes a normal or damaged portal bile duct in a dense lymphocytic infiltrate, sometimes organized as a lymph follicle (e.g. early primary biliary cirrhosis).

Pleomorphic cholangitis [25] refers to a normal or altered portal bile duct surrounded (or even infiltrated) by a mixed inflammatory infiltrate (e.g. in liver allograft rejection and graft-versus-host disease).

Granulomatous cholangitis [25] indicates the presence of a non-caseating epithelioid cell granuloma close to or around a damaged portal bile duct (e.g. in primary biliary cirrhosis and sarcoidosis with chronic cholestasis) (see Plate 4.1.13, facing p. 72). This lesion is also referred to as a florid bile duct lesion in primary biliary cirrhosis.

Fibro-obliterative cholangitis [25] corresponds to prominent layers of concentric dense connective tissue ('onion-skinning') around a portal bile duct, which may show features of atrophy and epithelial damage. The lesion indicates chronic irritation of the duct, but is not disease specific.

Purulent (suppurative) cholangitis [25] is characterized by the accumulation of polymorphs in the lumen and in the wall of bile ducts; destruction of the epithelial lining may proceed to the formation of cholangitic abscesses.

Paucity of intrahepatic bile ducts (ductopenia) is morphometrically defined as a portal bile duct to portal tract ratio of less than 0.5 (normal value 0.9–1.8) [33]. The disappearance of the ducts seems to result from pleomorphic cholangitis. The entity is part of the 'vanishing bile duct' disorders [34].

'Vanishing bile duct' disorders are recognized by the occurrence of portal tracts in which a portal bile duct of approximately the same size as the accompanying hepatic artery branch is missing [35]. These disorders include extrahepatic bile duct atresia, paucity of intrahepatic bile ducts, idiopathic adulthood ductopenia, primary biliary cirrhosis, autoimmune cholangiopathy, Hodgkin's disease, sarcoidosis with chronic cholestasis, primary sclerosing cholangitis, hepatic graft-versus-host disease, liver allograft rejection and some rare forms of prolonged drug-induced cholestasis [25,34].

The ductal plate is the primitive shape of intrahepatic bile ducts during embryonic development [34]. It corresponds to a partly double layer of bile duct epithelium around the primitive portal tracts (see Plate 4.1.14, facing p. 72). Its normal fate is to become remodelled into the normal network of portal bile ducts [36].

The ductal plate malformation represents a lack of remodelling of the embryonic ductal plate, with persistence of primitive bile duct structures [37]. It is observed in infantile polycystic disease, congenital hepatic fibrosis, Caroli's disease, Meckel syndrome and Von Meyenburg complexes (see Plate 4.1.15, facing p. 72). Ductal plate malformation associated with features of duct destruction and inflammation (pleomorphic cholangitis) is also part of early, severe forms of so-called extrahepatic bile duct atresia [34,38].

Ductular reaction ('cholangiolitis') refers to a periportal increase in the number of ductular profiles in histological sections. The ductules are accompanied by oedema and neutrophil polymorphs (inflammation of the ductules or cholangioles) (see Plate 4.1.16, facing p. 72). It is observed to a variable extent in all varieties of biliary disease [26,29,39].

In the case of acute, complete mechanical obstruction of larger bile ducts, the ductular reaction is mainly the result of ductular proliferation (so-called 'typical ductules', 'elongation type' of ductular proliferation or 'marginal bile duct proliferation') [40], resulting from multiplication of pre-existing ductules at the margin of portal tracts [39].

In the case of chronic, incomplete obstruction of larger bile ducts (e.g. in primary biliary cirrhosis, primary sclerosing cholangitis), the ductular reaction results from ductular

metaplasia of zone 1 hepatocytes and from activation, proliferation and differentiation of 'facultative stem cells' or progenitor cells (so-called 'atypical' or 'sprouting type' of ductular proliferation) [39].

Pericholangitis [41], reported as a hepatic complication of ulcerative colitis, corresponds to the 'isolated small duct sclerosing cholangitis' variant of primary sclerosing cholangitis [25].

Fibrosis

The term fibrosis indicates an increase in connective tissue in the liver; it may occur in various patterns.

Portal fibrosis describes increased density and fibrous enlargement of portal tracts.

Concentric periductal fibrosis is a synonym of fibro-(obliterating) cholangitis.

Periportal fibrosis refers to fibrous extensions radiating from portal tracts.

Centrolobular (acinar zone 3) fibrosis describes fibrous scarring around the terminal hepatic venules. When conspicuous, as in some forms of alcoholic liver disease, it has been described as 'sclerosing hyaline necrosis' [42].

Perivenular fibrosis [43] indicates a fibrous thickening of the wall of the terminal hepatic venule. The lesion comprises a fibrotic rim more than 4 mm in thickness involving at least two-thirds of the perimeter of hepatic venules.

In *pericellular or perisinusoidal fibrosis*, collagen is laid down around single liver cells or small groups of hepatocytes. It occurs mostly in acinar zone 3. In alcoholic liver disease, this pattern was described as 'chicken-wire fibrosis' [7,26].

Septal fibrosis indicates fibrosis in the form of fibrous sheets. It occurs in various topographical patterns (portal–portal septa, portal–central septa, central–central septa, incomplete septa, etc.) according to the type of vascular canals linked by the connective tissue membranes [22].

Active septa represent connective tissue sheets that are infiltrated by mononuclear inflammatory cells, with imprecise delineation from the adjacent parenchyma. They can be conceived as extensive degrees of piecemeal necrosis (see Plate 4.1.6, facing p. 72) [22].

Passive septa are fibrous membranes that are rich in fibres and poor in cells, with sharp delineation from the adjacent parenchyma (see Plate 4.1.17, facing p. 72). They derive from post-necrotic collapse and scarring after extensive confluent lytic necrosis [7,22]. Older (more than 6 months) passive septa contain elastic fibres, demonstrable by orcein or Victoria blue staining [44].

Primary collapse indicates post-necrotic collapse and scarring after confluent necrosis in a previously normal parenchyma; the topographical spacing of the approximated portal tracts and terminal hepatic veins is more or less preserved [9].

Secondary collapse refers to post-necrotic scarring following necrosis in abnormal parenchymal territories (e.g. in cirrhosis), resulting in irregular spacing of afferent and efferent vessels [9].

Hepatoportal sclerosis corresponds to phlebosclerosis of portal vein branches, as a result of organized mural thrombi or of portal hypertension, usually associated with some degree of portal and periportal fibrosis [7,9,12,26].

Biliary fibrosis is often confused with true biliary cirrhosis. It represents an advanced but potentially reversible state of chronic bile duct disease, characterized by periportal or portal–portal septa and garland-shaped parenchymal nodules; the basic lobular architecture and vascular relationships are preserved [9,25,29].

Cirrhosis is a diffuse type of septal fibrosis of the liver, associated with regenerative parenchymal nodules and disturbed intrahepatic circulation (see Chapter 7.1) [45].

Vascular changes

Hepatic artery

Obliterative endarteritis is a feature of chronic vascular rejection of a liver allograft. It consists of the obstruction of arteries by subintimal fibrosis or the accumulation of foamy lipid-loaded cells [12].

Afferent and efferent veins

Endothelialitis consists of lymphocytic infiltration of the portal or central vein endothelium, which appears to be damaged and lifted from its basement membrane. Endothelialitis is a helpful diagnostic feature in graft-versus-host disease and in acute liver allograft rejection [46].

Endophlebitis of the (terminal) hepatic veins consists of lymphocytic infiltration in the intima of the vessels. It is seen in acute (sub)massive necrosis in fulminant hepatitis. A lymphocytic phlebitis has been described in the (pre)cirrhotic stages of alcoholic liver disease [18].

Veno-occlusive disease corresponds to narrowing of the lumen of terminal hepatic venules and larger draining hepatic veins, due to subintimal fibrosis. First observed in bush tea intoxication (senecio and crotalaria alkaloids), it may result from several drugs, such as methotrexate and chemotherapy drugs used before a bone marrow transplantation, alcohol and irradiation [12,18,26].

Phlebosclerosis corresponds to fibrous thickening of the walls of veins, with or without an increase in elastic fibres. Phlebosclerosis of terminal hepatic venules occurs in several conditions, for example chronic passive congestion, alcoholic liver disease and graft-versus-host disease. Phlebosclerosis of portal vein branches is part of the lesion of hepatoportal sclerosis [12,18,26].

Prolapse of hepatocytes into terminal hepatic venules may result in partial occlusion and disruption of the wall of terminal hepatic venules. It has been reported in long-term anabolic–androgenic steroid therapy [18].

Sinusoids and the space of Disse

The space of Disse lies between the sinusoidal wall and the sinusoidal surface of the hepatocyte, from which abundant microvilli project into the space. The sinusoidal endothelium is discontinuous, extensively fenestrated and lacks a basement membrane. Therefore, the space of Disse is freely permeable to blood plasma and constitutes the immediate exchange area between blood and hepatocytes. The space of Disse contains collagen type 1 and 3, constituting the 'reticulin' framework of the liver. However, several other extracellular matrix components are also present, for instance collagen type 4, laminin and perlecan, in spite of the absence of a morphologically recognizable basement membrane.

Sinusoidal congestion occurs in acinar zone 3 as a result of venous outflow block; the sinusoids appear dilated and the parenchymal cells atrophic with pericellular fibrosis (see Plate 4.1.18, facing p. 72); all changes are variable according to the degree or duration, or both, of the venous congestion.

Sinusoidal dilatation in acinar zone 1 [47] may occur in patients using contraceptive steroids. It is often accompanied by slight perisinusoidal fibrosis in that area [48]. Sinusoidal dilatation lacking any particular zonal localization can be associated with neoplasms, mainly Hodgkin's disease, and granulomatous diseases [49].

Peliosis indicates irregular blood-filled cavities corresponding to sinusoidal dilatation without constant zonal topography. The dilatation may be huge, creating blood pools in which liver cells are missing [12,18,26].

Fibrin deposition in sinusoids is typically seen in acinar zone 1 in eclampsia (see Plate 4.1.19, facing p. 72) and in irregular topography in disseminated intravascular coagulopathy.

Capillarization of the sinusoids refers to important modifications of the space of Disse in fibrotic liver, as a morphologically distinct basement membrane-like structure appears, containing collagen type 4 and laminin. In addition, increased amounts of collagen types 1, 3, 5 and 6, fibronectin, tenascin and undulin are deposited along the sinusoids. These changes are associated with loss of fenestrations of endothelial cells, further impairing exchange between blood and hepatocytes [50]. Hepatic stellate cells (Ito cells) increase in number and acquire an activated myofibroblast-like phenotype.

Hairy cell leukaemia may produce a characteristic 'angiomatous' picture, consisting of dilated sinusoids lined by leukaemic cells that have replaced the sinusoidal lining cells. Hairy cells display a clear rim of cytoplasm and are positive for tartrate-resistant acid phosphatase and non-specific esterase [18].

Extramedullary haematopoiesis is recognized by the occurrence in sinusoids of clusters of haematopoietic precursor cells of the erythropoietic, granulopoietic and thrombopoietic series. Normoblasts and megakaryocytes are the most easily identifiable precursor cells [18].

Amyloidosis is characterized by the linear deposition of homogeneous eosinophilic material in vessel walls and in spaces of

Disse. Occasionally, globular deposition occurs. Advanced linear deposition of amyloid in parenchymal territories leads to atrophy of parenchymal cells. Amyloid is identified by the special stains Congo red and Sirius red, displaying characteristic green dichroism in polarized light [18].

Light chain (deposit) disease resembles amyloidosis with granular and fibrillar material in the spaces of Disse; the deposited material is PAS positive but does not stain as amyloid. Immunohistochemical stains for κ and λ light chains identify the deposits (see Plate 4.1.20, facing p. 72) [18].

Kupffer cell reaction and granuloma

Sinusoidal cell activation refers to excess sinusoidal cells, often of different type, including activated Kupffer cells and increased endothelial cells admixed with lymphocytes, monocytes and plasma cells [9].

Epithelioid granuloma. The term granuloma is not strictly defined; it refers to a focal accumulation of histiocytic cells, assuming epithelioid and multinucleated giant cell appearance in its most typical form (epithelioid granuloma). Histiocytic and epithelioid granulomas, with or without associated significant parenchymal inflammation (hepatitis), occur in numerous conditions [51].

Lipogranuloma describes the accumulation of histiocytes and mononuclear cells around a parenchymal cell with large droplet steatosis [47].

Mineral oil granulomas are a special form of foreign body granuloma, consisting of histiocytes and vacuolated macrophages around clear spaces (mineral oil deposits) in portal tracts and near terminal hepatic venules [18].

Doughnut granuloma (fibrin ring granuloma) has a characteristic appearance with a central empty-appearing fat globule surrounded by a collar of histiocytes sprinkled with some lymphocytes, neutrophils and sometimes eosinophils, and encircled by a ring of fibrin. Although highly characteristic of Q fever, this lesion is also observed in other conditions (for instance Hodgkin's disease, allopurinol hypersensitivity) [18].

Storage phenomena

Several metabolic diseases (storage diseases) are associated with deposition of metabolites in liver tissue [52]. Many of them require ultrastructural investigation for adequate identification. Their description is beyond the scope of this chapter.

Fat storage (steatosis, fatty metamorphosis) in hepatocytes is a feature common to numerous liver diseases. Neutral fat can be stained with oil red O or Sudan black in frozen sections; in paraffin-embedded tissue, fat appears as clear holes in parenchymal cells. The fat droplets may be small (microvesicular steatosis) with retained central position of the nucleus (see Plate 4.1.21, facing p. 72) or large (macrovesicular steatosis), in which case the nucleus is pushed to one side of the cell (see Plate 4.1.22, facing p. 72). The simultaneous presence of macro- and microvesicular steatosis indicates the presence of the inciting agent until the time of biopsy (e.g. alcohol abuse). Exclusive macrovesicular steatosis indicates a steady state of fat overload. Some special conditions with almost exclusive microvesicular steatosis have been emphasized (microvesicular fat diseases) [53], including Reye syndrome, acute fatty liver of pregnancy, Jamaican vomiting sickness and tetracycline and valproate intoxication.

Acute alcoholic foamy degeneration is a type of severe alcoholic liver damage with nearly exclusive microvesicular steatosis [54].

Morula cells or spongiocytes correspond to hepatocytes with microvesicular steatosis, observed in Labrea fever in the Amazon river basin, which appears to represent delta hepatitis superinfection of HBV carriers [9,55], perhaps by a more pathogenic strain [56].

Phospholipidosis is reflected in light microscopy in very small clear droplets and eosinophilic fine granules, often associated with Mallory bodies in some drug reactions (amiodarone, perhexiline maleate) [9,18].

Hepatic stellate cell hyperplasia (Ito cell hyperplasia) is recognized by an increased number of hepatic stellate cells (Ito cells, perisinusoidal cells); they appear as sinusoidal cells containing smaller or larger fat droplets indenting the nucleus (see Plate 23, facing p. 72). It is a diagnostic feature of vitamin A intoxication [8].

Iron storage (siderosis) is reflected in the accumulation of Prussian blue-positive haemosiderin granules in hepatocytes (parenchymal siderosis) (see Plate 4.1.24, facing p. 72) and/or in Kupffer cells and macrophages (reticuloendothelial siderosis) (see Plate 4.1.25, facing p. 72).

Copper storage is recognized by the accumulation of intrahepatocellular granules that stain positively with rhodamine (copper) and orcein or Victoria blue (copper-binding protein or metallothionein) [12,26].

Glycogen storage is reflected by a clear appearance of enlarged hepatocytes with accentuated cell walls (plant cell-like appearance), often associated with glycogen vacuolation of the nucleus [52].

α_1-*Antitrypsin storage* in the endoplasmic reticulum appears as eosinophilic inclusions of variable size in zone 1 hepatocytes. The inclusions are strongly PAS positive and diastase resistant (see Plate 4.1.26, facing p. 72), and can be identified by immunohistochemical stains and electron microscopy [52].

Fibrinogen storage may take the appearance of eosinophilic inclusions (resembling α_1-antitrypsin inclusions) or of ground-glass hepatocytes. The fibrinogen nature of the inclusions is ascertained by immunohistochemical staining [57].

Lipofuscin (wear and tear pigment) appears as brownish pericanalicular granules in acinar zone 3 hepatocytes, which represent the ageing cells of the liver acinus. The amount of lipofuscin may increase (lipofuscinosis), for example in abuse of analgesics.

The pigment in Dubin–Johnson syndrome (see Plate 4.1.27,

facing p. 72) resembles lipofuscinosis. The nature of this pigment (possibly melanin) is still debated [58].

Malaria pigment accumulates as dark granules in Kupffer cells in chronic malaria and schistosomiasis. The pigment is Prussian blue negative and birefringent in polarized light [18].

Ceroid pigment is an ill-defined material, appearing as granules and coarse clumps in hypertrophic Kupffer cells and macrophages ('ceroid macrophages') in all conditions associated with hepatocellular necrosis. The material represents phagocytosed debris from necrotizing liver cells. Ceroid macrophages thus attest to liver cell damage. They lie in the parenchyma in the early stages and migrate to portal tracts later on. Ceroid pigment is PAS positive, diastase resistant, stains partly with fat stains and is fluorescent under ultraviolet light.

Erythropoietic protoporphyria causes deposition of protoporphyrin as dark granules in hepatocytes and Kupffer cells and larger clumps of black material in dilated canaliculi and ductules. Under polarized light, the material is birefringent (appearing red in Maltese cross configuration in the larger deposits) and autofluorescent under ultraviolet light (see Plate 4.1.28, facing p. 72) [18].

Uroporphyrin crystals accumulate in hepatocytes in porphyria cutanea tarda. Difficult to recognize on haematoxylin- and eosin-stained sections, they are best visualized in unstained sections examined by polarizing microscopy (birefringence) or under ultraviolet light (red autofluorescence) [18].

Foreign material which may be stored in Kupffer cells includes talc, cellulose (in drug abusers), silica and anthracitic pigment (in coal workers), polyvinyl pyrrolidone (from plasma expanders), silicone (for instance from prosthetic heart valve devices) and thorotrast (a former contrast medium) [18].

Hepatitis (inflammation)

The term *liver cell pleomorphism* summarizes the complex set of histological changes of the liver parenchyma in several forms of acute viral- and drug-induced hepatitis (ballooning, acidophil condensation, apoptosis, regeneration). It is usually most marked in acinar zone 3 (see Plates 4.1.2 and 4.1.8, facing p. 72) [6].

Lobular disarray refers to the disruption of the normal regular arrangement of liver cell plates caused by liver cell pleomorphism and focal necrosis in acute hepatitis (see Plate 4.1.2 facing p. 72) [9].

Acute hepatitis is characterized by mononuclear cell infiltration in portal tracts (portal hepatitis) and in the parenchyma, associated with signs of parenchymal damage (see Plates 4.1.2 and 4.1.8, facing p. 72). The last depends on the severity of the hepatitis, corresponding to lobular disarray, liver cell pleomorphism and spotty necrosis in milder forms and various extents of confluent necrosis in severe cases [6].

Portal hepatitis refers to mononuclear cell infiltration in portal tracts. Portal hepatitis without significant parenchymal damage is the hallmark of mild chronic hepatitis, although of itself, it is a non-specific lesion [22].

Periportal hepatitis describes necroinflammatory changes in acinar zone 1 parenchyma around the portal tracts. It is a feature of viral hepatitis A. As a morphological descriptive term, it also refers to piecemeal necrosis (e.g. in moderate and severe chronic hepatitis) [59].

Central (centrolobular) hepatitis refers to necroinflammatory lesions in acinar zone 3.

Non-specific reactive hepatitis indicates mild inflammatory changes, combining portal hepatitis and mild focal necrosis without a demonstrable causative agent in the liver. It is observed in systemic and extrahepatic diseases, apparently due to circulating toxins and breakdown products [9,60].

Chronic lobular hepatitis is not a morphological entity. Histologically, it corresponds to a picture of mild acute hepatitis. The notion of chronicity relies on the clinical history [9,26].

Hepatitis B can be recognized in several cases by the presence of ground-glass hepatocytes. In acute episodes, liver cell pleomorphism is often marked, and hepatocyte degeneration tends to be of a ballooning or lytic type and is localized in acinar zone 3.

Features suggestive of *hepatitis C* include portal lymphoid aggregates or lymph follicles, bile duct damage, intra-acinar necroinflammatory changes with numerous apoptotic bodies, some steatosis and a mild degree of piecemeal necrosis [61].

Hepatitis D superinfection of chronic hepatitis B is usually characterized by severe lobular lesions with extensive piecemeal necrosis and rapid progression to cirrhosis. Marked panacinar inflammation with a morphology similar to hepatitis C is typical [62,63]. 'Morula cells' (hepatocytes with microvesicular steatosis) have been described in some instances [64].

Fibrosing cholestatic hepatitis, a peculiar morphological pattern of hepatitis B, was first observed after liver transplantation [65]. It is characterized by unusually high-level expression of intracytoplasmic HBsAg and HBcAg associated with only mild necrosis and inflammation. In addition, there is severe bilirubinostasis and a characteristic perisinusoidal fibrosis, encasing groups of liver cells or entire liver cell plates. It is apparently related to the immunosuppressed state of the patient, as it has also been reported in coinfection by HBV and human immunodeficiency virus (HIV) [66] and in renal transplant recipients [67,68].

Drug-induced chronic hepatitis can be suspected in some cases from the presence of small granulomas, eosinophilic infiltration and bile duct damage involving the finest biliary radicles.

Autoimmune hepatitis admittedly has no specific histopathology; however, a picture of severely active hepatitis including extensive piecemeal necrosis, bridging confluent necrosis, hepatitic liver cell rosettes and abundance of plasma cells is quite suggestive.

Wilson's disease is the result of tissue injury due to copper overload in the liver and other organs. Clinically as well as histopathologically, it may manifest itself as acute hepatitis mimicking acute viral hepatitis, as fulminant hepatitis, as chronic hepatitis indistinguishable from that due to viral and other aetiologies or as cirrhosis. Helpful differential clues in the diagnosis of Wilson's disease include the presence of steatosis, glycogenated nuclei, the presence of Mallory bodies in periportal liver cells and moderate to marked copper storage (best seen on rhodamine stain).

α₁-Antitrypsin deficiency can histologically resemble chronic hepatitis of viral and other aetiologies. Recently, a high prevalence of hepatotrophic viral infection (HCV and HBV) has been documented in predominantly heterozygote patients with chronic liver disease [69]. However, other studies suggest that α₁-antitrypsin deficiency *per se* may be the cause of chronic liver disease [70].

Immunohistochemical stains (immunofluorescence and immunoperoxidase methods) are based on the binding of antibodies to specific antigens in tissue sections. Several procedures are available, the two most commonly used at present being the peroxidase–antiperoxidase immune complex method and the biotin–avidin immunoenzymatic technique. In the latter procedure, the high affinity of avidin for biotin is used to couple the peroxidase label to the primary antibody. Their use in demonstrating viral antigens has enormously increased the diagnostic impact of liver biopsy in confirming or establishing the viral aetiology of hepatitis. Some of the most frequently used are for hepatitis B (HBsAg, HBcAg), C and D, herpes and cytomegalovirus. Demonstration of HBsAg and HBcAg on paraffin sections of liver biopsies from patients with chronic hepatitis B is helpful in determining whether the patient is still in the viral replicative phase, and hence a potential candidate for interferon therapy, or whether the patient has already evolved into the so-called viral integration phase [63].

In situ hybridization finds increasing application in diagnostic pathology in general [71]. It is applied to liver tissue for the assessment of viral replication in hepatitis A, B, C and D, cytomegalovirus hepatitis and Epstein–Barr viral hepatitis [72]. Combination of the *polymerase chain reaction* with *in situ* hybridization becomes possible, providing the pathologist with an extremely sensitive detection method.

Acute alcoholic hepatitis (*acute hepatitis of the alcoholic type, fatty liver hepatitis, steatohepatitis*) comprises several changes; there is no general agreement on minimum requirements. Usually, the histological changes comprise steatosis, Mallory bodies and satellitosis. In most cases, some degree of fibrosis (periportal, pericentral, pericellular) is also present. In the face of continuing alcohol abuse, the lesions may persist in the cirrhotic stage. It must be realized that, in a minority of cases, this lesion is not due to alcohol (e.g. diabetes and obesity, amiodarone and perhexiline maleate toxicity, abetalipoproteinaemia) [7,18] (see also Chapters 12.3 and 13).

Regeneration

Parenchymal giant cells (*multinucleated hepatocytes*) correspond to huge, often pale parenchymal cells with multiple nuclei; they result from fusion rather than from incomplete division of hepatocytes. They occur most typically in neonatal cholestasis (so-called neonatal hepatitis and bile duct atresia), but are occasionally observed in adults, for example in viral hepatitis C and some forms of drug-induced hepatitis [9].

Anisokaryosis refers to unequal size of the liver cell nuclei. It increases with advancing age, due to increasing ploidy of liver cell nuclei.

Liver cell dysplasia (*dysplastic liver cells*) [73] usually occurs in groups of hepatocytes. They are characterized by unequal size and shape and increased staining density (hyperchromatism) of their nuclei (see Plate 4.1.29, facing p. 72). Dysplasia seems to be related to HBV and HCV infection [74]; its presence heralds an increased risk of hepatocellular carcinoma [75]. Two types of liver cell dysplasia, small cell dysplasia and large cell dysplasia, are recognized.

Twin-cell plates. In the normal liver beyond the age of 5 years, hepatocytes are arranged in single-cell plates (muralium simplex). Plates of two or more cells in thickness (muralium duplex or multiplex) indicate regeneration (see Plate 4.1.17, facing p. 72).

Nodular regeneration refers to regenerative expansion of smaller or larger parenchymal territories.

Micronodules are conventionally defined as 3 mm or less in diameter. They comprise regenerative parenchymal masses that may correspond to different parts or combinations of architectural liver units, as follows [12,18,26,45]:
1 segments of simple acini dissected by portal–central septa (pseudolobular nodules without vascular landmarks);
2 segments of simple acini encircled by portal–portal septa, carrying a central draining venule (monolobular nodules in biliary fibrosis and cirrhosis);
3 complex acini delineated by central–central septa and centred by a portal tract (in congestive or cardiac cirrhosis).

Macronodules (more than 3 mm in diameter) consist of large areas of parenchyma equivalent to several acini, presumably regenerating acinar agglomerates (multilobular nodules). A macronodule reveals a substructure, identified by draining veins, often in excess of portal tracts, which may appear diminutive; these anatomical landmarks show a less regular distribution than in normal liver parenchyma [12,18,26,45].

Nodular regenerative hyperplasia is characterized by diffuse nodularity of the liver parenchyma, due to regeneration and hyperplasia of acinar zones 1 and 2, associated with parenchymal atrophy and compression in the intervening acinar zones 3, without obvious internodular septum formation [12,18,26].

References

1 Hadziyannis S, Gerber MA, Vissoulis C *et al.* (1973) Cytoplasmic hepatitis B antigen in 'ground-glass' hepatocytes of carriers. *Arch Pathol* 96, 327–330.
2 Bruguera M, Lamar C, Bernet M, Rodes J (1986) Hepatic disease associated with ground-glass inclusions in hepatocytes after cyanamide therapy. *Arch Pathol Lab Med* 110, 906–910.

3 Callea F, de Vos R, Togni R et al. (1986) Fibrinogen inclusions in liver cells: a new type of ground-glass hepatocyte. Immune light and electron microscopic characterization. *Histopathology* 10, 65–73.

4 Wisell J, Boitnott J, Haas M et al. (2006) Glycogen pseudoground glass change in hepatocytes. *Am J Surg Pathol* 30, 1085–1090.

5 Lefkowitch JH, Lobritto SJ, Brown RS Jr et al. (2006) Ground-glass, polyglucosan-like hepatocellular inclusions: A 'new' diagnostic entity. *Gastroenterology* 131, 713–718.

6 Bianchi L (1983) Liver biopsy interpretation in hepatitis. Part II: histopathology and classification of acute and chronic viral hepatitis/differential diagnosis. *Pathol Res Pract* 178, 180–213.

7 Bianchi L (1983) Liver biopsy interpretation in hepatitis. Part I. Presentation of critical morphologic features used in diagnosis (Glossary). *Pathol Res Pract* 178, 2–19.

8 Phillips MJ, Poucell S, Patterson J et al. (1987) *The Liver. An Atlas and Text of Ultrastructural Pathology.* New York: Raven Press, p. 524.

9 Popper H (1986) General pathology of the liver: light microscopic aspects serving diagnosis and interpretation. *Semin Liver Dis* 6, 175–184.

10 Albot G, Schlumberger CS, Faye CM et al. (1956) Enlarged liver in alcoholics: biological formula and two histological aspects. *Sem Hop* 32, 1705–1722.

11 Desmet VJ (1986) Current problems in diagnosis of biliary disease and cholestasis. *Semin Liver Dis* 6, 233–245.

12 MacSween RNM, Anthony PP, Scheuer PJ et al. (1994) *Pathology of the Liver.* Edinburgh: Churchill Livingstone.

13 Desmet VJ (1985) Alcoholic liver disease. Histological features and evolution. *Acta Med Scand Suppl* 703, 111–126.

14 Bruguera M, Bertran A, Bombi JA et al. (1977) Giant mitochondria in hepatocytes: a diagnostic hint for alcoholic liver disease. *Gastroenterology* 73, 1383–1387.

15 Lefkowitch JH, Arborgh BA, Scheuer PJ (1980) Oxyphilic granular hepatocytes. Mitochondrion-rich liver cells in hepatic disease. *Am J Clin Pathol* 74, 432–441.

16 Bianchi L, Gudat F (1976) Sanded nuclei in hepatitis B: eosinophilic inclusions in liver cell nuclei due to excess in hepatitis B core antigen formation. *Lab Invest* 35, 1–5.

17 Vanstapel MJ, Desmet VJ (1983) Cytomegalovirus hepatitis: a histological and immunohistochemical study. *Appl Pathol* 1, 41–49.

18 Ishak KG (1987) New developments in diagnostic liver pathology. In: Farber E, Phillips MJ, Kaufman N (eds) *Pathogenesis of Liver Diseases.* Baltimore: Williams & Wilkins, pp. 223–373.

19 Nakanuma Y, Ohta G, Matsubara F et al. (1982) Cytoplasmic blood plasma inclusions in human hepatocytes. *Liver* 2, 212–221.

20 Patel T, Gores GJ (1995) Apoptosis and hepatobiliary disease. *Hepatology* 21, 1725–1741.

21 Bianchi L (1986) Necroinflammatory liver diseases. *Semin Liver Dis* 6, 185–198.

22 International Group (1977) Acute and chronic hepatitis revisited. *Lancet* ii, 914–919.

23 Desmet VJ (1988) Liver lesions in hepatitis B viral infection. *Yale J Biol Med* 61, 61–83.

24 Christoffersen P, Poulsen H, Skeie E (1970) Focal liver cell necroses accompanied by infiltration of granulocytes arising during operation. *Acta Hepatosplenol* 17, 240–245.

25 Ludwig J (1987) New concepts in biliary cirrhosis. *Semin Liver Dis* 7, 293–301.

26 Scheuer PJ, Lefkowitch JH (1994) *Liver Biopsy Interpretation,* 5th edn. London: WB Saunders.

27 Nagore N, Howe S, Boxer L et al. (1989) Liver cell rosettes: structural differences in cholestasis and hepatitis. *Liver* 9, 43–51.

28 Desmet VJ, De Vos R (1984) Structural analysis of acute liver injury. In: Keppler D, Bianchi L, Reutter W (eds) *Mechanisms of Hepatocyte Injury and Death.* Lancaster: MTP Press, pp. 11–30.

29 Desmet VJ (1986) Current problems in diagnosis of biliary disease and cholestasis. *Semin Liver Dis* 6, 233–245.

30 Schmid M, Cueni B (1972) Portal lesions in viral hepatitis with submassive hepatic necrosis. *Hum Pathol* 3, 209–216.

31 Lefkowitch JH (1982) Bile ductular cholestasis: an ominous histopathologic sign related to sepsis and 'cholangitis lenta'. *Hum Pathol* 13, 19–24.

32 International Group (1983) Histopathology of the intrahepatic biliary tree. *Liver* 3, 161–175.

33 Alagille D, Odievre M, Gautier M et al. (1975) Hepatic ductular hypoplasia associated with characteristic facies, vertebral malformations, retarded physical, mental, and sexual development, and cardiac murmur. *J Pediatr* 86, 63–71.

34 Desmet VJ (1987) Cholangiopathies: past, present and future. *Semin Liver Dis* 7, 67–76.

35 Nakanuma Y, Ohta G (1979) Histometric and serial section observations of the intrahepatic bile ducts in primary biliary cirrhosis. *Gastroenterology* 76, 1326–1332.

36 Van Eyken P, Sciot R, Callea F et al. (1988) The development of the intrahepatic bile ducts in man: a keratin-immunohistochemical study. *Hepatology* 8, 1586–1595.

37 Jorgensen MJ (1977) The ductal plate malformation. *Acta Pathol Microbiol Scand Suppl* 257, 1–87.

38 Desmet VJ, Callea F (1996) Cholestatic syndromes of infancy and childhood. In: Zakim D, Boyer TD (eds) *Hepatology. A Textbook of Liver Disease,* Vol. 2, 3rd edn. Philadelphia: WB Saunders, pp. 1649–1698.

39 Desmet V, Roskams T, Van Eyken P (1995) Ductular reaction in the liver. *Pathol Res Pract* 191, 513–524.

40 Christoffersen P, Poulsen H (1970) Histological changes in human liver biopsies following extrahepatic biliary obstruction. *Acta Pathol Microbiol Scand Suppl* 212(Suppl.), 150.

41 Mistilis SP (1965) Pericholangitis and ulcerative colitis. I. Pathology, etiology, and pathogenesis. *Ann Intern Med* 63, 1–16.

42 Edmondson HA, Peters RL, Reynolds TB et al. (1963) Sclerosing hyaline necrosis of the liver in the chronic alcoholic. A recognizable clinical syndrome. *Ann Intern Med* 59, 646–673.

43 Van Waes L, Lieber CS (1977) Early perivenular sclerosis in alcoholic fatty liver: an index of progressive liver injury. *Gastroenterology* 73, 646–650.

44 Scheuer PJ, Maggi G (1980) Hepatic fibrosis and collapse: histological distinction by orecin staining. *Histopathology* 4, 487–490.

45 Anthony PP, Ishak KG, Nayak NC et al. (1978) The morphology of cirrhosis. *J Clin Pathol* 31, 395–414.

46 Snover DC, Freese DK, Sharp HL et al. (1987) Liver allograft rejection. An analysis of the use of biopsy in determining outcome of rejection. *Am J Surg Pathol* 11, 1–10.

47 Poulsen H, Christoffersen P (1979) *Atlas of Liver Biopsies.* Copenhagen: Munksgaard.

48 Winkler K, Poulsen H (1975) Liver disease with periportal sinusoidal dilatation. A possible complication to contraceptive steroids. *Scand J Gastroenterol* 10, 699–704.

49 Bruguera M, Aranguibel F, Ros E et al. (1978) Incidence and clinical significance of sinusoidal dilatation in liver biopsies. *Gastroenterology* 75, 474–478.

50 Martinez-Hernandez A, Martinez J (1991) The role of capillarization in hepatic failure: studies in carbon tetrachloride-induced cirrhosis. *Hepatology* 14, 864–874.

51 Denk H, Scheuer PJ, Baptista A *et al.* (1994) Guidelines for the diagnosis and interpretation of hepatic granulomas. *Histopathology* 25, 209–218.

52 Ishak KG (1986) Hepatic morphology in the inherited metabolic diseases. *Semin Liver Dis* 6, 246–258.

53 Sherlock S (1983) Acute fatty liver of pregnancy and the microvesicular fat diseases. *Gut* 24, 265–269.

54 Uchida T, Kao H, Quispe-Sjogren M *et al.* (1983) Alcoholic foamy degeneration – a pattern of acute alcoholic injury of the liver. *Gastroenterology* 84, 683–692.

55 Buitrago B, Popper H, Hadler SC *et al.* (1986) Specific histologic features of Santa Marta hepatitis: a severe form of hepatitis delta-virus infection in northern South America. *Hepatology* 6, 1285–1291.

56 Parana R, Gerard F, Lesbordes JL *et al.* (1995) Serial transmission of spongiocytic hepatitis to woodchucks (possible association with a specific delta strain). *J Hepatol* 22, 468–473.

57 Callea F (1987) In: Lowe GDO *et al.* (eds) *Fibrinogen 2, Biochemistry, Physiology and Clinical Relevance.* Amsterdam: Elsevier Science Publishers (Biomedical Division), p. 75.

58 Kitamura T, Alroy J, Gatmaitan Z *et al.* (1992) Defective biliary excretion of epinephrine metabolites in mutant (TR-) rats: relation to the pathogenesis of black liver in the Dubin-Johnson syndrome and Corriedale sheep with an analogous excretory defect. *Hepatology* 15, 1154–1159.

59 Baptista A, Bianchi L, De Groote J *et al.* (1988) The diagnostic significance of periportal hepatic necrosis and inflammation. *Histopathology* 12, 569–579.

60 Gerber MA, Thung SN (1987) Histology of the liver. *Am J Surg Pathol* 11, 709–722.

61 Dhillon AP, Dusheiko GM (1995) Pathology of hepatitis C virus infection. *Histopathology* 26, 297–309.

62 Bianchi L, Gudat F (1994) Chronic hepatitis. In: MacSween RNM, Anthony PP, Scheuer PJ *et al.* (eds) *Pathology of the Liver*, 3rd edn. Edinburgh: Churchill Livingstone, pp. 349–395.

63 Desmet VJ (1991) Immunopathology of chronic viral hepatitis. *Hepato-Gastroenterology* 38, 14–21.

64 Buitrago B, Popper H, Hadler SC *et al.* (1986) Specific histologic features of Santa Marta hepatitis. A severe form of hepatitis delta-virus infection in northern South America. *Hepatology* 6, 1285.

65 Davies SE, Portmann BC, O'Grady JG *et al.* (1991) Hepatic histological findings after transplantation for chronic hepatitis B virus infection, including a unique pattern of fibrosing cholestatic hepatitis. *Hepatology* 13, 150–157.

66 Fang JW, Wright TL, Lau JY (1993) Fibrosing cholestatic hepatitis in patient with HIV and hepatitis B. *Lancet* 342, 1175.

67 Chen CH, Chen PJ, Chu JS *et al.* (1994) Fibrosing cholestatic hepatitis in a hepatitis B surface antigen carrier after renal transplantation. *Gastroenterology* 107, 1514–1518.

68 Booth JC, Goldin RD, Brown JL *et al.* (1995) Fibrosing cholestatic hepatitis in a renal transplant recipient associated with the hepatitis B virus precore mutant. *J Hepatol* 22, 500–503.

69 Propst T, Propst A, Dietze O (1992) High prevalence of viral infection in adults with homozygous and heterozygous a1-antitrypsin deficiency and chronic liver disease. *Ann Intern Med* 117, 641–645.

70 Geller SA, Nichols WS, Kim S *et al.* (1994) Hepatocarcinogenesis is the sequel to hepatitis in Z#2 alpha 1-antitrypsin transgenic mice: histopathological and DNA ploidy studies. *Hepatology* 19, 389–397.

71 Crocker J (1994) *Molecular Biology in Histopathology.* Chichester: John Wiley & Sons.

72 Desmet V, Fevery J (1995) Liver biopsy. *Baillières Clin Gastroenterol* 9, 811–828.

73 Anthony PP, Vogel CL, Barker LF (1973) Liver cell dysplasia: a premalignant condition. *J Clin Pathol* 26, 217–223.

74 Lefkowitch JH, Schiff ER, Davis GL *et al.* (1993) Pathological diagnosis of chronic hepatitis C: a multicenter comparative study with chronic hepatitis B. *Gastroenterology* 104, 595–603.

75 Borzio M, Bruno S, Roncalli M *et al.* (1995) Liver cell dysplasia is a major risk factor for hepatocellular carcinoma in cirrhosis: a prospective study. *Gastroenterology* 108, 812–817.

4.2 Classifications, scoring systems and morphometry in liver pathology

Pierre Bedossa and Valerie Paradis

The changing pattern of liver biopsy reports: from a detailed analytical report to classification and scoring systems

Liver biopsy is a useful diagnostic tool for the hepatologist [1]. It can assess the effects of a noxious agent on the liver at a level of detail that cannot be reached by any other means including imaging techniques [2]. In addition to providing help in diagnosis or establishing the aetiology of a liver disease (complementary to clinical, biological and serological data), liver biopsy provides valuable information about the intensity of parenchymal destruction or any other direct effect of the noxious agent that governs the immediate prognosis. It also provides information about lobular disorganization and architectural disturbance that is of major importance for long-term prognosis in chronic liver diseases. All these data are usually put together in a comprehensive and detailed biopsy report, and some of them should also be included in an easily accessible and more understandable manner for the hepatologist, namely a scoring system. The development of efficient treatment in chronic liver diseases has also stimulated pathologists, in close association with hepatologists, to develop classifications and scoring systems that summarize the most important lesions in a standardized form, providing a useful tool for treatment decisions and for assessing treatment efficacy. However, these scoring systems should not replace an analytical biopsy report but must complement and summarize in a concise and easy-to-access manner those features of importance.

Advantages of scoring liver biopsy

Dissection of the mental process that leads the pathologist to the elaboration of a histopathologic diagnosis gives some clues to the advantages and limits of scoring systems. When evaluating a liver biopsy, the first step is the identification of elementary histopathologic features (steatosis, Mallory bodies, hyaline bodies, apoptotic bodies, etc.). Once recognized, these features must be quantified (percentage, semi-quantification). Then, these lesions have to be integrated into a pathological diagnosis according to clinical and biological data. In order to achieve these goals, the pathologist needs experience in shape recognition, objectivity for quantification and guidelines to integrate the features into a diagnosis. Scoring systems can provide the pathologist with the objectivity to score lesions and the guidelines to make a diagnosis. By providing clear and detailed descriptions for each each elementary lesion and details on how to associate them, any pathologist should, in theory, be able to recognize a particular lesion and evaluate it. That is probably why histological scores have been adopted so widely; there is no chronic liver disease for which a scoring system has not been proposed, including chronic viral hepatitis, cholestatic liver diseases, alcoholic steatohepatitis (ASH) and non-alcoholic steatohepatitis (NASH), iron overload and even cancerous and precancerous lesions.

A scoring system provides major advantages both for cohort studies and also for individuals:

• Scores are very useful for cohort studies. Scoring a disease allows standardization of lesion evaluation that increases the reliability of multicentre studies. By categorizing patients into homogeneous groups with the same extent and severity of a disease, scoring adds to the validity of large multicentric epidemiological studies or clinical trials.

• In clinical practice and at the level of individual patients, scoring systems are very useful to support medical decisions. The best example is the simplification of treatment decisions provided by scores of chronic viral hepatitis. In addition, scoring liver damage allows the follow-up of the disease progression in a given patient spontaneously or under treatment. The semi-quantification provided by scores renders the comparison of biopsies performed in the same patient easier than comparing detailed reports.

• A score makes a liver biopsy report more accessible to non-specialized physicians and also to non-specialized pathologists. A score is easier to understand than a formal report: it does not require knowledge of the underlying liver histopathology.

- Finally, numerical scores are also very useful for setting up and validating surrogate markers, and it must be borne in mind that non-invasive markers of fibrosis are ultimately surrogates of histological scores.

In this context, it is important to emphasize that although scoring simplifies statistical calculations, restrictions do apply. Even when expressed in numerical values, scores are only semi-quantitative categorical data and not continuous variables. Although they refer to the progression in the severity of a histopathological feature or of a group of features, scores should not be used as quantitative variables in statistical analysis.

Limitations of scoring systems in liver biopsies

Although very useful, scoring systems have some drawbacks that have to be borne in the minds of both clinicians and pathologists. Some are related to the liver biopsy procedure itself while others are related directly to scoring systems.

Scores and sampling variability

Even for chronic diseases supposed to be diffuse within the liver, sampling variability remains a major drawback and sampling error strongly influences the performance of a scoring system. Sampling variability refers to the possible heterogeneous distribution of a histopathological feature within the liver. A liver biopsy represents a very limited part (<0.0001–0.00002%) of the whole organ. Such a tiny piece might give a wrong reflection of any lesion if this feature is not uniformly distributed in the liver. This variability depends on the type of pathological feature. Taking chronic hepatitis as an example, inflammation and steatosis are relatively homogeneously distributed within the liver, fibrosis is much more heterogeneous [3]. To limit the extent of sampling variation, the use of biopsy samples of sufficient size plus a scoring system that is not 'overprecise' is recommended. It has been shown that when the biopsy is long, the risk of sampling variability is reduced [4]. The recommended minimum sample size is a length of 15 mm; the optimum size should be around 25 mm [4,5]. Even with these thresholds, and taking the whole liver as the reference, 25–30% of biopsies are wrongly scored when fibrosis is concerned [4]. Fortunately, most discrepancies are only one stage different from the reference value. It is noteworthy that the complexity of a scoring system increases the risk of sampling error. A scoring system in which histopathological features are too rarely represented or too accurately evaluated does not work well with the sampling limitations of a liver biopsy core. However, a too simplistic score, although less sensitive to sampling error, will not provide enough information for the clinician. Therefore an efficient score will be the one that has reached a delicate equilibrium between the amount of information in the scoring system and the sampling variability.

Scores and observer variation

Observer variation refers to differences in scoring between pathologists. Interobserver variation is a major limitation in semi-quantitative histopathology and is highly dependent on the scoring system [6,7]. Observer variation must be tested for any new classification or scoring system, and only scores with low or acceptable interobserver variation should be retained [8,9]. Evaluation of observer variation should include both interobserver (i.e. the divergence of scores between different pathologists assessing the same biopsy) and intraobserver variation (i.e. the divergence when one pathologist scores the same biopsy at two different times). In general, intraobserver variation is lower than interobserver variation. Observer variation is closely related to the scoring system. For observer variation to be low, the scoring system must relate to unambiguously well-defined pathological items with accurate definitions of each grade on the scale. Observer variation increases with the complexity of the scoring system. In order to rule out observer variation, scoring by two observers in a collective lecture or by two observers independently with resolution of discordances in a dual lecture are the methods of choice especially in the context of clinical trials. When several biopsies have been performed in the same patient, scoring of more recent ones should be performed in conjunction with rereading of the older ones. Finally, it is recommended that in the context of clinical trials, all biopsies should be scored by the same referent pathologist. A recent study from France has shown that observer variation is related not only to the scoring system but also to pathologist experience [10]. Observer variation is lower between senior pathologists specialized in liver pathology and working in an academic environment than between junior or general pathologists. Biopsy size or staining does matter but is less important.

Chronic hepatitis C as a paradigm of scoring systems

The worldwide prevalence of hepatitis C virus infection and its frequent evolution towards chronicity has provided an instructive demonstration of the advantages and limits of scoring systems of liver biopsy [11]. It has also demonstrated how a score can evolve with time according to better knowledge of the natural history of the disease, to the expectations of hepatologists and to a clearer understanding of the limitations of the liver biopsy procedure [12].

The international classification that was proposed by an international panel of pathologists in 1968 has been used for years. It made a distinction between chronic persistent and chronic aggressive (active) hepatitis [13,14]. This classification has been utilized worldwide due to its clarity and simplicity. However, it has several limitations:

- Low information value, with only two classes (chronic persistent and chronic aggressive hepatitis).

- A systematic link between the stage and the grade: chronic persistent hepatitis shows no (or low) activity and no fibrosis whereas aggressive hepatitis shows both. We now know that the intensity of grade and stage are often dissociated, especially in chronic hepatitis C where fibrosis is common and activity generally low.
- In clinical practice, 'persistent' and 'active' hepatitis have been associated with two different diseases; however, it is now well known that these two lesions are simply two stages of the same disease with possible evolution from one to another [15].

Because the different histopathological features in chronic hepatitis can display a linear spectrum in intensity and can change either spontaneously or because of treatment, it was therefore of major importance to have a semi-quantitative scoring system [16]. The histological index of activity (Knodell score) responded in part to this aim and has been widely introduced [17]. This was a major step forward because it was the first scoring system that dissociated the different histopathological features that make up chronic hepatitis. It provides a numerical score (from 0 to 22) that is easy to computerize, and this index has been well utilized in clinical trials. However, several criticisms have been raised [18–20]:

- a lack of reproducibility for some items;
- an inappropriate grading system for mild chronic hepatitis;
- a non-linearity in score: values should be considered as categorical not nominal in statistical evaluations.
- addition of scores in different categories ignores their different pathogenic mechanisms and prognostic significance.

In recent years, a great amount of literature has addressed these concerns, and other new classifications have been proposed [21,22]. Although they differ somewhat in their content and methods of evaluation, there is a consensus among pathologists on the following points:

- The classification of chronic hepatitis must be reproducible. Any scoring system must take into account sampling variability. A histological feature that shows a high sampling variability must be assessed with a global, not overaccurate, scoring system, or assessed only on a biopsy of sufficient size.
- Any classification of chronic hepatitis should assess separately the grade and the stage of the disease. Grading evaluates the intensity of necroinflammation (or activity) and staging the degree of liver fibrosis. These two features must be dissociated because they correspond to two different mechanisms in term of pathogenesis, chronology, disease evolution and drug sensitivity. Whether scoring of fibrosis is easy to define unambiguously, there is more uncertainty in the grading of necroinflammation.
- The accuracy of a scoring system of chronic hepatitis should only reflect what the pathologist can reliably evaluate by light microscopy. However, it must be informative enough to be useful in the management of patients.
- A classification of chronic hepatitis must be applicable to all the aetiologies, whether infectious, autoimmune or toxic.

Based on these guidelines, the classifications that were commonly used in chronic hepatitis have been critically reassessed

Table 1 METAVIR scoring system with algorithm for evaluation of grade of activity.

Stage of fibrosis
F0 = No fibrosis
F1 = Stellate enlargement of portal tract without septa
F2 = Stellate enlargement of portal tract with few septa (at least one on the biopsy)
F3 = Septal fibrosis without cirrhosis (more septa than portal tract without septa)
F4 = Cirrhosis
Grade of activity (a combination of periportal and lobular necrosis but not portal inflammation)
A0 = None
A1 = Mild activity
A2 = Moderate activity
A3 = Severe activity

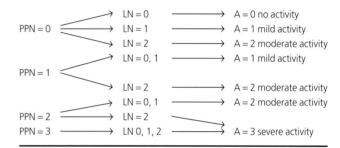

PPN, periportal necrosis; LN, lobular necrosis.

and new guidelines and classifications have been proposed [16,18,19,23,24]. They all satisfactorily meet the main criticisms outlined previously and differ only on minor points.

The METAVIR scoring system assesses fibrosis and necroinflammation separately and linearly [22]. A detailed algorithm that enables a global score of activity according to two elementary features (interface hepatitis and lobular inflammation) has been defined [25,26]. These scores have shown good reproducibility (excellent for score of fibrosis and acceptable for activity) and are widely adopted among pathologists and hepatologists. The detailed METAVIR scores are shown in Table 1. The simplicity and reproducibility of the METAVIR score make it useful both for routine practice and for clinical trials.

The Ishak scoring system is also commonly used [27]. It is a modification of the Knodell system that takes into account the major criticisms raised before. Both grade and stage are more detailed, which provides more information but to the detriment of reproducibility [28]. The Ishak scoring system is given in Table 2.

Although very useful, all these systems have limits. None of these scores assesses perisinusoidal fibrosis, and progress is still needed as regards the definition of activity. Which histological features are relevant to prognosis and to predicting response to treatment? A major criterion of acceptance for any classification will be its prognostic value, and data for this are still lacking. Better knowledge of the pathogenesis and natural history of liver

Table 2 The Ishak scoring system for grading and staging [27].

GRADING: Necroinflammatory scores	Score
A. Periportal or periseptal interface hepatitis (piecemeal necrosis)	
Absent	0
Mild (focal, few portal areas)	1
Mild/moderate (focal, most portal areas)	2
Moderate (continuous around 50% of tracts or septa)	3
Severe (continuous >50% of tracts or septa)	4
B. Confluent necrosis	
Absent	0
Focal confluent necrosis	1
Zone 3 necrosis in some areas	2
Zone 3 necrosis in most areas	3
Zone 3 necrosis + occasional portal–central (P-C) bridging	4
Zone 3 necrosis + multiple P-C bridging	5
Panacinar or multiacinar necrosis	6
C. Focal (spotty) lytic necrosis, apoptosis and focal inflammation	
Absent	0
One focus or less per 10× objective	1
Two to four foci per 10× objective	2
Five to ten foci per 10× objective	3
More than ten foci per 10× objective	4
D. Portal inflammation	
None	0
Mild, some or all portal areas	1
Moderate, some or all portal areas	2
Moderate/marked, all portal areas	3
Marked, all portal areas	4

STAGING: Architectural changes, fibrosis and cirrhosis	Score
No fibrosis	0
Fibrous expansion of some portal areas with or without short fibrous septa	1
Fibrous expansion of most portal areas with or without short fibrous septa	2
Fibrous expansion of most portal areas with occasional portal–portal bridging	3
Fibrous expansion of portal areas with marked portal–portal (P-P) and portal–central (P-C) bridging	4
Marked bridging (P-P and/or P-C) with occasional nodules (incomplete cirrhosis)	5
Cirrhosis, probable or definite	6

fibrosis and cirrhosis in chronic hepatitis would provide a firmer basis for a definitive classification of chronic hepatitis.

Scoring systems in other chronic hepatitides

The scoring systems described above have been developed mainly for chronic hepatitis C but they are also widely used for hepatitis B, although the pattern of necroinflammation is slightly different.

For autoimmune hepatitis, combined clinical and histopathological scoring systems have been proposed and recently reviewed [29]. They are useful to ascertain the diagnosis of autoimmune hepatitis and, to a lesser extent, to assess the severity. The various scores of chronic hepatitis described previously are also usable for this purpose.

Scoring systems in other chronic liver diseases

Alcoholic and non-alcoholic steatohepatitis (ASH and NASH)

Until the rise of metabolic syndrome and related liver diseases, there was no universal scoring system for alcoholic and non-alcoholic steatohepatitis [30]. Most authors used, for either clinical trials or research purposes, homemade scores or scores of fibrosis derived from the score of chronic hepatitis. Although this approach has been successful in several aspects, the physiopathology as well as key prognostic features of ASH and NASH are clearly different, rendering the use of these scores partly inappropriate. As an example, zone 3 and perisinusoidal fibrosis, which are cardinal features of ASH and NASH, are rarely encountered in the context of chronic hepatitis and never considered in scoring systems of chronic hepatitis [31]. In an attempt to take these features into account, a system for semi-quantitative evaluation of fibrosis that is more adapted to the unique lesions recognized in NASH was proposed by Brunt *et al.* and recently reviewed by Kleiner *et al.* (Table 3) [32,33].

The grading of liver cell lesions in NASH is far from easy mainly because the natural history of the disease remains partly unknown [34–36]. Therefore the choice of lesions to score and their quantification system remains uncertain and has to be tested and validated in prospective studies.

Cholestatic liver diseases

The scoring systems proposed by P. Scheuer and J. Ludwig *et al.* for primary biliary cirrhosis are the ones most widely accepted [37,38]. These two systems largely overlap. They are used both for individuals and for cohorts in clinical trials and are divided into four stages (Table 4). Because one characteristic of these diseases is the focal distribution of lesions, different stages might be present in a single liver simultaneously, thus diminishing the role of staging in cholestatic chronic liver diseases.

Table 3 Score of fibrosis in NASH [33].

0	None
1a	Mild zone 3 perisinusoidal fibrosis
1b	Moderate zone 3 perisinusoidal fibrosis
1c	Portal fibrosis only
2	Zone 3 perisinusoidal fibrosis and portal/periportal fibrosis
3	Bridging fibrosis (any bridging: i.e. central–central, central–portal, portal–portal)
4	Cirrhosis (probable and definite)

Table 4 Score of fibrosis in primary biliary cirrhosis [37].

Stage I	Florid lesion. Bile duct damage with inflammatory reaction
Stage II	Periportal fibrosis. Vanished bile ducts, portal and periportal inflammation and ductular proliferation
Stage III	Fibrosis. Portal fibrosis with periportal expansion and bridging fibrosis, typically without bile ducts
Stage IV	Cirrhosis

Morphometry as a step forward in scoring systems

When studying a liver biopsy, the hepatopathologist has two major tasks: shape recognition and shape quantification. Whereas shape recognition is an achievable goal with experience, quantification of individual histopathological items is more difficult, less suited to the working of the pathologist's eyes and brain. In order to gain more accuracy and objectivity in this matter, pathologists have developed a more sophisticated approach (i.e. morphometry) where the subjectivity of the eye–brain connection is replaced by a more objective and complex system that relies on image analysis [39]. Less expensive computer and image analysis hardware and better software and morphometric algorithms have been developed within the past 10 years and these developments have made morphometry more accessible and useful to pathologists [40]. It is of note that, even when using fully automated techniques, morphometry is very time-consuming and not recommended for routine practice. One of its most powerful applications is the evaluation of a drug in clinical trials.

There are several reasons to quantify features by morphometry:
• To decrease variability in quantifying features. Semi-quantification of morphological changes is dependent on observer variability. The sources of variability include the use of different visual templates, which arise from different educational or experiential backgrounds, and the fact that different pathologists emphasize the features differently. Morphometry potentially decreases this variability.
• To provide a finite quantitative scale. Scores are ordinal semi-quantitative assessments of changes to which numbers are typically assigned. However, these different scores are categories. Morphometric approaches to evaluating changes in tissue are linear and quantitative.
• To increase sensitivity in identifying minimal changes in features. Morphometry also offers the possibility of stratifying a disease process by an infinite number of categories, which cannot be done by visual estimation of the extent of change. This would permit a greater number of management and treatment options.
• To use as a research tool. Certain morphometric abnormalities, e.g. chromatin texture, area of fibrosis, correlate with biochemical and molecular changes [41,42].

Technical considerations

Morphometric studies are currently based on the analysis of two-dimensional structures – sections of cells and of tissue [43]. Three-dimensional (stereological) information can also be obtained from two-dimensional data, either by making assumptions about the three-dimensional structure regarding object size and shape or by directly assessing the third dimension by different means, such as confocal microscopy, or by reconstruction of serial sections or using computer-based image convolution techniques [44].

The choice of technique depends on the nature of the cells or tissue being analysed, the type of measurement being undertaken and the cost, measured in both time and money. Techniques can be categorized as manual, partially automated, automated with user interaction and fully automated. The rapid development of image analysis systems allowing fully automated analysis is now the method of choice. The principles are as follows:
• Obtain a digitized image from a histological slide. This is easily achieved through high-definition digital cameras or with software able to digitize analogue images obtained through high-definition video cameras. In some cases the digitized images are processed with the interaction of the pathologist to yield more accurate results.
• Thresholding the digitized image according to greyscale values provides the basis for segmenting the objects of interest.
• Segmentation to divide an image into two regions: the region that contains objects of interest for analysis (e.g. steatosis or fibrous tissue) and background data. In general, segmentation is based on the optical density of stained objects. Therefore highly contrasted staining is mandatory (such as picrosirius red for fibrosis).
• Measuring the structure of interest. Methods include point counting using a grid superimposed on microscopic sections or measuring the fractional area of interest using image analysis software, which provides a very high level of accuracy and allows complete automation of the process.

The main applications of morphometry are to measure linear distances (e.g. distance from a malignant tumour to a margin, or maximal two-dimensional size of a malignancy); object counting (e.g. counting mitoses or quantifying proliferation using immunohistochemistry to identify cycling cells for estimating the prognosis of tumours) [45]; measurement of fractional area (the fraction of tissue that consists of a particular structure or process); measurement of form factors – size and shape (sizes and shape of nuclei to identify disease and to predict the behaviour of cancer); and complex measurements (measure anisotropic biological structures that are not randomly oriented in tissue). For this approach, fractal geometry is the technique of choice [46]. Fractals are geometric patterns that retain their form at different scales of measurement [47]. Complex shapes, such as tumoral cell surfaces or areas of fibrosis, can be expressed as fractal dimensions [48,49].

Morphometry in liver diseases

In liver pathology, morphometry has been applied to quantify different but simple histological features. Despite the recent development of completely automated procedures, morphometry remains time-consuming, which prevents its use in routine practice. Therefore, morphometry has been used mainly for research purposes or to evaluate drug effects in clinical trials.

Steatosis

In several studies, objective computer-assisted methods and stereological point counting have been used to quantify the degree of steatosis [50,51]. The technique is simple and can be performed either by feeding images into the computer and using an overlay lattice, or supplying one eyepiece of the microscope with a graticule incorporating a point lattice and counting directly in the microscope [52].

Fibrosis

Digital image analysis rapidly provides objective quantitative results similar to but more precise than those determined by semi-quantitative scoring methods. With this approach the relative area of fibrosis is measured [53,54]. To be valuable, an interactive procedure with an experienced pathologist is needed before measuring to eliminate physiological fibrous tissue (e.g. Glisson's capsule, large proximal portal tracts). Falling costs and improvements in electronic and computer technology have enabled the implementation on personal computers of specific automatic applications for histology morphometry and fibrosis quantification [55,56]. Pilette *et al.* have demonstrated that the area of fibrosis, as determined by image analysis, and the semi-quantitative score are well correlated [54]. In addition to portal or septal fibrosis, morphometry allows rapid, reproducible and sensitive quantifications of perisinusoidal and perivenular fibrosis, features that are not usually assessed in semi-quantitative scores of fibrosis [57–60].

Another approach to assess fibrosis is fractal geometry. The fractional dimension of its irregular shape defines fibrosis as a natural fractal structure. The complex distribution of its components can be optimally quantified using a single numerical score that seems to be a better alternative to the semi-quantitative methods adopted so far [61,62].

A major advantage of morphometry in liver fibrosis is in the evaluation of antifibrotic treatments [63–65]. Because the changes induced by antifibrotic treatment are expected to be mild, the precision of fibrosis evaluation by morphometry is helpful [66]. However, because sampling error is a major drawback in fibrosis evaluation, morphometry should be performed in biopsies of at least 20mm in length [4]. Finally, due to its linearity and accuracy, measuring fibrosis with morphometry is the perfect reference to evaluate the performance of non-invasive methods.

Cirrhosis

In this context, three-dimensional structure reconstitution is of great interest in exploring the architectural reorganization accompanying cirrhosis. Several studies have used this approach to clarify the morphogenesis of cirrhotic nodules [67,68]. Morphometry enabled the demonstration that parenchyma consists of cirrhotic nodules centrifugally formed around the portal veins, and that their flows drain into the hepatic veins inside and around the nodule and nodule derived from the first. The latter was divided into the former by bridging fibrosis-induced intranodular septation.

Regeneration, benign and malignant liver tumours

Morphometric characterization of a variety of nuclear features provides the basis for distinguishing carcinoma cells from benign cells in liver tumours [69]. Combinations of morphometric features can be used for diagnosis and classification of tumours and especially hepatocellular carcinoma [70–73]. Morphological features of nuclei, including skewness of area, length of the major axis and nuclear roundness, provide the basis for distinguishing hepatocellular carcinoma from regenerative nodules. Based on these parameters, the positive predictive value of a neural net classifier of nuclear dimensions was 100%, and the negative predictive value was 85% in one study [74].

Cholestasis

Two- and three-dimensional reconstructions have been used to explore bile duct and bile-duct remodelling in several conditions including secondary biliary cirrhosis and bile duct ischaemia [75–77].

The limits of morphometry

There are many potential sources of error in morphometry. Some of the most important are:

• Error in identifying the object of interest. There is marked variability in the consistency with which observers identify objects. However, an image analysis system, which identifies objects by segmenting images, is also subject to variability. This can result either from the staining procedure, where staining can be too weak or lacking sufficient contrast or specificity to form a reliable basis for greyscale-based separation of object and background, or from the observer, who sets the threshold.

• Tissue processing. This involves multiple steps in which tissue components are chemically modified. The nature of the fixative and the conditions of fixation alter the dimensions of tissue components, which can lead to errors in counting objects. Whether such steps influence the relative fractional area of objects should be evaluated for each tissue constituent that is to be analysed.

• Errors in sampling. Is the sample size sufficiently large to obtain meaningful results? A morphometric analysis should sample the specimen to an extent sufficient to minimize variability [78,79]. The distribution of objects of interest is a consideration in sampling. Tissue-based studies have shown greater heterogeneity in feature distribution. Fibrosis or tumour vascularity is not uniformly distributed throughout a given section.

Conclusion

Semi-quantitative scoring systems are valuable tools for histopathological evaluation. They have been widely used in several chronic liver diseases although chronic viral hepatitis is probably the one that benefits most from this approach. Quantification techniques, which so far remain in the realm of research, might yield increasingly valuable information if the numerous problems inherent with the techniques can be solved.

References

1 Smetana HF (1954) The histologic diagnosis of viral hepatitis by needle biopsy. *Gastroenterology* 26, 612–625.

2 Bravo AA, Sheth SG, Chopra S (2001) Liver biopsy. *N Engl J Med* 344, 495–500.

3 Regev A, Berho M, Jeffers LJ et al. (2002) Sampling error and intra-observer variation in liver biopsy in patients with chronic HCV infection. *Am J Gastroenterol* 97, 2614–2816.

4 Bedossa P, Dargère D, Paradis V (2003) Sampling variability of liver fibrosis in chronic hepatitis C. *Hepatology* 38, 1449–1457.

5 Colloredo G, Guido M, Sonzogni A et al. (2003) Impact of liver biopsy size on histological evaluation of chronic viral hepatitis: the smaller the sample, the milder the disease. *J Hepatol* 39, 239–244.

6 Bedossa P, Poynard T, Naveau S et al. (1988) Observer variation in assessment of liver biopsies of alcoholic patients. *Alcoholism: Clin Exp Res* 12, 173–178.

7 Rozario R, Ramakrishna B (2003) Histopathological study of chronic hepatitis B and C: a comparison of two scoring systems. *J Hepatol* 38, 223–229.

8 METAVIR (1994) Quelle classification pour les hépatites chroniques? Les leçons du virus C. *Gastroentérol Clin Biol* 18, 403–406.

9 Brunt EM (2000) Grading and staging the histopathological lesions of chronic hepatitis: the Knodell histology activity index and beyond. *Hepatology* 31, 241–246.

10 Rousselet MC, Michalak S, Dupre F et al. (2005) Sources of variability in histological scoring of chronic viral hepatitis. *Hepatology* 41, 257–264.

11 Perrillo RP (1997) The role of liver biopsy in hepatitis C. *Hepatology* 26 Suppl., 57S–61S.

12 Goodman ZD, Ishak KG (1995) Histopathology of hepatitis C virus infection. *Semin Liver Dis* 15, 70–81.

13 DeGroote J, Desmet V, Gedigk P et al. (1968) A classification of chronic hepatitis. *Lancet* ii, 626–628.

14 Anon (1977) Review by an international group. Acute and chronic hepatitis revisited. *Lancet* ii, 914–919.

15 Fattovich G, Brollo L, Alberti A (1990) Chronic persistent hepatitis B can be a progressive disease when associated with sustained virus replication. *J Hepatol* 11, 29–33.

16 Scheuer PJ (1991) Classification of chronic viral hepatitis: a need for reassessment. *J Hepatol* 13, 372–374.

17 Knodell KG, Ishak KG, Black WC et al. (1981) Formulation and application of a numerical scoring system for assessing histological activity in asymptomatic chronic active hepatitis. *Hepatology* 1, 431–435.

18 Czaja AJ (1993) Chronic active hepatitis: the challenge for a new nomenclature. *Ann Intern Med* 119, 510–517.

19 Ludwig J (1993) The nomenclature of chronic active hepatitis: an obituary. *Gastroenterology* 105, 274–278.

20 Scheuer PJ (1995) The nomenclature of chronic hepatitis: time for a change. *J Hepatol* 22, 112–114.

21 Ludwig L (1994) Terminology of chronic hepatitis. *Am J Gastroenterol* 89, S177–1.

22 METAVIR cooperative group (1994) Inter- and intra-observer variation in the assessment of liver biopsy of chronic hepatitis C. *Hepatology* 20, 15–20.

23 Desmet VJ, Gerber M, Hoofnagle JH et al. (1994) Classification of chronic hepatitis: diagnosis, grading and staging. *Hepatology* 19, 1513–1519.

24 Ishak K (2000) Pathologic features of chronic hepatitis. A review and update. *Am J Clin Pathol* 113, 40–55.

25 METAVIR (1993) Proposition d'une grille de recueil des lésions histopathologiques dans l'hépatite chronique virale C. *Ann Pathol* 13, 260–265.

26 METAVIR cooperative study group (1996) An algorithm for the grading of activity in chronic hepatitis. *Hepatology* 24, 289–293.

27 Ishak K, Baptista A, Bianchi L et al. (1995) Histological grading and staging of chronic hepatitis. *J Hepatol* 22, 696–699.

28 Westin J, Lagging LM, Wejstal R et al. (1999) Interobserver study of liver histopathology using the Ishak score in patients with chronic hepatitis C virus infection. *Liver* 19, 183–187.

29 Czaja AJ, Carpenter HA (1996) Validation of a scoring system for the diagnosis of autoimmune hepatitis. *Dig Dis Sci* 41, 305–314.

30 Ludwig J, Viggiano TR, McGill DB et al. (1980) Nonalcoholic steatohepatitis: Mayo Clinic experiences with a hitherto unnamed disease. *Mayo Clin Proc* 55, 434–438.

31 Brunt EM (2004) Nonalcoholic steatohepatitis. *Semin Liver Dis* 24, 3–20.

32 Brunt EM, Janney CG, Di Bisceglie AM et al. (1999) Nonalcoholic steatohepatitis: a proposal for grading and staging the histological lesions. *Am J Gastroenterol* 94, 2468–2474.

33 Kleiner DE, Brunt EM, Van Natta M et al. (2005) Design and validation of a histological scoring system for nonalcoholic fatty liver disease. *Hepatology* 41, 1313–1321.

34 Angulo P, Keach JC, Batts KP et al. (1999) Independent predictors of liver fibrosis in patients with nonalcoholic steatohepatitis. *Hepatology* 30, 1356–1362.

35 Matteoni CA, Younossi ZM, Gramlich T et al. (1999) Nonalcoholic fatty liver disease: a spectrum of clinical and pathological severity. *Gastroenterology* 116, 1413–1419.

36 Dixon JB, Bhathal PS, O'Brien PE (2001) Nonalcoholic fatty liver disease: predictors of nonalcoholic steatohepatitis and liver fibrosis in the severely obese. *Gastroenterology* 121, 91–100.

37 Scheuer PJ (1967) Primary biliary cirrhosis. *Proc Roy Soc Med* 60, 1257–1260.

38 Ludwig J, Dickson ER, McDonald GS (1978) Staging of chronic non-suppurative destructive cholangitis. *Virchows Arch A* 379, 103–112.

39 Weibel ER (1979) *Stereological Methods: Practical Methods for Biological Morphometry*. San Diego, CA: Academic Press.

40 Dahab GM, Kheriza MM, El-Beltagi HM et al. (2004) Digital quantification of fibrosis in liver biopsy sections: description of a new method by Photoshop software. *J Gastroenterol Hepatol* 19, 78–85.

41 Liautaud RF, Teyssier JR, Ferre D et al. (1992) Can chromatin texture predict structural karyotypic changes in diploid cells from thyroid cold nodules? *Anal Cell Pathol* 4, 421–428.

42 Mulder J-WR, Offerhaus GJA, Feyter EP de et al. (1992) The relationship of quantitative nuclear morphology to molecular genetic alterations in the adenoma-carcinoma sequence of the large bowel. *Am J Pathol* 141, 797–804.

43 Wied CL, Bartels PH, Bibbo M et al. (1989) Image analysis in quantitative cytopathology and histopathology. *Hum Pathol* 20, 549–571.

44 Zhu Q, Tekola P, Baak JP *et al* (1994) Measurement by confocal laser scanning microscopy of the volume of epidermal nuclei in thick skin sections. *Anal Quant Cytol Histol* 16, 145–152.

45 Quinn CM, Wright NA (1990) The clinical assessment of proliferation and growth in human tumours: Evaluation of methods and applications as prognostic variables. *J Pathol* 160, 93–102.

46 Cross SS (1994) The application of fractal geometric analysis to microscopic images. *Micron* 25, 101–113.

47 Barnsley MF, Massopust P, Strickland H *et al.* (1987) Fractal modeling of biological structures. *Ann NY Acad Sci* 504, 179–194.

48 Keough KMW, Hyam P, Pink DA *et al.* (1991) Cell surfaces and fractal dimensions. *J Microsc* 163, 95–99.

49 Cross SS, Cotton DWK (1992) The fractal dimension may be a useful morphometric discriminant in histopathology. *J Pathol* 166, 409–411.

50 Auger J, Schoevaert D, Martin ED (1986) Comparative study of automated morphometric and semiquantitative estimations of alcoholic liver steatosis. *Anal Quant Cytol Histol* 8, 56–62.

51 Zaitoun AM, Al Mardini M, Record CO (1998) Stereology and morphometry of steatosis in human alcoholic (ALD) and non-alcoholic liver disease (NALD). *Acta Stereol* 17, 49–56.

52 Zaitoun AM, Al Mardini H, Awad S *et al.* (2001) Quantitative assessment of fibrosis and steatosis in liver biopsies from patients with chronic hepatitis C. *J Clin Pathol* 54, 461–465.

53 Ryoo JW, Buschmann RJ (1989) Morphometry of liver parenchyma in needle biopsy specimens from patients with alcoholic liver disease: Preliminary variables for the diagnosis and prognosis of cirrhosis. *Mod Pathol* 2, 382–389.

54 Pilette C, Rousselet MC, Bedossa P *et al.* (1998) Histopathological evaluation of liver fibrosis: quantitative image analysis vs semiquantitative scores. Comparison with serum markers. *J Hepatol* 28, 439–446.

55 O'Brien MJ, Keating NM, Elderiny S *et al.* (2000) An assessment of digital image analysis to measure fibrosis in liver biopsy specimens of patients with chronic hepatitis C. *Am J Clin Pathol* 114, 712–718.

56 Masseroli M, Caballero T, O'Valle F *et al.* (2000) Automatic quantification of liver fibrosis: design and validation of a new image analysis method: comparison with semi-quantitative indexes of fibrosis. *J Hepatol* 32, 453–464.

57 Promrat K, Lutchman G, Uwaifo GI *et al.* (2004) A pilot study of pioglitazone treatment for nonalcoholic steatohepatitis. *Hepatology* 39, 188–196.

58 Imamura H, Kawasaki S, Bandai Y *et al.* (1994) Morphometry of sinusoids and portal hypertension in non-alcoholic cirrhosis. *J Hepatol* 21, 167–173.

59 Moragas A, Allende H, Sans M (1998) Characteristics of perisinusoidal collagenization in liver cirrhosis: computer-assisted quantitative analysis. *Anal Quant Cytol Histol* 20, 169–177.

60 Zimmermann A, Zhao D, Reichen J (1999) Myofibroblasts in the cirrhotic rat liver reflect hepatic remodeling and correlate with fibrosis and sinusoidal capillarization. *J Hepatol* 30, 646–652.

61 Dioguardi N, Grizzi F, Bossi P *et al.* (1999) Fractal and spectral dimension analysis of liver fibrosis in needle biopsy specimens. *Anal Quant Cytol Histol* 21, 262–266.

62 Moal F, Chappard D, Wang J *et al.* (2002) Fractal dimension can distinguish models and pharmacologic changes in liver fibrosis in rats. *Hepatology* 36, 840–849.

63 Baroni GS, D'Ambrosio L, Curto P *et al.* (1996) Interferon gamma decreases hepatic stellate cell activation and extracellular matrix deposition in rat liver fibrosis. *Hepatology* 23, 1189–1199.

64 Bruck R, Hershkoviz R, Lider O *et al.* (1996) Inhibition of experimentally-induced liver cirrhosis in rats by a nonpeptidic mimetic of the extracellular matrix-associated Arg-Gly-Asp epitope. *J Hepatol* 24, 731–738.

65 Alpini G, Elias I, Glaser S *et al.* (1997) Gamma-interferon inhibits secretin-induced choleresis and cholangiocyte proliferation in a murine model of cirrhosis. *J Hepatol* 27, 371–380.

66 Neef M, Ledermann M, Saegesser H *et al.* (2006) Oral imatinib treatment reduces early fibrogenesis but does not prevent progression in the long term. *J Hepatol* 44, 167–175.

67 Sakata A, Takasaki S, Kawakami M (1999) Three-dimensional image analysis of the hepatic restructuring process in chronic active hepatitis. *Anal Quant Cytol Histol* 21, 245–249.

68 Vizzotto L, Vertemati M, Gambacorta M *et al.* (2002) Analysis of histological and immunohistochemical patterns of the liver in posthepatitic and alcoholic cirrhosis by computerized morphometry. *Mod Pathol* 15, 798–806.

69 Rubin EM, Martin AA, Thung SN *et al.* (1995) Morphometric and immunohistochemical characterization of human liver regeneration. *Am J Pathol* 147, 397–404.

70 Herman CJ, Vooijs GP, Baak JPA *et al.* (1984) Quantitative cytologic and histologic techniques to assist in cancer evaluation. *Methods Achiev Exp Pathol* 11, 73–95.

71 Hall TL, Fu YS (1985) Applications of quantitative microscopy in tumor pathology. *Lab Invest* 53, 5.

72 Ueda K, Terada T, Nakanuma Y, Matsui O (1992) Vascular supply in adenomatous hyperplasia of the liver and hepatocellular carcinoma: A morphometric study. *Hum Pathol* 23, 619–626.

73 Terayama N, Terada T, Nakanuma Y (1996) A morphometric and immunohistochemical study on angiogenesis of human metastatic carcinomas of the liver. *Hepatology* 24, 816–819.

74 Erler BS, Hsu L, Truong HM *et al.* (1994) Image analysis and diagnostic classification of hepatocellular carcinoma using neural networks and multivariate discriminant functions. *Lab Invest* 71, 446–451.

75 Ohara N, Schaffner T, Reichen J (1993) Structure-function relationship in secondary biliary cirrhosis in the rat: Stereologic and hemodynamic characterization of a model. *J Hepatol* 17, 155–162.

76 De Craemer D, Pauwels M, Van Den Branden C (1995) Regression of bile duct damage and bile duct proliferation in the non-rearterialized transplanted rat liver is associated with spontaneous graft rearterialization. *Hepatology* 21, 1353–1360.

77 Beaussier M, Wendum D, Fouassier L *et al.* (2005) Adaptive bile duct proliferative response in experimental bile duct ischemia. *J Hepatol* 42, 257–265.

78 Mathieu O, Cruz-Grive LM, Hoppeler H *et al.* (1981) Measuring error and sample variation in stereology: Comparison of the efficiency of various methods for planar image analysis. *J Microsc* 121, 75–88.

79 Collan Y, Torkkeli T, Kosma V-M *et al.* (1987) Sampling in diagnostic morphometry: The influence of variation sources. *Pathol Res Pract* 182, 401–406.

5 Investigation of hepatobiliary disease

5.1 Signs and symptoms of liver disease

Jürg Reichen

Signs and symptoms are nonspecific for either liver disease *per se* or for differentiating disease of the liver from that of other systems. Nevertheless, an adequate history, review of systems and physical examination can yield the clue to the diagnosis even in this age of advanced immunological, virological and biochemical testing – let alone the array of wonderful imaging techniques.

Symptoms

Weakness, fatigue and resulting decrease in quality of life

Close to 80% of the patients in my outpatient clinic complain of fatigue regardless of their underlying diagnosis. This is particularly frustrating for both patient and clinician as this symptom is notoriously difficult to treat.

This nonspecific symptom is said to be particularly prevalent in hepatitis C; an early study into this topic concluded that hepatitis C patients – as compared with healthy controls and patients with hepatitis B – had marked impairment in quality of life [1]. Changes in ^{1}H-magnetic resonance spectroscopy correlate well with cognitive impairment and decreased quality of life [2]. However, when other factors associated with fatigue such as depression, intravenous drug abuse and advanced liver disease are removed, the clinical relevance of impaired cognition becomes relatively minor [3].

Fatigue is also a relevant symptom in cholestatic liver disease, in particular in primary biliary cirrhosis [4]; rat experiments pioneered by Mark Swain have laid a pathophysiological basis for this phenomenon suggesting a central origin [5]. In a recent study, fatigue was present, albeit to a lesser degree, in patients with primary biliary cirrhosis but the impact on quality of life was minor; of particular interest was the fact that weakness (as assessed by grip strength) was not correlated with the self-assessment of fatigue by validated questionnaires [6]; indeed, a population-based survey has demonstrated a clear central effect for this symptom [7]. In contrast to primary biliary cirrhosis, patients with primary sclerosing cholangitis appear not to be fatigued [8].

Anorexia, dysgeusia and dysosmia

Lack of appetite is a prevalent symptom of acute liver disease of any cause. In endstage liver disease, anorexia is also prevalent. The reason(s) for anorexia are poorly understood. Research into satiety hormones may advance the field in the next few years. Support for this contention is the observation that the organism tries to correct reduced food intake by upregulating ghrelin [9].

Disordered taste and smell acuity are frequent in patients with acute and chronic liver disease but the reasons for this phenomenon remain unclear. Zinc defiency would be a plausible candidate for dysgeusia but this has not been borne out by a thorough investigation of different micronutrients [10]. Recently, a central origin for alterations in the sense of taste has been proposed [11].

Sicca syndrome

Dry gland syndrome is often not spontaneously reported and should be asked for. Measurement of tear flow with Schirmer's test or salivary flow should be performed in the appropriate settings. Although sicca syndrome is obviously strongly associated with primary biliary cirrhosis it can be seen in any cholestatic disorder resulting in ductopenia, including sarcoidosis [12] or drug-induced intrahepatic cholestasis. Another condition where sicca syndrome is quite frequent is chronic hepatitis C; Cacoub *et al.* reported an incidence of 11% [13]. Conversely, the presence of hepatitis C in patients presenting with sicca syndrome is also high at 19% [14]. Sicca syndrome can also be seen in chronic hepatitis B, albeit less frequently [15].

Abdominal pain and discomfort

Abdominal pain, particularly when it is localized to the right upper quadrant, may reflect stretching of the liver capsule.

This occurs when there is a rapid increase in liver volume due to, for example, swelling in right heart failure, hepatic vein occlusion in Budd–Chiari syndrome or the occurrence of a primary or metastatic liver tumour. Patients with chronic liver disease, in particular hepatitis C but also haemochromatosis, will often report a dull ache, which often occurs postprandially; one might speculate that this is due to swelling of the liver as a result of the osmotic load of a meal. This symptom often appears only once the patient has been told that there is something wrong with his or her liver. A careful history is of paramount importance when right upper quadrant pain is present; it might guide further evaluation by ultrasonography and/or oesophagogastroscopy.

A completely different issue is biliary pain – often misnamed biliary colic. The so-called biliary colic is not colicky at all but a constant pain lasting 30 min or more [16]. A meta-analysis clearly demonstrated that dyspeptic symptoms and fat intolerance are not related to gallstones [17]. Acute obstruction by gallstones in either the cystic duct or choledochus will last as long as the obstruction persists; biliary pain is often associated with nausea. In contrast, slowly developing obstruction is usually devoid of pain because the ducts are able to accommodate the slow increase in pressure by dilatation.

Abdominal discomfort with a feeling of abdominal swelling is most often due to intestinal gas, in particular when it is of short duration and/or waxing and waning. However, persistent discomfort with increased girth leading to changes in the size of clothes is most often due to ascites or marked organomegaly. In the latter case, the patient will also report a mass effect.

Bowel habits, stools and flatulence

Constipation is not a feature of liver disease but may aggravate or precipitate hepatic encephalopathy in patients with advanced liver disease.

Diarrhoea – a common symptom – should not be primarily attributed to acute or chronic liver disease but properly evaluated. It is, however, a frequently encountered presenting symptom in acute liver disease of viral or, particularly, alcoholic aetiology. Diarrhoea is seen in only 14% of patients with amoebic liver abscess [18]. In patients referred for workup of abnormal liver enzymes or a change in bowel habits to increased frequency and/or stool volume, several autoimmune diseases including primary sclerosing cholangitis, primary biliary cirrhosis, Behçet's disease and coeliac disease ought to be considered. A rare cause of liver disease and diarrhoea is amyloidosis – biopsy the intestine rather than the liver if suspicion is high!

Diarrhoea is of particular interest in the transplanted patient; there, nosocomial infections, antibiotic-induced diarrhoea and drug-induced diarrhoea ought to be considered [19]. Similar considerations apply to the HIV-positive patient. A classical but rare phenomenon is diarrhoea, sepsis and liver abscess due to iron-dependent microorganisms such as *Yersinia enterocolitica* in iron overload.

Changes in micturition and urine

Patients often notice that their urine gets darker before noticing scleral icterus; when questioning, one should ask whether the urine is like coca cola – lesser darkening is usually due to concentrated urine in dehydrated patients.

In the review of systems, symptoms of urinary tract infection (UTI) ought to be sought because UTIs are the second most frequent cause of bacterial infection in patients with endstage liver disease [20]. In contrast to some earlier reports, patients with primary biliary cirrhosis appear not to be prone to UTIs in precirrhotic stages [21].

Jaundice and pruritus

Profound jaundice will not be missed by patients; if it is accompanied by dark urine (see above), a hepatobiliary cause is very likely. Intermittent jaundice in a young patient with normally coloured urine is most probably the result of Gilbert syndrome.

Pruritus is an important sign of cholestatic liver disease but can also be seen in acute and chronic viral hepatitis. Pruritus is quite frequent in hepatitis C; different skin diseases – in particular eczema, urticaria, atopic dermatitis, cryoglobulinaemia and lichen planus – are often associated with hepatitis C [22,23].

The aetiology of pruritus of cholestasis has recently been reviewed by Bergasa [24]. Typically, it is more severe at night and affects the extremities more than the trunk. Painless jaundice together with pruritus in the elderly patient is often due to malignant obstruction but can also be caused by stones and even intrahepatic cholestasis, in particular primary biliary cirrhosis.

Muscle cramps

Cramps are a frequent symptom in endstage liver disease, occurring in close to two-thirds of patients with cirrhosis as compared with 7% in matched controls [25]. This symptom should be asked for and treatment considered because it is a major factor for the decreased quality of life in patients with endstage liver disease [26]. For such a frequent and painful symptom, amazingly little research has been done to elucidate the cause and optimal treatment.

Fever and shaking chills (rigors)

Fever is a frequent symptom in acute and chronic liver disease whereas shaking chills are rather rare. The latter – if liver is the leading diseased organ – should make you consider suppurative cholangitis or liver abscess.

Liver biopsy should be considered in all patients with fever of unknown origin and negative imaging studies.

Irritability, confusion, difficulties in concentration and sleep disturbance

The confused, disoriented patient with asterixis and known

cirrhosis is easily recognized as suffering from portosystemic encephalopathy (PSE). More subtle signs of PSE include a reversal in the diurnal rhythm [27], changes in personality – in particular irritability – which are often not recognized by the patient but can be elicited by asking close relatives.

Bleeding and bruising

Easy bruising and spontaneous bleeding from the nose or gums is a frequent symptom in endstage liver disease. Bleeding time in cirrhosis is prolonged concomitant with impairment of hepatic dysfunction and should therefore be measured in patients with advanced liver disease before invasive procedures [28].

Massive upper or lower gastrointestinal bleeding is, of course, a frequent first presentation of chronic liver disease and will be covered extensively in other chapters. Intra-abdominal bleeding can be a first manifestation of hepatocellular cancer and other malignant or even benign liver tumors.

Past medical history, family history and review of systems

Past medical history

I trust that all hepatologists will obtain a careful history of events that have occurred previously in the patient's life. Of particular interest for hepatology are previous episodes of jaundice, abdominal surgery and, in women, the course of pregnancy and the onset of menopause.

Family history

A history of relatives dying from liver disease may point to inherited diseases such as haemochromatosis, alpha-1-antitrypsin deficiency and others. Of note is that nonalcoholic steatohepatitis may run in families. Acquired liver diseases, in particular hepatitis B, might be revealed by an appropriate family history.

Review of systems

A thorough review of systems is mandatory. Particular attention should be paid to drugs and medicinal plants. It has to be realized that often megavitamins, a 'tea against the cold' (which in Europe may contain paracetamol) or phytotherapeutics are not considered 'drugs' by the patient. The heavily muscled young man who spends 6 hours per day in the gym will not tell you that he has been ingesting anabolic steroids. The elderly lady who has been taking a benzodiazepine for sleep for decades does not consider this a drug because she has been with it forever.

The review of systems should also consider work, hobbies and pets because these can be associated with exposure to toxins or infectious agents of which the patient is not aware.

Signs

Although modern imaging techniques have rendered many bedside skills 'obsolete', a thorough inspection and physical examination will still reveal many clues to the presence and even the aetiology of the underlying disease.

General appearance and vital signs

It goes without saying that the general appearance and the nutritional state should be recorded. Malnutrition – part of the original Child classification – has been shown to be related to the degree of liver failure [29]; onset of malnutrition is particularly important when considering the need for liver transplantation. Conversely, an elevated body mass index (BMI) will lead the physician to consider the presence of nonalcoholic fatty liver disease or steatohepatitis (NAFLD/NASH).

Decreased arterial pressure and a high heart rate are part of the hyperdynamic circulation syndrome in portal hypertension [30,31]. With liver function decreasing, pre-existing arterial hypertension often disappears. Conversely, arterial hypertension is part of the metabolic syndrome and therefore associated with NAFLD/NASH.

Dyspnoea and tachypnoea are frequent findings in advanced liver disease as a result of elevation and compression of the diaphragm by an enlarged liver, ascites or the presence of pleural effusions. Cystic fibrosis and alpha-1-antitrypsin deficiency obviously can affect both the lung and the liver; patients with alcoholic liver disease often smoke, and alcoholic liver disease is often associated with chronic obstructive pulmonary disease (COPD). Dyspnoea can also be a sign of portopulmonary hypertension; this will be covered in more depth in Chapter 7.7.

Fever is a hallmark of many acute viral and bacterial liver diseases, covered in Sections 9 and 10 respectively. Other liver infections usually associated with fever include suppurative cholangitis and liver abscess. Fever should be taken seriously in any patient with cirrhosis because infections are a leading cause of death in this population. Similarly, alarm bells should ring in the transplanted patient with fever (see Chapter 25.6). In the absence of infection, fever can be an accompanying symptom of any chronic liver disease, in particular of alcoholic hepatitis (see Chapter 12.4), hepatitis C and autoimmune liver diseases.

A particularly interesting situation is fever of unknown origin (FUO). A recent systematic review demonstrated that liver biopsy can be revealing in 14–17% of cases in this setting even when liver enzymes are normal [32]. My personal algorithm for this condition is to scan thorax and abdomen and, if this is negative, to proceed with liver biopsy.

Eyes

The obvious sign of liver disease to be sought in the eyes is scleral jaundice, which can be detected when serum bilirubin exceeds ~35 μmol/L. Red and dry conjunctivae might hint at the presence of sicca syndrome and should elicit further questioning and performance of Schirmer's test.

Rare, but delightful if you see it because it allows you to make a rapid diagnosis, is the presence of a Kayser–Fleischer ring – golden-brown to greenish pigment deposition in Descemet's membrane – which obviously makes you think of Wilson's disease [33]. In advanced cases, this might proceed to sunflower cataracts by copper deposition on the anterior capsule of the lens. Kayser–Fleischer ring is not pathognomonic for Wilson's disease but might be found in other conditions with severe copper overload.

Cataracts in young patients should make you think of galactosaemia, cerebrotendinous xanthomatosis or familial hyperferritinaemia [34]. A posterior embryotoxon is found in 95% of patients with Alagille syndrome where other ocular abnormalities also prevail [35].

Skin

The discussion of the skin is restricted to the most important and general signs of liver disease; for a more thorough discussion of this fascinating topic, the reader is referred to Chapter 21.6.

A thorough inspection of the whole integument can yield valuable clues; a pale skin can indicate anemia, in particular when verified by pallor of the lips and conjunctivae. Jaundice – initially best seen in the sclerae and frenulum of the tongue – is an obvious sign. Neil McIntyre, who wrote the first and second editions of this chapter, considered enoral jaundice an epiphenomenon of little clinical value; our hospital unfortunately puts our patients on yellow bed linen – using a white lamp, I find enoral jaundice a good sign and can detect the usual visual limit of 35 μmol/L.

Many plant dyes – mostly carotenes and lycopenes – can cause pseudojaundice; such substances are abundant in carrots, tomatoes and papaya. Differentiation can be made chemically or by inspection of the sclerae: these are spared in pseudojaundice. Longstanding jaundice leads to a characteristic grey-greenish discoloration of the whole integument.

Cyanosis is most often thought of as being associated with cardiac or pulmonary disease. Either can also affect the liver and lead to hepatomegaly and disturbed liver function tests. In the patient with known cirrhosis, cyanosis should lead to diagnostic workup of potential hepatopulmonary syndrome [36].

Haemochromatosis is labelled in old textbooks as 'bronze diabetes'; nowadays the diagnosis should be made earlier. The increased skin pigmentation in extreme iron overload is due to iron and melanin deposition [37].

Vitiligo – patchy discoloration of the skin due to local destruction of melanocytes – can be associated with autoimmune liver disease and chronic hepatitis C. Whether vitiligo can be provoked by interferon treatment has been claimed but not proven because it is clearly associated with hepatitis C *per se* [38].

Xanthelasmata and excoriations hint at a chronic cholestatic liver disease, most often primary biliary cirrhosis.

Palmar erythema

Palmar erythema is not specific for liver disease but is also associated with rheumatoid arthritis, haematological malignancies and pregnancy. Furthermore, certain drugs – in particular cytostatic agents – are well known to induce palmar erythema; in this case, there is often dysaesthesia, which is absent in patients with liver disease or other causes of palmar erythema. The origin of the phenomenon is postulated to be capillary dilatation, presumably as a consequence of the hyperdynamic circulation syndrome; however, blood flow to the skin in the forearm of cirrhotic patients is not increased.

Spider naevi

Spider naevi are considered a hallmark of alcoholic liver disease. They are typically lesions measuring 1 mm to 1 cm with a central artery and a spider's web of capillaries radiating from them, and they disappear with pressure applied by a transparent spatula. Most spiders (>99%) are seen above the waist. Certain investigators consider palmar erythema and spider naevi as common manifestations of hyperdynamic circulation and/or a hormonal imbalance. The latter is supported by the fact that spider naevi can also appear rapidly and in great number in pregnant women (who also exhibit a hyperdynamic circulation). The evidence for and history of spider naevi is amply referenced and, as always, thoughtfully and scholarly discussed in the series by Professor Adrian Reuben in *Hepatology* [39]. The number of spider naevi should be recorded, because some find their presence and number to be of prognostic importance [39–42].

Extremities

An inspection of the extremities can yield valuable clues to the presence and even aetiology of liver disease and associated conditions.

Dupuytren's disease
This is a thickening of the palmar and digital fascia that can lead to contracture of the digits. In a prospective study in the late 1980s, a clear association with alcohol consumption – but not alcoholic liver disease – was found [43]. However, the presence of Dupuytren's disease in a liver clinic should not prompt labelling of the patient as an alcoholic because the disease is fairly common, increasing from 4% in the general population to 20% in those older than 65. Moreover, clear associations also exist between Dupuytren's disease and diabetes and epilepsy; furthermore, there must be a genetic basis because it is seen almost exclusively in Caucasians [44].

Nails
Inspection of the fingernails or toenails may yield valuable clues to the presence of liver disease. Muehrcke's line – a white transverse line on the nail – was initially described as revealing

nephrotic syndrome but can also be seen in cirrhosis. Terry's nails is a white discoloration of the nail bed with a pink distal band, initially described in cirrhotic patients; it is also seen in heart failure, diabetes and with increasing age; it is thought to reflect telangiectasias [45] and therefore is probably a manifestation of the hyperdynamic circulation syndrome. Grey or blue discoloration of the lunulae may hint at an excess heavy metal burden, namely Wilson's disease or argyrosis.

Clubbing – a sign well known to pneumologists – can also be seen in cirrhosis and other diseases with portal hypertension. It should lead the physician to further explore the presence of pulmonary arterial hypertension [46].

Cardiopulmonary examination

The effect of cardiovascular disease on the liver is reported in Chapter 20.1; the converse, the effect of liver disease on the cardiovascular system, is detailed in Chapter 21.1. I would just state here that a thorough cardiopulmonary examination in a liver clinic is mandatory. Congested neck veins, wet rales or a third heart sound are clues to congestive heart failure, which might explain abnormal liver function tests for which the patient has been referred to the liver clinic. A paradoxical pulse may indicate constrictive pericarditis – a frequently overlooked cause of transsudative ascites [47].

The same holds true for percussion and auscultation of the lungs; pulmonary complications of portal hypertension are covered in Chapter 7.7. I am puzzled by young physicians searching for pleural effusions with ultrasound: they are easily detected by percussion and, in a liver clinic (and any other clinic), one should consider the possibility of hepatic hydrothorax – which accounts for 5–10% of pleural effusions [48]. A pronounced P2 should evoke the possibility of pulmonary hypertension, a not so rare complication of portal hypertension (see Chapter 7.7). Physical signs of COPD should be taken into consideration because liver tests are frequently abnormal in severe COPD and sleep apnoea [49,50].

Physical signs of emphysema in young patients should evoke the presence of alpha-1-antitrypsin deficiency or cystic fibrosis.

Inspection, palpation and percussion of the abdomen

Inspection

Inspection of the abdomen can reveal striae as signs of recent distension due to ascites, weight gain or, more joyfully in the appropriate sex, pregnancy. Fresh striae are also seen in patients on corticosteroids and patients with autoimmune hepatitis.

Dilatation of the epigastric veins hints at portal hypertension, particularly if the flow is in the physiological direction, that is, upwards above the umbilicus and downwards below it. Massive venous dilatation of epigastric veins, in particular on the side of the abdomen, is a clue to obstruction of the vena cava; in this condition, the flow is upwards throughout the venous system and there is often pronounced leg oedema. Collaterals are also often seen on the back of the patient.

Umbilical hernia may be an early indicator of ascites formation; if it is associated with a venous hum (Cruveilhier–Baumgarten syndrome), it indicates recanalization of the umbilical vein and portal hypertension. This syndrome is rather rare – but blue discoloration around the umbilicus due to distended veins is not.

Flank distension can indicate the presence of ascites. Some very big and hard livers (and spleens) can be seen with appropriate lighting. This is particularly true for metastatic and polycystic liver disease, but I have also 'seen' hepatic amyloidosis.

Palpation and percussion of the liver

The whole abdomen should be palpated in a liver clinic because masses can yield a clue to metastatic liver disease. You recognize an old-fashioned hepatologist by the fact that he or she will stand at the right side of the patient's bed. With respect to palpation of the liver and spleen, both should initially be sought in the pelvic area: massive hepatomegaly and/or splenomegaly can be missed if palpation is begun a handbreadth or two below the costal margin; this is particularly true if the organ is soft. Riedel's lobe is notoriously missed if you do not start palpation in the pelvic area and to the right of the midclavicular line. Riedel's lobe is a normal variant apparently increasing with age [51] and not deserving further workup.

I palpate the liver just to the right of the rectus sheet leading with my index finger; try to exert some pressure, in particular in muscular patients. Then, ask for a deep breath and you will feel the liver flipping over your leading finger. Once you have felt the edge to the right of the rectus abdominis, it will be easy to follow the remainder of the liver edge into the left side of the belly. In muscular patients, this might be impossible across the rectus abdominis. Palpation fares reasonably well in patients with liver cirrhosis: in a prospective study, correlation between palpation and sonography regarding liver span was excellent in patients with cirrhosis but poor in controls [52] (where liver span is not that interesting anyhow). Palpation will tell you something about the firmness of the organ. Personally, I cannot feel 'nodularity', for which ultrasound is certainly better. However, superficial tumors or cysts can often be palpated and might direct further workup.

The scratch test and liver percussion do not stand up to scrutiny when compared with imaging procedures for assessing organ size [53,54]. Personally, I still find them helpful in following patients, for instance with fulminant hepatic failure or congestive heart failure, where a decrease or increase, respectively, might indicate worsening of the condition. With the wide availability of ultrasonography, however, these tests are, or soon will be, history.

Pulsatile livers are reported to occur in tricuspid insufficiency [55] and constrictive pericarditis [56]. It is a rare event and you can call your students to observe a phenomenon they'll never see again. But kindly do not write a case report if you see it: it has been seen before.

The gallbladder may be palpated in cases of biliary obstruction (Courvoisier's sign). In such cases, it is most often a cystic, soft mass yielding to pressure in the right upper quadrant tending toward the umbilicus. In these days where a computerized tomography (CT) scan is obtained before a history is taken, the sign has probably lost its clinical usefulness as a clue to pancreatic/ampullary cancer in a patient with painless jaundice. Moreover, the gallbladder is enlarged to the same extent in patients with benign, as those with malignant, biliary obstruction [57].

Murphy's sign will be covered in the section on gallstone diseases (Chapter 19.3). Briefly, Murphy's sign can be suggestive of acute cholecystitis but, in this age of early imaging, more accurate results are obtained by ultrasound or CT. The sonographer, however, should report elicitation of the typical pain when touching the gallbladder. This may be a helpful sign in recurrent right upper quadrant pain, in particular in gallbladder dysfunction when the imaging techniques – except for biliary scintigraphy – are not revealing.

Palpation and percussion of the spleen

As for the liver, a spleen ought first to be sought in the pelvis. Big spleens are often reported by the patient as a mass. In the asymptomatic patient, single-handed palpation of the hypochondrium is not revealing in my experience: I prefer to start with a bimanual examination where the right hand is placed below the margin of the rib cage and exerts an upward and inward pressure. The right hand – with all digits deployed – is used to feel the spleen descending on a deep inspiration, accompanied by the mentioned movement of the left hand. This manoeuvre should be repeated with several different starting positions of the right hand. You will feel the spleen tip flipping over the most sensitive part of your right hand – the fingertips.

Other methods advocated in the times when clinical examination was still cherished included palpation with a similar position of the right hand as described above and moving the patient to a right lateral decubitus making use of gravity. If the first manoeuvre is unsuccessful and, if I have the time, I still use this method.

A nice study prospectively comparing different methods [58] concluded that percussion of Traube's space was best for raising suspicion of splenomegaly; if positive, it should be followed by any of the manoeuvres described above and a positive finding would be most likely in lean patients. Interestingly, ultrasound is also most revealing in lean patients. On the other hand, percussion is felt to be worthless for assessment of spleen size based on a critical analysis of the literature [54]. I beg to disagree – but I realise that clinical skills will be replaced by more objective imaging techniques.

Loins, kidneys and testicles

Kidneys can occasionally be felt in the loins – in particular if they are of the transplanted variety. Enlarged hard kidneys in either loin and, in particular, if they are also felt in the back are usually diagnostic of polycystic disease. I have given up on examining exactly how the organs move with inspiration to differentiate a big spleen from a big kidney – this is better answered by ultrasound.

Inguinal hernias should be sought in each and every patient, particularly in those with ascites. You'll miss them if you look for them with the patient lying down comfortably. Because you have moved to the nether regions of urinary tract organs, you might as well assess testicular size. 'Small testicles' are in the eye (hand?) of the beholder. But, if the patient confirms that they have shrunk, you should further explore alcohol consumption and rule out haemochromatosis.

Auscultation

Auscultation of the whole abdomen should be performed to check for bowel sounds or absence thereof, arterial bruits, venous hums and friction rubs.

Arterial bruits

Arterial bruits should be listened for while palpating the pulse and – because they are usually quite faint – during a breath-hold. Arterial bruits during systole in the epigastrium are frequent, particularly in young, lean subjects, and often disappear with a change in position. Occasionally, they can reflect stenosis of the superior mesenteric artery; such bruits are louder and longer, extending into diastole. Arterial bruits may be due to aortic disease such as aneurysms and aortitis. Splenic arterial bruits are located over the left hypochondrium or below the left ribcage. Such bruits can be heard with splenic artery compression due to pancreatic disease.

Arterial bruits over the liver are rare and usually due to aortovenous fistulae after trauma [59], including liver biopsy [60], in tumours [61] or in Osler–Weber–Rendu disease with hepatic involvement [62]. The prevalence of arterial bruits in hepatocellular cancer must be low although good data are missing – but, when you hear it in a patient with cirrhosis, the odds are high that imaging will reveal a hepatocellular cancer.

Venous hum

Even more difficult to hear, less frequent and probably completely unimportant in practice are venous hums. They are continuous, of low frequency and heard over the umbilicus in Cruveilhier–Baumgarten syndrome (see above) or occasionally over the portal vein. I still listen for them – and, when I hear one, I am pleased and call the medical students to listen for it. I also tell them that they probably will not hear it again and that they can forget it for the qualifying exams.

Rubs

Rubs can be heard over the liver in Fitz-Hugh–Curtis syndrome – pelvic inflammatory disease most often due to chlamydial infection [63] but also seen in other venereal and nonvenereal diseases including tuberculosis. Rubs can also be heard in uraemia and with hepatocellular cancer. The sign is rare in my experience and should be noted when present.

Ascites

Massive ascites is seen on inspection and does not require imaging or further clinical testing. In my experience, there is only one more or less unequivocal clinical sign of ascites, namely shifting dullness by percussion: have the patient lie supine and percuss on both sides and mark the region where dullness goes to resonance (due to floating bowels). Then, have the patient shift on one side, wait for about half a minute and percuss again. If there is more than 2 cm in shifting dullness you can be quite certain that there is ascites. This is supported by a 25-year-old study of a very limited number of patients [64].

I find 'fluid thrill' useless in detecting ascites (it is elicited by tapping the lateral abdominal wall on one side with the other hand waiting for the 'thrill' to arrive on the other side). Cattau and colleagues [64] have already called for ultrasound to prove the presence of ascites; it has to be pointed out, however, that the Child–Pugh classification is based on clinical detection of ascites.

Neurological examination

I have never had the patience to perform a thorough neurological examination on my patients – if I have the impression that something is wrong, I ask for a neurology consultation and have the big thinkers sort out what is wrong. This attitude is probably wrong because reversible focal deficits can be found in ~15% of patients with hepatic coma [65].

A few tests definitively belong in the hepatology clinic, namely signs hinting at hepatic encephalopathy, Wilson's disease (covered in Chapter 16.1.) and subtle signs of neuropathy – in particular loss of sense of vibration – which are frequent in endstage liver disease, particularly that originating from alcohol toxicity.

Encephalopathy

The time-proven sign of hepatic encephalopathy is flapping tremor or asterixis. It is elicited by having the patient dorsiflex his or her hands in prone rotation. Asterixis is seen as a rhythmic loss of tone appearing as a flapping movement of the hands, reminding one of flapping bird wings. In very weak patients, asterixis can be felt by asking the patient to hold both of your hands or by looking at the tongue, again asking for a lifting of the tongue. Further testing for hepatic encephalopathy is described in Chapter 7.8.

Neuropathy

Peripheral neuropathy is frequent in patients abusing alcohol [66] but also in advanced liver disease of any atiology [67]. It should be sought in hepatitis C patients with cryoglobulinaemia. In patients with longstanding cholestasis, it can be related to vitamin E deficiency.

References

1 Foster GR, Goldin RD, Thomas HC (1998) Chronic hepatitis C virus infection causes a significant reduction in quality of life in the absence of cirrhosis. *Hepatology* 27, 209–212.

2 Weissenborn K, Krause J, Bokemeyer M *et al.* (2004) Hepatitis C virus infection affects the brain – evidence from psychometric studies and magnetic resonance spectroscopy. *J Hepatol* 41, 845–851.

3 McAndrews MP, Farcnik K, Carlen P *et al.* (2005) Prevalence and significance of neurocognitive dysfunction in hepatitis C in the absence of correlated risk factors. *Hepatology* 41, 801–808.

4 Poupon RE, Chrétien Y, Chazouillères O *et al.* (2004) Quality of life in patients with primary biliary cirrhosis. *Hepatology* 40, 489–494.

5 Swain MG (2000) Fatigue in chronic disease. *Clin Sci* 99, 1–8.

6 Stanca CM, Bach N, Krause C *et al.* (2005) Evaluation of fatigue in US patients with primary biliary cirrhosis. *Am J Gastroenterol* 100, 1104–1109.

7 Goldblatt J, Taylor PJS, Lipman T *et al.* (2002) The true impact of fatigue in primary biliary cirrhosis: A population study. *Gastroenterology* 122, 1235–1241.

8 Björnsson E, Simren M, Olsson R, Chapman RW (2004) Fatigue in patients with primary sclerosing cholangitis. *Scand J Gastroenterol* 39, 961–968.

9 Marchesini G, Bianchi G, Lucidi P *et al.* (2004) Plasma ghrelin concentrations, food intake, and anorexia in liver failure. *J Clin Endocrinol Metab* 89, 2136–2141.

10 Madden AM, Bradbury W, Morgan MY (1997) Taste perception in cirrhosis: its relationship to circulating micronutrients and food preferences. *Hepatology* 26, 40–48.

11 Bergasa NV (1998) Hypothesis: taste disorders in patients with liver disease may be mediated in the brain: potential mechanisms for a central phenomenon. *Am J Gastroenterol* 93, 1209–1210.

12 Drosos AA, Constantopoulos SH, Psychos D *et al.* (1989) The forgotten cause of sicca complex: sarcoidosis. *J Rheumatol* 16, 1548–1551.

13 Cacoub P, Poynard T, Ghillani P *et al.* (1999) Extrahepatic manifestations of chronic hepatitis C. *Arthritis Rheum* 42, 2204–2212.

14 Jorgensen C, Legouffe MC, Perney P *et al.* (1996) Sicca syndrome associated with hepatitis C virus infection. *Arthritis Rheum* 39, 1166–1171.

15 Cacoub P, Saadoun D, Bourlière M *et al.* (2005) Hepatitis B virus genotypes and extrahepatic manifestations. *J Hepatol* 43, 764–770.

16 Diehl AK, Sugarek NJ, Todd KH (1990) Clinical evaluation for gallstone disease: usefulness of symptoms and signs in diagnosis. *Am J Med* 89, 29–33.

17 Kraag N, Thijs C, Knipschild P (1995) Dyspepsia—how noisy are gallstones? A meta-analysis of epidemiologic studies of biliary pain, dyspeptic symptoms, and food intolerance. Scand J Gastroenterol 30, 411–421.

18 Misra SP, Misra V, Dwivedi M *et al.* (2004) Factors influencing colonic involvement in patients with amebic liver abscess. *Gastrointest Endosc* 59, 512–516.

19 Ginsburg PM, Thuluvath PJ (2005) Diarrhea in liver transplant recipients: etiology and management. *Liver Transpl* 11, 881–890.

20 Navasa M, Rimola A, Rodés J (1997) Bacterial infections in liver disease. *Semin Liver Dis* 17, 323–333.

21 O'Donohue J, Workman MR, Rolando N *et al.* (1997) Urinary tract infections in primary biliary cirrhosis and other chronic liver diseases. *Eur J Clin Microbiol Infect Dis* 16, 743–746.

22 Cribier B, Samain F, Vetter D *et al.* (1998) Systematic cutaneous examination in hepatitis C virus infected patients. *Acta Derm Venereol (Stockh)* 78, 355–357.

23 Dega H, Frances C, Dupin N *et al.* (1998) Pruritus and the hepatitis C virus. The MULTIVIRC Unit. *Ann Dermatol Venereol* 125, 9–12.

24 Bergasa NV (2005) The pruritus of cholestasis. *J Hepatol* 43, 1078–1088.

25 Baskol M, Ozbakir O, Coskun R *et al.* (2004) The role of serum zinc and other factors on the prevalence of muscle cramps in non-alcoholic cirrhotic patients. *J Clin Gastroenterol* 38, 524–529.

26 Marchesini G, Bianchi G, Amodio P *et al.* (2001) Factors associated with poor health-related quality of life of patients with cirrhosis. *Gastroenterology* 120, 170–178.

27 Steindl PE, Finn B, Bendok B *et al.* (1995) Disruption of the diurnal rhythm of plasma melatonin in cirrhosis. *Ann Intern Med* 123, 274–277.

28 Blake JC, Sprengers D, Grech P *et al.* (1990) Bleeding time in patients with hepatic cirrhosis. *Br Med J* 301, 12–15.

29 Merli M, Riggio O, Dally L *et al.* (1996) Does malnutrition affect survival in cirrhosis? *Hepatology* 23, 1041–1046.

30 Abelmann WH (1994) Hyperdynamic circulation in cirrhosis: a historical perspective. *Hepatology* 20, 1356–1358.

31 Kowalski HJ, Abelmann WH (1953) The cardiac output at rest in Laennec's cirrhosis. *J Clin Invest* 32, 1025–1033.

32 Mourad O, Palda V, Detsky AS (2003) A comprehensive evidence-based approach to fever of unknown origin. *Arch Intern Med* 163, 545–551.

33 Kitzberger R, Madl C, Ferenci P (2005) Wilson disease. *Metab Brain Dis* 20, 295–302.

34 Beaumont C, Leneuve C, Deveaux I *et al.* (1995) Mutation in the iron responsive element of the L ferritin mRNA in a family with dominant hyperferritinemia and cataract. *Nature Genet* 11, 444–446.

35 Hingorani M, Nischal KK, Davies A *et al.* (1999) Ocular abnormalities in Alagille syndrome. *Ophthalmology* 106, 330–337.

36 Rodriquez-Roisin R, Krowka MJ, Herve P, Fallon MB (2005) Highlights of the ERS Task Force on pulmonary-hepatic vascular disorders (PHD). *J Hepatol* 42, 924–927.

37 Milman N (1991) Hereditary haemochromatosis in Denmark 1950–1985. Clinical, biochemical and histological features in 179 patients and 13 preclinical cases. *Dan Med Bull* 38, 385–393.

38 El-Serag HB, Hampel H, Yeh C, Rabeneck L (2002) Extrahepatic manifestations of hepatitis C among United States male veterans. *Hepatology* 36, 1439–1445.

39 Reuben A (2002) Along came a spider. *Hepatology* 35, 735–736.

40 Orrego H, Israel Y, Blake JE, Medline A (1983) Assessment of prognostic factors in alcoholic liver disease: toward a global quantitative expression of severity. *Hepatology* 3, 896–905.

41 Foutch PG, Sullivan JA, Gaines JA, Sanowski RA (1988) Cutaneous vascular spiders in cirrhotic patients: correlation with hemorrhage from esophageal varices. *Am J Gastroenterol* 83, 723–726.

42 Pilette C, Oberti F, Aubé C *et al.* (1999) Non-invasive diagnosis of esophageal varices in chronic liver diseases. *J Hepatol* 31, 867–873.

43 Attali P, Ink O, Pelletier G *et al.* (1987) Dupuytren's contracture, alcohol consumption, and chronic liver disease. *Arch Intern Med* 147, 1065–1067.

44 Hart MG, Hooper G (2005) Clinical associations of Dupuytren's disease. *Postgrad Med J* 8, 425–428.

45 Holzberg M, Walker HK (1984) Terry's nails: revised definition and new correlations. *Lancet* i, 896–899.

46 Martínez GP, Barberà JA, Visa J *et al.* (2001) Hepatopulmonary syndrome in candidates for liver transplantation. *J Hepatol* 34, 651–657.

47 Van der Merwe S, Dens J, Daenen W *et al.* (2000) Pericardial disease is often not recognised as a cause of chronic severe ascites. *J Hepatol* 32, 164–169.

48 Cardenas A, Kelleher T, Chopra S (2004) Review article: hepatic hydrothorax. *Aliment Pharmacol Ther* 20, 271–279.

49 Henrion J, Colin L, Schapira M, Heller FR (1997) Hypoxic hepatitis caused by severe hypoxemia from obstructive sleep apnea. *J Clin Gastroenterol* 24, 245–249.

50 Tanné F, Gagnadoux F, Chazouillères O *et al.* (2005) Chronic liver injury during obstructive sleep apnea. *Hepatology* 41, 1290–1296.

51 Gillard JH, Patel MC, Abrahams PH, Dixon AK (1998) Riedel's lobe of the liver: fact or fiction? *Clin Anat* 11, 47–49.

52 Zoli M, Magalotti D, Grimaldi M *et al.* (1995) Physical examination of the liver: is it still worth it? *Am J Gastroenterol* 90, 1428–1432.

53 Tucker WN, Saab S, Rickman LS, Mathews WC (1997) The scratch test is unreliable for detecting the liver edge. *J Clin Gastroenterol* 25, 410–414.

54 McGee SR (1995) Percussion and physical diagnosis: separating myth from science. *Dis Mon* 41, 641–692.

55 Cha SD, Desai RS, Gooch AS *et al.* (1982) Diagnosis of severe tricuspid regurgitation. *Chest* 82, 726–731.

56 Manga P, Vythilingum S, Mitha AS (1984) Pulsatile hepatomegaly in constrictive pericarditis. *Br Heart J* 52, 465–467.

57 Chen JJ, Changchien CS, Tai DI, Kuo CH (1994) Gallbladder volume in patients with common hepatic duct dilatation – an evaluation of Courvoisier's sign using ultrasonography. *Scand J Gastroenterol* 29, 284–288.

58 Barkun AN, Camus M, Green L *et al.* (1991) The bedside assessment of splenic enlargement. *Am J Med* 91, 512–518.

59 Isik FF, Greenfield AJ, Guben J *et al.* (1989) Iatrogenic arterioportal fistulae: diagnosis and management. *Ann Vasc Surg* 3, 52–55.

60 Okuda K, Musha H, Nakajima Y *et al.* (1978) Frequency of intrahepatic arteriovenous fistula as a sequela to percutaneous needle puncture of the liver. *Gastroenterology* 74, 1204–1207.

61 Clain D, Wartnaby K, Sherlock S (1966) Abdominal arterial murmurs in liver disease. *Lancet* ii, 516–519.

62 Bernard G, Mion F, Henry L *et al.* (1993) Hepatic involvement in hereditary hemorrhagic telangiectasia – clinical, radiological, and hemodynamic studies of 11 cases. *Gastroenterology* 105, 482–487.

63 Zeger W, Holt K (2003) Gynecologic infections. *Emerg Med Clin North Am* 21, 631–648.

64 Cattau EL, Benjamin SB, Knuff TE, Castell DO (1982) The accuracy of the physical examination in the diagnosis of suspected ascites. *J Am Med Assoc* 247, 1164–1166.

65 Cadranel JF, Lebiez E, Di Martino V *et al.* (2001) Focal neurological signs in hepatic encephalopathy in cirrhotic patients: an underestimated entity? *Am J Gastroenterol* 96, 515–518.

66 Zambelis T, Karandreas N, Tzavellas E *et al.* (2005) Large and small fiber neuropathy in chronic alcohol-dependent subjects. *J Peripher Nerv Syst* 10, 375–381.

67 Chaudhry V, Corse AM, O'Brian R *et al.* (1999) Autonomic and peripheral (sensorimotor) neuropathy in chronic liver disease: a clinical and electrophysiologic study. *Hepatology* 29, 1698–1703.

5.2 Biochemical investigations in the management of liver disease

Igino Rigato, J. Donald Ostrow and Claudio Tiribelli

Introduction

Due to the complex and multiple metabolic functions of the liver, there is no single, ideal biochemical test that can fully assess the nature and severity of hepatic dysfunction. Rather, individual biochemical tests can be applied to assess specific aspects of hepatic function. Thus, necrosis of hepatocytes can be assessed by measuring enzymes that have leaked into the blood through the damaged plasma membranes of the liver cells. The ability of the liver to synthesize plasma proteins produced selectively by the liver can be assessed from the plasma concentrations of these proteins, keeping in mind that the concentration of each protein is influenced also by its catabolism. Impairment of the excretory functions of the liver, including bile secretion and flow, can be indirectly assessed from increases in the plasma levels of endogenous compounds (e.g. bile salts and bilirubin) that are normally cleared by the liver and secreted in bile. The plasma levels, however, may also be affected by changes in the rates of production, intestinal absorption and enterohepatic circulation, and renal excretion of these compounds.

These distinctions among classes of 'liver function' tests are somewhat arbitrary, but examining the results of all of these markers together often reveals patterns typical of different pathophysiological conditions, and allows some assessment of the severity of the liver disease. In this chapter, we will describe tests for plasma constituents that are commonly measured in the evaluation of patients with hepatobiliary diseases. For each of them, we will describe the following features, when available: description of rationale and biochemical reactions for the test; a critical comparison of available methods; interpretation of the results; and clinical relevance.

Markers of hepatocellular damage

Aminotransferases: aspartate aminotransferase (AST) and alanine aminotransferase (ALT)

Nature of the enzymes and their reactions

The most frequently used indices of hepatocellular necrosis are activities in the serum of aspartate aminotransferase (AST, previously known as glutamic–oxaloacetic transaminase, GOT) and alanine aminotransferase (ALT, previously known as glutamic–pyruvic transaminase, GPT). These enzymes, which are involved in the pathways of gluconeogenesis, catalyse the enzymatic transfer of the α-amino group from an amino acid, aspartate or alanine, to the oxo- group of α-ketoglutarate, yielding glutamate plus, respectively, oxaloacetate or pyruvate.

Distribution and localization of the enzymes

ALT is localized exclusively in the cytosol and essentially restricted to the hepatocytes and renal tubular epithelium, although there is also slight activity in skeletal muscle and heart [1]. By contrast, AST is widely distributed throughout the body, with highest activity in the heart, liver, skeletal muscle, brain, gastric mucosa, kidney, pancreas, spleen and lung [2]; it is also detectable in erythrocytes. Inside the liver cell, AST is localized mainly in the mitochondrial membrane (80%), with the remainder in the cytosol [3]. In normal healthy people, cytosolic AST is the source of more than 90% of total serum AST activity [3]. The two isoforms (cytosolic and mitochondrial) can be separated by immunochemical methods or by chromatographic and electrophoretic techniques, but, as those methods are not available in most laboratories, the distinction in the activity of the two isoenzymes is seldom used clinically.

The aminotransferases are released into the blood when enzyme-containing cells are damaged, resulting in an increase in their concentrations and activity in plasma. AST is not detectable in the urine except during renal ischaemia [4]: measurement of urine AST was formerly used to detect kidney failure after renal tubular necrosis, but other enzymes are now more reliably employed for this purpose. AST and ALT were formerly assayed by colorimetric methods, which have now been superseded completely by spectrophotometric techniques.

Assays of enzyme activity

The older colorimetric methods involved addition of the substrates α-ketoglutarate plus aspartate (for AST) or alanine (for ALT) to a buffered plasma sample. Pyruvate, formed directly from ALT, or produced by subsequent decarboxylation of the oxaloacetate product of AST by addition of aniline citrate, was then treated with 2,4-dinitrophenylhydrazine. The hydrazone product turned brown in an alkaline solution, and was measured colorimetrically. The modern spectrophotometric AST method, recommended by the International Federation of Clinical Chemistry [5], is based on a simultaneous double reaction: reduction, with NADH and H^+, of the oxaloacetate formed by the aminotransferase reaction is catalysed by adding malate dehydrogenase, yielding L-malate and NAD^+. The absorbances at 365, 340 or 334 nm are used to quantify the loss of NADH or formation of NAD^+, which correlates directly with the content of AST in the sample. The spectrophotometric ALT assay utilizes a method analogous to that described for AST: L-alanine and α-ketoglutarate are transformed by ALT into pyruvate and L-glutamate. The pyruvate is then enzymatically converted to lactate by addition of lactic dehydrogenase and NADH, and the loss of NADH or formation of NAD^+ is monitored spectrophotometrically, as with the AST method.

Normal values and influencing factors

The normal serum transaminase levels in adults are below 40 U/L. Transaminases in serum specimens are stable for 3 days at room temperature and for 3 weeks in the refrigerator. In whole blood, by contrast, AST (but not ALT) increases during storage due to its release from spontaneous haemolysis of red cells.

The half-life of total AST in the blood is 17 ± 5 h whereas that of ALT is 47 ± 10 h. Within the normal range, the activities of AST and ALT in plasma vary with age and sex. AST and ALT activities increase from childhood to adulthood, then plateau at a steady level between the ages of 30 to 60. In adults, the enzymatic activity is higher in males than in females, and plasma levels of AST tend to be lower than ALT. Above age 60, AST levels rise slowly, whereas ALT levels decline after 60 [6]. AST is 15% higher in African–American men.

Abnormal values in hepatobiliary diseases

Aminotransferases in serum are usually elevated during hepatocellular injury of any cause. Marked elevations (8–20-fold above normal) suggest acute hepatocellular necrosis, due to viral hepatitis, drug- or toxin-induced liver damage or ischaemic hepatitis; ischaemic necrosis may lead to extreme elevations in aminotransferase levels (up to 100-fold). The degree of increase of serum levels, however, does not correlate with the extent of liver damage observed on liver biopsy, and does not predict mortality. Persistent, fluctuating, usually mild elevations of serum aminotransferase activities are observed during chronic liver injury caused by chronic viral hepatitis, alcoholic liver disease, nonalcoholic fatty liver disease (NAFLD), autoimmune hepatitis, haemochromatosis, Wilson's disease or liver cirrhosis. ALT and AST increase during extrahepatic obstruction, typically associated with elevation in serum of markers of cholestasis [alkaline phosphatase, γ-glutamyltransferase (γ-GT) and bilirubin].

Several patterns of increased aminotransferases have been touted as markers of specific liver diseases or different prognoses (Fig. 1). It was suggested that an AST/ALT ratio above 0.6 is associated with a poor outcome in cases of severe acute hepatitis [7]. The AST/ALT ratio is also increased in alcoholic liver damage (see below), exposure to various organic compounds (i.e. toluene, furan, methylene chloride), and in liver fibrosis. However, due to the wide spectrum of liver diseases associated with mildly elevated levels of aminotransferases, the AST/ALT ratio is of weak predictive value in defining the aetiology of liver disease. It is important to remember that, although elevations in aminotransferase levels may be the first or only marker of liver damage, significant liver damage may be present without any elevation of either AST or ALT, for example in chronic viral hepatitis, haemochromatosis or liver cirrhosis [8].

Drug-related hepatotoxicity engenders a significant increase in serum aminotransferase activity that usually is characterized by an elevated AST/ALT ratio; this aetiology should be considered every time an increased AST/ALT ratio is found in patients who do not consume alcohol. For this reason, aminotransferases are good markers of chemotherapy-induced hepatocellular necrosis. Aminotransferase activities are increased in 11–28% of patients undergoing anticonvulsant therapy [2].

Elevations of AST and/or ALT activity in alcoholic patients are generally mild (2–4 times the upper normal limits), but may be higher in acute alcoholic hepatitis. Intake of 3–4 g/kg body weight of alcohol by healthy subjects leads to an increase of aminotransferases within 24–48 h. In alcoholic liver disease, AST tends to be higher than ALT activity [9]. This is due to release of AST as a result of alcoholic damage to red cells, inhibition of the ALT reaction by alcohol and an increase in mitochondrial AST (mAST) during excessive alcohol consumption. It has been suggested that serum mAST activity, or the ratio of mAST/total AST activity, could be used to screen for excessive alcohol intake in the general population. In this setting, however, the specificity and sensitivity were low, and these indices have proven to be useful markers of alcoholic liver disease only in an inpatient setting [9].

Interestingly, although AST and ALT are both increased in NAFLD, serum aminotransferase activity is logarithmically related to body mass index irrespective of the aetiology of liver disease [10].

An inverse relationship has been described between serum AST activity and serum creatinine concentration. In uraemic patients, for unknown reasons, the AST level is decreased, irrespective of the analytical method and whether or not the patient is undergoing dialysis. Furthermore, in uraemic patients, AST may not increase when hepatic disease supervenes, rendering the AST determination an unreliable marker of hepatobiliary disease in such patients [11].

Abnormal values in other diseases

AST, in particular, is usually elevated in many nonhepatic diseases. AST is increased in acute myocardial infarction and with acute muscle damage that occurs in Duchenne's type muscular dystrophy, dermatomyositis, muscle trauma or surgery and

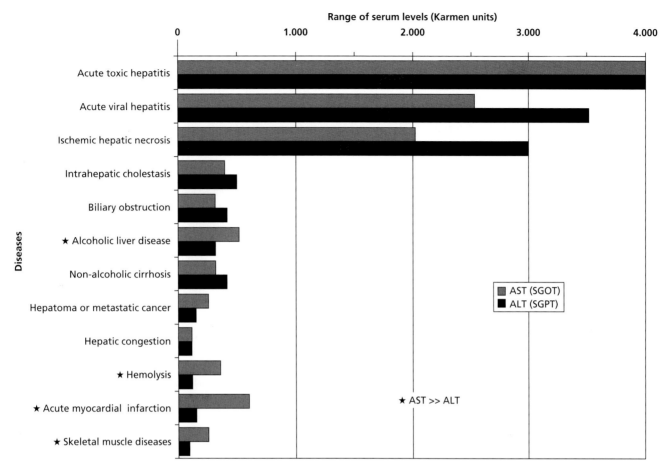

Fig. 1 Elevations of aspartate aminotransferase (AST) and alanine aminotransferase (ALT) in various diseases.

gangrene of the toes [12]. In children affected by rotaviral gastro-enteritis, AST of enterocyte origin can be increased in serum [13]. Elevated serum aminotransferases are typically observed in pre-eclampsia and HELLP (haemolysis, elevated liver enzymes, low platelets) syndrome during pregnancy.

Several other factors can affect the AST and ALT plasma activity: exercise can increase (up to threefold) the AST levels while ALT levels may decrease. The day-to-day variation is similar in liver disease and health, and is around 5–10% for AST and 10–30% for ALT [14]. Even if both AST and ALT activities are higher in red blood cells than in plasma, only severe haemolysis causes a significant increase in serum aminotransferase activity [2]. By an unknown mechanism, aminotransferase activity, especially ALT, is increased by heparin therapy, more frequently in males than females [2]. The mAST isoenzyme was suggested to be useful to assess myocardial damage after thrombolysis as it is not influenced by the reperfusion of the damaged tissue [15].

Lactate dehydrogenase

Nature of the enzyme and its reaction

Lactic dehydrogenase (LDH), an enzyme of the glycolytic cycle, catalyses the reversible conversion of lactate to pyruvate, utiliz-ing $NAD^+/NADH$ as a cofactor. LDH also catalyses the reduc-tion of other α-keto or α-γ-diketo groups. LDH enzyme is a tetramer that is constructed from two monomeric isoforms: type H from heart muscle and type M from liver. Various combinations of these two isoforms can yield five different isoenzymes, which have different tissue distributions. Increased release of LDH from damaged, dying or metabolically deranged cells in any of these tissues may cause an elevated serum LDH concentration.

Distribution and localization of the enzyme

LDH is highly expressed in kidney but it is also expressed in heart, skeletal muscle, spleen, liver, lung and erythrocytes. In liver, only LDH type 5 (the MMMM tetramer) is expressed. LDH5 is, however, also expressed in kidney, skeletal muscles and pancreas.

Assays of enzyme activity

Of the many different LDH assay techniques described, the most used and most accurate one for automated analysis is the photo-metric assessment of the oxidation rate of NADH, measured at 365 or 340 nm. The serum sample is incubated with standard concentrations of pyruvate and NADH, and the results are expressed as arbitrary units per litre. For greater tissue specificity, the different isoenzymes can be separated by electrophoresis on cellulose acetate membranes, and the individual protein bands incubated with lactate and NAD$^+$; the NADH product is then reacted with a tetrazolium salt to produce a coloured dye (formazan), which is quantitated by densitometry.

Normal values and influencing factors

Each laboratory must determine its own normal values. Age influences the serum LDH activity: the normal range is higher in children than adults, and it decreases progressively with aging, reaching an adult range at about age 14 years [16]. The proportions of the five isoenzymes detected in normal serum are:

- LDH1 (HHHH)   18–33%
- LDH2 (HHHM)   28–40%
- LDH3 (HHMM)   18–30%
- LDH4 (HMMM)   6–16%
- LDH5 (MMMM)   2–13%.

Abnormal values in hepatobiliary diseases

An increase in serum LDH activity is often observed during acute hepatitis or hepatocyte necrosis of any aetiology.

Abnormal values in other diseases

Because of its wide tissue distribution, serum LDH can be increased with myocardial diseases, haemolytic anaemia, myopathies, leukaemias and lymphomas, acute pancreatitis and nephropathies.

Summary of clinical usefulness

Elevations in serum LDH are not specific for active liver disease, and are less sensitive and specific than the elevations in serum transaminases in this situation. It may be useful in jaundiced subjects to determine if haemolysis is contributory, because elevations in LDH, AST and indirect bilirubin are usually more striking than elevations in ALT in this situation. It is more often used to evaluate myocardial damage in patients with suspected myocardial infarction, in which case electrophoretic analysis of isoenzyme activity is essential to pinpoint the source of the serum enzyme elevation.

Markers to assess hepatic synthetic function

Albumin

Nature of the protein and its function

Albumin is a single, unglycosylated polypeptide chain of 575 amino acids (molecular mass 69 kDa). It is synthesized exclusively by hepatocytes at a rate of about 14 g/day [17], and secreted into the plasma [18], where it normally constitutes 58–64% of total serum proteins. It has two principal functions in plasma: maintenance of osmotic pressure and reversible, noncovalent binding of a variety of substances, both endogenous

(e.g. bilirubin, bile salts, fatty acids and other organic anions and metal cations) and exogenous (drugs, contrast media). This transport function is essential for hydrophobic compounds that have low aqueous solubility.

The half-life of albumin in human serum is 14–21 days [19]. Hyperalbuminaemia is observed only with haemoconcentration during dehydration, whereas hypoalbuminaemia is a frequent condition, related to decreased synthesis, increased catabolism or excessive losses in the urine or stool (see below).

Assays

Many methods exist for measurement of the serum albumin concentration, including: precipitation, electrophoresis, immunochemical procedures and binding of dyes. Due to the ease of automation, binding of dyes, particularly bromocresol green (BCG), is most frequently used. In acid solution (pH 4.15), BCG has high affinity for albumin and little interaction with other serum proteins. The albumin–BCG complex has an absorbance maximum at 630 nm that avoids interference from the spectral peaks of haemoglobin or bilirubin. Some laboratories prefer bromocresol purple, which is more specific, because it reacts even less with serum globulin or transferrin [20]. With either dye, falsely low albumin levels may be obtained with jaundiced or haemolysed samples due to displacement of the dye from albumin by bilirubin or haemoglobin respectively.

Immunoassay techniques can be automated, but are more expensive. Electrophoresis on cellulose acetate membranes permits simultaneous measurement of the concentrations of all classes of serum proteins, but is difficult to automate.

Normal values

Serum albumin levels are typically low in neonates (2.8–4.4 g/dL), increasing progressively during the first week of life to normal adult concentrations (3.7–5.0 g/dL). By age 6 years, the values increase further (4.5–5.4 g/dL) and remain stable through young adulthood before decreasing again to the normal adult values. Further mild declines in serum albumin levels occur in old age, principally due to more rapid catabolism [19]. There is no significant difference between genders.

Influencing factors

Several conditions may influence albumin synthesis by a healthy liver. Despite adequate caloric intake, a strict vegetarian diet can impair albumin synthesis if it is not supplemented with soy proteins. High altitude can increase albumin synthesis, especially if the high altitude is reached by climbing. In addition, recovery from a period of intense physical exercise, in an upright position, can increase albumin synthesis. Albumin synthesis can increase by up to 30% when normoalbuminaemic patients are treated with haemodialysis [21].

Abnormal values in hepatobiliary diseases

The albumin concentration is decreased in liver cirrhosis, due to impaired hepatic synthesis, often aggravated by losses into

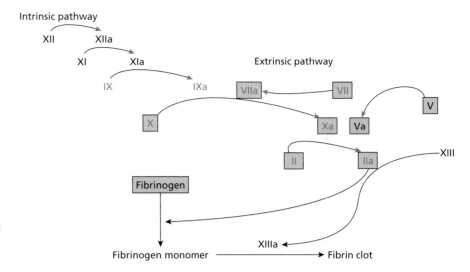

Fig. 2 The coagulation pathway. Highlighted factors are produced by the liver; vitamin K-dependent factors are shaded grey.

ascitic fluid due to leakage from hepatic lymphatics or exudation across the capsule of the liver [22].

Abnormal values in other diseases

Decreased albumin synthesis is also observed during malnutrition, and begins after only 24–48 hours of fasting [19]; for this reason, it is considered to be a good parameter to evaluate malnutrition, despite its poor sensitivity [23]. Every kind of 'stress' condition (major surgery, injury, severe infection or almost any severe, acute disease) may be associated with a decline in the serum albumin levels due to the release of cytokines and hormones (i.e. cortisone, thyroid hormones, growth hormone, insulin and sex hormones) that inhibit synthesis of this protein [23].

Hypoalbuminaemia may also result from excessive losses of serum albumin in the urine or stool. The nephrotic syndrome is characterized, by definition, by the presence of over 3.5 g/day of protein in the urine [24], the majority of which is represented by albuminuria. Leakage of protein from plasma into the gut lumen, with excessive faecal losses, characterizes protein-losing enteropathy, seen with Crohn's disease, sprue, kwashiorkor, Ménétrier's disease, eosinophilic gastroenteritis and radiation enteritis, among others [25]. Excessive intestinal protein loss may also occur secondary to high pressure in the portal capillaries, as in Budd–Chiari syndrome and constrictive pericarditis; it contributes to the hypoalbuminaemia of cirrhosis. With extensive burns or bed sores, exudation of albumin from the damaged skin can lead to severe hypoalbuminaemia [26].

Summary of clinical usefulness

Serum albumin concentration is one of the most important indices of residual hepatocytic synthetic function. When serum albumin concentration is decreased (<3.0 g/dL) in patients with liver disease, it strongly suggests the presence of cirrhosis. Serum albumin is an important parameter in both the Child–Pugh and MELD (model for end-stage liver disease) scores, the two most widely used systems to evaluate prognosis in chronic liver disease.

Prothrombin time (PT) and the international normalized ratio (INR)

Nature of the reaction

The one-stage prothrombin time (PT) reflects the presence or functional absence of those factors involved in the extrinsic clotting system. The cascade that leads to clot formation through the activation of the extrinsic pathway involves factors I, II, V, VII and X (Fig. 2). All those factors are produced in the liver and three of them (II, VII, X) require vitamin K as a cofactor for their synthesis. Low plasma levels of factors II, V and VII have been reported in patients with liver disease and therefore the PT can be considered an index of hepatocyte synthetic function [27].

Assay

The assay is based on the original method of Quick [28]. Sodium citrate is added to a blood sample, preventing coagulation by binding calcium. Afterwards tissue thromboplastin and calcium are added and the time to form a fibrin clot is registered. The results are expressed as the interval (in seconds) between the addition of calcium and the clot formation, compared with the time required for clot formation when the same reagents are added to a citrated pool of normal blood samples (control).

Normal values and influencing factors

The normal prothrombin time is usually below 12 s, with a ratio to the control time that is above 0.7. Storage in a refrigerator falsely shortens the PT, whereas storage at room temperature for up to 3 days does not influence the result. It is very important to completely fill the blood sample tube, because incomplete filling increases the PT. A high haematocrit leads to an increase in the PT [29].

The determination of PT is highly sensitive to the type of thromboplastin used (human-brain- or rabbit-brain-derived) and the PT may be 30–100% longer with different batches [30]. The PT is frequently used for monitoring subjects treated with anticoagulant drugs (warfarin, acenocoumarol). Because these drugs are administered for prolonged periods and patients may move from one lab to another, it is extremely important to be able to compare results from different laboratories in order to safely adjust the dose of the medicine. For this reason, the World Health Organization (WHO) introduced the international normalized ratio (INR) as a unit for comparison of results among laboratories everywhere. Each batch of commercial thromboplastin is assigned an international sensitivity index (ISI), which is derived by comparison of the PT obtained with the commercial batch with a standard thromboplastin. The PT of the laboratory sample is then multiplied by the ISI, yielding the INR, which, like the PT, is an index of residual hepatocytic synthetic function (see below). Correction of the PT using the ISI has a greater effect on the PT obtained during anticoagulant treatment than in subjects with liver disease, and a decrease in the ISI of the thromboplastin used may not engender a significant increase in the PT. This is probably related to different isoforms of prothrombin produced during vitamin K deficiency and/or liver failure [14]. The general recommendation, therefore, is to use the INR for monitoring anticoagulant therapy and the PT to assess hepatic synthetic function.

Abnormal values in hepatobiliary diseases

During liver disease, several pathological mechanisms may affect the coagulation cascade, lengthening the PT, including: (i) decreased synthesis of coagulation factors and (ii) decreased intake and/or absorption of vitamin K. The latter cofactor is lipid soluble and requires adequate concentrations of bile salts in the intestinal lumen in order to be absorbed. Decreased synthesis of bile salts in hepatocellular diseases, and/or decreased biliary secretion of bile salts in cholestatic disorders, may decrease the luminal concentration of bile salts below the critical micellar concentration necessary for normal absorption of lipids, including vitamin K. A third cause of a prolonged PT in liver failure is related to impaired ability of the hepatic Kupffer cells to remove activated clotting factors from the circulation. This may lead to intravascular coagulation, with consumption of clotting factors [31].

Impairment of the PT is roughly proportional to the degree of liver damage, so the PT is an excellent prognostic index of liver disease [32]. The sensitivity of the PT as a marker of acute as well as chronic liver disease is related to the fact that this test assesses the extrinsic coagulation pathway that begins with the activation of factor VII. Factor VII has the shortest half-life (3–5.5 h) of any of the coagulation factors, and so is the first to decline when synthesis of coagulation factors is impaired, either due to hepatocellar damage or vitamin K deficiency [31].

The injection of 10 mg of vitamin K for three consecutive days can help to discriminate between a decreased absorption of vitamin K (due to cholestasis or other causes) and decreased hepatic protein synthesis: if the PT returns to the normal range, the reduced availability of vitamin K was the cause of the prolonged coagulation time; if the PT decreases but still is above the upper normal limit, then a double cause (reduced absorption

and reduced liver synthetic function) should be considered; and if the PT hardly changes, it means that the PT was prolonged because of impaired liver function.

Abnormal values in other diseases

The PT may be prolonged in coeliac sprue due to malabsorption of vitamin K. It may, for unknown reasons, be abnormal in hepatic congestion related to right-sided heart failure.

Clinical usefulness

PT is an excellent prognostic factor in either acute or chronic liver failure. During acute viral or alcoholic hepatitis, the degree of elevation of the PT ratio is the best predictor of the risk of death. With paracetamol (acetaminophen) toxicity, however, only a persistent increase in the PT ratio heralds a fatal outcome [1]. In cirrhotic patients, the PT ratio is an important component of two commonly used prognostic indices, the Child–Pugh and MELD score; in both algorithms the PT ratio strongly influences the total score.

Although a key prognostic index in both acute and chronic liver disease, the PT has no value as a screening marker for liver disease. Rather it should be reserved to assess residual hepatic synthetic function for patients with known liver disease [33].

Plasma fibrinogen

Nature of the compound and its distribution

Fibrinogen is a homodimeric plasma protein that is synthesized in hepatocytes; each monomer is formed by three polypeptide chains: α, β and γ. In the final step of the coagulation cascade, fibrinogen is converted to fibrin monomers by the peptidase activity of thrombin. These in turn aggregate to form the insoluble polymer, fibrin gel, which is stabilized by activated factor XIII [34].

Assays for detection

The two most useful assays for quantitation of plasma fibrinogen are a clotting rate assay and an enzyme immunosorbent assay (EIA). Sodium citrate is used as anticoagulant to collect the plasma specimen. For the clotting rate assay, the plasma sample, diluted 10-fold, is incubated with thrombin; the resultant fibrin clot is suspended in 6.7 M alkaline urea, and the fibrinogen concentration is derived from the optical density at 280 nm, compared with standards containing known concentrations of fibrinogen. The EIA assay is performed using an immobilized monoclonal antibody against the carboxyl-terminal end of the fibrinogen α-chain to capture the fibrinogen. A monoclonal antibody against the amino-terminal end of the α-chain, complexed with horse radish peroxidase (HRP), is then added. The clot and EIA methods yield comparable results [35].

Normal values, factors influencing them and abnormal values in organ diseases other than liver

The normal range in plasma is 200–400 mg/dL, and this can

be influenced by several different pathological states. Fibrinogen is an 'acute phase protein', concentrations of which are often elevated in: severe infections, postsurgical states, collagenoses, rheumatoid arthritis and pregnancy. Decreases in the plasma concentration of fibrinogen can be due to a hereditary dysfibrinogenaemia, or to acquired conditions that decrease synthesis or increase consumption. Genetic hypofibrinogenaemia, present from birth, is related to gene mutations in either the α, β or γ chain [34]. Increased consumption of fibrinogen occurs in the syndrome of disseminated intravascular coagulation (DIC), in which fibrinogen levels are decreased due to increased degradation of fibrinogen to split products.

Abnormal values in hepatobiliary diseases

Plasma fibrinogen concentration is usually increased during fulminant hepatitis as an acute phase response. In such patients, the prognosis is poor if the fibrinogen concentration fails to rise or decreases, reflecting severely impaired protein synthesis [36] or development of DIC [37]. With chronic liver disease, fibrinogen levels usually remain within the normal range, decreasing only when severe liver dysfunction develops (Child class C patients) [35]. The decrease in plasma fibrinogen is a result of decreased protein synthesis and/or increased peripheral intravascular coagulation [38]. The latter is distinguished by increased plasma levels of fibrin split products.

Summary of clinical usefulness

Because plasma fibrinogen concentration decreases mainly in endstage liver failure, it has very limited predictive value in chronic liver disease [39] but suggests a poor prognosis in acute hepatic failure.

Pseudocholinesterase

Nature of the enzyme and its reaction

Pseudocholinesterase (PChE), or serum cholinesterase, is a family of 11 enzymes that hydrolyse acetylcholine and other choline esters to choline and an organic acid, for example acetic acid.

Distribution and localization of the enzyme

It is expressed in liver and to a lesser extent in small intestine, smooth muscle cells, heart, pancreas and adipocytes and it is present in plasma [40].

Assays of enzyme activity

Many different tests have been developed to detect PChE activity:
• detection of CO_2 produced (manometric method);
• assessment of the amount of acetic acid produced by monitoring the decrease in pH;
• direct measurement of acetic acid (titrimetric assay) by colorimetric or voltammeter detection.

In all of these techniques, the serum sample is incubated with 10 mM acetylcholine. This high concentration has two purposes:

(i) to produce sufficient concentrations of thiocholine and acetate to be detected by colorimetric methods, and (ii) to inhibit a different acetylcholinesterase in serum that can contribute to the enzymatic activity. This cholinesterase, which originates in erythrocytes, utilizes acetyl-β-methylcholine as its specific substrate.

Normal values and factors influencing them

Normal values are between 4000 and 12 000 U/L. Normal values in females are on average 15% lower than in males and fall even further during pregnancy [41]. PChE concentration can be lower in subjects without any disease who carry one or two atypical alleles (polymorphism) that have much less activity (serum levels <3000 U/L). Treatment with steroids (corticosteroids) can reduce the serum PChE activity [42].

Abnormal values in hepatobiliary diseases

PChE is an index of liver synthetic function and is depressed during either acute or chronic liver damage. During acute hepatitis, the degree of decrease is mild, but it may be lowered by 30–50% during severe necrosis. In liver cirrhosis, PChE decreases progressively to values as low as 50–70% of normal. In patients affected by chronic liver disease, this test is more sensitive than estimation of plasma albumin to detect impairment of protein synthesis in the liver [43].

Abnormal values in other diseases

Starvation and malnutrition can reduce the serum PChE activity as part of the general impairment in protein synthesis; the same effect is observed in patients with intestinal malabsorption, sepsis or severe burns [44]. Mild reduction of PChE activity is observed during myocardial infarction. A severe decrease (up to 60% lower than normal values) occurs with intoxication by organophosphate and carbamate pesticides. High serum activity is observed in obese patients, and in diabetic patients activity is positively correlated with high levels of triglycerides and inversely with insulin sensitivity; the reasons are unknown [40]. One person in 1500 has a deficit of PChE activity due to inheritance of an atypical variant of the enzyme; such subjects may suffer prolonged apnoea after treatment with succinylcholine during surgical procedures.

Summary of clinical usefulness

Serum PChE activity is an index of liver function although its advantage versus serum albumin is not proven. Therefore the routine use of PChE is not recommended.

Ammonia

Nature of the compound and its distribution

Ammonia (NH_3) is present in normal blood and derives from the metabolism of amino acids by the kidney and of amino acids and urea by intestinal bacteria. At the near neutral pH values of body fluids and cells, ammonia ($pK_a = 9.25$) exists mainly in the form of ammonium ions (NH_4^+), which cannot diffuse passively across membranes. Thus, only the small fraction of ammonia in the form of NH_3 is diffusible, and it will passively move along a pH gradient from a compartment with higher pH to a compartment with lower pH, due to being trapped as NH_4^+ in the lower pH compartment. Thus, the lower pH of the tissues compared with the blood favours diffusion of NH_3 into tissues, and the lower pH of the colon compared with blood tends to limit absorption of NH_3 from the intestine.

In the fasting state, the intestine (50%) and kidney (40%) are the two major sources of blood ammonia. The greatest fraction originates by passive absorption of NH_3 from the intestinal lumen, where it is derived from three sources: (i) NH_3 present in foods like meat and cheese; (ii) the deamination of ingested amino acids and deamidation of glutamine by the activity of intestinal bacteria; and (iii) the formation of NH_3 and CO_2 from urea, about 25% of which diffuses from the blood into the intestinal lumen on each circulation. The absorbed ammonia passes via the portal venous blood to the liver, where it is normally metabolized to produce urea or ligated to glutamate to produce glutamine. Skeletal muscles can also reversibly form glutamine from ammonia + glutamate.

Assays of blood ammonia

Two different principles are used to extract ammonia from the blood: one involves isothermal diffusion of NH_3, and the other utilizes ion-exchange resins. The former is performed in a vial with two chambers separated by a microfilter: after addition of potassium carbonate to the blood sample chamber, NH_4^+ is converted to NH_3, which diffuses across the microfilter and is trapped as NH_4^+ in the second chamber containing HCl. After 45 min, the remaining HCl is precipitated as $BaCl_2$ by addition of 0.01 N barium hydroxide. Measurement of the precipitated $BaCl_2$ by this method allows calculation of the amount of HCl consumed, and thus the quantity of ammonia that neutralized it. The other method is based on the reversible enzymatic reaction of glutamate dehydrogenase (GDH). In this method, the ammonium, trapped in the ion-exchange resin, is incubated with GDH, α-ketoglutarate and NADPH, resulting in the formation of L-glutamate and $NADP^+$; the decrease of spectral absorbance of NADPH at 340 nm is directly related to the concentration of ammonia.

Normal values and factors influencing them

The normal blood ammonia concentration is quite low: 40–80 µg/dL (23–46 µM). The blood ammonia determination is very sensitive to outside influences and variations in technique, so must be performed with extreme care. The blood sample should be arterial rather than venous. Red blood cells rapidly deaminate labile compounds (like glutamine). Studies with an ammonia electrode show that generation of ammonia by erythrocytes occurs rapidly from the moment the blood sample is drawn. To minimize spurious increases in ammonia concentration from this source, the sample must be put in ice immediately and analysed within 2 h. Cigarette smoke contains considerable

ammonia, so the laboratory and technician must be smoke-free and the patient should not smoke during the previous 8 h [44].

Blood ammonia rises markedly after eating protein and after gastrointestinal bleeding, both of which provide increased substrate for generation of ammonia by the intestinal flora. Acidosis increases renal ammonia synthesis and vigorous exercise increases the formation of ammonia from adenylic acid and glutamine in muscle.

Abnormal values in hepatobiliary diseases

Patients affected by either acute liver failure or chronic liver disease may suffer a decrease in hepatic urea synthesis and shunting of portal blood around the liver, resulting in increased ammonia concentrations in the peripheral blood. The consequent elevations in ammonia levels in the central nervous system may engender hepatic encephalopathy through both direct and indirect mechanisms [45]. There is, however, a poor correlation between arterial ammonia concentrations and the symptoms or severity of encephalopathy [46]. This may be related to the multiplicity of factors, other than ammonia, that may also affect CNS function in patients with hepatic failure or cirrhosis, as well as the technical problems with measurement of ammonia, discussed above.

Abnormal values in other diseases

Few other conditions increase blood ammonia concentrations. Infants may suffer encephalopathy due to rare congenital hyperammonaemias, caused by genetic deficiencies of enzymes involved in urea synthesis. The deficient enzymes are carbamoylphosphate synthase (type 1) and ornithine transcarbamylase (type 2). An increase of ammonia is occasionally observed in patients affected by severe pulmonary emphysema or carbon monoxide (CO) intoxication.

Summary of clinical usefulness

Blood ammonia is widely used to confirm the diagnosis of hepatic encephalopathy in patients with liver dysfunction. Its sensitivity and specificity for the diagnosis of hepatic encephalopathy are, however, only 85% and 29%, respectively, so this test is used less frequently now than in the past.

Cholesterol, phospholipids and triglycerides

All of these lipids are both synthesized and catabolized by the liver, as well as by other organs.

Abnormal values in hepatobiliary diseases

Modifications of both the amount and composition of plasma lipoproteins are common in all forms of hepatobiliary diseases, with different patterns according to the aetiology of the disease. In cholestatic disorders, either intra- or extrahepatic, there is commonly elevation of free cholesterol and phospholipids in plasma. This is due to: (i) inhibition of the conversion of cholesterol to bile salts; and (ii) regurgitation of cholesterol/lecithin vesicles from the bile, which combine with plasma albumin to form the abnormal lipoprotein, LP-X [47]. LP-X is specific for cholestasis and familial LCAT (lecithin-cholesterol acyltransferase) deficiency. Characteristically, in both intra- and extra-hepatic cholestasis, plasma high-density lipoprotein (HDL), apolipoprotein A-I (ApoA-I) and apolipoprotein A-II (ApoA-II) are increased also [48]. Treatment of primary biliary cirrhosis (PBC) with ursodiol usually decreases the plasma cholesterol concentration [49]. In patients with chronic excessive alcoholic intake, either with or without hepatic steatosis, it is common to observe hypertriglyceridaemia related to an increase of VLDL (very-low-density lipoproteins); increases in plasma cholesterol and phospholipids are frequent also. After alcohol withdrawal, triglyceride clearance is rapid while the cholesterol and phospholipid concentrations decrease more slowly. In cirrhosis, serum cholesterol and ApoB levels are progressively decreased in concert with the impairment of the liver function. The decrease in serum cholesterol concentration is mainly at the expense of the esterified fraction, associated with decreased concentrations of α- and pre-β-lipoproteins [50].

Summary of clinical usefulness

Measurement of plasma cholesterol can be useful in two different clinical situations: (i) an increase as a marker for the diagnosis and severity of cholestatic disorders, such as PBC; and (ii) a decrease as a marker of impaired liver function in cirrhosis. Triglycerides can be used as a marker for the follow-up of patients with suspected abuse of alcohol.

Markers to assess hepatic excretory function

Bilirubin

Structure and properties of bilirubin

Bilirubin is a yellow pigment present in serum in two different forms: unconjugated bilirubin (UCB), also called indirect bilirubin (see below), and conjugated bilirubin (CB), also called direct bilirubin. Both forms of bilirubin are potent antioxidants at low concentrations, and may play a role in protecting cells against diseases caused by oxidant damage [51]. At higher concentrations, however, the unconjugated form, which readily diffuses across cell membranes, may be cytotoxic.

UCB is produced in adults at a rate of approximately 3.8 mg/kg/day as the final product of the catabolism of the porphyrin ring of haem. It is a tetrapyrrole with two substituent propionic acid groups, each internally hydrogen-bonded to the >C=O and >N–H groups of the opposite dipyrrole half of the molecule. This endows the molecule with very low water solubility (<0.1 μM), requiring that it be transported in blood 99.9% bound to plasma albumin (90%) and apolipoprotein D (10%).

Distribution, transport and metabolism of bilirubin

UCB is produced mainly in the spleen from the catabolism of haem released when senescent red cells are destroyed by the reticuloendothelial cells. About one-fourth of UCB derives from ineffective erythropoiesis in the bone marrow and catabolism of other haem proteins, particularly cytochromes in the liver and myoglobin in muscle. UCB, delivered from the spleen via the splenic vein, undergoes uptake across the basolateral membrane of the hepatocyte by a facilitated diffusion process; the responsible carrier remains unclear [52]. In the hepatocyte cytosol, UCB is bound to ligandin and then diffuses into the microsomes, where it is conjugated with one or two molecules of glucuronic acid by a specific UDP-glucuronosyl transferase (UGT1A1). This renders the bilirubin soluble in water and CB is actively secreted in the bile by the multidrug resistance–associated protein 2 (MRP2) [53] membrane transporter at the canalicular membrane. After passing through the biliary tree and the small intestine, CB is deconjugated by coliforms in the small intestine and anaerobic bacteria in the terminal ileum and colon. The anaerobes then reduce UCB to form colourless urobilinogens that are mostly expelled with faeces. In adults and older children, small proportions of UCB and urobilinogens are reabsorbed from the intestine into the portal venous blood and return to the liver (enterohepatic circulation). The absence of the appropriate flora in newborns precludes formation of urobilinogens and enhances greatly the enterohepatic circulation of UCB.

Assays

The 'gold standard' is high-performance liquid chromatography of bilirubins in plasma, either native or after derivatization. Though very accurate and specific, these methods are expensive and not easily automated, and are thus not routinely available clinically. The method most commonly used is based on the reaction of bilirubin with diazotized sulfanilic acid, which splits the molecule into two dipyrroles, each coupled with the diazo reagent [54]. These azopigments, which are red in neutral solution and blue or green in strongly acid or alkaline solution, are measured spectrophotometrically. Due to the internal hydrogen-bonding, UCB couples only slowly with the diazo reagent, and the reaction essentially measures only 'direct-reacting' CB. Addition of an 'accelerator' (caffeine or diphylline) that breaks the hydrogen bonds of UCB, allows the UCB to react also, yielding the total bilirubin concentration. The total-direct bilirubin = 'indirect-reacting' bilirubin, which is a rough measure of UCB in the sample.

The method used nowadays was originally developed by Jendrassik and Grof. The serum or plasma sample is added to a solution of sodium acetate and caffeine–sodium benzoate, which stabilizes the bilirubin and buffers the pH when the very acid diazo-reagent is added; for the direct reaction, the caffeine is omitted. The diazo reagent, freshly prepared by addition of HCl and sodium nitrite to sulfanilic acid, is then added. After 10 min, addition of an alkaline solution stops the reaction and changes the colour of the azopigments from pink to blue–green, shifting the absorption maximum to 600 nm, well away from the absorption maxima of other coloured compounds in serum. Inclusion of ascorbic acid in the alkaline stop solution helps arrest the reaction and stabilize the azopigments. Unreactive blanks, prepared without nitrite or with ascorbic acid added before the diazo reagent, are used to correct for other coloured compounds in serum. The net A_{600} is then converted to bilirubin concentration by comparison with a standard curve prepared from a stock solution of bilirubin in serum.

A commercial modification of the diazo method (Kodak Ektachem, Rochester, NY) utilizes multilayered filters/adsorbants to separate the UCB, CB and δ-bilirubin (bilirubin covalently linked to albumin in cholestatic disorders), then measures the azopigments formed in each layer by reflectance spectroscopy.

In newborns, due to the very small amount of blood sample available, a direct spectrophotometric determination is often used. A blood sample is collected in heparinized capillary tubes; after centrifugation the plasma is removed and diluted in Tris buffer. The absorbance of this solution is measured spectrophotometrically at 453 and 575 nm or at 436 and 578 nm. The lower wavelength is near the peak of bilirubin absorbance, and the higher wavelength detects one of the multiple absorbance peaks of haem, which is commonly present in neonatal plasma due to haemolysis. Using constants determined from standard samples, total bilirubin concentration is calculated from the difference between the two absorbances:

$$\text{bilirubin (mg/dL)} = \text{dilution factor} \times (1.3A_{453} - 1.37A_{575}).$$

This method is feasible only in newborns because yellow carotenoids, which have absorbance maxima similar to bilirubin, are almost absent from plasma in the first week of life [55]. With this method it is not possible to differentiate between conjugated and unconjugated bilirubin.

Normal values and influencing factors

Normal serum bilirubin levels in adults range from 0.15 to 1.2 mg/dL (3–21 μM). Some factors may influence the accuracy of the measurement: it is important that the blood sample is collected after 8–12 h fasting, as the postprandial presence of chylomicrons and lipids in plasma renders the sample turbid, impairing the absorbance measurement. Haemolysed samples give falsely low values due to interference of haem with the diazo reaction. The sample should be kept in the dark or protected from direct light to minimize photo-oxidation of bilirubins to products that do not react with the diazo reagent.

It is also important to note that virtually all the bilirubin present in normal serum is in the unconjugated form [56]; the low level of direct-reacting bilirubin (<15% of the total) results from slow reaction of UCB even in the absence of added accelerator and possibly from endogenous accelerators in the plasma (caffeine, urea, bile salts). Unidentified diazo-reactive compounds present in the serum may falsely elevate the direct-reacting fraction [57].

Abnormal values in hepatobiliary diseases

The metabolism and excretion of bilirubin is impaired in almost all hepatobiliary disorders, giving rise to retention of the yellow pigments in the plasma and tissues (jaundice or icterus).

Jaundice can be divided into two major classes: an increase of (i) UCB, or (ii) CB + UCB. Type (ii) is readily distinguished by the presence of bilirubin in the urine, because the conjugated bilirubins are less tightly bound to plasma proteins and can filter at the glomerulus. Making this distinction is the first step in the differential diagnosis of jaundice.

Unconjugated hyperbilirubinaemia (<15% direct-reacting) may be caused by overproduction of bilirubin (haemolysis), shunting around the liver of portal blood (including the UCB-rich blood in the splenic vein), impaired hepatic uptake of UCB, and/or genetic deficiencies of the conjugating enzyme, UGT1A1. Almost all newborns are 'physiologically' jaundiced because of increased haemolysis and enterohepatic circulation of UCB, increasing the load on immature mechanisms for uptake and conjugation of UCB by the liver. Genetic impairment of conjugation by 60–70%, accompanied by impaired hepatic uptake and/or overproduction of UCB, causes Gilbert syndrome. Seen in 6–10% of adults, this harmless syndrome is characterized by mild indirect hyperbilirubinaemia without overt haemolysis or evidence of structural liver disease. The rare Crigler–Najjar syndromes (types 1 and 2) are due to the genetic absence (I) or very low (<10%) activity (II) of UGT1A1. Type 1 patients show very high serum levels of indirect bilirubin (20–30 mg/dL) without direct bilirubin; type 2 patients usually have 8–12 mg/dL indirect bilirubin in serum, with small proportions of direct bilirubin [58].

Conjugated hyperbilirubinaemia is accompanied by bilirubinuria, and is almost always indicative of significant hepatobiliary disease, even if as little as 30% of the serum bilirubin is direct-reacting. The retention of bilirubin conjugates is due to impaired canalicular secretion or biliary flow, with regurgitation of the bilirubin conjugates from the liver cell or bile back into the plasma. The significant concomitant elevation of indirect-reacting (unconjugated) bilirubin is due to: (i) deconjugation of the retained CB by β-glucuronidases in the tissues; and (ii) accompanying defects leading to retention of UCB, including impairment of hepatocytic uptake, portosystemic shunting, and haemolysis. It is important to realize that bilirubin conjugation is little impaired in hepatobiliary diseases except with severe acute or chronic liver failure.

Once conjugated hyperbilirubinaemia has been detected, the next step is to determine whether the problem is primarily due to hepatocellular injury or to impaired bile secretion and/or flow (cholestasis). Initial clues come from the age of the patients, the history of exposure to drugs, toxins or hepatitis viruses, the presence of biliary colic, and the symptom of pruritus (itching), which occurs in 75% of patients with cholestasis.

Elevations of serum transaminases and/or low levels of serum albumin point to hepatocellular diseases, and the diagnosis is further established by other serological and biochemical tests, often followed by liver biopsy. By contrast, an increase in serum alkaline phosphatase levels to more than three times the upper limit of normal values favours a cholestatic disorder; in this case, the next step is to distinguish between intrahepatic cholestasis and extrahepatic obstruction. This is usually achieved by visualization of the biliary tree, most often by endoscopic cholangiography. Because some hepatocellular diseases (e.g. drug-induced) may affect biliary secretion, and persistent cholestasis secondarily damages the hepatocytes (e.g. in primary biliary cirrhosis), a mixed clinical and laboratory picture is not uncommon. Nonetheless, 85–90% of cases of conjugated hyperbilirubinaemia can be correctly classified as primarily hepatocellular disease vs cholestasis, and intra- vs extra-hepatic cholestasis, utilizing only history, physical examination and routine serum biochemical tests.

Hereditary defects in MRP2, the canalicular exporter of conjugated bilirubins, cause the Dubin–Johnson and Rotor syndromes [53], typically marked by direct hyperbilirubinaemia with little or no increase of alkaline phosphatase and the other serum markers of cholestasis. Hereditary conjugated hyperbilirubinemias, due to genetic abnormalities in the canalicular transporters of bile salts or phospholipids, cause the syndromes of progressive familial intrahepatic cholestasis (PFIC) types 1–3, benign recurrent intrahepatic cholestasis, or cholestasis of pregnancy. Some of these defects are accompanied by significant elevations of γ-GT, which assists in their classification: PFIC type 3 is distinguished from the other familial cholestasis by significant elevations of the γ-GT levels in serum.

Abnormal values in other diseases

Serum UCB can be increased by haemolysis, due to increased production of bilirubin from the catabolism of haem. Haemolytic anaemia, by itself, rarely raises the total serum bilirubin above 4 mg/dL (68 μM). There is no increase of cholestatic markers (γ-GT, alkaline phosphatase or 5′-nucleotidase) or ALT, but release of LDH and AST from the damaged red cells can increase these enzymes in serum. The diagnosis is made from examination of erythrocyte ± bone marrow morphology, plus increases in serum haptoglobin and reticulocytes.

Clinical usefulness

Although the proportion of direct/total bilirubin tends to be higher in cholestatic than hepatocellular jaundice, it has been known for half a century that the overlap among disease categories is so great that the direct/total bilirubin ratio is of no diagnostic value except to distinguish unconjugated (<15%) from conjugated (>30%) hyperbilirubinaemia.

Total serum bilirubin is an important parameter in assessing the prognosis of both acute and chronic liver failure and in the decision to propose liver transplantation; an increased total serum bilirubin concentration is associated with a shorter life expectancy. In acute viral hepatitis, a serum total bilirubin concentration higher than 384 μM (22.5 mg/dL) predicts mortality with a positive predictive value of 0.80 and sensitivity of 0.80. Combination with total serum cholic acid and glycocholic acid levels enhances the predictive value even further [59]. In cirrhosis of the liver of any cause, total serum bilirubin is a key variable in the Child–Pugh and MELD scores, the two most widely used to predict long-term survival. The endstage of primary biliary cirrhosis (PBC), an autoimmune cholangiolitis, is characterized

by an increasing rise of serum bilirubin concentration. Total serum bilirubin greater than 150 μmol/L (8.8 mg/dL) is the best single indicator for orthotopic liver transplantation [60].

Alkaline phosphatase (ALP)

Nature of the enzyme and tissue distribution

Alkaline phosphatases constitute a group of membrane-bound, glycosylated metalloenzymes with low substrate specificity that catalyse the hydrolysis of a phosphoester bond at an alkaline pH, with the release of inorganic phosphate. The ALPs, whose physiological functions are unknown, comprise four classes of isoenzymes (tissue-nonspecific, intestinal, germ-cell and placental ALP), encoded by at least four different gene loci. Posttranslational modifications (e.g. in glycosylation) yield further isoforms, the most important of which are produced in bone and liver [61]. In normal subjects, the serum ALP activity is represented mainly by the intestinal, bone and liver isoenzymes, with at least half the activity represented by the liver isoforms. The placental isoenzyme becomes a major component during pregnancy. In the liver, ALP is expressed in both the sinusoidal and canalicular membranes of the hepatocyte, principally in the latter [62]. It is also localized in the brush borders of the epithelial cells of the renal proximal convoluted tubules, small intestine, pulmonary alveoli and the membrane bordering the bile canaliculus [63].

Assays of detection

ALP activity is assayed enzymatically, utilizing one of a panoply of phosphate esters that are substrates for ALP. The analytical methods can be divided into two general categories: detection of the released phosphate (from phosphate esters as β-glycerolphosphate), or measurement of the liberated alcohol (e.g. phenol from phenylphosphate).

Values obtained on individual specimens agree poorly among the various methods (Table 1), due to several factors: (i) different substrates vary in their affinity for the different isoenzymes; (ii) activities of the various isoforms and isoenzymes are profoundly and differently affected by reaction conditions (pH, temperature, type of phosphate ester, the concentration and nature of the metal activator, etc.) [63]. Conversion factors for comparison of average values from one test to another are poorly applicable to individual specimens. Thus, in everyday clinical practice, ALP activities obtained from different laboratories are best compared by expressing the results as the ratio to the upper limit of normal range of values for that facility.

Distinguishing isoenzyme activities

Several different physicochemical, electrophoretic and immunochemical techniques have been developed to distinguish the contributions of the different isoenzymes and isoforms to total ALP activity. Among the most common are:
• differences in sensitivity of isoenzymes to inactivation by elevated temperatures, alterations in pH, or concentratons of urea;

Table 1 Some assays used for determination of serum ALP activity. Modified from ref. 63 with permission of Williams & Wilkins Co.

Method	Substrate	Temp. (°C)	pH	Buffer	Unit	Normal range
Bessey–Lowry–Brock	p-Nitrophenyl phosphate	39	10.5	Glycine	1 mmol p-nitrophenol/L/60 min	0.8–3.0
Bodansky	β-Glycerophosphate	37	8.6	Diethyl barbiturate	1 mg Pi/100 mL/60 min	1.5–4.0
International	p-Nitrophenyl phosphate	37	10.5	2-Amino-2-methyl-1-propanol	1 µmol p-nitrophenol/L/min	21.0–85.0
International	Phenylphosphate	37	10.0	Sodium carbonate	1 mg phenol/100 mL/30 min	3.0–13.0
King–Armstrong	Phenylphosphate	37	9.3	Diethyl barbiturate	1 mg phenol/100 mL/30 min	3.0–13.0
Klein–Read–Babson	Phenolphthalein diphosphate	37	9.3	Tris	1 mg phenolphthalein/100 mL/30 min	1.0–4.0
Shinowara–Jones–Reinhart	β-Glycerolphosphate	37	9.3	Diethyl barbiturate	1 mg phenol/100 mL/60 min	2.2–8.6

Pi, inorganic phosphate.

- comparative reactivity to a panel of specific substrates;
- electrophoretic separation according to molecular weight or isoelectric point;
- removal of isoenzymes by specific immunoprecipitation.

These techniques are not commonly used because many: (i) are too cumbersome for a routine use; (ii) have low sensitivity; (iii) don't yield a quantitative result; and (iv) poorly resolve the bone and the liver isoforms (the most important distinction in clinical practice). For those reasons, the origin of the ALP activity in patients is usually inferred from the contemporaneous determination of serum γ-GT and/or 5′-nucleotidase activities, enzymes that originate mainly from the liver (see below). The absence of a contemporaneous increase of γ-GT [64] or 5′-nucleotidase activities suggests that the elevated serum ALP activity originates from bone or placenta; a pregnancy test can help confirm the latter possibility.

Influencing factors
Serum ALP activity increases markedly during the pubertal increase in height and bone growth, between 5 and 14 years of age in males and 5 and 12 years of age in females [65]. African American boys and girls, who have larger skeletal mass, have higher values than Caucasaians of the same age [66]. After puberty, activities decrease towards adult values, but tend to remain higher in males than in females [67].

In the elderly, the serum total ALP activity of both sexes increases with increasing age, especially above age 60 years. The same trends are seen in the non-bone isoforms (assumed to be largely from liver) (Fig. 3). By contrast, the activity of the bone isoenzyme (b-ALP) increases in women and decreases in men. The reason for the postmenopausal increase of b-ALP in women has been attributed to loss of the inhibitory effects of estrogen on bone turnover. In men, the decline in b-ALP activity with age correlates with decreases in the histomorphometric markers of bone formation [68].

Abnormal values in hepatobiliary diseases
Total ALP activity is increased in hepatobiliary diseases due to three mechanisms: (i) cleavage of the membrane-bound enzyme from its glycophospholipid anchor in the sinusoidal membrane

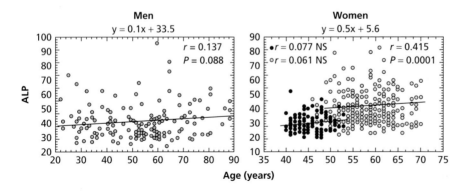

Fig. 3 Increase in total serum alkaline phosphatase (ALP) with age. The two r values at the left upper corner of the right panel for women are for (●) pre- and (○) post-menopausal women respectively. From ref. 68 with permission of American Association for Clinical Chemistry, Inc.

of the damaged hepatocyte; (ii) impaired trafficking of the enzyme from the sinusoidal to the apical membrane of the hepatocyte; and (iii) enhanced enzyme synthesis in the hepatocyte due to induction by retained bile acids [69]. The former concept that biliary secretion of the enzymes was impaired in cholestatic diseases has been negated by evidence that the hepatocyte does not excrete ALP into the bile [70].

The ALP activity is most strikingly increased in cholestatic and infiltrative liver diseases, less so in hepatocellular diseases. If ALP is not increased, the presence of cholestasis is unlikely, except for the cholestasis related to therapy with oestrogens or anabolic steroids; it is not known why there is little or no elevation of the serum ALP in the majority of such cases. With biliary tract obstruction, ALP activity is almost never normal and is at least three times the upper normal limit in over 90% of such cases. Elevation of the ALP is often the only abnormal 'liver function' test in patients with partial biliary obstruction (e.g. due to pancreatic or bile duct carcinomas, or sclerosing cholangitis) or multifocal intrahepatic duct obstruction by infiltrative diseases (e.g. hepatocellular or metastatic carcinoma, sarcoidosis, amyloidosis, or abscesses). ALP activity reportedly has a high sensitivity (90%) to detect metastatic malignancy [71].

It is important to understand that increased ALP activity is of no value in differentiating between intra- vs extrahepatic cholestasis, as it can be increased whenever bile flow is impaired, whether from obstructive lesions (tumours, primary biliary cirrhosis, sclerosing cholangitis) or hepatocellular damage (viral, drug or alcoholic hepatitis) [72].

Abnormal values in other diseases

Mild elevation of ALP levels of hepatic origin may occur in patients with stage I or II Hodgkin's disease, hypernephroma, congestive heart failure, myeloid metaplasia, peritonitis, diabetes, subacute thyroiditis or uncomplicated gastric ulcer [72].

During pregnancy, ALP activity of placental origin starts rising beyond the second trimester and reaches a peak of up to four times the normal range at the ninth month, then subsides to normal levels within 20 days after delivery.

Increased ALP activity originating from bone is observed in bone diseases whenever osteoblastic activity is increased (Paget's syndrome, healing fractures, rickets, osteomyelitis, bone metastases, osteoporosis, osteomalacia, primary hyperparathyroidism, etc.). Distinctively, in all those diseases, γ-GT and/or 5′-nucleotidase are usually normal. Patients affected by chronic renal failure, especially if treated with haemodialysis or peritoneal dialysis, can develop an increase of ALP activity related to the secondary bone or liver disease.

Several medications (Table 2) interfere directly with the measurement of ALP because they inhibit its enzymatic activity. Artefactual elevation of ALP activity has been described after albumin infusion because of the concomitant infusion of the active enzyme as a contaminant. This is possible because one of the sources of human albumin for infusion is the placenta and the ALP isoform in the placenta is resistant to the sterilization

Table 2 Drugs that can inhibit enzymatic activity of serum alkaline phosphatase (ALP). From ref. 73 with permission of Adis International.

Arsenicals	Lithium	Serum phosphorus
Beryllium salts	Serum magnesium	Potassium
Ethionamide	Nitrofurantoin	Sulfhydryl compounds
Fluorides	Oxalates	Zinc salts

process [73]. ALP can be increased after drug treatment because of induction of liver damage (e.g. paracetamol, azathiaprine, methotrexate, oral contraceptives) or by inactivation of vitamin D (as it occurs in 25% of children receiving anticonvulsant therapy).

As a curiosity we refer to a family with autosomal dominant inheritance of a 2–4× increase of serum ALP activity in the absence of disease [74]; the mechanism is unknown.

Gamma-glutamyltransferase (γ-GT)

Nature of the enzyme

γ-GT is a cell-surface glycoprotein that cleaves γ-glutamyl amide bonds. It catalyses the transfer of the γ-glutamyl group from the γ-glutamylpeptide to another peptide or amino acid. The most abundant physiological substrates for the enzyme are glutathione and glutathione conjugates.

Tissue distribution

γ-GT is expressed most strongly in the kidney (brush border membranes of proximal convoluted tubules), moderately in the liver and pancreas, and to some degree in the heart, intestine, lung and spleen [75]. In the liver, its activity is located mainly in the microsomal fraction of the intra- and extrahepatic bile duct epithelium.

Assays of detection

The method recommended by the International Federation of Clinical Chemistry is based on the original procedure, using γ-glutamyl-3-carboxy-4-nitroanilide as a substrate and glycylglycine as the acceptor of the γ-glutamyl group. The final products are L-glutamyl-glycylglycine and 5-amino-2-nitrobenzoate. The latter compound is chromogenic (yellow) and is measured spectrophotometrically at a wavelength of 405 nm [76].

Normal serum levels and factors affecting them

The reference range for serum γ-GT is 12–32 IU/L. Within the normal range, values are influenced by:
- sex (higher in male);
- age (increases with age above 40–50 years) [77];
- race (higher values in black people);
- smoking (higher levels in smokers);
- childbirth (higher levels at 5–10 days postpartum and greater increase after caesarean section).

Physical exercise does not influence the serum activity [78].

Serum levels in hepatobiliary diseases

Serum γ-GT activity may be increased in all types of liver disease, but is most strikingly increased with obstruction of either intra- or extrahepatic bile ducts, although not directly correlated with the serum bilirubin levels. In cholestasis, it is more liver-specific than alkaline phosphatase (ALP), but its sensitivity may be less. The main clinical value of γ-GT activity is that it is not elevated when the increased serum ALP activity is of osseous or placental origin [79]. Its activity is increased in viral acute hepatitis, usually reaching a peak from the second to the third week, whereas it remains slightly elevated in chronic viral hepatitis and cirrhosis, and it can be considered as an expression of intrahepatic cholestasis during hepatitis. During acute hepatitis, however, the aminotransferase levels are disproportionally increased suggesting that an ALT/γ-GT ratio may help in the discrimination between hepatitis and obstructive hepatic disease (<1.8) [79]. The detection of elevated γ-GT activity in patients with proven malignancy is highly suggestive for the presence of metastatic lesions localized in the liver [80]. Elevation in γ-GT activity may be useful to distinguish PFIC type 3 from types 1 and II.

Abnormal values in other diseases and clinical situations

Serum γ-GT activity can be increased by treatment with drugs, such as the anticonvulsants phenytoin and phenobarbitone, that induce microsomal enzymes; the γ-GT levels are only weakly correlated with the drug concentrations in plasma [81]. Other drugs (i.e. oral contraceptives, carbamazepine, valproate) or chemicals (i.e. DDT, hexachlorobenzene) likewise may increase serum γ-GT activity [64].

Persistent alcohol consumption engenders a progressive, dose-related increase in γ-GT levels, but a single dose of alcohol has no effect [82]. The apparent half-life of serum γ-GT after abstention from alcohol varies from 5 to 17 days [83], being longer in patients with chronic liver disease. In decompensated cirrhosis, γ-GT levels can remain elevated despite abstinence, because of severe liver fibrosis [84]. For the detection of alcohol intake, the sensitivity and specificity of elevated γ-GT levels range from 33 to 58% and from 70 to 87% respectively. Thus, γ-GT alone is inadequate to screen for excessive alcohol intake, but it can be useful for serially monitoring alcohol abuse by individual patients [64].

γ-GT increases with increases in body weight, and in particular body mass index or hip/waist ratio. γ-GT is frequently elevated in patients affected by the metabolic syndrome, especially in patients affected by hypertriglyceridaemia, hypercholesterolaemia and insulin resistance, and in most patients with nonalcoholic fatty liver disease (NASH). γ-GT is increased also in 20% of diabetic patients – particularly noninsulin-dependent diabetes mellitus (NIDDM). In all these situations, the increased serum levels of γ-GT may be related to the associated fatty liver. Amyloidosis is another infiltrative hepatic disorder in which γ-GT activity can be raised [85].

Other causes of elevated serum γ-GT activity are myocardial infarction, congestive heart failure, acute pancreatitis, obstructive lung disease and chronic kidney failure.

Summary of clinical usefulness

Elevated serum γ-GT activity is a highly sensitive marker of hepatobiliary disease, but its usefulness is limited because of low specificity, related to the wide spectrum of diseases in which this enzyme activity is elevated. In our opinion, measurement of γ-GT activity is of value only to exclude a hepatobiliary source for an increased serum ALP, and to monitor the response to treatment in patients with uncomplicated alcoholic liver disease or other liver disorders who presented initially with an increased γ-GT activity. It is also useful in the differential diagnosis of PFIC.

5′-Nucleotidase

Nature of the enzyme

5′-Nucleotidase is an alkaline phosphatase that specifically catalyses the hydrolysis of the phosphopurine nucleotides by releasing inorganic phosphate from carbon 5 of the ribose (pentose) ring.

Assays of detection

Two different techniques are available: the first is based on the measurement of the total ALP activity (as previously described) after adding adenosine-5′-monophosphate to the sample as a specific substrate, and again after inhibiting the 5′-nucleotidase activity by adding Ni^{2+} or Zn^{2+}. The difference between the two values represents the activity of the 5′-nucleotidase. The second method consists of measuring the total phosphatase activity with added nonspecific substrates (i.e. phenylphosphate or β-glycerolphosphate) ± the specific substrate (adenosine-5′-monophosphate). The difference is taken as the 5′-nucleotidase activity. The first method is preferred, because of the greater influence of the unpredictable activity of nonspecific phosphatases on the second method.

Distribution

5′-Nucleotidase is present in most tissues and cells but the serum enzyme activity is increased only during cholestasis. This specificity is supposedly related to the highly hydrophobic nature of the enzyme, which results in its tight binding to plasma membranes; it then becomes soluble only upon treatment with detergents, such as bile salts. The markedly higher levels of retained bile salts in the liver during cholestasis presumably explains the specificity of high levels of serum 5′-nucleotidase for cholestatic disorders [86].

Normal serum levels, factors affecting them and clinical usefulness

The normal values are from 2 to 17 U/L and are not altered by age or sex [42], nor elevated by pregnancy or bone diseases.

These features make this assay valuable in infancy, pregnancy or subjects with bone diseases to discriminate whether an increase of serum ALP activity is related in part to underlying hepatobiliary disease. Because serum γ-GT can discriminate if the ALP increase is related or not to a biliary disorder except in paediatric patients, 5′-nucleotidase activity should be used in anicteric or icteric infants and children when cholestasis is suspected. In adults, 5′-nucleotidase activity is more specific than γ-GT, but the sensitivity is lower. Thus, in subjects with an elevated serum ALP, 5′-nucleotidase is useful only to prove the presence of hepatobiliary disease when positive, whereas γ-GT is useful only to exclude hepatobiliary disease when it is normal.

Overall take-home message

Unlike the lucky nephrologists, we hepatologists don't have creatinine for liver diseases. This means that we need to combine different tests to figure out what is wrong in the liver. In addition, although several of the tests described above have been used for more than 30 years, we still lack a precise correlation between the test result and its value for prognosis of the underlying liver disease, bar a few exceptions (albumin and prothrombin time for cirrhosis and bilirubin for biliary disorders). Therefore, decisions about what test to use and when must be driven by clinical suspicion and the results interpreted within the same frame.

References

1 Dufour DR, Lott JA, Nolte FS *et al.* (2000) Diagnosis and monitoring of hepatic injury. II. Recommendations for use of laboratory tests in screening, diagnosis, and monitoring. *Clin Chem* 46, 2050–2068.

2 Rej R (1989) Aminotransferases in disease. *Clin Lab Med* 9, 667–687.

3 Rej R (1978) Aspartate aminotransferase activity and isoenzyme proportions in human liver tissues. *Clin Chem* 24, 1971–1979.

4 Kempe E, Laursen T (1960) Investigations of the excretion of enzymes in urine. *Scand J Clin Lab Invest* 12, 463–471.

5 Bergmeyer HU, Horder M, Rej R (1986) International Federation of Clinical Chemistry (IFCC) Scientific Committee, Analytical Section: approved recommendation (1985) on IFCC methods for the measurement of catalytic concentration of enzymes. Part 3. IFCC method for alanine aminotransferase (L-alanine:2-oxoglutarate aminotransferase, EC 2.6.1.2). *J Clin Chem Clin Biochem* 24, 481–495.

6 Siest G, Schiele F, Galteau MM *et al.* (1975) Aspartate aminotransferase and alanine aminotransferase activities in plasma: statistical distributions, individual variations, and reference values. *Clin Chem* 21, 1077–1087.

7 Gitlin N (1982) The serum glutamic oxaloacetic transaminase/serum glutamic pyruvic transaminase ratio as a prognostic index in severe acute viral hepatitis. *Am J Gastroenterol* 77, 2–4.

8 Chopra S, Griffin PH (1985) Laboratory tests and diagnostic procedures in evaluation of liver disease. *Am J Med* 79, 221–230.

9 Sharpe PC (2001) Biochemical detection and monitoring of alcohol abuse and abstinence. *Ann Clin Biochem* 38, 652–664.

10 Salvaggio A, Periti M, Miano L *et al.* (1991) Body mass index and liver enzyme activity in serum. *Clin Chem* 37, 720–723.

11 Warnock LG, Stone WJ, Wagner C (1974) Decreased aspartate aminotransferase ('SGOT') activity in serum of uremic patients. *Clin Chem* 20, 1213–1216.

12 Wroblewski F (1959) The clinical significance of transaminase activities of serum. *Am J Med* 27, 911–923.

13 Grimwood K, Coakley JC, Hudson IL *et al.* (1988) Serum aspartate aminotransferase levels after rotavirus gastroenteritis. *J Pediatr* 112, 597–600.

14 Dufour DR, Lott JA, Nolte FS *et al.* (2000) Diagnosis and monitoring of hepatic injury. I. Performance characteristics of laboratory tests. *Clin Chem* 46, 2027–2049.

15 Panteghini M (1990) Aspartate aminotransferase isoenzymes. *Clin Biochem* 23, 311–319.

16 Bierman HR, Hill BR, Reinhardt L, Emory E (1957) Correlation of serum lactic dehydrogenase activity with the clinical status of patients with cancer, lymphomas, and the leukemias. *Cancer Res* 17, 660–667.

17 Peters T Jr (1977) Serum albumin: recent progress in the understanding of its structure and biosynthesis. *Clin Chem* 23, 5–12.

18 Campbell PN (1975) The biosynthesis of serum albumin. *FEBS Lett* 54, 119–121.

19 Rothschild MA, Oratz M, Schreiber SS (1988) Serum albumin. *Hepatology* 8, 385–401.

20 Hill PG (1985) The measurement of albumin in serum and plasma. *Ann Clin Biochem* 22, 565–578.

21 De Feo P, Lucidi P (2002) Liver protein synthesis in physiology and in disease states. *Curr Opin Clin Nutr Metab Care* 5, 47–50.

22 Rothschild MA, Oratz M, Schreiber SS (1972) Albumin synthesis (second of two parts). *N Engl J Med* 286, 816–821.

23 Doweiko JP, Nompleggi DJ (1991) The role of albumin in human physiology and pathophysiology, Part III: Albumin and disease states. *J Parenter Enteral Nutr* 15, 476–483.

24 Lewith G, Gabriel R (1975) Biochemical anomalies of the nephrotic syndrome. *Curr Med Res Opin* 3, 199–202.

25 Murch S (2005) Protein-losing disorders of the gastrointestinal tract. In: Wilfred M, Weinstein CJ, Bosch J (eds) *Clinical Gastroenterology and Hepatology*. London: Elsevier Mosby, pp. 309–314.

26 Kim GH, Oh KH, Yoon JW *et al.* (2003) Impact of burn size and initial serum albumin level on acute renal failure occurring in major burn. *Am J Nephrol* 23, 55–60.

27 Walls WD, Losowsky MS (1971) The hemostatic defect of liver disease. *Gastroenterology* 60, 108–119.

28 Quick AJ (1949) The coagulation mechanism, with specific reference to the interpretation of prothrombin time and a consideration of the prothrombin consumption time. *Am J Clin Pathol* 19, 1016–1023.

29 Baglin T, Luddington R (1997) Reliability of delayed INR determination: implications for decentralized anticoagulant care with off-site blood sampling. *Br J Haematol* 96, 431–434.

30 Munoz SJ (1991) Prothrombin time in fulminant hepatic failure. *Gastroenterology* 100, 1480–1481.

31 Roberts HR, Cederbaum AI (1972) The liver and blood coagulation: physiology and pathology. *Gastroenterology* 63, 297–320.

32 Rybak M, Dyrhon V, Losticky C *et al.* (1988) Effect of liver damage on the level of coagulation factor II, X and VII in human and bovine plasma. *Thromb Res* 52, 79–85.

33 Eisenberg JM, Goldfarb S (1976) Clinical usefulness of measuring prothrombin time as a routine admission test. *Clin Chem* 22, 1644–1647.

34 Roberts HR, Stinchcombe TE, Gabriel DA (2001) The dysfibrinogenaemias. *Br J Haematol* 114, 249–257.

35 de Maat MP, Nieuwenhuizen W, Knot EA *et al.* (1995) Measuring plasma fibrinogen levels in patients with liver cirrhosis. The occurrence of proteolytic fibrin(ogen) degradation products and their influence on several fibrinogen assays. *Thromb Res* 78, 353–362.

36 Izumi S, Hughes RD, Langley PG *et al.* (1994) Extent of the acute phase response in fulminant hepatic failure. *Gut* 35, 982–986.

37 Mammen EF (1994) Coagulation defects in liver disease. *Med Clin North Am* 78, 545–554.

38 Coccheri S, Mannucci PM, Palareti G *et al.* (1982) Significance of plasma fibrinopeptide A and high molecular weight fibrinogen in patients with liver cirrhosis. *Br J Haematol* 52, 503–509.

39 Ballmer PE, Reichen J, McNurlan MA *et al.* (1996) Albumin but not fibrinogen synthesis correlates with galactose elimination capacity in patients with cirrhosis of the liver. *Hepatology* 24, 53–59.

40 Rustemeijer C, Schouten JA, Voerman HJ *et al.* (2001) Is pseudocholinesterase activity related to markers of triacylglycerol synthesis in Type II diabetes mellitus? *Clin Sci (Lond)* 101, 29–35.

41 Sanz P, Rodriguez-Vicente MC, Diaz D *et al.* Red blood cell and total blood acetylcholinesterase and plasma pseudocholinesterase in humans: observed variances. *J Toxicol Clin Toxicol* 29, 81–90.

42 Breen KJ, Schenker S (1971) Liver function tests. *CRC Crit Rev Clin Lab Sci* 2, 573–599.

43 Wilson A, Calvert RJ, Geoghegan H (1952) Plasma cholinesterase activity in liver disease: its value as a diagnostic test of liver function compared with flocculation tests and plasma protein determinations. *J Clin Invest* 31, 815–823.

44 Viby-Mogensen J, Hanel HK, Hansen E *et al.* (1975) Serum cholinesterase activity in burned patients. I: biochemical findings. *Acta Anaesthesiol Scand* 19, 159–168.

45 Butterworth RF (2000) Complications of cirrhosis III. Hepatic encephalopathy. *J Hepatol* 32(1 Suppl.), 171–180.

46 Lockwood AH (2004) Blood ammonia levels and hepatic encephalopathy. *Metab Brain Dis* 19, 345–349.

47 Simon JB, Poon RW (1978) Lipoprotein-X levels in extrahepatic versus intrahepatic cholestasis. *Gastroenterology* 75, 177–180.

48 Miller JP (1990) Dyslipoproteinaemia of liver disease. *Baillières Clin Endocrinol Metab* 4, 807–832.

49 Szalay F (2001) Treatment of primary biliary cirrhosis. *J Physiol Paris* 95, 407–412.

50 Baraona E, Lieber CS (1979) Effects of ethanol on lipid metabolism. *J Lipid Res* 20, 289–315.

51 Rigato I, Ostrow JD, Tiribelli C (2005) Bilirubin and the risk of common non-hepatic diseases. *Trends Mol Med* 11, 277–283.

52 Persico M, Persico E, Bakker CT *et al.* (2001) Hepatic uptake of organic anions affects the plasma bilirubin level in subjects with Gilbert's syndrome mutations in UGT1A1. *Hepatology* 33, 627–632.

53 Paulusma CC, Kothe MJ, Bakker CT *et al.* (2000) Zonal downregulation and redistribution of the multidrug resistance protein 2 during bile duct ligation in rat liver. *Hepatology* 31, 684–693.

54 Gambino R (1965) Bilirubin (modified Jendrassik and Grof). In: Meites S (ed.) *Standard Methods of Clinical Chemistry.* New York and London: Academic Press, pp. 55–64.

55 Richterich R (1969) Total bilirubin in the newborn: direct spectrophotometry. In: Karger S. (ed.) *Clinical Chemistry. Theory and Practice.* New York and London: Academic Press, pp. 416–418.

56 Blanckaert N, Kabra PM, Farina FA *et al.* (1980) Measurement of bilirubin and its monoconjugates and diconjugates in human serum by alkaline methanolysis and high-performance liquid chromatography. *J Lab Clin Med* 96, 198–212.

57 Lumeng L, O'Connor K (1986) Differential diagnosis of jaundice. In: Ostrow JD (ed.) *From Bile Pigments to Jaundice.* New York: Marcell Dekker, pp. 475–538.

58 Cekic D, Rigato I, Tiribelli C (2005) Disturbances of bilirubin metabolism. In: Weinstein WM, Hawkey CJ, Bosch J (eds) *Clinical Gastroenterology and Hepatology.* London: Elsevier Mosby, pp. 693–698.

59 Christensen E, Bremmelgaard A, Bahnsen M *et al.* (1984) Prediction of fatality in fulminant hepatic failure. *Scand J Gastroenterol* 19, 90–96.

60 Neuberger J (1997) Transplantation for primary biliary cirrhosis. *Semin Liver Dis* 17, 137–146.

61 Van Hoof VO, De Broe ME (1994) Interpretation and clinical significance of alkaline phosphatase isoenzyme patterns. *Crit Rev Clin Lab Sci* 31, 197–293.

62 Hagerstrand I (1975) Distribution of alkaline phosphatase activity in healthy and diseased human liver tissue. *Acta Pathol Microbiol Scand* [A] 83, 519–526.

63 Kaplan MM (1972) Alkaline phosphatase. *Gastroenterology* 62, 452–468.

64 Whitfield JB, Pounder RE, Neale G, Moss DW (1972) Serum-glutamyl transpeptidase activity in liver disease. *Gut* 13, 702–708.

65 Cherian AG, Hill JG (1978) Age dependence of serum enzymatic activities (alkaline phosphatase, aspartate aminotransferase, and creatine kinase) in healthy children and adolescents. *Am J Clin Pathol* 70, 783–789.

66 Bennett DL, Ward MS, Daniel WA Jr (1976) The relationship of serum alkaline phosphatase concentrations to sex maturity ratings in adolescents. *J Pediatr* 88, 633–636.

67 Eastman JR, Bixler D (1977) Serum alkaline phosphatase: normal values by sex and age. *Clin Chem* 23, 1769–1770.

68 Hsu SH, Tsai KS (1997) Different age-related trends of bone and nonbone forms of alkaline phosphatase in Chinese men and women. *Clin Chem* 43, 186–188.

69 Hatoff DE, Hardison WG (1979) Induced synthesis of alkaline phosphatase by bile acids in rat liver cell culture. *Gastroenterology* 77, 1062–1067.

70 Kaplan MM (1972) Alkaline phosphatase. *N Engl J Med* 286, 200–202.

71 Schaefer J, Schiff L (1965) Liver function tests in metastatic tumor of the liver: study of 100 cases. *Gastroenterology* 49, 360–363.

72 Breen KJ, Schenker S (1971) Liver function tests. *CRC Crit Rev Clin Lab Sci* 2, 573–599.

73 Sher PP (1982) Drug interference with clinical laboratory tests. *Drugs* 24, 24–63.

74 Wilson JW (1979) Inherited elevation of alkaline phosphatase activity in the absence of disease. *N Engl J Med* 301, 983–984.

75 Jacobs WL (1972) Gamma-glutamyl-transpeptidase in diseases of the liver, cardiovascular system and diabetes mellitus. *Clin Chim Acta* 38, 419–434.

76 Szasz G (1969) A kinetic photometric method for serum gamma-glutamyl transpeptidase. *Clin Chem* 15, 124–136.

77 Schiele F, Guilmin AM, Detienne H, Siest G (1977) Gamma-glutamyltransferase activity in plasma: statistical distributions, individual variations, and reference intervals. *Clin Chem* 23, 1023–1028.

78 Whitfield JB (2001) Gamma glutamyl transferase. *Crit Rev Clin Lab Sci* 38, 263–355.

79 Lum G, Gambino SR (1972) Serum gamma-glutamyl transpeptidase activity as an indicator of disease of liver, pancreas, or bone. *Clin Chem* 18, 358–362.

80 Cooper EH, Turner R, Steele L *et al.* (1975) The contribution of serum enzymes and carcinoembryonic antigen to the early diagnosis of metastatic colorectal cancer. *Br J Cancer* 31, 111–117.

81 Braide SA, Davies TJ (1987) Factors that affect the induction of gamma glutamyltransferase in epileptic patients receiving anti-convulsant drugs. *Ann Clin Biochem* 24, 391–399.

82 Nagaya T, Yoshida H, Takahashi H *et al.* (1999) Dose-response relationships between drinking and serum tests in Japanese men aged 40–59 years. *Alcohol* 17, 133–138.

83 Lamy J, Baglin MC, Aron E, Weill J (1975) Decrease in serum gamma-glutamyltranspeptidase following abstention from alcohol in cirrhotics. *Clin Chim Acta* 60, 97–101.

84 Silva IS, Ferraz ML, Perez RM *et al.* (2004) Role of gamma-glutamyl transferase activity in patients with chronic hepatitis C virus infection. *J Gastroenterol Hepatol* 19, 314–318.

85 McKenna JP, Moskovitz M, Cox JL (1989) Abnormal liver function tests in asymptomatic patients. *Am Fam Physician* 39, 117–126.

86 Goldberg DM (1973) 5′-Nucleotidase: recent advances in cell biology, methodology and clinical significance. *Digestion* 8, 87–99.

5.3 Hepatic removal kinetics: importance for quantitative measurements of liver function

Susanne Keiding and Michael Sørensen

Quantitative measurements of specific liver functions have been a challenge for hepatologists for many years. The many vital functions of the liver are not directly measurable, mainly because of the inaccessibility of sampling blood from the liver vessels. Several indirect tests have been proposed but few have proved clinically useful. A number of quantitative tests, each measuring particular metabolic functions or biliary excretory processes, are needed [1]. For successful design of such tests, it is most important to take into account the unique characteristics of liver structure, microcirculation, intracellular metabolism and biliary excretion.

The liver is ideally evolved for removal of substances from the circulation. Blood flows from the portal vein and the hepatic artery to the liver veins through a highly interconnected, spongelike system of sinusoids lined by hepatocytes. The endothelial cells are fenestrated, allowing large molecules, but not the corpuscular elements of the blood, direct access to the hepatocyte membrane, where numerous microvilli extend into the space of Disse. Bloodborne substances have direct access to a large area of the sinusoidal surface of the hepatocytes.

From a functional point of view, the bloodstream is unidirectional from the inlet to the outlet of the sinusoids. Substrate removal from the blood creates concentration gradients along the flow direction. This is in contrast to the *in vitro* test-tube experiment where all enzyme molecules are exposed to a uniform substrate concentration.

When describing the dynamics of hepatic removal of substances from the circulation, concepts developed *in vitro* must be adapted to the sinusoidal arrangement of hepatocyte anatomy and microcirculation. Model concepts should adequately express the complex physiological conditions in the intact organ. Parameters should, however, be limited to a few pertinent variables until experimental results justify the inclusion of further terms.

This review starts from enzyme kinetics *in vitro* and then transposes those concepts to the liver structure in terms of mathematical–physiological models. We describe *in vivo* Michaelis–Menten kinetics and discuss clearance measurements because these may be convenient estimates of liver blood flow or removal capacity for particular substances. Finally, we introduce the use of functional imaging by positron emission tomography (PET) as a unique technique for quantitative 3-D measurements of regional liver haemodynamics and metabolism.

In vitro Michaelis–Menten kinetics

In test-tube experiments, the enzymatic conversion of a substrate to a metabolite, viz. substrate removal, is characterized by Michaelis–Menten saturation kinetics; the relation between the conversion rate V and the substrate concentration c depends on the maximal conversion rate V_{max} and the half-saturation substrate concentration K_m (Fig. 1):

$$V = V_{max}\, c / (K_m + c) \tag{1}$$

At low substrate concentrations, that is $c \ll K_m$, an increase in c causes a proportional increase in V; the kinetics is first-order. At high concentrations, that is $c \gg K_m$, an increase in c causes only a small increase in V; the metabolism approximates saturation, and the kinetics is zero-order.

In vivo Michaelis–Menten kinetics

For the intact liver, we first consider the simplest possible physiological approach, the single equivalent sinusoidal perfusion model [2,3]: all sinusoids contain the same amount of enzyme and they are perfused by identical flow rates. Substrate is given as a constant intravenous (i.v.) infusion so that blood concentrations are constant with time (steady-state), and there is complete presinusoidal mixing of blood from the portal vein and the hepatic artery. Red blood cells have about the same diameter as the sinusoid and this causes complete mixing of the substrate within each cross-section of the sinusoid. Diffusion from the sinusoidal bulk through the space of Disse up to the hepatocyte membrane is much faster than the removal rate. The substrate concentration accordingly is similar throughout each transverse section of the sinusoid.

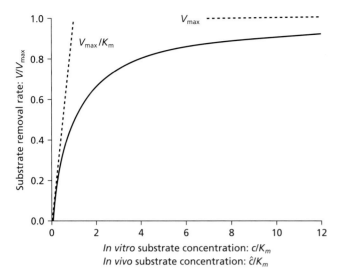

Fig. 1 Michaelis–Menten steady-state removal kinetics: $V = V_{max}c/(c + K_m)$, where V is the removal rate, c the substrate concentration, V_{max} the maximal substrate removal rate, and K_m is the half-saturation concentration. In the figure, V is normalized in respect to V_{max}, and c in respect to K_m. *In vitro*, all enzymes are exposed to the same concentration. *In vivo*, the hepatocytes lining the sinusoids are exposed to substrate concentration gradients along the blood-flow direction, decreasing from the inlet (c_i) to the outlet (c_o). In the sinusoidal perfusion model, $V = V_{max}\hat{c}/(\hat{c} + K_m)$, where the logarithmic average concentration $\hat{c} = (c_i - c_o)/\ln(c_i/c_o)$ accounts for the sinusoidal substrate gradient. At high concentrations, V approximates *in vivo* to V_{max}. At low concentrations, $V/\hat{c}$ approximates *in vivo* to V_{max}/K_m.

For the sinusoid, steady-state substrate removal rate, V, is:

$$V = F(c_i - c_o) \qquad (2)$$

where F is the blood flow rate, and c_i and c_o are the inlet and outlet substrate concentrations respectively. This relation is model-independent, being based on Fick's principle of mass conservation only.

Removal of substrate by the hepatocytes is assumed to be governed by irreversible Michaelis–Menten kinetics of the rate-limiting step, either due to transport into the cell, metabolic conversion within the cell, or biliary excretion. The removal kinetics is described in relation to the local sinusoidal blood (or rather plasma water) substrate concentration pertaining to the rate-limiting step. During the passage of blood through the sinusoid, substrate removal by the hepatocytes gradually depletes the substrate, and a concentration gradient develops along the flow direction [3].

For the whole liver, integration of Equations 1 and 2 for all sinusoids gives [2,3]:

$$V = V_{max}\hat{c}/(K_m + \hat{c}) \qquad (3)$$

where V, V_{max} and K_m now are parameters for the whole liver and $\hat{c} = (c_i - c_o)/\ln(c_i/c_o)$. As illustrated in Fig. 1, this is an *in vivo* Michaelis–Menten relation where the concentration $\hat{c}$ is the logarithmic mean of steady-state values of c_i and c_o; $\hat{c}$ is smaller than $(c_i + c_o)/2$ and larger than the integrated mean [3] and

accounts for decreasing sinusoidal concentration gradients. It is seen that the flow F does not appear in Equation 3. This flow-independence of the relation between V and $\hat{c}$ is a salient feature of the model and has been validated experimentally [4–7].

Direct *in vivo* estimates of V_{max} and K_m were obtained from sets of steady-state values of c_i, c_o and F (Equations 2 and 3) for galactose [3,8,9], ethanol [10], antipyrine [11] and the parathyroid hormone [12].

Approximate estimates of V_{max} can be obtained at near-saturating substrate concentrations since for $\hat{c} \gg K_m$, Equation 3 reduces to $V \approx V_{max}$. Such estimates of galactose V_{max} were obtained in humans, using constant i.v. infusion of galactose and liver vein blood samples, and confirmed the flow-independence of these V_{max} estimates [13]. The measurement of the galactose elimination capacity (GEC) is another example. In this test, galactose is injected intravenously and GEC calculated from the decreasing blood galactose concentration [14]. GEC is measured at quasi-steady-state galactose concentrations higher than 2 mmol/L [14,15]. At these concentrations, $c_i \approx \hat{c} > 10K_m$ [3,9], and GEC approximates galactokinase V_{max} by 85% or more. GEC has been shown to contain prognostic information for both acute liver failure [16] and chronic liver disease [17–20].

Urea is produced nearly exclusively in the liver, and the excretion into the urine during constant i.v. infusion of alanine at near-saturating concentrations is used to quantify the V_{max} of hepatic urea synthesis [21,22]. This value is reduced during liver disease [21,23] and is used in studies of liver nitrogen metabolism [23,24].

Clearance

It is not always possible to determine V_{max}, because high concentrations may be toxic or have unwanted haemodynamic effects. In this case, clearance measurements can be useful, employing lower concentrations. Clearance of a substance from the blood is defined as the substrate removal rate (V) divided by the substrate concentration (c) at first-order kinetics, that is $\hat{c} \ll K_m$, viz. $V \ll V_{max}$ (see Fig. 1). Before a substance is chosen for clearance measurements, its removal kinetics must be evaluated to ensure that it follows first-order at the concentrations used. The consequence of using a substance with kinetics deviating from first-order is that the calculated clearance value depends on the dose given and, furthermore, that it varies with changes in liver function in a not easily comprehensive way [29,30]. In the present context it is useful to distinguish between intrinsic and systemic clearance.

Intrinsic hepatic clearance

Intrinsic hepatic clearance, Cl_{int}, is a flow-independent clearance that depends only on the 'intrinsic' transport/enzymatic removal processes. It is defined in relation to the $\hat{c}$ substrate concentration, and for $\hat{c} \ll K_m$, Equation 3 reduces to:

$$Cl_{int} = V/\hat{c} \approx V_{max}/K_m \qquad (4)$$

It is seen that replacing V in Equation 4 by the term in Equation 2 and $\hat{c}$ by the term in Equation 3, we get:

$$Cl_{int} = -F \ln(1 - E) \qquad (5)$$

where $E = (c_i - c_o)/c_i$ is the hepatic extraction fraction related to the rate-limiting metabolic step at steady state. E is flow-dependent (see Equation 7 below) in such a way that Cl_{int} (Equation 5) is flow-independent. It is mathematically identical to that used in capillary physiology [25] but in the present context applies to steady-state substrate removal.

For some substances, intrinsic clearance may be used to assess liver function. For $\hat{c} \ll 0.1K_m$, the first-order approximation of intrinsic clearance Cl_{int} to V_{max}/K_m is 90% or better (Equations 3 and 4). Intrinsic clearance of indocyanine (ICG) may be used as a measure of the biliary excretion function [6] and its flow-independence has been validated in human [6]. As seen from Equation 4, intrinsic hepatic clearance reflects V_{max} of the rate-limiting step of the particular metabolic or biliary excretory process studied, provided K_m is not changed by the experimental or pathophysiological conditions studied. The importance of this requirement is illustrated by findings in the isolated perfused pig liver, where experimental hypoxia was followed by parallel reductions of galactose V_{max} and K_m, yielding unchanged Cl_{int} values in spite of reduction of V_{max} to 2/3 of control values [26].

Systemic clearance: classification according to V_{max}/FK_m

Systemic clearance (Cl) is based on measurements of peripheral blood concentration (c_i). This clearance expression is of special interest in many experimental and clinical situations because it is based on substrate concentration measurements in peripheral blood only. This advantage is, however, gained at the expense of introducing a number of theoretical and practical limitations [27]. As a first approach, we consider cases with steady-state concentrations, no extrahepatic removal, and complete presinusoidal mixing of blood from the hepatic artery and the portal vein. Then, the sinusoidal inlet concentration c_i equals the peripheral (arterial) blood concentration. For $V \ll V_{max}$ or $V/FK_m \ll 1$, Equations 2 and 3 give for the systemic clearance:

$$Cl = V/c_i \approx F(1 - e^{-V_{max}/FK_m}) \qquad (6)$$

It is seen that systemic clearance in general depends on both the removal capacity, in terms of V_{max}/K_m, and the liver blood flow F (Fig. 2). Depending on the specific test substance, blood flow and the physiological/pathophysiological conditions, systemic clearance can be used as an approximate estimate of either F or V_{max}/K_m.

Classification of substances for clearance measurements depends on the V_{max}/K_m ratio in relation to the blood flow, F. For substrates with high values of V_{max}/FK_m, Cl approximates F, and for low values of V_{max}/FK_m, Cl approximates V_{max}/K_m. The

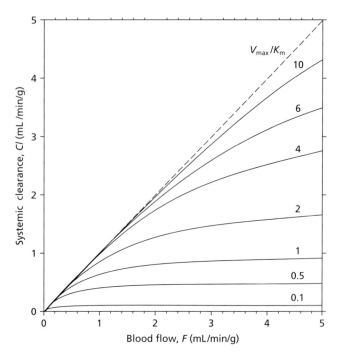

Fig. 2 Clearance of substances removed by the liver, Cl, in relation to liver blood flow, F, at different values of V_{max}/K_m. Clearance is flow-determined when $V_{max}/K_m \gg F$: $Cl \approx F$. Clearance is enzyme-determined when $V_{max}/K_m \ll F$: $Cl \approx V_{max}/K_m$ (see Table 1).

value of V_{max}/FK_m accordingly can be used for an unambiguous classification of clearance substances [27,28] (Fig. 3 and Table 1). For a substance with V_{max}/FK_m larger than 2.3, Cl approximates F by 90% or more (Equation 6). Systemic clearance is flow-determined and may be used as an estimate of F. For a substance with V_{max}/FK_m less than 0.10, Cl approximates V_{max}/K_m by 90% or more. Systemic clearance is enzyme-determined and may be used as an estimate of intrinsic clearance. For substances with V_{max}/FK_m within these limits, clearance depends on both F and V_{max}/K_m; the substance belongs to the intermediate clearance regime [27].

Previously, many test substances were classified according to their hepatic extraction fraction [31]. It is true that a high E generally indicates a high degree of flow-dependence, and that a low E indicates a high degree of enzyme-dependence. However, the effects of V_{max}/K_m and F cannot be separated, as seen from:

$$E = 1 - e^{-V_{max}/FK_m} \qquad (7)$$

Hence, E is not a suitable basis for classification of hepatic clearance substances.

Enzyme-determined systemic clearance

When V_{max} of a given substance is small in relation to FK_m, the general clearance relation (Equation 6) reduces to $Cl \approx V_{max}/K_m$, which is identical to intrinsic clearance (Equation 4). This enzyme-determined clearance does not vary with flow and is

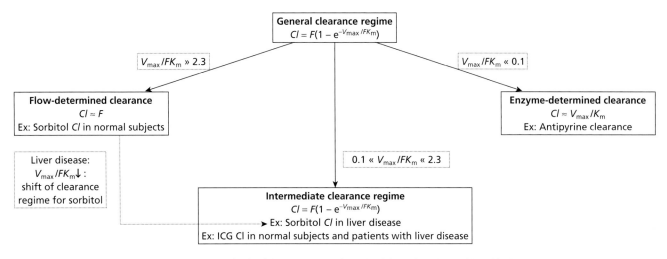

Fig. 3 Diagram of clearance regimes with example of shift of clearance regime for sorbitol during liver disease (dotted line).

Table 1 Clearance classification of substrates removed by the liver according to V_{max}/FK_m.

Test substrate	Experimental model	V_{max}/FK_m Mean (range)	Reference
Enzyme-determined clearance regimen: $V_{max}/FK_m < 0.1$			
Antipyrine (phenazone)	Normal pig, liver perfusion[a]	0.05 (0.03–0.08)	11
Caffeine	Normal human, breath test[c]	0.002	30
Caffeine	Cirrhosis human, breath test[c]	0.001	30
Flow-determined clearance regimen: $V_{max}/FK_m > 2.3$			
Sorbitol	Normal human, liver vein cath.[b]	3.6	38
Sorbitol	Normal human, liver vein cath.[b]	2.9	36
Sorbitol	Normal human, liver vein cath.[b]	2.8 (2.3–4.2)	35
Ethanol	Normal human, liver vein cath.[a]	7.4 (3.2–9.7)	10
Ethanol	Normal pig, liver vein cath.[a]	4.6 (1.9–11)	10
Galactose	Normal human, liver vein cath.[b]	2.5 (1.9–4.6)	40
Galactose	Normal pig, liver vein cath.[a]	4.1 (2.1–6.7)	9
Galactose	Normal cat, liver vein cath.[a]	3.2 (2.0–6.3)	8
Intermediate clearance regimen: $0.1 < V_{max}/FK_m < 2.3$			
Sorbitol	Cirrhosis human, liver vein cath.[b]	0.57	36
Sorbitol	Cirrhosis human, liver vein cath.[b]	1.9 (0.4–2.8)	35
Indocyanine green	Normal human, liver vein cath.[b]	0.70	36
Indocyanine green	Cirrhosis human, liver vein cath.[b]	0.20	36
Indocyanine green	Normal human, liver vein cath.[b]	0.9	34
Indocyanine green	Cirrhosis human, liver vein cath.[b]	0.4	34
Indocyanine green	Normal human, liver vein cath.[b]	1.7 (0.8–3.1)	35
Indocyanine green	Cirrhosis human, liver vein cath.[b]	0.9 (0.2–2.7)	35
Ethanol	Normal pig, liver perfusion[a]	1.5 (0.7–2.9)	10
Galactose	Normal pig, liver perfusion[a]	2.3 (1.5–3.6)	3

[a]Measurements of sets of steady-state c_i, c_o and F (Equation 3).
[b]Constant infusion at first-order kinetics with measurements of steady-state c_i and c_o: $E = (c_i - c_o)/c_i$; $V_{max}/FK_m = -\ln(1 - E)$ (Equation 5).
[c]Calculation of clearance from dose and concentration curve; liver flow assumed 1.2 L/min/70 kg body weight: $E = Cl/F$; $V_{max}/FK_m = -\ln(1 - E)$ (Equation 5).

proportional to V_{max}. Antipyrine (phenazone) is the only substance that has been thoroughly evaluated kinetically for its use as an enzyme-determined clearance substance. It is metabolized in the microsomes with first-order kinetics, has negligible extrahepatic elimination, and V_{max}/FK_m is about 0.05 in pigs [32] (Table 1). Antipyrine clearance was reduced in cirrhotic rats [33], and may provide prognostic information in patients with acute liver failure [16].

Flow-determined systemic clearance

When a substrate is removed in the liver by a process with a large amount of enzyme and a high affinity (low K_m) relative to hepatic blood flow, that is $V_{max}/FK_m \gg 1$, the general clearance relation (Equation 6) reduces to $Cl \approx F$. The removal is now entirely determined by the perfusion; all substrate is removed in a single pass. In subjects with no liver disease, V_{max}/FK_m for steady-state removal of sorbitol (corrected for urinary excretion) is >2.3 (Table 1) and extrahepatic metabolism is negligible [35–38]. In agreement with this, sorbitol clearance showed good agreement with flow measurements using ICG–Fick's principle (Equation 4) [35]. Sorbitol thus is an ideal test substance for clearance measurements of liver blood flow in healthy subjects. In subjects with liver disease, however, V_{max}/K_m is reduced [35,37] and sorbitol clearance shifts to the intermediate clearance regime (Table 1 and Fig. 2).

Galactose has been proposed as a clearance substance for measurement of liver blood flow because of a very high hepatic extraction fraction [39], but its use is hampered by significant extrahepatic elimination relative to that in the liver at low galactose concentrations [40]. The same is true for ethanol [10] (Table 1).

Some studies use systemic ICG clearance as a flow measurement, others as a measure of liver cell function. Neither is justified because ICG belongs to the intermediate clearance regime (Table 1).

PET measurements of regional liver metabolism

Positron emission tomography (PET) is an imaging modality that is new in the context of quantitative measurements of liver functions. The technique provides unique possibilities for measurements of regional liver blood perfusion and metabolism by means of i.v. injected radiolabelled tracers. PET tracers are positron-labelled natural substances, analogues thereof, drugs or receptor ligands. Combined PET/CT (computed tomography) cameras have the advantage of depicting functional PET images in CT-defined structures and allowing for noninvasive measurement of tracer supply through the liver blood vessels.

Clinical studies usually use PET images of the mean radioactivity concentration in a given time interval after tracer injection. Such images yield a visual impression of possible differences of metabolism between specific regions in the tissue. This provides the basis for the much used diagnostic detection of increased glucose metabolism in cancer nodules. Quantification of regional metabolic processes requires *dynamic* PET scanning, that is recordings of the time courses of tissue and blood radioactivity concentrations following tracer administration. Analysis of dynamic PET data comprises definition of a tissue region of interest (ROI) and analysis of the time course of tissue radioactivity concentrations in that region in relation to that in blood supplying the organ (see below). The kinetic modelling is based on a mathematical model of the metabolic diagram for the specific tracer used. In the case of ^{18}F-deoxy-2-glucose (FDG), metabolism can be described as illustrated in Figure 4.

Hepatic dual-input function

Following an i.v. injection of a tracer, the tracer is supplied to the liver via its dual blood supply. As seen in Figure 5, tracer radioactivity concentration in the hepatic artery rises steeply, reaches a peak and then decreases; the portal venous concentration curve is delayed and dispersed compared with that in the artery. The concentration resulting from the dual blood supply can be calculated as the flow-weighted average of the radioactivity concentrations in the hepatic artery and the portal vein. In experimental pig studies, estimates of kinetic parameters for the FDG kinetics (Fig. 4) using the liver dual-input function and nonlinear regression of the model to pig liver data gave parameter values that were comparable with independent estimates of flow and blood volume [41].

Because of difficulties in measuring the portal venous concentration, most PET studies of the liver ignore the dual blood supply, and kinetic parameter estimates rely on the use of an arterial input function. However, the importance of using dual-input function for determination of the kinetic parameters in the metabolic diagram (Figure 4) was demonstrated in pig studies using two glucose analogues, FDG [41,42] and ^{11}C-methylglucose [41].

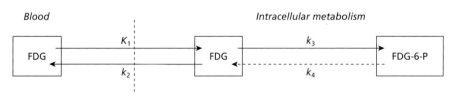

Fig. 4 Compartmental metabolic diagram for FDG (a glucose analogue) in the liver. Arrows indicate transport/metabolism of FDG. K_1 is the unidirectional clearance of FDG from blood to cell and k_2 the rate constant for the backflux; k_3 and k_4 are rate constants for phosphorylation and dephosphorylation. If the metabolism is irreversible, that is, k_4 is negligible, then the net metabolic clearance $K = K_1 k_3/(k_2 + k_3)$.

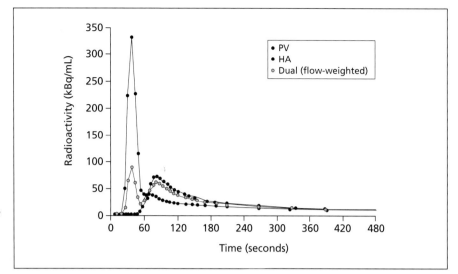

Fig. 5 Typical time-activity-curves for FDG in hepatic artery (HA), portal vein (PV) and flow-weighted dual-input blood. Initial 7 min are shown, when differences in shapes are most pronounced. The PV concentration is delayed and dispersed compared with the HA concentration as the result of the bolus passage through the intestinal vascular bed. After a few minutes, the three blood curves are similar. Blood data points are connected by straight lines.

In humans it is not possible to obtain successive blood samples from the portal vein or to measure the blood flow rates of the two supplying blood vessels. Work is in progress towards estimating the time courses of the radioactivity concentrations and the relative flow rates in the portal vein and hepatic artery by combined dynamic PET and contrast-CT for complete non-invasive measurement of the dual input [43–45]. However, a simpler but less informative analysis provided by the Gjedde–Patlak plot [46,47], using arterial concentration measurements only, can be very useful [41]. For substances with irreversible liver metabolism and negligible net removal in the intestines, the 'net metabolic clearance', K, can be used to describe steady-state irreversible clearance from blood to cell due to metabolism or biliary excretion. K is a simple mathematical combination of the kinetic rate constants as shown in Figure 4. K of FDG was used in experimental clinical studies to quantify differences in glucose metabolism between cholangiocarcinoma and nonmalignant liver tissue [48,49]. This relation has been used to measure pig liver metabolism of ammonia [55] and ^{18}F-deoxygalactose (M. Sørensen, unpublished data) as well as brain metabolism of ammonia during hepatic encephalopathy [56].

In routine clinical work it may be difficult to obtain series of arterial blood samples, and radioactivity concentration measurements from the abdominal aorta obtained from dynamic liver PET images may be used instead [43,50]. Furthermore, parametric images depicting pixel-by-pixel K values will often better distinguish between areas with increased metabolism due to tumour tissue or focal inflammation [49]. Thus, clinically useful parametric images of the net metabolic clearance can be produced based on totally noninvasive dynamic scans.

Compartment and microvascular models

Today, the standard kinetic model used for analysis of dynamic PET scans is most often a compartmental model (Fig. 4). This model regards tracer input to be instantaneously distributed in the capillaries/sinusoids and the transport/metabolism to take place at an identical input concentration all along the vascular path; it is an 'arterial equilibration model'. According to this modelling, mass is exchanged between well-mixed compartments as a function of time, and model parameters are rate constants that describe this exchange (Fig. 4). From a practical point of view, these models are often useful [41,51] but deviate obviously from liver physiology. Uncritical use of such models may lead to unphysiological parameter estimates [52,53]. We therefore have developed microvascular models to interpret PET data with a more physiological approach. When a tracer bolus passes through the capillary, time- and space-dependent concentration gradients develop [53], and by external detection the PET camera sees the spatial integral of the concentration at any time. These new microvascular models have been used to determine regional liver blood perfusion by dynamic $C^{15}O$ PET of pigs, validated by independent measurements using ultrasound transit-time flow-meters [53,54]. The models have not yet been developed for more complex metabolic diagrams, for example including backflux from cell to blood. In the next sections, we therefore restrict the discussion to the traditional 'hybrid' of using compartmental models but including expressions from classical capillary physiology to estimate flow and clearances (see also Chapter 5.8).

Physiological complexities

Sinusoidal heterogeneity

In the intact liver, the sinusoids form a highly interconnected, labyrinthine system. The sinusoids are not 'equivalent sinusoids'. Enzyme content of the hepatocytes may vary along the sinusoid, a phenomenon called sinusoidal zonation [57]. This phenomenon has been shown for metabolism of various amino acids [58], glucose [59] and ammonia [57,60], with ammonia metabolism being quantified *in vivo* by pig liver PET studies [61].

Heterogeneity between the sinusoids [62] lead to diminished efficiency of the overall removal, namely a diminished V_{max} as described in the distributed sinusoidal perfusion model [63].

Distribution of hepatic artery branches into acini is heterogeneous even in the normal liver as shown in rat studies [64]. In accordance with this, there was a remarkably higher variation of ^{13}N-ammonia trapped in the liver tissue as ^{13}N-glutamine in pig livers following ^{13}N-ammonia injection into the hepatic artery than following tracer injection into the portal or caval vein [65]. Thus, metabolic consequences of vascular heterogeneity could be quantified by dynamic liver PET. Similarly, measurements of the hepatic venous pressure gradient in two liver veins in subjects without liver disease showed a larger variation than can be attributed to measurement uncertainties [66]. The physiological importance of these variations remains to be elucidated.

Liver blood flow varies under different physiological conditions or pharmacological interventions. Food intake increases total flow [34,67] and e.g. vasopressin decreases it [13]. In agreement with the predicted flow-independence of V_{max}, neither of these flow changes changed the estimates of galactose V_{max} [13] or ICG intrinsic clearance [6]. Similarly, in perfused rat liver studies, galactose V_{max} was not influenced by flow changes as long as the perfusion rate was above 0.9 mL blood/min/g liver [68]. Similar results were found in the intact cat liver [8]. As the flow rate was gradually reduced, the effect of sinusoidal heterogeneity became more significant [69,70].

Hepatic first-pass elimination and systemic availability during saturation kinetics

The location of the liver between the portal and the systemic circulation means that substances absorbed from the gut have to pass through the liver before reaching the systemic circulation [61,71]. This constitutes the basis for the hepatic first-pass filter function.

For many orally taken drugs, for example acetylsalicylic acid [72], hepatic removal follows saturation kinetics and the systemic availability (the fraction of the absorbed dose that reaches the systemic circulation) depends on the dose (Fig. 6). Systemic availability approximates to unity at doses (V) approximating (or exceeding) the maximal removal capacity (V_{max}). In general, the lower the V_{max}/FK_m, the higher the systemic availability.

Systemic availability is very difficult to quantify *in vivo* because of the inaccessibility of portal venous blood. The dynamic PET/CT methods for noninvasive measurements of the hepatic dual-input function, as mentioned above, provide a promising methodological basis for a much-needed breakthrough in this research area.

Binding to circulating plasma proteins

Hydrophobic substances, such as long-chain fatty acids and organic anions like bilirubin and ICG, circulate in plasma bound to plasma proteins. It has been shown for several substances,

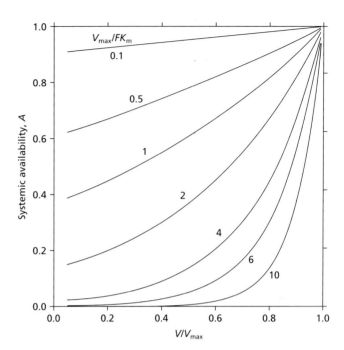

Fig. 6 Systemic availability at saturation removal kinetics: $A = 1 - E = e^{-V_{max}/FK_m}$. Curves show systemic availability in relation to dose, namely, V/V_{max} for different values of V_{max}/FK_m.

however, that more substrate is removed than corresponds to the unbound fraction [73–78]. This may be explained by diffusion barriers in the unstirred water layer adjacent to the hepatocyte plasma membrane [79,80]. The uptake of unbound substrate by the hepatocytes creates disequilibrium between bound and unbound substrate and the rate of dissociation of the protein–substrate complex becomes higher than the rate of complex formation within the unstirred water layer. Binding protein is not taken up by the hepatocytes: after unloading the drug, it returns to the sinusoidal bulk, where equilibrium between bound and unbound substrate molecules replenishes protein–substrate complex [81]. This model assumes no membrane binding of plasma proteins, but for free fatty acids there seems to be some albumin-mediated facilitation of the uptake process [82]. In liver vein catheterization studies using a constant i.v. infusion of ICG, experimental changes of plasma protein changed the removal of ICG in agreement with the codiffusion model in intact pigs [74] and in humans [77].

In perfused rat liver studies, backflux of dibromosulphthalein from the cells to the perfusate increased with increasing albumin concentration in the perfusate [83], which is also accounted for by the codiffusion phenomena.

Liver disease

Impaired liver-cell function

When hepatic metabolic functions are impaired due to liver disease, concepts of using V_{max} or enzyme-determined clearance measurements are still valid (Fig. 3). Diminished GEC [84,85], antipyrine clearance [32] and urea synthesis capacity [21] in liver patients reflect reduced liver cell metabolism. However, when transposing flow-determined clearance measurements to pathological conditions, it must be ensured that the requirements for flow-determined clearance remain fulfilled. The shift of sorbitol clearance from being flow-determined in healthy subjects to being in the intermediate clearance in cirrhotic patients illustrates this question [35] (Fig. 3).

Intra- and extrahepatic vascular shunting

Patients with cirrhosis often develop extra- and intrahepatic portal–hepatic venous vascular shunts [86] and capillarization of the sinusoids [87]. Loss of metabolic liver function and both types of shunts will diminish the hepatic first-pass removal of substances. Systemic availability will increase and may lead to drug toxicity or hepatic encephalopathy. The effect of extrahepatic shunting can be assessed by dynamic magnetic resonance (MR) scans or catheterization of the azygos vein, which drains oesophageal varices [88,89]. At present, the effects of intrahepatic shunting cannot be distinguished from reduced liver cell function [37].

Clinical use of quantitative liver function measurements

Hepatic failure is ultimately the major cause of death in patients with liver disease. It is, therefore, reasonable to assume that quantitative measurements of various specific liver functions as outlined above, or serial measurements thereof, may provide clinically valuable prognostic information. Table 2 gives an overview of tests used today. Numerous tests have been proposed, but unfortunately most have not proved clinically useful. This is probably related to the fact that they have not been founded on proper physiological and pathophysiological grounds. Also, properly performed prognostic studies are astonishingly scarce.

PET or PET/CT measurements of regional liver haemodynamics and metabolism have the potential of being clinically useful prognostic quantitative tests [49].

Acute liver disease

In fulminant hepatic failure, quantitative tests of liver function may provide information on short-term survival. GEC was of prognostic value in patients with acute liver failure due to viral hepatitis [90] or paracetamol intoxication [91]. Following an overdose of paracetamol, the aminopyrine breath test was also able to predict fatal outcome [92]. In alcoholic hepatitis, the aminopyrine breath test predicted survival with reasonable accuracy [93].

Chronic liver disease

In chronic liver disease, GEC provides information on long-term survival [17–20,94–96]. In patients with primary biliary cirrhosis, serial determinations of GEC provided prognostic information [85]. The aminopyrine breath test was one of the statistically significant predictors of death in patients with cirrhosis [97] or chronic hepatitis [98].

Assessment of surgical risk

Liver resection in patients with chronic liver disease is associated with an increased risk of severe postoperative liver impairment. In a large prospective study of the predictive value of various preoperative liver tests, GEC was a strong independent and valuable predictor for short- and long-term outcome in patients with primary and secondary hepatic tumours undergoing resection [99]. In the treatment of patients with primary liver tumours or liver metastases, it is often impossible to predict if the patient will tolerate treatment with resection, radiofrequency, stereotactic radiotherapy or chemotherapy.

Assessment of therapeutic response

Only a few studies have attempted to evaluate treatment effects and prognostic value of quantitative liver function measurements. Jansen and co-workers (100) found that following liver resection, the liver regained 75% of the volume and 100% of the galactose elimination capacity after 120 days. In two studies,

Table 2 Quantitative liver function tests.

Test	Provides an estimate of:	Reference
Galactose elimination capacity	V_{max} of cytosolic enzyme galactokinase	[15]
Urea synthesis capacity	V_{max} of alanine to urea synthesis	[21]
Antipyrine clearance	V_{max}/K_m of microsomal metabolism	[11,105]
Intrinsic clearance of indocyanine green	V_{max}/K_m of biliary excretion	[6,35]
Sorbitol clearance	Liver blood flow in healthy subjects	[35–38]
Caffeine clearance	Microsomal function	[29,30]
Aminopyrine breath test	Microsomal demethylation	[106]
Ketoisocaproic acid breath test	Mitochondrial decarboxylation	[107]

FDG PET was found to be useful for prediction of treatment response in patients treated with chemotherapy for colorectal metastases to the liver [101,102]. Recent FDG PET studies successfully evaluated the effect of experimental radiotherapy [103] and radiofrequency treatment [104] of pig livers. Quantitative dynamic PET studies may be of significant benefit for the patients and more studies need to be done.

References

1 Tygstrup N. (1990) Assessment of liver function: principles and practice. *J Gastroenterol Hepatol* 5, 468–482.

2 Bass L, Keiding S, Winkler K *et al.* (1976) Enzymatic elimination of substrates flowing through the intact liver. *J Theor Biol* 61, 393–409.

3 Keiding S, Johansen S, Winkler K *et al.* (1976) Michaelis-Menten kinetics of galactose elimination by the isolated perfused pig liver. *Am J Physiol* 230, 1302–1313.

4 Keiding S, Chiarantini E. (1978) Effect of sinusoidal perfusion on galactose elimination kinetics in perfused rat liver. *J Pharmacol Exp Ther* 205, 465–470.

5 Keiding S, Priisholm K. (1984) Current models of hepatic pharmacokinetics: flow effects on kinetic constants of ethanol elimination in perfused rat liver. *Biochem Pharmacol* 33, 3209–3212.

6 Keiding S, Skak C. (1988) Methodological limitations of the use of intrinsic hepatic clearance of ICG as a measure of liver cell function. *Eur J Clin Invest* 18, 507–511.

7 Krarup N, Larsen JA. (1976) The influence of dye infusion rate and hepatic plasma flow on indocyanine green clearance. *Scand J Clin Lab Invest* 36, 183–188.

8 Greenway CV, Burczynski FJ. (1987) Effects of liver blood flow on hepatic uptake kinetics of galactose in anesthetized cats: parallel tube model. *Can J Physiol Pharmacol* 65, 1193–1199.

9 Keiding S, Johansen S, Winkler K. (1982) Hepatic galactose elimination kinetics in the intact pig. *Scand J Clin Lab Invest* 42, 253–259.

10 Keiding S, Johansen S, Midtboll I *et al.* (1979) Ethanol elimination kinetics in human liver and pig liver *in vivo. Am J Physiol* 237, E316–E324.

11 Andreasen B, Tonnesen K, Rabol A *et al.* (1977) Michaelis–Menten kinetics of phenazone elimination in the perfused pig liver. *Acta Pharmacol Toxicol* 40, 1–13.

12 D'Amour P, Huet PM. (1989) Ca^{2+} concentration influences the hepatic extraction of bioactive human PTH-(1–34) in rats. *Am J Physiol* 256, E87–E92.

13 Jacobsen KR, Ranek L, Tygstrup N. (1969) Liver function and blood flow in normal man during infusion of vasopressin. *Scand J Clin Lab Invest* 24, 279–284.

14 Tygstrup N. (1977) Effect of sites of blood sampling in determination of the galactose elimination capacity. *Scand J Clin Lab Invest* 37, 333–338.

15 Tygstrup N. (1966) Determination of the hepatic elimination capacity (Lm) of galactose by single injection. *Scand J Clin Lab Invest Suppl* 18, 118–125.

16 Ranek L, Andreasen PB, Tygstrup N. (1976) Galactose elimination capacity as a prognostic index in patients with fulminant liver failure. *Gut* 17, 959–964.

17 Merkel C, Bolognesi M, Angeli P *et al.* (1989) Prognostic indicators of survival in patients with cirrhosis and esophageal varices, without previous bleeding. *Am J Gastroenterol* 84, 717–722.

18 Merkel C, Gatta A, Zoli M *et al.* (1991) Prognostic value of galactose elimination capacity, aminopyrine breath test, and ICG clearance in patients with cirrhosis. Comparison with the Pugh score. *Dig Dis Sci* 36, 1197–1203.

19 Merkel C, Marchesini G, Fabbri A *et al.* (1996) The course of galactose elimination capacity in patients with alcoholic cirrhosis: possible use as a surrogate marker for death. *Hepatology* 24, 820–823.

20 Jepsen P, Vilstrup H, Sørensen HT *et al.* (2004) Galactose elimination capacity and prognosis of patients with liver cirrhosis – a Danish registry-based cohort study with complete long-term follow-up. *J Hepatol* 40 (Suppl. 1), 69A.

21 Vilstrup H. (1980) Synthesis of urea after stimulation with amino acids: relation to liver function. *Gut* 21, 990–995.

22 Hamberg O, Vilstrup H. (1994) A rapid method for determination of hepatic amino nitrogen to urea nitrogen conversion ('the Functional Hepatic Nitrogen Clearance'). *Scand J Clin Lab Invest* 54, 377–383.

23 Hamberg O, Nielsen K, Vilstrup H. (1992) Effects of an increase in protein intake on hepatic efficacy for urea synthesis in healthy subjects and in patients with cirrhosis. *J Hepatol* 14, 237–243.

24 Grofte T, Wolthers T, Jorgensen JO *et al.* (1999) Hepatic amino- to urea-N clearance and forearm amino-N exchange during hypoglycemic and euglycemic hyperinsulinemia in normal man. *J Hepatol* 30, 819–825.

25 Crone C. (1963) The permeability of capillaries in various organs as determined by use of the 'indicator dilution' method. *Acta Physiol Scand* 58, 292–305.

26 Keiding S, Johansen S, Tygstrup N. (1990) Galactose removal kinetics during hypoxia in perfused pig liver: reduction of Vmax, but not of intrinsic clearance Vmax/Km. *Eur J Clin Invest* 20, 305–309.

27 Winkler K, Bass L, Keiding S *et al.* (1979) The physiologic basis for clearance measurements in hepatology. *Scand J Gastroenterol* 14, 439–448.

28 Keiding S. (1976) Hepatic elimination kinetics: the influence of hepatic blood flow on clearance determination. *Scand J Clin Lab Invest* 36, 113–118.

29 Bonati M, Latini R, Galletti F *et al.* (1982) Caffeine disposition after oral doses. *Clin Pharmacol Ther* 32, 98–106.

30 Renner E, Wietholtz H, Huguenin P *et al.* (1984) Caffeine: a model compound for measuring liver function. *Hepatology* 4, 38–46.

31 Wilkinson GR, Shand DG. (1975) Commentary: a physiological approach to hepatic drug clearance. *Clin Pharmacol Ther* 18, 377–390.

32 Andreasen PB, Ranek L, Statland BE *et al.* (1974) Clearance of antipyrine-dependence of quantitative liver function. *Eur J Clin Invest* 4, 129–134.

33 Buters JT, Zysset T, Reichen J. (1993) Metabolism of antipyrine *in vivo* in two rat models of liver cirrhosis. Its relationship to intrinsic clearance *in vitro* and microsomal membrane lipid composition. *Biochem Pharmacol* 46, 983–991.

34 Skak C, Keiding S. (1987) Methodological problems in the use of indocyanine green to estimate hepatic blood flow and ICG clearance in man. *Liver* 7, 155–162.

35 Keiding S, Engsted E, Ott P. (1998) Sorbitol as a test substance for measurements of liver plasma flow in humans. *Hepatology* 28, 50–56.

36 Molino G, Avagnina P, Ballare M *et al.* (1991) Combined evaluation of total and functional liver plasma flows and intrahepatic shunting. *Dig Dis Sci* 36, 1189–1196.

37 Ott P, Clemmesen O, Keiding S. (2000) Interpretation of simultaneous measurements of hepatic extraction fractions of indocyanine

green and sorbitol: evidence of hepatic shunts and capillarization? *Dig Dis Sci* 45, 359–365.

38 Zeeh J, Lange H, Bosch J *et al.* (1988) Steady-state extrarenal sorbitol clearance as a measure of hepatic plasma flow. *Gastroenterology* 95, 749–759.

39 Henderson JM, Kutner MH, Bain RP. (1982) First-order clearance of plasma galactose: the effect of liver disease. *Gastroenterology* 83, 1090–1096.

40 Keiding S. (1988) Galactose clearance measurements and liver blood flow. *Gastroenterology* 94, 477–481.

41 Munk OL, Bass L, Roelsgaard K *et al.* (2001) Liver kinetics of glucose analogs measured in pigs by PET: importance of dual-input blood sampling. *J Nucl Med* 42, 795–801.

42 Brix G, Ziegler SI, Bellemann ME *et al.* (2001) Quantification of [(18)F]FDG uptake in the normal liver using dynamic PET: impact and modeling of the dual hepatic blood supply. *J Nucl Med* 42, 1265–1273.

43 Keiding S, Munk OL, Schiott KM *et al.* (2000) Dynamic 2-[18F]fluoro-2-deoxy-D-glucose positron emission tomography of liver tumours without blood sampling. *Eur J Nucl Med* 27, 407–412.

44 Munk OL, Keiding S, Bass L. (2003) Impulse-response function of splanchnic circulation with model-independent constraints: theory and experimental validation. *Am J Physiol Gastrointest Liver Physiol* 285, G671–G680.

45 Munk OL. (2005) Hepatic metabolism of glucose analogs measured by dynamic positron emission tomography and interpreted by compartment models. PhD thesis, Faculty of Health Sciences, University of Aarhus, Denmark.

46 Gjedde A. (1982) Calculation of cerebral glucose phosphorylation from brain uptake of glucose analogs *in vivo*: a re-examination. *Brain Res* 257, 237–274.

47 Patlak CS, Blasberg RG. (1985) Graphical evaluation of blood-to-brain transfer constants from multiple-time uptake data. Generalizations. *J Cereb Blood Flow Metab* 5, 584–590.

48 Keiding S, Hansen SB, Rasmussen HH *et al.* (1998) Detection of cholangiocarcinoma in primary sclerosing cholangitis by positron emission tomography. *Hepatology* 28, 700–706.

49 Prytz H, Keiding S, Björnsson E *et al.* (2006) Dynamic FDG PET is useful for detection of cholangiocarcinoma in patients with PSC listed for liver transplantation. *Hepatology* 44, 1572–1580.

50 Germano G, Chen BC, Huang SC *et al.* (1992) Use of the abdominal aorta for arterial input function determination in hepatic and renal PET studies. *J Nucl Med* 33, 613–620.

51 Munk OL, Keiding S. (2002) Quantification of (18)F-FDG uptake in the liver using dynamic PET. *J Nucl Med* 43, 439–441.

52 Becker G, Müller-Schauenburg W, Spilker ME *et al.* (2005) *A priori* identifiability of a one-compartment model with two input functions for liver blood flow measurements. *Phys Med Biol* 50, 1393–1404.

53 Munk OL, Keiding S, Bass L. (2003) Capillaries within compartments: microvascular interpretation of dynamic positron emission tomography data. *J Theor Biol* 225, 127–141.

54 Munk OL, Bass L, Feng H *et al.* (2003) Determination of regional flow by use of intravascular PET tracers: microvascular theory and experimental validation for pig livers. *J Nucl Med* 44, 1862–1870.

55 Sørensen M, Keiding S. (2006) Ammonia metabolism in cirrhosis. In: Häussinger D, Kircheis G, Schless F (eds) *Proceedings of the 12th International Symposium of Hepatic Encephalopathy and Nitrogen Metabolism.* Springer Verlag, pp. 406–419.

56 Keiding S, Sørensen M, Bender D *et al.* (2006) Brain metabolism of ^{13}N-ammonia during acute hepatic encephalopathy in cirrhosis measured by PET. *Hepatology* 43, 42–50.

57 Haussinger D, Stoll B, Stehle T *et al.* (1989) Hepatocyte heterogeneity in glutamate metabolism and bidirectional transport in perfused rat liver. *Eur J Biochem* 185, 189–195.

58 Stoll B, McNelly S, Buscher HP *et al.* (1991) Functional hepatocyte heterogeneity in glutamate, aspartate and alpha-ketoglutarate uptake: a histoautoradiographical study. *Hepatology* 13, 247–253.

59 Gumucio JJ. (1989) Hepatocyte heterogeneity: the coming of age from the description of a biological curiosity to a partial understanding of its physiological meaning and regulation. *Hepatology* 9, 154–160.

60 Haussinger D, Lamers WH, Moorman AF. (1992) Hepatocyte heterogeneity in the metabolism of amino acids and ammonia. *Enzyme* 46, 72–93.

61 Keiding S, Munk OL, Roelsgaard K *et al.* (2001) Positron emission tomography of hepatic first-pass metabolism of ammonia in pig. *Eur J Nucl Med* 28, 1770–1775.

62 Lautt WW, Schafer J, Legare DJ. (1993) Hepatic blood flow distribution: consideration of gravity, liver surface, and norepinephrine on regional heterogeneity. *Can J Physiol Pharmacol* 71, 128–135.

63 Bass L, Robinson P, Bracken AJ. (1978) Hepatic elimination of flowing substrates: the distributed model. *J Theor Biol* 72, 161–184.

64 Richter S, Vollmar B, Mucke I *et al.* (2001) Hepatic arteriolo-portal venular shunting guarantees maintenance of nutritional microvascular supply in hepatic arterial buffer response of rat livers. *J Physiol* 531, 193–201.

65 Keiding S, Munk OL, Vilstrup H *et al.* (2005) Hepatic microcirculation assessed by positron emission tomography of first-pass ammonia metabolism in porcine liver. *Liver Int* 25, 171–176.

66 Keiding S, Vilstrup H. (2002) Intrahepatic heterogeneity of hepatic venous pressure gradient in human cirrhosis. *Scand J Gastroenterol* 37, 960–964.

67 Hansen HJ, Engell HC, Ring-Larsen H *et al.* (1977) Splanchnic blood flow in patients with abdominal angina before and after arterial reconstruction. A proposal for a diagnostic test. *Ann Surg* 186, 216–220.

68 Keiding S, Vilstrup H, Hansen L. (1980) Importance of flow and haematocrit for metabolic function of perfused rat liver. *Scand J Clin Lab Invest* 40, 355–359.

69 Brauer RW. (1963) Liver circulation and function. *Physiol Rev* 43, 115–213.

70 Lautt WW. (1977) Hepatic vasculature: a conceptual review. *Gastroenterology* 73, 1163–1169.

71 Keiding S. (1995) Drug administration to liver patients: aspects of liver pathophysiology. *Semin Liver Dis* 15, 268–282.

72 Levy G. (1965) Pharmacokinetics of salicylate elimination in man. *J Pharm Sci* 54, 959–967.

73 Forker EL, Luxon BA. (1983) Albumin-mediated transport of rose bengal by perfused rat liver. Kinetics of the reaction at the cell surface. *J Clin Invest* 72, 1764–1771.

74 Ott P, Keiding S, Bass L. (1992) Intrinsic hepatic clearance of indocyanine green in the pig: dependence on plasma protein concentration. *Eur J Clin Invest* 22, 347–357.

75 Weisiger RA, Zacks CM, Smith ND *et al.* (1984) Effect of albumin binding on extraction of sulfobromophthalein by perfused elasmobranch liver: evidence for dissociation-limited uptake. *Hepatology* 4, 492–501.

76 Weisiger RA. (1985) Dissociation from albumin: a potentially rate-limiting step in the clearance of substances by the liver. *Proc Natl Acad Sci USA* 82, 1563–1567.

77 Keiding S, Ott P, Bass L. (1993) Enhancement of unbound clearance of ICG by plasma proteins, demonstrated in human subjects and interpreted without assumption of facilitating structures. *J Hepatol* 19, 327–344.

78 Sorrentino D, Licko V, Weisiger RA *et al.* (1987) Phenobarbital specifically increases the hepatocellular uptake of sulfobromophthalein-glutathione. *Biochem Biophys Res Commun* 149, 921–926.

79 Bass L, Keiding S. (1988) Physiologically based models and strategic experiments in hepatic pharmacology. *Biochem Pharmacol* 37, 1425–1431.

80 Pond S, Bass L. (1988) The puzzle of rates of cellular uptake of protein-bound ligands. In: Pecile A, Rescigno A (eds) *Pharmacokinetics: Mathematical Approaches to Metabolism and Distribution of Chemicals and Drugs.* New York, London: Plenum Publishing, pp. 245–269.

81 Ott P, Weisiger RA. (1997) Nontraditional effects of protein binding and hematocrit on uptake of indocyanine green by perfused rat liver. *Am J Physiol* 273, G227–G238.

82 Weisiger RA, Pond SM, Bass L. (1989) Albumin enhances unidirectional fluxes of fatty acid across a lipid-water interface: theory and experiments. *Am J Physiol* 257, G904–G916.

83 Nijssen HM, Pijning T, Meijer DK *et al.* (1992) Influence of albumin on the net sinusoidal efflux of the organic anion dibromosulfophthalein from rat liver. *Hepatology* 15, 302–309.

84 Tygstrup N. (1964) The galactose elimination capacity in relation to clinical and laboratory findings in patients with cirrhosis. *Acta Med Scand* 175, 291–300.

85 Reichen J, Widmer T, Cotting J. (1991) Accurate prediction of death by serial determination of galactose elimination capacity in primary biliary cirrhosis: a comparison with the Mayo model. *Hepatology* 14, 504–510.

86 Popper H, Elias H, Petty DE. (1952) Vascular pattern of the cirrhotic liver. *Am J Clin Pathol* 22, 717–729.

87 Huet PM, Goresky CA, Villeneuve JP *et al.* (1982) Assessment of liver microcirculation in human cirrhosis. *J Clin Invest* 70, 1234–1244.

88 Sugano S, Yamamoto K, Takamura N *et al.* (1999) Azygos venous blood flow while fasting, postprandially, and after endoscopic variceal ligation, measured by magnetic resonance imaging. *J Gastroenterol* 34, 310–314.

89 Bendtsen F, Henriksen JH, Sorensen TI. (1991) Long-term effects of oral propranolol on splanchnic and systemic haemodynamics in patients with cirrhosis and oesophageal varices. *Scand J Gastroenterol* 26, 933–939.

90 Ramsoe K, Andreasen PB, Ranek L. (1980) Functioning liver mass in uncomplicated and fulminant acute hepatitis. *Scand J Gastroenterol* 15, 65–72.

91 Schmidt LE, Ott P, Tygstrup N. (2004) Galactose elimination capacity as a prognostic marker in patients with severe acetaminophen-induced hepatotoxicity: 10 years' experience. *Clin Gastroenterol Hepatol* 2, 418–424.

92 Saunders JB, Wright N, Lewis KO. (1980) Predicting outcome of paracetamol poisoning by use of 14C-aminopyrine breath test. *Br Med J* 280, 279–280.

93 Schneider JF, Baker AL, Haines NW *et al.* (1980) Aminopyrine N-demethylation: a prognostic test of liver function in patients with alcoholic liver disease. *Gastroenterology* 79, 1145–1150.

94 Merkel C, Bolognesi M, Finucci GF *et al.* (1989) Indocyanine green intrinsic hepatic clearance as a prognostic index of survival in patients with cirrhosis. *J Hepatol* 9, 16–22.

95 Merkel C, Bolognesi M, Bellon S *et al.* (1992) Aminopyrine breath test in the prognostic evaluation of patients with cirrhosis. *Gut* 33, 836–842.

96 Merkel C, Morabito A, Sacerdoti D *et al.* (1998) Updating prognosis of cirrhosis by Cox's regression model using Child-Pugh score and aminopyrine breath test as time-dependent covariates. *Ital J Gastroenterol Hepatol* 30, 276–282.

97 Villeneuve JP, Infante-Rivard C, Ampelas M *et al.* (1986) Prognostic value of the aminopyrine breath test in cirrhotic patients. *Hepatology* 6, 928–931.

98 Lashner BA, Jonas RB, Tang HS *et al.* (1988) Chronic hepatitis: disease factors at diagnosis predictive of mortality. *Am J Med* 85, 609–614.

99 Redaelli CA, Dufour JF, Wagner M *et al.* (2002) Preoperative galactose elimination capacity predicts complications and survival after hepatic resection. *Ann Surg* 235, 77–85.

100 Jansen PL, Chamuleau RA, van Leeuwen DJ *et al.* (1990) Liver regeneration and restoration of liver function after partial hepatectomy in patients with liver tumors. *Scand J Gastroenterol* 25, 112–118.

101 Bender H, Bangard N, Metten N *et al.* (1999) Possible role of FDG-PET in the early prediction of therapy outcome in liver metastases of colorectal cancer. *Hybridoma* 18, 87–91.

102 Dimitrakopoulou-Strauss A, Strauss LG, Rudi J. (2003) PET-FDG as predictor of therapy response in patients with colorectal carcinoma. *Q J Nucl Med* 47, 8–13.

103 Antoch G, Kaiser GM, Mueller AB *et al.* (2004) Intraoperative radiation therapy in liver tissue in a pig model: monitoring with dual-modality PET/CT. *Radiology* 230, 753–760.

104 Antoch G, Vogt FM, Veit P *et al.* (2005) Assessment of liver tissue after radiofrequency ablation: findings with different imaging procedures. *J Nucl Med* 46, 520–525.

105 Poulsen HE, Loft S. (1988) Antipyrine as a model drug to study hepatic drug-metabolizing capacity. *J Hepatol* 6, 374–382.

106 Bircher J, Kupfer A, Gikalov I *et al.* (1976) Aminopyrine demethylation measured by breath analysis in cirrhosis. *Clin Pharmacol Ther* 20, 484–492.

107 Lauterburg BH, Liang D, Schwarzenbach FA *et al.* (1993) Mitochondrial dysfunction in alcoholic patients as assessed by breath analysis. *Hepatology* 17, 418–422.

5.4 Immunological investigations in liver diseases

Elmar Jaeckel and Michael P. Manns

Introduction to the hepatic immune system

The hepatic immune system is capable of responding to and eliminating pathogenic microorganisms, toxins and tumour cells. At the same time, hepatic defence mechanisms are so tightly regulated that the induction of tolerance is favoured over the induction of immunity. The hepatic immune system is equipped with a specialized repertoire of cells that can selectively modulate various immune effector functions or tolerance. Hepatic antigen-presenting cells (APCs), such as Kupffer cells (liver-resident macrophages), dendritic cells and liver sinusoidal endothelial cells, can induce either tolerance or immunity via the selective release of proinflammatory cytokines, such as interleukin (IL)-6 or IL-12, or regulatory cytokines such as IL-10 or transforming growth factor (TGF)-β [1]. Additionally, hepatocytes, biliary epithelial cells and other liver cells release a complex array of lymphocyte growth, differentiation and activation factors. The presence of lymphocytes within the liver has, until recently, largely been dismissed as inflammatory infiltrates that enter the liver via the blood to respond to pathogenic stimuli. They were used, in part, to diagnose inflammatory conditions such as autoimmune and viral liver disease. However, recent studies have shown that healthy human liver contains large numbers of lymphocytes (approximately 10^{10}) that appear to be resident rather than circulating [2]. The liver contains various conventional lymphocytes such as αβ-T cells, B cells and natural killer (NK) cells. Many express mature/activated phenotypes, suggesting that, even in the healthy liver, they are mediating routine immunosurveillant functions [2,3]. Besides these, there are a large number of unconventional lymphocytes such as αβ- or γδ-natural killer T cells (NKT), which are much more abundant in the liver than in peripheral blood (Fig. 1) [2,4]. Many of these cells have roles in innate immunity, as evidenced by their ability to recognize common, conserved antigenic structures, their ability to mediate killing of target cells and/or their capacity to release cytokines that activate and regulate subsequent adaptive immune responses.

Immune responses against viruses, pathogens, toxins and self usually involve both the innate and the adaptive immune response. One problem in examining this immune response stems from the fact that we usually just have access to peripheral blood mononuclear cells and not to the site of inflammation. Even when analysing a patient's liver biopsy, this is restricted to the surface phenotype of infiltrating leukocytes. Although this might be helpful in assessment of the activity of viral hepatitis, autoimmune hepatitis and in the diagnosis of acute transplant rejection and/or graft-versus-host disease, most of

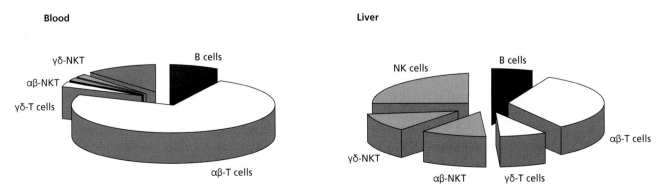

Fig. 1 Distribution of lymphocyte subpopulations in healthy human blood and liver.

the histopathological patterns are unspecific. Furthermore, specific immunological tests cannot be performed on fixed tissue specimens. Systemic cytokine levels have been evaluated in various hepatic disease conditions and especially after liver transplantation to identify acute rejection. However, cytokine levels simply reflect the extent of the immune activation, and no cytokine pattern has yet been described to be disease specific. Therefore, systemic measurement of cytokine levels – besides the problem of preanalytical stability of the serum sample – has no role in clinical hepatology so far [5]. Likewise, measurement of caspase activity in serum has been used to evaluate the extent of hepatic inflammation in steatosis, hepatitis C virus (HCV) infection and autoimmunity, but the source of the caspases (lymphocytes or hepatocytes) and their clinical significance remains uncertain [6,7].

On the other hand, the analysis of T-cell responses against hepatitis B virus (HBV) and HCV has provided interesting insights into the pathophysiology of acute and chronic viral infections of the liver [8]. Similarly, analysis of T-cell responses was crucial in our understanding of autoimmune liver diseases [9]. However, because of the large variability of the human major histocompatibility complex (MHC), the heterogeneity of the hepatotropic viruses and the variation in the antigen experience of the human T-cell repertoire between individuals, there is no clinical role for the analysis of T-cell responses in clinical practice.

The most constant and easiest to determine immunological measures in human viral and autoimmune liver diseases are provided by the humoral immune response [10]. Antibodies produced during HBV infection are markers of the immune status, and antibodies in hepatitis A virus (HAV) and HCV infection are important signs of the contact of the pathogen with the host's immune system (described elsewhere in this book). Besides this humoral immune response against viral proteins, measurement of response against self-antigens is a valuable scientific and clinical tool for our understanding of autoimmune liver diseases [10]. This response may also accompany inflammation caused by pathogens or toxins.

Autoantibodies and autoantigens in autoimmune hepatitis

Autoimmune hepatitis (AIH) represents a chronic, mainly periportal, hepatitis upon histology, which is characterized by female predominance, hypergammaglobulinaemia and circulating autoantibodies and benefits from immunosuppressive treatment (Table 1). The diagnosis of AIH is based on clinical, serological and immunological features as well as on the exclusion of other hepatobiliary diseases with and without autoimmune phenomena. These include disease entities such as chronic viral hepatitis, primary biliary cirrhosis (PBC), primary sclerosing cholangitis (PSC) and the so-called overlap or outlier syndromes. The revised AIH diagnostic score contributes to the establishment of the diagnosis in difficult cases by calculating a probability expressed as a numeric score [11].

Ever since the first description of AIH in 1950 by Waldenström [12], serological findings have attracted considerable attention, not only for the diagnosis of this chronic liver disease but also as a means of studying and eventually understanding its pathophysiology [13–15]. Waldenström described a disease predominantly affecting women and characterized by amenorrhoea, jaundice and elevated gammaglobulins leading to cirrhosis of the liver. It was recognized that patients with AIH displayed antinuclear antibodies (ANA), which led to the designation 'lupoid' hepatitis [16,17]. However, the term lupoid hepatitis has long been abandoned as AIH is not part of the syndrome of systemic lupus erythematosus (SLE). Autoantibodies have been the driving force of research aimed at elucidating the underlying mechanisms of AIH. They also serve as a means of serological subclassification of AIH [18,19].

Table 1 Prevalence of autoantibodies in autoimmune liver diseases.

Criterion	AIH	PBC	PSC
Female:male ratio	4:1	9:1	1:2
Serum Ig elevation	IgG	IgM	Variable
Autoantibodies			
ANA	60–85%	20–50%	7–77%
SMA	60–80%	10%	13–20%
LKM-1	5%	–	–
SLA	30–58%	0%	0%
pANCA	30–75%	18%	26–87% (atypical)
AMA	20%	95%	–
Diagnosis	AIH score > 15	AMA-M2, cholestatic serum enzyme pattern, histology	Cholangiography, cholestatic serum enzyme pattern, ulcerative colitis, pANCA

AIH, autoimmune hepatitis; PBC, primary biliary cirrhosis; PSC, primary sclerosing cholangitis; Ig, immunoglobulin; ANA, antinuclear antibody; SMA, smooth muscle antibody; LKM, Liver–kidney microsomal antibody; SLA, soluble liver antigen; AMA, antimitochondrial antibody; pANCA, perinuclear antineutrophil cytoplasmic antibody.

Table 2 Characterization of the major autoantibodies in autoimmune hepatitis.

Antibody	kDa	Target antigen	Disease
Autoantigens of the endoplasmic reticulum (microsomal autoantigens)			
LKM-1	50	Cytochrome P-450 2D6	Autoimmune hepatitis type 2, hepatitis C
LKM-2	50	Cytochrome P-450 2C9	Ticrynafen-induced hepatitis
LKM-3	55	UGTIA	Hepatitis D-associated autoimmunity
LKM	50	Cytochrome P-450 2A6	Autoimmune hepatitis type 2
			Autoimmune polyendocrine syndrome type 1 (APS-1)
			Hepatitis C
LM	52	Cytochrome P-450 1A2	Dihydralazine-induced hepatitis
			Hepatitis with autoimmune polyendocrine syndrome type 1 (APS-1)
	57	Disulphidisomerase	Halothane hepatitis
	59	Carboxylesterase	Halothane hepatitis
	35	?	Autoimmune hepatitis
	59	?	Chronic hepatitis C
	64	?	Autoimmune hepatitis
	70	?	Chronic hepatitis C
Soluble autoantigens of the cytoplasm			
LC-1	58–62	Formiminotransferase	Autoimmune hepatitis type 2
		cyclodeaminase	Autoimmune hepatitis
			Hepatitis C?
SLA/LP	50	UGA repressor tRNA-associated protein	Autoimmune hepatitis (type 3)

LC-1, anti-cytosol type 1; LM, liver microsomal.

Although this classification remains controversial, three subtypes can be distinguished based on the presence of serum autoantibodies. The classic form of AIH, AIH type 1, displays ANA. Research in the 1970s and 1980s led to the realization that autoantibodies in some patients are directed against antigens expressed in the endoplasmic reticulum (ER) [20–24]. These antimicrosomal autoantibodies were later identified as possessing specificity against cytochrome P-450 (CYP) mono-oxygenases expressed in the ER, which were identifiable in the microsomal fraction of cells (Table 2). Antimicrosomal antibodies directed against CYP 2D6, expressed not only in the liver but also in the kidney (LKM), characterized a second form of AIH (LKM-1) [24]. Finally, the analysis of serum from a patient with AIH by radioimmunoassay identified an antibody directed against a protein present in the 100 000-*g* supernatant of liver homogenate that was termed anti-SLA/LP [25–27]. These autoantibodies have recently been identified as being directed against a UGA repressor tRNA-associated protein [28–31]. The third serological group of AIH (AIH type 3) is clinically similar to AIH type 1 and, therefore, some researchers believe it does not represent a distinct subentity of its own [32]. The serological diversity of autoantibodies found in AIH supports the aforementioned subclassification and provides a framework for the scientific analysis of this heterogeneous disease group [33]. It also demonstrates that AIH is not a single disease with a single underlying mechanism, but is most likely a group of diseases with a similar clinical presentation.

Autoantibodies in autoimmune hepatitis type 1

When AIH is classified according to the presence of serological markers, ANA characterize AIH type 1. In most cases, smooth muscle autoantibodies (SMAs) are also present. The clinical profile of ANA-positive AIH shows hypergammaglobulinaemia in 97% of patients with an elevated immunoglobulin G. This form of AIH represents 80% of all cases of AIH, making it the most prevalent subclass. ANA-positive AIH was first described as lupoid, classical or idiopathic AIH by Cowling and colleagues [16]. Seventy per cent of patients are women, with a peak incidence between the ages of 16 and 30 years. It is noteworthy that 50% are older than 30 years. An association with other immune syndromes is observed in 48% of cases, with autoimmune thyroid disease, synovitis and ulcerative colitis as leading associations. The clinical course is usually not fulminant or clinically spectacular, and an acute onset is very rare. However, in rare cases, AIH may start as fulminant hepatitis. About 25% of patients have cirrhosis at the time of diagnosis.

ANA

ANA show specificity for both functional and structural proteins in the cell nucleus. They can be directed against nuclear membranes or even DNA [34–38]. Unfortunately, for diagnostic reasons, the target antigens are heterogeneous and incompletely defined, and heterogeneous even within a single disease such

Table 3 Differentiation between pANCA, cANCA and ANA.

Autoantibody	Ethanol-fixed granulocytes	Formalin-fixed granulocytes	Hep-2 cell
cANCA	Cytoplasmic	Cytoplasmic	None
pANCA	Nuclear/perinuclear	Nuclear/perinuclear	None
ANA	Nuclear/perinuclear	Reduced/none	Nuclear

as AIH. For the diagnostic workup of AIH, the molecular characterization of target antigen specificity does not supply important additional information to increase diagnostic precision. Screening determinations of ANA are routinely performed by indirect immunofluorescence on cryostat sections of rat liver and on Hep2 cell slides. Most commonly, a homogeneous or speckled immunofluorescence pattern is demonstrable. ANA have been found to be reactive with an array of antigens that include centromeres, ribonucleoproteins and cyclin A. They represent the most common autoantibody in AIH and occur in high titres, usually exceeding 1:160. However, the titre does not correlate with disease course, prognosis, progression, requirement for transplantation or disease activity.

SMA

SMA autoantibodies are also determined by indirect immunofluorescence on cryostat sections of rat stomach and kidney [39]. SMA are directed against cytoskeletal proteins such as actin, troponin and tropomyosin [40,41]. They frequently occur in high titres in association with ANA. They are not highly specific for AIH and have been shown to occur in advanced liver diseases of other aetiologies and in infectious diseases and rheumatic disorders (Table 1). In these cases, titres are often lower than 1:80. In paediatric patients, SMA autoantibodies may be the only marker of AIH type 1. When present in very young patients with AIH type 1, the titres may be as low as 1:40. SMAs have been found to be generally associated with the human leukocyte antigen (HLA) A1-B8-DR3 haplotype and, possibly as a reflection of this HLA status, the affected patients are younger and have a poorer prognosis [42]. Moreover, antibodies to actin identify a subgroup of patients with SMA who have disease at an earlier age and a poorer response to corticosteroid therapy [40].

Asialoglycoprotein receptor

The asialoglycoprotein receptor (ASGPR) is a liver-specific glycoprotein of the cell membrane. Autoimmunity targeting this antigen is observed in 88% of AIH patients [43]. However, anti-ASGPR antibodies are also found in chronic hepatitis B and C, alcoholic liver disease and PBC. The levels of anti-ASGPR antibodies vary according to inflammatory activity of the disease and could play a role as a marker to monitor therapeutic efficacy [44]. Anti-ASGPR appears to be a general marker of liver autoimmunity, and routine clinical determination is not recommended on account of the low specificity.

Antineutrophil cytoplasmic autoantibodies

Antineutrophil cytoplasmic autoantibodies (ANCA) are detected in 30–75% of sera [45,46]. Care has to be taken that high titres of ANAs are not misdiagnosed as perinuclear antineutrophil cytoplasmic autoantibodies (pANCA) on ethanol-fixed granulocytes. Additional stainings on formalin-fixed granulocytes and Hep2 cells can usually solve this problem (Table 3). pANCAs are rare in AIH type 2. The role of ANCA in AIH is not clear, and their routine determination is not recommended. However, these antibodies can be of diagnostic value for those patients with AIH type 1 who have been tested negative for ANA/SMA.

Autoantibodies in autoimmune hepatitis type 2

AIH type 2 is a rare disorder that affects up to 20% of AIH patients in Europe but only 4% in the United States [22,47]. There is a predominance in women. The average age at onset is around 10 years, but AIH type 2 is also observed in adults, especially in Europe. AIH type 2 carries a higher risk of progression to cirrhosis and of a fulminant course. When AIH type 2 is diagnosed in children, cirrhosis is very frequently present at the time of diagnosis.

LKM-1

The ER of the cell harbours two critical enzyme families that are the main players in phase I and phase II metabolism: the CYPs and the uridine diphosphate (UDP)-glucuronosyltransferases (UGT) [48]. Phase I metabolism leads to the oxidative modification of compounds, usually by the addition of functional groups such as hydroxylation [49]. Phase II metabolism leads to the conjugation with polar prosthetic groups such as glucuronic acid (glucuronidation) [50]. In the case of the UGTs, glucuronidation leads to a water-soluble glucuronide that is targeted for renal or biliary elimination [51]. Both enzyme families are preferred targets of a B-cell response in autoimmune liver diseases (Fig. 2, Table 2). Indirect immunofluorescence first led to the description of autoantibodies reactive with the proximal renal tubule and the hepatocellular cytoplasm in 1973 [52]. These autoantibodies, termed LKM-1, were associated with a second form of ANA-negative AIH. Between 1988 and 1991, the 50-kDa antigen of LKM-1 autoantibodies was identified as CYP 2D6 [20–25]. LKM-1 autoantibodies recognize a major linear epitope between amino acids 263 and 270 of the CYP 2D6 protein [53]. These autoantibodies inhibit CYP 2D6 activity

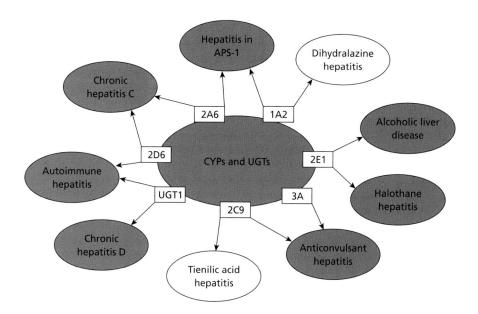

Fig. 2 Autoantibodies against enzymes of phase I and II metabolism in autoimmune liver disease. APS-1, autoimmune polyglandular syndrome type 1.

in vitro and are capable of activating liver-infiltrating T lymphocytes [54, 55], indicating the combination of B- and T-cell activity is involved in the autoimmune process. In addition to linear epitopes [53], LKM-1 autoantibodies have also been shown to recognize conformation-dependent epitopes [56]. However, the recognition of epitopes located between amino acids 257 and 269 appears to be a specific autoimmune reaction of AIH and is discriminatory against LKM-1 autoantibodies associated with chronic HCV infection [57–59].

LKM-3

LKM-3 autoantibodies are directed against UGT proteins with a molecular weight of 55 kDa. They occur in 10% of patients with AIH type 2 (Table 2). They are described further below.

LC-1

Anti-cytosol type 1 (anti-LC-1) antibodies are viewed as a second marker of AIH type 2, in which they have been detected in up to 50% of LKM-positive sera [62]. Other data indicate their occurrence in combination with ANA and SMA autoantibodies and also in chronic hepatitis C [63]. In contrast to LKM autoantibodies, LC-1 autoantibodies appear to correlate with disease activity. The molecular antigen target has been identified as formiminotransferase cyclodeaminase [64]. Their clinical significance is not yet completely defined, but some rare cases may present with anti-LC-1 as the sole marker of AIH.

Autoantibodies in autoimmune hepatitis type 3

AIH type 3 is serologically defined by the presence of soluble liver antigen (SLA)/liver–pancreas (LP) autoantibodies (Table 2).

However, 74% of patients also have other serological markers of autoimmunity, including SMA and ANA. AIH type 3 has a lower prevalence than AIH type 2, affects female patients in 90% of cases and has an age maximum between 20 and 40 years. This subclass of AIH is based solely on the autoantibody profile and clinically resembles AIH type 1 [17]. Autoantibodies that target a soluble liver and pancreas antigen (anti-SLA/LP) exhibit a high specificity for AIH. They are detectable in about 10–30% of all patients with AIH [26,29–31]. In 1992, specific autoantibodies were identified in patients with a severe form of autoimmune chronic active hepatitis. These antibodies precipitated a UGA suppressor serine tRNA–protein complex that is likely to be involved in co-translational selenocysteine incorporation in human cells [29]. The screening of cDNA expression libraries confirmed these findings and identified a previously unknown amino acid sequence, which presumably encodes a UGA suppressor tRNA-associated protein, as target antigen of SLA antibodies [30,31]. In addition, it was demonstrated that anti-SLA and the independently described anti-LP are identical, and the designation anti-SLA/LP has replaced anti-SLA and anti-LP [27,30]. Recent data confirmed the previous finding that patients with anti-SLA/LP display a more severe course of AIH [65–67]. Regarding the disease specificity, anti-SLA/LP may be linked to the pathogenesis of the autoimmune process; however, the exact function and its role in autoimmunity are so far unclear.

Autoantibodies in primary biliary cirrhosis

Primary biliary cirrhosis (PBC) is an inflammatory, primarily T cell-mediated, chronic destruction of intrahepatic small bile ducts of unknown aetiology. In 90% of cases, it affects women who exhibit elevated immunoglobulin M, antimitochondrial antibodies (AMAs) directed against the E2 subunit of pyruvate dehydrogenase (PDH-E2) and a cholestatic liver enzyme profile leading to cirrhosis over the course of years or decades (Table 1). A prominent feature is the presence of extrahepatic immune-mediated disease associations, including autoimmune thyroid disease, Sjögren syndrome, rheumatoid arthritis, inflammatory bowel disease and, less frequently, coeliac disease and CREST syndrome (calcinosis, Raynaud's disease, oesophageal motility disorders, sclerodactyly and telangiectasis). Extrahepatic syndromes frequently precede hepatic disease manifestation [68,69].

AMA

Antimitochondrial antibodies are found in approximately 95% of patients with PBC and are considered a serological hallmark of this disease. The targets of AMAs in PBC sera are members of an enzyme family, the 2-oxo acid dehydrogenase complexes (2-OADC, AMA-M2), which are located on the inner membrane of the mitochondria and catalyse the oxidative decarboxylation of various α-keto acid substrates. Components of 2-OADC include the E2 subunit of PDC (PDC-E2), the E2 subunit of the 2-oxoglutarate dehydrogenase complex (OGDC-E2), the E2 subunit of the branched-chain 2-oxo acid dehydrogenase complex (BCOADC-E2) and the dihydrolipoamide dehydrogenase-binding protein (E3BP) [70]. The most predominant reactivity of AMAs in sera from PBC patients is directed against PDC-E2. Reactivity against OGDC-E2 and BCOADC-E2 is lower, around 50–70%. Antibodies to PDC-E1-α are present in lower titres. Approximately 10% of patients react only to OGDC-E2 or BCOADC-E2, or to both [71,72].

ANA

Antinuclear antibodies (ANAs) have been identified in more than 50% of patients with PBC, and some ANA reactivities have a high specificity for PBC. In AMA-negative patients, they can be the only diagnostic marker suggestive of PBC [34]. These include antibodies against the nuclear pore protein, gp120, which are found in 25% of patients with AMA-positive PBC and in up to 50% of patients with AMA-negative PBC. The disease specificity for the detection of such antibodies by immunoblotting is more than 90% [73]. Other autoantigens include the nuclear pore protein p62, which is recognized by PBC sera in 32% of cases [74]. In about 20–30% of PBC patients, autoantibodies are directed against the nucleoprotein Sp100, which appears to have a high specificity for PBC [75]. Less than 1% of PBC patients present antibodies to the lamin B receptor (LBR), an inner nuclear membrane protein. These autoantibodies, although rare, also have a high disease specificity for PBC [76]. In summary, the presence of PBC-associated ANAs in AMA-negative patients may be the only immunological finding for establishing the diagnosis of PBC.

Autoantibodies in primary sclerosing cholangitis

Primary sclerosing cholangitis (PSC) is a chronic cholestatic liver disease involving the destruction of larger biliary ducts, which is frequently associated with ulcerative colitis [77]. A cholestatic liver enzyme pattern, typical cholangiographic findings and a compatible histology are mandatory to establish the diagnosis (Table 1). Autoantibodies can be helpful in early cases in which cholangiographic findings are mild [78]. However, it is unclear whether PSC represents a classical autoimmune disease with lack of adaptive tolerance to a disease-specific antigen, as there are no disease-specific autoantibodies and no response to immunosuppressive therapies [77]. The alternative hypothesis on the pathogenesis proposes PSC as an immune-mediated inflammatory disease. In this model, tissue destruction would result from an interplay between innate and adaptive immune effector mechanisms, resulting in the generation of proinflammatory cytokines such as tumour necrosis factor (TNF)α [77,79]. Tissue specificity in this model would be explained by continued homing of inflammatory cells to target tissue secreting specific chemokines.

pANCA

Between 30% and 88% of PSC patients, with or without ulcerative colitis, have atypical perinuclear-staining, antineutrophil cytoplasmic antibodies (pANCAs) [77,80]. Autoantibodies in PSC, irritable bowel disease (IBD) and AIH are rather atypical, in that they are not reacting with cytoplasmic actin, catalase or enolase antigens [81]. Instead, they react with the nuclear envelope and not cytoplasmic antigens. Therefore, the term peripheral antineutrophil nuclear antibodies (pANNAs) was introduced [81]. Western blotting has shown that 92% of atypical pANCAs in patients with IBD or hepatobiliary diseases react with a 50-kDa myeloid-specific nuclear envelope protein [82]. The putative autoantigen was identified as tubulin-β isotype 5. The role of pANNAs in the immunopathogenesis of PSC remains speculative as the myeloid-specific tubulin autoantigen is recognized by autoantibodies from patients with either PSC or AIH. The presence of atypical pANNAs also correlates with certain clinical features of PSC, including biliary complications [83] and intrahepatic rather than extrahepatic strictures [84], and higher titres are associated with cirrhosis [45]. However, none of these studies was appropriately powered to assess clinical correlations.

Autoantibodies in autoimmune polyglandular syndrome type 1

Autoimmune polyglandular syndrome type 1 [APS-1, autoimmune polyendocrinopathy–candidiasis–ectodermal dystrophy (APECED)] combines hypoparathyroidism, mucocutaneous fungal infections, adrenal insufficiency and a number of other immune-mediated syndromes, such as nail dystrophy, vitiligo and alopecia. AIH is found in 10% of patients with APS-1 [85–87]. LKM autoantibodies against CYP 1A2 and CYP 2A6 are found in patients with APS-1 and hepatic involvement [86–88]. Anti-CYP 2A6 autoantibodies also occur in HCV infection [57,89]. LM autoantibodies, which are characterized by an immunofluorescence pattern selectively staining the hepatocellular cytoplasm but not the kidney, have been found to be directed against CYP 1A2 [90–92]. These autoantibodies are also found in APS-1 syndrome with hepatic involvement and occur in dihydralazine-induced hepatitis [86,93] (Fig. 2). APS-1 is associated with the presence of mutations within a single gene, the autoimmune regulator gene (*AIRE*) [94,95]. However, patients with AIH in the absence of APS-1 do not display mutations of the *AIRE* gene and are therefore genetically distinct from this form of AIH [96].

Autoantibodies in chronic HCV infection

Hepatitis C is associated with an array of extrahepatic manifestations, including mixed cryoglobulinaemia, membranoproliferative glomerulonephritis, polyarthritis, porphyria cutanea tarda, Sjögren syndrome and autoimmune thyroid disease [97–100]. Not surprisingly, numerous autoantibodies are associated with chronic hepatitis C. Similar to AIH, ANA, SMA, LKM and antithyroid antibodies are found with a high prevalence. An HCV-specific autoantibody, designated anti-GOR, that is present in at least 80% of sera from patients with hepatitis C, has been described [101]. However, anti-GOR seems to be anti-hepatitis C core antibodies cross-reacting with a nuclear self-antigen rather than being a proper autoantibody. This assumption is based on the fact that anti-GOR disappears once HCV replication has stopped. The examination of LKM autoantibodies in HCV patients revealed that, although anti-CYP 2D6 titres are similar to titres in AIH type 2, differences exist regarding the epitopes recognized by LKM autoantibodies [58,102–104]. In patients with AIH type 2, the epitope of amino acids 257–269 is recognized with a significantly higher prevalence than in chronic hepatitis C [103]. In addition, the immune reaction seems to be more heterogeneous than in AIH, as indicated by recognized protein targets of 59 kDa and 70 kDa [105]. The presence of anti-LKM-1 autoantibodies may also represent a HCV infection in patients with underlying AIH-2. In such cases, interferon (IFN)-α therapy can exacerbate the disease, and immunosuppression should be considered instead [57].

Another autoantibody was detected in patients infected with HCV and the hepatitis G virus (HGV)/GB virus subtype C. About 2% of HCV-positive sera in general and 7.5% of LKM-1-positive HCV sera recognize CYP 2A6. This autoantibody appears to occur more frequently in HCV-infected patients with LKM-1 autoantibodies. Interestingly, anti-CYP 2A6 autoantibodies are not detected in patients with AIH type 2 who exhibit high titres

of LKM-1 autoantibodies. The clinical relevance of this finding remains to be determined [89]. Anti-CYP 2A6 autoantibodies have also been detected in patients with APS-1 [86].

Autoantibodies in chronic HDV infection

LKM-3 autoantibodies are directed against UGT proteins with a molecular weight of 55 kDa. They occur in 6–14% of patients with hepatitis D in addition to 10% of patients with AIH type 2. In contrast to LKM-1 and LKM-2 autoantibodies, which, on immunofluorescence, stain liver and kidney tissue only, with LKM-3 autoantibodies, additional fluorescence signals may be present in tissue from the pancreas, adrenal gland, thyroid and stomach. Western blot assay revealed several molecular targets around 55 kDa [60,61]. The molecular targets of the LKM-3 autoantibody were identified as UGTs of family 1 [60,61]. LKM-3 autoantibodies are not detected in sera from patients with chronic hepatitis B, chronic hepatitis C, PBC, PSC or lupus erythematosus [60]. Autoantibody titres in patients with chronic HDV infection are usually lower than they are in patients with AIH type 2 [61].

Overlap syndromes

The term overlap syndrome describes variant forms of the major hepatobiliary autoimmune diseases AIH, PBC and PSC. Patients present with both hepatitic and cholestatic biochemical patterns and histological features of AIH/PBC and/or PSC [106]. Autoantibodies characteristic of more than one of the disease phenotypes may strengthen the diagnosis. AIH/PBC overlaps have been reported in 10% of adult patients. Up to 8% of patients have an overlap of AIH and PSC. It remains unclear whether these overlaps represent distinct disease entities or just variants of AIH, PBC or PSC [107,108]. A standardization of diagnostic criteria does not exist, and the term overlap syndrome is often misused in clinical practice.

Conclusions

Much progress has been made in characterizing autoantibody/autoantigen systems in chronic liver diseases, and particularly in autoimmune liver diseases. Despite the fact that none of the autoantigenic targets discussed is expressed in a tissue-specific fashion and just a few are disease specific, their occurrence is very important for the diagnosis and classification of autoimmune liver diseases. Although the classification of AIH based on serological findings is still controversial, it does indicate the diversity of the mechanisms underlying AIH and gives us an indication of a complex aetiology. Autoantigen/autoantibody characterization continues to be an attractive model to gain insight into the as yet unresolved mystery of how tolerance of the liver is given up and autoimmunity ensues.

References

1 Doherty DG, O'Farrelly C (2001) Dendritic cells: regulators of hepatic immunity or tolerance? *J Hepatol* 34, 156–160.

2 Norris S, Collins C, Doherty DG *et al.* (1998) Resident human hepatic lymphocytes are phenotypically different from circulating lymphocytes. *J Hepatol* 28, 84–90.

3 Doherty DG, O'Farrelly C. (2000) Innate and adaptive lymphoid cells in the human liver. *Immunol Rev* 174, 5–20.

4 Tsukahara A, Seki S, Iiai T *et al.* (1997) Mouse liver T cells: their change with aging and in comparison with peripheral T cells. *Hepatology* 26, 301–309.

5 Maher JJ (1999) Cytokines: overview. *Semin Liver Dis* 19, 109–115.

6 Seidel N, Volkmann X, Langer F *et al.* (2005) The extent of liver steatosis in chronic hepatitis C virus infection is mirrored by caspase activity in serum. *Hepatology* 42, 113–120.

7 Bantel H, Lugering A, Heidemann J *et al.* (2004) Detection of apoptotic caspase activation in sera from patients with chronic HCV infection is associated with fibrotic liver injury. *Hepatology* 40, 1078–1087.

8 Rehermann B, Nascimbeni M (2005) Immunology of hepatitis B virus and hepatitis C virus infection. *Nature Rev Immunol* 5, 215–229.

9 Ichiki Y, Aoki CA, Bowlus CL *et al.* (2005) T cell immunity in autoimmune hepatitis. *Autoimmun Rev* 4, 315–321.

10 Moritoki Y, Lian ZX, Ohsugi Y *et al.* (2006) B cells and autoimmune liver diseases. *Autoimmun Rev* 5, 449–457.

11 Alvarez F, Berg PA, Bianchi FB *et al.* (1999) International Autoimmune Hepatitis Group Report: review of criteria for diagnosis of autoimmune hepatitis. *J Hepatol* 31, 929–938.

12 Waldenström J (1950) Leber, Blutproteine und Nahrungseiweisse. *Dtsch Gesellsch Verd Stoffw* 15, 113–119.

13 Manns MP, Vogel A (2006) Autoimmune hepatitis, from mechanisms to therapy. *Hepatology* 43, S132–144.

14 (2000) *Immunology and the Liver*. Boston, MA: Kluwer.

15 Strassburg CP, Obermayer-Straub P, Manns MP (2000) Autoimmunity in liver diseases. *Clin Rev Allergy Immunol* 18, 127–139.

16 Cowling DC, Mackay IR, Taft LI (1956) Lupoid hepatitis. *Lancet* 271, 1323–1326.

17 Mackay IR (1983) Immunological aspects of chronic active hepatitis. *Hepatology* 3, 724–728.

18 Manns MP, Strassburg CP (2001) Autoimmune hepatitis: clinical challenges. *Gastroenterology* 120, 1502–1517.

19 Czaja AJ, Manns MP (1995) The validity and importance of subtypes in autoimmune hepatitis: a point of view. *Am J Gastroenterol* 90, 1206–1211.

20 Zanger UM, Hauri HP, Loeper J *et al.* (1988) Antibodies against human cytochrome P-450db1 in autoimmune hepatitis type II. *Proc Natl Acad Sci USA* 85, 8256–8260.

21 Gueguen M, Meunier-Rotival M, Bernard O *et al.* (1988) Anti-liver kidney microsome antibody recognizes a cytochrome P450 from the IID subfamily. *J Exp Med* 168, 801–806.

22 Homberg JC, Abuaf N, Bernard O *et al.* (1987) Chronic active hepatitis associated with antiliver/kidney microsome antibody type 1: a second type of 'autoimmune' hepatitis. *Hepatology* 7, 1333–1339.

23 Manns M, Meyer zum Buschenfelde KH, Slusarczyk J *et al.* (1984) Detection of liver–kidney microsomal autoantibodies by radioimmunoassay and their relation to anti-mitochondrial antibodies in inflammatory liver diseases. *Clin Exp Immunol* 57, 600–608.

24 Manns MP, Johnson EF, Griffin KJ *et al.* (1989) Major antigen of liver kidney microsomal autoantibodies in idiopathic autoimmune hepatitis is cytochrome P450db1. *J Clin Invest* 83, 1066–1072.

25 Manns M, Gerken G, Kyriatsoulis A *et al.* (1987) Characterisation of a new subgroup of autoimmune chronic active hepatitis by autoantibodies against a soluble liver antigen. *Lancet* 1, 292–294.

26 Berg PA, Stechemesser E, Strienz J (1981) Hyper-gammglobulinaemische chronisch aktive Hepatitis mit Nachweis von Leber-Pankreas-spezifischen komplementbindenden Antikörpern. *Verh Dtsch Ges Inn Med* 87.

27 Stechemesser E, Klein R, Berg PA (1993) Characterization and clinical relevance of liver-pancreas antibodies in autoimmune hepatitis. *Hepatology* 18, 1–9.

28 Costa M, Rodriguez-Sanchez JL, Czaja AJ *et al.* (2000) Isolation and characterization of cDNA encoding the antigenic protein of the human tRNP(Ser)Sec complex recognized by autoantibodies from patients withtype-1 autoimmune hepatitis. *Clin Exp Immunol* 121, 364–374.

29 Gelpi C, Sontheimer EJ, Rodriguez-Sanchez JL (1992) Autoantibodies against a serine tRNA-protein complex implicated in cotranslational selenocysteine insertion. *Proc Natl Acad Sci USA* 89, 9739–9743.

30 Wies I, Brunner S, Henninger J *et al.* (2000) Identification of target antigen for SLA/LP autoantibodies in autoimmune hepatitis. *Lancet* 355, 1510–1515.

31 Volkmann M, Martin L, Baurle A *et al.* (2001) Soluble liver antigen: isolation of a 35-kd recombinant protein (SLA-p35) specifically recognizing sera from patients with autoimmune hepatitis. *Hepatology* 33, 591–596.

32 Kanzler S, Weidemann C, Gerken G *et al.* (1999) Clinical significance of autoantibodies to soluble liver antigen in autoimmune hepatitis. *J Hepatol* 31, 635–640.

33 Obermayer-Straub P, Strassburg CP, Manns MP (2000) Autoimmune hepatitis. *J Hepatol* 32, 181–197.

34 Strassburg CP, Manns MP (1999) Antinuclear antibody (ANA) patterns in hepatic and extrahepatic autoimmune disease. *J Hepatol* 31, 751.

35 Strassburg CP, Alex B, Zindy F *et al.* (1996) Identification of cyclin A as a molecular target of antinuclear antibodies (ANA) in hepatic and non-hepatic autoimmune diseases. *J Hepatol* 25, 859–866.

36 Tan EM (1991) Autoantibodies in pathology and cell biology. *Cell* 67, 841–842.

37 Czaja AJ, Nishioka M, Morshed SA *et al.* (1994) Patterns of nuclear immunofluorescence and reactivities to recombinant nuclear antigens in autoimmune hepatitis. *Gastroenterology* 107, 200–207.

38 Czaja AJ, Ming C, Shirai M *et al.* (1995) Frequency and significance of antibodies to histones in autoimmune hepatitis. *J Hepatol* 23, 32–38.

39 Bottazzo GF, Florin-Christensen A, Fairfax A *et al.* (1976) Classification of smooth muscle autoantibodies detected by immunofluorescence. *J Clin Pathol* 29, 403–410.

40 Czaja AJ, Cassani F, Cataleta M *et al.* (1996) Frequency and significance of antibodies to actin in type 1 autoimmune hepatitis. *Hepatology* 24, 1068–1073.

41 Toh BH (1979) Smooth muscle autoantibodies and autoantigens. *Clin Exp Immunol* 38, 621–628.

42 Strassburg CP, Manns MP (2002) Autoantibodies and autoantigens in autoimmune hepatitis. *Semin Liver Dis* 22, 339–352.

43 Poralla T, Treichel U, Lohr H *et al.* (1991) The asialoglycoprotein receptor as target structure in autoimmune liver diseases. *Semin Liver Dis* 11, 215–222.

44 Treichel U, Gerken G, Rossol S *et al.* (1993) Autoantibodies against the human asialoglycoprotein receptor: effects of therapy in autoimmune and virus-induced chronic active hepatitis. *J Hepatol* 19, 55–63.

45 Mulder AH, Horst G, Haagsma EB *et al.* (1993) Prevalence and characterization of neutrophil cytoplasmic antibodies in autoimmune liver diseases. *Hepatology* 17, 411–417.

46 Targan SR, Landers C, Vidrich A *et al.* (1995) High-titer antineutrophil cytoplasmic antibodies in type-1 autoimmune hepatitis. *Gastroenterology* 108, 1159–1166.

47 Czaja AJ, Manns MP, Homburger HA (1992) Frequency and significance of antibodies to liver/kidney microsome type 1 in adults with chronic active hepatitis. *Gastroenterology* 103, 1290–1295.

48 Obermayer-Straub P, Strassburg CP, Manns MP (2000) Target proteins in human autoimmunity: cytochromes P450 and UDP-glucuronosyltransferases. *Can J Gastroenterol* 14, 429–439.

49 Tukey RH, Johnson EF (1990) Molecular aspects of drug metabolizing enzymes. In: Pratt W, Taylor P (eds) *Principles of Drug Action*. New York: Churchill Livingstone, pp. 423–468.

50 Tukey RH, Strassburg CP (2000) Human UDP-glucuronosyltransferases: metabolism, expression, and disease. *Annu Rev Pharmacol Toxicol* 40, 581–616.

51 Tukey RH, Strassburg CP (2001) Genetic multiplicity of the human UDP-glucuronosyltransferases and regulation in the gastrointestinal tract. *Mol Pharmacol* 59, 405–414.

52 Rizzetto M, Swana G, Doniach D (1973) Microsomal antibodies in active chronic hepatitis and other disorders. *Clin Exp Immunol* 15, 331–344.

53 Manns MP, Griffin KJ, Sullivan KF *et al.* (1991) LKM-1 autoantibodies recognize a short linear sequence in P450IID6, a cytochrome P-450 monooxygenase. *J Clin Invest* 88, 1370–1378.

54 Manns M, Zanger U, Gerken G *et al.* (1990) Patients with type II autoimmune hepatitis express functionally intact cytochrome P-450 db1 that is inhibited by LKM-1 autoantibodies in vitro but not in vivo. *Hepatology* 12, 127–132.

55 Lohr HF, Schlaak JF, Lohse AW *et al.* (1996) Autoreactive CD4+ LKM-specific and anticlonotypic T-cell responses in LKM-1 antibody-positive autoimmune hepatitis. *Hepatology* 24, 1416–1421.

56 Duclos-Vallee JC, Hajoui O, Yamamoto AM *et al.* (1995) Conformational epitopes on CYP2D6 are recognized by liver/kidney microsomal antibodies. *Gastroenterology* 108, 470–476.

57 Dalekos GN, Wedemeyer H, Obermayer-Straub P *et al.* (1999) Epitope mapping of cytochrome P4502D6 autoantigen in patients with chronic hepatitis C during alpha-interferon treatment. *J Hepatol* 30, 366–375.

58 Ma Y, Peakman M, Lobo-Yeo A *et al.* (1994) Differences in immune recognition of cytochrome P4502D6 by liver kidney microsomal (LKM) antibody in autoimmune hepatitis and chronic hepatitis C virus infection. *Clin Exp Immunol* 97, 94–99.

59 Yamamoto AM, Cresteil D, Boniface O *et al.* (1993) Identification and analysis of cytochrome P450IID6 antigenic sites recognized by anti-liver-kidney microsome type-1 antibodies (LKM1). *Eur J Immunol* 23, 1105–1111.

60 Philipp T, Durazzo M, Trautwein C *et al.* (1994) Recognition of uridine diphosphate glucuronosyl transferases by LKM-3 antibodies in chronic hepatitis D. *Lancet* 344, 578–581.

61 Strassburg CP, Obermayer-Straub P, Alex B *et al.* (1996) Autoantibodies against glucuronosyltransferases differ between viral hepatitis and autoimmune hepatitis. *Gastroenterology* 111, 1576–1586.

62 Lenzi M, Manotti P, Muratori L *et al.* (1995) Liver cytosolic 1 antigen-antibody system in type 2 autoimmune hepatitis and hepatitis C virus infection. *Gut* 36, 749–754.

63 Martini E, Abuaf N, Cavalli F *et al.* (1988) Antibody to liver cytosol (anti-LC1) in patients with autoimmune chronic active hepatitis type 2. *Hepatology* 8, 1662–1666.

64 Lapierre P, Hajoui O, Homberg JC *et al.* (1999) Formiminotransferase cyclodeaminase is an organ-specific autoantigen recognized by sera of patients with autoimmune hepatitis. *Gastroenterology* 116, 643–649.

65 Baeres M, Herkel J, Czaja AJ *et al.* (2002) Establishment of standardised SLA/LP immunoassays: specificity for autoimmune hepatitis, worldwide occurrence, and clinical characteristics. *Gut* 51, 259–264.

66 Ma Y, Okamoto M, Thomas MG *et al.* (2002) Antibodies to conformational epitopes of soluble liver antigen define a severe form of autoimmune liver disease. *Hepatology* 35, 658–664.

67 Czaja AJ, Donaldson PT, Lohse AW (2002) Antibodies to soluble liver antigen/liver pancreas and HLA risk factors for type 1 autoimmune hepatitis. *Am J Gastroenterol* 97, 413–419.

68 Giorgini A, Selmi C, Invernizzi P *et al.* (2005) Primary biliary cirrhosis: solving the enigma. *Ann NY Acad Sci* 1051, 185–193.

69 Jones DE, Watt FE, Metcalf JV *et al.* (1999) Familial primary biliary cirrhosis reassessed: a geographically-based population study. *J Hepatol* 30, 402–407.

70 Ishibashi H, Shimoda S, Gershwin ME (2005) The immune response to mitochondrial autoantigens. *Semin Liver Dis* 25, 337–346.

71 Manns MP, Kruger M (1994) Immunogenetics of chronic liver diseases. *Gastroenterology* 106, 1676–1697.

72 Nishio A, Keeffe EB, Gershwin ME (2002) Immunopathogenesis of primary biliary cirrhosis. *Semin Liver Dis* 22, 291–302.

73 Bandin O, Courvalin JC, Poupon R *et al.* (1996) Specificity and sensitivity of gp210 autoantibodies detected using an enzyme-linked immunosorbent assay and a synthetic polypeptide in the diagnosis of primary biliary cirrhosis. *Hepatology* 23, 1020–1024.

74 Wesierska-Gadek J, Hohenuer H, Hitchman E *et al.* (1996) Autoantibodies against nucleoporin p62 constitute a novel marker of primary biliary cirrhosis. *Gastroenterology* 110, 840–847.

75 Szostecki C, Krippner H, Penner E *et al.* (1987) Autoimmune sera recognize a 100 kD nuclear protein antigen (sp-100). *Clin Exp Immunol* 68, 108–116.

76 Courvalin JC, Lassoued K, Worman HJ *et al.* (1990) Identification and characterization of autoantibodies against the nuclear envelope lamin B receptor from patients with primary biliary cirrhosis. *J Exp Med* 172, 961–967.

77 O'Mahony CA, Vierling JM (2006) Etiopathogenesis of primary sclerosing cholangitis. *Semin Liver Dis* 26, 3–21.

78 Charatcharoenwitthaya P, Lindor KD (2006) Primary sclerosing cholangitis: diagnosis and management. *Curr Gastroenterol Rep* 8, 75–82.

79 Mayer L (2003) Redefining autoimmunity. *Gastroenterology* 125, 1574.

80 Worthington J, Cullen S, Chapman R (2005) Immunopathogenesis of primary sclerosing cholangitis. *Clin Rev Allergy Immunol* 28, 93–103.

81 Terjung B, Worman HJ (2001) Anti-neutrophil antibodies in primary sclerosing cholangitis. *Best Pract Res Clin Gastroenterol* 15, 629–642.

82 Terjung B, Spengler U, Sauerbruch T *et al.* (2000) 'Atypical p-ANCA' in IBD and hepatobiliary disorders react with a 50-kilodalton nuclear envelope protein of neutrophils and myeloid cell lines. *Gastroenterology* 119, 310–322.

83 Pokorny CS, Norton ID, McCaughan GW *et al.* (1994) Anti-neutrophil cytoplasmic antibody: a prognostic indicator in primary sclerosing cholangitis. *J Gastroenterol Hepatol* 9, 40–44.

84 Bansi DS, Bauducci M, Bergqvist A *et al.* (1997) Detection of anti-neutrophil cytoplasmic antibodies in primary sclerosing cholangitis: a comparison of the alkaline phosphatase and immunofluorescent techniques. *Eur J Gastroenterol Hepatol* 9, 575–580.

85 Obermayer-Straub P, Perheentupa J, Braun S *et al.* (2001) Hepatic autoantigens in patients with autoimmune polyendocrinopathy–candidiasis–ectodermal dystrophy. *Gastroenterology* 121, 668–677.

86 Clemente MG, Obermayer-Straub P, Meloni A *et al.* (1997) Cytochrome P450 1A2 is a hepatic autoantigen in autoimmune polyglandular syndrome type 1. *J Clin Endocrinol Metab* 82, 1353–1361.

87 Clemente MG, Meloni A, Obermayer-Straub P *et al.* (1998) Two cytochromes P450 are major hepatocellular autoantigens in autoimmune polyglandular syndrome type 1. *Gastroenterology* 114, 324–328.

88 Gebre-Medhin G, Husebye ES, Gustafsson J *et al.* (1997) Cytochrome P450IA2 and aromatic L-amino acid decarboxylase are hepatic autoantigens in autoimmune polyendocrine syndrome type I. *FEBS Lett* 412, 439–445.

89 Dalekos G, Obermayer-Straub P, Maeda T *et al.* (1998) Antibodies against cytochrome P450 2A6 in patients with chronic viral hepatitis are mainly linked to hepatitis C virus infection. *Digestion* 59, S36.

90 Manns MP, Griffin KJ, Quattrochi LC *et al.* (1990) Identification of cytochrome P450IA2 as a human autoantigen. *Arch Biochem Biophys* 280, 229–232.

91 Bourdi M, Larrey D, Nataf J *et al.* (1990) Anti-liver endoplasmic reticulum autoantibodies are directed against human cytochrome P-450IA2. A specific marker of dihydralazine-induced hepatitis. *J Clin Invest* 85, 1967–1973.

92 Sacher M, Blumel P, Thaler H *et al.* (1990) Chronic active hepatitis associated with vitiligo, nail dystrophy, alopecia and a new variant of LKM antibodies. *J Hepatol* 10, 364–369.

93 Bourdi M, Gautier JC, Mircheva J *et al.* (1992) Anti-liver microsomes autoantibodies and dihydralazine-induced hepatitis: specificity of autoantibodies and inductive capacity of the drug. *Mol Pharmacol* 42, 280–285.

94 Aaltonen J, Bjorses P, Sandkuijl L *et al.* (1994) An autosomal locus causing autoimmune disease: autoimmune polyglandular disease type I assigned to chromosome 21. *Nature Genet* 8, 83–87.

95 Rinderle C, Christensen HM, Schweiger S *et al.* (1999) AIRE encodes a nuclear protein co-localizing with cytoskeletal filaments: altered sub-cellular distribution of mutants lacking the PHD zinc fingers. *Hum Mol Genet* 8, 277–290.

96 Vogel A, Liermann H, Harms A *et al.* (2001) Autoimmune regulator AIRE: evidence for genetic differences between autoimmune hepatitis and hepatitis as part of the autoimmune polyglandular syndrome type 1. *Hepatology* 33, 1047–1052.

97 Agnello V, Chung RT, Kaplan LM (1992) A role for hepatitis C virus infection in type II cryoglobulinemia. *N Engl J Med* 327, 1490–1495.

98 Cacoub P, Lunel-Fabiani F, Du LT (1992) Polyarteritis nodosa and hepatitis C virus infection. *Ann Intern Med* 116, 605–606.

99 Haddad J, Deny P, Munz-Gotheil C *et al.* (1992) Lymphocytic sialadenitis of Sjogren's syndrome associated with chronic hepatitis C virus liver disease. *Lancet* 339, 321–323.

100 Johnson RJ, Gretch DR, Yamabe H *et al.* (1993) Membrano-proliferative glomerulonephritis associated with hepatitis C virus infection. *N Engl J Med* 328, 465–470.

101 Michel G, Ritter A, Gerken G *et al.* (1992) Anti-GOR and hepatitis C virus in autoimmune liver diseases. *Lancet* 339, 267–269.

102 Yamamoto AM, Cresteil D, Homberg JC *et al.* (1993) Characterization of anti-liver-kidney microsome antibody (anti-LKM1) from hepatitis C virus-positive and -negative sera. *Gastroenterology* 104, 1762–1767.

103 Muratori L, Lenzi M, Ma Y *et al.* (1995) Heterogeneity of liver/kidney microsomal antibody type 1 in autoimmune hepatitis and hepatitis C virus related liver disease. *Gut* 37, 406–412.

104 Yamamoto AM, Johanet C, Duclos-Vallee JC *et al.* (1997) A new approach to cytochrome CYP2D6 antibody detection in auto-immune hepatitis type-2 (AIH-2) and chronic hepatitis C virus (HCV) infection: a sensitive and quantitative radioligand assay. *Clin Exp Immunol* 108, 396–400.

105 Durazzo M, Philipp T, Van Pelt FN *et al.* (1995) Heterogeneity of liver-kidney microsomal autoantibodies in chronic hepatitis C and D virus infection. *Gastroenterology* 108, 455–462.

106 Beuers U, Rust C (2005) Overlap syndromes. *Semin Liver Dis* 25, 311–320.

107 Poupon R (2003) Autoimmune overlapping syndromes. *Clin Liver Dis* 7, 865–878.

108 Czaja AJ (1996) The variant forms of autoimmune hepatitis. *Ann Intern Med* 125, 588–598.

5.5 Biopsy and laparoscopy

Arthur Zimmermann

Liver biopsy: its indications and contraindications

The issues of liver biopsy and laparoscopy have been extensively addressed in several recent textbooks and reviews [1–5]. As liver biopsy is an invasive manoeuvre planned subsequent to previous clinical, functional and imaging procedures, biopsy candidates must be carefully selected in accordance with distinct indications. An indication for biopsy should not only be based on a suspected liver disorder, but also on knowing what can reasonably be detected in a small liver tissue sample, and how findings can be interpreted [6–7]. The main indications for a liver biopsy (nongrafted livers) are summarized in Table 1.

In addition to the indications listed in Table 1, biopsy in the case of chronically elevated liver enzymes may be considered [8–12], but it will frequently be nondiagnostic. The main

Table 1 Indications for a liver biopsy.

Chronic fibrosing liver disease/liver cirrhosis
Chronic viral hepatitis (grading and staging)
Unexplained hepatomegaly
Suspected fatty liver disease (including ALD and NASH)
Cholestasis of unknown origin
Grading and staging of autoimmune biliary disorders
Diagnosis of space-occupying liver lesions (hyperplastic, dysplastic, neoplastic)
Unexplained multifocal liver disease (mainly granulomatous hepatitis and metastases)
Metabolic liver disease (haemochromatosis)
Specific infections (in particular mycobacterioses, fungi, CMV and EBV)
Hepatic venous outflow disorders
Suspected multisystem disease with liver involvement
Liver injury due to drugs or toxins
Fever of unknown origin (FUO)
Staging of malignancy
Assessment of response to treatment

ALD, alcoholic liver disease; CMV, cytomegalovirus; EBV, Epstein–Barr virus; NASH, non-alcoholic steatohepatitis.

contraindications of liver biopsies include impaired haemostasis, severe anaemia, tense ascites, high-grade extrahepatic biliary obstruction with or without bacterial cholangitis, local infections, hepatic lesions with suspected high risk of bleeding, certain tumours (risk of seeding), suspected echinococcal cysts and cystic lesions that may cause bile leakage upon puncture, and severely sick or uncooperative patients. Hepatic amyloidosis is now regarded as a relative contraindication only [13].

What is an adequate, and what is a normal, liver biopsy?

A needle biopsy of the liver is a 'sample' in the proper sense of this term, usually representing about 1/50 000 of the organ mass, which of course raises concern about how representative a needle biopsy can be [14]. Against the background of such a limited sample, three major lesional patterns can be represented and visualized: diffuse lesions (e.g. steatosis); focal lesions (in part with anisotropic distribution, e.g. granulomas, multiple metastases and microabscesses; Fig. 1); and structural lesions (fibrosing hepatopathy with remodelling/cirrhosis). The presence of one of these patterns, or combinations thereof, has a marked impact on the required sample size. In the case of chronic hepatitis it has been shown that 'the smaller the sample, the milder the disease' [15]. The diagnostic yield of the sample also depends on the puncture sites – for example, inflammation may vary between the two liver lobes [16,17]. Furthermore, the interpretation of a sample of variable size is subject to intra-observer and interobserver variations, specifically in grading and staging [18].

What, then, is an adequate liver biopsy? Although a consensus has not been reached so far, a biopsy specimen should be at least 2.5 cm in length and contain at least 10 completely represented portal tract areas. Should more than one pass be recommended? Obtaining more than one core of liver tissue can augment the diagnostic yield, but morbidity increases with the number of passes, in particular when three or more consecutive samples are taken [19], and in the presence of older age and malignancy [20].

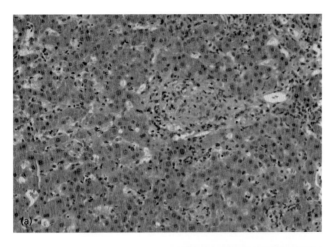

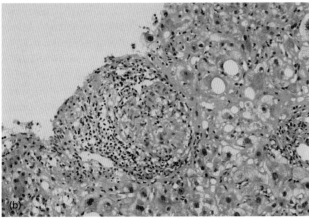

Fig. 1 Sampling of small focal liver lesions. (a) There is a small (early) granuloma in the parenchyma (to the right of the middle). Such intralobular granulomas seem to be randomly distributed, and their detection in biopsies depends on their number in relation to the sample size. It has been estimated that many millions of these lesions must be present in the liver for them to be reliably represented in a tissue section. (b) Granuloma located near a portal tract space. In contrast to (a), the spatial distribution of such granulomas depends on a pre-existent, highly ordered hepatic structure.

What is a normal liver biopsy? Liver biopsies present the interpreter with the question of what is normal, and what the range of normality is. This refers to several parameters, such as the overall tissue geometry and the mutual relationship of tissue compartments (portal tracts vs. elements of the vascular outflow tract), the configuration of liver cell plates, sinusoids and the perisinusoidal space, normal fat and other constituents in hepatocytes, the amount of connective tissue in portal tracts, the number of ducts and ductules (see Plate 5.5.1, facing p. 000), and the physiological amount of infiltrated cells (the liver-associated lymphoid tissue). Biopsies erroneously classified as normal frequently concern macronodular cirrhosis, regenerative nodular hyperplasia, and noncirrhotic portal hypertension; avoiding such errors requires sufficient knowledge of normal histological tissue relationships. However, data on normal liver histology are relatively sparse, owing to the difficulty of obtaining reference material that is not biased in regard to selection of individuals with apparently undamaged livers [21]. The shapes, diameters and densities of portal tracts detected in needle biopsies have systematically been studied [22]. This study has shown that there is a significant correlation of aggregate biopsy length with the number of portal tracts. In regard to 'normal' infiltrates, one study observed grade 1 or 2 inflammatory lesions in two-thirds of biopsies of patients with Gilbert's disease only [23], suggesting that there is a background of infiltrates that has to be taken into account.

Liver biopsy techniques and methods of processing

Liver biopsies are obtained percutaneously as a core with distinct biopsy needles, as needle biopsies performed during laparoscopy or laparotomy, as a wedge biopsy, or transvenously, usually via a transjugular route. Percutaneous liver biopsies are classified according to the site of entry, whether performed blind or guided, and whether the track is plugged after entry. A transjugular liver biopsy is chiefly indicated for patients with severly compromised haemostasis, liver failure, and/or marked ascites. Each method has advantages and disadvantages, and criteria for choosing a given technique, the different yields to be expected, and issues of imaging assistance for performing a biopsy have been discussed in detail [24,25].

The percutaneous approach is, in regard to the size and quality of the sample thus obtained, preferable. Transjugular biopsy specimens are thinner than Menghini cores, are advanced only 1–2 cm into liver substance, are sometimes fragmented, and contain fewer assessable portal tracts, but they may excellently serve to analyse parenchymal disease and the extent of hepatocyte damage. In contrast, wedge biopsies are not recommended, except for instances where a focal lesion is seen during laparoscopy or laparotomy. The reason is that, although the sample may be impressive as to its size, it will only represent a peripheral (subcapsular) part of the liver that is usually not representative. For instance, connective tissue pillars that normally extend from the capsule into the liver substance may mimic septal fibrosis, lymphoid cells are known to accumulate in the subcapsular compartment in the absence of relevant liver inflammation, and hepatocyte iron distribution is different in core vs. peripheral areas of the liver [26]. Therefore, a needle biopsy should also be performed during laparoscopy or laparotomy.

Upon harvesting, the biopsy should promptly be transferred into buffered neutral formalin (ideally 4%), as any delay will rapidly cause drying and then severe autolytic change of liver tissue. In case electron microscopy is planned, small samples must be preserved in glutaraldehyde, in accordance with the local laboratory's requirements. Samples must not be placed on paper or cloth towel, or gauze, which rapidly dehydrate the sample, but in a saline-moisturized plastic foil. Immersion of samples in saline must be avoided, as this causes extraction of cellular constituents and cell swelling.

Recommendations for staining vary considerably in the literature, but minimum requirements for adequate diagnosis include the haematoxylin and eosin stain, a reliable connective tissue stain (trichrome stains; a stain containing sirius red; or chromotrope aniline stains), a reticulin stain (Gomori stain; essential for the assessment of liver cell plate thickness and the recognition of nodular regenerative hyperplasia), the periodic acid–Schiff (PAS) stain (preferably with and without diastase pretreatment), and an iron stain (Perls stain). As so much depends on the high quality of histology stains, staining procedures should be subjected to quality management programmes. It is highly advisable to produce sufficient extra sections in the first run of cutting (preferably on Superfrost Plus slides or a similar product), as any secondary cutting will inevitably result in tissue loss from the blocks. Apart from paraffin-embedded biopsies, frozen sections of native or fixed tissue may be required in distinct situations, but this approach requires special skill to produce thin sections based on sparse material. Intraoperative frozen sections are mainly indicated for the assessment of liver graft quality (in particular steatosis and small focal lesions), and for the typing of (unexpected) smaller nodular lesions during liver resections. Frozen sections also hold a crucial place in the reliable diagnosis of microvesicular fatty change.

Although an adequate evaluation of biopsies will be possible by use of conventionally stained preparations in most instances, immunohistochemistry (IHC) plays an increasing role. IHC is nowadays, with few exceptions, performed employing formalin-fixed tissue. Particularly important and helpful immunostains comprise those for microbial antigens – mainly hepatitis B virus (HBV)-, cytomegalovirus (CMV)- and herpes simplex virus (HSV)-associated antigens – the selective demonstration of bile duct and ductular cells (cytokeratins 7 and 19), the assessment of proliferative activity (e.g. Ki-67) and ubiquitin (detection of Mallory bodies) (Fig. 2 and Plates 5.5.2 and 5.5.3, facing p. 72). Tumour typing (primary or secondary hepatic neoplasms) will require an extended palette of antibodies, as in other tumour locations.

Liver biopsies are increasingly used for molecular biology examinations, specifically *in situ* hybridization (ISH; e.g. for EBV and CMV), fluorescence *in situ* hybridization (FISH), and polymerase chain reaction (PCR). As, for example, PCR may require several tissue sections of increased thickness (typically 10 μm) in order to obtain a sufficient amount of DNA, it is advisable to clarify the requirements before the biopsy is performed and processed. The same organizational steps have to be planned in case part of the biopsy material should be preserved for tissue banking, which usually requires tissue freezing in liquid nitrogen, and/or the storage of DNA, RNA or proteins (proteomics).

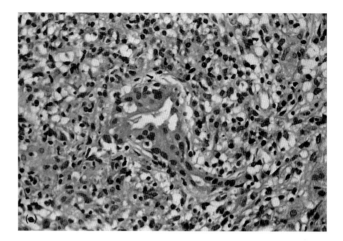

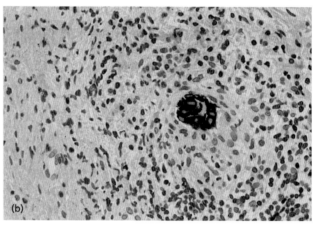

Fig. 2 Immunohistochemistry in liver biopsies: assessment of bile duct injury. (a) In this H&E-stained preparation, a florid bile duct lesion occurring in primary biliary cirrhosis (PBC) is seen (centre of the figure). (b) Bile duct lesion in PBC, demonstrated by cytokeratin-19 immunostaining. The details of the duct lesion are better seen, and this stain may uncover discrete changes that are not easily detectable in routine stains. Note the ductocentric granuloma.

Selected situations for bioptic assessment of disease

Alcoholic and non-alcoholic fatty liver disease

Macrovesicular steatosis (macrosteatosis; fatty liver disease, FLD; Fig. 3), defined as visible steatosis exceeding 5%, is increasingly prevalent, mainly related to obesity and excessive weight (body mass index ≥ 25 kg/m^2), type 2 (non-insulin-dependent) diabetes mellitus and hyperlipidaemia, and is a frequent indication for liver biopsy. FLD is broadly classified into two categories, namely, alcoholic liver disease (ALD; or alcoholic fatty liver disease, AFLD; see Plate 5.5.4, facing p. 72) and non-alcoholic fatty liver disease (NAFLD). It is estimated that NAFLD affects 10–25% of the general population in various countries. The histological criteria for the diagnosis of these major groups have been defined and reviewed [27]. The histological

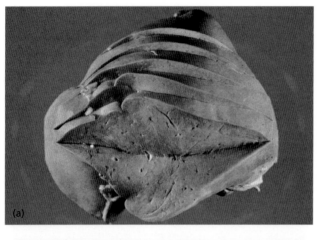

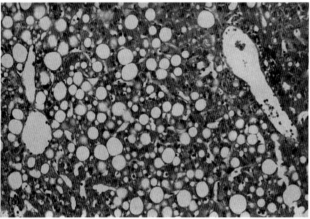

Fig. 3 Fatty liver disease. (a) Macroscopic features of marked diffuse fatty liver disease. In regard to biopsy sampling it is easily seen that steatosis will be represented histologically irrespective of the place of the biopsy. (b) Macrovesicular steatosis of the liver (macrosteatosis). In this biopsy, steatosis is a single pathological feature, resulting in a rather broad differential diagnosis (H&E stain).

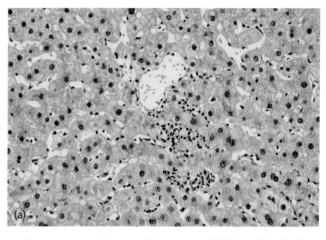

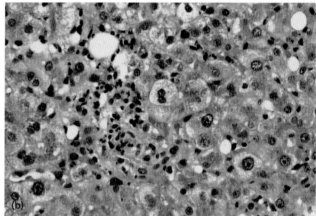

Fig. 4 Viral hepatitis. (a) The histology of acute viral hepatitis is characterized by cell damage and a lymphocyte-predominant lobular infiltrate, indicating the immune response directed against viral antigens (H&E stain). (b) At higher magnification, the features of the infiltrate are better resolved. Note that some of the lymphocytes look distorted, owing to their polarization in the course of locomotion/migration to antigen-containing cells. In this case, marked cholestasis is in evidence (cholestatic variant of acute viral hepatitis) (H&E stain).

spectrum of macrosteatosis comprises non-alcoholic fatty liver (NAFL), alcoholic fatty liver (AFL) and steatohepatitis (alcoholic steatohepatitis, ASH; see Plate 5.5.4a, facing p. 72; and nonalcoholic steatohepatitis, NASH). NASH is recognized as the progressive form of NAFLD with histological similarities to ASH [28]. NASH is associated with obesity, hyperlipidaemia and insulin resistance syndromes (and hence is a hepatic manifestation of syndrome X), but also causes progressive fibrotic liver disease [29]. In the latter context, and similar to chronic viral liver disease, grading and staging of NASH is necessary, grading reflecting the degree of steatosis and associated necroinflammatory changes, and staging estimating the extent of fibrosis and remodelling [30]. Several systems for grading and staging of NASH have been proposed [31]. In regard to biopsy requirements for the diagnosis of these disorders, the confirmation of fatty liver and early steatohepatitis as diffuse lesions is possible with small samples, while fibrosing lesions require the same staging samples as chronic viral hepatitis [32].

Chronic viral hepatitis: grading and staging

Liver biopsy has a central role in the assessment of disease activity and progression in chronic viral hepatitis [33]. A first reproducible semiquantitative approach to score liver biopsies with chronic hepatitis goes back to 1981, which resulted in a histological activity index (HAI) [34]. Later systems more clearly separated grade from stage, grade referring to the degree of inflammatory activity (or the immune reaction directed against viral antigens), and stage to the degree of fibrosis and hepatic remodelling. The histological features that should be included in grading and staging (Figs 4–9 and Plates 5.5.5 and 5.5.6, facing p. 72) have been reviewed in detail [35]. As the manifestations of chronic viral hepatitis are markedly heterogeneous within the liver, sampling to obtain an adequate biopsy specimen is particularly crucial in grading and staging; for example, it has been suggested that

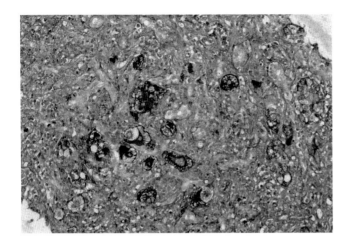

Fig. 5 Fulminant viral hepatitis (massive necrosis). In this periodic acid–Schiff (PAS) stain, the hepatic architecture is completely effaced, and only a few PAS-positive, viable-looking hepatocytes are still present.

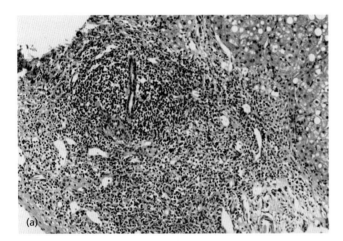

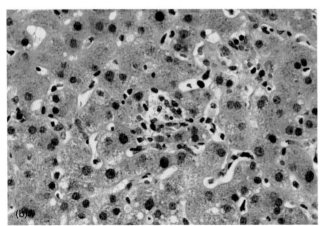

Fig. 6 Chronic viral hepatitis. (a) Chronic hepatitis C. The activity of the process manifests in the form of a dense portal tract infiltration, in part ductocentric. Around the bile duct (upper half), a lymph follicle has developed (H&E stain). (b) The intralobular component of the inflammation may be more discrete, and presents in the form of a focal macrophage and lymphocyte reaction (H&E stain).

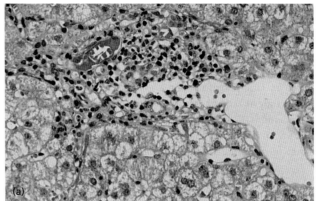

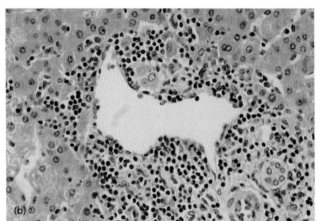

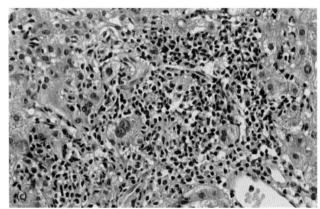

Fig. 7 Chronic viral hepatitis: grading. (a–c) Increasing levels of inflammatory activity in portal tracts and periportal parenchyma. These and other visible features of the immune reactions and their sequelae form the grading of lesions.

adequacy entails a sample that is 2.5 cm or more in length containing more than 10 complete portal tracts, but there is still no consensus [14]. The earlier Knodell classification has, over the past decade, been replaced by other systems, although what is the 'best' assessment procedure remains unresolved [36]. Well-known systems now include the Ishak modification of HAI, the Scheuer system, the Ludwig system, and the algorithm devised by the METAVIR group in France (for review see ref. 35). As any

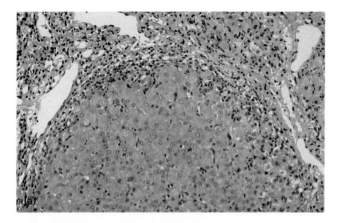

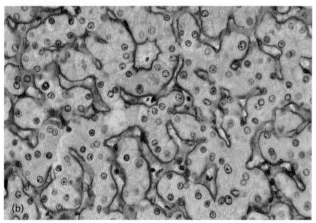

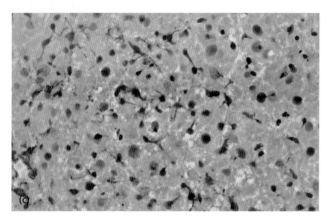

Fig. 8 Chronic viral hepatitis: staging. (a) A cirrhotic nodule representing a stage 4 lesion is seen (upper half). Note that interface lesions indicating activity of the process involve this nodule (H&E stain). (b) Cirrhosis is associated with a distinct change of the perisinusoidal matrix. In this collagen type 4 immunostain, the perisinusoidal space shows a linear red contour representing the establishment of a sinusoidal basement membrane (capillarization). (c) Cells critical for the fibrosing process are hepatic stellate cells (HSC), here demonstrated by use of a desmin immunostain (frozen section).

such scoring approach will be prone to intra- and interobserver errors, the systems should have an appropriate sensitivity together with an acceptably low level of complexity, plus well-defined and easily identifiable histological criteria.

Metabolic liver disease

Apart from fatty liver, hepatic iron storage disorders are the most important metabolic conditions to be assessed by biopsy. Among these, the now diverse forms of hereditary haemochromatosis [37] are regularly approached using biopsies, liver biopsy still being regarded as the gold standard for grading and, in particular, staging of disease (Fig. 10). In addition to haemochromatosis and other, much rarer, hereditary disorders, any interpretation of liver biopsies with hepatocyte iron overload has to consider an increasing spectrum of acquired disorders. A rather novel hepatic iron overload situation is observed in patients with NASH and insulin resistance, the so-called metabolic syndrome or syndrome X [38]. The assessment of biopsies with hepatocyte iron overload requires a biopsy from deeper parts of the liver (as iron is not uniformly distributed in this organ), a description of stainable iron distribution, and an estimation of the amount of iron that has progressively accumulated. Frequently employed semiquantitative estimations of iron overload include the Brissot score [39] and the Deugnier score/histological hepatic iron index [40]. For a quantitative assessment, the reference limits for iron in liver biopsies have been defined [41]. This allows the determination of the hepatic iron index (HII) calculated by the hepatic iron concentration (μg iron per gram dry weight) divided by the atomic weight of iron (55.846) times the patient's age in years, or μmol/g dry weight divided by the patient's age in years. An HII greater than 1.9 strongly suggests haemochromatosis, but not all haemochromatosis patients have an HII >1.9, related to the timing of biopsy and the variable penetrance of the disease. In case fresh tissue is employed for quantitative iron determination, the samples must be transported in iron-free containers, and not in saline, as this may extract part of the iron. Does the determination of the HII always require fresh tissue? It has been shown that an accurate measurement of the iron concentration in deparaffinized biopsy specimens is possible, provided the sample is ≥ 0.4 mg [42].

The role of the biopsy in liver transplantation

Because in the context of liver transplantation (LTX), clinical signs and liver function tests do not reflect well the status of the graft, liver biopsy has a significant place in graft monitoring and in the timely detection of complications [43]. The most frequent biopsies in LTX are usually termed 'null', 'protocol' and 'indicated' biopsies. So-called null biopsies, i.e. needle biopsies performed during or immediately after LTX, serve in some centres as a measure to assess eventual pre- or peritransplantation liver lesions (such as preservation injury), the identification of donor lesions (unrecognized inflammatory or fibrotic lesions), and as a baseline for comparing later histological findings with the original status of the graft. There is still no consensus as to whether, and when, such biopsies should be performed. Indicated graft biopsies are performed at any time when

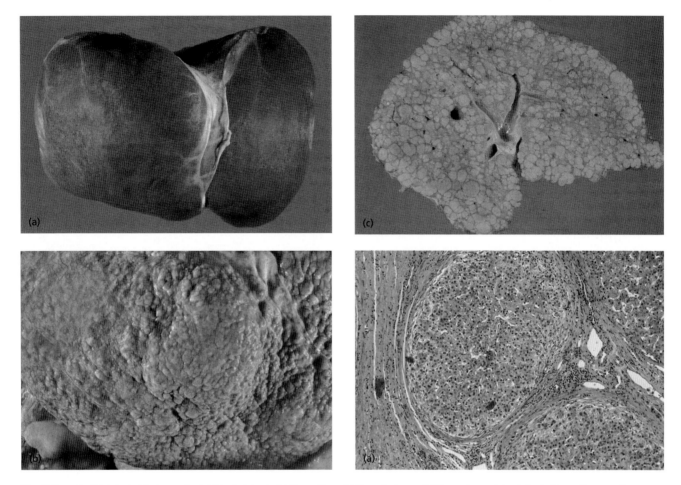

Fig. 9 Gross and histological features of established cirrhosis. (a) Normal liver. (b) Gross features of diffuse micronodular cirrhosis. The entire organ is replaced by densely placed regenerative nodules. (c) Cut surface of fully developed cirrhosis in chronic viral hepatitis. (d) Histology of the liver shown in (c). Note that a needle biopsy will need to be big enough to represent adequately both the nodules and their spatial relation to fibrotic areas (H&E stain).

abnormal graft function requires histological assessment. Conversely, the indications and the timing of so-called protocol biopsies (if performed) seem to still be controversial. A fourth, but not systematically performed, type of biopsy, is the donor organ biopsy, done in order to assess graft quality, specifically in regard to macrosteatosis, which is now established to adversely affect graft function, or in case of other suspected grossly identifiable lesions of unknown significance. Such biopsies can be processed as an intraoperative frozen section.

The histopathological alterations detectable in post-LTX liver biopsies may be divided into four main groups:
• changes directly associated with grafting (sequelae of ischaemia; rejection; Fig. 11a); infections (Figs 11b, 11c); adverse drug reactions; sequelae of technical complications;
• recurrence of the original liver disease (particularly viral hepatitis);
• *de novo* hepatic disease;
• unexpected donor lesions not recognized so far.

In the context of graft lesions related to preservation injury and rejection, grading systems have been developed. Acute rejection is graded according to the rejection activity score (RAI), and European and Banff classifications are available [44]. Similarly, criteria for staging chronic rejection have been worked out [45]. If microbiological examinations using hepatic biopsy material are planned, these procedures should be organized according to the local microbiology laboratory's requirements.

Complications of liver biopsy

Several large series (>20 000 interventions) have summarized the prevalence of minor and major complications directly related to liver biopsy. Overall, relevant or severe morbidity is estimated at 0.1–0.2%, while fatality rates range from 0% to 0.2%. Most complications (about 60%) become manifest within the first 3 hours after biopsy [46–48]. The most frequent adverse event is pain (usually resolving in 1–2 days), reported to occur in up to 50% of the patients, but only about half of them will require analgesia. Whereas minor bleeding is frequent, significant haemorrhage, sometimes requiring transfusion, is

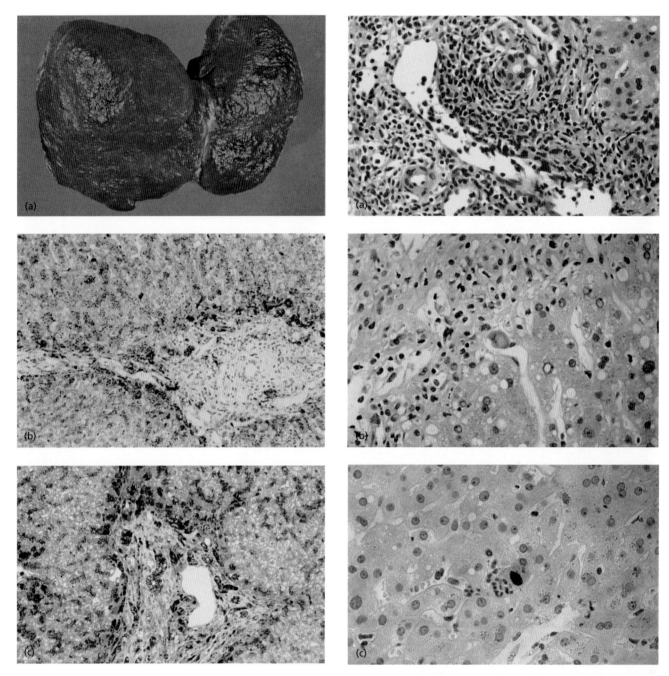

Fig. 10 Haemochromatosis. (a) Gross features of liver cirrhosis in haemochromatosis. This cirrhotic liver shows diffuse discoloration caused by the massive iron overload (pigment cirrhosis). (b) In an iron stain, the preferential localization of stainable iron (darker areas) in hepatocytes is seen. Note the typical zonation of iron overload. (c) At higher magnification, iron overload in cell systems other than hepatocytes (bile ducts, macrophages) is in evidence.

Fig. 11 Biopsy in liver transplantation. (a) Acute graft rejection. Three key features – a marked infiltration of portal tracts, venous endothelitis, and bile duct damage are observed (H&E stain). (b) Cytomegalovirus infection of a liver allograft. Note the markedly enlarged (cytomegalic) endothelial cell in the middle of the figure (H&E stain). (c) Immunostaining is particularly suited to detect cytomegalovirus (CMV) hepatitis. In this liver allograft, a typical nuclear (dark spot) inclusion body is seen, associated with a neutrophil accumulation (microabscess).

estimated to occur in 0.2% only, but is the most common cause of biopsy-associated death. Bile leakage with subsequent bile peritonitis is a high-risk complication, but should be avoidable if the typical contraindication of high-grade extrahepatic bile duct obstruction is respected. Other complications include right-sided pneumothorax or haemothorax (<0.5%), haemobilia (<0.2%), hepatic arteriovenous fistula (up to 5%), sepsis (<0.1%), subcutaneous emphysema (<0.2%), adverse anaesthetic reactions (<0.3%), needle break (≈0.02%), and puncture

Table 2 Indications for diagnostic laparoscopy.

Chronic fibrosing liver disease (in particular, staging)
Primary hepatic tumours, both benign and malignant
Nodular precursor lesions of the liver
Metastatic liver disease
Lymphomatous involvement of the liver
Evaluation of unclear abdominal masses
Staging of primarily extrahepatic malignancies
Ascites of unknown cause
Infection of the peritoneal cavity
Hepatic parasitoses
Chronic abdominal pain
Hepatomegaly or hepatosplenomegaly of unknown cause
Liver disease in renal failure
Liver involvement in multiorgan failure
Subfulminant liver failure
Assessment for liver transplantation
Patients at increased risk for other bioptic procedures

injury to other intra-abdominal organs (overall <0.5%). Intra-abdominal seeding of neoplastic cells upon puncture of hepatic malignancy is a possible complication that caused reluctance to perform such biopsies. In recent studies, needle tract implantation of hepatocellular carcinoma was found to range in prevalence from 1.6% to 5.1% [49,50], hence requiring a careful risk–benefit analysis when planning a tumour biopsy.

Laparoscopy

Diagnostic laparoscopy has an important place in the assessment of liver disease, albeit for a restricted spectrum of indications [51]. These are summarized in Table 2. Diagnostic laparoscopy is probably one of the most accurate measures for the diagnostic evaluation of specific forms of chronic liver disease. In this approach, the surgeon becomes a visual anatomist [52] whose macroscopic information will help the pathologist in the histopathological diagnosis (Fig. 12). Laparoscopic liver

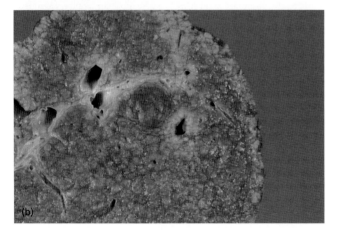

Fig. 12 Laparoscopic liver biopsy. (a) Laparoscopic biopsy is indicated in lesions of uncertain aetiology and in patients with increased risk (e.g. bacterial infection). In this case, a patient with infectious cholangitis and small focal liver lesions, the biopsy shows purulent cholangitis with bile duct rupture and leakage of bile (H&E stain). (b) Precursor lesions of hepatocellular carcinoma can be reliably assessed by use of laparoscopy. This excision shows a so-called bulging nodule, histologically representing a dysplastic nodule.

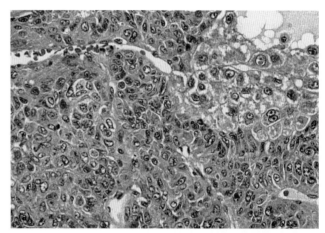

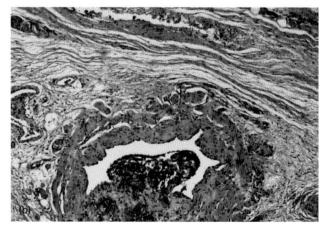

Fig. 13 Laparoscopic liver biopsy. (a) Hepatocellular carcinoma (HCC), trabecular type. Owing to their highly aggressive and invasive phenotype, HCC are regarded as a risk factor for needle biopsies (needle tract seeding), therefore laparoscopic biopsy is preferable (H&E stain). (b) In an excisional biopsy, the prognostically important feature, angioinvasion, has an increased chance of being detected (H&E stain).

biopsy is frequently used, in particular for patients with compromised haemostasis and for whom the transjugular procedure is not available. In some centres it is performed on an outpatient basis, and it seems to have a similar complication rate and mortality as percutaneous liver biopsy [51,53]. For certain lesions, this procedure seems to be more specific, in particular for staging chronic fibrosing liver disease in case of macronodularity [54,55]. Even minilaparoscopy (laparoscopy with a small-diameter telescope) offers the possibility of assessing macroscopic liver features and of coagulation of the biopsy site [56,57]. Laparoscopy associated with laparoscopic ultrasonography and biopsy plays an increasing role in the evaluation of patients with suspected liver tumours and hepatic tumour staging procedures [58,59,60,61], and allows better control of the circumstances that may favour tumour cell seeding (Fig. 13), but it also offers an approach for the treatment of liver tumours [62].

References

1 McGill DB (2001) Liver biopsy: when, how, by whom, and where? *Curr Gastroenterol Rep* 3, 19–23.

2 Geller SA, Pitman MB (2002) Morphological diagnostic procedures (liver biopsy). In: MacSween RNM, Burt AD, Portmann BC *et al.* (eds) *Pathology of the Liver*, 4th edn. London: Churchill Livingstone, pp. 943–960.

3 Reddy KR, Mallat DB, Jeffers LJ (2003) Evaluation of the liver: Liver biopsy and laparoscopy. In: Schiff ER, Sorrell MF, Maddrey WC (eds) *Schiff's Disease of the Liver*, 9th edn. Philadelphia: Lippincott Williams & Wilkins, Vol. 1, pp. 257–280.

4 Campbell MS, Reddy KR (2004) Review article: the evolving role of liver biopsy. *Aliment Pharmacol Ther* 20, 249–259.

5 Siegel CA, Silas AM, Suriawinata AA *et al.* (2005) Liver biopsy 2005: when and how? *Cleve Clin J Med* 72, 199–201.

6 Grant A, Neuberger J (1999) Guidelines on the use of liver biopsy in clinical practice. *Gut* 45 (Suppl. IV), IV1–IV11.

7 Bravo AA, Sheth SG, Chopra S (2001) Liver biopsy. *N Engl J Med* 344, 495–500.

8 Spycher C, Zimmermann A, Reichen J (2001) The diagnostic value of liver biopsy. *BMC Gastroenterol* 1, 12.

9 Friedman LS (2004) Controversies in liver biopsy: Who, where, when, how, why? *Curr Gastroenterol Rep* 6, 30–36.

10 Van Ness NM, Diehl AM (1989) Is liver biopsy useful in the evaluation of patients with chronically elevated liver enzymes? *Ann Intern Med* 111, 473–478.

11 Sorbi D, McGill DB, Thistle JL (2000) An assessment of the role of liver biopsies in asymptomatic patients with chronic liver test abnormalities. *Am J Gastroenterol* 95, 3206–3210.

12 Bianchi L (2001) Liver biopsy in elevated liver function tests? An old question revisited. *J Hepatol* 35, 290–294.

13 Stauffer MH, Gross JB, Foulk WT *et al.* (1961) Amyloidosis: diagnosis with needle biopsy of the liver in 18 patients. *Gastroenterology* 41, 92–96.

14 Guido M, Rugge M (2004) Liver biopsy sampling in chronic viral hepatitis. *Semin Liver Dis* 24, 89–97.

15 Colloredo G, Guido M, Sonzogni A *et al.* (2003) Impact of liver biopsy size on histological evaluation of chronic viral hepatitis: the smaller the sample, the milder the disease. *J Hepatol* 39, 239–244.

16 Regev A, Berho M, Jeffers LJ *et al.* (2002) Sampling error and intraobserver variation in liver biopsy in patients with chronic HCV infection. *Am J Gastroenterol* 97, 2614–2618.

17 Siddique I, El-Naga HA, Madda JP *et al.* (2003) Sampling variability on percutaneous liver biopsy in patients with chronic hepatitis C virus infection. *Scand J Gastroenterol* 38, 427–432.

18 METAVIR Cooperative Study Group (1994) Intraobserver and interobserver variations in liver biopsy interpretation in patients with chronic hepatitis C. *Hepatology* 20, 15–20.

19 Maharaj B, Bhoora IG (1992) Complications associated with percutaneous needle biopsy of the liver when one, two, or three specimens are taken. *Postgrad Med J* 68, 964–967.

20 McGill DB, Rakela J, Zinsmeister AR *et al.* (1990) A 21-year experience with major haemorrhage after percutaneous liver biopsy. *Gastroenterology* 99, 1396–1400.

21 Hilden M, Christoffersen P, Juhl E *et al.* (1977) Liver histology in a 'normal' population – examination of 503 consecutive fatal traffic casualties. *Scand J Gastroenterol* 12, 593–597.

22 Cawford AR, Lin XZ, Crawford JM (1998) The normal adult human liver biopsy: a quantitative reference standard. *Hepatology* 28, 323–331.

23 Kay EW, O'Dowd J, Thomas R *et al.* (1997) Mild abnormalities in liver histology associated with chronic hepatitis: distinction from normal liver histology. *J Clin Pathol* 50, 929–931.

24 Lebrec D (1996) Various approaches to obtaining liver tissue – choosing the biopsy technique. *J Hepatol* 25 (Suppl. 1), 20–24.

25 McCormack G, Nolan N, McCormack PA (2001) Transjugular liver biopsy: a review. *Ir Med J* 94, 11–12.

26 Petrelli M, Scheuer PJ (1967) Variation in subcapsular liver structure and its significance in the interpretation of wedge biopsies. *J Clin Pathol* 20, 743–748.

27 Sanyal AJ (2002) AGA technical review on nonalcoholic fatty liver disease. *Gastroenterology* 123, 1705–1725.

28 Brunt EM, Tiniakos DG (2002) Pathology of steatohepatitis. *Best Pract Res Clin Gastroenterol* 16, 691–707.

29 Neuschwander-Tetri BA, Caldwell SH (2003) Nonalcoholic steatohepatitis: summary of an AASLD single topic conference. *Hepatology* 37, 1202–1219.

30 Zafrani ES (2004) Non-alcoholic fatty liver disease: an emerging pathological spectrum. *Virchows Arch* 444, 3–12.

31 Mendler MH, Kanel G, Govindarajan S (2005) Proposal for a histological scoring and grading system for non-alcoholic fatty liver disease. *Liver International* 25, 294–304.

32 Goldstein NS, Hastah F, Galan MV *et al.* (2005) Fibrosis heterogeneity in nonalcoholic steatohepatitis and hepatitis C virus needle core biopsy specimens. *Am J Clin Pathol* 123, 382–387.

33 Gebo KA, Herlong HF, Torbenson MS *et al.* (2002) Role of liver biopsy in management of chronic hepatitis C – a systematic review. *Hepatology* 36, S161–S172.

34 Knodell RG, Ishak KG, Black WC *et al.* (1981) Formulation and application of a numerical scoring system for assessing histological activity in asymptomatic chronic active hepatitis. *Hepatology* 1, 431–435.

35 Brunt EM (2000) Grading and staging the histopathological lesions of chronic hepatitis: the Knodell histology activity index and beyond. *Hepatology* 31, 241–246.

36 Scheuer PJ (2003). Assessment of liver biopsies in chronic hepatitis: how is it best done? *J Hepatol* 38, 240–242.

37 Franchini M, Veneri D (2005) Recent advances in hereditary hemochromatosis. *Ann Hematol* 84, 347–352.

38 Moirand R, Mendler MH, Guillygomarc'h A *et al.* (2000) Non-alcoholic steatohepatitis with iron: part of insulin resistance-associated hepatic iron overload? *J Hepatol* 33, 1024–1026.

39 Brissot P, Bourel M, Herry D *et al.* (1981) Assessment of liver iron content in 271 patients: a reevaluation of direct and indirect methods. *Gastroenterology* 80, 557–565.

40 Deugnier YM, Turlin B, Powell LW *et al.* (1993) Differentiation between heterozygotes and homozygotes in genetic hemochromatosis by means of a histological hepatic iron index: a study of 192 cases. *Hepatology* 17, 30–34.

41 Nuttall KL, Palaty J, Lockitch G (2003) Reference limits for copper and iron in liver biopsies. *Ann Clin Lab Sci* 33, 443–450.

42 Olynyk JK, O'Neill R, Britton RS *et al.* (1994) Determination of hepatic iron concentration in fresh and paraffin-embedded tissue: diagnostic implications. *Gastroenterology* 106, 674–677.

43 Sebagh M, Samuel D (2004) Place of the liver biopsy in liver transplantation. *J Hepatol* 41, 897–901.

44 Demetris AJ (1997) International Panel. Banff schema for grading liver allograft rejection: an international consensus document. *Hepatology* 25, 658–663.

45 Demetris A, Adams D, Bellamy C *et al.* (2000) Update of the International Banff Schema for liver allograft rejection: working recommendations for the histopathologic staging and reporting of chronic rejection. An International Panel. *Hepatology* 31, 792–799.

46 Piccinino F, Sagnelli E, Pasquale G *et al.* (1986) Complications following percutaneous liver biopsy. A multicentre retrospective study on 68276 biopsies. *J Hepatol* 2, 165–173.

47 Garcia-Taso G, Boyer JL (1993) Outpatient liver biopsy: how safe is it? *Ann Intern Med* 118, 150–153.

48 Terjung B, Lemnitzer I, Dumoulin FL *et al.* (2003) Bleeding complications after percutaneous liver biopsy. An analysis of risk factors. *Digestion* 67, 138–145.

49 Takamori R, Wong LL, Dang C *et al.* (2000) Needle-tract implantation from hepatocellular cancer: is needle biopsy of the liver always necessary? *Liver Transpl* 6, 67–72.

50 Kosugi C, Furuse J, Ishii H *et al.* (2004) Needle tract implantation of hepatocellular carcinoma and pancreatic carcinoma after ultrasound-guided percutaneous puncture: clinical and pathologic characteristics and the treatment of needle tract implantation. *World J Surg* 28, 29–32.

51 Haydon GH, Hayes PC (1997) Diagnostic laparoscopy by physicians: we should do it. *QJM* 90, 297–304.

52 Schwaitzberg SD (2002) Diagnostic laparoscopy. *Semin Laparoscop Surg* 9, 10–23.

53 Lightdale CJ, Das L (1997) Difficult liver biopsies: only for radiologists? *Am J Gastroenterol* 92, 364–365.

54 Jalan RJ, Hayes PC (1995) Laparoscopy in the diagnosis of chronic liver disease. *Br J Hosp Med* 53, 81–86.

55 Helmreich-Becker I, Schirmacher P, Denzer U *et al.* (2003) Minilaparoscopy in the diagnosis of cirrhosis: superiority in patients with Child-Pugh A and macronodular disease. *Endoscopy* 35, 55–60.

56 Orlando R, Lirussi F (2003) Laparoscopy and guided liver biopsy in the diagnosis of cirrhosis: conventional technique vs. minilaparoscopy. *Endoscopy* 35, 1079–1080.

57 Denzer U, Helmreich-Becker I, Galle PR *et al.* (2003) Liver assessment and biopsy in patients with marked coagulopathy: value of minilaparoscopy and control of bleeding. *Am J Gastroenterol* 98, 893–900.

58 Berber E, Garland AM, Engle KL *et al.* (2004) Laparoscopic ultrasonography and biopsy of hepatic tumors in 310 patients. *Am J Surg* 187, 213–218.

59 White RR, Pappas TN (2004) Laparoscopic staging for hepatobiliary carcinoma. *J Gastrointest Surg* 8, 920–922.

60 Kim RD, Nazarey P, Katz E *et al.* (2004) Laparoscopic staging and tumor ablation for hepatocellular carcinoma in Child C cirrhotics evaluated for orthotopic liver transplantation. *Surg Endosc* 18, 39–44.

61 Grobmeyer SR, Fong Y, D'Angelica M *et al.* (2004) Diagnostic laparoscopy prior to planned hepatic resection for colorectal metastases. *Arch Surg* 139, 1326–1330.

62 Teramoto K, Kawamura T, Takamatsu S *et al.* (2005) Laparoscopic and thoracoscopic approaches for the treatment of hepatocellular carcinoma. *Am J Surg* 189, 474–478.

5.6 Imaging of the liver

5.6.1 Ultrasonography

Luigi Bolondi, Valeria Camaggi and Fabio Piscaglia

Ultrasonography (US) is the first-line imaging technique for the examination of the hepatobiliary system and other abdominal organs. The main advantages of US are low cost, broad availability, non-invasiveness, safety, repeatability and efficacy. US guidance provides an easy way for performing interventional procedures, such as percutaneous treatments for hepatic malignancies and biopsy. Its weakness is the difficulty in exploring the entire liver in cases of abundant intestinal gas and in obese or uncooperative patients. It is an operator-dependent technique, especially Doppler US, which requires thorough training to obtain good intra- and interobserver reproducibility.

Overview of the physical principles of US

The properties of ultrasound are used to create a real-time image of the insonated structures. Ultrasound consists of sound waves of frequencies beyond the range of human hearing (>20 kHz). When an ultrasound beam, generated by the US transducer, crosses an interface between two structures with different acoustic impedance, waves are partially reflected and received by the transducer, which translates them into electric pulses. A bidimensional real-time image is obtained by coding these pulses into a grey-scale panel of signals.

Human organs contain several acoustic interfaces both at a macroscopic (vessels, masses, etc.) and microscopic level (differences in cellular content and mesenchymal stroma) that are the basis for the US representation of the human body. A big difference in acoustic impedance between two adjacent structures (i.e. parenchyma and gas or bones) causes the near complete reflection of the US beam thereby preventing evaluation of the structures behind. This 'posterior acoustic shadowing' hampers liver examination when generated by ribs or intestinal gas, but may aid the correct diagnosis in other cases (e.g. gallstones). The key terms in the description of conventional US features are reported in Table 1.

Doppler US allows a non-invasive assessment of blood flow by the application of the Doppler physical principle: when

Table 1 Key terms in conventional US.

Term	Description	Examples
Anechoic or echo-free	Homogenous structure without internal interfaces, so that no echoes are returned. It appears black	Liquid filled structures (vessels, gallbladder, cysts), ascites
Echoic or reflective	Every structure that returns echoes. It can assume every gradation of grey up to white	Parenchyma, biliary sludge
Hypoechoic	A structure that is less echoic than the background, so that it appears darker	Several types of liver lesion (neoplasm, abscesses)
Hyperechoic	A structure that is more echoic than the background, so that it appears brighter	Small haemangiomas, some HCC, some metastases
Isoechoic	A structure that is as echoic as the background	Some liver masses (typically FNH)
Posterior acoustic shadowing	Absence of echoes behind a structure that reflects the US beam almost completely	Gallstones, bones, intestinal gas, calcifications
Posterior acoustic enhancement	Increased echogenicity behind a homogeneous structure that presents low attenuation of the US beam	Liquid-filled structure (cysts), fluid-rich lesions (haemangiomas)

FNH, focal nodular hyperplasia; HCC, hepatocellular carcinoma.

Table 2 Indications for US.

Indication	What to evaluate
Alteration in liver laboratory exams	Signs of diffuse liver disease
	Mass liver lesions
	Bile-duct dilatations, gallbladder pathology
Signs of PTH (ascites, oesophageal varices)	Signs of cirrhosis, portal and hepatic vein patency
	Doppler evaluation of splanchnic circulation
Jaundice	Bile-duct dilatations and cause of biliary obstruction
	Signs of diffuse liver disease
Abdominal pain	Biliary tract disease
	Portal thrombosis
	Extrahepatic causes of pain
Abdominal trauma	Hepatic haematoma
	Lesions of other abdominal organs (especially spleen)
Staging of known chronic hepatitis	Signs of progression to cirrhosis and PTH
Surveillance of cirrhotic patients (every 6 months)	Detection and characterization of mass lesions (HCC?)
Staging and follow-up in patients with known extrahepatic neoplasm	Detection and characterization of mass lesions (metastases?)
	Routine CEUS can be useful to disclose small lesions
Characterization of mass liver lesions	Conventional US appearance, presence and characteristics of vascular signals, pattern at CEUS. Assessment of resectability
Presurgical assessment for OLT	Confirmation of endstage liver disease
	Detection of HCC, portal thrombosis, wide collaterals
Follow-up after OLT	Vascular and biliary complications

HCC, hepatocellular carcinoma; OLT, orthotopic liver transplantation; PTH, portal hypertension.

ultrasound is reflected by a moving target, such as blood cells flowing in the vessels, the frequency of the reflected waves differs from that of the incident waves: it increases when the target is moving towards the transducer and decreases when the target is moving away. The difference between the incident and the reflected frequency is the *Doppler frequency*.

The Doppler frequencies can be represented by different modalities: *colour Doppler* displays a map of vascular structures in a selected portion of the real-time US scan, providing qualitative information about the presence and direction of blood flow by means of a colour code. Sensitivity in detecting slow flow can be increased by using *power Doppler*, which displays the integrated amplitude of the Doppler signal instead of its frequency. *Doppler spectral analysis* visualizes the velocity distribution of blood cells in a time function, giving quantitative and semiquantitative information about flow velocity and features. Impedance indices (i.e. resistance index, RI) and frequency peak are important in the characterization of mass liver lesions and splanchnic haemodynamics. Unfortunately, very small vessels (as in tumoral lesions) and deeply located structures are poorly recognized by Doppler US.

A revolutionary advance in US was the introduction of *contrast-enhanced US* (CEUS). US contrast media are gas-filled microbubbles dissolved in water. After injection in a peripheral vein, microbubbles reach the liver through both the hepatic artery and portal vein in subsequent phases, so that an arterial (10–30 s after injection), a portal (30–120 s) and a late phase are recognizable.

As no enhancement is detectable with conventional US, CEUS requires contrast-specific imaging modes, known as harmonic imaging techniques, that visualize exclusively the nonlinear tissue echoes generated by microbubbles, nullifying the linear tissual echoes. Whereas the first-generation contrast media, i.e. Levovist (Schering AG, Berlin, Germany), permit only intermittent visualization of focal lesions, the second-generation contrast media, such as SonoVue (Bracco, Milan, Italy), allow continuous, real-time evaluation of hepatic structures. Thanks to this advantage, real-time CEUS, or perfusional angiosonography, has become the reference standard in this setting [1]. Clinical indications for US are summarized in Table 2.

Diffuse liver disease

Normal liver parenchyma gives a homogeneous pattern of low-level echoes in which vessels appear as anechoic tubular structures (Fig. 1). The size, morphology, echo-pattern and surface characteristics of the liver have to be assessed.

US has a sensitivity of up to 95% in distinguishing normal from abnormal liver, but the accuracy in discriminating different stages of chronic liver diseases is limited, with the exception of overt cirrhosis [2].

Acute hepatitis

Acute hepatitis does not produce specific US findings. The 'starry-night liver pattern', resulting from a decreased parenchymal

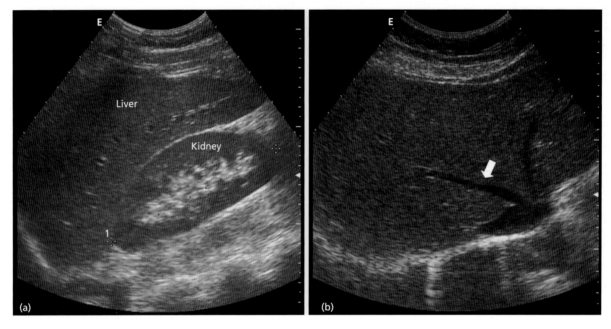

Fig. 1 The normal liver parenchyma is isoechoic or slightly hyperechoic in comparison with the right renal cortex (a); it is crossed by vessels, which appear anechoic (b, arrow).

echogenicity enhancing the hyperechoic periportal structures, has been associated with acute hepatitis, but its specificity and sensitivity are low. Hepatomegaly is a frequent finding.

Hepatic steatosis

Fatty infiltration produces an increased reflectivity of hepatic parenchyma, known as 'bright liver pattern' (Fig. 2). This feature

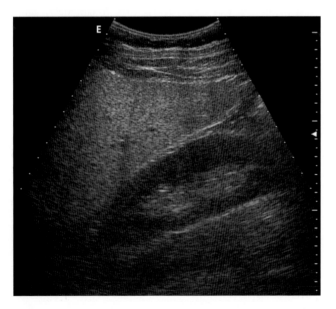

Fig. 2 Hepatic steatosis: the liver is brighter than the cortex of the right kidney.

can be assessed by comparing liver parenchyma with the right kidney's cortex, which normally presents an echogenicity equal to or slightly lower than that of the liver (Fig. 1a). Severe steatosis produces a strong attenuation in the deepest liver sections, resulting in poor explorability. The liver is frequently enlarged, with rounded profiles. US is unable to differentiate simple fatty liver from steatohepatitis.

Steatosis frequently presents an inhomogeneous distribution, appearing as 'patchy' hyperechoic areas, sometimes with a segmental distribution, or as hypoechoic areas frequently located near the gallbladder or the portal bifurcation. CEUS may help in distinguishing inhomogeneous steatosis from mass lesions by disclosing an isoechoic pattern in all the perfusional phases.

Chronic liver disease: from chronic hepatitis to cirrhosis

Chronic liver disease produces a broad continuous spectrum of US anomalies, from a near normal aspect in mild chronic hepatitis to overt alterations in cirrhosis. The progression from chronic hepatitis to compensated cirrhosis is difficult to evaluate with biochemical parameters, imaging techniques or even hepatic biopsy, as an underestimation is possible due to sampling error. Nevertheless, the diagnosis of cirrhosis at an early stage is useful because specific follow-up programmes are instituted for cirrhotic patients (i.e. surveillance for hepatocellular carcinoma and endoscopic evaluation for oesophageal varices).

As fibrosis progresses, US shows an increasingly coarsened echo-pattern and an increased echogenicity of the liver. A relative enlargement of the left lobe may take place, but the liver

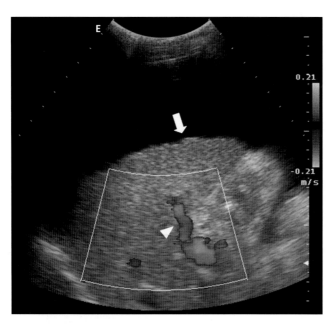

Fig. 3 Decompensated cirrhosis. Ascites enhances the visualization of the nodular liver surface (arrow). Colour Doppler shows a patent portal system with hepatopetal flow (arrow head).

surface still appears smooth and no signs of portal hypertension are detectable. Small lengthened adenopathies are often detected at the hepatic hilum in viral and autoimmune hepatitis.

The more sensitive and specific sign of progression to cirrhosis is the emergence of an irregular or nodular liver surface (Fig. 3), especially when associated with a reduction in portal flow velocity at Doppler examination [3]. Other findings suggesting cirrhosis are marked hypertrophy of the left and caudate lobes, atrophy of the right lobe and the onset of ascites. Doppler US can show signs of portal hypertension, as described below.

Portal hypertension

Doppler US and upper gastrointestinal endoscopy are the first-line exams when portal hypertension (PHT) is suspected. The aim of Doppler US is to disclose signs suggesting PHT and its cause.

US diagnosis of PHT

Many conventional US signs of PHT, namely splenomegaly and enlargement of the portal, splenic and superior mesenteric veins, present poor sensitivity and specificity. Instead, the absence of the normal calibre variation of splenic and superior mesenteric veins during forced inspiration–expiration (<40% reduction) is sensitive (up to 80%) and specific [4].

Doppler examination adds a significant contribution to the diagnosis of PHT by characterizing splanchnic haemodynamics. A reduction in portal flow velocity suggests PHT, but is not totally specific. The normal postprandial increase in portal flow velocity is reduced. An inversion in portal flow direction is rare but specific for PHT [4].

Collateral portosystemic pathways are a highly specific sign of PHT. They can be visualized by conventional US as tortuous channels, but Doppler US greatly increases the confidence in their recognition, confirming their vascular nature and showing traces indicative of turbulent venous flow. One of the most frequent collaterals is the recanalization of umbilical or paraumbilical veins, running from the left intrahepatic portal branch to the abdominal wall. Spontaneous splenorenal shunts connecting the splenic vein with the left renal vein are located at the lower spleen pole and are generally massive. Other sites of portosystemic shunts are the left gastric vein behind the left hepatic lobe (considered a sign of PHT only in case of reversed flow), the short gastric veins near the upper spleen pole, the gallbladder wall and retroperitoneum. Direct visualization of oesophageal varices is rare.

The width and location of collaterals can affect the flow characteristics in the portal system. Large splenorenal shunts reduce or even reverse the flow in the splenic and portal veins, probably decreasing the gastro-oesophageal bleeding risk. Umbilical vein patency can increase portal flow, which is mainly diverted into the collateral with a reduction or inversion of the right portal branch flow.

PHT affects the impedance of several arterial vessels [4]. The intraparenchymal branches of the splenic artery show increased impedance indices at Doppler evaluation (RI > 0.63), irrespective of spleen size. Impedance indices can also increase in intrarenal arterioles (RI > 0.70), due to renal vasoconstriction. In contrast, the superior mesenteric artery impedance is reduced as a consequence of cirrhotic hyperdynamic circulation.

Causes of PHT

US can identify the cause of PHT by showing signs of advanced chronic liver disease (intrahepatic PHT), portal thrombosis or splenic arteriovenous fistulae (prehepatic PHT), Budd–Chiari syndrome or cardiac liver (posthepatic PHT). US findings in cirrhosis, the most frequent cause of PHT, have been already described.

Portal vein thrombosis is frequently related to intrahepatic PHT, but it can be the primary cause. A recent thrombus is generally echo-poor, so that it may be undetectable at conventional US. Colour Doppler shows the absence of flow in the whole vessel (complete thrombosis) or in part of it (partial or mural thrombosis). The optimal setting of the equipment and the use of power Doppler allow the detection of very slow flow in the portal system that could have raised the suspicion of thrombosis at a first examination. As the thrombus organizes, it becomes visible as echoic material filling the lumen. Cavernous transformation in longstanding portal thrombosis appears as several tortuous vessels with turbulent flow at the porta hepatis.

Budd–Chiari syndrome is characterized by occlusion of the hepatic veins. Conventional US shows hepatomegaly, enlargement

Table 3 US features of the commonest liver masses.

Lesion	Conventional US	Colour Doppler signals	Spectral analysis of arterial signals		Contrast-enhanced US	
			Resistance index	Peak frequency	Arterial phase	Portal-late phase
Cysts	Anechoic with posterior enhancement	Absent	–	–	Anechoic	Anechoic
Haemangioma	Hyperechoic	Scarce or absent	Low	Low	Centripetal globular filling (slow)	Isoechoic
Focal nodular hyperplasia	Isoechoic with central scar	Rich spoke-wheel vascularization	Low	High	Early CE from central artery	Isoechoic
Dysplastic nodules on cirrhotic liver	Generally hypoechoic	Scarce or absent	Low	Low	Isoechoic	Isoechoic
Hepatocellular carcinoma	Variable	Present	Very high	High	Early CE	Slightly hypoechoic or isoechoic
Metastasis	Variable	Scarce or absent	High	High	Peripheral CE	Markedly hypoechoic

CE, contrast enhancement.

of the caudate lobe and ascites. Hepatic veins are not detectable or appear as fibrotic bands. In other cases, they are dilated and tortuous with nonvisualization of their confluence with the inferior vena cava (IVC), and Doppler examination discloses a flat waveform without the normal phasic variations. The latter sign is nonspecific, as it can also be found in advanced cirrhosis. Reversed flow in hepatic veins is pathognomonic albeit rare. The IVC is often obstructed or narrowed, with continuous and sometimes reversed flow in its lower portion.

Liver masses

US is the first-line exam for suspected liver masses and often detects incidental lesions when performed for other indications. Most benign and clinically irrelevant lesions (i.e. cyst, haemangioma and focal nodular hyperplasia) can often be diagnosed solely by using Doppler US and ultimately CEUS (Table 3). In other instances, US represents a complementary source of information, used in addition to other imaging techniques. Moreover, US can guide biopsy and visualizes the relationship between lesions and vascular and biliary structures, which is fundamental in assessing the resectability of liver tumours.

The clinical setting is useful in suggesting diagnosis (e.g. cirrhosis and hepatocellular carcinoma [5], a known extrahepatic malignancy and metastases, oral contraceptive use and adenoma, otherwise healthy subjects and haemangioma or focal nodular hyperplasia).

Liver cyst

Simple liver cyst is a common incidental US finding without any clinical relevance. Conventional US is diagnostic: cysts appear as anechoic, round-to-oval lesions with posterior acoustic enhancement.

Polycystic liver disease is an inherited condition characterized by multiple cysts throughout the liver, often associated with autosomal dominant polycystic kidney disease. Hepatic cysts generally arise in puberty and increase in number and size with time. In the case of very numerous or large cysts, the patient may become symptomatic for abdominal discomfort, early satiety or dyspnoea.

Echinococcal cyst

The liver is the most frequent site of hydatid disease. Echinococcal cysts are characterized by a thick wall, sometimes with two distinct layers and focal or circumferential calcifications. Inner daughter cysts and intraluminal debris may be present. Inactive lesions appear completely calcified or display the so-called 'waterlily sign', characterized by linear echoes floating into the cyst.

A classification based on the US appearance has been approved by the World Health Organization to guide the approach to treatment.

Liver abscess

Pyogenic liver abscesses present a great variability in US appearance even in the same patient, as their aspect may change over time. They frequently appear as slightly irregular hypoechoic lesions with distal enhancement. A hyperechoic pattern is possible especially in the initial phases.

Amoebic abscesses produce similar features, but they are generally round, and in a subcapsular location. Occasionally, a cystic area persists after recovery.

Haematoma

Haematoma, related to abdominal trauma or to interventional procedures such as biopsy, is usually hyperechoic in the very early phase and then becomes hypoechoic. Large subcapsular haematomas can appear hypo- to anechoic even in the early phase. A residual fibrous scar or a cystic area may persist after resolution.

Haemangioma

Haemangioma, the commonest benign hepatic tumour, is generally an incidental finding. Haemangiomas <3 cm in diameter typically appear as hyperechoic, well-demarcated lesions, often adjacent to liver vessels. Such lesions can cast a posterior acoustic enhancement. Larger lesions can present atypical features, for example an inhomogeneous or hypoechoic texture. If steatosis is present, haemangioma can be less evident or even appear hypoechoic.

Doppler US detects little or no blood flow within the lesion, because of the low flow velocity inside it.

Haemangioma presents a typical CEUS pattern, namely a peripheral globular enhancement with centripetal filling, so that in the late phase it appears isoechoic or even hyperechoic [6]. Large haemangiomas may present thrombosed areas that remain hypoechoic.

Focal nodular hyperplasia (FNH)

FNH generally appears as an isoechoic mass at conventional US. The presence of a central hyperechoic scar is infrequent, but highly suggestive for FNH.

Colour Doppler discloses a highly vascularized pattern often with a distinctive 'spoke-wheel' distribution. Spectral analysis shows both central and peripheral arterial waveforms characterized by high peak frequencies and low impedance [7]. The differential diagnosis with other hypervascular lesions (i.e. hepatocellular carcinoma or adenomas) is based on the central scar and the above-mentioned Doppler features.

At CEUS, FNH presents an early homogeneous filling in the arterial phase. It subsequently becomes isoechoic [6].

Hepatocellular adenoma

Adenoma is a rare lesion, more common in females using oral contraceptives. Its recognition is important despite the benign nature, as adenoma can cause significant morbidity (e.g. haemorrhage). In particular, adenoma should be differentiated from FNH, which shows similar features but is clinically irrelevant. If diagnostic clues for FNH are lacking, differential diagnosis is difficult and not always possible even for experienced US operators. Guided biopsy may be required.

Adenoma appears as an isohypoechoic inhomogeneous lesion characterized by rich peri- and intralesional vascularization without the spoke-wheel distribution observed in FNH. Both venous and arterial signals are detectable, the latter with high peak frequency and low impedance.

No large series are available about the accuracy of CEUS in adenoma. Like FNH, it usually presents an early flush-like enhancement in the arterial phase and an isoechoic aspect in the portal-late phase.

Metastases

Metastases are the most common malignant liver lesions in developed countries. Unfortunately, US appearance is extremely variable and does not show a significant relationship with the primary tumour. A hypoechoic mass is the most frequent presentation and may be seen in any type of malignancy. Hyperechoic lesions, often with a peripheral hypoechoic halo or a target aspect, are more frequently related to gastrointestinal or urogenital cancers.

Vascular signals are absent or rare with both colour and power Doppler US. Where observed, vascularization is irregular with high impedance and high peak frequency arterial signals.

Conventional US sensitivity in detecting hepatic metastases is relatively poor compared with contrast-enhanced computerized tomography (CT) and magnetic resonance imaging (MRI). In contrast, CEUS visualizes small metastases missed at conventional US and is thought to have a sensitivity similar or even slightly superior to CT in detecting small lesions [8].

The typical pattern of metastases at CEUS is a markedly hypoechoic aspect in the portal-late phase, due to poor contrast uptake with respect to the surrounding parenchyma. A peripheral or homogeneous enhancement is sometimes detected during the arterial phase.

Lymphoma

Both Hodgkin's and non-Hodgkin's lymphomas can affect the liver, assuming a diffuse or more rarely a focal pattern. Occasionally the liver can be the primary and unique site. A generalized decrease in hepatic echogenicity can be detected in diffuse infiltration. Circumscribed lymphoma appears as a markedly hypoechoic focal lesion with rare vascular signals. After contrast medium injection it is hypoechoic in the portal-late phase.

Cholangiocellular carcinoma (CCC)

No characteristic US and Doppler appearance is described for CCC. It appears as a mass located at the hepatic hilum with intrahepatic bile duct dilatation (Klatskin tumour) or as a focal lesion within the liver parenchyma (peripheral CCC), often with small satellite nodules. Portal invasion is a frequent finding.

Generally, CCC appears hypervascularized in the arterial phase and hypoechoic in the portal-late phase at CEUS.

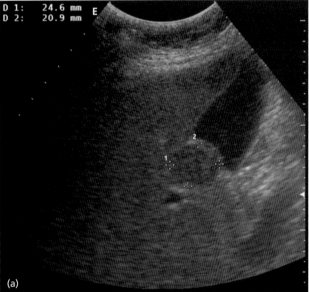

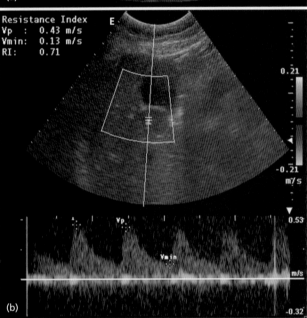

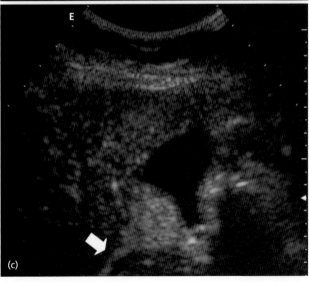

Mass lesions on cirrhotic liver: hepatocellular carcinoma (HCC) and non-malignant nodules

Surveillance programmes for cirrhotic patients have made the US detection of small nodules on cirrhotic liver a frequent event [5], pointing out the problem of differential diagnosis between HCC and nonmalignant macronodules [9]. Arterial hypervascularization is the hallmark of HCC [10] and differentiates it from large regenerative and dysplastic nodules. More recently, contrast medium washout in the portal–late phase has been recognized as a characteristic feature of HCC. The AASLD guideline [11] stated that, in the case of a nodule >2 cm found on US screening of a cirrhotic liver, the detection of both arterial contrast enhancement and venous washout on one imaging technique (out of CE, MRI, and CEUS) is diagnostic for HCC. Two concordant imaging techniques showing this pattern are required if the nodule is 1–2 cm in diameter.

Even if a cirrhotic patient may be affected by any one of the already described lesions, the detection of a nodule on cirrhotic liver should always raise the suspicion of HCC. It presents variable features at conventional US. HCCs <5 cm are usually hypoechoic, while larger lesions are hyperechoic or have a mixed echo-pattern. Nevertheless, up to 20–30% of HCCs <2 cm are hyperechoic.

The aim of Doppler and CEUS is the disclosure of arterial hypervascularization (Fig. 4). Doppler examination shows arterial signals with high peak frequencies and high impedance within or at the periphery of the nodule [7]. CEUS is more sensitive than Doppler US in detecting hypervascularization in small nodules: HCC appears hyperechoic in the early arterial phase and becomes isoechoic or slightly hypoechoic in the portal-late phase due to contrast medium washout [6]. Nonneoplastic nodules are isoechoic in all the phases.

HCC has a strong tendency to infiltrate portal vessels, which appear filled by echoic tissue. The detection of arterial signals within the thrombus at Doppler US or hypervascularization at CEUS confirms the suspicion of neoplastic thrombosis.

Biliary disease

In fasting patients, the gallbladder is distended by anechoic bile, which facilitates the detection of stones and wall abnormalities. The gallbladder wall appears as a single smooth reflective line <2 mm thick.

Gallstones

A stone in the gallbladder appears as a hyperechoic intraluminal structure with posterior acoustic shadowing [12]. Its position is gravity-dependent, so that it moves as the patient changes their decubitus. Changing a patient's position can reveal small stones previously hidden in the gallbladder neck. If the gallbladder is

Fig. 4 (*opposite*) Hepatocellular carcinoma: appearances on
(a) conventional US, (b) Doppler US and (c) CEUS (arterial phase).
Note the feeding artery (arrow) disclosed by CEUS.

scleroatrophic, gallstones appear separated from the gallbladder wall by only a thin hypoechoic rim.

Gravity-dependent echoes lacking distal shadowing within the gallbladder are named biliary sludge or echogenic bile. Aggregations of biliary sludge can mimic a soft-tissue mass. Differential diagnosis is aided by the absence of Doppler signals and by movement of the echoes under gravity.

Acute cholecystitis

The prompt recognition of acute cholecystitis is important due to the recent spread of early cholecystectomy within 72 hours of admission. There is no single absolutely specific US sign for acute cholecystitis [12], but the simultaneous finding of several signs increases US specificity up to 88–94%.

Thickened gallbladder wall is a common finding, but it can be present in several other conditions (i.e. PHT, haematological diseases or physiologically in the postprandial phase). The detection of an echo-poor halo around the gallbladder or focal hypoechoic zones in the wall, both ascribed to oedema, is more specific and is regarded as a major sign of acute cholecystitis. Other major signs are the presence of gallstones (acute cholecystitis is acalculous only in 5–10% of cases, generally related to severe systemic illnesses), the 'ultrasonic Murphy's sign' (compression of the gallbladder fundus by the US transducer elicits pain), and the presence of gas in the gallbladder wall (suggesting emphysematous cholecystitis). Minor signs are gallbladder wall thickening (>4 mm) without oedema, enlargement of the gallbladder, which assumes a rounded shape (transverse diameter >4.5 cm), the presence of pericholecystic fluid or intraluminal nonshadowing echoes related to pus or debris.

Gallbladder polyps and carcinoma

Cholesterol polyps appear as small (few millimetres) hyperechoic masses fixed to the gallbladder wall, without acoustic shadowing.

Gallbladder carcinoma is usually discovered in an advanced stage. In case of early, generally incidental, diagnosis, it appears as an irregular thickening of the gallbladder wall or an inhomogeneous echoic mass that partly or almost totally fills the lumen. In more advanced stages the gallbladder is hardly recognizable and a solid mass is instead visualized in the gallbladder fossa. The presence of stones within the mass facilitates the diagnosis [12].

Bile duct dilatation

US is essential in the diagnostic workup of jaundice as it promptly recognizes bile duct dilatation, the hallmark of obstructive jaundice, and can reveal the cause of obstruction (e.g. a mass at the porta hepatis, a stone within the common bile duct or a pancreatic neoplasm).

When investigating the common bile duct, it should be considered that its diameter increases with age (the upper normal value in millimetres is equal to the patient's decades of life) and after cholecystectomy.

Intrahepatic bile ducts are normally too small to be visualized. When dilated, they appear as anechoic tubular structures running adjacent to portal vein branches. This is known as the 'parallel channel sign'. Dilated bile ducts can be distinguished from vessels as they do not display flow at Doppler examination and converge towards the porta hepatis with a stellate pattern (whereas portal vessels present a branching pattern).

Liver transplant

US examination is useful both in the preoperative assessment of candidates for orthotopic liver transplantation (OLT) and in the postoperative follow-up.

Preoperative assessment

Firstly, US examination can confirm the indication for OLT by showing signs of endstage liver disease and PHT, fulminant hepatitis, or Budd–Chiari syndrome. The detection and staging of HCC is particularly important, as it should not exceed the accepted transplantation criteria, and many transplant centres grant a priority in the waiting list in case of HCC. Vascular and biliary invasion must be ruled out, as they are absolute contraindications to OLT. US also provides a guide for percutaneous treatments to prevent tumour growth beyond transplantation criteria.

Another important task of US examination is to assess portal vein patency. In case of portal occlusion, vascular anastomosis can be accomplished onto the superior mesenteric vein; if this vessel is also obstructed, OLT is not feasible according to the classical procedure and most centres reject such candidates.

Finally, the presence of wide portosystemic collaterals, especially splenorenal shunts, has to be assessed, because they can dramatically decrease portal perfusion after OLT.

Postoperative follow-up

The aim of post-transplantation US follow-up is the prompt recognition of vascular and biliary complications [13]. Moreover, US shows the disappearance of many haemodynamic alterations observed in decompensated cirrhosis [14]. Portal vein flow velocity and renal and splenic impedance return to normal. Spleen size decreases but generally does not return to normal values. Collateral vessels persist long after OLT.

Early arterial occlusion is the most frequent and threatening vascular complication [15], as it causes massive hepatic necrosis. Right and left intrahepatic branches of the hepatic artery and, if possible, the extrahepatic artery should be investigated with colour Doppler and spectral analysis. Failure to identify arterial signals requires urgent angiography to confirm the occlusion. A dampened spectrum with very low velocity flow and increased time between the beginning of systole and systolic peak (known as 'tardus-parvus' profile) is suspicious for either thrombosis or critical upstream stenosis. Angiography is advised to confirm the diagnosis, and eventually percutaneous angioplasty can be performed. US can show further complications caused by ischaemic damage, such as intrahepatic abscess and biliary leaks or strictures. Biliary strictures are disclosed by the presence of bile duct dilatations.

The portal vein should be studied to exclude portal thrombosis or significant anastomotic stenosis, which causes a focal flow acceleration. The portal vein flow velocity is typically increased over the normal value in the first month after OLT [14]. It subsequently decreases to normal levels.

The classical surgical procedure for OLT includes resection of the recipient's retrohepatic IVC and double anastomosis with the donor's vena cava. In the case of superior anastomosis stenosis, a focal flow acceleration is observed and hepatic vein flow is flattened.

Piggy-back OLT is a technical variant that preserves the recipient's IVC. An anastomotic stenosis or kinking causes an obstacle to outflow through hepatic veins; in this case Doppler US will disclose accelerated and turbulent flow through piggy-back anastomosis.

There are no reliable conventional and Doppler US signs related to acute or chronic rejection.

References

1 Albrecht T, Blomley M, Bolandi L et al. (2004) Guidelines for the use of contrast agents in ultrasound. *Ultrashall Med* 25, 249–256.

2 Tchelepi H, Ralls PW, Radin R et al. (2002) Sonography of diffuse liver disease. *J Ultrasound Med* 21, 1023–1032.

3 Gaiani S, Gramantieri L, Venturoli N et al. (1997) What is the criterion for differentiating chronic hepatitis from compensated cirrhosis? A prospective study comparing ultrasonography and percutaneous liver biopsy. *J Hepatol* 27, 979–985.

4 Piscaglia F, Donati G, Serra C et al. (2001) Value of splanchnic Doppler ultrasound in the diagnosis of portal hypertension. *Ultrasound Med Biol* 27, 893–899.

5 Bolondi L, Sofia S, Siringo S et al. (2001) Surveillance programme of cirrhotic patients for early diagnosis and treatment of hepatocellular carcinoma: a cost-effectiveness analysis. *Gut* 48, 251–259.

6 Von Herbay A (2004) Real-time imaging with the sonographic contrast agent SonoVue. *J Ultrasound Med* 23, 1557–1568.

7 Gaiani S, Volpe L, Piscaglia F et al. (2001) Vascularity of liver tumors and recent advances in Doppler ultrasound. *J Hepatol* 34, 474–482.

8 Hohmann J, Albrecht T, Oldenburg A et al. (2004) Liver metastases in cancer: detection with contrast-enhanced ultrasonography. *Abdom Imaging* 29, 669–681.

9 Bolondi L, Gaiani S, Selli N et al. (2005) Characterization of small nodules in cirrhosis by assessment of vascularity. The problem of hypovascular hepatocellular carcinoma. *Hepatology* 42, 27–34.

10 Bruix J, Sherman M, Liovet JM et al. (2001) Clinical management of hepatocellular carcinoma. Conclusions of the Barcelona-2000 EASL conference. *J Hepatol* 35, 421–430.

11 Bruix J, Sherman M (2005) Management of hepatocellular carcinoma. *Hepatology* 42, 1208–1236.

12 Gandolfi L, Torresan F, Solmi L et al. (2003) The role of ultrasound in biliary and pancreatic diseases. *Eur J Ultrasound* 16, 141–159.

13 Kok T, Slooff MJ, Thijn CJ et al. (1998) Routine Doppler ultrasound for the detection of clinically unsuspected vascular complications in the early postoperative phase after orthotopic liver transplantation. *Transpl Int* 11, 272–276.

14 Piscaglia F, Zironi G, Gaiani S et al. (1999) Systemic and splanchnic hemodynamic changes after liver transplantation for cirrhosis: a long-term prospective study. *Hepatology* 30, 58–64.

15 De Gaetano AM, Cotroneo AR, Maresca G et al. (2000) Colour Doppler sonography in the diagnosis and monitoring of arterial complications after liver transplantation. *J Clin Ultrasound* 28, 373–380.

5.6.2 Computerized tomography imaging of the liver

Daniel T. Cohen and Dushyant V. Sahani

The exponential advance in computerized tomography (CT) imaging technology over the last decade, arguably, has been faster than improvements in any other imaging modality. The pixelated single-slice axial images from the first CT scanner in 1972 have progressed to 64-detector helical scanners with true isotropic resolution [1]. More importantly, CT is also the temporally fastest modality with cross-sectional capabilities (compared with ultrasound or magnetic resonance imaging). The addition of multiphase contrast enhancement to CT allows superior lesion characterization compared with non-contrast ultrasound. Although magnetic resonance imaging (MRI) may provide superior contrast resolution and tissue characterization capabilities even compared with CT, MRI remains a 'problem-solving' modality because of its high cost and long imaging times. The combination of ready availability, speed and high spatial resolution with three-dimensional capabilities has made CT imaging the *de facto* workhorse of liver imaging.

The indications for CT imaging of the hepatobiliary system can be classified as either targeted or non-targeted and incidental. For example, if a patient has a known hepatoma, CT may be performed for targeted liver evaluation and assessment of tumour size and multiplicity. Alternatively, if a patient presents to the emergency department with episodic right upper quadrant-flank pain and suspected renal colic, a CT scan may be performed for evaluation of the abdominal pelvic urinary tract. This examination will also necessarily image the liver and potentially discover incidental hepatic pathology (Fig. 1). This latter example represents non-targeted, or incidental, imaging of the liver. This distinction is not merely 'academic'. With the marked advances in CT technology, the CT protocol and the technical parameters of an individual examination can vary dramatically depending on indication. In this way, the clinical history provided at the time of imaging can significantly alter the CT protocol and the technical parameters that must be optimized to answer the clinical question.

As illustrated by the thickness of this entire volume, the pathophysiology of the liver is both broad and complex. Most of these hepatic conditions are amenable to radiological imaging,

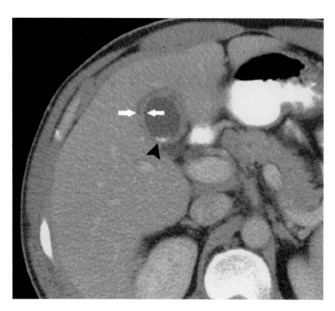

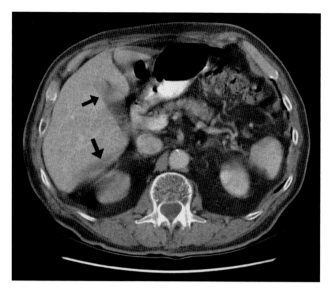

Fig. 1 Contrast-enhanced axial computerized tomography (CT) image. Arrowhead denotes hyperdense (white) calcified gallstones layering in the gallbladder. Gallbladder wall thickening is denoted by the white arrows. Pericholecystic low-density fluid is also present.

Fig. 2 Contrast-enhanced axial CT image degraded by respiratory motion. Black arrows denote blurring of the liver edges caused by liver motion secondary to diaphragmatic movement. In contrast, the vertebral body, which does not move during respiration, shows crisp edges.

frequently with CT. A comprehensive discussion of computerized tomography imaging techniques, protocols, normal variant and pathological imaging is beyond the scope of this chapter. This chapter will introduce several key concepts of CT technology and technique so that the non-imaging clinician can appreciate the benefits and limitations of a CT examination when utilizing hepatic CT imaging as part of clinical care. CT imaging can not only detect many hepatic abnormalities but also often characterize them into benign or malignant aetiologies. The latest generation of multidetector CT also provides angiographic quality assessment of the hepatic vasculature. In addition to presenting classic examples of benign lesions that can be confidently characterized by hepatic CT imaging, this chapter will also focus on detection and characterization of hepatocellular carcinoma (hepatoma) and hepatic metastases. Common hepatic metastases frequently present with either hypervascular or hypo-enhancing characteristics and thus require different imaging techniques.

CT imaging technique

At the basic level, computerized tomography still relies on the physical principles that govern plain radiography, the attenuation of an X-ray beam by the relative density differences within a patient. However, CT imaging has the marked advantage of cross-sectional depiction of the body. Early-generation scanners would generate 'thick slices'; each CT image represented a relatively large amount of body tissue and often appeared coarse [1]. Long imaging times made the images susceptible to motion; respiratory movements would frequently cause significant blurring of the liver (Fig. 2). Current scanners have multiple detector

elements acquiring X-rays simultaneously (detector numbers range from 4 to 64). Additionally, all multidetector computerized tomography (MDCT) scanners also operate with a helical motion; this allows rapid overlapping coverage of the patient. Improvements in hardware and software capabilities have led to dramatic reductions in imaging times. During a patient's breath hold, the liver can be imaged multiple times (approximately 5–10 s per pass) allowing multiphase contrast imaging. This spatial resolution and rapid imaging speed must be coupled with intravenous (i.v.) contrast to allow appropriate opacification of and distinction between hepatic arteries, portal and hepatic veins, and the hepatic parenchyma; this is known as 'contrast resolution'. Intravenous contrast is unambiguously required for the detection and characterization of nearly all hepatic lesions.

Iodinated i.v. contrast is categorized based on its osmolarity relative to plasma. Most radiology departments utilize low osmolar or iso-osmolar contrast agents because of the reduced risk of allergic reaction and contrast-induced nephropathy [2]. For dedicated liver imaging, the i.v. contrast must be injected at a rapid rate to allow for separate imaging of the hepatic arteries without portal venous opacification on the initial series. With an injection of the standard 150 mL at a rate of approximately 2 mL/s and a modern MDCT, this hepatic arterial phase (HAP) occurs at approximately 30 s after the end of bolus injection. At approximately 60–70 s, there is peak opacification of the portal veins, hepatic veins and interposed liver parenchyma; this is the portal-venous phase (PVP). At longer time intervals, often 2 min, 'delayed' phase images can be obtained that represent additional recirculation of the intravascular i.v. contrast and more homogeneous opacification of the liver parenchyma. This sequence of arterial, portal-venous and delayed phase series constitutes the 'triple phase' protocol liver CT (see Figs 11 and 19). An unenhanced series of the liver before contrast injection may demonstrate calcification or acute haemorrhage, which are hyperdense relative to the unopacified liver. The diagnostic role of these multiple phases will be discussed in the following sections as they apply to hepatic pathology detection and characterization.

The high spatial resolution of MDCT imaging allows for isotropic data sets; imaging resolution is nearly equivalent in all directions. The images can be presented in any coordinate system (sagittal, coronal and three-dimensional re-formations) in addition to the traditional axial image sets. CT angiography with three-dimensional (3-D) re-formations now replaces diagnostic catheter angiography in many institutions. With arterial phase imaging, the aorto-coeliac-hepatic arterial tree can be optimally opacified without venous contamination. Three-dimensional manipulation can present these data in various forms to aid surgeons in preoperative planning. The relationship of intrahepatic tumours to major vascular structures can be easily visualized in multiple planes (Figs 3 and 4). Additional 3-D techniques include surface and volume rendering for assessment of relative hepatic lobar volumes (Fig. 5). MDCT with multiphase imaging and 3-D data reconstruction provides comprehensive presurgical imaging for living related liver donors and hepatic tumour patients assessed for partial hepatectomy [3,4].

Continued dramatic improvements in CT technology are expected. CT perfusion, a technique pioneered in cerebral imaging of occlusive stroke patients, can also be utilized to assess any pathological state that causes alterations in liver parenchyma vascularity. In the future, CT perfusion will probably play a role in assessing tumour treatment therapy by monitoring changes in tumour neovascularity [5].

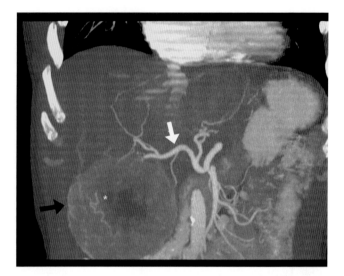

Fig. 4 Coronal maximum intensity projection from MDCT axial data. Black arrow denotes a large metastatic (colon cancer) lesion in the inferior right liver lobe. The relationship of the tumour to the hepatic artery (white arrow) is clearly seen. Prominent tumour neovascularity is also identified (asterisk).

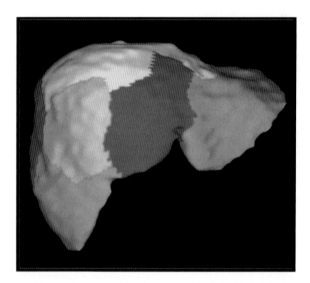

Fig. 5 Three-dimensional volume render of MDCT axial data, originally with colour coding of liver volumes. Subtle surface nodularity can be seen suggesting cirrhosis.

Normal hepatic anatomy

The unenhanced liver demonstrates intermediate density compared with other soft tissues of the body, between 50 and 75 Hounsfield units. (A Hounsfield unit, HU, is the standard CT measurement of density ranging from −1000 to 1000, with water measuring 0 HU and cortical bone approximately 300 HU.) The normal liver density closely matches the spleen. This liver–spleen relationship can provide a qualitative reference standard for assessing diffuse hepatic parenchymal changes on an unenhanced CT. The major vascular structures are hypodense to the

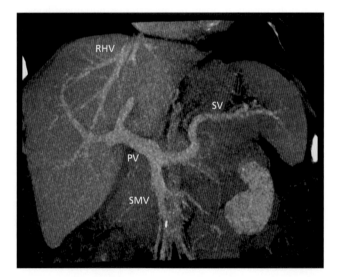

Fig. 3 Coronal maximum intensity projection from MDCT axial data demonstrates the portal–venous system. RHV, right hepatic vein; PV, portal vein; SMV, superior mesenteric vein; SV, splenic vein.

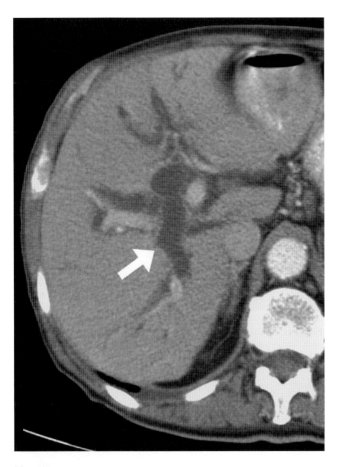

(a)

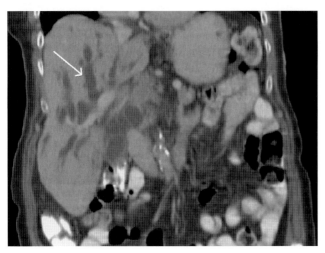

(b)

Fig. 6 (a) Contrast-enhanced axial CT image. (b) Coronal maximum intensity projection from MDCT axial data. Arrows denote low-density dilated intrahepatic biliary ducts adjacent to contrast-enhanced portal veins. Biliary dilatation was secondary to a pancreatic head mass (not pictured).

normal unenhanced liver. On contrast injection, the common hepatic artery (HA) and its major branches can be identified as they ramify into the liver. Peak HA enhancement occurs around 30 s after standard contrast injection, the HA phase. Variant hepatic arterial branches, such as a replaced right hepatic artery from the coeliac artery, are easily identified, especially with 3-D re-formations. Portal venous (PV) and hepatic venous (HV) opacification is less pronounced than HA and peaks at around 70 s, the PV phase. Seventy per cent of liver blood flow is via the portal venous system. In this way, liver parenchyma enhancement is maximized when PV and HV enhancement is optimal. Thus, the PV phase is the default imaging time for most liver and general abdominal pelvic imaging indications. The main portal and hepatic veins are key landmarks in localizing a hepatic lesion according to the eight Couinaud segments (Figs 3–5).

Computerized tomography provides an excellent rapid assessment of the biliary tree including the gallbladder. The density of bile is low, approximately 0–20 HU. Biliary dilatation, intra- or extrahepatic, is easily seen and measured especially following contrast administration (Fig. 6). Often, CT will identify the aetiology of biliary obstruction as well. Many of the classic ultrasound 'signs' of acute cholecystitis can be assessed with MDCT including gallbladder wall thickening, pericholecystic fluid and radio-opaque gallstones (Fig. 1). Nevertheless, rapid acquisition time and large field of view allow CT to rival ultrasound (US) in cholecystitis assessment, especially in an uncooperative, obtunded or obese patient.

Diffuse hepatic disease

Diffuse, or non-focal, hepatic disease must induce gross, detectable morphological change in order to be successfully diagnosed or monitored by CT. Along with the rise in body mass index in western society, there has been a similar rise in the frequency of steatohepatitis [6]. Steatohepatitis, or 'fatty liver', is also seen with alcohol and medication use. From a CT imaging perspective, the aetiology is rarely apparent. On an unenhanced examination, the liver with steatohepatitis will demonstrate lower density compared with the 'internal standard', the spleen (a >10 HU difference) [7]. Qualitatively, if there is sufficient fatty infiltration, the liver parenchyma will appear less dense than the blood vessels, mimicking contrast enhancement (Fig. 7). Fatty infiltration of the liver can also present as focal geographic areas of hypodensity, particularly adjacent to the falciform ligament and gallbladder fossa (Fig. 8). Conversely, when there is a background of steatohepatitis, these same areas can demonstrate relative absence of the fatty infiltration and will appear relatively hyperdense compared with the remainder of the liver. This is termed 'focal fatty sparing'. The location, geographical nature and absence of mass effect are often nearly diagnostic for these 'inverse' entities. Magnetic resonance with fat saturation techniques can provide the most definitive non-invasive imaging of steatohepatitis as well as focal fatty infiltration and sparing.

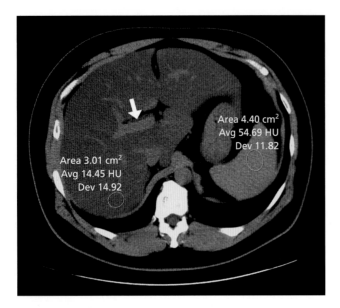

Area 4.40 cm²
Avg 54.69 HU
Dev 11.82

Area 3.01 cm²
Avg 14.45 HU
Dev 14.92

Fig. 7 Unenhanced axial CT image. Qualitatively, the liver is less dense compared with the spleen. Quantitatively, the liver measures 14 HU compared with 55 HU of the spleen consistent with diffuse fatty infiltration. Hepatic vasculature appears dense (arrow) mimicking contrast enhancement.

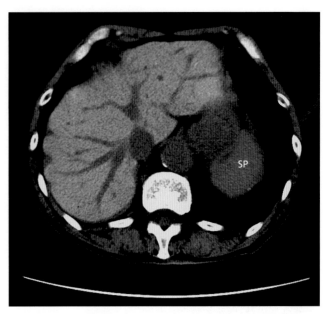

SP

Fig. 9 Unenhanced axial CT image. In this patient with long-term amiodarone use, the liver parenchyma demonstrates marked hyperdensity compared with the superior portion of the spleen (SP).

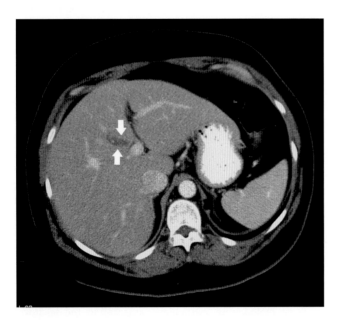

Fig. 8 Contrast-enhanced axial CT image. Focal area of hypodensity (arrows) adjacent to falciform ligament and portal vein is consistent with focal fatty infiltration.

Acute and chronic hepatitis, regardless of aetiology, can often be undetectable by CT. When the hepatitis is fulminant in severity, the liver may demonstrate overall decreased density with the influx of excess oedema water into the hepatic extra-cellular space. Accompanying periportal oedema may present as a low-density halo surrounding the portal venous tributaries.

Generalized, upper abdominal ascites may be present and is reactive in nature.

Most common diffuse hepatic parenchymal diseases present on CT as hepatic hypodensity. In contrast, the relatively short differential diagnosis for diffuse increased hepatic density includes haemochromatosis, Gaucher's disease, Wilson's disease and amiodarone toxicity (Fig. 9). Haemochromatosis represents abnormal accumulation of iron in the hepatocytes. This dense metal raises the native liver density to greater than 75 HU on an unenhanced scan and is the 'inverse' of steatohepatitis; the liver appears markedly denser than the spleen. In Gaucher's disease, secondary to glucocerebrosidase deficiency, abnormal accumulation of ceramide in reticuloendothelial cells raises the liver density, and hepatomegaly and splenomegaly will also be present. Focal hypodense lesions typically represent infarcts. When there is hepatic involvement, the myriad glycogen storage diseases can increase hepatic CT density. In Wilson's disease, abnormal copper accumulation leads to hyperdensity. Finally, long-term amiodarone use can lead to increased iodine deposition in hepatocytes with resultant diffuse hepatic CT hyperdensity [8]. In comparison with the other aetiologies for hyperdense liver parenchyma, amiodarone does not generally lead to gross morphological changes in the liver [9].

Benign focal liver lesions

'Non-targeted' contrast-enhanced imaging of the abdomen is routinely performed during the portal–venous phase of contrast enhancement. This PVP provides homogeneous enhancement

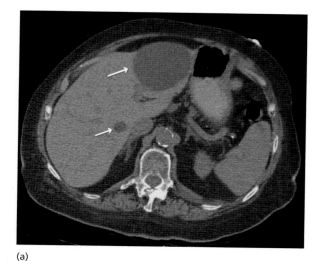

(a)

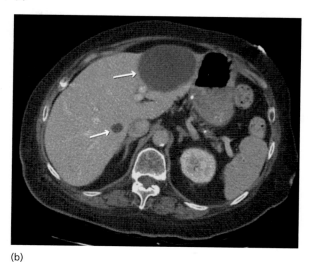

(b)

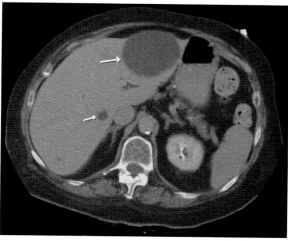

(c)

of the liver, the other abdominal parenchymal organs and the bowel wall. Although this phase of enhancement is generally sensitive for both liver and extrahepatic pathology, it often lacks specificity. Many radiologists will recommend 'targeted' multi-phase hepatic CT imaging for further characterization despite adequate visualization of a lesion with portal venous CT imaging. The addition of non-contrast, arterial and delayed phase imaging can often triage a lesion between benign, malignant and indeterminate aetiologies.

Hepatic cysts are frequent incidental findings on CT. With low-density appearance (<20 HU), they appear as well-circumscribed, homogeneous masses without enhancement. Delayed phase imaging is necessary to ensure the absence of late enhancement, which suggests a solid internal structure (Fig. 10). Small cysts may appear to have higher density because of partial volume averaging with denser adjacent liver parenchyma; often, these small lesions may be too small to characterize by any imaging modality (CT, MR or US). If clinically relevant, watchful waiting and repeat imaging may be the only option. Unlike renal cyst classification, the presence of septations generally does not predict a higher risk of malignancy. However, some infectious aetiologies can present with septated cystic lesions, for example echinococcal hydatid cyst. Patients with polycystic syndromes may demonstrate dramatic macroscopic replacement of the liver with cysts with amazingly preserved hepatic function [10].

The rapid imaging speed of modern CT scanners now allows confident diagnosis of most hepatic haemangiomas by multi-phase contrast-enhanced imaging. Cavernous haemangiomas are the most common liver tumour and frequently are incidental findings on both 'targeted' hepatic CT and 'non-targeted' abdominal pelvic CT. Haemangiomas appear as well-circumscribed lesions that are hypodense to surrounding unenhanced liver and may appear similar to benign cysts. Calcification within a haemangioma is unusual and can have a myriad of appearances [11]. Cavernous haemangiomas have a typical enhancement pattern (on both CT and MR), which allows confident diagnosis by imaging. On arterial phase imaging, the haemangiomas demonstrate peripheral, but discontinuous, nodular enhancement. There is progressive centripetal contrast filling of the entire lesion on the PV and delayed phases of contrast imaging. This 'fill-in' combined with nodular enhancement is considered pathognomonic for a typical cavernous haemangioma (Fig. 11). The discontinuous nodularity of haemangiomas allows for confident distinction between this benign lesion and hepatic metastasis, which can demonstrate a continuous peripheral rim of enhancement and also delayed homogeneous enhancement,

Fig. 10 (*opposite*) (a) Non-contrast axial CT image. (b) Portal–venous phase contrast-enhanced axial CT image. (c) Delayed phase contrast-enhanced axial CT image. Hepatic cysts (arrows) are low density on non-contrast imaging and show no evidence of vascular enhancement on contrast administration. Delayed imaging confirms absence of late tumour enhancement.

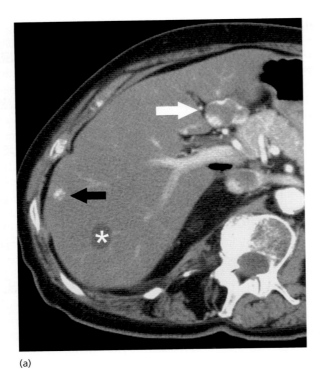

(a)

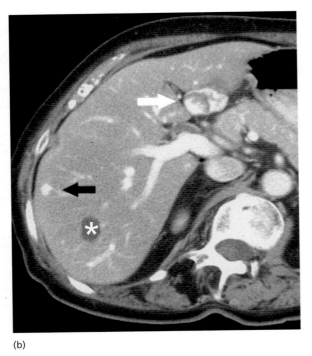

(b)

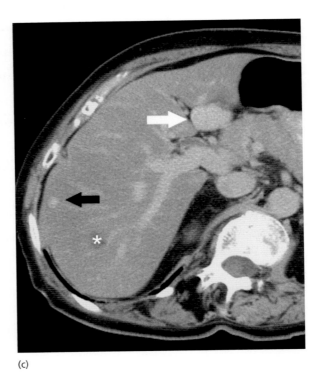

(c)

Fig. 11 (a) Hepatic arterial phase (HAP) contrast-enhanced axial CT image. (b) Portal–venous phase (PVP) contrast-enhanced axial CT image. (c) Delayed phase contrast-enhanced axial CT image. Classic haemangioma (white arrow) demonstrates characteristic peripheral nodular appearance on arterial phase, with progressive central fill on PVP and homogeneous enhancement on delayed phase (c). A small right liver lobe enhancing focus (black arrow) is also probably a small haemangioma but is too small to characterize by imaging and is without the classic peripheral nodular enhancement. A non-enhancing cyst is seen (asterisk).

or 'fill', of the lesion. Qualitatively, the degree of vascular enhancement within the haemangioma characteristically matches that of the aorta. In the early arterial phase, the peripheral nodular areas demonstrate intense arterial enhancement. During the portal–venous phase, the 'fill' of the haemangioma is slightly less intense, matching both the portal vein and the aorta density.

Small haemangiomas will frequently show intense and uniform enhancement during the arterial phase and persistent homogeneous density during the PV phase [12]. Unfortunately, without the classic peripheral nodular enhancement, these small haemangiomas may be confused with other hypervascular liver tumours such as hepatoma, focal nodular hyperplasia, adenoma and hypervascular metastases (Fig. 11). In these cases, the absence of a history of cirrhosis or primary malignancy is an important factor in suggesting haemangioma, and short-interval follow-up imaging documenting stability in size may obviate the need for invasive biopsy. The relatively rare giant haemangioma generally measures >5 cm. Giant haemangiomas will often show atypical enhancement patterns such as persistent central hypodense areas even on delayed phases and may show central calcification (Fig. 12). Capsular retraction secondary to haemangioma is possible, although this feature generally suggests a malignant lesion [13].

Focal nodular hyperplasia (FNH), a benign entity without malignant potential, is the second most common tumour of the

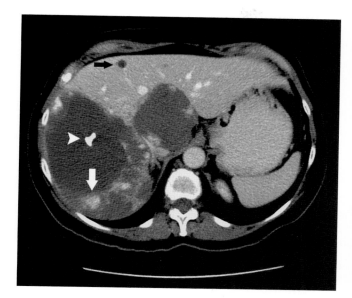

Fig. 12 Contrast-enhanced axial CT image. The giant haemangioma of the right liver lobe demonstrates some areas of peripheral nodular enhancement (white arrow). There is central tumour calcification (arrowhead). An incidental non-enhancing cyst is seen (black arrow).

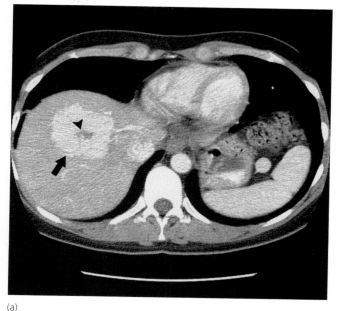

(a)

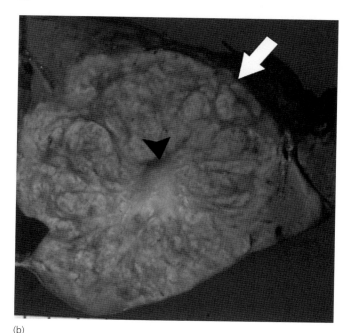

(b)

Fig. 13 (a) Contrast-enhanced axial CT image. Right liver lobe focal nodular hyperplasia (arrow) demonstrates classic peripheral enhancement with hypodense central scar (arrowhead). (b) Photograph from gross resection. Pathological findings mimic the CT imaging appearance: white arrow denotes tumour edge and black arrowhead shows the pearly white fibrosis of central scar region.

liver, generally asymptomatic and usually found incidentally as a solitary lesion. The classic distinguishing feature of FNH, both radiologically and pathologically, is the presence of a central scar of fibrous tissue (Fig. 13). On non-contrast examination, FNH is hypodense or isodense and may show occasional mass effect and lobulated contours. On multiphase contrast enhancement (Fig. 14), the classic FNH shows transient intense enhancement of the lesion during the arterial phase with rapid change to isodensity of the lesion during PV and delayed phases [14]. In this way, the lesion can easily be obscured by surrounding hepatic parenchyma if an arterial phase series is not performed. The key to characterization lies in identifying the central scar, which will be hypodense on arterial phase with progressive enhancement until the scar becomes hyperdense compared with the surrounding lesion and liver on delayed phase. When possible, classic FNH lesions should be characterized by triple-phase contrast imaging so as to avoid unnecessary biopsy and follow-up imaging. Atypical FNH may be larger than classic FNH or present as multiple lesions. An atypical FNH may show less arterial enhancement, absence of a central scar and the presence of an enhancing pseudocapsule. In these situations, a broader differential diagnosis must be considered and biopsy or excision may be indicated.

Hepatic adenomas are rare liver tumours composed of atypical hepatocytes (without bile ducts or Kupffer cells as seen in FNH). With a strong association with oral contraceptives, anabolic steroids and glycogen storage diseases, adenomas are most often found in young women. Large adenomas may cause symptoms secondary to mass effect. Clinically, adenomas carry a risk of spontaneous intraperitoneal haemorrhage with hypo-

volaemic shock. Intratumoral haemorrhage can cause acute right upper quadrant pain. Adenomas, even those stable over many years, may degenerate into hepatocellular carcinoma [15]. Adenomas are usually 5–10 cm in diameter and present as hypodense or isodense lesions on non-contrast imaging. An adenoma

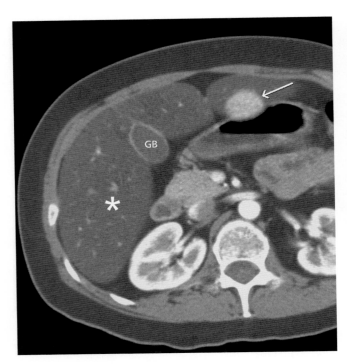

Fig. 14 Portal–venous phase contrast-enhanced axial CT image. Homogeneous enhancement of the left liver lobe hepatic adenoma (arrow) appears more prominent because of the background diffuse fatty infiltration of the liver (asterisk). The density of this liver is so low as to match the low-density bile seen in the gallbladder (GB).

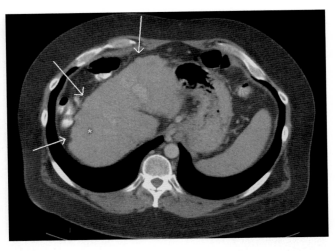

Fig. 15 Contrast-enhanced axial CT image. Liver surface nodularity (arrows) consistent with cirrhosis is easily seen. Incidental non-enhancing cyst is noted (asterisk).

is generally well circumscribed because of the presence of a capsule. Prior haemorrhage may show focal areas of precontrast hyperdensity. During the arterial phase of contrast imaging and owing to subcapsular feeding arterioles, there may be peripheral intense enhancement with centripetal 'fill' of contrast. Unlike haemangiomas, this peripheral enhancement is not nodular in character. Because the adenomas are composed of hepatocytes, they subsequently match the surrounding liver enhancement on portal–venous and delayed phases. As with FNH, larger adenomas can give atypical presentations leading to diagnostic uncertainty. Because of the overlap of imaging characteristics between adenoma, fibrolamellar hepatoma, atypical FNH and hypervascular metastasis, most lesions will eventually require percutaneous biopsy or excision.

Cysts, haemangioma, FNH and adenoma account for a large portion of the benign focal lesions that will be encountered either incidentally or on targeted liver imaging. The clinical history will often dictate the appropriate differential diagnosis; for example, multiple hypodense lesions in a febrile immunocompromised patient will add abscess to the list of possibilities. Magnetic resonance imaging, with improved contrast resolution compared with CT, will occasionally provide additional characterization of lesions that are indeterminate by CT. Finally, the morbidity associated with image-guided focal liver biopsy is generally low and, on occasion, definitive characterization may require a pathologist.

Cirrhosis, nodular hyperplasia and hepatocellular carcinoma

The anatomical resolution of MDCT is well suited to diagnosing the three main pathological characteristics of moderately advanced cirrhosis: fibrosis, nodular regeneration and hepatic architecture distortion [16]. Classic segmental lobar hypertrophy and atrophy can be easily appreciated; in fact, 3-D re-formations can provide accurate hepatic volume measurements (Fig. 5). A caudate to right lobe ratio >0.65 is suggestive of cirrhosis. The liver surface appears irregular and nodular (Fig. 15). The wide field of view afforded by MDCT will illustrate many of the secondary changes of cirrhosis and portal hypertension including portosystemic collateral varices, splenomegaly and ascites (Figs 16–18). Additionally, multiphase MDCT, particularly with thin-section series, can confidently diagnose portal vein thrombosis, a common and unfortunate complication of portal hypertension and cirrhosis [17]. Hepatic fibrosis and architectural distortion lead to alterations in hepatic perfusion, which can be seen as geographical, segmental and focal areas of either hyperperfusion/enhancement or hypoperfusion/hypodensity on contrast administration. These perfusion abnormalities, often in the absence of an underlying focal lesion, can create diagnostic uncertainty when searching for arterially enhancing hepatomas.

The two main types of cirrhosis, chronic sclerosing and nodular, demonstrate different morphological and, thus, CT appearances. In the former, the liver is small with minimal regenerative hepatocyte activity. In nodular cirrhosis, the liver may hypertrophy as a result of the innumerable small regenerating nodules or larger macronodules. The nodules represent foci of hypertrophied liver parenchyma surrounded by areas of fibrosis. Siderotic, iron-containing, regenerative nodules may be noted as hyperdense areas on the non-contrast examination. Macroregenerating nodules (>3 mm in size) may be visualized

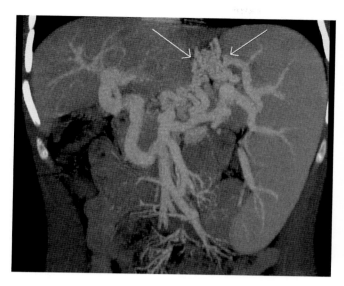

Fig. 16 Coronal maximum intensity projection from MDCT axial data. Arrows denote the prominent and tortuous gastrosplenic varices resulting from portal hypertension. Massive splenomegaly is also present.

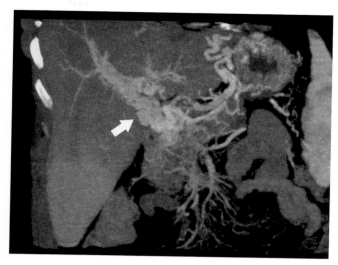

Fig. 18 Coronal maximum intensity projection from MDCT axial data. Arrow denotes the prominent and tortuous portal vein radicals resulting from portal hypertension and cavernous transformation of the hepatic hilum.

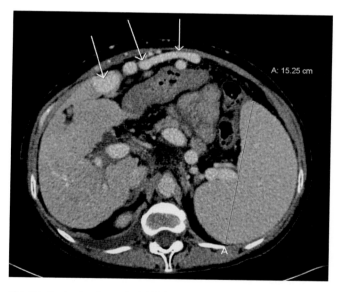

Fig. 17 Contrast-enhanced axial CT image. A recanalized umbilical vein is present secondary to liver cirrhosis and portal hypertension (arrows). Splenomegaly at 15 cm is noted.

by distortion of the liver capsule or intrahepatic vasculature (Fig. 15). However, the enhancement of regenerating nodules mimics that of the surrounding fibrotic liver and these nodules do not show arterial hyperenhancement. Thus, small regenerating nodules are rarely confidently diagnosed by MDCT, even with multiphase imaging [18].

Dysplastic nodules differ from regenerating nodules by the presence of cellular atypia and non-triadal arterial vessels [19]. Despite this increased arterialization on imaging, many dysplastic nodules do not show discernible arterial enhancement above the baseline surrounding liver parenchyma and otherwise match hepatic density on other phases. Thus, as with regenerating nodules, most dysplastic nodules cannot be distinguished from the cirrhotic liver background with MDCT. Comparatively, magnetic resonance offers superior hepatocellular nodular detection through utilization of multiple pulse sequences (e.g. T1- and T2-weighted series) in addition to similar i.v. contrast multiphase imaging with gadolinium enhancement. Unfortunately, a minority of small dysplastic nodules may show a mild degree of arterial enhancement similar to hepatocellular carcinoma [20].

When the arterial–portal venous perfusion ratio shifts even further away from portal flow, multiphase MDCT can detect the arterial neovascularization that is characteristic of classic hepatocellular carcinoma (HCC) (Fig. 19). With the majority of blood flow to the HCC from hepatic artery radicals, these, now frankly malignant, lesions classically demonstrate marked arterial enhancement compared with the cirrhotic liver background. On portal–venous phase, the HCC will be hyperdense – or isodense to the liver – and is frequently hypodense on delayed phase. This transition from hyper- to hypoenhancement has been called 'washout'. More than 90% of HCC lesions will show this arterial enhancement and approximatley three-quarters will demonstrate contrast 'washout' [21]. Whether employing CT or MR imaging for the detection of HCC, a rapid contrast bolus injection and fast imaging speed are necessary to confidently detect the HCC arterial blush. About 15% of HCCs will also demonstrate an enhancing capsular lesion; in some cases, this capsule may help to distinguish HCC from FNH, which is usually without a capsule. These 'classic' imaging characteristics apply more frequently to small HCC foci (<1.5 cm). As the

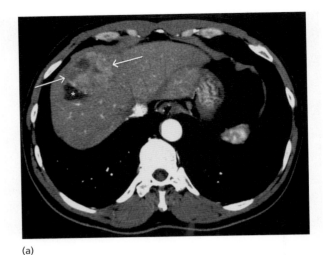

(a)

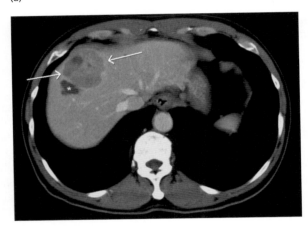

(b)

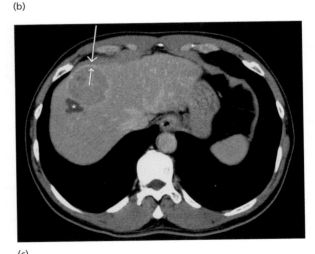

(c)

Fig. 19 (a) Hepatic arterial phase (HAP) contrast-enhanced axial CT image. (b) Portal–venous phase (PVP) contrast-enhanced axial CT image. (c) Delayed phase contrast-enhanced axial CT image. The hepatocellular carcinoma (HCC; arrows) shows arterial enhancement (a, HAP) and is isodense on PVP (b). The HCC is hypodense relative to the surrounding liver on delayed phase but shows delayed enhancement of its capsule (arrows). Incidental non-enhancing cyst is noted (asterisk).

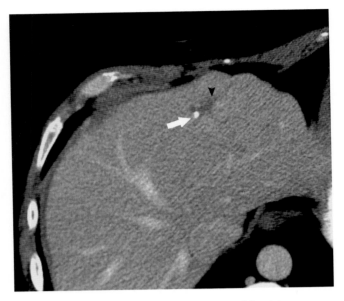

Fig. 20 Contrast-enhanced axial CT image. A small left liver lobe fibrolamellar HCC is seen. The central scar is hypodense (arrowhead) and internal calcification is present (white arrow).

lesions grow in size, 'non-classic' features such as mosaic patterns of enhancement as well as central necrosis may be seen. Diffuse infiltration by HCC may be difficult to detect on a background of cirrhotic fibrosis with altered hepatic perfusion. Calcification is also present in about 25% of HCC lesions with an increased frequency (40%) in the fibrolamellar subtype. Fibrolamellar HCC typically presents in a younger and non-cirrhotic patient population as a lobulated heterogeneous mass with a central scar (Fig. 20). Other hepatic lesions with scar must also be considered in the differential diagnosis, as discussed previously. MR may be an adjuvant modality to differentiate these possibilities.

Despite optimization of modern contrast-enhanced MDCT techniques, CT studies with pathological correlation in transplant patients demonstrate an overall sensitivity of approximately 65% for the presence of HCC and approximately 40% for the total number of lesions [18]. It is clinically important to identify and characterize these focal lesions as accurately as possible. Outcomes from treatment of small HCC lesions are superior to larger, more conspicuous lesions. The Milan criteria, discussed in Section 23, govern a patient's ranking on the US United Network for Organ Sharing (UNOS) transplantation lists. The presence, size and number of HCC lesions can both elevate a patient's rank and also disqualify a patient from transplant. MDCT can accurately screen the post-transplant patient for disease recurrence and transplant complication.

Hepatic metastasis

Metastatic disease is the most common neoplasm in the adult liver and is the second most common focal liver lesion following hepatic cysts. The liver may be the only metastatic site in some colorectal carcinomas, HCC and neuroendocrine tumours. Most metastases (~70%) present as multiple foci in both lobes with only approximately 10% as single foci [22]. They are generally iso- or hypodense to the surrounding liver in the non-contrast, arterial and portal–venous phases. A peripheral, complete ring of arterial enhancement may be seen. During the PV phase, a slightly thicker rind of enhancement can be noted; but this rind is still hypodense compared with the surrounding liver. Late enhancement of the centre of the metastatic lesion, isodense to liver on delayed phase, is common. This delayed, 'centripetal' fill-in is also a characteristic of haemangiomas. However, as discussed above, the classic haemangioma can be distinguished by its peripheral, nodular enhancement. The margins of metastasis may be irregular or illdefined; this is not a strict criterion, and a surrounding capsule is unusual. Central necrosis may account for the low-density centre in larger lesions, which outstrip their neovascular blood supply (Fig. 21). Mucinous gastrointestinal, ovarian, breast, lung, renal and thyroid cancer metastases may demonstrate variable degrees of calcification. Similarly, all metastases may show dystrophic calcification following active therapy.

A subset of hepatic metastases are hypervascular and will show homogeneous hyperenhancement relative to the liver during arterial phase imaging. The primary tumours include melanoma, renal cell carcinoma, sarcoma, neuroendocrine (carcinoid and pancreatic islet cell), choriocarcinoma and thyroid cancers (Fig. 22). Often, these metastases will be isodense or hypodense to the surrounding liver on all other, non-arterial, imaging phases. In this way, they are only detectable with MDCT or MR arterial phase contrast imaging. These hypervascular

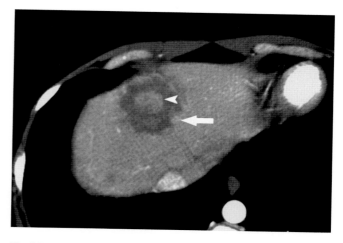

Fig. 22 Hepatic arterial phase contrast-enhanced axial CT image. Carcinoid hepatic metastasis demonstrates both central (arrowhead) and peripheral (arrow) arterial hyperenhancement.

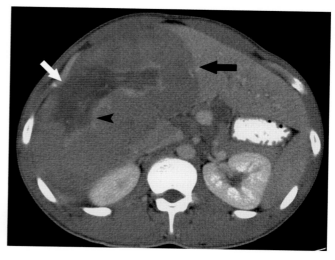

Fig. 23 Delayed phase contrast-enhanced axial CT image. Large primary liver lymphoma (black arrow denotes tumour edge) shows delayed enhancement (arrowhead) adjacent to an area of central necrosis. There is also retraction of the right liver lobe capsule (white arrow).

metastases, particularly when solitary, can create a diagnostic dilemma [23]. Many small haemangiomas demonstrate a homogeneous arterial enhancement, without the classic peripheral nodular rim. These haemangiomas also show a washout similar to hypervascular metastasis [24]. Capsular retraction adjacent to a mass is highly suggestive of malignancy [25] (Fig. 23).

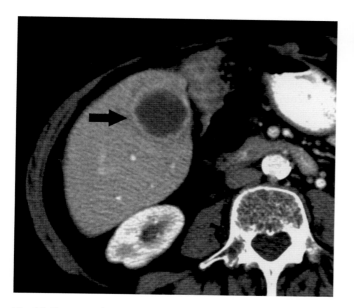

Fig. 21 Contrast-enhanced axial CT image. Right liver lobe cholangiocarcinoma (arrow) demonstrates prominent central low density consistent with central necrosis.

Colorectal carcinoma hepatic metastasis

Colorectal carcinoma (CRC) metastases deserve special mention. Although CRC metastasis imaging features are not significantly

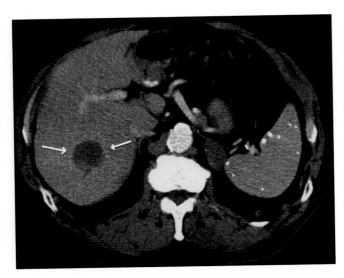

Fig. 24 Contrast-enhanced axial CT image. A right liver lobe colon cancer metastasis (arrows) demonstrates mild peripheral enhancement and central low density. Incidental splenic calcifications are seen, possibly from prior granulomatous disease.

different from other hepatic metastases, the clinical management of metastatic CRC has evolved (Fig. 24). Previously, hepatic CRC metastases were treated solely with chemotherapy with a dismal 5-year survival of approximately 5%. Patients who undergo hepatic CRC metastasis resection now experience 5-year survival ranging from 25% to 48%, with long-term disease-free survival approaching 12–19% [26]. These survival figures are predicated on primary colonic tumour removal and technically successful CRC hepatic metastasis resection, as well as the absence of known additional metastatic sites. Currently, many oncology surgeons will resect single CRC metastases or even multiple foci if they are confined to a localized hepatic region; adequate margins of resection must allow for preserved liver function following surgery (e.g. all foci confined to one lobe or resectable segment). MDCT remains the dominant imaging modality for screening for CRC metastasis both within the liver as well as extrahepatic abdominal pelvic sites. MDCT can achieve a sensitivity of >90% for hepatic CRC metastasis >1 cm in diameter and a sensitivity of 56% for smaller lesions [27]. The combination of positron emission tomography (PET) with MDCT 'fuses' the specificity of MDCT anatomical resolution to the sensitivity of PET physiological metabolic imaging [28]. It is important to identify the total number and sites of CRC metastasis in order to spare patients from a futile and potentially morbid hepatic resection in the presence of extensive hepatic or extrahepatic metastases. Conversely, as mentioned in the section on imaging technique, MDCT with appropriate angiographic technique and 3-D re-formation can provide all the necessary anatomical information for the oncology surgeon to plan a complete and safe CRC metastasis resection when appropriate.

Conclusion

Modern multidetector computerized tomography with isotropic high-resolution imaging is a highly sensitive modality for detecting both diffuse and focal hepatic pathology. Rapid imaging speed and multiphase intravenous contrast-enhanced imaging allow for characterization of many focal liver lesions. Benign hepatic lesions such as cysts, haemangiomas, focal nodular hyperplasia and adenomas can frequently be distinguished from hepatocellular carcinoma and hepatic metastases. Atypical lesions can be triaged between follow-up imaging and biopsy or excision. Advanced computer techniques yield three-dimensional display of hepatic pathology for non-invasive hepatic vascular assessment and presurgical planning. Of the advanced radiological imaging modalities, multidetector computerized tomography with multiphase contrast enhancement provides the most consistent, rapid and, overall, comprehensive assessment of liver pathology.

References

1 Husband J, Dombrowe G (2005) X-ray computed tomography – a truly remarkable medical development. *Br J Radiol* 78, 97–98.

2 Michael A, Bettmann MD (2004) Frequently asked questions: iodinated contrast agents. *Radiographics* 24, S3–S10.

3 Sahani D, Mehta A, Blake M *et al.* (2004) Preoperative hepatic vascular evaluation with CT and MR angiography: implications for surgery. *Radiographics* 24, 1367–1380.

4 Pomfret EA, Pomposelli JJ, Lewis WD *et al.* (2001) Live donor adult liver transplantation using right lobe grafts: donor evaluation and surgical outcome. *Arch Surg* 136, 425–433.

5 Pandharipande PV, Krinsky GA, Rusinek H, Lee VS (2005) Perfusion imaging of the liver: current challenges and future goals. *Radiology* 234, 661–673.

6 Bray GA (2004) Medical consequences of obesity. *J Clin Endocrinol Metab* 89, 2583–2589.

7 Jacobs JE, Birnbaum BA, Shapiro MA *et al.* (1998) Diagnostic criteria for fatty infiltration of the liver on contrast-enhanced helical CT. *Am J Roentgenol* 171, 659–664.

8 Goldman IS, Winkler ML, Raper SE *et al.* (1985) Increased hepatic density and phospholipidosis due to amiodarone. *Am J Roentgenol* 144, 541–546.

9 Mergo PJ, Ros PR (1998) Imaging of diffuse liver disease. *Radiol Clin North Am* 36, 365–375.

10 Everson GT, Scherzinger A, Berger-Leff N *et al.* (1988) Polycystic liver disease: quantitation of parenchymal and cyst volumes from computed tomography images and clinical correlates of hepatic cysts. *Hepatology* 8, 1627–1634.

11 Mitsudo K, Watanabe Y, Saga T *et al.* (1995) Nonenhanced hepatic cavernous hemangioma with multiple calcifications: CT and pathologic correlation. *Abdom Imaging* 20, 459–461.

12 Vilgrain V, Boulos L, Vullierme MP *et al.* (2000) Imaging of atypical hemangiomas of the liver with pathologic correlation. *Radiographics* 20, 379–397.

13 Yang DM, Yoon MH, Kim HS *et al.* (2001) Capsular retraction in hepatic giant hemangioma: CT and MR features. *Abdom Imaging* 26, 36–38.

14 Carlson SK, Johnson CD, Bender CE, Welch TJ (2000) CT of focal nodular hyperplasia of the liver. *Am J Roentgenol* 174, 705–712.

15 Foster JH, Berman MM (1994) The malignant transformation of liver cell adenomas. *Arch Surg* 129, 712–717.

16 Gupta AA, Kim DC, Krinsky GA, Lee VS (2004) CT and MRI of cirrhosis and its mimics. *Am J Roentgenol* 183, 1595–1601.

17 Kang HK, Jeong YY, Choi JH *et al.* (2002) Three-dimensional multidetector row CT portal venography in the evaluation of portosystemic collateral vessels in liver cirrhosis. *RadioGraphics* 22, 1053–1061.

18 Baron RL, Peterson MS (2001) Screening the cirrhotic liver for hepatocellular carcinoma with CT and MR imaging: opportunities and pitfalls. *RadioGraphics* 21, S117–S132.

19 International Working Party (1995) Terminology of nodular hepatocellular lesions. *Hepatology* 22, 983–993.

20 Jeong YY, Mitchell DG, Kamishima T (2002) Small (<20 mm) enhancing hepatic nodules seen on arterial phase MR imaging of the cirrhotic liver: clinical implications. *Am J Roentgenol* 178, 1327–1334.

21 Lee KH, O'Malley ME, Haider MA, Hanbidge A (2004) Triple-phase MDCT of hepatocellular carcinoma. *Am J Roentgenol* 182, 643–649.

22 Sica GT, Ji H, Ros PR (2000) CT and MR imaging of hepatic metastases. *Am J Roentgenol* 174, 691–698.

23 Hanafusa K, Ohashi I, Himeno Y *et al.* (1995) Hepatic hemangioma: findings with two-phase CT. *Radiology* 196, 465–469.

24 Leslie DF, Johnson CD, Johnson CM *et al.* (1995) Distinction between cavernous hemangiomas of the liver and hepatic metastases on CT: value of contrast enhancement patterns. *Am J Roentgenol* 164, 625–629.

25 Soyer P, Bluemke DA, Vissuzaine C *et al.* (1994) CT of hepatic tumors: prevalence and specificity of retraction of the adjacent liver capsule. *Am J Roentgenol* 162, 1119–1122.

26 Headrick JR, Miller DL, Nagorney DM *et al.* (2001) Surgical treatment of hepatic and pulmonary metastases from colon cancer. *Ann Thorac Surg* 71, 975–979.

27 Kuszyk BS, Bluemke DA, Urban BA *et al.* (1996) Portal-phase contrast-enhanced helical CT for the detection of malignant hepatic tumors: sensitivity based on comparison with intraoperative and pathologic findings. *Am J Roentgenol* 166, 91–95.

28 Cohade C, Osman M, Leal J, Wahl RL (2003) Direct comparison of (18)F-FDG PET and PET/CT in patients with colorectal carcinoma. *J Nucl Med* 44, 1797–1803.

5.6.3 Magnetic resonance imaging

Christoforos Stoupis

The major advantage of magnetic resonance imaging (MRI) compared with the other cross-sectional imaging techniques is its ability to detect as well to characterize focal liver lesions due to the superior soft-tissue contrast of this modality compared with irradiating and other non-irradiating imaging techniques [1].

Technical aspects

The MR equipment and its field strength is the first important hardware issue for liver imaging. Soft-tissue contrast between hepatic lesions and the normal hepatic parenchyma correlates with the field strength. The most acceptable field strength is 1.5 T (tesla).

The second most important issue regarding the equipment is the coils. For many years MRI of the liver has been commonly performed using a whole-volume body coil; however, phased-array surface multicoil systems have been developed for improved signal-to-noise ratio and high-resolution MR liver imaging. The phased-array technology has demonstrated the potential to significantly improve lesion-to-liver contrast, lesion detection and image definition.

The imaging protocol must be tailored to the clinical problem being considered. Both T1-weighted and T2-weighted image sequences are essential and justified for liver imaging [1]. T1-weighted imaging analyses the normal anatomy whereas T2-weighted imaging is of major importance for the characterization of focal lesions. Both sequences are generally used for transvessel imaging of the liver using a slice thickness ranging from 4 to 8 mm to cover the whole organ. Today, fast spin echo sequences are used mainly with breath-hold imaging techniques in order to obtain multiple images in one breath hold similar to the techniques used in computerized tomography (CT). Breath-hold T1- and T2-weighted images of the liver enable shorter imaging time with a higher contrast:noise ratio compared with conventional techniques.

In case of diffuse liver diseases, specifically in case of focal or diffused steatosis, a specific imaging technique has been developed called fat-suppressed imaging. The most commonly used technique is the chemical shift imaging method, which is sensitive to differences in resonance frequency between water and triglyceride protons. The opposed phase imaging technique is the most commonly used chemical shift imaging method; it is based on signal cancellation within a voxel that contains both water and triglyceride. This means that areas that contain both water and triglycerides (such as steatotic liver areas) will reduce their signal intensity in the opposed phase sequence while areas of malignancy, containing only water, will not change their signal. This imaging technique is proposed in case of focal or diffused steatosis of the liver in order to differentiate inhomogeneous parenchyma from metastatic disease. A second technique for faster imaging is the short time inversion recovery technique (STIR); remember, however, that this sequence suppresses signals from any tissue that has relaxation values similar to that of fat. Although the signal-to-noise ratio in the sequence is relatively low, in case of a focal liver lesion there is high lesion-to-liver contrast value available, and therefore it could be used for lesion detection.

An important technical advantage of MRI is the potential for vascular imaging using flow-sensitive MR sequences in order to depict and image hepatic vessels. The time of flight imaging angiography allows non-invasive imaging of the portal and the hepatic venous system without administration of contrast agent; using a flow-sensitive sequence, blood flowing into an image section that has higher longitudinal magnetization than the partially saturated stationary tissues within the section can easily be detected. Phase-contrast angiographic imaging is based on the detection of changes in phase secondary to flow; however, this complicated encoding process is time consuming and the images are sensitive to motion artifacts. Therefore, phase-contrast imaging is not in daily use.

Three-dimensional contrast-enhanced MR angiography (MRA) is nowadays available for regular application; it uses a three-dimensional (3-D) gradient echo sequence on magnets with high-performance gradient systems; high-resolution 3-D volume of image data acquisition can be accomplished in a single breath hold of the patient (Fig. 1). A paramagnetic contrast medium is injected intravenously and the image data are collected as the contrast circulates through the vascular territory of interest using different phases and acquisition of contrast agent circulation (early and late arterial phase, hepatic parenchymal phase, etc.). Compared with other angiography techniques, contrast-enhanced MRA has the advantage of non-iodinated contrast agent with less risk of anaphylactic reactions. There is no nephrotoxicity and the volume injected for angiography is 20–30 mL as opposed to 80–100 mL with computerized tomography angiography. The reconstruction of images from MRA is similar to other imaging techniques.

MR liver imaging has the advantage of allowing 'all-in-one imaging', including transverse sectional imaging of the liver (MRI), magnetic resonance angiography in different phases (MRA) and MR cholangiopancreatography (MRCP; see Chapter 5.6.5), all in the same imaging session in a non-invasive way.

Contrast enhancement

Several contrast agents have been investigated and are in use for specific MR imaging of the liver. These contrast agents can be categorized as paramagnetic (increasing signal intensity in T1-weighted images) or superparamagnetic (decreasing the signal density of the normal hepatic parenchyma in T2-weighted images). According to their biochemical behaviour, they can be characterized as extracellular, reticuloendothelial system-directed agents or hepatocyte-specific contrast agents [2].

Extracellular agents

The gadolinium chelates are the most widely used MR contrast agents. These agents include gadoterate dimeglumine and gadopentetate dimeglumine (ionic agents), as well as gadodiamide and gadoteridol (non-ionic contrast agents). Because these extracellular agents display a rapid equilibration in the interstitial spaces, a dynamic MR imaging technique (bolus injection, rapid acquisition) that provides a high temporary resolution is essential to demonstrate differences in enhancement pattern between the normal hepatic parenchyma and the potential focal liver lesion. Similar to CT during arterial portography, gadolinium chelates have also been delivered to the liver via the superior mesenteric artery (MR imaging during arterial portography) providing the highest parenchymal enhancement,

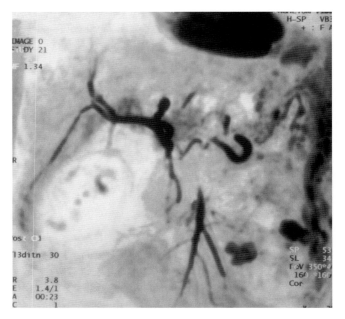

(a)

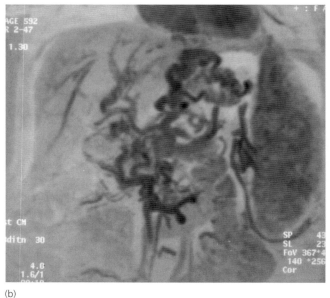

(b)

Fig. 1 MR angiography. (a) 3-D contrast-enhanced MR angiography after intravenous administration of gadolinium demonstrates the vessels in the arterial and early portal inflow phase. Note active bleeding within the gallbladder. This examination was done in a patient with renal insufficiency. (b) Contrast-enhanced MR angiography in hepatic parenchymal phase demonstrates collaterals by portal hypertension along the common ways of portosystemic circulation. Note the splenomegaly.

excellent lesion-to-liver contrast and high sensitivity for lesion detection although non-tumoral perfusion abnormalities and invasiveness are drawbacks of this technique. Extracellular gadolinium chelates, if given with the power injector, can be used in the initial injection phase for MR angiography acquisition, again demonstrating the potential for both angiographic and late arterial hepatic phase and hepatic venous phase of the liver parenchyma similar to the phases seen by multidetector CT.

Superparamagnetic contrast agents such as Endorem (Advanced Magnetics Inc., Cambidge, MA, USA) or Resovist (Schering AG, Berlin, Germany) are phagocytes by the reticuloendothelial system. Because signal reduction of normal hepatic parenchyma, secondary to the administration of superparamagnetic contrast agent, is more pronounced on T2-weighted gradient echo images than on conventional T2-weighted images, gradient echo sequences (so called T*) are more sensitive in demonstrating focal liver lesion diseases. Lesions that do not contain reticuloendothelial system cells will not demonstrate a signal intensity drop as opposed to the normal hepatic parenchyma.

Hepatobiliary agents

Several hepatocyte-specific paramagnetic contrast agents are available. Mangafodipir trisodium (Mn-DPDP) is a typical example of this group. T1-weighted images are essential after the administration of these contrast agents because they affect the T1 relaxation times and therefore the T1 contrast (high signal intensity in the area of contrast accumulation). Two gadolinium chelates (gadolinium BOPTA and gadolinium EOB-DTPA) can also be used as hepatobiliary contrast agents. These two agents display extracellular activity; however, there is uptake by the hepatocytes followed by hepatobiliary secretion. Representative commercial products include Multihance (Bracco, Milan, Italy) and Primovist (Schering AG, Berlin, Germany) [3,4].

MR imaging of focal liver lesions

Benign hepatic tumours

Benign tumours of the liver are classified pathologically by their cell origin. Lesions of mesenchymal origin include haemangiomas, angiomyolipomas and lipomas. Lesions of epithelial origin include focal nodular hyperplasia (FNH), hepatocellular adenomas, hepatic cysts and biliary hamartomas. Determination of tumour extent and tissue characterization is provided by T1- and T2-weighted images as well as after intravenously administered contrast agents such as extracellular agents, reticuloendothelial system (RES)-directed contrasts or hepatobiliary secreted agents. Knowledge of the underlying gross and microscopic pathological features of benign liver masses leads to a better understanding of their MR imaging appearances [1,5].

Hepatic cysts are common and mostly asymptomatic, representing incidental finding by MR imaging of the liver. Most are unilocular but occasionally they have a multilocular appearance. On MR imaging they have a homogeneous well-defined appearance demonstrating low signal intensity on T1-weighted and high signal intensity on T2-weighted images reflecting their simple nature. After gadolinium administration cysts do not demonstrate any enhancement (Fig. 2). Complicated cysts

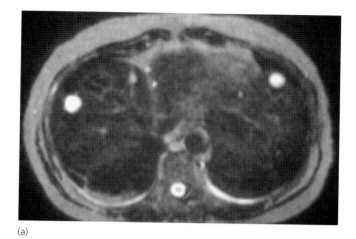

(a)

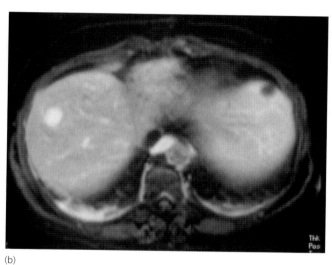

(b)

Fig. 2 Use of contrast agent to differentiate cystic from other lesions. (a) T2-weighted image demonstrates multiple lesions in the liver with high signal intensity. Further differentiation of those lesions is not possible. (b) T1-weighted image after gadolinium administration demonstrates that the lesion in the right lobe of the liver is a haemangioma whereas the other lesions do not enhance, representing simple cysts.

might demonstrate high signal intensity on T1- and low signal intensity on T2-weighted images.

Biliary hamartomas are benign, solitary or multiple biliary malformations of small size (<1 cm). Similar to cysts, they have low signal intensity on T1- and high signal intensity on T2-weighted images. However, after contrast administration they demonstrate rim enhancement; this feature might cause difficulties in differentiating them from metastatic lesions.

Angiomyolipoma of the liver is an uncommon tumour of mesenchymal origin often seen in patients with tuberous sclerosis. On MR imaging they often demonstrate high signal intensity on T1-weighted images due to their fatty content, which is well suppressed on T1 fat-suppressed images. Usually they do have moderate to high signal intensity on T2-weighted images. They demonstrate diffuse and heterogeneous enhancement

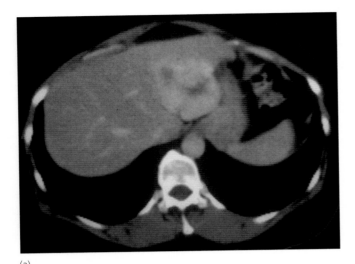

(a)

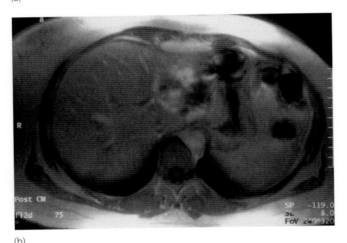

(b)

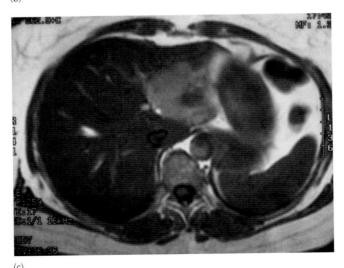

(c)

Fig. 3 Behaviour of contrast agents in haemangiomas. (a) Typical enhancement pattern by CT after injection of iodinated contrast agent. (b) The same patient after administration of gadolinium chelates with a typical peripheral enhancement of the lesion. (c) The same patient after superparamagnetic contrast agent administration with typical high signal intensity within the lesion because of pooling of the agent.

after gadolinium administration, which poses difficulties in differentiating them from hepatocellular carcinomas.

Haemangioma is the most common benign tumour of the liver; symptoms and complications are discussed in Chapter 18.1.1. Haemangiomas are well-defined round or lobular lesions with low signal intensity on T1-weighted and high signal intensity on T2-weighted images. Due to their large vascular lakes and channels they demonstrate peripheral enhancements with a typical cottonwool appearance (Fig. 3). If they are large they might contain central areas of fibrosis, which do not enhance after contrast administration. Unfortunately, areas of calcifications that can be seen by CT cannot be demonstrated by means of MRI. If the haemangioma is small and hypervascular, the typical features of peripheral nodular enhancement with centripetal progression to homogeneity are not seen. Instead immediate homogeneous enhancement might be present, which can be difficult to differentiate from hypervascular metastases. Haemangiomas can be differentiated from metastases by RES-directed contrast agents (SPIO, superparamagnetic iron oxide). In haemangioma there is pooling of the contrast agent in T2-weighted imaging. Signal intensity is high in T2 images before and after contrast administration, whereas the pooling produces a high signal intensity in T1-weighted images after contrast administration (Fig. 3). Metastases remain hypointense in T1-weighted images after SPIO administration. In case of hepatobiliary-directed contrast agents there is enhancement due to the vascularity of the lesion in the late arterial phase; however, in the delayed phase there is no pooling of this agent, similar to the metastatic lesions where no enhancement is seen. Giant haemangiomas might be difficult to differentiate from aggressive malignant lesions due to their large size. However, even with the presence of fibrosis, with the typical persistent central hypointense area after gadolinium administration, the peripheral nodular enhancement with a centripetal progression is typical and well demonstrated in those lesions [6].

Liver cell adenomas are benign tumours of hepatocellular origin; their clinical presentation is discussed in Chapter 18.1.2. Liver cell adenomas are composed of hepatocytes that might contain substantial amounts of glycogen or fat; therefore, T1-weighted images produce high signal intensity, which can be suppressed in fat-suppressed T1 images. If any complications are present, such as haemorrhage, causing high signal intensity in T1-weighted images similar to that of fat, differentiation between blood and fat can be accomplished by fat-suppressed techniques (blood remains bright, fat darkens its signal intensity). On T2-weighted images adenomas are seen as intermediate signal intensity lesions. After contrast administration they demonstrate a high vascularity; this sometimes produces difficulties in distinguishing adenomas from hepatocellular carcinomas. Therefore, if imaging appearance suggests adenoma and the lesion is solitary, surgical resection is suggested. Hepatocyte-specific contrast agents as well as iron oxide particulate agents demonstrate uptake, because adenomas accumulate contrast agents due to the presence of hepatocytes and RES cells [6,7].

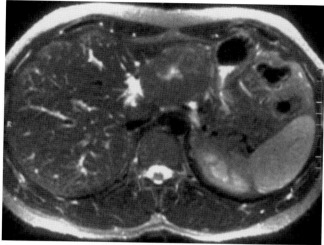

(a)

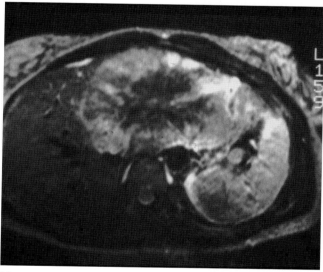

(b)

Fig. 4 Differentiation of focal nodular hyperplasia (FNH) from fibrolamellar carcinoma using the T2-weighted image. (a) Typical flow within the central scar of the FNH with high signal intensity on T2-weighted image. (b) In case of fibrolamellar carcinoma there is no flow within the central scar, which represents fibrous tissue. Around the fibrotic tissue note septae and necrotic oedematous changes with high signal intensity.

Focal nodular hyperplasia (FNH) is the second most common benign hepatic tumour after haemangioma. It is thought to be a hyperplastic response to an underlying congenital arterial venous malformation. The central fibrous scar contains the arterial venous malformation; this feature demonstrates high signal intensity on T2-weighted images (Fig. 4). Various appearances on T1- and T2-weighted images are described. After intravenous administration of gadolinium the lesions demonstrate prompt and marked enhancement higher than that of the liver, particularly in the late arterial phase. If the extracellular contrast agents do not reveal the underlying pathology in a small hypervascular lesion suspected of being FNH, cell-specific contrast agents can demonstrate the benign origin of the lesion. This can also be used to distinguish them from other lesions with a central scar such as fibrolamellar carcinoma. A specific type of FNH has been described as a telangiectatic focal nodular hyperplasia, an entity that does not demonstrate the typical scar and has an appearance similar to that of hepatocellular adenoma or carcinoma. Cell-specific contrast agents demonstrate the typical hepatocyte and Kupffer cell activities and allow for differentiation from carcinoma and adenoma.

Malignant hepatic tumours

Fibrolamellar carcinoma (FLC) is a malignant hepatocellular tumour with clinical and pathological features distinct from HCC. On MR imaging fibrolamellar carcinomas are typically of low signal intensity on T1-weighted images with the exception of bleeding, where hyperintense areas are seen. On T2-weighted images signal intensity is low; this low-intensity central scar differentiates FLC from FNH, where a high signal intensity on T2-weighted images within the scar is seen (Fig. 4). Radiating septae with low signal intensity in both T1- and T2-weighted images are also seen (Fig. 4). After gadolinium enhancement there is a heterogeneous enhancement of the lesion as opposed to the homogeneous enhancement of FNH. The central scar is due to true fibrotic tissue and remains hypointense after contrast administration [1].

Hepatocellular carcinoma (HCC) occasionally arises in patients without any pre-existing hepatic abnormalities; however, it is mostly seen in a previously damaged liver as in the case of hepatitis or fibrosis and cirrhosis (Figs 5 and 6). On MRI HCC generally has a variable appearance depending on its growth pattern. Vascular invasion, if present, is well displayed with thrombosis of the hepatic or portal vein branches. The ability of MRI to depict vascular invasion makes this technique essential for the diagnosis of a suspected lesion. On T1-weighted images, hepatocellular carcinoma has a variable appearance, depending on the presence of haemorrhage or steatosis, which produce high signal intensity. Haemorrhage can be differentiated from fat by the fat-suppression technique. On T2-weighted images the lesions may demonstrate a hyperintensity relative to the normal liver with areas of increased signal intensity in case of necrosis. In case of encapsulated HCC there is often a low signal intensity rim on T1-weighted images representing the fibrotic tumour capsule. After intravenous extracellular agent administration the tumours demonstrate enhancement due to their hypervascular nature [8,9].

Diagnostic problems abound when imaging of liver cirrhosis demonstrates regenerative and dysplastic nodules, as opposed to HCC. There are many studies and papers demonstrating the potential of MRI to differentiate between regenerative and dysplastic nodules and HCC; however, in general, the majority of HCC nodules are of slightly higher signal intensity

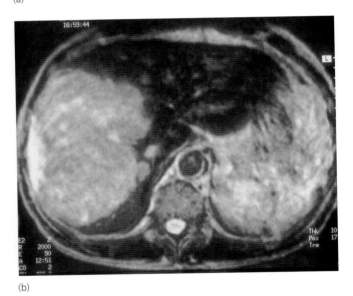

(a)

(b)

Fig. 5 Superparamagnetic contrast agent for detection of liver lesions. (a) T2-weighted image without contrast administration is unable to clearly delineate the HCC lesions in this patient. (b) After contrast administration note the darkening of the normal hepatic parenchyma. The HCC, which contains no reticuloendothelial system (RES) cells in this case, retains high signal intensity and therefore can be easily detected and delineated.

and regenerative nodules are of lower signal intensity on T2-weighted images, compared with the liver parenchyma. The degree of vascularity might be useful in demonstrating the high vascularity of HCC and the very fast washout compared with the other lesions. A published study demonstrated that, in the case of cirrhotic liver, many areas of hypervascularity could be seen in the late arterial phase. Of those areas that were visualized, only those whose size exceeded 2 cm were suspected hepatocellular carcinoma. Lesions in the periphery smaller than 1 cm were often due to intrahepatic shunts. Lesions between 1 and 2 cm should be followed up by re-examination; most often they are of benign regenerative origin [10].

Although the use of hepatospecific contrast agents (hepatocyte- or Kupffer cell-directed) suggested a higher degree of characterization of HCC, this remains problematic in the case of well-differentiated HCC, where both phagocytosis of SPIO particles and hepatocytic activity with uptake is demonstrated. In general, in the case of hypervascular lesions in a cirrhotic patient, even if these lesions are of low signal intensity on T2-weighted images, hepatocellular carcinoma must be considered in the differential diagnosis, and follow-up examination is essential. On the other hand attention needs to be paid in case the hepatocellular carcinoma is not hypervascular; other imaging features such as the high signal intensity in T2-weighted images and the presence of a pseudocapsule might guide the correct diagnosis.

Intrahepatic cholangiocarcinoma is the second most common primary malignant hepatic neoplasm after HCC. As opposed to the vascular enhancement of HCC, in cholangiocarcinoma there is encasement of large vessels without invasion. Areas of necrosis and haemorrhage can been seen with the typical changes on T1- and T2-weighted images. On MR imaging intrahepatic cholangiocarcinoma appears as a large heterogeneous mass, often encasing large vessels such as the portal vein and the hepatic veins without tumour thrombus as seen in HCC. On T1-weighted images the lesion is hypointense compared with the normal liver and on T2-weighted images the variable periphery is hyperintense with respect to normal liver, with central areas of hypointensity corresponding to fibrosis [1,11]. The use of gadolinium chelates demonstrates concentric enhancement with sparing of central areas due to the presence of central fibrosis (Fig. 7).

In extrahepatic cholangiocarcinoma, unlike intrahepatic cholangiocarcinoma, there is no space-occupying lesion but a stenosis of the involved bile duct segment (Fig. 8), while the additional use of gadolinium might demonstrate a rim enhancement in the area of the stenotic bile duct. MRCP is essential in the diagnosis and 'all-in-one MRI' could help in the further evaluation of the disease.

Biliary cystadenoma and cystadenocarcinoma represent two points on a disease spectrum; they are uncommon and present as large multilocular intrahepatic cystic masses that contain proteinaceous fluid material. On MR imaging the multilocular cystic masses have an irregular wall. On T1-weighted images the locules appear with variable signal intensity depending on their protein content. A similar appearance is seen in T2-weighted images, where the signal intensity seen is not that of clear fluid, demonstrating locules with lower signal intensity due to the content, that is, tinged bile. After gadolinium administration there is a variable enhancement seen in the irregular septae. The presence of solid components and mural nodules demonstrates cystadenocarcinoma [1]. Again, unlike CT, calcifications cannot be demonstrated by means of MRI.

Angiosarcoma is a rare malignancy seen specifically after exposure to different toxins. Haemorrhage and a heterogeneous appearance of the lesions is commonly seen. On MR imaging

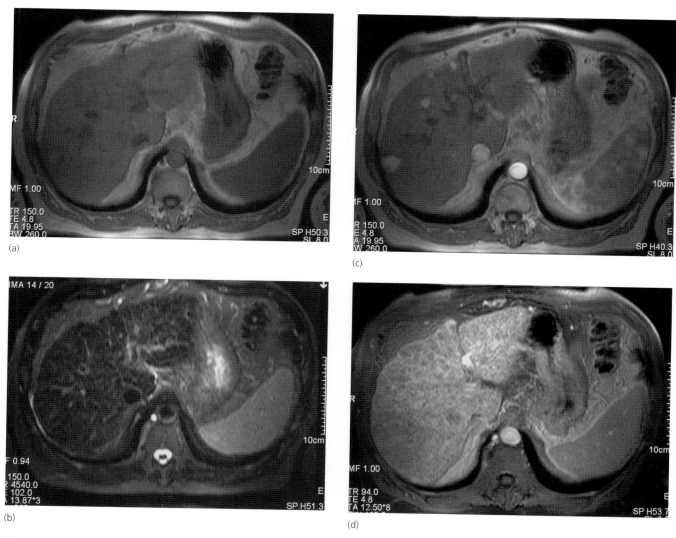

Fig. 6 Use of dynamic imaging to depict and characterize lesions in case of hepatic cirrhosis. (a) Non-enhanced T1-weighted image of the liver does not demonstrate any focal liver lesions. Note the irregular surface of the liver parenchyma due to cirrhosis. (b) T2-weighted image is unable to detect any liver lesions. (c) Arterial phase after intravenous administration of gadolinium. Note several lesions in the right and left lobes of the liver; based on the size of the lesions the one in the right lobe must be suspected HCC. (d) Late parenchymal phase reveals multiple lesions; however, regenerative nodules and HCC cannot be differentiated in this phase.

angiosarcoma is hypointense in relation to the normal liver parenchyma on T1-weighted images although areas of haemorrhage represent hyperintensity, similar to that of adenoma. An inhomogeneous appearance can be seen on T2-weighted images where normally, if not complicated, the lesion demonstrates high signal intensity. The intravenous administration of extracellular contrast agents demonstrates peripheral enhancement, sometimes similar to that seen with haemangioma [1].

Liver metastases

Examination for liver metastasis is one of the most common indications for liver MR imaging. However, differentiation of detected lesions in an oncology patient is necessary to exclude liver metastases specifically if, after chemotherapy, diffuse fatty change of the liver has occurred. Similarly to CT, depending upon the pattern of vascularization, liver metastases have been classified as hypovascular or hypervascular. A specific group has been described that is known to be of near isovascularity and demonstrates the particular appearance of those lesions if imaging targets to the vascularization pattern [3,4].

Hypovascular metastases have a non-specific pattern in MRI, demonstrating low signal intensity on T1-weighted images and similar signal intensity to the normal hepatic parenchyma on T2-weighted images. Because of the characteristic signal and relaxation changes after gadolinium enhancement, even hypovascular metastases demonstrate a peripheral rim enhancement

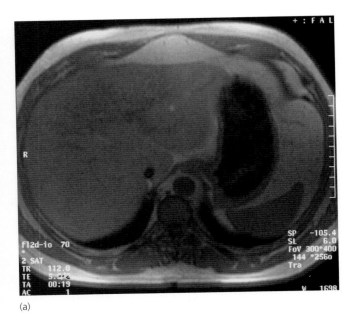

(a)

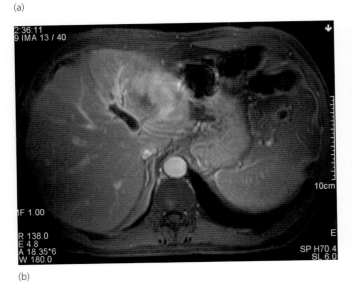

(a)

(b)

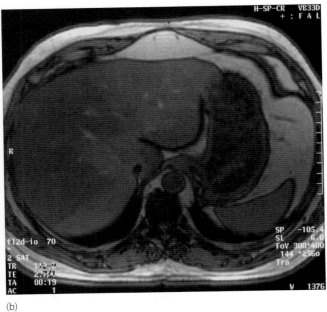

(b)

Fig. 7 Intrahepatic cholangiocarcinoma. (a) Coronal T2-weighted image demonstrates a space-occupying lesion within the left lobe. The adjacent intrahepatic bile ducts are dilated. (b) Contrast-enhanced T1-weighted image demonstrates the lesion in the left lobe with obstruction of the intrahepatic bile ducts.

Fig. 8 Diffuse hepatic liver steatosis. Chemical shift imaging. (a) T1-weighted in-phase image demonstrates no abnormalities of the liver parenchyma. (b) T1-weighted out-of-phase image demonstrates drop of signal intensity in the areas where steatosis is evident. Liver segment I and part of the left lobe do not demonstrate a signal intensity decrease; hence there is no steatosis.

in the late arterial hepatic phase; however; these lesions typically demonstrate low signal intensity in the hepatic venous phase. Although hypovascular metastases may sometimes mimic hepatic cysts, delayed enhancement of the liver demonstrates a slightly peripheral enhancement in the metastases, a finding that is not seen with cysts.

Hypervascular metastases, similar to CT, are seen in the early and late hepatic arterial phases, therefore dynamic MR imaging must be applied in the case of suspected hypervascular metastasis even if there is no high signal intensity on T2-weighted images.

Near isovascular metastases, as the name implies, do enhance when using an extracellular contrast agent, and appear similar to the liver in early and late arterial phases. Because of this peculiar pattern of enhancement, attention needs to be paid to the non-enhanced T1-weighted images, where the lesions are conspicuous and there is at least the potential of differentiation from other lesions.

As discussed previously, the use of extracellular contrast agents to detect and differentiate metastases from other lesions might produce diagnostic problems because of the different vascularity patterns of metastases. Therefore, in this situation, agents other than gadolinium chelates can be applied in order to demonstrate the number, location and extent of metastatic disease in the liver. One group of substances that can be administered intravenously and can be used for specific detection of metastases of a known primary tumour are the superparamagnetic contrast agents, which can be given either by drip infusion (Endorem) or by means of a bolus technique (Resovist). These agents target the absence of reticuloendothelial system cells within the metastatic lesions. On T2-weighted images there is a signal intensity increase in the normal liver compared with the non-enhanced images while metastatic lesions remain unchanging in their signal intensity and therefore appear much brighter in the post-contrast images as opposed to the precontrast images. Superparamagnetic contrast agents demonstrate a higher sensitivity than CT in detecting metastatic lesions, independent of the vascularity of those metastases. In addition to the superparamagnetic contrast agents, a specific extracellular contrast agent that demonstrates partial hepatocyte uptake and excretion through the biliary system can also be used for detection of metastases [12,13]. Two products are used routinely: Multihance and Primovist. Both agents can be used initially as extracellular agents to detect vascularity; thereafter, some 20–40 min after injection, a proportion of the contrast agent is taken up by the hepatocytes. Hence, in T1-weighted images, the normal liver becomes more intense compared with the images before the contrast administration, whereas metastatic lesions do not take up contrast and are darker than in the precontrast images. A similar contrast characteristic is produced after the use of Mn-DPDP. Although various different contrast agents have been introduced for detecting metastatic liver disease, attention needs to be paid to their utility in differentiating metastases from other focal liver lesions, specifically benign hypervascular lesions such as hypervascular haemangiomas and FNH. Furthermore, differentiation of small hypervascular lesions and small intrahepatic vessels is not always easy. Finally, the imaging of small capsular liver metastases in the case of peritoneal metastatic disease is an unsolved issue.

MR imaging of diffuse liver disease

Hepatic steatosis

Diffuse hepatic steatosis is not uncommon. It is known that CT examination of the liver can detect fatty liver changes if non-enhanced imaging is performed. The most sensitive MR technique to detect fatty change of the liver is the use of specific gradient echo pulse sequences, particularly chemical shift imaging (Fig. 8). Using 1.5 T at an echo time of 4.2 ms, water and lipid protons are in phase and their signal intensities are additive. However, using an echo time of half this value (i.e. 2.1 ms), water and lipid protons are out of phase and their signal intensities cancel each other. Hence, in steatotic areas of the liver the signal intensity decreases when out of phase compared to when in phase, whereas in areas of the liver with less fat the signal intensity out of phase remains similar to that when in phase. This simple imaging technique can be used not only to detect fatty changes of the liver parenchyma but also to differentiate fatty changes from other focal or diffuse entities of the liver such as liver metastases. This technique can be used to differentiate specific focal lesions that could mimic liver masses such as focal fatty infiltration and/or focal fatty sparing, specifically in liver segment IV. These changes are more pronounced in T1-weighted sequences; however, they can be manifest in T2-weighted images specifically with a fast spin echo technique. Therefore, in and out (opposed) phase gradient echo images must be used in every liver MRI examination in order to detect or to exclude focal changes and differentiate those from other potential focal liver lesions [14–16].

Hepatic iron deposition

Haemochromatosis of the liver can be genetic in origin or be caused by transfusional iron overload. In both entities the iron deposition within the liver decreases the signal intensity in both T1- and T2-weighted images. However, the findings are more pronounced in T2-weighted images, where the liver appears very dark. Differentiation between genetic and transfusional iron overload can be accomplished using the signal intensity of the spleen: in the first case the spleen is spared because it comprises dysfunctional reticuloendothelial cells, whereas with transfusional iron overload, iron is found in the Kupffer cells of the spleen and therefore the spleen decreases its signal intensity. A specific sequence, called a T2-weighted gradient echo image, is employed to detect and semi-quantify abnormal iron deposition in the liver, specifically exploiting the sensitivity of iron in the magnetic field. The same sequence can be used to detect hepatocellular carcinoma in patients with haemochromatosis, because iron does not accumulate in hepatoma and therefore those lesions can be seen within the liver using this T2-weighted gradient echo sequence [17,18].

Inflammatory liver diseases

Hepatic abscess

Ultrasonography and CT are the primary diagnostic tools for detecting pyogenic and amoebic abscesses in the liver with high sensitivity, and to guide treatment by means of interventional radiology and drainage of abscesses. Therefore MR imaging should not be the first imaging choice where a liver abscess is suspected. MR imaging is used as a secondary tool for this diagnosis. Biogenic abscesses have a non-specific appearance on MR imaging and may mimic malignant neoplasms. On T1-weighted images the lesions are of low signal intensity and in T2 they have high signal intensity. Following administration of gadolinium an abscess shows a peripheral rim of enhancement surrounding the centre filled with necrotic debris of low signal intensity. In the case of amoebic abscess, similar to the findings on CT, a zone of hyperintensity might be seen around the abscess on T2-weighted images with enhancement after gadolinium administration, demonstrating the surrounding oedematous non-infected liver parenchyma [19].

Hydatid disease

As with other infectious diseases, MR imaging is not a primary tool for detecting and evaluating hepatic echinococcosis. Due to the inability of MRI to detect calcifications, this technique is not suggested as a primary tool to detect and differentiate cystic lesions, specifically echinococcosis, from other cystic lesions of the liver. The MR imaging features of hydatid cysts are those of hypointense lesions on T1-weighted imaging and of hyperintense lesions on T2-weighted images. In case of calcification a low signal intensity is evident on T1- or T2-weighted images. Dotted cysts may be seen within the lesion with similar signal intensity on T1- and T2-weighted images, hence they cannot be easily detected by MRI. A specific entity that may produce differential diagnostic problems is echinococcus alveolaris. In this case the lesion presents as a mass of low signal intensity in T1-weighted images and intermediate to high signal intensity in T2-weighted images, mimicking malignant tumours, whereas after contrast administration the lesion does not enhance, appearing as a necrotic area similar to that of a tumour. Therefore in cases where hydatid disease is suspected the method of choice is CT examination and not MRI because, specifically in case of echinococcus alveolaris, MRI may suggest the wrong differential diagnosis.

MR imaging of the bile system

One of the major advantages of MRI is the potential for imaging the bile duct system due to the signal intensity of slow-moving liquid within the intra- and extrahepatic bile ducts. Using T2-weighted images it is possible to darken the signal intensity of the liver, to avoid the appearance of the hepatic vessels and to demonstrate only the branches of the intra- and extrahepatic ducts depending upon the quantity of bile within the biliary system. This technique enables the delineation of the anatomy of the biliary system, demonstrating specifically potential variations of the bile duct system, an important issue before surgery. It is the method of choice to detect intra- and extrahepatic stones, although compared with endoscopic retrograde cholangiopancreatography (ERCP), it might miss stones that are smaller than

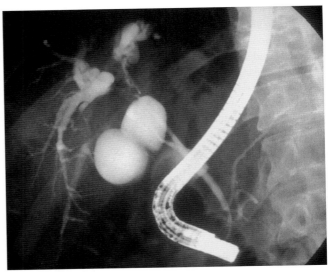

(a)

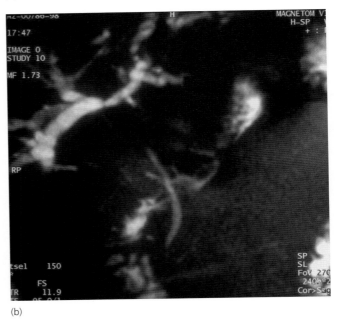

(b)

Fig. 9 Extrahepatic cholangiocarcinoma. Correlation of two different imaging techniques. (a) ERCP demonstrates the stenosis in the proximal part of the extrahepatic bile duct. Note the intrahepatic bile duct dilatation. (b) In the same patient MRCP reveals similar findings with proximal stenosis of the bile duct due to extrahepatic cholangiocarcinoma.

3 mm. However, MRCP has the potential to detect cholangiocarcinoma of the extrahepatic bile ducts (Fig. 9). Irregular changes of the intrahepatic bile duct system with additional periductal enhancement from contrast agent help to detect primary sclerosing cholangitis and differentiate this entity from other diffuse diseases of the liver that might deform the hepatic parenchyma.

In the future, the implementation of stronger and faster gradient systems, as in 3 T units, ushers in the potential for faster acquisition times and acquisition of a complete data set in one measurement (single-shot techniques). Echo planar imaging and diffusion imaging are potential imaging techniques that could be applied to specific aspects of liver imaging, targeting perfusional and functional features of the hepatic parenchyma. However, these exciting techniques are still under development.

References

1 Powers C, Ros PR, Stoupis C *et al.* (1994) Primary liver neoplasms: MR imaging with pathologic correlation. *Radiographics* 14, 459–482.

2 Semelka RC, Helmberger TK (2001) Contrast agents for MR imaging of the liver. *Radiology* 218, 27–38.

3 Ji H, Ros PR (2002) Magnetic resonance imaging. Liver-specific contrast agents. *Clin Liver Dis* 6, 73–90.

4 Balci NC, Semelka RC (2005) Contrast agents for MR imaging of the liver. *Radiol Clin North Am* 43, 887–898.

5 Motohara T, Semelka RC, Nagase L (2002) MR imaging of benign hepatic tumors. *Magn Reson Imaging Clin North Am* 10, 1–14.

6 Kim MJ, Kim JH, Chung JJ *et al.* (2003) Focal hepatic lesions: detection and characterization with combination gadolinium- and superparamagnetic iron oxide-enhanced MR imaging. *Radiology* 228, 719–726.

7 Scharitzer M, Schima W, Schober E *et al.* (2005) Characterization of hepatocellular tumors: value of mangafodipir-enhanced magnetic resonance imaging. *J Comput Assist Tomogr* 29, 181–190.

8 Hussain SM, Zondervan PE, IJzermans JN *et al.* (2002) Benign versus malignant hepatic nodules: MR imaging findings with pathologic correlation. *Radiographics* 22, 1023–1036.

9 Taouli B, Losada M, Holland A, Krinsky G (2004) Magnetic resonance imaging of hepatocellular carcinoma. *Gastroenterology* 127, S144–S152.

10 Shimizu A, Ito K, Koike S *et al.* (2003) Cirrhosis or chronic hepatitis: evaluation of small (≤2-cm) early-enhancing hepatic lesions with serial contrast-enhanced dynamic MR imaging. *Radiology* 226, 550–555.

11 Park MS, Kim TK, Kim KW *et al.* (2004) Differentiation of extrahepatic bile duct cholangiocarcinoma from benign stricture: findings at MRCP versus ERCP. *Radiology* 233, 234–240.

12 Ros PR, Freeny PC, Harms SE *et al.* (1995) Hepatic MR imaging with ferumoxides: a multicenter clinical trial of the safety and efficacy in the detection of focal hepatic lesions. *Radiology* 196, 481–488.

13 Tanimoto A, Wakabayashi G, Shinmoto H *et al.* (2005) Superparamagnetic iron oxide-enhanced MR imaging for focal hepatic lesions: a comparison with CT during arterioportography plus CT during hepatic arteriography. *J Gastroenterol* 40, 371–380.

14 Mergo PJ, Ros PR, Buetow PC, Buck JL (1994) Diffuse disease of the liver: radiologic-pathologic correlation. *Radiographics* 14, 1291–1307.

15 Itai Y, Saida Y (2002) Pitfalls in liver imaging. *Eur Radiol* 12, 1162–1174.

16 Siegelman ES, Rosen MA (2001) Imaging of hepatic steatosis. *Semin Liver Dis* 21, 71–80.

17 Siegelman ES, Mitchell DG, Rubin R *et al.* (1991) Parenchymal versus reticuloendothelial iron overload in the liver: distinction with MR imaging. *Radiology* 179, 361–366.

18 Gandon Y, Guyader D, Heautot JF *et al.* (1994) Hemochromatosis: diagnosis and quantification of liver iron with gradient-echo MR imaging. *Radiology* 193, 533–538.

19 Ralls PW, Henley DS, Colletti PM *et al.* (1987) Amebic liver abscess: MR imaging. *Radiology* 165, 801–804.

5.6.4 Hepatic angiography

Sanjeeva P. Kalva and Dushyant V. Sahani

The current role of angiography in the investigation of liver disease is limited due to technical advances in cross-sectional imaging. Computerized tomography (CT) and magnetic resonance imaging (MRI) are very useful in the diagnosis of hepatic parenchymal and vascular disorders. However, angiography is useful in a few specific circumstances and is part of various interventional procedures. This chapter summarizes the current indications, techniques and findings of hepatic angiography in liver disease. Angiography of the liver can be divided into three sections: hepatic arteriography, portal venography and hepatic venography.

Hepatic arteriography

Hepatic arteriography, the study of hepatic arteries by catheter angiography, is indicated in the following circumstances [1].
• To study the hepatic arterial anatomy before liver resection and intra-arterial chemotherapy pump placement.
• As part of various interventional procedures such as chemoembolization, embolization following trauma and as a part of planning before intra-arterial therapy with radioactive particles (such as SIRSpheres, Sirtex Medical, Lake Forest, IL, USA).
• Assessment of hepatic vascular disorders such as vasculitis, aneurysms, arteriovenous fistulae.
• To diagnose the source of haemobilia.
• Rarely to diagnose primary or metastatic neoplasms.
• As a part of CT arterioportography.
• Evaluation of vascular complications following hepatic transplantation.

Technique

With a transfemoral antegrade approach, a Cobra or Sidewinder catheter is used to cannulate the coeliac axis. If an axillary or brachial arterial approach is used, a Davis or multipurpose catheter can be used to cannulate the coeliac axis. In general, a coeliac arteriogram is performed to obtain a global view of coeliac axis anatomy. Then, selective cannulation of hepatic artery is performed using a hydrophilic guide wire or a coaxial technique. Cannulation of branches of the proper hepatic artery usually requires coaxial catheters. The complications of hepatic arteriography include injury to hepatic arteries (dissection, rupture, occlusion) due to catheter manipulation, access site complications such as haematoma, pseudoaneurysm and infection, and contrast material-related complications.

Standard hepatic arterial anatomy

A standard hepatic arterial anatomy is found in 55–60% of the population [2,3]. The common hepatic artery (CHA) arises from the coeliac axis (CA) and divides into the proper hepatic artery (PHA) and gastroduodenal arteries (GDA). The proper hepatic artery divides into right and left hepatic arteries. The right hepatic artery (RHA) supplies the right lobe of the liver through right ventrocranial and right dorsocaudal branches. The caudate lobe receives blood supply from the right hepatic artery. The left hepatic artery supplies the left lobe through medial and lateral segmental branches. The lateral branch bifurcates into superior and inferior segmental arteries, which give the characteristic fork-like configuration to the left hepatic artery. The artery supplying the medial segment of the left lobe is often called the middle hepatic artery (segment IV artery).

Variant hepatic arterial anatomy

A variant hepatic arterial anatomy occurs in 40–45% of the population. In general, the following comments can be made. A portion of or the entire right lobe or the entire liver can get its blood supply from the superior mesenteric artery. Similarly, part or all of the left lobe may be supplied from the left gastric artery (LGA). The proper or common hepatic artery can arise directly from the aorta or from the superior mesenteric artery (Fig. 1). The segmental arteries may arise directly from the common hepatic artery in 25% of individuals. A maximum of

Table 1 Variations in hepatic artery anatomy and their incidence.

Anatomical variation	Incidence (%)
Variant common hepatic artery (CHA)	
Origin from SMA	2.5
Origin from aorta	2.0
Variant proper hepatic artery	
Replaced RHA from SMA	12–14
Accessory RHA from SMA	6–8
RHA from aorta or CA or CHA	<2
Replaced LHA from LGA	11–12
Accessory LHA from LGA	11–12
LHA/LGA common trunk from aorta	1–2

CA, coeliac axis; LGA, left gastric artery; LHA, left hepatic artery; RHA, right hepatic artery; SMA, superior mesenteric artery.

three hepatic arteries supply the liver. The variations and their incidence are listed in Table 1 [4].

Collateral pathways for the hepatic artery

In the event of stenosis or occlusion of the coeliac axis or the common hepatic artery, the proper hepatic artery is perfused through retrograde flow from the gastroduodenal artery through the pancreatico-duodenal arcades. Similarly, the accessory or replaced hepatic arteries provide excellent collateral pathways. Additionally, collateral pathways exist between phrenic and hepatic arteries at the liver capsule. Hepatocellular carcinomas can derive blood supply from the internal mammary, gastroepiploic, intercostal, phrenic and oesophageal arteries. The intrahepatic arteries are end arteries and collateral pathways within the intrahepatic segments are scant and imperfect [5].

Portal venography

Portal venography can be performed by placing a catheter in the portal vein (direct portal venography) or by other means without directly cannulating the portal vein (indirect portal venography). Portal vein patency and flow direction can be reliably imaged on colour Doppler sonography. CT and MRI are also useful in the detection of portal vein thrombus or tumour in the portal vein. The current indications for indirect portal venography are as follows:
• To assess patency of the portal vein before portosystemic shunt surgery.
• To assess patency of a portosystemic shunt (such as a splenorenal shunt).
• To study the portal haemodynamics (hepatopetal vs hepatofugal flow) when other imaging studies are inconclusive.
• Evaluation of portal vein for suspected vascular compromise following liver transplantation.

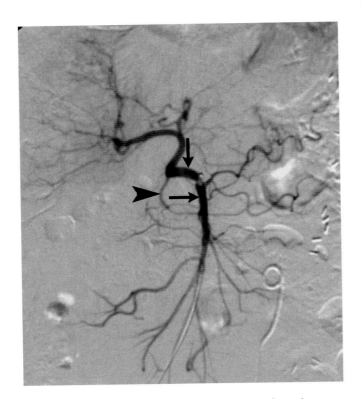

Fig. 1 Variant hepatic arterial anatomy. Superior mesenteric arteriogram demonstrates common hepatic artery (vertical arrow) arising from proximal superior mesenteric artery (horizontal arrow). The gastroduodenal artery is marked with an arrowhead.

The indications for direct portal venography are as follows:
• All the indications of indirect portal venography when the results of indirect portal venography are inconclusive.
• To obtain portal vein pressures.
• As part of other interventional procedures such as portal vein embolization before liver surgery, autologous islet cell transplantation, embolization of gastric and oesophageal varices, and as part of transjugular intrahepatic portosystemic shunt (TIPS) procedure.
• Venous sampling for localization of endocrine tumours.

Techniques of portal venography

Direct portal venography can be performed via a percutaneous transhepatic approach, a transjugular transhepatic venous approach or by cannulating a patent umbilical vein in retrograde fashion. These are discussed in separate sections. The methods of indirect portal venography are arterial portography, splenoportography and wedged hepatic venography in patients with portal hypertension.

Arterial portography

During this study, either the superior mesenteric or the splenic artery is catheterized (through a femoral artery or brachial artery approach) and imaging is continued during the venous phase of arteriography (Fig. 2) [6]. This study requires a large volume of contrast material (40–60 mL injected at a rate of 6–8 mL/s) and filming is continued for 30–60 s. The drawbacks of this procedure include poor or inadequate opacification of the portal vein in patients with splenomegaly or due to hepatofugal flow in the portal vein. Another limitation is that a partial filling defect may be seen in the portal vein simulating a thrombus due to inflow from splenic vein during superior mesenteric artery (SMA) arterial portography or vice versa.

Splenoportography

Percutaneous splenoportography is performed by puncturing the spleen in the posterior axillary line with a 20–22 G needle and injecting contrast material into the spleen [7]. Portal pressures can be obtained by directly connecting the needle to a manometer as the splenic pulp pressure corresponds to portal pressure. During contrast injection the splenic and portal veins are opacified. The presence of portosystemic collaterals, oesophageal or fundal varices or hepatofugal flow may result in inadequate opacification of the portal vein. In addition, inflow of non-opacified blood from superior mesenteric or inferior mesenteric veins may simulate a thrombus in the splenic or portal veins. The main complications of this procedure are bleeding, which may require transfusions or splenectomy, injury to bowel, kidney or lung, and splenic artery aneurysms or arteriovenous fistulae. Embolization of the needle tract with Gelfoam (Pfizer Inc., New York, USA) decreases bleeding complications [8].

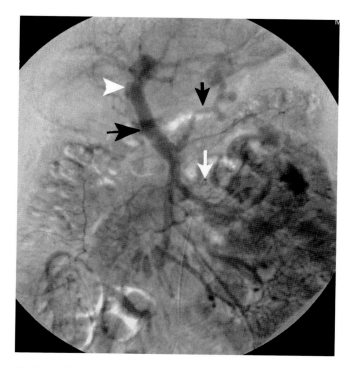

Fig. 2 Arterial portography. The superior mesenteric artery is catheterized (white arrow). The venous phase of the arteriogram depicts the portal vein (horizontal black arrow). The coronary vein (vertical black arrow) and gastric varices are also seen. The right portal vein is occluded (arrowhead) due to thrombus from a hepatoma.

Wedged hepatic venography

In patients with portal hypertension, wedged hepatic venography provides good opacification of the portal vein. This procedure is performed by placing a catheter in a hepatic vein tributary (through either a transjugular or femoral vein approach), such that the catheter wedges in the lumen of the hepatic vein, and contrast material is injected through the catheter. As an alternative, a balloon catheter can be used to occlude the hepatic vein. In patients with no portal hypertension, the contrast material opacifies other hepatic veins through hepatic venous collaterals. However, in patients with portal hypertension, the portal vein is opacified (Fig. 3). A hepatofugal flow may opacify the splenic, mesenteric veins and portosystemic collaterals. The degree of portal vein opacification depends on portal venous pressure and flow direction. In addition, the use of less viscous contrast material (such as CO_2) rather than the highly viscous iodinated contrast material provides better opacification of the portal vein [9]. The normal wedged hepatic venous pressure is <10 mmHg. The wedged hepatic venous pressure roughly equals the portal vein pressure. However, in patients with well-developed portosystemic collaterals, the wedged hepatic venous pressure may be less than the portal vein pressure. The wedged hepatic venous pressure is normal in patients with presinusoidal or extrahepatic types of

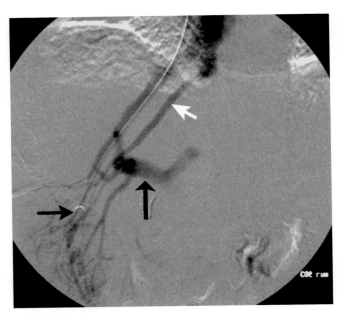

Fig. 3 Wedged hepatic venography in a patient with moderate portal hypertension. A balloon occlusion catheter is placed in the right hepatic vein (horizontal black arrow) and CO_2 venography is performed. There is opacification of the right (vertical black arrow) and left portal veins. There is also opacification of other hepatic veins (white arrow).

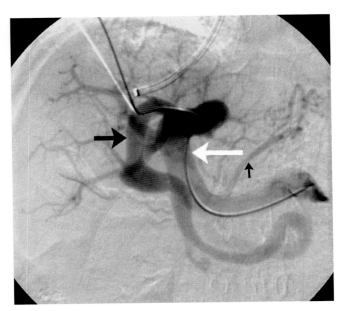

Fig. 4 Portography through umbilical vein catheterization. The umbilical vein (horizontal black arrow) is catheterized and the catheter tip is in the splenic vein. The coronary vein (vertical black arrow) and the portal vein (white arrow) are well seen.

portal hypertension. A falsely elevated wedged hepatic venous pressure may be recorded if pressure measurements are obtained after contrast material injection. The complications of wedged hepatic venography are minimal and include access site haematoma, injury to hepatic veins, haemorrhagic infarction and hepatic perforation [10].

Portal venography through patent umbilical vein

A patent umbilical vein, especially in patients with portal hypertension, provides a route for direct access to the portal vein [11]. The umbilical vein can be catheterized through the anterior abdominal wall under ultrasound guidance. Direct pressure measurements in the portal vein and portography can be performed (Fig. 4). The main limitation is that the umbilical vein is patent in only a few patients with portal hypertension. The complications are minimal and include bleeding and injury to liver, pleura and pericardium.

Percutaneous transhepatic portal venography

Percutaneous transhepatic portal venography is performed from the right midaxillary line at the 9–10th intercostal space using a 22 G Chiba needle. Generally, the right portal vein is opacified and the needle is exchanged for a catheter, which is placed in the main portal vein. Pressure measurements are obtained and portal venography undertaken. The catheter tract is usually embolized with Gelfoam upon completion of the study [12]. The main complications of the procedure are haemorrhage, injury to the pleura or intestine, traumatic pseudoaneurysm of the hepatic artery, and infection.

Transjugular transhepatic portal venography

Transjugular transhepatic portal venography is usually a part of the TIPS (transjugular intrahepatic portosystemic shunt) procedure [13]. Once the hepatic vein is cannulated through a transjugular route, access to the portal vein is obtained using a Colapinto needle. The portal vein is opacified and the needle is exchanged for a catheter over a wire. Portal venography and pressure measurements are performed (Fig. 5). The complications of this procedure are bleeding, traumatic pseudoaneurysm of the hepatic artery, injury to gallbladder, bile leak, injury to intestine and infection.

Normal portal venous anatomy

The splenic and superior mesenteric veins join at the pancreatic head to form the main portal vein. In the porta hepatis the main portal vein lies anterior to the common bile duct and to the right of the hepatic artery. As it enters the liver, it divides into right and left portal veins. The branching pattern is dichotomous and follows the branching pattern of the hepatic artery.

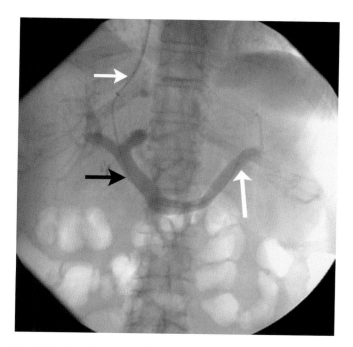

Fig. 5 Transjugular portography. The portal vein (black arrow) was catheterized through transjugular access. There is a large sheath in the hepatic vein (horizontal white arrow) and the catheter's tip is in the splenic vein (vertical white arrow).

Portosystemic collateral pathways

Multiple communications exist between the portal venous circulation and systemic veins that serve as collateral pathways in patients with portal hypertension [14]. These are listed in Table 2.

Hepatic venography

Hepatic vein catheterization and venography are indicated in the following circumstances.
• Measurement of free hepatic vein pressure and wedged hepatic vein pressure in patients with portal hypertension.

• During wedged hepatic venography to document patency and flow reversal in patients with portal hypertension.
• To detect occlusion or thrombus in hepatic veins.
• As a part of other interventional procedures such as transjugular liver biopsy and transjugular intrahepatic portosystemic shunt procedure.

Techniques of hepatic venography

There are several methods to opacify the hepatic veins.
• The hepatic veins can be catheterized through either the transjugular approach or femoral vein approach. Other approaches include subclavian vein or antecubital vein.
• Inferior venacavography with the Valsalva manoeuvre results in reflux of the contrast material into the hepatic veins.
• Percutaneous transhepatic venography can be performed if other methods are unsuccessful. In this method, a 22 G Chiba needle is used to inject 10–15 mL of contrast material into the hepatic parenchyma. In normal liver, this produces a dense parenchymal stain and, later, multiple hepatic veins are opacified. The portal vein radicals and hepatofugal flow may be seen in patients with portal hypertension.

Complications of hepatic venography

Hepatic venography is a safe procedure and complications are minimal. The complications include intrahepatic haematoma, focal haemorrhagic infarcts and hepatic perforation with subcapsular injection of contrast medium (especially during wedged hepatic venography).

Pathology

Angiography is rarely performed as a diagnostic test for evaluation of focal or diffuse liver disease. However, lesions may be detected on angiography performed for other indications, and it is important to know the angiographic appearances of various focal and diffuse liver diseases. The following sections describe briefly the imaging appearances of various diseases on angiography.

Table 2 Connections between the portal venous system and systemic veins that can serve as collaterals in portal hypertension.

Portal vessels	Connect to
Portal vein tributary (normally drains into the portal vein)	Systemic vein tributary (drains into SVC/IVC)
Oesophageal, gastric cardiac veins	Oesophageal veins of azygos, hemiazygos veins
Oesophageal, gastric cardiac veins	Left phrenic vein, which drains into left renal vein
Superior haemorrhoidal veins of inferior mesenteric vein	Middle and inferior rectal haemorrhoidal veins, which drain into internal pudendal veins
Splenic vein	Retroperitoneal veins such as renal, adrenal and phrenic veins
Recanalized umbilical vein (communicates with left portal vein)	Epigastric veins in the anterior abdominal wall
Mesenteric vein tributaries	Retroperitoneal veins
Patent ductus venosus (communicates left portal vein directly to IVC)	IVC

IVC, inferior vena cava; SVC, superior vena cava.

Neoplasms

Angiography plays an important role in the management of liver malignancies. It is part of interventional procedures such as transcatheter tumour embolization, and portal vein embolization to induce liver hypertrophy before liver resection. Angiography may also be used to detect focal hypervascular liver tumours that are not visible or incompletely characterized on other modalities. Angiography is also useful in characterizing suspected perfusion abnormalities detected on CT or MRI. Angiography may also be used to evaluate the hepatic arterial anatomy before chemotherapy pump placement or hepatic resection. CT arteriography and CT arterioportography require selective cannulation of the hepatic artery and splenic or mesenteric artery respectively. These two procedures are performed for the workup of hepatomas and metastases and for detecting small tumours in the liver.

Hepatic tumours are of either hepatocyte origin or nonhepatocyte origin. Tumours can also be divided into benign and malignant. Tumours of hepatocyte origin are supplied by the hepatic artery and tend to be hypervascular. The angiographic appearance depends on the size of the tumour, presence of haemorrhage or necrosis within the tumour and prior therapy. The angiographic findings of tumours (Fig. 6) in general are as follows:

- tumour neovascularity;
- arteriovenous shunting;
- tumour stain;
- contrast pooling or 'lakes';
- displacement of vessels;
- enlargement of feeding artery;
- vascular ingrowth or invasion or occlusion.

The angiographic appearances of various liver tumours are listed in Table 3 [15,16].

Trauma

CT is the initial imaging test for blunt and penetrating trauma. CT is useful for diagnosing subcapsular haematoma, liver contusion and laceration. Angiography is indicated in suspected major arterial injury in patients with acute trauma, for evaluation of haemobilia following trauma (especially following biliary interventions), suspected traumatic pseudoaneurysm on CT, and in the evaluation of traumatic haematoma in the liver. Hepatic arteriography may show active extravasation of contrast material at the site of laceration or amputation or occlusion of hepatic arteries, pseudoaneurysm (Fig. 7) or arterioportal or arteriobiliary fistulae [17]. Intrahepatic haematoma appears as a focal defect during the parenchymal phase with displacement of hepatic arteries. An infected haematoma may show peripheral rim enhancement. Mycotic aneurysms may be seen in association with infected haematomas. Subcapsular haematomas result in characteristic curvilinear configuration to the liver edge during the parenchymal phase. Embolization of the hepatic artery can be successfully performed for traumatic injuries using Gelfoam, particles or coils [18]. Portal vein patency should be assessed prior to embolizing the hepatic artery. Injuries to the portal vein are rarely encountered in practice as these result in profound haemodynamic instability and such patients are usually taken for immediate surgery. In major trauma, inferior vena cavography should also be performed to assess injury to the intrahepatic portion of the inferior vena cava.

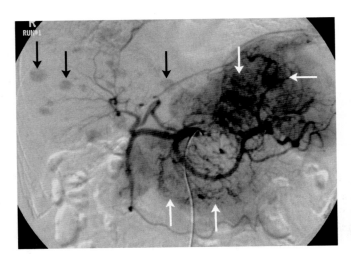

Fig. 6 Multicentric hepatoma. Coeliac axis angiogram shows multiple hypervascular liver lesions in the right lobe (black arrows). A large lesion in the left lobe (white arrows) demonstrates neovascularity, arteriovenous shunting and tumour stain.

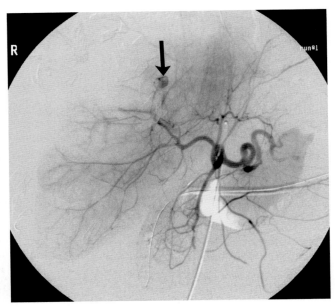

Fig. 7 Post-traumatic hepatic artery pseudoaneurysm. Coeliac axis angiogram in a 20-year-old male with hepatic laceration on CT following a motor vehicle accident. There is a pseudoaneurysm (arrow) arising from a branch of the right hepatic artery. This was successfully embolized.

Table 3 Angiographic appearances of liver tumours.

Tumour	Appearance during hepatic arteriography
Hepatic adenoma	Round, well-circumscribed hypervascular lesion with enlarged hepatic artery that is displaced to the periphery of the tumour; tumour vessels in the periphery of the lesion; diffuse parenchymal stain; focal areas of hypovascularity if the lesion is complicated by haemorrhage and necrosis
Focal nodular hyperplasia	Well-circumscribed hypervascular liver lesion that is subcapsular in location; 'spoke-wheel pattern' in small tumours as the hepatic artery enters the tumour centrally and divides into branches; enlarged displaced hepatic artery in large lesions; fine granular appearance in parenchymal phase with radiolucent septae or scar
Capillary haemangioma	Enlarged hepatic artery that divides into a capillary network; tumour stain
Cavernous haemangioma	Normal sized hepatic artery, splaying of hepatic artery if the tumour is large; irregular, nodular contrast pooling ('lakes') occurring in the periphery of the lesion and progressively moving towards the centre of the lesion and persisting during the venous phase; occasional phleboliths
Peliosis hepatis	Appearance similar to cavernous haemangioma; however, the 'contrast pooling' is not as dense and nodular as in cavernous haemangioma, and does not progress to the centre of the lesion
Regenerating nodule	No neovascularity; lesions isodense or hypodense to liver in parenchymal phase; hepatic artery branch at the centre of the lesion; displaced portal vein and hepatic vein branches if the lesion is large
Haemangioendothelioma	Enlarged hepatic artery; hypervascular lesion with no neovascularity; contrast pooling similar to haemangiomas with early washout; arteriovenous shunting
Hepatocellular carcinoma	Solitary or multicentric or diffuse; enlarged hepatic artery; hypervascular lesion with neovascularity; dense tumour stain; arterioportal shunting (Fig. 6); vascular encasement; vascular ingrowth into the portal vein or the hepatic vein; extrahepatic arterial supply from phrenic, intercostal, internal mammary and gastroduodenal arteries
Metastases	Angiographic appearance depends on the size and histology of the tumour; hypervascular metastases (carcinoid, islet cell, choriocarcinoma, renal cell, thyroid) demonstrate neovascularity, tumour stain and vascular encasement Hypovascular metastases demonstrate vascular displacement, tumour stain. Portal venography may show amputation or encasement of portal vein branches
Cholangiocarcinoma	Encasement; displacement of hepatic artery branches and portal vein; absent or minimal tumour stain
Hepatoblastoma	Enlarged hepatic artery; hypervascular tumour with neovascularity; tumour stain and arteriovenous shunting

Infections and inflammatory disorders

Angiography is rarely performed in the evaluation of hepatic infections and inflammatory disorders. Ultrasound and CT are the imaging tests for diagnosis of various focal infections. Angiographic appearances of abscesses and hepatitis are of historic interest. Abscesses may show displacement of vessels with focal defects in the parenchymal phase of the hepatic arteriogram. A peripheral rim enhancement may be seen. A few abscesses are hypervascular and show dilated tortuous vessels in the periphery with arteriovenous shunting. In acute hepatitis, the intrahepatic arteries are stretched and splayed with slow flow and dense inhomogeneous hepatogram.

Cirrhosis

Although angiography is not a diagnostic test in the evaluation of cirrhosis of the liver, angiographic appearances are characteristic and may help stage the disease [19]. The morphological changes in vessels and flow patterns are secondary to parenchymal fibrosis and increased portal venous pressure. During the early stage, hepatic arterial flow may be normal or the arteries may demonstrate delayed filling. The arteries may show stretching with a normal hepatogram. The portal venous flow is hepatopetal with normal morphology. Wedged hepatic venography shows an inhomogeneous sinusoidal pattern with no portal vein opacification. During the advanced stages, the arteries show enlargement with increased flow to the liver and occasional portal vein filling during the venous phase. The intrahepatic arteries demonstrate a corkscrew appearance (Fig. 8) with dense hepatogram. The portal vein radicals show change in calibre with tortuosity and hepatofugal or bidirectional flow pattern. The umbilical vein may be recanalized (Cruveilhier–Baumgarten syndrome) and other portosystemic collaterals may be seen. Wedged hepatic venography shows preferential filling of the portal vein with minimal or no opacification of hepatic veins.

Portal hypertension

Portal hypertension is classified based on the location of obstruction to normal portal venous flow. The types are presinusoidal (either extrahepatic or intrahepatic), sinusoidal or postsinusoidal. The indications for angiographic evaluation of portal hypertension are as follows [19]:

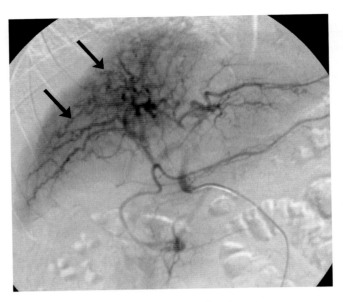

Fig. 8 Arteriographic appearance of cirrhotic liver. Late phase common hepatic arteriogram demonstrates corkscrew appearance (arrows) of intrahepatic arteries with dense hepatogram predominantly affecting the right lobe.

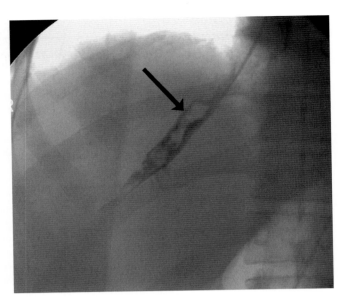

Fig. 9 Hepatic vein thrombosis in a patient with Budd–Chiari syndrome. Hepatic venography with catheter in the right hepatic vein demonstrates multiple filling defects (arrow) consistent with thrombus.

- To assess the severity of portal hypertension by pressure measurements and haemodynamic evaluation.
- To differentiate various types of portal hypertension.
- To evaluate patency of the portal venous system, surgical portosystemic shunts and TIPS.
- To demonstrate and embolize gastric and oesophageal varices.

The classification of portal hypertension is covered in Chapter 7.2. and its assessment is considered in Chapter 7.4

Budd–Chiari syndrome

Budd–Chiari syndrome is due to hepatic venous outflow obstruction. The obstruction may be in the hepatic veins – due to thrombus (Fig. 9) or tumour – or suprahepatic either in the inferior vena cava (thrombus, web, tumour) or in the heart (right heart failure, constrictive pericarditis). The intrahepatic type is common in women. Hepatic venography fails to demonstrate a main hepatic vein and multiple venous collaterals may be seen in spiderweb fashion during percutaneous hepatic venography [20,21]. Thrombi in the hepatic veins may be seen as filling defects. The hepatic wedge pressure is elevated. A web, thrombus, tumour or extrinsic impression may be demonstrable during inferior vena cavography. Portal venography shows bidirectional or hepatofugal flow with portosystemic collaterals. Hepatic arteriography may show stretching and splaying of hepatic arterial branches with inhomogeneous hepatogram due to congestive hepatomegaly.

Portosystemic shunts

Angiography of portosystemic shunts or TIPS is indicated when shunt malfunction is suspected and endovascular therapy is planned. During the evaluation of these shunts, pressure gradients across the anastomosis and contrast venography are obtained. Angioplasty and stent insertion may be performed whenever indicated.

Diseases of blood vessels

Aneurysms, arteriovenous fistulae, atherosclerosis, emboli, dissection and vasculitis may affect the hepatic arteries. Aneurysms are often post-traumatic and are usually intrahepatic. Atherosclerotic hepatic aneurysms affect the extrahepatic arteries (Fig. 10) and have a high risk of rupture [22]. Mycotic aneurysms are secondary to infected haematomas or abscesses. Multiple intrahepatic aneurysms may be seen in systemic vasculitis syndromes such as polyarteritis nodosa. Arteriography is indicated for diagnosis and treatment planning. Endovascular therapy may be attempted in intrahepatic aneurysms using particles or coils. Extrahepatic aneurysms are usually treated surgically. Atherosclerotic disease of the hepatic arteries is part of systemic arterial disease, and calcified and non-calcified plaques, vessel narrowing and occlusions may be seen affecting the extrahepatic arteries. Embolic occlusion is rare and is often due to emboli from the heart. Dissection of hepatic arteries is iatrogenic during catheter manipulation during selective hepatic arteriography. These dissections appear as focal or diffuse

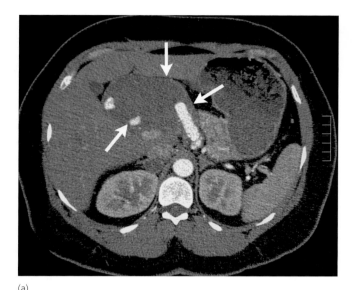

(a)

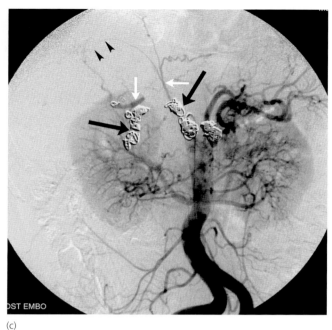

(c)

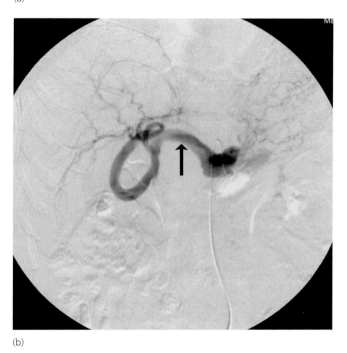

(b)

Fig. 10 Aneurysm of common hepatic artery. (a) CT scan of the abdomen shows a large aneurysm (arrows) affecting the common hepatic artery. There is thrombus within the aneurysm. (b) Angiography with catheter in the common hepatic artery shows a large false lumen (arrow) that communicates with the true lumen and fills intrahepatic arteries. (c) After embolization with coils (black arrows), the aneurysm is no longer filling. The intrahepatic arteries are seen (vertical white arrow) filling through capsular collaterals (arrowheads) from the right phrenic artery (horizontal white arrow).

narrowing, vessel occlusion and may resolve without any treatment. Fibromuscular dysplasia may affect the common hepatic artery, and the artery appears 'beaded' with multiple areas of focal narrowing and dilatation on arteriography. Various systemic vasculitis syndromes may affect the hepatic arteries and the angiographic appearance is non-specific with areas of diffuse or focal smooth narrowing and multiple aneurysms [23].

Evaluation of transplanted liver

Angiographic evaluation of a transplanted liver is indicated when liver function tests are abnormal and vascular compromise is suspected. Angiographic evaluation is usually preceded by non-invasive evaluation with ultrasound or MRI [24]. Aortography and selective arteriography are performed when arterial anastomotic stenosis or hepatic artery thrombosis is suspected. A pressure gradient across the anastomosis may be obtained. In the immediate postoperative period, treatment is surgical. Transluminal angioplasty may be performed during the late postoperative period [25]. When hepatic venous anastomotic stricture is suspected, MRI is usually sufficient; however, selective hepatic venography may be performed and the pressure gradient may be measured when MRI results are equivocal. Transjugular liver biopsy may be performed in acute and chronic rejections.

References

1 Dittman W (1982) Hepatic angiography. *Semin Liver Dis* 2, 41–48.

2 Covey AM, Brody LA, Maluccio MA *et al.* (2002) Variant hepatic arterial anatomy revisited: digital subtraction angiography performed in 600 patients. *Radiology* 224, 542–547.

3 Jones RM, Hardy KJ (2001) The hepatic artery: a reminder of surgical anatomy. *J R Coll Surg Edinb* 46, 168–170.

4 Bonn J (1996) Diagnostic visceral normal and variant anatomy – celiac, superior mesenteric and inferior mesenteric arteries. In: Haskal ZJ, Kerlan RK, Trerotola SO (eds) *Thoracic and Visceral Vascular Interventions*. SCVIR syllabus. Fairfax, VI: Society of Cardiovascular and Interventional Radiology, pp. 153–163.

5 Charnsangavej C, Chuang VP, Wallace S *et al.* (1982) Angiographic classification of hepatic arterial collaterals. *Radiology* 144, 485–494.

6 Herlinger H (1978) Arterioportography. *Clin Radiol* 29, 255–275.

7 Zamir O, Mogle P, Lernau O, Nissan S (1984) Splenoportography – a reappraisal. *Am J Gastroenterol* 79, 283–286.

8 Brazzini A, Hunter DW, Darcy MD *et al.* (1987) Safe splenoportography. *Radiology* 162, 607–609.

9 Martinez-Cuesta A, Elduayen B, Vivas I *et al.* (2000) CO(2) wedged hepatic venography: technical considerations and comparison with direct and indirect portography with iodinated contrast. *Abdom Imaging* 25, 576–582.

10 Castaneda-Zuniga WR, Jauregui H, Rysavy JA *et al.* (1978) Complications of wedge hepatic venography. *Radiology* 126, 53–56.

11 Pochaczevsky R, Calem WS, Richter RM (1967) Umbilical vein portography. Its value in the diagnosis of extrahepatic portal vein obstruction and in other applications. *Radiology* 89, 868–873.

12 Burcharth F (1979) Percutaneous transhepatic portography. I. Technique and application. *AJR Am J Roentgenol* 132, 177–182.

13 Stanley AJ, Jalan R, Forrest EH *et al.* (1996) Longterm follow up of transjugular intrahepatic portosystemic stent shunt (TIPSS) for the treatment of portal hypertension: results in 130 patients. *Gut* 39, 479–485.

14 Ahn J, Cooper JM, Silberzweig JE, Mitty HA (1997) Venographic appearance of portosystemic collateral pathways. *Br J Radiol* 70, 1302–1306.

15 Freeny PC (1983) Angiography of hepatic neoplasms. *Semin Roentgenol* 18, 114–122.

16 Watson RC, Baltaxe HA (1971) The angiographic appearance of primary and secondary tumors of the liver. *Radiology* 101, 539–548.

17 Schorn L, Coln D (1977) Hepatic angiographic changes after trauma. *Am J Surg* 134, 754–757.

18 Mohr AM, Lavery RF, Barone A *et al.* (2003) Angiographic embolization for liver injuries: low mortality, high morbidity. *J Trauma* 55, 1077–1081.

19 Kadir S (1986) Angiography of the liver, spleen and pancreas. In: Kadir S (ed.) *Diagnostic Angiography*. Philadelphia: WB Saunders.

20 Maguire R, Doppman JL (1977) Angiographic abnormalities in partial Budd-Chiari syndrome. *Radiology* 122, 629–635.

21 Wilson MW, Ring EJ, LaBerge JM *et al.* (1996) Percutaneous transhepatic venography in the delineation and treatment of Budd-Chiari syndrome. *J Vasc Interv Radiol* 7, 133–138.

22 Abbas MA, Fowl RJ, Stone WM *et al.* (2003) Hepatic artery aneurysm: factors that predict complications. *J Vasc Surg* 38, 41–45.

23 Herskowitz MM, Flyer MA, Sclafani SJ (1993) Percutaneous transhepatic coil embolization of a ruptured intrahepatic aneurysm in polyarteritis nodosa. *Cardiovasc Intervent Radiol* 16, 254–256.

24 Nghiem HV, Tran K, Winter TC 3rd *et al.* (1996) Imaging of complications in liver transplantation. *Radiographics* 16, 825–840.

25 Abbasoglu O, Levy MF, Vodapally MS *et al.* (1997) Hepatic artery stenosis after liver transplantation – incidence, presentation, treatment, and long term outcome. *Transplantation* 63, 250–255.

5.6.5 Endoscopic retrograde cholangiopancreatography

Alan J. Wigg and James Toouli

Introduction

Since the first descriptions of therapeutic endoscopic retrograde cholangiography (ERCP) in 1975, this technique has gained rapid and widespread acceptance in the diagnosis and management of a variety of biliary and pancreatic diseases. With advances in alternative techniques, the role of ERCP has changed now mostly to a therapeutic one. However, it should be noted that expertise in ERCP remains the most widely available, and newer approaches to therapy and diagnosis described below remain unavailable in many centres. In this chapter, we focus on the role of ERCP in the diagnosis and therapy of some common biliary diseases and also on important current controversies. The role of ERCP in sphincter of Oddi dysfunction is covered elsewhere in this book, and its role in pancreatic diseases is not discussed in this chapter.

ERCP in diagnosis

Bile duct stones

The sensitivity and specificity of clinical, biochemical and transabdominal ultrasound variables (fever, cholangitis, pancreatitis, abnormal liver function tests, dilated bile ducts) is poor. Mathematical models using combinations of these variables may improve the ability to predict the presence of bile duct stones, but they remain too imprecise for routine clinical use [1]. This problem has previously led to the routine use of ERCP in the diagnosis of suspected bile duct stones. Although ERCP has the obvious advantage of enabling definitive therapy to be performed immediately following the diagnosis of bile duct stones, this approach exposes a significant number of patients, without bile duct stones, to the risks associated with this invasive procedure. In the commonly encountered clinical situation in which there are associated gallstones, our approach is to proceed to laparoscopic cholecystectomy and use intra-operative cholangiography for diagnosis of suspected common bile duct stones. However, in instances in which the gallbladder stones may not be the primary candidate for suspecting bile duct pathology or where patient comorbidities make laparoscopic cholecystectomy high risk, a less invasive approach for diagnosis is justified. The emergence of sensitive and specific non-invasive biliary imaging modalities including magnetic resonance cholangiopancreatography (MRCP), endoscopic ultrasound (EUS) and computerized tomographic cholangiography (CTC) are now changing the role of diagnostic ERCP in this setting.

The performance characteristics of these new modalities have been compared with ERCP by multiple investigators. However, a number of problems hamper the interpretation of these studies. First, ERCP has frequently been used as the gold standard to measure sensitivity, specificity, positive predictive and negative predictive values of the alternative diagnostic test. As ERCP may also have false-positive and false-negative findings in the diagnosis of bile duct stones, most of these studies measure only concordance with ERCP findings, and the results can only be worse than ERCP. Most studies have also suffered from small size and therefore inadequate power to detect what appear to be small differences in performance characteristics between the various tests.

MRCP, using state of the art technology, experienced radiologists and single breath-hold techniques, has demonstrated good concordance with ERCP in the diagnosis of bile duct stones (see Fig. 1). Sensitivities and specificities for MRCP in this setting have both been higher than 90% in most studies [2,3]. In one study, where endoscopic or surgical stone extraction was used as the gold standard rather than ERCP images, the sensitivity of ERCP (100%) was shown to be superior to that of MRCP (91%), but specificities were the same (both 100%) [4]. As the resolution of MRCP currently remains less than that of good-quality fluoroscopic ERCP images, a reduced sensitivity of MRCP due to lack of detection of smaller bile duct stones (< 5 mm) has been suggested by several authors [4–6].

The use of EUS in the diagnosis of bile duct stones was first described in 1992 [7]. The superior sensitivity of EUS compared with conventional transabdominal ultrasound and computerized tomography (CT) has been demonstrated [8], and nine reasonable quality studies have reported results comparing the performance characteristics of EUS vs. ERCP in the detection of bile duct stones [2]. In most of these studies, independent gold standards have been available as a result of endoscopic or surgical stone removal following both EUS and ERCP. The sensitivities of both techniques have been similar in these studies ranging from 84% to 96% for EUS and 79% to 100% for ERCP. Specificities have also been very similar in all studies ranging from 97% to 100% for EUS and 87% to 100% for ERCP. Significantly different differences in performance characteristics between the tests have not been reported.

CTC has also been proposed as a non-invasive alternative to ERCP for the diagnosis of bile duct stones. Comparison studies with ERCP are difficult to interpret because of differences in the choice of gold standard and the variety of contrast techniques used (none, oral, intravenous). In studies with independent reference standards, sensitivities appear to be lower than those for ERCP, ranging from 71% to 88% [9–12]. Specificities were 95% and above for three of these four studies. These studies provide an impression of lower sensitivity of CTC for the detection of bile duct stones, but more rigorous comparison is not possible.

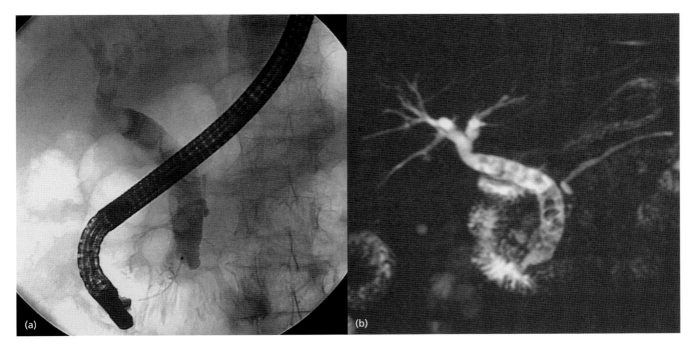

Fig. 1 Cholangiography of the same patient with ERCP (a) and MRCP (b) showing multiple filling defects due to bile duct stones.

On the basis of current evidence, the diagnostic performance of ERCP, MRCP and EUS appears to be equivalent in patients with suspected bile duct stones. However, the use of these tests is also determined by other important factors, including the probability of therapy and local expertise. In situations in which the probability of therapy is high, non-invasive diagnostic tests are likely to increase the expense and time required to treat patients with bile duct stones. Conversely, where the probability of therapy is lower, the use of non-invasive diagnostic tests has been shown to reduce the numbers of unnecessary ERCPs, morbidity and costs associated with the investigation of suspected bile duct stones [5,13,14]. The choice of non-invasive diagnostic test will vary according to available expertise. Proponents of EUS have advocated an approach in which EUS is performed immediately prior to ERCP, thus enabling avoidance of ERCP in those without stones demonstrated by EUS [13]. For most institutions, the logistics of such an approach are prohibitive. We favour MRCP in this setting as the technique is more widely available, is non-invasive with negligible morbidity and mortality and can be performed in an outpatient setting. The greatest use of MRCP in the diagnosis of bile duct stones is likely to be in the evaluation of patients with low to intermediate probability of bile duct stones who do not require cholecystectomy. Neither MRCP nor ERCP should be used routinely to rule out stones prior to laparoscopic cholecystectomy, as intraoperative cholangiography in this setting is the most cost-effective and efficient means.

Biliary strictures

Biliary strictures causing obstruction have a variety of benign (inflammatory, chronic pancreatitis) and malignant causes (pancreatic and gallbladder cancer, cholangiocarcinoma, portal metastases). Definitive diagnosis of such strictures and differentiation between a benign and a malignant process is a common challenge confronting clinicians. The role of ERCP in diagnosis appears to be changing following the introduction of several alternative diagnostic techniques.

Studies investigating the ability of MRCP and direct cholangiography to differentiate benign from malignant pancreaticobiliary strictures that have used independent reference standards (subsequent histology or follow-up) have demonstrated equivalent accuracy [15,16]. Initial MRCP also has a number of advantages in the setting of biliary obstruction. It avoids the risk of infection following contrast injection and incomplete subsequent drainage at ERCP. In conjunction with abdominal magnetic resonance imaging (MRI), it can provide useful information about surrounding abdominal structures that is not provided by ERCP. Proximal ducts beyond a stricture may be more easily seen, allowing more careful planning of future stent placements. Failure to obtain a cholangiogram is rare with MRCP and occurs less commonly than unsuccessful ERCP. MRCP can also be performed in patients with Roux-en-Y choledochojejunostomy or Bilroth II gastroenterostomy.

Multislice or multidetector CT, in which rapid 1- to 1.5-mm sections are performed, is another technique that is useful in the assessment of biliary obstruction due to strictures. It has been widely used in the evaluation of pancreatic neoplasms and their resectability. It may also be a reasonable alternative or complementary to MRCP in the evaluation of malignant obstruction, with high sensitivity and specificity for malignant obstruction reported in one study [17].

With suspected malignant strictures, tissue sampling techniques using ERCP have been the mainstay of definitive diagnosis. Such techniques have included brush cytology, bile or pancreatic juice aspiration for cytology, forceps biopsy and fine-needle aspiration (FNA) cytology. The technical difficulties associated with forceps biopsy and FNA cytology and the poor sensitivity of juice aspiration cytology have meant that most endoscopists use brush cytology alone. The sensitivity of brush cytology alone, however, remains poor with most studies reporting sensitivities between 30% and 70%. Techniques such as the use of microsatellite markers or DNA image analysis, when combined with brush cytology, may have the potential to improve the sensitivity of this technique, but are not currently widely available [18,19].

To improve the accuracy of tissue sampling, EUS-guided FNA of biliary strictures has been evaluated by a number of groups, with varying reported sensitivities for the diagnosis of malignancy. In one study directly comparing ERCP and brush biopsy with EUS-guided FNA, sensitivities were similar for both modalities (46% and 43% respectively) [20]. It is likely that EUS-guided FNA will be more useful as an adjunct to ERCP, following non-diagnostic ERCP intraductal tissue sampling. Higher sensitivities (86–89%) for the diagnosis of malignancy, leading to significant impacts on patient management, have been described using such an approach [21,22].

Intraductal ultrasound (IDUS) has also been proposed as a useful adjunct during ERCP to improve sensitivity in the diagnosis of malignant bile duct strictures. With this technique, a high-frequency ultrasound catheter is passed over a guidewire and into the bile duct during ERCP. Although this technique does not provide tissue, a number of ultrasonographic criteria have been proposed which suggest malignancy. In the hands of enthusiasts, the combination of ERCP and IDUS has been reported to be as sensitive than ERCP and ERCP biopsy techniques alone for the diagnosis of malignant strictures [23,24].

In summary, the diagnosis of biliary strictures often remains difficult. Where available, the use of abdominal MRI and MRCP is a useful initial strategy with less morbidity and equivalent diagnostic performance to ERCP. It also frequently enables proper planning of subsequent therapeutic procedures. Diagnostic (to obtain tissue specimens) and therapeutic ERCP will also frequently be required. Failure to obtain a tissue diagnosis with intraluminal biopsy techniques is a common problem due to the low sensitivity of ERCP tissue sampling methods. In this setting, the use of complementary testing including EUS-guided FNA or IDUS should be considered if available.

ERCP in therapy

Bile duct stones

Bile duct stones (choledocholithiasis) are associated with symptomatic gallbladder stones in 10–15% of cases. The majority of bile duct stones are formed in the gallbladder and then migrate to the bile duct. Bile duct stones may also form in the bile duct. These 'primary' bile duct stones are more common in Asian populations and may be associated with biliary stasis and infection. Symptoms and complications from bile duct stones are more frequent than with gallstones so, when discovered, their removal is usually indicated. Common clinical manifestations of bile duct stones and the role of ERCP in each are discussed below. ERCP removal of bile duct stones is performed following endoscopic sphincterotomy using balloon catheters or baskets (see Figs 2 and 3).

Synchronous gallbladder and bile duct stones

A common clinical scenario is that of a patient with symptomatic gallstones requiring cholecystectomy and with a high suspicion of bile duct stones. A number of options exist in this setting including split therapeutic approaches (pre- or postoperative ERCP and cholecystectomy) or a one-stage laparoscopic cholecystectomy and bile duct clearance. Laparoscopic common duct exploration techniques have evolved rapidly since their introduction in the 1990s. The bile duct can be visualized intraoperatively via insertion of catheters into the cystic duct and subsequently explored usually by the transcystic route. Exploration via the more invasive transductal route (choledo-

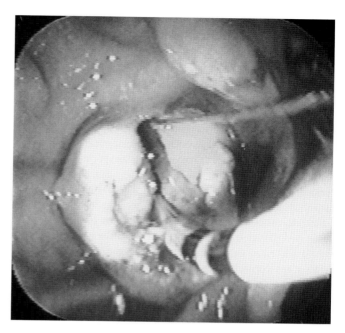

Fig. 2 Endoscopic sphincterotomy of the ampulla of Vater.

chotomy) is usually reserved for when removal of larger stones is being considered. Using a variety of techniques, similar to endoscopic stone removal, successful duct clearance has been reported in approximately 95% of cases in most recent large series with morbidity and mortality similar to the range described for ERCP [25]. Limited randomized control data comparing split and one-stage approaches have shown similar rates of duct clearance and morbidity [26,27]. Cost-effectiveness

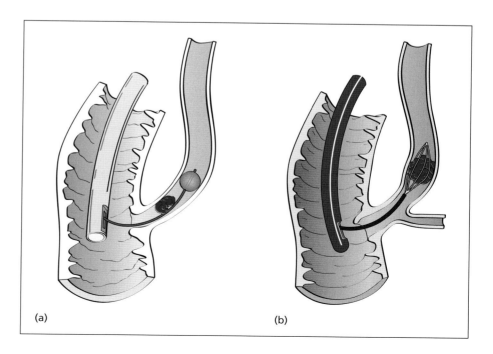

Fig. 3 Methods of endoscopic stone extraction using a balloon (a) or a basket (b).

(a) (b)

data, however, appear to favour a one-stage laparoscopic approach [28]. Therefore, in situations in which patients require laparoscopic cholecystectomy and there is a suspicion of bile duct stones, we favour the one-stage laparoscopic cholecystectomy with intraoperative cholangiography (IOC) and laparoscopic bile duct clearance of visualized stones.

A number of important caveats exist to the routine use of this approach. The most significant obstacle to the widespread adoption of this one-stage laparoscopic approach is its lack of availability. In addition, outcomes by inexperienced surgeons are likely to be less impressive than those described by experienced, high-volume centres. Therefore, in the many centres without access to surgeons experienced in laparoscopic bile duct clearance techniques, other treatment options must be considered. Patient comorbidity can also influence the approach to synchronous gallbladder and bile duct stones. Patients with significant comorbidities, which increase the risks associated with laparoscopic cholecystectomy, should be considered for ERCP and sphincterotomy alone, particularly if bile duct stones are primarily responsible for symptoms.

Important indications for urgent preoperative ERCP include severe cholangitis and severe gallstone pancreatitis, and these are discussed below. However, in the absence of these indications, the role of preoperative ERCP for bile duct stones appears to be limited. While the routine use of preoperative ERCP should be discouraged, its use in situations where there is a high suspicion of bile duct stones also remains problematic. Efforts to tighten the selection criteria for suspected bile duct stones using models based on clinical, radiological and ultrasound variables still remain imprecise, and as many as 50% of ERCPs in this setting will not demonstrate stones [1,29]. Avoiding the morbidity and cost of unnecessary ERCPs is best achieved by selecting patients for postoperative ERCP using IOC. When bile duct stones are discovered at IOC and cannot be dealt with laparoscopically, an alternative to postoperative ERCP is conversion to an open duct exploration. However, this surgery is associated with added morbidity, and postoperative ERCP should be favoured in centres with expert endoscopists. To facilitate postoperative ERCP extraction of bile duct stones, a biliary stent may be placed in the bile duct and through the sphincter of Oddi into the duodenum. The stent can subsequently be used by the ERCP endoscopist to gain access to the bile duct prior to sphincterotomy and stone removal. Good-quality data examining the cost and risk benefits of the above algorithms for the management of bile duct stones around the time of laparoscopic cholecystectomy are lacking and are an important priority for future research.

Post-cholecystectomy stones

Another common clinical scenario is of symptomatic retained or recurrent bile duct stones in patients following cholecystectomy. In this setting, ERCP is the most practical option and avoids the morbidity and expense of surgery. Although such an approach is routine in clinical practice, prospective randomized trials confirming the superiority of ERCP over surgery in post-cholecystectomy patients are lacking. It is unlikely that such trials will be done as the differences between these two approaches are marked and obvious.

Cholangitis

Cholangitis is frequently associated with bile duct stones, which enhance bacterial colonization and become coated with a bacterial biofilm. This bacterial biofilm on stones is often activated by cytokines from the bile duct epithelium when stones cause obstruction of bile ducts [30]. The severity of cholangitis varies greatly. In mild to moderate cases, patients can often be treated conservatively with appropriate resuscitation and antibiotics and bridged to elective, definitive procedures involving both laparoscopic cholecystectomy and laparoscopic or endoscopic bile duct clearance. A proportion of patients with more severe cholangitis (hypotension on presentation, deterioration despite conservative therapy) will require urgent biliary decompression. Controlled trial data have established ERCP as the preferred treatment for urgent biliary decompression in the setting of severe cholangitis, with significantly less mortality than open biliary surgery [31].

Gallstone pancreatitis

The role of early ERCP in gallstone pancreatitis has been investigated by four randomized controlled studies. In two of these studies, significant reductions in complications were observed in the endoscopically treated group compared with the conservatively treated group, and the benefit was greatest in those with more severe pancreatitis [32,33]. Non-significant trends towards reduced mortality were also observed in these studies. A third study, published in abstract form only, found significant reductions in both complications and mortality for patients with gallstone pancreatitis who were treated with early ERCP and stone removal [34]. In this study, benefits of early ERCP were seen for both mild and severe pancreatitis. In the most recent study, early ERCP was not associated with any reduction in either complications or mortality [35]. An important difference between this study and previous randomized controlled trials was the exclusion of patients likely to benefit from ERCP (including those with associated cholangitis or jaundice). Two meta-analyses of these trials have reached slightly different conclusions. The first suggested that early ERCP and endoscopic sphincterotomy when required reduced both morbidity and mortality in acute biliary pancreatitis [36]. A more recent meta-analysis, which excluded the unpublished study by Nowak, found that ERCP with or without sphincterotomy reduced complications in severe gallstone pancreatitis but had no benefit in milder pancreatitis or on mortality in any subgroup [37].

On the basis of the above data, those patients presenting with severe pancreatitis (based on modified Glasgow scale, APACHE scores or Ranson criteria) should undergo early ERCP with sphincterotomy and stone removal when present. Patients with associated biliary obstruction or who deteriorate in hospital despite an initial mild attack should also be considered for urgent ERCP. Biliary sphincterotomy disconnects the pancreatic and bile ducts and may provide some protection from recurrent bouts of gallstone pancreatitis. However, unless contraindications exist, most patients should also undergo cholecystectomy during the same admission to prevent further stone formation in the gallbladder (the usual site of origin of stones), with subsequent migration to the bile duct. Milder forms of pancreatitis are best managed conservatively with spontaneous improvement due to passage of stones occurring in the majority of such patients. Owing to the high recurrence rate of biliary pancreatitis in those with persistent gallstones, patients with milder forms of pancreatitis should also be considered for elective laparoscopic cholecystectomy with intraoperative cholangiography at the time of surgery to confirm passage of bile duct stones.

Malignant biliary obstruction

Malignant biliary obstruction may result from a variety of causes including pancreatic and gallbladder carcinoma, cholangiocarcinomas, hilar metastases and ampullary neoplasia. Frequently, malignancies in this region are unresectable, and therapeutic ERCP has an important palliative role in this setting via the relief of symptoms (jaundice, pruritus, pain) and improvement in the quality of life. Important controversies surrounding therapeutic ERCP in the management of malignant biliary obstruction are discussed below.

Preoperative biliary decompression

Owing to its widespread availability, ERCP and stenting are frequently performed early in the evaluation of patients with malignant jaundice. In those patients who, on subsequent staging, are shown to have resectable disease, the value of preoperative biliary decompression has been examined by multiple studies [38,39]. Studies comparing outcomes following preoperative decompression with no decompression have been of generally poor quality and have given conflicting results. While preoperative stent insertion has consistently demonstrated an improvement in bilirubin and liver function tests, it has not demonstrated improvements in significant clinical outcomes such as perioperative mortality. Concerns about increased infectious complications following ERCP and implantation metastases due to stenting have also been raised. On the basis of currently available data, it therefore seems unnecessary to decompress patients who are about to undergo surgery, which highlights the need for thorough staging investigations before ERCP is contemplated. Preoperative decompression may be more appropriate in a number of situations other than cholangitis. Decompression in patients with prolonged waiting times for surgery because of preoperative chemoradiotherapy may permit

improvements in nutritional status. Patients with prolonged, severe jaundice may also be at higher risk of poorer postoperative outcomes [40]. Patients with poor cardiac function may also benefit from biliary decompression via decreases in levels of atrial natriuretic peptide and reductions in left ventricular systolic work [41]. However, clinical data demonstrating improvements in these subsets of patients following preoperative decompression are currently lacking.

Endoscopic vs. surgical palliation

Palliation of malignant biliary obstruction can be achieved with endoscopic stenting or surgical bypass, usually performed with hepaticojejunostomy. Percutaneous transhepatic stenting can also be performed, but increased mortality and less frequent technical success rates have been reported when compared with the less invasive endoscopic approach [42]. Five studies (three randomized controlled trials, two retrospective studies) have compared outcomes between endoscopic and surgical bypass [38]. These data have not demonstrated a survival advantage for either approach. An increased perioperative morbidity in the surgery group and an increased need for readmission and stent changes in the ERCP group have been consistent findings. More relevant trials, comparing minimally invasive surgical bypass techniques with longer patency expandable metal stents, have not been done and would be helpful in defining the preferred approach. In the absence of such definitive data, patient management needs to be individualized. A reasonable approach is to perform stenting with an expandable metal stent and to reserve surgical bypass for those patients in whom stenting cannot be achieved or who have unresectable disease found at the time of operation. In addition, patients who may have difficulty accessing expert endoscopic services, such as those from remote locations, may be better served by the surgical approach.

Plastic vs. metal stents

A significant drawback associated with the use of plastic (polyethylene) stents is stent occlusion due to bacterial biofilms clogging the internal stent lumen. Consequently, the median plastic stent patency is only around 4 months. Stent occlusion is usually heralded by recurrent jaundice and cholangitis. To avoid stent occlusion, many endoscopists will schedule elective stent changes 3- to 6-monthly, an approach that increases the costs of care. An alternative approach has been to perform stent changes only when clinically indicated; however, this approach may expose the patient to the risks of cholangitis.

The most promising current strategy to reduce the problem of stent occlusion is the use of expandable metal stents. Several controlled trials have compared the use of metal vs. plastic stents [43–46]. Conclusions from these studies have been that metal stents are associated with significantly longer patency rates and a reduction in costs associated with stent dysfunction. Median patency rates for metal stents are reported to be from

8 to 12 months in most studies. Therefore, in patients with an anticipated longer life expectancy, the higher initial costs of metallic stent insertion seem justifiable. In those patients with life expectancies less than 4 months, usually because of liver metastases, the use of plastic stents is more appropriate [46].

Although the use of metal stents appears to represent an advance in some settings, a number of problems associated with their use have been described. Tumour ingrowth and overgrowth are common causes of metal stent occlusion. As metal stents are not removable, further stent placement inside the initial stent is then required. Efforts to overcome such problems are being actively pursued and include the use of covered stents, removable metal stents and metal stents with antitumour activity.

Proximal lesions

Effective palliation of malignant obstruction involving the hilum or proximal extrahepatic bile ducts (see Fig. 4) is more difficult to achieve endoscopically than for distal lesions [47]. The use of multiple stents to provide adequate drainage to both liver lobes and prevent cholangitis following ERCP has been advocated. Despite the increased difficulties, proximal lesions

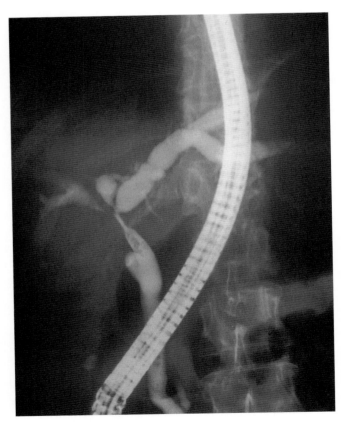

Fig. 4 Malignant hilar stricture at the bifurcation of the left and right hepatic ducts.

can frequently be managed successfully with the use of single metal stents and careful preprocedure planning. Using unilateral metal stents, successful palliation of hilar obstruction has been reported in 97% of cases in one study and in 77% in another [48,49]. MRI can be particularly useful in helping to identify which lobes or segments require decompression and to avoid stenting atrophic segments. Although encouraging, some caution is required, as such an approach requires a high degree of technical expertise and stent occlusion rates are also higher for proximal lesions compared with distal lesions [47]. Percutaneous stenting using expandable metal stents is an alternative option in these patients and one that we usually prefer. In patients with very poor life expectancies, avoiding the expense and potential morbidity of biliary stenting can also be a sensible option.

References

1 Soltan HM, Kow L, Toouli J (2001) A simple scoring system for predicting bile duct stones in patients with cholelithiasis. *J Gastrointest Surg* 5(4), 434–437.

2 Mark DH, Flamm CR, Aronson N (2002) Evidence-based assessment of diagnostic modalities for common bile duct stones. *Gastrointest Endosc* 56(Suppl. 6).

3 Fulcher AS (2002) MRCP and ERCP in the diagnosis of common bile duct stones. *Gastrointest Endosc* 56(Suppl. 6).

4 Sugiyama M, Atomi Y, Hachiya J (1998) Magnetic resonance cholangiography using half-Fourier acquisition for diagnosing choledocholithiasis. *Am J Gastroenterol* 93(10), 1886–1890.

5 Griffin N, Wastle ML, Dunn WK *et al.* (2003) Magnetic resonance cholangiopancreatography versus endoscopic retrograde cholangiopancreatography in the diagnosis of choledocholithiasis. *Eur J Gastroenterol Hepatol* 15(7), 809–813.

6 Laokpessi A, Bouillet P, Sautereau D *et al.* (2001) Value of magnetic resonance cholangiography in the preoperative diagnosis of common bile duct stones. *Am J Gastroenterol* 96(8), 2354–2359.

7 Edmundowicz SA, Aliperti G, Middleton WD (1992) Preliminary experience using endoscopic ultrasonography in the diagnosis of choledocholithiasis. *Endoscopy* 24(9), 774–778.

8 Amouyal P, Amouyal G, Levy P *et al.* (1994) Diagnosis of choledocholithiasis by endoscopic ultrasonography (see comment). *Gastroenterology* 106(4), 1062–1067.

9 Ishikawa M, Tagami Y, Toyota T *et al.* (2000) Can three-dimensional helical CT cholangiography before laparoscopic cholecystectomy be a substitute study for endoscopic retrograde cholangiography? *Surg Laparosc Endosc Percutan Techn* 10(6), 351–356.

10 Polkowski M, Palucki J, Regula J *et al.* (1999) Helical computed tomographic cholangiography versus endosonography for suspected bile duct stones: a prospective blinded study in non-jaundiced patients. *Gut* 45(5), 744–749.

11 Neitlich JD, Topazian M, Smith RC *et al.* (1997) Detection of choledocholithiasis: comparison of unenhanced helical CT and endoscopic retrograde cholangiopancreatography (see comment). *Radiology* 203(3), 753–757.

12 Jimenez Cuenca I, del Olmo Martinez L, Pérez Homs M *et al.* (2001) Helical CT without contrast in choledocholithiasis diagnosis. *Eur Radiol* 11(2), 197–201.

13 Buscarini E, Tansini P, Vallisa D et al. (2003) EUS for suspected chole-docholithiasis: do benefits outweigh costs? A prospective, controlled study. Gastrointest Endosc 57(4), 510–518.

14 Kaltenthaler E, Vergel YB, Chilcott J et al. (2004) A systematic review and economic evaluation of magnetic resonance cholangiopancre-atography compared with diagnostic endoscopic retrograde cholan-giopancreatography. Health Technol Assess 8(10), 1–89.

15 Rosch T, Meining A, Fruhmorgen S et al. (2002) A prospective comparison of the diagnostic accuracy of ERCP, MRCP, CT, and EUS in biliary strictures. Gastrointest Endosc 55(7), 870–876.

16 Park MS, Kim TK, Kim KW et al. (2004) Differentiation of extra-hepatic bile duct cholangiocarcinoma from benign stricture: findings at MRCP versus ERCP. Radiology 233(1), 234–240.

17 Ahmetoglu A, Kosucu P, Kul S et al. (2004) MDCT cholangiography with volume rendering for the assessment of patients with biliary obstruction. Am J Roentgenol 183(5), 1327–1332.

18 Khalid A, Pal R, Sasatomi E et al. (2004) Use of microsatellite marker loss of heterozygosity in accurate diagnosis of pancreaticobiliary malignancy from brush cytology samples (see comment). Gut 53(12), 1860–1865.

19 Krishnamurthy S, Katz RL, Shumate A et al. (2001) DNA image ana-lysis combined with routine cytology improves diagnostic sensitivity of common bile duct brushing. Cancer 93(3), 229–235.

20 Rosch T, Hofrichter K, Frimberger E et al. (2004) ERCP or EUS for tissue diagnosis of biliary strictures? A prospective comparative study. Gastrointest Endosc 60(3), 390–396.

21 Eloubeidi MA, Chen VK, Jhala NC et al. (2004) Endoscopic ultrasound-guided fine needle aspiration biopsy of suspected cholangiocarcinoma (see comment). Clin Gastroenterol Hepatol 2(3), 209–213.

22 Fritscher-Ravens A, Broering DC, Knoefel WT et al. (2004) EUS-guided fine-needle aspiration of suspected hilar cholangiocarcinoma in potentially operable patients with negative brush cytology. Am J Gastroenterol 99(1), 45–51.

23 Farrell RJ, Agarwal B, Brandwein SL et al. (2002) Intraductal US is a useful adjunct to ERCP for distinguishing malignant from benign biliary strictures. Gastrointest Endosc 56(5), 681–687.

24 Domagk D, Poremba C, Dietl KH et al. (2002) Endoscopic transpapil-lary biopsies and intraductal ultrasonography in the diagnostics of bile duct strictures: a prospective study. Gut 51(2), 240–244.

25 Dorman JP, Franklin ME Jr, Glass JL (1998) Laparoscopic common bile duct exploration by choledochotomy. An effective and efficient method of treatment of choledocholithiasis. Surg Endosc 12(7), 926–928.

26 Cuschieri A, Croce E, Faggioni A et al. (1996) EAES ductal stone study. Preliminary findings of multi-center prospective randomized trial comparing two-stage vs single-stage management (see comment). Surg Endosc 10(12), 1130–1135.

27 Sgourakis G, Karaliotas K (2002) Laparoscopic common bile duct exploration and cholecystectomy versus endoscopic stone extraction and laparoscopic cholecystectomy for choledocholithiasis. A prospect-ive randomized study. Minerva Chir 57(4), 467–474.

28 Urbach DR, Khajanchee YS, Jobe BA et al. (2001) Cost-effective man-agement of common bile duct stones: a decision analysis of the use of endoscopic retrograde cholangiopancreatography (ERCP), intra-operative cholangiography, and laparoscopic bile duct exploration. Surg Endosc 15(1), 4–13.

29 Tham TC, Lichtenstein DR, Vandervoort J et al. (1998) Role of endoscopic retrograde cholangiopancreatography for suspected choledocholithiasis in patients undergoing laparoscopic cholecystec-tomy. Gastrointest Endosc 47, 50–56.

30 Ko CW, Lee SP (2002) Epidemiology and natural history of common bile duct stones and prediction of disease. Gastrointest Endosc 56(Suppl. 6).

31 Lai EC, Mok FP, Tan ES et al. (1992) Endoscopic biliary drainage for severe acute cholangitis (see comment). N Engl J Med 326(24), 1582–1586.

32 Neoptolemos JP, Carr-Locke DL, London NJ et al. (1988) Controlled trial of urgent endoscopic retrograde cholangiopancreatography and endoscopic sphincterotomy versus conservative treatment for acute pancreatitis due to gallstones. Lancet 2(8618), 979–983.

33 Fan ST, Lai EC, Mok FP et al. (1993) Early treatment of acute biliary pancreatitis by endoscopic papillotomy (see comment). N Engl J Med 328(4), 228–232.

34 Nowak A, Nowakowska-Dulawa E, Marek T et al. (1995) Final results of a prospective, randomized, controlled study on endoscopic sphinc-terotomy versus conventional management in acute biliary pancreatitis. Gastroenterology 108, A380.

35 Folsch UR, Nitsche R, Ludtke R et al. (1997) Early ERCP and pap-illotomy compared with conservative treatment for acute biliary pancreatitis. The German Study Group on Acute Biliary Pancreatitis (see comment). N Engl J Med 336(4), 237–242.

36 Sharma VK, Howden CW (1999) Metaanalysis of randomized con-trolled trials of endoscopic retrograde cholangiography and endo-scopic sphincterotomy for the treatment of acute biliary pancreatitis. Am J Gastroenterol 94(11), 3211–3214.

37 Ayub K, Imada R, Slavin J (2004) Endoscopic retrograde cho-langiopancreatography in gallstone-associated acute pancreatitis. Cochrane Database Syst Rev 4.

38 Flamm CR, Mark DH, Aronson N (2002) Evidence-based assessment of ERCP approaches to managing pancreaticobiliary malignancies. Gastrointest Endosc 56(Suppl. 6).

39 Strasberg SM (2002) ERCP and surgical intervention in pancreatic and biliary malignancies. Gastrointest Endosc 56(Suppl. 6).

40 Su CH, Tsay SH, Wu CC et al. (1996) Factors influencing postoper-ative morbidity, mortality, and survival after resection for hilar chol-angiocarcinoma. Ann Surg 223(4), 384–394.

41 Padillo J, Puente J, Gomez M et al. (2001) Improved cardiac function in patients with obstructive jaundice after internal biliary drainage: hemodynamic and hormonal assessment. Ann Surg 234(5), 652–656.

42 Speer AG, Cotton PB, Russell RC et al. (1987) Randomised trial of endoscopic versus percutaneous stent insertion in malignant obstruc-tive jaundice. Lancet 2(8550), 57–62.

43 Knyrim K, Wagner HJ, Pausch J et al. (1993) A prospective, random-ized, controlled trial of metal stents for malignant obstruction of the common bile duct. Endoscopy 25(3), 207–212.

44 Davids PH, Groen AK, Rauws EA et al. (1992) Randomised trial of self-expanding metal stents versus polyethylene stents for distal malignant biliary obstruction (see comment). Lancet 340(8834–8835), 1488–1492.

45 Prat F, Chapat O, Ducot B et al. (1998) A randomized trial of endo-scopic drainage methods for inoperable malignant strictures of the common bile duct (see comment). Gastrointest Endosc 47(1), 1–7.

46 Kaassis M, Boyer J, Dumas R et al. (2003) Plastic or metal stents for malignant stricture of the common bile duct? Results of a randomized prospective study. Gastrointest Endosc 57(2), 178–182.

47 Becker CD, Glattli A, Maibach R *et al.* (1993) Percutaneous palliation of malignant obstructive jaundice with the Wallstent endoprosthesis: follow-up and reintervention in patients with hilar and non-hilar obstruction. *J Vasc Interv Radiol* 4(5), 597–604.

48 De Palma GD, Pezzullo A, Rega M *et al.* (2003) Unilateral placement of metallic stents for malignant hilar obstruction: a prospective study. *Gastrointest Endosc* 58(1), 50–53.

49 Freeman ML, Overby C (2003) Selective MRCP and CT-targeted drainage of malignant hilar biliary obstruction with self-expanding metallic stents. *Gastrointest Endosc* 58(1), 41–49.

5.7 Interventional radiology in hepatobiliary diseases

José Ignacio Bilbao Jaureguízar, Concepció Bru, Joan Falcó Fages and Lluís Donoso

Unlike other applications of diagnostic imaging, the main emphasis in interventional radiology is on the procedure, and this makes it especially amenable to innovation. Image-guided, minimally invasive therapies will continue to grow in importance as current techniques of delivering various forms of energy for ablation evolve towards non-invasiveness and methods are developed to deliver genes, gene products and drugs to specific target sites in order to control angiogenesis and other biological processes.

Percutaneous techniques have proved their usefulness in the management of hepatic pathology and have become the treatment of choice in a wide variety of diseases. The next few paragraphs will explain to what extent and in which situations interventional techniques are useful in treating problems deriving from hepatic haemorrhaging, hepatic tumours (in particular hepatocellular carcinoma) and bile duct obstruction.

Gastrointestinal bleeding of hepatic origin

Introduction

From the vascular viewpoint, the liver is unique in its double afferent vascularization. The hepatic artery, a branch of the coeliac trunk with a wide range of anatomical variants, accounts for 30% of the vascular flow to the liver. Apart from supplying the bile tract, this artery practically exclusively feeds liver tumours, whether primary or metastatic in origin. The portal vein, which supplies the remaining 70% of flow, is a closed system made up of mesenteric and splenic veins, and is connected to the systemic circulation through multiple collateral (fundamentally gastro-oesophageal, splenorenal and haemorrhoidal) vessels. The venous drainage of the liver is achieved through a single system (hepatic veins), which, like the arteries, can present multiple anatomical variants.

Arterial haemorrhaging

A lesion in the hepatic artery can manifest itself by bleeding freely into the peritoneal cavity, as in intrahepatic, subcapsular lesions or haemobilia, which may ultimately lead to gastrointestinal haemorrhage. This type of bleeding can be difficult to identify and distinguish from other types of intestinal haemorrhages. If the lesion is in the extravisceral part of the common hepatic artery, the haemorrhage is usually massive and difficult to control. It is normally caused by a pseudoaneurysm related to previous surgery (e.g. liver transplant) with or without associated infection. Percutaneous treatment consists of selective embolization, stopping the bleeding in the affected area. It is highly recommended that the permeability of the gastroduodenal artery should be maintained to ensure hepatic arterial perfusion. If embolization is not possible, for whatever reason, then, in isolated cases, the repair of the lesion should be done by placing a covered endovascular stent, which will seal the point of haemorrhage but at the same time maintain the hepatic arterial flow.

Morphologically speaking, vascular lesions causing gastrointestinal haemorrhage can be divided into four types [1–4]:

1 Small terminal vessel lesions. Usually caused by biopsy needles or biliary catheters, these can lead to major haemorrhage.

2 Vascular lacerations, almost always caused by a drainage catheter, injury or laceration trauma. Such cases need to be treated at both the proximal and the distal levels. The artery should be embolized using coils, first in the distal part of the lesion to avoid reperfusion through intrahepatic collaterals, after which the proximal artery should be embolized.

3 Vascular lesions with arterial–portal shunt – the traumatic/iatrogenic arterial–portal shunt is sometimes the only angiographic manifestation of intermittent haemobilia. The closing of the connection between the portal vein and hepatic artery will also seal the point of bleeding.

4 Vascular laceration with a pseudoaneurysm. The example most frequently seen is a lesion in the right hepatic artery or the common hepatic artery after surgery, especially after a laparoscopic cholecystectomy. In large pseudoaneurysms, just as in vascular lacerations, the most adequate percutaneous treatment is the occlusion of both the distal and the proximal arteries with the aim of excluding the arterial lesion and preserving the distal flow. Occasionally, this procedure is not technically possible or is ineffective and, for that reason, it is better to resort to other possibilities such as the direct treatment of the lesion by direct puncture and thrombosis using coils, fibrin sponges or thrombin.

Haemorrhage due to portal hypertension

Whatever the circumstances that increase the gradient of the portal system (the difference in pressure between the portal system and the central blood pressure), more than a 10–15 mmHg increase will develop into a possible rupture of the collateral vessels, which leads to the fluid from the portal system entering the systemic vascularization. The cause of this increase in gradient has multiple aetiologies and depends upon a number of factors. The origin may be in the liver parenchyma (e.g. cirrhosis) or in the venous outflow, as in the Budd–Chiari syndrome, or in the venous inflow as in portal vein thrombosis.

The endovascular procedures applied in interventional radiology have shown their effectiveness in the three above-mentioned cases. We continue to discuss the different possible techniques (palliative as well as curative) using interventional radiology in the treatment of patients with portal hypertension and bleeding.

Venous outflow obstruction

This can be due to Budd–Chiari syndrome, congenital membranous obstructive disease or postsurgical complications, particularly those arising after liver transplantation (Fig. 1). In these cases, the percutaneous transhepatic access – guided by echography – of the blocked or obstructed vein followed by angioplasty or the placement of a metallic endoprosthesis offers good long-term results and may sometimes be curative. The rate of restenosis of the treated lesion is very low (permeability at 3 years is 90%), and complications of the procedure are infrequent but severe when thy occur [5].

Treatment of diseases causing portal hypertension by affecting liver parenchyma

Independent of whether the lesion is presinusoidal, sinusoidal or postsinusoidal, the percutaneous treatment in these cases is palliative. The transjugular intrahepatic portosystemic shunt (TIPS) procedure involves a percutaneous approach that connects the hepatic with the portal vein [6]. When it was first described in 1969, it opened up new and different possibilities for percutaneous intervention, which allowed direct connection between the two blood vessels. Since then, it has been incorporated into various different technical aspects and has become a widely used procedure for treating patients with portal hypertension. The success rate of the technique is 90%; patients with acute haemorrhage have a survival rate of more than 70% after 1 month when the liver function is maintained (Child–Pugh A/B) [7–9]. The most frequent complications are hepatic encephalopathy (13%) and intraprosthetic stenosis, which often recurs.

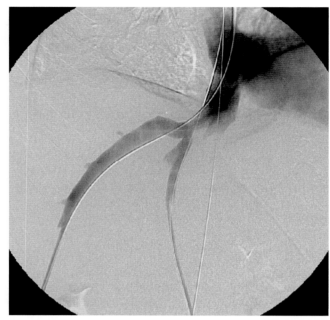

(a)

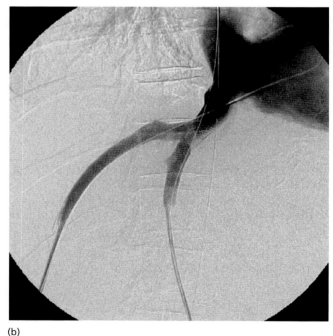

(b)

Fig. 1 Liver transplant performed 2 months ago. Patient with ascites; ultrasound (US) shows a severe slowing down of hepatic vein flow. (a) After the percutaneous catheterization of the right and middle hepatic veins, a phlebography is performed showing moderate stenosis of the surgical venous connection. Stenosis is crossed with angiographical wires. Hepatic vein–right atrial pressure gradient is 7 mmHg. (b) Image obtained after co-locating two metallic autoexpandible prostheses. The pressure gradient has diminished to 1 mmHg.

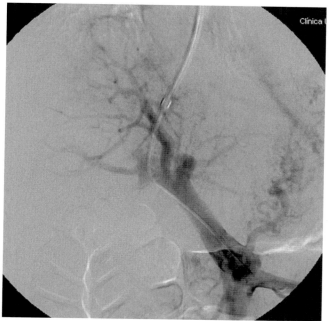

(a)

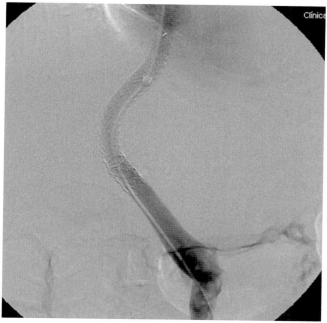

(b)

Fig. 2 Patient with cirrhosis and recurrent bleeding due to gastro-oesophageal varices, in spite of being treated with endoscopic sclerotherapy. (a) Transjugular portography using catheters placed in a transparietal approach. Portosystemic gradient is 21 mmHg. Note hepatofugal flow into gastro-oesophageal varices. (b) Metallic prosthesis covered with PTFE between portal and right hepatic veins. Gradient is now 8 mmHg.

The uncovered prostheses are very effective in creating a channel deriving directly from the portal vein, but they have a tendency to occlusion. There are a variety of reasons, one of which is the intraductal 'contamination' of biliary material due to the transection of the biliary canaliculus in the TIPS procedure. To avoid restenosis, two alternative approaches have been developed: first, the creation of extrahepatic portosystemic percutaneous connections and, secondly, the implanting of a covered prosthesis of a non-permeable material [polytetrafluoroethylene (PTFE)] [10] (Fig. 2). With these advances, the permeability of TIPS has changed radically, from 50% to 90% in the year 2005. Therefore, in patients with portal hypertension and gastrointestinal bleeding, in whom pharmacological and endoscopic treatments have failed, treatment with TIPS is the best alternative.

Lesions of the portal vein

There are various causes that can generate portal hypertension as result of alterations in the portal vein and its tributaries. Among these are inflammatory stenosis and obstructions (pancreatic, pylophlebitis, etc.) as well as surgical causes (e.g. after liver transplant). In the absence of associated liver disease, the most appropriate treatment is angioplasty, preferably with the placement of an endoprosthesis, with direct transhepatic portal access (Fig. 3). There is a high permeability rate in the following 3–5 years after placement [11,12].

Hepatocellular carcinoma percutaneous treatment

Introduction

Hepatocellular carcinoma (HCC) develops in liver cirrhosis of any aetiology, being more frequent in advanced cirrhosis and the final cause of death in more than 50% of these patients.

The possibility of detecting the tumour at an early stage [13], when curative treatments can be applied, will represent the possibility of increasing survival in patients with HCC, who will otherwise have a really dismal prognosis.

To propose one or other therapy, we use the BCLC system [14], which links staging with treatment indication. Classification as well as diagnosis criteria are explained in Chapter 18.2.1.

Unfortunately, curative therapies can be applied only in 30–40% of the patients corresponding to stage A [15]. Most of the patients with HCC are diagnosed at stage B, and the only option that has been shown to have a positive impact on survival is transarterial chemoembolization (TACE).

Percutaneous treatments

Destruction or ablation of tumour cells can be achieved by the injection of chemical substances [ethanol (PEI), acetic acid (PAI)] or by inserting a probe that modifies local tumour

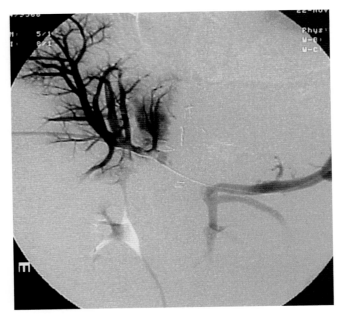

(a)

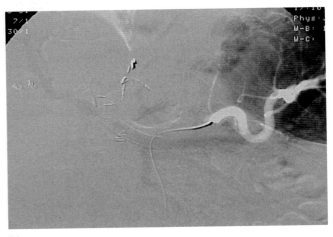

(b)

Fig. 3 A 45-year-old patient with recurrent pancreatitis requiring several surgical interventions with actual large varices due to a portal vein occlusion. (a) After a percutaneous transparietal puncture of the portal vein, a vascular introducer is placed in the right portal vein and a catheter, crossing the obstruction in the splenic vein. (b) Images obtained after co-locating a prosthesis in the obstructed area. It corresponds to an indirect portography after the administration of contrast into the splenic artery. It shows a good inner flow through the prosthesis without opacity of collateral veins.

temperature [cryotherapy, laser, radiofrequency (RF) and microwaves (MW)].

Percutaneous ablation is considered the best option for patients with early HCC who are ineligible for resection or transplantation [5] or who are on a waiting list for a liver transplant.

A few years ago, PEI was the most frequently employed technique as it is inexpensive, requires simple technology and – with expertise in fine-needle puncture of the liver – has a low rate of complications: < 3% morbidity with 0.5% mortality [16,17]. PEI aims at imbibing the tumour completely with ethanol, resulting in coagulative necrosis of the tissue and thrombosis of the small surrounding vessels. PEI is usually performed under ultrasound (US) guidance, which allows control of the diffusion of the alcohol by observing small bright spots spreading into the tumour and flowing in the nearby vessels. This permits exact control of the diffusion and change in the position of the needle if the tissue does not retain the alcohol. This characteristic can only be detected with US when injecting alcohol, which preserves a small amount of air that acts as a contrast. When using computerized tomography (CT), the diffusion of alcohol cannot be controlled, and a large amount of alcohol can reach a vessel producing non-desired thrombosis. PEI has to be repeated on separate days, and it achieves complete tumour necrosis in 90–100% of HCCs < 2 cm in diameter. This is reduced to 70% in tumours of 2–3 cm and to 50% in tumours of 3–5 cm. The 5-year survival of Child–Pugh A candidates with a complete response is more than 50% [16,17,29]. The presence of septa prevents the diffusion of ethanol into the whole tumour volume and, hence, complete necrosis is rarely achieved in tumours larger than 3 cm [17].

The injection of acetic acid (PAI) represents an alternative. It is painless, and comparative studies have shown that PAI needed fewer sessions than PEI, producing wide areas of necrosis. PAI has been employed mainly in China and Japan [18,19].

The introduction of RF in the late 1990s replaced PEI/PAI in most instances, PEI/PAI being reserved for some selected cases or as an adjuvant to RF [20] or TACE. This is particularly true for tumours near great vessels; vessels larger than 3 mm result in rapid dissipation of the heat by blood flow. In such cases, PEI in the area close to the vessel permits the achievement of complete necrosis. In superficial lesions, or those close to the gallbladder or intestinal structures, the risk of complications such as seeding or perforation is increased, but they are easily treated with PEI.

In a recent series [22,26], there are almost no criteria of exclusion for RF, but the incidence of complications is not negligible. RF is nowadays the ablative therapy used most frequently (Fig. 4). It can be applied through different kinds of electrodes, percutaneously, laparoscopically or intraoperatively. The main drawbacks of RF ablation are its higher cost, a morbidity of 8–10% and a mortality of close to 1% [23–25]. Studies comparing antitumoral efficacy of RF and PEI showed a clear advantage for RF [21–22]. RF is usually performed under US guidance, but CT or magnetic resonance imaging (MRI) with adequate needles can be used.

While PEI can be performed in an outpatient setting, RF needs a minimum of 24 hours in hospital and strong sedation or anaesthesia to support the therapy.

A post-RF syndrome consisting of pain, malaise and fever related to necrosis can appear, but should be over after 1 week. If it persists, the presence of complications must be suspected.

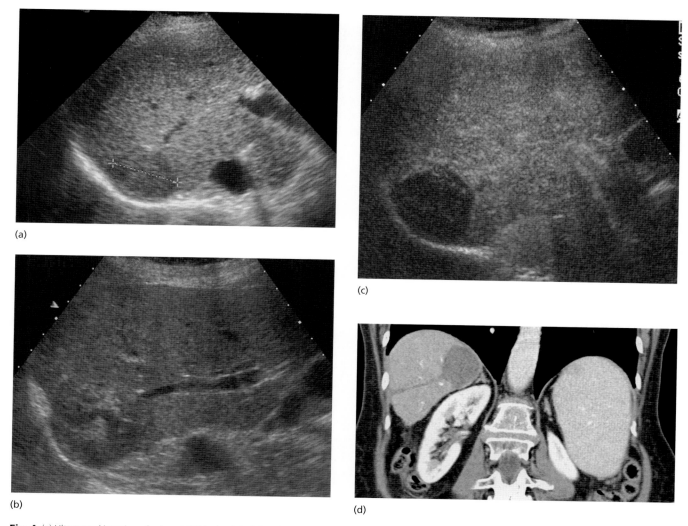

Fig. 4 (a) Ultrasound imaging of a 4 cm HCC in the right lobe of the liver. (b) Changes in echostructure after radiofrequency ablation performed with US control. (c) In the arterial phase of ultrasound contrast, no perfusion of the treated area is detected. (d) Coronal plane of CT showing the ablated area and the coagulation of the needle traject.

Control of efficacy

The degree of ablation is assessed at 1 month by dynamic contrast-enhanced ultrasound (CEUS), CT or MRI. The absence of contrast uptake in the tumour reflects tumour necrosis, while the recognition of contrast uptake indicates incomplete treatment. CEUS is useful during treatment as it detects persistence of tumour in areas that have not been reached by alcohol, or 24 hours after RF to assess technical adequacy or complications [27,28].

If CT or MRI is performed early after the treatment, the hyperaemia induced by the therapy all round the tumour can generate confusion with respect to the efficacy of the intervention: persistence of tumour or recurrence are usually partial and in a nodular shape; also, any enlargement of the lesion will suggest tumoral growth. CT or MRI will be useful in detecting new lesions and should be performed every 4 months in the first 2 years.

The recurrence rate after percutaneous ablation is similar to that detected after surgical resection and can occur within the vicinity of the treated nodule or in separate segments of the liver. Tumours initially classified as completely necrosed may present intratumoral recurrence later on, and this should be considered as a treatment failure that was not detectable in the early follow-up on imaging techniques. Nevertheless, initial complete necrosis obtained with either alcohol or RF will produce a significant increase in survival in Child A or B patients [29].

Other percutaneous therapies

Microwave ablation (MW) is an emerging modality [30,31] that consists of introducing a special needle (antennas) – usually under sonographic guidance – generating microwaves inside the tumour. Thereby, wide areas of complete necrosis similar to those obtained with RF are attained for single tumours < 3 cm. Newer antennas with different shapes or combination with embolization have been tried to increase efficacy for larger tumours. There are no limitations in terms of proximity to large vessels, but prospective studies are needed to establish the safety of the procedure.

High-intensity focused ultrasound (HIFU)

This method is well established for prostate cancer. The advantages of this method include non-invasiveness and preservation of the nearby structures. Recently, this method has been reported in a series of patients with HCC [32]. The main limitation is the small area of necrosis produced, which can mean up to 8 hours' treatment for small lesions.

Transarterial chemoembolization (TACE) for HCC treatment

Occlusion of hepatic artery blood flow to HCC results in extensive tumour necrosis and has been a therapeutic option for years. Extrahepatic disease and absence of portal blood flow (secondary to portal vein obstruction with thrombosis or tumour, portosystemic anastomosis or hepatofugal flow) constitute the main contraindications. Patients with advanced disease (Child–Pugh C) should also be excluded because of the risk of acute liver failure.

Gelfoam is the most frequently used agent for arterial obstruction, but polyvinyl alcohol, beads, alcohol, starch microspheres, blood clots and metallic coils have also been used. Hepatic artery occlusion (transarterial embolization; TAE) is an angiographic procedure in which the catheter is advanced into the hepatic artery, attempting interruption of arterial inflow as close to the tumour as possible. In the treatment of multifocal HCC involving both hepatic lobes, the main branches of the hepatic artery may be safely occluded in patients with well-preserved liver function. During injection, it is important to avoid the backward flow of particles to avoid embolization of arterial vessels outside the liver (e.g. ischaemic cholecystitis).

TAE has been largely abandoned in favour of TACE, i.e. transarterial chemoembolization, in which the arterial occlusion is combined with injection of cytostatic drugs such as doxorubicin, mitomycin or cisplatin. The chemotherapeutic agents are suspended in lipiodol; some centres inject 25% of chemotherapy into the remaining liver, in the hope of eliminating undetected tumour cells.

The main side-effect of TACE is the 'post-embolization syndrome' observed in 50% of patients; it consists of fever, abdominal pain and a moderate degree of ileus. It is usually self-limited, and most patients can be discharged within 48–72 hours. Prophylactic antibiotics are not routinely used as post-

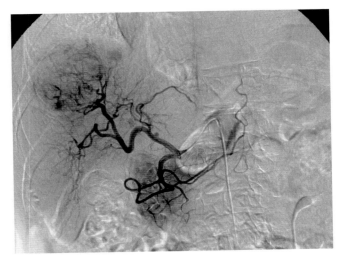

(a)

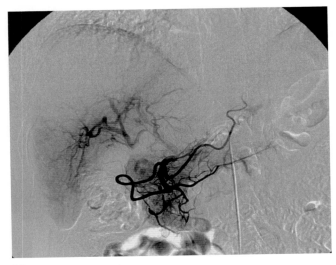

(b)

Fig. 5 (a) Arteriography performed prior to TACE. Hypervascularized big nodule in the right lobe of the liver and a daughter nodule in the periphery. (b) After two sessions of TACE, complete ischaemia of the tumoral area is obtained, preserving the arterial vascularization of the remaining non-tumoral liver.

procedure fever reflects tumour necrosis. If fever persists, severe infectious complications such as a hepatic abscess or cholecystitis associated with ischaemia should be ruled out.

Therapeutic efficacy is 15–55%, as defined by delayed tumour progression and vascular invasion. However, the residual tumour typically recovers its blood supply, and repeated treatments are necessary (Fig. 5). The results of two randomized trials show a beneficial effect of TACE in selected patients [33,34]; however, patient selection and the most active agents remain to be defined.

PEI, RF and, more recently, MW have been used prior to or after TACE to add the effects of both therapies, suggesting that they can be employed in patients with intermediate stage tumours [14,35].

Local radiation therapy

The potential of conventional radiation therapy of the liver is limited because of the high sensitivity of hepatocytes. The potential of local application of iodine-131, yttrium-90, rhenium-188 or holmium-166 incorporated into lipiodol or microspheres through TAE appears to be promising, but formal trials have yet to be performed before such interventions can be incorporated into clinical practice.

Percutaneous management of bile duct obstruction due to malignant or benign strictures

Since the early 1970s, percutaneous techniques such as percutaneous transhepatic cholangiography (PTC) [39] and percutaneous treatment of cholecystolithiasis [40,41] have become popular. Recent developments such as polyurethane endoprostheses or expandable metallic stents have changed the palliative management of tumours causing obstructive jaundice [42–44].

Stenting in obstructive jaundice due to malignancy

Biliary obstruction due to a tumour in the biliary tree should be diagnosed by non-invasive modalities such as multidetector computerized tomography (MDCT), magnetic resonance cholangiography (MRCP) or endoscopic ultrasound (EUS). Invasive techniques such as PTC or endoscopic retrograde cholangiopancreatography (ERCP) should be reserved for therapeutic interventions.

The main indication for the use of endoprostheses or stents is the palliation of obstructive jaundice due to biliary malignancy where resection is not possible, which applies to 70–80% of patients at the time of diagnosis [45]. Although some authors believe that surgery is the best palliative technique [46], the use of stents has become more popular [47].

The choice between PTC and ERCP to access the extrahepatic biliary tree should be determined by expertise and local availability. Only in complex high-level obstruction is the percutaneous radiological approach the first-line option.

For some authors, the only indication for surgical intervention is the presence of both malignant biliary and duodenal obstruction. Combined self-expandable metal stenting for simultaneous palliation of malignant biliary and duodenal obstruction may provide a safe and less invasive alternative to surgical palliation and should be considered as a treatment option for patients who are poor candidates for surgery [48] (Fig. 6).

Palliation – who are the right candidates?

Both procedures, percutaneous biliary drainage (PBD) and bil-

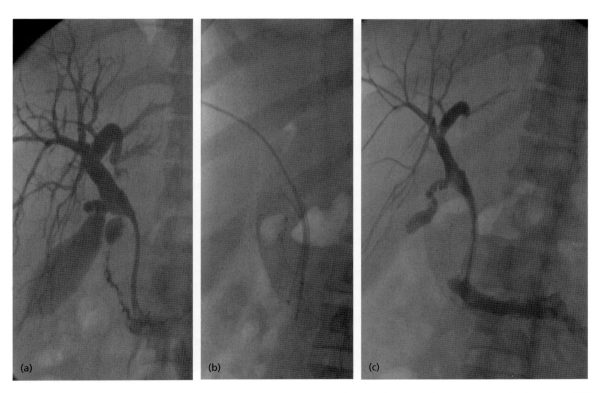

Fig. 6 Neoplasm of the pancreas with duodenal involvement. (a) Incomplete resolution of biliary obstruction after percutaneous implantation of biliary stent. Marked infiltration of duodenum. (b and c) Complete resolution after peroral implantation of duodenal stent.

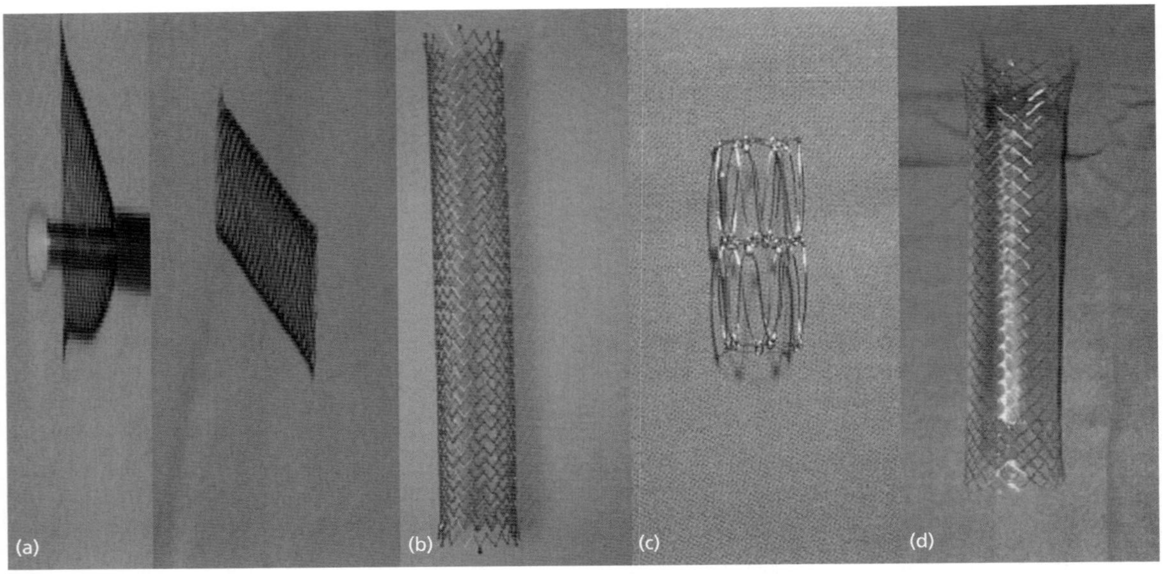

Fig. 7 Metallic stents. (a) Autoexpandable Wallstent. (b) Absolute nitinol stent. (c) Gianturco Z-stent. (d) Covered Wallstent.

iary endoprosthesis, can be considered for adequate palliation. The main objection to the use of an endoprosthesis has been the fact that they are likely to become occluded in patients with a relatively long life expectancy [42]. The use of PBD is associated with an increase in infection, biliary leakage and pain at the skin entry site.

In the past, the endoprostheses used were plastic stents made of polyethylene or polyurethane. Their high obstruction rate and other complications were due to the use of large-bore devices; the main reason for obstruction was not tumour growth but bile encrustation [50]. Neither Teflon, hydrourethane nor hydrophilic coating could improve the patency [51].

This was changed by the introduction of metallic stents in the late 1980s. There are basically two broad categories, i.e. balloon-expandable stents (Palmaz or Strecker stents) or autoexpandable stents (Wallstent, Gianturco Z-stent, Zilver stent or Absolute nitinol stents; Fig. 7).

Their main advantage is that they can be introduced through a very small-calibre track (6 Fr), but can be expanded to a large internal lumen of 10 mm. However, they are still prone to obstruction; the true incidence of occlusion is difficult to establish because follow-up of patients in many series is incomplete. In a recent series of 142 consecutive patients managed with Wallstent, mean survival was 186 days with a need for reintervention in 12% [47]. Similar results were reported with nitinol alloy devices [52] or with drug-eluting or covered stents.

Achieving clinical success

We insist on aggressively achieving normalization of coagulation and broad-spectrum antibiotic coverage. Accurate selection of the puncture site and a decision about uni- or bilobar drainage is based on MRCP. Real-time ultrasound permits the identification of the most appropriate entry site (Fig. 8). To avoid haemobilia, selection of the most peripheral intrahepatic duct is mandatory. In our centre, we always use a micropuncture set, Acoustic (Boston Scientific Corporation) or Cruiser (PBN Medicals Denmark) with a coaxial sheath and a 0.38-inch stiff guidewire.

In biliary strictures without involvement of the ampulla of Vater, a stent with the end 1–2 cm above the ampulla is preferable to prevent ascending cholangitis [53]. In high-level obstruction, a bilobar drainage is accomplished with a single puncture and two stents in a Y arrangement, but our preference is a double puncture with two stents side by side (Fig. 9). When the ampulla is involved, a long stent from the hilum through the ampulla projecting just 1 cm into the duodenum is recommended to avoid mucosal damage.

Stent occlusion

Despite large-bore stents and new materials now available, stent occlusion remains a major problem. With plastic endoprostheses, bile incrustation and infection were the main problems. With the metal stents, problems of tumour growth are a major problem, but also fibrotic mucosal hyperplasia is well documented. In a palliative situation, the placement of a new stent provides adequate palliation.

Percutaneous treatment of benign biliary strictures

The treatment of benign strictures is no longer dependent on surgical techniques, with radiological and endoscopic approaches being used as alternatives, in particular for the following groups:

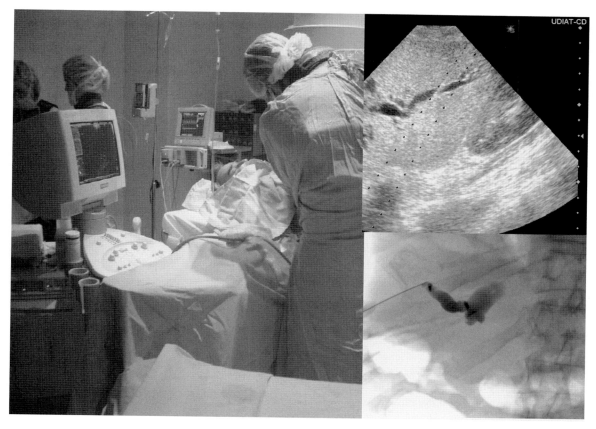

Fig. 8 PBD performed with peripheral puncture under US guidance. Note correlation between US image and cholangiography.

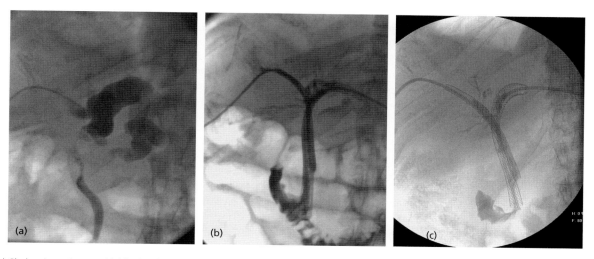

Fig. 9 (a) Cholangiocarcinoma with hilar involvement. (b and c) Bilateral bile duct puncture with a double stent in a side-by-side arrangement. Good drainage through the papilla.

1 Iatrogenic or traumatic bile duct lesions after cholecystectomy or liver transplantation.
2 Non-traumatic: sclerosing cholangitis, recurrent pyogenic cholangitis and Mirizzi syndrome. In this group, imaging diagnosis can be difficult, and histology is mandatory to differentiate benign causes from malignant strictures.

Criteria for selection of a radiological approach

The best results for surgical treatment are better than any published results for radiological management and, in specialist surgical centres, the treatment of choice for strictures of the extrahepatic ducts should be surgery.

Apart from local expertise, the following factors adversely affect the outcome of surgical stricture repair [55]. The presence of one or more of these factors favours the selection of a radiological approach:

1 Multiple previous operative attempts at repair.
2 Stricture of intrahepatic ducts or their confluence, associated or not with stones.
3 Presence of portal hypertension.

Access and technique for percutaneous dilation

The transhepatic route provides the most adequate access to repair biliary strictures, in particular in the presence of a biliodigestive anastomosis with a Roux loop. An alternative approach without hepatic puncture is possible when a surgical superficially fixed Roux loop is fixed to the anterior abdominal wall. The afferent fixed loop is marked with metal clips to facilitate radiological puncture and retrograde access to the biliary tree [56]. The technique for gaining transhepatic access is the standard for PTC.

Strictures are dilated using angioplasty balloon catheters with a diameter between 6 and 12 mm and a length of 2–6 cm. Inflation pressures of 12 atm are usual, but there is sometimes extensive fibrosis requiring high-pressure balloons with a pressure of 17–20 atm. The number and duration of inflations are variable, and the endpoint of the procedure is to restore a normal lumen with no residual wasting of the balloon. In our experience, the best results are accomplished with a catheter or plastic stent left in place for 4–6 weeks after dilation. Following this, the catheter is removed if there is no evidence of restenosis at cholangiographic control. Approximately 20–30% of benign stenoses will present a restenosis at follow-up [57]. Recently, the use of commercially available cutting balloons (Fig. 10) with small blades has increased the technical success rate of percutaneous management of transplant biliary strictures, with only 10% restenosis [58].

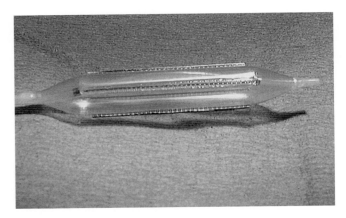

Fig. 10 Expandable balloon angioplasty into which four longitudinally orientated small blades are incorporated.

Is the use of metallic stents advisable in benign biliary strictures?

In spite of relatively good initial results with Gianturco stents [59,60], long-term follow-up of metallic stents is not encouraging with a high failure rate of more than 50% [60]. Metallic biliary stents should be used only for the treatment of benign biliary strictures in selected cases, where repeated balloon dilation has failed and the patient is a poor candidate for surgery.

References

1 Bilbao JI, Torres E, Martínez-Cuesta A (2002) Non-traumatic abdominal emergencies: imaging and intervention in gastrointestinal hemorrhage and ischemia. *Eur Radiol* 12, 2161–2171.

2 Hidalgo F, Narvaez JA, Rene M *et al.* (1995) Treatment of hemobilia with selective hepatic artery embolization. *J Vasc Interv Radiol* 6, 793–798.

3 Tarazov PG (1993) Intrahepatic arterioportal fistulae: role of transcatheter embolization. *Cardiovasc Interv Radiol* 16, 368–373.

4 Nicholson T, Travis S, Ettles D *et al.* (1999) Hepatic artery angiography and embolization for hemobilia following laparoscopic cholecystectomy. *Cardiovasc Interv Radiol* 22, 20–24.

5 Zhang CO, Fu LN, Xu L *et al.* (2003) Long-term effect of stent placement in 115 patients with Budd–Chiari syndrome. *World J Gastroenterol* 9, 2587–2591.

6 Bilbao JI, Quiroga J, Herrero JI *et al.* (2002) Transjugular intrahepatic portosystemic shunt (TIPS): current status and future possibilities. *Cardiovasc Interv Radiol* 25, 251–269.

7 Rossle M, Olschewski M, Siegerstetter V *et al.* (2004) The Budd–Chiari syndrome: outcome after treatment with the transjugular intrahepatic portosystemic shunt. *Surgery* 135, 394–403.

8 Boyer TD, Haskal ZJ (2005) The role of transjugular intrahepatic portosystemic shunt in the management of portal hypertension. *Hepatology* 41, 386–400.

9 Rossle M, Grandt D (2004) TIPS: an update. *Best Pract Res Clin Gastroenterol* 18, 99–123.

10 Bureau C, García-Pagán JC, Otal P *et al.* (2004) Improved clinical outcome using polytetrafluoroethylene-coated stents for TIPS: results of a randomized study. *Gastroenterology* 126, 469–475.

11 Rossle M, Mullen KD (2004) Long-term patency is expected with covered TIPS stents: this effect may not always be desirable! *Hepatology* 40, 495–497.

12 Wang JF, Zhai RY, Wei BJ *et al.* (2006) Percutaneous intravascular stents for treatment of portal venous stenosis after liver transplantation: midterm results. *Transplant Proc* 38, 1461–1462.

13 Sangiovanni A, Del Ninno E, Fasani P *et al.* (2004) Increased survival of cirrhotic patients with a hepatocellular carcinoma detected during surveillance. *Gastroenterology* 126(4), 1005–1014.

14 Llovet JM, Bru C, Bruix J (1999) Prognosis of hepatocellular carcinoma: the BCLC staging classification. *Semin Liver Dis* 19(3), 329–338.

15 Llovet JM, Bruix J (2003) Systematic review of randomized trials for unresectable hepatocellular carcinoma: chemoembolization improves survival. *Hepatology* 37(2), 429–442.

16 Ebara M, Akabe S, Kita K *et al.* (2005) Percutaneous ethanol injection for small hepatocellular carcinoma: therapeutic efficacy based on 20-year observation. *J Hepatol* 43, 458–464.

17 Vilana R, Bruix J, Bru C *et al.* (1993) Tumor size determines the efficacy of percutaneous ethanol injection for the treatment of small hepatocellular carcinoma. *Hepatology* 16, 353–357.

18 Ohnishi K (1998) Comparison of percutaneous acetic acid injection and percutaneous ethanol injection for small hepatocellular carcinoma. *Hepatogastroenterology* 45, 1254–1258.

19 Lin SM, Lin CJ, Lin CC *et al.* (2005) Randomised controlled trial comparing percutaneous radiofrequency thermal ablation, percutaneous ethanol injection, and percutaneous acetic acid injection to treat hepatocellular carcinoma of 3 cm or less. *Gut* 54, 1151.

20 Vallone P, Catalano O, Izzo F *et al.* (2006) Combined ethanol injection therapy and radiofrequency ablation therapy in percutaneous treatment of hepatocellular carcinoma larger than 4 cm. *Cardiovasc Interv Radiol* 29, 544–541.

21 Livraghi T, Goldberg SN, Lazzaroni S *et al.* (1999) Small hepatocellular carcinoma: treatment with radio-frequency ablation versus ethanol injection. *Radiology* 210(3), 655–661.

22 Shiina S, Teratami T, Obis S *et al.* (2005) A randomized controlled trial of radiofrequency ablation with ethanol injection for small HCC. *Gastroenterology* 129, 122–130.

23 Rhim HYK, Lee JM *et al.* (2003) Major complications after radio-frequency thermal ablation of hepatic tumors: spectrum of imaging findings. *RadioGraphics* 23, 123–136.

24 de Baere T, Risse O, Kuoch V *et al.* (2003) Adverse events during radiofrequency treatment of 582 hepatic tumors. *AJR Am J Roentgenol* 181, 695–700.

25 Jaskolka JD, Asch MR, Kachiura JR *et al.* (2005) Needle tract seeding after radiofrequency ablation of hepatic tumors. *J Vasc Interv Radiol* 16, 485–491.

26 Teratani T, Yoshida H, Shiina S *et al.* (2006) Radiofrequency ablation for hepatocellular carcinoma in so-called high-risk locations. *Hepatology* 43, 1101–1108.

27 Vilana R, Bianch IL, Varela M *et al.* (2006) Is microbubble-enhanced ultrasonography sufficient for assessment of response to percutaneous treatment in patients with early hepatocellular carcinoma? *Eur Radiol* 16, 2454–2462.

28 Meloni MF, Livraghi T, Filice C *et al.* (2006) RF ablation of liver tumors: the role of microbubble ultrasound contrast agents. *Ultrasound Quarterly* 22, 41–47.

29 Sala M, Llovet JM, Vilana R *et al.* (2004) Initial response to percutaneous ablation predicts survival in patients with hepatocellular carcinoma. *Hepatology* 40(6), 1352–1360.

30 Lu MD, Xu HX, Xie XY *et al.* (2005) Percutaneous microwave and radiofrequency ablation for hepatocellular carcinoma: a retrospective study. *J Gastroenterol* 40, 1054–1060.

31 Dong B, Liang P, Yu X *et al.* (2003) Percutaneous sonographically guided microwave coagulation therapy for HCC: results in 234 patients. *AJR Am J Roentgenol* 180, 1547–1555.

32 Wu F, Wang ZB, Chem WZ *et al.* (2004) Extracorporeal high intensity focused ultrasound ablation in the treatment of patients with large hepatocellular carcinoma. *Am Surg Oncol* 11, 1061–1069.

33 Llovet JM, Real MI, Montanya X *et al.* (2002) Arterial embolization, chemoembolization versus symptomatic treatment in patients with unresectable hepatocellular carcinoma: a randomized controlled trial. *Lancet* 359, 1734–1739.

34 Lo CM, Ngan H, Tso WK *et al.* (2002) Randomized controlled trial of transarterial lipiodol chemoembolization for unresectable hepatocellular carcinoma. *Hepatology* 35(5), 1164–1171.

35 Livraghi T, Meloni F, Morabito A (2004) Multimodality image-guided tailored therapy of early and intermediate hepatocellular carcinoma: long-term survival in the experience of a single radiological referral centre. *Liver Transpl* 10, S98–106.

36 Veltri A, Moretto P, Doriguzzi A *et al.* (2006) Radiofrequency thermal ablation (RFA) after transarterial chemoembolization (TACE) as a combined therapy for unresectable non-early hepatocellular carcinoma (HCC). *Eur Radiol* 16, 661–669.

37 Lu DS, Lu NC, Raman SS *et al.* (2005) Percutaneous radiofrequency ablation for hepatocellular carcinoma as a bridge for liver transplantation. *Hepatology* 41, 130–137.

38 Bruix J, Hessheimer AJ, Forner A *et al.* (2006) New aspects of diagnosis and therapy of hepatocellular carcinoma. *Oncogene* 25, 3848–3856.

39 Ferrucci JT Jr, Wittenberg J, Sarno RA *et al.* (1976) Fine needle transhepatic cholangiography: a new approach to obstructive jaundice. *AJR Am J Roentgenol* 127(3), 403–407.

40 Mazzariello RM (1976) Residual biliary tract stones: nonoperative treatment of 570 patients. *Surg Annu* 8, 113–144.

41 Burhenne HJ (1980) Percutaneous extraction of retained biliary tract stones: 661 patients. *AJR Am J Roentgenol* 134(5), 889–898.

42 Mueller PR, Ferrucci JT Jr, Teplick SK *et al.* (1985) Biliary stent endoprosthesis: analysis of complications in 113 patients. *Radiology* 156(3), 637–639.

43 Lammer J (1985) [Percutaneous transhepatic bile duct endoprosthesis. Choice of material, technique, clinical results]. *Rofo* 142(3), 243–253 (in German).

44 Coons HG, Carey PH (1983) Large-bore, long biliary endoprostheses (biliary stents) for improved drainage, *Radiology* 148(1), 89–94.

45 Connolly MM, Dawson PJ, Michelassi F *et al.* (1987) Survival in 1001 patients with carcinoma of the pancreas. *Ann Surg* 206, 366–376.

46 Blumgart LH, Hadjis NS, Benjamín IS *et al.* (1984) Surgical approaches to cholangiocarcinoma. At confluence of hepatic ducts. *Lancet* 14, 66–70.

47 Adam A, Cheetty N, Roddie M *et al.* (1991) Self-expandable stainless steel endoprostheses for the treatment of malignant bile duct obstruction. *Am J Radiol* 156, 321–325.

48 Kaw M, Singh S, Gagneja H (2003) Clinical outcome of simultaneous self-expandable metal stents for palliation of malignant biliary and duodenal obstruction. *Surg Endosc* 17(3), 457–461.

49 Sohn TA, Yeo CJ, Cameron JL *et al.* (2000) Do preoperative biliary stents increase postpancreaticoduodenectomy complications? *J Gastrointest Surg* 4(3), 258–267; discussion 267–268.

50 Moss AC, Morris E, MacMathuna P (2006) Palliative biliary stents for obstructing pancreatic carcinoma. *Cochrane Database Syst Rev* 19(2).

51 Han YH, Kim MY, Kim SY *et al.* (2006) Percutaneous insertion of Zilver stent in malignant biliary obstruction. *Abdom Imaging* 20, [epub ahead of print].

52 Okamoto T, Fujioka S, Yanagisawa S *et al.* (2006) Placement of a metallic stent across the main duodenal papilla may predispose to cholangitis. *Gastrointest Endosc* 63(6), 792–796.

53 Park do H, Kim MH, Choi JS *et al.* (2006) Covered versus uncovered wallstent for malignant extrahepatic biliary obstruction: a cohort comparative analysis. *Clin Gastroenterol Hepatol* 4(6), 790–796.

54 Blumgart LH, Kelley CJ, Benjamin IS (1984) Benign bile duct stricture following cholecystectomy: critical factors in management. *Br J Surg* 71(11), 836–843.

55 Hutson DG, Russell E, Schiff E *et al.* (1984) Balloon dilation of biliary strictures through a choledochojejuno-cutaneous fistula. *Ann Surg* 199(6), 637–647.

56 Gibson RN, Adam A, Yeung E *et al.* (1988) Percutaneous techniques in benign hilar and intrahepatic benign biliary strictures. *J Interv Radiol* 3, 125–130.

57 Saad WE, Davies MG, Saad NE *et al.* (2006) Transhepatic dilation of anastomotic biliary strictures in liver transplant recipients with use of a combined cutting and conventional balloon protocol: technical safety and efficacy. *J Vasc Interv Radiol* 17(5), 837–843.

58 Rossi P, Bezzi M, Salvatori FM *et al.* (1997) Clinical experience with covered wallstents for biliary malignancies: 23-month follow-up. *Cardiovasc Interv Radiol* 20(6), 441–447.

59 Irving JD, Adam A, Dick R *et al.* (1989) Gianturco expandable metallic biliary stents: results of a European clinical trial. *Radiology* 172(2), 321–326.

60 Hausegger KA, Kugler C, Uggowitzer M *et al.* (1996) Benign biliary obstruction: is treatment with the Wallstent advisable? *Radiology* 200(2), 437–441.

5.8 Positron emission tomography of the liver

Michael Sørensen and Susanne Keiding

For the hepatologist, positron emission tomography (PET) provides unique possibilities for the direct quantification of regional liver blood perfusion and metabolism of substances *in vivo*. Furthermore, PET is used in the clinical management of patients with malignancies in the liver.

Before a PET scan the patient inhales or receives an intravenous injection of a positron-labelled tracer. Tracers are natural substances, analogues hereof, drugs or receptor ligands. The most commonly used positron-emitters with different physical half-lives are: ^{15}O (2 min), ^{13}N (10 min), ^{11}C (20 min) and ^{18}F (109 min). Within the body, an emitted positron travels a few millimetres and then is annihilated by an electron, which leads to simultaneous emission of two 511-keV photons travelling in 180° opposing directions. The photons are recorded by the PET camera and data reconstructed into three-dimensional images of tracer concentrations in Bq/mL tissue.

Contemporary PET cameras are available as whole-body cameras, high-resolution brain cameras, small animal PET systems, and PET cameras combined with computerized tomography (CT). Combined PET/CT cameras have the advantage of aligning PET images of metabolic processes with detailed CT images of anatomical structures. For most purposes, PET/CT is performed with a low-dose CT scan, but, if indicated, it may comprise diagnostic CT, contrast-enhanced CT and respiratory-gated recordings. At present, combined PET/ magnetic resonance (MR) cameras are being developed.

Regional liver metabolism

Dynamic PET recordings are used for quantification of metabolic processes. Starting at the time of tracer injection, data acquisition comprises recordings of the time courses of radioactivity concentrations in tissue and in the blood supply to the organ. The time course of the tissue concentration is analysed as a function of the time course of the blood input radioactivity concentration by fitting a kinetic model of the metabolic scheme for the tracer to the data. This provides clearance values and rate constants for the metabolic processes.

The dual tracer input to the liver has to be taken into account when performing detailed calculations of the kinetic parameters [1–3]. The time course of the blood radioactivity concentration in the hepatic artery following an i.v. bolus injection shows a high, narrow peak, whereas in the portal vein the peak is dispersed and delayed due to the passage of the bolus through the intestinal vascular bed (see Fig. 5 in Chapter 5.3). However, for a substance with irreversible liver metabolism and negligible elimination in the intestines, calculation of the net metabolic clearance of the tracer, K (mL blood/min/mL tissue) using arterial blood concentrations, can be used [1]. The constant K characterizes irreversible steady-state net transfer of the tracer from blood into intracellular metabolites. Munk *et al.* [1] showed that this calculation was applicable for the metabolism of the glucose analogue, 2-deoxy-2-[^{18}F]fluoro-deoxy-glucose (^{18}FDG) in the pig liver. The method can be made non-invasive by replacing arterial blood sampling by scan data of arterial blood radioactivity concentration from the aorta [4–5]. This makes the procedure completely non-invasive. In order to estimate the dual tracer input from both supplying vessels, current studies are exploring the use of combined dynamic PET and dynamic contrast-enhanced CT scans [6]. This will allow for non-invasive evaluation of kinetic properties of the initial tracer distribution, such as blood perfusion and blood-to-cell transfer processes.

The PET camera measures only total radioactivity concentration in the tissue. Kinetic models must embody the fact that the PET camera cannot separate un-metabolized tracer from possible radio-labelled metabolites. The models accordingly are based on metabolic schemes understood from biochemistry but may be validated by measurements of radio-labelled metabolites in tissue samples following tracer injection [7–8]. Similarly, the blood may contain both un-metabolized tracer and radio-labelled metabolites. However, these can often be accounted for by direct measurements in blood samples [9–11].

Table 1 shows examples of metabolic processes in the liver that have been studied by PET. Glucose analogues were used to study the importance of the dual tracer supply to the liver, using ^{18}FDG [1–3] as a substance transported across the cell membrane and metabolized within the cells and ^{11}C-methyl-glucose,

Table 1 Examples of PET studies of liver metabolism.

PET tracer	Experimental model	Metabolism studied	References
[18]FDG	Pig and human liver	Glucose	[1–3,12,13]
[11]C-methyl-glucose	Pig liver	Glucose	[1]
[124]I-iodoinsulin	Rat liver	Insulin receptors	[14]
[13]N-ammonia	Pig and human liver	Ammonia	[16–19]
[11]C-glutamate	Rat liver	Amino acid	[15]
[11]C-glutamine			
[11]C-aspartate			
L-methyl-^{11}C-methionine	Rat, pig, and human liver	Protein synthesis	[9,20]
L-[1-^{11}C]-methionine			
14(R,S)-[^{18}F]-6-thia-heptadecanoic acid	Rat, pig, and human liver	Fatty acid	[21–26]
15-^{18}F-fluoro-3-oxa-entadecanoate			
1-^{11}C-octanoate			
^{15}O-CO	Pig liver	Blood perfusion	[28]

which is transported across the cell membrane in a similar way to [18]FDG but not metabolized. Other studies of liver glucose metabolism have shown that glucose ingestion inhibits the [18]FDG uptake by the liver [12] and that insulin increases hepatic glucose uptake [13]. In agreement with these findings, Iozzo et al. [14] demonstrated insulin receptors in rat liver PET studies, using [124]I-labelled human insulin.

Transport of three amino acids across the liver cell membrane was studied in rats [15]. The high first-pass liver metabolism of ammonia was quantified in pigs by means of a kinetic model of zonation sinusoidal distribution, with periportal urea production and perivenous glutamine production [16]. In a subsequent paper [17], comparison of the first-pass metabolism of ^{13}N-ammonia into the portal vein or the hepatic artery suggested that heterogeneous distribution of the arterial branches gives rise to heterogeneous tissue ammonia metabolism. Interestingly, a human study [18] found that liver ^{13}N-ammonia net metabolic clearance of ammonia, K, was similar in patients with cirrhosis and healthy subjects, may be of pathogenetic importance. Contrary to what was believed hitherto, recent dynamic ^{13}N-ammonia brain studies have shown that the permeability of the blood–brain membrane barrier is not significantly changed in patients with hepatic encephalopathy when compared with patients with cirrhosis without hepatic encephalopathy and healthy controls [10,19]. Brain metabolism of ammonia was increased corresponding to the increased blood ammonia [10]. PET studies may give new insight into the role of ammonia in the development of hepatic encephalopathy and catabolic stress in patients with liver failure.

Liver protein synthesis [9,20] and fatty acid oxidation [21–26] are important liver functions that have also been measured by PET (Table 1). Figure 1 gives an example of the PET measurements of ^{11}C-methionine uptake in a pig liver with production of ^{11}C-labelled protein released into the blood after a delay of approx. 15 min (S. Lausten, unpublished data, December 2006).

Metabolic schemes are most often represented by compartmental models in which tracer input concentration throughout the capillaries is assumed to equal the input concentration, i.e. in the present context, that in the mixed hepatic arterial and portal venous inlet. Such models ignore substrate concentration gradients along the vascular paths of the organ and in surrounding cells. By utilizing the high spatial and temporal resolution of contemporary PET technology, Munk et al. recently [27], developed models of microcirculation that account for the concentration gradients of a vascular tracer along the blood flow direction as a tracer bolus passes through the capillary. Application of the model in subsequent pig experiments with dynamic ^{15}O-CO PET gave values of the liver blood perfusion comparable with independent measurements [28] (see also Chapter 5.3).

Liver tumours

PET, with the glucose analogue [18]FDG, has proven very successful in the diagnostic evaluation of patients with cancer, and it is currently used routinely worldwide [29]. This is based on the fact that most malignant cells have increased glucose metabolism. [18]FDG enters the cells through the same Glut-1 membrane transporters as glucose and is phosphorylated by the rate-limiting hexokinase or, in the hepatocytes, by glucokinase to [18]FDG-6-phosphate. Both membrane transport and phosphorylation are up-regulated in cancer cells (Fig. 2). [18]FDG-6-phosphate is not a substrate for hexose-6-P-isomerase and therefore it accumulates in the cells. In the hepatocytes, but not in non-hepatocyte-derived tumour cells and bile duct cells, [18]FDG-6-phosphate can be de-phosphorylated by glucose-6-phosphatase. Compared with surrounding non-malignant liver tissue, [18]FDG-6-phosphate accumulates in cholangiocarcinoma and metastases in the liver. Hence, these metabolic characteristics make [18]FDG PET especially suitable for detection of such tumours (Fig. 2). Consequently, tumour nodules are seen as

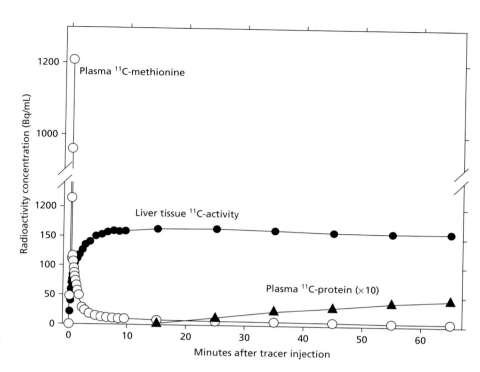

Fig. 1 Time courses of ^{11}C-radioactivity concentrations in pig liver tissue (PET) and plasma after intravenous injection of ^{11}C-methionine. Plasma radioactivity was separated into ^{11}C-methionine and ^{11}C-protein (radio HPLC).

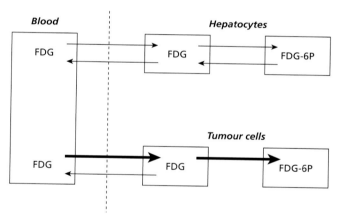

Fig. 2 Compartmental model showing the key differences between [18]FDG metabolism in hepatocytes and tumour cells, which form the basis for using [18]FDG PET in the diagnosis of liver metastases. Bold arrows indicate enhanced membrane transport and enzymatic phosphorylation of [18]FDG in malignant cells.

focal areas of increased radioactivity concentrations, so-called hotspots (Fig. 3).

Because the tumour-to-liver background tissue ratio is higher during fasting than after food intake, [18]FDG PET is usually performed after a fasting period of 6–8 h [30]. This is of especial importance for liver studies, as physiologic hyperinsulinemia stimulates [18]FDG uptake in normal liver tissue [13]. Furthermore, PET recordings typically take place at least 1 h after the [18]FDG injection, as the contrast between tumour and surrounding tissue is higher than at earlier time points [31–33]. This

so-called static scan yields images of the mean radioactivity concentrations in the time period of the recordings. The concentrations are often normalized with respect to injected dose and body weight, yielding images of the standardized uptake value (SUV). This normalization procedure may be useful for defining criteria for ascribing hotspots to malignancies [33–34] and for comparison of PET results between individuals and evaluation of response to treatment in individual patients. The diagnostic accuracy for tumour diagnostics is better in combined PET/CT than in PET or contrast-enhanced CT alone [35]. The radiation dose given to the patient is in of the order of the yearly background radiation.

Cholangiocarcinoma

[18]FDG PET is useful for the detection of cholangiocarcinoma. In a series of 36 consecutive patients who underwent [18]FDG PET for suspected cholangiocarcinoma [36], 31 patients had cholangiocarcinoma and five did not. Sensitivity for nodular morphology (mass 1 cm) was 85% but only 18% for infiltrating morphology. Reinhardt *et al.* [33] found a cutoff SUV of 3.6 for the detection of malignancy. In the study by Delbeke *et al.* [34], each of eight cholangiocarcinomas was classified correctly compared to pathological diagnosis. Similarly, each of eight cholangiocarcinomas was clearly visualised in an early [18]FDG PET study by our group [37].

Patients with primary sclerosing cholangitis (PSC) are at risk of developing cholangiocarcinoma [38] and a simple, reliable screening method for early detection of tumours would benefit these patients considerable. A key question is, if [18]FDG PET can

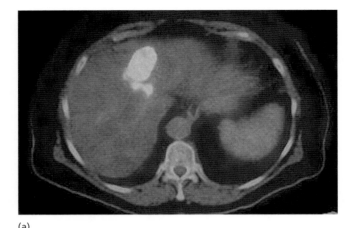

(a)

(b)

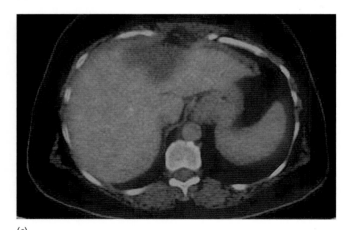

(c)

Fig. 3 [18]FDG PET/CT scan of a patient treated for colorectal cancer revealed synchronous liver metastases (a). The patient was treated with radiofrequency ablation (RFA). [18]FDG PET/CT 4 weeks later showed RFA-induced necrosis but also residual tumour (b). The patient was treated with RFA again, this time resulting in complete ablation of the tumour tissue (c).

distinguish between malignant tissue and local cholangitis. In a recent study, Prytz *et al.* [39] performed dynamic [18]FDG PET scans of 24 consecutive PSC patients listed for liver transplantation and with no signs of liver malignancies on CT or ultrasonography. PET results were compared with pathological diagnosis of the explanted liver in a double-blind study design. The scans were performed as dynamic studies, and parametric images of the net metabolic clearance K of [18]FDG were retrieved. By using a cutoff value of lesion-to-normal liver tissue ratio of K, PET diagnosed three out of four cholangiocarcinomas correctly, and it correctly classified hotspots with smaller K-ratios as being caused by local cholangitis. The procedure missed one case with high-grade hilar bile duct dysplasia. However, this was diagnosed by endoscopic cholangiography with brush cytology. Thus, dynamic [18]FDG PET seems to have a role as a supplement to CT in pre-transplant diagnostic work-up of liver patients. Dynamic [18]FDG PET may further prove to be useful in surveillance programs of patients with PSC.

Hepatocellular carcinoma

Similar to ultrasonography and CT, [18]FDG PET detects only two-thirds of known hepatocellular carcinoma (HCC) [40–43]. This is ascribed to similarities between [18]FDG metabolism in normal and malignant hepatocytes [42]. Nevertheless, in a study comprising 91 HCC patients, Wudel *et al.* [43] found that [18]FDG PET had significant impact on treatment in half of the patients with positive PET results, corresponding to 28% of all patients. Furthermore, [18]FDG PET was found useful for detection of extrahepatic metastases [44]. Even so, there is a need for improved diagnostic methods, and in order to comply with this, multi-tracer PET approaches have been investigated. In a PET study comprising 39 patients with HCC [45], ^{11}C-acetate was found to complement [18]FDG for the detection of hotspots. However, the ^{11}C-radioactivity tumour-to-reference tissue ratio was relatively low and highly variable, on average 1.96 ± 0.63 ($\pm$SD). Similarly, PET using ^{13}N-ammonia did not supplement [18]FDG PET well enough to be clinically useful [46, S. Keiding, unpublished data, December 2006]. Consequently the search for more useful PET tracers needs to continue.

Colorectal cancer liver metastases

[18]FDG PET is an established tool in the clinical management of liver metastases from colorectal cancers [47–59]. Delbeke and co-workers [34] found that, validated by pathology, static [18]FDG PET correctly classified each of 60 colorectal cancer liver metastases and each of 23 benign hepatic lesions by using a cut-off value of 2 for the lesion-to-liver background tissue or a cutoff SUV of 3.5. PET changed diagnostic or therapeutic management of patients with colorectal cancer liver metastases in 20–50% [51–54], mainly by detecting previously unknown extrahepatic and/or hepatic disease. The utility of [18]FDG PET in patients with rising or elevated blood carcinoembryogenic antigen (CEA) is

discussed by Wiering *et al.* [49] and Liu *et al.* [50]. ^{18}FDG PET/CT does not replace CT and MR for preoperative anatomical evaluation of primary colorectal cancer but is a useful tool for pre-treatment evaluation of possible spread of the disease of known or suspected recurrence.

^{18}FDG PET is suitable for differentiating between benign and malignant lesions, viz. residual or relapse malignancy versus scarred liver tissue following resection or local ablative treatment [55]. Figure 3 shows an example of ^{18}FDG PET/CT findings in the course of a series of radiofrequency ablation (RFA) of a patient with colorectal liver metastases. Finally, comparison of ^{18}FDG PET results before and after chemotherapy of patients with colorectal liver metastases was predictive for outcome [56,57]. Thus, ^{18}FDG PET or PET/CT may prove useful for early detection of treatment failure and lead to revision of the therapeutic strategy.

Liver metastases from other tumours

Systematic studies of the use of ^{18}FDG PET or PET/CT in the therapeutic management of patients with tumour spread to the liver are scarce, but the technique seems suitable for the diagnosis and staging of liver metastases from breast, malignant melanoma, pancreatic, gastric and oesophageal cancer [58,59]. Liver metastases from neuroendocrine tumours cannot be unambiguously visualized by ^{18}FDG, but ^{11}C-hydroxy-tryptophan or ^{18}F-DOPA seem to be promising PET tracers [60].

References

1 Munk OL, Bass L, Roelsgaard K *et al.* (2001) Liver kinetics of glucose analogs measured in pigs by PET: importance of dual-input blood sampling. *J Nucl Med* 42, 795–801.

2 Brix G, Ziegler SI, Bellemann ME, Doll J *et al.* (2001) Quantification of [(18)F]FDG uptake in the normal liver using dynamic PET: impact and modeling of the dual hepatic blood supply. *J Nucl Med* 42, 1265–1273.

3 Munk OL, Keiding S (2002) Quantification of (18)F-FDG uptake in the liver using dynamic PET. *J Nucl Med* 43, 439–441.

4 Germano G, Chen BC, Huang SC *et al.* (1992) Use of the abdominal aorta for arterial input function determination in hepatic and renal PET studies. *J Nucl Med* 33, 613–620.

5 Keiding S, Munk OL, Schiott KM *et al.* (2000) Dynamic 2-[^{18}F]fluoro-2-deoxy-D-glucose positron emission tomography of liver tumours without blood sampling. *Eur J Nucl Med* 27, 407–412.

6 Munk OL (2005) Hepatic metabolism of glucose analogs measured by dynamic positron emission tomography and interpreted by compartment models. PhD thesis, Faculty of Health, University of Aarhus, Aarhus, Denmark.

7 Bender D, Munk OL, Feng HQ *et al.* (2001) Metabolites of (18)F-FDG and 3-O-(11)C-methylglucose in pig liver. *J Nucl Med* 42, 1673–1678.

8 Ishiwata K, Yamaguchi K, Kameyama M *et al.* (1989) 2-Deoxy-2-[^{18}F]fluoro-D-galactose as an in vivo tracer for imaging galactose metabolism in tumors with positron emission tomography. *Int J Rad Appl Instrum B* 16, 247–254.

9 Ishiwata K, Vaalburg W, Elsinga PH *et al.* (1988) Comparison of L-[1–^{11}C]methionine and L-methyl-[^{11}C]methionine for measuring in vivo protein synthesis rates with PET. *J Nucl Med* 29, 1419–1427.

10 Keiding S, Sørensen M, Bender D *et al.* (2006) Brain metabolism of ^{13}N-ammonia during acute hepatic encephalopathy in cirrhosis measured by PET. *Hepatology* 43, 42–50.

11 Nieves E, Rosenspire K, Filc-Dericco S *et al.* (1986) High-performance liquid chromatographic on-line flow-through radioactivity detector system for analyzing amino acids and metabolites labeled with nitrogen-13. *J Chromatogr* 383, 325–337.

12 Choi Y, Hawkins RA, Huang SC *et al.* (1994) Evaluation of the effect of glucose ingestion and kinetic model configurations of FDG in the normal liver. *J Nucl Med* 35, 818–823.

13 Iozzo P, Geisler F, Oikonen V *et al.* (2003) Insulin stimulates liver glucose uptake in humans: an ^{18}F-FDG PET Study. *J Nucl Med* 44, 682–689.

14 Iozzo P, Osman S, Glaser M *et al.* (2002) In vivo imaging of insulin receptors by PET: preclinical evaluation of iodine-125 and iodine-124 labelled human insulin. *Nucl Med Biol* 29, 73–82.

15 Wu F, Orlefors H, Bergstrom M *et al.* (2000) Uptake of ^{14}C- and ^{11}C-labeled glutamate, glutamine and aspartate in vitro and in vivo. *Anticancer Res* 20, 251–256.

16 Keiding S, Munk OL, Roelsgaard K *et al.* (2001) Positron emission tomography of hepatic first-pass metabolism of ammonia in pig. *Eur J Nucl Med* 28, 1770–1775.

17 Keiding S, Munk OL, Vilstrup H *et al.* (2005) Hepatic microcirculation assessed by positron emission tomography of first-pass ammonia metabolism in porcine liver. *Liver Int* 25, 171–176.

18 Sørensen M, Keiding S (2006) Ammonia metabolism in cirrhosis. In Häussinger D, Kircheis G, Schliess F (eds) *Hepatic Encephalopathy and Nitrogen Metabolism*. Dordrecht, The Netherlands: Springer, pp. 406–419.

19 Ahl B, Weissenborn K, van den Hoff J *et al.* (2004) Regional differences in cerebral blood flow and cerebral ammonia metabolism in patients with cirrhosis. *Hepatology* 40, 73–79.

20 Keiding S, Lausten S, Buus S *et al.* (2006) Liver protein synthesis measured in humans by dynamic ^{11}C-methionine PET: Validation of methodology in rat and pig studies. *Hepatology* 44 (Suppl.1), 488A.

21 Yamamura N, Magata Y, Kitano H *et al.* (1998) Evaluation of [1–^{11}C]octanoate as a new radiopharmaceutical for assessing liver function using positron emission tomography. *Nucl Med Biol* 25, 467–472.

22 DeGrado TR, Wang S, Rockey DC (2000) Preliminary evaluation of 15-[^{18}F]fluoro-3-oxa-pentadecanoate as a PET tracer of hepatic fatty acid oxidation. *J Nucl Med* 41, 1727–1736.

23 Iozzo P, Turpeinen AK, Takala T *et al.* (2003) Liver uptake of free fatty acids in vivo in humans as determined with 14(R, S)-[^{18}F]fluoro-6-thia-heptadecanoic acid and PET. *Eur J Nucl Med Mol Imaging* 30, 1160–1164.

24 Iozzo P, Takala T, Oikonen V *et al.* (2004) Effect of training status on regional disposal of circulating free fatty acids in the liver and skeletal muscle during physiological hyperinsulinemia. *Diabetes Care* 27, 2172–2177.

25 Iozzo P, Turpeinen AK, Takala T *et al.* (2004) Defective liver disposal of free fatty acids in patients with impaired glucose tolerance. *J Clin Endocrinol Metab* 89, 3496–3502.

26 Guiducci L, Järvisalo M, Kiss J *et al.* (2006) [^{11}C]palmitate kinetics across the splanchnic bed in arterial, portal and hepatic venous plasma during fasting and euglycemic hyperinsulinemia. *Nucl Med Biol* 33, 521–528.

27 Munk OL, Keiding S, Bass L (2003) Capillaries within compartments: microvascular interpretation of dynamic positron emission tomography data. *J Theor Biol* 225, 127–141.

28 Munk OL, Bass L, Feng H *et al.* (2003) Determination of regional flow by use of intravascular PET tracers: microvascular theory and experimental validation for pig livers. *J Nucl Med* 44, 1862–1870.

29 Reske SN, Kotzerke J (2001) FDG-PET for clinical use. Results of the 3rd German Interdisciplinary Consensus Conference, 'Onko-PET III', 21 July and 19 September 2000. *Eur J Nucl Med* 28, 1707–1723.

30 Choi Y, Hawkins RA, Huang SC *et al.* (1994) Evaluation of the effect of glucose ingestion and kinetic model configurations of FDG in the normal liver. *J Nucl Med* 35, 818–823.

31 Chen YK, Kao CH (2005) Metastatic hepatic lesions are detected better by delayed imaging with prolonged emission time. *Clin Nucl Med* 30, 455–456.

32 Nishiyama Y, Yamamoto Y, Monden T *et al.* (2005) Evaluation of delayed additional FDG PET imaging in patients with pancreatic tumour. *Nucl Med Commun* 26, 895–901.

33 Reinhardt MJ, Strunk H, Gerhardt T *et al.* (2005) Detection of Klatskin's tumor in extrahepatic bile duct strictures using delayed 18F-FDG PET/CT: preliminary results for 22 patient studies. *J Nucl Med* 46, 1158–1163.

34 Delbeke D, Martin WH, Sandler MP *et al.* (1998) Evaluation of benign vs malignant hepatic lesions with positron emission tomography. *Arch Surg* 133, 510–515.

35 Roman CD, Martin WH, Delbeke D (2005) Incremental value of fusion imaging with integrated PET-CT in oncology. *Clin Nucl Med* 30, 470–477.

36 Anderson CD, Rice MH, Pinson CW *et al.* (2004) Fluorodeoxyglucose PET imaging in the evaluation of gallbladder carcinoma and cholangiocarcinoma. *J Gastrointest Surg* 8, 90–97.

37 Keiding S, Hansen SB, Rasmussen HH *et al.* (1998) Detection of cholangiocarcinoma in primary sclerosing cholangitis by positron emission tomography. *Hepatology* 28, 700–706.

38 Boberg KM, Bergquist A, Mitchell S *et al.* (2002) Cholangiocarcinoma in primary sclerosing cholangitis: risk factors and clinical presentation. *Scand J Gastroenterol* 37, 1205–1211.

39 Prytz H, Keiding S, Björnsson E *et al.* (2006) Dynamic FDG PET is useful for detection of cholangiocarcinoma in patients with PSC listed for liver transplantation. *Hepatology* 44, 1572–1580.

40 Jeng LB, Changlai SP, Shen YY *et al.* (2003) Limited value of 18F-2-deoxyglucose positron emission tomography to detect hepatocellular carcinoma in hepatitis B virus carriers. *Hepatogastroenterology* 50, 2154–2156.

41 Khan MA, Combs CS, Brunt EM *et al.* (2000) Positron emission tomography scanning in the evaluation of hepatocellular carcinoma. *J Hepatol* 32, 792–797.

42 Torizuka T, Tamaki N, Inokuma T *et al.* (1995) In vivo assessment of glucose metabolism in hepatocellular carcinoma with FDG-PET. *J Nucl Med* 36, 1811–1817.

43 Wudel LJ, Jr., Delbeke D, Morris D *et al.* (2003) The role of [18F]fluorodeoxyglucose positron emission tomography imaging in the evaluation of hepatocellular carcinoma. *Am Surg* 69, 117–124.

44 Sugiyama M, Sakahara H, Torizuka T *et al.* (2004) 18F-FDG PET in the detection of extrahepatic metastases from hepatocellular carcinoma. *J Gastroenterol* 39, 961–968.

45 Ho CL, Yu SC, Yeung DW (2003) ^{11}C-acetate PET imaging in hepatocellular carcinoma and other liver masses. *J Nucl Med* 44, 213–221.

46 Shibata T, Yamamoto K, Hayashi N (1988) Dynamic positron emission tomography with ^{13}N-ammonia in liver tumors. *Eur J Nucl Med* 14, 607–611.

47 Boykin KN, Zibari GB, Lilien DL *et al.* (1999) The use of FDG-positron emission tomography for the evaluation of colorectal metastases of the liver. *Am Surg* 65, 1183–1185.

48 Delbeke D, Martin WH (2004) PET and PET-CT for evaluation of colorectal carcinoma. *Semin Nucl Med* 34, 209–223.

49 Wiering B, Ruers TJ, Oyen WJ (2004) Role of FDG-PET in the diagnosis and treatment of colorectal liver metastases. *Expert Rev Anticancer Ther* 4, 607–613.

50 Liu FY, Chen JS, Changchien CR *et al.* (2005) Utility of 2-fluoro-2-deoxy-D-glucose positron emission tomography in managing patients of colorectal cancer with unexplained carcinoembryonic antigen elevation at different levels. *Dis Colon Rectum* 48, 1900–1912.

51 Wiering B, Krabbe PF, Jager GJ *et al.* (2005) The impact of fluor-18-deoxyglucose-positron emission tomography in the management of colorectal liver metastases. *Cancer* 15, 2658–2670.

52 Lejeune C, Bismuth MJ, Conroy T (2005) Use of a decision analysis model to assess the cost-effectiveness of 18F-FDG PET in the management of metachronous liver metastases of colorectal cancer. *J Nucl Med* 46, 2020–2028.

53 Selzner M, Hany TF, Wildbrett P *et al.* (2004) Does the novel PET/CT imaging modality impact on the treatment of patients with metastatic colorectal cancer of the liver? *Ann Surg* 240, 1027–1034.

54 Truant S, Huglo D, Hebbar M *et al.* (2005) Prospective evaluation of the impact of [18F]fluoro-2-deoxy-D-glucose positron emission tomography of resectable colorectal liver metastases. *Br J Surg* 92, 362–369.

55 Bender H, Bangard N, Metten N *et al.* (1999) Possible role of FDG-PET in the early prediction of therapy outcome in liver metastases of colorectal cancer. *Hybridoma* 18, 87–91.

56 Vitola JV, Delbeke D, Meranze SG *et al.* (1996) Positron emission tomography with F-18-fluorodeoxyglucose to evaluate the results of hepatic chemoembolization. *Cancer* 78, 2216–2222.

57 Dimitrakopoulou-Strauss A, Strauss LG *et al.* (2004) Prognostic aspects of 18F-FDG PET kinetics in patients with metastatic colorectal carcinoma receiving FOLFOX chemotherapy. *J Nucl Med* 45, 1480–1487.

58 Khandani AH, Wahl RL (2005) Applications of PET in liver imaging. *Radiol Clin North Am* 43, 849–860.

59 Kinkel K, Lu Y, Both M *et al.* (2002) Detection of hepatic metastases from cancers of the gastrointestinal tract using noninvasive imaging methods (US, CT, MR imaging, PET): a meta-analysis. *Radiology* 224, 748–756.

60 Mottaghy FM, Reske SN (2006) Functional imaging of neuroendocrine tumours with PET. *Pituitary* 9, 237–242.

5.9 Splanchnic haemodynamic investigations

Didier Lebrec and Richard Moreau

Introduction

In general, the circulatory system is evaluated by determination of blood flow, pressure and volume. In the splanchnic territory, portal pressure and splanchnic blood flow may be measured; vascular resistance is calculated by the ratio between pressure and blood flow. Portal pressure depends on two factors: portal intrahepatic vascular resistance (and vascular resistance of the portosystemic collateral when portal hypertension is present); and portal tributary blood flow (the sum of gastrointestinal, colic, splenic, mesenteric and pancreatic blood flow). Splanchnic blood flow or hepatic blood flow is the sum of portal tributary blood flow and hepatic arterial blood flow. In portal hypertension, splanchnic blood flow may be higher than hepatic blood flow as only a fraction of the portal blood reaches the systemic circulation by passing through the liver.

The haemodynamic investigation of the splanchnic circulation consists of the measurements of pressure and blood flow. In man, while pressures may be measured, there is no simple method for measuring either portal and hepatic arterial blood flows or the circulation in the collateral vessels. Regional blood flow can, however, be measured in animals. Finally, as it is altered in portal hypertension, the systemic circulation must also be evaluated.

In this chapter, the main haemodynamic methods used in man are described. It must be emphasized, however, that the results reported are those measured in fasted, conscious patients in a supine position. Results obtained in other conditions may differ widely from those reported below.

Measurement of portal pressure

The measurement of pressure in the portal venous system is the main method used to define and characterize portal hypertension. Normally, portal pressure ranges from 7 to 12 mmHg, and the pressure gradient between portal pressure and vena cava territory pressure ranges from 1 to 4 mmHg. Portal hypertension is present when portal pressure is higher than 12 mmHg or when the pressure gradient is higher than 4 mmHg. If the pressure in the vena cava territory increases, portal hypertension develops, but not collateral circulation. Portal pressure may be evaluated either directly or indirectly. Direct measurement of portal pressure is more invasive than the indirect method but is more valid, especially with cases of presinusoidal or extrahepatic portal hypertension.

Direct methods

During abdominal surgery, portal pressure may be measured directly by introducing a needle into the lumen of the portal vein or by inserting a catheter into a small ileal vein. These values differ from those measured without surgery, however, as anaesthetic agents modify splanchnic and systemic circulation. The catheterization of the umbilical vein also allows direct measurement of portal pressure. As the last invasive technique necessitates both general anaesthesia and surgery, it is not used regularly.

The most common direct technique is the percutaneous transhepatic puncture of the portal vein with a thin needle (Chiba needle). The portal vein may be located by ultrasonography [1]. Larger needles may also be used and, in this case, a catheter may be inserted in the lumen of the portal vein in order to cannulate different veins. If ascites or coagulation defects are present, these methods are contraindicated. The portal vein may be catheterized through a hepatic vein in the same manner as with a transvenous liver biopsy procedure [2]. This method allows measurement of the pressure in the inferior vena cava. It may cause abdominal pain.

Indirect methods

Intrasplenic pressure

Although splenic pressure, measured with a needle, has been widely used, this technique has a high risk of intraperitoneal haemorrhage. Splenic pulp pressure is similar to splenic vein pressure.

Intrahepatic pressure

It has been claimed that pressure in the hepatic tissue reflects sinusoidal pressure. This intrahepatic pressure measurement is performed blindly by introducing a needle percutaneously in the hepatic parenchyma [3]. While this pressure may be 'sinusoidal', it may also be intra-arterial, portal or that of the hepatic vein or the biliary tract.

Hepatic venous pressures

As it is simple and safe, measurement of wedged and free hepatic venous pressure is the most common procedure used to evaluate portal pressure indirectly. A radio-opaque catheter is introduced into a hepatic vein (usually the right vein) with an approach through a jugular, femoral or humeral vein under local anaesthesia. This procedure is performed under radioscopic control [4]. The tip of the catheter is wedged to block the circulation in a small hepatic venule. The wedged position is verified by the absence of reflux of radio-opaque dye. Wedged hepatic venous pressure is similar to the occluded pressure obtained with a balloon catheter. Free hepatic venous pressure is measured with the tip of the catheter placed in the hepatic vein close to the inferior vena cava. Recently, a divergence of pressure measurements between different hepatic veins has been demonstrated [5]. The investigator's experience plays a major role in ensuring that the technique is performed properly [6].

The hepatic venous pressure gradient (wedged minus free hepatic venous pressure) ranges from 1 to 4 mmHg in normal subjects. The hepatic venous pressure gradient remains normal in cases of extrahepatic portal hypertension and in certain cases of presinusoidal portal hypertension such as schistosomiasis [7]. In presinusoidal portal hypertension, the pressure gradient may be elevated, in general to no more than 13 mmHg, thus indicating two blocks (presinusoidal and sinusoidal). In chronic liver disease with extensive fibrosis, as well as in non-cirrhotic portal hypertension, the hepatic venous pressure gradient is increased from 5 to 20 mmHg but remains lower than portal pressure. This increase in the pressure gradient is also observed in several acute liver diseases such as fulminant hepatitis [8].

In alcoholic cirrhosis and in hepatitis-B-related cirrhosis, wedged hepatic venous pressure is similar to portal pressure [4]. The hepatic venous pressure gradient exhibits a circadian variation with two peaks (09.00 h and 23.00 h), and it may also increase during physical exercise. Among these patients, the hepatic venous pressure gradient may differ widely from 10 to 30 mmHg. This value is correlated with the severity of cirrhosis as estimated by the Child–Pugh classification [9]. Liver lesions of acute alcoholic hepatitis increase the hepatic venous pressure gradient [10]. The value for hepatic venous pressure gradient is correlated with the extent of fibrosis and the amount of liver cell necrosis. In patients with cirrhosis, it has also been observed that the presence of hepatocellular carcinoma may markedly increase the hepatic venous pressure gradient to more than 30 mmHg, and that it may be heterogeneous from one vein to another [11]. In patients with alcoholic cirrhosis with a hepatic venous pressure

gradient of more than 12 mmHg, the pressure gradient is not associated with either the development of oesophageal varices or the risk of gastrointestinal bleeding [12]. When the hepatic venous pressure gradient is less than 12 mmHg, it has been established that rupture of oesophageal varices does not occur.

A hepatic venous pressure gradient of more than 4 mmHg indicates sinusoidal portal hypertension, but the mechanism causing this increase is not clear. It depends mainly on the reduction in hepatic vascular space, which increases intrahepatic vascular resistance [13]. This pressure gradient also depends on several other factors such as portal pressure, portal tributary blood flow and hepatic arterial blood flow.

Finally, in patients with alcoholic cirrhosis, a pharmacological decrease in the hepatic venous pressure gradient indicates a reduction in portal pressure [4]. In this case, however, the reduction in hepatic venous pressure gradient may be more marked than the decrease in portal pressure.

Oesophageal variceal pressures

In patients with portal hypertension and oesophageal varices, during oesophageal endoscopy, variceal pressures may be measured by different techniques. A first approach consists of puncturing the lumen of a varix with a needle [14]. This procedure should be performed before sclerotherapy because it may precipitate variceal bleeding. When measured by this technique, variceal pressure is elevated in cases with portal hypertension, but no correlation with portal pressure or hepatic venous pressure gradient has been reported. Intravariceal pressure seems to correlate with the size of the varix and with a previous history of ruptured oesophageal varices.

A second approach uses an endoscopic gauge allowing the measurement of variceal pressure without puncturing varices [15]. This non-invasive method uses a hemispheric pressure gauge with a small chamber fed with a constant flow of gas. This chamber is covered by a latex membrane. When the gauge is placed over a varix, the pressure needed to fill the gauge, as measured by a pressure transducer, is equal to the variceal pressure. It is assumed that the pressure needed to compress a varix equals the pressure inside the varix. It has been demonstrated recently that this technique is reproducible and can be used to assess variceal pressure regularly and evaluate the effects of pharmacological therapy [16].

A third endoscopic method has been described more recently using a transparent plastic balloon fixed to the tip of a gastroscope and observation of the pressure equilibrium between varices and the balloon [17]. The pressure values obtained with this technique correlate well with those measured by needle puncture or with direct portal pressure measurements [18].

Measurement of blood flow

Portal and hepatic arterial blood flows

During abdominal surgery, portal and hepatic arterial blood flow may be measured separately by means of an electromagnetic flow-meter. The results of this invasive method are erroneous because it is performed under general anaesthesia. The ratio between portal and hepatic arterial blood flows can also be calculated by measuring hepatic radioactivity after the injection of a radioactive substance into a peripheral vein. A gamma camera may evaluate both hepatic arterial and the portal radioactivity. This method cannot be widely used because renal and pulmonary radioactivity interferes with hepatic and portal radioactivity; moreover, it is difficult to dissociate arterial and portal curves.

Measurement of hepatic blood flow

Indicator dilution method

Hepatic blood flow can be estimated with the indicator dilution method [19]. The indicator is injected into either the hepatic artery or the portal vein, and blood is drawn into a hepatic vein. Analysis of the hepatic curve gives the hepatic blood flow. This invasive technique is not widely used because there is inadequate mixing between the indicator and the blood. This method has been used, however, to evaluate hepatic microcirculation, transit time and distribution volume [20].

Hepatic clearance method

The clearance method is the most widely used technique at present for estimating hepatic blood flow in man. It is based on the Fick principle [21]. The hepatic clearance (Cl) depends on hepatic blood flow (HBF) and the extraction (E) of a substance by the liver:

$$Cl = HBF \times E$$

Hence:

$$HBF = Cl/E$$

Absolute hepatic clearance can be calculated by the continuous infusion method. When the peripheral concentration (C_p) of the substance has reached a plateau, the amount of substance removed by the liver is equal to the amount of perfused solution Q:

$$Cl = Q/C_p$$

Extraction depends on afferent (C_{aff}) and efferent (C_{eff}) concentrations of the substance. Thus:

$$E = (C_{aff} - C_{eff})/C_{aff}$$

If this substance is captured only by the liver, afferent concentration is equal to peripheral vein or arterial concentration of this substance. Efferent concentration is obtained from blood drawn from a hepatic vein. Therefore, hepatic vein catheterization is necessary to measure hepatic blood flow by the clearance method. Hepatic clearance is hepatic blood flow only if extrac-

tion reaches 100%. If extraction is lower than 10%, the values of hepatic blood flow are not calculated as it is considered that a slight change in extraction induces large variation in hepatic blood flow. Thus, the clearance method cannot evaluate hepatic blood flow in patients with severe liver disease. Moreover, a decrease in hepatic clearance does not indicate a decrease in hepatic blood flow as extraction may also decrease, leaving hepatic blood flow constant.

Fraction clearance (K) may also be used for the calculation of hepatic blood flow:

$$K = Cl/\text{Blood volume}$$

This method, using a bolus injection, is similar to the continuous infusion method.

Substances used for the clearance method should meet three criteria: they should be devoid of toxicity, should diffuse only within the vascular space and should be removed only by the liver. Two types of substance can be used: those cleared by hepatocytes [bromsulphthalein (BSP), indocyanine cardiogreen (ICG)] and those cleared by the Kupffer cells (colloid labelled with radiogold, denaturated labelled albumin).

Galactose clearance has been proposed for the estimation of hepatic blood flow as hepatic extraction of this substance is more than 90% in normal subjects [22]. In patients with liver disease, however, this extraction is markedly decreased and, hence, hepatic blood flow is not properly evaluated by galactose clearance. Moreover, it has been demonstrated recently that extrahepatic uptake of galactose occurs in cirrhotic patients. These findings clearly indicate that galactose clearance can be used neither for measurement of hepatic blood flow nor for studying variations in hepatic blood flow.

Values of hepatic blood flow

In normal fasted conscious subjects in the supine position, hepatic blood flow ranges from 1 to 2 L/min, i.e. 1 mL/min per g of liver tissue. In man, it is accepted, but has not been clearly demonstrated, that one-third of hepatic blood flow comes from the hepatic artery and two-thirds from the portal vein. In patients with liver diseases, hepatic blood flow may differ widely from one patient to another [23]. In patients with cirrhosis, hepatic blood flow may be low, normal or elevated. In particular, acute alcoholic hepatitis increases hepatic blood flow [24]. In patients with acute hepatitis, hepatic blood flow may be increased, while hepatic blood flow is low in patients with extrahepatic portal hypertension [25]. In patients with cirrhosis, no correlation has been found between hepatic blood flow and liver failure, nor has hepatic blood flow been correlated with portal pressure [26]. This observation is not surprising as, in portal hypertensive patients, a certain percentage of the portal blood does not reach the liver but bypasses this organ through the collateral circulation. Hence, portal pressure may decrease without a change in hepatic blood flow. In this case, the reduction in portal pressure depends on a decrease in portal tributary blood flow.

Measurement of portal blood flow

Several invasive methods have been described for measuring portal blood flow. However, they necessitate the insertion of a catheter into the lumen of the portal vein. Portal blood flow can be measured by the continuous thermodilution method or by means of a catheter with an electromagnetic flow-meter.

The most common method for the evaluation of portal blood flow is by Doppler sonography [27]. This non-invasive procedure measures the velocity of red blood cells. At present, however, the pulsed Doppler method is not accurate in man for the following reasons:

1 The mean angle between the Doppler beam and the axis of the portal vein may be too large, reaching up to 60°. In this case, a slight error in the angle results in a large variation in the cosine angle, which is related to flow velocity.

2 The ultrasound diffraction between the skin and the portal vein is not taken into consideration.

3 The measurement of maximal velocity in one area of the portal vein may differ from one position to another.

4 As the measurement of blood flow depends on the cross-sectional area of the portal vein, a slight error in the estimated diameter of the portal vein results in a large variation in this value.

The pulsed Doppler method has not yet been validated in man. The Doppler technique may, however, be used to assess the presence and direction of portal blood flow. In addition, in the same individual, physiological or pharmacological variations in blood velocity in the portal vein may be evaluated. Its accuracy and reproducibility are still in question [28].

In normal subjects, the portal blood flow goes towards the liver and has a continuous spectrum, with mild waves. In patients with portal hypertension, there is a continuous flow towards the liver. In some cases, alterations in portal blood flow appear as an absence of end-diastolic, arterialized flow or bidirectional flow. Reversed flow is rarely observed in the portal vein. Portal vein diameter and blood flow changes are not, however, correlated with the hepatic venous pressure gradient in patients with cirrhosis [29].

Estimation of blood flow in the collateral circulation

Quantification of portosystemic circulation

The percentage of portal venous inflow shunted through portosystemic collaterals may be estimated by comparing the area of an isotope dilution curve recorded from the hepatic vein after injecting an isotope into the superior mesenteric or splenic artery with the curve obtained after injecting an isotope into the hepatic artery [30]. In normal subjects, no shunting was detected but, in patients with cirrhosis, shunting of mesenteric or splenic flow ranged from zero to 100%. A similar estimation may be obtained after intrasplenic injection of a radioactive indicator.

The comparison of bioavailability of drugs after oral and intravenous administration allows the measurement of the shunt fraction of portal inflow [31]. The liver must remove 100% of these substances. The systemic availability of oral glyceryl trinitrate has been used. In this case, drug concentrations in plasma were replaced by assessments of pharmacological effects using digital plethysmography [32]. None of these invasive and non-invasive methods, however, could be used to predict the complication of portal hypertension.

Azygos blood flow

The superior portosystemic collateral circulation can be estimated by measuring blood flow in the azygos vein [33]. This vein essentially drains the splenogastric collateral circulation. Azygos blood flow is measured by the local continuous thermodilution method. Under fluoroscopic control, a continuous thermodilution catheter with a curved tip is introduced into the azygos vein up to approximately 5 cm from its junction with the superior vena cava. Its position is verified by injection of a contrast medium into the catheter. During routine haemodynamic investigation, catheterization of the azygos vein may be performed either from the femoral vein or from the right internal jugular vein. In normal subjects, azygos blood flow is approximately 100 mL/min. In patients with portal hypertension, azygos blood flow is six times higher than in normal subjects and ranges from 200 to 1500 mL/min.

An elevated azygos blood flow indirectly confirms the increased portal tributary blood flow observed in portal hypertensive animals. Azygos blood flow is correlated with portal pressure and depends on the severity of cirrhosis. Azygos blood flow is not correlated with either the presence and size of the oesophageal varices or the risk of ruptured varices [34]. Finally, azygos blood flow is a more sensitive measurement than the hepatic venous pressure gradient for evaluating the change in splanchnic circulation after portal hypotensive drug administration. Thus, the measurement of azygos blood flow seems to be the most viable method for the evaluation of portal hypertension.

Preliminary results showed that cine phase-contrast magnetic resonance angiography is a practical non-invasive method for measuring absolute azygos blood flow and provides a non-invasive method of monitoring portal hypertension [35].

References

1 Burcharth F, Joyce F (1987) Percutaneous transhepatic catheterization of the portal venous system. *J Gastroenterol Hepatol* 2, 569–587.

2 Lebrec D, Goldfarb G, Degott C et al. (1982) Transvenous liver biopsy. An experience based on 1000 hepatic tissue samplings with this procedure. *Gastroenterology* 83, 338–340.

3 Fenyves D, Pomier-Layrargues G, Willems B et al. (1988) Intrahepatic pressure measurement: not an accurate reflection of portal vein pressure. *Hepatology* 8, 211–216.

4 Valla D, Bercoff E, Menu Y *et al.* (1984) Discrepancy between wedged hepatic venous pressure and portal venous pressure after acute propranolol administration in patients with alcoholic cirrhosis. *Gastroenterology* 86, 1400–1403.

5 Keiding S, Vilstrup H (2002) Intrahepatic heterogeneity of hepatic venous pressure gradient in human cirrhosis. *Scand J Gastroenterol* 37, 960–964.

6 Groszmann RJ, Wongcharatrawee S (2004) The hepatic venous pressure gradient: Anything worth doing should be done right. *Hepatology* 39, 280–282.

7 Lebrec D, Benhamou JP (1986) Noncirrhotic intrahepatic portal hypertension. *Semin Liver Dis* 6, 332–340.

8 Valla D, Fléjou JF, Lebrec D *et al.* (1989) Portal hypertension and ascites in acute hepatitis. Clinical, hemodynamic and histological correlations. *Hepatology* 10, 482–487.

9 Braillon A, Calès P, Valla D *et al.* (1986) Influence of the degree of liver failure on systemic and splanchnic haemodynamics and on response to propranolol in patients with cirrhosis. *Gut* 27, 1204–1209.

10 Poynard T, Degott C, Munoz C *et al.* (1987) Relationship between degree of portal hypertension and liver histologic lesions in patients with alcoholic cirrhosis. Effect of acute alcoholic hepatitis on portal hypertension. *Dig Dis Sci* 32, 337–344.

11 Lee SS, Koshy A, Hadengue A *et al.* (1990) Heterogeneous hepatic venous pressures in patients with liver cancer. *J Clin Gastroenterol* 12, 53–56.

12 Lebrec D, de Fleury P, Rueff B *et al.* (1980) Portal hypertension size of esophageal varices, and risk of gastrointestinal bleeding in alcoholic cirrhosis. *Gastroenterology* 79, 1139–1144.

13 Lee SS, Hadengue A, Girod C *et al.* (1987) Reduction of intrahepatic vascular space in the pathogenesis of portal hypertension. In vitro and in vivo studies in the rat. *Gastroenterology* 93, 157–161.

14 Staritz M, Poralla T, Meyer Zum Buschenfelde H (1985) Intravascular oesophageal variceal pressure (IOVP) assessed by endoscopic fine needle puncture under basal conditions, Valsalva's manoeuvre and after glyceryltrinitrate application. *Gut* 26, 525–530.

15 Bosch J, Bordas JM, Rigau J *et al.* (1986) Noninvasive measurement of the pressure of esophageal varices using an endoscopic gauge: comparison with measurements by variceal puncture in patients undergoing endoscopic sclerotherapy. *Hepatology* 6, 667–672.

16 Nevens F, Sprengers D, Feu F *et al.* (1996) Measurement of variceal pressure with an endoscopic pressure sensitive gauge: validation and effect of propranolol therapy in chronic conditions. *J Hepatol* 24, 66–73.

17 Gertsch P, Fischer G, Kleber G *et al.* (1993) Manometry of esophageal varices: comparison of an endoscopic balloon technique with needle puncture. *Gastroenterology* 105, 1159–1166.

18 Brensing KA, Neubrand M, Textor J *et al.* (1998) Endoscopic manometry of esophageal varices: evaluation of a balloon technique compared with direct portal pressure measurement. *J Hepatol* 29, 94–102.

19 Cohn JN, Khatri IM, Groszmann RJ *et al.* (1972) Hepatic blood flow in alcoholic liver disease measured by an indicator dilution technique. *Am J Med* 53, 704–722.

20 Huet P-M, Pomier-Layrargues G, Villeneuve J-P *et al.* (1986) Intrahepatic circulation in liver disease. *Semin Liver Dis* 6, 277–286.

21 Caesar J, Shaldon S, Chiandussi L *et al.* (1961) The use of indocyanine green in the measurement of hepatic blood flow and as a test of hepatic function. *Clin Sci* 21, 43–57.

22 Keiding S (1988) Galactose clearance measurements and liver blood flow. *Gastroenterology* 94, 477–481.

23 Gadano A, Hadengue A, Vachiery F *et al.* (1997) Relationship between hepatic blood flow, liver tests, haemodynamic values and clinical characteristics in patients with chronic liver disease. *J Gastroenterol Hepatol* 12, 167–171.

24 Cohn JN, Khatri IM, Groszmann RJ *et al.* (1972) Hepatic blood flow in alcoholic liver disease measured by an indicator dilution technique. *Am J Med* 53, 704–722.

25 Lebrec D, Bataille C, Bercoff E *et al.* (1983) Hemodynamic changes in patients with portal venous obstruction. *Hepatology* 3, 550–553.

26 Lebrec D, Sicot C, Benhamou JP (1973) Débit sanguin hépatique, hypertension portale et insuffisance hépatocellulaire chez les malades atteints de cirrhose alcoolique. *Arch Fr Mal App Dig* 62, 465–471.

27 Burns p, Taylor K, Blei AT (1987) Doppler flowmetry and portal hypertension. *Gastroenterology* 92, 824–826.

28 Bolondi L, Gaiani S, Barbara L (1991) Accuracy and reproducibility of portal flow measurement by Doppler US. *J Hepatol* 13, 269–273.

29 Choi YJ, Baik SK, Park DH *et al.* (2003) Comparison of Doppler ultrasonography and the hepatic venous pressure gradient in assessing portal hypertension in liver cirrhosis. *J Gastroenterol Hepatol* 18, 424–429.

30 Groszmann R, Kotelanski B, Cohn JN *et al.* (1972) Quantitation of portasystemic shunting from the splenic and mesenteric beds in alcoholic liver disease. *Am J Med* 53, 715–722.

31 Nordlinger R, Parquet M, Infante R *et al.* (1982) Noninvasive measurement of nutrient portal blood shunting: an experimental study with [^{14}C]ursodeoxycholic acid. *Hepatology* 2, 412–419.

32 Porchet H, Bircher J (1982) Noninvasive assessment of portal-systemic shunting: evaluation of a method to investigate systemic availability of oral glyceryl trinitrate by digital plethysmography. *Gastroenterology* 92, 629–637.

33 Bosch J, Groszmann RJ (1984) Measurement of azygos venous blood flow by a continuous thermal dilution technique: an index of blood low through gastroesophageal collaterals in cirrhosis. *Hepatology* 4, 424–429.

34 Calès P, Braillon A, Jiron MI *et al.* (1984) Superior portosystemic collateral circulation estimated by azygos blood flow in patients with cirrhosis. Lack of correlation with oesophageal varices and gastro-intestinal bleeding. Effect of propranolol. *J Hepatol* 1, 37–46.

35 Lomas DL, Hayball MP, Jones DP *et al.* (1995) Non-invasive measurement of azygos venous blood flow using magnetic resonance. *J Hepatol* 22, 399–403.

5.10 The Cochrane Hepatobiliary Group

Christian Gluud, on behalf of the Cochrane Hepatobiliary Group*

Introduction

On 20 May 1747, the Scottish naval surgeon James Lind studied six interventions for 12 sailors with scurvy. The patients all had putrid gums, spots and lassitude. They shared a room and meals. Lind divided them into six groups: two patients were given sea water, two cider, two vinegar, two elixir vitriol, two a concoction of spices, garlic and mustard seeds, and two oranges and lemons. Within six days, the two patients given oranges and lemons became fit for duty or well enough to be appointed nurse for the remaining patients – see The James Lind Library (http://www.jameslindlibrary.org) and the European Clinical Research Infrastructures Network (http://www.ecrin.org). Lind reported this clinical trial in 1753. It took about another 150 years until we discovered vitamin C and understood the effect of oranges and lemons in scurvy. It took about another 200 years until we rediscovered the idea of conducting bias-free comparative trials (http://www.jameslindlibrary.org). Researchers began to use randomization at the time of the Second World War. The methods of conducting randomized trials have been refined since then. Such trials remain the most reliable way to test the effects of interventions [1].

Hepatobiliary randomized trials started to appear in 1955 [2]. Thomas C Chalmers and co-workers conducted the first two factorial-designed trials on diet, rest and physical reconditioning for acute infectious hepatitis [2]. In these trials, 260 patients and 200 patients were randomized [2]. Several other early trials in liver diseases have been reviewed [3]. It took a while before hepatobiliary controlled trials started to appear regularly (Fig. 1). Presently about 550 publications on hepatobiliary randomized trials are published each year (Fig. 1). This corresponds to about three publications per working day appearing in more than 1000 different journals. Nobody can any longer claim to be a specialist in all hepatobiliary diseases. The workload of keeping up to date has become so heavy that we have to collaborate and divide the tasks among ourselves. The first task is to conduct the randomized trials. The second task is to systematically review these trials. The third task is to implement the evidence from the systematic reviews into clinical practice.

In this chapter we describe the evidence hierarchy that may guide evidence-based clinical practice. We assess the proportion of hepatobiliary randomized trials with sample size estimation, the achieved sample size, and the proportion with adequate quality components. We compare the quality of hepatobiliary randomized trials to that of trials from all medical fields. Finally, The Cochrane Collaboration and the Cochrane Hepatobiliary Group (CHBG) are described.

The evidence hierarchy

The hierarchy of evidence is well established [4–6]. It is based on the estimated risks of bias in the different study designs. Randomized trials are internationally considered the gold standard for intervention comparisons [1–13]. The results from randomized trials form the basis for determining which drugs and devices are effective. Historically controlled studies, cohort studies and case–control studies are unreliable designs unless the intervention effect is dramatic [13,14]. Dramatic intervention effects are rare. Expert opinions, case reports and experimental models may be misleading and rank lowest in the evidence hierarchy [4–6]. Study designs other than randomized trials remain important for diagnostic [6,15] and prognostic [16,17] studies as well as for assessing rare adverse events [18,19] – but they cannot replace randomized trials in assessing beneficial effects of interventions.

Randomized trials are increasingly being used to guide evidence-based clinical practice. You need to address a central question before you consider using the results for patient care:

---

* Members of the Cochrane Hepatobiliary Group Editorial Team are: Bodil Als-Nielsen, Editor (Denmark), Gennaro D'Amico, Editor (Italy), Christian Gluud, Co-ordinating Editor (Denmark), Lise Lotte Gluud, Editor (Denmark), Saboor Khan, Editor (UK), Sarah L. Klingenberg, Hand Search Coordinator (Denmark), Ronald L. Koretz, Editor (USA), Rob Myers, Editor (Canada), Luigi Pagliaro, Editor (Italy), Rosanna Simonneti, Editor (Italy), Robert Sutton, Editor (UK), Dimitrinka Nikolova, Review Group Co-ordinator (Denmark) and Nader Salas, Data Manager (Denmark).

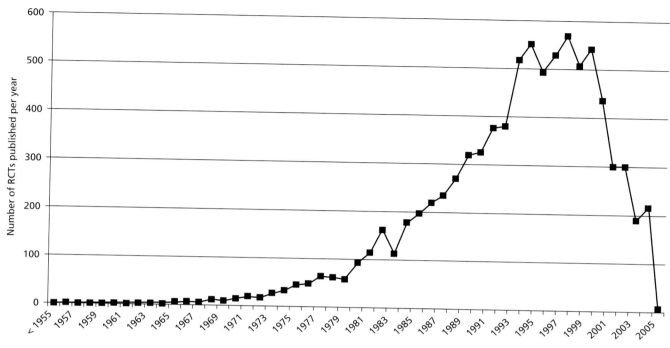

Fig.1 Number of publications on randomized trials and controlled clinical trials during the period 1955 to 2005 according to the Cochrane Hepatobiliary Group Controlled Trial Register [56]. The decline since 2001 is most likely due to a backlog in identification and registration. RCT, randomized controlled trial.

Table 1 Components used to assess the methodological quality of randomized trials

	Adequate	Inadequate
Generation of allocation sequence	Computer-generated random numbers, table of random numbers, or similar	Not described or inadequate methods
Allocation concealment	Central randomization, sealed envelopes, or similar	Not described or inadequate (by an open table or similar)
Double blinding	Identical placebo tablets or similar	Inadequate (e.g. tablets versus injection), not described, or no double blinding

are the results valid? The validity depends on the internal validity of the trial. The internal validity of a trial depends on the risks of *random errors* [10,20] and the risks of *systematic errors* (i.e. bias) [8–13,20,21]. Conducting randomized trials with many participants and outcomes decreases the risks of random errors [10,20]. Conducting randomized trials with high methodological quality, avoiding selection, performance, assessment, attrition and other biases, decreases the risks of systematic errors [8–13,20,21]. Methodological quality has been defined as 'the confidence that the trial design, conduct, and analysis has minimized or avoided biases in its treatment comparison' [9]. The methodological quality of a trial can be assessed as described in Table 1. The external validity of a trial should only be considered if the internal validity is considered adequate. If the internal validity is inadequate, the external validity becomes irrelevant.

A single randomized clinical trial may give misleading results due to random errors or bias. It is essential that independent groups conduct trials on the same therapeutic question, to establish firm evidence for an intervention effect [22–26]. Several trials on the same intervention for the same type of patients may reach more or less concurring conclusions. Conducting a meta-analysis will increase power and increase precision [27–29]. Systematic reviews with meta-analyses of several randomized trials have become an important tool for clinical decision-making [30] – see also The Cochrane Collaboration website (www.cochrane.org). The tendency not to publish trials with neutral or negative intervention effects leads to publication bias [31–34]. It is important that all trials are registered before inclusion of the first patient [35]. Here, details of the trial protocol as well as any amendments to the protocol should be registered. After the end of follow-up of the last patient and analysis, anonymous data from the trial should also be registered [35]. This reduces publication bias [31–34], bias due to post hoc changes of primary outcomes [36,37], and other biases.

Table 2 Number of randomized trials, the proportion of randomized trials reporting sample size calculations, and number of participants per intervention arm in four hepatobiliary journals [7,38–40]

	Liver	Journal of Hepatology	Hepatology	Gastroenterology[a]
Number of trials	32	171	235	383
Sample size calculations	7%	19%	26%	ND[b]
Number of participants per intervention arm				
Median	18	19	26	23
Interquartile range	10–36	11–31	14–44	10–50
Range	2–169	5–519	3–542	1–1107

[a]Includes trials on both hepatobiliary and other gastroenterology topics. There were no major differences between hepatobiliary trials and trials on other gastroenterology topics regarding sample size, but sample size varied significantly between the different disease areas examined (Kjaergard LL, Frederiksen S, Gluud C, unpublished observations).
[b]ND, not determined.

Table 3 Number of randomized trials and the proportion of randomized trials with adequate generation of the allocation sequence, allocation concealment, and double blinding in four journals publishing many hepatobiliary trials [7,38–40]

	Liver	Journal of Hepatology	Hepatology	Gastroenterology[a]
Number of trials	32	171	235	383
Adequate generation of the allocation sequence	21%	28%	52%	42%
Adequate allocation concealment	5%	13%	34%	39%
Adequate double blinding	28%	30%	34%	62%

[a]Includes trials on both hepatobiliary and other gastroenterology topics. There were no major differences between hepatobiliary randomized trials and randomized trials on other gastroenterology topics regarding methodological quality, but methodological quality varied significantly between the different disease areas examined (Kjaergard LL, Frederiksen S, Gluud C, unpublished observations).

Table 4 Comparison of 616 hepatobiliary randomized trials from 12 journals on MEDLINE [41] and 519 randomized trials from PubMed [44] regarding sample size and adequacy of methodological components

Variable	Randomized hepatobiliary clinical trials published from 1985 to 1996 [41]	Randomized trials from all disease areas published in December 2000 [44]
Median number of participants per intervention arm (10th to 90th percentiles participants per intervention arm)	23 participants (7–102 participants)	32 participants (12–159 participants)
Proportion with adequate generation of the allocation sequence	48%	21%
Proportion with adequate allocation concealment	38%	18%
Proportion with adequate double blinding	34%	38%

Most hepatobiliary randomized trials are too small and have methodological deficiencies [7,14,38–41] (Tables 2–4). Cumulative meta-analyses (i.e. adding each new trial to the meta-analyses when the trial is published) of interventions preventing oesophageal variceal bleeding and rebleeding, and of other interventions, have demonstrated that therapeutic recommendations in textbooks lag behind the available evidence [42,43]. Therefore we need a regular systematic review of the intervention literature.

Sample size estimation in randomized trials

In a trial with a dichotomous primary outcome, the sample size is determined from four pieces of information [20]:
• prior knowledge of the intervention effect (expected minimal relevant difference);
• the expected proportion of patients with the primary outcome during the trial in the control arm;

- alpha or the risk of committing a type 1 error (usually set to 0.05);
- beta or the risk of committing a type 2 error (usually set to 0.20 or 0.10) [20].

The sample size in a trial with a continuous outcome measure is determined from knowledge of the mean and standard deviation of the outcome instead of the expected proportion in the control arm [20]. Sample size estimation should be based on the primary outcome measure of the trial [20,36,37].

It is important to know the targeted sample size when we evaluate the internal validity of a randomized trial. Otherwise, we do not know whether the data of the trial are reported before, at, or after the targeted sample size was reached.

Some 7–26% of hepatobiliary randomized trials report a sample size calculation, depending on the journal in which they were published (Table 2). In a study including PubMed-indexed randomized trials from all disease areas, the figure was 27% [44].

Sample size of randomized trials

The number of patients included in hepatobiliary randomized trials varied only a little depending on the journal in which they were published (Table 2). The median number of participants per intervention arm was 23 (10th to 90th percentiles from 7 to 102) in hepatobiliary trials published in 12 different journals during 1985 to 1996 [41] (Table 4). In PubMed-indexed randomized trials from all disease areas, the median number was 32 participants per intervention arm (10th to 90th percentiles from 12 to 159) [44] (Table 4).

Small sample sizes are worrying, because they are connected with large risks of type 1 and type 2 errors [20,41,44]. With a small sample size, important prognostic variables may be unevenly distributed. This could lead to observation of significant 'intervention effects' simply due to the distribution of prognostic variables. A two-group comparison with 23 patients in each arm has 26% power to detect a difference between event rates of 30% in the control group and 10% in the experimental group at the 0.05 significance level. The difference in intervention effect corresponds to a relative risk of 0.33 or a relative risk reduction of 67%. Such intervention effects are rarely discovered. The power to detect smaller differences is less than 26%.

Random errors are a real problem in hepatobiliary and other types of randomized trials. These problems can only be overcome by developing more effective interventions (the molecular-genetic 'revolution' may give some hope) or by clinical researchers realizing that being a small part of a large trial is more important than being a large part of a small trial.

Methodological quality of randomized trials

Conducting randomized trials with high methodological quality, avoiding selection, performance, assessment, attrition and other biases, decreases the risks of systematic errors [8–13,20,21]. We have examined the methodological quality of hepatobiliary randomized trials (Tables 3 and 4), and have found that several trials have methodological deficiencies [7, 38–41,44–46].

The low methodological quality raises the question of whether biased estimates of intervention effects have occurred. A systematic review of the evidence may answer this question. The methodological quality of a trial is related to the number of centres involved [7], the therapeutic area [7,38,40,41] and whether the trial was sponsored [41]. We found no significant difference between the quality of trials sponsored by for-profit or not-for-profit organizations [41].

The proportion of hepatobiliary randomized trials with adequate generation of the allocation sequence varies from 21% to 52%, depending on the journal in which they were published (Table 3). About every second trial reported adequate generation of the allocation sequence among hepatobiliary trials published in 12 different journals during 1985–1996 [41]. The proportion was 21% in PubMed-indexed randomized trials from all disease areas [44] (Table 4).

The proportion of hepatobiliary randomized trials with adequate allocation concealment varies from 5% to 39%, depending on the journal in which they were published (Table 3). A total of 38% of trials reported adequate allocation concealment among hepatobiliary trials published in 12 different journals during 1985–1996 [41]. This proportion was higher in some areas of hepatology (e.g. primary biliary cirrhosis) and lower in others (e.g. hepatitis B and C) [41]. The proportion was 18% in PubMed-indexed randomized trials from all disease areas [44] (Table 4). Trials with unclear or inadequate allocation concealment are associated with a 20–30% exaggeration of the intervention effect [8–12,21]. Some studies have found that unclear reporting of allocation concealment does not necessarily mean inadequate conduct of allocation concealment, but these studies have been on small and select groups of trials [47–49]. Other studies observed unclear reporting of allocation concealment connected with unclear or inadequate methodology in about 80% of trials [50,51].

The proportion of hepatobiliary trials with adequate double blinding varies from 28% to 62%, depending on the journal in which they were published (Table 3). A total of 34% of trials were double blind among hepatobiliary randomized trials published in 12 different journals during 1985–1996 [41]. In PubMed-indexed randomized trials from all disease areas, 38% were double blind [44] (Table 4). Due to the nature of many interventions (e.g. endoscopy for portal hypertension, gallbladder surgery), double blinding (i.e. blinding of both patient and caregivers) may not be feasible. Only blinding of all involved in a trial can secure that reporting bias, performance bias, assessment bias, attrition bias and other biases do not occur. In trials where control interventions cannot be blinded with a placebo or a sham, you can always use blinded outcome assessment. This may reduce assessment and attrition bias.

The Cochrane Collaboration

The Cochrane Collaboration works to facilitate the preparation, maintenance and dissemination of systematic reviews of randomized trials and systematic reviews of other evidence evaluating health care. The Cochrane Collaboration is named after Archie Cochrane (1909–1988), the epidemiologist who first emphasized that reliable information from randomized trials is vital for making sound decisions in health care and research [52].

The Cochrane Collaboration started in 1993 and has since grown rapidly [52,53]. By 2005, 12 Cochrane Centres and 49 collaborative review groups were registered as part of the Collaboration. The infrastructure for covering all areas of health care is now in place. The tasks of the collaborative review groups are to:

• search the specialist literature for randomized trials, controlled clinical trials, and meta-analyses;
• establish and continuously update databases of these articles;
• prepare protocols for the systematic reviews;
• prepare the systematic reviews as well as continually updating them.

The protocols and the systematic reviews are peer-refereed by international experts before acceptance. Once accepted, the protocols and the systematic reviews are included in the Cochrane Database of Systematic Reviews in The Cochrane Library (http://www.cochrane.org). The Cochrane Library is disseminated electronically on CD-ROMs and via the internet (http://www.cochrane.org). The Cochrane Library contains the Cochrane Central Register of Controlled Trials. This register contains more than 450 000 references to abstracts or articles on controlled clinical trials. Further, The Cochrane Library contains about 20 reviews on methodology, a register of about 7000 articles on methodological issues, and references to different Methods Groups and Fields.

In 2005, more than 4000 protocols for systematic reviews and 2500 systematic reviews were published in The Cochrane Library. The Library also offers the *Cochrane Handbook for Systematic Reviews of Interventions* [29]. This *Handbook* describes the steps one has to take during formulating a protocol for a systematic review and when conducting the systematic review. It is available free of charge from http://www.cochrane.org or as part of the free software RevMan Analyses.

The Cochrane systematic review process is dynamic. The review is modified, as new information becomes available. If you want to contest something in a Cochrane review, you may send an e-mail to the Editorial Team and the authors. In this way, mistakes can be corrected and additional information included. The Cochrane Collaboration still has much to improve [53,54].

The scope of the Cochrane Hepatobiliary Group

The CHBG is one of the 49 collaborative review groups of The Cochrane Collaboration. The CHBG became registered in 1996 [55,56], and its scope is to perform the tasks of the Cochrane Collaboration within hepatobiliary diseases [55,56].

By 2005, the CHBG comprised more than 900 hepatologists, gastroenterologists, hepatobiliary surgeons and biostatisticians from more than 80 countries. Its members have expertise in clinical trials, clinical epidemiology and clinical practice related to hepatobiliary diseases.

The CHBG has the task of full-text searching the specialist journals for randomized trials and controlled clinical trials. Members of the CHBG are involved in searching 26 out of 159 identified specialist journals that need hand searching.

The productivity of the Cochrane Hepatobiliary Group

The CHBG has performed searches in a number of databases for randomized trials, controlled clinical trials, and meta-analyses pertinent to patients with hepatobiliary disorders. Millions of references have been identified and scanned. About 20 000 of these seem relevant for the work of the CHBG (Fig. 2). Of these, almost 9000 are articles on randomized trials (Fig. 2), published from 1955 until now (Fig. 1). These references are submitted to The Collaboration and included in the Cochrane Central Register of Controlled Trials in The Cochrane Library.

More than 200 titles for systematic reviews have been registered with the CHBG and more than 120 CHBG protocols have been published in The Cochrane Library. Of these protocols, 50 have turned into CHBG systematic reviews. Abstracts of these reviews are available free of charge via PubMed or http://www.cochrane.org. Total reviews are available free of charge in Australia, South Africa, a number of European countries, and in low-income countries via the WHO Health InterNetwork Access to Research Initiative.

How you can participate

You can participate as a hand searcher for randomized trials, an author of systematic reviews, or peer-referee of reviews by contacting the Editorial Team office. Interested parties can obtain information as to which specialist journals need full-text searching or which titles need to be reviewed or updated. You can also register a title for a new systematic review. For further information, please contact the CHBG Editorial Team Office, Copenhagen Trial Unit, Center for Clinical Intervention Research, Department 7102, Rigshospitalet, Copenhagen University Hospital, Blegdamsvej 9, DK-2100 Copenhagen, Denmark. Tel. +45 35457175; fax +45 35457101; e-mail dnikolov@ctu.rh.dk; home page http://inet.uni2.dk/~ctucph/chbg/.

The past and the future of clinical research

We have witnessed a dramatic increase in the number of randomized trials during the last 50 years (Fig. 1). The trial size and

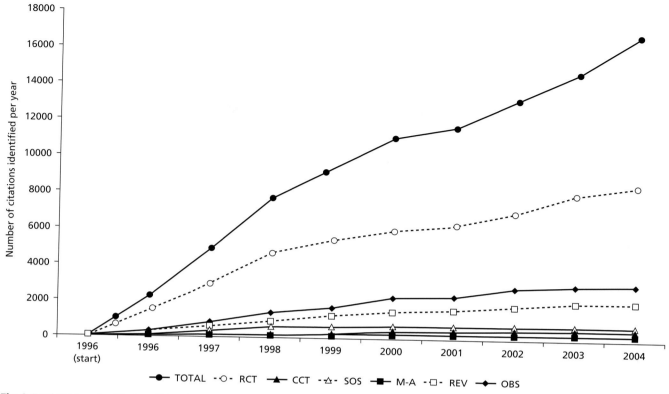

Fig. 2 Total number of publications (TOTAL) and number of publications on randomized trials (RCT), controlled clinical trials (CCT), second opinion ought to be sought (SOS), meta-analysis (MA), reviews (REV), and observational studies (OBS) registered in the Cochrane Hepatobiliary Group Controlled Trial Register from 1996 to 2005 [56].

methodological quality seem to leave a lot to be desired – and progress on this front has been slow or absent [7–13,29,38–41,44–46,52]. We need to improve education in clinical epidemiology and systematic reviewing. We need to pay more attention to adequate statistical power and adequate design of randomized trials. The recommendations of the CON-SORT statement (http://www.consort-statement.org) and the Cochrane Collaboration [54] may serve as guides to future research. We need more research into how to organize large randomized trials and how to reduce dropouts and insufficient follow-up. We need more research into analyses of randomized clinical trials. For example, logistic regression analyses seem to dramatically increase rather than decrease the risks of over- and underestimation of intervention effects [13]. We also need more independent evaluation of interventions [22–26]. Additional research in methods for systematic reviewing is also important, for instance how best to conduct trial sequential analysis with trial sequential boundaries in order to reduce the risk of committing type 1 errors [57–59]. Finally, we need to bridge the gaps between clinical research and clinical practice [60,61]. These tasks may be achieved – with investment and dedicated collaboration.

References

1 Chalmers I (2001) Comparing like with like: some historical milestones in the evolution of methods to create unbiased comparison groups in therapeutic experiments. *Int J Epidemiol* 30, 1156–1164.

2 Chalmers TC, Eckhardt RD, Reynolds WE *et al.* (1955) The treatment of acute infectious hepatitis. Controlled studies of the effects of diet, rest, and physical reconditioning on the acute course of the disease and on the incidence of relapses and residual abnormalities. *J Clin Invest* 34, 1163–1235.

3 Chalmers TC (1976) Randomized controlled clinical trials in diseases of the liver. *Prog Liver Dis* 5, 450–456.

4 Sackett DL, Straus SE, Richardson WS *et al.* (2000) *Evidence-Based Medicine; How to Practise and Teach EBM*, 2nd edn. Edinburgh: Churchill Livingstone.

5 Hayward R (ed.) (2002) Users' Guides Interactive. Chicago: JAMA Publishing Group. URL http://www.usersguides.org.

6 Gluud C, Gluud LL (2005) Evidence based diagnostics. *Br Med J* 330, 724–726.

7 Kjaergard LL, Nikolova D, Gluud C (1999) Randomized trials in hepatology: predictors of quality. *Hepatology* 30, 1134–1138.

8 Schulz KF, Chalmers I, Hayes RJ, Altman DG (1995) Empirical evidence of bias. Dimensions of methodological quality associated with estimates of treatment effects in controlled trials. *JAMA* 273, 408–412.

9 Moher D, Pham B, Jones A et al. (1998) Does quality of reports of randomized trials affect estimates of intervention efficacy reported in meta-analyses? Lancet 352, 609–613.

10 Kjaergard LL, Villumsen J, Gluud C (2001) Reported methodological quality and discrepancies between large and small randomized trials in meta-analyses. Ann Intern Med 135, 982–989.

11 Balk EM, Boris PA, Moskowitz H et al. (2002) Correlation of quality measures with estimates of treatment effect in meta-analyses of randomized controlled trials. JAMA 287, 2973–2982.

12 Als-Nielsen B, Chen W, Gluud LL et al. (2004) Are trial size and quality associated with treatment effects in randomized trials? Observational study of 523 randomized trials [abstract]. 12th International Cochrane Colloquium. Ottawa: The Cochrane Collaboration, pp. 102–103. http://www.cochrane.org/colloquia/abstracts/ottawa/P-003.htm

13 Deeks JJ, Dinnes J, D'Amico R et al. (2003) Evaluating non-randomized intervention studies. Health Technol Assess 7, 1–173.

14 Kjaergard LL, Liu J, Als-Nielsen B, Gluud C (2003) Artificial and bioartificial support systems for acute and acute-on-chronic liver failure: a systematic review. JAMA 289, 217–222.

15 Tatsioni A, Deborah AZ, Aronson N et al. (2005) Challenges in systematic reviews of diagnostic technologies. Ann Intern Med 142, 1048–1055.

16 D'Amico G, Morabito A, Pagliaro L, Marubini E (1986) Survival and prognostic indicators in compensated and decompensated cirrhosis. Dig Dis Sci 31, 468–475.

17 Christensen E (2004) Prognostic models including the Child-Pugh, MELD and Mayo risk scores – where are we and where should we go? J Hepatol 41, 344–350.

18 Ioannidis JP, Evans SJ, Gotzsche PC et al. (2004) Better reporting of harms in randomized trials: an extension of the CONSORT statement. Ann Intern Med 141, 781–788.

19 Chou R, Helfand M (2005) Challenges in systematic reviews that assess treatment harms. Ann Intern Med 142, 1090–1099.

20 Pocock SJ (1996) Clinical Trials – A Practical Approach. Chichester: John Wiley & Sons.

21 Als-Nielsen B, Gluud LL, Gluud C (2004) Methodological quality and treatment effects in randomized trials – a review of six empirical studies [abstract]. 12th International Cochrane Colloquium. Ottawa: The Cochrane Collaboration, pp. 88–89. http://www.cochrane.org/colloquia/abstracts/ottawa/O-072.htm

22 Kjaergard LL, Als-Nielsen B (2002) Association between competing interests and authors' conclusions: epidemiological study of randomized trials published in the BMJ. Br Med J 325, 249–252.

23 Als-Nielsen B, Chen W, Gluud C, Kjaergard LL (2003) Association of funding and conclusions in randomized drug trials: a reflection of treatment effect or adverse events? JAMA 290, 921–928.

24 Bekelman JE, Li Y, Gross CP (2003) Scope and impact of financial conflicts of interest in biomedical research: a systematic review. JAMA 289, 454–465.

25 Lexchin J, Bero LA, Djulbegovic B, Clark O (2003) Pharmaceutical industry sponsorship and research outcome and quality: systematic review. Br Med J 326, 1167–1170.

26 House of Commons Health Committee (2005) The Influence of the Pharmaceutical Industry. Fourth Report of Session 2004–05, Vol. I. URL http://www.publications.parliament.uk/pa/cm200405/cmselect/cmhealth/42/4202.htm.

27 Friedman HP, Goldberg JD (1996) Meta-analysis: An introduction and point of view. Hepatology 23, 917–928.

28 Egger M, Jüni P, Bartlett C et al. (2003) How important are comprehensive literature searches and the assessment of trial quality in systematic reviews? Empirical study. Health Technol Assess 7, 1–76.

29 Higgins JPT, Green S (eds) (2005) Cochrane Handbook for Systematic Reviews of Interventions 4.2.4 [updated March 2005]. In: The Cochrane Library, Issue 2, 2005. Chichester: John Wiley & Sons.

30 Santaguida PL, Helfand M, Raina P (2005) Challenges in systematic reviews that evaluate drug efficacy or effectiveness. Ann Intern Med 142, 1066–1072.

31 Simes RJ (1986) The case for an international registry of clinical trials. J Clin Oncol 4, 1529–1541.

32 Dickersin K (1988) Report from the panel on the case for registers of clinical trials at the Eighth Annual Meeting of the Society for Clinical Trials. Control Clin Trials 9, 76–81.

33 Gluud C (1998) 'Negative trials' are positive! J Hepatol 28, 731–733.

34 Dickersin K, Rennie D (2003) Registering clinical trials. JAMA 290, 516–523.

35 Krleza-Jeric K, Chan A-W, Dickersin K et al. (2005) Principles for international registration of protocol information and results from human trials of health related interventions: Ottawa statement (part 1). Br Med J 330, 956–958.

36 Chan A-W, Hrobjartsson A, Haahr MT et al. (2004) Empirical evidence for selective reporting of outcomes in randomized trials: comparison of protocols to published articles. JAMA 291, 2457–2465.

37 Chan A-W, Krleza-Jeric K, Schmid I, Altman DG (2004) Outcome reporting bias in randomized trials funded by the Canadian Institutes of Health Research. CMAJ 171, 735–740.

38 Gluud C (1999) Evidence based medicine in liver. Liver 19, 1–2.

39 Gluud C, Nikolova D (1998) Quality assessment of reports on clinical trials in the Journal of Hepatology. J Hepatol 29, 321–327.

40 Kjaergard LL, Frederiksen SL, Gluud C (2002) Validity of randomized trials in Gastroenterology from 1964–2000. Gastroenterology 122, 1157–1160.

41 Kjaergard LL, Gluud C (2002) Funding, disease area, and internal validity of hepatobiliary randomized trials. Am J Gastroenterol 97, 2708–2713.

42 Pagliaro L, D'Amico G, Pasta L et al. (1996) Efficacy and efficiency of treatments in portal hypertension. In: De Franchis R (ed.) Portal Hypertension II. Proceedings of the Second Baveno International Consensus Workshop on Definitions, Methodology and Therapeutic Strategies. Oxford: Blackwell Science, pp. 159–179.

43 Antman EM, Lau J, Kupelnick B et al. (1991) A comparison of results of meta-analyses of randomized control trials and recommendations of clinical experts. Treatments for myocardial infarction. JAMA 268, 240–248.

44 Chan A-W, Altman DG (2005) Epidemiology and reporting of randomized trials published in PubMed journals. Lancet 365, 1159–1162.

45 Gluud C (1999) Trials and errors in clinical research. Lancet 354, SIV59.

46 Wang J, Gluud C (eds) (2002) Evidence-Based Medicine and Clinical Practice. Beijing: Science Publisher.[in Chinese].

47 Hill CL, LaValley MP, Felson DT (2002) Discrepancy between published report and actual conduct of randomized trials. J Clin Epidemiol 55, 783–786.

48 Devereaux PJ, Choi PT, El-Dika S et al. (2004) An observational study found that authors of randomized controlled trials frequently use concealment of randomization and blinding, despite the failure to report these methods. J Clin Epidemiol 57, 1232–1236.

49 Soares HP, Daniels S, Kumar A *et al.* (2004) Bad reporting does not mean bad methods for randomized trials: observational study of randomized controlled trials performed by the Radiation Therapy Oncology Group. *Br Med J* 328, 22–24.

50 Liberati A, Himel HN, Chalmers TC (1986) A quality assessment of randomized control trials of primary treatment of breast cancer. *J Clin Oncol* 4, 942–951.

51 Pildal J, Chan A-W, Hróbjartsson A *et al.* (2005) Comparison of descriptions of allocation concealment in trial protocols and the published reports: cohort study. *Br Med J* 330, 1049.

52 Maynard A, Chalmers I (eds) (1997) *Non-random Reflections on Health Services Research. On the 25th Anniversary of Archie Cochrane's Effectiveness and Efficiency.* London: BMJ Publishing Group.

53 Olsen O, Middleton P, Ezzo J *et al.* (2001) Quality of Cochrane reviews: assessment of sample from 1998. *Br Med J* 323, 829–832.

54 Moja LP, Telaro E, D'Amico R *et al.* (2005) Assessment of methodological quality of primary studies by systematic reviews: results of the metaquality cross sectional study. *Br Med J* 330, 1053.

55 Gluud C, on behalf of the Cochrane Hepatobiliary Editorial Team (1999) The Cochrane Hepatobiliary Group. In: Bircher J, Benhamou JP, McIntyre N *et al.* (eds) *Oxford Textbook of Clinical Hepatology*, 2nd edn. Oxford: Oxford University Press, pp. 2145–2148.

56 Gluud C, Als-Nielsen B, D'Amico G *et al.* (2005) *The Cochrane Hepatobiliary Group. About The Cochrane Collaboration (Collaborative Review Groups (CRGs)).* The Cochrane Library, Issue 2. Chichester: John Wiley & Sons.

57 Wetterslev J, Thorlund K, Brok J, Gluud C (2005) Trial sequential analyses of six Cochrane Neonatal Review Group meta-analyses using actual information size (I). Abstract 24. *Clinical Trials* 2 (Suppl. 1), 32–33.

58 Brok J, Thorlund K, Gluud C, Wetterslev J (2005) Trial sequential analyses of six Cochrane Neonatal Review Group meta-analyses considering adequacy of allocation concealment (II). Abstract P35. *Clinical Trials* 2 (Suppl. 1), 61–62.

59 Thorlund K, Wetterslev J, Brok J, Gluud C (2005) Trial sequential analyses of six Cochrane Neonatal Review Group meta-analyses considering heterogeneity and trial weight (III). Abstract P36. *Clinical Trials* 2 (Suppl. 1), 62.

60 Gluud C, Afroudakis AP, Caballeria J *et al.* (1993) Diagnosis and treatment of alcoholic liver disease in Europe. First report. *Gastroenterol Int* 6, 221–230.

61 Kürstein P, Gluud LL, Kjellberg J *et al.* (2005) Agreement between reported use of interventions for liver diseases and research evidence in Cochrane systematic reviews. *J Hepatol* 43, 984–989.

6 Cirrhosis

6.1 The evolution of cirrhosis

John P. Iredale and I. Neil Guha

Introduction

Fibrosis is part of the innate wound healing response that occurs in injured tissues. Within the liver, fibrosis is characterized by the deposition of extracellular matrix. Current evidence indicates that net deposition of matrix is the result of a balance between synthesis and degradation and constitutes a dynamic process. The progression of fibrosis to cirrhosis has a number of sequelae. First, it will distort hepatic architecture and vasculature; second, it will have a deleterious effect on hepatic function; and third, it will increase the propensity for neoplastic transformation. Therefore, the evolution of fibrosis to cirrhosis represents a change in the morphology, haemodynamics and function of the liver. This chapter will focus on the mechanisms of progression and whether this process is potentially reversible.

Defining cirrhosis

The detailed histological description of fibrosis and cirrhosis can be found in Chapter 1.2. The definition of cirrhosis remains morphological, described by a working party for the World Health Organization (WHO) in 1978 as: 'a diffuse process characterized by fibrosis and the conversion of normal liver architectures into structurally abnormal nodules' [1]. Although nodularity is a prerequisite for the definition, regeneration is not. Regeneration is an important process in the development of cirrhosis but also occurs following virtually any insult to the liver that results in hepatocellular death. Another important aspect of the definition is that it does not include vascular changes associated with cirrhosis. However, these changes are an important component of the pathophysiology and progression of cirrhosis, and may determine the reversibility of fibrosis and cirrhosis, as discussed later in this chapter.

Mechanisms of progression

Iterative injury

It is self evident that iterative injury is an important and common mechanism by which fibrosis progresses to cirrhosis. This is exemplified by clinical paradigms in which the injurious insult is removed. In alcoholic liver disease, abstinence from alcohol not only prevents disease progression but may be associated with regression. Similarly, antiviral treatment in hepatitis B and hepatitis C infection and venesection in haemochromatosis are therapeutic strategies that can prevent the development of cirrhosis.

Apoptosis and collapse

Reduced hepatic cell mass is a key feature of advancing liver disease; apoptosis and collapse both contribute to this.

Toxic injury to hepatocytes can initiate 'programmed' cell death, a process known as apoptosis. However, apoptosis may also augment inflammation by the direct release of cellular contents such as cytokines or by the signals that induce apoptosis also co-stimulating inflammatory cascades [2]. Apoptosis results in the fragmentation of cells into membrane-bound bodies called apoptotic bodies. The clearance of apoptotic bodies has classically been viewed as not inducing inflammation but, in certain liver models, it has been shown to be fibrogenic [3]. Additionally, secondary necrosis can supervene in the context of massive apoptosis when clearance mechanisms are overwhelmed. Therefore, apoptosis not only causes a loss of hepatocytes but also contributes to inflammation and fibrosis, which in turn leads to further apoptosis. Finally, the complex interaction between apoptosis and fibrosis is highlighted by the role of apoptosis in the resolution of fibrosis, as discussed below.

Collapse of architecture results in the approximation of portal veins to hepatic veins, and it has been postulated that this results from vascular obstruction. A study of non-alcoholic hepatitis has demonstrated that 20% of hepatic veins were obstructed in fibrosis stage 0. This increased to 45% in stage 3–4 fibrosis [4]. These figures suggest that vascular obstruction is an important pathological process even in the milder stages of disease. Furthermore, collapse of architecture and disruption of sinusoidal blood flow results in hypoxia of the hepatic parenchyma with resulting accentuation of inflammation and fibrosis (see section below on angiogenesis).

Inflammation

Inflammation involves the processes of cellular exudation and increased vascular permeability. The presence or absence of inflammation in the liver is usually determined by histology. While the majority of chronic liver diseases are associated with inflammation, in others, e.g. haemochromatosis, histological evidence of inflammation may not be prominent. To subdivide fibrosis into 'inflammatory' and 'non-inflammatory' processes is oversimplistic as the two processes have a great deal of overlap. Furthermore, histological examination offers a 'snapshot' view of events and is also limited by sample size. Moreover, there may be evidence of release of cytokines associated with injury and inflammation even in the absence of a cellular infiltrate. Therefore, the absence of inflammatory cells on a biopsy does not always exclude an inflammatory aetiology. However, by using this classification, one can highlight some of the proposed mechanisms for the development and progression of fibrosis.

Inflammatory mechanisms of progression

Tissue fibrosis is mediated by fibroblasts and myofibroblasts. Potential contributors to the hepatic myofibroblast population in areas of inflammation include the hepatic stellate cell (HSC), portal myofibroblast and myofibroblast derived from stem cells. Of these, the HSC is the most thoroughly studied.

The HSC represents one of the principal components in the initiation, orchestration, progression and resolution of liver fibrosis (see Chapter 1.6). We will recap some of the important aspects of HSC activation and perpetuation below.

Stellate cell activation

Activation involves the transdifferentiation of the quiescent, retinoid-storing HSC, lying in the space of Disse, into the activated, contractile 'myofibroblast'. In the activated state, HSCs enter the cell cycle, leading to an accumulation of HSCs in areas of injury. There are a number of potential initiators for HSC activation, including soluble signals released by sinusoidal endothelium, hepatocytes, Kupffer cells, platelets and leukocytes. They are able to interact with the HSC using a variety of mediators ranging from fibronectin release from damaged endothelium [5] to platelet-derived growth factor (PDGF), transforming growth factor (TGF)-β1 and epidermal growth factor from platelets [6].

Kupffer cells, which are resident macrophages in the liver, have a significant interaction with HSCs. They are able to activate stellate cells and stimulate matrix synthesis via the release of cytokines, in particular TGF-β1, and reactive oxygen intermediates. Kupffer cells also secrete matrix metalloproteinases (MMPs), tissue inhibitors of metalloproteinases (TIMPs) and

anti-inflammatory cytokines such as interleukin (IL)-10, which may be important in fibrosis resolution (see below).

Perpetuation of stellate cell activation

The activation and proliferation of stellate cells has a number of effects. First, there is a direct increase in the amount of matrix produced, in particular collagen I but also collagen IV and collagen III.

Secondly, the HSC is a source of both MMPs and TIMPs. Studies in animal and human models have indicated that interstitial collagenase activity decreases with progression of liver fibrosis, an effect mediated by TIMPs. Therefore, activation of HSCs not only results in matrix accumulation, but matrix degradation is prevented through the expression of TIMPs. Proliferation of HSCs is promoted by PDGF released in a paracrine fashion from macrophages [7] and also in an autocrine manner from HSCs [8]. Other mitogens present in the inflammatory lesion include thrombin, insulin growth factor 1, TGF-α, endothelin-1, fibroblast growth factor (FGF) and vascular endothelial growth factor (VEGF) [9,10].

Studies have demonstrated a positive correlation between the degree of fibrosis and the accumulation of activated HSCs in the damaged liver [11,12]. Conversely, the resolution of acute liver injury following paracetamol overdose has been shown to be associated with a reduction in α-smooth muscle actin-positive activated HSCs [13].

A number of additional mechanisms may mediate both the activation and the perpetuation of activated HSCs, including chemotactic loops, retinoid loss and signalling and cytokine release. These are discussed in greater detail in Chapters 1.6 and 6.2.

The HSC has a central role in the inflammatory process, but there is a complex interaction with the other cell types, including Kupffer cells and T-lymphocyte cells, largely through cytokine mediators. T-cell subtype has been demonstrated to be important; for example, a type 2 T helper (Th2) response, in comparison to a Th1 response, promotes fibrogenesis [14]. This dichotomy of response may have evolved as a response to parasites, which classically elicit a Th2-driven response. Finally, there is emerging interest in the relative contribution to fibrosis from other myofibroblasts, i.e. portal myofibroblasts and myofibroblasts of bone marrow origin [15].

Extracellular matrix

The matrix components present in hepatic fibrosis include collagens (predominantly interstitial but including other collagen components, e.g. type 4 collagen), proteoglycans and matrix glycoproteins (see Chapter 2.4.3). In turn, this neomatrix may regulate progression. The normal basement membrane-type matrix (rich in collagen IV) and its replacement with a matrix rich in type I collagen, associated with inflammation and fibrosis, is likely to critically alter cell–matrix interactions, resulting in activation and perpetuation of activation of HSCs. Some studies demonstrate increased activation of HSCs cultured on the EDA isoform of fibronectin [5], whereas there is inhibition of activation of HSCs cultured on a membrane analogous to normal basement membrane [16].

Recent evidence indicates that contact with the type I collagen-rich matrix and specific integrin-derived signals associated with the turnover of type I collagen in a pericellular manner may be associated with stellate cell survival and proliferation respectively. In contrast, degradation of type I-rich matrix may be associated with stellate cell apoptosis; indeed, disruption of specific integrin signals has also been demonstrated to result in stellate cell apoptosis. Thus, aspects of the activated stellate cell–matrix interaction in the presence of established fibrosis can be viewed as perpetuating the fibrotic response in a manner that leads to the persistence of fibrosis.

The matrix may also provide a reservoir for the mediators of fibrogenesis/fibrolysis, for example by binding cytokines, MMPS and TIMPs [17].

Non-inflammatory mechanisms of progression

Contractility

The teleological reason for contractility is the necessity for the body to close wounds, an integral part of healing. In common with wound healing processes in other tissues, the myofibroblast population in hepatic areas determines contractile activity. The contraction of activated myofibroblasts may have a contributory role in the development of portal hypertension. Endothelin concentrations, a powerful stimulation for contraction of HSCs, rise after fibrotic injury. To confound this, nitric oxide, which antagonizes the effect of endothelin and is derived from endothelial cells, is reduced in injury. Receptors for endothelin-1 and other less potent factors, including eicosanoids, prostaglandins, vasopressin, adenosine, thrombin, platelet-activating factor (PAF) and angiotensin 11, have been found on activated HSCs [18].

Angiogenesis

The endothelial lining of sinusoids becomes non-fenestrated with the development of perisinusoidal fibrosis. This 'capillarization' of the sinusoids leads to functional shunting of the blood across the lobule, resulting in a deficient supply of nutrients and oxygen. Relative hypoxia of the parenchyma can result in the release of angiogenic factors, as evidenced by animal models [19,20]. The release of these factors may then contribute to the development of vascular structures within the fibrous tissue connecting portal to portal tract or, more significantly, connecting portal tract to central vein. Therefore, both functional and anatomic shunting of blood occurs within the lobule, causing the development of a vicious circle encompassing hypoxia and fibrosis. Furthermore, vascular thrombosis also contributes

to the vascular insufficiency. Imaging studies have demonstrated a significant proportion of portal vein thrombosis in cirrhotic patients [21–23] and, when explanted livers of this group are examined at autopsy, occlusion of the portal and hepatic vein is found in 36% and 70% of patients respectively [24].

Models of non-inflammatory progression

The most widely used example of non-inflammatory progression is haemochromatosis. Pronounced inflammatory cell infiltration is not a frequent feature seen in liver biopsy specimens from patients with genetic haemochromatosis. Therefore, other mechanisms of hepatic fibrogenesis have been proposed. Iron is involved in lipid peroxidation resulting in reactive oxygen species (ROS). Products of ROS, including isoprostanes and malondialdehyde, have been found in hepatic tissue in animal and human models of iron overload respectively [25,26]. These products of ROS may cause Kupffer cell activation or act directly on stellate cells. However, despite the absence of overt inflammation, an immunological/inflammatory aetiology cannot be entirely excluded. Studies have shown differences in immunological phenotypes including T-cell subsets and cytokine expression of IL-10 and interferon (IFN)-γ in patients with haemochromatosis [27,28]. Additionally, at least one study has shown that areas of intense iron deposition do not correspond with HSC activation as determined by immunostaining for α-smooth muscle actin [28]. Thus, the relative contribution of the immunological and oxidative stress pathways in producing fibrosis has yet to be definitively elucidated.

Studies of liver histology from patients with alcoholic liver disease have demonstrated that steatosis alone may be associated with the development of fibrosis [29]. There is some evidence that acetaldehyde, produced by the metabolism of ethanol, could also be directly fibrogenic by stimulating collagen production in HSCs [30]. However, this effect may require the stellate cells to be activated initially by an independent mechanism [31]. Furthermore, there is clear evidence that the development of inflammation in the context of alcoholic injury is associated with the progression to fibrosis and cirrhosis in comparison with individuals in whom alcoholic hepatitis does not supervene.

Taken together, these examples suggest that inflammation is a powerful stimulus for the fibrotic response and, as noted above, represents the most prevalent interactive injury in worldwide terms. However, there is significant overlap and synergy of the different mechanisms responsible for the progression of fibrosis.

Clinical factors influencing progression

In general, the progression of fibrosis requires the presence of ongoing stimulus over months to years. There are exceptions to this including neonatal fibrosis and veno-occlusive disease, which follow a more fulminant course for reasons that are not entirely clear [32,33]. The rate of progression varies within and between diseases. In hepatitis C, factors found to influence the progression of fibrosis include male sex, duration of infection, acquisition of infection at an older age (> 40 years), long-term excessive alcohol intake, immunosuppression, co-infection with human immunodeficiency virus (HIV) or hepatitis B virus (HBV) and non-response to antiviral therapy. Additionally, longitudinal studies have suggested that the degree of necroinflammation at the first biopsy may predict future fibrosis [34,35] and have added weight to the concept that fibrosis progresses in a non-linear fashion. In hepatitis B, ongoing inflammation, influenced by host and viral factors, correlates with fibrosis [36,37]. The risk factors for progression in non-alcoholic steato-hepatitis (NASH) are still being defined but include obesity, insulin resistance and age [38].

While some of the risk factors are intuitive, such as continuing inflammation and dual pathology, others are less so. In hepatitis C virus (HCV) and NASH, why does the age of acquisition of disease influence fibrosis progression? Is there a significant difference in the wound healing response with increasing age, perhaps determined by cellular senescence, or does this simply reflect a higher starting point resulting from subclinical fibrosis? Large studies to date have not shown that viral genotype has a role in fibrosis progression in HCV, yet this clearly influences response to treatment [39]. There is, however, increasing evidence for the role of the host genotype in fibrosis, e.g. polymorphisms including TGF-β and angiotensinogen [40] (see also Chapters 3.3.1 and 3.3.3). Recently, the genetic factor V Leiden mutation has also been shown to be associated with rapid progression of fibrosis in hepatitis C [41].

The progression of fibrosis may therefore be through a series of common pathways, but a multitude of factors determine to what extent and how quickly the final stage of cirrhosis is reached.

Cell and molecular events mediating perpetuation of the fibrotic response

While iterative injury and the persistence of inflammation will clearly continue to drive fibrosis, there are certain aspects of activated stellate cell behaviour and phenotype, described above, that will perpetuate the response and, in turn, may perpetuate fibrosis even in the absence of injury. Additionally, stellate cells can mediate inflammation. One recent observation is that senescent stellate cells may develop a proinflammatory phenotype. Senescence develops after prolonged periods of replication when critical shortening of telomeres prevents further replication and induces a specific phenotype of a given cell. One might anticipate that, in iterative injury in which stellate cells are driven to relentless cycles of proliferation, the development of senescence might indeed supervene and, in turn, be associated with the perpetuation of the inflammatory and fibrotic response.

Is fibrosis reversible?

The reversibility of fibrosis has been demonstrated in a spectrum of diseases including autoimmune hepatitis treated with steroids,

haemochromatosis responding to venesection, hepatitis C treated with antiviral therapy and biliary decompression for secondary biliary fibrosis [42–46].

Animal models demonstrating the reversal of fibrosis also exist including biliary obstruction and carbon tetrachloride toxicity [47]. In the carbon tetrachloride model, biological mechanisms for this reversal have been proposed. Rats previously exposed to carbon tetrachloride for 4 weeks demonstrated evidence of loss of activated HSCs mediated by apoptosis in the recovery phase of fibrosis. Additionally, mRNA levels of the metalloprotease inhibitors, TIMP-1 and TIMP-2, decreased during the recovery phase in comparison with collagenase levels, which remained relatively constant. These findings, in conjunction with other experiments, suggest that the reversal of fibrosis is a result of reduced inhibition of collagenases, secondary to HSC apoptosis, thus tipping the balance towards matrix degradation [48]. Proof of concept is demonstrated by administration of gliotoxin, a fungal metabolite that induces apoptosis in activated HSCs, causing an improvement in the severity of fibrosis in the carbon tetrachloride rat model [49].

The role of macrophages/Kupffer cells in fibrosis is complex. Macrophages may play opposing roles in fibrosis during injury and recovery. Using an animal model in which macrophages are selectively depleted, fibrosis was attenuated and associated with reduced numbers of HSCs when depletion occurred during injury. In contrast, if depletion occurred during recovery, there was a failure of fibrosis resolution but not a significant diminution in HSCs [50]. The question remains whether the resolution of fibrosis was due to macrophage-mediated HSC fibrolysis or HSC-mediated fibrolysis in combination with direct matrix degradation by macrophages.

Is cirrhosis reversible?

This is a controversial area and opinions on this topic are certainly not united. There are clinical examples of 'reversal' of fibrosis within cirrhosis in a number of diseases. Poynard et al. [51] demonstrated a reduction in metavir scoring in patients with HCV infection, including patients with stage F4 representing cirrhosis, following combination treatment with pegylated interferon and ribavarin. However, whether this represents 'reversal' of cirrhosis is open to question. A major problem lies in the obvious propensity of needle biopsy to result in a sampling error, an effect potentially confounded by the limitations of semi-quantitative histological scoring. There is a body of evidence in both animal and clinical models that resolution of cirrhosis is associated with the transformation of micronodular cirrhosis into macronodular cirrhosis. As the fibrous bands surrounding macronodules are often not included in the biopsy specimen, the more subtle aspects of regenerating parenchyma can be misinterpreted as normal or near normal hepatic architecture. When larger specimens of liver are examined, such as liver explants, there is evidence of regression of micronodular cirrhosis into not only macronodular cirrhosis but also incomplete septal fibrosis [52]. Remodelling has also been shown in a rat model of cirrhosis, studied over 366 days of recovery [53]. This model confirmed both a retreat from a micronodular to an attenuated macronodular cirrhosis as well as demonstrating that elements of the macronodular cirrhosis were essentially irreversible. Residual septae that were not remodelled were characterized by matrix cross-linking and, in certain cases, neoangiogenesis. This raises the intriguing possibility that cross-linking of collagen is a factor in determining the reversibility of cirrhosis. These examples also highlight the difficulty in trying to characterize a process that can take a prolonged and variable length of time. Certainly there is evidence for an improvement in fibrosis, although the balance of current evidence suggests that true cirrhosis is not entirely reversible. Whether this partial regression is sufficient to restore effective hepatocyte function is at present unknown.

A further problem with demonstrating reversal of cirrhosis lies in its definition. It is a morphological definition, yet cirrhosis also encompasses haemodynamic changes depicted above, and whether an improvement in fibrosis within the context of cirrhosis is associated with reversal of neovasculature is also unknown.

If histological reversal of cirrhosis is so contentious, is there any evidence of functional improvement in hepatocellular function as a surrogate measure? Clearly, no single surrogate marker will indicate reversal of cirrhosis in its entirety. For example, it may be possible to demonstrate an improvement in hepatic synthetic function but, in the presence of continued portal hypertension, this change is unlikely to represent a reversal of cirrhosis. In patients with cirrhosis secondary to hepatitis B, investigators have found an improvement in histological scores and clinical parameters of portal hypertension following treatment with lamivudine [54]. Similarly, in the HCV treatment trial quoted above, reduced rates of bleeding in association with improved liver parameters were found in patients treated with combination therapy. Using functional assessment is a useful tool for patients and clinicians alike, but alone cannot substitute for a histological definition for the reversal of cirrhosis.

Conclusion

The evolution of fibrosis to cirrhosis is critically dependent on the perpetuation/resolution of the underlying injury, the type of disease and host factors including specific genetic traits. A greater understanding of which factors have the greatest influence on progression and how they interact will give us insights into the prevention of this process.

Fibrosis is a dynamic process, and there is strong evidence that elements of fibrosis are completely reversible. The activation of hepatic stellate cells and the recruitment of other myofibroblast cells and the interaction of these cells with their environment and the inflammatory milieu may all determine the propensity of a given fibrotic lesion to resolve. Current evidence indicates that there are certain irreversible components of cirrhosis and,

while there can be significant histological improvement with regression of cirrhosis, complete resolution with a return to normal architecture seems unlikely. Whether the improvements that may occur spontaneously or as a result of antifibrotic intervention would cause sufficient regression of fibrosis to be associated with clinical change in hepatic function is currently unknown. It is intriguing to suggest that the effect of antifibrotic therapy might be sufficient to obviate the need for liver transplantation by leaving a patient with adequate hepatocellular function. In this patient, complications such as portal hypertension could be managed piecemeal by band ligation or shunts introduced by radiological or surgical means.

References

1 Anthony PP, Ishak KG, Nayak NC *et al.* (1978) The morphology of cirrhosis. Recommendations on definition, nomenclature, and classification by a working group sponsored by the World Health Organization. *J Clin Pathol* 31(5), 395–414.

2 Canbay A, Friedman S, Gores GJ (2004) Apoptosis: the nexus of liver injury and fibrosis. *Hepatology* 39(2), 273–278.

3 Canbay A, Taimr P, Torok N *et al.* (2003) Apoptotic body engulfment by a human stellate cell line is profibrogenic. *Lab Invest* 83(5), 655–663.

4 Wanless IR, Shiota K (2004) The pathogenesis of nonalcoholic steatohepatitis and other fatty liver diseases: a four-step model including the role of lipid release and hepatic venular obstruction in the progression to cirrhosis. *Semin Liver Dis* 24(1), 99–106.

5 Jarnagin WR, Rockey DC, Koteliansky VE *et al.* (1994) Expression of variant fibronectins in wound healing: cellular source and biological activity of the EIIIA segment in rat hepatic fibrogenesis. *J Cell Biol* 127(6 Pt 2), 2037–2048.

6 Bachem MG, Melchior R, Gressner AM (1989) The role of thrombocytes in liver fibrogenesis: effects of platelet lysate and thrombocyte-derived growth factors on the mitogenic activity and glycosaminoglycan synthesis of cultured rat liver fat storing cells. *J Clin Chem Clin Biochem* 27(9), 555–565.

7 Nagaoka I, Honma S, Someya A *et al.* (1992) Differential expression of the platelet-derived growth factor-A and -B genes during maturation of monocytes to macrophages. *Comp Biochem Physiol B* 103(2), 349–356.

8 Marra F, Choudhury GG, Pinzani M *et al.* (1994) Regulation of platelet-derived growth factor secretion and gene expression in human liver fat-storing cells. *Gastroenterology* 107(4), 1110–1117.

9 Friedman SL (2000) Molecular regulation of hepatic fibrosis, an integrated cellular response to tissue injury. *J Biol Chem* 275(4), 2247–2250.

10 Pinzani M, Marra F (2001) Cytokine receptors and signaling in hepatic stellate cells. *Semin Liver Dis* 21(3), 397–416.

11 Ballardini G, Degli ES, Bianchi FB *et al.* (1983) Correlation between Ito cells and fibrogenesis in an experimental model of hepatic fibrosis. A sequential stereological study. *Liver* 3(1), 58–63.

12 Knittel T, Kobold D, Piscaglia F *et al.* (1999) Localization of liver myofibroblasts and hepatic stellate cells in normal and diseased rat livers: distinct roles of (myo-)fibroblast subpopulations in hepatic tissue repair. *Histochem Cell Biol* 112(5), 387–401.

13 Mathew J, Hines JE, James OF *et al.* (1994) Non-parenchymal cell responses in paracetamol (acetaminophen)-induced liver injury. *J Hepatol* 20(4), 537–541.

14 Shi Z, Wakil AE, Rockey DC (1997) Strain-specific differences in mouse hepatic wound healing are mediated by divergent T helper cytokine responses. *Proc Natl Acad Sci USA* 94(20), 10663–10668.

15 Forbes SJ, Russo FP, Rey V *et al.* (2004) A significant proportion of myofibroblasts are of bone marrow origin in human liver fibrosis. *Gastroenterology* 126(4), 955–963.

16 Friedman SL, Arthur MJ (1989) Activation of cultured rat hepatic lipocytes by Kupffer cell conditioned medium. Direct enhancement of matrix synthesis and stimulation of cell proliferation via induction of platelet-derived growth factor receptors. *J Clin Invest* 84(6), 1780–1785.

17 Benyon RC, Arthur MJ (2001) Extracellular matrix degradation and the role of hepatic stellate cells. *Semin Liver Dis* 21(3), 373–384.

18 Rockey DC (2001) Hepatic blood flow regulation by stellate cells in normal and injured liver. *Semin Liver Dis* 21(3), 337–349.

19 Corpechot C, Barbu V, Wendum D *et al.* (2002) Hypoxia-induced VEGF and collagen I expressions are associated with angiogenesis and fibrogenesis in experimental cirrhosis. *Hepatology* 35(5), 1010–1021.

20 Rosmorduc O, Wendum D, Corpechot C *et al.* (1999) Hepatocellular hypoxia-induced vascular endothelial growth factor expression and angiogenesis in experimental biliary cirrhosis. *Am J Pathol* 155(4), 1065–1073.

21 Okuda K, Ohnishi K, Kimura K *et al.* (1985) Incidence of portal vein thrombosis in liver cirrhosis. An angiographic study in 708 patients. *Gastroenterology* 89(2), 279–286.

22 Belli L, Romani F, Sansalone CV *et al.* (1986) Portal thrombosis in cirrhotics. A retrospective analysis. *Ann Surg* 203(3), 286–291.

23 Gaiani S, Bolondi L, Li BS *et al.* (1991) Prevalence of spontaneous hepatofugal portal flow in liver cirrhosis. Clinical and endoscopic correlation in 228 patients. *Gastroenterology* 100(1), 160–167.

24 Wanless IR, Wong F, Blendis LM *et al.* (1995) Hepatic and portal vein thrombosis in cirrhosis: possible role in development of parenchymal extinction and portal hypertension. *Hepatology* 21(5), 1238–1247.

25 Houglum K, Ramm GA, Crawford DH *et al.* (1997) Excess iron induces hepatic oxidative stress and transforming growth factor beta1 in genetic hemochromatosis. *Hepatology* 26(3), 605–610.

26 Dabbagh AJ, Mannion T, Lynch SM *et al.* (1994) The effect of iron overload on rat plasma and liver oxidant status *in vivo*. *Biochem J* 300 (Pt 3), 799–803.

27 Porto G, Vicente C, Teixeira MA *et al.* (1997) Relative impact of HLA phenotype and CD4–CD8 ratios on the clinical expression of hemochromatosis. *Hepatology* 25(2), 397–402.

28 Ramm GA, Crawford DH, Powell LW *et al.* (1997) Hepatic stellate cell activation in genetic haemochromatosis. Lobular distribution, effect of increasing hepatic iron and response to phlebotomy. *J Hepatol* 26(3), 584–592.

29 Reeves HL, Burt AD, Wood S *et al.* (1996) Hepatic stellate cell activation occurs in the absence of hepatitis in alcoholic liver disease and correlates with the severity of steatosis. *J Hepatol* 25(5), 677–683.

30 Moshage H, Casini A, Lieber CS (1990) Acetaldehyde selectively stimulates collagen production in cultured rat liver fat-storing cells but not in hepatocytes. *Hepatology* 12(3 Pt 1), 511–518.

31 Friedman SL (1990) Acetaldehyde and alcoholic fibrogenesis: fuel to the fire, but not the spark. *Hepatology* 12(3 Pt 1), 609–612.

32 Sato Y, Asada Y, Hara S *et al.* (1999) Hepatic stellate cells (Ito cells) in veno-occlusive disease of the liver after allogeneic bone marrow transplantation. *Histopathology* 34(1), 66–70.

33 El Youssef M, Mu Y, Huang L *et al.* (1999) Increased expression of transforming growth factor-beta1 and thrombospondin-1 in congenital hepatic fibrosis: possible role of the hepatic stellate cell. *J Pediatr Gastroenterol Nutr* 28(4), 386–392.

34 Ryder SD, Irving WL, Jones DA *et al.* (2004) Progression of hepatic fibrosis in patients with hepatitis C: a prospective repeat liver biopsy study. *Gut* 53(3), 451–455.

35 Fontaine H, Nalpas B, Poulet B *et al.* (2001) Hepatitis activity index is a key factor in determining the natural history of chronic hepatitis C. *Hum Pathol* 32(9), 904–909.

36 Lindh M, Horal P, Dhillon AP *et al.* (2000) Hepatitis B virus DNA levels, precore mutations, genotypes and histological activity in chronic hepatitis B. *J Viral Hepat* 7(4), 258–267.

37 Merican I, Guan R, Amarapuka D *et al.* (2000) Chronic hepatitis B virus infection in Asian countries. *J Gastroenterol Hepatol* 15(12), 1356–1361.

38 Angulo P, Keach JC, Batts KP *et al.* (1999) Independent predictors of liver fibrosis in patients with nonalcoholic steatohepatitis. *Hepatology* 30(6), 1356–1362.

39 Poynard T, Bedossa P, Opolon P (1997) Natural history of liver fibrosis progression in patients with chronic hepatitis C. The OBSVIRC, METAVIR, CLINIVIR, and DOSVIRC groups. *Lancet* 349(9055), 825–832.

40 Powell EE, Edwards-Smith CJ, Hay JL *et al.* (2000) Host genetic factors influence disease progression in chronic hepatitis C. *Hepatology* 31(4), 828–833.

41 Wright M, Goldin R, Hellier S *et al.* (2003) Factor V Leiden polymorphism and the rate of fibrosis development in chronic hepatitis C virus infection. *Gut* 52(8), 1206–1210.

42 Dufour JF, DeLellis R, Kaplan MM (1998) Regression of hepatic fibrosis in hepatitis C with long-term interferon treatment. *Dig Dis Sci* 43(12), 2573–2576.

43 Shiratori Y, Imazeki F, Moriyama M *et al.* (2000) Histologic improvement of fibrosis in patients with hepatitis C who have sustained response to interferon therapy. *Ann Intern Med* 132(7), 517–524.

44 Dufour JF, DeLellis R, Kaplan MM (1997) Reversibility of hepatic fibrosis in autoimmune hepatitis. *Ann Intern Med* 127(11), 981–985.

45 Hammel P, Couvelard A, O'Toole D *et al.* (2001) Regression of liver fibrosis after biliary drainage in patients with chronic pancreatitis and stenosis of the common bile duct. *N Engl J Med* 344(6), 418–423.

46 Powell LW, Kerr JF (1970) Reversal of 'cirrhosis' in idiopathic haemochromatosis following long-term intensive venesection therapy. *Australas Ann Med* 19(1), 54–57.

47 Abdel-Aziz G, Lebeau G, Rescan PY *et al.* (1990) Reversibility of hepatic fibrosis in experimentally induced cholestasis in rat. *Am J Pathol* 137(6), 1333–1342.

48 Iredale JP, Benyon RC, Pickering J *et al.* (1998) Mechanisms of spontaneous resolution of rat liver fibrosis. Hepatic stellate cell apoptosis and reduced hepatic expression of metalloproteinase inhibitors. *J Clin Invest* 102(3), 538–549.

49 Wright MC, Issa R, Smart DE *et al.* (2001) Gliotoxin stimulates the apoptosis of human and rat hepatic stellate cells and enhances the resolution of liver fibrosis in rats. *Gastroenterology* 121(3), 685–698.

50 Duffield JS, Forbes SJ, Constandinou CM *et al.* (2005) Selective depletion of macrophages reveals distinct, opposing roles during liver injury and repair. *J Clin Invest* 115(1), 56–65.

51 Poynard T, McHutchison J, Manns M *et al.* (2002) Impact of pegylated interferon alfa-2b and ribavirin on liver fibrosis in patients with chronic hepatitis C. *Gastroenterology* 122(5), 1303–1313.

52 Wanless IR, Nakashima E, Sherman M (2000) Regression of human cirrhosis. Morphologic features and the genesis of incomplete septal cirrhosis. *Arch Pathol Lab Med* 124(11), 1599–1607.

53 Issa R, Zhou X, Constandinou CM *et al.* (2004) Spontaneous recovery from micronodular cirrhosis: evidence for incomplete resolution associated with matrix cross-linking. *Gastroenterology* 126(7), 1795–1808.

54 Villeneuve JP, Condreay LD, Willems B *et al.* (2000) Lamivudine treatment for decompensated cirrhosis resulting from chronic hepatitis B. *Hepatology* 31(1), 207–210.

6.2 Cellular and molecular pathobiology of liver fibrosis and its pharmacological intervention

Scott L. Friedman

Introduction

Many significant advances in the investigation of hepatic fibrosis have led to a new understanding of how the liver generates scar in response to injury, and pointed to new approaches to its treatment. These advances have included the isolation and characterization of fibrogenic cell types in liver, elucidation of pathogenic mechanisms and clarification of mediators. This chapter will review the substantial progress in understanding the pathophysiology of hepatic fibrosis, and how this has led to a rational new template for antifibrotic therapy. Mechanisms underlying reversibility of fibrosis are summarized in Chapter 6.1 (Evolution of cirrhosis), whereas clinical features of cirrhosis are detailed in Chapter 6.3 (Clinical aspects of cirrhosis). In addition, emerging genetic determinants of fibrosis progression are reviewed in Chapters 3.3.1 (Polymorphisms) and 3.3.3 (Genetic determinants).

Hepatic fibrosis refers to the accumulation of interstitial or 'scar' extracellular matrix that follows either acute or chronic liver injury. Cirrhosis, the endstage of progressive fibrosis, is characterized by septum formation and scar surrounding nodules of hepatocytes. The composition of extracellular matrix molecules in fibrotic liver is similar to those of other fibrosing parenchyma including lung and kidney, and also similar among different aetiologies of liver disease. Typically, fibrosis requires years or decades to become clinically apparent, but notable exceptions in which cirrhosis develops over months may include paediatric liver disease (e.g. biliary atresia), drug-induced liver disease and viral hepatitis associated with immunosuppression following liver transplantation.

Cellular sources of extracellular matrix in normal and fibrotic liver

The *hepatic stellate cell* (previously called lipocyte, Ito, fat-storing or perisinusoidal cell) is the primary source in normal and fibrotic liver. In addition, related mesenchymal cell types from a variety of sources may also make minor contributions to total matrix accumulation, including classical portal fibroblasts [1–3]

(especially in biliary fibrosis), bone marrow-derived cells [4], as well as fibroblast-derived epithelial–mesenchymal transition (EMT) [5]. EMT is a well-characterized response of the kidney [5] to injury, but its role in liver injury has been less convincing.

Hepatic stellate cells are resident perisinusoidal cells in the subendothelial space between hepatocytes and sinusoidal endothelial cells (for reviews, see [6,7]). As the primary storage site for retinoids (vitamin A compounds), stellate cells can be recognized by their vitamin A autofluorescence, perisinusoidal orientation and by expression of the cytoskeletal proteins desmin and glial acidic fibrillary protein.

The concept of 'stellate cells' may actually represent a heterogeneous population of mesenchymal cells with respect to cytoskeletal phenotype, vitamin A content and localization [8]. Moreover, remarkable plasticity of stellate cell phenotype has been documented *in vivo* and in culture, precluding a strict definition based only on cytoskeletal phenotype [9,10]. In addition, stellate cells with fibrogenic potential are not confined to liver and have been identified in pancreas, for example, where they contribute to desmoplasia in chronic pancreatitis [11] and carcinoma [12]. A common origin of hepatic and pancreatic stellate cells is strongly suggested by the remarkable similarity of their transcriptional profiles [13].

Stellate cell activation, a central event in hepatic fibrosis

'*Activation*' of stellate cells refers to a continuum of cellular and molecular changes in which stellate cells undergo a transition from a quiescent vitamin A-rich cell to a highly fibrogenic cell characterized by enlargement of rough endoplasmic reticulum, diminution of vitamin A droplets, ruffled nuclear membrane, appearance of contractile filaments and proliferation. Cells with features of both quiescent and activated cells are often called 'transitional cells'. Stellate cells have now been characterized in many human liver diseases. Alcoholic liver disease is the best studied example, with numerous reports documenting features of activation *in situ* (for review, see [14]); activation may even occur in the presence of steatosis alone without inflammation

[15]. Activated stellate cells have also been identified in viral hepatitis [16] and hepatocellular carcinoma, where they contribute to the deposition of tumour-associated stroma [17]. Stellate cells have additionally been characterized in a number of other human diseases, including vascular disease, haematological malignancy, biliary disease, mucopolysaccharidosis, paracetamol overdose, leishmaniasis and allograft rejection, and in drug abusers.

Extracellular matrix production by sinusoidal endothelial cells, while less than that of stellate cells, is nonetheless an important component of early fibrosis. Like stellate cells, there is considerable heterogeneity of sinusoidal endothelium in normal and fibrotic liver. Endothelial cells from normal liver produce types 3 and 4 collagen, laminin, syndecans and fibronectin [18]. Following acute liver injury, increased expression of cellular isoforms of fibronectin by these cells is a key early event [19], because their appearance creates a microenvironment that activates stellate cells.

Pathways of stellate cell activation (Fig. 1)

Stellate cell activation is conceptualized in two major phases of progression, *initiation* (also called a *preinflammatory stage*) and *perpetuation* [6], as well as a key stage of resolution (see Chapter 6.1). *Initiation* refers to early changes in gene expression and phenotype that render the cells responsive to other cytokines and stimuli, whereas perpetuation results from the effects of these stimuli on maintaining the activated phenotype and genera-

ting fibrosis. Initiation is largely due to paracrine stimulation, whereas perpetuation involves autocrine as well as paracrine loops.

Initiation of stellate cell activation

The earliest changes in stellate cells are likely to result from paracrine stimulation by all neighbouring cell types, including sinusoidal endothelium, Kupffer cells, hepatocytes and platelets. As noted above, early injury to endothelial cells stimulates the production of cellular fibronectin, which has an activating effect on stellate cells [20]. Endothelial cells are also likely to participate in the conversion of transforming growth factor (TGF)-β from the latent to the active, profibrogenic form. Sinusoidal endothelial cells, normally fenestrated to allow rapid bidirectional transport of solutes between sinusoidal blood and parenchymal cells, may rapidly lose their fenestrations upon injury and express proinflammatory molecules including intercellular adhesion molecule (ICAM)-1, vascular endothelial growth factor (VEGF) and adhesion molecules [21,22]. Together with stellate cells, they activate angiogenic pathways in response to hypoxia associated with local injury or malignancy [22–25].

Early stimulation of stellate cells by lipid peroxides contributes to many forms of liver fibrosis, particularly hepatitis C, non-alcoholic steatohepatitis (NASH) and iron overload [26]. In fact, there is an increased prevalence of heterozygosity for mutation of the haemochromatosis gene in patients with NASH, suggesting a potentially synergistic relationship between fat and iron overload [27]. Additionally, fibrosis is more likely among

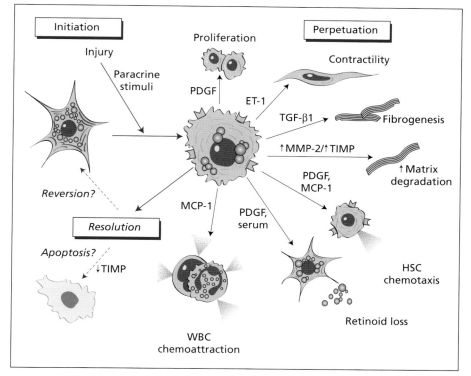

Fig. 1 Phenotypical features of hepatic stellate cell activation during liver injury and resolution. Following liver injury, hepatic stellate cells undergo 'activation', during which they are transformed from quiescent vitamin A-rich cells into proliferative, fibrogenic and contractile myofibroblasts. The major phenotypical changes after activation include proliferation, contractility, fibrogenesis, matrix degradation, chemotaxis, retinoid loss and white blood cell (WBC) chemoattraction. Key mediators underlying these effects are shown. The fate of activated stellate cells during the resolution of liver injury is uncertain but may include reversion to a quiescent phenotype or selective clearance by apoptosis. ECM, extracellular matrix; cFn, cellular fibronectin; PDGF, platelet-derived growth factor; ET-1, endothelin-1; TGF-β1, transforming growth factor β1; MMP-2, matrix metalloproteinase-2; MCP-1, monocyte chemoattractant protein-1; HSC, hepatic stellate cell (from ref. 94, with permission.)

patients with NASH who are obese, which correlates with increased hepatic steatosis [28]. Panels of biochemical markers have been developed to enhance the prediction of fibrosis in patients with NASH [29,30]. Because antioxidant levels are typically depleted in cirrhotic liver, as fibrosis advances, their loss could further amplify the injurious effects of lipid peroxides.

Hepatocytes, as the most abundant cell type in liver, are a potent source of these fibrogenic lipid peroxides. There is a correlation *in situ* between the presence of aldehyde adducts and collagen gene expression by stellate cells [31], and peroxides stimulate collagen synthesis by cultured stellate cells [32]. Steatosis in NASH and hepatitis C virus (HCV) infection correlates with increased stellate cell activation and fibrogenesis [33], possibly because fat represents an enhanced source of lipid peroxides. In culture, activation of stellate cells is provoked by the generation of free radicals and is blocked by antioxidants [34].

Whereas hepatocyte necrosis associated with lipid peroxidation is considered a classical inflammatory and fibrogenic stimulus, recent findings also implicate apoptosis, or programmed cell death, in the fibrogenic response [35]. Apoptotic fragments released from hepatocytes are fibrogenic towards cultured stellate cells, in part through induction of nicotinamide adenine dinucleotide phosphate hydrogenase (NADPH) oxidase [36,37], and also activate Kupffer cells [38]. Additionally, Fas-mediated hepatocyte apoptosis *in vivo* in experimental animals is fibrogenic [39].

Platelets are a potent source of growth factors in liver injury [40], yet their potential contribution has been largely overlooked. Potentially important platelet mediators include platelet-derived growth factor (PDGF), TGF-β1 and epidermal growth factor (EGF).

Perpetuation of stellate cell activation

Perpetuation of stellate cell activation reflects distinct alterations in cell behaviour that include: (i) proliferation; (ii) chemotaxis; (iii) fibrogenesis; (iv) contractility; (v) matrix degradation; (vi) retinoid loss; (vii) white blood cell (WBC) chemoattractant and cytokine release. Either directly or indirectly, the net effect of these changes is to increase the accumulation of extracellular matrix. For example, proliferation and chemotaxis lead to increased numbers of collagen-producing cells, but there is also more matrix production per cell. Cytokine release by stellate cells can amplify the inflammatory and fibrogenic tissue responses, and matrix proteases may hasten the replacement of normal matrix with one typical of the wound 'scar'.

Proliferation

PDGF is the most potent stellate cell mitogen that has been identified [41]. Induction of PDGF receptors early in stellate cell activation increases responsiveness to this potent mitogen [42]. Downstream pathways of PDGF signalling have been well characterized in stellate cells [43]. PDGF also stimulates Na^+/H^+ exchange, providing a potential site for therapeutic intervention by blocking ion transport [44]. Transgenic expression of PDGF-C in mice leads to both hepatic fibrosis and carcinoma

[45], raising a potential role for the cytokine in carcinogenesis as well as fibrosis. Other compounds with mitogenic and/or fibrogenic activity in stellate cells include VEGF [24], thrombin and its receptor [46,47], EGF, TGF-β, keratinocyte growth factor [48] and basic fibroblast growth factor (bFGF) [49]. Signalling pathways for these and other mitogens have been greatly clarified in stellate cells [43].

Chemotaxis

Stellate cells can migrate towards cytokine chemoattractants [23,43] mediated by a number of transmembrane receptors [43,50–53], which is characteristic of wound-infiltrating mesenchymal cells in other tissues as well. Chemotaxis of stellate cells explains in part why stellate cells align within inflammatory septae *in vivo*.

Fibrogenesis

Increased matrix production by each fibrogenic cell contributes significantly to matrix accumulation in hepatic fibrosis. Regulation of the collagen I gene in stellate cells provides an important paradigm for understanding the pathophysiology of stellate cell fibrogenesis (see also Chapter 2.4.3, Function and metabolism of collagen and other extracellular matrix proteins). The most potent stimulus to collagen I production is TGF-β1, which is derived from both paracrine and autocrine sources; TGF-β1 also stimulates the production of other matrix components, including cellular fibronectin and proteoglycans [54]. TGF-β1 stimulates collagen in stellate cells through a hydrogen peroxide-, p38 MAPK- and C/EBPβ-dependent mechanism [55,56]. TGF-β expression is increased in patients with chronic hepatitis C, emphasizing the potential importance of this cytokine in chronic liver disease [57]. Similarly, serum levels of TGF-β correlate with the risk of veno-occlusive disease following bone marrow transplantation [58]. Also, stellate cell responsiveness to TGF-β1 is increased during activation by enhanced ligand binding to its cognate receptors [54].

Signals downstream of TGF-β1 include a family of bifunctional molecules known as Smads, upon which many extracellular and intracellular signals converge to fine tune and additionally enhance TGF-β's effects during fibrogenesis, downstream of its receptors [59,60]. The response of Smads in stellate cells differs between acute and chronic injury to further favour matrix production [61,62]. Smads 2 and 3 elicit distinct signalling responses that promote stellate cell activation and fibrogenesis [43], whereas Smad 7 is inhibitory, making it an attractive molecule to use in antifibrotic therapies [63] (see section on Pharmacological intervention in hepatic fibrosis).

Continued understanding of collagen gene transcription, translation and mRNA stability have emphasized the many sites of regulation that may affect collagen production [64–67].

Lipid peroxidation products are recognized as important stimuli for extracellular matrix production [68], particularly when derived from hepatocytes [34]. Their effects may be amplified by loss of antioxidant capacity of stellate cells as they become activated [69]. These important insights have provoked efforts to use antioxidants as therapy for hepatic fibrosis (see section on Pharmacological intervention in hepatic fibrosis). Stimulation of fibrogenesis may be especially critical in the pathogenesis of NASH, in which fat provides a large reservoir of potential reactive oxygen species [70–72]. In addition to TGF-β1, connective tissue growth factor (now referred to as CCN2) is also a potent TGF-β-regulated fibrogenic cytokine [73,74].

Contractility

Contractility of stellate cells may be a major determinant of early and late increases in portal resistance during liver fibrosis. Activated stellate cells impede portal blood flow by both constricting individual sinusoids and contracting the cirrhotic liver, as the collagenous bands typical of endstage cirrhosis contain large numbers of activated stellate cells [75].

As stellate cells become contractile, expression of the cytoskeletal protein α-smooth muscle actin is increased. Detection of α-actin appears to be an important clinical predictor of subsequent fibrosis, particularly in NASH [76] or following liver transplantation [77–79].

The major contractile stimulus for stellate cells is endothelin-1, whose receptors are expressed on both quiescent and activated stellate cells but whose subunit composition may vary [75]. Unlike PDGF receptors, endothelin receptor expression does not increase with stellate cell activation, but there is a shift in the type of endothelin receptor that predominates, combined with increased sensitivity to autocrine endothelin-1 [80,81]. Increased endothelin levels result from increased endothelin-converting enzyme (ECE) activity resulting from stabilization of the ECE mRNA [82]. Contractility of stellate cells in response to endothelin-1 has also been documented *in vivo* as well as in culture [83].

Another key contractile mediator in activated stellate cells is angiotensin II, which is synthesized by activated stellate cells in an NADPH-dependent pathway [84–86]. These findings are particularly relevant to human disease, because antagonism of this pathway is an attractive antifibrotic therapy using a variety of safe, well-tolerated medications that are already available (see below) [87]. Contraction may also be induced in activated stellate cells by vasopressin [88], substance P [89] and atrial natriuretic peptide [90].

Locally produced vasodilator substances may counteract the constrictive effects of endothelin-1 [91,92]. Nitric oxide, which is also produced by stellate cells, is a well-characterized endogenous antagonist to endothelin. During acute endotoxaemia, stellate cell production of nitric oxide is increased. *In vivo* studies suggest that carbon monoxide also mediates sinusoidal relaxation through its effects on stellate cells [81,93].

Matrix degradation

Quantitative and qualitative changes in matrix protease activity play an important role in extracellular matrix remodelling accompanying fibrosing liver injury and resolution (for details, see Chapter 6.1).

Retinoid loss and nuclear receptor signalling

As stellate cells activate, they lose their characteristic perinuclear retinoid (vitamin A) droplets and acquire a more fibroblastic appearance. In culture, retinoid is stored as retinylesters, whereas stellate cells activate the retinoid released outside the cell as retinol, suggesting that there is intracellular hydrolysis of esters prior to export [94]. However, it is unknown whether retinoid loss is required for stellate cells to activate, and which retinoids might accelerate or prevent activation *in vivo*.

Several nuclear retinoid receptors have been identified in stellate cells [95–98]. This class of molecules binds intracellular retinoid ligands and regulates gene expression, but it is uncertain what regulatory role they play in fibrogenesis. This question has important clinical implications, as methods to use retinoids therapeutically are being considered (see below).

Recently, peroxisome proliferator-activated receptors (PPAR), in particular PPARγ, have been identified in stellate cells, and their expression increases with activation [96]. Ligands for this newly identified nuclear receptor family downregulate stellate cell activation [96,99]. Similarly, farnesoid X receptor (FXR) not only regulates a range of genes involved in choleresis but, in stellate cells, may drive antifibrotic pathways alone or by converging with PPARγ signalling [95,100,101]. In contrast, PPARβ ligands stimulate stellate cell proliferation [97].

Inflammatory signalling and WBC chemoattraction

Stellate cells are assuming an increasingly central role in our understanding of hepatic inflammation. They can amplify the inflammatory response by inducing infiltration of mono- and polymorphonuclear leukocytes, and chemokines secreted by bile duct epithelium may accelerate stellate cell activation during cholestasis [102]. Activated stellate cells produce chemokines that include MCP-1 [91], CCL21 [16] RANTES and CCR5 [103]. They also express Toll-like receptors (TLR) [104], indicating a capacity to interact with bacterial lipopolysaccharide and other exogenous ligands including possibly viral proteins and/or nucleic acids. TLR activation stimulates stellate cells [105], and a complete characterization of this receptor family and their potential roles in stellate cell biology is anticipated.

Stellate cells can also function as antigen-presenting cells [106] which can stimulate lymphocyte proliferation or apoptosis [107]. Stellate cells produce neutrophil chemoattractants including CINC [108], which could contribute to the neutrophil accumulation characteristic of alcoholic liver disease.

In addition to regulating leukocyte behaviour, stellate cells may in turn be affected by specific lymphocyte populations. For example, CD8 cells harbour more fibrogenic activity towards stellate cells than CD4 cells [109], which may explain in part the increased hepatic fibrosis seen in patients with hepatitis C virus (HCV)/HIV coinfection, in whom CD4/CD8 ratios are reduced, than in patients monoinfected with HCV alone. Apoptosis of hepatic stellate cells through stimulation by intrahepatic natural killer (NK) cells has also been identified and could reduce stellate cell numbers during resolution of fibrosis [110].

Transcriptional regulation of stellate cell activation

There have been significant advances in understanding intracellular signalling and transcriptional gene regulation in activated hepatic stellate cells [111,112]. A growing number of transcription factors and signalling molecules may regulate stellate cell behaviour, including p70S6K [113], PPARα, β and γ [97,114,115], CRP-2 [116], retinoid receptors [117], NFκB [104], Jun D [111], Krüppel-like factor 6 [118], Foxf1 [119], Lhx2 [120] and MEF2 [121], among others [111,114].

Disease-specific mechanisms regulating hepatic fibrosis – NASH and HCV

NASH is associated with an increasing incidence of advanced fibrosis and cirrhosis with accelerated mortality [28,122]. Leptin, a circulating adipogenic hormone whose serum concentration reflects adipose mass, has been clearly tied to stellate cell fibrogenesis [123–125] and requires sympathetic neurotransmission [126]. Sources are likely to be both endocrine and autocrine, associated with enhanced signalling through the leptin receptor, which is upregulated during stellate cell activation [123,127].

In contrast to leptin, downregulation of adiponectin in obesity, a counter-regulatory hormone, may amplify the fibrogenic activity of leptin. Rapid advances in our understanding of these adipokines in liver disease reflect their growing significance in liver fibrosis, particularly NASH [127–129]. For example, mice lacking adiponectin have enhanced fibrosis following toxic liver injury [130], and patients with NASH have reduced expression of adiponectin and its receptors [131].

Advances in HCV biology have uncovered a potential direct fibrogenic activity of the virus. Activated stellate cells might be infectable by HCV because they express candidate viral receptors, including CD80, LDL receptor and C1q [132]. Additionally, adenoviral transduction of HCV non-structural and core proteins induces stellate cell proliferation and release of inflammatory signals [132]. The E2 protein of HCV can interact directly with CD81, a stellate cell plasma membrane receptor [133]. Moreover, hepatocytes in culture that support HCV replication generate paracrine factors that also stimulate stellate cells [134]. In HCV-infected liver, chemokines and their receptors are upregulated, stimulating lymphocyte recruitment [16].

HCV proteins may also interact directly with sinusoidal endothelium [135]. A ductular reaction with portal expansion also correlates with fibrosis progression [136]. Steatosis and apoptosis in HCV may accelerate fibrosis [137], even in patients without NASH, and steatosis has emerged as an important determinant of fibrosis progression in HCV [138,139].

Pharmacological intervention in hepatic fibrosis

Thus far, no drugs are approved as antifibrotic agents in humans, although a number of agents are in clinical trials. There are several essential considerations in developing a safe, effective antifibrotic to be approved for clinical use: (i) therapies will need to be well tolerated over decades; (ii) there must be good targeting to liver and few adverse effects on other tissues; (iii) combination therapies may prove synergistic rather than additive, but agents must first be tested individually to establish safety and 'proof-of-principle'; (iv) it is uncertain whether antifibrotic therapies will require intermittent or continuous administration; (v) for potentially effective agents, evidence of a direct antifibrotic effect must be established in experimental models rather than only an indirect effect by attenuating the injury that drives the fibrogenic response; (vi) candidate therapies must be effective in a liver that is already damaged (as in clinical liver disease) rather than only before the onset of injury; (vii) antifibrotic therapies also carry the theoretical concern that inhibiting the scarring response will prevent the encapsulation of injured regions, leading to extension of tissue damage. In reality, however, antifibrotic therapies need only downregulate the scar response to be effective and, in patients with cirrhosis, it is the scarring, not injury, which usually leads to liver failure.

Antifibrotic therapies – rationale and specific agents

The paradigm of stellate cell activation provides an important framework to define sites of antifibrotic therapy (Table 1) (for review, see [6]). These include: (i) curing the primary disease to prevent injury; (ii) reducing inflammation or the host response in order to avoid stimulating stellate cell activation; (ii) directly downregulating stellate cell activation; (iv) neutralizing proliferative, fibrogenic, contractile and/or proinflammatory responses of stellate cells; (v) stimulating apoptosis of stellate cells; (vi) increasing the degradation of scar matrix by stimulating cells that produce matrix proteases, downregulating their inhibitors or by direct administration of matrix proteases.

Curing the primary disease

The most effective way to eliminate hepatic fibrosis is to clear the primary cause of liver disease. This includes abstinence in alcoholic liver disease, removal of excess iron or copper in precirrhotic genetic haemochromatosis or Wilson's disease, clearance of HBV or HCV in chronic viral hepatitis, eradication of organisms in schistosomiasis or decompression in mechanical bile duct obstruction. Not to be overlooked, weight loss in patients with NASH [140], or even those with HCV who are overweight, may improve histology and is a simple recommendation. Similarly, reversal of jejunoileal bypass-related hepatic fibrosis and cessation of methotrexate may also prevent progression to cirrhosis. Identification of the pathogenetic mechanisms

Table 1 Current and proposed pharmacological interventions for hepatic fibrosis.

Reducing injury and inflammation
Antiviral therapy for viral hepatitis
Antihelminthic therapy for schistosomiasis
Chelation/venesection, treatment of metabolic disease
Angiotensin II type 1 receptor antagonists, ACE inhibitors
Hepatoprotectants:
    Caspase inhibitors
    HGF/HGF mimetics
Attenuating stellate cell activation
Alpha interferon
Antioxidants
    Vitamin E, PDTC
    Angiotensin II type 1 receptor antagonists
Cytokine-directed therapy
    TGF-β antagonists
    Endothelin receptor antagonists
    HGF
PPARγ agonists
FXR agonists
Aldosterone antagonists
Pentoxifylline
Inhibiting properties of activated stellate cells
Antiproliferative
    PDGF receptor antagonists
    Sodium exchange inhibitors
    HMG CoA reductase inhibitors
    Plasmin/thrombin receptor antagonists
Anticontractile
    Endothelin/endothelin receptor antagonists
    Nitric oxide donors
Antifibrogenic
    Collagen synthesis inhibitors
    TGF-β inhibitors (soluble receptors, neutralizing antibodies)
    HGF/HGF mimetics
    AT receptor antagonists
    ACE inhibitors
    Integrin
    CTGF/CCN antagonists
    Smad 7 agonists
Promoting specific apoptosis of hepatic stellate cells
Gliotoxin
NGF agonists
TIMP antagonists
Degrading scar matrix
Direct collagenase administration
Inhibitors of transglutaminase or collagen cross-linking
TIMP antagonists
TGF-β inhibitors

ACE, angiotensinogen-converting enzyme; AT, angiotensin; CCN, cysteine-rich 61/connective tissue growth factor, neuroblastoma overexpressed; FXR, farnesyl X receptor; HGF, hepatocyte growth factor; HMG CoA, 3-hydroxy-3-methyl-glutaryl coenzyme A; NGF, nerve growth factor; NOV, nephroblastoma overexpressed; PDGF, platelet-derived growth factor; PDTC, pyrrolidine dithiocarbamate; PPAR, peroxisome proliferator-activated receptor; Smad, mothers against DPP homologue 7; TIMP, tissue inhibitor of metalloproteinase; TGF-β, transforming growth factor beta.

underlying primary biliary cirrhosis and sclerosing cholangitis could lead to elimination of bile duct injury and periductular fibrosis.

Reducing inflammation and immune response

Reduced fibrosis has been reported in HCV patients successfully treated with pegylated α-interferon and ribavirin [141], presumably through their effect on viral replication and liver injury. Sustained viral clearance will probably be associated with marked regression of fibrosis, so that long-term follow-up of patients successfully cleared of HCV may show more dramatic reversal of disease than at early time points. Importantly, some antifibrotic effect is observed even in the absence of viral clearance [142]. In experimental biliary fibrosis, α-interferon also reduces fibrosis [143], raising the possibility of a direct antifibrotic mechanism in addition to its antiviral effect.

A number of agents have anti-inflammatory activity *in vitro* and *in vivo*, which may eliminate the stimuli necessary for stellate cell activation. Corticosteroids have been used for decades to treat several types of liver disease, in particular autoimmune hepatitis [144]. Their activity is solely as anti-inflammatory agents, with no direct antifibrotic effect on stellate cells. Antagonists to tumour necrosis factor (TNF)α, or NFκB modulators have some rationale, as do a growing number of biologically active agents currently used in other chronic inflammatory diseases, in particular inflammatory liver disease. Pentoxifylline may exert its antifibrotic activity by downregulating TNFα signalling [145]. Other efforts to neutralize inflammatory cytokines include RGD (Arg-Gly-Asp) antagonists, which may limit immunological injury [146,147].

The renin–angiotensin system may also amplify inflammation through the generation of oxidative stress and, therefore, either angiotensin-converting enzyme antagonists and/or angiotensinogen II type 1 receptor antagonists may have anti-inflammatory as well as antifibrogenic activity [148,149].

Ursodeoxycholic acid has a beneficial effect on fibrosis in primary biliary cirrhosis [150,151], possibly in part because of its anti-inflammatory activity. Similarly, a nitric oxide-releasing derivative of ursodeoxycholic acid reduces inflammation, fibrosis and portal pressure in an animal model [152].

A new class of drugs, broadly referred to as 'hepatoprotectants', is showing considerable promise in preclinical and clinical studies, including hepatocyte growth factor (HGF), HGF deletion variants and HGF synthetic mimetics [153–155], as well as insulin-like growth factor [156] and a small-molecule caspase inhibitor that improves aspartate aminotransferase (AST) levels in patients with chronic HCV and is currently in clinical trials [157]. The exact mechanism of HGF's antifibrotic activity is uncertain, but may include inhibition of TGF-β1 activity or upregulation of bone morphogenic proteins (BMPs). Trials in large animals are under way, and those in humans are anticipated, with careful monitoring planned to screen for potential hepatocarcinogenesis, as HGF is a hepatocyte mitogen.

Inhibiting stellate cell activation

Reducing the transformation of quiescent stellate cells to activated myofibroblasts is a particularly attractive target given its central role in the fibrotic response. The most practical approach is to reduce oxidative stress, which is an important stimulus for activation. Antioxidants, including alpha-tocopherol (vitamin E) suppress fibrogenesis in some [158], but not all [159], studies of experimental fibrogenesis. Other antioxidants can also reduce stellate cell activation in culture [160], which provides a rationale for antioxidant trials in humans although, as noted above, more potent formulations than those currently available may be required.

Silymarin, a natural flavonoid component of the milk thistle *Silybum marianum*, has sparked interest as a potential antifibrotic therapy. The compound functions as an antioxidant and may decrease hepatic injury via both cytoprotection and inhibition of Kupffer cell function [160,161]. A single human trial in cirrhotics has reported a slight survival advantage in alcoholic cirrhotics in those with Child's A disease [162], but larger, carefully controlled studies are under way to assess its efficacy.

The cytokine definitive γ-interferon has inhibitory effects on stellate cell activation in animal models of fibrosis [163]. A clinical trial of γ-interferon did not show the expected antifibrotic benefit in patients with HCV, however, possibly because only patients with advanced fibrosis were enrolled and the treatment period (1 year) may have been too short.

Alpha-interferon, in addition to its antiviral effect, can downregulate stellate cell activation and fibrogenesis directly through well-defined molecular pathways and suppress experimental fibrosis [164]. Current long-term, low-dose α-interferon trials in HCV non-responders, including HALT-C [165], are based in part on this mechanism of action and, if these trials succeed, the drug may emerge as the first *bona fide* antifibrotic in humans. Inhibition of collagen gene expression in experimental models may also be accomplished using synthetic olignucleotides to inhibit collagen promoter activity [166].

Great excitement was generated by an uncontrolled trial of IL-10, which reported an antifibrotic effect in patients with advanced HCV [167]. The finding was particularly exciting because of parallel studies in animals and cultured stellate cells suggesting a direct antifibrotic activity for this agent [168–171]. However, a controlled clinical trial showed no benefit, possibly because the drug markedly increased HCV viral load [172].

PPARγ nuclear receptors are expressed in stellate cells, and synthetic PPARγ ligands (thiazolidinediones) downregulate stellate cell activation [96,173]. Given their widespread use in diabetes, second- and third-generation thiazolidinediones (i.e. lacking the hepatotoxicity seen with first-generation agents such as troglitazone) are now being tested in clinical trials in both NASH and other fibrotic liver diseases. FXR ligands appear to have similar effects, and small-molecule agonists are under study in preclinical models with evidence of antifibrotic activity [100].

Leptin is produced by activated stellate cells [174], which not only affects lipid metabolism, but can directly influence wound healing. In fact, animals deficient in leptin have reduced hepatic injury and fibrosis [175,176]. Based on this finding, the discovery of adiponectin, a natural counter-regulator to leptin, may lead to the use of this agent in fibrosis, particularly associated with NASH [127,130].

Progress in understanding transcriptional regulation has offered the opportunity to block stellate cell activation by inhibiting the activity of histone deacetylases (HDACs), enzymes critical for modifying chromatin during gene transcription [177]. Highly specific HDAC inhibitors offer the potential for selective blocking of stellate cell activation with tolerable safety and good efficacy [178], but none has reached clinical use. Similarly, modulation of intracellular proteins including transcription factors remains an elusive target for antifibrotic therapy.

Herbal therapies and products derived from natural compounds that are commonly used in the Far East are increasingly being tested under controlled, scientifically rigorous conditions [179], and some show promise of efficacy, in particular Sho-Saiko-To [180], salvia miltiorrhiza [181] and a green tea polyphenol [182].

Neutralizing proliferative, fibrogenic, contractile and/or proinflammatory responses of stellate cells

Significant advances in growth factor biology will benefit the treatment of hepatic fibrosis through the development of antagonists to cytokines and their receptors. In particular, many proliferative cytokines including PDGF, FGF and TGF-α signal through tyrosine kinase receptors, inhibitors of which are already undergoing clinical trials in other tissues [183]. Because the intracellular signalling pathways for these receptors are well understood, inhibitors to signalling models are being explored *in vivo* or in cultured stellate cells, including γ-linoleic acid and lipoxygenase inhibitors [184], and PPARγ pathway inhibitors (see above). Others include inhibitors of HMG CoA reductase [185], pentoxifylline, which inhibits PDGF receptor signalling [186], and compounds that elevate intracellular cyclic adenosine monophosphate (AMP) [187] or block ion transporters, including perfenidone [44,188].

The recent success in developing Gleevec, a safe, effective small-molecule tyrosine kinase antagonist in human leukaemia and mesenchymal cell tumours [189,190], augurs well for the potential of oral small-molecule therapies for other indications, including liver fibrosis. In fact, Gleevec is antifibrotic in experimental liver fibrosis [191,192]. Other orally available, low-molecular-weight small molecules to block cytokine receptor or intracellular signalling are under development. One such compound is a selective inhibitor of Rho-mediated focal adhesions, which can reduce experimental liver fibrosis [193]. Antisense mRNA to the PDGF B-chain as well as dominant-negative or soluble PDGF beta receptors also block stellate cell activation or experimental hepatic fibrosis [194–196]. As siRNA (small interfering RNA) technology has become clinically applicable, this approach will also merit further evaluation.

Inhibition of matrix production has been the primary target of most antifibrotic therapies to date. This has been attempted directly by blocking matrix synthesis and processing or indirectly by inhibiting the activity of TGF-β1, the major fibrogenic cytokine. Inhibitors of collagen synthesis such as HOE 077, which blocks the enzyme prolyl hydroxylase, were among the first antifibrotic compounds tested in liver, but success with this agent has been modest. The emerging importance of translational regulation of collagen gene expression [64,197–199] could lead to specific translational inhibitors with therapeutic value. Colchicine generated excitement at one time because of its apparent efficacy in a small group of patients [200]; however, a more recent study in alcoholic cirrhosis showed no benefit [201].

TGF-β antagonists are being tested extensively because neutralizing this potent cytokine would have the dual effect of inhibiting matrix production and accelerating its degradation (see [54]). Animal and culture studies using soluble TGF-β receptors or other means of neutralizing the cytokine including monoclonal antibodies and protease inhibitors to block TGF-β activation have established proof-of-principle [6,202,203]. Concerns that inhibiting TGF-β may alter hepatocellular growth or apoptosis will need to be considered as these antagonists reach clinical trials but, in other tissues, there is great promise for this approach. A number of even newer TGF-β antagonists are also being developed and may undergo testing soon. These could include recombinant Smad 7, which antagonizes TGF-β activity in stellate cells [204].

Rapamycin, an immunosuppressive drug used following liver transplantation, has the added benefit of inhibiting stellate cell proliferation [205], which could attenuate the accelerated fibrosis progression in patients with recurrent HCV; however, enthusiasm for using rapamycin has been tempered by a reported increase in hepatic artery thrombosis [206].

Relaxin, a natural peptide hormone that mediates parturition, has been developed as an agent to decrease collagen synthesis by stellate cells and increase matrix degradation in vitro and in vivo [207]. Stellate cells also express relaxin receptors [208], which might represent an attractive target for antagonism.

Because endothelin-1 is an important regulator of wound contraction and blood flow regulation mediated by stellate cells, antagonists have been tested as both antifibrotic and portal hypotensive agents. Bosentan, a mixed endothelin A and B receptor antagonist, has antifibrotic activity and reduces stellate cell activation in experimental hepatic fibrosis [209]. This and other endothelin antagonists remain attractive drug development targets [210]. Alternatively, delivery of nitric oxide to injured liver may have the same therapeutic effect as inhibiting endothelin-1 [152,211].

Halofuginone, an anticoccidial compound, has antifibrotic activity by blocking collagen expression and has been used in a number of models of tissue fibrosis, including liver [212].

The potential utility of retinoids (vitamin A) as antifibrotic therapy has been limited by inadequate knowledge about their regulatory role in stellate cell activation and by toxicity concerns. Although stellate cells export retinoid as they activate, it does not follow that restoration of cellular retinoid will prevent activation. In fact, some retinoids may accelerate fibrosis by augmenting membrane injury as in hypervitaminosis A [213].

Stimulating stellate cell apoptosis (see also Chapter 6.1) Attention is increasingly focused on how liver fibrosis regresses and, in particular, the fate of activated stellate cells as fibrosis recedes. Mounting evidence indicates that both reversal of the activated stellate cell phenotype and apoptosis are possible. In particular, as liver fibrosis is decreased, there is selective cell death of activated stellate cells [214]. This exciting observation has led to animal studies using gliotoxin, which provokes selective apoptosis of stellate cells in culture and in vivo, leading to reduced fibrosis [215,216]. A TIMP-1 neutralizing antibody has antifibrotic activity in experimental liver fibrosis [217]. Similarly, inhibition of Ikk, whose net effect is to increase NFκB signalling in stellate cells, may accelerate apoptosis [218]. Apoptosis can also be provoked by disruption of integrin-mediated adhesion [147] or through the use of TRAIL ligands [219]. Stellate cells contain several families of apoptotic mediators, including Fas/FasL, TNF receptors, nerve growth factor receptors [220] and Bcl/Bax, so that additional targets for promoting apoptosis will probably be exploited in the future [221].

Increasing the degradation of scar matrix
This component of treatment is very important, because antifibrotic therapy in human liver disease will need to provoke resorption of existing matrix in addition to preventing the deposition of new scar. As noted above, TGF-β antagonists have the advantage of stimulating matrix degradation by downregulating TIMPs and increasing the net activity of interstitial collagenase (for review, see [222]). Retinoids may also stimulate matrix degradation, but concerns over toxicity limit their utility. Relaxin can directly increase matrix degradation [223].

Direct expression of metalloproteinases in animal models of hepatic fibrosis has begun to confirm that matrix can be resorbed by the expression of exogenous enzymes [224,225]. While this may seem impractical in humans, the data establish an important proof-of-principle that matrix is responsive to degradation. Moreover, an experimental study has affirmed the importance of matrix degradation in the regression of hepatic fibrosis by demonstrating that a genetically altered mouse expressing mutant collagen resistant to degradation displays delayed regression of fibrosis following liver injury [226].

Conclusions

While the prospect of treating fibrosis is not new, current strategies of antifibrotic therapies are far more rational and mechanism based. In view of mounting proof of fibrosis regression in humans following successful treatment of the underlying liver disease, continued progress is certain. Therapies will increasingly be tailored to host genotype and disease-specific features, and given in combination. Methods of defining fibrosis progression risk and the likelihood of treatment response will be established. The two most immediate hurdles – the development of better diagnostics to clarify endpoints in clinical trials and the need to establish that an antifibrotic can halt or regress fibrosis even when the underlying disease is unchecked – will be important milestones for future trials of antifibrotic therapies.

References

1 Wells RG, Kruglov E, Dranoff JA (2004) Autocrine release of TGF-beta by portal fibroblasts regulates cell growth. *FEBS Lett* 559, 107–110.

2 Kinnman N, Housset C (2002) Peribiliary myofibroblasts in biliary type liver fibrosis. *Front Biosci* 7, D496–503.

3 Kruglov EA, Jain D, Dranoff JA (2002) Isolation of primary rat liver fibroblasts. *J Invest Med* 50, 179–184.

4 Forbes SJ, Russo FP, Rey V *et al.* (2004) A significant proportion of myofibroblasts are of bone marrow origin in human liver fibrosis. *Gastroenterology* 126, 955–963.

5 Kalluri R, Neilson EG (2003) Epithelial-mesenchymal transition and its implications for fibrosis. *J Clin Invest* 112, 1776–1784.

6 Friedman SL (2004) Mechanisms of hepatic fibrosis and therapeutic implications. *Nature Clin Pract Gastroenterol Hepatol* 1, 98–105.

7 Friedman SL (2003) Liver fibrosis – from bench to bedside. *J Hepatol* 38 (Suppl 1), S38–53.

8 Geerts A (2001) History, heterogeneity, developmental biology, and functions of quiescent hepatic stellate cells. *Semin Liver Dis* 21, 311–335.

9 Magness ST, Bataller R, Yang L *et al.* (2004) A dual reporter gene transgenic mouse demonstrates heterogeneity in hepatic fibrogenic cell populations. *Hepatology* 40, 1151–1159.

10 Friedman SL (2004) Stellate cells: a moving target in hepatic fibrogenesis. *Hepatology* 40, 1041–1043.

11 Apte MV, Wilson JS (2004) Mechanisms of pancreatic fibrosis. *Dig Dis* 22, 273–279.

12 Bachem MG, Schunemann M, Ramadani M *et al.* (2005) Pancreatic carcinoma cells induce fibrosis by stimulating proliferation and matrix synthesis of stellate cells. *Gastroenterology* 128, 907–921.

13 Buchholz M, Kestler HA, Holzmann K *et al.* (2005) Transcriptome analysis of human hepatic and pancreatic stellate cells: organ-specific variations of a common transcriptional phenotype. *J Mol Med* 83, 795–805.

14 Friedman SL (ed.) (2001) *The Hepatic Stellate Cell.* New York: Thieme.

15 Reeves HL, Burt AD, Wood S *et al.* (1996) Hepatic stellate cell activation occurs in the absence of hepatitis in alcoholic liver disease and correlates with the severity of steatosis. *J Hepatol* 25, 677–683.

16 Bonacchi A, Petrai I, Defranco RM *et al.* (2003) The chemokine CCL21 modulates lymphocyte recruitment and fibrosis in chronic hepatitis C. *Gastroenterology* 125, 1060–1076.

17 Faouzi S, Lepreux S, Bedin C *et al.* (1999) Activation of cultured rat hepatic stellate cells by tumoral hepatocytes. *Lab Invest* 79, 485–493.

18 Arthur MJ (2000) Fibrogenesis II. Metalloproteinases and their inhibitors in liver fibrosis. *Am J Physiol Gastrointest Liver Physiol* 279, G245–249.

19 George J, Wang SS, Sevcsik AM *et al.* (2000) Transforming growth factor-beta initiates wound repair in rat liver through induction of the EIIIA-fibronectin splice isoform. *Am J Pathol* 156, 115–124.

20 Jarnagin WR, Rockey DC, Koteliansky VE *et al.* (1994) Expression of variant fibronectins in wound healing: cellular source and biological activity of the EIIIA segment in rat hepatic fibrogenesis. *J Cell Biol* 127, 2037–2048.

21 LeCouter J, Moritz DR, Li B *et al.* (2003) Angiogenesis-independent endothelial protection of liver: role of VEGFR-1. *Science* 299, 890–893.

22 Olaso E, Salado C, Egilegor E *et al.* (2003) Proangiogenic role of tumor-activated hepatic stellate cells in experimental melanoma metastasis. *Hepatology* 37, 674–685.

23 Marra F (2002) Chemokines in liver inflammation and fibrosis. *Front Biosci* 7, d1899–1914.

24 Yoshiji H, Kuriyama S, Yoshii J *et al.* (2003) Vascular endothelial growth factor and receptor interaction is a prerequisite for murine hepatic fibrogenesis. *Gut* 52, 1347–1354.

25 Ankoma-Sey V, Wang Y, Dai Z (2000) Hypoxic stimulation of vascular endothelial growth factor expression in activated rat hepatic stellate cells. *Hepatology* 31, 141–148.

26 Parola M, Robino G (2001) Oxidative stress-related molecules and liver fibrosis. *J Hepatol* 35, 297–306.

27 Bonkovsky HL, Jawaid Q, Tortorelli K *et al.* (1999) Non-alcoholic steatohepatitis and iron: increased prevalence of mutations of the HFE gene in non-alcoholic steatohepatitis. *J Hepatol* 31, 421–429.

28 Angulo P (2002) Nonalcoholic fatty liver disease. *N Engl J Med* 346, 1221–1231.

29 Imbert-Bismut F, Ratziu V, Pieroni L *et al.* (2001) Biochemical markers of liver fibrosis in patients with hepatitis C virus infection: a prospective study. *Lancet* 357, 1069–1075.

30 Ratziu V, Giral P, Charlotte F *et al.* (2000) Liver fibrosis in overweight patients. *Gastroenterology* 118, 1117–1123.

31 Paradis V, Mathurin P, Kollinger M *et al.* (1997) In situ detection of lipid peroxidation in chronic hepatitis C: correlation with pathological features. *J Clin Pathol* 50, 401–406.

32 Nieto N, Friedman SL, Cederbaum AI (2002) Stimulation and proliferation of primary rat hepatic stellate cells by cytochrome P450 2E1-derived reactive oxygen species. *Hepatology* 35, 62–73.

33 Clouston AD, Jonsson JR, Purdie DM *et al.* (2001) Steatosis and chronic hepatitis C: analysis of fibrosis and stellate cell activation. *J Hepatol* 34, 314–320.

34 Nieto N, Friedman SL, Cederbaum AI (2002) Cytochrome P450 2E1-derived reactive oxygen species mediate paracrine stimulation of collagen I protein synthesis by hepatic stellate cells. *J Biol Chem* 277, 9853–9864.

35 Canbay A, Friedman S, Gores GJ (2004) Apoptosis: the nexus of liver injury and fibrosis. *Hepatology* 39, 273–278.

36 Canbay A, Taimr P, Torok N *et al.* (2003) Apoptotic body engulfment by a human stellate cell line is profibrogenic. *Lab Invest* 83, 655–663.

37 Zhan S-S, Wu J, Halsted C *et al.* (2006) Phagocytosis of apoptotic bodies by hepatic stellate cells induces NADPH oxidase and is associated with liver fibrosis in vivo. *Hepatology* 43, 435–443.

38 Canbay A, Feldstein AE, Higuchi H *et al.* (2003) Kupffer cell engulfment of apoptotic bodies stimulates death ligand and cytokine expression. *Hepatology* 38, 1188–1198.

39 Canbay A, Higuchi H, Bronk SF *et al.* (2002) Fas enhances fibrogenesis in the bile duct ligated mouse: a link between apoptosis and fibrosis. *Gastroenterology* 123, 1323–1330.

40 Bachem MG, Melchior R, Gressner AM (1989) The role of thrombocytes in liver fibrogenesis: effects of platelet lysate and thrombocyte-derived growth factors on the mitogenic activity and glycosaminoglycan synthesis of cultured rat liver fat storing cells. *J Clin Chem Clin Biochem* 27, 555–565.

41 Pinzani M (2002) PDGF and signal transduction in hepatic stellate cells. *Front Biosci* 7, d1720–1726.

42 Wong L, Yamasaki G, Johnson RJ *et al.* (1994) Induction of beta-platelet-derived growth factor receptor in rat hepatic lipocytes during cellular activation in vivo and in culture. *J Clin Invest* 94, 1563–1569.

43 Pinzani M, Marra F (2001) Cytokine receptors and signaling in hepatic stellate cells. *Semin Liver Dis* 21, 397–416.

44 Di Sario A, Bendia E, Taffetani S *et al.* (2003) Selective Na+/H+ exchange inhibition by cariporide reduces liver fibrosis in the rat. *Hepatology* 37, 256–266.

45 Campbell JS, Hughes SD, Gilbertson DG *et al.* (2005) Platelet-derived growth factor C induces liver fibrosis, steatosis, and hepatocellular carcinoma. *Proc Natl Acad Sci USA* 102, 3389–3394.

46 Marra F, Grandaliano G, Valente AJ *et al.* (1995) Thrombin stimulates proliferation of liver fat-storing cells and expression of monocyte chemotactic protein-1: potential role in liver injury. *Hepatology* 22, 780–787.

47 Marra F, DeFranco R, Grappone C *et al.* (1998) Expression of the thrombin receptor in human liver: up-regulation during acute and chronic injury. *Hepatology* 27, 462–471.

48 Steiling H, Muhlbauer M, Bataille F *et al.* (2004) Activated hepatic stellate cells express keratinocyte growth factor in chronic liver disease. *Am J Pathol* 165, 1233–1241.

49 Yu C, Wang F, Jin C *et al.* (2003) Role of fibroblast growth factor type 1 and 2 in carbon tetrachloride-induced hepatic injury and fibrogenesis. *Am J Pathol* 163, 1653–1662.

50 Efsen E, Grappone C, DeFranco RM *et al.* (2002) Up-regulated expression of fractalkine and its receptor CX3CR1 during liver injury in humans. *J Hepatol* 37, 39–47.

51 Mazzocca A, Carloni V, Sciammetta S *et al.* (2002) Expression of transmembrane 4 superfamily (TM4SF) proteins and their role in hepatic stellate cell motility and wound healing migration. *J Hepatol* 37, 322–330.

52 Ikeda K, Wakahara T, Wang YQ *et al.* (1999) In vitro migratory potential of rat quiescent hepatic stellate cells and its augmentation by cell activation. *Hepatology* 29, 1760–1767.

53 Kinnman N, Hultcrantz R, Barbu V *et al.* (2000) PDGF-mediated chemoattraction of hepatic stellate cells by bile duct segments in cholestatic liver injury. *Lab Invest* 80, 697–707.

54 Gressner AM, Weiskirchen R, Breitkopf K *et al.* (2002) Roles of TGF-beta in hepatic fibrosis. *Front Biosci* 7, D793–807.

55 Varela-Rey M, Montiel-Duarte C, Oses-Prieto JA *et al.* (2002) p38 MAPK mediates the regulation of alpha1(I) procollagen mRNA levels by TNF-alpha and TGF-beta in a cell line of rat hepatic stellate cells (1). *FEBS Lett* 528, 133–138.

56 Garcia-Trevijano ER, Iraburu MJ, Fontana L *et al.* (1999) Transforming growth factor beta1 induces the expression of alpha1(I) procollagen mRNA by a hydrogen peroxide-C/EBPbeta-dependent mechanism in rat hepatic stellate cells. *Hepatology* 29, 960–970.

57 Marek B, Kajdaniuk D, Mazurek U *et al.* (2005) TGF-beta1 mRNA expression in liver biopsy specimens and TGF-beta1 serum levels in patients with chronic hepatitis C before and after antiviral therapy. *J Clin Pharm Ther* 30, 271–277.

58 Anscher MS, Peters WP, Reisenbichler H *et al.* (1993) Transforming growth factor beta as a predictor of liver and lung fibrosis after autologous bone marrow transplantation for advanced breast cancer. *N Engl J Med* 328, 1592–1598.

59 Tsukada S, Westwick JK, Ikejima K *et al.* (2005) SMAD and p38 MAPK signaling pathways independently regulate alpha1(I) collagen gene expression in unstimulated and transforming growth factor-beta-stimulated hepatic stellate cells. *J Biol Chem* 280, 10055–10064.

60 Bonacchi A, Romagnani P, Romanelli RG *et al.* (2001) Signal transduction by the chemokine receptor CXCR3: activation of Ras/ERK, Src, and phosphatidylinositol 3-kinase/Akt controls cell migration and proliferation in human vascular pericytes. *J Biol Chem* 276, 9945–9954.

61 Tahashi Y, Matsuzaki K, Date M *et al.* (2002) Differential regulation of TGF-beta signal in hepatic stellate cells between acute and chronic rat liver injury. *Hepatology* 35, 49–61.

62 Uemura M, Swenson ES, Gaca MD *et al.* (2005) Smad2 and Smad3 play different roles in rat hepatic stellate cell function and {alpha}-smooth muscle actin organization. *Mol Biol Cell* 16, 4214–4224.

63 Dooley S, Hamzavi J, Breitkopf K *et al.* (2003) Smad7 prevents activation of hepatic stellate cells and liver fibrosis in rats. *Gastroenterology* 125, 178–191.

64 Stefanovic B, Stefanovic L, Schnabl B *et al.* (2004) TRAM2 protein interacts with endoplasmic reticulum Ca2+ pump Serca2b and is necessary for collagen type I synthesis. *Mol Cell Biol* 24, 1758–1768.

65 Yata Y, Scanga A, Gillan A *et al.* (2003) DNase I-hypersensitive sites enhance alpha1(I) collagen gene expression in hepatic stellate cells. *Hepatology* 37, 267–276.

66 Novitskiy G, Potter JJ, Rennie-Tankersley L *et al.* (2004) Identification of a novel NF-kappaB-binding site with regulation of the murine alpha2(I) collagen promoter. *J Biol Chem* 279, 15639–15644.

67 Dranoff JA, Ogawa M, Kruglov EA *et al.* (2004) Expression of P2Y nucleotide receptors and ectonucleotidases in quiescent and activated rat hepatic stellate cells. *Am J Physiol Gastrointest Liver Physiol* 287, G417–424.

68 Galli A, Svegliati-Baroni G, Ceni E *et al.* (2005) Oxidative stress stimulates proliferation and invasiveness of hepatic stellate cells via a MMP2-mediated mechanism. *Hepatology* 41, 1074–1084.

69 Whalen R, Rockey DC, Friedman SL *et al.* (1999) Activation of rat hepatic stellate cells leads to loss of glutathione S-transferases and their enzymatic activity against products of oxidative stress. *Hepatology* 30, 927–933.

70 George J, Pera N, Phung N *et al.* (2003) Lipid peroxidation, stellate cell activation and hepatic fibrogenesis in a rat model of chronic steatohepatitis. *J Hepatol* 39, 756–764.

71 MacDonald GA, Bridle KR, Ward PJ *et al.* (2001) Lipid peroxidation in hepatic steatosis in humans is associated with hepatic fibrosis and occurs predominately in acinar zone 3. *J Gastroenterol Hepatol* 16, 599–606.

72 Carmiel-Haggai M, Cederbaum AI, Nieto N (2005) A high-fat diet leads to the progression of non-alcoholic fatty liver disease in obese rats. *FASEB J* 19, 136–138.

73 Rachfal AW, Brigstock DR (2003) Connective tissue growth factor (CTGF/CCN2) in hepatic fibrosis. *Hepatol Res* 26, 1–9.

74 Gao R, Brigstock DR (2003) Low density lipoprotein receptor-related protein (LRP) is a heparin-dependent adhesion receptor for connective tissue growth factor (CTGF) in rat activated hepatic stellate cells. *Hepatol Res* 27, 214–220.

75 Housset C, Rockey DC, Bissel DM (1993) Endothelin receptors in rat liver: lipocytes as a contractile target for endothelin 1. *Proc Natl Acad Sci USA* 90, 9266–9270.

76 Kim WR, Gores GJ, Benson JT *et al.* (2005) Mortality and hospital utilization for hepatocellular carcinoma in the United States. *Gastroenterology* 129, 486–493.

77 Gawrieh S, Papouchado BG, Burgart LJ *et al.* (2005) Early hepatic stellate cell activation predicts severe hepatitis C recurrence after liver transplantation. *Liver Transpl* 11, 1207–1213.

78 Carpino G, Morini S, Ginanni Corradini S *et al.* (2005) Alpha-SMA expression in hepatic stellate cells and quantitative analysis of hepatic fibrosis in cirrhosis and in recurrent chronic hepatitis after liver transplantation. *Dig Liver Dis* 37, 349–356.

79 Russo MW, Firpi RJ, Nelson DR *et al.* (2005) Early hepatic stellate cell activation is associated with advanced fibrosis after liver transplantation in recipients with hepatitis C. *Liver Transpl* 11, 1235–1241.

80 Shao R, Rockey DC (2002) Effects of endothelins on hepatic stellate cell synthesis of endothelin-1 during hepatic wound healing. *J Cell Physiol* 191, 342–350.

81 Rockey DC (2003) Vascular mediators in the injured liver. *Hepatology* 37, 4–12.

82 Shao R, Yan W, Rockey DC (1999) Regulation of endothelin-1 synthesis by endothelin-converting enzyme-1 during wound healing. *J Biol Chem* 274, 3228–3234.

83 Zhang JX, Pegoli W, Jr, Clemens MG (1994) Endothelin-1 induces direct constriction of hepatic sinusoids. *Am J Physiol* 266, G624–632.

84 Bataller R, Sancho-Bru P, Gines P *et al.* (2003) Activated human hepatic stellate cells express the renin-angiotensin system and synthesize angiotensin II. *Gastroenterology* 125, 117–125.

85 Bataller R, Gines P, Nicolas JM *et al.* (2000) Angiotensin II induces contraction and proliferation of human hepatic stellate cells. *Gastroenterology* 118, 1149–1156.

86 Bataller R, Schwabe R, Choi Y *et al.* (2003) NADPH oxidase signal transduces angiotensin II in hepatic stellate cells and is critical in hepatic fibrosis. *J Clin Invest* 112, 1383–1394.

87 Bataller R, Brenner DA (2005) Liver fibrosis. *J Clin Invest* 115, 209–218.

88 Bataller R, Nicolas JM, Gines P *et al.* (1997) Arginine vasopressin induces contraction and stimulates growth of cultured human hepatic stellate cells. *Gastroenterology* 113, 615–624.

89 Sakamoto M, Ueno T, Kin M *et al.* (1993) Ito cell contraction in response to endothelin-1 and substance P. *Hepatology* 18, 978–983.

90 Gorbig MN, Gines P, Bataller R *et al.* (1999) Atrial natriuretic peptide antagonizes endothelin-induced calcium increase and cell contraction in cultured human hepatic stellate cells. *Hepatology* 30, 501–509.

91 Marra F, Pinzani M (2002) Role of hepatic stellate cells in the pathogenesis of portal hypertension. *Nefrologia* 22 (Suppl 5), 34–40.

92 Svegliati-Baroni G, Saccomanno S, van Goor H *et al.* (2001) Involvement of reactive oxygen species and nitric oxide radicals in activation and proliferation of rat hepatic stellate cells. *Liver* 21, 1–12.

93 Suematsu M, Goda N, Sana T *et al.* (1995) Carbon monoxide: an endogenous mediator of sinusoidal tone in the perfused liver. *J Clin Invest* 96, 2431–2437.

94 Friedman SL (2000) Molecular regulation of hepatic fibrosis, an integrated cellular response to tissue injury. *J Biol Chem* 275, 2247–2250.

95 Fiorucci S, Rizzo G, Antonelli E *et al.* (2005) Crosstalk between farnesoid X-receptor (FXR) and peroxisome proliferator-activated receptor (PPAR){gamma} contributes to the anti-fibrotic activity of FXR

96 Marra F, Efsen E, Romanelli RG *et al.* (2000) Ligands of peroxisome proliferator-activated receptor gamma modulate profibrogenic and proinflammatory actions in hepatic stellate cells. *Gastroenterology* 119, 466–478.

97 Hellemans K, Michalik L, Dittie A *et al.* (2003) Peroxisome proliferator-activated receptor-beta signaling contributes to enhanced proliferation of hepatic stellate cells. *Gastroenterology* 124, 184–201.

98 Ohata M, Lin M, Satre M *et al.* (1997) Diminished retinoic acid signaling in hepatic stellate cells in cholestatic liver fibrosis. *Am J Physiol* 272, G589–596.

99 Hazra S, Xiong S, Wang J *et al.* (2004) Peroxisome proliferator-activated receptor gamma induces a phenotypic switch from activated to quiescent hepatic stellate cells. *J Biol Chem* 279, 11392–11401.

100 Fiorucci S, Antonelli E, Rizzo G *et al.* (2004) The nuclear receptor SHP mediates inhibition of hepatic stellate cells by FXR and protects against liver fibrosis. *Gastroenterology* 127, 1497–1512.

101 Fiorucci S, Rizzo G, Antonelli E *et al.* (2005) A FXR-SHP regulatory cascade modulates TIMP-1 and MMPs expression in HSCs and promotes resolution of liver fibrosis. *J Pharmacol Exp Ther* 314, 584–595.

102 Kruglov EA, Nathanson RA, Nguyen T *et al.* (2005) Secretion of MCP-1/CCL2 by bile duct epithelia induces myofibroblastic trans-differentiation of portal fibroblasts. *Am J Physiol Gastrointest Liver Physiol* 290, G765–G771.

103 Schwabe RF, Bataller R, Brenner DA (2003) Human hepatic stellate cells express CCR5 and RANTES to induce proliferation and migration. *Am J Physiol Gastrointest Liver Physiol* 285, G949–958.

104 Paik YH, Schwabe RF, Bataller R *et al.* (2003) Toll-like receptor 4 mediates inflammatory signaling by bacterial lipopolysaccharide in human hepatic stellate cells. *Hepatology* 37, 1043–1055.

105 Brun P, Castagliuolo I, Pinzani M *et al.* (2005) Exposure to bacterial cell wall products triggers an inflammatory phenotype in hepatic stellate cells. *Am J Physiol Gastrointest Liver Physiol* ??, 000–000.

106 Vinas O, Bataller R, Sancho-Bru P *et al.* (2003) Human hepatic stellate cells show features of antigen-presenting cells and stimulate lymphocyte proliferation. *Hepatology* 38, 919–929.

107 Kobayashi S, Seki S, Kawada N *et al.* (2003) Apoptosis of T cells in the hepatic fibrotic tissue of the rat: a possible inducing role of hepatic myofibroblast-like cells. *Cell Tissue Res* 311, 353–364.

108 Maher JJ, Lozier JS, Scott MK (1998) Rat hepatic stellate cells produce cytokine-induced neutrophil chemoattractant in culture and in vivo. *Am J Physiol* 275, G847–853.

109 Safadi R, Ohta M, Alvarez CE *et al.* (2004) Immune stimulation of hepatic fibrogenesis by CD8 cells and attenuation by transgenic interleukin-10 from hepatocytes. *Gastroenterology* 127, 870–882.

110 Melhem A, Mohanna N, Bishara A *et al.* (2006) Anti-fibrotic activity of NK cells in experimental liver injury through killing of activated HSC. *J Hepatol* 45, 60–71.

111 Mann DA, Smart DE (2002) Transcriptional regulation of hepatic stellate cell activation. *Gut* 50, 891–896.

112 Rippe RA (1999) Role of transcriptional factors in stellate cell activation. *Alcohol Clin Exp Res* 23, 926–929.

113 Gabele E, Reif S, Tsukada S *et al.* (2005) The role of p70S6K in hepatic stellate cell collagen gene expression and cell proliferation. *J Biol Chem* 280, 13374–13382.

114 She H, Xiong S, Hazra S *et al.* (2005) Adipogenic transcriptional regulation of hepatic stellate cells. *J Biol Chem* 280, 4959–4967.

ligands in rodent models of liver cirrhosis. *J Pharmacol Exp Ther* 315, 58–68.

115 Yavrom S, Chen L, Xiong S *et al.* (2005) Peroxisome proliferator-activated receptor gamma suppresses proximal alpha1(I) collagen promoter via inhibition of p300-facilitated NF-I binding to DNA in hepatic stellate cells. *J Biol Chem* 280, 40650–40659.

116 Weiskirchen R, Moser M, Weiskirchen S *et al.* (2001) LIM-domain protein cysteine- and glycine-rich protein 2 (CRP2) is a novel marker of hepatic stellate cells and binding partner of the protein inhibitor of activated STAT1. *Biochem J* 359, 485–496.

117 Hellemans K, Verbuyst P, Quartier E *et al.* (2004) Differential modulation of rat hepatic stellate phenotype by natural and synthetic retinoids. *Hepatology* 39, 97–108.

118 Ratziu V, Lalazar A, Wong L *et al.* (1998) Zf9, a Kruppel-like transcription factor up-regulated in vivo during early hepatic fibrosis. *Proc Natl Acad Sci USA* 95, 9500–9505.

119 Kalinichenko VV, Bhattacharyya D, Zhou Y *et al.* (2003) Foxf1+/− mice exhibit defective stellate cell activation and abnormal liver regeneration following CCl4 injury. *Hepatology* 37, 107–117.

120 Wandzioch E, Kolterud A, Jacobsson M *et al.* (2004) Lhx2−/− mice develop liver fibrosis. *Proc Natl Acad Sci USA* 101, 16549–16554.

121 Wang X, Tang X, Gong X *et al.* (2004) Regulation of hepatic stellate cell activation and growth by transcription factor myocyte enhancer factor 2. *Gastroenterology* 127, 1174–1188.

122 Adams LA, Lymp JF, St Sauver J *et al.* (2005) The natural history of nonalcoholic fatty liver disease: a population-based cohort study. *Gastroenterology* 129, 113–121.

123 Ikejima K, Takei Y, Honda H *et al.* (2002) Leptin receptor-mediated signaling regulates hepatic fibrogenesis and remodeling of extracellular matrix in the rat. *Gastroenterology* 122, 1399–1410.

124 Leclercq IA, Farrell GC, Schriemer R *et al.* (2002) Leptin is essential for the hepatic fibrogenic response to chronic liver injury. *J Hepatol* 37, 206–213.

125 Saxena NK, Saliba G, Floyd JJ *et al.* (2003) Leptin induces increased alpha2(I) collagen gene expression in cultured rat hepatic stellate cells. *J Cell Biochem* 89, 311–320.

126 Oben JA, Roskams T, Yang S *et al.* (2004) Hepatic fibrogenesis requires sympathetic neurotransmitters. *Gut* 53, 438–445.

127 Ding X, Saxena NK, Lin S *et al.* (2005) The roles of leptin and adiponectin: a novel paradigm in adipocytokine regulation of liver fibrosis and stellate cell biology. *Am J Pathol* 166, 1655–1669.

128 Schaffler A, Scholmerich J, Buchler C (2005) Mechanisms of disease: adipocytokines and visceral adipose tissue – emerging role in non-alcoholic fatty liver disease. *Nature Clin Pract Gastroenterol Hepatol* 2, 273–280.

129 Musso G, Gambino R, Durazzo M *et al.* (2005) Adipokines in NASH: postprandial lipid metabolism as a link between adiponectin and liver disease. *Hepatology* 42, 1175–1183.

130 Kamada Y, Tamura S, Kiso S *et al.* (2003) Enhanced carbon tetrachloride-induced liver fibrosis in mice lacking adiponectin. *Gastroenterology* 125, 1796–1807.

131 Jonsson JR, Moschen AR, Hickman IJ *et al.* (2005) Adiponectin and its receptors in patients with chronic hepatitis C. *J Hepatol* 43, 929–936.

132 Bataller R, Paik YH, Lindquist JN *et al.* (2004) Hepatitis C virus core and nonstructural proteins induce fibrogenic effects in hepatic stellate cells. *Gastroenterology* 126, 529–540.

133 Mazzocca A, Cappadona Sciammetta S, Carloni V *et al.* (2004) Binding of hepatitis C virus envelope protein E2 to CD81 up-regulates MMP-2 in human hepatic stellate cells. *J Biol Chem* 280, 11329–11339.

134 Schulze-Krebs A, Preimel D, Popov Y *et al.* (2005) Hepatitis C virus-replicating hepatocytes induce fibrogenic activation of hepatic stellate cells. *Gastroenterology* 129, 246–258.

135 Pohlmann S, Zhang J, Baribaud F *et al.* (2003) Hepatitis C virus glycoproteins interact with DC-SIGN and DC-SIGNR. *J Virol* 77, 4070–4080.

136 Clouston AD, Powell EE, Walsh MJ *et al.* (2005) Fibrosis correlates with a ductular reaction in hepatitis C: roles of impaired replication, progenitor cells and steatosis. *Hepatology* 41, 809–818.

137 Walsh MJ, Vanags DM, Clouston AD *et al.* (2004) Steatosis and liver cell apoptosis in chronic hepatitis C: a mechanism for increased liver injury. *Hepatology* 39, 1230–1238.

138 Monto A (2002) Hepatitis C and steatosis. *Semin Gastrointest Dis* 13, 40–46.

139 Harrison SA (2005) Steatosis and chronic hepatitis C infection: mechanisms and significance. *Clin Gastroenterol Hepatol* 3, S92–96.

140 Dixon JB, Bhathal PS, Hughes NR *et al.* (2004) Nonalcoholic fatty liver disease: improvement in liver histological analysis with weight loss. *Hepatology* 39, 1647–1654.

141 Poynard T, McHutchison J, Manns M *et al.* (2002) Impact of pegylated interferon alfa-2b and ribavirin on liver fibrosis in patients with chronic hepatitis C. *Gastroenterology* 122, 1303–1313.

142 Shiratori Y, Imazeki F, Moriyama M *et al.* (2000) Histologic improvement of fibrosis in patients with hepatitis C who have sustained response to interferon therapy. *Ann Intern Med* 132, 517–524.

143 Moreno MG, Muriel P (1995) Remission of liver fibrosis by interferon-alpha 2b. *Biochem Pharmacol* 50, 515–520.

144 Czaja AJ, Carpenter HA (2004) Progressive fibrosis during corticosteroid therapy of autoimmune hepatitis. *Hepatology* 39, 1631–1638.

145 Raetsch C, Jia JD, Boigk G *et al.* (2002) Pentoxifylline downregulates profibrogenic cytokines and procollagen I expression in rat secondary biliary fibrosis. *Gut* 50, 241–247.

146 Kotoh K, Nakamuta M, Kohjima M *et al.* (2004) Arg-Gly-Asp (RGD) peptide ameliorates carbon tetrachloride-induced liver fibrosis via inhibition of collagen production and acceleration of collagenase activity. *Int J Mol Med* 14, 1049–1053.

147 Iwamoto H, Sakai H, Kotoh K *et al.* (1999) Soluble Arg-Gly-Asp peptides reduce collagen accumulation in cultured rat hepatic stellate cells. *Dig Dis Sci* 44, 1038–1045.

148 Ramalho LN, Ramalho FS, Zucoloto S *et al.* (2002) Effect of losartan, an angiotensin II antagonist, on secondary biliary cirrhosis. *Hepatogastroenterology* 49, 1499–1502.

149 Kurikawa N, Suga M, Kuroda S *et al.* (2003) An angiotensin II type 1 receptor antagonist, olmesartan medoxomil, improves experimental liver fibrosis by suppression of proliferation and collagen synthesis in activated hepatic stellate cells. *Br J Pharmacol* 139, 1085–1094.

150 Degott C, Zafrani ES, Callard P *et al.* (1999) Histopathological study of primary biliary cirrhosis and the effect of ursodeoxycholic acid treatment on histology progression. *Hepatology* 29, 1007–1012.

151 Pares A, Rodes J (2003) Natural history of primary biliary cirrhosis. *Clin Liver Dis* 7, 779–794.

152 Fiorucci S, Antonelli E, Morelli A (2003) Nitric oxide and portal hypertension: a nitric oxide-releasing derivative of ursodeoxycholic acid that selectively releases nitric oxide in the liver. *Dig Liver Dis* 35(Suppl), 61–69.

153 Kim WH, Matsumoto K, Bessho K *et al.* (2005) Growth inhibition and apoptosis in liver myofibroblasts promoted by hepatocyte growth factor leads to resolution from liver cirrhosis. *Am J Pathol* 166, 1017–1028.

154 Ueki T, Kaneda Y, Tsutsui H *et al.* (1999) Hepatocyte growth factor gene therapy of liver cirrhosis in rats. *Nature Med* 5, 226–230.

155 Masunaga H, Fujise N, Shiota A *et al.* (1998) Preventive effects of the deleted form of hepatocyte growth factor against various liver injuries. *Eur J Pharmacol* 342, 267–279.

156 Sanz S, Pucilowska JB, Liu S *et al.* (2005) Expression of insulin-like growth factor I by activated hepatic stellate cells reduces fibrogenesis and enhances regeneration after liver injury. *Gut* 54, 134–141.

157 Valentino KL, Gutierrez M, Sanchez R *et al.* (2003) First clinical trial of a novel caspase inhibitor: anti-apoptotic caspase inhibitor, IDN-6556, improves liver enzymes. *Int J Clin Pharmacol Ther* 41, 441–449.

158 Pietrangelo A, Borella F, Casalgrandi G *et al.* (1995) Antioxidant activity of silybin in vivo during long-term iron overload in rats. *Gastroenterology* 109, 1941–1949.

159 Brown KE, Poulos JE, Li L *et al.* (1997) Effect of vitamin E supplementation on hepatic fibrogenesis in chronic dietary iron overload. *Am J Physiol* 272, G116–123.

160 Kawada N, Seki S, Inoue M *et al.* (1998) Effect of antioxidants, resveratrol, quercetin, and N-acetylcysteine, on the functions of cultured rat hepatic stellate cells and Kupffer cells. *Hepatology* 27, 1265–1274.

161 Dehmlow C, Erhard J, de Groot H (1996) Inhibition of Kupffer cell functions as an explanation for the hepatoprotective properties of silibinin. *Hepatology* 23, 749–754.

162 Ferenci P, Dragosics B, Dittrich H *et al.* (1989) Randomized controlled trial of silymarin treatment in patients with cirrhosis of the liver. *J Hepatol* 9, 105–110.

163 Rockey DC, Chung JJ (1994) Interferon gamma inhibits lipocyte activation and extracellular matrix mRNA expression during experimental liver injury: implications for treatment of hepatic fibrosis. *J Invest Med* 42, 660–670.

164 Inagaki Y, Nemoto T, Kushida M *et al.* (2003) Interferon alfa down-regulates collagen gene transcription and suppresses experimental hepatic fibrosis in mice. *Hepatology* 38, 890–899.

165 Lee WM, Dienstag JL, Lindsay KL *et al.* (2004) Evolution of the HALT-C Trial: pegylated interferon as maintenance therapy for chronic hepatitis C in previous interferon nonresponders. *Control Clin Trials* 25, 472–492.

166 Cheng K, Ye Z, Guntaka RV *et al.* (2005) Biodistribution and hepatic uptake of triplex-forming oligonucleotides against type alpha1(I) collagen gene promoter in normal and fibrotic rats. *Mol Pharm* 2, 206–217.

167 Nelson DR, Lauwers GY, Lau JY *et al.* (2000) Interleukin 10 treatment reduces fibrosis in patients with chronic hepatitis C: a pilot trial of interferon nonresponders. *Gastroenterology* 118, 655–660.

168 Louis H, Van Laethem JL, Wu W *et al.* (1998) Interleukin-10 controls neutrophilic infiltration, hepatocyte proliferation, and liver fibrosis induced by carbon tetrachloride in mice. *Hepatology* 28, 1607–1615.

169 Thompson K, Maltby J, Fallowfield J *et al.* (1998) Interleukin-10 expression and function in experimental murine liver inflammation and fibrosis (see comments). *Hepatology* 28, 1597–1606.

170 Wang SC, Tsukamoto H, Rippe RA *et al.* (1998) Expression of interleukin-10 by in vitro and in vivo activated hepatic stellate cells. *J Biol Chem* 273, 302–308.

171 Mathurin P, Xiong S, Kharbanda KK *et al.* (2002) IL-10 receptor and coreceptor expression in quiescent and activated hepatic stellate cells. *Am J Physiol Gastrointest Liver Physiol* 282, G981–990.

172 Nelson DR, Tu Z, Soldevila-Pico C *et al.* (2003) Long-term interleukin 10 therapy in chronic hepatitis C patients has a proviral and anti-inflammatory effect. *Hepatology* 38, 859–868.

173 Galli A, Crabb DW, Ceni E *et al.* (2002) Antidiabetic thiazolidinediones inhibit collagen synthesis and hepatic stellate cell activation in vivo and in vitro. *Gastroenterology* 122, 1924–1940.

174 Saxena NK, Titus MA, Ding X *et al.* (2004) Leptin as a novel profibrogenic cytokine in hepatic stellate cells: mitogenesis and inhibition of apoptosis mediated by extracellular regulated kinase (Erk) and Akt phosphorylation. *FASEB J* 18, 1612–1614.

175 Saxena NK, Ikeda K, Rockey DC *et al.* (2002) Leptin in hepatic fibrosis: evidence for increased collagen production in stellate cells and lean littermates of ob/ob mice. *Hepatology* 35, 762–771.

176 Ikejima K, Honda H, Yoshikawa M *et al.* (2001) Leptin augments inflammatory and profibrogenic responses in the murine liver induced by hepatotoxic chemicals. *Hepatology* 34, 288–297.

177 Wade PA (2001) Transcriptional control at regulatory checkpoints by histone deacetylases: molecular connections between cancer and chromatin. *Hum Mol Genet* 10, 693–698.

178 Niki T, Rombouts K, De Bleser P *et al.* (1999) A histone deacetylase inhibitor, trichostatin A, suppresses myofibroblastic differentiation of rat hepatic stellate cells in primary culture. *Hepatology* 29, 858–867.

179 Geerts A, Rogiers V (1999) Sho-saiko-To: the right blend of traditional Oriental medicine and liver cell biology. *Hepatology* 29, 282–284.

180 Sakaida I, Hironaka K, Kimura T *et al.* (2004) Herbal medicine Sho-saiko-to (TJ-9) increases expression matrix metalloproteinases (MMPs) with reduced expression of tissue inhibitor of metalloproteinases (TIMPs) in rat stellate cell. *Life Sci* 74, 2251–2263.

181 Oh SH, Nan JX, Sohn DW *et al.* (2002) *Salvia miltiorrhiza* inhibits biliary obstruction-induced hepatocyte apoptosis by cytoplasmic sequestration of p53. *Toxicol Appl Pharmacol* 182, 27–33.

182 Sakata R, Ueno T, Nakamura T *et al.* (2004) Green tea polyphenol epigallocatechin-3-gallate inhibits platelet-derived growth factor-induced proliferation of human hepatic stellate cell line LI90. *J Hepatol* 40, 52–59.

183 Wiedmann MW, Caca K (2005) Molecularly targeted therapy for gastrointestinal cancer. *Curr Cancer Drug Targets* 5, 171–193.

184 Beno DW, Mullen J, Davis BH (1995) Lipoxygenase inhibitors block PDGF-induced mitogenesis: a MAPK-independent mechanism that blocks fos and egr. *Am J Physiol* 268, C604–610.

185 Rombouts K, Kisanga E, Hellemans K *et al.* (2003) Effect of HMG-CoA reductase inhibitors on proliferation and protein synthesis by rat hepatic stellate cells. *J Hepatol* 38, 564–572.

186 Preaux AM, Mallat A, Rosenbaum J *et al.* (1997) Pentoxifylline inhibits growth and collagen synthesis of cultured human hepatic myofibroblast-like cells. *Hepatology* 26, 315–322.

187 Shimizu E, Kobayashi Y, Oki Y *et al.* (1999) OPC-13013, a cyclic nucleotide phosphodiesterase type III inhibitor, inhibits cell proliferation and transdifferentiation of cultured rat hepatic stellate cells. *Life Sci* 64, 2081–2088.

188 Di Sario A, Bendia E, Svegliati Baroni G *et al.* (2002) Effect of pirfenidone on rat hepatic stellate cell proliferation and collagen production. *J Hepatol* 37, 584–591.

189 Demetri GD, von Mehren M, Blanke CD *et al.* (2002) Efficacy and safety of imatinib mesylate in advanced gastrointestinal stromal tumors. *N Engl J Med* 347, 472–480.

190 Druker BJ, Sawyers CL, Kantarjian H *et al.* (2001) Activity of a specific inhibitor of the BCR-ABL tyrosine kinase in the blast crisis of chronic myeloid leukemia and acute lymphoblastic leukemia with the Philadelphia chromosome. *N Engl J Med* 344, 1038–1042.

191 Kinnman N, Goria O, Wendum D *et al.* (2001) Hepatic stellate cell proliferation is an early platelet-derived growth factor-mediated cellular event in rat cholestatic liver injury. *Lab Invest* 81, 1709–1716.

192 Yoshiji H, Noguchi R, Kuriyama S *et al.* (2005) Imatinib mesylate (STI-571) attenuates liver fibrosis development in rats. *Am J Physiol Gastrointest Liver Physiol* 288, G907–913.

193 Tada S, Iwamoto H, Nakamuta M *et al.* (2001) A selective ROCK inhibitor, Y27632, prevents dimethylnitrosamine-induced hepatic fibrosis in rats. *J Hepatol* 34, 529–536.

194 Borkham-Kamphorst E, Herrmann J, Stoll D *et al.* (2004) Dominant-negative soluble PDGF-beta receptor inhibits hepatic stellate cell activation and attenuates liver fibrosis. *Lab Invest* 84, 766–777.

195 Borkham-Kamphorst E, Stoll D, Gressner AM *et al.* (2004) Inhibitory effect of soluble PDGF-beta receptor in culture-activated hepatic stellate cells. *Biochem Biophys Res Commun* 317, 451–462.

196 Borkham-Kamphorst E, Stoll D, Gressner AM *et al.* (2004) Antisense strategy against PDGF B-chain proves effective in preventing experimental liver fibrogenesis. *Biochem Biophys Res Commun* 321, 413–423.

197 Stefanovic B, Schnabl B, Brenner DA (2002) Inhibition of collagen a1(I) expression by the 5' stem-loop as a molecular decoy. *J Biol Chem* 277, 18229–18237.

198 Lindquist JN, Parsons CJ, Stefanovic B *et al.* (2004) Regulation of alpha1(I) collagen messenger RNA decay by interactions with alphaCP at the 3'-untranslated region. *J Biol Chem* 279, 23822–23829.

199 Stefanovic L, Stephens CE, Boykin D *et al.* (2005) Inhibitory effect of dicationic diphenylfurans on production of type I collagen by human fibroblasts and activated hepatic stellate cells. *Life Sci* 76, 2011–2026.

200 Kershenobich D, Vargas F, Garcia-Tsao G *et al.* (1988) Colchicine in the treatment of cirrhosis of the liver. *N Engl J Med* 318, 1709–1713.

201 Cortez-Pinto H, Alexandrino P, Camilo ME *et al.* (2002) Lack of effect of colchicine in alcoholic cirrhosis: final results of a double blind randomized trial. *Eur J Gastroenterol Hepatol* 14, 377–381.

202 George J, Roulot D, Koteliansky VE *et al.* (1999) In vivo inhibition of rat stellate cell activation by soluble transforming growth factor beta type II receptor: a potential new therapy for hepatic fibrosis. *Proc Natl Acad Sci USA* 96, 12719–12724.

203 Okuno M, Akita K, Moriwaki H *et al.* (2001) Prevention of rat hepatic fibrosis by the protease inhibitor, camostat mesilate, via reduced generation of active TGF-beta. *Gastroenterology* 120, 1784–1800.

204 Dooley D, Hamzavi J, Breitkopf K *et al.* (2003) Smad7 prevents activation of hepatic stellate cells and liver fibrosis in rats. *Gastroenterology* 125, 178–191.

205 Zhu J, Wu J, Frizell E *et al.* (1999) Rapamycin inhibits hepatic stellate cell proliferation in vitro and limits fibrogenesis in an in vivo model of liver fibrosis. *Gastroenterology* 117, 1198–1204.

206 Trotter JF (2003) Sirolimus in liver transplantation. *Transplant Proc* 35, 193S–200S.

207 Williams EJ, Benyon RC, Trim N *et al.* (2001) Relaxin inhibits effective collagen deposition by cultured hepatic stellate cells and decreases rat liver fibrosis in vivo. *Gut* 49, 577–583.

208 Bennett RG, Mahan KJ, Gentry-Nielsen MJ *et al.* (2005) Relaxin receptor expression in hepatic stellate cells and in cirrhotic rat liver tissue. *Ann NY Acad Sci* 1041, 185–189.

209 Rockey DC, Chung JJ (1996) Endothelin antagonism in experimental hepatic fibrosis. Implications for endothelin in the pathogenesis of wound healing. *J Clin Invest* 98, 1381–1388.

210 Rockey DC (2005) Antifibrotic therapy in chronic liver disease. *Clin Gastroenterol Hepatol* 3, 95–107.

211 Fiorucci S, Antonelli E, Morelli O *et al.* (2001) NCX-1000, a NO-releasing derivative of ursodeoxycholic acid, selectively delivers NO to the liver and protects against development of portal hypertension. *Proc Natl Acad Sci USA* 98, 8897–8902.

212 Gnainsky Y, Spira G, Paizi M *et al.* (2004) Halofuginone, an inhibitor of collagen synthesis by rat stellate cells, stimulates insulin-like growth factor binding protein-1 synthesis by hepatocytes. *J Hepatol* 40, 269–277.

213 Geubel AP, De Galocsy C, Alves N *et al.* (1991) Liver damage caused by therapeutic vitamin A administration: estimate of dose-related toxicity in 41 cases. *Gastroenterology* 100, 1701–1709.

214 Iredale JP, Benyon RC, Pickering J *et al.* (1998) Mechanisms of spontaneous resolution of rat liver fibrosis. Hepatic stellate cell apoptosis and reduced hepatic expression of metalloproteinase inhibitors. *J Clin Invest* 102, 538–549.

215 Dekel R, Zvibel I, Brill S *et al.* (2003) Gliotoxin ameliorates development of fibrosis and cirrhosis in a thioacetamide rat model. *Dig Dis Sci* 48, 1642–1647.

216 Wright MC, Issa R, Smart DE *et al.* (2001) Gliotoxin stimulates the apoptosis of human and rat hepatic stellate cells and enhances the resolution of liver fibrosis in rats. *Gastroenterology* 121, 685–698.

217 Parsons CJ, Bradford BU, Pan CQ *et al.* (2004) Antifibrotic effects of a tissue inhibitor of metalloproteinase-1 antibody on established liver fibrosis in rats. *Hepatology* 40, 1106–1115.

218 Oakley F, Meso M, Iredale JP *et al.* (2005) Inhibition of inhibitor of kappaB kinases stimulates hepatic stellate cell apoptosis and accelerated recovery from rat liver fibrosis. *Gastroenterology* 128, 108–120.

219 Taimr P, Higuchi H, Kocova E *et al.* (2003) Activated stellate cells express the TRAIL receptor-2/death receptor-5 and undergo TRAIL-mediated apoptosis. *Hepatology* 37, 87–95.

220 Elsharkawy AM, Oakley F, Mann DA (2005) The role and regulation of hepatic stellate cell apoptosis in reversal of liver fibrosis. *Apoptosis* 10, 927–939.

221 Fallowfield JA, Iredale JP (2004) Targeted treatments for cirrhosis. *Expert Opin Ther Targets* 8, 423–435.

222 Iredale JP (2001) Hepatic stellate cell behavior during resolution of liver injury. *Semin Liver Dis* 21, 427–436.

223 Unemori EN, Pickford LB, Salles AL *et al.* (1996) Relaxin induces an extracellular matrix-degrading phenotype in human lung fibroblasts in vitro and inhibits lung fibrosis in a murine model in vivo. *J Clin Invest* 98, 2739–2745.

224 Siller-Lopez F, Sandoval A, Salgado S *et al.* (2004) Treatment with human metalloproteinase-8 gene delivery ameliorates experimental rat liver cirrhosis. Gastroenterology 126, 1122–1133; discussion 1949.

225 Iimuro Y, Nishio T, Morimoto T *et al.* (2003) Delivery of matrix metalloproteinase-1 attenuates established liver fibrosis in the rat. *Gastroenterology* 124, 445–458.

226 Issa R, Zhou X, Trim N *et al.* (2003) Mutation in collagen-1 that confers resistance to the action of collagenase results in failure of recovery from CCl4-induced liver fibrosis, persistence of activated hepatic stellate cells, and diminished hepatocyte regeneration. *FASEB J* 17, 47–49.

6.3 Clinical and diagnostic aspects of cirrhosis

I. Neil Guha and John P. Iredale

Definition

Cirrhosis is defined as the pathological findings of diffuse fibrosis and conversion of normal liver architecture into nodules. In the fifth century BC, Hippocrates recognized that hardening of the liver was a poor prognostic sign in the presence of icterus. The term cirrhosis is credited to René Laënnec and derived from the Greek kirrhos, meaning orange-yellow. It described the autopsy appearance of the liver in a patient with cirrhosis that also demonstrated nodules and an irregular edge. The definition has been refined over the years, notably by a consensus conference in La Habana 1956 and a working party sponsored by the World Health Organization (WHO) in 1978 [1], to give us the basis for the present definition. Despite its morphological definition, cirrhosis also implies a disturbance of hepatic and posthepatic haemodynamics, which may play a significant role in the evolution of fibrosis (see Chapter 6.1) and the clinical sequelae.

Classification

Cirrhosis may be classified by three differing morphologies: micronodular cirrhosis, macronodular cirrhosis and mixed (see also Section 4).
• *Micronodular:* this is characterized by small nodules, usually less than 3 mm in size, distributed uniformly throughout the liver and contained by thick, regular septa. An example of micronodular cirrhosis is that induced by alcohol.
• *Macronodular:* this term is used to describe the presence of septa and nodules of varying size. The larger nodules may contain portal tracts; the close proximity of three or more portal tracts is suggestive of architectural collapse.
• *Mixed:* the combination of micronodular and macronodular cirrhosis is termed mixed cirrhosis. The proportion of each subtype may vary but is usually equal. There are examples of micronodular cirrhosis converting to macronodular cirrhosis in time [2].

Aetiology

The causes of cirrhosis are legion and Table 1 lists the major underlying diseases and disease associations. More detailed descriptions of these diseases may be found in specific chapters.

Epidemiology

The number of deaths from cirrhosis in different regions is graphically illustrated in Figure 1. These figures are based on estimates made by the WHO report for 2002.

The precise prevalence of cirrhosis is difficult to ascertain for a number of reasons. Firstly, cirrhosis is often clinically silent and a significant proportion of patients with undiagnosed cirrhosis have been found at autopsy studies [3,4]. Secondly, the reliance on death certification for the rates of cirrhosis is dependent on having the infrastructure to collect these data. Additionally, even if these resources are in place, the stigmata of documenting cirrhosis and its aetiology will influence reporting. Differences in prevalence exist not only between continents but also within individual countries. For example, Corrao et al. found a difference in mortality between northern and southern Europe [5] whilst Lessa reported different prevalence rates within Brazil [6].

Autopsy studies, even when randomized, have an inherent bias because cirrhosis carries a risk of mortality. Furthermore, death rate may not always be a valid surrogate for prevalence and the relationship is not always linear. For example, if treatment significantly improves, the prevalence of the condition in the community will rise but the death rate from the condition, depending on how data are collected and documented, may appear to fall if these subjects subsequently die from an unrelated condition. Currently, the absence of accurate, validated, noninvasive tools for the diagnosis of cirrhosis makes population screening a difficult proposition (see Chapter 6.2).

The epidemiology of individual aetiologies of cirrhosis will be discussed in greater detail in the relevant chapters. Generally, viral hepatitis is the leading cause of cirrhosis in the developing world. Alcohol, hepatitis C and, more recently, nonalcoholic steatohepatitis associated with the metabolic syndrome are the most significant causes of cirrhosis in the developed world.

Table 1 Main causes of cirrhosis.

Aetiology	Examples
Infectious	Hepatitis B, C, D
	Schistosomiasis
	Syphilis
	HIV (sclerosing cholangitis)
Metabolic/inherited	Nonalcoholic steatohepatitis (NASH) in association with the metabolic syndrome
	Wilson's disease
	Haemochromatosis
	Alpha-1-antitrypsin deficiency
	Glycogen storage disease
	Cystic fibrosis
	Tyrosinaemia
	Galactosaemia
	Fructose intolerance
	Byler's disease
	Mucopolysaccharidosis
	Abetalipoproteinaemia
	Porphyria
	Wolman's disease
Biliary disease	Extrahepatic obstruction
	Intrahepatic obstruction
Immunological	Autoimmune hepatitis
	Primary biliary cirrhosis
	Primary sclerosing cholangitis
Vascular	Veno-occlusive disease
	Budd–Chiari syndrome
	Cardiac failure
	Hereditary haemorrhagic telangiectasia
Drugs and toxins	Alcohol
	Amiodarone
	Dantrolene
	Halothane
	Isoniazid
	Methotrexate
	Methyldopa
	Aflatoxin
	Diclofenac
	Hypervitaminosis A
Miscellaneous	Indian childhood
	Malnutrition
	Sarcoidosis
	Ischaemia
	Graft vs. host disease

Clinical features of cirrhosis

The visible signs and symptoms of cirrhosis are summarized in Table 2.

Compensated cirrhosis

Cirrhosis may progress insidiously without clinical signs or symptoms, giving rise to the term compensated cirrhosis.

Compensated cirrhosis can continue for a variable length of time before the development of complications, hepatocellular carcinoma or hepatic failure. The appearance of these complications is referred to as decompensated cirrhosis. As stated earlier in this chapter, quantifying the numbers of asymptomatic cirrhotics is difficult because of the bias of autopsy studies and lack of noninvasive diagnostic tools.

Decompensated cirrhosis (see also Section 7)

Portal hypertension

Portal hypertension is defined by an elevated portal pressure greater than the normal value of 1–5 mmHg. In general, portal pressure becomes clinically significant above a level of 12 mmHg. The major complications of portal hypertension include ascites, gastrointestinal haemorrhage and renal dysfunction. Of these, gastrointestinal haemorrhage is the most dramatic and occurs frequently. Prospective studies suggest that 90% of patients with cirrhosis will develop oesophageal varices and a third of these will bleed [7]. Furthermore, gastrointestinal haemorrhage has been reported to carry a short-term mortality rate as high as 50% in the group with most severe liver dysfunction [8].

Ascites

In the presence of ascites, a diagnostic tap may help distinguish the possible aetiologies. Traditionally, these were subdivided into exudative and transudative on the basis of protein in ascites being greater than 25 g/L. More recently, a newer classification based on the serum–ascites albumin gradient has been proposed [9]. A gradient greater than 1.1 g/dL suggests nonperitoneal disease, including portal hypertension. This can help exclude some of the peritoneal causes of ascites, which have a gradient less than 1.1 g/dL, including malignancy, granulomatous peritonitis and vasculitis. For a more detailed account see Chapter 7.5.

Hypersplenism

This occurs in the context of portal hypertension and results in a variable pancytopenia with sequestration of red blood cells, white blood cells and platelets in the splenic tissues. This will affect oxygen delivery, coagulation and the immune response. The extent of thrombocytopaenia does not correlate directly with splenic size and rarely leads to spontaneous bleeding, but it may complicate bleeding from other sites such as varices.

Renal dysfunction

In cirrhosis there is abnormal renal handling of sodium and this in combination with abnormal haemodynamics results in a spectrum of disease culminating in hepatorenal syndrome (HRS). Patients with cirrhosis who are free of ascites, termed preascitic cirrhotics, have been shown to have a positive sodium balance after being fed a high-salt diet for one week compared with normal healthy controls [10]. There is increasing evidence from vascular studies in the supine and upright position that abnormal salt retention is the initiating event rather than a

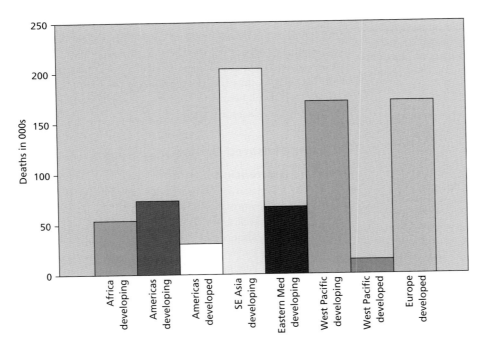

Fig. 1 Number of deaths from cirrhosis of the liver according to region. Data taken from www.who.int/healthinfo/bodgb2002original/en/

consequence of the hyperdynamic circulation [11,12]. The progression to hepatorenal syndrome is associated with splanchnic vasodilatation, increased cardiac output, decreased peripheral resistance and renal vasoconstriction, as discussed in detail in Chapter 7.6.

Prognosis is dependent on the subtype of HRS, as defined by the International Ascites Club, with type 2 HRS developing more insidiously and being associated with increased survival compared with type 1 (Table 3). Treatment options include pharmacological intervention with albumin and vasopressors, transjugular intrahepatic portosystemic shunts (TIPS), dialysis procedures and orthotopic liver transplantation (OLT) as discussed in Chapter 7.6.

Clinical features of portal hypertension

Clinical manifestations of portal hypertension include ascites, collateral circulation and splenomegaly (see Table 2).

The collateral circulation can manifest on the abdominal surface. For example, dilated veins around the umbilicus are known as caput medusae, and are derived from portal blood via the recannalized umbilical vein and paraumbilical veins. The distribution of blood flow on the abdominal surface is away from the umbilicus in all directions, a feature that can help differentiate this diagnosis from occlusion of the inferior vena cava.

Splenomegaly in the context of portal hypertension can lead to a pancytopenia with consequences for immunity and coagulation as discussed previously. Ascites may be clinically detectable after the accumulation of 2 L of fluid. Where clinical doubt remains, ultrasound can be a useful investigation. Abdominal distension will generally cause discomfort with large volumes of ascites. The presence of underlying infection should be excluded by performing a diagnostic ascitic tap. Pleural effusions can be associated with ascites in approximately 10% of cases [13]; the majority of effusions are right sided and are due to defects in the diaphragm.

Gastrointestinal haemorrhage from gastric or oesophageal varices will usually be self-evident. Endoscopy will provide a diagnostic and therapeutic tool. Rarely, bleeding is from other sites of portosystemic anastomoses including rectal and periumbilical varices. These can be more difficult to treat and often require radiological embolization and/or TIPS insertion.

Hepatopulmonary syndrome (HPS)

This is a disorder of pulmonary oxygenation occurring in the context of liver disease or portal hypertension. It is not exclusive to cirrhosis but, in this setting, studies have shown HPS has a prevalence of 24% and is an independent risk factor for mortality [14]. The pathophysiology is thought to relate to nitric oxide production as evidenced by increased levels of endothelial nitric oxide synthetase (eNOS) and inducible nitric oxide synthetase (iNOS) [15,16]. This may cause microvasular dilatation and contribute to intrapulmonary shunts with resultant hypoxaemia. Diagnosis involves the exclusion of other causes of cardiopulmonary disease and the demonstration of dependent hypoxaemia and pulmonary shunts using microbubble echocardiography. Hitherto, there have only been anecdotal or case reports or small uncontrolled trials of success with medical treatment. OLT remains the only effective long-term treatment [17,18], although HPS will also increase the anaesthetic risks associated with transplantation.

Clinical features

Patients with HPS may complain of dyspnoea on exertion and have objective evidence of decreased oxygen saturation.

Table 2 Clinical stigmata directly or indirectly associated with cirrhosis.

Stigmata	Comments
Palmar erythema	This condition also occurs in pregnancy, rheumatoid arthritis, leukaemia, chronic febrile illness and thyrotoxicosis
Leuconychia	Related to hypoalbuminaemia
Finger clubbing	Not specific to cirrhosis
Dupuytren's contracture	Thickening of the palmar fascia; occurs in, but not exclusive to, excess alcohol intake
Asterixis	Suggests underlying hepatic encephalopathy
Spider angiomas	Related to disturbance of oestrogen metabolism
Foetor hepaticus	Distinctive aroma thought to be of intestinal origin
Jaundice	May be the result of endstage liver disease, decompensation, cholestasis or haemolysis
Collateral veins and caput medusae	Direction of flow will differentiate portal hypertension from inferior vena caval (IVC) obstruction
Bruising	Results from abnormalities in platelets, coagulation pathways or both
Parotid gland enlargement	Raises the suspicion of alcohol as aetiology of cirrhosis
Kayser–Fleischer rings	Occurs in the context of Wilson's disease. Absence does not exclude diagnosis
Xanthelasma	May occur in hyperlipidaemia associated with primary biliary cirrhosis
Wernicke's encephalopathy	Triad of symptoms including ophthalmoplegia, ataxia and confusion caused by thiamine deficiency and invariably associated with alcoholic liver disease
Splenomegaly	Caused by portal hypertension; often the first clinical sign of cirrhosis.
Ascites	Can be clinically detected after approximately 2 L
Cachexia	Occurs in the context of malnutrition in cirrhosis but may also be associated with the development of HCC
Muscle cramps	Nonspecific feature and often difficult to treat
Hypertrophic osteoarthropathy	Occurs in cirrhosis but classically associated with carcinoma of the bronchus
Arthritis	Rheumatoid arthritis may indicate underlying autoimmune disease; haemochromatosis can cause chondrocalcinosis and osteoarthritis
Pigmentation	'Bronze diabetes' caused by excess ACTH following pituitary failure in haemochromatosis
Hypotension, bounding pulse and warm peripheries	Reduced peripheral resistance in the context of the hyperdynamic circulation
Striae	May be related to steroid use for autoimmune hepatitis; also occurs in pregnancy
Central obesity with raised waist to hip ratio	These patients are at increased risk of developing NASH and subsequent fibrosis/cirrhosis
Pulsatile liver	Classically found in tricuspid regurgitation. Long-term hepatic congestion may lead to cirrhosis
Gynaecomastia	Result from oestrogen imbalance but also a side effect of spironolactone
Scratch marks	Consequence of pruritus; if irretractable, an indication for OLT in PBC
Testicular atrophy	Occurs as a result of cirrhosis but also a direct effect of alcohol
Cyanosis	Raises the suspicion of underlying hepatopulmonary syndrome
Hair loss	As part of the loss of secondary sexual characteristics
'Emphysematous' chest	Exclude alpha-1-antitrypsin deficiency
Cushingoid appearance	Related to steroid therapy
Telangiectasia	Hereditary haemorrhagic telangiectasia is a rare cause of cirrhosis

ACTH, adrenocorticotropic hormone; HCC, hepatocellular carcinoma; NASH, nonalcoholic steatohepatitis; OLT, orthotopic liver transplantation; PBC, primary biliary cirrhosis.

Significant disease will result in central cyanosis. Other contributory factors to dyspnoea in the cirrhotic patient include anaemia, marked ascites and intrinsic pulmonary disease.

Cirrhotic cardiomyopathy

The affect of alcohol and iron on cardiac function have long been recognized. More recently, there has been increasing evidence of the effect of cirrhosis *per se* on the myocardium and the term 'cirrhotic cardiomyopathy' was described in 1989 by Lee [19]. The features include increased baseline cardiac output, attenuated systolic contractility and diastolic relaxation in response to inotropic and chronotropic stimuli and the absence of florid left ventricular failure. There can be associated electrophysiological abnormalities such as repolarization anomalies but morphological changes are often not pronounced. The exact pathophysiology is not completely understood but possibilities include alterations in beta-adrenergic receptors, membrane function, calcium channels, nitric oxide and carbon monoxide [20]. OLT has been shown to improve this condition [21].

Clinical features

The absence of overt signs of heart failure, which forms part of the definition, makes this a difficult clinical diagnosis. The condition is sometimes revealed when the patient undergoes acute

Table 3 Classification of hepatorenal syndrome (HRS).

Subtypes of HRS
Type 1: Progressive renal impairment defined by a doubling of initial serum creatinine above 2.5 mg/dL in less than 2 weeks
Type 2: Stable or slowly progressive renal impairment

Critical exclusions/features for the above:
Absence of shock, ongoing bacterial infection, fluid loss and no treatment with nephrotoxic drugs
Absence of obstructive uropathy and intrinsic renal disease
Serum creatinine concentration >1.5 mg/dL or 24-hour creatinine clearance <40 mL/min
No sustained improvement following removal of diuretic and fluid challenge

haemodynamic changes such as major surgery or TIPS insertion. An attenuated response to inotropic agents in the intensive care setting can also be a clue but in this situation there are often confounding factors, such as sepsis, causing alterations to myocardial function. A low index of suspicion and awareness of the condition are therefore key to making the diagnosis.

Hepatocelluar carcinoma (see also Chapter 18.2.1)
Cirrhosis remains the commonest cause for the development of hepatocellular carcinoma (HCC); it has been estimated that 80% of tumours occur in this setting [22]. The aetiology and the global location of disease are important determinants of the risk of cirrhosis progressing to HCC. For example, the annual risk of developing HCC in patients with hepatits C virus (HCV) is estimated to be 3–8% [23]. The 5-year cumulative incidence of HCC on the background of HCV is reported to be as high as 30% in Japan compared with 17% in the West. Comparing aetiologies, the rates decrease in the following order: haemochromatosis, hepatitis B infection, alcohol and biliary disease [24]. Interestingly, HCC is an uncommon complication of autoimmune hepatitis [25]. Regardless of aetiology, independent risk factors for HCC include gender, age, severity of compensated cirrhosis at presentation and sustained activity of liver disease [24].

The development of HCC may be heralded by symptoms of pain, bleeding, general decompensation or screening (see 'Follow-up and screening' below). The pathology and management of HCC will be discussed in greater detail in Chapter 18.2.1.

Clinical features
Right upper quadrant pain and abdominal distension with bloody ascites, on the background of cirrhosis, are very suggestive of rupture of an underlying HCC into the peritoneal cavity. However, this occurs infrequently and usually late in the disease. Often there are few signs of underlying malignancy; for example, cachexia may not change the physical appearance of the patient because of the underlying malnutrition. Cirrhotic patients that decompensate suddenly, either clinically or biochemically, without obvious cause, should always prompt the search for HCC.

Encephalopathy
Hepatic encephalopathy (HE) on the background of cirrhosis can occur in a subclinical, acute or chronic setting. The prevalence of subclinical encephalopathy (SCE) in patients with cirrhosis has reached 84% in some studies [26]. As there may be no compromise in routine daily life, SCE may only come to light upon psychometric testing using number connection tests, block reception tests and reaction times. Acute hepatic encephalopathy can be precipitated by sepsis, sedatives, dehydration, haemorrhage, etc. but it may also occur with no obvious precipitants in the presence of terminal liver failure. Chronic encephalopathy is usually due to the formation of portosystemic shunts, as part of the disease or iatrogenically as a consequence of TIPS insertion. In 2002, a working party created a new classification of hepatic encephalopathy (Table 4) [27]. Encephalopathy occurring in chronic liver disease was defined as episodic or persistent, and subclinical encephalopathy replaced with the term minimal encephalopathy. For a more detailed description of the pathophysiology, diagnosis and treatment of encephalopathy see Chapter 7.8.

Clinical features
Reversal of the day/night sleep pattern and somnolence during the day is a subtle clinical sign of underlying HE. As the HE progresses, the patient may become withdrawn, confused and

HE type	Nomenclature	Subcategory	Subdivisions
A	Encephalopathy associated with acute liver failure		
B	Encephalopathy associated with portosystemic shunts and no intrinsic hepatic disease		
C	Encephalopathy associated with cirrhosis and portal hypertension/or portosystemic shunts	Episodic HE	Precipitated Spontaneous Recurrent
		Persistent HE	Mild Severe Treatment dependent
		Minimal HE	

Table 4 Proposed nomenclature of hepatic encephalopathy (HE) by working party at 11th World Congress of Gastroenterology, 1998.

agitated before finally becoming unconscious. The clinical sign of asterixis (Table 2) usually represents established HE. The waveforms demonstrated by an electroencephalogram (EEG) in hepatic encephalopathy are not highly specific to this condition, as they can also occur in the context of other metabolic encephalopathies, but nonetheless can be a useful investigation. The presence of new HE should prompt the clinician to exclude precipitating factors such as new medications, underlying sepsis, occult haemorrhage and electrolyte disturbances. In severe cases of HE, the patient may need to be ventilated, especially if there is compromise to respiratory function.

Malnutrition

Cirrhosis is a catabolic state and, in combination with dietary insufficiency, can lead to significant malnutrition. Additionally, malabsorption, hypermetabolism and resistance to growth factors such as insulin and growth factor contribute to the pathophysiology. In hospitalized patients with liver disease, the prevalence of malnutrition is estimated to be as high as 20% in compensated disease rising to 60% with severe liver insufficiency [28]. Studies have shown that nourishment, measured by parameters such as skin-fold thickness and midarm muscle circumference, is an independent predictor of survival at 2 years [29].

Measures of anthropometry, such as skin-fold thickness, may be distorted by fluid retention and occur late in malnutrition. Thus, there has been interest in finding accurate tools for assessing nutritional status. This has led to the creation of measures such as the subjective global assessment tool (SGA), prognostic nutritional index (PNI) and hand grip strength (HGS). A recent study found that the prevalence of malnutrition was 63% in patients with Childs A cirrhosis using HGS, compared with a prevalence of 28% and 19% detected by SGA and PNI respectively [30].

Clinical features

In severe cases the patient will appear cachectic. Profound muscle wasting may manifest by a proximal myopathy and the inability of the patient to stand up. Diagnosis of less advanced cases requires objective assessment using one or more of the tools discussed above. Relying on simple weight measurements may be inaccurate – for example, the presence of ascites may disguise muscle weight loss.

Sepsis

It has been estimated that sepsis is present in 30–50% of hospital admissions due to cirrhosis [31]. Once sepsis has developed there is a higher rate of mortality, up to 30%, and this is independent of the severity of liver disease [32,33].

There are a number of reasons for increased susceptibility to sepsis in this group. Bacterial translocation (BT) is the migration of bacteria or their products from the intestinal lumen to mesenteric lymph nodes. BT has been shown to be significantly increased in patients with Childs C cirrhosis compared with the less severe Childs stages [34]. Moreover, not only does the

antigen load increase but also there are changes in immunity, both within the local lymph nodes and systemically, which also determine whether there is progression to sepsis. Studies have shown a reduced phagocytic and killing capacity of the immune system [35,36] and reduced opsonization relating to low complement levels in ascites [37].

Sepsis results in a spectrum of physiological outcomes including the systemic inflammatory response syndrome (SIRS), septic shock and multiorgan failure [38]. The inflammatory response associated with sepsis is mediated by the cytokine cascade. Activation of Toll-like receptors by bacterial products, including lipopolysaccharide (LPS), is one such mechanism of activating the innate immune system. Investigators have found that the expression of Toll-like receptor 2 (TLR2) is increased on peripheral blood mononuclear cells in patients with cirrhosis but Toll-like receptor 4 (TLR4) is unaltered or downregulated [39,40]. Furthermore, the same study showed raised serum levels of tumour necrosis factor alpha (TNFα) levels correlating with TLR2. Thus, the cytokine response may be influenced by the amount and type of bacterial product presented and also the relative expression of the corresponding receptors.

It has been postulated that sepsis has a major aetiological role in disturbances of coagulation, haemodynamics and variceal bleeding. It is a predictor of variceal rebleeding, and patients with controlled bleeding have lower rates of sepsis than those with uncontrolled bleeding [41]. In the presence of variceal haemorrhage, cirrhotic patients given prophylactic antibiotic therapy have been shown to have improved survival rates [42]. Optimizing haemodynamic state is also important in cirrhotics with sepsis. In spontaneous bacterial peritonitis, survival has been shown to improve if albumin is administered with intravenous antibiotic compared with antibiotics alone [43]. Additionally, parameters of haemodynamics such as renin levels and renal function also improved in the group administered albumin. The alterations in coagulation may be due to increased amounts of heparinoid substances [44] and may augment the deficiencies in clotting factors because of hepatic insufficiency.

Clinical features

The characteristic features of sepsis in the previously healthy individual, such as hypotension, tachycardia and warm peripheries, often occur in cirrhotics with no evidence of sepsis because of the hyperdynamic circulation (see Table 2). Additionally, aetiologies such as alcoholic hepatitis cause the release of inflammatory cytokines, resulting in a low-grade pyrexia and raised peripheral white cell count. Thus, supervening sepsis in these individuals can be difficult to distinguish. The possibility of sepsis should be explored in unexplained decompensation or patients slow to respond to treatment with supportive measures. Often, confirmation of microbial infection by culture is not possible, particularly in the context of fungal sepsis, necessitating the use of broad-spectrum antibiotics. Expert advice should be sought at an early stage in these situations.

Haematological complications

Reduced platelets

The reduction of platelet count in cirrhosis is largely due to the effects of hypersplenism causing increased splanchnic pooling as discussed above. In health, 30% of the total platelet population is sequestered in the spleen but this can rise to 90% in portal hypertension. Additionally, there may be reduced bone marrow production particularly in alcoholic liver disease and viral hepatitis. Not only are absolute numbers of platelets reduced but also there may be deficiencies in function, particularly aggregation, and membrane composition.

Anaemia

A macrocytic, microcytic or normochromic anaemia can be found in cirrhosis. Macrocytic anaemia, secondary to folate deficiency, is often due to poor nutrition particularly in the context of alcoholic liver disease. Macrocytosis also occurs as a result of poor membrane function and is associated with advanced cirrhosis. Increased destruction of red blood cells occurs because of increased fragility, as a consequence of membrane defects. Damaged red blood cells are then extracted by the spleen. Haemolysis is also associated with certain autoimmune liver diseases, Wilson's disease, Zieve syndrome (alcoholic hepatitis and hypercholesterolaemia) and following the placement of uncovered stents inserted at TIPS. Reduced bone marrow production further contributes to lower red cell numbers.

Impaired coagulation

The liver is responsible for the production of both coagulants and anticoagulants. Disruption of synthetic function can disturb the homeostatic balance of these two pathways. Commonly, patients have impaired coagulation and, in combination with quantitative and qualitative deficiencies in platelets, this leads to complications of bleeding. Factors II, VII, IX and X, labile factor V, factor VIII, contact factors XI and XII, fibrinogen and fibrin-stabilizing factor XIII are vitamin K dependent. Vitamin K is produced by the intestinal bacteria and requires bile salts for absorption. Therefore, cholestatic conditions, in particular biliary obstruction, will also contribute to impaired coagulation.

Clinical features of haematological disturbance

Bruising in a patient with cirrhosis will often signify an underlying bleeding diathesis. In some cases, the bruising also may bring to light less obvious causes of internal bleeding. For example, a subdural haemorrhage in a patient with alcoholic liver disease may cause the patient to have further falls and external bruising. Haemolysis will cause a rise in unconjugated bilirubin and, if significant, result in jaundice (see Table 2).

Endocrine disturbance

Because the liver plays a major role in the metabolism of hormones it is unsurprising that cirrhosis affects a variety of endocrine pathways.

Feminization and hypogonadism

Feminization in men is reflected by a loss of libido, reduced secondary sexual hair and gynaecomastia. Testicular atrophy may be a consequence of alcohol rather than liver disease itself. In women, hypogonadism manifests as sterility, erratic or absent menstruation and loss of feminine characteristics in premenopausal women. Although there may be changes in plasma testosterone and oestradiol, they are insufficient to account for the degree of feminization or hypogonadism. Thus, a variety of mechanisms may be important.

Dysfunction of the hypothalamic–pituitary axis is suggested by normal levels of gonadotropins even in the presence of testicular or ovarian failure [45]. Oestradiol and testosterone are bound to sex hormone-binding globulin (SHBG); increasing levels of SHBG seen in cirrhosis can lead to a lower unbound fraction and subsequent decreased biological effect. The liver is responsible for the uptake and metabolism of oestrogen and testosterone; the concentration of receptors, blood delivery and conjugation process will all be altered by cirrhosis. Finally, increased peripheral conversion of the androgenic hormones into oestrogens may account for local effects.

The metabolic syndrome (see also Chapter 13)

The link between liver disease and the metabolic syndrome, previously known as syndrome X, has become more clearly established over recent years. The metabolic syndrome is characterized by insulin resistance, obesity, hyperlipidaemia and hypertension. Its associated liver condition, nonalcoholic fatty liver disease (NAFLD), represents a spectrum of disease from steatosis to hepatic necroinflammation (nonalcoholic steatohepatitis, or NASH) to cirrhosis. The diagnosis requires the presence of hepatic steatosis, usually macrovesicular, and the absence of excessive alcohol consumption. The progression of fibrosis within NAFLD has been estimated at 30% and evolution of NASH to cirrhosis estimated at 10–20% [46–48]. The true incidence of cirrhosis related to NAFLD is difficult to know precisely because of the indolent and asymptomatic nature of the disease. Moreover, with advancing disease, the steatosis is replaced by fibrotic tissue and therefore there may be few clues of NAFLD histologically. It is thought that a significant proportion of patients provisionally diagnosed with cryptogenic cirrhosis have underlying NAFLD. This is evidenced by studies showing a greater incidence of diabetes and obesity in cryptogenic cirrhosis compared with cirrhosis of other causes [49–51].

The exact pathophysiological mechanisms of NAFLD are incompletely understood. The interplay of insulin resistance and hepatic steatosis has a major role, with one worsening the other. Triglyceride accumulation is thought to result from excess free fatty acid influx into the liver. The 'second hit' may come from a variety of sources, including oxidative stress, endotoxins and cytokines, and leads to necroinflammation.

The production of hormones and cytokines from fat depots, termed adipokines, is also thought to have a role in the evolution of NASH. Individuals with NASH have been shown to have low levels of adiponectin and high levels of TNFα [52]. Whilst TNFα promotes insulin resistance and liver inflammation, adiponectin antagonizes fatty acid oxidation and reduces the production and activity of TNFα. In addition, adiponectin is antifibrotic. The hormone leptin has been shown to be important in the development of fibrogenesis in animal models. The fibrotic response, absent in leptin-deficient mice, becomes apparent once leptin is restored by exogenous injection [53]. Also, higher serum leptin concentrations are found in patients with NASH compared with controls [54]. Research continues into the pathogenic roles of the adipokines and how they interact in patients with NASH. A more comprehensive review of the pathophysiology, treatment and management of NAFLD is given in Chapter 13.

Clinical features of endocrine disturbance

The endocrine stigmata of cirrhosis include spider angiomas and palmar erythema (Table 2). Spider angiomas are classically described as lying in the distribution of the vascular territory of the superior vena cava, but occasionally they occur outside this area. They consist of a central arteriole surrounded by smaller vessels. When sufficiently large, they can be seen or felt to pulsate. The lesion can be seen to disappear by applying pressure to the central region. Occasionally they may grow to cover a large area when the diagnosis may be mistaken. Their aetiology is thought to be related to oestrogen metabolism and can occur in other conditions including pregnancy, rheumatoid arthritis and oestrogen therapy.

Palmar erythema manifests with a bright-red coloration of the thenar and hypothenar eminences and pulps of the fingers. The soles of the feet may also be affected. Palmar erythema can coexist with spider angiomas but the two conditions also appear independently. The reason for the development of palmar erythema is obscure. White nails (leuconychia) occur due to an opacity of the nail bed. A small pink zone at the tip of the nail is preserved. The condition occurs bilaterally.

Foetor hepaticus is a sweet, faecal smell on the breath. It may represent a failure of hepatic detoxication function and is likely to have an intestinal origin, being more pronounced when there is an extensive collateral circulation and lessening after the use of broad-spectrum antibiotics.

In patients with the clinical suspicion of NASH, certain phenotypic features may be present. A history of type 2 diabetes and hypertension is suggestive of the presence of the underlying metabolic syndrome. Central obesity, and in particular an enlarged waist to hip ratio, is a risk factor for the presence of underlying steatohepatitis. Striae can occur with the use of steroids and pregnancy, but may also occur in rapid weight loss; the latter is a risk factor for NASH.

Miscellaneous features of cirrhosis

The patient with cirrhosis may have nonspecific symptoms such as fatigue, weight loss and depression. Furthermore, conditions such as gallstones and peptic ulcers have been reported to be higher in this patient subgroup [55,56].

Finger clubbing, hypertrophic osteoarthropathy, Dupuytren's contractures, parotid gland enlargement and muscle cramps may also be seen in cirrhosis although they are not specific to this condition (Table 2).

Diagnosis

The diagnosis of cirrhosis is based on a histological definition and therefore liver biopsy has been regarded as the 'gold standard'. But liver biopsy is not without its problems (see below). In practical clinical terms, a diagnosis of 'cirrhosis' is sometimes made in the presence of indicative clinical features, with serum and imaging results which map to a diagnosis (e.g. primary biliary cirrhosis). Therefore, the utilization of clinical, biochemical, haematological, endoscopic and radiological tools is vital in the diagnosis of cirrhosis and its associated complications (see also Chapter 6.2).

Clinical

A careful history and examination is important to ascertain aetiological clues and assess the severity of disease. A history of thyroid disease or family history of autoimmune conditions may suggest a predisposition to autoimmune liver disease. Medication is of relevance as certain drugs may directly cause hepatotoxicity (see Table 1) or may be prescribed for conditions that can be associated with fibrosis and cirrhosis: for example, oral hypoglycaemics prescribed in the context of type 2 diabetes. Furthermore, a thorough clinical examination will not only give rise to aetiological clues but may also indicate how far fibrosis has progressed. For example, a middle-aged man presenting with a history of intravenous drug abuse and signs of portal hypertension raises the clinical suspicion of chronic hepatitis C that has progressed to possible cirrhosis. In the history, careful attention to ethnic background, occupation, family history, blood transfusions, history of sexual contacts, history of participation in mass inoculation programmes, recreational drug use, alcohol consumption and medications is important. These details will influence the diagnostic tests requested and augment their findings.

Biochemical and haematological investigations in the clinical setting

A detailed description of blood tests used to diagnose and monitor liver disease is given in Chapter 5.2. The following section will address investigations of particular relevance to cirrhosis. It should be stated that individual haematological and biochemical tests are not diagnostic of cirrhosis but certain patterns do suggest significant underlying disease. The term 'liver function tests', traditionally used for the biochemical description of transaminases, γ-glutamyl transferase and alkaline phosphatase, is something of a misnomer. It could be argued that serum albumin and prothrombin time are a better reflection of underlying synthetic function and hence truer liver function tests.

Transaminases

Alanine aminotransferase (ALT) and aspartate aminotransferase (AST) can be depressed, normal or elevated in cirrhosis. It has been proposed that an AST/ALT ratio of >1 can be helpful in diagnosing cirrhosis in nonalcoholic liver disease [57]. In hepatitis C, the specificity of this ratio appears to be better than the sensitivity [58]. In alcoholic liver disease, the ratio of AST/ALT is >1, independent of the development of cirrhosis. Although usually elevated in cirrhosis, both AST and ALT can be normal in up to 10% and 35% of cases respectively [59].

γ-Glutamyltransferase (γ-GT)

This test is often nonspecifically raised in cirrhosis. Alcoholic liver disease and cholestasis are thought to have a more profound effect on this enzyme compared with other aetiologies.

Alkaline phosphatase

This enzyme is not infrequently raised in cirrhosis; a level greater than threefold the upper limit of normal suggests either intra- or extrahepatic cholestatic aetiology.

Serum albumin

Diminished serum albumin levels are a hallmark of cirrhosis. Hypoalbuminaemia results from a combination of decreased synthesis, haemodilution and decreased secretion. However, care needs to be taken in the interpretation of hypoalbuminaemia. For example, intervening sepsis can produce fluctuations in serum albumin.

Hypoglycaemia

This usually is associated with fulminant liver failure, but also with acute alcohol ingestion.

Renal dysfunction

Hyponatraemia is a common finding in cirrhosis. The intrinsic water- and salt-handling abilities of the kidneys are impaired in cirrhosis (Table 5); the appearance of hyponatraemia represents a poor prognostic sign [60]. The injudicious, inappropriate or insufficient use of fluids during hospital admission and use of diuretics will additionally influence serum sodium levels.

Urea and creatinine levels are influenced by underlying muscle mass and protein metabolism. Both urea and creatinine

Table 5 Features of hyponatraemia in cirrhosis.

Splanchnic arterial vasodilatation
Arterial underfilling
Nonosmotic release of vasopressin
Impaired water excretion
Dilutional hyponatraemia

levels can be depressed in cirrhosis. This has particular relevance in monitoring renal function, because a serum creatinine within the 'normal range' may be indicative of significant deterioration in glomerular function.

Serum globulin

There is a polyclonal increase in immunoglobulins in cirrhosis. The subtype of immunoglobulins increased will depend on the aetiology of disease, for example, increased IgA in alcoholic cirrhosis, IgG in autoimmune cirrhosis and IgM in biliary cirrhosis.

Prothrombin time

This is a useful marker of synthetic function in cirrhosis. Alone or in combination with other serum tests it has been used in screening tests for cirrhosis. The prothrombin time (PT) is the best day-to-day parameter of hepatic function because of the half-life of clotting factors. The PT is also exquisitely sensitive to conditions of vitamin K deficiency, and this may supervene in the ill cirrhotic patient, particularly after extensive malnourishment. Thus, the PT should be measured in the context of replete vitamin K levels.

The above are general biochemical and haematological investigations. In addition, specific investigations to find the cause of the underlying liver disease may be required, for example antimitochondrial antibody in primary biliary cirrhosis, urinary copper excretion in Wilson's disease, transferrin saturation in haemochromatosis, antibodies to and RNA levels of hepatitis C virus, etc. (see Chapter 5.4 for more details).

Imaging techniques valuable in cirrhosis
(see also Chapter 6.2)

Ultrasound

Ultrasound is a relatively noninvasive method of assessing the size, texture and vascular patency of the liver and for detecting space-occupying lesions in the liver. The former parameters may change in cirrhosis, but unfortunately are not specific to the condition. The cirrhotic liver may be enlarged (e.g. nonalcoholic steatohepatitis), normal or reduced in size. The echo pattern of the liver is frequently described as coarse (increased irregular echogenicity) in cirrhosis but can alternatively be small and nodular. Care must be taken in the interpretation of these findings as they are subjective and, additionally, conditions such as fatty infiltration, granulomatous disease and diffuse malignant infiltration can produce a similar textural appearance. Ultrasound is able to detect certain complications of cirrhosis, such as ascites and splenomegaly. Additionally, it is a useful, initial investigation in the patient with liver disease and jaundice to exclude extrahepatic causes of biliary obstruction.

Doppler ultrasound provides a technique to measure blood flow in the portal vein, hepatic artery and hepatic veins. It measures the frequency differences between the ultrasound signal emitted from the transducer and returned from the vessel to

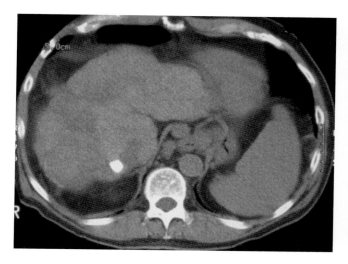

Fig. 2 CT image of a hepatocellular carcinoma, enhanced by lipiodal, on the background of a cirrhotic liver.

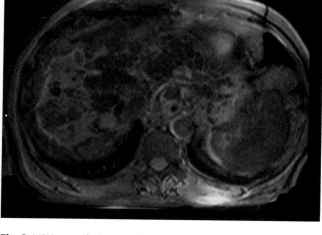

Fig. 3 MRI image of a liver showing dense uptake of Resovist® by a nodule on the background of cirrhosis.

generate direction and velocity of flow. The major vascular changes seen in cirrhosis reflect underling portal hypertension. They include reversal of portal vein blood from hepatopetal to hepatofugal, flattening of the Doppler waveform in hepatic veins and enlargement of the portal vein to greater than 15 mm.

Ultrasound has a further role in detecting the development of HCC on the background of cirrhosis. Isolated nodules larger than 2 cm are detected with good sensitivity but lower specificity. In combination with an elevated alpha-fetoprotein, the presence of HCC can be suspected (see 'Follow-up and screening' below). The performance of ultrasound in the presence of diffuse malignancy is poor.

Computed tomography (CT)

CT also has a role in assessing parenchymal disease in cirrhosis. The density of liver parenchyma is usually within the normal range but can vary depending on aetiology – for instance, it increases in haemochromatosis and decreases in fatty infiltration. The advantage of CT is that it provides cross-sectional anatomy. With the advent of multislice CT scanning, detailed information about space-occupying lesions can be gleaned. Furthermore, the addition of contrast agents such as lipiodal may improve detection of HCC. Helical CT can also visualize vascular anomalies of lesions by obtaining images in the arterial or portal phase. For example, HCC typically will have a brisk enhancement during the arterial phase (Fig. 2) but appears hypodense during the portal phase. Direct catheterization of the superior mesenteric artery and hepatic artery can also be used in combination with CT to improve diagnostic accuracy. Therefore, CT in isolation or in combination with arteriography is able to provide a 'road map', highlighting the blood supply of lesions or vascular anomalies that occur in the context of cirrhosis.

Magnetic resonance imaging (MRI)

This modality represents an emerging tool in liver disease. Dramatic and remarkably clear images of cirrhosis can be obtained in advanced disease (Fig. 3). There is evidence for the use of MRI in assessing hepatic iron concentration [61] and differentiating small benign nodules and HCC [62]. Injection of Resovist® may help distinguish lesions of focal nodular hyperplasia and HCC. MRI spectroscopy is currently an experimental tool but may yet emerge to provide a measure of metabolic changes within the liver; its role in the assessment of cirrhosis is hitherto unproven.

Arteriography

Arteriography does not a have a major diagnostic role in cirrhosis *per se*. It may be a useful additional investigation for HCC and remains the gold standard for the delineation of hepatic vasculature. Occasionally, the attenuated and tortuous arterial patterns seen in cirrhosis are observed when arteriography is performed for another indication, a finding that can be diagnostically useful.

Miscellaneous

Radionuclide scans and positron emission tomography (PET) scans are both emerging examples of other imaging modalities for cirrhosis. Neither technique has yet become widespread. PET imaging based on metabolic changes, particularly in ammonia and glucose metabolism, has been effectively focused on changes in the brain related to encephalopathy.

The role of radiology also extends to the diagnosis of complications arising in the presence of cirrhosis. For example, patients with cirrhosis have a higher incidence of gallstones. Gallstones within the common bile duct are not adequately visualized by ultrasound and mild intrahepatic biliary duct dilatation may be more difficult to detect within a cirrhotic liver. Thus, magnetic resonance cholangiopancreatography (MRCP) is a useful non-invasive tool. If gallstones are found, patients can then be selected for endoscopic retrograde cholangiopancreatography (ERCP) or cholecystectomy for therapeutic intervention. Radiology is also valuable in the diagnosis of specific malignant complications of fibrotic and cirrhotic processes, such as the presence of a dominant stricture or cholangiocarcinoma on the background of primary sclerosing cholangitis. A combination of investigations including helical CT, MRCP and ERCP may be required, depending on the site of the lesion, to reach a diagnosis.

Endoscopy

It is not uncommon for the cirrhosis to present initially with gastrointestinal haemorrhage. Portal hypertension may be suspected at endoscopy by the presence of varices. Although these can occur at the site of any collateral circulation, they commonly occur in the lower oesophagus and gastric fundus. Bleeding, particularly in the context of a coaguloapthy, may also occur from portal gastropathy, which typically gives a 'snake-skin appearance' to the gastric mucosa. It is important to remember that approximately 50% of upper gastrointestinal bleeding episodes in a patient with cirrhosis may arise from lesions other than varices.

Histology

As alluded to earlier in this chapter, histological analysis remains the 'gold standard', and arguably from the purist's standpoint, the only method of diagnosing cirrhosis. Various histological classifications exist for the grading of fibrosis and cirrhosis including Scheuer, Ishak, Knodell and Metavir [63–65]; the majority of scores were originally validated for hepatitis C. A more detailed account of histological analysis and classification is given in Section 4.

The method for obtaining a liver biopsy can vary from the blind versus image-guided transabdominal approach, transjugular approach, laparoscopic approach and open approach at operation or post mortem. The choice of route will depend on factors such as body habitus, clotting abnormalities, the presence of ascites, available expertise and the quantity of specimen required (see Chapter 5.5 for more details).

The biopsy provides information in three major areas. Firstly, it can elucidate aetiology: for example, marked accumulation of iron in the hepatic parenchyma suggests haemochromatosis whereas biliary duct damage associated with granulomas raises the suspicion of primary biliary cirrhosis. Secondly, it stages the severity of fibrosis and presence of cirrhosis. Thirdly, it can also act as a prognostic indicator. For example, in the context of hepatitis C, inflammation in the biopsy is suggestive of future fibrosis [66].

Liver biopsy does have its limitations and some have questioned whether it truly represents a 'gold standard' reference test. In large studies of patients undergoing biopsy, pain has been reported in 20% and severe complications reported in 0.57% [67]. Sampling error exists, which is unsurprising considering the average biopsy specimen represents just 1/50 000th of the organ. Studies have shown discordance rates of up to 30% or more when right and left lobes are sampled laparoscopically, even in homogeneously distributed disease [68]. Interpretation of the biopsy is open both to intra- and interobserver error [69,70]. Morphometry allows an automated assessment of fibrosis, but hitherto the finer points of staging disease by pathologists have been difficult to replicate.

Surrogate markers

There has been considerable interest in finding surrogate markers of cirrhosis and liver fibrosis as an alternative to liver biopsy. Serum tests include markers of matrix turnover such as hyaluronic acid and procollagen of PIIINP [71–73]; more recently, panels of serum tests that produce a continuous score using algorithms have been published [74–78]. A systematic review of serum tests in the context of hepatitis C suggested that these markers, particularly panel markers, showed promise [79]. The tests in general are more robust in distinguishing cirrhosis from mild disease whereas they are less effective in differentiating more subtle variations such as moderate versus mild fibrosis.

The surrogate markers, however, still have significant limitations even in the context of cirrhosis. They are unable to provide aetiological clues to disease and, whilst this may not be required in diseases with good diagnostic tests such as hepatitis C, it may be more relevant in cases of cryptogenic cirrhosis or where there is a question concerning dual aetiology. The subtle aspects of architectural disturbance, fibrosis distribution and neovascular formation can only be seen on biopsy. On the positive side, surrogate markers largely offer a continuous scale for the diagnosis of fibrosis and cirrhosis, although the thresholds with high sensitivities and specificities tend to occur at the extremes of the scale and are not applicable to the majority of the population tested. The correlation of serum markers to clinical outcomes may overcome some of the limitations of using liver biopsy as a gold standard. Furthermore, surrogate markers may prove most useful in the serial monitoring of an individual or in the assessment of the effectiveness of intervention (e.g. antifibrotic trial).

Despite reservations, there is a continuing search for surrogate markers using more powerful technologies and varying combinations of markers. For example, it may be possible to bring serum markers together with imaging in an algorithm that gives clinically valuable sensitivities and specificities for the diagnosis and monitoring of cirrhosis.

Differential diagnosis

The differential diagnosis will depend on the mode of presentation. This is best illustrated by the use of clinical examples.

A patient presents with marked jaundice and signs of portal hypertension. The causes of jaundice are multiple (see Table 2) and include haemolysis, biliary obstruction, decompensated liver disease and fulminant liver failure. Tests that will diagnose haemolysis include unconjugated/conjugated bilirubin, reticulocyte count, haptoglobulin, a Coombs test and blood film. The presence of signs of encephalopathy – decreased conscious level, rapidly deteriorating synthetic function (occasionally seen early after presentation) and hypoglycaemia – is highly suggestive of fulminant hepatic failure. Finally, radiological investigation with ultrasound, CT and MRCP may be required to exclude the presence of a supervening HCC, cholangiocarcinoma or biliary tract disease.

A patient presents with ascites and deranged liver function tests. The causes of ascites need to be considered. A diagnostic ascitic tap is required for microbiology, cytology and the serum–ascites albumin gradient to be calculated. A gradient of 2 g/dL with findings of portal hypertension on ultrasound may then narrow the diagnosis to cirrhosis, veno-occlusive disease (VOD), congestive heart failure and constrictive pericarditis. The last two differentials potentially could be excluded by clinical findings or, where doubt remains, by echocardiography. This leaves VOD and cirrhosis, which may require more detailed radiology or a liver biopsy to disentangle.

The final example is a patient presenting with an acute upper gastrointestinal haemorrhage and jaundice. An endoscopy shows bleeding oesophageal varices suggesting portal hypertension. Clinical findings of emaciation and parotid gland enlargement accompanying biochemical test results of a raised γ-GT and AST/ALT ratio of >1 would further suggest alcohol as the major aetiological factor. If this patient also had recurrent attacks of pancreatitis, the possibility of portal vein thrombosis would need to be excluded by radiological investigation. If portal vein thrombosis was present, three differentials could still exist: alcoholic cirrhosis with secondary portal vein thrombosis, portal vein thrombosis secondary to pancreatic inflammation and/or liver disease but not cirrhosis, and cirrhosis accompanying a portal vein thrombosis caused by pancreatic inflammation. Detailed histological and radiological assessment will therefore be required to reach the final diagnosis.

Prognosis

The prognosis will depend on the underlying aetiology of disease, the continuing presence or cessation of aetiological factors, stage of disease progression and underlying residual capacity of the liver. For example, in patients with alcoholic liver disease, if they are able to maintain abstinence over time they will have a prognosis similar to healthy individuals. If symptoms of decompensation have occurred, prognosis is adversely affected. In alcoholic liver disease, 5-year survival is 90% in compensated cirrhosis but falls to 30% in decompensated disease [80].

Prognostic models are either generalized or more disease specific. Examples of disease-specific prognostic scores include the Mayo model of primary biliary cirrhosis. Generalized prognostic models include the Child–Turcotte score and the modified Child–Pugh score [81]. The original purpose of the score was to assess the operative risks of patients undergoing

Table 6 Criteria for Child–Turcotte classification.

	A	B	C
Serum bilirubin (mg/100 mL)	<2.0	2.0–3.0	>3.0
Serum albumin (g/100 mL)	>3.5	3.0–3.5	<3.0
Ascites	None	Easily controlled	Poorly controlled
Neurological disorders	None	Minimal	Severe, coma
Nutrition	Excellent	Good	Poor, 'wasting'

Table 7 Criteria for modified Child–Pugh.

	1	2	3
Serum bilirubin (mg/100 mL)	<2.0	2.0–3.0	>3.0
Serum albumin (g/100 mL)	>3.5	2.8–3.5	<2.8
Prothrombin (seconds prolonged)	1–4	4–6	>6
Encephalopathy (grade)	None	1 and 2	3 and 4
Ascites	Absent	Slight	Moderate
For primary biliary cirrhosis:			
Bilirubin (mg/100 mL)	1–4	4–10	>10
Bilirubin (µmol/L)	17–68	68–170	>170

Each parameter is assigned a score from 1 to 3:
Child's A: 0–6
Child's B: 7–9
Child's C: 10–15

portosystemic shunts, but it has evolved into a model for assessing prognosis in liver disease. Tables 6 and 7 show the parameters that constitute the score.

More recently the Model for End-Stage Liver Disease (MELD) has been developed to guide prioritization in liver transplantation. There are parallels to the Child–Pugh score as the MELD was originally developed to predict survival in patients undergoing TIPS. It has subsequently been validated in different disease aetiologies and centres [82,83]. The formula for the MELD score is:

$$3.8 \log_e[\text{bilirubin (mg/dL)}] + 11.2*\log_e(\text{INR})$$
$$+ 9.6 \log_e[\text{creatinine (mg/dL)}]$$
$$+ 6.4 \text{ (aetiology: 0 cholestatic or alcoholic, 1 otherwise)}$$

The advantages of MELD over the Child–Pugh score include the use of objective parameters and its greater discriminatory ability; it is rapidly gaining acceptance as a method for prioritizing patients awaiting transplantation.

Treatment

General

Ultimately the goal in cirrhotic liver disease is identification of the aetiology and, when possible, to treat the underlying disease to prevent the progression and promote the reversal of disease. Patients generally present when disease is advanced and important supportive measures may be required.

Nutrition

Nutritional management must be active. As discussed above and in Chapter 23.2, patients with cirrhosis are catabolic and, particularly alcoholics, may have profound nutritional deficiencies. In the short term, a reduction in caloric intake has been shown to be an independent risk factor for mortality [84]. This study observed that enteral feeding was often initiated late and to patients who had advanced liver dysfunction. Overnight nasogastric feeding (ng) can be a useful measure, allowing patients to eat meals during the day. By feeding patients in an upright position, gastro-oesophageal reflux and pulmonary aspiration can be reduced. Enteral nutrition may be in the form of a polymeric diet, hypercaloric diet, hyperproteinic diet or a combination of these depending on nutritional requirements. Previously, there was a school of thought advocating the avoidance of high-protein diets in cirrhotic patients to prevent hepatic encephalopathy. This view is no longer widely held and nutritional repletion should be considered paramount. In individuals for whom protein feeding is associated with encephalopathy, the dietary/supplemental intake can be adjusted.

Nutritional support has also been shown to have beneficial effects in specific conditions. For example, in a randomized controlled trial of patients with alcoholic hepatitis, patients in the enteral nutrition arm had similar short-term survival and improved 1-year survival compared with the corticosteroid arm [85].

Haemodynamic consequences of cirrhosis

The complications of variceal haemorrhage will require endoscopic, pharmacological and radiological intervention in isolation or combination as discussed in Chapter 7.3. The prevention of ascites by vigilance over salt and water intake may be possible during the earlier stages of disease. However, in more advanced disease, specific intervention may be required in the form of large volume paracentesis or TIPS. Large multicentre controlled trials are divided about the benefit of TIPS versus paracentesis [86–89], as discussed in Section 7.5, but it seems likely that a consensus on TIPS as a treatment for ascites will emerge in the near future.

Orthotopic liver transplant (see Section 25)

The indications for liver transplantation will depend on the underlying aetiology and presence of complications such as diuretic resistance ascites, encephalopathy, hepatorenal syndrome, etc. Liver transplantation offers potentially curative treatment in toxic and metabolic conditions such as alcoholic liver disease and Wilson's disease. However, in the context of viral hepatitis or NASH, recurrence can frequently occur and may take a more aggressive form with rapid progression to fibrosis. There are also limits on resources, even when the evolving practice of living donor transplantation is taken into consideration. The complications listed above, which may be the indication for orthotopic liver transplantation (OLT), will also influence the success and postoperative recovery. Thus, OLT, whilst still offering the best available treatment for endstage liver disease, is not universally available, or without its problems, including those associated with long-term immunosuppression. See Chapter 25 for a more detailed review.

Antifibrotic drugs

There are a number of antifibrotic agents, as discussed in detail in Section 6.2. There have been a small number of published trials utilizing specific antifibrotic strategies (e.g. colchicine, interferon-gamma and peroxisome proliferator-activated receptor (PPAR) ligands) in patients with fibrosis [90]. Although the data from these trials are encouraging, the consensus opinion is that an effective, inexpensive and safe antifibrotic is so far unavailable. There are ongoing randomized controlled trials looking at novel targets, both in the context of fibrosis and cirrhosis. Patients with established cirrhosis are the most difficult to treat yet they may have the most to gain because of dwindling hepatic reserve. The other interesting question posed is what constitutes a success in treatment in this group – reversal in histological parameters, clinical outcomes, or both (see Chapter 6.1 for discussion of reversal of cirrhosis).

Follow-up and screening

Patients with compensated cirrhosis are at risk of developing the complications listed above. Careful follow-up may help to prevent or detect them at an early stage. Of particular relevance are the issues of upper gastrointestinal varices and HCC. Elective endoscopy to detect varices remains the gold standard diagnostic test, although there has been interest in noninvasive tests [91]. In the presence of varices, primary prophylaxis is recommended by either pharmacological means (e.g. beta-blockers) or band ligation in those intolerant to medication.

Screening for HCC remains controversial (see Chapter 18.2). The majority of HCC (80–90%) arise on the background of cirrhosis [92], and it has been estimated that the annual risk of developing HCC in this context is 1–5% per year. Therefore, it could be argued that this represents a good population to screen. Additionally, the screening tools of ultrasound and alpha-fetoprotein (AFP) are widely available and have a negligible morbidity. The sensitivity and specificity of these tests varies from 60 to 90%. Ultrasound has a subjective element and is operator dependent whilst the specificity of AFP is reduced by regeneration, which occurs in the context of cirrhosis and fluctuating viral replication. However, there is no substantive evidence that screening using ultrasound and AFP reduces mortality and there is no consensus that screening is cost effective [93]. The reasons for this may be due to, firstly, the inability to detect tumours at a stage that is amenable to treatment. Secondly, although there are a number of treatment modalities, including resection, chemoembolization and radiotherapy ablation, only OLT prevents *de novo* HCC from arising in the future. The latter is limited by resources, and by the time an appropriate graft is available the disease may have progressed. Despite the lack of firm evidence, many clinicians choose to screen patients with cirrhosis on a 6-monthly basis with ultrasound and AFP. With improving diagnostics and therapy, there may be stronger evidence for screening in the future.

The transition from compensated disease into decompensated disease will usually be self-evident and often requires emergency admission. There will also be cases of insidious progression with reducing reservoirs of hepatic function. In these cases, the timing of liver transplantation is crucial and careful attention to clinical, nutritional and biochemical trends is required over a period of time.

References

1 Anthony PP, Ishak KG, Nayak NC *et al.* (1978) The morphology of cirrhosis. Recommendations on definition, nomenclature, and classification by a working group sponsored by the World Health Organization. *J Clin Pathol* 31, 395–414.

2 Chedid A (2000) Regression of human cirrhosis. *Arch Pathol Lab Med* 124, 1591–1593.

3 Graudal N, Leth P, Marbjerg L, Galloe AM (1991) Characteristics of cirrhosis undiagnosed during life: a comparative analysis of 73 undiagnosed cases and 149 diagnosed cases of cirrhosis, detected in 4929 consecutive autopsies. *J Intern Med* 230, 165–171.

4 Haellen J, Norden J (1964) Liver cirrhosis unsuspected during life: a series of 79 cases. *J Chronic Dis* 17, 951–958.

5 Corrao G, Ferrari P, Zambon A *et al.* (1997) Trends of liver cirrhosis mortality in Europe, 1970–1989: age-period-cohort analysis and changing alcohol consumption. *Int J Epidemiol* 26, 100–109.

6 Lessa I (1996) [Liver cirrhosis in Brazil: mortality and productive years of life lost prematurely]. *Bol Oficina Sanit Panam* 121, 111–122.

7 The North Italian Endoscopic Club for the Study and Treatment of Esophageal Varices (1988) Prediction of the first variceal hemorrhage in patients with cirrhosis of the liver and esophageal varices. A prospective multicenter study. *N Engl J Med* 319, 983–989.

8 D'Amico G, Pagliaro L, Bosch J (1995) The treatment of portal hypertension: a meta-analytic review. *Hepatology* 22, 332–354.

9 Runyon BA, Montano AA, Akriviadis EA *et al.* (1992) The serum-ascites albumin gradient is superior to the exudate-transudate concept in the differential diagnosis of ascites. *Ann Intern Med* 117, 215–220.

10 Wong F, Liu P, Allidina Y, Blendis L (1995) Pattern of sodium handling and its consequences in patients with preascitic cirrhosis. *Gastroenterology* 108, 1820–1827.

11 Bernardi M, Trevisani F, Gasbarrini G (1993) Hyperdynamic circulation in cirrhosis: physiology or pathophysiology? *Gastroenterology* 104, 1579–1580.

12 Pozzi M, Grassi G, Redaelli E *et al.* (2001) Patterns of regional sympathetic nerve traffic in preascitic and ascitic cirrhosis. *Hepatology* 34, 1113–1118.

13 Johnston RF, Loo RV (1964) Hepatic hydrothorax: studies to determine the source of the fluid and report of thirteen cases. *Ann Intern Med* 61, 385–401.

14 Schenk P, Schoniger-Hekele M, Fuhrmann V *et al.* (2003) Prognostic significance of the hepatopulmonary syndrome in patients with cirrhosis. *Gastroenterology* 125, 1042–1052.

15 Fallon MB, Abrams GA, Luo B *et al.* (1997) The role of endothelial nitric oxide synthase in the pathogenesis of a rat model of hepatopulmonary syndrome. *Gastroenterology* 113, 606–614.

16 Nunes H, Lebrec D, Mazmanian M *et al.* (2001) Role of nitric oxide in hepatopulmonary syndrome in cirrhotic rats. *Am J Respir Crit Care Med* 164, 879–885.

17 Taille C, Cadranel J, Bellocq A *et al.* (2003) Liver transplantation for hepatopulmonary syndrome: a ten-year experience in Paris, France. *Transplantation* 75, 1482–1489.

18 Swanson KL, Wiesner RH, Krowka MJ (2005) Natural history of hepatopulmonary syndrome: impact of liver transplantation. *Hepatology* 41, 1122–1129.

19 Lee SS (1989) Cardiac abnormalities in liver cirrhosis. *West J Med* 151, 530–535.

20 Liu H, Song D, Lee SS (2002) Cirrhotic cardiomyopathy. *Gastroenterol Clin Biol* 26, 842–847.

21 Myers RP, Lee SS (2000) Cirrhotic cardiomyopathy and liver transplantation. *Liver Transpl* 6(4 Suppl. 1), S44–S52.

22 Velazquez RF, Rodriguez M, Navascues CA *et al.* (2003) Prospective analysis of risk factors for hepatocellular carcinoma in patients with liver cirrhosis. *Hepatology* 37, 520–527.

23 Tsukuma H, Hiyama T, Tanaka S *et al.* (1993) Risk factors for hepatocellular carcinoma among patients with chronic liver disease. *N Engl J Med* 328, 1797–1801.

24 Fattovich G, Stroffolini T, Zagni I, Donato F (2004) Hepatocellular carcinoma in cirrhosis: incidence and risk factors. *Gastroenterology* 127(5 Suppl. 1), S35–S50.

25 Park SZ, Nagorney DM, Czaja AJ (2000) Hepatocellular carcinoma in autoimmune hepatitis. *Dig Dis Sci* 45, 1944–1948.

26 Quero JC, Schalm SW (1996) Subclinical hepatic encephalopathy. *Semin Liver Dis* 16, 321–328.

27 Ferenci P, Lockwood A, Mullen K *et al.* (2002) Hepatic encephalopathy – definition, nomenclature, diagnosis, and quantification: final report of the working party at the 11th World Congresses of Gastroenterology, Vienna, 1998. *Hepatology* 35, 716–721.

28 Italian Multicentre Cooperative Project on Nutrition in Liver Cirrhosis (1994) Nutritional status in cirrhosis. *J Hepatol* 21, 317–325.

29 Alberino F, Gatta A, Amodio P *et al.* (2001) Nutrition and survival in patients with liver cirrhosis. *Nutrition* 17, 445–450.

30 Alvares-da-Silva MR, Reverbel DS (2005) Comparison between hand-grip strength, subjective global assessment, and prognostic nutritional index in assessing malnutrition and predicting clinical outcome in cirrhotic outpatients. *Nutrition* 21, 113–117.

31 Navasa M, Fernandez J, Rodes J (1999) Bacterial infections in liver cirrhosis. *Ital J Gastroenterol Hepatol* 31, 616–625.

32 Borzio M, Salerno F, Piantoni L *et al.* (2001) Bacterial infection in patients with advanced cirrhosis: a multicentre prospective study. *Dig Liver Dis* 33, 41–48.

33 Caly WR, Strauss E (1993) A prospective study of bacterial infections in patients with cirrhosis. *J Hepatol* 18, 353–358.

34 Cirera I, Bauer TM, Navasa M *et al.* (2001) Bacterial translocation of enteric organisms in patients with cirrhosis. *J Hepatol* 34, 32–37.

35 Hassner A, Kletter Y, Jedvab M *et al.* (1979) Impaired monocyte function in liver cirrhosis. *Lancet* i, 329–330.

36 Rajkovic IA, Williams R (1986) Abnormalities of neutrophil phagocytosis, intracellular killing and metabolic activity in alcoholic cirrhosis and hepatitis. *Hepatology* 6, 252–262.

37 Runyon BA, Morrissey RL, Hoefs JC, Wyle FA (1985) Opsonic activity of human ascitic fluid: a potentially important protective mechanism against spontaneous bacterial peritonitis. *Hepatology* 5, 634–637.

38 Wong F, Bernardi M, Balk R *et al.* (2005) Sepsis in cirrhosis: report on the 7th meeting of the International Ascites Club. *Gut* 54, 718–725.

39 Riordan SM, Skinner N, Nagree A *et al.* (2003) Peripheral blood mononuclear cell expression of toll-like receptors and relation to cytokine levels in cirrhosis. *Hepatology* 37, 1154–1164.

40 Iredale JP (2003) Regulating hepatic inflammation: pathogen-associated molecular patterns take their toll. *Hepatology* 37, 979–982.

41 Bernard B, Cadranel JF, Valla D *et al.* (1995) Prognostic significance of bacterial infection in bleeding cirrhotic patients: a prospective study. *Gastroenterology* 108, 1828–1834.

42 Bernard B, Grange JD, Khac EN *et al.* (1999) Antibiotic prophylaxis for the prevention of bacterial infections in cirrhotic patients with gastrointestinal bleeding: a meta-analysis. *Hepatology* 29, 1655–1661.

43 Sort P, Navasa M, Arroyo V *et al.* (1999) Effect of intravenous albumin on renal impairment and mortality in patients with cirrhosis and spontaneous bacterial peritonitis. *N Engl J Med* 341, 403–409.

44 Goulis J, Patch D, Burroughs AK (1999) Bacterial infection in the pathogenesis of variceal bleeding. *Lancet* 353, 139–142.

45 Bannister P, Handley T, Chapman C, Losowsky MS (1986) Hypogonadism in chronic liver disease: impaired release of luteinising hormone. *Br Med J (Clin Res Ed)* 293, 1191–1193.

46 Powell EE, Cooksley WG, Hanson R *et al.* (1990) The natural history of nonalcoholic steatohepatitis: a follow-up study of forty-two patients for up to 21 years. *Hepatology* 11, 74–80.

47 Caldwell SH, Crespo DM (2004) The spectrum expanded: cryptogenic cirrhosis and the natural history of non-alcoholic fatty liver disease. *Journal of Hepatology* 40(4), 578–584.

48 Harrison SA, Torgerson S, Hayashi PH (2003) The natural history of nonalcoholic fatty liver disease: a clinical histopathological study. *Am J Gastroenterol* 98, 2042–2047.

49 Caldwell SH, Oelsner DH, Iezzoni JC *et al.* (1999) Cryptogenic cirrhosis: clinical characterization and risk factors for underlying disease. *Hepatology* 29, 664–669.

50 Poonawala A, Nair SP, Thuluvath PJ (2000) Prevalence of obesity and diabetes in patients with cryptogenic cirrhosis: a case-control study. *Hepatology* 32, 689–692.

51 Sakugawa H, Nakasone H, Nakayoshi T *et al.* (2003) Clinical characteristics of patients with cryptogenic liver cirrhosis in Okinawa, Japan. *Hepatogastroenterology* 50, 2005–2008.

52 Hui JM, Hodge A, Farrell GC *et al.* (2004) Beyond insulin resistance in NASH: TNF-alpha or adiponectin? *Hepatology* 40, 46–54.

53 Leclercq IA, Farrell GC, Schriemer R, Robertson GR (2002) Leptin is essential for the hepatic fibrogenic response to chronic liver injury. *J Hepatol* 37, 206–213.

54 Chitturi S, Farrell G, Frost LC *et al.* (2002) Serum leptin in NASH correlates with hepatic steatosis but not fibrosis: a manifestation of lipotoxicity? *Hepatology* 36, 403–409.

55 Bouchier IA (1969) Postmortem study of the frequency of gallstones in patients with cirrhosis of the liver. *Gut* 10, 705–710.

56 Kirk AP, Dooley JS, Hunt RH (1980) Peptic ulceration in patients with chronic liver disease. *Dig Dis Sci* 25, 756–760.

57 Williams AL, Hoofnagle JH (1988) Ratio of serum aspartate to alanine aminotransferase in chronic hepatitis. Relationship to cirrhosis. *Gastroenterology* 95, 734–739.

58 Park GJ, Lin BP, Ngu MC *et al.* (2000) Aspartate aminotransferase: alanine aminotransferase ratio in chronic hepatitis C infection: is it a useful predictor of cirrhosis? *J Gastroenterol Hepatol* 15, 386–390.

59 Ellis G, Goldberg DM, Spooner RJ, Ward AM (1978) Serum enzyme tests in diseases of the liver and biliary tree. *Am J Clin Pathol* 70, 248–258.

60 Borroni G, Maggi A, Sangiovanni A *et al.* (2000) Clinical relevance of hyponatraemia for the hospital outcome of cirrhotic patients. *Dig Liver Dis* 32, 605–610.

61 Gandon Y, Olivie D, Guyader D *et al.* (2004) Non-invasive assessment of hepatic iron stores by MRI. *Lancet* 363, 357–362.

62 Macdonald GA, Peduto AJ (2000) Magnetic resonance imaging (MRI) and diseases of the liver and biliary tract. Part 1. Basic principles, MRI in the assessment of diffuse and focal hepatic disease. *J Gastroenterol Hepatol* 15, 980–991.

63 Bedossa P, Poynard T (1996) An algorithm for the grading of activity in chronic hepatitis C. The METAVIR Cooperative Study Group. *Hepatology* 24, 289–293.

64 Knodell RG, Ishak KG, Black WC *et al.* (1981) Formulation and application of a numerical scoring system for assessing histological activity in asymptomatic chronic active hepatitis. *Hepatology* 1, 431–435.

65 Scheuer PJ, Standish RA, Dhillon AP (2002) Scoring of chronic hepatitis. *Clin Liver Dis* 6, 335–347, v–vi.

66 Ryder SD, Irving WL, Jones DA *et al.* (2004) Progression of hepatic fibrosis in patients with hepatitis C: a prospective repeat liver biopsy study. *Gut* 53, 451–455.

67 Cadranel JF, Rufat P, Degos F (2000) Practices of liver biopsy in France: results of a prospective nationwide survey. For the Group of Epidemiology of the French Association for the Study of the Liver (AFEF). *Hepatology* 32, 477–481.

68 Regev A, Berho M, Jeffers LJ *et al.* (2002) Sampling error and intra-observer variation in liver biopsy in patients with chronic HCV infection. *Am J Gastroenterol* 97, 2614–2618.

69 Bedossa P, Dargere D, Paradis V (2003) Sampling variability of liver fibrosis in chronic hepatitis C. *Hepatology* 38, 1449–1457.

70 The French METAVIR Cooperative Study Group (1994) Intraobserver and interobserver variations in liver biopsy interpretation in patients with chronic hepatitis C. *Hepatology* 20, 15–20.

71 Patel K, Lajoie A, Heaton S *et al.* (2003) Clinical use of hyaluronic acid as a predictor of fibrosis change in hepatitis C. *J Gastroenterol Hepatol* 18, 253–257.

72 Pares A, Deulofeu R, Gimenez A *et al.* (1996) Serum hyaluronate reflects hepatic fibrogenesis in alcoholic liver disease and is useful as a marker of fibrosis. *Hepatology* 24, 1399–1403.

73 Nojgaard C, Johansen JS, Christensen E *et al.* (2003) Serum levels of YKL-40 and PIIINP as prognostic markers in patients with alcoholic liver disease. *J Hepatol* 39, 179–186.

74 Imbert-Bismut F, Ratziu V, Pieroni L *et al.* (2001) Biochemical markers of liver fibrosis in patients with hepatitis C virus infection: a prospective study. *Lancet* 357, 1069–1075.

75 Forns X, Ampurdanes S, Llovet JM *et al.* (2002) Identification of chronic hepatitis C patients without hepatic fibrosis by a simple predictive model [see comment]. *Hepatology* 36, 986–992.

76 Wai CT, Greenson JK, Fontana RJ *et al.* (2003) A simple noninvasive index can predict both significant fibrosis and cirrhosis in patients with chronic hepatitis C [see comment]. *Hepatology* 38, 518–526.

77 Sud A, Hui JM, Farrell GC *et al.* (2004) Improved prediction of fibrosis in chronic hepatitis C using measures of insulin resistance in a probability index. *Hepatology* 39, 1239–1247.

78 Rosenberg WM, Voelker M, Thiel R *et al.* (2004) Serum markers detect the presence of liver fibrosis: a cohort study. *Gastroenterology* 127, 1704–1713.

79 Gebo KA, Herlong HF, Torbenson MS *et al.* (2002) Role of liver biopsy in management of chronic hepatitis C: a systematic review. *Hepatology* 36(5 Suppl. 1), S161–S172.

80 Alexander JF, Lischner MW, Galambos JT (1971) Natural history of alcoholic hepatitis. II. The long-term prognosis. *Am J Gastroenterol* 56, 515–525.

81 Pugh RN, Murray-Lyon IM, Dawson JL *et al.* (1973) Transection of the oesophagus for bleeding oesophageal varices. *Br J Surg* 60, 646–649.

82 Kamath PS, Wiesner RH, Malinchoc M *et al.* (2001) A model to predict survival in patients with end-stage liver disease. *Hepatology* 33, 464–470.

83 Botta F, Giannini E, Romagnoli P *et al.* (2003) MELD scoring system is useful for predicting prognosis in patients with liver cirrhosis and is correlated with residual liver function: a European study. *Gut* 52, 134–139.

84 Campillo B, Richardet JP, Scherman E, Bories PN (2003) Evaluation of nutritional practice in hospitalized cirrhotic patients: results of a prospective study. *Nutrition* 19, 515–521.

85 Cabré E, Rodriguez-Iglesias P, Caballerzia J *et al.* (2000) Short- and long-term outcome of severe alcohol-induced hepatitis treated with steroids or enteral nutrition: a multicenter randomized trial. *Hepatology* 32, 36–42.

86 Rossle M, Ochs A, Gulberg V *et al.* (2000) A comparison of paracentesis and transjugular intrahepatic portosystemic shunting in patients with ascites. *N Engl J Med* 342, 1701–1707.

87 Gines P, Uriz J, Calahorra B *et al.* (2002) Transjugular intrahepatic portosystemic shunting versus paracentesis plus albumin for refractory ascites in cirrhosis. *Gastroenterology* 123, 1839–1847.

88 Sanyal AJ, Genning C, Reddy KR *et al.* (2003) The North American Study for the Treatment of Refractory Ascites. *Gastroenterology* 124, 634–641.

89 Salerno F, Merli M, Riggio O *et al.* (2004) Randomized controlled study of TIPS versus paracentesis plus albumin in cirrhosis with severe ascites. *Hepatology* 40, 629–635.

90 Rockey DC (2005) Antifibrotic theapy in chronic liver disease. *Clin Gastroenterol Hepatol* 3, 95–107.

91 Pilette C, Oberti F, Aube C *et al.* (1999) Non-invasive diagnosis of esophageal varices in chronic liver diseases. *J Hepatol* 31, 867–873.

92 Simonetti RG, Camma C, Fiorello F *et al.* (1991) Hepatocellular carcinoma. A worldwide problem and the major risk factors. *Dig Dis Sci* 36, 962–972.

93 Di Bisceglie AM (2004) Issues in screening and surveillance for hepatocellular carcinoma. *Gastroenterology* 127(5 Suppl. 1), S104–S107.

7 Portal hypertension and its complications

7.1 Anatomy of the portal venous system in portal hypertension

J. Michael Henderson

Normal anatomy of the portal system

Embryology [1]

The development of the portal circulation builds around the two vitelline veins bringing blood from the yolk sac and the two umbilical veins returning the blood from the placenta. The vitelline veins intercommunicate in the septum transversum which is the site of development of the liver sinusoids. The extrahepatic portal venous system develops primarily from the left vitelline vein, which is later joined by the splenic vein to join the portal vein. Portions of both the right and left vitelline veins disappear and the remnant of the right vitelline vein continues as the right branch of the intrahepatic portal vein, while the left branch of the intrahepatic portal vein is formed from the left vitelline vein. The right umbilical vein atrophies; the left maintains its patency and communicates with the liver sinusoids but is directly connected to the sinus venosus. The ductus venosus communicates directly to a large common hepatic vein, bypassing much of the hepatic sinusoids in the fetal circulation, allowing most of the placental blood to bypass the developing liver. Despite this complex development, there are surprisingly few congenital anomalies of the portal venous system.

Gross anatomy [2]

The adult portal venous system includes all the veins that collect blood from the abdominal portion of the alimentary tract, the spleen and the pancreas. The portal vein itself is formed behind the neck of the pancreas by the confluence of the superior mesenteric and splenic veins. It is approximately 6–8 cm long, 1–1.2 cm in diameter, and passes superiorly from the upper margin of the pancreas, behind the duodenum, in the free edge of the lesser omentum, to terminate at the right end of the portahepatis.

The superior mesenteric vein is primarily formed by all the veins draining the small bowel, with significant further contributions of the ileocolic, right colic and middle colic veins. It runs in the root of the mesentery, in front of the third portion of the duodenum to unite with the splenic vein behind the neck of the pancreas. The splenic vein originates at the splenic hilus and runs on the posterior surface of the pancreas transversely to join the superior mesenteric vein behind the neck of the pancreas. The splenic vein receives numerous small feeding branches from the body and tail of the pancreas. The short gastric veins enter the spleen pulp superior to the origin of the splenic vein as does the left end of the gastroepiploic arcade. The third vein to contribute to portal venous inflow is the inferior mesenteric vein which drains blood from the rectum and the left colon. It enters the splenic vein in approximately two-thirds of patients within 1–2 cm of the splenic veins union with the superior mesenteric vein. In one-third of subjects, the inferior mesenteric vein enters directly into the superior mesenteric vein or at its confluence with the splenic vein. Finally, the left gastric, or coronary vein, has a variable entry into the portal venous system usually within 1–2 cm of the confluence, entering the splenic vein approximately 50% of the time and the portal vein in the other 50%.

The portal system carries all the blood from the alimentary tract to the liver and, thus, in the normal subject, all of the above named veins have blood flow directed towards the liver. This is of particular pertinence in portal hypertension because, in these patients, some of these vessels show reversal of blood flow with blood going away from the liver to collateral veins, which shunt directly to the systemic circulation [3].

The gastro-oesophageal junction

The normal venous anatomy of the gastro-oesophageal junction and lower oesophagus is particularly relevant to this chapter on portal hypertension [4–7]. This has been extensively studied by Vianna and colleagues [4]. Their work used the three techniques of radiological study, corrosion casting and morphometry. These studies were performed in specimens of a block of tissue that comprised the lower two-thirds of the oesophagus and the entire intra-abdominal portal circulation. Injections for corrosion casting and for radiographic studies were made by cannulating the splenic vein, ligating obviously leaking sites in the tissue block and proceeding to injection with the test substance.

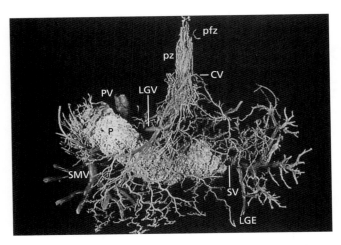

Fig. 1 A corrosion cast of the portal venous system, with emphasis of the upper stomach and lower oesophagus. P, pancreas; SMV, superior mesenteric vein; PV, portal vein; LGV, left gastric vein; LGE, left gastric epiploeic vein; SV, splenic vein; pz, palisade zone; pfz, perforating zone. This corrosion cast of normal blood vessels illustrates how the portal venous system condenses at the gastric fundus to form a tight longitudinal plexus of veins through the lower oesophagus in the palisade zone. (From ref. 4, with permission)

The morphometric studies examined 1-cm slices in the region of interest to document luminal areas of the main venous channels.

These studies documented four distinct zones of venous drainage:

1 The gastric zone, which extends for 2–3 cm just below the gastro-oesophageal junction, is the junctional zone between the stomach and lower oesophagus; the veins are longitudinal rather than the irregular network seen in the rest of the stomach. These veins are in the submucosa and lamina propria and come together at the lower (gastric) end to drain into the short gastric and left gastric veins. This configuration can be seen in Figures 1 and 2 marked as GZ.

2 The palisade zone extends 2–3 cm superiorly from the gastric zone into the lower oesophagus. The veins are uniformly distributed, parallel and run longitudinal in four groups which correspond to the oesophageal mucosal folds. The corrosion casting and radiological imaging of this zone (PZ) are illustrated in Figures 1 and 2. There are multiple anastomoses between these veins, which occupy the lamina propria as illustrated in Figure 3. There are no perforating veins in the palisade zone linking the intrinsic and extrinsic veins of the distal oesophagus. Morphometric study shows that the cross sectional area of the veins at this level is increased compared to other levels. These observations strongly support the palisade zone as being the watershed between the portal and systemic circulation. This is the anatomic location of the lower oesophageal sphincter – a region of the oesophagus of major physiological importance in swallowing and in control of gastro-oesophageal reflux.

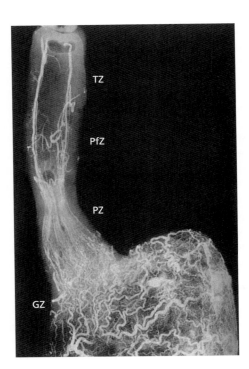

Fig. 2 A postmortem radiograph study of the venous anatomy at the gastro-oesophageal junction in a normal subject. The vessels have been injected with a barium gelatine solution to demonstrate the venous anatomy. GZ, gastric zone; PZ, palisade zone; PfZ, perforating zone; TZ, truncal zone. The network of veins in the gastric fundus condense just below the gastro-oesophageal junction and come together with longitudinal channels in the palisade zone. The perforating veins in the perforating zone can be identified. (From ref. 4, with permission.)

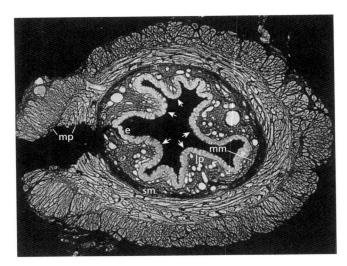

Fig. 3 A morphometric study of a transverse section of the distal oesophagus in a normal subject. This specimen has been injected with barium gelatine and transected 3 cm above the gastro-oesophageal junction. lp, lamina propria; sm, submucosa; mm, muscularis mucosa; e, epithelium; mp, muscularis propria. The white channels in the lamina propria represent the venous channels of the palisade zone which can clearly be seen to congregate in the longitudinal folds of the oesophagus. (From ref. 4, with permission.)

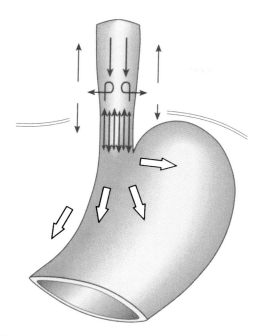

Fig. 4 Diagrammatic representation of the postulated pattern of normal venous drainage of the lower oesophagus. Venous drainage from the gastric fundus and lesser curvature is inferiorly to the portal vein. In the palisade zone, there is to/fro flow that is probably respiration dependent. The perforating veins connect the intrinsic and extrinsic oesophageal plexuses. Flow in the truncal zone is inferior to the perforating zone. (From ref. 4, with permission.)

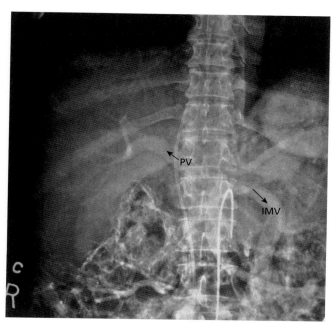

Fig. 5 Venous phase of a superior mesenteric artery injection in a patient with cirrhosis. PV, portal vein; IMV, inferior mesenteric vein. The inferior mesenteric vein fills in a retrograde pattern indicating blood flow away from the liver in this patient with portal hypertension. This large inferior mesenteric vein fills pararectal varices and anastomosis to the haemorrhoidal veins.

3 The perforating zone extends approximately 2 cm further up the oesophagus above the palisade zone. The organized longitudinal structure is lost, with veins looping and forming a network. The main feature of this zone is perforating veins through the muscle wall of the oesophagus linking the internal and external veins. These perforating veins occur circumferentially around the oesophageal wall and are best illustrated in Figure 2.

4 The truncal zone is 8–10 cm long and is characterized by four or five longitudinal veins in the lamina propria, as illustrated in Figure 2. Perforating veins penetrate from the submucosa at irregular intervals to the external oesophageal venous plexus.

The summary of these zones is schematically illustrated in Figure 4, as conceptualized by Vianni and colleagues [4]. This diagram represents the blood flow directions in the four zones described above.

Changes with portal hypertension

Obstruction of portal venous flow, whatever the aetiology, results in a rise in portal venous pressure. The first response to increased venous pressure is the development of a collateral circulation diverting the obstructed portal flow to the systemic

veins [8]. The sites and extent of these collaterals' paths vary and are illustrated in some of the following figures. While some of these collaterals are relatively 'benign', clinically the most important and dangerous are gastro-oesophageal varices. The patterns of development and anatomic variations of these will be described in more detail.

Collateral pathways

Figure 5 illustrates a large inferior mesenteric vein shown at angiography in a patient with cirrhosis and portal hypertension. The flow in this vein is away from the liver towards the rectum and anal canal, which is one of the natural portal–systemic collateral sites. Retrograde flow in the inferior mesenteric vein is a consistent finding in portal hypertension, but only occasionally does the vein enlarge to the size illustrated in this figure.

Figure 6 illustrates a large umbilical vein in a patient with cirrhosis and portal hypertension. The umbilical vein can enlarge from its vestigial size up to 2 cm in diameter and this always communicates with the left portal vein. It runs in the falciform ligament and may give rise to the clinical finding of a caput medusae at the umbilicus. Although the umbilical vein may not always be visualized at angiography, a prominent dye pattern in

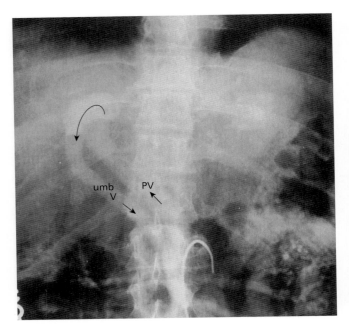

Fig. 6 This venous phase superior mesenteric artery injection demonstrates prograde flow in the portal vein (PV) and hepatofugal flow in the umbilical vein (umb V) carrying blood away from the liver towards the umbilicus. This patient had a caput medusae fed by this large umbilical vein.

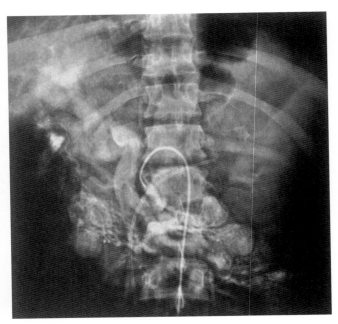

Fig. 8 Venous phase superior mesenteric artery study of cavernous transformation of the portal vein in a patient with portal vein thrombosis. Three large collateral venous channels can be seen in the region of the portal vein and have developed from the obstructed superior mesenteric vein to the low pressure sinusoids in this normal liver.

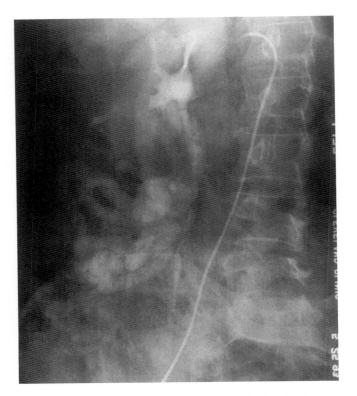

Fig. 7 Venous phase of a superior mesenteric artery injection showing large retroperitoneal collaterals around the terminal ileum, cecum and the right pelvis.

the left portal vein is usually due to the origin of an umbilical vein. Flow in this is again away from the liver depriving the liver sinusoids of portal flow.

Figure 7 illustrates retroperitoneal collaterals with spontaneous shunting to the gonadal vessels. This is more common in female patients where the retroperitoneal collaterals will often communicate with larger ovarian vessels and spontaneously shunt into the iliac veins.

Figure 8 illustrates a patient with portal vein thrombosis and cavernous transformation of the portal vein. Rather than a single portal vein going to this liver, there are three or four very large channels, which demonstrate the preferred collateralization route when there is portal vein thrombosis. It is easier for the obstructed, high pressure superior mesenteric vein to collateralize to the low pressure sinusoids in the liver than to seek the more complex routes illustrated above. A clinical correlation with this abnormality is that an ultrasound exam may demonstrate an apparently good portal flow to the liver, when in reality one is only visualizing one of the large collateral vessels.

Gastro-oesophageal varices

This collateral pathway is of particular clinical importance because of the propensity of these abnormal veins to bleed. In total, 30% of patients identified with compensated cirrhosis and 60% of patients with decompensated cirrhosis have gastro-oesophageal varices at the time of presentation. The risk of

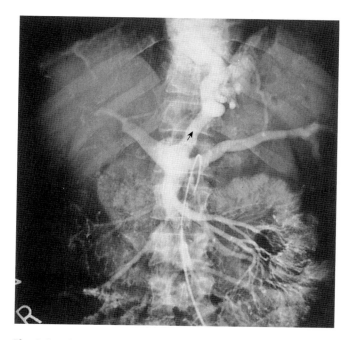

Fig. 9 Superior mesenteric artery injection in a patient with cirrhosis in whom there is no prograde portal flow into the liver although the portal vein is patent. Virtually all of the superior mesenteric venous flow is diverted into a large left gastric vein (↑) filling varices at the gastric fundus (gastric zone) and large paraoesophageal varices around the oesophagus. Note that there is also retrograde filling of the splenic vein.

bleeding from gastro-oesophageal varices is 30% in the first year after their identification [9]. An understanding of the pathophysiology leading to the development of varices and of the anatomic changes around the gastro-oesophageal junction provide some basis for therapies used to reduce the risk of bleeding.

There are two main inflows to gastro-oesophageal varices. The first of these is the left gastric or coronary vein. This may be a major contributor to variceal inflow as illustrated in Figure 9 where virtually all the portal venous flow is diverted into the left gastric vein to gastric fundal and oesophageal varices. In contrast, the patient illustrated in Figure 10 also had a major bleed from gastro-oesophageal varices, yet the left gastric vein is of a very small calibre.

The other major route of inflow for gastro-oesophageal varices is from the splenic hilus through the short gastric veins. This is illustrated in Figure 11, where the dominant venous outflow from the spleen is into gastric varices. The splenic vein is open in this patient with cirrhosis. However, the finding of isolated gastric fundus varices raises the question of isolated splenic vein thrombosis, where all the splenic outflow traverses the short gastric veins to the gastric fundus. The importance of identifying these patients is that they have a normal liver and are

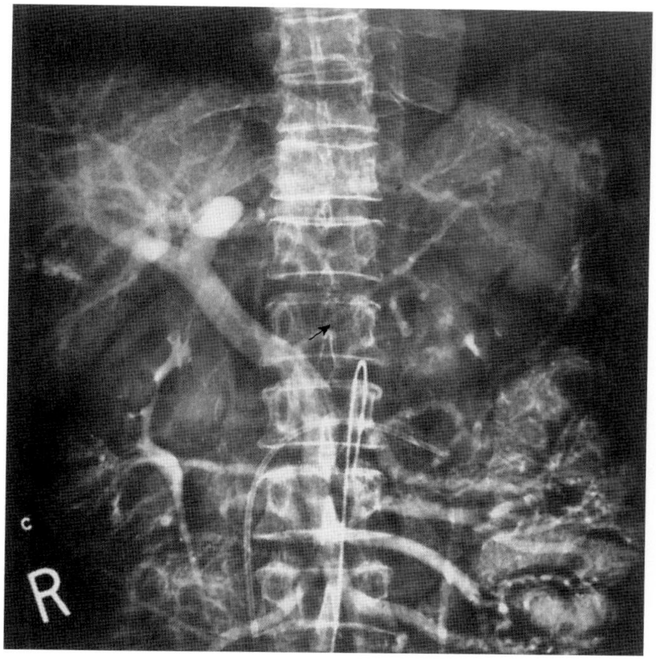

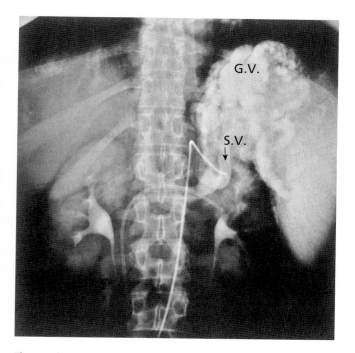

Fig. 11 The venous phase of a splenic artery injection in this patient with cirrhosis demonstrates a tortuous splenic vein (S.V.) and large gastric fundal varices (G.V.). It should be noted that these gastric varices drain through the retroperitoneum into a spontaneous splenorenal shunt with faint visualization of the inferior vena cava. The lower catheter is in the left renal vein which can be seen to drain some of the contrast on this venous phase study.

Fig. 10 Superior mesenteric venous phase study in a patient with cirrhosis who still has good prograde portal flow to the liver. The increased density in the left branch of the portal vein is probably the origin of a large umbilical vein. The arrow indicates a small left gastric vein filling small gastric fundal varices. It should be noted that this patient had significant variceal bleeding.

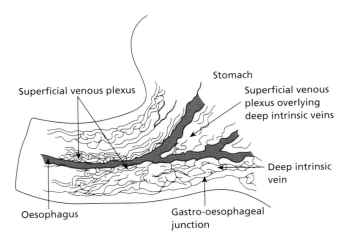

Fig. 12 Schematic representation of a resin cast of the lower oesophagus and upper stomach in a patient with portal hypertension. This cast has been partially dissected with the anterior wall removed to demonstrate the enlarged superficial venous plexus of veins as well as large deep intrinsic veins. These intercommunicate in the gastric zone. (Reprinted from ref. 10, with permission.)

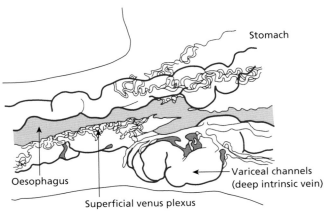

Fig. 13 A resin cast of the lower oesophagus and upper stomach at a later stage of dissection. Two very large, tortuous deep intrinsic variceal channels are demonstrated with overlying superficial venous plexus. For this dissection, some of the superficial venous plexus illustrated in the previous figure has been removed. (Reprinted from ref. 10, with permission.)

cured by splenectomy. The impact of these inflow changes on the venous anatomy at the gastro-oesophageal junction has been studied with the same techniques as those described previously for normal anatomy. The gastric, palisade perforating and truncal zones can again be identified, but undergo significant change in portal hypertension. The two main features of adaptation are dilatation and tortuosity, which are highly variable and do not occur in any constant or regular manner. Dilatation of the veins in the palisade zone is the most clinically problematic as this is the commonest site of rupture and bleeding. In contrast, enlargement of the paraoesophageal varices has less clinical consequence in terms of bleeding risk, but has physiological significance in terms of diverting portal flow.

Resin cast studies by Kitano and coworkers [10] demonstrate the dilatation and tortuosity of both the deep and superficial venous plexuses and are illustrated in Figures 12 and 13. When the deep veins become very large, they can displace the superficial veins and lie immediately beneath the mucosa as illustrated in Figure 13.

Further interesting data were generated by Spence et al. [11] who showed blood-filled channels in the oesophageal squamous epithelium as illustrated in Figure 14. These are apparently fed by communicating channels which erode into the epithelium. The precise relationship of each of these anatomic abnormalities to the event of variceal bleeding has not been fully clarified.

The main vascular patterns that develop in portal hypertension, demonstrated by these various studies, can be summarized as:

1 Varices in the fundus of the stomach are predominantly fed by the short gastric veins but may also be fed by the left gastric vein. From a clinical perspective, gastric varices may either occur 'in continuity' with oesophageal varices or be 'isolated' in the fundus. The latter group have a higher propensity to bleed and are particularly problematic in management.

2 Varices in the gastric and palisade zones form most of the varices seen in clinical practice, are markedly tortuous, numerous and dilated. They run longitudinally in these two zones and are usually in continuity. Because there are no perforating veins in the palisade zone, the submucosal veins are particularly prone to rupture and bleeding. This is the main anatomical site for the clinical problem of bleeding gastro-oesophageal varices.

3 Varices at the perforating and truncal zones – the perforating vessels above the palisade zone – provide a communication between the paraoesophageal varices and the submucosal varices. These perforating pathways can increase the pressure in the submucosal varices and in some patients flow to submucosal vessels will increase the risk of bleeding. Doppler ultrasound studies of perforating veins in patients with portal hypertension have suggested that these may be incompetent and there may be bidirectional flow through the perforators [12]. It has been speculated that turbulence of flow through these incompetent perforators is a risk factor in further bleeding.

4 Paraoesophageal varices are not at risk of bleeding but may develop as very large veins with significant flow. This flow can be measured clinically as azygos blood flow. These channels become important when there are incompetent perforators allowing this high flow to increase submucosal venous pressure and flow.

Anatomic studies of the portal circulation, and particularly the detailed studies of the gastro-oesophageal junction, have increased knowledge as to why and how gastro-oesophageal varices form. This information also provides pointers as to the therapeutic options.

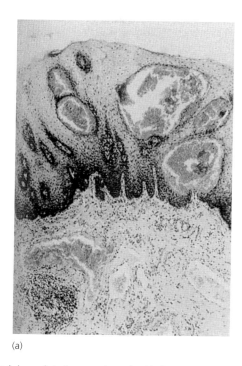
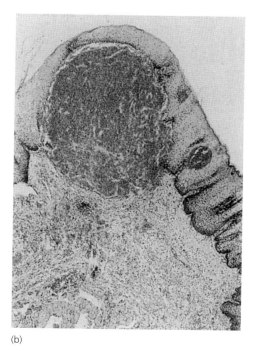

(a)   (b)

Fig. 14 (a) Blood-filled channels in the oesophageal epithelium in a patient with portal hypertension. In addition, there are dilated vessels in the lamina propria. Magnification × 40. (b) A large subepithelial blood-filled channel in a patient with portal hypertension. The smaller intraepithelial channel appears to be arising from papillary capillary present to the right of the larger lesions. Magnification × 26. (Reproduced from ref. 11, with permission.)

References

1 Davies DV, Davies F (1962) *Gray's anatomy – descriptive and applied*. Longmans, Green and Co.

2 Douglas BE, Baggenstoss AH, Hollinshead WH (1979) The anatomy of the portal vein and its tributaries. *Surg Gynecol Obstet* 91, 562–576.

3 Salam AA, Warren WD (1974) Anatomic basis of the surgical treatment of portal hypertension. *Surg Clin North Am* 54(6), 1247–1257.

4 Vianna A, Hayes PC, Moscoso G *et al.* (1987) Normal venous circulation of the gastroesophageal junction. A route to understanding varices. *Gastroenterology* 93(4), 876–889.

5 Butler H (1951) The veins of oesophagus. *Thorax* 6, 276–96.

6 Kegaries D (1934) The venous plexus of the oesophagus. *Surg Gynecol Obstet* 58, 46–51.

7 Noda T (1984) Angioarchitectural study of esophageal varices. With special reference to variceal rupture. *Virchows Archiv A Pathol Anat Histopathology* 404(4), 381–392.

8 Sikuler E, Kravetz D, Groszmann RJ (1985) Evolution of portal hypertension and mechanisms involved in its maintenance in a rat model. *Am J Physiol* 248, G618–625.

9 The North Italian Endoscopic Club for the Study and Treatment of Esophageal Varices (1988) Prediction of the first variceal hemorrhage in patients with cirrhosis of the liver and esophageal varices. A prospective multicenter study. *N Engl J Med* 319(15), 983–989.

10 Kitano S, Terblanche J, Kahn D *et al.* (1986) Venous anatomy of the lower oesophagus in portal hypertension: practical implications. *Br J Surg* 73(7), 525–531.

11 Spence RA, Sloan JM, Johnston GW (1984) Histologic factors of the esophageal transection ring as clues to the pathogenesis of bleeding varices. *Surg Gynecol Obstet* 159(3), 253–259.

12 McCormack TT, Rose JD, Smith PM *et al.* (1983) Perforating veins and blood flow in oesophageal varices. *Lancet* ii, 1442–1444.

7.2 Pathogenesis of portal hypertension

Roberto J. Groszmann and Juan G. Abraldes

Introduction

Portal hypertension is the haemodynamic abnormality most frequently associated with cirrhosis of the liver, although it is also recognized less commonly in a variety of hepatic and extra-hepatic diseases. Many of the most lethal complications of liver cirrhosis are related to the presence of portal hypertension, including haemorrhage from gastro-oesophageal varices, hepatic encephalopathy, ascites and functional renal failure, bacterial infections and hepatopulmonary syndrome. A thorough knowledge of the pathogenesis leading to portal hypertension sets the framework for a rational approach to treatment and is, therefore, central in the management of the patient with liver cirrhosis and in devising rational investigational strategies. This chapter is an overview of the basic pathophysiological mechanisms of the intrahepatic, splanchnic and systemic circulatory derangements involved in the genesis of portal hypertension.

Pathogenesis of portal hypertension: resistance and flow

Ohm's law states that changes in pressure ($P1-P2$) along a blood vessel are a function of the interplay between blood flow (Q) and vascular resistance (R):

$$P1 - P2 = Q \times R$$

It follows that portal hypertension may develop as the result of an increase in portal blood flow, an increase in resistance to portal blood flow, or both. The pathophysiology of portal hypertension is best approached by analysing these components separately, although mathematical formulas necessarily oversimplify the complex and dynamic interactions that exist in biological systems. Resistance to the flow in vessels can be expressed by Poiseuille's law:

$$R = (8nL)/\pi r^4$$

where n is the coefficient of viscosity, L the length of the vessel and r its radius. Under physiological conditions, resistance is mainly a function of changes in r, which have a dramatic influence because these are taken to the fourth power. In contrast, L and n are basically constant because neither the length of a vessel nor the viscosity of blood vary greatly under usual circumstances. The liver is the main site of resistance to portal blood flow, but the liver itself has no active role in regulating portal inflow; this function is provided by resistance vessels at the splanchnic arteriolar level. Hence, the normal liver is a passive recipient of fluctuating amounts of blood flow that, because of its huge and distensible vascular network, can encompass a wide range of portal blood flow with minimal effect on pressure in the portal system. Thus, an increase in portal venous inflow, *per se*, does not induce portal hypertension. This means that the primary and necessary factor for the development of portal hypertension is an increased resistance to portal blood flow [1]. However, once portal hypertension develops, a series of mechanisms (not yet fully characterized) leads to an increase in portal venous inflow, which contribute to perpetuate and aggravate portal hypertension.

Hepatic vascular resistance

In liver cirrhosis, the most frequent cause of portal hypertension in western countries, marked morphological aberrations, characterized by fibrous tissue and regenerative nodules, result in vascular obliteration that leads to increased resistance to blood flow. In the early stages of liver fibrosis, sinusoidal capillarization is probably the initial factor that induces portal hypertension. Capillarized sinusoids are characterized by the accumulation of extracellular matrix in the space of Disse, and sinusoidal endothelial cells that lose their fenestrations and their typical phenotype. This, *per se*, may limit the ability of the sinusoids to accommodate variations in blood flow. In viral hepatitis, this occurs initially in the periportal area, while in alcoholic liver disease, it is predominant at the pericentral area. Later, the development of fibrous septae and regenerative nodules markedly alters the hepatic angioarchitecture. Additionally, it was suggested recently that thrombosis of the small portal and hepatic venules [2] could contribute to increase hepatic resistance and could be an important factor in the progression of the architectural disturbances of cirrhosis. Although these morphological changes are undoubtedly the most important factor, functional factors leading to an increase in intrahepatic vascular tone also contribute to increased hepatic resistance in cirrhosis. The initial demonstration that vasodilators could decrease hepatic resistance in cirrhosis was the key study by Bhathal and Grossman [3], in which the use of the isolated and perfused liver model allowed the evaluation of the changes in hepatic resistance independently from the changes in systemic haemodynamics. It was suggested that up to 30% of the increase in hepatic resistance in cirrhosis is due to an increased vascular tone. There are no convincing studies that have quantified the magnitude of this functional component in patients with cirrhosis, and it is not well known whether its importance changes during the natural history of cirrhosis. This finding set the rationale for the treatment of portal hypertension with vasodilators.

The dynamic component in the increase in hepatic resistance reflects the existence of contractile structures in the liver that modulate hepatic resistance in response to endogenous or pharmacological vasoactive substances. In the normal liver, it has been demonstrated that the hepatic sinusoids can contract, and that changes in sinusoidal calibre colocalize with hepatic stellate cells (HSCs) [4]. These cells, located in the space of Disse, normally act as a deposit for retinoids and regulate the extracellular matrix turnover, but their contractile properties allow HSCs to behave as tissue pericytes that regulate microcirculation through capillary contraction [5]. The contractile capacity of HSCs, already present in the normal liver [4], is particularly important after liver injury, when HSCs acquire an activated phenotype, with increased proliferative, synthetic and contractile capacity, behaving as myofibroblasts [5]. Also, in the normal liver, it has been demonstrated that portal venules contract in response to vasoactive substances [6], but it is unknown whether this contributes to the increased hepatic resistance in cirrhosis. In that regard, data from a rat model of cirrhosis suggest that presinusoidal resistance is decreased in cirrhosis [7]. The same study suggests that the contraction of the postsinusoidal vascular bed could contribute to the increase in hepatic resistance and to ascites formation in cirrhosis. It is uncertain whether these results could be generalized to human cirrhosis.

Several vasoconstrictors and vasodilators have been shown to modify hepatic resistance. These substances can be of hepatic origin and act in a paracrine fashion [nitric oxide (NO), prostacyclin, endothelin, locally produced angiotensin II, thromboxane and leukotrienes], can arrive in the liver from the systemic circulation (circulating angiotensin II, vasopressin or norepinephrine) or can be of neural origin (norepinephrine). It is not known which of these systems is more relevant, but it is clear that in cirrhosis there is an imbalance between vasoconstrictive and vasodilating forces, characterized by an abundance of vasoconstrictors and a deficient production of and deficient response to vasodilators. These abnormalities are amplified by the fact that, compared with the normal liver, the hepatic vascular bed of the

cirrhotic liver exhibits an increased response to vasoconstrictors and a deficient response to vasodilators. In addition, most vasoconstrictors have profibrogenic actions, whereas vasodilators have antifibrogenic properties, so the effects of this imbalance go beyond the increase in intrahepatic vascular tone.

Deficit and hyporesponse to vasodilators

In the early 1990s, it was demonstrated that NO regulates intrahepatic resistance in the normal liver [8]. In the normal liver, sinusoidal endothelial cells respond to increases in shear stress with an increase in NO production. This allows the normal liver to accommodate physiological changes in portal blood flow with minimal changes in portal pressure. In contrast, the cirrhotic liver exhibits endothelial dysfunction, characterized by an insufficient production of NO, that contributes to an increase in hepatic vascular tone (and, thus, to the development and progression of portal hypertension) and a decreased capacity to accommodate increases in flow [9–11] (Fig. 1). The physiological increases in portal blood flow, such as those occurring after the ingestion of a meal, result in marked increases in portal pressure in cirrhotic patients [12]. Recent work in experimental models of cirrhosis have validated hepatic NO deficiency as a useful therapeutic target in cirrhosis, showing that it is possible to improve portal haemodynamics by increasing NO bioavailability in the liver circulation, either by transfection of the liver with adenovirus encoding nitric oxide synthase (NOS) [13] or by the administration of a liver-selective NO donor [14].

The mechanisms leading to the insufficient production of NO in cirrhosis have not been fully clarified. Endothelial nitric oxide synthase (eNOS) expression has been found to be normal [10,11] or decreased [13], while eNOS activity has been found to be consistently decreased. This is due to abnormalities in the complex posttranslational regulation of the enzyme, which include protein–protein interactions, phosphorylation and intracellular localization. Among other mechanisms, interaction with caveolin-1 reduces the activity of eNOS, while Akt-dependent eNOS phosphorylation increases eNOS activity. In the cirrhotic liver, an increase in caveolin-1 expression has been found and increased interaction of this protein with eNOS, with ensuing decreased activity of eNOS [11]. Also, a decrease in Akt-dependent eNOS phosphorylation has been found in the cirrhotic rat liver [15]. The status in the cirrhotic liver of other posttranslational regulatory mechanisms of eNOS has not been explored so far.

On the other hand, the response of the liver circulation to NO is impaired [16]. The mechanisms involved in this abnormality are not well understood, but could involve increased degradation of NO before the molecule reaches its targets (i.e. by increased oxidative stress and superoxide production [17]) or abnormalities at the downstream signal pathways of NO (the most relevant being the cGMP pathway) [18].

Carbon monoxide is another endogenous vasodilator that has been shown to modulate hepatic resistance in the normal

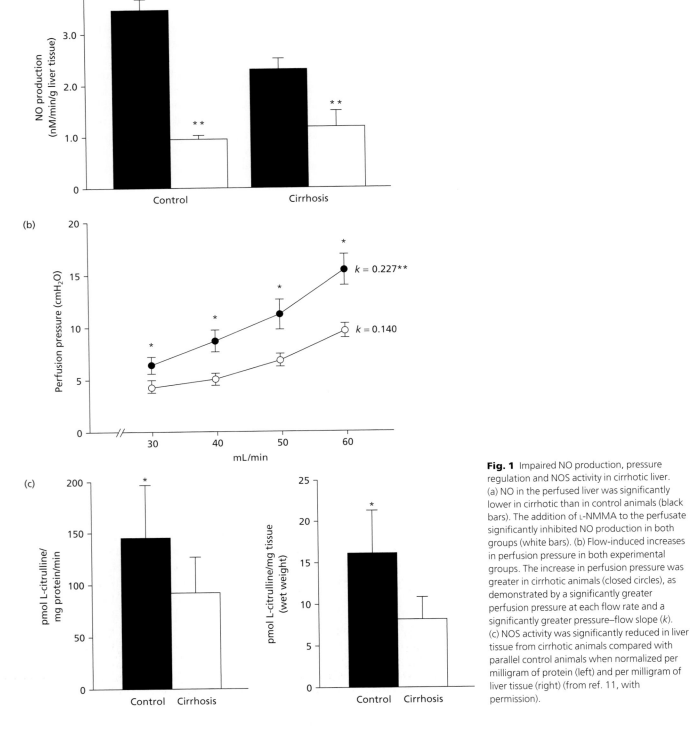

Fig. 1 Impaired NO production, pressure regulation and NOS activity in cirrhotic liver. (a) NO in the perfused liver was significantly lower in cirrhotic than in control animals (black bars). The addition of L-NMMA to the perfusate significantly inhibited NO production in both groups (white bars). (b) Flow-induced increases in perfusion pressure in both experimental groups. The increase in perfusion pressure was greater in cirrhotic animals (closed circles), as demonstrated by a significantly greater perfusion pressure at each flow rate and a significantly greater pressure–flow slope (k). (c) NOS activity was significantly reduced in liver tissue from cirrhotic animals compared with parallel control animals when normalized per milligram of protein (left) and per milligram of liver tissue (right) (from ref. 11, with permission).

liver [19]. In the cirrhotic liver, an increased expression of haemoxygenase-1 (the enzyme responsible for carbon monoxide synthesis) has been demonstrated [20], but its relevance in the pathogenesis of portal hypertension has not been addressed so far.

Increased production and response to vasoconstrictors

As discussed previously, both the normal and the cirrhotic liver vasculatures have contractile capacity. Consequently, infusion of vasoconstrictors increases intrahepatic resistance in the isolated liver [21–23]. In the cirrhotic liver, there is an increase both in local vasoconstrictors produced in the liver itself and in circulating levels of vasoconstrictors [24–26]. Further, the cirrhotic liver exhibits an enhanced response to certain vasoconstrictors with respect to normal liver [7,21,23,27]. This hyper-response has been attributed to different abnormalities, namely an increase in the amount of contractile tissue (proliferation of myofibroblast and activation of HSCs), a deficient production of vasodilators, changes in the expression and sensitivity of the receptors and amplification of the vasoconstrictive response by secondary production of vasoconstrictors. While the first two mechanisms would be non-specific and apply to every vasoconstrictor, the other two would be associated with changes in the signalling pathways of specific vasoconstrictors.

Endothelin

This is the vasoconstrictor that has been most thoroughly studied in the hepatic circulation. However, its role in portal hypertension remains unclear. There is evidence that circulating and intrahepatic levels of endothelin are increased in cirrhosis [25,28], and that endothelin can increase intrahepatic resistance in the isolated liver [29]. Endothelin acts through two receptors: ET-A and ET-B. The former mediates vasoconstriction, while the latter can mediate both vasoconstriction and vasodilation. The vasoconstrictive response of the cirrhotic liver vasculature to endothelin has been found to be both increased [29] and decreased [22] compared with the normal liver, while the vasoconstrictive response to selective ET-B agonists has been shown to be uniformly increased in cirrhosis [22]. On the other hand, activation of HSCs is associated with a change in endothelin receptor pattern from a predominance of ET-A receptors in normal subjects to a predominance of ET-B receptors in cirrhosis [25], which could suggest a change in the sensitivity of HSCs to endothelin. *In vivo* studies have not contributed to the clarification of the role of endothelin in portal hypertension. Acute administration of a mixed ET-A/ET-B receptor blocker seems to decrease portal pressure, whereas chronic administration does not modify portal pressure. On the contrary, chronic selective blockade of ET-A receptor decreases collagen accumulation in a secondary biliary cirrhosis model, whereas acute ET-A blockade to cirrhotic rats does not lower portal pressure [30]. Preliminary results in humans have shown that neither ET-A nor ET-B blockers are able to decrease portal pressure in cirrhotic patients, and that ET-A blockers induce marked hypotension [31]. Therefore, although these results suggest that endothelin might regulate hepatic resistance in the normal and cirrhotic liver, endothelin does not seem to be a useful pharmacological target in portal hypertension in cirrhosis.

Angiotensin II

In patients with advanced cirrhosis, there is a marked activation of the renin–angiotensin system (RAS), which correlates with the severity of portal hypertension [26]. In experimental studies in the isolated liver, angiotensin II infusion increases intrahepatic resistance [21,22], and infusion of angiotensin II through the portal vein of cirrhotic patients increases portal pressure and decreases hepatic blood flow. These effects are probably mediated by the contraction of HSCs which, once activated, express angiotensin II type 1 receptors and contract in response to angiotensin II [32]. Further, HSCs express all the components of the RAS [33], which suggests that not only circulating angiotensin but also locally produced angiotensin II has a role in the increased resistance in cirrhosis. Activation of RAS, however, is a homeostatic process that contributes to maintaining arterial pressure in advanced cirrhosis [34] and, therefore, RAS blockade induces marked hypotension in these patients without a significant decrease in portal pressure [35]. This means that angiotensin II is probably not a useful target for the treatment of portal hypertension, at least in advanced cirrhosis.

Cysteinyl-leukotrienes

These are potent vasoconstrictors that are derived from arachidonic acid through the 5-lipoxygenase (5-LO) pathway. Cysteinyl-leukotriene production is increased in livers from cirrhotic rats, which show an increase in 5-LO expression [24,27]. The isolated cirrhotic liver responds to leukotrienes with a marked increase in intrahepatic resistance, and 5-LO blockade decreases hepatic resistance in cirrhotic livers [27]. There is no information on the *in vivo* haemodynamic effects of 5-LO blockers.

Alpha-adrenergic stimulus

This increases hepatic resistance [21], and this effect is higher in cirrhotic than in normal liver [7,9,23]. This finding cannot be fully explained by a decreased production of NO in the cirrhotic liver [23]. A recent study demonstrated that the cirrhotic liver responds to alpha-adrenergic agonists with an increased endothelial production of thromboxane A_2 mediated by COX-1, which amplifies its vasoconstrictive effect [23,36]. This expands the concept of endothelial dysfunction in cirrhosis, characterized not only by insufficient production of NO but also by increased production of vasoconstrictive prostanoids (Fig. 2). *In vivo* studies have shown that alpha-adrenergic blockade decreases intrahepatic resistance in patients with cirrhosis, but the use of these agents in portal hypertension is hampered by the fact that, like most vasodilators, they not only act in the hepatic circulation, but also induce hypotension [30].

In summary, the cirrhotic liver exhibits a dysregulation in the production of and response to a number of vasconstrictors and vasodilators, and it is likely that more than a single target needs to be hit to effectively decrease intrahepatic resistance in cirrhosis.

Collateral resistance

The development of collaterals in portal hypertension is the key event that leads to severe complications such as variceal bleeding and hepatic encephalopathy. Collaterals develop as a consequence of the pressure increase in the portal system,

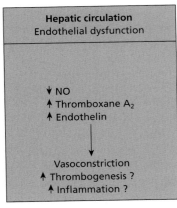

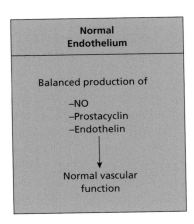

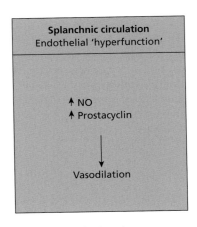

Fig. 2 The endothelium has a central role in the pathophysiology of portal hypertension. In the normal endothelium, a balanced production of vasoconstrictive and vasodilatory substances maintains a normal vascular tone and an anti-inflammatory and antithrombotic environment. In cirrhosis, endothelial dysfunction develops in the intrahepatic circulation, characterized by a decreased production of nitric oxide and an increased production of vasoconstrictive prostanoids and endothelin. This results in an increase in the intrahepatic vascular tone, and probably contributes to create a prothrombogenic and proinflammatory environment. In contrast, in the splanchnic circulation, there is an increase in the endothelial production of nitric oxide, which contributes to splanchnic vasodilation and the ensuing increase in portal blood inflow that maintains and worsens portal hypertension.

allowing the decompression of the portal territory to vascular beds of low pressure. However, this decompression is ineffective, not because these collaterals have a very high resistance but because, in parallel with the development of collaterals, an increase in portal blood inflow maintains portal hypertension.

Collateral formation results in part from the opening and dilation of preformed channels. Additionally, an active angiogenesis process intervenes in collateral formation, and this process is vascular endothelial growth factor (VEGF) dependent. VEGF expression increases in the intestine and mesentery of rats with prehepatic portal hypertension, and VEGF blockade reduces by 50% the development of collaterals in this model [37]. Additional studies showed that collateral formation is also NO dependent [38], raising the possibility that VEGF acts upstream of NO in the collateralization process.

Because as much as 90% of portal blood flow could be shunted through portosystemic collaterals in advanced portal hypertension, changes in collateral resistance can modify portal pressure. A number of studies performed in a model in which the collateral bed is perfused *in situ* have demonstrated that these vessels have functional receptors for vasopressin, endothelin, serotonin and alpha- and beta-adrenergic receptors, and respond to NO with vasodilation [39,40].

Increase in hepatic blood flow: the hyperdynamic circulation

In 1953, Kowalski and Abelman first demonstrated that cirrhosis is associated with a hyperdynamic circulatory syndrome, characterized by a marked decrease in systemic vascular resistance, arterial hypotension and increased cardiac output. These profound alterations in peripheral circulation in liver cirrhosis contribute to the development of complications such as ascites,

hepatorenal syndrome and hepatopulmonary syndrome. Additionally, in the 1970s, a series of studies in patients with liver cirrhosis suggested that the splanchnic circulation was also hyperdynamic, and that not only an increase in hepatic resistance but also an increase in portal blood flow contributed to portal hypertension in cirrhosis [41]. This was unequivocally demonstrated in subsequent studies in rodent models of portal hypertension [42], and set the rationale for the use of vasoconstrictors in the treatment of portal hypertension. The hyperdynamic circulatory state in portal hypertension is the consequence of two pathophysiological phenomena: arterial vasodilation and plasma volume expansion. The presence of both is required for the expression of the hyperdynamic state [34,43,44].

Splanchnic and peripheral vasodilation

At least three mechanisms are thought to contribute to vasodilatation in portal hypertension: (i) increased concentration of circulatory vasodilators; (ii) increased endothelial production of local vasodilators; and (iii) decreased vascular responsiveness to endogenous vasoconstrictors. The last mechanism is probably due to the effect of the first two components.

Circulatory vasodilators

Glucagon Initial studies focused on circulating mediators that would be increased as a result of deficient removal by the liver because of deteriorated liver function and/or portosystemic shunting. Glucagon is probably the humoral vasodilator for which there is the most evidence of a significant role in promoting splanchnic hyperaemia in portal hypertension. Many studies have demonstrated that plasma glucagon levels are elevated in cirrhosis. Hyperglucagonism results, in part, from decreased hepatic clearance but, more importantly, from an increased secretion by pancreatic alpha cells [45]. Support for a role for glucagon in modulating the splanchnic blood flow comes from studies showing that the normalization of the circulating levels of glucagon partially reverses the increased splanchnic blood flow, and this can be prevented by a concomitant glucagon infusion [46]. However, some studies showed no correlation between glucagon levels and splanchnic blood flow, thus questioning a major role for hyperglucagonism in portal hypertension. Glucagon release is clearly implicated in postprandial hyperaemia which, in patients with cirrhosis, is associated with marked increases in portal pressure [47]. Collectively, these data provided the rationale for the use of somatostatin and octreotide in the treatment of patients with portal hypertension, although it has been demonstrated recently that these drugs promote vasoconstriction by mechanisms independent of those of glucagon inhibition [48].

Endocannabinoids In rats and in patients with advanced cirrhosis, there is an increase in the production of the endogenous cannabinoid anandamide by monocytes [49,50], and the specific blockade of the peripheral cannabinoid receptor CB1 attenuates the hyperdynamic circulation [49,50] and decreases portal pressure [49]. It has been postulated that cannabinoids would act through an increase in NO production [49], but results are contradictory [50]. The mechanisms that would induce anandamide production are not clear, but could be related to the frequent endotoxaemia observed in cirrhosis.

Several other circulating vasodilators, such as calcitonin gene-related peptide (CGRP), adrenomedullin and carbon monoxide, have also been linked to the pathogenesis of vasodilation in portal hypertension, but evidence is still scarce.

Local vasodilators

The implication of NO in portal hypertension was initially suggested by Vallance and Moncada [51]. Several lines of evidence confirmed the central role of NO in the development of the hyperdynamic circulation. On one hand, patients with cirrhosis have increased levels of nitrites and nitrates [52], the degradation products of NO. In experimental animals, it was demonstrated that NO production is increased in the splanchnic vascular bed of portal hypertensive rats, and this accounts for the hyporesponse to vasoconstrictors characteristic of portal hypertension [53]. Furthermore, inhibition of NO production reduces portal pressure, portosystemic shunting and prevents (although not completely) the development of the hyperdynamic circulation [54,55]. This last finding, together with the fact that double eNOS/inducible NOS (iNOS) knockout mice still develop the hyperdynamic circulation after the induction of portal hypertension [56], suggests that NO is the principal, but not the only, mediator of vasodilation.

A number of studies have characterized at the molecular level the mechanisms leading to increased NO production in portal hypertension. At odds with the original hypothesis, which suggested that endotoxaemia present in cirrhosis would upregu-

late iNOS [51], overwhelming data suggest that increased NO in portal hypertension is mediated by eNOS [57]. Preliminary data suggest that neuronal NOS (nNOS) activation could also have a role in the increased NO production that occurs in portal hypertension [58], but this role would be far outweighed by that of eNOS [59].

The most powerful stimulus for eNOS upregulation is shear stress. Indeed, shear stress is increased in portal hypertension once the hyperdynamic circulation is established. Furthermore, the superior mesenteric vascular bed from portal hypertensive rats shows an enhanced production of NO in response to shear stress [53]. Bacterial translocation also contributes to increased NO production in advanced cirrhosis, but the mechanism involves an upregulation of eNOS, not iNOS [60]. Finally, portosystemic shunt, *per se*, can induce NO-mediated vasodilation [61]. However, sequential studies in the portal vein ligated model have shown that eNOS activation occurs before any of these three mechanisms is present [62,63]. This indicates, on the one hand, that increased eNOS production is a primary factor in the development of vasodilation and, on the other hand, that different mechanisms from those mentioned above activate eNOS in the very early phases of portal hypertension. Recent data indicate that the initial eNOS upregulation occurs at the small arterioles of the intestinal mucosa, and that it is secondary to VEGF upregulation [64], raising the possibility that the first stimulus that upregulates eNOS is intestinal hypoxia secondary to congestion or to superior mesenteric artery (SMA) reflex vasoconstriction in response to increased portal pressure [63]. In keeping with these findings, it was demonstrated recently that blocking VEGF action from the onset of portal hypertension markedly attenuates the development of the hyperdynamic circulation and decreases portal blood inflow by 50% [65]. Whether these mechanisms account for the development of the hyperdynamic circulation in human cirrhosis needs to be confirmed.

When looking at the signalling level, molecular studies have shown that, in the early stages of portal hypertension, increased eNOS activity is detected before the increase in eNOS expression. This is due to activation of eNOS at the posttranslational level, mediated by increased Akt-dependent eNOS phosphorylation [66]. In the more advanced stages of portal hypertension, NO production increases as a result of both an increase in eNOS expression [60] and an increase in eNOS activity related to changes at the posttranslational level. This latter mechanism involves an increased interaction of eNOS with the molecular chaperone Hsp90 [67]. Also, it has been shown that bacterial translocation activates eNOS through a tumour necrosis factor (TNF)α-dependent increase in tetrahydrobiopterin (BH$_4$) [60,68], an essential cofactor of eNOS. Taken together, these studies show that different mechanisms upregulate eNOS (Fig. 3) and that the relative importance of these mechanisms varies during the evolution of portal hypertension.

In summary, in striking contrast to what occurs in the intrahepatic circulation, in which there is a deficit in NO production,

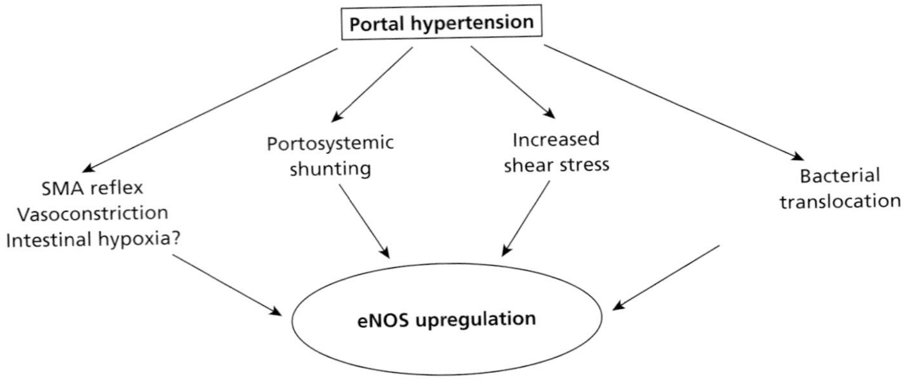

Portal hypertension

SMA reflex
Vasoconstriction
Intestinal hypoxia?

Portosystemic
shunting

Increased
shear stress

Bacterial
translocation

eNOS upregulation

Fig. 3 Portal hypertension activates different mechanisms that ultimately lead to eNOS upregulation.

in the splanchnic circulation, there is an increase in NO production (Fig. 2) [57]. This paradox poses enormous difficulties in developing NO-based therapies for portal hypertension. However, it must be taken into account that the primary defect is the increase in intrahepatic resistance, and splanchnic vasodilation is a secondary alteration. Therefore, it is likely that, by improving the increase in hepatic resistance, some of the alterations in the splanchnic circulation can be reverted [15].

Another local vasodilator that has been linked to splanchnic hyperaemia in portal hypertension is prostacyclin [69,70], but the available evidence is less extensive than that for NO. Systemic and splanchnic production of prostacyclin is increased in portal hypertension as a consequence of an increased expression of COX-1 and COX-2 [71]. Blocking any of the two isoforms increases the response of the splanchnic vasculature to vasoconstrictors, but the effect of COX-2 blockade is more intense [71]. Further, COX blockade has been shown to attenuate the hyperdynamic circulation in portal hypertension [72,73].

Plasma volume expansion

For many years, plasma volume expansion has been recognized in a wide variety of portal hypertensive liver diseases. In conditions of constant peripheral vascular resistance, an increase in circulatory blood volume results in increased venous return and cardiac output. However, expansion of blood volume leads to stress relaxation of the vasculature and, after this initial increase, cardiac output returns to normal. This demonstrates that blood volume expansion alone is not sufficient in itself to maintain a hyperkinetic circulatory state. It is the combination of arterial vasodilation and blood volume expansion that produces optimal conditions for maintaining the hyperdynamic circulatory state in portal hypertension.

Sodium retention is the earliest and most frequent abnormality of renal function associated with portal hypertension. Sodium restriction markedly attenuates the development of the hyperdynamic circulation in portal hypertensive rats, normalizing cardiac output and portal venous inflow [74]. On the other hand, it has been demonstrated that diuretics such as spironolactone decrease (although mildly) portal pressure [75]. The initial stimulus for sodium retention is arterial vasodilation

[76,77], which leads to arterial underfilling and subsequent activation of baroreceptors. This leads to the activation of the sympathetic nervous system, renin–angiotensin system and vasopressin secretion. The final result is sodium and water retention by the kidneys and plasma volume expansion (Fig. 4).

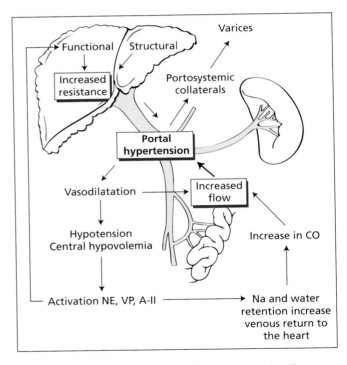

Fig. 4 Summary of the pathophysiology of portal hypertension. The increase in hepatic resistance leads to an increase in portal pressure. This leads to a cascade of disturbances in the splanchnic and systemic circulation characterized by vasodilation, sodium and water retention and plasma volume expansion, which are major players in the pathogenesis of ascites and hepatorenal syndrome. Additionally, these alterations lead to an increase in portal blood inflow that contributes to maintaining and aggravating portal hypertension. Another characteristic feature is the development of portosystemic collaterals that are responsible for complications such as variceal bleeding and hepatic encephalopathy. CO, cardiac output; NE, norepinephrine; VP, vasopressin; A-II, angiotensin II; Na, sodium.

This has been called the peripheral arterial vasodilation hypothesis [34], and not only explains the pathophysiology of the hyperdynamic circulation in portal hypertension, but also many aspects of other complications of portal hypertension such as ascites and hepatorenal syndrome [43].

Summary and conclusions

The primary event leading to portal hypertension in liver cirrhosis is increased hepatic resistance. This is due not only to the architectural disturbances in liver vasculature associated with the cirrhotic process, but also to an increased intrahepatic vascular tone that results from an imbalance between excessive vasoconstrictors and deficient vasodilators. Besides, portal hypertension induces marked alterations in the systemic and splanchnic circulation, characterized by a decrease in systemic vascular resistance, arterial hypotension, increased cardiac output and plasma volume expansion, and is known as the hyperdynamic circulatory state. This leads to an increase in portal blood inflow that contributes to maintain and aggravate portal hypertension (Fig. 4). These concepts provide the rationale for understanding the pharmacological treatments of portal hypertension in cirrhosis.

References

1 Sikuler E, Groszmann RJ (1986) Interaction of flow and resistance in maintenance of portal hypertension in a rat model. *Am J Physiol* 250, G205–G212.

2 Wanless IR, Wong F, Blendis LM *et al.* (1995) Hepatic and portal vein thrombosis in cirrhosis: possible role in development of parenchymal extinction and portal hypertension. *Hepatology* 21, 1238–1247.

3 Bhathal PS, Grossman HJ (1985) Reduction of the increased portal vascular resistance of the isolated perfused cirrhotic rat liver by vasodilators. *J Hepatol* 1, 325–337.

4 Zhang JX, Pegoli W Jr, Clemens MG (1994) Endothelin-1 induces direct constriction of hepatic sinusoids. *Am J Physiol (Gastrointest Liver Physiol)* 29, G624–G632.

5 Pinzani M, Gentilini P (1999) Biology of hepatic stellate cells and their possible relevance in the pathogenesis of portal hypertension in cirrhosis. *Semin Liver Dis* 19, 397–410.

6 Kaneda K, Sogawa M, Matsumara A *et al.* (1998) Endothelin-1 induced vasoconstriction causes a significant increase in portal pressure of rat liver: localized constrictive effect on the distal segment of preterminal portal venules as revealed by light and electron microscopy and serial reconstruction. *Hepatology* 27, 735–747.

7 Loureiro-Silva MR, Cadelina GW, Groszmann RJ (2003) Deficit in nitric oxide production in cirrhotic rat livers is located in the sinusoidal and postsinusoidal areas. *Am J Physiol Gastrointest Liver Physiol* 284, G567–G574.

8 Mittal MK, Gupta TK, Lee FY *et al.* (1994) Nitric oxide modulates hepatic vascular tone in normal rat liver. *Am J Physiol* 267, G416–G422.

9 Gupta TK, Toruner M, Chung MK *et al.* (1998) Endothelial dysfunction and decreased production of nitric oxide in the intrahepatic microcirculation of cirrhotic rats. *Hepatology* 28, 926–931.

10 Rockey DC, Chung JJ (1998) Reduced nitric oxide production by endothelial cells in cirrhotic rat liver: endothelial dysfunction in portal hypertension. *Gastroenterology* 114, 344–351.

11 Shah V, Toruner M, Haddad F *et al.* (1999) Impaired endothelial nitric oxide synthase activity associated with enhanced caveolin binding in experimental cirrhosis in the rat. *Gastroenterology* 117, 1222–1228.

12 Bellis L, Berzigotti A, Abraldes JG *et al.* (2003) Low doses of isosorbide mononitrate attenuate the postprandial increase in portal pressure in patients with cirrhosis. *Hepatology* 37, 378–384.

13 Van de CM, Omasta A, Janssens S *et al.* (2002) In vivo gene transfer of endothelial nitric oxide synthase decreases portal pressure in anaesthetised carbon tetrachloride cirrhotic rats. *Gut* 51, 440–445.

14 Loureiro-Silva MR, Cadelina GW, Iwakiri Y *et al.* (2003) A liver-specific nitric oxide donor improves the intra-hepatic vascular response to both portal blood flow increase and methoxamine in cirrhotic rats. *J Hepatol* 39, 940–946.

15 Morales-Ruiz M, Cejudo-Martn P, Fernandez-Varo G *et al.* (2003) Transduction of the liver with activated Akt normalizes portal pressure in cirrhotic rats. *Gastroenterology* 125, 522–531.

16 Dudenhoefer AA, Loureiro-Silva MR, Cadelina GW *et al.* (2002) Bioactivation of nitroglycerin and vasomotor response to nitric oxide are impaired in cirrhotic rat livers. *Hepatology* 36, 381–385.

17 Van De Casteele M, Van Pelt JF, Nevens F *et al.* (2003) Low NO bioavailability in CCl4 cirrhotic rat livers might result from low NO synthesis combined with decreased superoxide dismutase activity allowing superoxide-mediated NO breakdown: a comparison of two portal hypertensive rat models with healthy controls. *Comp Hepatol* 2, 2.

18 Loureiro-Silva MR, Iwakiri Y, Abraldes JG *et al.* (2006) Increased phosphodiesterase-5 expression is involved in the decreased vasodilator response to nitric oxide in cirrhotic rat livers. *J Hepatol* 44, 886–893.

19 Suematsu M, Goda N, Sano T *et al.* (1995) Carbon monoxide: an endogenous modulator of sinusoidal tone in the perfused rat liver. *J Clin Invest* 96, 2431–2437.

20 Makino N, Suematsu M, Sugiura Y *et al.* (2001) Altered expression of heme oxygenase-1 in the livers of patients with portal hypertensive diseases. *Hepatology* 33, 32–42.

21 Ballet F, Chretien Y, Rey C *et al.* (1988) Differential response of normal and cirrhotic liver to vasoactive agents. A study in the isolated perfused rat liver. *J Pharmacol Exp Ther* 244, 233–235.

22 Rockey DC, Weisiger RA (1996) Endothelin induced contractility of stellate cells from normal and cirrhotic rat liver: implications for regulation of portal pressure and resistance. *Hepatology* 24, 233–240.

23 Graupera M, Garcia-Pagan JC, Abraldes JG *et al.* (2003) Cyclooxygenase-derived products modulate the increased intrahepatic resistance of cirrhotic rat livers. *Hepatology* 37, 172–181.

24 Titos E, Claria J, Bataller R *et al.* (2000) Hepatocyte-derived cysteinyl leukotrienes modulate vascular tone in experimental cirrhosis. *Gastroenterology* 119, 794–805.

25 Pinzani M, Milani S, De Franco R *et al.* (1996) Endothelin 1 is overexpressed in human cirrhotic liver and exerts multiple effects on activated hepatic stellate cells. *Gastroenterology* 110, 534–548.

26 Bosch J, Arroyo V, Betriu A *et al.* (1980) Hepatic hemodynamics and the renin-angiotensin-aldosterone system in cirrhosis. *Gastroenterology* 78, 92–99.

27 Graupera M, Garcia-Pagan JC, Titos E *et al.* (2002) 5-lipoxygenase inhibition reduces intrahepatic vascular resistance of cirrhotic rat livers: a possible role of cysteinyl-leukotrienes. *Gastroenterology* 122, 387–393.

28 Asbert M, Gines A, Gines P et al. (1993) Circulating levels of end-othelin in cirrhosis. Gastroenterology 104, 1485–1491.

29 Elliot AJ, Vo LT, Grossman VL et al. (1997) Endothelin-induced vaso-constriction in isolated perfused liver preparations from normal and cirrhotic rats. J Gastroenterol Hepatol 12, 314–318.

30 Bosch J, Abraldes JG, Groszmann RJ (2003) Current management of portal hypertension. J Hepatol 38, S54–S68.

31 Tripathi D, Therapondos G, Ferguson JW et al. (2006) Endothelin-1 contributes to the maintenance of systemic but not portal haemody-namics in patients with early cirrhosis: a randomised controlled trial. Gut 55, 1290–1295.

32 Bataller R, Gines P, Nicolas JM et al. (2000) Angiotensin II induces contraction and proliferation of human hepatic stellate cells. Gastroenterology 118, 1149–1156.

33 Bataller R, Sancho-Bru P, Gines P et al. (2003) Activated human hep-atic stellate cells express the renin–angiotensin system and synthesize angiotensin II. Gastroenterology 125, 117–125.

34 Schrier RW, Arroyo V, Bernardi M et al. (1988) Peripheral arterial vasodilation hypothesis: a proposal for the initiation of renal sodium and water retention in cirrhosis. Hepatology 8, 1151–1157.

35 Gonzalez-Abraldes J, Albillos A, Banares R et al. (2001) Randomized comparison of long-term losartan versus propranolol in lowering portal pressure in cirrhosis. Gastroenterology 121, 382–388.

36 Graupera M, March S, Engel P et al. (2005) Sinusoidal endothelial COX-1-derived prostanoids modulate the hepatic vascular tone of cirrhotic rat livers. Am J Physiol Gastrointest Liver Physiol 288, G763–G770.

37 Fernandez M, Vizzutti F, Garcia-Pagan JC et al. (2004) Anti-VEGF receptor-2 monoclonal antibody prevents portal-systemic collateral vessel formation in portal hypertensive mice. Gastroenterology 126, 886–894.

38 Sieber CC, Sumanovski LT, Stumm M et al. (2001) In vivo angiogenesis in normal and portal hypertensive rats: role of basic fibroblast growth factor and nitric oxide. J Hepatol 34, 644–650.

39 Mosca P, Lee FY, Kaumann AJ et al. (1992) Pharmacology of portal–systemic collaterals in portal hypertensive rats: role of endothe-lium. Am J Physiol 263, G544–G550.

40 Chan CC, Wang SS, Lee FY et al. (2001) Endothelin-1 induces vaso-constriction on portal–systemic collaterals of portal hypertensive rats. Hepatology 33, 816–820.

41 Kotelanski B, Groszmann R, Cohn JN (1972) Circulation times in the splanchnic and hepatic beds in alcoholic liver disease. Gastroenterology 63, 102–111.

42 Vorobioff J, Bredfeldt J, Groszmann RJ et al. (1983) Hyperdynamic circulation in a portal hypertensive rat model: a primary factor for maintenance of chronic portal hypertension. Am J Physiol 244, G52–G56.

43 Groszmann RJ (1994) Hyperdynamic circulation of liver disease 40 years later: pathophysiology and clinical consequences. Hepatology 20, 1359–1363.

44 Iwakiri Y, Groszmann RJ (2006) The hyperdynamic circulation in chronic liver diseases: from the Patient to the Molecule. Hepatology 43(2 Suppl. 1), S121–131.

45 Gomis R, Fernandez-Alvarez J, Pizcueta P et al. (1994) Impaired func-tion of pancreatic islets from rats with portal hypertension resulting from cirrhosis and partial portal vein ligation. Hepatology 19, 1257–1261.

46 Kravetz D, Bosch J, Arderiu MT et al. (1988) Effects of somatostatin on splanchnic hemodynamics and plasma glucagon in portal hyper-tensive rats. Am J Physiol 254, G322–G328.

47 Albillos A, Rossi I, Iborra J et al. (1994) Octreotide prevents postpran-dial splanchnic hyperemia in patients with portal hypertension. J Hepatol 21, 88–94.

48 Wiest R, Tsai MH, Groszmann RJ (2001) Octreotide potentiates PKC-dependent vasoconstrictors in portal-hypertensive and control rats. Gastroenterology 120, 975–983.

49 Batkai S, Jarai Z, Wagner JA et al. (2001) Endocannabinoids acting at vascular CB1 receptors mediate the vasodilated state in advanced liver cirrhosis. Nature Med 7, 827–832.

50 Ros J, Claria J, To-Figueras J et al. (2002) Endogenous cannabinoids: a new system involved in the homeostasis of arterial pressure in experi-mental cirrhosis in the rat. Gastroenterology 122, 85–93.

51 Vallance P, Moncada S (1991) Hyperdynamic circulation in cirrhosis: a role for nitric oxide? Lancet 337, 776.

52 Guarner C, Soriano G, Tomas A et al. (1993) Increased serum nitrite and nitrate levels in patients with cirrhosis: relationship to endotox-emia. Hepatology 18, 1139–1143.

53 Hori N, Wiest R, Groszmann RJ (1998) Enhanced release of nitric oxide in response to changes in flow and shear stress in the superior mesenteric arteries of portal hypertensive rats. Hepatology 28, 1467–1473.

54 Lee FY, Colombato LA, Albillos A et al. (1993) Administration of N omega-nitro-L-arginine ameliorates portal-systemic shunting in portal-hypertensive rats. Gastroenterology 105, 1464–1470.

55 García-Pagán JC, Fernandez M, Bernadich C et al. (1994) Effects of continued nitric oxide inhibition on the development of the portal hypertensive syndrome following portal vein stenosis in the rat. Am J Physiol 30, 984–990.

56 Iwakiri Y, Cadelina G, Sessa WC et al. (2002) Mice with targeted deletion of eNOS develop hyperdynamic circulation associated with portal hypertension. Am J Physiol Gastrointest Liver Physiol 283, G1074–G1081.

57 Wiest R, Groszmann RJ (2002) The paradox of nitric oxide in cirrhosis and portal hypertension: too much, not enough. Hepatology 35, 478–491.

58 Jurzik L, Froh M, Straub RH et al. (2005) Up-regulation of nNOS and associated increase in nitrergic vasodilation in superior mesenteric arteries in pre-hepatic portal hypertension. J Hepatol 43, 258–265.

59 Kwon SY, Groszmann RJ, Iwakiri Y (2007) Increased neuronal nitric oxide synthase interaction with soluble guanylate cyclase contributes to the splanchnic arterial vasodilation in portal hypertensive rats. Hepatol Res (in press).

60 Wiest R, Das S, Cadelina G et al. (1999) Bacterial translocation in cirrhotic rats stimulates eNOS-derived NO production and impairs mesenteric vascular contractility. J Clin Invest 104, 1223–1233.

61 Bernadich C, Bandi JC, Piera C et al. (1997) Circulatory effects of graded diversion of portal blood flow to the systemic circulation in rats: role of nitric oxide. Hepatology 26, 262–267.

62 Wiest R, Shah V, Sessa WC et al. (1999) NO overproduction by eNOS precedes hyperdynamic splanchnic circulation in portal hypertensive rats. Am J Physiol 276, G1043–G1051.

63 Tsai MH, Iwakiri Y, Cadelina G et al. (2003) Mesenteric vasoconstric-tion triggers nitric oxide overproduction in the superior mesenteric artery of portal hypertensive rats. Gastroenterology 125, 1452–1461.

64 Abraldes JG, Iwakiri Y, Loureiro-Silva et al. (2006) Mild increases in portal pressure upregulate vascular endothelial growth factor and endothelial nitric oxide synthase in the intestinal microcirculatory bed, leading to a hyperdynamic state. Am J Physiol Gastrointest Liver Physiol 290, G980–G987.

65 Fernandez M, Mejias M, Angermayr B *et al.* (2005) Inhibition of VEGF receptor-2 decreases the development of hyperdynamic splanchnic circulation and portal-systemic collateral vessels in portal hypertensive rats. *J Hepatol* 43, 98–103.

66 Iwakiri Y, Tsai MH, McCabe TJ *et al.* (2002) Phosphorylation of eNOS initiates excessive NO production in early phases of portal hypertension. *Am J Physiol Heart Circ Physiol* 282, H2084–H2090.

67 Shah V, Wiest R, Garcia-Cardena G *et al.* (1999) Hsp90 regulation of endothelial nitric oxide synthase contributes to vascular control in portal hypertension. *Am J Physiol* 277, G463–G468.

68 Wiest R, Cadelina G, Milstien S *et al.* (2003) Bacterial translocation up-regulates GTP-cyclohydrolase I in mesenteric vasculature of cirrhotic rats. *Hepatology* 38, 1508–1515.

69 Guarner C, Soriano G, Such J *et al.* (1992) Systemic prostacyclin in cirrhotic patients. Relationship with portal hypertension and changes after intestinal decontamination. *Gastroenterology* 102, 303–309.

70 Sitzmann JV, Bulkley GB (1989) Role of prostacyclin in the splanchnic hyperemia contributing to portal hypertension. *Ann Surg* 209, 322–327.

71 Potenza MA, Botrugno OA, De Salvia MA *et al.* (2002) Endothelial COX-1 and -2 differentially affect reactivity of MVB in portal hypertensive rats. *Am J Physiol Gastrointest Liver Physiol* 283, G587–G594.

72 Fernandez M, Garcia-Pagan JC, Casadevall M *et al.* (1996) Acute and chronic cyclooxygenase blockade in portal hypertensive rats. Influence on nitric oxide biosynthesis. *Gastroenterology* 110, 1529–1535.

73 Bruix J, Bosch J, Kravetz D *et al.* (1985) Effects of prostaglandin inhibition on systemic and hepatic hemodynamics in patients with cirrhosis of the liver. *Gastroenterology* 88, 430–435.

74 Genecin P, Polio J, Groszmann RJ (1990) Na restriction blunts expansion of plasma volume and ameliorates hyperdynamic circulation in portal hypertension. *Am J Physiol* 259, G498–G503.

75 Garcia-Pagan JC, Salmeron JM, Feu F *et al.* (1994) Effects of low-sodium diet and spironolactone on portal pressure in patients with compensated cirrhosis. *Hepatology* 19, 1095–1099.

76 Albillos A, Colombato LA, Groszmann RJ (1992) Vasodilatation and sodium retention in prehepatic portal hypertension. *Gastroenterology* 102, 931–935.

77 Colombato LA, Albillos A, Groszmann RJ (1996) The role of central blood volume in the development of sodium retention in portal hypertensive rats. *Gastroenterology* 110, 193–198.

7.3 Clinical manifestations and management of bleeding episodes in cirrhotics

Jaime Bosch, Juan G. Abraldes and Juan Carlos García-Pagán

Introduction

Variceal bleeding is one of the commonest and most severe complications of liver cirrhosis. Even with the current best medical care, mortality from variceal bleeding is still around 20%. Moreover, variceal bleeding often leads to deterioration in liver function, and it is a common trigger for other complications of cirrhosis, such as bacterial infections or hepatorenal syndrome. In this chapter, we will review the natural history of varices in patients with cirrhosis, the primary and secondary prevention of acute variceal bleeding, and the medical management of the bleeding episode.

The natural history and clinical course of variceal bleeding

Development of oesophageal varices

When cirrhosis is diagnosed, varices are present in about 30–40% of compensated patients and in 60% of those who present with ascites [1]. In those cirrhotic patients who present without varices, the annual incidence of new varices is about 5–10% [2–6]. An hepatic venous pressure gradient (HVPG) over 10 mmHg [6] is a strong predictor for the development of varices. This is in keeping with the role of portal pressure as the driving force for the development of collaterals. No other factors have been associated with the development of varices [5,7].

Progression of oesophageal varices from small to large

Once developed, varices increase in size from small to large before they eventually rupture and bleed. Studies assessing the progression from small to large varices are controversial, showing rates of progression of varices ranging from 5% to 30% per year [1,5,8,9]. The most likely reason for such variability is the different patient selection and follow-up endoscopy schedule across studies (7). The factor that has been most consistently associated with variceal progression is baseline Child–Pugh or

its worsening during follow-up [5,8,10]. Other reported factors were alcoholic aetiology of cirrhosis and the presence of red wale markings [5]. It has been shown that changes in HVPG [either 'spontaneous' or caused by drug therapy or transjugular intrahepatic portosystemic shunts (TIPS)] are usually accompanied by parallel variations in the size of the oesophageal varices, which are significantly reduced when HVPG falls below 12 mmHg [11,12]. Thus, an increased HVPG plays a key role in both the development and the progression of the varices.

Incidence and risk indicators of first bleeding from oesophageal varices

Once varices have been diagnosed, the overall incidence of variceal bleeding is of the order of 25% at 2 years in non-selected patients [13]. Many efforts have been made to define risk criteria for the development of variceal bleeding. The most important predictive factors are variceal size, severity of liver dysfunction expressed by the Child–Pugh classification and red wale marks [14]. These risk indicators have been combined in the North Italian Endoscopic Club (NIEC) index, which allows the classification of patients into different groups with predicted 1-year bleeding risk ranging from 6% to 76% [14]. Overall, variceal size remains the most useful predictor for variceal bleeding [15]. This is the variable used in clinical practice to decide whether a patient should be given prophylactic therapy or not. The risk of bleeding is very low (between 1% and 2%) in patients without varices at the first examination, and increases to about 5% per year in those with small varices, and to 15% per year in those with medium or large varices at diagnosis [1].

The course of the acute bleeding episode

Prognostic factors

Ruptured oesophageal varices cause 70% of all upper gastrointestinal bleeding episodes in patients with portal hypertension [16]. Thus, in any cirrhotic patient with acute upper gastrointestinal bleeding, a variceal origin should be suspected. Clinical features are those of upper gastrointestinal bleeding (often massive), combined with those of liver cirrhosis. The incidence of variceal bleeding shows a diurnal rhythm, with two peak incidences at 08.00–10.00 and 20.00–22.00 [17,18]. This rhythmicity is probably related to circadian variations in portal pressure [18]. Variceal bleeding is often intermittent, which should be taken into account in its diagnostic approach. Diagnosis is established at emergency endoscopy based on observing one of the following: (i) active bleeding from a varix (observation of blood spurting or oozing from the varix) (nearly 20% of patients); (ii) white nipple or clot adherent to a varix; (iii) presence of varices without other potential sources of bleeding.

Initial control of bleeding

Because variceal bleeding is frequently intermittent, it is difficult to assess when the bleeding stops and when a new haematemesis or melaena should be considered an episode of rebleeding. Several consensus conferences have addressed this issue and set definitions for events and timing of events related to episodes of variceal bleeding [19]. By using these definitions, data from placebo-controlled clinical trials have shown that variceal bleeding is spontaneously controlled in 40–50% of patients [13]. With currently available treatments, control of bleeding increases to about 80% of the patients [16].

Early rebleeding

The incidence of early rebleeding ranges between 30% and 40% in the first 6 weeks. The risk peaks in the first 5 days, with 40% of all rebleeding episodes occurring in this very early period, remains high during the first 2 weeks and then declines slowly in the next 4 weeks. After 6 weeks, the risk of further bleeding becomes virtually equal to that before bleeding [20]. Currently available treatments have reduced 6-week rebleeding to 20% [16]. Early rebleeding is a strong predictor of death within 6 weeks, indicating that its prevention should be a priority in the management of variceal bleeding. Prognostic indicators for early rebleeding were assessed in most studies together with initial failure to control bleeding and 5-day risk of death, confirming a composite endpoint referred to as '5-day failure'. Bacterial infection [21–23], active bleeding at emergency endoscopy [16,22,24], Child–Pugh class or score [16,22], aspartate aminotransferase (AST) levels [16], the presence of portal vein thrombosis [16] and an HVPG > 20 mmHg measured shortly after admission [25,26] have been reported as significant predictors of risk for 5-day failure.

Mortality

Mortality from variceal bleeding has greatly decreased in the last two decades from 42% mortality registered in the Graham and Smith study in 1981 [20] to the current 15–20% [16,27]. This decrease results from the implementation of effective treatments, such as endoscopic and pharmacological therapies and TIPS, as well as improved general medical care (i.e. antibiotic prophylaxis). As it may be difficult to assess the true cause of death (i.e. bleeding vs. liver failure or other adverse events), the

general consensus is that any death occurring within 6 weeks from hospital admission for variceal bleeding should be considered as a bleeding-related death [19].

Immediate mortality from uncontrolled bleeding is in the range of 4–8% [3,4,16]. Prehospital mortality from variceal bleeding might be around 3% [28]. Like the risk of rebleeding, the risk of mortality peaks in the first days after bleeding, slowly declines thereafter and, after 6 weeks, becomes constant and virtually equal to that before bleeding [13,20]. Nowadays, only 40% of deaths are directly related to bleeding, while 50% are caused by liver failure and hepatorenal syndrome [16]. Thus, although there is still room for improving haemostatic treatments to substantially decrease mortality from variceal bleeding, therapies should be able to prevent liver and renal function deterioration.

Accurate indicators of risk of early death, available at hospital admission, could allow selection of patients for more aggressive therapies, such as emergency shunt or TIPS, before their conditions deteriorate, hampering further therapy. Unfortunately, the indicators of risk so far identified are also indicators of poor outcomes after derivative treatments and, consequently, are of limited clinical value. On hospital admission, the most consistently reported death risk indicators are Child–Pugh classification or its components, blood urea nitrogen (BUN) or creatinine, active bleeding on endoscopy, hypovolaemic shock and hepatocellular carcinoma [16,20,21,29–31]. Additionally, an HVPG > 20 mmHg [25] has been reported as a strong indicator of treatment failure. Conceivably, it is also associated with a higher risk of death, although its specific prognostic role for 6-week mortality has not been assessed. Prognostic indicators gathered in the early follow-up period are of no help in selecting immediate therapy, but do aid in developing a more focused and rational management of the patient. The most important among late prognostic indicators are early rebleeding [24,30], bacterial infection [23] and renal failure [30,31]. From these data, it is clear that management of the bleeding cirrhotic patient should be aimed not only at controlling the bleeding, but also at preventing early rebleeding, infection and renal failure.

Long-term recurrent bleeding from oesophageal varices and mortality

Patients surviving a first episode of variceal bleeding have a very high risk of rebleeding and death. Median rebleeding incidence within 1–2 years in untreated patients is around 60%, while mortality is around 33% [13]. Because of these high risks, all patients surviving a variceal bleeding should be treated for prevention of rebleeding independently of other risk indicators [32,33]. Randomized controlled trials (RCTs) for the prevention of rebleeding suggest that risk indicators of rebleeding and death are variceal size, Child–Pugh class, continued alcohol abuse and hepatocellular carcinoma [13]. An HVPG > 20 mmHg is significantly associated with a higher risk of 1-year mortality [25]. A spontaneous decrease in portal pressure after alcohol abstinence or the pharmacological reduction of portal pressure by more than 20% of baseline values or below 12 mmHg are associated with a sustained decrease in the risk of rebleeding [11,34,35], indicating that effective portal pressure reduction can reverse the natural history of portal hypertension [35] (see below).

The management of portal hypertension

Rational basis for the treatment of portal hypertension

A very important concept, which has been strongly substantiated in recent years, is that the major factor determining the development of the complications and the clinical significance of portal hypertension is that portal pressure (assessed in clinical practice by the HVPG) increases above a critical threshold value. Varices do not develop until HVPG increases to ≥ 10 mmHg, and the HVPG should be of at least 12 mmHg for the appearance of other complications, such as variceal bleeding and ascites [36–38]. Implicit in this concept is that preventing the HVPG from increasing above these values will prevent the development of the complications of portal hypertension. Further, if HVPG is reduced below these thresholds by means of pharmacological treatment [12,34] or spontaneously as a result of an improvement

in liver disease [11], variceal bleeding is totally prevented and varices decrease in size. Besides, even if this target is not achieved, a 20% decrease from baseline HVPG offers an almost total protection from variceal bleeding [34,35,39–43]. Such a reduction in HVPG, below 12 mmHg or of more than 20% of baseline, is now accepted as a therapeutic target in the treatment of portal hypertension. Achievement of these targets has also been shown to be associated with a decreased risk of developing ascites, spontaneous bacterial peritonitis, hepatorenal syndrome and death [35]. This provides the proof-of-concept of the reversibility of the portal hypertensive syndrome by means of portal pressure reduction.

A basic knowledge of the pathophysiology of portal hypertension is required to understand the pharmacological treatment of portal hypertension (Fig. 1). The initial factor that leads to portal hypertension is the increase in vascular resistance to portal blood flow. In cirrhosis, this increase in resistance occurs at the hepatic microcirculation (sinusoidal portal hypertension). It is important to emphasize that, contrary to what was traditionally thought, increased hepatic vascular resistance in cirrhosis is not only a mechanical consequence of the hepatic architectural disorder caused by the liver disease, but there is also a dynamic (and therefore reversible) component secondary to an increased intrahepatic vascular tone. This provides a rationale for the use of vasodilators in portal hypertension. Another way of

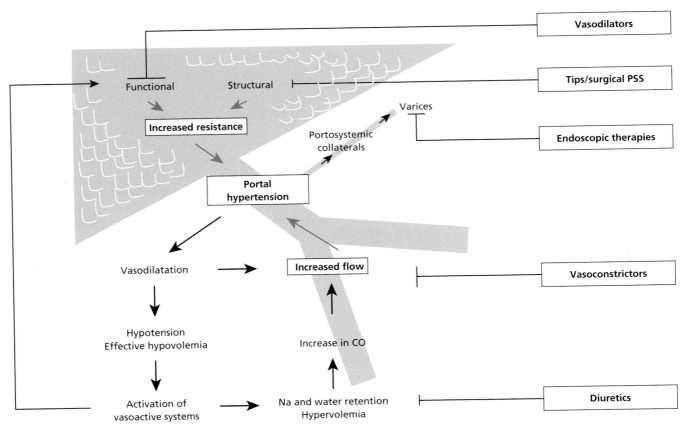

Fig. 1 Rationale for the treatment of portal hypertension (see text for details). CO, cardiac output; Na, sodium; PSS, portosystemic shunt.

overcoming the increased resistance through the cirrhotic liver is by means of portosystemic shunt surgery and TIPS. These procedures are highly effective in decreasing portal pressure, but have the detrimental effect that, by further decreasing portal blood flow through the liver and by increasing portosystemic shunting, they may enhance liver failure and facilitate hepatic encephalopathy.

A second factor contributing to portal hypertension is an increased blood flow through the portal venous system due to splanchnic arteriolar vasodilatation. Splanchnic hyperaemia contributes by aggravating the increase in portal pressure, and this explains why portal hypertension persists despite the establishment of an extensive network of portosystemic collaterals that may divert over 80% of the portal blood flow. The increased portal venous inflow can be corrected pharmacologically by means of splanchnic vasoconstrictors, such as vasopressin and its derivatives, somatostatin and its analogues and non-selective beta-adrenergic blockers, which are the drugs that have been more widely used in the treatment of portal hypertension. Splanchnic vasodilatation is accompanied by increased cardiac index and hypervolaemia, representing the hyperkinetic circulatory syndrome associated with portal hypertension [44,45]. An expanded blood volume is necessary to maintain the hyperdynamic circulation, which provides a rationale for the use of a low-sodium diet and spironolactone to attenuate the hyperkinetic syndrome and the portal pressure elevation in patients with cirrhosis [46].

Combined pharmacological therapy consists of associating vasoconstrictive drugs, which act by decreasing portal blood inflow, and vasodilators, which reduce the intrahepatic and portocollateral vascular resistance, in an attempt to enhance the reduction in portal pressure caused by the former.

Local treatments at the varices complete the spectrum of treatments for complications of portal hypertension. These treatments do not decrease portal pressure and therefore have no potential for preventing other complications of portal hypertension. Endoscopic therapy is directed at 'eradicating' the varices either by injecting a variety of irritating substances into or around the varices to promote thrombosis and fibrosis or by ligating the varices using elastic bands. It is possible that the efficacy of endoscopic therapy could be enhanced if combined with an agent that effectively lowers portal pressure [47]. Finally, haemostatic agents, such as recombinant activated factor VII, are being explored as adjuvants to conventional therapy to arrest variceal bleeding [48].

Prevention and treatment of the bleeding episodes

The treatment of portal hypertension includes the prevention of variceal haemorrhage in patients who have varices but never bled, the treatment of the acute bleeding episode and the prevention of rebleeding in patients who have survived a bleeding episode from oesophageal or gastric varices. So far, there is no effective treatment to prevent the development of varices ('preprimary prophylaxis') [6].

The main difference between these scenarios is that natural history and prognosis are very different from one to another. The previous considerations about the natural history of each of these situations should guide the selection of therapies, as the haemostatic or prophylactic efficacy of the available treatments are inversely proportional to their invasiveness and adverse effects.

Prevention of first bleeding from oesophageal varices

Screening for oesophageal varices

The aim of screening for oesophageal varices is to detect those patients with varices that will benefit from prophylactic treatment. The current consensus is that every cirrhotic patient should be screened endoscopically for varices at the time of diagnosis [19]. Although several studies indicate that non-invasive tests (particularly platelet count and data obtained from abdominal ultrasound) may have a potential use in selecting a group of patients with a high risk of varices [49–52], so far none of these has proved to be accurate enough in independent samples so that endoscopy can safely be omitted in patients with negative non-invasive indicators.

Cost-effectiveness decision analysis has challenged universal endoscopy screening in cirrhosis [53,54]. In these reports, it is suggested that empiric beta-blocker therapy for all patients without endoscopic screening is more cost-effective than universal screening and primary prophylaxis only in patients with large varices. A third study also suggested that empiric beta-blocker therapy is more cost-effective, but only in patients with decompensated cirrhosis [55]. However, the major drawbacks of beta-adrenergic blockers are patient adherence and side-effects (and thus quality of life), which are difficult to account for fully in decision analysis studies. The lack of effectiveness of beta-adrenergic blockers in preventing the development of varices and the high rate of side-effects observed even in well-compensated patients [6] severely compromise the use of beta-adrenergic blockers without screening.

In patients without varices on initial endoscopy, a second (follow-up) evaluation should be performed after 2–3 years to detect the development of varices before these bleed [19]. In those centres in which hepatic haemodynamic studies are available, it is advisable to measure HVPG. An HVPG over 10 mmHg indicates a more rapid progression to complications of cirrhosis and calls for shorter surveillance intervals [6]. In patients with small varices on initial endoscopy, the aim of subsequent evaluations is to detect the progression of small to large varices because of the important prognostic and therapeutic implications. Based on an expected 10–15% per year rate of progression of variceal size, endoscopy should be repeated every 1–2 years in patients with small varices [19]. In patients with advanced cirrhosis, red wale marks or alcoholic aetiology of cirrhosis, a 1-year interval might be recommended [5,7]. Once the patient is started on beta-adrenergic blockers, there is no need for further endoscopic surveillance.

Treatments for the prevention of first bleeding

Pharmacological therapy The modern era of drug therapy for portal hypertension started in 1980 with the first publication of the use of propranolol for the prevention of recurrent variceal bleeding [56]. Since then, the efficacy of non-selective beta-adrenergic blockers has been assessed in a number of RCTs that consistently showed a significant reduction in the bleeding risk, both in the prophylaxis of first bleeding and in the prevention of rebleeding.

Non-selective beta-adrenergic blockers reduce portal pressure by decreasing portal venous inflow. Also, by reducing portal blood inflow, these drugs reduce portocollateral blood flow. This means that beta-adrenergic blockers can be beneficial in the prevention of variceal bleeding even in the absence of a decrease in portal pressure. The decrease in splanchnic blood flow is the result of a decrease in cardiac output due to the blockade of cardiac beta-1 adrenoceptors, and of splanchnic vasoconstriction due to the beta-2 receptor blockade, which leads to unopposed alpha-adrenergic activity [57].

Both propranolol and nadolol have been proven effective in the prevention of variceal bleeding [13]. Nadolol may be more convenient as it is administered once a day and, on account of its low lipid solubility, may have lower potential for central side-effects [58]. Timolol also has low liposolubility [58] and has the greatest beta-2 adrenoceptor blocking effect [59], but this drug was only tested in one randomized trial evaluating the prevention of the development of varices, with negative results [6]. Therefore, there is no evidence to support the use of timolol for the prevention of variceal bleeding.

The dose of beta-adrenergic blockers is determined by stepwise increases in dose until reaching the maximum tolerated. This approach is probably more effective than titrating against heart rate to achieve a reduction of about 25% [35]. Propranolol is commonly initiated at a dose of 20–40 mg b.i.d., while nadolol is initiated at a dose of 40 mg/day. The most common side-effects are lightheadedness, fatigue, shortness of breath, impotence and sleep disorders. Although severe events are rare, these side-effects often result in lack of compliance. About 10–15% of patients develop intolerance that results in treatment withdrawal [60]. In addition, up to 15–20% of cirrhotic patients with varices present contraindications that preclude the use of beta-blockers [61]. Absolute contraindications are congestive heart failure, asthma, chronic obstructive pulmonary disease, second- or third-degree heart block and peripheral vascular disease. Insulin-dependent diabetes and portopulmonary hypertension are relative contraindications.

A total of 12 trials have been conducted assessing beta-adrenergic blockers for the prevention of first bleeding. Meta-analysis of these studies shows that continued propranolol or nadolol therapy markedly reduces the bleeding risk, from 25% with non-active treatment to 15% with beta-adrenergic blockers over a median follow-up period of 2 years [13]. Mortality was only slightly reduced from 27% to 23%; this effect barely approached the level of statistical significance. The benefit of therapy has been proved in patients with moderate/large varices (> 5 mm), either with or without ascites or with good or poor liver function [13,62]. A recent trial demonstrated that beta-adrenergic blockers reduce the rate of progression from small to large varices, and decrease the incidence of variceal bleeding in patients with small varices [9]. Although confirmatory double-blind trials are required before a definite recommendation can be given [63], this suggests that the indication of beta-adrenergic blockers could be extended to patients with small varices, especially to those in Child class B and C. Therapy with beta-adrenergic blockers should be maintained indefinitely because, when they are withdrawn, the risk of variceal haemorrhage returns to what would be expected in an untreated population [64].

The addition of isosorbide mononitrate increases the portal pressure reduction of beta-adrenergic blockers [65,66]. However, it is not clear whether this translates into a greater clinical efficacy. An open trial comparing nadolol vs. nadolol plus isosorbide mononitrate demonstrated a significantly lower rate of first bleeding in the combination group, which was maintained after 55 months of follow-up, without survival advantage [67,68]. However, a large, randomized, double-blind study failed to confirm these results [60]. The current consensus does not recommend this combination therapy in primary prophylaxis [19]. Isosorbide mononitrate administered alone, despite its mild portal pressure-lowering effect, is ineffective in the prevention of variceal bleeding [61].

Endoscopic therapy Endoscopic band ligation is also effective in preventing the first variceal bleeding in patients with medium to large varices [69]. Twelve trials have compared endoscopic band ligation with beta-adrenergic blockers as first-line option for primary prophylaxis of variceal bleeding [70–81]. The meta-analysis of theses trials shows a clear but marginal advantage of endoscopic band ligation over beta-adrenergic blockers in terms of prevention of first bleeding, with no differences in mortality (Figs 2 and 3). However, the performance of beta-adrenergic blockers in the two trials showing a significant benefit of endoscopic band ligation was extremely poor [74,78]. Five of these trials are only available in abstract form, which makes it difficult to evaluate their quality. An additional concern is that, in the largest study [72], there was a 7% incidence of bleeding from ligation-induced ulcers, and two patients died as a direct consequence of this complication (treatment-related mortality of 2.6%). Further, because of the short duration of follow-up in most of these studies, the long-term safety and benefits of prophylactic endoscopic band ligation are still uncertain. On the contrary, the long-term safety and efficacy of prophylactic therapy using non-selective beta-adrenergic blockers has been established in a large number of trials [64,82]. On this basis, the current recommendation is to restrict

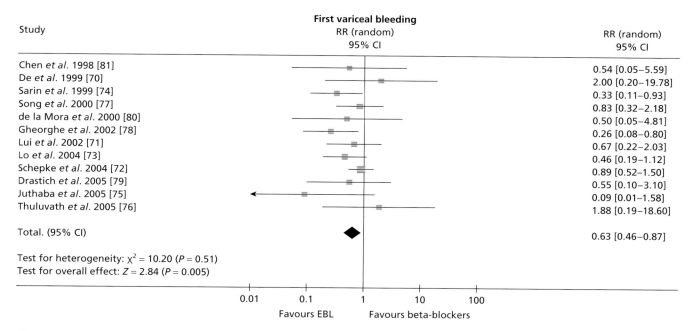

Fig. 2 Prevention of first variceal bleeding. Meta-analysis (random effects model) of randomized controlled trials comparing endoscopic band ligation (EBL) with beta-adrenergic blockers in the prevention of first variceal bleeding. EBL achieves a marginal improvement in the risk of developing a first variceal bleeding. RR, relative risk.

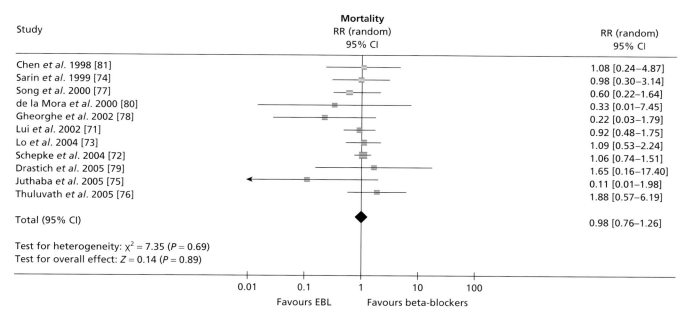

Fig. 3 Prevention of first variceal bleeding. Meta-analysis (random effects model) of randomized controlled trials comparing endoscopic band ligation (EBL) with beta-adrenergic blockers in the prevention of first variceal bleeding. EBL does not improve mortality. RR, relative risk.

the use of endoscopic band ligation to those patients with contraindications or intolerance to beta-adrenergic blockers (Fig. 4) [19]. Even in this case, the use of band ligation is controversial, as a recent trial comparing band ligation with no treatment in this subgroup of patients was stopped because of a high rate (12%) of iatrogenic bleeding in the band ligation group [83].

The combination of endoscopic band ligation plus beta-adrenergic blockers appears to offer no benefit in terms of prevention of first bleeding when compared with endoscopic band ligation alone, but more studies are required [84]. There is a lower rate of recurrence of varices in patients treated with endoscopic band ligation plus propranolol, but at the expense of more side-effects.

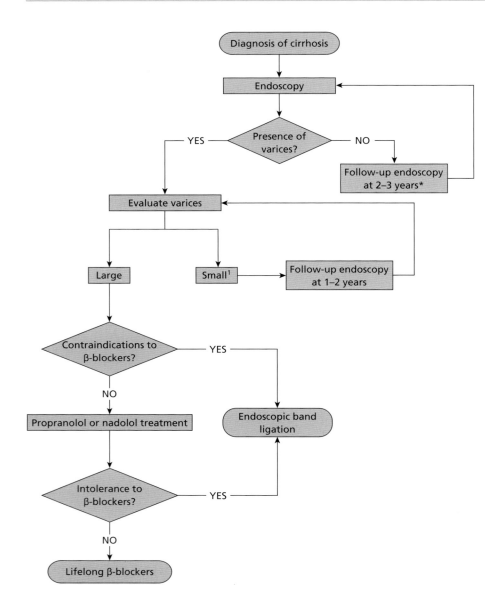

Fig. 4 Algorithm with recommendations for the prevention of first variceal bleeding in patients with cirrhosis. *Beta-adrenergic blockers might be initiated in patients with small varices. This would be especially indicated in patients in Child class B and C or with red signs at the varices.

Prevention of recurrent bleeding from oesophageal varices

Because of the extremely high risk of rebleeding in untreated patients, all patients surviving a variceal bleeding should receive active treatments for the prevention of rebleeding [19,32,85]. In addition, those with poor liver function or with other recurrent complications of portal hypertension should be considered for liver transplantation.

Drug therapy

Pharmacological treatment is based on the use of non-selective beta-adrenergic blockers [86]. Meta-analyses consistently found a marked benefit from beta-adrenergic blockers, in terms of both rebleeding (from 63% in control subjects to 42% under beta-adrenergic blockers) and mortality (from 27% to 20%) [13]. Controversy exists over whether nitrates should be added

to beta-adrenergic blockers. Two trials are available [87,88], with one of them double-blind and placebo-controlled, but only published in abstract form [87]. These studies failed consistently to show a benefit from combination therapy in terms of rebleeding or survival. However, combination therapy has been used as 'optimal' pharmacological therapy for comparisons with band ligation. Whenever possible, it is recommended to assess the haemodynamic response to beta-adrenergic blockers. If a 20% decrease in baseline HVPG or a decrease to ≤ 12 mmHg is not achieved, isosorbide mononitrate may be added, which results in achieving the target reduction in portal pressure in a third of non-responders to beta-adrenergic blockers alone ('à la carte' treatment) [89].

Endoscopic therapy

Endoscopic injection sclerotherapy of oesophageal varices also

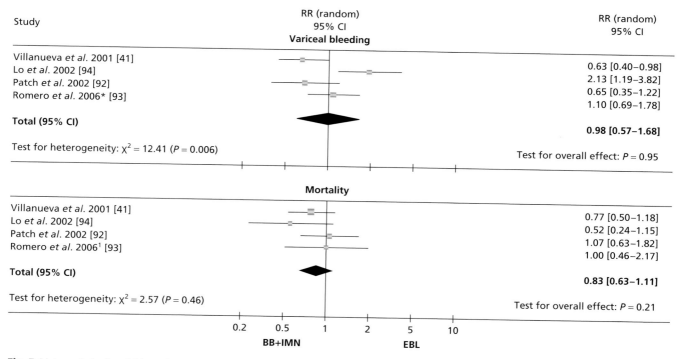

Fig. 5 Meta-analysis of available randomized controlled trials comparing pharmacological treatment [beta-adrenergic blockers plus nitrates (BB + IMN)] with endoscopic banding ligation (EBL) to prevent rebleeding. There were no differences between the two therapies in terms of variceal rebleeding and survival. *In the trial by Romero *et al.* [93], low-volume sclerotherapy was added to banding ligation.

reduces both rebleeding and death [90], but has been replaced by endoscopic band ligation, which is superior to sclerotherapy in terms of efficacy and complications [90,91]. The meta-analysis of the four available trials comparing optimal endoscopic treatment (band ligation) vs. optimized pharmacological treatment (the combination of beta-blockers and isosorbide mononitrate) [41,92–94] shows comparable results with the two therapies, but significant heterogeneity exists in the reported risk of variceal rebleeding (Fig. 5). Therefore, both beta-adrenergic blockers ± nitrates or banding ligation can be used as first-line treatments for the prevention of variceal rebleeding. If the patient bleeds while on primary prophylaxis with beta-adrenergic blockers, then the choice should be to add banding ligation, maintaining beta-adrenergic blockers (Fig. 6).

Two recent trials have shown that the association of beta-adrenergic blockers and endoscopic band ligation fares better than band ligation alone [47,95], suggesting that treatment with band ligation alone should be restricted to patients with contraindications to beta-adrenergic blockers.

Transjugular intrahepatic portosystemic shunt (TIPS)

A large corpus of consistent data indicates that TIPS is more effective than endoscopic therapy in preventing rebleeding [96]. A single trial demonstrated that it is also better than pharmacological therapy with propranolol and isosorbide mononitrate [97]. However, TIPS is associated with an increased rate of encephalopathy, does not increase survival [96] and is more

expensive than drug therapy [97]. Thus, TIPS should only be used as rescue therapy for patients experiencing repeated or significant episodes of rebleeding while being treated with beta-adrenergic blockers ± isosorbide mononitrate or endoscopic band ligation. An open question is whether TIPS should be preferred to surgical shunts in patients with good liver function (Child A or 'good' B). Two RCTs have addressed this issue so far. One compared TIPS with an 8-mm prosthetic H-graft portocaval shunt, showing a lower rate of rebleeding, death and liver transplantation in the surgical group [98]. Another trial including 140 patients compared TIPS and distal splenorenal shunt in endoscopic and/or pharmacological failures [99]. There were no significant differences in rebleeding, hepatic encephalopathy or death. Patients with TIPS required more reinterventions to maintain portal decompression, on account of the well-known tendency of TIPS to dysfunction over time. The use of polytetrafluoroethylene (PTFE)-covered stents has dramatically decreased the rate of TIPS dysfunction, clinical relapses and the need for reinterventions [100], overcoming the main drawback of traditional bare stents without increasing the risk of hepatic encephalopathy and liver failure. Therefore, PTFE-covered stents should be the choice for TIPS placement.

Treatment of acute variceal bleeding

The management of acute variceal bleeding should be undertaken in an intensive care setting by a team of experienced

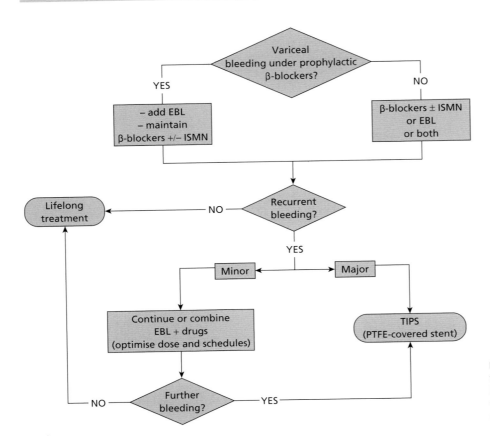

Fig. 6 Algorithm with recommendations for the prevention of rebleeding in patients who had recovered from an episode of acute variceal bleeding. EBL, endoscopic band ligation; ISMN, isosorbide mononitrate.

medical staff, including well-trained nurses, clinical hepatologists, endoscopists, interventional radiologists and surgeons. Lack of these facilities demands immediate referral. Decision-making should follow the guidelines set up in a written protocol developed to optimize the resources of each centre.

Acute variceal bleeding is defined as either active bleeding at endoscopy (emanating blood from a varix oozing or sprouting) or signs of an upper gastrointestinal bleeding (haematemesis, intragastric blood or coagulated blood, melaena) when active bleeding cannot be detected by endoscopy.

General management

The general management of the bleeding patient is aimed at correcting hypovolaemic shock (with judicious volume replacement and transfusion) and preventing complications associated with gastrointestinal bleeding (such as renal failure, hepatic decompensation, hepatic encephalopathy and bacterial infections). These goals, which are independent of the cause of the haemorrhage, demand immediate management.

Blood volume replacement should be initiated as soon as possible, aiming at maintaining the haematocrit around 24% (haemoglobin 8 g/L). The avoidance of prolonged hypovolaemic shock is particularly important in preventing complications such as infection and renal failure, which are associated with the risk of rebleeding and death [4,31]. Overtransfusion should be avoided, not only because of the risks inherent with

blood transfusion, but also because there may be a rebound increase in portal pressure with a consequent risk of continued bleeding or rebleeding [101,102]. Although the role of transfusion of platelets in patients with a platelet count less than 50 000/μL and of administration of fresh frozen plasma in patients with coagulopathy has not been assessed in clinical studies, these agents are frequently used. Initial reports demonstrated that recombinant activated factor VII (rVIIa, Novoseven) corrects prothrombin time in cirrhotics, both in non-bleeders [103] and in the acute variceal bleeding setting [104]. A recent double-blind, multicentre RCT showed that rFVIIa administration may significantly improve the results of conventional therapy in patients with moderate and advanced liver failure (stages B and C of the Child–Pugh classification), in whom variceal bleeding carries a more severe prognosis, without increasing the incidence of adverse events [48], but these results must be confirmed in new trials focusing on this target population.

Infection is a strong prognostic indicator in acute variceal bleeding [22,105]. The more frequent infections are spontaneous bacterial peritonitis (50%), urinary tract infections (25%) and pneumonia (25%). The use of antibiotics in acute variceal bleeding has been shown to reduce both the risk of rebleeding [106] and mortality [107]. Therefore, antibiotics should be given to all patients from admission. Norfloxacin, 400 mg/12 h, is the first choice on account of its simpler administration and lower cost [108]. In high-risk patients (hypovolaemic shock, ascites, jaundice or malnutrition), intravenous ceftriaxone has recently been shown to be superior to oral norfloxacin [109].

Bronchial aspiration of gastric contents and blood is a particular risk, especially in encephalopathic patients, which may be further exacerbated by endoscopic procedures. Endotracheal intubation is mandatory if there is any concern about the safety of the airway. Variceal bleeding can trigger hepatic encephalopathy. Lactulose can be given orally or by enema to prevent hepatic encephalopathy, although this has not been evaluated in randomized trials.

Specific therapy for control of bleeding

Specific therapy for acute variceal bleeding includes vasoactive drugs, endoscopic therapy and portosystemic shunts, either surgical or TIPS.

Pharmacological therapy

The action of vasoactive drugs is to reduce variceal pressure by decreasing variceal blood flow. The selection of the drug depends on the local resources. Terlipressin should be the first choice if available, as it is the only drug shown to improve survival [110]. Somatostatin, octreotide or vapreotide are the second choice [13,111]. If these drugs are not available, vasopressin plus transdermal nitroglycerin is an acceptable option [13].

Vasopressin was the first drug used, but was abandoned 25 years ago because of the severity of its cardiovascular adverse events. The association of vasopressin infusion plus nitroglycerin resulted in an enhanced fall in portal pressure and less marked systemic effects, and has been shown to be more effective and safer than vasopressin [13]. Vasopressin is started at 0.2–0.4 units/min and can be increased to a maximum of 0.8 units/min. Nitroglycerin is most commonly administered transdermally (20 mg/12 h). This combination is still used in countries were neither terlipressin nor somatostatin is available, but should not be maintained for more than 48 h because of an increased incidence of side-effects.

Terlipressin is a long-acting triglycyl lysine derivative of vasopressin. On top of its own vasoactive effects, terlipressin is slowly transformed to vasopressin by enzymatic cleavage of the triglycyl residues by tissue peptidases [112]. Clinical studies have consistently shown less frequent and severe side-effects with terlipressin than with vasopressin, even when vasopressin is associated with nitroglycerin. It has been speculated that this increased safety may be related to the combination of high tissue concentration with low circulating levels consequent to the slow release of vasopressin [112]. Terlipressin should be used with great caution in the rare cirrhotic patient with ischaemic heart disease or peripheral vascular disease. The most common side-effects are abdominal pain and hyponatraemia. Serious side-effects such as peripheral or myocardial ischaemia occur in less than 3% of patients [113].

Terlipressin may be initiated as early as variceal bleeding is suspected at a dose of 2 mg/4 h for the first 48 h, and it may be maintained for up to 5 days at a dose of 1 mg/4 h to prevent rebleeding [113]. Compared with placebo or non-active treatment, terlipressin significantly improves the rate of control of bleeding and survival [114]. This is the only treatment that has been shown to improve the prognosis of variceal bleeding in placebo-controlled RCTs and meta-analysis [13,114]. Terlipressin is as effective as any other effective therapy, including endoscopic injection sclerotherapy (EIS), and is safer than vasopressin plus nitroglycerin and EIS [13,113,114]. The overall efficacy of terlipressin in controlling acute variceal bleeding at 48 h is 75–80% across trials [114] and 67% at 5 days [113]. Terlipressin is also useful in hepatorenal syndrome [115]. Thus, the use of terlipressin for variceal bleeding may prevent renal failure, which is frequently precipitated by variceal bleeding [31].

Somatostatin has been used for over two decades [116] in the treatment of acute variceal bleeding, based on its ability to decrease portal pressure and collateral blood flow [117]. The usual scheme for somatostatin administration is an initial bolus of 250 μg followed by a 250 μg/h infusion that is maintained until the achievement of a 24-h bleed-free period. The bolus injection can be repeated up to three times in the first hour if bleeding is uncontrolled. Therapy may be maintained for up to 5 days to prevent early rebleeding [118]. The use of higher doses (500 μg/h) has been shown to translate into increased clinical efficacy in the subset of patients with more difficult bleedings (those with active bleeding at emergency endoscopy) [119]. Major side-effects with somatostatin are negligible. Minor side-effects, such as nausea and vomiting, occur in up to 25% of patients [120] and hyperglycaemia in 2–4% [118,119,121]. Several RCTs have shown that somatostatin significantly improves the rate of control of bleeding compared with placebo or non-active treatment [13,111]. However, despite the beneficial effect on control of bleeding, somatostatin did not reduce mortality [13]. Somatostatin has been compared with terlipressin, and no differences were found for failure to control bleeding, rebleeding, mortality or in the incidence of adverse events in both treatment groups [13].

Octreotide is a somatostatin analogue with a longer half-life. However, this is not associated with longer haemodynamic effects than somatostatin [122]. The optimal doses are not well determined. It is usually given as an initial bolus of 50 μg, followed by an infusion of 25 or 50 μg/h [111]. As with somatostatin, therapy can be maintained for 5 days to prevent early rebleeding. The safety profile of octreotide is similar to that of somatostatin. The efficacy of octreotide as a single therapy for variceal bleeding is controversial. No benefit from octreotide was found in the only trial using octreotide or placebo as initial treatment [123], which may be due to rapid development of tachyphylaxis [122]. However, RCTs using octreotide on top of sclerotherapy or ligation have shown a significant benefit in terms of reducing early rebleeding [124]. It has been speculated that this may be related to its sustained ability to prevent postprandial increase in portal pressure [111]. However, mortality was not affected [13,124]. These results suggest that octreotide may improve the results of endoscopic therapy but has no or little effect if used alone. When compared with other vasoactive drugs, octreotide was better than vasopressin and equivalent to terlipressin, again suggesting a clinical value from the use of octreotide [13]. Side-effects were less frequent and severe with octreotide than with either vasopressin or terlipressin, but the difference was significant only for vasopressin [13].

Endoscopic therapy

Both sclerotherapy and band ligation have been shown to be effective in the control of acute variceal bleeding [90]. Two randomized trials specifically compared band ligation and sclerotherapy in acute variceal bleeding [125,126]. In one of them, all patients received pharmacological therapy (somatostatin) [126]. Additional information can be drawn from eight trials in which these two modalities were compared for both acute bleeding and the prevention of rebleeding [90]. The meta-analysis of these data shows that endoscopic band ligation is better than sclerotherapy in the initial control of bleeding and is associated with less adverse events and improved mortality (Fig. 7). Additionally, it has been shown that sclerotherapy, but not band ligation, induces a sustained increase in portal pressure [127], a factor associated with increased risk of treatment failure [25]. Therefore, band ligation should be the endoscopic therapy of

choice in acute variceal bleeding, although injection sclerotherapy is acceptable if band ligation is not available or is technically difficult. Endoscopic therapy can be performed at the time of diagnostic endoscopy, soon after admission. However, if there is no active bleeding and the patient is stable, endoscopic treatment can probably be delayed until the next working day. This approach allows endoscopic therapy to be performed in the best conditions by a skilled endoscopist and an experienced nursing team, instead of the commonly less skilled physicians on duty. This may reduce the complications and the burden from emergency endoscopic procedures.

Current recommendations for initial treatment

The current recommendation is to combine these two approaches, starting vasoactive drug therapy early (ideally during the transfer to the hospital, even if active bleeding is only suspected) and performing endoscopic band ligation (or injection sclerotherapy if band ligation is technically difficult) after initial resuscitation (Fig. 8a). The rationale for this comes from a number of RCTs demonstrating that early administration of a vasoactive drug facilitates endoscopy and improves the control of bleeding and 5-day rebleeding [110,128,129]. Drug therapy also improves the results of endoscopic treatment if started just

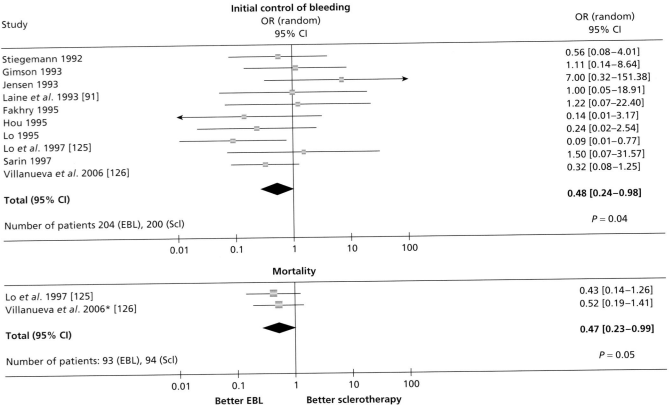

Fig. 7 Endoscopic therapy in acute variceal bleeding. Meta-analysis of studies comparing endoscopic band ligation (EBL) with endoscopic injection sclerotherapy (EIS). Note than EBL is better than sclerotherapy in terms of initial control of bleeding and mortality (update of the meta-analysis by de Franchis and Primignani [90]). OR, odds ratio.
*All patients received somatostatin.

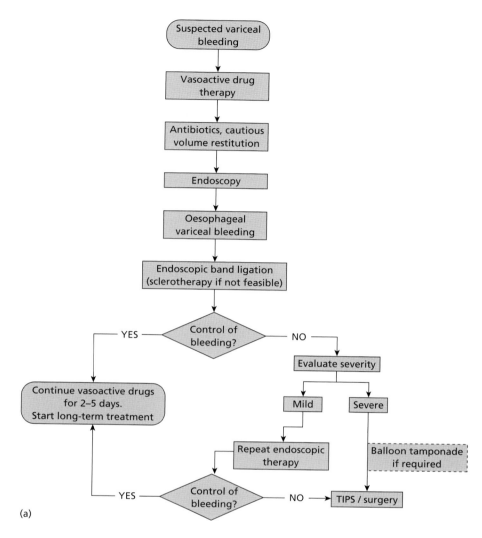

Fig. 8 Algorithm with recommendations for the treatment of acute variceal bleeding. (a) Bleeding from oesophageal varices.

(a)

after sclerotherapy or band ligation [13,111,124]. Moreover, the association with endoscopic therapy may improve the efficacy of vasoactive treatment [121]. However, this combined approach failed to improve 6-week mortality compared with endoscopic therapy [130] or a vasoactive drug [121] alone. On the other hand, single vasoactive therapy is as effective as endoscopic therapy, but with significantly fewer side-effects [131]. The optimal duration of drug therapy is not well established and requires evaluation. The current recommendation is to maintain the drug for 2–5 days. The rationale for this would be to cover the period of maximum risk of rebleeding [19].

Rescue therapies: tamponade, surgery and TIPS

In 10–20% of patients, variceal bleeding is unresponsive to initial endoscopic and/or pharmacological treatment. If bleeding is mild and the patient is stable, a second endoscopic therapy might be attempted. If this fails, or bleeding is severe, the patient should be promptly offered a derivative treatment before further deterioration in the clinical status of the patient occurs. Balloon tamponade achieves haemostasis in 60–90% of variceal bleedings [85] but should only be used in the case of massive bleeding,

for a short period of time (less than 24 h) as a temporary 'bridge' until definite treatment is instituted. These treatments include implantation of a TIPS and surgical shunts. Both are extremely effective in controlling variceal bleeding (control rate approaches 95%), but invasiveness and side-effects (mainly encephalopathy and worsening of liver function) result in high mortality [85,132,133]. TIPS is the first choice, as most patients have advanced liver disease [134]. In patients with sepsis, inotropic support, ventilation after aspiration and deterioration of liver and renal function [132], mortality after TIPS placement is nearly 100%. This clearly indicates that some patients do not benefit from TIPS in this setting, and it is usually not difficult to make a clinically based decision. Rarely, if ever, will a patient with a Child–Pugh score over 13 survive TIPS. Prognostic scores [135] may provide objective parameters to ease the decision of not offering invasive treatments in some cases.

It was suggested recently that some high-risk patients might benefit from TIPS implantation as a first-line therapy. This suggestion comes from a single study showing that patients with high portal pressure (> 20 mmHg) who underwent early TIPS

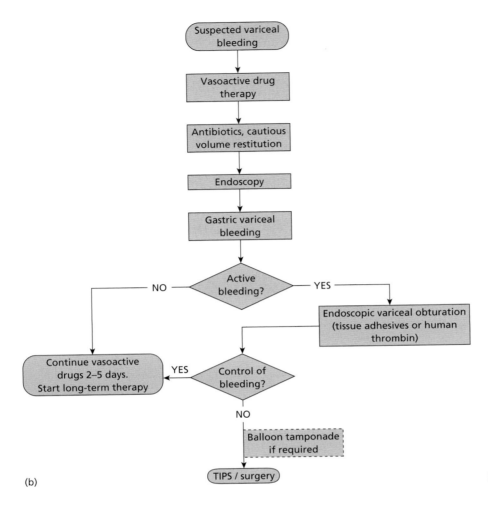

(b)

Fig. 8 (b) Bleeding from gastric varices.

placement after endoscopy had significantly fewer treatment failures and lower mortality rates than patients undergoing standard therapy [26]. If further studies, preferably with clinical criteria of high risk of failure, confirm this finding, TIPS may become an integral part of treatment for acute variceal bleeding according to individual risk factors.

Gastric varices

Gastric varices develop in approximately 20% of patients with portal hypertension [136]. They are the source of 5–10% of all upper digestive bleeding episodes in patients with cirrhosis. The risk of gastric variceal bleeding is lower than that of oesophageal variceal bleeding, but gastric variceal bleeding, in particular that from fundal varices, tends to be more severe, to require more transfusions and to have a higher mortality rate [136].

The optimal treatment of gastric varices has not been determined, as there are only a few RCTs and most data come from retrospective series and case reports. Although no RCT has been conducted until now, it seems reasonable to use non-selective beta-adrenergic blockers in patients with gastric varices to prevent the first bleeding episode. Also, the optimal treatment of acute

gastric variceal bleeding is not known. The initial treatment is similar to that of oesophageal variceal bleeding, including the administration of a vasoactive drug (terlipressin, somatostatin or a somatostatin analogue) and general management for haemodynamic stabilization and the prevention of complications (Fig. 8b). However, the efficacy of vasoactive drugs has not been assessed. Balloon tamponade, with the Linton–Nachlas tube, has been used with limited success [137,138], but may serve as a bridge to derivative treatments in massive bleedings.

Some endoscopic therapies are promising, but quality information is scarce. Sclerotherapy, glue injection, thrombin, elastic band ligation and ligation with large detachable snares have been reported [139]. In most uncontrolled series, cyanoacrylate is highly effective, in the order of 90% [140–142]. A recent RCT confirmed that endoscopic obturation using cyanoacrylate was more effective and safer than band ligation in the management of bleeding gastric varices [143]. Also, in another RCT by Sarin and coworkers, cyanoacrylate was better than alcohol injection at achieving initial haemostasis and at achieving faster variceal obliteration [144]. Novel endoscopic therapies are under evaluation. Among them, the use of human thrombin injection [145,146] seems the most promising, as this treatment does not cause mucosal damage and ulceration. These techniques need expertise and may not be feasible in massive bleedings.

TIPS is very effective in the treatment of bleeding gastric varices, with a more than 90% success rate for initial haemostasis and a low rebleeding rate [147,148]. In these patients, many centres associate TIPS with the embolization of the collateral vessels that feed the varices. Derivative and devascularization surgery is also effective, but with limited applicability in advanced cirrhosis.

The authors' recommendation is to start with a vasoactive drug. If bleeding is not controlled and an expert endoscopist is available, endoscopic treatment (cyanoacrylate or human thrombin) should be attempted. In cases of massive bleeding or after failure of previous therapies, TIPS (or surgical shunt in Child A patients) is mandatory. In some patients, especially in those with massive initial bleeding or in centres with reduced endoscopic experience in the treatment of gastric varices, TIPS may be used even before attempting endoscopic therapy.

Portal hypertensive gastropathy (PHG)

Portal hypertensive gastropathy is a macroscopic finding of a characteristic mosaic-like pattern of the gastric mucosa ('mild' PHG), red point lesions, cherry red spots and/or black–brown spots ('severe' PHG) [149]. However, these lesions are not entirely specific, i.e. they can occur in the absence of portal hypertension. In PHG, there is marked dilatation of the vasculature of the gastric mucosa and submucosa, together with an increased blood flow and a tendency towards decreased acid secretion. PHG is unrelated to *Helicobacter pylori* infection. In the largest study on the natural history of PHG, the overall prevalence of this condition was 80% in patients with cirrhosis [149]. Its prevalence is strongly correlated with the severity of portal hypertension and ranges between 11% and 80%. The incidence of acute bleeding is low (< 3% at 3 years) with a mortality of 12.5%; for chronic bleeding, the incidence is around 10–15% at 3 years. Chronic PHG bleeding usually manifests as chronic iron deficiency anaemia. Iron supplementation might be enough to keep a normal haemoglobin level. If not, beta-adrenergic blockers are the only treatment that has proved effective in these patients [150]. In acute PHG bleeding, beta-adrenergic blockers, somatostatin, octreotide, vasopressin, terlipressin and estrogens have been proposed based on their ability to decrease gastric perfusion in this condition [151–154]. However, only one uncontrolled study has so far evaluated one of these drugs (somatostatin) in the treatment of acute bleeding from PHG [155], achieving haemostasis in all patients. Propranolol has been found to reduce recurrent bleeding from PHG in a randomized trial [150]. The role of derivative treatments is controversial. Reported results with shunt surgery and TIPS suggest that these treatments are effective [156–158] but, because of a lack of randomized studies, the fluctuating nature of PHG and, possibly, unreported failures, both TIPS and shunt surgery should be considered only as rescue therapies for the uncommon patient who has repeated bleeding from PHG despite propranolol treatment. Liver transplantation reverses portal hypertension and therefore effectively treats PHG.

References

1 D'Amico G (2004) Esophageal varices: from appearance to rupture; natural history and prognostic indicators. In: Groszmann RJ, Bosch J (eds) *Portal Hypertension in the 21st Century*. Dordrecht: Kluwer Academic Publishers, pp. 147–154.

2 Christensen E, Fauerholdt L, Schlichting P *et al.* (1981) Aspects of the natural history of gastrointestinal bleeding in cirrhosis and the effect of prednisone. *Gastroenterology* 81, 944–952.

3 D'Amico G, Luca A (1997) Natural history. Clinical–haemodynamic correlations. Prediction of the risk of bleeding. *Baillieres Clin Gastroenterol* 11, 243–256.

4 de Franchis R, Primignani M (2001) Natural history of portal hypertension in patients with cirrhosis. *Clin Liver Dis* 5, 645–663.

5 Merli M, Nicolini G, Angeloni S *et al.* (2003) Incidence and natural history of small esophageal varices in cirrhotic patients. *J Hepatol* 38, 266–272.

6 Groszmann RJ, Garcia-Tsao G, Bosch J *et al.* (2005) Beta-blockers to prevent gastro-esophageal varices in patients with cirrhosis. *N Engl J Med* 353, 2254–2261.

7 De Franchis R (2003) Evaluation and follow-up of patients with cirrhosis and oesophageal varices. *J Hepatol* 38, 361–363.

8 Zoli M, Merkel C, Magalotti D *et al.* (2000) Natural history of cirrhotic patients with small esophageal varices: a prospective study. *Am J Gastroenterol* 95, 503–508.

9 Merkel C, Marin R, Angeli P *et al.* (2004) A placebo-controlled clinical trial of nadolol in the prophylaxis of growth of small esophageal varices in cirrhosis. *Gastroenterology* 127, 476–484.

10 Cales P, Desmorat H, Vinel JP *et al.* (1990) Incidence of large oesophageal varices in patients with cirrhosis: application to prophylaxis of first bleeding. *Gut* 31, 1298–1302.

11 Vorobioff J, Groszmann RJ, Picabea E *et al.* (1996) Prognostic value of hepatic venous pressure gradient measurements in alcoholic cirrhosis: a 10-year prospective study. *Gastroenterology* 111, 701–709.

12 Groszmann RJ, Bosch J, Grace ND *et al.* (1990) Hemodynamic events in a prospective randomized trial of propranolol versus placebo in the prevention of a first variceal hemorrhage (see comments). *Gastroenterology* 99, 1401–1407.

13 D'Amico G, Pagliaro L, Bosch J (1999) Pharmacological treatment of portal hypertension: an evidence-based approach. *Semin Liver Dis* 19, 475–505.

14 NIEC (1988) Prediction of the first variceal hemorrhage in patients with cirrhosis of the liver and esophageal varices. A prospective multicenter study. The North Italian Endoscopic Club for the Study and Treatment of Esophageal Varices (see comments). *N Engl J Med* 319, 983–989.

15 Merkel C, Zoli M, Siringo S *et al.* (2000) Prognostic indicators of risk for first variceal bleeding in cirrhosis: a multicenter study in 711 patients to validate and improve the North Italian Endoscopic Club (NIEC) index (in process citation). *Am J Gastroenterol* 95, 2915–2920.

16 D'Amico G, De Franchis R (2003) Upper digestive bleeding in cirrhosis. Post-therapeutic outcome and prognostic indicators. *Hepatology* 38, 599–612.

17 Merican I, Sprengers D, McCormick PA et al. (1993) Diurnal pattern of variceal bleeding in cirrhotic patients. J Hepatol 19, 15–22.

18 Garcia-Pagan JC, Feu F, Castells A et al. (1994) Circadian variations of portal pressure and variceal hemorrhage in patients with cirrhosis. Hepatology 19, 595–601.

19 de Franchis R (2005) Evolving consensus in portal hypertension. Report of the Baveno IV Consensus Workshop on methodology of diagnosis and therapy in portal hypertension. J Hepatol 43, 167–176.

20 Graham D, Smith J (1981) The course of patients after variceal hemorrhage. Gastroenterology 80, 800–806.

21 Bernard B, Cadranel JF, Valla D et al. (1995) Prognostic significance of bacterial infection in bleeding cirrhotic patients: a prospective study. Gastroenterology 108, 1828–1834.

22 Goulis J, Armonis A, Patch D et al. (1998) Bacterial infection is independently associated with failure to control bleeding in cirrhotic patients with gastrointestinal hemorrhage. Hepatology 27, 1207–1212.

23 Vivas S, Rodriguez M, Palacio MA et al. (2001) Presence of bacterial infection in bleeding cirrhotic patients is independently associated with early mortality and failure to control bleeding. Dig Dis Sci 46, 2752–2757.

24 Ben Ari Z, Cardin F, McCormick AP et al. (1999) A predictive model for failure to control bleeding during acute variceal haemorrhage. J Hepatol 31, 443–450.

25 Moitinho E, Escorsell A, Bandi JC et al. (1999) Prognostic value of early measurements of portal pressure in acute variceal bleeding. Gastroenterology 117, 626–631.

26 Monescillo A, Martinez-Lagares F, Ruiz-del-Arbol L et al. (2004) Influence of portal hypertension and its early decompression by TIPS placement on the outcome of variceal bleeding. Hepatology 40, 793–801.

27 Carbonell N, Pauwels A, Serfaty L et al. (2004) Improved survival after variceal bleeding in patients with cirrhosis over the past two decades. Hepatology 40, 652–659.

28 Nidegger D, Ragot S, Berthelemy P et al. (2003) Cirrhosis and bleeding: the need for very early management. J Hepatol 39, 509–514.

29 Gatta A, Merkel C, Amodio P et al. (1994) Development and validation of a prognostic index predicting death after upper gastrointestinal bleeding in patients with liver cirrhosis: a multicenter study. Am J Gastroenterol 89, 1528–1536.

30 del Olmo JA, Pena A, Serra MA et al. (2000) Predictors of morbidity and mortality after the first episode of upper gastrointestinal bleeding in liver cirrhosis. J Hepatol 32, 19–24.

31 Cardenas A, Gines P, Uriz J et al. (2001) Renal failure after upper gastrointestinal bleeding in cirrhosis: incidence, clinical course, predictive factors, and short-term prognosis. Hepatology 34, 671–676.

32 Grace ND, Groszmann RJ, Garcia-Tsao G et al. (1998) Portal hypertension and variceal bleeding: an AASLD single topic symposium. Hepatology 28, 868–880.

33 de Franchis R (2000) Updating consensus in portal hypertension: report of the Baveno III Consensus Workshop on definitions, methodology and therapeutic strategies in portal hypertension. J Hepatol 33, 846–852.

34 Feu F, Garcia-Pagan JC, Bosch J et al. (1995) Relation between portal pressure response to pharmacotherapy and risk of recurrent variceal haemorrhage in patients with cirrhosis. Lancet 346, 1056–1059.

35 Abraldes JG, Tarantino I, Turnes J et al. (2003) Hemodynamic response to pharmacological treatment of portal hypertension and long-term prognosis of cirrhosis. Hepatology 37, 902–908.

36 Viallet A, Marleau D, Huet M et al. (1975) Hemodynamic evaluation of patients with intrahepatic portal hypertension. Relationship between bleeding varices and the portohepatic gradient. Gastroenterology 69, 1297–1300.

37 Garcia-Tsao G, Groszmann RJ, Fisher RL et al. (1985) Portal pressure, presence of gastroesophageal varices and variceal bleeding. Hepatology 5, 419–424.

38 Casado M, Bosch J, Garcia-Pagan JC et al. (1998) Clinical events after transjugular intrahepatic portosystemic shunt: correlation with hemodynamic findings. Gastroenterology 114, 1296–1303.

39 Merkel C, Bolognesi M, Sacerdoti D et al. (2000) The hemodynamic response to medical treatment of portal hypertension as a predictor of clinical effectiveness in the primary prophylaxis of variceal bleeding in cirrhosis. Hepatology 32, 930–934.

40 Villanueva C, Balanzo J, Novella MT et al. (1996) Nadolol plus isosorbide mononitrate compared with sclerotherapy for the prevention of variceal rebleeding. N Engl J Med 334, 1624–1629.

41 Villanueva C, Minana J, Ortiz J et al. (2001) Endoscopic ligation compared with combined treatment with nadolol and isosorbide mononitrate to prevent recurrent variceal bleeding. N Engl J Med 345, 647–655.

42 Escorsell A, Bordas JM, Castaneda B et al. (2000) Predictive value of the variceal pressure response to continued pharmacological therapy in patients with cirrhosis and portal hypertension. Hepatology 31, 1061–1067.

43 Villanueva C, Lopez-Balaguer JM, Aracil C et al. (2004) Maintenance of hemodynamic response to treatment for portal hypertension and influence on complications of cirrhosis. J Hepatol 40, 757–765.

44 Schrier RW, Arroyo V, Bernardi M et al. (1988) Peripheral arterial vasodilation hypothesis: a proposal for the initiation of renal sodium and water retention in cirrhosis. Hepatology 8, 1151–1157.

45 Groszmann RJ (1994) Hyperdynamic circulation of liver disease 40 years later: pathophysiology and clinical consequences. Hepatology 20, 1359–1363.

46 Garcia-Pagan JC, Salmeron JM, Feu F et al. (1994) Effects of low-sodium diet and spironolactone on portal pressure in patients with compensated cirrhosis. Hepatology 19, 1095–1099.

47 de la Pena J, Brullet E, Sanchez-Hernandez E et al. (2005) Variceal ligation plus nadolol compared with ligation for prophylaxis of variceal rebleeding: a multicenter trial. Hepatology 41, 572–578.

48 Bosch J, Thabut D, Bendtsen F et al. (2004) Recombinant factor VIIa for upper gastrointestinal bleeding in patients with cirrhosis: a randomized, double-blind trial. Gastroenterology 127, 1123–1130.

49 Zaman A, Hapke R, Flora K et al. (1999) Factors predicting the presence of esophageal or gastric varices in patients with advanced liver disease. Am J Gastroenterol 94, 3292–3296.

50 Chalasani N, Imperiale TF, Ismail A et al. (1999) Predictors of large esophageal varices in patients with cirrhosis. Am J Gastroenterol 94, 3285–3291.

51 Madhotra R, Mulcahy HE, Willner I et al. (2002) Prediction of esophageal varices in patients with cirrhosis. J Clin Gastroenterol 34, 81–85.

52 Giannini E, Botta F, Borro P et al. (2003) Platelet count/spleen diameter ratio, proposal and validation of a non-invasive parameter to predict the presence of oesophageal varices in patients with liver cirrhosis. Gut 52, 1200–1205.

53 Saab S, DeRosa V, Nieto J et al. (2003) Costs and clinical outcomes of primary prophylaxis of variceal bleeding in patients with hepatic cirrhosis: a decision analytic model. Am J Gastroenterol 98, 763–770.

54 Spiegel BM, Targownik L, Dulai GS *et al.* (2003) Endoscopic screening for esophageal varices in cirrhosis: is it ever cost effective? *Hepatology* 37, 366–377.

55 Arguedas MR, Heudebert GR, Eloubeidi MA *et al.* (2002) Cost-effectiveness of screening, surveillance, and primary prophylaxis strategies for esophageal varices. *Am J Gastroenterol* 97, 2441–2452.

56 Lebrec D, Nouel O, Corbic M *et al.* (1980) Propranolol – a medical treatment for portal hypertension? *Lancet* 2, 180–182.

57 Kroeger RJ, Groszmann RJ (1985) Effect of selective blockade of beta 2-adrenergic receptors on portal and systemic hemodynamics in a portal hypertensive rat model. *Gastroenterology* 88, 896–900.

58 Gengo FM, Huntoon L, McHugh WB (1987) Lipid-soluble and water-soluble beta-blockers. Comparison of the central nervous system depressant effect. *Arch Intern Med* 147, 39–43.

59 Wang T, Kaumann AJ, Brown MJ (1996) (–)-Timolol is a more potent antagonist of the positive inotropic effects of (–)-adrenaline than of those of (–)-noradrenaline in human atrium. *Br J Clin Pharmacol* 42, 217–223.

60 Garcia-Pagan J, Morillas RM, Bañares R *et al.* (2003) Propranolol plus placebo vs propranolol plus isosorbide-5-mononitrate in the prevention of the first variceal bleed. A double blind RCT. *Hepatology* 37, 1260–1266.

61 Garcia-Pagan JC, Villanueva C, Vila MC *et al.* (2001) Isosorbide mononitrate in the prevention of first variceal bleed in patients who cannot receive beta-blockers. *Gastroenterology* 121, 908–914.

62 Poynard T, Cales P, Pasta L *et al.* (1991) Beta-adrenergic-antagonist drugs in the prevention of gastrointestinal bleeding in patients with cirrhosis and esophageal varices. An analysis of data and prognostic factors in 589 patients from four randomized clinical trials. Franco-Italian Multicenter Study Group. *N Engl J Med* 324, 1532–1538.

63 Bosch J (2005) Is treatment with nadolol effective against the growth of small esophageal varices in patients with cirrhosis? *Nature Clin Pract Gastroenterol Hepatol* 2, 18–19.

64 Abraczinskas DR, Ookubo R, Grace ND *et al.* (2001) Propranolol for the prevention of first esophageal variceal hemorrhage: a lifetime commitment? *Hepatology* 34, 1096–1102.

65 Garcia-Pagan JC, Feu F, Bosch J *et al.* (1991) Propranolol compared with propranolol plus isosorbide-5-mononitrate for portal hypertension in cirrhosis. A randomized controlled study. *Ann Intern Med* 114, 869–873.

66 Merkel C, Sacerdoti D, Bolognesi M *et al.* (1997) Hemodynamic evaluation of the addition of isosorbide-5-mononitrate to nadolol in cirrhotic patients with insufficient response to the beta-blocker alone. *Hepatology* 26, 34–39.

67 Merkel C, Marin R, Enzo E *et al.* (1996) Randomised trial of nadolol alone or with isosorbide mononitrate for primary prophylaxis of variceal bleeding in cirrhosis. Gruppo-Triveneto per L'ipertensione portale (GTIP) (see comments). *Lancet* 348, 1677–1681.

68 Merkel C, Marin R, Sacerdoti D *et al.* (2000) Long-term results of a clinical trial of nadolol with or without isosorbide mononitrate for primary prophylaxis of variceal bleeding in cirrhosis. *Hepatology* 31, 324–329.

69 Imperiale TF, Chalasani N (2001) A meta-analysis of endoscopic variceal ligation for primary prophylaxis of esophageal variceal bleeding. *Hepatology* 33, 802–807.

70 De BK, Ghoshal UC, Das T *et al.* (1999) Endoscopic variceal ligation for primary prophylaxis of oesophageal variceal bleed: preliminary report of a randomized controlled trial. *J Gastroenterol Hepatol* 14, 220–224.

71 Lui HF, Stanley AJ, Forrest EH *et al.* (2002) Primary prophylaxis of variceal hemorrhage: a randomized controlled trial comparing band ligation, propranolol, and isosorbide mononitrate. *Gastroenterology* 123, 735–744.

72 Schepke M, Kleber G, Nurnberg D *et al.* (2004) Ligation versus propranolol for the primary prophylaxis of variceal bleeding in cirrhosis. *Hepatology* 40, 65–72.

73 Lo GH, Chen WC, Chen MH *et al.* (2004) Endoscopic ligation vs. nadolol in the prevention of first variceal bleeding in patients with cirrhosis. *Gastrointest Endosc* 59, 333–338.

74 Sarin SK, Lamba GS, Kumar M *et al.* (1999) Comparison of endoscopic ligation and propranolol for the primary prevention of variceal bleeding (see comments). *N Engl J Med* 340, 988–993.

75 Jutabha R, Jensen DM, Martin P *et al.* (2005) Randomized study comparing banding and propanolol to prevent initial variceal hemorrhage in cirrhotics with high-risk esophageal varices. *Gastroenterology* 128, 870–881.

76 Thuluvath PJ, Maheshwari A, Jagannath S *et al.* (2005) A randomized controlled trial of beta-blockers versus endoscopic band ligation for primary prophylaxis: a large sample size is required to show a difference in bleeding rates. *Dig Dis Sci* 50, 407–410.

77 Song H, Shin JW, Kim HI *et al.* (2000) A prospective randomized trial between the prophylactic endoscopic variceal ligation and propranolol administration for prevention of first bleeding in cirrhotic patients with high risk esophageal varices. *J Hepatol* 32 (Suppl. 2), 41A.

78 Gheorghe C, Gheorghe L, Vadan R *et al.* (2002) Prophylactic banding ligation of high-risk esophageal varices in patients on the waiting list for liver transplantation: an interim analysis. *J Hepatol* 36 (Suppl. 1), 38A.

79 Drastich P, Lata J, Petrtyl J *et al.* (2005) Endoscopic variceal band ligation in comparison with propranolol in prophylaxis of first variceal bleeding in patients with liver cirrhosis. *J Hepatol* 42, 202a.

80 de la Mora, Farca-Belsaguy AA, Uribe M *et al.* (2000) Ligation vs propranolol for primary prophylaxis of variceal bleeding using multiple band ligator and objective measurements of treatment adequacy: preliminary results. *Gastroenterology* 118, 6511A.

81 Chen CY, Sheu MZ, Su SY (1998) Prophylactic endoscopic variceal ligation for esophageal varices. *Gastroenterology* 114, 1224A.

82 Turnes J, García-Pagán JC, Abraldes JG *et al.* (2003) Pharmacological reduction of portal pressure and long term risk of first variceal bleeding in patients with cirrhosis. *Hepatology* 38, 219A.

83 Triantos C, Vlachogiannakos J, Armonis A *et al.* (2005) Primary prophylaxis of variceal bleeding in cirrhotics unable to take beta-blockers: a randomized trial of ligation. *Aliment Pharmacol Ther* 21, 1435–1443.

84 Sarin SK, Wadhawan M, Agarwal SR *et al.* (2005) Endoscopic variceal ligation plus propranolol versus endoscopic variceal ligation alone in primary prophylaxis of variceal bleeding. *Am J Gastroenterol* 100, 797–804.

85 D'Amico G, Pagliaro L, Bosch J (1995) The treatment of portal hypertension: a meta-analytic review. *Hepatology* 22, 332–354.

86 Lebrec D, Nouel O, Bernuau J *et al.* (1981) Propranolol in prevention of recurrent gastrointestinal bleeding in cirrhotic patients. Lancet 1, 920–921.

87 Pasta L, D'Amico G, Patti R (1999) Isosorbide mononitrate (IMN) with nadolol compared with nadolol alone for prevention of recurrent bleeding in cirrhosis. a double-blind placebo-controlled randomised trial. *J Hepatol* 30, 81A.

88 Gournay J, Masliah C, Martin T et al. (2000) Isosorbide mononitrate and propranolol compared with propranolol alone for the prevention of variceal rebleeding. Hepatology 31, 1239–1245.

89 Bureau C, Peron JM, Alric L et al. (2002) 'A la carte' treatment of portal hypertension: adapting medical therapy to hemodynamic response for the prevention of bleeding. Hepatology 36, 1361–1366.

90 de Franchis R, Primignani M (1999) Endoscopic treatments for portal hypertension. Semin Liver Dis 19, 439–455.

91 Laine L, el Newihi HM, Migikovsky B et al. (1993) Endoscopic ligation compared with sclerotherapy for the treatment of bleeding esophageal varices. Ann Intern Med 119, 1–7.

92 Patch D, Sabin CA, Goulis J et al. (2002) A randomized, controlled trial of medical therapy versus endoscopic ligation for the prevention of variceal rebleeding in patients with cirrhosis. Gastroenterology 123, 1013–1019.

93 Romero G, Kravetz D, Argonz J et al. (2006) Comparative study between nadolol and 5-isosorbide mononitrate vs. endoscopic band ligation plus sclerotherapy in the prevention of variceal rebleeding in cirrhotic patients: a randomized controlled trial. Aliment Pharmacol Ther 24, 601–611.

94 Lo GH, Chen WC, Chen MH et al. (2002) Banding ligation versus nadolol and isosorbide mononitrate for the prevention of esophageal variceal rebleeding. Gastroenterology 123, 728–734.

95 Lo GH, Lai KH, Cheng JS et al. (2000) Endoscopic variceal ligation plus nadolol and sucralfate compared with ligation alone for the prevention of variceal rebleeding: a prospective, randomized trial. Hepatology 32, 461–465.

96 Burroughs AK, Vangeli M (2002) Transjugular intrahepatic portosystemic shunt versus endoscopic therapy: randomized trials for secondary prophylaxis of variceal bleeding: an updated meta-analysis. Scand J Gastroenterol 37, 249–252.

97 Escorsell A, Banares R, Garcia-Pagan JC et al. (2002) TIPS versus drug therapy in preventing variceal rebleeding in advanced cirrhosis: a randomized controlled trial. Hepatology 35, 385–392.

98 Rosemurgy AS, Serafini FM, Zweibel BR et al. (2000) Transjugular intrahepatic portosystemic shunt vs. small-diameter prosthetic H-graft portacaval shunt: extended follow-up of an expanded randomized prospective trial. J Gastrointest Surg 4, 589–597.

99 Henderson JM, Boyer TD, Kutner MH et al. (2006) Distal splenorenal shunt versus transjugular intrahepatic portal systematic shunt for variceal bleeding: a randomized trial. Gastroenterology 130, 1643–1651.

100 Bureau C, Garcia-Pagan JC, Otal P et al. (2004) Improved clinical outcome using polytetrafluoroethylene-coated stents for tips: results of a randomized study. Gastroenterology 126, 469–475.

101 McCormick PA, Jenkins SA, McIntyre N et al. (1995) Why portal hypertensive varices bleed and bleed: a hypothesis. Gut 36, 100–103.

102 Castaneda B, Morales J, Lionetti R et al. (2001) Effects of blood volume restitution following a portal hypertensive-related bleeding in anesthetized cirrhotic rats. Hepatology 33, 821–825.

103 Bernstein DE, Jeffers L, Erhardtsen E et al. (1997) Recombinant factor VIIa corrects prothrombin time in cirrhotic patients: a preliminary study. Gastroenterology 113, 1930–1937.

104 Ejlersen E, Melsen T, Ingerslev J et al. (2001) Recombinant activated factor VII (rFVIIa) acutely normalizes prothrombin time in patients with cirrhosis during bleeding from oesophageal varices. Scand J Gastroenterol 36, 1081–1085.

105 Vivas S, Rodriguez M, Palacio MA et al. (2001) Presence of bacterial infection in bleeding cirrhotic patients is independently associated with early mortality and failure to control bleeding. Dig Dis Sci 46, 2752–2757.

106 Hou MC, Lin HC, Liu TT et al. (2004) Antibiotic prophylaxis after endoscopic therapy prevents rebleeding in acute variceal hemorrhage: a randomized trial. Hepatology 39, 746–753.

107 Bernard B, Grange JD, Khac EN et al. (1999) Antibiotic prophylaxis for the prevention of bacterial infections in cirrhotic patients with gastrointestinal bleeding: a meta-analysis. Hepatology 29, 1655–1661.

108 Rimola A, Garcia-Tsao G, Navasa M et al. (2000) Diagnosis, treatment and prophylaxis of spontaneous bacterial peritonitis: a consensus document. International Ascites Club. J Hepatol 32, 142–153.

109 Fernandez J, Ruiz del Arbol L, Serradilla R et al. (2006) Norfloxacin vs ceftriaxone in the prophylaxis of infections in cirrhotics with advanced cirrhosis and hemorrhage. Gastroenterology 131, 1049–1056.

110 Levacher S, Letoumelin P, Pateron D et al. (1995) Early administration of terlipressin plus glyceryl trinitrate to control active upper gastrointestinal bleeding in cirrhotic patients. Lancet 346, 865–868.

111 Abraldes JG, Bosch J (2002) Somatostatin and analogues in portal hypertension. Hepatology 35, 1305–1312.

112 Bosch J, Lebrec D, Jenkins SA (1998) Development of analogues: successes and failures. Scand J Gastroenterol Suppl 226, 3–13.

113 Escorsell A, Ruiz d'A, Planas R et al. (2000) Multicenter randomized controlled trial of terlipressin versus sclerotherapy in the treatment of acute variceal bleeding: the TEST study. Hepatology 32, 471–476.

114 Ioannou GN, Doust J, Rockey DC (2003) Systematic review: terlipressin in acute oesophageal variceal haemorrhage. Aliment Pharmacol Ther 17, 53–64.

115 Uriz J, Gines P, Cardenas A et al. (2000) Terlipressin plus albumin infusion: an effective and safe therapy of hepatorenal syndrome. J Hepatol 33, 43–48.

116 Tyden G, Sammegard H, Thulin L et al. (1978) Treatment of bleeding esophageal varices with somatostatin. N Engl J Med 299, 1466–1467.

117 Bosch J, Kravetz D, Rodes J (1981) Effects of somatostatin on hepatic and systemic hemodynamics in patients with cirrhosis of the liver: comparison with vasopressin. Gastroenterology 80, 518–525.

118 Escorsell A, Bordas JM, del Arbol LR et al. (1998) Randomized controlled trial of sclerotherapy versus somatostatin infusion in the prevention of early rebleeding following acute variceal hemorrhage in patients with cirrhosis. Variceal Bleeding Study Group. J Hepatol 29, 779–788.

119 Moitinho E, Planas R, Bañares R et al. (2001) Multicenter randomized controlled trial comparing different schedules of somatostatin in the treatment of acute variceal bleeding. J Hepatol 35, 712–718.

120 Valenzuela JE, Schubert T, Fogel MR et al. (1989) A multicenter, randomized, double-blind trial of somatostatin in the management of acute hemorrhage from esophageal varices (see comments). Hepatology 10, 958–961.

121 Villanueva C, Ortiz J, Sabat M et al. (1999) Somatostatin alone or combined with emergency sclerotherapy in the treatment of acute esophageal variceal bleeding: a prospective randomized trial. Hepatology 30, 384–389.

122 Escorsell A, Bandi JC, Andreu V et al. (2001) Desensitization to the effects of intravenous octreotide in cirrhotic patients with portal hypertension. Gastroenterology 120, 161–169.

123 International Octreotide Varices Study Group and Burroughs AK (1996) Double blind RCT of 5 day octreotide versus placebo, associated with sclerotherapy for trial failures. Hepatology 24, 352A.

124 Corley DA, Cello JP, Adkisson W *et al.* (2001) Octreotide for acute esophageal variceal bleeding: a meta-analysis. *Gastroenterology* 120, 946–954.

125 Lo GH, Lai KH, Cheng JS *et al.* (1997) Emergency banding ligation versus sclerotherapy for the control of active bleeding from esophageal varices. *Hepatology* 25, 1101–1104.

126 Villanueva C, Morales J, Lionetti R *et al.* (2001) A randomized controlled trial comparing ligation and sclerotherapy as emergency endoscopic treatment added to somatostatin in acute variceal bleeding. *J Hepatol* 45, 560–567.

127 Avgerinos A, Armonis A, Stefanidis G *et al.* (2004) Sustained rise of portal pressure after sclerotherapy, but not band ligation, in acute variceal bleeding in cirrhosis. *Hepatology* 39, 1623–1630.

128 Avgerinos A, Nevens F, Raptis S *et al.* (1997) Early administration of somatostatin and efficacy of sclerotherapy in acute oesophageal variceal bleeds: the European Acute Bleeding Oesophageal Variceal Episodes (ABOVE) randomised trial. *Lancet* 350, 1495–1499.

129 Cales P, Masliah C, Bernard B *et al.* (2001) Early administration of vapreotide for variceal bleeding in patients with cirrhosis. French Club for the Study of Portal Hypertension. *N Engl J Med* 344, 23–28.

130 Banares R, Albillos A, Rincon D *et al.* (2002) Endoscopic treatment versus endoscopic plus pharmacologic treatment for acute variceal bleeding: a meta-analysis. *Hepatology* 35, 609–615.

131 D'Amico G, Pietrosi G, Tarantino I *et al.* (2003) Emergency sclerotherapy versus vasoactive drugs for variceal bleeding in cirrhosis: a Cochrane meta-analysis. *Gastroenterology* 124, 1277–1291.

132 Burroughs AK, Patch D (1999) Transjugular intrahepatic portosystemic shunt. *Semin Liver Dis* 19, 457–473.

133 Bosch J (2001) Salvage transjugular intrahepatic portosystemic shunt: is it really life-saving? *J Hepatol* 35, 658–660.

134 Henderson JM (2001) Salvage therapies for refractory variceal hemorrhage. *Clin Liver Dis* 5, 709–725.

135 Patch D, Nikolopoulou V, McCormick A *et al.* (1998) Factors related to early mortality after transjugular intrahepatic portosystemic shunt for failed endoscopic therapy in acute variceal bleeding. *J Hepatol* 28, 454–460.

136 Sarin SK, Lahoti D, Saxena SP *et al.* (1992) Prevalence, classification and natural history of gastric varices: a long-term follow-up study in 568 portal hypertension patients. *Hepatology* 16, 1343–1349.

137 Teres J, Cecilia A, Bordas JM *et al.* (1978) Esophageal tamponade for bleeding varices. Controlled trial between the Sengstaken–Blakemore tube and the Linton–Nachlas tube. *Gastroenterology* 75, 566–569.

138 Panes J, Teres J, Bosch J *et al.* (1988) Efficacy of balloon tamponade in treatment of bleeding gastric and esophageal varices. Results in 151 consecutive episodes. *Dig Dis Sci* 33, 454–459.

139 Sarin SK, Agarwal SR (2001) Gastric varices and portal hypertensive gastropathy. *Clin Liver Dis* 5, 727–767, x.

140 Huang YH, Yeh HZ, Chen GH *et al.* (2000) Endoscopic treatment of bleeding gastric varices by N-butyl-2-cyanoacrylate (Histoacryl) injection: long-term efficacy and safety. *Gastrointest Endosc* 52, 160–167.

141 Lee YT, Chan FK, Ng EK *et al.* (2000) EUS-guided injection of cyanoacrylate for bleeding gastric varices. *Gastrointest Endosc* 52, 168–174.

142 Kind R, Guglielmi A, Rodella L *et al.* (2000) Bucrylate treatment of bleeding gastric varices: 12 years' experience. *Endoscopy* 32, 512–519.

143 Lo GH, Lai KH, Cheng JS *et al.* (2001) A prospective, randomized trial of butyl cyanoacrylate injection versus band ligation in the management of bleeding gastric varices. *Hepatology* 33, 1060–1064.

144 Sarin SK, Jain AK, Jain M *et al.* (2002) A randomized controlled trial of cyanoacrylate versus alcohol injection in patients with isolated fundic varices. *Am J Gastroenterol* 97, 1010–1015.

145 Heneghan MA, Byrne A, Harrison PM (2002) An open pilot study of the effects of a human fibrin glue for endoscopic treatment of patients with acute bleeding from gastric varices. *Gastrointest Endosc* 56, 422–426.

146 Yang WL, Tripathi D, Therapondos G *et al.* (2002) Endoscopic use of human thrombin in bleeding gastric varices. *Am J Gastroenterol* 97, 1381–1385.

147 Chau TN, Patch D, Chan YW *et al.* (1998) 'Salvage' transjugular intrahepatic portosystemic shunts: gastric fundal compared with esophageal variceal bleeding. *Gastroenterology* 114, 981–987.

148 Barange K, Peron JM, Imani K *et al.* (1999) Transjugular intrahepatic portosystemic shunt in the treatment of refractory bleeding from ruptured gastric varices. *Hepatology* 30, 1139–1143.

149 Primignani M, Carpinelli L, Preatoni P *et al.* (2000) Natural history of portal hypertensive gastropathy in patients with liver cirrhosis. The New Italian Endoscopic Club for the study and treatment of esophageal varices (NIEC). *Gastroenterology* 119, 181–187.

150 Perez-Ayuso RM, Pique JM, Bosch J *et al.* (1991) Propranolol in prevention of recurrent bleeding from severe portal hypertensive gastropathy in cirrhosis. *Lancet* 337, 1431–1434.

151 Panes J, Bordas JM, Pique JM *et al.* (1993) Effects of propranolol on gastric mucosal perfusion in cirrhotic patients with portal hypertensive gastropathy. *Hepatology* 17, 213–218.

152 Panes J, Pique JM, Bordas JM *et al.* (1994) Reduction of gastric hyperemia by glypressin and vasopressin administration in cirrhotic patients with portal hypertensive gastropathy. *Hepatology* 19, 55–60.

153 Panes J, Pique JM, Bordas JM *et al.* (1994) Effect of bolus injection and continuous infusion of somatostatin on gastric perfusion in cirrhotic patients with portal-hypertensive gastropathy. *Hepatology* 20, 336–341.

154 Panes J, Casadevall M, Fernandez M *et al.* (1994) Gastric microcirculatory changes of portal-hypertensive rats can be attenuated by long-term estrogen–progestagen treatment. *Hepatology* 20, 1261–1270.

155 Kouroumalis EA, Koutroubakis IE, Manousos ON (1998) Somatostatin for acute severe bleeding from portal hypertensive gastropathy. *Eur J Gastroenterol Hepatol* 10, 509–512.

156 Orloff MJ, Orloff MS, Orloff SL *et al.* (1995) Treatment of bleeding from portal hypertensive gastropathy by portacaval shunt. *Hepatology* 21, 1011–1017.

157 Urata J, Yamashita Y, Tsuchigame T *et al.* (1998) The effects of transjugular intrahepatic portosystemic shunt on portal hypertensive gastropathy. *J Gastroenterol Hepatol* 13, 1061–1067.

158 Kamath PS, Lacerda M, Ahlquist DA *et al.* (2000) Gastric mucosal responses to intrahepatic portosystemic shunting in patients with cirrhosis. *Gastroenterology* 118, 905–911.

7.4 Haemodynamic assessment of portal hypertension

Juan Carlos García-Pagán, Juan Turnes and Jaime Bosch

Portal hypertension is a frequent clinical syndrome defined by a pathological increase in the portal venous pressure, which is responsible for the more frequent and severe complications of cirrhosis: gastrointestinal bleeding from gastro-oesophageal varices, ascites, renal dysfunction and hepatic encephalopathy. Because of the combined impact of these complications, portal hypertension represents the main cause of death and liver transplantation in patients with cirrhosis [1].

Measurement of portal pressure

Introduction and scientific basis

Measurement of the portal pressure is still the single most important haemodynamic measurement in portal hypertension. Other methods, such as the endoscopy assessment of the existence of oesophageal or gastric varices or the visualization of portal collateral circulation by imaging techniques, provide additional information but are not substitutes for the measurement of portal pressure.

The first published measurement of portal pressure in humans was that of Thompson *et al.* in 1937 [2] who recorded portal venous pressure during abdominal surgery. But it was in 1951 that Myers and Taylor [3], inspired by Dexter *et al.*'s experience with pulmonary capillary pressure for measuring left auricular pressure [4], developed the measurement of wedged hepatic venous pressure (WHVP) as an indirect index of portal venous pressure. The scientific basis is that, when blood flow in a hepatic vein is stopped by a 'wedged' small catheter, a continuous column of blood between the catheter and the sinusoid is formed, resulting in a pressure reading that is equal to the sinusoidal pressure. Thus, WHVP is a measurement of the hepatic sinusoidal pressure and not of the portal pressure itself. However, many studies have demonstrated that WHVP adequately reproduces portal pressure in alcoholic liver disease and hepatitis C- and hepatitis B-related cirrhosis [5,6]. These entities are by far the most frequent aetiologies of chronic liver disease in developed countries. It was soon evident that hepatic vein catheterization constituted a safe and relatively simple technique

for performing accurate measurements of portal pressure in patients with liver disease [7,8]. However, it took five decades of broad experience with the technique before hepatic vein pressure measurements were recognized as a useful tool in the clinical management of patients with cirrhosis and portal hypertension. A limitation of this technique is that it does not reproduce the portal pressure in presinusoidal causes of portal hypertension such as portal vein thrombosis, early primary biliary cirrhosis, idiopathic portal hypertension or schistosomiasis. In these cases, a direct assessment of the portal pressure is mandatory.

Portal pressure should be expressed in terms of the portal pressure gradient, defined as the difference between WHVP and free hepatic venous pressure (FHVP), the so-called hepatic venous pressure gradient or HVPG, which has the advantage of not being modified by changes in intra-abdominal pressure such as those occurring in the presence of tense ascites or after total-volume paracentesis [9]. Increased intra-abdominal pressure will increase both the WHVP and the FHVP, but will not significantly modify the HVPG.

Description of the technique

Portal pressure may be measured by either direct or indirect methods.

Direct measurements of portal pressure

Direct measurement of portal pressure involves invasive techniques based on the surgical, percutaneous transhepatic or transvenous (transjugular) catheterization of the portal vein. In these techniques, except for the transjugular approach, the measurement of inferior vena cava (IVC) pressure requires the additional, simultaneous puncture of a hepatic vein to be able to determine the portal pressure gradient [10]. Because of this inconvenience and the associated surgical or haemorrhagic risk, direct measurements of portal pressure are reserved for cases of suspected presinusoidal portal hypertension.

The safety of either the percutaneous transhepatic or transjugular catheterization of the portal vein may be increased by

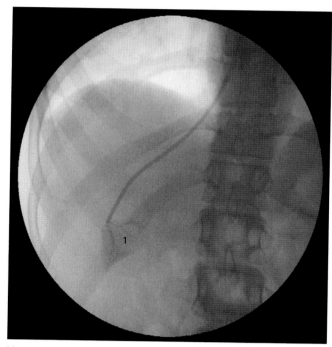

(a)

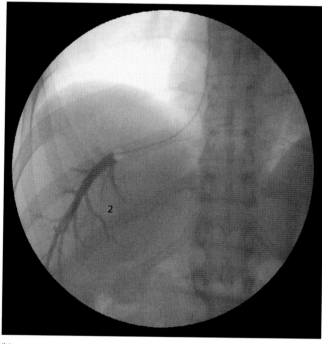

(b)

Fig. 1 The catheter (a) is advanced until it becomes 'wedged' into a small branch of the hepatic vein. Injection of contrast dye shows a small area of liver parenchyma draining to the vein where the catheter is wedged (1). The balloon-tipped catheter (b) allows occlusion of the blood flow in a larger segment of the liver (2), and allows repeat measurements of WHVP and FHVP in the same position.

performing the procedures under ultrasonographic guidance. The haemorrhagic risk is greater in the percutaneous procedure, which precludes its use in patients with impaired coagulation. This can be partly overcome by using a thin needle and by occluding the intrahepatic tract with gelatine sponge particles or coils passed through the catheter while withdrawing it from the liver.

Other drawbacks of the technique are the risk of causing portal vein thrombosis due to local trauma, capsular laceration with haemoperitoneum and subcapsular haematoma.

Indirect measurements of portal pressure: hepatic vein catheterization

This is the most commonly used technique to evaluate portal pressure [11] and has become a routine test in many hospitals. Basically, it consists of introducing, by the Seldinger technique, a venous introducer into the femoral or jugular vein under local anaesthesia and conscious sedation. A 5 or 7 French balloon-tipped catheter is then advanced into a hepatic vein, usually the main right hepatic vein, under fluoroscopic control. Before balloon inflation, the pressure measured is the FHVP, which reflects the IVC pressure (indeed, the difference between both should be less than 2 mmHg). WHVP is measured by occluding the hepatic vein, either by inflating the balloon at the tip of the catheter ('occluded' pressure) or by advancing the catheter until it becomes 'wedged' into a small branch of a hepatic vein (Fig. 1). The wedged/occluded position is confirmed by a slow injection of 5 mL of contrast dye through the catheter. If wedging is complete, the contrast outlines a portion of the hepatic venous tree distal to the catheter tip. Otherwise, the contrast flows back along the catheter or washout through communications with other hepatic veins (Fig. 2). The catheter should be carefully rinsed with 5% dextrose before measuring pressures. The balloon catheter is preferred on account of the lower variability of measurements as the pressure obtained represents the average of a wider vascular area of the liver [12]. In addition, the balloon catheter technique has the advantage of allowing repeated measurements from the same hepatic vein, which otherwise requires advancing and withdrawing the catheter for each HVPG measurement.

Although it is easy and simple to perform, accurate HVPG measurements require specific training, because the procedure differs from that used in heart catheterization laboratories and intensive care units. The following are useful tips to ensure adequate measurements:

• The transducer should be calibrated against known external pressures before starting measurements (e.g. 13.6 cmH$_2$O should read 10 mmHg and 27.2 cmH$_2$O should read 20 mmHg). Transducers that do not calibrate exactly should be discarded.

• The transducer should be placed at the level of the right atrium (midaxillary line), and the 'zero' pressure (the atmospheric pressure with the transducer open to the air) should match the 'zero' line in the pressure tracing.

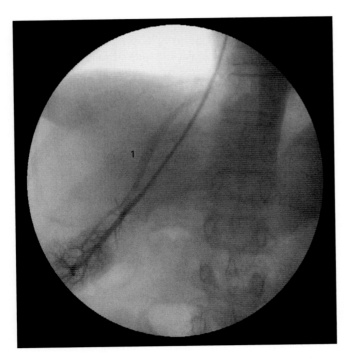

Fig. 2 In the presence of a communicating hepatic vein (1), WHVP will not reflect the actual portal pressure in this patient unless in a different hepatic vein there are no communicating vessels. This finding is more frequent in instances of presinusoidal intrahepatic portal hypertension, such as 'idiopathic' portal hypertension.

• Use an appropriate scale to be able to sense small changes. The scales used for arterial pressure measurements are not adequate. The scale should be set, at least, at 1 mmHg = 1 mm of paper.
• Digital readings on the screen are instantaneous readings and may not reliably reflect the true pressure. Therefore, paper recordings should be used, allowing for the independent review of pressure tracings (Fig. 3).
• Venous pressures should be allowed to stabilize over a period of at least 1 min for WHVP and 15 s for FHVP (some patients may require longer). A slow paper speed (< 5 mm/s) should be used in the recorder.
• FHVP should be measured with the catheter tip introduced less than 5 cm into the hepatic vein. FHVP should not be more than 2 mmHg greater than the IVC pressure, measured at the level of the hepatic veins. If the difference is greater, a hepatic outflow problem should be investigated.
• Check that inflating the distal balloon totally occludes the hepatic vein before measuring WHVP.
• For each measurement, also obtain a 'mean' pressure by 'filtering' the tracing or by selecting this option in the recorder.
• Do all measurements in duplicate (or triplicate if the pressures differ by more than 1 mmHg).
• Any event that may cause an artifact, such as coughing or moving, should be noted.

In addition to pressure measurements, hepatic vein catheterization allows for the performance of a wedged hepatic retrograde portography using CO_2 as a contrast agent (Fig. 4). This will demonstrate the portal vein in most instances. In fact, an inability to demonstrate the portal vein on CO_2 retrograde portography strongly suggests the presence of presinusoidal portal hypertension [13]. Hepatic vein catheterization also allows for the performance of a transjugular liver biopsy, which adds very little time, discomfort and risk to the procedure, and can be done on a day-hospital basis.

Indications
The principal applications of HVPG measurements are discussed below.

Classification of portal hypertension
Findings at hepatic vein catheterization may help to identify the cause of portal hypertension. Causes of portal hypertension may be classified into presinusoidal, sinusoidal or postsinusoidal. In patients with clinical manifestations of portal hypertension who have normal WHVP, a presinusoidal source of portal hypertension should be suspected. In these cases, WHVP underestimates the true portal pressure because the catheter is recording the pressure of the normal sinusoid but not of the obstructed area. In liver cirrhosis, the increased WHVP is nearly equal to portal venous pressure [5,6]. In postsinusoidal portal hypertension resulting from Budd–Chiari syndrome, IVC obstruction, right heart failure or constrictive pericarditis, both FHVP and WHVP are increased, while HVPG remains usually normal [14] (Fig. 5).

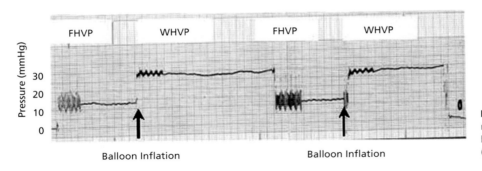

Fig. 3 Typical reading of correct measurements of hepatic venous pressures before (FHVP) and after balloon inflation (WHVP).

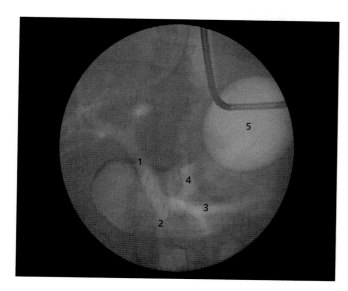

Fig. 4 Wedged retrograde portography using CO_2 as a contrast agent showing patent portal (1), mesenteric (2) and splenic veins (3). Retrograde portography also showed an extensive collateralization (4) in a patient with HCV-related cirrhosis in which a Sengstaken tube (5) was placed to treat a variceal bleeding episode.

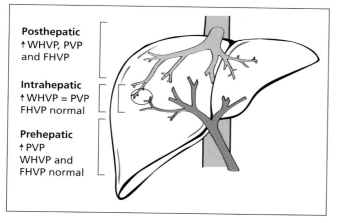

Fig. 5 Intrahepatic causes of portal hypertension may be classified into presinusoidal, sinusoidal or postsinusoidal according to the position of blood flow obstruction.

Evaluation of portal hypertension and assessment of the response to pharmacological therapy

The normal HVPG value is up to 5 mmHg. Oesophageal varices do not develop until the HVPG increases to 10–12 mmHg, and the HVPG should be at least 12 mmHg for the appearance of complications of portal hypertension, such as variceal bleeding and ascites [15,16]. Furthermore, longitudinal studies have demonstrated that, if HVPG is decreased below 12 mmHg by means of pharmacological treatment [17,18] or spontaneously due to an improvement in liver disease [19], variceal bleeding is totally prevented and varices may decrease in size. Therefore, patients with a HVPG below 12 mmHg are at negligible or no risk of experiencing portal hypertension-related complications. Besides, even if this target is not achieved, a decrease in HVPG of at least 20% [18] from baseline levels offers an almost total protection from variceal bleeding. Lack of achievement of these targets (reduction below 12 mmHg or more than 20% from baseline) constitutes the strongest independent predictor of variceal bleeding or rebleeding [18,20–22]. Therefore, tailoring the treatment of portal hypertension by measuring the individual portal pressure response to therapy would allow us to predict whether the treatment is likely to offer optimal or adequate protection from the risk of bleeding at short- and long-term (up to 8 years) follow-up [22,23]. However, whether the HVPG response to 'à la carte' treatment is cost-effective must be evaluated in specifically designed clinical trials [24].

Prognostic evaluation during variceal bleeding

Early measurements of HVPG within 48 h of admission for acute variceal bleeding provides useful prognostic information regarding the outcome of the bleeding episode and 1-year survival [25]. Patients with an HVPG > 20 mmHg are five times more likely to experience failure to control acute variceal bleeding or early rebleeding, require significantly more blood transfusions and days in the intensive care unit and have a higher mortality on follow-up. In addition, recent work has suggested that the early use of transjugular intrahepatic portosystemic shunts (TIPS) in these high-risk patients improves the control of bleeding and reduces early rebleeding and mortality [26].

Preoperative evaluation of resection risk in patients with small hepatocellular carcinoma

HVPG measurement may provide useful prognostic information in patients undergoing partial hepatectomy for small (< 5 cm) hepatocellular carcinoma. Patients with an HVPG > 10 mmHg and/or increased bilirubin levels have an increased risk of hepatic decompensation after surgical resection of hepatocellular carcinoma [27], even in cases with well-preserved liver function (Child–Pugh A). In a recent study, more than 50% of Child–Pugh class A patients had hepatic decompensation after surgery. This decompensation not only affected quality of life but was also associated with reduced long-term survival [27,28]. Surgical resection should therefore be restricted to patients with an HVPG below 10 mmHg. Otherwise, liver transplantation or local ablative therapies should be preferred.

Evaluation of progression of chronic liver disease

It has been suggested that, in the setting of severe chronic hepatitis C, HVPG could be considered a dynamic marker of fibrosis progression [29]. Thus, HVPG measurements may be considered as an adjunctive for the therapeutic evaluation of the response to antiviral therapy [29,30]. However, prospective trials in this area are needed to clarify the role of HVPG in the management of these patients.

Contraindications

Past episodes of allergic reaction to radiographic contrast medium constitute the only major contraindication to hepatic vein catheterization. Coagulation disorders are usually seen in cirrhotic patients, but the evidence of complications associated with severe thrombocytopenia or low prothrombin time is limited. Therefore, we do not use supportive therapy for routine HVPG measurements.

Complications

The measurement of the HVPG is a reproducible method that can be repeated because it carries very little discomfort. Performed under slight conscious sedation that does not modify haemodynamic measurements (midazolam 0.02 mg/kg i.v.) [31], its acceptability is comparable to that of upper gastrointestinal endoscopy, and the cost is similar to that of conventional venography. The complications reported occur in less than 1% of patients [32], and major complications are usually limited to local injury of the femoral or jugular vein (arteriovenous fistulae, leakage or rupture of venous introducers), Horner syndrome and transient brachial paralysis. These complications are greatly reduced by performing the venous puncture under Doppler ultrasonography guidance. Passage of the catheter through the right atrium may cause arrhythmias that are usually transient or easily corrected. Transjugular liver biopsies may rarely be complicated by intraperitoneal bleeding due to capsular perforation and subcapsular haematomas. The authors have observed no fatalities in over 10 000 studies. Because of the many clinical applications, hepatic vein catheterization is becoming a routine test in many hospitals.

Hepatic blood flow

The portal hypertension syndrome is characterized by the development of a hyperdynamic circulation with increased cardiac output and decreased systemic vascular resistance that leads to splanchnic vasodilatation with increased portal blood flow. Under normal circumstances, total hepatic blood flow represents approximately 25% of the cardiac output; a third is supplied by the hepatic artery and the remainder by the portal venous system. A reduction in portal blood flow results in an increase in hepatic artery flow up to 100% from baseline. This 'hepatic artery buffer response' is very important in cases in which portal blood flow decreases dramatically, such as in portal vein thrombosis or portocaval shunts. In contrast, the portal venous system is thought to be a passive vascular bed receiving the venous blood draining from the stomach, intestines, pancreas, spleen and omentum. Therefore, factors that regulate portal venous flow are those that control the arterial supply of blood to these organs. Contrary to what happens in the hepatic artery, there is no portal venous buffer hyperaemia in response to decreased hepatic arterial flow.

Measurement of hepatic blood flow is usually performed by means of clearance techniques. These techniques require the injection of dyes or radiolabelled particles that are avidly extracted by the liver. If a substance is totally extracted by the liver in a single pass, its plasma clearance will be equal to total hepatic blood flow. However, no substance possesses this property. Because of that, it is necessary to measure the hepatic extraction of the test compound directly (the fractional uptake in a single passage through the liver), which requires sampling blood simultaneously from a hepatic vein and a peripheral artery once the steady-state concentration for this substance has been reached. This is particularly true in the setting of clinical liver disease, in which extraction of the indicator is frequently diminished [33]. The most commonly used indicator is the albumin-bound dye indocyanine green, which is removed only by the liver, and its plasma clearance rate represents the hepatic clearance of the compound [34]. The extrarenal sorbitol clearance has been reported to be a safe, non-invasive and reliable means of measuring 'parenchymal' or 'effective' liver blood flow in patients with normal or diseased livers [35]. Other techniques have been described such as the indicator dilution technique and the inert gas washout, but these are invasive methods requiring catheterization of the hepatic artery and/or the portal vein, as well as of the hepatic vein.

The main application of measurements of hepatic blood flow is in the setting of studies aimed at assessing changes in the hepatic blood flow following the administration of vasoactive drugs and evaluating the accommodation of the hepatic vascular bed to increases in blood flow such as that produced by meals.

Measurement of azygos blood flow

Superior portal–systemic collaterals, including gastro-oesophageal varices, drain mainly into the azygos venous system. Therefore, measurement of the azygos blood flow represents an index of blood flow through the gastro-oesophageal collaterals and oesophageal varices in portal hypertension [36]. Patients with portal hypertension have an increased portocollateral blood flow, leading to an increased azygos blood flow. Values in normal subjects range from 100 to 250 mL/min, whereas mean values in patients with portal hypertension average 650–700 mL/min [36]. The azygos blood flow is also increased in patients with non-cirrhotic portal hypertension. Measurement of azygos blood flow requires the retrograde catheterization of the azygos vein using a continuous thermal dilution catheter. The procedure is simple and may be done in the course of routine haemodynamic investigations. Blood flow is measured by the thermodilution technique, applying Fick's principle.

It is important to note that this technique does not allow the separation of how much of the increase in azygos blood flow is contributed by oesophageal varices and how much by peri-oesophageal collaterals, which also drain into the azygos vein. In addition, in 25% of the cases, these gastro-oesophageal collaterals drain into other thoracic veins (subclavian, innominate and pulmonary), different from the azygos vein. Therefore, a normal azygos blood flow does not necessarily indicate the absence of oesophageal varices.

The main application of measurements of azygos blood flow is in the monitoring of the effects of pharmacological therapy in portal hypertension. Azygos blood flow is markedly reduced by the use of vasoconstrictive drugs such as vasopressin [37], somatostatin [38], octreotide [39–41], terlipressin [40] and beta-blockers [42]. The ability of the technique to quantify changes in portocollateral blood flow has allowed a better understanding of the beneficial effects of vasoactive drugs currently used in the medical treatment of portal hypertension. It has been demonstrated that some splanchnic vasoconstrictors, such as propranolol, cause greater decreases in azygos blood flow than in portal pressure [42], suggesting that they may have specific effects at the collaterals, which cannot be evaluated by the isolated measurement of portal pressure [42,43].

Finally, promising results have been obtained measuring portal and azygos blood flow non-invasively using phase-contrast magnetic resonance imaging (MRI) angiography [44,45] and, recently, with dynamic contrast material-enhanced MRI [46]. Endoscopic ultrasonography has also been proposed [47], although it is less accurate.

Measurement of variceal pressure

Several endoscopic findings, such as the size of the varices and the presence of red colour signs, show a significant correlation with the risk of bleeding [48]. These are some of the main determinants of variceal wall tension [49], which is believed to play a key role in determining variceal rupture [50,51]. According to Laplace's law, variceal wall tension is directly related to the radius of the varix and inversely related to its wall thickness [49]. The other direct determinant of variceal wall tension is the transmural pressure at the varices, the difference between intravariceal pressure and oesophageal luminal pressure.

Variceal pressure can be accurately measured at endoscopy by puncturing the varices or by means of pressure gauges or low-resistance balloons [52–54]. The endoscopic pressure gauge is the method that has been used most commonly in prospective studies. The technique is based on the assumption that, because of their thin walls and lack of external tissue support, the varices behave as an elastic structure; thus, the pressure needed to compress a varix equals the pressure inside the varix. It consists of using a pressure-sensitive capsule, attached to the tip of an endoscope, that has a small chamber covered by a thin latex membrane, which is continuously perfused with a constant flow of nitrogen. It is assumed that, when the gauge is applied to the varix, the pressure needed to perfuse the gauge equals the pressure inside the varix. The difference between the pressure measured when applying the gauge over a varix and the pressure recorded when the gauge is free in the oesophageal lumen equals the transmural variceal pressure, which is the value used to express the results using this technique [50,53,55].

Variceal pressure correlates significantly with portal pressure [53]. Despite this correlation, variceal pressure is significantly lower than portal pressure, probably because a significant resistance along the collaterals feeding the varices causes a pressure drop from the portal vein to the varix [50]. Variceal pressure is of clinical interest because patients who have bled from varices have significantly greater variceal pressure than those who have not [56,57]. Several clinical studies have demonstrated that variceal pressure measurements using the endoscopic pressure gauge have prognostic value with regard to the evolution of an acute variceal bleeding episode [58], the development of the first variceal haemorrhage [59] and the risk of variceal rebleeding in patients receiving pharmacological therapy [60]. In addition, variceal pressure measurement may be used to assess the effects of pharmacological treatment [57,60,61]. A fall in variceal pressure after pharmacological therapy of at least 20% from baseline was associated with a very low risk of variceal bleeding on follow-up (the actuarial probability of variceal bleeding was only 7% at 3 years, whereas this was 46% in patients failing to achieve this target [60]). The prognostic value of the variceal pressure response to treatment was as powerful as that of the HVPG response. The two methods identify different populations of patients with a favourable outcome; therefore, they should be considered complementary rather than mutually exclusive [60].

Unfortunately, measurements of variceal pressure are difficult and prone to artifacts resulting from oesophageal peristalsis. In addition, the technique is not feasible in every patient; about 25% of patients initially scheduled to have variceal pressure measurements must be excluded because of technical difficulties, mainly in patients with small varices [60]. Variceal pressure measurements are considered satisfactory only when fulfilling the following predetermined criteria: (i) stable intra-oesophageal pressure; (ii) absence of artifacts caused by oesophageal peristalsis; and (iii) correct placement of the capsule over the varix, as shown by the fine fluctuations of the pressure tracing according to heart cycle and respiration, for at least 12 s [60]. These conditions are easily met when the procedure is performed by a skilled endoscopist in a cooperative patient. However, it should be kept in mind that endoscopic measurements are not exactly non-invasive, although certainly less so than HVPG measurements. Finally, the variability of the measurement and the training required for correct measurements exceed, by far, those of HVPG. Because of these limitations, it is highly unlikely that it might be used in routine clinical practice.

References

1 Bosch J, Abraldes JG, Groszmann RJ (2003) Current management of portal hypertension. *J Hepatol* 38, S54–S68.

2 Thompson W, Caughey J, Whippel A *et al.* (1937) Splenic vein pressure in congestive splenomegaly (Banti's syndrome). *J Clin Invest* 16, 571.

3 Myers JD, Taylor WJ (1951) An estimation of portal venous pressure by occlusive catheterization of an hepatic venule. *J Clin Invest* 30, 662.

4 Dexter L, Dow J, Haynes F (1950) Studies of the pulmonary circulation in man at rest, normal variations and the inter-relations between increased pulmonary blood flow, elevated pulmonary arterial pressure, and high pulmonary 'capillary' pressure. J Clin Invest 29, 602–613.

5 Perello A, Escorsell A, Bru C et al. (1999) Wedged hepatic venous pressure adequately reflects portal pressure in hepatitis C virus-related cirrhosis. Hepatology 30(6), 1393–1397.

6 Deplano A, Migaleddu V, Pischedda A et al. (1999) Portohepatic gradient and portal hemodynamics in patients with cirrhosis due to hepatitis C virus infection. Dig Dis Sci 44(1), 155–162.

7 Reynolds TB, Geller HM, Kuzma OT et al. (1960) Spontaneous decrease in portal pressure with clinical improvement in cirrhosis. N Engl J Med 263, 734–739.

8 Viallet A, Joly JG, Marleau D et al. (1970) Comparison of free portal venous pressure and wedged hepatic venous pressure in patients with cirrhosis of the liver. Gastroenterology 59(3), 372–375.

9 Luca A, Feu F, Garcia-Pagan JC et al. (1994) Favorable effects of total paracentesis on splanchnic hemodynamics in cirrhotic patients with tense ascites. Hepatology 20(1 Pt 1), 30–33.

10 Pomier-Layrargues G, Kusielewicz D, Willems B et al. (1985) Presinusoidal portal hypertension in non-alcoholic cirrhosis. Hepatology 5(3), 415–418.

11 Groszmann RJ, Glickman M, Blei AT et al. (1979) Wedged and free hepatic venous pressure measured with a balloon catheter. Gastroenterology 76(2), 253–258.

12 Groszmann RJ, Wongcharatrawee S (2004) The hepatic venous pressure gradient: anything worth doing should be done right. Hepatology 39(2), 280–282.

13 Debernardi-Venon W, Bandi JC, Garcia-Pagan JC et al. (2000) CO(2) wedged hepatic venography in the evaluation of portal hypertension. Gut 46(6), 856–860.

14 Groszmann RJ, Atterbury CE (1982) The pathophysiology of portal hypertension: a basis for classification. Semin Liver Dis 2(3), 177–186.

15 Garcia-Tsao G, Groszmann RJ, Fisher RL et al. (1985) Portal pressure, presence of gastroesophageal varices and variceal bleeding. Hepatology 5(3), 419–424.

16 Casado M, Bosch J, Garcia-Pagan JC et al. (1998) Clinical events after transjugular intrahepatic portosystemic shunt: correlation with hemodynamic findings. Gastroenterology 114(6), 1296–1303.

17 Groszmann RJ, Bosch J, Grace ND et al. (1990) Hemodynamic events in a prospective randomized trial of propranolol versus placebo in the prevention of a first variceal hemorrhage. Gastroenterology 99(5), 1401–1407.

18 Feu F, Garcia-Pagan JC, Bosch J et al. (1995) Relation between portal pressure response to pharmacotherapy and risk of recurrent variceal haemorrhage in patients with cirrhosis. Lancet 346(8982), 1056–1059.

19 Vorobioff J, Groszmann RJ, Picabea E et al. (1996) Prognostic value of hepatic venous pressure gradient measurements in alcoholic cirrhosis: a 10-year prospective study. Gastroenterology 111(3), 701–709.

20 Merkel C, Bolognesi M, Sacerdoti D et al. (2000) The hemodynamic response to medical treatment of portal hypertension as a predictor of clinical effectiveness in the primary prophylaxis of variceal bleeding in cirrhosis. Hepatology 32(5), 930–934.

21 Abraldes JG, Tarantino I, Turnes J et al. (2003) Hemodynamic response to pharmacological treatment of portal hypertension and long-term prognosis of cirrhosis. Hepatology 37(4), 902–908.

22 Bureau C, Peron JM, Alric L et al. (2002) 'A la carte' treatment of portal hypertension: adapting medical therapy to hemodynamic response for the prevention of bleeding. Hepatology 36, 1361–1366.

23 Bosch J, Garcia-Pagan JC (2003) Prevention of variceal rebleeding. Lancet 361(9361), 952–954.

24 de Franchis R (2005) Evolving Consensus in Portal Hypertension Report of the Baveno IV Consensus Workshop on methodology of diagnosis and therapy in portal hypertension. J Hepatol 43(1), 167–176.

25 Moitinho E, Escorsell A, Bandi JC et al. (1999) Prognostic value of early measurements of portal pressure in acute variceal bleeding. Gastroenterology 117(3), 626–631.

26 Monescillo A, Martinez-Lagares F, Ruiz-del-Arbol L et al. (2004) Influence of portal hypertension and its early decompression by TIPS placement on the outcome of variceal bleeding. Hepatology 40(4), 793–801.

27 Bruix J, Castells A, Bosch J et al. (1996) Surgical resection of hepatocellular carcinoma in cirrhotic patients: prognostic value of preoperative portal pressure. Gastroenterology 111(4), 1018–1022.

28 Llovet JM, Fuster J, Bruix J (1999) Intention-to-treat analysis of surgical treatment for early hepatocellular carcinoma: resection versus transplantation. Hepatology 30(6), 1434–1440.

29 Burroughs AK, Groszmann R, Bosch J et al. (2002) Assessment of therapeutic benefit of antiviral therapy in chronic hepatitis C: is hepatic venous pressure gradient a better end point? Gut 50(3), 425–427.

30 Groszmann RJ (1996) The hepatic venous pressure gradient: has the time arrived for its application in clinical practice? Hepatology 24(3), 739–741.

31 Steinlauf AF, Garcia-Tsao G, Zakko MF et al. (1999) Low-dose midazolam sedation: an option for patients undergoing serial hepatic venous pressure measurements. Hepatology 29(4), 1070–1073.

32 Trejo R, Alvarez W, Garcia-Pagan JC et al. (1996) [The applicability and diagnostic effectiveness of transjugular liver biopsy]. Med Clin (Barc) 107(14), 521–523.

33 Navasa M, Bosch J, Mastai R et al. (1991) Measurement of hepatic blood flow, hepatic extraction and intrinsic clearance of indocyanine green in cirrhosis. Comparison of a non-invasive pharmacokinetic method with measurements using hepatic vein catheterization. Eur J Gastroenterol Hepatol 3, 305–312.

34 Groszmann RJ (1983) The measurement of liver blood flow using clearance techniques. Hepatology 3(6), 1039–1040.

35 Zeeh J, Lange H, Bosch J et al. (1988) Steady-state extrarenal sorbitol clearance as a measure of hepatic plasma flow. Gastroenterology 95(3), 749–759.

36 Bosch J, Feu F, Garcia-Pagan JC (1991) Measurement of azygos blood flow. In: Okuda K, Benhamou JP (eds) Portal Hypertension. Tokyo: Springer-Verlag, pp. 139–150.

37 Bosch J, Mastai R, Kravetz D et al. (1985) Measurement of azygos venous blood flow in the evaluation of portal hypertension in patients with cirrhosis. Clinical and haemodynamic correlations in 100 patients. J Hepatol 1(2), 125–139.

38 Cirera I, Feu F, Luca A et al. (1995) Effects of bolus injections and continuous infusions of somatostatin and placebo in patients with cirrhosis: a double-blind hemodynamic investigation. Hepatology 22(1), 106–111.

39 McCormick PA, Biagini MR, Dick R et al. (1992) Octreotide inhibits the meal-induced increases in the portal venous pressure of cirrhotic patients with portal hypertension: a double-blind, placebo-controlled study. Hepatology 16(5), 1180–1186.

40 Escorsell A, Bandi JC, Moitinho E et al. (1997) Time profile of the haemodynamic effects of terlipressin in portal hypertension. J Hepatol 26(3), 621–627.

41 Escorsell A, Bandi JC, Andreu V *et al.* (2001) Desensitization to the effects of intravenous octreotide in cirrhotic patients with portal hypertension. *Gastroenterology* 120(1), 161–169.

42 Bosch J, Mastai R, Kravetz D *et al.* (1984) Effects of propranolol on azygos venous blood flow and hepatic and systemic hemodynamics in cirrhosis. *Hepatology* 4(6), 1200–1205.

43 Mastai R, Bosch J, Navasa M *et al.* (1987) Effects of alpha-adrenergic stimulation and beta-adrenergic blockade on azygos blood flow and splanchnic haemodynamics in patients with cirrhosis. *J Hepatol* 4(1), 71–79.

44 Debatin J, Zahner B, Meyenberger C *et al.* (1996) Azygos blood flow: phase contrast quantitation in volunteers and patients with portal hypertension pre- and postintrahepatic shunt placement. *Hepatology* 24, 1109–1115.

45 Wu MT, Pan HB, Chen C *et al.* (1996) Azygos blood flow in cirrhosis: measurement with MR imaging and correlation with variceal hemorrhage. *Radiology* 198(2), 457–462.

46 Annet L, Materne R, Danse E *et al.* (2003) Hepatic flow parameters measured with MR imaging and Doppler US: correlations with degree of cirrhosis and portal hypertension. *Radiology* 229(2), 409–414.

47 Nishida H, Giostra E, Spahr L *et al.* (2001) Validation of color Doppler EUS for azygos blood flow measurement in patients with cirrhosis: application to the acute hemodynamic effects of somatostatin, octreotide, or placebo. *Gastrointest Endosc* 54(1), 24–30.

48 NIEC (1988) Prediction of the first variceal hemorrhage in patients with cirrhosis of the liver and esophageal varices. A prospective multicenter study. The North Italian Endoscopic Club for the Study and Treatment of Esophageal Varices. *N Engl J Med* 319(15), 983–989.

49 Polio J, Groszmann RJ (1986) Hemodynamic factors involved in the development and rupture of esophageal varices: a pathophysiologic approach to treatment. *Semin Liver Dis* 6(4), 318–331.

50 Rigau J, Bosch J, Bordas JM *et al.* (1989) Endoscopic measurement of variceal pressure in cirrhosis: correlation with portal pressure and variceal hemorrhage. *Gastroenterology* 96(3), 873–880.

51 Escorsell A, Bosch J (2004) Pathophysiology of variceal bleeding. In: Groszmann RJ, Bosch J (eds) *Portal Hypertension in the 21st Century*. Dordrecht: Kluwer Academic Publishers, pp. 155–166.

52 Mosimann R (1982) Nonaggressive assessment of portal hypertension using endoscopic measurement of variceal pressure. Preliminary report. *Am J Surg* 143(2), 212–214.

53 Bosch J, Bordas JM, Rigau J *et al.* (1986) Noninvasive measurement of the pressure of esophageal varices using an endoscopic gauge: comparison with measurements by variceal puncture in patients undergoing endoscopic sclerotherapy. *Hepatology* 6(4), 667–672.

54 Gertsch P, Fischer G, Kleber G *et al.* (1993) Manometry of esophageal varices: comparison of an endoscopic balloon technique with needle puncture. *Gastroenterology* 105(4), 1159–1166.

55 Escorsell A, Bordas JM, Feu F *et al.* (1997) Endoscopic assessment of variceal volume and wall tension in cirrhotic patients: effects of pharmacological therapy. *Gastroenterology* 113(5), 1640–1646.

56 Nevens F, Sprengers D, Feu F *et al.* (1996) Measurement of variceal pressure with an endoscopic pressure sensitive gauge: validation and effect of propranolol therapy in chronic conditions. *J Hepatol* 24(1), 66–73.

57 Feu F, Bordas JM, Luca A *et al.* (1993) Reduction of variceal pressure by propranolol: comparison of the effects on portal pressure and azygos blood flow in patients with cirrhosis. *Hepatology* 18(5), 1082–1089.

58 Ruiz del Arbol L, Martin de Argila C, Vázquez M *et al.* (1992) Endoscopic measurement of variceal pressure during hemorrhage from esophageal varices. *Hepatology* 16, 147.

59 Nevens F, Bustami R, Scheys I *et al.* (1998) Variceal pressure is a factor predicting the risk of a first variceal bleeding: a prospective cohort study in cirrhotic patients. *Hepatology* 27(1), 15–19.

60 Escorsell A, Bordas JM, Castaneda B *et al.* (2000) Predictive value of the variceal pressure response to continued pharmacological therapy in patients with cirrhosis and portal hypertension. *Hepatology* 31(5), 1061–1067.

61 Bosch J, Bordas JM, Mastai R *et al.* (1988) Effects of vasopressin on the intravariceal pressure in patients with cirrhosis: comparison with the effects on portal pressure. *Hepatology* 8(4), 861–865.

7.5 Pathogenesis, diagnosis and treatment of ascites in cirrhosis

Vicente Arroyo, Carlos Terra and Luis Ruiz-del-Arbol

Aetiology and diagnosis of ascites

Causes

Many diseases are known to lead to the formation of free fluid within the peritoneal cavity. Basically, the causes of ascites may be grouped into those conditions in which the pathological process does not directly affect the peritoneum and those in which the peritoneum itself is involved. The first group includes diseases associated with sinusoidal portal hypertension, hypoalbuminaemia and a variety of disorders that may cause ascites through different mechanisms, such as myxoedema, ovarian diseases, chronic pancreatitis, biliary tract leakage, diseases affecting the lymphatic system of the splanchnic area and chronic renal failure. In the second group, ascites is formed as a consequence of primary peritoneal disease or as a result of peritoneal involvement in systemic processes; tuberculous, fungal, parasitic and granulomatous peritonitis, primary or metastatic peritoneal tumours, vasculitis, eosinophilic gastroenteritis and Whipple's disease are the most characteristic causes of ascites in this group. By far the most frequent cause of ascites in Europe and in North America is hepatic cirrhosis, followed by neoplasms and, to a lesser extent, congestive heart failure and tuberculous peritonitis. These four conditions account for more than 90% of the ascites in these areas [1].

Detection

The diagnosis of ascites is simple when large amounts of fluid accumulate in the peritoneal cavity. However, the diagnosis is much more difficult by physical examination when there is a small volume of ascitic fluid. It has been suggested that minimal amounts of ascites (less than 500 mL) can be detected by an exploratory manoeuvre that combines percussion and auscultation of the abdomen [2]. After 5 min in the prone position, the patient is asked to assume a position on hands and knees so that the middle portion of the abdomen is dependent. One flank is percussed by repeated, light flicking at a constant intensity, with the stethoscope being over the most dependent portion of the abdomen (the area of the ascitic 'puddle'). The stethoscope is then gradually moved towards the flank opposite the percussion site. A positive sign indicating the presence of ascites consists of a marked change in the intensity and character of the percussion note as the stethoscope is moved from the ascitic puddle to the flank opposite the point of percussion, where ascites is not present. A point of demarcation between the ascitic puddle and the area without intraperitoneal fluid can be obtained, correlating with the amount of ascitic fluid present. Nevertheless, in a prospective study in which five physical signs (bulging flanks, flank dullness, shifting dullness, fluid wave and puddle sign) were compared with the ultrasonographic demonstration of ascites (which can detect as little as 100–200 mL of intraperitoneal fluid) in patients in whom the bedside diagnosis of ascites was in question, the puddle sign did not show greater specificity and sensitivity for the detection of intra-abdominal fluid than the other signs of ascites [3].

Peripheral oedema (oedema in the lower extremities) is common in patients with cirrhosis. In many cases, it precedes the development of ascites by weeks or months, but it may also appear simultaneously with, or following, the accumulation of fluid within the abdomen. Massive peripheral oedema without ascites is occasionally seen in cirrhotic patients with severe hepatic insufficiency and a surgical portocaval shunt. Peripheral oedema in cirrhosis decreases or disappears with nocturnal rest and increases with ambulation. It is postulated that hypoalbuminaemia and increased venous pressure in the lower extremities due to constriction of the intrahepatic segment of the inferior vena cava or to the high intra-abdominal pressure caused by the presence of ascites are the main factors causing peripheral oedema in cirrhosis.

Ultrasonography, computerized tomography (CT) and magnetic resonance imaging (MRI) are very useful in the assessment of patients with ascites [4–7]. In addition to their sensitivity in detecting minimal amounts of ascites, they may suggest its cause, based on the characteristics of the intra-abdominal organs and vessels and the appearance of the intra-abdominal fluid. Ultrasonography is the best of these methods as it is not expensive, is as reliable as CT and is free of radiation hazards.

Intraperitoneal fluid resulting from portal hypertension appears as homogeneous, echo-free areas surrounding and interposed between the loops of bowel and viscera in a relatively uniform manner. When the amount of ascites is small, the fluid tends to collect in the flanks and the superior right paracolic gutter, around the liver and in the lowest peritoneal reflection in the pelvis. Rectal and transvaginal echography are particularly sensitive in the detection of small volumes of intra-abdominal fluid, the transvaginal approach being able to detect less than 50 mL of ascitic fluid [8]. Atypical sonographic characteristics, such as the presence of multiple fine echoes (indicating the presence of debris) or septations and fibrous strands within the ascitic fluid, may be seen in exudative ascites. Matted loops of bowel, plastering of the liver to surrounding structures and loculation of fluid, when present, are very suggestive of malignant ascites [9]. Peritoneal thickening, lymphadenopathy and bowel thickening in the ileocaecal junction are suggestive of a tuberculous aetiology [10].

Characteristics of cirrhotic ascites

The ascitic fluid in cirrhotics is transparent and yellow/amber in colour. Traditionally, ascites in these patients is considered to have the characteristics of a transudate, with a total protein concentration of less than 2.5 g/dL and with relatively few cells. However, cirrhotics with ascites do not constitute a homogeneous population with respect to the characteristics of the ascitic fluid. Total ascitic protein concentration ranges between 0.5 and more than 6 g/dL [11] and is greater than 3 g/dL ('exudative ascites') in up to 30% of patients with otherwise uncomplicated cirrhosis [12–14]. The proportions of albumin and globulins in the total protein concentration are approximately 45% and 55% respectively [12,14]. There is a close, direct correlation between ascitic albumin and globulin concentrations, indicating that proteins in ascitic fluid in cirrhosis derive from capillaries with relatively large pores, such as the hepatic sinusoids [14,15]. This contention is also supported by the observation of a similar ascites:plasma ratio for albumin and globulins (approximately 0.3 for both types of proteins) [12,14,15]. However, although ascitic proteins may come mainly from the extremely permeable hepatic sinusoids, the relative contribution of the hepatic microvasculature and the splanchnic capillaries to the formation of ascites may vary markedly from patient to patient, as the ascitic fluid:plasma ratios for total proteins, albumin and globulins range between 0.04 and 1.03 in patients with cirrhosis and ascites [12,14–16]. The total protein, albumin and globulin concentrations in ascitic fluid in cirrhosis correlate directly with the corresponding plasma concentrations and inversely with portal pressure [14]. The mobilization of ascites with diuretics increases the concentration of proteins in the ascitic fluid [17]. The total protein concentration in ascitic fluid in cirrhosis is an important predictive factor for spontaneous bacterial peritonitis. Spontaneous bacterial peritonitis usually occurs in cirrhotics with a low total protein concentration in ascitic fluid (< 1 g/dL),

whereas it is infrequent in cirrhotics with higher protein concentrations in ascitic fluid and in patients with cardiac or malignant ascites, who generally have a protein concentration over this limit. The ascitic fluid has opsonic and bactericidal activity, which seems to be mediated by complement and fibronectin [18,19]. The total protein concentration in ascitic fluid correlates with the concentration of these proteins with antibacterial activity; the predictive value of the total protein concentration in ascitic fluid for the development of spontaneous bacterial peritonitis is probably a consequence of this relation [20,21].

The ascitic fluid in the cirrhotic without spontaneous bacterial peritonitis usually has fewer than 300–500 white blood cells/μL; nevertheless 10–15% may have more than 500 cells and 5% more than 1000 cells [12,22,23]. More than 70% of these white cells are mononuclear leukocytes. In contrast, in cirrhotic patients with spontaneous bacterial peritonitis, the ascitic fluid usually contains more than 500 white blood cells/μL (frequently more than 2000), with more than 70% of them being polymorphonuclear leukocytes [23,24]. The pH and the concentration of lactate in ascitic fluid in otherwise uncomplicated cirrhosis is similar to that in plasma [25]. Patients with spontaneous bacterial peritonitis have a significantly lower pH and higher lactate concentration in ascitic fluid than in plasma [26,27]. As with the total protein concentration, the absolute concentration of white cells in ascitic fluid increases during diuretic treatment, while the concentration of polymorphs remains unchanged [28]. Therefore, the percentage of polymorphs over the total leukocyte content of the ascitic fluid actually decreases during the mobilization of ascites with diuretics. The concentration of red blood cells in cirrhotic ascites is usually lower than 1000 cells/μL, although higher concentrations may occasionally be detected. In fact, bloody ascitic fluid, which indicates more than 50 000 red cells/μL (haematocrit of about 0.5%), occurs in approximately 2% of cirrhotics [22]. In one-third of these patients, bloody ascites is secondary to a superimposed hepatocellular carcinoma bleeding into the peritoneal cavity [29]. However, in as many as 50% of patients, no apparent cause of bloody ascites can be detected. The hepatic and the thoracic lymph of cirrhotics is often bloody also [30]. The mechanism of bloody ascites in cirrhotics without hepatocellular carcinoma could, therefore, be related to the leakage of bloody lymph from the liver lymphatics.

Alterations in the coagulation-related proteins in ascites have been reported in cirrhotic patients. The concentration of fibrinogen and plasminogen in ascitic fluid is lower than that expected from their molecular weights, whereas the concentrations of plasminogen activators and fibrin/fibrinogen degradation products are higher than in plasma [31]. This suggests that fibrinolysis is occurring within the peritoneal cavity. In addition, there is apparently intraperitoneal coagulation in cirrhotic patients as the concentration of fibrin monomers in ascitic fluid is almost 10 times higher than in plasma [32]. Therefore, the alterations in the coagulation-related proteins in cirrhotic ascites are probably the consequence of a complex coagulation disturbance within the ascitic fluid, resulting in intraperitoneal coagulation and primary and secondary fibrinolysis. The infusion of ascitic fluid into the general circulation, either directly or by the insertion of a peritoneovenous shunt, is often associated with disseminated intravascular coagulation, as manifested by a marked reduction in platelet count, prothrombin time and fibrinogen concentration, and an increase in the plasma concentrations of fibrin degradation products, thus confirming the procoagulant activity of ascitic fluid [33,34]. This coagulopathy is clinically significant in 20–50% of patients treated with a peritoneovenous shunt and sometimes requires ligation of the prosthesis. Several substances present in the ascites, such as tissue thromboplastin, endotoxin, collagen, activated clotting factors and fibrin degradation products, have been implicated in the procoagulant activity of the ascitic fluid.

Cirrhotic patients with ascites have a very high concentration of interleukin (IL)-6 in ascitic fluid. The ascitic fluid:plasma concentration ratio of IL-6 is approximately 100 in these patients, indicating intra-abdominal production of this cytokine [35,36]. The concentration of tumour necrosis factor (TNF) is also higher in ascitic fluid than in plasma in cirrhotic patients, although the differences are much less impressive than with IL-6 [36]. Significant concentrations of soluble TNF receptors have also been detected in the ascitic fluid of cirrhotic patients with and without spontaneous bacterial peritonitis, the significance of which is still unknown. Activated peritoneal macrophages could be the origin of the intra-abdominal production of cytokines. Spontaneous bacterial peritonitis is associated with a marked increase in cytokines in the ascitic fluid [37]. Intra-abdominal cytokines escape into the systemic circulation, and this may explain some of the complications observed in patients with spontaneous bacterial peritonitis, particularly the impairment in circulatory and renal function [37]. The concentration of leptin and vascular endothelial growth factor (VEGF) is also higher in ascitic fluid than in plasma [38,39].

The biochemical and cytological characteristics of ascitic fluid in other diseases causing intrahepatic sinusoidal portal hypertension, such as acute alcoholic hepatitis, fulminant or subacute viral or toxic hepatitis and massive metastatic infiltration of the liver, are similar to those found in cirrhotic ascites.

Differential diagnosis of cirrhotic ascites

Malignant ascites

The macroscopic appearance of malignant ascites is generally similar to that of cirrhotic ascites (less than 10% of malignant ascites are macroscopically bloody) [40]. Thus, the differential diagnosis must be based on exploratory findings and laboratory tests. Measurement of the total protein concentration of the ascitic fluid (generally over 3 g/dL in malignant ascites) and its cytological examination for malignant cells, which were the laboratory tests first used to differentiate malignant ascites from that secondary to portal hypertension, are still the most common methods used [40,41].

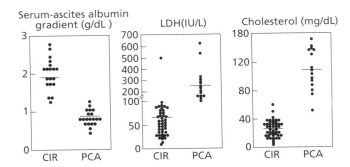

Fig. 1 Serum–ascites albumin gradient and ascitic fluid concentration of lactic dehydrogenase (LDH) and cholesterol in patients with cirrhosis (CIR) and peritoneal carcinomatosis (PCA).

Standard cytological examination is 60–90% accurate in the diagnosis of malignant ascites, especially when adequate volumes of fluid (at least several hundred millilitres) and concentration techniques are used [42]. False-positive results are rare in skilled hands. The greatest source of confusion is the differentiation of malignant cells from atypical mesothelial cells. The use of immunocytochemical techniques with monoclonal or polyclonal antibodies against numerous tumour markers is helpful in differentiating malignant from non-malignant ascites in these cases. These techniques may also help to differentiate primary (mesothelioma) from metastatic peritoneal malignancy. False-negative results on standard cytological examinations are the rule when ascites is due to portal hypertension secondary to massive liver metastases with little peritoneal involvement [40]. In this type of ascites, the total ascitic protein concentration is usually lower than 2.5 g/dL.

The serum–ascitic fluid gradient for albumin improves the diagnostic accuracy of the total protein concentration in ascitic fluid (Fig. 1) [40,41,43]. The concentration of lactic dehydrogenase in malignant ascites is higher than the corresponding values in plasma because of leakage of the enzyme from the malignant cells lining the peritoneum, whereas the reverse is the rule for cirrhotic ascites [44]. The concentration of lactic dehydrogenase in ascitic fluid and its ascitic fluid:plasma ratio are, therefore, useful for differentiating malignant from cirrhotic ascites, although they do not improve the results obtained with the ascitic fluid:plasma albumin gradient (Fig. 1) [40,44]. Other measurements in ascitic fluid that have proved to be of value in differentiating malignant from cirrhotic ascites include total lipids, free fatty acids, cholesterol, fibronectin, carcinoembryonic antigen and other tumour-associated antigens, urokinase, tissue plasminogen activator, plasminogen activator inhibitor and fibrin/fibrinogen degradation products, and human chorionic gonadotropin-β [40,43–48]. Of these, the cholesterol concentration of ascitic fluid, which is higher in most malignant ascites than in cirrhotic ascites owing to higher permeability to lipoproteins (Fig. 1), seems to be the most interesting because of its simplicity and cost-effectiveness [43,44]. Laparoscopy and direct biopsy of the peritoneal metastases is a useful approach to confirm the diagnosis of malignant ascites in those cases with negative cytology [49].

Chylous ascites

Chylous ascites is an infrequent feature in patients with cirrhosis. In some cases, it develops in the postoperative period after splenorenal shunt but, in most instances, it appears spontaneously [50]. Chylous ascites is macroscopically turbid and white ('milky' ascites), and separates into layers on standing. These characteristics are due to a high concentration of chylomicrons very rich in triglycerides. The diagnosis of chylous ascites is based on triglyceride concentration in ascitic fluid, which is usually over 110 mg/dL and always higher than the corresponding value in plasma [51]. The concentration of cholesterol and phospholipids in ascitic fluid is, however, similar to that of non-chylous ascites. Gross milkiness of chylous ascites correlates poorly with absolute triglyceride concentrations because turbidity also reflects the size of the chylomicrons [51]. The proportion of lipids in chylous ascites is very similar to that in human intestinal and thoracic duct lymph after the ingestion of a fat meal [52]. As patients with cirrhosis usually have elevated pressure within the splanchnic lymph vessels, it has been suggested that spontaneous chylous ascites in these patients may be a consequence of the rupture of these lymph vessels, leading to the leakage of whole intestinal lymph into the peritoneal cavity [52]. Chylous ascites after splenorenal shunt is probably secondary to injury to retroperitoneal lymphatics [53]. In fact, chylous ascites is a well-recognized postoperative complication in patients submitted for renal transplantation, aortic aneurysmectomy, retroperitoneal lymph adenectomy and pancreatoduodenectomy [51]. Hepatic cirrhosis is a relatively infrequent cause of chylous ascites. Primary abnormalities of the lymphatics (lymphangiectasia) and the obstruction of the lymphatic system due to malignancies, especially lymphomas, are by far the most common causes in adults [51]. Other diseases associated with chylous ascites in adults include portal vein thrombosis, sarcoidosis, nephrotic syndrome, tuberculosis, pancreatitis, abdominal trauma, constrictive pericarditis, encapsulating peritonitis and pulmonary fibrosis with thoracic duct obstruction. Congenital malformations of the lymphatic system, including stenosis or atresia of the lymphatics and lymphatic mesenteric cysts, are the main causes of chylous ascites in children. Chylous ascites should be differentiated from pseudochylous ascites in which, although the macroscopic appearance may be identical, the triglyceride concentration is lower than 110 mg/dL. Clinically, chylous ascites is usually silent except for the distension of the abdomen.

Tuberculous peritonitis

The differential diagnosis between cirrhotic ascites and ascites due to tuberculous peritonitis is particularly important as alcoholic cirrhosis may predispose to peritoneal tuberculosis. Clinically, tuberculous peritonitis is characterized by fever, abdominal pain, anorexia, weight loss, abdominal tenderness and ascites. However, none of these symptoms is invariably present. The proportion of patients with pleural or pulmonary tuberculosis or with a reactive tuberculin skin test ranges between 21% and 78% and between 30% and 89%, respectively, in the different series [54,55]. In females without active pulmonary tuberculosis, peritoneal tuberculosis may represent the local extension of a tuberculous salpingitis. However, in many cases, no active focus of tuberculosis, apart from the peritoneal disease, can be detected. Ultrasonography and CT may suggest the diagnosis of tuberculous peritonitis. Findings frequently seen in tuberculous peritonitis include diffuse, regular peritoneal thickening, infiltration of the greater omentum, ascites with fine, mobile septation or floating debris on ultrasonography, loculation of ascites, bowel thickening, particularly in the ileocaecal area, retroperitoneal lymph node enlargement, lesions in solid organs (pelvic, adrenal, hepatic, splenic), cold abscesses and adhesions [55]. Results of examination of the peritoneal fluid are also suggestive of tuberculous infection if there is an increased concentration of proteins (over 3 g/dL) and lymphocytes. However, it has been shown that the ascitic fluid may be a transudate, particularly in cirrhotics with ascites and tuberculous peritonitis [56]. Ziehl–Nielsen-stained smears usually fail to show acid-fast bacilli. The proportion of cultures of ascitic fluid positive for *Mycobacterium tuberculosis* varies markedly from series to series (from 8% to 69%), probably reflecting technical differences. It has been suggested that the proportion of positive cultures may be increased up to 80% by concentrating 1 L of the fluid by centrifugation. Nevertheless, the diagnosis of tuberculous peritonitis cannot be based on cultures of ascitic fluid as the usual techniques of culturing acid-fast bacilli may require several weeks to obtain a definite result. The activity of lactic dehydrogenase in ascitic fluid is greater in tuberculous peritonitis than in cirrhosis. As in malignant ascites, the concentration of this enzyme in tuberculous ascites is higher than in plasma [56]. The activity of adenosine deaminase in the peritoneal fluid is a proven sensitive and specific test for tuberculous peritonitis [54,57] (Fig. 2). This is an enzyme involved in the catabolism of purine bases (catalysing the deamination of adenosine with the formation of inosine). It participates in the proliferation and differentiation of lymphocytes, and increases in tuberculous effusions, probably as a consequence of the stimulation of cell-mediated immunity and T lymphocytes. The concentration of adenosine deaminase in ascitic fluid in tuberculous peritonitis correlates directly with the total protein concentration in ascites. It is therefore not surprising that the number of false-negative results for adenosine deaminase in tuberculous peritonitis is higher in cirrhotic patients than in patients without chronic liver diseases [58].

Open peritoneal biopsy during a laparotomy or minilaparotomy, blind needle biopsy of the peritoneum and laparoscopy with direct biopsy of the affected areas have been used to confirm the diagnosis of tuberculous peritonitis [59,60]. Laparoscopy with direct peritoneal biopsy is the best of these methods [61]. The peritoneum characteristically shows scattered or confluent miliary nodules of uniform size, with

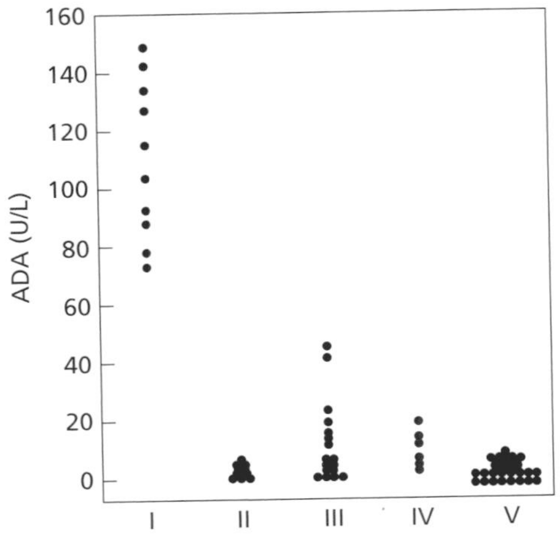

Fig. 2 Ascitic fluid concentration of adenosine deaminase (ADA) in different groups of patients with ascites: group I, tuberculous peritonitis; group II, non-tuberculous septic peritonitis; group III, malignant ascites; group IV, miscellaneous; group V, cirrhosis (reproduced with permission from ref. 56).

adhesions between bowel loops, liver capsule and abdominal walls. The histological appearance is characterized by the presence of caseating granulomas. In some instances, tubercle bacilli may be seen by staining with auramine–rhodamine and microscopy under ultraviolet light. *Mycobacterium tuberculosis* can be cultured from the biopsy specimen of the peritoneum. The macroscopic and microscopic appearances of tuberculous peritonitis are similar to those of other conditions causing granulomatous peritonitis, such as sarcoidosis, Crohn's disease and iatrogenic granulomatous peritonitis. The last condition occurs after 0.15% of abdominal operations and is usually caused by a cell-mediated immune response to starch, talc, cotton fibres and wood fibres originating from disposable surgical gowns and drapes [62]. Iatrogenic granulomatous peritonitis appears 2–9 weeks postoperatively and is characterized by abdominal pain, tenderness and fever, and frequently by the accumulation of ascites. The observation of starch granules in the ascitic fluid obtained by paracentesis can be diagnostic.

The detection of DNA of *Mycobacterium tuberculosis* by means of polymerase chain reaction (PCR) assay of ascitic fluid is very rapid and appears to be as sensitive as culture. To date, however, there are no controlled studies of PCR in patients with tuberculous peritonitis. Moreover, false-negative results have been reported, justifying the administration of antituberculous treatment in patients with clinical and histological features characteristic of peritoneal tuberculosis, even in cases with negative results from culture and PCR analysis [63]. The ligase chain reaction (LCR) DNA amplification method has recently been introduced into practice. This assay provides rapid information for the diagnosis of extrapulmonary tuberculosis with a higher diagnostic accuracy than PCR [64]. Further studies are needed to determine the clinical use of PCR and/or LCR in the diagnosis of tuberculous peritonitis.

Ascites due to hepatic venous outflow block

Ascites secondary to postsinusoidal portal hypertension generally shows a total protein concentration and ascitic fluid:plasma albumin gradient similar to that reported in malignant ascites and tuberculous peritonitis [65]. The diagnosis can, however, be established by considering the clinical condition of the patient and the concentrations of leukocytes, lactic dehydrogenase, cholesterol and adenosine deaminase in the ascitic fluid, which are lower in ascites secondary to hepatic outflow block. Patients with ascites due to constrictive pericarditis often lack symptoms of congestive heart failure. It is therefore important to seek physical findings characteristic of this entity in any patient with exudative ascites and no evidence of liver disease. Clear lung fields on radiographic examination and low voltage of the electrocardiogram suggest constrictive pericarditis. The diagnosis is confirmed by cardiac echography or catheterization. In patients with ascites due to a congenital web in the inferior vena cava, a cava-to-cava collateral circulation can be observed on the abdomen or back. The final diagnosis is based on inferior vena cavography. The differential diagnosis between chronic Budd–Chiari syndrome and cirrhosis is often difficult on clinical grounds. The protein concentration in ascitic fluid may be low in some of these patients as a result of the capillarization of the hepatic sinusoids. On the other hand, they may have hepatic stigmata, abnormal liver function tests, splenomegaly and oesophageal varices. If major hepatic veins are not visualized by CT and ultrasonography, this may suggest Budd–Chiari syndrome. The liver scintiscan sometimes shows a marked increase in isotope uptake centrally, possibly because of hypertrophy of the caudate lobule related to its autonomous venous drainage directly into the vena cava. However, in most cases, the diagnosis is made by liver biopsy. Ascites with a high protein concentration is frequently found in the postoperative period of liver transplantation. It is usually due to postsinusoidal portal hypertension secondary to deficient venous drainage from the implanted liver. Ascites due to obstructed hepatic venous outflow has also been reported in patients with polycystic liver disease.

Bile ascites

The leakage of bile into the peritoneal cavity may lead to two different clinical pictures [66]. Some patients develop signs and symptoms of acute peritonitis. Others have essentially no symptoms other than those caused by the accumulation of large quantities of bile ascites in the abdominal cavity. In both circumstances, paracentesis yields a green ascitic fluid with a bilirubin concentration considerably higher than in plasma. Between these two extremes, there is a wide spectrum of symptoms. Why intraperitoneal leakage of bile induces these two clinical pictures is unknown. Bile ascites usually occurs after biliary tract surgery (mainly cholecystectomy), percutaneous diagnostic procedures (liver biopsy and percutaneous transhepatic cholangiography) and trauma with injuries to the gallbladder, common bile duct, hepatic duct or liver. In contrast, the most common cause of bile peritonitis is spontaneous perforation of the gallbladder or bile ducts due to erosion by stones or cholecystitis [66].

Pancreatic ascites

Pancreatic ascites occurs in approximately 3% of patients with chronic pancreatitis as a result of the leakage of fluid from a ruptured pancreatic duct, or from a pancreatic pseudocyst, into the peritoneal cavity [67]. Other, less frequent causes include acute haemorrhagic pancreatitis, abdominal trauma and pancreatic cancer [68]. As most patients with chronic pancreatitis are alcoholics and may develop massive ascites with little or no abdominal tenderness, the differential diagnosis of pancreatic from cirrhotic ascites may be difficult on clinical grounds. Laboratory analyses are therefore essential to establish a correct diagnosis. In virtually all cases, ascitic fluid amylase and lipase are dramatically increased. The concentration of pancreatic enzymes in ascitic fluid is between 5 and 20 times greater than the plasma concentrations obtained simultaneously. The protein concentration in ascitic fluid is generally over 3 g/dL, and the fluid is usually serous, but can be serosanguineous, turbid or chylous. The concentration of methaemalbumin in ascites is markedly increased in patients with haemorrhagic pancreatitis and has prognostic significance. The concentration of leukocytes in ascitic fluid ranges between 70 and 2200/µL, 80% being lymphocytes [69]. Ultrasonography and CT are important diagnostic procedures for pancreatic ascites as they may detect the presence of a pseudocyst. Pseudocysts in patients with pancreatic ascites are usually small, due to continuous leakage of the cystic fluid into the peritoneal space.

Other types of ascites

Other causes of ascites easily differentiated from cirrhotic ascites include nephrogenic ascites, myxoedema and Meig syndrome. Nephrogenic ascites may become a severe problem in approximately 5% of patients maintained on chronic haemodialysis [70]. The pathogenesis of ascites in these patients is unknown. The protein concentration in ascitic fluid is usually over 3 g/dL, and the white blood cell count ranges between 30 and 1500/µL. The amylase and lactic dehydrogenase activities in ascitic fluid are lower than the plasma concentrations obtained simultaneously. Peritoneal biopsies show only minor inflammation or fibrosis. The diagnosis of nephrogenic ascites is one of exclusion, so that it is important to rule out other causes.

Myxoedema is an infrequent cause of gross ascites (about 3–4% of cases of myxoedema develop significant ascites). As the systemic changes of myxoedema may be mild, it may not be identified as the cause of the ascites, thus leading to unnecessary diagnostic procedures. The ascitic fluid in myxoedema may be serous or gelatinous and characteristically has a high protein concentration. The pathogenesis of myxoedematous ascites is unknown.

Meig syndrome consists of the association of ascites and hydrothorax with various types of benign ovarian tumours (fibroma, cystadenoma, struma ovarii). A 'modern' type of Meig

syndrome is the ovarian hyperstimulation syndrome occurring in patients treated with clomiphene and human menopausal gonadotrophins to induce ovulation. This syndrome is characterized by massive ascites, pleural effusions, signs of hypovolaemia (tachycardia, haemoconcentration, oliguria), enlarged ovaries (more than 10 cm in diameter), marked arterial vasodilation and activation of the renin–aldosterone and sympathetic nervous systems and antidiuretic hormone [71].

Cirrhotic hydrothorax

Pleural effusions, in the absence of primary pulmonary, pleural or cardiac disease, occur in approximately 5% of patients with hepatic cirrhosis [72]. Clinical ascites is almost always evident, and the pleural effusion is usually right-sided. Occasionally, however, effusion develops in the left pleura, on both sides or in the absence of detectable ascites. The pathogenesis of cirrhotic hydrothorax involves, in most cases, the direct passage of ascitic fluid from the abdomen through acquired defects in the diaphragm into the pleural space (Fig. 3) [73,74]. The driving force leading to the peritoneal–pleural transfer of fluid is the hydrostatic gradient between the positive intra-abdominal pressure and the negative intrathoracic pressure. In cases of cirrhotic hydrothorax without detectable ascites, the transport of fluid into the pleural space probably equals the rate of production of ascites. The presence of direct communications between the peritoneal and pleural cavities can be demonstrated by radioisotopic studies. The intraperitoneal injection of tracer amounts of [^{99m}Tc]sulphur colloid is followed by the rapid appearance of the isotope in the pleural cavity. The communications can be visualized by ultrafast echo MRI. The biochemical and cytological characteristics of the pleural fluid are similar to those of the ascitic fluid obtained simultaneously. It is not unusual, however, to find slightly higher concentrations of total protein, albumin, cholesterol and total lipids in pleural than in ascitic fluid, probably related to a higher rate of water reabsorption from the pleural compartment. However, if there are marked differences in

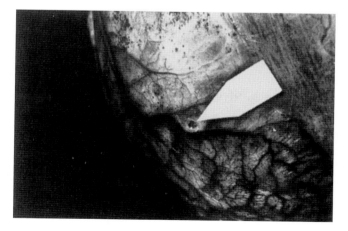

Fig. 3 Hole of 1 mm diameter in the right hemidiaphragm in a cirrhotic patient with right pleural effusion (reproduced with permission from ref. 74).

the biochemical or cytological characteristics between the pleural and the ascitic fluids, one should search for another cause of the pleural effusion. Spontaneous bacterial empyema due to Gram-negative bacilli is a frequent complication in patients with cirrhotic hydrothorax. The pathogenesis of this complication is similar to that of spontaneous bacterial peritonitis [75]. Videothoracoscopy has been used effectively to localize and close the diaphragmatic defects causing cirrhotic hydrothorax [76].

Factors involved in ascites formation in cirrhosis

Portal hypertension

In patients with liver disease, portal hypertension is essential for the formation of ascites. The accumulation of fluid within the peritoneal cavity is a common complication in diseases causing sinusoidal portal hypertension, for example Budd–Chiari syndrome, hepatic veno-occlusive disease, cirrhosis and severe acute hepatitis of toxic, viral or alcoholic origin. In contrast, it is extraordinarily infrequent in liver diseases in which the block to portal flow occurs before the sinusoids. Similarly, when portal hypertension develops as a consequence of an extrahepatic blockage of the hepatic or portal blood flow, ascites only occurs in those circumstances in which the vascular blockade increases sinusoidal pressure (right heart failure, constrictive pericarditis, obstruction of the inferior vena cava by congenital membranous webs), but not when the portal or the splenic veins are occluded. The relation between sinusoidal portal hypertension and the formation of ascites is also evident from experimental studies. Obstruction of the thoracic inferior vena cava or the hepatic veins is followed by rapid accumulation of fluid within the abdominal cavity. Ascites also occurs in several experimental models of cirrhosis (induced by carbon tetrachloride, dimethylnitrosamine or chronic ligation of the bile duct). In contrast, partial or even complete obstruction of the portal vein is not followed by the formation of ascites.

Effect of sinusoidal portal hypertension on trans-sinusoidal fluid exchange

Differences in anatomical and functional characteristics between the hepatic and splanchnic microvasculature have been proposed to explain why ascites only develops in circumstances of sinusoidal portal hypertension. The hepatic sinusoids are structurally unique among microvessels as they do not have a basement membrane. They are lined by three main types of cells: endothelial, Kupffer and fat storing (Ito or stellate cells). The endothelial cells are by far the main component of the sinusoidal wall. Kupffer cells also contribute to the wall, although they are most often found within the lumen, attached by processes to the endothelial cells. Ito cells are found in the space of Disse, between the endothelial and liver cells. The endothelial cells form a very porous sinusoidal wall with large apertures, ranging

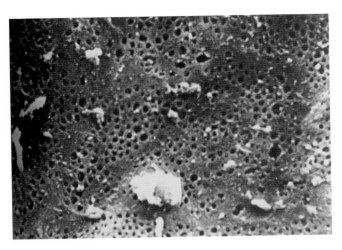

Fig. 4 Surface view of the endothelial lining of a liver sinusoid, as seen by scanning electron microscopy. Numerous fenestrae, with a pore size of 100–500 nm radius, are observed.

from 100 to 500 nm in radius (Fig. 4). Occasionally, microvilli from the hepatocytes cross the space of Disse and pass through these gaps in the endothelial membrane, thus reaching the sinusoidal lumen. This extremely porous membrane is almost completely permeable to macromolecules, including plasma proteins. These special characteristics of the sinusoidal wall are not surprising considering that the main function of the hepatic sinusoids is to promote intimate contact between the blood entering the liver and the hepatocytes. The space of Disse is relatively inconspicuous in normal conditions. It includes sparse bundles of collagen, glycosaminoglycans, occasional particles of very-low-density lipoprotein, Ito cells and hepatocyte microvilli. As no lymph vessels can be identified within the hepatic lobule, it has been suggested that the fluid in the space of Disse, in free communication with the interstitial spaces at the portal and central venous ends of the sinusoid, enters the lymphatics present in the portal tracts and in the central venous area as liver lymph. The highly porous nature of the sinusoidal wall explains why, in the normal liver, the protein concentration of hepatic lymph is approximately 95% that of plasma measured simultaneously [77]. A consequence of this high permeability is that the trans-sinusoidal oncotic gradient is virtually zero. Liver lymph is principally drained by vessels leaving at the liver hilus, although a small proportion passes through vessels accompanying the hepatic veins into the chest [78]. Lymph from the hilus, as well as that from other organs including the pancreas, spleen, kidney, adrenals, stomach, large and small intestines, gallbladder and mesentery, all drains via the para-aortic plexus and cisterna chyli into the thoracic duct [78]. This duct is a lymphatic channel 36–45 cm long that begins at the upper end of the cisterna chyli near the lower border of the 12th thoracic vertebra, passes through the diaphragm and ascends in the posterior mediastinum in close relation to the aorta and azygos vein. It passes into the neck behind the aortic arch and then curves laterally, joining the left subclavian or internal jugular vein. The anatomical arrangement of the terminal thoracic duct is extremely variable. Only occasionally does it drain into the right jugular or subclavian vein alone. Usually, there are many anastomotic sites between it and the venous system in the left side of the neck. In normal humans, the thoracic lymph flow may reach 800–1000 mL/day.

Constriction of the suprahepatic inferior vena cava or the hepatic veins in experimental animals has been the model most frequently used to investigate the effect of sinusoidal portal hypertension on fluid exchange through the sinusoidal wall. The increased pressure in the hepatic veins is almost completely transmitted back to the hepatic sinusoids, indicating that capillary pressure is not autoregulated in the liver [79]. In addition, because of the high permeability to plasma proteins of the sinusoidal wall, no oncotic force opposes the increase in hydrostatic sinusoidal pressure. Consequently, elevation of hepatic venous pressure is followed by a dramatic increase in the passage of fluid with a protein concentration similar to that of plasma, from the sinusoidal lumen to the space of Disse [79–81]. The relation between sinusoidal pressure and the hepatic production of lymph is such that an increase of 60% in lymph production occurs for every millimetre rise in sinusoidal pressure [80]. The macroscopic consequence of this phenomenon is a marked enlargement of the liver. However, the compliance of the liver, that is the relation between interstitial pressure and interstitial volume, is very low [82]. This means that little interstitial fluid can accumulate without altering interstitial pressure. It has been estimated that, for venous pressures between zero and 30 mmHg, approximately 65% of the rise in hepatic venous pressure is transmitted to the hepatic interstitium [83]. The remaining 35% is absorbed by the increase in intravascular and interstitial volume. This high interstitial pressure explains the two major consequences of experimental sinusoidal portal hypertension: a striking increase in lymph flow through the liver lymphatics and thoracic duct; and the direct passage of hepatic lymph with very high protein concentrations from the liver surface into the peritoneal cavity, forming ascites [79,81].

Results of studies in cats with experimental constriction of the thoracic inferior vena cava strongly support the hypothesis that the ascitic fluid produced during acute experimental blockage of the hepatic outflow is mainly derived from the hepatic microvascular compartment. Greenway and Lautt [80] investigated the effect of increasing hepatic venous pressure on the formation of hepatic lymph in anaesthetized cats. The livers of these animals, with venous and arterial inflow intact, were inserted into a plethysmograph. The sequence of events occurring after the elevation in hepatic venous pressure consisted of a transient increase in hepatic volume, followed by a rapid accumulation of fluid with a protein concentration of approximately 80% of the plasma concentrations within the plethysmograph. With obstruction of the hepatic lymphatics, the rate of fluid filtration through the liver surface was directly proportional to the sinusoidal pressure. Freeman [84] and Mallet-Guy et al. [85] repositioned the liver supradiaphragmatically and subsequently

constricted the thoracic inferior vena cava. Ascites only developed in the thoracic cavity. When a cellophane bag was placed around the liver, ascitic fluid only accumulated in the bag.

Effects of portal hypertension on splanchnic transmicrovascular fluid exchange

The structural and functional characteristics of the microvasculature of the stomach and small and large intestines are very different from those of the liver. First, the splanchnic capillaries are much less porous than the hepatic sinusoids and have a well-defined basement membrane. Although most splanchnic capillaries are fenestrated, the estimated pore size, 3.7–12 nm in radius, is between 50 and 100 times less than that of the hepatic sinusoids. The oncotic reflection coefficient (ORC), which describes the fraction of the total protein oncotic pressure generated across a capillary membrane (impermeable proteins generate 100% of their maximum oncotic pressure, ORC = 1, whereas freely permeable proteins generate no oncotic pressure, ORC = 0) has been estimated as 0 in the normal liver and 0.78, 0.92 and 0.85 in the stomach, small intestine and colon respectively [80,86]. Consequently, any increase in filtration in the splanchnic capillaries is quickly counterbalanced by an increase in the oncotic pressure difference between the capillary lumen and interstitial space. This may explain the infrequency of ascites in presinusoidal portal hypertension.

Three other factors may contribute to the infrequency of ascites when the blockage to portal flow occurs before the sinusoids. First, the gastric and intestinal interstitium is much more compliant than the hepatic interstitium, and considerable interstitial fluid can accumulate in these organs without causing any major changes in interstitial pressure [82]. Secondly, the intestines have a very efficient lymphatic system for removing interstitial oedema. In this respect, it is interesting that, in normal conditions, approximately 20% of the fluid absorbed by the small intestine is carried out into the general circulation by the lymphatics. The abrupt elevation in portal venous pressure increases lymph flow from the stomach, small intestine and colon [86,87]. Because of the low permeability of intestinal capillaries to plasma proteins, the ratio between protein concentrations in the intestinal lymph and in plasma in conditions of portal hypertension is characteristically low (20%) [77]. Finally, as most splanchnic capillaries are located within the submucosa [82] and the hydraulic conductance (permeability to submucosal interstitial fluid) of the muscular and serosal layers of the stomach, small bowel and colon is probably low, it is not surprising that partial occlusion of the portal vein produces marked accumulation of fluid in the submucosa with no major changes in the serosal and muscular layers. This also explains why transudation of fluid out of the gut in this condition occurs mainly into the lumen and not into the intraperitoneal space. In fact, net fluid and electrolyte secretion into the lumen of the small bowel occurs in animal models following acute elevation of portal pressure [83].

Source of ascites in cirrhosis

All the findings discussed above offer a rational explanation for the absence of ascites in patients and experimental animals with presinusoidal portal hypertension. They also suggest that an imbalance between hepatic lymph production and the capacity of the lymphatic system of the liver and thoracic duct to return the hepatic lymph to the general circulation may be the predominant mechanism of ascites formation in experimental blockade of the hepatic venous outflow and in patients with constrictive pericarditis, Budd–Chiari syndrome and hepatic veno-occlusive disease, who have increased lymph flow in the thoracic duct and ascites with a high protein content [82,88]. However, as hepatic cirrhosis differs in many respects from experimental blockade of the hepatic venous outflow, the pathogenesis of ascites in patients with chronic liver disease may vary from that in experimental sinusoidal portal hypertension.

First, it is well established that there are marked structural changes in the hepatic microvasculature in cirrhosis, the most characteristic being capillarization of the hepatic sinusoids. This abnormality has been extensively investigated by Huet *et al.* [89]. These workers showed that the marginal areas of the regenerative nodules were perfused with capillaries rather than sinusoids, whereas sinusoids were present in the central areas of the micronodules. The sinusoids were fenestrated in a normal fashion and lacked a basement membrane. In contrast, capillaries exhibited a continuous endothelial lining lacking fenestrae, supported by a basement membrane and collagenous tissue. The structure was such that, along a single vascular pathway, capillary and sinusoidal structures were encountered in sequence. Variations in the degree of capillary change were found from patient to patient. Huet *et al.* also investigated the functional consequences in cirrhotic patients of this alteration in liver microcirculation by using a multiple indicator dilution technique. Labelled red blood cells and albumin were injected simultaneously into the portal vein or hepatic artery and the outflow dilution pattern was obtained from hepatic venous blood. In the normal liver, labelled red cells occupy the intravascular compartment, whereas the volume of distribution of albumin, which gains access to the space of Disse, includes both the intravascular and the interstitial compartments. This explains why, in normal livers, the volume of distribution of albumin exceeds that of red cells by 60%. In contrast, in organs with less permeable capillaries in which no significant albumin exchange occurs during the time of a single passage, the difference between the volume of distribution of these two markers is only 7%. In cirrhotic patients, the calculated volume of distribution of albumin within the liver exceeded that of red cells by 7–60%. Some patients showed a pattern similar to that expected in the normal liver, while in others the hepatic sinusoids were almost impermeable to albumin.

Second, there is evidence that, contrary to what occurs in other vascular territories, the intestinal microvasculature does not autoregulate its capillary pressure or the capillary filtration coefficient in cirrhosis. Portal hypertension in cirrhotic patients and in animals with experimental cirrhosis is not associated with an increased splanchnic arteriolar resistance but, rather, with a generalized splanchnic arteriolar vasodilation [90]. As discussed later, the simultaneous occurrence of increased portal venous pressure and arterial blood inflow to the splanchnic microcirculation leads to a marked increase in splanchnic microvascular hydrostatic pressure and permeability, explaining why interstitial oedema in the mucosal, muscular and serosal layers is prominent in human cirrhosis. The serosal oedema is manifested by a fivefold increase in the thickness of the jejunal peritoneum in cirrhotic patients compared with control subjects [91].

Third, the total protein content in hepatic and thoracic duct lymph and in ascitic fluid is remarkably lower in cirrhosis than in experimental blockage of the hepatic outflow. Increased flow of thoracic duct lymph (usually 8–9 L/day) is a characteristic finding in cirrhosis, whether or not ascites is present [92]. This is associated with a marked enlargement of the thoracic duct and an elevation in duct pressure, which has been attributed to the presence of valves and endothelial folds at the duct–venous junction, making the flow of lymph into the venous system of the neck difficult. The number, size and thickness of lymphatics in the hilum of the liver, and in the mucosal and serosal layers of the intestine and mesentery, are markedly increased in cirrhosis. The hepatic lymph:plasma ratio for total proteins in cirrhosis with ascites ranges between 20% and 80% [93]. This low protein concentration of hepatic lymph is probably a consequence of the capillarization of hepatic sinusoids. The total protein content of intestinal lymph in cirrhotics with ascites is generally under 20% of that in plasma [93]. Finally, the thoracic duct lymph and the total protein concentration of ascitic fluid in these patients are between those of the hepatic and intestinal lymph [77,93]. It is therefore very likely that ascites in cirrhosis derives from both hepatic and splanchnic vascular compartments.

Studies evaluating the escape of radiolabelled albumin from the intravascular to the extravascular compartment and to the intraperitoneal space (which estimates the fluid dynamics through the capillary wall and peritoneum and liver surface respectively) indicate that the lymphatic system is extremely efficient in returning most of the excessive hepatic and splanchnic lymph to the general circulation in cirrhotic patients with ascites [16]. The transvascular escape rate of radiolabelled albumin in these patients is remarkably high (8.5% of the total intravascular mass of albumin per hour). The fraction of the transvascular escape of albumin passing into the peritoneal cavity is, however, very low (0.21%). Ascites formation is therefore the consequence of a small spillover of the increased rate of formation of hepatic and splanchnic lymph, most of which is returned directly to the circulation through the lymphatic system.

Effects of portal hypertension on splanchnic arteriolar circulation

In addition to increasing hepatic and splanchnic lymph production, portal hypertension induces a profound alteration in the splanchnic circulation. Classically, portal hypertension was considered to be due solely to an increased resistance to portal venous flow. However, it is now clear that the pathogenesis of portal hypertension is much more complex and that increased portal venous inflow secondary to a generalized splanchnic arteriolar vasodilation also plays an important part in the increased portal pressure [90,94–98]. This high portal venous inflow may explain why, in experimental animals, portal pressure remains increased despite the development of a marked collateral circulation. The mechanism by which portal hypertension induces splanchnic arteriolar vasodilation and increased portal venous inflow is not entirely understood. There is strong evidence suggesting that an increased local production of vasodilatory substances (i.e. nitric oxide) is the most probable mechanism of splanchnic arterial vasodilation associated with portal hypertension. This enhanced production of local vasodilators also explains the decreased sensitivity of the gastric and intestinal microvasculature to endogenous vasoconstrictor systems, which also contribute to the splanchnic hyperaemia associated with portal hypertension [99].

There is indirect evidence that splanchnic arteriolar vasodilation also occurs in patients with cirrhosis and portal hypertension. Under normal conditions, almost all the flow circulating in the splanchnic bed reaches the liver, so the hepatic equals the splanchnic blood flow. In patients with cirrhosis and portal hypertension, because there is important shunting of blood through the portosystemic collateral circulation, the hepatic blood flow represents only a part of the splanchnic blood flow. Between 60% and 80% of the mesenteric and splenic blood flow is shunted through the collateral circulation in cirrhotic patients [100,101]. As several investigations have shown that the hepatic blood flow is normal or even increased in most such patients [102–104], it follows that in these there must be a marked increase in splanchnic blood flow secondary to arteriolar vasodilation. The observation that the mean transit time in the splanchnic vascular bed is substantially reduced in alcoholic cirrhotics further indicates the occurrence of splanchnic arteriolar vasodilation in these patients [105].

Renal functional abnormalities

Sodium retention is the most common abnormality of renal function in cirrhosis. It is constantly present in patients with ascites and plays a major role in the pathogenesis of this complication. Ascites disappears in most patients when sodium retention is inhibited by diuretics. Conversely, diuretic withdrawal or a high sodium diet leads to the reaccumulation of ascites. The degree of sodium retention in cirrhosis with ascites varies considerably from one patient to another, being practically nonexistent in some patients, but relatively high in others [106]. The observation that ascites might disappear in the latter patients only by reducing sodium intake below sodium excretion is a further argument for the importance of sodium retention in the pathogenesis of ascites. Experimental studies have shown that

sodium retention precedes ascites formation in cirrhosis [107]. The impairment of sodium excretion in most cirrhotics occurs in the setting of a normal glomerular filtration rate. Therefore, the predominant mechanism for sodium retention in these patients is an increased tubular sodium reabsorption.

Patients with compensated cirrhosis do not have sodium retention. However, they present subtle abnormalities of sodium metabolism. For example, these patients are unable to excrete an acute intravenous salt load normally [108–110]. On the other hand, compensated cirrhotics with severe portal hypertension may not 'escape' from an exogenously administered mineralocorticoid hormone. If a normal individual ingesting a diet containing a constant amount of sodium is given a salt-retaining mineralocorticoid daily, a transient period of sodium retention is experienced, and limited weight gain occurs, reflecting the expansion of the extracellular fluid volume. After 3–5 days, however, sodium excretion increases and equals dietary intake, so that no further weight gain or extracellular volume expansion occurs. In contrast, compensated cirrhotics with high portal pressure may not escape from the sodium-retaining effect of mineralocorticoids, and they develop continuous renal fluid and sodium retention, leading to the formation of ascites and oedema [111,112]. Finally, it has been shown that compensated cirrhotics retain sodium while they are in an upright posture, whereas they show an exaggerated natriuresis during bedrest [113,114].

The oral or the intravenous (as 5% glucose solution) administration of a water overload of 20 mL/kg body weight over 45 min to a normal individual is followed after a period of between 30 and 60 min by the excretion of hypotonic urine (60–110 mosm/kg), at a rate of 8–14 mL/min. The volume of water excreted per minute by this individual can ideally be divided into two parts. The first consists of water, which dissolves urinary solutes iso-osmotically with respect to plasma (osmolar clearance). The second part consists of water free of solutes (free-water clearance, C_{H_2O}). As osmolar clearance in normal individuals is 1.5–2.5 mL/min, free-water clearance after a water overload in these subjects ranges between 6 and 12 mL/min. This means that a healthy person is able to maintain total body water within normal limits even if water ingestion is 10 L or more per day.

C_{H_2O} after a water overload is normal in compensated cirrhotics and reduced in most patients with cirrhosis and ascites [115–117]. The degree of impairment of water excretion in cirrhosis with ascites also varies markedly from patient to patient (Fig. 5). Thus, whereas in some cirrhotics with ascites, C_{H_2O} after a water overload is only slightly reduced, others present very low C_{H_2O} or may be unable to dilute the urine after the water load (negative C_{H_2O}). These patients with very low (< 1 mL/min) or negative C_{H_2O} retain most water taken in with the diet, causing a dilution of the interior milieu, hyponatraemia and hypo-osmolality [118]. Hyponatraemia in cirrhosis with ascites is, therefore, a consequence of an excess of water and not of sodium deficiency. This concept is important from a

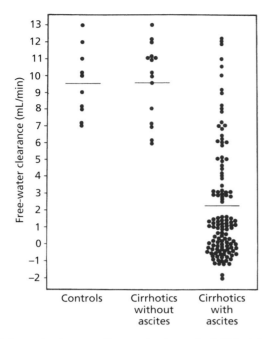

Fig. 5 Free-water clearance after an oral water overload of 20 mL/kg body weight in normal subjects and in patients with hepatic cirrhosis with and without ascites.

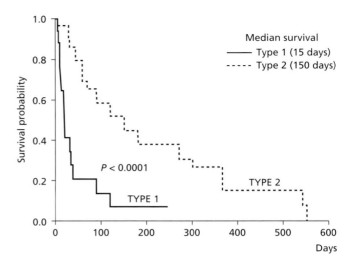

Fig. 6 Survival of patients with cirrhosis after the diagnosis of type 1 or type 2 HRS [reproduced with permission from Ginès P (2003) *Lancet* 362, 1819–1827].

therapeutic point of view. The incidence of hyponatraemia in cirrhotic patients with ascites is approximately 35% [118].

Hepatorenal syndrome is a peculiar type of functional renal failure that occurs in patients with acute liver failure and cirrhosis with ascites. It is due to reduced renal perfusion and, in most cases, renal histology is normal or presents minor abnormalities. Retrospective studies indicate that it is present in approximately 17% of patients admitted to hospital with ascites and in more than 50% of the cirrhotics who die [119]. The probability of developing hepatorenal syndrome 2 and 5 years after the onset of ascites in patients with cirrhosis is 32% and 41% respectively [120]. Hepatorenal syndrome represents the most accurate prognostic index in patients with cirrhosis and ascites: most of these patients die within weeks or months after the onset of the syndrome, independently of the degree of hepatic insufficiency [121,122]. There are two distinct types of hepatorenal syndrome in cirrhosis [122,123]. Type 1 hepatorenal syndrome is characterized by a rapid increase in blood urea nitrogen (BUN) and serum creatinine, which reach extremely high levels within days after the onset of renal failure (over 100 mg/dL and 5 mg/dL respectively). Most of these patients also present progressive oliguria, dilutional hyponatraemia (often below 120 mEq/L) and hyperkalaemia. This rapidly progressive renal impairment always occurs in patients with extremely poor hepatic function who, in addition to ascites, often present other complications of the underlying cirrhosis, such as jaundice or hepatic encephalopathy. Type 1 hepatorenal syndrome is commonly observed in alcoholic cirrhotics with superimposed severe alcoholic hepatitis or in any aetiological type of cirrhosis with ascites

in which hepatic function deteriorates rapidly as a consequence of a serious bacterial infection, gastrointestinal haemorrhage or a major surgical procedure. The development of type 1 hepatorenal syndrome carries an ominous prognosis as most of these patients die within days or weeks after the onset of the syndrome. Type 2 hepatorenal syndrome is characterized by a moderate increase in BUN and serum creatinine (usually lower than 60 mg/dL and 2 mg/dL respectively), which remains steady for months [122,123]. It is important to realize, however, that in cirrhosis a small increase in BUN or serum creatinine represents a marked fall in glomerular filtration rate (GFR). In fact, GFR in patients with type 2 hepatorenal syndrome is reduced by more than 50%. Type 2 hepatorenal syndrome usually occurs in cirrhotics with a relatively preserved hepatic function, whose main clinical problem is an ascites refractory to diuretic treatment [122]. Survival of these patients, however, is considerably less than that of non-azotaemic cirrhotics with ascites (Fig. 6).

Mechanisms of renal function abnormalities in cirrhosis

Several neurohumoral systems and endogenous substances with sodium- or water-retaining activities, or vasoactive properties, have been implicated in the pathogenesis of renal dysfunction in cirrhosis, including the renin–angiotensin–aldosterone and the sympathetic nervous systems, antidiuretic hormone, prostaglandins, leukotrienes, natriuretic peptides, endothelin, nitric oxide, carbon monoxide, endogenous cannabinoids, natriuretic hormone, the renal–kallikrein–kinin system, glomerulopressin, endotoxin, false neurotransmitters, platelet-activating factor, estrogens and vasoactive intestinal peptide. It is important to point out, however, that more than 100 different compounds with significant effects on renal function have been isolated in human urine. Therefore, the systems and substances cited above probably represent only a small fraction of the neurohumoral factors that may affect renal function in cirrhotics with ascites. In addition, alterations in intrarenal haemodynamics may also participate in the pathogenesis of sodium and water retention in these patients. Here, we summarize the extensive data presently available implicating the renin–angiotensin–aldosterone system, sympathetic nervous system, antidiuretic hormone and arachidonic acid metabolites in the pathogenesis of renal dysfunction in cirrhosis. Readers should consult other articles and chapters to review the potential role of other vasoactive substances, such as natriuretic peptides, nitric oxide and endothelin.

The renin–angiotensin–aldosterone system

Through the secretion of renin, the kidney exerts powerful control over arterial pressure, extracellular fluid volume (including blood volume), sodium and potassium excretion and the electrolyte composition of the body [124]. Renin is produced in the kidney by specialized cells of the juxtaglomerular apparatus, the granular cells of the wall of the afferent arteriola, which are in intimate contact with the macula densa in the ascending limb of the loop of Henle. The vascular and tubular components of the juxtaglomerular apparatus are richly innervated by sympathetic nerves. Renin is an enzyme with no biological activity and acts on an α-globulin (renin substrate or angiotensinogen), synthesized by the liver, releasing the inactive decapeptide angiotensin I (A-I).

Three major mechanisms control renin release from the kidney: the renal baroreceptor mechanism sensitive to changes in renal perfusion pressure; the macula densa mechanism, which responds to changes in sodium delivery or transport within the ascending limb of the loop of Henle; and the renal sympathetic nervous activity, which directly stimulates renin release by operating upon β1-receptors present in the juxtaglomerular apparatus. These three mechanisms operate in concert, as they are influenced in the same direction when there are changes in effective circulating blood volume or arterial pressure.

A-I is subsequently transformed to the octapeptide A-II by the action of the specific converting enzyme dipeptidyl carboxypeptidase. As the largest concentration of this converting enzyme is found in the lung, it was believed that conversion of A-I to A-II was primarily systemic rather than intrarenal. However, the converting enzyme is also present in the juxtaglomerular apparatus, and significant amounts of A-II are generated locally within the kidney.

A-II is one of the active components of the renin–angiotensin–aldosterone system. It is among the most active of the endogenous vasoconstrictors so far identified. The renal vasculature is especially sensitive to the vasoconstrictor effect of A-II because a striking reduction in renal blood flow occurs with doses of A-II well below those required to induce a pressor response. A-II also reduces the glomerular filtration rate. The latter effect is related to both a decrease in renal perfusion and a direct contractile effect on glomerular mesangial cells. Finally, the interaction of A-II with AT1 receptors in the adrenal glomerulosa cells stimulates the aldosterone biosynthetic pathway and increases the release of this hormone to the circulation [124].

The second active component of the renin–angiotensin–aldosterone system is aldosterone, an important regulator of sodium, potassium and acid–base balance [124]. The collecting tubule is the nephron segment responsive to aldosterone. The principal cells, located predominantly in the cortical segments, probably mediate the aldosterone-regulated sodium reabsorption and potassium secretion, whereas the intercalated cells, which predominate in the inner stripe of the outer medulla, participate in the aldosterone-regulated hydrogen ion transport. Aldosterone diffuses freely across the basolateral membrane of the principal cells and binds to a cytoplasmic receptor. The steroid–receptor complex is transported into the nuclear compartment and binds to specific promoters of a number of genes that are under aldosterone regulation. The interaction of the steroid–receptor complex with the promoter leads to the transcription of mRNAs which are, in turn, translated into their respective proteins, mediators of the sodium transport process. Among these proteins, the amiloride-sensitive sodium channel and the Na^+-K^+ATPase are of particular importance in the antinatriuretic effect of aldosterone. The sodium channels are inserted into the luminal membrane and favour the passive transport of sodium from the tubular lumen to the intracellular space. The Na^+-K^+ATPase (or sodium pump) molecules are located in the basolateral membrane and promote the active transport of intracellular sodium to the extracellular compartment and the entry of potassium from the extracellular to the intracellular space. The kaliuretic effect of aldosterone is related to its stimulatory effect on Na^+-K^+ATPase and probably also to the activation of luminal membrane potassium channels. The synthesis of the proteins activated by aldosterone takes time, and the half-life of these proteins is relatively prolonged. This explains the delay between the administration or withdrawal of spironolactone, a drug that competitively inhibits the binding of aldosterone to the cytosolic receptor, and the onset or finalization of the diuretic action.

The renin–angiotensin–aldosterone system is activated in most cirrhotics with ascites with marked sodium retention (urinary sodium excretion lower than 5 mEq/L) and in all patients with hepatorenal syndrome (Fig. 7). In many of these patients, the plasma levels of renin and aldosterone reach extraordinarily high values. In cirrhotic patients with ascites and moderate sodium retention, the plasma levels of renin and aldosterone may be normal or only slightly elevated (Fig. 7). Plasma renin activity and aldosterone are normal or reduced in compensated cirrhotics [125,127]. Several lines of evidence indicate that aldosterone plays a major role in the pathogenesis of sodium retention in cirrhosis. Urinary sodium excretion in cirrhotics with ascites correlates closely with the degree of hyperaldosteronism, plasma aldosterone levels being higher in cirrhotics with marked sodium retention [128]. On the other hand, sodium retention can be reversed in most of these patients following the

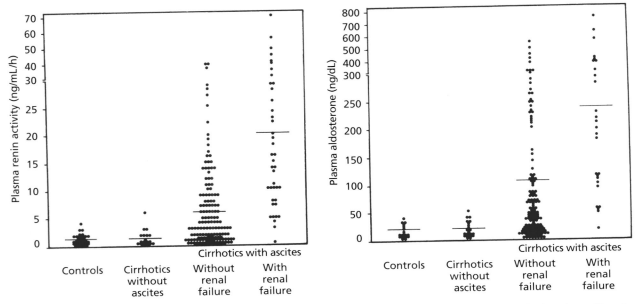

Fig. 7 Plasma renin activity and plasma aldosterone concentration in healthy subjects, cirrhotic patients without ascites and cirrhotic patients with ascites with and without hepatorenal syndrome. Measurements were made after 5 days on a 50-mEq sodium diet and without diuretics. Plasma renin activity was measured after incubating for 1 h.

blockade of the renal tubular effect of aldosterone with spirono-lactone [129]. The observation that cirrhotics with ascites may present sodium retention in the absence of hyperaldosteronism is generally considered to be an indication that factors other than aldosterone are involved in the excessive tubular sodium reabsorption [126]. However, cirrhotics with moderate sodium retention and normal plasma aldosterone concentration are extremely sensitive to spironolactone [128]; these patients may have an increased tubular sensitivity to aldosterone.

Studies using pharmacological agents that interrupt the renin–angiotensin–aldosterone system (inhibitors of the converting enzyme and structural analogues that competitively antagonize A-II at the vascular AT1 receptor) have been important in our understanding of the activation of the renin–angiotensin–aldosterone system in patients with cirrhosis and ascites. These patients present a systemic circulatory dysfunction characterized by low arterial pressure, hypervolaemia, high cardiac output and low peripheral resistance, findings consistent with marked arteriolar vasodilation [122,129–132]. Inhibition of the endogenous renin–angiotensin–aldosterone system in cirrhotic patients with increased plasma levels of renin by the intravenous injection of saralasin, a specific antagonist of A-II, or by converting enzyme inhibitors is associated with a further decrease in arterial pressure and peripheral resistance; this may be striking in patients with marked overactivity of the renin–angiotensin–aldosterone system [133]. The systemic circulatory disturbance of these patients would, therefore, be much more intense if endogenous A-II was not acting at the peripheral vasculature to maintain arterial pressure at normal or near-normal levels. Renin release in cirrhotics with ascites is, therefore, a

homeostatic mechanism to maintain systemic haemodynamics, with arterial hypotension being the most likely mechanism of hyper-reninism in these patients.

Plasma renin activity is particularly elevated in patients with hepatorenal syndrome (Fig. 7) [134,135]. On the other hand, plasma renin activity in non-azotaemic cirrhotic patients with ascites is an independent predictor of hepatorenal syndrome development [120]. Therefore, it is reasonable to presume that endogenous A-II is involved in the pathogenesis of the active vasoconstriction, causing hepatorenal syndrome in cirrhosis.

The sympathetic nervous system

The sympathetic nervous system is another important endogenous mechanism controlling systemic haemodynamics and renal function in man. This system is influenced by high-pressure baroreceptors located in the carotid sinus and aortic arch and low-pressure baroreceptors (volume receptors) present in the cardiac atria and pulmonary veins. High-pressure baroreceptors are quiescent below an arterial pressure of 80 mmHg and show a progressive excitation with increasing arterial pressure up to approximately 180 mmHg. The activity from these receptors elicits a reflex inhibition of the sympathetic outflow and thus provides the afferent limb of the buffer reflexes that stabilize arterial pressure. When compared with the sympathetic activity directed to other visceral structures, efferent renal nerve activity appears to be particularly sensitive to inhibition by arterial baroreceptors [136]. Low-pressure baroreceptors are activated by distension of the cardiac atria and pulmonary veins and, therefore, function as intravascular volume receptors. Afferent impulses arising from high- and low-pressure baroreceptors travel via the glossopharyngeal and vagus nerves to an integrative site in the medulla, which alters the sympathetic nervous outflow according to the information received. Afferent impulses from high- and low-pressure baroreceptors are also sent to the supraoptic and paraventricular nuclei of the hypothalamus, thus modifying antidiuretic hormone secretion [137]. Therefore, three neurohormonal vasoactive systems, the sympathetic nervous system, the renin–angiotensin–aldosterone system and antidiuretic hormone, are closely interrelated and operate simultaneously to regulate arterial pressure and intravascular volume.

The kidney is richly innervated by sympathetic noradrenergic fibres, which reach the afferent and efferent arterioles, juxtaglomerular apparatus, proximal and distal convoluted tubules, thick ascending limb of the loop of Henle and distal and collecting tubules [138]. In contrast, there is neither physiological nor anatomical evidence supporting the existence of sympathetic cholinergic vasodilator fibres in the kidney. Direct electrical stimulation of the renal nerves produces a decrease in renal blood flow and GFR, and stimulates sodium reabsorption in the proximal tubule, loop of Henle and distal nephron [139]. These effects, which can also be demonstrated when the renal sympathetic nervous system is reflexively activated through high- and low-pressure baroreceptors, are mediated by α1-adrenoreceptors [139]. The effect of the sympathetic nervous system on renal sodium metabolism is independent of its haemodynamic effect, as it can be observed with subpressor nerve stimulation in the absence of changes in renal perfusion and GFR.

The most commonly used method to assess sympathetic nervous activity in man is by measuring the plasma levels of noradrenaline (nonepinephrine), as most noradrenaline circulating in plasma is derived from that released as a transmitter at postsynaptic sympathetic nerve terminals. Many studies have been performed using this method in patients with cirrhosis with and without ascites or hepatorenal syndrome; they demonstrate that the plasma noradrenaline concentration in peripheral venous samples is normal in compensated cirrhosis, and usually increased in patients showing sodium retention and ascites (see Fig. 8) [130,134,135,140,141]. In normal subjects, the plasma concentration of noradrenaline in renal vein samples is similar to, or lower than, that in arterial samples, the renal venous–arterial difference, therefore, being zero or slightly negative. In contrast, in cirrhotics with ascites, this difference is usually positive, indicating an increased activity of the renal sympathetic nervous system [141]. By using radiotracer techniques, it has been shown that both total body and renal release of noradrenaline was elevated in parallel in these patients [142]. Direct evidence of a generalized overactivity of the sympathetic nervous system in cirrhosis has been provided by measuring the sympathetic nerve discharge rates from a peripheral muscular nerve. Muscular sympathetic nerve activity is markedly increased in patients with ascites and normal in patients without ascites, and correlates directly with plasma noradrenaline.

As the sympathetic nervous activity stimulates sodium reabsorption and is a vasoconstrictor in the renal circulation, it has

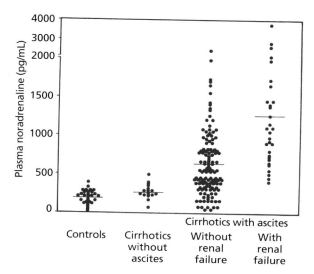

Fig. 8 Plasma noradrenaline concentration in healthy subjects, cirrhotic patients without ascites and cirrhotic patients with ascites with and without hepatorenal syndrome. Measurements were made after 5 days on a 50-mEq sodium diet without diuretics.

been implicated in the pathogenesis of sodium retention and hepatorenal syndrome in cirrhosis. There is evidence supporting this contention. Plasma noradrenaline and total noradrenaline spillover are normal in compensated cirrhotics, and usually increased in patients with ascites and sodium retention. In the latter group, sodium excretion correlates inversely with these measurements [140]. Acute bilateral renal surgical denervation is followed by increased urine volume and sodium excretion in bile duct-ligated miniature swine with cirrhosis and ascites; in conscious cirrhotic rats with ascites, it improves renal excretion of both an intravenous and an oral sodium load. Such direct evidence has also been presented in patients with cirrhosis, in whom anaesthetic blockade of the lumbar sympathetic nervous system, a manoeuvre that reduces the renal sympathetic nervous activity, improves sodium excretion [143]. Among cirrhotics with ascites, patients with hepatorenal syndrome have the highest plasma concentration of noradrenaline (Fig. 8) [131]. Moreover, the acute inhibition of the renal sympathetic outflow with clonidine in patients with cirrhosis is associated with a reduction in renal vascular resistance and an increase in GFR, indicating that the activation of the sympathetic nervous system participates in the pathogenesis of the renal vasoconstriction of cirrhosis.

Factors other than the sympathetic nervous activity and aldosterone are involved in sodium retention in cirrhosis [126]. A series of non-azotaemic patients with ascites, moderate to intense sodium retention and normal recumbent levels of plasma renin activity, aldosterone and noradrenaline were studied in an upright position and during moderate physical exercise and compared with a group of normal subjects and a group of patients with compensated cirrhosis. There were no significant differences in plasma renin activity, aldosterone and noradrenaline between the three groups in any of the study conditions. Interestingly enough, the cirrhotic patients with ascites showed high circulating levels of atrial natriuretic peptide, indicating that sodium retention may occur in cirrhosis in the absence of detectable activation of the renin–angiotensin–aldosterone system and sympathetic nervous system and despite increased circulating levels of natriuretic peptides.

Antidiuretic hormone

Antidiuretic hormone (ADH) is produced by magnocellular neurones arising bilaterally in the supraoptic nuclei of the hypothalamus [137]. These neurones project medially to merge in the pituitary stalk and continue to form the posterior lobe of the pituitary gland. The neurones terminate as bulbous enlargements on capillary networks scattered through the stalk and body of the neurohypophysis. Biosynthesis of ADH occurs from the peptide precursor propressophysin, which is composed of ADH and the vasopressin-binding protein neurophysin. The precursor is synthesized in cell bodies in the supraoptic nuclei, packed in secretory granules and cleaved progressively as it moves down to the axon to yield neurophysin and ADH. In the nerve terminals, ADH and neurophysin are stored in secretory granules and secreted.

The most important physiological stimulus for ADH secretion is the osmotic pressure of body water, which induces changes in the water content of a group of neurones (osmoreceptors) concentrated in the anterior hypothalamus near the supraoptic nuclei [137]. The functional properties of these neurones resemble those of a set-point receptor. Plasma osmolality below a threshold level suppresses ADH to low or undetectable levels. Above that point, plasma ADH rises steeply in direct proportion to plasma osmolality. Secretion of ADH is also affected by changes in systemic haemodynamics [137]. Small decreases (< 10%) in blood volume or arterial pressure have little effect on plasma ADH. However, beyond that point, plasma ADH rises at a rapidly increasing rate. The ADH responses to haemodynamic changes are mediated by neurogenic stimuli that arise from high- and low-pressure baroreceptors. Changes in blood volume or pressure large enough to affect ADH secretion do not interfere with osmoreceptor regulation of the hormone but, rather, raise or lower the threshold level of hormone secretion. For example, in the presence of hypovolaemia, plasma ADH secretion can be suppressed if plasma osmolality falls, but the set-point at which ADH decreases in response to hypo-osmolality is lower than under normal conditions. This concept is of importance in explaining the relationship between ADH and plasma osmolality in circumstances, such as cirrhosis, with simultaneous changes in systemic haemodynamics and extracellular osmolality.

The two major biological effects of ADH are to increase water permeability in the cortical and medullary collecting tubules (hydro-osmotic effect), thus allowing water to be reabsorbed passively from the tubular lumen to the isotonic cortical and hypertonic medullary interstitium, and to produce contraction of the vascular smooth muscle cells (vasoconstrictor effect)

[137]. The hydro-osmotic effect of ADH is mediated by the insertion of water channels (aquaporin-2), which are stored in cytoplasmic vesicles near the tubular lumen, in the luminal membrane of the collecting tubule epithelial cells [144,145]. In the unstimulated state, this membrane is almost impermeable to water because of a lack of water channels. In contrast, the basocellular membrane, which is very rich in aquaporin-3 (a different water channel that also transports non-ionic solutes such as urea), is highly permeable to water. The hydro-osmotic effect of ADH is initiated by the binding of the hormone to a V_2 receptor on the basolateral membrane of the collecting duct epithelial cells. This receptor is coupled to adenylate cyclase by a guanine nucleotide-binding protein (Gs), which stimulates the enzyme. Adenylate cyclase stimulation results in the insertion of aquaporin-2 molecules into the luminal membrane. The vasoconstrictor effect of ADH is initiated by the interaction of the hormone with V_1 receptors placed in the plasma membrane of the vascular smooth muscle cells. The vascular effect of ADH is particularly striking in the splanchnic, muscular and cutaneous vasculature, with renal circulation being much less sensitive to its vasoconstrictor action.

The production of free water within the kidney occurs in the ascending limb of the loop of Henle by a process involving the reabsorption of sodium chloride without a concomitant reabsorption of water (this segment of the nephron is almost impermeable to water) [146]. Free-water formation is, therefore, the result of a reabsorption of electrolytes from the tubular fluid rather than of an addition of water. In normal conditions, the kidney is continuously producing a hypotonic tubular fluid in the ascending limb of the loop of Henle. The final osmolality of the urine, therefore, depends on the degree of water reabsorption in the cortical and medullary collecting tubules, which is influenced by ADH [146].

Impairment in free-water excretion in cirrhosis was initially considered to be the result of reduced delivery of sodium chloride to the ascending limb of the loop of Henle due to low GFR and increased sodium reabsorption in the proximal tubule. Recent studies, however, have presented data indicating that ADH plays a major role in the impairment of free-water excretion in cirrhosis. Plasma levels of ADH are increased in most cirrhotics with ascites and correlate closely with the reduction in free-water excretion (Fig. 9) [140,147]. Longitudinal studies in rats with experimental cirrhosis and ascites have shown that impairment of water excretion appears in close chronological relationship to the onset of ADH hypersecretion. Brattleboro rats (rats with a congenital deficiency of ADH) with cirrhosis do not develop an impairment in water excretion [148]. Kidneys from cirrhotic rats with ascites show increased gene expression of aquaporin-2, the ADH-regulated water channel. The blockade of V_2 receptors with specific peptide and non-peptide ADH antagonists returns the impaired renal water excretion to normal in rats with carbon tetrachloride-induced cirrhosis and ascites [149] and in patients with cirrhosis, ascites and dilutional hyponatraemia [150–152]. This effect has also been observed

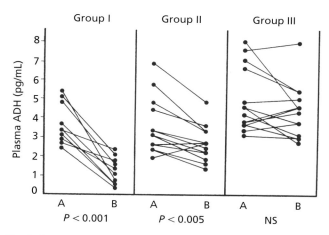

Fig. 9 Plasma antidiuretic hormone (ADH) concentration after 16 h of water restriction (A) and following a water overload of 20 mL/kg body weight (B). Group I includes normal subjects (free-water clearance 9.6 ± 0.8 mL/min). Group II includes cirrhotic patients with ascites who were able to generate free water after the overload (free-water clearance 3.6 ± 0.6 mL/min). Group III includes cirrhotic patients with ascites who were unable to generate free water after the overload (free-water clearance 0.37 ± 0.07 mL/min). (Reproduced with permission from ref. 147.) NS, not significant.

following the administration of niravoline (RU-51599), a kappa opioid agonist that inhibits the release and the tubular effect of ADH, to rats with cirrhosis and patients with ascites [153]. Plasma levels of ADH in patients with cirrhosis and ascites also correlate with renal perfusion and GFR, patients with hepatorenal syndrome having higher levels of ADH [147]. Therefore, ADH might contribute to the active renal vasoconstriction in hepatorenal syndrome.

The increased plasma ADH concentration in cirrhosis is due to an increased hypothalamic synthesis and not to a reduced systemic clearance of the peptide. Evidence indicates that this increased synthesis of ADH is related to a non-osmotic haemodynamic stimuli. Most patients with high plasma levels of ADH have a degree of hyponatraemia that would suppress the release of this hormone in normal subjects [147]. Moreover, ADH in cirrhotic patients with ascites correlates with plasma renin activity and noradrenaline, and is suppressed by manoeuvres that increase effective arterial blood volume, such as head-out water immersion or peritoneovenous shunting [140,147]. Finally, the blockade of V_1 receptors with specific ADH antagonists in rats with experimental cirrhosis, ascites and ADH hypersecretion is followed by a significant decrease in arterial pressure, an effect not observed in control animals [149]. This indicates that ADH hypersecretion contributes to the maintenance of arterial pressure in cirrhotics and suggests that the most likely mechanism of ADH hypersecretion in decompensated cirrhosis is arterial hypotension.

Arachidonic acid metabolites

The kidneys are able to synthesize substances that act locally to regulate renal function. Among these substances, the most

extensively studied are prostaglandins (PGs), which are derived from arachidonic acid metabolism. The initial step in the formation of these compounds is the interaction of a stimulus, commonly a hormone, with a receptor on the cell surface, leading to an activation of phospholipase A_2. The net effect of this process is an increase in free arachidonic acid concentration, normally quite low, within the cell. The second step is the synthesis of the endoperoxides PGG_2 and PGH_2 from arachidonic acid. This is a complex process catalysed by a cyclo-oxygenase. Cyclo-oxygenase exists in two isoforms. Cyclo-oxygenase-1 (COX-1) is constitutively expressed in most of the tissues and is involved in the physiological production of PGs. Activation of COX-1 leads, for instance, to the production of PGI_2 which, when released by the renal vasculature, contributes to the maintenance of renal perfusion and GFR and, when released by the gastric mucosa, is cytoprotective [154]. The inducible form, cyclo-oxygenase-2 (COX-2), is present in cells exposed to pro-inflammatory agents, including cytokines, and is expressed during certain inflammatory processes. Inhibition of inducible COX-2 by non-steroidal anti-inflammatory drugs (NSAIDs) explains the therapeutic utility of these drugs as anti-inflammatory agents, whereas inhibition of constitutive COX-1 explains their unwanted side-effects on the stomach and the kidneys. The recent development of new drugs with selective action on COX-2 has opened a new field in the pharmacology of the inflammatory process, particularly in patients who require PGs to maintain vital functions. PGG_2 and PGH_2 are extremely unstable intermediates that are rapidly converted through various enzymes to the active compounds $PGF_{2\alpha}$, PGE_2, PGI_2 (or prostacyclin), PGD_2 and thromboxane A_2 by the action of specific enzymes.

The kidney contains several structures capable of synthesizing PGs. Glomeruli predominantly produce PGI_2 with lesser amounts of PGE_2, thromboxane A_2 and $PGF_{2\alpha}$; afferent and efferent arterioles produce PGI_2 and PGE_2, and medullary interstitial cells and collecting duct epithelial cells produce PGE_2. PGs are rapidly metabolized to products with no biological activity. Because of their rapid degradation, their biological actions are exerted at the site of synthesis. Therefore, PGI_2 and PGE_2 synthesized by the arterioles and glomeruli are thought to regulate renal perfusion and GFR; PGE_2 synthesized by the collecting duct epithelial cells is involved in the tubular handling of sodium and water in the distal nephron [155].

PGs are involved in the control of renal haemodynamics. PGE_2 and PGI_2 have powerful vasorelaxant effects on the renal arterioles and the glomerular mesangium [156]. In contrast, thromboxane A_2 and leukotrienes C4 and D4 produce contraction of the mesangial cells and possibly also the renal arterioles [156]. A-II and ADH, by interacting with ATI and V1 receptors, respectively, in vascular smooth muscle and mesangial cells, stimulate phospholipase A_2, which releases arachidonic acid from membrane phospholipids and enhances the renal synthesis of PGI_2 and PGE_2. Noradrenaline and efferent renal nerve activity also stimulate the renal synthesis of PGs, an effect that

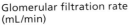
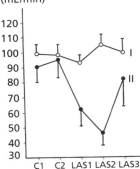
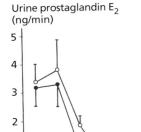
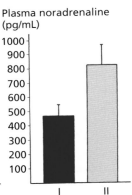

Fig. 10 Glomerular filtration rate and urinary excretion of prostaglandin E_2 (mean ± SEM) before and after the intravenous injection of 450 mg of lysine acetylsalicylate in 19 patients with cirrhosis and ascites. Patients were divided into two groups according to whether they developed renal insufficiency (II; 11 patients) or not (I; 8 patients) after the administration of the drug. C1 and C2 represent two 30-min periods before the administration of lysine acetylsalicylate. LAS1, LAS2 and LAS3 represent three 30-min periods after the administration of lysine acetylsalicylate. Values of plasma noradrenaline correspond to those of samples obtained before lysine acetylsalicylate injection. (Reproduced with permission from ref. 135.)

is mediated by α-receptors. PGE_2 and PGI_2 antagonize the renal vasoconstrictor effect of these endogenous vasoactive compounds. Finally, cyclo-oxygenase inhibition by NSAIDs potentiates the renal vasoconstrictor effect of A-II, noradrenaline, ADH and renal nerve stimulation, and impairs renal blood flow and GFR in circumstances of low effective blood volume, in which there is activation of the renin–angiotensin–aldosterone system, sympathetic nervous system and ADH. In these conditions, the renal production of PGs is increased, probably as a homeostatic response to antagonize the renal vascular effects of these systems. Renal PGE_2 and PGI_2 therefore regulate renal haemodynamics by modulating the renal vascular effects of endogenous vasoconstrictors.

PGE$_2$ also modulates the renal tubular action of ADH [156]. ADH stimulates the production of PGE_2 by cortical and medullary collecting duct epithelial cells. This effect appears to be secondary to the interaction of ADH with V1 receptors present in these cells. On the other hand, PGE_2 inhibits the hydro-osmotic effect of ADH. Finally, inhibition of PGs with NSAIDs enhances the tubular effect of ADH. A negative feedback therefore exists, in which ADH itself stimulates the synthesis of its antagonist PGE_2 in the collecting duct epithelial cells.

The following points support the suggestion that PGs play an important role in the homeostasis of renal blood flow and GFR in cirrhotic patients with ascites:

1 The urinary excretion of PGE_2 and 6-keto-$PGF_{1\alpha}$ (a stable metabolite of PGI_2), which is thought to estimate the renal production of PGE_2 and PGI_2, respectively, is increased in non-azotaemic cirrhotics with ascites, whereas it is reduced in patients with hepatorenal syndrome [134,135,157,158].

2 Non-azotaemic cirrhotics with ascites also show high urinary excretion of thromboxane B_2 (a stable metabolite of thromboxane A_2) and $PGF_{2\alpha}$ [157,158], which suggests that the stimulus promoting synthesis of PGs in these patients acts at the initial step of the arachidonic acid cascade, thus increasing the synthesis of all prostaglandins.

3 The administration of NSAIDs induces a profound decrease in renal blood flow and GFR in non-azotaemic cirrhotics with

increased activity of the renin–angiotensin–aldosterone system and sympathetic nervous system and marked sodium retention. In contrast, PG inhibition with these drugs in patients with ascites and normal plasma renin activity and plasma noradrenaline is not associated with significant changes in renal perfusion and GFR (Fig. 10) [15,159,160]. These findings are the most persuasive arguments indicating that renal PGs are important factors in the maintenance of renal blood flow and GFR in non-azotaemic cirrhotics with ascites, and that an equilibrium between the degree of activity of endogenous vasoconstrictors and the renal synthesis of vasodilator PGs is of crucial importance in the homeostasis of renal haemodynamics in these patients.

4 In patients with compensated cirrhosis, the urinary excretion of PGs is similar to that in normal subjects [135,158,161]. On the other hand, there have been several studies showing that renal perfusion and GFR are normal in these patients and that PG inhibition with NSAIDs is not associated with significant changes in renal function [135,159,162]. These studies therefore indicate that PGs are not involved in the regulation of renal perfusion during the initial phases of cirrhosis, prior to the appearance of ascites. This feature is not surprising as it is well known that PGs are important in the maintenance of renal perfusion only in conditions of activated endogenous renal vasoconstrictors.

The increased renal production of PGE_2 in non-azotaemic cirrhotics with ascites, by antagonizing the hydro-osmotic effect of ADH, also contributes to the maintenance of free-water excretion in these patients. Most cirrhotic patients with ascites can dilute the urine after a water load despite inadequate suppression of ADH, indicating a relative resistance to the tubular effect of this hormone [147]. This renal resistance to ADH is related to increased renal production of PGE_2, as PG inhibition in these patients is associated with marked impairment in free-water excretion, occurring in the absence of changes in plasma ADH and independent of changes in renal blood flow and GFR [147].

Studies in experimental animals with cirrhosis and ascites and a recent investigation in patients with cirrhosis, ascites and increased activity of the renin–angiotensin system show that COX-2 inhibitors do not impair renal function in decompensated cirrhosis [163]. The PG synthetic pathway participating in the maintenance of renal function in decompensated cirrhosis is, therefore, that related to COX-1.

Circulatory dysfunction in cirrhosis: role in the pathogenesis of renal function abnormalities in cirrhosis

Splanchnic arterial vasodilation: the peripheral arterial vasodilation hypothesis of renal dysfunction in cirrhosis

Renal dysfunction in patients with cirrhosis occurs in the setting of a circulatory dysfunction characterized by a marked arterial vasodilation [104,164] (Fig. 11). There is evidence that the site of this arterial vasodilation is the splanchnic circulation as there is vasoconstriction in all the other major vascular territories such as the kidneys, muscle and skin and brain [142,165,166]. In contrast, in the splanchnic circulation, there is vasodilation, which increases the inflow of blood into the portal venous system [167].

The mechanism of the decreased splanchnic arterial vascular resistance associated with portal hypertension in cirrhosis is not completely understood. For many years, arterial vasodilation in cirrhosis has been attributed to increased circulating plasma levels of vasodilators such as glucagon, prostaglandins, adrenomedullin and natriuretic peptide. However, because the site of arterial vasodilation is the splanchnic circulation, a local mechanism (increased release of a vasodilator substance within the splanchnic area) is a more likely hypothesis. Results of subsequent studies suggesting that nitric oxide, a vasodilator

substance that acts in a paracrine manner, is important in the pathogenesis of splanchnic arterial vasodilation in cirrhosis is consistent with this hypothesis. Increased activity of nitric oxide synthase in the splanchnic circulation has been reported in experimental cirrhosis [168–170]. On the other hand, inhibition of nitric oxide normalizes circulatory function in experimental cirrhosis [170]. Two hypotheses have been raised to explain the mechanism of the increased production of nitric oxide in the splanchnic circulation. The first is that it is secondary to bacterial translocation from the intestinal lumen to the interstitial intestinal space. Endotoxin and the increased cytokine production would stimulate the activity of nitric oxide synthase in the endothelial and vascular smooth muscle cells [169,171]. The second hypothesis considers that there is a stimulation of the non-adrenergic, non-cholinergic nervous system secondary to portal hypertension [169,172]. This is a sensitive system that, when activated, releases numerous vasodilatory neurotransmitters, including nitric oxide, calcitonin gene-related peptide, substance P and vasoactive intestinal peptide [173,174]. Non-adrenergic, non-cholinergic terminals are abundant not only in the gastrointestinal smooth muscle but also in the vascular smooth muscle cells. It may be possible that portal hypertension induces changes in the intestinal wall (increase in interstitial pressure and interstitial oedema) that stimulate this system and cause splanchnic arterial vasodilation and an inhibitory effect on the gastrointestinal smooth muscle cells. In fact, the gastrointestinal transit time is greatly prolonged in patients with cirrhosis [175].

At the initial stages of cirrhosis, the circulatory dysfunction induced by the splanchnic arterial vasodilation is compensated by the development of a hyperdynamic circulation. Plasma volume, cardiac output and heart rate increase and the circulatory

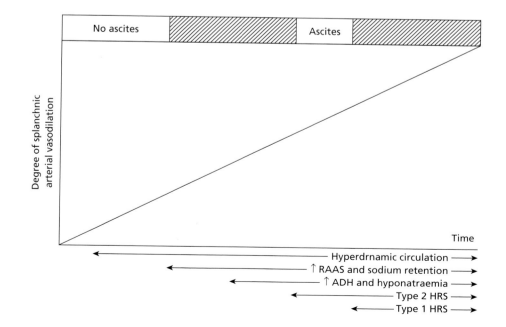

Fig. 11 Time course of the circulatory, neurohormonal and renal function abnormalities in cirrhosis. ADH, antidiuretic hormone; HRS, hepatorenal syndrome; RAAS, renin–angiotensin–aldosterone system.

transit time decreases. The incidence of arterial hypertension in cirrhotic patients with portal hypertension is very low because of this circulatory abnormality. With the progression of the liver disease and the accentuation of portal hypertension and splanchnic arterial vasodilation, patients develop sodium retention and ascites. In the initial phases of ascites, the renin–angiotensin and the sympathetic nervous systems are not stimulated, and the mechanism of sodium retention in this period is unknown. Later during the course of the disease, the renin–angiotensin–aldosterone system and the sympathetic nervous system become progressively activated in parallel with a more intense reduction in urinary sodium excretion. Patients with ascites and normal plasma renin activity and aldosterone concentration, in general, have urinary sodium excretion over 10 mEq/day, and they easily respond to low diuretic dosage. In contrast, most patients with high renin and aldosterone show a urinary sodium excretion lower than 5 mEq/day (in many cases almost zero) and need high diuretic dosage to achieve a natriuretic response. Hypersecretion of antidiuretic hormone occurs at later stages of the disease. This explains why hyponatraemia is a late event in decompensated cirrhosis. This is probably related to the fact that antidiuretic hormone is less sensitive than the sympathetic nervous system and the renin–angiotensin system to changes in the effective circulating blood volume. Hepatorenal syndrome (HRS) develops in the very late stages of the disease, always in the setting of a significant arterial hypotension and an intense activation of the renin–angiotensin and sympathetic nervous systems and antidiuretic hormone.

These different phases of circulatory and renal dysfunction in cirrhosis correlate closely with the progression of portal hypertension and splanchnic arterial vasodilation. In patients with cirrhosis, there is a strong direct relationship between the degree of portal hypertension, plasma levels of renin, aldosterone and norepinephrine and the intensity of sodium retention. Arterial pressure is lower in patients with cirrhosis and ascites than in those with compensated cirrhosis. Finally, among patients with ascites, those with HRS present the lowest arterial pressure and the highest plasma levels of renin, norepinephrine and antidiuretic hormone.

Renal and other extrasplanchnic regional circulations in cirrhosis

Traditional studies with para-aminohippurate clearance and recent investigations with the echo Doppler technique have shown increased intrarenal vascular resistance in patients with cirrhosis and ascites prior to the development of HRS. HRS is therefore the extreme expression of an impairment in renal circulatory function starting at earlier stages. Renal plasma flow, intrarenal vascular resistance and GFR in cirrhosis with ascites correlate closely with the degree of stimulation of the renin–angiotensin system and the sympathetic nervous system [135]. Patients with normal or moderately increased plasma levels of renin and norepinephrine usually show normal renal perfusion and GFR,

whereas these substances are markedly increased in patients with HRS. These data have led to the contention that HRS in cirrhosis is caused by renal vasoconstriction related to the activation of these systems [176]. However, this hypothesis is too simple and, at present, there is evidence that intrarenal mechanisms may also participate in the regulation of renal perfusion.

The kidneys synthesize vasodilator substances. As discussed previously, renal PGE$_2$ and prostacyclin antagonize the vasoconstrictor effect of angiotensin II and norepinephrine and, by this mechanism, play an essential role in the maintenance of renal perfusion and GFR in decompensated cirrhosis. A syndrome similar to HRS can be produced in patients with non-azotaemic cirrhosis and ascites by the administration of NSAIDs, which inhibit prostaglandin synthesis [135,159]. Investigations in experimental animals with cirrhosis and ascites have shown that the renal production of nitric oxide also participates in the maintenance of renal perfusion [177]. Finally, the administration of antagonists of the vascular receptors of natriuretic peptides in animals with cirrhosis and ascites induces an impairment in renal function that mimics HRS [178]. Therefore, intrarenal and circulating vasodilatory substances contribute to the maintenance of renal perfusion in cirrhosis with ascites. HRS would develop when the renal production of these substances is insufficient to antagonize the renal effects of the endogenous vasoconstrictor systems. This can occur when there is a stimulation of the vasoconstrictor systems, a reduction in the synthesis of vasodilators or both.

The kidney produces vasoconstrictor substances, such as angiotensin-II, endothelin and adenosine. The production of these substances is stimulated in conditions of renal hypoperfusion. Therefore, these substances could also participate in the pathogenesis of HRS. If fact, it has been proposed that, when severe renal hypoperfusion develops in cirrhosis with ascites, there could be a reduction in the intrarenal synthesis of vasodilators and a stimulation of the renal synthesis of vasoconstrictors secondary to renal ischaemia, thus creating vicious circles that lead to a rapidly progressive impairment in renal perfusion and GFR (type 1 HRS).

Doppler studies of the brachial and femoral arteries, which supply blood mainly to skin and muscles, and of the middle cerebral artery, which supplies approximately 75% of the blood in the cerebral hemispheres, in patients with cirrhosis and ascites have also shown the presence of vasoconstriction in these vascular territories [165]. This vasoconstriction is correlated with the renal blood flow (Fig. 12). Because cutaneous, muscular and cerebral vascular resistance in patients with cirrhosis and ascites parallels renal vascular resistance and correlates closely with the degree of activity of the renin–angiotensin and sympathetic nervous systems, it is clear that changes in these regional circulations in decompensated cirrhosis represent a homeostatic response to maintain the arterial pressure.

Finally, the circulatory dysfunction induced by the splanchnic arterial vasodilation could contribute to the increased resistance

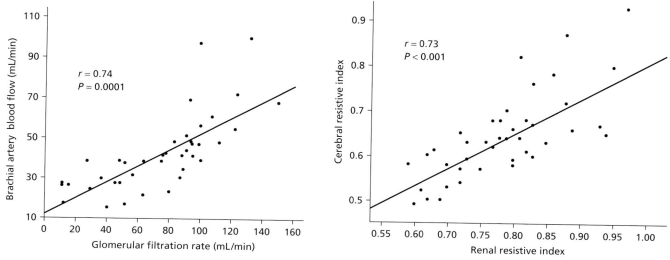

Fig. 12 Left graph: relationship between brachial artery blood flow and glomerular filtration rate. Right graph: relationship between renal resistive index and the resistive index in the middle cerebral artery in cirrhotic patients (reproduced with permission from refs 140 and 166).

to the portal venous flow and to portal hypertension. It is well known that, although the distortion of the liver vascular architecture caused by fibrosis and nodule formation is the most important mechanism in the increased intrahepatic vascular resistance in cirrhosis, there is a functional component of portal hypertension due to an increase in the intrahepatic vascular tone. The contractile intrahepatic vascular elements include the vascular smooth muscle cells from the small hepatic and portal venules and the hepatic stellate cells that surround the sinusoids. In cirrhosis, these stellate cells undergo a phenotypical transformation acquiring receptors for numerous endogenous vasoactive substances, including angiotensin II, norepinephrine, antidiuretic hormone and endothelin, and contractile properties. Therefore, the circulatory dysfunction in cirrhosis and the secondary activation of these endogenous vasoactive substances may result in an increase in the intrahepatic resistance to the portal venous flow and portal pressure. Three types of evidence support this contention. First, portal pressure in cirrhosis correlates closely with the plasma levels of renin and norepinephrine. Second, angiotensin-II blockage is associated with a decrease in portal pressure in the absence of changes in hepatic blood flow, indicating a decrease in intrahepatic vascular resistance. Finally, circulatory dysfunction associated with spontaneous bacterial peritonitis (SBP)-related type 1 HRS induces an acute and marked increase in portal pressure and a reduction in hepatic blood flow [176,179].

Splanchnic arterial vasodilation persists in decompensated cirrhosis despite the marked stimulation of the renin–angiotensin and sympathetic nervous systems and the non-osmotic hypersecretion of antidiuretic hormone. This phenomenon is related to a marked resistance of the splanchnic arterioles to the vasoconstrictor effect of angiotensin II, noradrenaline and vasopressin.

Data on experimental cirrhosis suggest that the resistance is caused by increased local synthesis of nitric oxide, because inhibition of nitric oxide synthase normalizes the response of the splanchnic circulation to these vasoconstrictors. Therefore, splanchnic arterial vasodilation in cirrhosis progresses with the increase in portal hypertension, increases the activity of the endogenous vasoconstrictor systems and leads to vasoconstriction in the extrasplanchnic vascular territories. Because the splanchnic circulation in cirrhosis has little capacity to participate in the homeostasis of arterial pressure due to the lack of response vasoconstrictors, muscular and cutaneous blood flow is very low under resting conditions, and the cerebral circulation is regulated by a very effective mechanism, the maintenance of circulatory function in cirrhosis relies mainly on the renal circulation. This explains why cirrhotic patients with ascites are very prone to the development of renal impairment and HRS in conditions associated with an impairment in circulatory function, such as bacterial infections, paracentesis, haemorrhage and diuretic treatment.

Cardiac dysfunction in cirrhosis: a second important mechanism of circulatory and renal dysfunction and ascites

Research on circulatory function in cirrhosis has been focused for many years on the peripheral arterial circulation. However, recent studies suggest that, in cirrhosis, there is also a cardiac dysfunction that could be of major importance in the deterioration of circulatory and renal function and in the pathogenesis of ascites and HRS [176,179]. As indicated previously, arterial vasodilation in the splanchnic circulation increases during the course of the disease, leading to homeostatic activation of the

	NA-1	NA-2	Type 2 HRS
Mean arterial pressure (mmHg)*	88 ± 9	86 ± 10	79 ± 7
Plasma renin activity (ng/mL/h)*	3 ± 2	7.5 ± 3.7	11.9 ± 4.8
Norepinephrine (pg/mL/h)*	221 ± 256	412 ± 155	628 ± 320
Systemic vascular resistance (dyn/s/cm^{-5})	962 ± 256	1058 ± 265	1014 ± 276
Cardiac output (L/min)*	7.2 ± 1.8	6.2 ± 1.4	5.8 ± 1.2
Heart rate (b.p.m.)	87 ± 15	84 ± 12	80 ± 14

Table 1 Chronological changes in vasoactive systems and cardiovascular function from non-azotaemic cirrhosis with ascites (NA) to type 2 HRS.

NA-1: Baseline measurement in non-azotaemic cirrhotic patients who did not develop hepatorenal syndrome in the follow-up.
NA-2: Baseline measurement in non-azotaemic cirrhotic patients who developed type 2 hepatorenal syndrome in the follow-up.
*$P < 0.01$.

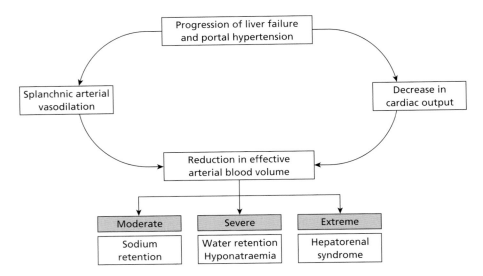

Fig. 13 Liver failure and portal hypertension.

renin–angiotensin and sympathetic nervous systems to maintain arterial pressure. This progressive decrease in cardiac afterload should be followed by an increase in cardiac output and heart rate. However, this is not the case (Table 1). Heart rate in patients with non-azotaemic cirrhosis, ascites and normal or slightly increased activity of the renin–angiotensin and sympathetic nervous systems is similar to that in non-azotaemic patients with increased activity of these systems or with HRS, indicating a severe impairment in cardiac chronotropic function. On the other hand, the cardiac output, although higher than normal in most cases, decreases progressively during the course of the disease. The mechanisms of circulatory dysfunction in cirrhosis may, therefore, be more complex than that proposed by the peripheral arterial vasodilation hypothesis (Fig. 13). In patients with compensated cirrhosis, the splanchnic arterial vasodilation would be compensated by an appropriated cardiac response, with increased heart rate, left ventricular systolic ejection fraction and cardiac output. However, with

the progression of liver failure and portal hypertension, this compensatory mechanisms fails. The increased arterial vasodilation is not followed by an increase in heart rate. On the other hand, the cardiac output decreases rather than increases. Arterial pressure homeostasis is, therefore, solely dependent on the stimulation of the endogenous vasoconstrictor systems (renin–angiotensin system, sympathetic nervous system and antidiuretic hormone), which has deleterious effects on renal perfusion and on the perfusion of other organs and produces sodium retention and ascites formation.

Cardiac chronotropic dysfunction in cirrhosis is probably related to a downregulation of β-adrenergic receptors owing to the overactivity of the sympathetic nervous system. The decrease in cardiac output is probably related to a reduction in cardiac preload [176]. There is a cirrhotic cardiomyopathy characterized by an impaired left ventricular diastolic function and cardiac hypertrophy [180]. However, it is unlikely that it plays a significant role in the decrease in cardiac function because, in decompensated cirrhosis, cardiac output increases following manoeuvres that expand the central blood volume (head-out water immersion, plasma volume expansion, therapeutic paracentesis and insertion of a peritoneovenous or a transjugular intrahepatic portocaval shunt), indicating a preserved cardiac reserve. Cardiac dysfunction in cirrhosis, therefore, appears to be a functional disorder unrelated to the structural changes in the heart.

Pathogenesis of ascites

The forward theory

The traditional concept of ascites formation in cirrhosis considers hepatic oedema to be a direct consequence of the 'backward' increase in hydrostatic pressure in the hepatic sinusoids and splanchnic capillaries due to the sinusoidal portal hypertension [92,93,181]. This feature, together with the hypoalbuminaemia, would alter the Starling equilibrium within the hepatic and splanchnic microcirculation, leading to the accumulation of fluid in the interstitial space of these vascular territories. Leakage of fluid from the interstitial space to the peritoneal cavity would occur when the formation of interstitial oedema overcomes the capacity of the abdominal lymphatic system to return the hepatic and splanchnic lymph to the systemic circulation. Renal dysfunction in cirrhosis would be a consequence of a reduction in the circulating blood volume secondary to the formation of ascites. The fact that the blood volume is constantly increased in patients with cirrhosis would not invalidate this hypothesis, as the effective blood volume would be reduced as a result of an enlargement of the intravascular venous compartment promoted by the increased portal pressure. During the last decade, data have been presented indicating that ascites formation in cirrhosis could be better explained on a 'forward' basis, as follows:

1 As indicated above, splanchnic arteriolar vasodilation is a constant finding in cirrhosis with ascites and portal hypertension. It is the primary event in the hyperdynamic circulation (hypervolaemia, high cardiac output, low peripheral vascular resistance, arterial hypotension) that characterizes patients with compensated and decompensated cirrhosis prior to HRS. Arteriolar vasodilation is also the primary event in the stimulation of the renin–aldosterone and sympathetic nervous systems and ADH, and renal dysfunction (sodium and water retention and HRS) in patients with ascites [182].

2 Investigations on portal vein-ligated rats have demonstrated that the increased hydrostatic pressure in the splanchnic microcirculation in chronic portal hypertension is predominantly due to the increased inflow of blood to this vascular territory, secondary to the splanchnic arteriolar vasodilation [97,183,184]. This increased inflow of blood into the splanchnic microcirculation increases not only the capillary hydrostatic pressure but also the filtration coefficient, leading to a marked increase in intestinal lymph flow [97]. Splanchnic arteriolar vasodilation

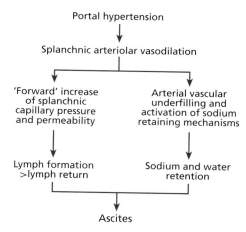

Fig. 14 The forward theory of ascites formation.

is therefore the predominant mechanism of increased lymph formation during chronic portal hypertension.

3 Portal hypertension is higher in cirrhosis than in prehepatic portal hypertension. In experimental animals with chronic ligation of the portal vein, portal pressure averages 15 mmHg, whereas it approaches 25–30 mmHg in experimental cirrhosis [97]. Among cirrhotic patients, the degree of portal hypertension is also higher in those with rather than without ascites [104]. Splanchnic arteriolar vasodilation is also higher in patients with decompensated than compensated cirrhosis, as they have a similar decrease in peripheral vascular resistance in the setting of marked overactivity of endogenous vasoconstrictor systems [104].

These data suggest that the pathogenesis of ascites could be satisfactorily explained on the basis of the changes in the arterial circulation induced by portal hypertension (Fig. 14) [185]. The hypothesis (forward theory of ascites formation) considers that the accumulation of fluid within the abdomen is a consequence of the splanchnic arteriolar vasodilation, which would simultaneously produce arteriolar vascular underfilling and a 'forward' increase in the splanchnic capillary pressure and filtration coefficient. In patients with compensated cirrhosis or with prehepatic portal hypertension, the degree of portal hypertension and of splanchnic arteriolar vasodilation is moderate. Their arterial vascular underfilling can be compensated for by transient and undetectable episodes of sodium and water retention that increase the plasma volume and cardiac index and refill the dilated arterial vascular bed [182]. The lymphatic system is able to return the moderate increase in lymph produced to the systemic circulation, thus preventing leakage of fluid into the abdominal cavity. As cirrhosis progresses, however, portal hypertension and the secondary fall in splanchnic vascular resistance are more intense and, on the other hand, the heart is unable to maintain an appropriate hyperdynamic circulation to compensate for the progression in the splanchnic hyperaemia. The maintenance of arterial pressure then requires persistent activation of the renin–aldosterone system, the sympathetic nervous system and ADH, which produces continuous water and sodium retention. The retained fluid is, however, ineffective in refilling the dilated arterial vascular bed because it escapes from the intravascular compartment, due to an imbalance between the excessive lymph production and the ability of the lymphatic system to return it to the systemic circulation. The final consequence of both disorders is continuous leakage of fluid into the abdominal cavity and the formation of ascites.

Reabsorption of ascites

Although the above discussion has exclusively emphasized factors involved in the formation of ascites, the amount of ascites present at any given time reflects the balance between the rates of formation and reabsorption. Information on reabsorption is limited. It appears that the lymphatics on the undersurface of the diaphragm are especially important in removing ascitic fluid from the peritoneal cavity. Electron microscopic studies of the diaphragmatic peritoneum have demonstrated an anatomical arrangement that facilitates absorption from the peritoneal cavity. The peritoneal surface of the diaphragm is covered by a single layer of two different populations of mesothelial cells (cuboidal and extremely flattened) [186,187]. These cells rest on a connective tissue matrix within which lies a rich plexus of terminal lymphatic vessels (lymphatic lacunae). Cuboidal mesothelial cells are usually over the lymphatic lacunae, and the submesothelial connective tissue between them is scant or even absent. The remaining areas of the diaphragm, which lack submesothelial lymphatic lacunae, are mainly covered by flattened cells. Areas with cuboidal and flattened cells differ markedly in the structure of their intercellular (lateral) surfaces. Flattened cells form a layer with no discontinuity between adjacent cells. In contrast, numerous gaps are present between the cuboidal mesothelial cells, large enough to allow the passage of particles of Indian ink, colloidal carbon and of erythrocytes. Basically, two types of structurally different intercellular gaps may be found between the cuboidal cells. One type, which is formed by interlacing filamentous processes from adjacent mesothelial cells, represents a 'true intercellular gap' and overlies a thin layer of connective tissue. The other type, which represents a 'stoma', consists of a circular pore formed among several mesothelial cells whose cell membranes form adhesions with the underlying lymphatic endothelium. This results in a well-defined channel leading directly from the peritoneal cavity to the lumen of the lymphatic lacunae. The submesothelial plexus of lymphatic vessels intercommunicates at regular intervals by way of transverse anastomoses that drain into a deeper plexus of valved collecting vessels, which penetrate connective tissue septa of the muscular fibres of the diaphragm. Drainage from the deeper lymphatics of the diaphragm is mainly via parasternal trunks on the ventral thoracic wall, right lymphatic duct and right subclavian or internal jugular veins [188]. The lymphatic drainage of the diaphragm is therefore independent of the thoracic duct. The periodic respiratory movements of the diaphragm may be important in the passage of ascites into the lymphatic system and general circulation [188]. During inspiration, intercellular gaps and stomata close, intraperitoneal pressure is increased, and the lacunae are emptied through the combined effects of local compression and increased intra-abdominal and reduced intrathoracic pressures. During expiration, the gaps and stomata are opened, and free communication is re-established. The importance of diaphragmatic lymphatics in the reabsorption of intraperitoneal fluid has been demonstrated in animal studies showing that particles and cells of various sizes are rapidly removed from the peritoneal cavity by the lymphatics of the diaphragm; the obliteration of these diaphragmatic lymphatics by abrasion significantly delays the absorption of serum from the peritoneal cavity and increases the propensity of portal hypertension to produce ascites [186].

Reabsorption of ascites from the peritoneal cavity into the general circulation is a rate-limited phenomenon. The average fractional reabsorption rate of radiolabelled albumin from the peritoneal cavity into the general circulation in cirrhotics with ascites has been estimated as 1.27% of the intraperitoneal protein mass per hour, corresponding to a rate of ascitic fluid reabsorption of 1.4 L/24 h [16]. The rate of reabsorption of ascitic fluid, as estimated by the transport of radiolabelled proteins from the abdominal cavity into the circulating plasma, varies markedly from patient to patient [16,189]. Henriksen *et al.* [16] reported a range of reabsorption rates of 0.57–4.42 L/24 h in six cirrhotics with a mean ascitic fluid volume of 6.2 L. The values obtained by Buhac *et al.* [189] in 12 patients with an average volume of ascitic fluid of 9.95 L ranged from 1.0 to 5.3 L/24 h (mean 2.25 L/24 h). The time of appearance of radioactivity in plasma after the injection of radiolabelled albumin into the ascitic fluid in these patients was, on average, 0.5 h (range 0.1–1.2 h). This time lag between the intraperitoneal injection of tracer and the appearance of tracer in plasma suggests that the transport of ascitic fluid into the general circulation is slow and through tubes (lymphatic vessels) and not a transperitoneal absorption [16]. There are very few data on the factors influencing the reabsorption rate of ascitic fluid. Animal studies have demonstrated a positive relation between intra-abdominal pressure and reabsorption of intraperitoneal fluid. However, this relation was not observed in cirrhotic patients, in whom a decrease in intra-abdominal pressure did not lead to significant changes in the reabsorption of ascitic fluid from the peritoneal cavity [189]. The low rates of ascites formation and reabsorption of ascitic fluid in cirrhotics with ascites should not be taken as an indication that, in these patients, the intraperitoneal cavity is a segregated compartment isolated from the rest of the body. In fact, the transperitoneal exchange of water and water-soluble substances (for example antibiotics not bound to proteins) by diffusion is very rapid in cirrhotics with ascites. It has been demonstrated that the water content of ascitic fluid enters and leaves the peritoneal cavity very rapidly, approximating 40–80%/h.

Prognosis of patients with cirrhosis and ascites

The appearance of ascites in patients with cirrhosis carries a poor prognosis. The probability of survival 1 and 5 years after the first episode of ascites has been estimated as 50% and 20% respectively [190]. Among cirrhotics with ascites, those with hepatorenal syndrome have the shortest survival. They usually die within weeks or months after the onset of renal failure, independent of the degree of hepatic insufficiency [120]. Studies in non-azotaemic cirrhotics with ascites have shown that sodium excretion and plasma renin activity have prognostic significance [191]. Non-azotaemic cirrhotics with elevated plasma renin activity or with marked sodium retention (urinary sodium excretion lower than 10 mEq/day) have a significantly lower survival than those with normal plasma renin concentrations or relatively high urinary sodium excretion. Two investigations have evaluated the prognostic value in cirrhotics with ascites of numerous variables based on history, physical examination, hepatic biochemical tests (including galactose elimination capacity), renal function tests, systemic and splanchnic haemodynamics and endogenous vasoactive systems. Among 38 variables considered in the series by Llach *et al.* [121], composed of 139 patients in hospital for the treatment of an episode of ascites, only seven had independent prognostic value, including mean arterial pressure, plasma noradrenaline, glomerular filtration rate, urinary sodium excretion, nutritional status, hepatomegaly and serum albumin (Fig. 15). In the multivariate analysis by Tage-Jensen *et al.* [192] in 81 alcoholic cirrhotics with and without ascites, among the 25 variables considered, only the presence of ascites, the plasma noradrenaline concentration, portal pressure and serum bilirubin were independent predictors of survival. Thus, both studies indicate that measures estimating systemic and portal haemodynamics and renal function are better predictors of survival than those used to estimate hepatic function in patients with cirrhosis and ascites. Other variables with prognostic significance in cirrhotic patients with ascites include the Child–Pugh score, the ascitic protein concentration, a history of spontaneous bacterial peritonitis, the presence of dilutional hyponatraemia and the resistance of the ascites to diuretic therapy [118,193–198].

Treatments for ascites

Bedrest and low-sodium diet

The assumption of an upright posture by patients with cirrhosis and ascites is associated with a striking activation of the renin–angiotensin–aldosterone and sympathetic nervous systems, a reduction in GFR and sodium excretion and a decreased response to loop diuretics. These effects are even more striking when upright posture is associated with moderate physical exercise [126,199]. Therefore, from a theoretical point of view, bedrest could be useful for the treatment of ascites in cirrhosis, particularly in patients who respond poorly to diuretics.

The aim of the medical treatment of ascites is to mobilize the intra-abdominal fluid by creating a net negative balance of sodium. In approximately 10–20% of cirrhotics with ascites, those who spontaneously excrete relatively high amounts of sodium in the urine, this can be obtained simply by reducing the sodium content in the diet to 60–90 mEq/day [106,200,201]. A more intense dietary sodium restriction is not practical, as it is difficult to accomplish and may worsen the anorexia and malnutrition commonly present in these patients. In the remaining cases with marked sodium retention, a negative sodium balance cannot be obtained without the aid of diuretics to increase urinary sodium excretion over intake. However, even in these patients, dietary sodium restriction is very important as it reduces the diuretic requirements. In cirrhotics responding poorly to diuretic treatment, a negative sodium balance cannot be obtained unless sodium intake is limited. A frequent cause of diuretic-resistant ascites is inadequate sodium restriction. This 'apparently intractable' ascites should be suspected in any patient whose ascites does not decrease despite a good natriuretic response to diuretics. In this respect, it is important to note that many drugs, particularly antibiotics, may contain relatively high amounts of sodium. Once ascites has disappeared, many cirrhotics continue to require a strict sodium diet and diuretics to avoid its reaccumulation. Other cases can, however, be maintained without ascites by moderate sodium restriction and low doses of diuretics. Finally, some patients may even recover their ability to excrete sodium normally and may be free of ascites despite normal sodium intake and no diuretics. Therefore, the long-term management of cirrhotics with ascites varies markedly from patient to patient, and every effort should be made to adjust sodium intake and diuretic dosage to individual requirements during the course of the disease.

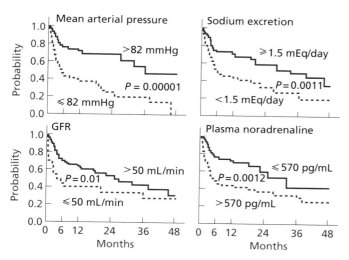

Fig. 15 Probability of survival in 136 cirrhotic patients with ascites classified according to mean arterial pressure, plasma noradrenaline concentration, urinary sodium excretion and glomerular filtration rate (GFR) (reproduced with permission from ref. 121).

Diuretics

Loop diuretics, in particular furosemide, and distal diuretics, especially spironolactone, are the drugs most commonly used in the treatment of ascites in cirrhosis. Loop diuretics inhibit chloride and sodium reabsorption in the ascending limb of the loop of Henle but have no effect on the distal nephron (distal and collecting tubules) [202,203]. They must reach the tubular lumen to be effective. Loop diuretics are all organic acids and are highly bound to plasma proteins. As a consequence, they can only reach the lumen by being actively secreted from the blood into the urine via the organic acid transport pathway of the straight segment of the proximal tubule. Once in the luminal compartment, furosemide is carried with the luminal fluid to the ascending limb of the loop of Henle, where it inhibits a specific cotransport system, the Na^+-$2Cl^-$-K^+ carrier, located in the luminal membrane of the ascending limb cells. It is therefore not surprising that the urinary concentration of furosemide correlates best with the response. Loop diuretics also increase the renal synthesis of prostaglandins, and anti-inflammatory drugs reduce their natriuretic effect. Renal prostaglandins therefore appear to be involved in the natriuretic response to loop diuretics.

Loop diuretics such as furosemide are the most powerful diuretics presently available. High dosage of furosemide can increase sodium excretion up to 30% of the filtered sodium in normal individuals. This high natriuretic potency can be attributed to two features. Firstly, between 20% and 50% of the filtered sodium is reabsorbed in the loop of Henle. Secondly, in the absence of hyperaldosteronism, the distal and collecting tubules, which are downstream from the loop of Henle, have a limited capacity for sodium reabsorption and are not capable of mitigating the diuresis induced by loop diuretics. Furosemide is rapidly absorbed from the gut. The onset of action is extremely rapid (within 30 min of oral administration), with peak effects occurring within 1–2 h; most of the natriuretic activity has finished in 3–4 h.

Spironolactone and other distal diuretics (triamterene, amiloride) have a much lower intrinsic natriuretic potency than loop diuretics. They are able to increase sodium excretion up to 2% of the filtered sodium in normal individuals [202,203]. Spironolactone undergoes extensive metabolism in man, leading to numerous biologically active compounds, including canrenone, 6-β-hydroxy-7-α-thiomethylspironolactone and 7-α-thiomethylspironolactone [204]. The antimineralocorticoid effect of spironolactone has traditionally been attributed to its major metabolite, canrenone. However, recent studies show that canrenone only accounts for 10–25% of the antimineralocorticoid activity. Other metabolites are therefore important in its diuretic effect. Spironolactone metabolites are tightly bound to plasma proteins, from which they are released slowly to the kidney and other target organs; the half-life of these metabolites in healthy individuals has been estimated to range between 10 and 35 h after single or multiple doses of spironolactone. This

explains the 24- to 48-h delay between drug withdrawal and the end of the natriuretic effect. Spironolactone metabolism is impaired in cirrhosis, so that the terminal half-lives of spironolactone and its metabolites are increased when compared with values in normal individuals [205].

Spironolactone metabolites act by competitively inhibiting the tubular effect of aldosterone on the distal nephron. The activity of spironolactone and spironolactone metabolites does not depend on their filtration or tubular secretion but, rather, on their plasma concentrations because they act on the capillary side of the collecting tubular cells. They enter the basolateral membrane and interact with the mineralocorticoid cytosolic receptor. However, contrary to what occurs with aldosterone, the interaction of spironolactone with the receptor does not result in the exposure of the high-affinity DNA region. Therefore, spironolactone acts as a specific antagonist of aldosterone. This explains why spironolactone is effective in increasing sodium excretion in patients with primary or secondary hyperaldosteronism and in healthy people on a low-sodium diet; however, it has no effect on patients with adrenalectomy or healthy people on a high-sodium diet. The half-life of the aldosterone-induced proteins (sodium channels and Na^+-K^+ATPase molecules) is relatively prolonged, explaining the lag of 2 days between the beginning of spironolactone treatment and the onset of the natriuretic effect. The effective dosage of spironolactone depends on the plasma aldosterone concentration. Patients with moderately increased plasma aldosterone require low doses (100–150 mg/day), but as much as 500 mg/day may be required to antagonize the tubular effect of aldosterone in cases with marked hyperaldosteronism [128].

The administration of standard doses of loop diuretics to non-azotaemic cirrhotics with ascites gives rise to a good natriuretic response in only 50% of patients [128]. The mechanism of this poor diuretic effect is not well established. The bioavailability of furosemide is reportedly normal in cirrhotics with ascites, indicating that the renal resistance to the drug cannot be explained by impaired intestinal absorption [206]. On the other hand, although there is one study that shows impaired tubular secretion of furosemide in cirrhotics with ascites [207], others suggest that the pharmacokinetics and renal handling of furosemide in such patients are similar to those in healthy individuals [206–209]. Therefore, the most likely mechanism for diuretic resistance to furosemide in cirrhosis with ascites is pharmacodynamic in nature; that is, furosemide does not increase sodium excretion either because the delivery of fluid to the loop of Henle is reduced, owing to enhanced proximal sodium reabsorption [210], or because most sodium not reabsorbed in the loop of Henle by the action of furosemide is subsequently taken up in the convoluted distal and collecting tubules, owing to secondary hyperaldosteronism. The latter proposal is supported by several studies showing that non-azotaemic cirrhotics with ascites who have renal resistance to furosemide or other loop diuretics are those with higher plasma aldosterone concentrations [128,206].

Treatment of non-azotaemic cirrhotics with ascites with spironolactone is followed by a good natriuretic response in most patients. Therefore, contrary to what would be expected on the basis of their intrinsic natriuretic potencies, spironolactone is more effective than furosemide in non-azotaemic cirrhotics with ascites, which was also the conclusion in the only published, randomized study comparing furosemide with spironolactone in these patients [128]. The most rational treatment of cirrhotics with ascites is spironolactone alone or with furosemide. The simultaneous administration of furosemide and spironolactone increases the natriuretic effect of both drugs and reduces the incidence of the hypo- or hyperkalaemia frequently observed when these agents are given alone.

Two different approaches are commonly employed in the treatment of cirrhotic ascites with diuretics. The 'step care' medical treatment consists of progressive implementation of the therapeutic measures currently available [210,211]. Treatment is begun with a low-sodium diet; if there is no response, spironolactone is given at increasing dosage (starting with 100 mg/day) until a satisfactory diuresis is achieved. Where there is no response to the highest dosage of spironolactone (400 mg/day), furosemide is added, also at increasing dosage (40–160 mg/day). A more rapid therapeutic schedule, which may be particularly indicated in patients with tense ascites and avid sodium retention, is the 'combined treatment' [212]. It begins with the simultaneous administration of 40 mg/day furosemide and 100 mg/day spironolactone. If there is no response after 4–5 days, the dosage is increased stepwise up to 160 mg/day furosemide and 400 mg/day spironolactone. A recent randomized controlled trial has shown that the step care and the combined treatment approaches are similar regarding response rate, rapidity of ascites mobilization and incidence of complications [213]. There is general agreement that patients not responding to this programme should be considered to have diuretic-resistant ascites (see below). The best way to assess the effectiveness of diuretic therapy is by monitoring body weight. The goal of diuretic treatment should be to achieve a weight loss of 300–500 g/day. Once ascites has been mobilized, diuretic treatment should be adjusted to maintain the patient free of ascites. In most non-azotaemic cirrhotics, this can be achieved with low doses of spironolactone (100–200 mg/day). The most important predictor of diuretic response in cirrhotic patients with ascites is the degree of impairment of circulatory and renal function. Patients with a low glomerular filtration rate and/or high plasma concentrations of renin, aldosterone and noradrenaline require a high diuretic dosage or do not respond to medical treatment [128,210,211].

Complications of diuretic treatment in cirrhosis

The use of diuretics in cirrhotics with ascites may be associated with complications related to the effect of these drugs on the kidney and on extrarenal organs. Approximately 20% of these patients develop azotaemia due to depletion of intravascular volume [122]. This diuretic-induced renal failure is usually moderate and always reversible after diuretic withdrawal; it is the consequence of an imbalance between the intravascular fluid loss caused by the diuretics and the net passage of fluid (ascites reabsorption minus ascites formation) from the peritoneal cavity into the general circulation [214]. If diuretic therapy produces a loss of fluid above the net passage of ascitic fluid into the intravascular compartment, a contraction in circulating blood volume and a concomitant decrease in glomerular filtration rate will occur. Interstitial fluid accumulated as oedema is more easily reabsorbed than ascites. This explains why diuretic-induced renal failure occurs less frequently in patients with both ascites and oedema than in those with only ascites.

Hyponatraemia, occasionally severe, is another common complication of diuretic therapy in cirrhotics with ascites [215,216]. Although the pathogenesis of this abnormality is multifactorial, impairment of the renal ability to excrete free water induced by these drugs is probably the most important mechanism. Free-water formation in the kidney occurs in the ascending limb of the loop of Henle, where sodium chloride is reabsorbed without a concomitant reabsorption of water, leading to hypotonic urine. The second factor in water excretion is ADH, which regulates water reabsorption in the collecting tubules. Loop diuretics inhibit chloride and sodium reabsorption in the ascending limb of the loop of Henle. Moreover, the intravascular volume depletion produced by diuretic therapy increases fluid reabsorption in the proximal tubule, thus diminishing the delivery of sodium chloride to the loop of Henle. Both mechanisms impair the formation of free water in the diluting segment of the nephron. Finally, diuretic-induced hypovolaemia stimulates the release of ADH.

The distal nephron (distal and collecting tubules) plays a critical part in regulating acid balance. Sodium reabsorption in this segment generates a lumen-negative voltage that promotes passive potassium and H^+ excretion into the lumen. In cirrhotics with ascites, the inhibition of sodium reabsorption by spironolactone or other distally acting diuretics, such as triamterene or amiloride, may therefore produce metabolic acidosis. The administration of loop diuretics alone markedly increases potassium excretion and may produce serious hypokalaemia. This is not due to a specific direct effect on potassium transport but to increased potassium secretion by the distal nephron promoted by a high delivery of fluid to this segment. Spironolactone, triamterene and amiloride increase the serum potassium and may produce severe hyperkalaemia when used at high doses. This complication is particularly common in cirrhotics with hepatorenal syndrome. Spironolactone-induced hyperkalaemia is generally considered to be due to a reduction in urinary potassium excretion secondary to the inhibition of distal sodium reabsorption. However, studies on cirrhotics with ascites have shown that spironolactone produces a small but significant increase in potassium excretion [128]. An alternative mechanism may be a shift of potassium from the intracellular to extracellular space due to inhibition of the aldosterone effect on internal potassium balance or to metabolic acidosis.

The most important complication of diuretic therapy is hepatic encephalopathy, which has been estimated to occur in approximately 25% of cirrhotic patients admitted to hospital with tense ascites and treated with diuretics [215,216]. Diuretic-induced hepatic encephalopathy was traditionally considered to be secondary to hyperammonaemia because of increased renal ammonia production following diuretic-induced hypokalaemia and alkalosis. However, more recent studies show that some diuretics may also impair the urea cycle, leading to reduced hepatic transformation of ammonia to urea. Finally, other more recent studies suggest that, in cirrhotic patients with ascites, there is an increase in arteriolar vascular resistance in the cerebral circulation that may result in a reduction in cerebral blood flow. As cerebral arterial vascular resistance correlates closely with renal vascular resistance in these patients, the hypothetical mechanism of cerebral vasoconstriction in decompensated cirrhosis is arterial vascular underfilling. Because diuretic therapy may impair effective arterial blood volume, a further deterioration in cerebral blood flow could contribute to diuretic-induced hepatic encephalopathy.

Perhaps the most frequent side-effects of spironolactone in cirrhotics with ascites are those related to its antiandrogenic activity. Chronic spironolactone treatment is often associated with decreased libido, impotence and gynaecomastia in men, and menstrual irregularities in women. The origin of these abnormalities is probably related to alterations in sex steroid metabolism. At high dosage, spironolactone reduces testosterone biosynthesis and increases the peripheral conversion of testosterone to estradiol. In addition, *in vitro* experiments have shown that spironolactone inhibits the binding of testosterone to the cytosolic and nuclear receptors in the target organs.

Finally, cirrhotic patients treated with diuretics over a long period frequently complain of intense muscle cramps. They usually appear during the night, affect both the lower extremities and the hands and disappear rapidly either following assumption of the upright position or spontaneously. The mechanism of diuretic-induced muscle cramps is unknown. They are clearly related to the reduced effective arterial blood volume present in these patients as muscle cramps occur particularly in cases with low mean arterial pressure and high plasma renin activity, and their frequency can be drastically reduced if diuretic treatment is combined with plasma volume expansion with albumin [217]. The oral administration of quinine reduces the frequency of muscle cramps [218].

Refractory ascites

Although the term refractory ascites (or intractable ascites, resistant ascites or problematic ascites) was introduced in the 1950s to define ascites not responding to sodium restriction and diuretics, there has been major confusion concerning the use of this term during the last few decades. For this reason, the International Ascites Club recently organized a consensus conference to elaborate a new definition and the diagnostic criteria

for refractory ascites in cirrhosis [123]. This conference extended the concepts proposed by a consensus conference held in Rome during the 13th International Congress of Gastroenterology in 1988.

According to this organization, 'refractory ascites' is that which cannot be mobilized or the early recurrence of which (i.e. after therapeutic paracentesis) cannot be satisfactorily prevented by medical therapy. Two different subtypes of refractory ascites can be identified: (i) 'diuretic-resistant ascites' is that which cannot be mobilized or the early recurrence of which cannot be prevented because of a lack of response to dietary sodium restriction and intensive diuretic treatment; (ii) 'diuretic-intractable ascites' is that which cannot be mobilized or the early recurrence of which cannot be prevented because of the development of diuretic-induced complications that preclude the use of an effective diuretic dosage.

The following criteria were considered to be important for the diagnosis of refractory ascites:

1 Ascites: the term ascites in these definitions refers to grade 2 or 3 clinically detectable ascites (grade 1, mild; grade 2, moderate; grade 3, massive or tense).

2 Mobilization of ascites: decrease of ascites to at least grade 1.

3 Treatment period to define refractory ascites: patients must have been on intensive diuretic treatment for at least 1 week.

4 Lack of response: mean loss of body weight of less than 200 g/day during the past 4 days on intensive diuretic therapy and urinary sodium excretion of less than 50 mEq/day.

5 Dietary sodium restriction: a 60- to 90-mEq sodium diet.

6 Intensive diuretic treatment: spironolactone, 400 mg/day, plus furosemide, 160 mg/day (bumetanide, 4 mg/day, or equivalent doses of other loop diuretics).

7 Early ascites recurrence: reappearance of grade 2–3 ascites within 4 weeks of initial mobilization; reaccumulation of ascites within 2–3 days of paracentesis must not be considered as early recurrence because it represents a shift of interstitial fluid into the intraperitoneal space.

8 Diuretic-induced complications: diuretic-induced hepatic encephalopathy is the development of hepatic encephalopathy in the absence of other precipitating factors. Diuretic-induced renal failure is an increase in serum creatinine by greater than 100% to a value above 2 mg/dL in patients with ascites responding to diuretic treatment. Diuretic-induced hyponatraemia is a decrease in serum sodium by greater than 10 mEq/L to a concentration lower than 125 mEq/L. Diuretic-induced hypo- or hyperkalaemia are, respectively, a decrease in serum potassium to less than 3 mEq/L or an increase to more than 6 mEq/L despite appropriate measures to normalize potassium concentrations.

'Recidivant ascites' is defined as ascites that recurs frequently (on three or more occasions within a 12-month period) despite dietary sodium restriction and adequate diuretic dosage, and is not to be considered as a true refractory ascites [123].

Most cirrhotics with diuretic-resistant ascites have type 2 hepatorenal syndrome [123], or lesser, although significant, degrees of impairment in renal perfusion and glomerular filtration rate (increased serum creatinine to between 1.2 and 1.5 mg/dL) [106,200,203] It is important to stress that the inverse relation between glomerular filtration rate and serum creatinine concentration is hyperbolic. This means that a small increase in creatinine over normal represents a marked impairment of renal haemodynamics and glomerular filtration rate. The mechanism whereby ascites is resistant to diuretic therapy in cirrhotics with renal failure is probably related to alterations in both the pharmacokinetics and the pharmacodynamics. The access of loop diuretics to the organic acid secretory site, and of spironolactone to the aldosterone receptors, which is mainly determined by the amount of blood flowing to the proximal tubule and distal nephron, respectively, may be impaired in cirrhotics with functional renal failure due to the low renal perfusion. Moreover, the delivery of sodium chloride to the loop of Henle and distal nephron, the sites where furosemide and spironolactone inhibit sodium reabsorption, may be markedly reduced in cirrhotics with functional renal failure secondary to a low glomerular filtration rate and enhanced sodium reabsorption in the proximal tubule [210]. Therefore, both impaired access of diuretics to the effective sites on the tubular cells and a reduced substrate for the diuretic action are presumably the most important mechanisms of refractory ascites in cirrhosis. Additional factors that may contribute to the renal resistance to diuretics in cirrhotics with functional renal failure are hypoalbuminaemia, which reduces the delivery of diuretics to the kidney, and the increased activity of endogenous systems with sodium-retaining effects (renin–angiotensin–aldosterone and sympathetic nervous systems), which may inhibit the natriuretic effect of diuretics.

NSAIDs depress the diuretic response to furosemide and spironolactone in cirrhotics with ascites by a mechanism unrelated to the impairment in renal haemodynamics [219,220]. Evidence for the possible use of these agents should therefore be carefully sought in any cirrhotic patient not responding to sodium restriction and an adequate diuretic regimen.

Therapeutic paracentesis

Treatment with a low-sodium diet and diuretics is very effective in mobilizing ascites in cirrhosis. However, it has several limitations. First, approximately 10–20% of patients do not respond to diuretics (diuretic-resistant ascites). Second, diuretic treatment is frequently associated with complications, particularly when high doses of diuretics have to be used. Finally, the mobilization of ascites with diuretics is a slow process. This problem, which is not relevant in the care of patients with moderate ascites, who are usually treated as outpatients, is very important in patients with massive ascites, most of whom need prolonged hospitalization for diuretic therapy.

The demonstration in 1987 that large-volume paracentesis associated with plasma volume expansion is a rapid, effective and safe treatment for ascites in cirrhosis has considerably simplified the treatment of patients admitted to hospital with tense ascites [221]. Therapeutic paracentesis is considered to be the therapy of choice for tense ascites in cirrhosis [201]. It considerably shortens hospital stay and therefore the cost of treatment, and the incidence of complications during hospitalization is significantly lower among patients treated with paracentesis than among patients treated with diuretics [221–223]. In patients with moderate ascites, diuretics should be preferred to paracentesis.

Although paracentesis is a very simple procedure, several precautions should be taken to avoid complications. Therapeutic paracentesis can be performed either as repeated large-volume paracentesis (4–6 L/day until complete disappearance of ascites) or as total paracentesis (complete removal of ascites in only one paracentesis session). Total paracentesis is the best method because it is faster and associated with a lower incidence of local complications [221–223]. Ascites leakage through the skin or within the abdominal wall is relatively frequent after partial paracentesis, because a significant volume of ascites remains in the peritoneal cavity after the procedure. On the other hand, although complications related to the insertion of the needle are exceptional, the incidence increases with the number of taps. Paracentesis should be performed under strictly sterile conditions with specially designed needles. There are commercial kits for paracentesis using different types of needles with bluntedged cannulas and side holes. With the patient under local anaesthesia, the needle is inserted into the left lower abdominal quadrant. The inner part is removed, and the cannula is connected to a large-capacity suction pump. The physician should remain at the bedside throughout the procedure. With this technique, the duration of treatment ranges from 30 to 60 min, depending on the amount of ascitic fluid removed. Total paracentesis procedures are finished when the flow from the cannula becomes intermittent despite gentle mobilization of the cannula within the peritoneal cavity and turning the patient to the left side. Peripheral oedema is rapidly reabsorbed after the mobilization of ascites in most patients and usually disappears within the first 2 days after treatment. Most of the fluid goes to the abdominal cavity as ascites. It is therefore not infrequent for patients with marked peripheral oedema to need a second procedure after complete mobilization of ascites at the initial paracentesis. Patients treated by means of repeated large-volume paracentesis should recline for 2 h on the side opposite the paracentesis site to prevent the leakage of ascitic fluid.

When paracentesis is performed without plasma volume expansion, there are no apparent major changes in circulatory function. Arterial pressure decreases slightly, but this also occurs when paracentesis is performed with plasma volume expansion. The pulse rate does not increase, and the patient does not experience any symptoms other than those related to the disappearance of ascites [222,224]. In addition, if serum creatinine and serum electrolytes are measured within the first days after paracentesis, no changes are observed in most patients. For this reason, some investigators have suggested that therapeutic paracentesis does not adversely affect circulatory function and that, consequently, plasma volume expansion is not necessary in the care of patients with cirrhosis and ascites treated with this procedure.

However, when circulatory function is assessed by sensitive direct and indirect measures, marked changes are detected [222]. Immediately after paracentesis, circulatory function improves with a marked increase in cardiac output and stroke volume, a reduction in cardiopulmonary pressure and a suppression of the renin–angiotensin and sympathetic nervous systems [222]. These effects, which persist for approximately 12 h and have been attributed to mechanical factors (reduction in intrathoracic pressure and increase in venous return), are followed by opposing haemodynamic changes, including a reduction in cardiac output to baseline value and marked activation of the renin–angiotensin and sympathetic nervous systems over levels before paracentesis [224]. Renal function also improves during the first hours after paracentesis and may worsen 24–48 h after the procedure. The impairment in circulatory function induced by paracentesis is not related, as proposed initially, to a decrease in circulating blood volume secondary to a rapid reaccumulation of ascites, but rather to an accentuation of the arterial vasodilation already present in these patients (Fig. 16). The mechanism by which paracentesis induces reduction in peripheral vascular resistance and the site where this vasodilation occurs are unknown. An important observation is that the circulatory dysfunction induced by paracentesis is not spontaneously reversible [223]. Once plasma renin activity and plasma norepinephrine concentration increase, they remain elevated throughout the course of the disease. The cause of this phenomenon is unknown.

Plasma renin activity is a very sensitive marker of circulatory function and is the parameter used to detect impairment in circulatory function after paracentesis in most studies.

Paracentesis-induced circulatory dysfunction has been defined as a 50% increase in plasma renin activity over baseline on the sixth day after treatment up to a value greater than 4 ng/mL/h (upper normal limit) [223,224]. According to this criterion, the incidence of spontaneous circulatory dysfunction among patients with cirrhosis admitted to hospital because of tense ascites and not receiving any treatment during 1 week of hospitalization was 16% (unpublished observations). The incidence of paracentesis-induced circulatory dysfunction has been estimated to be 75% among patients not undergoing plasma volume expansion, 33–38% in patients receiving polygeline (saline solution, 8 g/L ascitic fluid removed), dextran-70 (dextrose solution, 8 g/L ascitic fluid removed) or saline and 11–18% among patients receiving albumin (salt-poor solution, 8 g/L ascitic fluid removed) [223]. Similar findings have been reported in a recent trial comparing albumin with saline in patients with ascites treated by total paracentesis [225]. The incidence of paracentesis-induced circulatory dysfunction was 33.3% in patients receiving saline and 11.4% in those receiving albumin.

The amount of ascitic fluid removed is a predictor of paracentesis-induced circulatory dysfunction (Fig. 17). When the amount of ascitic fluid removed is less than 5 L, the incidence of circulatory dysfunction is similar among patients treated with albumin and those treated with synthetic plasma expanders (16% vs. 18%). However, when the amount is between 5 and 9 L, the incidence of circulatory dysfunction is higher among patients receiving synthetic plasma expanders (19% vs. 30%). Differences are particularly marked when the volume of paracentesis is greater than 9 L. In this case, the incidence of paracentesis-induced circulatory dysfunction is 21% among patients receiving albumin and 60% in those receiving synthetic plasma expanders [223].

These data indicate the following: (i) paracentesis-induced circulatory dysfunction is very frequent when the plasma volume is not expanded; (ii) plasma volume expansion with synthetic colloids is effective in reducing the incidence of circulatory dysfunction after paracentesis; (iii) plasma volume expansion with albumin almost totally prevents paracentesis-induced

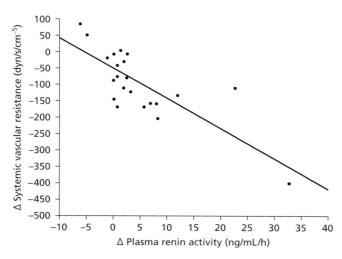

Fig. 16 Direct negative correlation between the increase in plasma renin activity (Δ PRA) and the decrease in systemic vascular resistance (Δ SVR) following therapeutic paracentesis in cirrhosis (reproduced with permission from ref. 224).

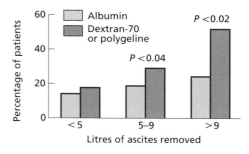

Fig. 17 Incidence of paracentesis-induced circulatory dysfunction in cirrhotic patients with ascites divided according to the volume of ascitic fluid removed and the type of plasma expander used (reproduced with permission from ref. 223).

circulatory dysfunction; (iv) among patients with an ascitic fluid volume of less than 5 L, the incidence of paracentesis-induced circulatory dysfunction is low and independent of the type of plasma expander used; (v) when the amount of ascitic fluid volume removed is more than 5 L, the incidence of circulatory dysfunction increases with the volume of paracentesis in patients receiving synthetic plasma expanders but not in patients receiving albumin.

Despite being asymptomatic, paracentesis-induced circulatory dysfunction adversely affects the clinical course of the disease. The incidence of hyponatraemia (3.8% vs. 17%) and renal impairment (0 vs. 11%) within a few days after paracentesis is significantly lower among patients receiving albumin infusions than among those not receiving plasma expanders. The time to first readmission to hospital is significantly shorter for patients with circulatory dysfunction after paracentesis than among those who do not have this complication. Finally, the probability of survival is also lower among patients with circulatory dysfunction after paracentesis [223].

The mechanism by which deterioration in circulatory function impairs the clinical course and the prognosis for patients with cirrhosis and ascites is probably multifactorial. Circulatory dysfunction is associated with an increase in circulating levels of vasoconstrictors that impair renal haemodynamics and the renal response to diuretics. Angiotensin-II and norepinephrine are important mechanisms of HRS, which is associated with poor survival. These substances also induce vasoconstriction of intrahepatic vascular resistance, which may reduce liver perfusion, impair hepatic function and increase portal pressure. These changes may further deteriorate circulatory function and create vicious circles that accelerate the course of the disease. One study has shown that the hepatic venous pressure gradient (an estimation of the intrahepatic vascular resistance) increases after paracentesis in patients in whom circulatory dysfunction develops but not in patients who do not have this complication [224].

Therefore, there is substantial evidence indicating that paracentesis-induced circulatory dysfunction is a relevant complication that should be prevented. The best way to do this is to expand the plasma volume with albumin when the volume of ascitic fluid removed is more than 5 L. When the volume is less than 5 L, less expensive synthetic plasma expanders can be used. The amount of albumin given in most centres is 8 g/L ascitic fluid removed, which represents the approximate amount of albumin removed with the paracentesis. We infused 50% of the dose immediately after paracentesis and 50% 6 h later. The patient may then leave hospital with diuretics to prevent the reaccumulation of ascites. Patients with normal BUN and serum creatinine require a standard diuretic dosage (200 mg/day spironolactone or 40 mg/day furosemide plus 100 mg/day spironolactone). However, higher diuretic dosages are required in patients with abnormal BUN or serum creatinine concentration, or in patients with ascites that is refractory before treatment.

Peritoneovenous shunting

In 1974, LeVeen and associates [226] introduced the peritoneovenous shunt for the treatment of cirrhotics with diuretic-resistant ascites. This device consists of a perforated intra-abdominal tube connected through a one-way, pressure-sensitive valve to a silicone tube that traverses the subcutaneous tissue up to the neck, where it enters one of the jugular veins (usually the internal jugular). The tip of the intravenous tube is located in the superior vena cava near the right atrium or in the right atrium itself. The aim of the shunt is to produce sustained expansion of the circulating blood volume by the continuous passage of ascites from the peritoneal cavity to the general circulation. Whenever a pressure gradient of 3 cmH$_2$O or more exists between the abdominal cavity and the superior vena cava, the valve remains open, and ascitic fluid flows into the central venous system. If this gradient diminishes, the valve closes, thus preventing blood from reflushing into the venous limb of the shunt. The insertion of a LeVeen shunt is technically simple and can be performed under local anaesthesia. It is advisable to assess the correct placement of the venous tip by chest radiography in the operating room. Although the LeVeen is the most widely used peritoneovenous shunt, other types are available. The Denver shunt has a valvular system with a pumping mechanism. The valvular system opens at low pressure gradients (1 cmH$_2$O) or when the pump chamber, placed in an intercostal space, is pressed externally. The Denver shunt was designed to reduce the high incidence of shunt obstruction observed with the LeVeen. It was thought that the compression of the pump chamber would avoid the formation of thrombi at, and within, the tip of the intravenous segment and the deposition of fibrin within the valve. However, a randomized study comparing LeVeen and Denver shunts in cirrhotics with medically intractable ascites showed a higher probability of shunt obstruction in patients treated with the Denver shunt, probably as a consequence of the reflux of blood into the valve during the release phase of the pumping cycle [227]. To avoid this problem, a double-valve Denver shunt was later developed. Whether this new valvular system is effective in preventing shunt obstruction is unknown.

Numerous studies show that the peritoneovenous shunt is capable of correcting most abnormalities thought to be involved in the pathogenesis of ascites. It produces a striking increase in circulating blood volume and cardiac output. As arterial pressure does not rise, there is a concomitant reduction in peripheral vascular resistance. These haemodynamic changes are associated with an increase in the plasma concentration of atrial natriuretic factor and a suppression of the plasma concentrations of renin, aldosterone, noradrenaline and ADH. Urine volume and free-water clearance increase in most patients, as is seen with the serum sodium in cases with dilutional hyponatraemia. However, there is significant natriuresis in less than half the patients. In cirrhotics with moderate functional renal failure, the peritoneovenous shunt may improve renal blood flow and glomerular filtration rate [228]. Finally, a marked reduction in portal pressure and intrahepatic vascular resistance, as estimated by the wedged-to-free hepatic venous pressure gradient, has been reported after the insertion of a peritoneovenous shunt. The mechanism of this last effect is unknown. Follow-up studies show that these haemodynamic and hormonal changes persist in most cases and that a significant proportion of patients remain with minimal or no ascites despite a moderate sodium restriction and low diuretic dosage. Additionally, the nutritional status, as estimated by the arm muscle circumference, improved significantly in patients successfully treated with a peritoneovenous shunt.

Unfortunately, the procedure is associated with a high rate of complications, which may occur early in the postoperative period or at any time during follow-up. Acute bacterial infection, generally caused by *Staphylococcus* spp., is the most serious early complication [229]. The prosthesis is usually colonized and, in most cases, the infection cannot be eradicated unless the shunt is removed. The prophylactic administration of anti-staphylococcal antibiotics 24 h before and for 48 h after surgery reduces the incidence of early postoperative infections [229]. Postoperative fever, probably related to the passage of endotoxin contained in the ascitic fluid into the general circulation, is almost inevitable and disappears spontaneously within the second postoperative week [230]. Practically every cirrhotic patient treated with a peritoneovenous shunt develops biochemical signs of intravascular coagulation within the early postoperative period, including a decrease in plasma fibrinogen and platelets, prolongation of prothrombin, thrombin and partial thromboplastin times and a rise in the plasma concentrations of fibrin and fibrinogen degradation products [231,232]. The mechanism of this complication is unknown, but it may possibly be secondary to the massive passage of tissue thromboplastin and clotting factors, plasminogen activators, endotoxin, fibrin split products and collagen, which are present in the ascitic fluid, into the general circulation. The incidence of symptomatic intravascular coagulation was relatively high (25%) within the years immediately following the introduction of the shunt when the shunt was inserted without prior removal of ascitic fluid. At that time, the mortality rate attributed to intravascular coagulation was 5%. However, at present, with the widespread acceptance of the need to evacuate ascitic fluid preoperatively, or during surgery before inserting the shunt, the rate of symptomatic intravascular coagulation after peritoneovenous shunting has decreased dramatically. Some investigators have suggested the removal of all ascitic fluid and its replacement with normal saline before insertion of the prosthesis. Antiplatelet therapy with aspirin (300 mg/day) and dipyridamole (400 mg/day) in the immediate pre- and postoperative periods prevented intravascular coagulation after peritoneovenous shunting [233]. Other postoperative complications, such as bleeding from oesophagogastric varices and congestive heart failure, which are related to the acute expansion in the circulating blood volume, can also be prevented by reducing the volume of ascitic fluid before inserting the shunt. Postoperative mortality

(within the first month after surgery) ranges between 0% and 26% [229].

Obstruction of the shunt is the most common complication during follow-up [229]. It occurs in more than 30% of patients and is usually due to deposition of fibrin within the valve or around the intravenous catheter, thrombotic obstruction of the venous limb of the prosthesis or thrombosis of the superior vena cava or right atrium initiated at the venous end of the shunt or in damaged endothelium [229]. Although the thrombosis of the superior vena cava is usually incomplete, total occlusion may occur, resulting in the development of a superior vena cava syndrome. Vascular thrombosis may result in pulmonary embolism. Obstruction of the shunt is frequently, but not necessarily, followed by reaccumulation of ascites. In these cases, Doppler ultrasonography or ^{99m}Tc scintigraphy after intraperitoneal injection of radioisotope will show the absence of flow through the shunt. When obstruction is confirmed by these techniques, a shuntogram after the injection of contrast medium into the proximal subcutaneous limb of the shunt should be performed in order to identify its exact site. Patients with obstruction at the venous limb of the shunt require venography or digital angiography to rule out vascular thrombosis. It has been suggested that the insertion of a titanium tip 3 cm long into the venous end of the LeVeen shunt prevents thrombotic obstruction of its venous limb and the development of thrombosis in the superior vena cava. Titanium is highly thromboresistant, a characteristic that has been exploited extensively in intravascular devices such as prosthetic heart valves. The titanium tip was also designed to provide gradual, streamlined flow convergence of ascites and blood. Finally, the weight and design of the tip may limit endothelial damage and mural thrombus formation in the superior vena cava. Unfortunately, in a study on a large series of patients, Ginès *et al.* [234] were not able to confirm that the titanium tip reduces the incidence of obstruction in peritoneovenous shunts.

Bacterial infections, particularly bacteraemia and spontaneous peritonitis, are also common complications during follow-up [229]. Bacteraemia can be successfully treated with antibiotics. Early recurrence indicates colonization of the shunt or bacterial endocarditis. Removal of the shunt has been recommended in patients with peritonitis, although some have successfully treated patients with bacterial peritonitis without this [229]. To prevent bacterial infections in patients with peritoneovenous shunts, prophylactic antibiotics should be administered whenever an invasive manoeuvre is to be performed.

Finally, another long-term complication of peritoneovenous shunting is small bowel obstruction, which occurs in approximately 10% of patients [235]. The small bowel is compressed and kinked inside multiple 'cocoons' and cysts consequent to marked peritoneal fibrosis. The shunt is usually not ensnared in the fibrosed areas but remains free. The cause is unknown.

Because of the high incidence of shunt-related complications, peritoneovenous shunting should be restricted to patients with refractory ascites. However, these patients often have endstage liver disease and an extremely poor prognosis, which cannot be modified by successful treatment of ascites. In fact, an overall analysis of the four prospective, randomized trials comparing peritoneovenous shunting with conventional medical treatment in patients with refractory ascites does not disclose any benefit in terms of survival [236–239]. The role of peritoneovenous shunting in the management of patients with hepatorenal syndrome is also unclear: a beneficial effect has been observed in single cases, but the results obtained in the only two randomized trials published so far seem to indicate that peritoneovenous shunting, although preventing the progression of functional renal failure, does not improve the chances of survival. The reintroduction of therapeutic paracentesis has led to a decline in the use of peritoneovenous shunting. In the two randomized, controlled trials comparing paracentesis with the LeVeen shunt in patients with refractory ascites, shunting was superior in the long-term control of ascites, as estimated by the time to first readmission for ascites, the number of readmissions for ascites and diuretic requirements [234,240]. However, these advantages had little impact on the natural course of the disease as patients treated in both groups did not differ significantly in their time to first readmission for any reason, total time in hospital during follow-up and probability of survival. Furthermore, frequent reoperations were required in the surgical group because of shunt obstruction. At present, many groups consider paracentesis to be the treatment of choice in patients with refractory ascites, peritoneous shunting being indicated only in those intolerant of frequent paracentesis. The morbidity and survival of cirrhotics treated with the LeVeen shunt correlate with the degree of impairment of liver and renal function, patients with severe hepatic and renal failure having a higher incidence of complications and lower survival. Therefore, the best results with this procedure should be expected in those very few patients with diuretic-resistant ascites and preserved hepatic function.

Surgical portocaval anastomosis and transjugular intrahepatic portacaval shunt (TIPS)

Ascites and its complications (hepatorenal syndrome and spontaneous bacterial peritonitis) are rare in cirrhotic patients submitted to end-to-side portocaval anastomosis for the treatment of variceal bleeding, and the surgical relief of portal hypertension, either by end-to-side or side-to-side portocaval anastomosis, is an apparently effective treatment for ascites. It is therefore not surprising that portocaval anastomosis has been proposed as a treatment for refractory ascites. In 1970, Orloff [241], reviewing the literature on the surgical treatment of ascites, was able to collect data for 71 cirrhotics with ascites treated with end-to-side portocaval anastomoses and for 131 patients treated with side-to-side portocaval shunts. In most of these cases, ascites was refractory to diuretic treatment. Twenty-three patients treated with end-to-side shunts (32%) and 24 treated with side-to-side anastomoses (18%) died in the postoperative period. Of the

surviving patients, 39 (81%) in the end-to-side group and 100 (90%) in the side-to-side group remained free of ascites during a follow-up period ranging from months to more than 10 years, despite a normal sodium diet and no diuretics. Subsequently, it was shown that, in cirrhotics treated with end-to-side portocaval shunts, the development of ascites during follow-up usually occurs in those cases who maintain a relatively high sinusoidal pressure and hepatic arterial blood flow. More recently, Franco [242] reported his experience with 41 patients submitted to side-to-side or end-to-side portocaval anastomoses for the treatment of refractory ascites. Almost all these patients had previously been treated with a LeVeen shunt that had to be removed because of complications such as thrombosis of the superior vena cava, infections or gastrointestinal haemorrhage. The operative mortality (within 2 months of surgery) was exceptionally low (two patients, 4.8%), probably related to the relatively well-preserved hepatic function presented by most cases. Every patient reaccumulated ascites in the immediate postoperative period, and 12 developed renal failure. However, ascites and renal impairment disappeared a few days after the operation in all but two cases. Only one of the survivors developed ascites during follow-up. The probability of survival 1 and 3 years after surgery was 73% and 39% respectively. However, the incidence of severe chronic hepatic encephalopathy (36%) was very high. Other studies have shown that side-to-side portocaval shunting may be followed by a return to normal renal function in patients with hepatorenal syndrome. The disappearance of ascites and renal failure in patients treated with portocaval shunts is associated with a return to normal plasma concentrations of renin and aldosterone. These data suggest that, although portocaval anastomosis is an effective treatment for refractory ascites in patients with cirrhosis and preserved hepatic function, it is associated with a high postoperative mortality and a high incidence of incapacitating chronic hepatic encephalopathy. As no controlled trials have compared the portocaval shunt with other treatments such as the LeVeen shunt or therapeutic paracentesis, its role in the management of refractory ascites is unconfirmed. Nevertheless, it is important to point out that only a few patients with refractory ascites are suitable candidates for surgical portocaval shunts as they usually present with a severe hepatic insufficiency that precludes any major surgical procedure.

The development of the transjugular intrahepatic portacaval shunt (TIPS) for the treatment of gastrointestinal haemorrhage in cirrhosis has reintroduced the idea of treating ascites and its complications (hepatorenal syndrome and refractory ascites) by reducing portal pressure. TIPS works as a side-to-side portocaval shunt and, from a theoretical point of view, it should correct the two principal mechanisms in the pathogenesis of ascites [243]. By doing so, it should suppress the endogenous vasoconstrictor system, improve renal perfusion and GFR and increase the response to diuretics. On the other hand, by decompressing both the splanchnic and the hepatic microcirculation, TIPS should decrease the formation of lymph both in the liver and in the other splanchnic organs.

A review of the records of the first 358 reported patients with refractory ascites treated with TIPS clearly indicated that this therapeutic procedure is extremely effective in improving circulatory and renal function and in the management of ascites in these patients [243]. TIPS induces a marked increase in cardiac output, a decrease in systemic vascular resistance and an elevation in right atrial pressure, pulmonary artery pressure and pulmonary wedge pressure [243]. These changes, which are similar to those following peritoneovenous shunting, are probably caused by an increase in venous return resulting from the presence of portocaval fistulas. The decrease in systemic vascular resistance, which is also a constant feature in patients treated by peritoneovenous shunting, is probably a physiological response to accommodate the increase in cardiac output.

Because it increases the hyperdynamic circulation, it has been suggested that TIPS impairs the systemic haemodynamics in cirrhosis. However, the results of studies of the effects of TIPS on the endogenous vasoactive systems do not support this concept. The results indicate that effective arterial blood volume is markedly improved following TIPS in patients with cirrhosis and ascites. As indicated earlier, the maintenance of arterial pressure in patients with advanced cirrhosis and ascites is critically dependent on a marked overactivity of the renin–angiotensin system, sympathetic nervous system and antidiuretic hormone. If TIPS enhances arterial vasodilation, a further increase in the degree of stimulation of these vasoconstrictor systems should occur. In contrast, TIPS insertion is associated with marked suppression of the plasma levels of renin, aldosterone, norepinephrine and antidiuretic hormone [243]. Suppression of the renin–angiotensin–aldosterone system occurs within the first week following TIPS insertion and persists during the follow-up period. Suppression of norepinephrine and antidiuretic hormone appears to require a longer period of time.

Deterioration in circulatory function should also be associated with a further impairment in renal function after TIPS; however, TIPS insertion induces a rapid increase in urinary sodium excretion, which is already observed within the first 1–2 weeks and persists during the follow-up period [243]. A significant increase in serum sodium concentration and GFR is also observed, indicating an improvement in renal perfusion and free-water clearance. However, these changes require 1–3 months to occur.

TIPS induces a marked decrease in the portocaval gradient. In the aforementioned review of the care of 358 patients with refractory ascites treated by TIPS, the mean decrease was from 20.9 to 10 mmHg [243]. Portal venous pressure also decreased markedly, from 29.4 to 21.8 mmHg. However, TIPS only partially decompresses the portal venous system; portal venous pressure in most healthy subjects is less than 5 mmHg. Although suppression of the renin–aldosterone system is evident, the plasma levels of renin and aldosterone do not decrease to normal levels. Improvement in splanchnic and systemic haemodynamics is associated with disappearance of ascites or partial response (no need for paracentesis) in most patients. Only 10% of cases do not respond to TIPS. Ascites characteristically resolves very slowly (within 1–3 months). Continuous diuretic treatment is required in more than 95% of cases, either for the management of ascites or to reduce the peripheral oedema that frequently occurs in patients treated with TIPS. The persistence of portal hypertension and hyperaldosteronism may be the explanation for this phenomenon.

Hepatic encephalopathy is the most important complication among patients with cirrhosis with refractory ascites managed with TIPS [243]. More than 40% of patients have this complication. In most cases, hepatic encephalopathy responds to standard therapy. However, it occasionally requires a decrease in stent size. Although hepatic encephalopathy before TIPS is a predictor of encephalopathy after TIPS, new or worsening hepatic encephalopathy develops in approximately 30% of cases. Shunt dysfunction is also a major problem, occurring in approximately 40% of cases within the first year. This is an important limitation of TIPS requiring frequent retreatments. However, the recent introduction of covered stents, which is associated with a very low rate of shunt dysfunctions, has solved this problem. The 1-year probability of survival among patients with cirrhosis with refractory ascites treated with TIPS is extremely poor. Early mortality (within 30 days after TIPS) is approximately 12% and late mortality 40%. Predictors of survival are the Child–Pugh score, age and the presence of HRS prior to TIPS [243].

Five randomized, controlled trials have been reported comparing TIPS and therapeutic paracentesis [244–248] (Table 2). Two included patients with recidivant and refractory ascites, and three included only patients with refractory ascites. The five trials clearly show that TIPS is better than paracentesis in the long-term control of ascites. Three trials showed significantly higher incidence of hepatic encephalopathy in patients treated

Table 2 TIPS vs. paracentesis for refractory ascites: a summary.

	Control	HRS	Hepatic encephalopathy	Cost	Survival
Lebrec et al. [244]	Better with TIPS	–	No difference	–	Worse with TIPS
Rossle et al. [245]	Better with TIPS	–	No difference	–	Better with TIPS?
Gines et al. [247]	Better with TIPS	Less frequent with TIPS	Worse with TIPS	Greater with TIPS	No difference
Sanyal et al. [248]	Better with TIPS	–	Worse with TIPS	–	No difference
Salerno et al. [246]	Better with TIPS	–	Worse with TIPS	–	Better with TIPS

with TIPS. An improvement in survival in the TIPS group was only observed in the trials including patients with recidivant ascites. The total time in hospital during follow-up was similar in both groups owing to the high incidence of shunt obstruction requiring new hospitalization for the treatment of complications related to portal hypertension and/or restenting. In one of these trials, the quality of life was assessed, and changes were similar in the two therapeutic groups [249]. These results indicate that TIPS changes the course of cirrhosis from ascites to hepatic encephalopathy without improving the overall results of paracentesis in relation to length of hospitalization and survival.

Treatment of hyponatraemia in cirrhosis with ascites

Aquaretic drugs

Dilutional hyponatraemia is the most common abnormality of serum electrolytes in patients with cirrhosis and ascites. Traditionally, hyponatraemia has been considered a minor problem in cirrhosis, as it is usually asymptomatic, even in patients with a markedly reduced serum sodium. On the other hand, the presence of hyponatraemia does not contraindicate diuretic treatment in patients with cirrhosis and ascites. In fact, most cirrhotics with ascites and hyponatraemia respond satisfactorily to diuretics without a further reduction in serum sodium. For these reasons, the use of aggressive procedures for the treatment of hyponatraemia in cirrhosis, such as the insertion of a LeVeen shunt or a TIPS, has never been justified. However, recent studies suggest that hyponatraemia may be more relevant than previously thought. It is associated with very poor prognosis. The probability of hepatic encephalopathy is significantly higher in patients with hyponatraemia than in those with comparable deterioration of hepatic function but with normal serum sodium concentration. Finally, the incidence of severe neurological events after liver transplantation in patients with dilutional hyponatraemia, probably related to the rapid correction of extracellular osmolality during the operation, is relatively high [250]. Therefore, treatment of hyponatraemia could be beneficial in patients with decompensated cirrhosis.

Studies using isotopic techniques have shown that total body sodium is markedly increased in cirrhotic patients with ascites and hyponatraemia, indicating that the reduced serum sodium is the result of a dilution of body fluids secondary to the impairment of free-water excretion. Consequently, the treatment of hyponatraemia should be directed towards reducing total body water. The administration of sodium may produce a transient increase in serum sodium, but at the expense of increasing the rate of ascites formation. Classically, the treatment of dilutional hyponatraemia consisted of water restriction. However, this therapy is difficult to carry out and is rarely effective. Demeclocycline, a tetracycline that inhibits the tubular effect of ADH, has been shown to correct water retention and hyponatraemia in cirrhotics with ascites, but its usefulness in

these patients is limited by the high incidence of renal failure that it produces [251,252].

During the last two decades, a great effort has been made to develop specific antagonists of the tubular effect of ADH that could act as aquaretic agents and be used for the treatment of dilutional hyponatraemia in cirrhosis with ascites, and in congestive heart failure. The initial approach was to develop analogues of the ADH molecule with affinity for the V_2 receptors but lacking hydro-osmotic activity. Unfortunately, although several peptides with aquaretic activity in experimental animals were developed, they disclosed ADH agonistic activity when given to humans. It is interesting that the administration of one of these analogues to rats with carbon tetrachloride-induced cirrhosis, ascites and dilutional hyponatraemia was associated with a normalization of renal water metabolism with polyuria and an increase in free-water excretion [149].

The investigation of non-peptidic substances with aquaretic effects has had very promising results, and several types of aquaretic agents have been developed that are effective in experimental animals as well as in man. The first renal ADH antagonist identified was a benzazepine derivative named OPC-31260, which is 100 times more selective for V_2 receptors than for V_1 receptors. It is active after oral and intravenous administration, has no agonistic effect and increases the urine volume in normal rats and in rats treated with ADH without increasing urinary solute excretion, but not in Brattleboro rats with congenital diabetes insipidus. In normal man, OPC-31260 also induces a marked increase in urine volume (it may be as high as that obtained with furosemide) with a decrease in urine osmolality towards very low values (it may reach concentrations below 100 mosmol/kg), resulting in a remarkable increase in free water, with minor effects on electrolyte excretion [253]. The peak effects on urine volume and osmolality are observed between 1 and 2 h and last for 4 h. With the highest single dose used in normal individuals, the aquaretic effect is so marked that it is associated with a significant increase in serum osmolality and sodium. The plasma ADH also increases in these individuals. Other non-peptide V_2 antagonists have been developed (VPA-985, SR-121463, OPC-41061 and YMD-087) and are currently being investigated.

There are several studies assessing the effects of V_2 antagonists in human and experimental cirrhosis. Tsuboi et al. [254] examined the role of OPC-31260 in rats with carbon tetrachloride-induced cirrhosis and control rats. Water excretion after a water load increased fourfold and minimal urinary osmolality decreased by 30% after the administration of this agent. Additionally, serum sodium and urinary sodium excretion increased significantly when compared with the control group. However, in another study by Bosch-Marcé et al. [255], the maximum effect of this drug was limited to the first 2 days of treatment, probably due to the development of tachyphylaxis. Jimenez et al. [256] reported the long-term (10 days) efficacy of SR-121463 in cirrhotic rats with ascites and impaired water excretion after a water load. The administration of the drug led

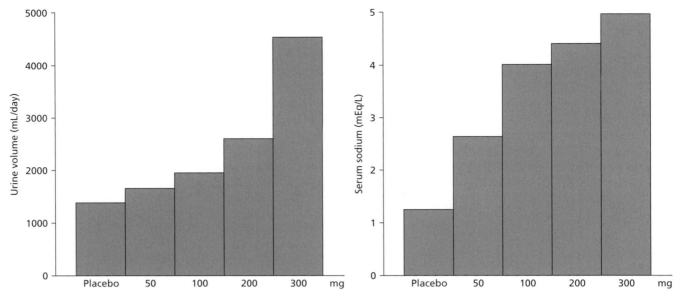

Fig. 18 Urine volume and serum sodium after a single dose of VPA-985 in cirrhotic patients with ascites (reproduced with permission from ref. 264.

to a significant increase in urine volume and reduced urine osmolality when compared with a vehicle. This also resulted in a great renal ability to excrete a water load and normalization of serum sodium and osmolality. In contrast to OPC-31260, the effects of SR-121463 were sustained, and there was no tachyphylaxis. Finally, Fernández-Varo *et al.* [257] in 2003 reported the effects of conivaptan, a combined receptor V_{1a}/V_2 antagonist, on renal water handling and systemic haemodynamics in cirrhotic rats with ascites. In this study, the chronic administration (10 days) of this agent to rats with severe water retention and ascites produced an acute increase in urine volume and a reduction in urine osmolality; the aquaretic effect lasted for only 5 days. Interestingly, there was a remarkable improvement in sodium excretion, which was probably due to the effect of conivaptan on the renin–angiotensin system. Most importantly, these effects occurred without affecting creatinine clearance or arterial pressure, an effect that could be expected because of the vasoactive action that the V_{1a} receptor exerts over blood vessels mediating vasoconstriction.

Inoue *et al.* [258] reported in 1998 the first study in humans examining the therapeutic effect of OPC-31260 in patients with cirrhosis and ascites. The administration of 30 mg/day p.o. to eight patients with cirrhosis and ascites without hyponatraemia was associated with an increase in the urine volume and solute-free water clearance at 2 and 4 h, respectively, and a decrease in urine osmolality at 2 h after administration. However, as patients did not have hyponatraemia at baseline, the effect on serum sodium was not assessed. Furthermore, neither the normal serum sodium rise nor urinary sodium excretion changed. In 2002, Guyader *et al.* [259] reported the pharmacodynamics, safety and pharmacokinetics of ascending single doses of VPA-985 (25–300 mg) in 27 patients with cirrhosis and ascites in

a phase II randomized, double-blind, placebo-controlled trial. VPA-985 produced a marked dose-related rise in urinary output and a dose-related decrease in urine osmolality when given at 300 mg/day. Urine volume increased significantly with the 300-mg dose. Solute-free water clearance increased to levels greater than 3 mL/min for doses of 100 mg and higher. In addition, significant increases in urine sodium excretion and serum osmolality, sodium and vasopressin levels were observed (Fig. 18). In this pharmacodynamic study, the authors only demonstrated the potential of VPA-985 as a therapeutic agent for water retention in cirrhosis. But, as the main endpoint was to evaluate the safety and efficacy of this compound, they did not examine its role in managing patients with dilutional hyponatraemia; in fact, all patients had serum sodium levels above 130 mEq/L. Both agents (VPA-985 and OPC-31260) in the above studies were clinically well tolerated and did not produce any significant side-effects or changes in systemic haemodynamics.

Two multicentre, randomized, placebo-controlled trials published in 2003 evaluated the use of VPA-985 in cirrhotic patients with dilutional hyponatraemia. In the first trial, Wong *et al.* [260] investigated the effects of VPA-985 on serum sodium during a 7-day period in 44 hospitalized patients with dilutional hyponatraemia [33 with cirrhosis, five with congestive heart failure and five with syndrome of inappropriate secretion of ADH (SIADH)]. Patients with cirrhosis and congestive heart failure were kept on diuretics, and an escalating dose of VPA-985 ranging from 50 to 500 mg/day was given. VPA-985 had a significant aquaretic response compared with placebo in those on diuretic therapy as well as in patients not on diuretics (SIADH group). There was a dose-related increase in the net fluid volume (urine output-minus fluid intake) and solute-free water clearance, leading to significant increases in serum sodium and serum

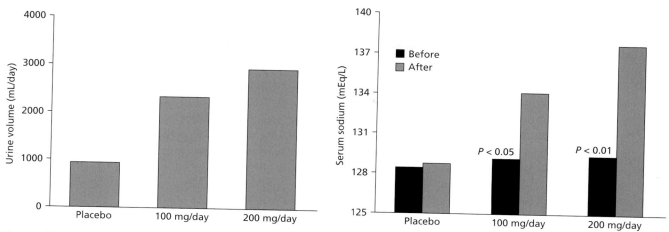

Fig. 19 Effects of V_2 receptor antagonist (VPA-985) on urine volume and serum sodium in patients with cirrhosis and hyponatraemia (reproduced with permission from ref. 261).

osmolality. Unfortunately, there was a high dropout rate (12 patients or 27%; six due to dehydration and the other half for other reasons). The highest doses of the drug (250–500 mg/day) were poorly tolerated and associated with dehydration, as assessed by systemic postural hypotension, increased thirst and marked sodium elevation. As a result, half the patients on the 500-mg/day dose had the medication withheld on several occasions. VPA-985 was most effective and safe when given at a dose of 125–250 mg/day. The second study by Gerbes *et al.* [261] included 60 patients with cirrhosis and dilutional hyponatraemia on fluid restriction who were randomly assigned to receive 100 or 200 mg/day VPA-985 or placebo for 7 days. There was a significant dose-dependent increase in serum sodium concentration and urine volume as well as a significant reduction in urine osmolality and body weight in both groups receiving VPA-985, whereas no changes in these parameters were found in the placebo arm (Fig. 19). Complete response, defined by reaching serum sodium $\geq$ 136 mEq/L, was observed in 27% on the 100-mg dose and 50% on the 200-mg dose. Thirst sensation was the main side-effect in the 200-mg group, but not in the other groups. Two problems with this study were the small number of patients in each group (around 20) and the effects of VPA-985 were only evaluated until serum sodium normalized with no information on long-term response.

A recent report in abstract form of the use of satavaptan (SR-12146) in patients with cirrhosis, ascites and dilutional hyponatraemia at baseline showed that it had significant effects on improvement in serum sodium [152]. In this randomized, double-blind, placebo-controlled study, the drug was administered in fixed doses of 5, 12.5 and 25 mg in 110 cirrhotic patients with ascites who received spironolactone treatment (100 mg/day). The percentage of patients with improvement in serum sodium at day 5 (defined as serum sodium $\geq$ 135 mEq/L or an increase of $\geq$ 5 mEq/L) was higher for the 5-mg, 12.5-mg and 25-mg doses (61%, 54% and 64% respectively) compared with the placebo (19%; $P < 0.05$ for all).

The findings of these studies suggest that the effects of V_2 receptor antagonists seem to be independent of sodium reabsorption proximal to the renal collecting tubules. This compound was administered in combination with diuretics without any significant problems. In fact, other aquaretics such as tolvaptan and conivaptan have a significant natriuretic effect in disease states such as congestive heart failure. This makes V_2 receptor antagonists attractive drugs for potential combination therapy with diuretics in diseases where there is concomitant sodium retention and dilutional hyponatraemia, such as cirrhosis and ascites. Nonetheless, caution would be needed when administering V_2 receptor antagonists and diuretics such as furosemide because this combination could produce a marked diuretic effect and lead to volume depletion and subsequent dehydration and/or renal failure. Currently, studies with V_2 receptor antagonists in patients with cirrhosis and dilutional hyponatraemia demonstrate that these drugs have a dose-related response when correcting hyponatraemia over 1 week. Results of further phase III trials will certainly help to define the usefulness of V_2 receptor antagonists in clinical practice.

A second type of aquaretic agent that may be relevant for the treatment of dilutional hyponatraemia in oedematous conditions are the κ-opioid agonists (ketazocine, ethylketazocine, bremazocine, R-84760, E-2078, U-62,066E, CI-997 and RU-51599), which increase urine volume in man and experimental animals with a reduction in urine osmolality and without changes in electrolyte excretion. The mechanism of this aquaretic effect is complex but clearly mediated through κ-receptors as it is blocked by κ-opioid receptor antagonists. The κ-opioid agonists act on the central nervous system, inhibiting the release of ADH from the neurohypophysis. The observation that these substances increase urine flow in the isolated perfused kidney suggests the existence of a local, intrarenal mechanism of action. The efficacy of κ-opioid agonists in the treatment of water retention in human and experimental cirrhosis was recently evaluated by Gadano *et al.* [262] and by Bosch-Marcé *et al.*

[153]. The acute subcutaneous administration of RU-51599 (niravoline) to rats with cirrhosis, ascites and impaired free-water excretion was associated with normalization of renal water metabolism. The plasma concentrations of ADH decreased after the administration of the drug, but did not reach normal values The acute intravenous administration of RU-51599 to patients with cirrhosis and ascites induced a marked (five to seven times) increase in urine volume during the first 2–3 h, associated with a reduction in urine osmolality to values lower than plasma osmolality and a significant increase in serum sodium. Personality disorders and mild confusion were detected in only two of the eight patients treated and disappeared within 8 h.

There is only one study assessing the effect of these two different types of aquaretic drugs given long term (10 days). This is a comparative study of OPC-31260 and RU-51599 in rats with experimental cirrhosis [255]. The aquaretic effect of OPC-31260 was transitory, occurring only during the first 2 days. In contrast, RU-51599 showed an aquaretic effect throughout the whole study period. There are no such studies recorded in humans.

Drug-induced renal impairment in cirrhosis

Antibiotics

Patients with cirrhosis and ascites are predisposed to aminoglycoside nephrotoxicity, the reported incidence of which (32%) [263] is much higher than that found by other investigators in the general population (3–11%). In that study, aminoglycoside nephrotoxicity was associated with a marked deterioration in renal function. A study of the risk factors in aminoglycoside toxicity found that the presence of liver disease was an independent predictor of nephrotoxicity [264]. The mechanism of this high incidence of aminoglycoside nephrotoxicity in cirrhosis is not known. In the study by Cabrera *et al.* [263], gentamicin or tobramycin was administered in association with cephalothin, which is known to increase the nephrotoxicity of aminoglycosides. However, this was not the case in the study by Moore *et al.* [264]. Another possibility is that patients with decompensated cirrhosis are prone to develop this complication; they frequently have impaired renal blood flow and glomerular filtration rates, and renal accumulation of aminoglycosides is greater with renal impairment. Cabrera *et al.* [263] found that aminoglycoside nephrotoxicity was five times more frequent in patients with renal failure before treatment than in those with a normal baseline serum creatinine.

The diagnosis of aminoglycoside nephrotoxicity in cirrhotics with serious infection is difficult because these patients may also develop functional renal failure. The determination of urinary sodium concentration, fractional sodium excretion and urine:plasma osmolality and creatinine ratios is not useful in differentiating functional renal failure from acute tubular necrosis in cirrhotic patients with ascites. The differential diagnosis, however, is of clinical importance. Aminoglycosides must be interrupted when nephrotoxicity develops, whereas careful dosage adjustment is necessary in the presence of functional renal failure. Furthermore, dialysis is indicated in cirrhotics with acute tubular necrosis, but not in patients with functional renal failure. The measurement of other urinary markers of tubular damage, such as β_2-microglobulin and tubular enzymes, may help in differentiating these disorders. The urinary concentration of β_2-microglobulin in alcoholic cirrhotics with superimposed acute alcoholic hepatitis, severe renal failure and deep jaundice (serum bilirubin greater than 20 mg/dL) may be similar to that commonly observed in acute tubular necrosis, suggesting a spontaneous development of tubular damage in these patients. Therefore, urinary β_2-microglobulin and tubular enzymes may not be useful in the diagnosis of aminoglycoside nephrotoxicity in patients with terminal hepatic and renal failure.

Non-steroidal anti-inflammatory drugs

The initial studies showing that patients with cirrhosis and ascites develop renal failure after cyclo-oxygenase inhibition with NSAIDs were made almost 20 years ago [159,265,266]. The first group of investigators observed that the oral administration of indomethacin (50 mg every 6 h for a total of four doses) produced a significant reduction in renal plasma flow and glomerular filtration rate in a large series of cirrhotics with ascites, but not in patients without ascites. Zipser *et al.* [266] gave indomethacin (200 mg for 1 day) or ibuprofen (2 mg for 1 day) to 12 cirrhotics with ascites and eight normal individuals; both drugs induced a marked decrease in urinary PGE_2 excretion and creatinine clearance in all patients, but they caused no change in creatinine clearance in normal individuals. Finally, Arroyo *et al.* [265] gave an intravenous bolus of 450 mg of lysine acetylsalicylate (equivalent to 250 mg of acetylsalicylic acid) to five normal individuals, nine cirrhotics who had never had ascites and 19 cirrhotics with ascites; it did not alter renal function in normal individuals and cirrhotics without ascites, but it reduced the glomerular filtration rate in 11 of the 19 patients with ascites. Urinary PGE_2 was decreased in all individuals after lysine acetylsalicylate. In these three studies, the degree of impairment in renal function after NSAIDs correlated with baseline values of urine sodium excretion and plasma renin and noradrenaline; patients with lower sodium excretion and higher plasma renin activity and noradrenaline concentrations developed greater reductions in renal plasma flow and glomerular filtration rate. These studies therefore indicate that cirrhotics with increased activity of the renin–angiotensin and sympathetic nervous systems and marked sodium retention are especially predisposed to develop renal failure after cyclo-oxygenase inhibition. The results of these three studies have been confirmed by subsequent investigations in cirrhotic patients with ascites receiving indomethacin, naproxen, lysine acetylsalicylate and sulindac, and in dogs with cirrhosis secondary to common bile duct ligation. The decline in glomerular filtration rate and renal blood flow in the dogs with ligated common bile ducts and cirrhosis was preventable by prior administration of saralasin or captopril [267], confirming that overactivity of endogenous vasoconstrictor systems as well as inhibition of renal prostaglandin synthesis is a major determinant of renal failure after NSAID administration.

Some investigators have suggested that non-acetylated salicylates are less effective in inhibiting renal synthesis of prostaglandins than other NSAIDs, and do not impair renal function or the renal response to furosemide in patients and experimental animals with cirrhosis and ascites. On the other hand, there are several experimental studies and one investigation in human cirrhosis showing that pharmacological doses of COX-2 inhibitors (celecoxib), given during a short period of time (3 days), do not affect renal function or the renal response to diuretics in patients with ascites and increased plasma renin activity [268–270]. Further studies are needed to confirm these findings.

The most important practical conclusion of these investigations is that NSAIDs should be used with great caution, if ever, in patients with cirrhosis and ascites because they may induce renal failure, water retention and dilutional hyponatraemia, and diuretic-resistant ascites. Although these adverse renal effects have always been rapidly reversible after drug withdrawal, it is important to note that, in these studies, NSAIDs were given as an investigative tool, at low dosage and for 1 or 2 days only. Whether renal impairment would also be quickly reversible after long-term treatment with therapeutic dosages of these drugs is unknown.

Drugs used in the treatment of portal hypertension

Reports on the renal effects of somatostatin, a drug used for the treatment of acute variceal bleeding, are conflicting. One study [271] shows a significant decrease in glomerular filtration rate, sodium excretion and free-water clearance during the acute infusion of somatostatin. Conversely, another study [272] shows an increase in urine volume and creatinine clearance in patients with ascites who received octreotide, a synthetic analogue of somatostatin.

Propranolol, the drug used most extensively in the prophylaxis of variceal bleeding and rebleeding, has significant effects on systemic and splanchnic haemodynamics and on the endogenous vasoactive systems. It reduces cardiac output, increases systemic vascular resistance and circulating noradrenaline and reduces plasma renin activity and aldosterone in patients with cirrhosis with and without ascites. However, it has no significant effects on renal function in these patients [273].

Nitrates have been introduced for the prophylaxis of variceal rebleeding, given alone or in combination with propranolol. They reduce portal pressure mainly by decreasing hepatic vascular resistance, whereas propranolol is effective by reducing portal venous inflow and acting on the portocollateral circulation. This difference might explain the additive effects of the combined treatment in reducing portal pressure. The acute oral administration of isosorbide-5-mononitrate in cirrhotic patients with and without ascites is associated with a significant reduction in cardiac output, systemic vascular resistance and arterial pressure, an increase in plasma renin activity and aldosterone concentration, a suppression of the plasma concentrations of atrial natriuretic peptide and a reduction in renal blood flow, glomerular filtration rate, free-water clearance and sodium excretion [274]. These effects were particularly marked in the patients with ascites. These findings were later confirmed [275] in a study that observed the same changes after the acute administration of isosorbide-5-mononitrate in 21 patients with and without ascites. Interestingly, Salerno et al. [275] also found a significant reduction in arterial pressure, urine volume and sodium excretion during long-term administration of the drug in the patients with ascites. Therefore, acute and chronic administration of nitrates alone impairs renal function in decompensated cirrhosis. The effect of the combined treatment (propranolol plus nitrates) on renal function is more controversial. Vorobioff et al. [276] compared patients chronically treated with propranolol alone with those treated with propranolol plus isosorbide dinitrate. Eight of the 14 patients with ascites or a history of ascites receiving propranolol plus isosorbide dinitrate showed impairment in renal function and sodium metabolism, as reflected by the clinical development or worsening of ascites and a need for higher diuretic dosage. This high frequency of renal impairment did not occur in patients receiving propranolol alone, In contrast, others did not observe any detrimental effects on renal function after 3 or 6 months of therapy with a combination of isosorbide-5-mononitrate and β-blockers [277,278].

Prazosin is another drug investigated as a possible treatment for portal hypertension. It is an α-adrenergic blocker that reduces portal pressure by decreasing intrahepatic vascular resistance. Long-term administration of prazosin to compensated cirrhotic patients with portal hypertension caused vasodilation of the systemic circulation, which led to ascites or oedema formation in a significant number of patients [279].

References

1 Berner C, Davis JS, Riggs S et al. (1964) Diagnostic probabilities in patients with conspicuous ascites. *Arch Intern Med* 113, 687–690.

2 Lawson JD, Weissbein AS (1959) The puddle sign – an aid in the diagnosis of minimal ascites. *N Engl J Med* 260, 652–654.

3 Cattau EL, Benjamin SB, Knuff TE et al. (1982) The accuracy of the physical examination in the diagnosis of suspected ascites. *JAMA* 247, 1164–1166.

4 Branney SW, Wolfe RE, Moore EE et al. (1995) Quantitative sensitivity of ultrasound in detecting free intraperitoneal fluid. *J Trauma Injury Infect Crit Care* 39, 375–380.

5 Huning R (1973) Ultrasonic diagnosis of Wilms tumor. *Fortschritte Gebiete Rontgenstrahl Nuklearmed* 158–159.

6 Wall SD, Hricak H, Bailey GD et al. (1986) MR imaging of pathological abdominal fluid collections. *J Comp Assist Tomogr* 10, 746–750.

7 Proto AV, Lane EJ (1976) Visualization of differences in soft-tissue densities – liver in ascites. *Radiology* 121, 19–23.

8 Steinkampf MP, Blackwell RE, Younger JB (1991) Visualization of free peritoneal fluid with transvaginal sonography – a preliminary study. *J Reprod Med* 36, 729–730.

9 Edell SL, Gefter WB (1979) Ultrasonic differentiation of types of ascitic fluid. *Am J Roentgenol* 133, 111–114.

10 Kedar RP, Shah PP, Shivde RS *et al.* (1994) Sonographic findings in gastroenterology and peritoneal tuberculosis. *Clin Radiol* 49, 24–29.

11 Runyon BA, Montano AA, Akriviadis EA *et al.* (1992) The serum ascites albumin gradient is superior to the exudate–transudate concept in the differential diagnosis of ascites. *Ann Intern Med* 117, 215–220.

12 Wilson JAP, Suguitan EA, Cassidy WA *et al.* (1979) Characteristics of ascitic fluid in the alcoholic cirrhotic. *Dig Dis Sci* 24, 645–648.

13 Sampline RE, Iber FL (1974) High protein ascites in patients with uncomplicated hepatic cirrhosis. *Am J Med Sci* 267, 275–279.

14 Hoefs JC (1983) Serum protein concentration and portal pressure determine the ascitic fluid protein concentration in patients with chronic liver disease. *J Lab Clin Med* 102, 260–273.

15 Henriksen JH (1983) Permselectivity of the liver blood lymph (ascitic fluid) barrier to macromolecules in decompensated cirrhosis – relation to calculated pore size. *Clin Physiol* 3, 163–171.

16 Henriksen JH, Lassen NA, Parving HH *et al.* (1980) Filtration as the main transport mechanism of protein exchange between plasma and the peritoneal-cavity in hepatic cirrhosis. *Scand J Clin Lab Invest* 40, 503–513.

17 Runyon BA, Vanepps DE (1986) Diuresis of cirrhotic ascites increases its opsonic activity and may help prevent spontaneous bacterial peritonitis. *Hepatology* 6, 396–399.

18 Fromkes JJ, Thomas FB, Mekhjian HS *et al.* (1977) Antimicrobial activity of human ascitic fluid. *Gastroenterology* 73, 668–672.

19 Simberkoff MS, Moldover NH, Weiss G (1978) Bactericidal and opsonic activity of cirrhotic ascites and nonascitic peritoneal fluid. *J Lab Clin Med* 91, 831–839.

20 Runyon BA, Morrissey RL, Hoefs JC *et al.* (1985) Opsonic activity of human ascitic fluid – a potentially important protective mechanism against spontaneous bacterial peritonitis. *Hepatology* 5, 634–637.

21 Such J, Guarner C, Enriquez J *et al.* (1988) Low C-3 in cirrhotic ascites predisposes to spontaneous bacterial peritonitis. *J Hepatol* 6, 80–84.

22 Barmeir S, Lerner E, Conn HO (1979) Analysis of ascitic fluid in cirrhosis. *Dig Dis Sci* 24, 136–144.

23 Conn HO, Fessel JM (1971) Spontaneous bacterial peritonitis in cirrhosis – variations on a theme. *Medicine* 50, 161–197.

24 Hoefs JC, Runyon BA (1985) Spontaneous bacterial peritonitis. *Disease-A-Month* 31, 1–48.

25 Gitlin N, Stauffer JL, Silvestri RC (1982) The Ph of ascitic fluid in the diagnosis of spontaneous bacterial peritonitis in alcoholic cirrhosis. *Hepatology* 2, 408–411.

26 Stassen WN, McCullough AJ, Bacon BR *et al.* (1986) Immediate diagnostic-criteria for bacterial-infection of ascitic fluid – evaluation of ascitic fluid polymorphonuclear leukocyte count, Ph, and lactate concentration, alone and in combination. *Gastroenterology* 90, 1247–1254.

27 Garciatsao G, Conn HO, Lerner E (1985) The diagnosis of bacterial peritonitis – comparison of Ph, lactate concentration and leukocyte count. *Hepatology* 5, 91–96.

28 Hoefs JC (1981) Increase in ascites white blood cell and protein concentrations during diuresis in patients with chronic liver disease. *Hepatology* 1, 249–254.

29 Desitter L, Rector WG (1984) The significance of bloody ascites in patients with cirrhosis. *Am J Gastroenterol* 79, 136–138.

30 Dumont AE, Mulholland JH (1960) Flow rate and composition of thoracic-duct lymph in patients with cirrhosis. *N Engl J Med* 263, 471–474.

31 Buo L, Karlsrud TS, Dyrhaug G *et al.* (1995) The fibrinolytic system in human ascites. *Scand J Gastroenterol* 30, 1101–1107.

32 Hoefs J, Barnes T, Halle P (1981) Intraperitoneal coagulation in chronic liver disease ascites. *Dig Dis Sci* 26, 518–522.

33 Wilkinson SP, Henderson J, Davidson AR *et al.* (1975) Ascites reinfusion using rhodiascit apparatus – clinical experience and coagulation abnormalities. *Postgrad Med J* 51, 583–587.

34 Leveen HH, Ahmed N, Hutto RB *et al.* (1987) Coagulopathy post peritoneovenous shunt. *Ann Surg* 205, 305–311.

35 Bac DJ, Pruimboom WM, Mulder PGH *et al.* (1995) High interleukin-6 production within the peritoneal-cavity in decompensated cirrhosis and malignancy-related ascites. *Liver* 15, 265–270.

36 Zeni F, Tardy B, Vindimian M *et al.* (1993) High levels of tumor necrosis factor alpha and interleukin-6 in the ascitic fluid of cirrhotic patients with spontaneous bacterial peritonitis. *Clin Infect Dis* 17, 218–223.

37 Navasa M, Follo A, Filella X *et al.* (1998) Tumor necrosis factor and interleukin-6 in spontaneous bacterial peritonitis in cirrhosis: relationship with the development of renal impairment and mortality. *Hepatology* 27, 1227–1232.

38 Cejudo P, Jimenez W, Ros J *et al.* (2001) Increased production of vascular endothelial growth factor in peritoneal macrophages of cirrhotic patients with spontaneous bacterial peritonitis. *Hepatology* 34, 184A.

39 Giannini E, Romagnoli P, Tenconi GL *et al.* (2004) High ascitic fluid leptin levels in patients with decompensated liver cirrhosis and sterile ascites: relationship with TNF-alpha levels. *Dig Dis Sci* 49, 275–280.

40 Runyon BA, Hoefs JC, Morgan TR (1988) Ascitic fluid analysis in malignancy-related ascites. *Hepatology* 8, 1104–1109.

41 Rector WG, Reynolds TB (1984) Superiority of the serum ascites albumin difference over the ascites total protein concentration in separation of transudative and exudative ascites. *Am J Med* 77, 83–85.

42 Garcia LW, Ducatman BS, Wang HH (1994) The value of multiple fluid specimens in the cytological diagnosis of malignancy. *Mod Pathol* 7, 665–668.

43 Prieto M, Gomezlechon MJ, Hoyos M *et al.* (1988) Diagnosis of malignant ascites – comparison of ascitic fibronectin, cholesterol, and serum-ascites albumin difference. *Dig Dis Sci* 33, 833–838.

44 Gerbes AL, Jungst D, Xie YN *et al.* (1991) Ascitic fluid analysis for the differentiation of malignancy-related and nonmalignant ascites – proposal of a diagnostic sequence. *Cancer* 68, 1808–1814.

45 Castaldo G, Oriani G, Cimino L *et al.* (1994) Total discrimination of peritoneal malignant ascites from cirrhosis-associated and hepatocarcinoma-associated ascites by assays of ascitic cholesterol and lactate dehydrogenase. *Clin Chem* 40, 478–483.

46 Hafter R, Klaubert W, Gollwitzer R *et al.* (1984) Crosslinked fibrin derivatives and fibronectin in ascitic fluid from patients with ovarian cancer compared to ascitic fluid in liver cirrhosis. *Thromb Res* 35, 53–64.

47 Gerbes AL, Hoermann R, Mann K et al. (1996) Human chorionic gonadotropin-beta in the differentiation of malignancy-related and nonmalignant ascites. Digestion 57, 113–117.

48 Lee CM, Changchien CS, Shyu WC et al. (1992) Serum ascites albumin concentration gradient and ascites fibronectin in the diagnosis of malignant ascites. Cancer 70, 2057–2060.

49 Chu CM, Lin SM, Peng SM et al. (1994) The role of laparoscopy in the evaluation of ascites of unknown origin. Gastrointest Endosc 40, 285–289.

50 Rector WG (1984) Spontaneous chylous ascites of cirrhosis. J Clin Gastroenterol 6, 369–372.

51 Press OW, Press NO, Kaufman SD (1982) Evaluation and management of chylous ascites. Ann Intern Med 96, 358–364.

52 Malagela JR, Iber FL, Linschee WG (1974) Origin of fat in chylous ascites of patients with liver cirrhosis. Gastroenterology 67, 878–886.

53 Maywood BT, Goldstein L, Busuttil RW (1978) Chylous ascites after a Warren shunt. Am J Surg 135, 700–702.

54 Lingenfelser T, Zak J, Marks IN et al. (1993) Abdominal tuberculosis – still a potentially lethal disease. Am J Gastroenterol 88, 744–750.

55 Lundstedt C, Nyman R, Brismar J et al. (1996) Imaging of tuberculosis. 2. Abdominal manifestations in 112 patients. Acta Radiol 37, 489–495.

56 Shakil AO, Korula J, Kanel GC et al. (1996) Diagnostic features of tuberculous peritonitis in the absence and presence of chronic liver disease: a case control study. Am J Med 100, 179–185.

57 Martinezvazquez JM, Ocana I, Ribera E et al. (1986) Adenosine deaminase activity in the diagnosis of tuberculous peritonitis. Gut 27, 1049–1053.

58 Hillebrand DJ, Runyon BA, Yasmineh WG et al. (1996) Ascitic fluid adenosine deaminase insensitivity in detecting tuberculous peritonitis in the United States. Hepatology 24, 1408–1412.

59 Wolfe JHN, Behn AR, Jackson BT (1979) Tuberculous peritonitis and role of diagnostic laparoscopy. Lancet 1, 852–853.

60 Delope CR, Joglar GSM, Romero FP (1982) Laparoscopic diagnosis of tuberculous ascites. Endoscopy 14, 178–179.

61 Bhargava DK, Shriniwa S, Chopra P et al. (1992) Peritoneal tuberculosis – laparoscopic patterns and its diagnostic accuracy. Am J Gastroenterol 87, 109–112.

62 Holmes EC, Eggleston JC (1972) Starch granulomatous peritonitis. Surgery 71, 85–90.

63 Schwake L, von Herbay A, Junghanss T et al. (2003) Peritoneal tuberculosis with negative polymerase chain reaction results: report of two cases. Scand J Gastroenterol 38, 221–224.

64 Gamboa F, Dominguez J, Padilla E et al. (1998) Rapid diagnosis of extrapulmonary tuberculosis by ligase chain reaction amplification. J Clin Microbiol 36, 1324–1329.

65 Runyon BA (1988) Cardiac ascites – a characterization. J Clin Gastroenterol 10, 410–412.

66 Ackerman NB, Sillin LF, Suresh K (1985) Consequences of intraperitoneal bile – bile ascites versus bile peritonitis. Am J Surg 149, 244–246.

67 Sankaran S, Walt AJ (1976) Pancreatic ascites – recognition and management. Arch Surg 111, 430–434.

68 Maringhini A, Ciambra M, Patti R et al. (1996) Ascites, pleural, and pericardial effusions in acute pancreatitis – a prospective study of incidence, natural history, and prognostic role. Dig Dis Sci 41, 848–852.

69 Boyer TD, Kahn AM, Reynolds TB (1978) Diagnostic value of ascitic fluid lactic-dehydrogenase, protein, and WBC levels. Arch Intern Med 138, 1103–1105.

70 Hammond TC, Takiyyuddin MA (1994) Nephrogenic ascites – a poorly understood syndrome. J Am Soc Nephrol 5, 1173–1177.

71 Balasch J, Arroyo V, Fabregues F et al. (1994) Neurohormonal and hemodynamic-changes in severe cases of the ovarian hyperstimulation syndrome. Ann Intern Med 121, 27–33.

72 Lieberman F, Hidemura R, Peters RL et al. (1966) Pathogenesis and treatment of hydrothorax complicating cirrhosis with ascites. Ann Intern Med 64, 341–351.

73 Lieberman F, Peters RL (1970) Cirrhotic hydrothorax. Further evidence that an acquired diaphragmatic defect is at fault. Arch Intern Med 125, 114.

74 Singer JA, Kaplan MM, Katz RL (1977) Cirrhotic pleural effusion in absence of ascites. Gastroenterology 73, 575–577.

75 Xiol X, Castellvi JM, Guardiola J et al. (1996) Spontaneous bacterial empyema in cirrhotic patients: a prospective study. Hepatology 23, 719–723.

76 Mouroux J, Perrin C, Venissac N et al. (1996) Management of pleural effusion of cirrhotic origin. Chest 109, 1093–1096.

77 Witte MH, Witte CL, Dumont AE (1981) Estimated net transcapillary water and protein flux in the liver and intestine of patients with portal-hypertension from hepatic cirrhosis. Gastroenterology 80, 265–272.

78 Gnepp D (1984) Lymphatics. In: Staub N, Taylor AE (eds) Edema. New York: Raven Press, pp. 263–298.

79 Laine GA, Hall JT, Laine SH et al. (1979) Trans-sinusoidal fluid-dynamics in canine liver during venous hypertension. Circ Res 45, 317–323.

80 Greenway CV, Lautt WW (1970) Effects of hepatic venous pressure on transsinusoidal fluid transfer in liver of anesthetized cat. Circ Res 26, 697–703.

81 Granger DN, Miller T, Allen R et al. (1979) Permselectivity of cat liver blood–lymph barrier to endogenous macromolecules. Gastroenterology 77, 103–109.

82 Granger DN, Barrowman J (1984) Gastroenterology and liver edema. In: Staub N, Taylor AE (eds) Edema. New York: Raven Press, pp. 615–656.

83 Iber FL (1974) Normal and pathologic physiology of the liver. In: Sodeman W, Sodeman WJ (eds) Pathologic Physiology. Philadelphia: Saunders, pp. 790–817.

84 Freeman S (1953) Recent progress in the physiology and biochemistry of the liver. Med Clin N Am 1, 109–124.

85 Mallet-Guy P, Devic G, Feroldi J et al. (1954) Experimental study of ascites: posthepatic venous stenosis and transposition of the liver into the thorax. Lyon Chir 49, 153–172.

86 Richardson PDI, Granger DN, Mailman D et al. (1980) Permeability characteristics of colonic capillaries. Am J Physiol 239, G300–G305.

87 Mortillaro NA, Taylor AE (1976) Interaction of capillary and tissue forces in cat small-intestine. Circ Res 39, 348–358.

88 Witte CL, Witte MH, Dumont AE (1980) Lymph imbalance in the genesis and perpetuation of the ascites syndrome in hepatic cirrhosis. Gastroenterology 78, 1059–1068.

89 Huet PM, Goresky CA, Villeneuve JP et al. (1982) Assessment of liver microcirculation in human cirrhosis. J Clin Invest 70, 1234–1244.

90 Vorobioff J, Bredfeldt JE, Groszmann RJ (1984) Increased blood flow through the portal system in cirrhotic rats. Gastroenterology 87, 1120–1126.

91 Buhac I, Jarmolych J (1978) Histology of intestinal peritoneum in patients with cirrhosis of liver and ascites. Am J Dig Dis 23, 417–422.

92 Witte MH, Witte CL, Dumont AE (1971) Progress in liver disease – physiological factors involved in causation of cirrhotic ascites. *Gastroenterology* 61, 742–750.

93 Witte CL, Witte MH, Cole WR *et al.* (1969) Dual origin of ascites in hepatic cirrhosis. *Surg Gynecol Obstet/Int Abstracts Surg* 129, 1027–1033.

94 Vorobioff J, Bredfeldt JE, Groszmann RJ (1983) Hyperdynamic circulation in portal-hypertensive rat model – a primary factor for maintenance of chronic portal-hypertension. *Am J Physiol* 244, G52–G57.

95 Bosch J, Enriquez R, Groszmann RJ *et al.* (1983) Chronic bile-duct ligation in the dog – hemodynamic characterization of a portal hypertensive model. *Hepatology* 3, 1002–1007.

96 Sugita S, Ohnishi K, Saito M *et al.* (1987) Splanchnic hemodynamics in portal hypertensive dogs with portal fibrosis. *Am J Physiol* 252, G748–G754.

97 Korthuis RJ, Kinden DA, Brimer GE *et al.* (1988) Intestinal capillary filtration in acute and chronic portal-hypertension. *Am J Physiol* 254, G339–G345.

98 Benoit JN, Granger DN (1986) Splanchnic hemodynamics in chronic portal hypertension. *Semin Liver Dis* 6, 287–298.

99 Kiel JW, Pitts V, Benoit JN *et al.* (1985) Reduced vascular sensitivity to norepinephrine in portal-hypertensive rats. *Am J Physiol* 248, G192–G195.

100 Benoit JN, Korthuis RJ, Granger DN *et al.* (1990) Splanchnic hemodynamics in acute and chronic portal hypertension. In: Bomzon A, Blendis L (eds) *Cardiovascular Complications of Liver Disease*. Boca Raton: CRC Press, pp. 179–206.

101 Groszmann RJ (1995) Mechanisms of portal hypertension. In: Arrovo V, Bosch J, Rodes J (eds) *Treatments in Hepatology*. Barcelona: Masson SA, pp. 3–8.

102 Huet PM, Pomierlayrargues G, Villeneuve JP *et al.* (1986) Intrahepatic circulation in liver disease. *Semin Liver Dis* 6, 277–286.

103 Bosch J, Mastai R, Kravetz D *et al.* (1985) Measurement of azygous venous blood flow in the evaluation of portal hypertension in patients with cirrhosis – clinical and hemodynamic correlations in 100 patients. *J Hepatol* 1, 125–139.

104 Bosch J, Arroyo V, Betriu A *et al.* (1980) Hepatic hemodynamics and the renin–angiotensin–aldosterone system in cirrhosis. *Gastroenterology* 78, 92–99.

105 Kotelanski B, Groszman R, Cohn JN (1972) Circulation times in splanchnic and hepatic beds in alcoholic liver disease. *Gastroenterology* 63, 102–111.

106 Arroyo V, Rodes J (1975) Rational approach to treatment of ascites. *Postgrad Med J* 51, 558–562.

107 Jimenez W, Martinezpardo A, Arroyo V *et al.* (1985) Temporal relationship between hyper-aldosteronism, sodium retention and ascites formation in rats with experimental cirrhosis. *Hepatology* 5, 245–250.

108 Caregaro L, Lauro S, Angeli P *et al.* (1985) Renal water and sodium handling in compensated liver-cirrhosis – mechanism of the impaired natriuresis after saline loading. *Eur J Clin Invest* 15, 360–364.

109 Naccarato R, Messa P, Dangelo A *et al.* (1981) Renal handling of sodium and water in early chronic liver-disease – evidence for a reduced natriuretic activity of the cirrhotic urinary extracts in rats. *Gastroenterology* 81, 205–210.

110 Wong F, Massie D, Hsu P *et al.* (1994) Renal response to a saline load in well-compensated alcoholic cirrhosis. *Hepatology* 20, 873–881.

111 Wilkinson SP, Smith IK, Moodie H *et al.* (1979) Studies on mineralo-corticoid escape in cirrhosis. *Clin Sci* 56, 401–406.

112 Lavilla G, Salmeron JM, Arroyo V *et al.* (1992) Mineralocorticoid escape in patients with compensated cirrhosis and portal hypertension. *Gastroenterology* 102, 2114–2119.

113 Trevisani F, Bernardi M, Gasbarrini A *et al.* (1992) Bed-rest-induced hypernatriuresis in cirrhotic-patients without ascites – does it contribute to maintain compensation? *J Hepatol* 16, 190–196.

114 Bernardi M, Dimarco C, Trevisani F *et al.* (1993) Renal sodium retention during upright posture in preascitic cirrhosis. *Gastroenterology* 105, 188–193.

115 Papper S, Rosenbaum JD (1952) Abnormalities in the excretion of water and sodium in compensated cirrhosis of the liver. *J Lab Clin Med* 40, 523–530.

116 Shear L, Hall PW, Gabuzda GJ (1965) Renal failure in patients with cirrhosis of liver. 2. factors influencing maximal urinary flow rate. *Am J Med* 39, 199–209.

117 Epstein M (1985) Derangements of renal water handling in liver disease. *Gastroenterology* 89, 1415–1425.

118 Arroyo V, Rodes J, Gutierrezlizarraga MA *et al.* (1976) Prognostic value of spontaneous hyponatremia in cirrhosis with ascites. *Am J Dig Dis* 21, 249–256.

119 Rodes J, Brugera M, Teres J *et al.* (1970) Terminal functional renal insufficiency (TFRI) in liver cirrhosis with ascites. *Rev Clin Esp* 117, 475–482.

120 Gines A, Escorsell A, Gines P *et al.* (1993) Incidence, predictive factors, and prognosis of the hepatorenal-syndrome in cirrhosis with ascites. *Gastroenterology* 105, 229–236.

121 Llach J, Gines P, Arroyo V *et al.* (1988) Prognostic value of arterial pressure, endogenous vasoactive systems, and renal function in cirrhotic patients admitted to the hospital for the treatment of ascites. *Gastroenterology* 94, 482–487.

122 Rodes J, Arroyo V, Bosch J (1975) Clinical types and drug therapy of renal impairment in cirrhosis. *Postgrad Med J* 51, 492–497.

123 Arroyo V, Gines P, Gerbes AL *et al.* (1996) Definition and diagnostic criteria of refractory ascites and hepatorenal syndrome in cirrhosis. *Hepatology* 23, 164–176.

124 Laragh J, Sealey JE (1992) Renin–angiotensin–aldosterone system and the regulation of sodium, potassium and blood pressure homeostasis. In: Windhager E (ed.) *Handbook of Physiology: Renal Physiology*. New York: Oxford University Press, pp. 1409–1542.

125 Simon MA, Diez J, Prieto J (1991) Abnormal sympathetic and renal response to sodium restriction in compensated cirrhosis. *Gastroenterology* 101, 1354–1360.

126 Salo J, Gines A, Anibarro L *et al.* (1995) Effect of upright posture and physical exercise on endogenous neurohormonal systems in cirrhotic patients with sodium retention and normal supine plasma renin, aldosterone, and norepinephrine levels. *Hepatology* 22, 479–487.

127 Wilkinson SP, Jowett TP, Slater JDH *et al.* (1979) Renal sodium retention in cirrhosis – relation to aldosterone and nephron site. *Clin Sci* 56, 169–177.

128 Perezayuso RM, Arroyo V, Planas R *et al.* (1983) Randomized comparative study of efficacy of furosemide versus spironolactone in nonazotemic cirrhosis with ascites – relationship between the diuretic response and the activity of the renin–aldosterone system. *Gastroenterology* 84, 961–968.

129 Kotelanski B, Groszman R, Cohn JN (1972) Circulation times in splanchnic and hepatic beds in alcoholic liver disease. *Gastroenterology* 63, 102–111.

130 Nicholls KM, Shapiro MD, Vanputten VJ *et al.* (1985) Elevated plasma norepinephrine concentrations in decompensated cirrhosis – association with increased secretion rates, normal clearance rates, and suppressibility by central blood volume expansion. *Circ Res* 56, 457–461.

131 Henriksen J, Ring-Larsen H, Christensen N (1985) Circulating noradrenaline and central haemodynamics in patients with cirrhosis. *Scand J Gastroenterol* 20, 1185–1190.

132 Lieberman F, Reynolds TB (1967) Plasma volume in cirrhosis of liver – its relation to portal hypertension ascites and renal failure. *J Clin Invest* 46, 1297–1308.

133 Arroyo V, Bosch J, Mauri M *et al.* (1981) Effect of angiotensin-II blockade on systemic and hepatic hemodynamics and on the renin-angiotensin-aldosterone system in cirrhosis with ascites. *Eur J Clin Invest* 11, 221–229.

134 Perezayuso RM, Arroyo V, Camps J *et al.* (1984) Renal kallikrein excretion in cirrhotics with ascites – relationship to renal hemodynamics. *Hepatology* 4, 247–252.

135 Arroyo V, Planas R, Gaya J *et al.* (1983) Sympathetic nervous activity, renin–angiotensin system and renal excretion of prostaglandin-e2 in cirrhosis – relationship to functional renal failure and sodium and water excretion. *Eur J Clin Invest* 13, 271–278.

136 Tobey JC, Weaver LC (1987) Pressoreceptor modulation of renal but not splenic sympathetic reflexes. *Am J Physiol* 252, R26–R33.

137 Robertson GL (1992) Regulation of vasopressin secretion. In: Seldin D, Giebisch G (eds) *The Kidney: Physiology and Pathophysiology*. New York: Raven Press, pp. 1595–1614.

138 Barajas L, Muller J (1973) Innervation of juxtaglomerular apparatus and surrounding tubules – quantitative-analysis by serial section electron microscopy. *J Ultrastruct Res* 43, 107–132.

139 Kopp U, DiBona G (1992) Neural control of renal function. In: Seldin D, Giebisch G (eds) *The Kidney: Physiology and Pathophysiology*. New York: Raven Press, pp. 1157–1204.

140 Bichet DG, Vanputten VJ, Schrier RW (1982) Potential role of increased sympathetic activity in impaired sodium and water excretion in cirrhosis. *N Engl J Med* 307, 1552–1557.

141 Ringlarsen H, Hesse B, Henriksen JH *et al.* (1982) Sympathetic nervous activity and renal and systemic hemodynamics in cirrhosis – plasma norepinephrine concentration, hepatic extraction, and renal release. *Hepatology* 2, 304–310.

142 Maroto A, Gines P, Arroyo V *et al.* (1993) Brachial and femoral artery blood flow in cirrhosis – relationship to kidney dysfunction. *Hepatology* 17, 788–793.

143 Solisherruzo JA, Duran A, Favela V *et al.* (1987) Effects of lumbar sympathetic block on kidney function in cirrhotic patients with hepatorenal syndrome. *J Hepatol* 5, 167–173.

144 Ishikawa S, Schrier RW (2003) Pathophysiological roles of arginine vasopressin and aquaporin-2 in impaired water excretion. *Clin Endocrinol* 58, 1–17.

145 Ishikawa S, Saito T, Kasono K (2004) Pathological role of aquaporin-2 in impaired water excretion and hyponatremia. *J Neuroendocrinol* 16, 293–296.

146 Jamison R, Gehrig JJ (1992) Urinary concentration and dilution. In: Windhager E (ed.) *Handbook of Physiology: Section 8, Renal Physiology*. New York: Oxford University Press, pp. 1219–1280.

147 Perezayuso RM, Arroyo V, Camps J *et al.* (1984) Evidence that renal prostaglandins are involved in renal water metabolism in cirrhosis. *Kidney Int* 26, 72–80.

148 Linas SL, Anderson RJ, Guggenheim SJ *et al.* (1981) Role of vasopressin in impaired water-excretion in conscious rats with experimental cirrhosis. *Kidney Int* 20, 173–180.

149 Claria J, Jimenez W, Arroyo V *et al.* (1989) Blockade of the hydroosmotic effect of vasopressin normalizes water excretion in cirrhotic rats. *Gastroenterology* 97, 1294–1299.

150 Gerbes AL, Golberg V, Gines P *et al.* (2003) Therapy of hyponatremia in cirrhosis with a vasopressin receptor antagonist: a randomized double-blind multicenter trial. *Gastroenterology* 124, 933–939.

151 Wong F, Blei AT, Blendis LM *et al.* (2003) A vasopressin receptor antagonist (VPA-985) improves serum sodium concentration in patients with hyponatremia: a multicenter, randomized, placebo-controlled trial. *Hepatology* 37, 182–191.

152 Gines P, Wong F, Milutinovic S *et al.* (2006) Effects of satavaptan (SR121463B), a selective vasopressin V2 receptor antagonist, on serum sodium concentration and ascites in patients with cirrhosis and hyponatremia. *J Hepatol* 44(2), S270.

153 Bosch-Marcé M, Jimenez W, Angeli P *et al.* (1995) Aquaretic effect of the kappa-opioid agonist Ru-51599 in cirrhotic rats with ascites and water retention. *Gastroenterology* 109, 217–223.

154 Smith WL (1992) Prostanoid biosynthesis and mechanisms of action. *Am J Physiol* 263, F181–F191.

155 Schnermann J, Briggs JP (1981) Participation of renal cortical prostaglandins in the regulation of glomerular filtration rate. *Kidney Int* 19, 802–815.

156 Conrad K, Dunn M (1992) Renal prostaglandins and other eicosanoids. In: Windhager E (ed.) *Handbook of Physiology: Section 8, Renal Physiology*. New York: Oxford University Press, pp. 1708–1757.

157 Rimola A, Gines P, Arroyo V *et al.* (1986) Urinary excretion of 6-keto-prostaglandin F1-alpha, thromboxane B-2 and prostaglandin-E2 in cirrhosis with ascites – relationship to functional renal failure (hepatorenal syndrome). *J Hepatol* 3, 111–117.

158 Moore K, Ward PS, Taylor GW *et al.* (1991) Systemic and renal production of thromboxane-A2 and prostacyclin in decompensated liver disease and hepatorenal syndrome. *Gastroenterology* 100, 1069–1077.

159 Boyer TD, Zia P, Reynolds TB (1979) Effect of indomethacin and prostaglandin-A1 on renal function and plasma renin activity in alcoholic liver disease. *Gastroenterology* 77, 215–222.

160 Lianos EA, Alavi N, Tobin M *et al.* (1982) Angiotensin-induced sodium-excretion patterns in cirrhosis – role of renal prostaglandins. *Kidney Int* 21, 70–77.

161 Wong F, Massie D, Hsu P, Dudley F (1993) Indomethacin-induced renal dysfunction in patients with well-compensated cirrhosis. *Gastroenterology* 104, 869–876.

162 Lianos EA, Alavi N, Tobin M *et al.* (1982) Angiotensin-induced sodium-excretion patterns in cirrhosis – role of renal prostaglandins. *Kidney Int* 21, 70–77.

163 Claria J, Kent JD, Lopez-Parra M *et al.* (2005) Effects of celecoxib and naproxen on renal function in nonazotemic patients with cirrhosis and ascites. *Hepatology* 41, 579–587.

164 Abelmann WH (1994) Hyperdynamic circulation in cirrhosis – a historical perspective. *Hepatology* 20, 1356–1358.

165 Fernandez-Seara J, Prieto J, Quiroga J *et al.* (1989) Systemic and regional hemodynamics in patients with liver cirrhosis and ascites with and without functional renal-failure. *Gastroenterology* 97, 1304–1312.

166 Guevara M, Bru C, Gines P *et al.* (1998) Increased cerebrovascular resistance in cirrhotic patients with ascites. *Hepatology* 28, 39–44.

167 Morales-Ruiz M, Tugues S, Cejudo-Martin P et al. (2005) Ascites from cirrhotic patients induces angiogenesis through the phosphoinositide 3-kinase/Akt signaling pathway. *J Hepatol* 43, 85–91.

168 Wiest R, Das S, Cadelina G et al. (1999) Bacterial translocation in cirrhotic rats stimulates eNOS-derived NO production and impairs mesenteric vascular contractility. *J Clin Invest* 104, 1223–1233.

169 Xu LM, Carter EP, Ohara M et al. (2000) Neuronal nitric oxide synthase and systemic vasodilation in rats with cirrhosis. *Am J Physiol (Renal Physiol)* 279, F1110–F1115.

170 Martin PY, Ohara M, Gines P et al. (1998) Nitric oxide synthase (NOS) inhibition for one week improves renal sodium and water excretion in cirrhotic rats with ascites. *J Clin Invest* 101, 235–242.

171 Wiest R, Groszmann RJ (2002) The paradox of nitric oxide in cirrhosis and portal hypertension: too much, not enough. *Hepatology* 35, 478–491.

172 Li Y, Song D, Zhang Y et al. (2003) Effect of neonatal capsaicin treatment on haemodynamics and renal function in cirrhotic rats. *Gut* 52, 293–299.

173 Gupta S, Morgan TR, Gordan GS (1992) Calcitonin gene-related peptide in hepatorenal-syndrome – a possible mediator of peripheral vasodilation. *J Clin Gastroenterol* 14, 122–126.

174 Fernandezrodriguez CM, Prieto J, Quiroga J et al. (1995) Plasma levels of substance P in liver cirrhosis – relationship to the activation of vasopressor systems and urinary sodium excretion. *Hepatology* 21, 35–40.

175 Chang CS, Chen GH, Lien HC et al. (1998) Small intestine dysmotility and bacterial overgrowth in cirrhotic patients with spontaneous bacterial peritonitis. *Hepatology* 28, 1187–1190.

176 Ruiz-del-Arbol L, Monescillo A, Arocena C et al. (2005) Circulatory function and hepatorenal syndrome in cirrhosis. *Hepatology* 42, 439–447.

177 Ros J, Claria J, Jimenez W et al. (1995) Role of nitric oxide and prostacyclin in the control of renal perfusion in experimental cirrhosis. *Hepatology* 22, 915–920.

178 Angeli P, Jimenez W, Arroyo V et al. (1994) Renal effects of natriuretic peptide receptor blockade in cirrhotic rats with ascites. *Hepatology* 20, 948–954.

179 Ruiz-del-Arbol W, Urman J, Fernandez J et al. (2003) Systemic, renal, and hepatic hemodynamic derangement in cirrhotic patients with spontaneous bacterial peritonitis. *Hepatology* 38, 1210–1218.

180 Moller S, Henriksen JH (2002) Cirrhotic cardiomyopathy: a pathophysiological review of circulatory dysfunction in liver disease. *Heart* 87, 9–15.

181 Witte CL, Witte MH, Dumont AE (1980) Lymph imbalance in the genesis and perpetuation of the ascites syndrome in hepatic cirrhosis. *Gastroenterology* 78, 1059–1068.

182 Schrier RW, Arroyo V, Bernardi M et al. (1988) Peripheral arterial vasodilation hypothesis – a proposal for the initiation of renal sodium and water-retention in cirrhosis. *Hepatology* 8, 1151–1157.

183 Benoit JN, Barrowman JA, Harper SL et al. (1984) Role of humoral factors in the intestinal hyperemia associated with chronic portal-hypertension. *Am J Physiol* 247, G486–G493.

184 Benoit JN, Granger DN (1988) Intestinal microvascular adaptation to chronic portal hypertension in the rat. *Gastroenterology* 94, 471–476.

185 Arroyo V, Gines P (1992) Arteriolar vasodilation and the pathogenesis of the hyperdynamic circulation and renal sodium and water-retention in cirrhosis. *Gastroenterology* 102, 1077–1079.

186 Leak LV, Rahil K (1978) Permeability of diaphragmatic mesothelium – ultrastructural basis for stomata. *Am J Anat* 151, 557–593.

187 Tsilibary EC, Wissig SL (1977) Absorption from peritoneal-cavity – SEM study of mesothelium covering peritoneal surface of muscular portion of diaphragm. *Am J Anat* 149, 127–133.

188 Yoffey J, Courtice F (1970) Lymph flow and regional lymphatics. In: Arnold E (ed.) *Lymphatics, Lymph and Lymphomyeloid Complex.* New York: Academia, pp. 356–443.

189 Buhac I, Flesh L, Kishore R (1984) Intraabdominal pressure and resorption of ascites in decompensated liver cirrhosis. *J Lab Clin Med* 104, 264–270.

190 Arroyo V, Gines P, Planas R et al. (1986) Management of patients with cirrhosis and ascites. *Semin Liver Dis* 6, 353–369.

191 Arroyo V, Bosch J, Gayabeltran J et al. (1981) Plasma renin activity and urinary sodium excretion as prognostic indicators in nonazotemic cirrhosis with ascites. *Ann Intern Med* 94, 198–201.

192 Tage-Jensen U, Henriksen JH, Christensen E et al. (1988) Plasma catecholamine level and portal venous pressure as guides to prognosis in patients with cirrhosis. *J Hepatol* 6, 350–358.

193 Salerno F, Borroni G, Moser P et al. (1993) Survival and prognostic factors of cirrhotic patients with ascites – a study of 134 outpatients. *Am J Gastroenterol* 88, 514–519.

194 Guardiola J, Xiol X, Escriba JM et al. (1995) Prognosis assessment of cirrhotic patients with refractory ascites treated with a peritoneovenous shunt. *Am J Gastroenterol* 90, 2097–2102.

195 Ruf AE, Kremers WK, Chavez LL et al. (2005) Addition of serum sodium into the MELD score predicts waiting list mortality better than MELD alone. *Liver Transplant* 11, 336–343.

196 Heuman DM, Abou-assi SG, Habib A et al. (2004) Persistent ascites and low serum sodium identify patients with cirrhosis and low MELD scores who are at high risk for early death. *Hepatology* 40, 802–810.

197 Schepke M, Roth F, Koch L et al. (2003) Prognostic impact of renal impairment and sodium imbalance in patients undergoing transjugular intrahepatic portosystemic shunting for the prevention of variceal rebleeding. *Digestion* 67, 146–153.

198 Borroni G, Maggi A, Sangiovanni A et al. (2000) Clinical relevance of hyponatraemia for the hospital outcome of cirrhotic patients. *Dig Liver Dis* 32, 605–610.

199 Salo J, Guevara M, FernandezEsparrach G et al. (1997) Impairment of renal function during moderate physical exercise in cirrhotic patients with ascites: relationship with the activity of neurohormonal systems. *Hepatology* 25, 1338–1342.

200 Gines P, Arrovo V, Rodes J (1992) Pharmacotherapy of ascites associated with cirrhosis. *Drugs* 43, 316–332.

201 Moore KP, Wong F, Gines P et al. (2003) The management of ascites in cirrhosis: report on the consensus conference of the international ascites club. *Hepatology* 38, 258–266.

202 Suki W, Eknoyan G (1992) Physiology of diuretic action. In: Seldin D, Giebisch G (eds) *The Kidney: Physiology and Pathophysiology,* 2nd edn. New York: Raven, pp. 3629–3670.

203 Puschett J, Winaver J (1992) Effects of diuretics on renal function. In: Windhager E (ed.) *Handbook of Physiology: Section 8, Renal Physiology.* New York: Oxford University Press, pp. 2335–2407.

204 Karim A (1986) Spironolactone metabolism in man revisited. In: Brumer H (ed.) *Contemporary Trends in Diuretic Therapy.* Amsterdam: Excerpta Medica, pp. 23–27.

205 Sungaila I, Bartle WR, Walker SE et al. (1992) Spironolactone pharmacokinetics and pharmacodynamics in patients with cirrhotic ascites. *Gastroenterology* 102, 1680–1685.

206 Sawhney VK, Gregory PB, Swezey SE *et al.* (1981) Furosemide disposition in cirrhotic patients. *Gastroenterology* 81, 1012–1016.

207 Pinzani M, Daskalopoulos G, Laffi G *et al.* (1987) Altered furosemide pharmacokinetics in chronic alcoholic liver disease with ascites contributes to diuretic resistance. *Gastroenterology* 92, 294–298.

208 Traeger A, Hantze R, Penzlin M *et al.* (1985) Pharmacokinetics and pharmacodynamic effects of furosemide in patients with liver cirrhosis. *Int J Clin Pharmacol Therapeut* 23, 129–133.

209 Villeneuve JP, Verbeeck RK, Wilkinson GR *et al.* (1986) Furosemide kinetics and dynamics in patients with cirrhosis. *Clin Pharmacol Therapeut* 40, 14–20.

210 Gatta A, Angeli P, Caregaro L *et al.* (1991) A pathophysiological interpretation of unresponsiveness to spironolactone in a stepped-care approach to the diuretic treatment of ascites in nonazotemic cirrhotic patients. *Hepatology* 14, 231–236.

211 Bernardi M, Laffi G, Salvagnini M *et al.* (1993) Efficacy and safety of the stepped care medical treatment of ascites in liver cirrhosis – a randomized controlled clinical trial comparing 2 diets with different sodium content. *Liver* 13, 156–162.

212 Forns X, Gines A, Gines P *et al.* (1994) Management of ascites and renal failure in cirrhosis. *Semin Liver Dis* 14, 82–96.

213 Santos J, Planas R, Pardo A *et al.* (2003) Spironolactone alone or in combination with furosemide in the treatment of moderate ascites in nonazotemic cirrhosis. A randomized comparative study of efficacy and safety. *J Hepatol* 39, 187–192.

214 Shear L, Ching S, Gabuzda GJ (1970) Compartmentalization of ascites and edema in patients with hepatic cirrhosis. *N Engl J Med* 282, 1391-&.

215 Sherlock S, Senewira B, Scott A *et al.* (1966) Complications of diuretic therapy in hepatic cirrhosis. *Lancet* 1, 1049–1052.

216 Strauss E, de Sa M, Laut C (1985) Standardization of therapeutic approach for ascites due to chronic liver disease. A prospective study of 100 cases. *Gastroenterol Endosc Dig* 4, 79–86.

217 Angeli P, Albino G, Carraro P *et al.* (1996) Cirrhosis and muscle cramps: evidence of a causal relationship. *Hepatology* 23, 264–273.

218 Lee FY, Lee SD, Tsai YT *et al.* (1991) A randomized controlled trial of quinidine in the treatment of cirrhotic-patients with muscle cramps. *J Hepatol* 12, 236–240.

219 Planas R, Arroyo V, Rimola A *et al.* (1983) Acetylsalicylic acid suppresses the renal hemodynamic effect and reduces the diuretic action of furosemide in cirrhosis with ascites. *Gastroenterology* 84, 247–252.

220 Mirouze D, Zipser RD, Reynolds TB (1983) Effect of inhibitors of prostaglandin synthesis on induced diuresis in cirrhosis. *Hepatology* 3, 50–55.

221 Gines P, Arroyo V, Quintero E *et al.* (1987) Comparison of paracentesis and diuretics in the treatment of cirrhotics with tense ascites – results of a randomized study. *Gastroenterology* 93, 234–241.

222 Gines P, Tito L, Arroyo V *et al.* (1988) Randomized comparative study of therapeutic paracentesis with and without intravenous albumin in cirrhosis. *Gastroenterology* 94, 1493–1502.

223 Gines A, FernandezEsparrach G, Monescillo A *et al.* (1996) Randomized trial comparing albumin, dextran 70, and polygeline in cirrhotic patients with ascites treated by paracentesis. *Gastroenterology* 111, 1002–1010.

224 Ruiz-del-Arbol L, Monescillo A, Jimenez W *et al.* (1997) Paracentesis-induced circulatory dysfunction: mechanism and effect on hepatic hemodynamics in cirrhosis. *Gastroenterology* 113, 579–586.

225 Sola-Vera J, Minana J, Ricart E *et al.* (2003) Randomized trial comparing albumin and saline in the prevention of paracentesis-induced circulatory dysfunction in cirrhotic patients with ascites. *Hepatology* 37, 1147–1153.

226 LeVeen HH, Christou G, Ip M *et al.* (1974) Peritoneo-venous shunting for ascites. *Ann Surg* 180, 580–591.

227 Fulenwider JT, Galambos JD, Smith RB *et al.* (1986) Denver peritoneovenous shunts for intractable ascites of cirrhosis – a randomized, prospective trial. *Arch Surg* 121, 351–355.

228 Schroeder ET, Anderson GH, Smulyan H (1979) Effects of a portacaval or peritoneovenous shunt on renin in the hepatorenal syndrome. *Kidney Int* 15, 54–61.

229 Smadja C, Franco D (1985) The Leveen shunt in the elective treatment of intractable ascites in cirrhosis – a prospective study on 140 patients. *Ann Surg* 201, 488–493.

230 Lund RH, Moritz MW (1982) Complications of Denver peritoneovenous shunting. *Arch Surg* 117, 924–928.

231 Harmon DC, Demirjian Z, Ellman L *et al.* (1979) Disseminated intravascular coagulation with the peritoneovenous shunt. *Ann Intern Med* 90, 774–776.

232 Stein SF, Fulenwider JT, Ansley JD *et al.* (1981) Accelerated fibrinogen and platelet destruction after peritoneovenous shunting. *Arch Intern Med* 141, 1149–1151.

233 Tang HH, Salem HH, Wood LJ *et al.* (1992) Coagulopathy during ascites reinfusion – prevention by antiplatelet therapy. *Gastroenterology* 102, 1334–1339.

234 Ginès A, Planas R, Angeli P *et al.* (1995) Treatment of patients with cirrhosis and refractory ascites using leveen shunt with titanium tip – comparison with therapeutic paracentesis. *Hepatology* 22, 124–131.

235 Greenlee HB, Stanley MM, Reinhardt GF (1981) Intractable ascites treated with peritoneovenous shunts (LeVeen) – a 24-month to 64-month follow-up of results in 52 alcoholic cirrhotics. *Arch Surg* 116, 518–524.

236 Wapnick S, Grosberg SJ, Evans MI (1979) Randomized prospective matched pair study comparing peritoneovenous shunt and conventional therapy in massive ascites. *Br J Surg* 66, 667–670.

237 Bories P, Garcia Compean D, Michel H *et al.* (1986) The treatment of refractory ascites by the LeVeen shunt. A multi-centre controlled trial (57 patients). *J Hepatol* 3, 212–218.

238 Ringlarsen H, Siemssen O, Krintel JJ *et al.* (1988) Diuretic resistant ascites in cirrhosis treated with peritoneo-venous shunt – a randomized controlled trial. *Hepatology* 8, 1353.

239 Stanley MM, Ochi S, Lee KK *et al.* (1989) Peritoneovenous shunting as compared with medical-treatment in patients with alcoholic cirrhosis and massive ascites. *N Engl J Med* 321, 1632–1638.

240 Gines P, Arroyo V, Vargas V *et al.* (1991) Paracentesis with intravenous infusion of albumin as compared with peritoneovenous shunting in cirrhosis with refractory ascites. *N Engl J Med* 325, 829–835.

241 Orloff MJ (1970) Pathogenesis and surgical treatment of intractable ascites associated with alcoholic cirrhosis. *Ann NY Acad Sci* 170, 213.

242 Franco D (1983) Treatment of intractable ascites in cirrhotic-patients by portal–systemic shunt. *Gastroenterol Clin Biol* 7, 533–539.

243 Arrovo V, Cardenas A (1999) TIPS in the treatment of refractory ascites. In: Arrovo V, Bosch J, Bruguera M *et al.* (eds) *Treatment of Liver Diseases*. Barcelona: Masson, pp. 43–51.

244 Lebrec D, Giuily N, Hadengue A *et al.* (1996) Transjugular intrahepatic portosystemic shunts: comparison with paracentesis in patients with cirrhosis and refractory ascites: a randomized trial. *J Hepatol* 25, 135–144.

245 Rossle M, Ochs A, Gulberg V *et al.* (2000) A comparison of paracentesis and transjugular intrahepatic portosystemic shunting in patients with ascites. *N Engl J Med* 342, 1701–1707.

246 Salerno F, Merli M, Riggio O *et al.* (2004) Randomized controlled study of TIPS versus paracentesis plus albumin in cirrhosis with severe ascites. *Hepatology* 40, 629–635.

247 Gines P, Uriz J, Calahorra B *et al.* (2002) Transjugular intrahepatic portosystemic shunting versus paracentesis plus albumin for refractory ascites in cirrhosis. *Gastroenterology* 123, 1839–1847.

248 Sanyal AJ, Genning C, Reddy KR *et al.* (2003) The North American study for the treatment of refractory ascites. *Gastroenterology* 124, 634–641.

249 Campbell NS, Brensinger CM, Sanyal AJ *et al.* (2005) Quality of life in refractory ascites: transjugular intrahepatic portal–systemic shunting versus medical therapy. *Hepatology* 42, 635–640.

250 Londono MC, Guevara M, Rimola A *et al.* (2006) Hyponatremia impairs early posttransplantation outcome in patients with cirrhosis undergoing liver transplantation. *Gastroenterology* 130, 1135–1143.

251 Carrilho F, Bosch J, Arroyo V *et al.* (1977) Renal failure associated with demeclocycline in cirrhosis. *Ann Intern Med* 87, 195–197.

252 Perezayuso RM, Arroyo V, Camps J *et al.* (1984) Effect of demeclocycline on renal-function and urinary prostaglandin-E2 and kallikrein in hyponatremic cirrhotics. *Nephron* 36, 30–37.

253 Ohnishi A, Orita Y, Okahara R *et al.* (1993) Potent aquaretic agent – a novel nonpeptide selective vasopressin-2 antagonist (Opc-31260) in men. *J Clin Invest* 92, 2653–2659.

254 Tsuboi Y, Ishikawa SE, Fujisawa G *et al.* (1994) Therapeutic efficacy of the nonpeptide AVP antagonist Opc-31260 in cirrhotic rats. *Kidney Int* 46, 237–244.

255 Bosch-Marcé M, Poo JL, Jimenez W *et al.* (1999) Comparison of two aquaretic drugs (niravoline and OPC-31260) in cirrhotic rats with ascites and water retention. *J Pharmacol Exp Therapeut* 289, 194–201.

256 Jimenez W, Serradeil-Le Gal C, Ros J *et al.* (2000) Long-term aquaretic efficacy of a selective nonpeptide V-2-vasopressin receptor antagonist, SR121463, in cirrhotic rats. *J Pharmacol Exp Therapeut* 295, 83–90.

257 Fernández-Varol G, Ros J, Cejudo-Martin P *et al.* (2003) Effect of the V-1a/V-2-AVP receptor antagonist, conivaptan, on renal water metabolism and systemic hemodynamics in rats with cirrhosis and ascites. *J Hepatol* 38, 755–761.

258 Inoue T, Ohnishi A, Matsuo A *et al.* (1998) Therapeutic and diagnostic potential of a vasopressin-2 antagonist for impaired water handling in cirrhosis. *Clin Pharmacol Therapeut* 63, 561–570.

259 Guyader D, Patat A, Ellis-Grosse EJ *et al.* (2002) Pharmacodynamic effects of a nonpeptide antidiuretic hormone V2 antagonist in cirrhotic patients with ascites. *Hepatology* 36, 1197–1205.

260 Wong F, Blei AT, Blendis LM *et al.* (2003) A vasopressin receptor antagonist (VPA-985) improves serum sodium concentration in patients with hyponatremia: a multicenter, randomized, placebo-controlled trial. *Hepatology* 37, 182–191.

261 Gerbes AL, Golberg V, Gines P *et al.* (2003) Therapy of hyponatremia in cirrhosis with a vasopressin receptor antagonist: a randomized double-blind multicenter trial. *Gastroenterology* 124, 933–939.

262 Gadano A, Moreau R, Pessione F *et al.* (2000) Aquaretic effects of niravoline, a kappa-opioid agonist, in patients with cirrhosis. *J Hepatol* 32, 38–42.

263 Cabrera J, Arroyo V, Ballesta AM *et al.* (1982) Aminoglycoside nephrotoxicity in cirrhosis – value of urinary beta-2-microglobulin to discriminate functional renal failure from acute tubular damage. *Gastroenterology* 82, 97–105.

264 Moore RD, Smith CR, Lipsky JJ *et al.* (1983) Analysis of risk for development of aminoglycoside nephrotoxicity. *Clin Res* 31, A251.

265 Arroyo V, Perezayuso RM, Camps J *et al.* (1983) Evidence that renal prostaglandin-E2 (Pge2) plays a major role in the maintenance of water excretion in cirrhosis. *Hepatology* 3, 856.

266 Zipser RD, Hoefs JC, Speckart PF *et al.* (1979) Prostaglandins – modulators of renal function and pressor resistance in chronic liver disease. *J Clin Endocrinol Metab* 48, 895–900.

267 Levy M, Wexler MJ, Fechner C (1983) Renal perfusion in dogs with experimental hepatic cirrhosis – role of prostaglandins. *Am J Physiol* 245, F521–F529.

268 Bosch-Marce M, Claria J, Titos E *et al.* (1999) Selective inhibition of cyclooxygenase 2 spares renal function and prostaglandin synthesis in cirrhotic rats with ascites. *Gastroenterology* 116, 1167–1175.

269 Lopez-Parra M, Claria J, Planaguma A *et al.* (2002) Cyclooxygenase-1 derived prostaglandins are involved in the maintenance of renal function in rats with cirrhosis and ascites. *Br J Pharmacol* 135, 891–900.

270 Lopez-Parra M, Claria J, Titos E *et al.* (2005) The selective cyclooxygenase-2 inhibitor celecoxib modulates the formation of vasoconstrictor eicosanoids and activates PPAR gamma. Influence of albumin. *J Hepatol* 42, 75–81.

271 Gines A, Salmeron JM, Gines P *et al.* (1992) Effects of somatostatin on renal function in cirrhosis. *Gastroenterology* 103, 1868–1874.

272 Mountokalakis T, Kallivretakis N, Mayopoulousymvoulidou D *et al.* (1988) Enhancement of renal-function by a long-acting somatostatin analog in patients with decompensated cirrhosis. *Nephrol Dialys Transplant* 3, 604–607.

273 Bernardi M, Depalma R, Trevisani F *et al.* (1989) Renal function and effective beta-blockade in cirrhosis with ascites – relationship with baseline sympathoadrenergic tone. *J Hepatol* 8, 279–286.

274 Salmeron JM, Delarbol LR, Gines A *et al.* (1993) Renal effects of acute isosorbide-5-mononitrate administration in cirrhosis. *Hepatology* 17, 800–806.

275 Salerno F, Borroni G, Lorenzano E *et al.* (1996) Long-term administration of isosorbide-5-mononitrate does not impair renal function in cirrhotic patients. *Hepatology* 23, 1135–1140.

276 Vorobioff J, Picabea E, Gamen M *et al.* (1993) Propranolol compared with propranolol plus isosorbide dinitrate in portal-hypertensive patients – long-term hemodynamic and renal effects. *Hepatology* 18, 477–484.

277 Morillas RM, Planas R, Cabre E *et al.* (1994) Propranolol plus isosorbide-5-mononitrate for portal hypertension in cirrhosis – long-term hemodynamic and renal effects. *Hepatology* 20, 1502–1508.

278 Merkel C, Gatta A, Donada C *et al.* (1995) Long-term effect of nadolol or nadolol plus isosorbide-5-mononitrate on renal function and ascites formation in patients with cirrhosis. *Hepatology* 22, 808–813.

279 Albillos A, Lledo JL, Rossi I *et al.* (1995) Continuous prazosin administration in cirrhotic-patients – effects on portal hemodynamics and on liver and renal function. *Gastroenterology* 109, 1257–1265.

7.6 Hepatorenal syndrome

Pere Ginès and Mónica Guevara

Renal failure is a frequent complication of patients with advanced cirrhosis [1,2]. Its occurrence usually entails a poor prognosis because of the combined detrimental effect of renal and liver failure. In some instances, renal failure in cirrhosis is due to aetiological factors that may also lead to renal failure in patients without liver disease, such as volume depletion, shock or administration of nephrotoxic drugs, or it is the consequence of an intrinsic renal disease, such as glomerulonephritis. However, in other instances, renal failure in cirrhosis occurs in the absence of these aetiological factors and with a normal renal histology. This unique condition, known as hepatorenal syndrome (HRS), is due to marked abnormalities in circulatory function that lead to an intense vasoconstriction of the renal circulation, which causes a striking reduction in glomerular filtration rate (GFR) [1–5]. In recent years, significant advances have been made in the knowledge of HRS. The aim of this chapter is to provide an updated revision of HRS, with special emphasis on clinical features, diagnosis and management.

Definition

HRS is a clinical condition that usually occurs in patients with advanced liver disease and portal hypertension and is characterized by a combination of disturbances in circulatory and kidney functions [6]. The major abnormality in the systemic circulation is arterial hypotension due to markedly reduced total systemic vascular resistance. Kidney function is markedly impaired because of severe reduction of renal blood flow. HRS occurs predominantly in the setting of cirrhosis, but it may also develop in other types of severe chronic liver diseases, such as alcoholic hepatitis, or in acute liver failure [7–9].

Pathogenesis

The pathophysiological hallmark of HRS is vasoconstriction of the renal circulation [1,2,4,6,10–15]. The mechanism of this vasoconstriction is incompletely understood and possibly multifactorial, involving disturbances in the circulatory function and activity of systemic and renal vasoactive mechanisms. In the systemic circulation, there is severe arterial underfilling due to a marked arterial vasodilation located in the splanchnic circulation, which is related to the presence of portal hypertension. In contrast, in the kidney, there is marked vasoconstriction.

The theory that best fits with the observed alterations in the renal and circulatory function in HRS is the arterial vasodilation theory, which proposes that HRS is the result of the effect of vasoconstrictor systems (i.e. the renin–angiotensin and the sympathetic nervous systems) acting on the renal circulation activated as a homeostatic response to improve the extreme underfilling of the arterial circulation [6,15–17]. As a result of this increased activity of the vasoconstrictor systems, renal perfusion and GFR are markedly reduced, but tubular function is preserved. Most available data suggest that the arterial underfilling is due to a marked vasodilation of the splanchnic circulation related to an increased splanchnic production of vasodilator substances, particularly nitric oxide [18,19]. In the early phases of decompensated cirrhosis, renal perfusion is maintained within normal levels because of an increased synthesis of renal vasodilator factors (mainly prostaglandins). In later phases of the disease, renal perfusion is not maintained because of the extreme arterial underfilling causing maximal activation of vasoconstrictor systems and/or decreased production of renal vasodilator factors, and HRS develops. The marked activation of vasoconstrictor systems results in vasoconstriction of some vascular beds other than the kidneys, including lower and upper extremities and brain [20–23]. The splanchnic area escapes from the effect of vasoconstrictors probably because of a markedly enhanced local production of vasodilators. Several recent studies suggest a role for a decreased cardiac function in the pathogenesis of the arterial underfilling leading to HRS [24–27]. A schematic illustration of the proposed pathogenesis of HRS is shown in Figure 1.

Clinical and laboratory findings

HRS usually occurs in the late stages of cirrhosis when patients have developed some of the major complications of the disease, especially ascites. Low urine sodium and dilutional hyponatraemia are the major risk factors for the development of HRS in patients with ascites [28]. The presence of ascites is

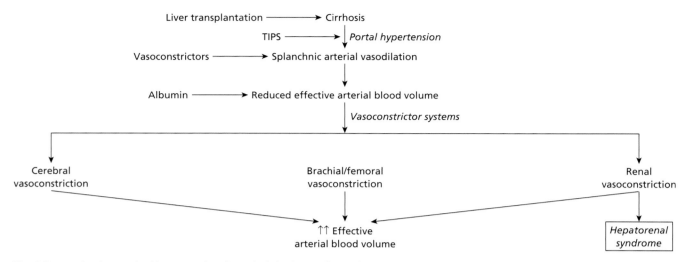

Fig. 1 Proposed pathogenesis of hepatorenal syndrome in cirrhosis according to the arterial vasodilation theory and effective therapeutic interventions. TIPS, transjugular intrahepatic portosystemic shunts.

universal in patients with HRS, so that the lack of ascites in a patient with cirrhosis and renal failure argues against HRS being the cause of renal failure and points towards other causes, particularly prerenal failure due to volume depletion because of excessive diuresis.

Precipitating factors

In some instances, HRS develops spontaneously without any apparent triggering event, whereas, in others, it occurs in close chronological relationship to some precipitating factors that can impair circulatory function [1,3,15,29]. The most common precipitating factors are bacterial infections, particularly spontaneous bacterial peritonitis (SBP), although the frequency of HRS after SBP has decreased markedly (from 33% to 10%) since the introduction of albumin in the management of patients with SBP (see below) [30,31]. Another well-known precipitating factor of HRS is large-volume paracentesis without plasma expansion [32]. Up to 15% of patients with ascites develop HRS when large volumes of ascitic fluid (more than 5 L) are removed without the administration of a plasma expander. Finally, renal failure occurs in about 10% of patients with cirrhosis and gastrointestinal bleeding [33,34]. However, it should be pointed out that a large proportion of episodes of renal failure after gastrointestinal bleeding are probably due to acute tubular necrosis related to hypovolaemic shock and not to HRS [34]. Intravascular volume depletion (i.e. diuretic-induced, extrarenal fluid losses) has been classically considered as a triggering factor for HRS [1], but no convincing evidence has been reported to support this pathogenetic relationship.

Renal function

In the past, HRS was generally diagnosed because of the development of oligoanuria [1,35–37]. Currently, however, with the widespread use of frequent biochemical monitoring for both outpatients and, especially, inpatients, HRS is most frequently first diagnosed by a finding of increased concentrations of serum creatinine and/or blood urea nitrogen (BUN). In some patients, there is a rapid rise in serum creatinine and BUN to very high values [3,37,38]. In other patients, the increases in serum creatinine and BUN levels are moderate with no (or very little) tendency to progress over time, at least in the short term [38–40]. These two different patterns of progression of renal failure define two different clinical types of HRS, type 1 and type 2 HRS [6,38]. The rate of progression used to define HRS type 1 has been arbitrarily set as a 100% increase in serum creatinine reaching a value greater than 2.5 mg/dL (221 μmol/L) in less than 2 weeks [6]. Patients not meeting these criteria of progression are considered to have type 2 HRS. Some patients with type 2 HRS eventually develop a sudden progression of renal failure after weeks or months of stable serum creatinine levels and may then meet the criteria for type 1 HRS. In patients with type 1 HRS, GFR is very low, commonly below 20 mL/min, and serum creatinine levels are high, with average values around 4 mg/dL – 356 μmol/L [38]. In contrast, patients with type 2 HRS have less severely abnormal GFR and creatinine concentrations (average around 2 mg/dL or 178 μmol/L) [38]. The predominant clinical feature of patients with type 1 HRS is severe renal failure, while that of patients with type 2 HRS is recurrent ascites because of poor or no response to diuretics due to the combination of reduced GFR and marked activation of antinatriuretic systems [6,38]. A major clinical difference between the two types of HRS is that patients with type 1 HRS have a very poor short-term outcome compared with that of patients with type 2 HRS (Fig. 2) [38].

Besides renal failure, patients with HRS have marked sodium retention with features of salt and water overload. Urine sodium is lower than 10 mEq/L in most patients [6,15,29,38]. The subsequently enhanced positive sodium balance results in weight gain due to an increase in ascites volume and peripheral oedema.

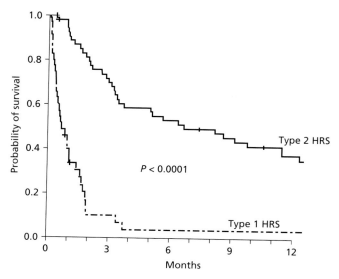

Fig. 2 Survival of patients with cirrhosis after the diagnosis of type 1 or type 2 hepatorenal syndrome (reproduced with permission from ref. 38).

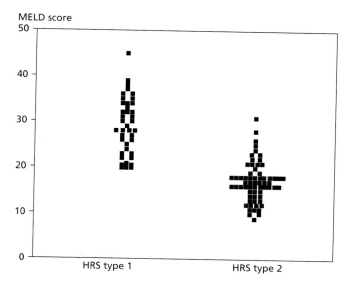

Fig. 3 Individual values of MELD score in patients with type 1 and type 2 hepatorenal syndrome (reproduced with permission from ref. 38).

Serum sodium concentration is low in patients with HRS, and most patients have hyponatraemia (serum sodium lower than 130 mEq/L) [6,38]. If serum sodium concentration in a patient with cirrhosis and renal failure is normal (> 135 mEq/L), the diagnosis of HRS is unlikely, and the patient should be investigated for a different cause of renal failure, particularly an intrinsic renal disease. Hyperkalaemia is also common but usually moderate. High rates of increase in plasma potassium levels are infrequent. Nevertheless, potassium levels should be monitored frequently and hyperkalaemia treated aggressively, if present, to avoid cardiac complications. Severe metabolic acidosis is also uncommon in HRS except for patients who develop a severe infection.

Cardiovascular function

Cardiovascular function is severely affected in patients with HRS. The total systemic vascular resistance is markedly reduced despite a striking activation of major vasoconstrictor systems, such as the renin–angiotensin and the sympathetic nervous systems [2,6,15–17,20,21,27,41–44]. Cardiac output may be increased, normal or reduced [15,20,21,27,42–45]. Recent studies have reported a reduction in cardiac output in some patients with HRS, which may be due to cardiomyopathy associated with cirrhosis [24–27]. Arterial pressure is usually low but stable (average mean arterial pressure around 70 mmHg). When haemodynamic instability exists, sepsis should be suspected. Except for arterial hypotension, the other cardiovascular abnormalities mentioned are not recognized unless invasive vascular monitoring is done and vasoconstrictor factors are measured. Nevertheless, these procedures are not required in the diagnosis or management of patients with HRS. Pulmonary oedema, which is a common and severe complication of acute renal

failure in the absence of liver disease, is very rare in patients with HRS except in patients with very low urine volume who are treated aggressively with plasma expanders.

Liver function

Most patients with HRS show signs and symptoms of advanced liver failure and portal hypertension, particularly jaundice, coagulopathy, malnutrition and hepatic encephalopathy, yet a small proportion may develop HRS in the setting of only moderate liver insufficiency [38]. Because of this, most patients belong to the Child–Pugh C class, although some patients belong to class B. Model for Endstage Liver Disease (MELD) scores of patients with HRS are high (average MELD score 22) owing to the combined effect of liver and renal failure. Patients with type 1 HRS have MELD scores higher than those of patients with type 2 HRS (Fig. 3).

Severe bacterial infections, especially septicaemia (either spontaneous or related to intravenous catheters), SBP and pneumonia, are common in patients with HRS and constitute a frequent cause of death [28,38,46,47]. Both the renal failure and advanced liver disease probably account for an increased susceptibility to the infections.

Diagnosis

The initial step in the diagnosis of HRS is the demonstration of the existence of renal failure. The serum creatinine concentration is usually considered a better marker of GFR than the BUN concentration, but this has not been specially assessed. On the other hand, serum creatinine concentration is not an ideal marker of GFR in cirrhosis because it is usually lower than expected for any given level of GFR as a result of a low

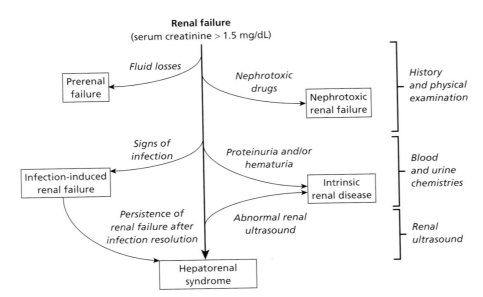

Fig. 4 Diagnostic flow chart of HRS (modified from ref. 75).

endogenous production of creatinine related to the reduced muscle mass that frequently occurs in advanced cirrhosis [48,49]. Nevertheless, as the use of more sensitive clearance techniques to evaluate GFR is expensive and not available in all settings, serum creatinine concentration is currently considered the method of choice to estimate GFR in cirrhosis [6]. There is consensus to establish the diagnosis of HRS when serum creatinine has increased above 1.5 mg/dL (133 μmol/L), which approximately corresponds to an average GFR of 30 mL/min [6,29]. In patients with increased serum creatinine concentration receiving diuretics, measurement of serum creatinine should be repeated after diuretic withdrawal because the use of diuretics may increase serum creatinine levels.

Because of the lack of specific diagnostic tests, the diagnosis of HRS must always be made after exclusion of other conditions that may cause renal failure in cirrhosis [6]. An algorithm for the diagnosis of HRS is shown in Figure 4. Acute renal failure of prerenal origin due to gastrointestinal fluid losses (vomiting, diarrhoea, nasogastric aspiration) or renal fluid losses (overdiuresis due to an excessive diuretic treatment) should be investigated by history and physical examination in all patients with cirrhosis and renal failure. If renal failure is secondary to volume depletion, renal function improves rapidly after volume expansion, whereas no improvement occurs in patients with HRS. The existence of shock before the onset of renal failure precludes the diagnosis of HRS and points towards the existence of acute tubular necrosis. Hypovolaemic shock due to gastrointestinal bleeding is easily recognized. However, septic shock may be more difficult to diagnose in the early phases because of the paucity of symptoms of bacterial infections in some patients with cirrhosis and because arterial hypotension due to sepsis may be erroneously attributed to the advanced liver disease. Therefore, a bacterial infection should always be ruled out by physical examination, laboratory tests and other procedures (i.e. chest X-ray) before the diagnosis of HRS is made. On the

other hand, some patients with cirrhosis and bacterial infections (either SBP or sepsis) develop transient renal failure, which may resolve after resolution of the infection [30,50]. In these patients, the diagnosis of HRS should be made if renal failure persists after complete resolution of the infection. Patients with cirrhosis are at high risk of developing renal failure during treatment with non-steroidal anti-inflammatory drugs or aminoglycosides [51]. Therefore, treatment with these drugs in the previous days or weeks before the initiation of renal failure should always be ruled out before the diagnosis of HRS is made. Renal failure due to the administration of radiocontrast agents is very uncommon [52]. Finally, patients with cirrhosis may also develop renal failure due to intrinsic renal diseases, particularly glomerulonephritis [53,54]. These cases may be recognized by the existence of proteinuria and/or haematuria. The diagnosis may be confirmed by renal biopsy in selected cases.

No published information exists as to the comparative frequency of the different causes of renal failure in patients with cirrhosis. In a prospective ongoing study of renal failure in patients with cirrhosis being carried out at our unit, which so far includes 320 episodes of renal failure diagnosed over a 3-year period, the frequency of the different causes of renal failure is as follows: (i) bacterial infections, 38%; (ii) hypovolaemia, 26%; (iii) intrinsic renal diseases, 13%; (iv) HRS, 12%; (v) mixed, 7%; and (vi) nephrotic drugs, 3% (P. Ginès, unpublished).

Prognosis

Patients with type 1 HRS have an extremely poor outcome, with a median survival of only 1 month [38]. Survival in patients with type 1 HRS is independent of the MELD score. Patients with type 2 HRS have a better prognosis than that of patients with type 1, with a median survival of 7 months. In patients with type 2 HRS, survival is dependent on MELD score (Figs 2 and 5) [38].

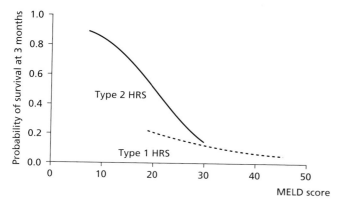

Fig. 5 Three-month survival probability in patients with type 1 and type 2 HRS according to MELD score (reproduced with permission from ref. 38).

Management

Type 1 hepatorenal syndrome

Patients with suspected type 1 HRS should have vital signs, urine output and blood chemistries monitored closely. Because most patients have dilutional hyponatraemia, total fluid intake [both oral and intravenous (i.v.) fluids] should be restricted to 1000 mL/day to avoid a positive fluid balance, which would cause a further reduction in serum sodium concentration. The administration of saline solutions may increase ascites and oedema markedly because of the presence of severe renal sodium retention, and therefore is not recommended. For this same reason and the lack of severe metabolic acidosis in most patients, the routine administration of sodium bicarbonate is also not advisable. Potassium-sparing diuretics should be withheld because of the risk of inducing severe hyperkalaemia. Early identification of infections and treatment with broad-spectrum antibiotics is fundamental, as severe infections are common and contribute to death in these patients. The efficacy of antibiotic prophylaxis for the prevention of infections in patients with HRS has not been assessed.

Several therapeutic approaches, which are discussed below, can be used in the management of type 1 HRS (Table 1).

Table 1 Recommendations for the management of type 1 hepatorenal syndrome.

Evaluate the patient for liver transplantation
Set up high priority for transplantation in candidate patients
Start vasoconstrictors plus i.v. albumin
Consider TIPS in patients without severe liver failure in whom vasoconstrictors have failed
Consider renal replacement therapy if there is pulmonary oedema, severe hyperkalaemia or metabolic acidosis not responding to medical therapy

TIPS, transjugular intrahepatic portosystemic shunt.

Liver transplantation

Liver transplantation is the treatment of choice for patients with cirrhosis and type 1 HRS because it allows the cure of both liver disease and the associated renal failure [55,56]. The most frequent contraindications for transplantation in these patients are advanced age, active alcoholism and infection. The main problem in the use of liver transplantation for type 1 HRS is that a significant proportion of patients die before transplantation is possible because of the short survival expectancy and prolonged waiting times in most transplant centres. This issue can be solved by assigning these patients a high priority for transplantation from a cadaveric donor. Because patients with type 1 HRS have high MELD scores (Fig. 3), the use of MELD score as a system for organ allocation for liver transplantation may improve the probability of transplantation in this patient population [57]. On the other hand, patients with type 1 HRS may probably benefit from treatment with vasoconstrictors before transplantation. This may improve renal function and help reduce the (moderately) higher morbidity and mortality reported in patients transplanted with HRS compared with those of patients transplanted without HRS [58–60]. In fact, patients with HRS treated with vasoconstrictors before transplantation have an outcome after transplantation that is no different from that of patients transplanted without HRS [61]. The use of combined liver–kidney transplantation for patients with HRS does not seem to improve the overall results obtained with liver transplantation alone and should not be used [62].

Vasoconstrictors

The administration of vasoconstrictors represents the only effective medical therapy currently available for the management of HRS. The rationale behind this therapy is to improve circulatory function by causing vasoconstriction of the extremely dilated splanchnic arterial bed, which subsequently improves arterial underfilling, suppresses the activity of the endogenous vasoconstrictor systems and increases renal perfusion (Fig. 1) [24]. Two types of drugs can be used, vasopressin analogues (terlipressin) or alpha-adrenergic agonists (noradrenaline or midodrine), which act on V_1 vasopressin receptors and α-1-adrenergic receptors, respectively, present in vascular smooth muscle cells (Table 2). In most studies, vasoconstrictors have been given in combination with i.v. albumin to further improve the arterial underfilling. Terlipressin is the vasoconstrictor that has been used more frequently in HRS [46,47,63–65]. The administration of terlipressin (0.5–2 mg/4–6 h i.v.) is associated with a complete renal response (reduction of serum creatinine below 1.5 mg/dL) in 50–75% of patients. The improvement in GFR occurs slowly over several days and, despite a marked improvement, GFR usually remains below normal values at the end of treatment. Recurrence of HRS after treatment withdrawal in responders is uncommon (approximately 15% of patients), and retreatment is usually effective. The incidence of ischaemic side-effects requiring the discontinuation of treatment ranges between 5% and 10%. The survival of responders to terlipressin

Table 2 Drugs used in the therapy of hepatorenal syndrome.

Drug	Dose range	Maximum duration of therapy (days)	Potential side-effects
Terlipressin[a]	0.5–2 mg/4 h i.v. bolus	15	Peripheral, splanchnic or cardiac ischaemia
Noradrenaline[b]	0.5–3 mg/h i.v. perfusion	15	Peripheral, splanchnic or cardiac ischaemia
Midodrine[c]	7.5–12.5 mg/8 h p.o.	Indefinite?	Not reported

[a]From refs 46, 47, and 63–65.
[b]From ref. 66.
[c]From refs 43 and 44.

is greater than that of non-responders [46,47]. There are two major shortcomings of the treatment with terlipressin, lack of availability in some countries and high cost, the latter being a major limiting factor for its use in some areas of the world. Alpha-adrenergic agonists (noradrenaline, midodrine) represent an attractive alternative to terlipressin because of their very low cost, wide availability and apparently similar efficacy compared with that of terlipressin [43,44,66]. However, information on the efficacy and side-effects of alpha-adrenergic agonists in patients with type 1 HRS is still very limited.

Transjugular intrahepatic portosystemic shunts

Only a few studies have reported the effects of transjugular intrahepatic portosystemic shunt (TIPS) in patients with type 1 HRS [67,68]. In patients with type 1 HRS, TIPS improves circulatory function and reduces the activity of vasoconstrictor systems. This is associated with a slow reduction in serum creatinine levels in approximately 60% of patients. Median survival after TIPS in patients with type 1 HRS ranges between 2 and 4 months [67,68]. TIPS is considered to be contraindicated in patients with severe liver failure (high serum bilirubin levels and/or Child–Pugh score greater than 12) or severe hepatic encephalopathy. Before comparative studies between TIPS and vasoconstrictors become available, it appears that vasoconstrictors are the treatment of choice in type 1 HRS because of an apparent similar efficacy, wider availability and lower costs compared with TIPS.

Other therapeutic methods

Renal replacement therapy (i.e. haemodialysis) is frequently used in the management of patients with type 1 HRS, especially in those who are candidates for liver transplantation, in an attempt to maintain patients alive until liver transplantation is performed or a spontaneous improvement in renal function occurs [69]. Unfortunately, the potential beneficial effect of this approach has not been unequivocally demonstrated. It is the clinical experience that most patients do not tolerate the haemodialysis and develop important side-effects, including arterial hypotension, bleeding and infections that may contribute to death during treatment. Moreover, findings that indicate the need for renal replacement therapy (severe fluid overload, acidosis or hyperkalaemia) are uncommon, at least

in the early stages of type 1 HRS. Therefore, the initial therapy for these patients should probably include measures aimed at improving circulatory function (vasoconstrictors, TIPS) before haemodialysis is started.

Recently, extracorporeal albumin dialysis, a system that uses an albumin-containing dialysate that is recirculated and perfused through charcoal and anion-exchanger columns, has been reported to improve renal function and survival in a small series of patients with HRS, but these results require confirmation in larger series of patients [70].

Type 2 hepatorenal syndrome

Unlike patients with type 1 HRS, patients with type 2 HRS can be managed as outpatients unless they develop complications that require hospitalization. The most frequent clinical finding in these patients is refractory ascites. Diuretics should be given only if they cause a significant natriuresis (i.e. urine sodium > 30 mEq/day). Care should be taken with the use of spironolactone in these patients because of the risk of development of hyperkalaemia. Repeated paracentesis with i.v. albumin is probably the method of choice for the treatment of episodes of large ascites in these patients [71]. If dilutional hyponatraemia is present, total fluid intake should be restricted to approximately 1000 mL/day. Bacterial infections should be diagnosed and treated early because of the risk of precipitating type 1 HRS. The usefulness of prophylactic antibiotics in patients with type 2 HRS has not been assessed and would be worthy of study. Recommendations for the management of patients with type 2 HRS are outlined in Table 3.

Liver transplantation is the treatment of choice for candidate patients. As for patients with type 1 HRS, the use of MELD score for organ allocation in liver transplantation may be useful in reducing mortality on the waiting list. There is limited information on the use of vasoconstrictors in the treatment of patients with type 2 HRS, but it appears that their administration improves renal function in these patients [47,72]. However, more information is required before a definitive conclusion about this therapeutic approach can be drawn. The use of TIPS in patients with type 2 HRS is associated with an improvement in renal function, better control of ascites and reduced risk of progression from type 2 to type 1 HRS [71,73]. However, TIPS

Table 3 Recommendations for the management of patients with type 2 hepatorenal syndrome.

Evaluate the patient for liver transplantation. Establish priority for transplantation
Use diuretics for management of ascites only if they cause significant natriuresis (> 30 mEq/day). Restrict dietary sodium intake
Use repeated paracentesis plus i.v. albumin to treat recurrent large/tense ascites
Restrict fluid intake if hyponatraemia is present
Consider vasoconstrictors or TIPS before liver transplantation

does not improve survival in these patients compared with treatment with repeated paracentesis and i.v. albumin [74]. Therefore, the beneficial effects of TIPS in reducing ascites recurrence rate and progression to type 1 HRS in patients with type 2 HRS should be weighed against the lack of improvement in survival, increased risk of encephalopathy and high costs.

Prevention

Until very recently, no effective methods for the prevention of HRS existed. However, two recent studies have shown that HRS can be prevented effectively in two specific clinical settings: SBP and alcoholic hepatitis. In patients with SBP, the administration of albumin (1.5 g/kg i.v. at the diagnosis of the infection and 1 g/kg i.v. 48 h later) together with antibiotics markedly reduces the occurrence of HRS compared with the standard treatment with antibiotics alone (10% in the albumin group vs. 33% in the non-albumin group) [31]. Moreover, hospital mortality is also lower in patients receiving albumin (10% vs. 29% respectively). The beneficial effect of albumin is probably related to its capacity to prevent arterial underfilling and subsequent activation of vasoconstrictor systems during the infection. In patients with alcoholic hepatitis, the administration of pentoxifylline (400 mg t.i.d.) reduces the occurrence of HRS and mortality (8% and 24% respectively) with respect to a control group (35% and 46% respectively) [9]. The beneficial effect of pentoxifylline is probably related to its capacity to inhibit tumour necrosis factor production. Although the beneficial effects obtained in these two clinical trials require confirmation in other studies, they represent the first big step forward towards effective prevention of HRS in patients with endstage liver disease.

References

1 Papper S (1983) Hepatorenal syndrome. In: Epstein M (ed.) *The Kidney in Liver Disease*. New York: Elsevier Biomedical, pp. 87–106.
2 Ginès P, Rodes J (1999) Clinical disorders of renal function in cirrhosis with ascites. In: Arroyo V, Ginès P, Rodes J et al. (eds) *Ascites and Renal Dysfunction in Liver Disease, Pathogenesis, Diagnosis and Treatment*. Malden: Blackwell Science, pp. 36–62.
3 Hecker R, Sherlock S (1956) Electrolyte and circulatory changes in terminal liver failure. *Lancet* 271 (6953), 1121–1125.
4 Epstein M, Berk DP, Hollenberg NK et al. (1970) Renal failure in the patient with cirrhosis. The role of active vasoconstriction. *Am J Med* 49 (2), 175–185.
5 Arroyo V, Hecker R, Sherlock S (2002) Electrolyte and circulatory changes in terminal liver failure [*Lancet* (1956) 2, 1221–1225]. *J Hepatol* 36 (3), 315–320.
6 Arroyo V, Ginès P, Gerbes AL et al. (1996) Definition and diagnostic criteria of refractory ascites and hepatorenal syndrome in cirrhosis. International Ascites Club. *Hepatology* 23(1), 164–176.
7 Wilkinson SP, Blendis LM, Williams R (1974) Frequency and type of renal and electrolyte disorders in fulminant hepatic-failure. *Br Med J* 1 (5900), 186–189.
8 O'Grady JG (2005) Clinical disorders of renal function in acute liver failure. In: Arroyo V, Ginès P, Rodes J et al. (eds) *Ascites and Renal Dysfunction in Liver Disease*. Malden: Blackwell Publishing, pp. 383–393.
9 Akriviadis E, Botla R, Briggs W et al. (2000) Pentoxifylline improves short-term survival in severe acute alcoholic hepatitis: a double-blind, placebo-controlled trial. *Gastroenterology* 119 (6), 1637–1648.
10 Schroeder ET, Shear L, Sancetta SM et al. (1967) Renal failure in patients with cirrhosis of the liver. Evaluation of intrarenal blood flow by para-aminohippurate extraction and response to angiotensin. *Am J Med* 43 (6), 887–896.
11 Kew MC, Brunt PW, Varma RR et al. (1971) Renal and intrarenal blood-flow in cirrhosis of the liver. *Lancet* 2 (7723), 504–510.
12 Ring-Larsen H (1977) Renal blood flow in cirrhosis: relation to systemic and portal haemodynamics and liver function. *Scand J Clin Lab Invest* 37 (7), 635–642.
13 Platt JF, Marn CS, Baliga PK et al. (1992) Renal dysfunction in hepatic disease: early identification with renal duplex Doppler US in patients who undergo liver transplantation. *Radiology* 183 (3), 801–806.
14 Dagher L, Moore K (2001) The hepatorenal syndrome. *Gut* 49 (5), 729–737.
15 Arroyo V, Guevara M, Ginès P (2002) Hepatorenal syndrome in cirrhosis: pathogenesis and treatment. *Gastroenterology* 122 (6), 1658–1676.
16 Schrier RW, Arroyo V, Bernardi M et al. (1988) Peripheral arterial vasodilation hypothesis: a proposal for the initiation of renal sodium and water retention in cirrhosis. *Hepatology* 8 (5), 1151–1157.
17 Schrier RW, Niederberger M, Weigert A et al. (1994) Peripheral arterial vasodilatation: determinant of functional spectrum of cirrhosis. *Semin Liver Dis* 14 (1), 14–22.
18 Martin PY, Ginès P, Schrier RW (1998) Nitric oxide as a mediator of hemodynamic abnormalities and sodium and water retention in cirrhosis. *N Engl J Med* 339 (8), 533–541.
19 Wiest R, Groszmann RJ (1999) Nitric oxide and portal hypertension: its role in the regulation of intrahepatic and splanchnic vascular resistance. *Semin Liver Dis* 19 (4), 411–426.
20 Fernandez-Seara J, Prieto J, Quiroga J et al. (1989) Systemic and regional hemodynamics in patients with liver cirrhosis and ascites with and without functional renal failure. *Gastroenterology* 97 (5), 1304–1312.
21 Maroto A, Ginès P, Arroyo V et al. (1993) Brachial and femoral artery blood flow in cirrhosis: relationship to kidney dysfunction. *Hepatology* 17 (5), 788–793.
22 Guevara M, Bru C, Ginès P et al. (1998) Increased cerebrovascular resistance in cirrhotic patients with ascites. *Hepatology* 28 (1), 39–44.
23 Sugano S, Yamamoto K, Atobe T et al. (2001) Postprandial middle cerebral arterial vasoconstriction in cirrhotic patients. A placebo, controlled evaluation. *J Hepatol* 34 (3), 373–377.

24 Ginès P, Guevara M (2002) Good news for hepatorenal syndrome. *Hepatology* 36 (2), 504–506.

25 Lee SS (2003) Cardiac dysfunction in spontaneous bacterial peritonitis: a manifestation of cirrhotic cardiomyopathy? *Hepatology* 38 (5), 1089–1091.

26 Ruiz-del-Arbol L, Urman J, Fernandez J et al. (2003) Systemic, renal, and hepatic hemodynamic derangement in cirrhotic patients with spontaneous bacterial peritonitis. *Hepatology* 38 (5), 1210–1218.

27 Ruiz-del-Arbol L, Monescillo A, Arocena C et al. (2005) Circulatory function and hepatorenal syndrome in cirrhosis. *Hepatology* 42 (2), 439–447.

28 Ginès A, Escorsell A, Ginès P et al. (1993) Incidence, predictive factors, and prognosis of the hepatorenal syndrome in cirrhosis with ascites. *Gastroenterology* 105 (1), 229–236.

29 Bataller R, Ginès P, Guevara M et al. (1997) Hepatorenal syndrome. *Semin Liver Dis* 17 (3), 233–247.

30 Follo A, Llovet JM, Navasa M et al. (1994) Renal impairment after spontaneous bacterial peritonitis in cirrhosis – incidence, clinical course, predictive factors and prognosis. *Hepatology* 20 (6), 1495–1501.

31 Sort P, Navasa M, Arroyo V et al. (1999) Effect of intravenous albumin on renal impairment and mortality in patients with cirrhosis and spontaneous bacterial peritonitis. *N Engl J Med* 341 (6), 403–409.

32 Ginès P, Tito L, Arroyo V et al. (1988) Randomized comparative study of therapeutic paracentesis with and without intravenous albumin in cirrhosis. *Gastroenterology* 94 (6), 1493–1502.

33 Del Olmo JA, Pena A, Serra MA et al. (2000) Predictors of morbidity and mortality after the first episode of upper gastrointestinal bleeding in liver cirrhosis. *J Hepatol* 32 (1), 19–24.

34 Cardenas A, Ginès P, Uriz J et al. (2001) Renal failure after upper gastrointestinal bleeding in cirrhosis: incidence, clinical course, predictive factors, and short-term prognosis. *Hepatology* 34, 671–676.

35 Epstein M (1996) Hepatorenal syndrome. In: Epstein M (ed.) *The Kidney in Liver Disease*. Philadelphia: Hanley & Belfus, pp. 75–108.

36 Papper S, Belsky JL, Bleifer KH (1959) Renal failure in Laennecs cirrhosis of the liver. 1. Description of clinical and laboratory features. *Ann Intern Med* 51 (4), 759–773.

37 Shear L, Kleinerman J, Gabuzda GJ (1965) Renal failure in patients with cirrhosis of the liver. I. Clinical and pathologic characteristics. *Am J Med* 39:184–198.

38 Alessandria C, Ozdogan O, Guevara M et al. (2005) MELD score and clinical type predict prognosis in hepatorenal syndrome: relevance to liver transplantation. *Hepatology* 41 (6), 1282–1289.

39 Rodes J, Arroyo V, Bosch J (1975) Clinical types and drug-therapy of renal impairment in cirrhosis. *Postgrad Med J* 51(598), 492–497.

40 Vesin P (1962) Late functional renal failure in cirrhosis with ascites: pathophysiology, diagnosis and treatment. In: Martinin GA, Sherlock S (eds) *Aktuelle Probleme der Hepatologie*. Stuttgart: Georg Thieme Verlag, pp. 98–109.

41 Maroto A, Ginès A, Salo J et al. (1994) Diagnosis of functional kidney failure of cirrhosis with doppler sonography – prognostic value of resistive index. *Hepatology* 20 (4), 839–844.

42 Guevara M, Ginès P, Fernandez-Esparrach G et al. (1998) Reversibility of hepatorenal syndrome by prolonged administration of ornipressin and plasma volume expansion. *Hepatology* 27 (1), 35–41.

43 Angeli P, Volpin R, Gerunda G et al. (1999) Reversal of type 1 hepatorenal syndrome with the administration of midodrine and octreotide. *Hepatology* 29 (6), 1690–1697.

44 Wong F, Pantea L, Sniderman K (2004) Midodrine, octreotide, albumin, and TIPS in selected patients with cirrhosis and type 1 hepatorenal syndrome. *Hepatology* 40 (1), 55–64.

45 Tristani FE, Cohn JN (1967) Systemic and renal hemodynamics in oliguric hepatic failure: effect of volume expansion. *J Clin Invest* 46 (12), 1894–1906.

46 Moreau R, Durand F, Poynard T et al. (2002) Terlipressin in patients with cirrhosis and type 1 hepatorenal syndrome: a retrospective multicenter study. *Gastroenterology* 122 (4), 923–930.

47 Ortega R, Ginès P, Uriz J et al. (2002) Terlipressin therapy with and without albumin for patients with hepatorenal syndrome: results of a prospective, nonrandomized study. *Hepatology* 36 (4 Pt 1), 941–948.

48 Caregaro L, Menon F, Angeli P et al. (1994) Limitations of serum creatinine level and creatinine clearance as filtration markers in cirrhosis. *Arch Intern Med* 154 (2), 201–205.

49 Papadakis MA, Arieff AI (1987) Unpredictability of clinical evaluation of renal function in cirrhosis – prospective study. *Am J Med* 82 (5), 945–952.

50 Terra C, Guevara M, Torre A et al. (2005) Renal failure in patients with cirrhosis and sepsis unrelated to spontaneous bacterial peritonitis: value of MELD score. *Gastroenterology* 129, 1944–1953.

51 Salerno F, Badalamenti S (2005) Drug-induced renal failure in cirrhosis. In: Arroyo V, Ginès P, Rodes J et al. (eds) *Ascites and Renal Dysfunction in Liver Disease*. Philadelphia: Blackwell Science Malden, pp. 372–382.

52 Guevara M, Fernandez-Esparrach G, Alessandria C et al. (2004) Effects of contrast media on renal function in patients with cirrhosis: a prospective study. *Hepatology* 40 (3), 646–651.

53 Lhotta K (2002) Beyond hepatorenal syndrome: glomerulonephritis in patients with liver disease. *Semin Nephrol* 22 (4), 302–308.

54 Poole B, Schrier RW, Jani A (2005) Glomerular disease in cirrhosis. In: Ginès P, Arroyo V, Rodes J et al. (eds) *Ascites and Renal Dysfunction in Liver Disease*. Malden: Blackwell Publishing, pp. 360–370.

55 Gonwa TA, Morris CA, Goldstein RM et al. (1991) Long-term survival and renal function following liver transplantation in patients with and without hepatorenal syndrome–experience in 300 patients. *Transplantation* 51 (2), 428–430.

56 Rimola A, Navasa M, Grande L et al. (2005) Liver transplantation for patients with cirrhosis and ascites. In: Arroyo V, Ginès P, Rodes J et al. (eds) *Ascites and Renal Dysfunction in Liver Disease*, 2nd edn. Oxford: Blackwell Publishing, pp. 271–285.

57 Wiesner R, Edwards E, Freeman R et al. (2003) Model for end-stage liver disease (MELD) and allocation of donor livers. *Gastroenterology* 124 (1), 91–96.

58 Rimola A, Gavaler JS, Schade RR et al. (1987) Effects of renal impairment on liver transplantation. *Gastroenterology* 93 (1), 148–156.

59 Gonwa TA, Klintmalm GB, Levy M et al. (1995) Impact of pretransplant renal-function on survival after liver-transplantation. *Transplantation* 59 (3), 361–365.

60 Nair S, Verma S, Thuluvath PJ (2002) Pretransplant renal function predicts survival in patients undergoing orthotopic liver transplantation. *Hepatology* 35 (5), 1179–1185.

61 Restuccia T, Ortega R, Guevara M et al. (2004) Effects of treatment of hepatorenal syndrome before transplantation on posttransplantation outcome. A case–control study. *J Hepatol* 40 (1), 140–146.

62 Jeyarajah DR, Gonwa TA, McBride M et al. (1997) Hepatorenal syndrome: combined liver kidney transplants versus isolated liver transplant. *Transplantation* 64 (12), 1760–1765.

63 Uriz J, Ginès P, Cardenas A *et al.* (2000) Terlipressin plus albumin infusion: an effective and safe therapy of hepatorenal syndrome. *J Hepatol* 33 (1), 43–48.

64 Mulkay JP, Louis H, Donckier V *et al.* (2001) Long-term terlipressin administration improves renal function in cirrhotic patients with type 1 hepatorenal syndrome: a pilot study. *Acta Gastroenterol Belg* 64 (1), 15–19.

65 Halimi C, Bonnard P, Bernard B *et al.* (2002) Effect of terlipressin (Glypressin) on hepatorenal syndrome in cirrhotic patients: results of a multicentre pilot study. *Eur J Gastroenterol Hepatol* 14 (2), 153–158.

66 Duvoux C, Zanditenas D, Hezode C *et al.* (2002) Effects of noradrenalin and albumin in patients with type I hepatorenal syndrome: a pilot study. *Hepatology* 36 (2), 374–380.

67 Brensing KA, Textor J, Perz J *et al.* (2000) Long term outcome after transjugular intrahepatic portosystemic stent-shunt in non-transplant cirrhotics with hepatorenal syndrome: a phase II study. *Gut* 47 (2), 288–295.

68 Guevara M, Ginès P, Bandi JC *et al.* (1998) Transjugular intrahepatic portosystemic shunt in hepatorenal syndrome: effects on renal function and vasoactive systems. *Hepatology* 28 (2), 416–422.

69 Wong LP, Blackley MP, Andreoni KA *et al.* (2005) Survival of liver transplant candidates with acute renal failure receiving renal replacement therapy. *Kidney Int* 68 (1), 362–370.

70 Mitzner SR, Stange J, Klammt S, *et al.* (2000) Improvement of hepatorenal syndrome with extracorporeal albumin dialysis MARS: results of a prospective, randomized, controlled clinical trial. *Liver Transpl* 3, 277–286.

71 Moore KP, Wong F, Ginès P *et al.* (2003) The management of ascites in cirrhosis: report on the consensus conference of the International Ascites Club. *Hepatology* 38 (1), 258–266.

72 Alessandria C, Venon WD, Marzano A *et al.* (2002) Renal failure in cirrhotic patients: role of terlipressin in clinical approach to hepatorenal syndrome type 2. *Eur J Gastroenterol Hepatol* 14 (12), 1363–1368.

73 Ginès P, Uriz J, Calahorra B *et al.* (2002) Transjugular intrahepatic portosystemic shunting versus paracentesis plus albumin for refractory ascites in cirrhosis. *Gastroenterology* 123 (6), 1839–1847.

74 Albillos A, Bañares R, Gonzalez M *et al.* (2005) A meta-analysis of transjugular intrahepatic portosystemic shunt versus paracentesis for refractory ascites. *J Hepatol* 43, 990–996.

75 Ginès P *et al.* (2003) Hepatorenal syndrome. *Lancet* 362, 1819–1827.

7.7 Pulmonary complications of portal hypertension

Michael J. Krowka

Introduction

Pulmonary complications of portal hypertension can be grouped broadly into two major categories: pulmonary vascular abnormalities and pleural/diaphragm effects of ascites. The pulmonary vascular abnormalities include hepatopulmonary syndrome, portopulmonary hypertension and pulmonary emboli. Ascites can result in pleural effusions (hepatic hydrothorax) and subsequent effects on pulmonary function test results. This chapter will focus on the clinical presentations, diagnostic essentials and important treatment considerations, especially for liver transplantation candidates, when these pulmonary complications exist.

Pulmonary vascular complications

Hepatopulmonary syndrome (HPS)

First reported by Hoffbauer and Rydell in 1956, the classic triad of chronic liver disease, arterial hypoxaemia on room air and intrapulmonary vascular dilatation characterizes HPS [1]. A consensus statement emanating from a task force co-sponsored by the European Respiratory Society (ERS) and the European Association for the Study of the Liver (EASL) has summarized current thinking regarding diagnosis, epidemiology, pathophysiology and therapeutic advances (Table 1) [2].

Table 1 Diagnostic criteria for hepatopulmonary syndrome (HPS).[a]

---

1. Liver disease (usually portal hypertension)
2. $P_aO_2 < 80$ mmHg or alveolar–arterial oxygen gradient > 15 mmHg
3. Pulmonary vascular dilatation documented by either
   a. 'positive' contrast enhanced transthoracic echocardiogram;[b] or
   b. brain uptake > 6% following lung perfusion scanning with [99mTc] macroaggregated albumin

---

[a]Modified from the ERS–EASL task force report.
[b]Microbubbles were detected in the left atrium between three and six cardiac cycles after visualization of microbubbles in the right atrium.

The clinical presentation of HPS includes dyspnoea and fatigue (manifestations of hypoxaemia at rest, with exertion and during sleep) [2]. The physical examination findings associated with HPS are nail bed and lip cyanosis, as well as skin spider angiomas. Screening for arterial hypoxaemia can be accomplished by either finger pulse oximetry or arterial blood gas analysis. Patients with finger pulse oximetry saturations less than 94% or arterial blood gas $P_aO_2 < 80$ mmHg while breathing room air in the sitting position should undergo testing for pulmonary vascular dilatations [2]. It is common in HPS to document worsening dyspnoea (platypnoea) and arterial oxygen (orthodeoxia) as the patient moves from the supine to sitting to standing position [3]. This phenomenon is presumably due to a combination of decreasing cardiac output and redistribution of blood flow to vascular dilatations in the lung bases as one assumes the standing position.

With the evolution of HPS over months and years, profound hypoxaemia ($P_aO_2 < 50$ mmHg) is not uncommon [3]. Spontaneous resolution of the syndrome with normalization of arterial oxygenation can occur, but is rare. Although varying degrees of hypoxaemia are common (40–50%) in the setting of chronic liver disease, the reported prevalence of this uncommon syndrome as a reason for hypoxaemia has varied as a function of cutoffs for arterial hypoxaemia [4]. Approximately 5% of patients referred annually to the Mayo Clinic liver transplant programme have HPS (using criteria of $P_aO_2 < 70$ mmHg) due to documented pulmonary vascular dilatations by contrast echocardiography [3].

Non-invasive methods used to determine the existence of pulmonary vascular dilatations are based upon the concept of either microbubbles (10–90 μm in diameter) or technetium-labelled macroaggregated albumen ([99mTc]-MAA 20–90 μm in size) traversing dilated pulmonary vessels (> 8 μm) [2,5]. Following peripheral arm vein injection of hand-agitated saline, the microbubbles are created and can be detected in the left heart by transthoracic echocardiography. Similarly, peripherally injected [99mTc]-MAA can be measured over the brain by radionuclide scintigraphy. The echocardiography test is qualitative and more sensitive in detecting pulmonary vascular dilatation than

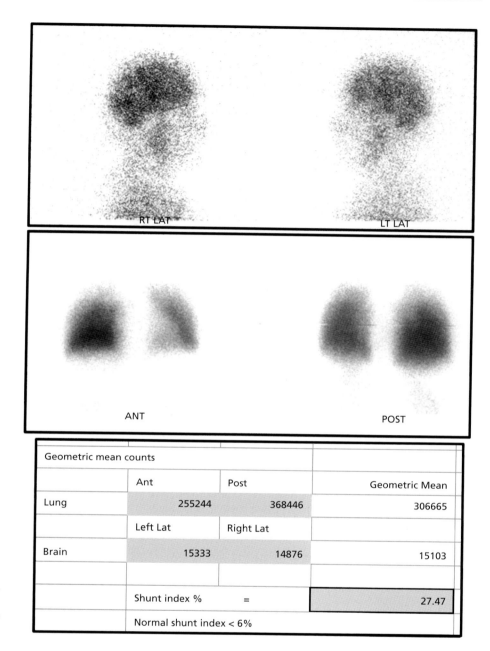

Geometric mean counts			
	Ant	Post	Geometric Mean
Lung	255244	368446	306665
	Left Lat	Right Lat	
Brain	15333	14876	15103
	Shunt index % =		27.47
	Normal shunt index < 6%		

Fig. 1 Lung perfusion scan with ^{99m}Tc-MAA and quantitative measurement of uptake over the brain in a patient with HPS. Abnormal uptake estimated the intrapulmonary shunt to be 27.5% (normal < 6%).

the lung perfusion test [2,5]. However, the lung perfusion study with brain uptake gives a quantitative, reproducible measure of the degree of pulmonary vascular dilatation (Fig. 1).

Pulmonary angiography as a means of documenting (or further characterizing) pulmonary vascular dilatation is not necessary in most cases [3]. However, angiography is advised in HPS patients when the degree of hypoxaemia is severe (P_aO_2 < 50 mmHg) and the response to 100% inspired oxygen is poor (< 300 mmHg). The reason for proceeding to angiography is to identify and treat (with vascular embolization) discrete arteriovenous communications. Such discrete lesions are quite uncommon; most patients with HPS have either normal or diffuse, bilateral spongy lesions noted on pulmonary angiography that are not usually amenable to embolization.

Approximately 20–30% of HPS patients may have other comorbidities that can cause significant hypoxaemia [i.e. ascites, hydrothorax, pneumonia, pulmonary fibrosis and chronic obstructive pulmonary disease (COPD)] [3,6]. The ^{99m}Tc-MAA lung scan is extremely helpful in discerning vascular dilatation (abnormal brain uptake ≥ 6%) vs. non-vascular reasons (normal brain uptake < 6%) for hypoxaemia in the setting of liver disease. This distinction is of clinical importance when discussing expectations of modifying arterial hypoxaemia when liver transplantation is considered.

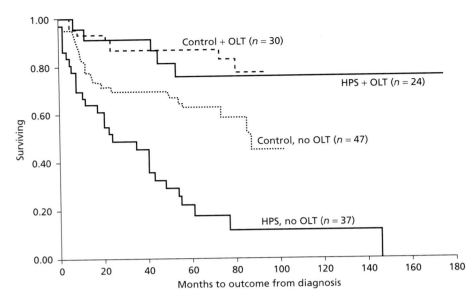

Fig. 2 Survival curves for patients with hepatopulmonary syndrome. Patients who underwent OLT had statistically similar baseline P_aO_2 levels, MELD scores and Child scores compared with those who did not undergo OLT. Survival for HPS patients who did not undergo OLT was significantly worse than for HPS patients who underwent OLT ($P < 0.001$).

Human and animal studies suggest that the pathophysiology of HPS may be related to circulating mediators that result in excess local effects of nitric oxide and bacterial translocation, upregulate pulmonary endothelium endothelin B receptors causing vasodilatation and pulmonary capillary proliferation via angiogenesis [2]. Yet, no proven medical treatments exist for HPS other than nasal cannula oxygen supplementation. There is no proven role for transjugular intrahepatic portosystemic shunts (TIPS). As the definitive treatment for HPS, orthotopic liver transplantation (OLT; cadaveric or living donor) is strongly advised assuming that no other major comorbidities complicate advanced liver disease [7–9]. Complications following OLT are not uncommon and appear to be related to the severity of hypoxaemia prior to transplantation. Some series have reported a 30–38% mortality within 12 months of OLT [5,6] and 16% transplant hospitalization mortality [7,10]. In addition, preliver transplant ^{99m}Tc-MAA lung perfusion scanning with brain uptake > 20% is associated with higher post-OLT mortality [11] However, complete resolution of HPS can occur even in the setting of severe hypoxaemia prior to OLT, and the time to resolution (usually many months) is related to the severity of hypoxaemia.

HPS alone is a risk factor for poor prognosis in patients with cirrhosis [11]. Long-term survival once the diagnosis of HPS has been established is related to the severity of hypoxaemia and whether liver transplantation can be successfully accomplished. The 5-year survivals with and without liver transplantation are 76% vs. 23% respectively. P_aO_2 < 50 mmHg with or without OLT is associated with worse survival compared with P_aO_2 > 50 mmHg (Fig. 2) [13]. Deterioration in P_aO_2 while awaiting OLT (approximately 5–10 mmHg per year) is well documented [13].

Portopulmonary hypertension (POPH)

Beginning with the 1951 report by Mantz and Craige, clinicians have recognized that patients with portal hypertension are predisposed to pulmonary arterial changes indistinguishable from those seen in idiopathic pulmonary artery hypertension [14]. The Venice 2003 Conference on Pulmonary Hypertension recognized POPH as one of the proven reasons for pulmonary artery hypertension [15]. The ERS–EASL consensus report estimated that fewer than 10% of patients referred for liver transplantation had true POPH based upon current right heart catheterization (RHC) diagnostic criteria (Table 2) [2].

Table 2 Diagnostic criteria for portopulmonary hypertension.

1. Presence of portal hypertension (clinical diagnosis)
2. Mean pulmonary artery pressure (MPAP) > 25 mmHg[a]
3. Pulmonary artery occlusion pressure (PAOP) < 15 mmHg[a]
4. Pulmonary vascular resistance (PVR) > 240 dynes/s/cm[5b]

[a]MPAP and PAOP are measured pressures obtained during right heart catheterization (RHC). MPAP is the measured mean arterial pressure of the systolic and diastolic pressures obtained from a distal catheter transducer in the main pulmonary artery. PAOP is the pressure obtained via the distal catheter transducer when the catheter is advanced peripherally with balloon occlusion to impede arterial flow. This measurement provides an estimate of pulmonary venous pressure. Hence, a pressure gradient (MPAP–PAOP) is obtained. Cardiac output (CO) is measured to give an estimate of blood *flow*. The pressure gradient and flow are used to calculate the pulmonary vascular resistance to flow (PVR).

[b]PVR is a calculated number obtained via the following formula (multiplier 80 is used to keep units consistent):

PVR = [(MPAP–PAOP) × 80]/CO

Table 3 Mayo Clinic classification of pulmonary hypertension in the setting of portal hypertension.[a]

Type	MPAP	PAOP	CO	PVR
I. Pulmonary artery high flow state	↑	n or ↓	↑↑	↓
II. Excess pulmonary venous volume	↑	↑	↑	↓
III. Portopulmonary hypertension[b]				
a. pulmonary vascular obstruction; normal volume[c]	↑↑↑	n or ↓	↑	↑↑↑
b. pulmonary vascular obstruction; excess volume	↑↑	↑	↑	↑

[a]Based upon right heart catheterization measurements (MPAP, CO, PAOP) and calculations (PVR).
[b]All patients with portopulmonary hypertension have increased transpulmonary pressure gradients (MPAP–PAOP > 12 mmHg); most will have (a) normal (n) PAOP, but some will have (b) increased PAOP.
[c]PAOP < 15 mmHg.

RHC is essential to make the diagnosis of POPH as there are several reasons for increased pulmonary artery pressures in patients with portal hypertension (Table 3). For example, the high flow–hyperdynamic circulatory state (increased cardiac output) is common in portal hypertension. Such a state frequently results in increased pulmonary artery pressures, yet the actual resistance to flow is normal. In addition, increased central volume may contribute to increased pulmonary artery pressure [16]. It is the patient with increased pulmonary artery pressure (MPAP), increased pulmonary vascular resistance (PVR) to flow and normal central volume (PAOP) who is the most problematic [17]

The clinical presentation of POH includes exertional dyspnoea (the earliest symptom) and later complaints of chest pain, palpitations and even syncope. Signs and symptoms of hypoxaemia are uncommon in POPH [2]. Sudden death due to cardiovascular events is not uncommon. Chest radiographic abnormalities (enlarged central pulmonary arteries and cardiomegaly) and electrocardiogram changes (right ventricle strain with T-wave inversion in the anterior chest leads V1–V4) are late signs of at least moderate to severe POPH [2].

In the early liver transplant era, the diagnosis of POPH was initially made in the operating room in 65% of patients who underwent liver transplant surgery [18]. Subsequent mortality was 36% and was deemed unacceptable, and efforts began to screen all liver transplant candidates for POPH [18]. The American Association for the Study of Liver Diseases (AASLD) now advises transthoracic Doppler echocardiography to screen for pulmonary artery systolic pressures by estimating right ventricular systolic pressures (RVsys) as a practice guideline [19]. Patients with elevated pressures are advised to undergo RHC to confirm the diagnosis of POPH [2,19]. This is crucial for liver transplant candidates. Thresholds for proceeding to RHC have varied, but recent data suggest that up to 34% of those with RVsys > 50 mmHg simply have a high flow state (low calculated PVR at RHC) and do not satisfy accepted criteria for POPH (increased PVR); 66% have the true problem of POPH [20]. The correlation between Doppler echo and RHC pressures worsens when RVsys > 50 mmHg [21,22].

The pathophysiology of POPH is poorly understood. No animal models for POPH exist to date. Intuitively, it is suspected, but not proven, that circulating mediators (such as increased endothelin, a potent vasoconstrictor and stimulus for smooth muscle proliferation) associated with portal hypertension, and mediators resulting from abnormal hepatic metabolism, may initiate the pulmonary endothelium injury [2,23]. Endothelial proliferation, smooth muscle proliferation, *in situ* thromboses, platelet aggregation, vascular remodelling (plexogenic arteriopathy) and subsequent obstruction to pulmonary arterial flow results [2]. The natural history of POPH is that of progressive right heart failure and death. Unlike HPS, spontaneous resolution of POPH has never been reported. The resolution of hepatopulmonary and subsequent development of pulmonary artery hypertension has occurred both spontaneously and following the transplant resolution of HPS [2].

In the current era of liver transplantation, POPH has resulted in intraoperative death and increased transplant hospitalization mortality [17,24]. Multicentre, retrospective analysis evidence indicates that a preoperative MPAP > 35 mmHg serves as a threshold for increased risk of death. MPAP values between 35 and 50 mmHg predispose to a 50% increased risk of death [18]. Some investigators suggest that MPAP values alone should not be considered absolute and, in a recent multicentre study, patients with MPAP > 50 mmHg survived OLT without pre-OLT pulmonary vasodilator therapy; however, very few centres have transplanted patients in this range [10,25]. Despite poor outcomes, persistence of POPH and the *de novo* development of pulmonary artery hypertension after liver transplantation, many case reports of post-OLT improvement in POPH exist [2].

In the pre-OLT and prostacyclin therapy era, mean and median survival following diagnosis was 15 and 6 months, respectively, with half of the deaths related to pulmonary hypertension [26]. In the current OLT era, limited data suggest 5-year survivals of 53% and 28% for POPH patients with and without OLT respectively [26]. Worse survival trends appear to be associated with selected haemodynamic cutoffs such as the transpulmonary gradient (TPG = MPAP–PAOP > 30 mmHg), MPAP (> 50 mmHg) and PVR (> 400 dynes/s/cm^5). The role of living donor OLT in the setting of POPH has yet to be determined [27].

Pre-OLT treatment with continuous intravenous infusions of prostacyclin may confer a survival advantage after OLT [28–31]. However, no large standardized protocols or randomized trials have addressed the issue of which agent may be the optimal pulmonary vasomodulating therapy in the setting of POPH or for those POPH patients considered for OLT. Single case reports and small series do suggest improved pulmonary haemodynamics with the use of newer pulmonary vascular modulating agents such as inhaled prostacyclin (iloprost) [32], dual endothelin receptor antagonists (bosentan) [33–35] and phosphodi-esterase-5 inhibitors (sildenafil) [36]. Long-term survival data collection in cohorts of POPH patients treated with pulmonary vasodilators (with and without OLT) will be informative. It is likely that surrogate measures of right heart function (sequential echocardiography and plasma levels of B-type natriuretic peptide to assess right ventricular strain) will play an important role in patient prognosis and management [2].

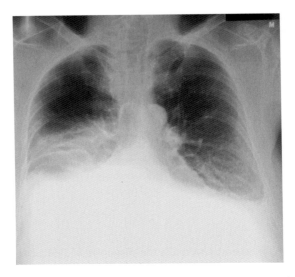

Fig. 3 Hepatic hydrothorax associated with massive ascites. Compressive atelectasis of right lower lobe of the lung resulted in significant hypoxemia (P_aO_2 = 43 mmHg in the supine position).

Pulmonary emboli

Acute or chronic pulmonary emboli in the setting of portal hypertension are rare. Most case reports follow surgical procedures, prolonged bed rest or coagulopathies associated with Budd–Chiari syndrome. Although most patients with advanced liver disease have some component of coagulopathy due to hepatic synthetic dysfunction in synthesizing coagulation factors II, VII, IX and X, the increased risk of deep venous thrombosis and pulmonary embolism rarely exists as a result of inability to produce protein C, protein S and antithrombin III [37]. Post-mortem pulmonary arterial thromboses associated with portopulmonary hypertension are thought to be related to platelet aggregation, *in situ* clot formation due to low flow or emboli that have originated from portosystemic vascular shunts [2,15]. Asymptomatic radiopaque pulmonary emboli following endoscopic injection sclerotherapy for oesophagogastric variceal bleeding can occur. No management interventions are necessary [38].

Pleural/diaphragm effects of ascites

The effects of ascites can lead to clinically significant dyspnoea for two reasons. First, with massive ascites, the upward stretch and displacement of the hemidiaphragms cause a restrictive pulmonary physiology, in which the total lung capacity (TLC) and forced vital capacity (FVC) are reduced [39,40]. Ventilation of the lungs is restricted and dyspnoea follows. Within 2 h of performing large-volume paracentesis in patients with tense ascites, dyspnoea can be ameliorated as the diaphragms move to a more normal position followed by immeasurable, improved ventilatory function [40]. Secondly, when ascitic fluid traverses the hemidiaphragms with any degree of ascites and fills either or both the pleural spaces ('hepatic hydrothorax'), the underlying

lung may become atelectatic, causing a physiological shunt (no ventilation with persistent perfusion) that leads to hypoxaemia (Fig. 3) [41]. The movement of ascitic fluid from the peritoneal cavity to the pleural space is thought to occur via lymphatic drainage and/or small hemidiaphragm anatomical defects. This movement is facilitated by the positive hydrostatic pressure in the peritoneal cavity combined with the negative pleural pressure with inspiration. If necessary to prove the abdominal origin of pleural fluid, scintigraphy can demonstrate the abnormal presence of thoracic activity within 90 min following intraperitoneal injection of ^{99m}Tc-sulphur-colloid radioisotope [41].

Hepatic hydrothorax (occurring in up to 12% of cases with portal hypertension) is usually transudative [low protein, low lactate dehydrogenase (LDH)], yellow in colour and not associated with pain or fever [41]. Chylous effusions (triglyceride levels > 110 mg/dL) are not infrequent [42]. A serum–pleural fluid albumen gradient of > 1.2 g/dL suggests a transudative pleural effusion in the setting of marked diuretic use. Although commonly bilateral, such pleural effusions can be right sided only, left sided only and may occur in the absence of clinical ascites on account of the negative pleural pressure that accompanies each inspiration. Most effusions occupy less than 25% of the hemithorax, but massive pleural effusions can occur causing a cardiac tamponade physiology as a result of collapse of the right ventricle. Infected hepatic hydrothorax (spontaneous bacterial empyema) is associated with 20% mortality without chest tube drainage; approximately 50% of cases are not associated with spontaneous bacterial peritonitis [43]. Aggressive medical management which includes dietary salt restriction and combination diuretics (including spironolactone) frequently reduces the symptoms resulting from hepatic hydrothorax.

Table 4 Summary of therapeutic and liver transplant considerations for hepatopulmonary syndrome (HPS) and portopulmonary hypertension (POPH). UNOS, United Network for Organ Sharing.

	HPS	POPH
High risk for OLT (↑mortality)	$P_aO_2 < 50$ mmHg ^{99m}Tc-MAA brain uptake > 20%	MPAP > 35 mmHg
UNOS 'indication' for OLT	Yes	No
Higher priority for OLT	Yes, if $P_aO_2 < 60$ mmHg	No
Syndrome deterioration awaiting OLT	Yes	Yes
Sudden death due to syndrome	No	25%
5-year survival without OLT	23%	30%
5-year survival with OLT	55%	No data
Pharmacological treatment without OLT prolongs survival	Not proven	Not proven
Pharmacologic treatment prior to OLT helpful	Not proven	Strongly suggested
Intraoperative death	Not reported	Yes
Transplant hospitalization mortality	16%	35%
Post-OLT syndrome resolution	Very common	Extremely variable

Therapeutic and diagnostic transthoracic thoracentesis may be necessary when dyspnoea is debilitating or if the clinical situation suggests neoplasm (pain) or infection within the pleural space (fever with or without pain). Chest tube insertion in the absence of infection for continual pleural fluid drainage is not advised because of the development of renal dysfunction, electrolyte imbalances and infection. Increased mortality in patients with prolonged chest tube drainage (> 5 days) has been associated with increased total bilirubin levels, encephalopathy and Child's C severity of liver disease [44].

When medical management fails, placement of a TIPS can reduce the amount of pleural fluid and improve symptoms in 60–80% of patients with hepatic hydrothorax [45,46]. TIPS can acutely worsen right heart function, but the effects usually improve within weeks [46]. Video-assisted thoracoscopy with hemidiaphragm defect closure can successfully eliminate the accumulation of pleural fluid in selected cases [41]. Refractory hepatic hydrothorax is considered to be an indication for liver transplantation [48].

Implications for liver transplantation

Understanding the distinctions between pulmonary vascular complications of portal hypertension are important, especially when OLT is considered (Table 4). No doubt, a subgroup of HPS patients poses a higher post-transplant risk of mortality (those with $P_aO_2 < 50$ mmHg breathing room air), but syndrome resolution over months is well documented even in those situations. For patients with POPH, the increased cardiopulmonary risk of the transplant procedure itself, transplant hospitalization complications and expected postliver transplant normalization of pulmonary haemodynamics remains problematic. Such patients remain an area of active clinical research with the advent of prospective screening [49] and POPH clinical trials that incorporate new pulmonary vasomodulating drugs. Complete resolution of hepatic hydrothorax and

pulmonary effects of massive ascites can be expected within weeks of successful OLT.

The experience of several liver transplant centres has culminated in the recommendation to obtain chest radiographs, measures of arterial oxygenation (pulse oximetry or arterial blood gases) and sequential screening by transthoracic Doppler echocardiography for any patient being considered for liver transplantation [19]. In selected patients, complete pulmonary function testing should be accomplished: (i) in those with smoking histories and (ii) in any patient whose portal hypertension is associated with an abnormal antitrypsin phenotype.

Summary

Clinically significant pulmonary complications are estimated to occur in 5–10% of patients with portal hypertension. These pulmonary vascular complications result from the downstream effect of absent/excessive blood levels of circulating mediators (HPS and POPH) with poor correlation with the degree of portal hypertension. The pleural/diaphragm complications (hepatic hydrothorax and restrictive lung mechanics) result from direct anatomical effects of ascites production. Importantly, treating hepatic dysfunction (with combinations of diuretics, TIPS and OLT) and using pulmonary vasomodulating drugs (in the case of POPH) may dramatically improve the pulmonary symptoms and enhance survival associated with these complications.

References

1 Rydell R, Hoffbauer FW (1956) Multiple pulmonary atriovenous fistulas in juvenile cirrhosis. *Am J Med* 21, 450–459.

2 Rodrigeuz-Roisin R, Krowka MJ, Fallon MB *et al.* (2004) Pulmonary-hepatic vascular disorders: report of a task force. *Eur Respir J* 24, 861–880.

3 Krowka MJ, Wiseman GA, Burnett OL *et al.* (2000) Hepatopulmonary syndrome: a prospective study of relationships between severity of

liver disease, PaO2 response to 100% oxygen, and brain uptake after (99m)Tc MAA lung scanning. *Chest* 118, 615–624.

4 Schenk P, Fuhrmann V, Madl C *et al.* (2002) Hepatopulmonary syndrome: prevalence and predictive value of various cut offs for arterial oxygenation and their clinical consequences. *Gut* 51, 853–859.

5 Abrams GA, Nanda NC, Dubovsky EV *et al.* (1998) Use of macroaggregated albumin lung perfusion scan to diagnose hepatopulmonary syndrome: a new approach. *Gastroenterology* 114, 305–310.

6 Martinez G, Barbera JA, Navasa M *et al.* (1999) Hepatopulmonary syndrome associated with cardiorespiratory disease. *J Hepatol* 30, 882–889.

7 Krowka MJ, Porayko MK, Plevak D *et al.* (1997) Hepatopulmonary syndrome with progressive hypoxemia as an indication for liver transplantation: case reports and review of the literature. *Mayo Clin Proc* 72, 44–53.

8 Egawa H, Kasahara M, Inomata Y *et al.* (1999) Long-term outcome of living related liver transplantation for patients with intrapulmonary shunting and strategy for complications. *Transplantation* 67, 712–717.

9 Taille C, Cadranel J, Bellocq A *et al.* (2003) Liver transplantation for hepatopulmonary syndrome. A ten-year experience in Paris, France. *Transplantation* 75, 1482–1489.

10 Krowka MJ, Mandell MS, Ramsay MA *et al.* (2004) Hepatopulmonary syndrome and portopulmonary hypertension: a report of the multicenter liver transplant database. *Liver Transpl* 10, 174–182.

11 Arguedas M, Abrams G, Krowka M *et al.* (2003) Prospective evaluation of outcomes and predictors of mortality in patients with hepatopulmonary syndrome undergoing liver transplantation. *Hepatology* 37, 192–197.

12 Schenk P, Schoniger-Hekele M, Fuhrmann V *et al.* (2003) Prognostic significance of the hepatopulmonary syndrome in patients with cirrhosis. *Gastroenterology* 125, 1042–1052.

13 Swanson KL, Wiesner RH, Krowka MJ (2005) Natural history of hepatopulmonary syndrome: impact of liver transplantation. *Hepatology* 41, 1122–1129.

14 Mantz FA, Craige E (1951) Portal axis thrombosis with spontaneous portacaval shunt and resultant cor pulmonale. *Arch Pathol* 52, 91–97.

15 Simmoneau G, Galie N, Rubin LJ *et al.* (2004) Clinical classification of pulmonary hypertension. *J Am Coll Cardiol* 43 (Suppl), 5S–12S.

16 Castro M, Krowka MJ, Schroeder DR *et al.* (1996) Frequency and clinical implications of increased pulmonary artery pressures in liver transplant patients. *Mayo Clin Proc* 71, 543–551.

17 Ramsay M, Simpson B, Nguyen A *et al.* (1997) Severe pulmonary hypertension in liver transplant candidates. *Liver Transpl Surg* 3, 494–500.

18 Krowka MJ, Plevak DJ, Findlay JY *et al.* (2000) Pulmonary hemodynamics and perioperative cardiopulmonary-related mortality in patients with portopulmonary hypertension undergoing liver transplantation. *Liver Transpl* 6, 443–450.

19 Murray KF, Carithers RL (2005) AASLD Practice Guidelines: evaluation of the patients for liver transplantation. *Hepatology* 41, 1407–1432.

20 Krowka MJ, Swanson KL, Frantz RP *et al.* (2006) Portopulmonary hypertension: results of a 10-year screening algorithm. *Hepatology* 44, 1502–1510.

21 Kim W, Krowka M, Plevak D *et al.* (2000) Accuracy of Doppler echocardiography in the assessment of pulmonary hypertension in liver transplant candidates. *Liver Transpl* 6, 453–458.

22 Cotton C, Gandhi S, Vaitkus P *et al.* (2002) Role of echocardiography in detecting portopulmonary hypertension in liver transplant candidates. *Liver Transpl* 8, 1051–1054.

23 Benjaminov FS, Prentice M, Sniderman KW *et al.* (2003) Portopulmonary hypertension in decompensated cirrhosis with refractory ascites. *Gut* 52, 1355–1362.

24 DeWolf AM, Gasior T, Kang Y (1991) Pulmonary hypertension in a patient undergoing liver transplantation. *Transpl Proc* 23, 2000–2110.

25 Starkel P, Vera A, Gunson B *et al.* (2002) Outcome of liver transplantation for patients with pulmonary hypertension. *Liver Transpl* 8, 382–388.

26 Robalino BD, Moodie DS (1991) Association between primary pulmonary hypertension and portal hypertension: analysis of its pathophysiology and clinical, laboratory and hemodynamic manifestations. *J Am Coll Cardiol* 17, 492–498.

27 Swanson KL, McGoon MD, Krowka MJ (2003) Survival in portopulmonary hypertension with the use of intravenous epoprostenol. *Am J Respir Crit Care Med* 167, A683.

28 Plotkin J, Kuo P, Rubin L *et al.* (1998) Successful use of chronic epoprostenol as a bridge to liver transplantation in severe portopulmonary hypertension. *Transplantation* 65, 457–459.

29 Krowka MJ, Frantz RF, McGoon MD *et al.* (1999) Improvement if pulmonary hemodynamics during intravenous epoprostenol (prostacyclin): a study of 15 patients with moderate to severe portopulmonary hypertension. *Hepatology* 30, 641–648.

30 Tan HP, Markowitz JS, Montgomery RA *et al.* (2001) Liver transplantation in patients with severe portopulmonary hypertension treated with preoperative chronic intravenous epoprostenol. *Liver Transpl* 7, 745–749.

31 Minder S, Fischier M, Muelhaupt B *et al.* (2004) Intravenous iloprost bridging to orthotopic liver transplantation in portopulmonary hypertension. *Eur Respir J* 24, 703–707

32 Halank M, Marx C, Miehlke S *et al.* (2004) Use of inhaled iloprost in the treatment of portopulmonary hypertension. *J Gastroenterol* 39, 1222–1223.

33 Hoeper MM, Halank M, Marx G *et al.* (2005) Bosentan for the treatment of portopulmonary hypertension. *Eur Respir J* 25, 502–508.

34 Halank M, Miehlke S, Hoeffken G *et al.* (2004) Use of oral endothelin-receptor antagonist bosentan in the treatment of portopulmonary hypertension. *Transplantation* 77, 1775–1776.

35 Kuntzen C, Gulberg V, Gerbes AL (2005) Use of a mixed endothelin receptor antagonist in portopulmonary hypertension: a safe and effective therapy? *Gastroenterology* 128, 164–168.

36 Makisalo H, Koivusalo A, Vakkuri A *et al.* (2004) Sildenafil for portopulmonary hypertension in a patient undergoing liver transplantation. *Liver Transpl* 10, 945–950.

37 Espiritu JD (2000) Pulmonary embolism in a patient with coagulopathy from end-stage liver disease. *Chest* 117, 924–925.

38 Marco de Lucas E, Fifalgo I, Garcia-Baron PL *et al.* (2004) Radiopaque pulmonary arteries in chest radiology. *J Thorac Imag* 19, 264–266.

39 Angueira CE, Kadakia SC (1994) Effects of large-volume paracentesis on pulmonary function in patients with tense ascites. *Hepatology* 20, 825–828.

40 Chang SCX, Chang HI, Chen FJ *et al.* (1997) Therapeutic effects of diuretics and paracentesis on lung function in patients with non-alcoholic cirrhosis and tense ascites. *J Hepatol* 833–838.

41 Garcia N, Jr, Mihas AA (2004) Hepatic hydrothorax: pathophysiology, diagnosis, and management. *J Clin Gastroenterol* 38, 52–58.

42 Romero S, Martin C, Hernandez L *et al.* (1998) Chylothorax in cirrhosis of the liver: analysis of its frequency and clinical characteristics. *Chest* 114, 154–159.

43 Xiol X, Castellvi JM, Guardiola J *et al.* (1996) Spontaneous bacterial empyema. *Hepatology* 64, 341–351.

44 Liu LU, Haddadin HA, Bodian CA *et al.* (2004) Outcome analysis of cirrhotic patients undergoing chest tube placement. *Chest* 126, 142–148.

45 Gordon FD, Anastopoulus HT, Crenshaw W *et al.* (1997) The successful treatment of refractory hepatic hydrothorax with transjugular intrahepatic portosystemic shunt. *Hepatology* 25, 1366–1369.

46 Boyer T, Haskal (2005) AASLD practice guideline: the role of transjugular intrahepatic portosystemic shunt in the management of portal hypertension. *Hepatology* 41, 386–400.

47 Van der Linden P, Le Moine O *et al.* (1996) Pulmonary hypertension after transjugular intrahepatic shunt: effects on right ventricular function. *Hepatology* 23, 982–987.

48 Jeffries MA, Kazanjian S, Wilson M *et al.* (1998) Transjugular intrahepatic portosystemic shunts and liver transplantation for refractory hepatic hydrothorax. *Liver Transpl Surg* 4, 416–423.

49 Colle I, Moreau R, Godinho E *et al.* (2003) Diagnosis of portopulmonary hypertension in candidates for liver transplantation: a prospective study. *Hepatology* 37, 401–409.

7.8 Hepatic encephalopathy

Dieter Häussinger and Andres T. Blei

Definition and classification

Hepatic encephalopathy, defined in broad terms as changes in neurological function that result from liver disease, encompasses a wide range of neuropsychiatric signs and symptoms that are associated with both acute and chronic liver failure [1–3]. The term is not used when specific liver diseases exhibit discrete neurological findings (e.g. Wilson's disease, Zellweger syndrome or bilirubin encephalopathy in Crigler–Najjar syndrome). Rather, it focuses on the changes in mental state seen in cirrhosis and fulminant hepatic failure. The development of encephalopathy carries important prognostic implications in such patients. In acute liver failure, individuals with deep encephalopathy can succumb from neurological complications such as brain oedema and intracranial hypertension. In cirrhosis, the grade of encephalopathy is one of the five elements included in the Child–Pugh classification, a prognostic tool [4].

Two major alterations underlie the development of encephalopathy in acute and chronic liver disease: on the one hand, hepatic insufficiency and, on the other, portal–systemic shunting, in which the opening of collateral vessels as a result of portal hypertension allows elements in the portal blood to gain access to the systemic circulation. In acute liver failure, liver function is lost while extrahepatic portal–systemic shunting is not present. In patients with cirrhosis and hepatic encephalopathy, the degree of hepatic failure and the extent of portal–systemic shunts are variable. In addition, even with similar degrees of shunting, flow through larger and wider collaterals increases the rate of delivery of substances from the portal blood to the systemic circulation [5]. Still, the separation between liver function and portal–systemic shunting should not be a rigid one as there is an interplay between both elements: extensive and longstanding portal–systemic shunting (seen after a non-selective portocaval anastomosis) can result in liver atrophy, while the ability of the liver with cirrhosis to extract substances from the portal vein decreases with worsening liver function [6]. In acute liver failure, portal blood flowing through a necrotic liver can also be viewed as a total portal–systemic shunt.

These considerations have led to a classification of hepatic encephalopathy that is based on the clinical setting in which symptoms occur (Table 1) [7]. The encephalopathy of acute liver failure shares clinical characteristics with that of cirrhosis, but also exhibits unique features (see below). Although not fully proven, there is agreement that the pathogenesis of hepatic encephalopathy in both conditions has similar underpinnings. In cirrhosis, three major syndromes can be present:

Table 1 Classification of hepatic encephalopathy.

	Hepatic failure	Extrahepatic portal–systemic shunting	Special features
Acute liver failure	Maximal	Absent	Development of brain oedema and intracranial hypertension
Cirrhosis			Low-grade cerebral oedema without overt signs of intracranial hypertension
Episodic encephalopathy	Variable	Variable	Precipitant induced
Persistent encephalopathy	Variable	Generally large	Most often seen after portocaval surgery or TIPS
Minimal encephalopathy	Variable	Variable	Requires neuropsychological/neurophysiological testing

TIPS, transjugular intrahepatic portosystemic shunt.

1 Episodic (precipitant-induced) encephalopathy, commonly seen in the hospital setting, where a superimposed event is a key factor.

2 Persistent (chronic) encephalopathy, seen with extensive portal–systemic shunts and after portocaval shunt surgery or placement of transjugular intrahepatic portosystemic shunt (TIPS).

3 Minimal (subclinical) encephalopathy reflects alterations in cognitive function in patients who clinically exhibit a normal mental state. Its diagnosis requires the use of neuropsychological or neurophysiological testing; many subjects with cirrhosis (up to 70%) appear to exhibit such deficits.

With the advent of surgical techniques to decompress the portal hypertensive territory, the term 'portal–systemic encephalopathy' had been coined to highlight the importance of the anatomical rearrangement [8]. The term can also be applied to patients who exhibit clinical and structural changes in the brain with extensive portal–systemic shunts in the absence of parenchymal liver damage [9], also referred to as type B encephalopathy [7]. Patients with congenital portal-systemic shunts exhibit abnormalities of neuropsychological tests and magnetic resonance spectroscopy (MRS) similar to those observed in liver cirrhosis [10,11].

Pathogenesis

Seldom has an area of hepatology been so full of controversy as the study of the pathogenesis of hepatic encephalopathy. Several hypotheses have been postulated over several decades [12–15]. However, most of these hypotheses, such as the false neurotransmitter hypothesis [16] or the γ-aminobutyric acid (GABA) hypothesis [17,18], could only explain some, but not all, findings in hepatic encephalopathy. The difficulties in obtaining information on human neurochemistry have led to the use of animal models that reproduce some features of the human counterpart but do not replicate the picture in its entirety [19]. As in many other neurological conditions, the response to specific therapeutic measures has been one arbiter of the validity of a postulated hypothesis. However, with the availability of modern techniques of cell and molecular biology, on the one hand, and the advances in human non-invasive brain imaging and quantification. on the other, such as magnetic resonance imaging (MRI) and MRS, positron emission tomography (PET) scanning and magnetencephalography (MEG), considerable progress has been made in the understanding of the pathogenesis of hepatic encephalopathy. Although many questions are still open, the emerging pathogenetic picture largely integrates previous experimental findings with clinical observations. With regard to the latter, pathogenetic concepts need to explain the remarkable dynamics and diversity of encephalopathy symptoms and why episodes of hepatic encephalopathy are precipitated in patients with cirrhosis by very heterogeneous conditions such as drugs, electrolyte disturbances, bleeding, trauma or infections. The following cornerstones for the understanding of the pathogenesis of hepatic encephalopathy will be reviewed, before an attempt is made to integrate this knowledge into a pathogenetic picture:

1 ammonia and other circulating neurotoxins;
2 neuroanatomical changes;
3 brain water homeostasis;
4 neurotoxins, astrocyte swelling and astrocyte function;
5 oxidative and nitrosative stress;
6 energy metabolism;
7 alterations in neurotransmission; and
8 disturbances of oscillatory networks in the brain.

Ammonia and other circulating neurotoxins

In the 1950s, it was postulated that the liver synthesizes compounds that are critical for brain function, such as cytidine and uridine [20]. From this perspective, hepatic encephalopathy could be viewed as arising from the lack of production of such compounds by a diseased liver. However, experimental and clinical evidence does not support this concept. Cross-perfusion experiments in a rat model of hepatic liver failure showed that depuration of its blood through a normal liver is far more critical for an adequate mental state than the provision of liver-derived blood from a normal animal [21]. For many years, the controversy has centred around the nature of gut-derived toxins. The clinical evidence that supports the existence of such toxins can be surmised from the response to therapy in cirrhosis. They are of nitrogenous origin, as witnessed by the precipitation of encephalopathy with different nitrogenous substances [22]. While constipation can precipitate encephalopathy, increased catharsis is a cornerstone of treatment. The main source of this activity appears to be the colon, as drugs that act at that level (non-absorbable disaccharides) are used to improve mental state. Intestinal bacteria appear to be involved in the generation of the toxins, as non-absorbable antibiotics (e.g. neomycin) are used therapeutically. The toxins must be present in high concentrations in portal blood, as the construction of a portocaval anastomosis can precipitate encephalopathy. Several gut-derived neurotoxins have been implicated, of which ammonia plays a key role.

Ammonia

In the early 1930s, it had already been noted that ammonia salts would induce neurological changes in patients with cirrhosis [23]. A role for ammonia in the pathogenesis of encephalopathy has been evaluated extensively over many years, and much is known about its metabolism and mode of action.

Ammonia is generated in the intestine via two major mechanisms: as a result of the breakdown of urea by bacteria in the colonic lumen and from the metabolism of glutamine by small bowel mucosa [24]. It is absorbed via non-ionic diffusion and exhibits a high concentration in the portal vein, almost 10-fold higher than arterial levels [6]. In the liver, both portal-derived ammonia and that derived from amino acid metabolism are taken up by periportal hepatocytes and used as a substrate for urea synthesis, in a reaction that exhibits a low affinity but a high capacity for ammonia metabolism. In downstream perivenous hepatocytes, ammonia combines with glutamate to form glutamine, a reaction catalysed by glutamine synthetase and exhibiting a high affinity but a low capacity for ammonia metabolism [25]. The cells that contain glutamine synthetase have been termed perivenous scavenger cells [26], because they eliminate with high affinity the ammonia not used by the upstream urea-synthesizing compartment. They are of crucial importance for the maintenance of non-toxic ammonia levels in the hepatic vein: selective damage of perivenous scavenger cells does not impair upstream urea synthesis, but leads to hyperammonaemia due to a failure of scavenger function [27]. The net effect of the two metabolic systems in series is a tight control of the levels of ammonia in the hepatic vein (see Chapter 2.3.7).

In patients with cirrhosis, multiple mechanisms contribute to the development of hyperammonaemia. The absorption rate from the intestine may be higher in view of the increased splanchnic inflow seen in the portal hypertensive state [28]. In view of the high hepatic extraction of ammonia, portal–systemic shunts, both extra- and intrahepatic, will result in an increased systemic bioavailability. A reduction in hepatic mass will decrease the capacity to synthesize urea [29] and glutamine [30]. Furthermore, extrahepatic sites also contribute to the development of hyperammonaemia. The synthesis of glutamine in muscle, an important alternative site for ammonia metabolism,[24,31], may be decreased in patients who lose muscle mass, a common finding in advanced cirrhosis with ascites. Generation of ammonia by the kidney may be increased in the face of respiratory alkalosis, an alteration that arises from primary hyperventilation seen in cirrhosis [32], and as a result of potassium deficiency [33], a frequent finding in cirrhosis irrespective of the use of diuretic therapy.

Studies using $^{13}NH_3$-PET scanning have shown an increased uptake of circulating ammonia into the brain in patients with cirrhosis, [34] and the increased permeability–surface product seen on PET scanning suggests that either the blood–brain barrier is more permeable to ammonia or an increased capillary surface is present, a finding that could be explained by cerebral vasodilatation and increased cerebral blood flow. Ammonia uptake by the brain may involve aquaporin 9, which is expressed in astrocytes [35] and was shown to mediate NH_3 and/or NH_4^+ uptake [36]. Ammonia taken up by the brain is trapped, at least in part, by glutamine synthesis, as evidenced by high glutamine signals in ^{1}H-MRS derived from the brain in patients with cirrhosis [37–39] and those with acute liver failure [40–41]. Ammonia-induced glutamine accumulation in the brain is probably one major event in the development of cerebral oedema in patients with hepatic encephalopathy (see below) [38,42,43]. Measurements of glutamine in the cerebrospinal fluid (CSF) of patients with hepatic encephalopathy correlate reasonably well with the degree of alteration in the mental state [44].

Once inside neural tissue, ammonia may exert deleterious effects at many levels [45–46]. Brain glucose and energy metabolism may be affected [47–51]. Specific alterations may be present in neurons, astrocytes and the interactions between both cell types [52,53]. Direct effects on cortical neurons include inhibition of chloride extrusion, affecting postsynaptic inhibitory potentials [54]. In addition, ammonia may decrease the activity of the tricarboxylic acid cycle via inhibition of α-ketoglutarate dehydrogenase [55]. The multiple effects of ammonia on astrocytes, which also involve changes in astrocyte hydration, morphology and the generation of oxidative/nitrosative stress, are discussed below.

A wide range of medical disorders that affect mental state are also associated with hyperammonaemia. These include urea cycle enzyme deficiencies, Reye syndrome and toxicity from drugs such as sodium valproate [53]. Medications that reduce ammonia levels (e.g. lactulose or sodium benzoate) or increase the activity of the urea cycle (zinc, ornithine–aspartate) have been reported to improve the altered mental state in all these conditions, including hepatic encephalopathy.

Although ammonia is widely accepted as a key factor in the pathogenesis of hepatic encephalopathy, hyperammonaemia cannot be equated with hepatic encephalopathy. Not all ammonium salts induce encephalopathy. Overt seizures, common in congenital hyperammonaemias [53], are seldom observed in subjects with cirrhosis and hepatic encephalopathy. The lack of correlation between circulating ammonia levels and the degree of encephalopathy has been a classic criticism; however, in the presence of an increased passage of ammonia into the brain, as seen in humans with hyperammonaemia [34], a direct relationship between blood and brain levels need not necessarily be present. A recent study showed a better correlation between mean values of PNH_3 and stages of encephalopathy [56], not confirmed by other authors [57].

Other neurotoxins

Other products of colonic bacterial metabolism may act synergistically with ammonia to aggravate encephalopathy. In experimental animals receiving intravenous doses of ammonia, the administration of mercaptans, such as methanethiol and dimethyldisulphide, reduced the dose of ammonia that resulted in coma [58]. Mercaptans are sulphur-containing products of methionine metabolism and have been implicated in the genesis of fetor hepaticus, a unique odour detected in the breath of encephalopathic patients. In one study, there was no relationship between the levels of methanethiol and the presence of encephalopathy [59]. However, administration of methionine to patients with cirrhosis can result in an altered mental state [60]. The mechanisms by which mercaptans may affect brain function have not been studied extensively. Phenols, derived from the catabolism of phenylalanine and tyrosine, are another category of compounds that may affect mental state [61]; their role is uncertain. Likewise, the role of indoles, which originate from bacterial tryptophan metabolism, remains to be settled.

Oxindol has neurodepressive effects [62], and its plasma levels are increased in acute liver failure in experimental animals [63].

Short-chain and medium-chain fatty acids may also potentiate the effects of ammonia on the brain [64]. Production of octanoic acid and C_3–C_5 short-chain fatty acids (such as propionate, butyrate and valerate) is reduced with therapy of hepatic encephalopathy using non-absorbable disaccharides [65].

Infections may synergistically modulate ammonia effects on the brain [66] in line with the longstanding experience that infections can trigger or exacerbate episodes of hepatic encephalopathy in patients with cirrhosis. Increased levels of inflammatory cytokines such as tumour necrosis factor α (TNFα), interleukin-1 and -6, oxidative stress and haemodynamic alterations may underlie this condition [67], as in sepsis-associated encephalopathy [68]. A relationship between plasma TNFα levels and the severity of hepatic encephalopathy was reported in cirrhotics [69].

Amino acid-derived neurotoxins may also be generated within the brain tissue itself. An increased transfer of neutral amino acids, such as phenylalanine and tryptophan, across the blood–brain barrier has been observed in experimental models [70]. It was explained by an increased exchange with glutamine [71], coupled with a plasma amino acid imbalance characterized by elevated plasma levels of aromatic amino acids (phenylalanine, tyrosine), but decreased levels of branched-chain amino acids [72] in chronic liver disease [73]. It was hypothesized that, in the presence of high aromatic amino acid levels in the brain, 'false neurotransmitters' such as octopamine, tyramine and β-phenylethanolamine are increasingly synthesized. However, measurements of brain catecholamines in postmortem samples from cirrhotic patients have shown a decrease in brain octopamine with normal noradrenaline/adrenaline (norepinephrine/epinephrine) values [74], and an increased entry of aromatic amino acids into brain was not confirmed in a group of patients with cirrhosis [75]. Also, clinical attempts at re-establishing the normal plasma aromatic/branched-chain amino acid ratio, which is also seen in patients without encephalopathy, have given inconclusive results.

Like the false neurotransmitter hypothesis, the 'gut-derived GABA hypothesis', proposed in the early 1980s [17,18] has essentially been abandoned. According to this view, GABA, a potent inhibitory neurotransmitter, which can also be generated within the intestine from the decarboxylation of glutamate, would gain access to the brain in the presence of liver failure and/or portal–systemic shunting and induce neuroinhibition after binding to GABA receptors, whose number is increased. Many tenets of this hypothesis have been refuted, as methodological problems were identified with regard to the measurements of GABA receptor density [76] and determination of GABA in plasma, hampered by cross-reactivity with other amino acids [77]. Furthermore, an increased permeability of the normally impermeable blood–brain barrier to GABA was not found in all animal models [78], and no alterations in GABA levels [79] or binding [80] were seen in human postmortem brain tissue.

Nonetheless, an alteration in GABAergic neurotransmission may still be present in hepatic encephalopathy. An increased concentration of compounds that bind to the GABA receptor (but not GABA itself) have been described in the plasma, CSF and brain of patients with acute and chronic liver failure [81]. These compounds have been termed 'endogenous' or 'natural' benzodiazepines, as they cross-react in a benzodiazepine radioreceptor assay but do not appear to exhibit the structure of this group of pharmacological agents. Animals without any lifetime exposure to exogenous benzodiazepines also have measurable levels of this activity [82,83]. A small fraction corresponds to known benzodiazepine compounds [84], but the source and nature of the greater fraction are unclear. It has been proposed that precursors of these compounds are produced by specific intestinal micro-organisms [85]. More recently, neurosteroids with positive allosteric modulatory properties at the $GABA_A$ receptor complex were identified in brain from patients with hepatic coma [86]. Animal studies showed that the synthesis of pregnenolone, which is a precursor of neurosteroids, is increased in hyperammonaemia and acute liver failure, probably as the result of activation of peripheral benzodiazepine receptors [87,88]. Ammonia may also synergistically interfere with GABAergic neurotransmission by increasing GABA-induced chloride currents in cultured neurons, ligand binding to the GABA receptor complex and inhibition of GABA uptake by astrocytes [89].

Neuroanatomical changes

With the exception of brain oedema, the brain of patients dying from acute liver failure in hepatic coma is surprisingly devoid of gross abnormalities. The only consistent change is the diffuse hyperplasia of astrocytes of the cerebral cortex, subcortical nuclei (such as the dentate and lenticular nucleus) and other brainstem nuclei [52]. Other parenchymal structures are minimally involved. In animal models of fulminant hepatic failure, astrocyte swelling (Fig. 1a) is a prominent pathological feature in practically all preparations [19,90,91]. Morphometric studies in patients with cirrhosis dying in hepatic coma indicate an increase in the size of astrocyte nuclei [92]. A characteristic appearance, the so-called Alzheimer type 2 astrocyte [93], is commonly observed in brains examined after immersion–fixation (Fig. 1b). It is characterized by enlarged pale nuclei with peripheral margination of chromatin and often prominent nucleoli. Human retinal glial cells undergo similar changes [94]. The changes can be reproduced in the experimental setting after administration of ammonia [95], and appear to be related to ammonia itself, as they can still be detected after inhibition of ammonia detoxification with methionine–sulphoximine, an inhibitor of glutamine synthetase [96]. They are also seen in congenital hyperammonaemic conditions [97]. Coupled with other evidence of astrocyte pathology, such as loss of glial fibrillary acidic protein, an intermediate filament [98,99], these changes highlight the need to consider a dysfunction of

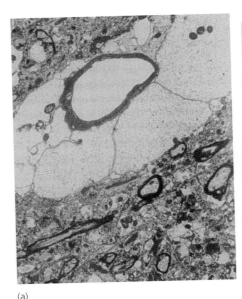

(a)

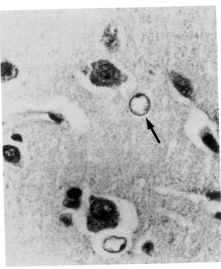

(b)

Fig. 1 Alterations in astrocytic morphology in liver failure. (a) Hydropic foot processes of astrocytes surround a cerebral capillary from the cerebral cortex in a rabbit with galactosamine-induced fulminant hepatic failure (courtesy of Dr Mauro dal Canto, Northwestern University). (b) An Alzheimer type 2 astrocyte (arrow), with a large nucleus and its chromatin displaced to the side (courtesy of Dr Roger Butterworth, Université de Montreal, Canada).

this cell in any theory of the pathogenesis of encephalopathy [100].

Cortical atrophy can be seen on neuroradiological imaging [101,102], but may also reflect the additive effects of alcohol, ageing or other non-liver-related processes. It is viewed as a minor player, if any, in the symptomatology of hepatic encephalopathy. Discrete macroscopic changes can be detected in the so-called hepatocerebral degeneration [103]. This entity is characterized by a patchy but diffuse, spongy degeneration of the cortex, in which, histologically, neuronal degeneration of the deep cortical layer can be observed. Microcavitation can be seen in the striatum [104], a lesion that is also observed in Wilson's disease, and hence the term 'acquired hepatolenticular degeneration' is also used to define this condition. This is a feature of longstanding portal–systemic shunting, and can be seen many years after portocaval shunt surgery. Very rarely, spinal demyelination can occur after shunt surgery, with a symmetrical and variable loss of axons beginning in the spinal cord and becoming more conspicuous at lower levels. It predominates in the lateral pyramidal tracts and can give rise to a syndrome of spastic paraparesis [105].

More recently, MRI has raised the possibility that abnormalities of the basal ganglia may be more widespread than previously thought. A symmetrical hyperintense globus pallidus (Fig. 2) on T1-weighted MR spin echo sequences can be observed in more than 70% of stable subjects with cirrhosis, even without evidence of encephalopathy [106,107]. It has been related to plasma ammonia levels, portal–systemic shunting and liver function [108–110]. It persists (at least) over a 2-year period [111] and is reversible after hepatic transplantation. Quantitative T1 mapping with partial inversion recovery showed a relationship between T1 in the globus pallidus and the severity of hepatic encephalopathy; however, the signal is affected by both man-

ganese and cerebral water content in opposite directions [112]. Direct measurements of the human brain at autopsy indicate that the accumulation of manganese could explain the hyperintensity seen on MR [113,114]. Manganese intoxication is a discrete neurological entity characterized by the development of similar changes in basal ganglia [115]. Manganese is neurotoxic, and possible pathogenic mechanisms include oxidative stress and excitotoxicity [116,117], inhibition of glutamate uptake in cultured astrocytes [118] and upregulation of binding sites for peripheral benzodiazepine receptor ligands [119]. In liver disease, portal–systemic shunting and biliary excretory failure could contribute to hypermanganesaemia [110,120]. The reasons for selective brain deposition of manganese are unclear, although a recent study suggests that hyperintensity seen at MR may be more widespread than a sole change in basal ganglia [121].

Brain water homeostasis

Whereas cerebral oedema is a frequent complication of fulminant liver failure [122], patients with cirrhosis and hepatic encephalopathy usually show no clinical signs of overt cerebral oedema and increased intracranial pressure, except for a few cases at the terminal stage [123]. Nonetheless, recent evidence suggests the presence of a low-grade cerebral oedema (without clinically overt signs of increased intracranial pressure) in patients with cirrhosis, which is even found in minimal hepatic encephalopathy and is considered to be of pathogenetic relevance [38–42]. The first indication for the presence of a low-grade cerebral oedema in patients with cirrhosis was derived from ^{1}H-MRS studies on the human brain *in vivo*, which identified the myoinositol signal as reflecting an osmosensitive myoinositol pool [38]. The brain from patients with hepatic

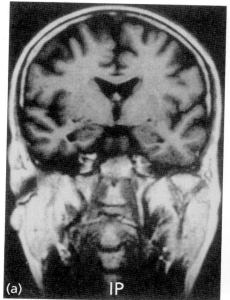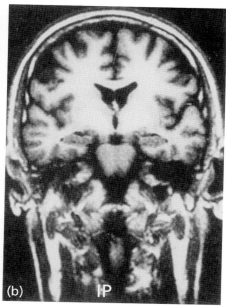

Fig. 2 Radiological alterations in cirrhosis. MR examination of a normal control subject (a) is compared with that of a cirrhotic individual (b), with conspicuous changes in the area of the basal ganglia. A hyper-resonant globus pallidus is seen (reproduced from ref. 108, with permission).

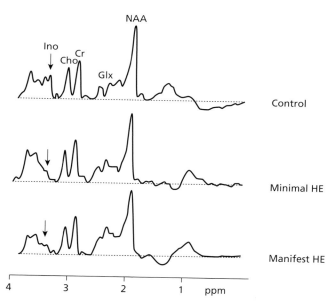

Fig. 3 Parietal ¹H-MR spectra from a healthy person (control) and patients with posthepatitic cirrhosis and minimal hepatic encephalopathy (HE) or manifest grade I–II HE. Note the decrease in myoinositol (Ino) signal and the increase in the glutamine/glutamate (Glx) signal. Other peaks refer to choline (Cho), creatine (Cr) and N-acetylaspartate (NAA) (reproduced from ref. 38, with permission).

explained, at least in part, by an osmotically active intracellular accumulation of glutamine in response to hyperammonaemia and counteraction of the resulting astrocyte swelling by myoinositol depletion. In addition to myoinositol, other organic osmolytes such as taurine and α-glycerophosphorylcholine are also depleted in order to counteract astrocyte swelling [127,129,130]. However, ammonia-induced glutamine accumulation may not be the only mechanism by which astrocyte swelling is triggered in hepatic encephalopathy. Astrocyte swelling occurs *in vitro* not only under the influence of ammonia in a methionine–sulphoximine-sensitive way [131], but also in response to hyponatraemia [132,133], some neurotransmitters [132,134,135], cytokines [136] and benzodiazepines [137]. The above-mentioned ¹H-MRS findings are also induced in the rat following porto-caval shunting [138], are aggravated following institution of a TIPS [38] and largely normalize following liver transplantation [139,140]. There is a good correlation between the extent of these ¹H-MRS changes and the clinical severity of hepatic encephalopathy (Fig. 3) [124]. The existence of a low-grade cerebral oedema in patients with cirrhosis *in vivo* was meanwhile confirmed in studies on magnetization transfer ratios [140–141] and by quantitative cerebral water mapping based on a new MRI method for fast quantitative mapping of T1 and water content (see the chapter by Shah in ref. 3).

Whereas hepatic encephalopathy in patients with cirrhosis is characterized by a low-grade cerebral oedema without clinical signs of a rise in intracranial pressure, the development of severe brain swelling in acute liver failure is frequent and a major complication. Brain oedema in acute liver failure is thought to involve cytotoxic and vasogenic components. A cytotoxic (or cellular) oedema results from an increase in intracellular osmolarity, and sodium and glutamine have been proposed as possible osmolytes. In the case of sodium, circulating inhibitors

encephalopathy consistently shows a depletion of this osmolyte (myoinositol) pool, which is accompanied by an increase in the glutamine/glutamate signal (Fig. 3) [38,124–126]. In view of the role of myoinositol as an organic osmolyte in astrocytes [127,128], these MRS findings suggested a disturbance of astrocyte volume homeostasis in the brain [43], supportive of a cellular (cytotoxic, but not vasogenic) oedema. This can be

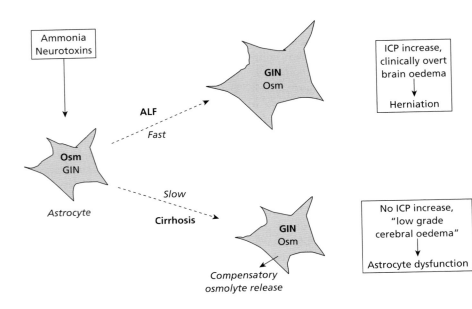

Fig. 4 Astrocyte volume homeostasis. Astrocyte swelling in acute liver failure (ALF) involves intracellular glutamine (GLN) accumulation, which is accompanied by an insufficient compensatory osmolyte release. Severe brain oedema with clinical signs of intracranial pressure (ICP) increase can develop. Glutamine also accumulates in the astrocytes of cirrhotic patients, but only a clinically inapparent low-grade cerebral oedema without signs of ICP increase develops due to a volume-regulatory osmolyte release. However, the mild increase in astrocyte water content may trigger astrocyte dysfunction.

of Na^+-K^+ATPase activity [142], whose presence can be determined indirectly, would enter brain tissue and prevent the exit of intracellular sodium. However, the existence of such inhibitors is controversial, and inhibition of brain Na^+-K^+ATPase has not been demonstrated convincingly in animal models. On the other hand, there is little doubt that the accumulation of glutamine, especially in astrocytes, plays a major role. Glutamine accumulation in the brain has been demonstrated in human postmortem tissue [79,143]. Inhibition of glutamine synthesis in animals infused with ammonia prevents the development of brain oedema [144,145]. There is clinical evidence that other acute conditions, such as chemotherapy-associated hyperammonaemia, are associated with brain swelling [146]. Interestingly, ^{1}H-MRS revealed that cerebral glutamine accumulation in acute liver failure was associated with unchanged myoinositol levels [141], while an increase in glutamine and a reduction in myoinositol are characteristic features of MRS in cirrhosis [37,38]. This suggests that, in contrast to the situation in liver cirrhosis, a compensatory osmolyte efflux in response to intracellular glutamine accumulation is compromised in the patient with acute liver failure, which results in more severe brain swelling (Fig. 4). The reasons underlying this difference between chronic and acute liver failure are unclear, but they may relate to different kinetics and time requirements of intracerebral glutamine accumulation, on the one hand, and the onset of volume-regulatory adaptations, on the other.

A vasogenic component ('vasogenic' oedema) would imply a disrupted blood–brain barrier. However, indirect evidence suggests that a gross disruption, as in cerebral tumours or trauma, is not seen in acute liver failure. Computerized tomography (CT) shows minimal changes [147] or, when present, subtle but diffuse changes in the cerebral cortex [148]; patchy involvement of both grey and white matter is noted in areas where the blood–brain barrier is broken. Brain biopsies of patients who had died with brain oedema showed intact tight junctions in the capillary endothelial cells [149]. On the other hand, there is evidence in experimental models of alterations of blood–brain barrier permeability towards the end of their clinical course [19]. It is unclear whether these arise from specific alterations in endothelial cell function or from changes in the cerebral circulation.

The fact that hepatic encephalopathy is associated with astrocyte swelling in both acute and chronic liver disease and that astrocytes are targets of neurotoxin action makes this cell type a central element in the pathogenesis of hepatic encephalopathy.

Neurotoxins, astrocyte swelling and astrocyte function

Astrocytes are the most abundant cellular element in the brain [150,151]. Their name reflects their stellar-like anatomy, with a small cellular body and extensive foot processes that surround capillary endothelial cells and neurons as well as axons. Functionally, this anatomical arrangement results in several key roles: neuronal function is optimized by controlling the extracellular environment (via mechanisms for the uptake of critical compounds such as CO_2, potassium and glutamate) [152,153]. Furthermore, astrocytes are components of the blood–brain barrier, which does not exhibit signs of gross disruption in liver disease [91,149,154]; however, alterations in distinct transport processes may be present [75]. Astrocytes also affect the function of the endothelial cells; in isolated preparations, coculturing with astrocytes allows endothelial cells to express blood–brain barrier properties, such as impermeable tight junctions [155]. Astrocytes are the only cellular elements containing glutamine synthetase, the sole mechanism that the brain possesses to detoxify ammonia [156].

Neurotoxin-induced alterations in astrocyte function have been studied in cultured astrocytes and experimental animals. Such alterations may be induced directly by neurotoxins and/or indirectly by the astrocyte swelling triggered by such neurotoxins. Changes in the cellular water content, i.e. cell hydration or the degree of cell swelling, have been identified in recent years as an independent signal that regulates function and gene expression through osmosensing and osmosignalling pathways in almost every cell type [157,158]. Thus, small increases in astrocyte water content, present in hepatic encephalopathy, may have important functional consequences despite the absence of clinically overt increases in intracranial pressure. Many, but not all, effects of ammonia on cultured astrocytes can be mimicked by swelling the astrocytes slightly in hypo-osmotic media. Like ammonia exposure, hypo-osmotic swelling of astrocytes activates extracellularly regulated protein kinases [132], upregulates the peripheral-type benzodiazepine receptor (PBR) [159], elevates the intracellular calcium concentration [160], affects multiple ion channels and amino acid transport [161] and increases the pH in endocytotic vesicles [162], i.e. a compartment that is involved in receptor/ligand sorting. Also, the increased deposition of glycogen in astrocytes in animal models of chronic hepatic encephalopathy can be explained by cell swelling [163]. Hyperammonaemia depresses glucose consumption in rat brain [164]. This and other metabolic effects of ammonia intoxication were shown to depend upon ammonia-induced glutamine synthesis, but not upon the presence of ammonia *per se* [165,166]. This points to a critical role for ammonia-induced astrocyte swelling, because inhibition of glutamine synthesis prevents ammonia-induced astrocyte swelling (see the chapter by Norenberg in ref. 167). Both ammonia and hypo-osmotic astrocyte swelling activate *N*-methyl-D-aspartate (NMDA) receptors and induce oxidative/nitrosative stress (see below). Astrocyte swelling leads to a release of cellular taurine, which has antioxidant properties. Taurine was shown to induce longlasting enhancement of corticostriatal neurotransmission [168], and taurine depletion may therefore affect synaptic plasticity [169]. Further, taurine depletion in mice was shown to upregulate GABA$_A$ receptors in various brain regions [170], and increased GABAergic tone may be found in the brain of patients with hepatic encephalopathy.

However, not all ammonia effects on astrocytes are triggered by ammonia-induced cell swelling. For example, ammonia, but not hypo-osmotic exposure, induces haem oxygenase-1 expression in cultured astrocytes [171]. An increased haem oxygenase-1 expression was also found in the brains from ammonia-intoxicated [171] and portocaval-shunted rats [172] and may play a role in the pathogenesis of cerebral hyperaemia found in acute liver failure, through the increased formation of the vasodilator carbon monoxide [173].

Genechip studies have revealed profound effects of ammonia and portocaval shunting on gene expression in astrocytes and the cerebral cortex. The genes involved comprise components of signal transduction, antiapoptosis, oxidative stress defence and genes for various receptor and transport systems [172]. Ammonia effects on the expression of glutamate transport systems were studied in detail. Ammonia downregulates the astrocytic glutamate transporters GLAST and GLT-1 [174,175] and the activity of the neuronal glutamate transporter EAAT3 [176]. Thus, acute ammonia intoxication inhibits glutamate uptake and contributes to the established increase in extracellular brain glutamate, which may be responsible for hyperexcitability in acute liver failure or acute ammonia intoxication.

Ammonia impairs axonal growth in cultured embryonic rat brain cell aggregates, a finding not observed in mature cultures [177,178]. This disturbance is accompanied by a decrease in phosphocreatine and creatine, and is prevented by creatine supplementation. Such phenomena may contribute to the irreversible neurological damage that is observed in inborn hyperammonaemic syndromes, such as urea cycle defects.

Oxidative and nitrosative stress

A role for oxidative and nitrosative stress in the pathogenesis of hepatic encephalopathy is largely derived from *in vitro* and animal studies, whereas little direct evidence is available in humans. Indirect support arises from some beneficial therapeutic measures in hepatic encephalopathy that exhibit antioxidant properties together with the increased amounts of lipofuscin in the brains from patients who died with hepatic encephalopathy [133,179]. In cultured astrocytes, ammonia induces an oxidative stress response [180,181], which is also seen when astrocytes undergo hypo-osmotic swelling [182] or are treated with benzodiazepines [183] or inflammatory cytokines such as TNFα or interferons (newly published [406]). These oxidative stress responses are mediated by an activation of NMDA receptors, but the exact mechanism of this activation is unclear [133]. Possibilities include a swelling-induced glutamate release from astrocytes and a deinhibition of NMDA receptors due to a depolarization-induced Mg^{2+} removal. There is a close relationship between astrocyte swelling, NMDA receptor activation and oxidative stress. On the one hand, astrocyte swelling induces oxidative stress through an NMDA receptor and Ca^{2+}-dependent mechanism [182] and, on the other, NMDA receptor activation triggers astrocyte swelling [184]. This points to an autoamplification signalling loop allowing mutual amplification of cell swelling and oxidative stress [133]. Ammonia and astrocyte swelling also induce nitrosative stress, probably through an NMDA receptor and Ca^{2+}/calmodulin-dependent activation of constitutive nitric oxide synthases (NOS). In addition, in cultured astrocytes, ammonia (but not hyponatraemia) upregulates inducible NOS [181]. Increased cerebral NO formation may contribute to cerebral vasodilatation after ammonia intoxication [122], and a pathogenetic role for ammonia-induced oxidative/nitrosative stress is suggested by the finding that NMDA receptor antagonists and inhibitors of NOS ameliorate ammonia toxicity in animal models [185–187].

One consequence of oxidative/nitrosative stress induced by ammonia, astrocyte swelling, benzodiazepines and inflammatory cytokines is a covalent modification of tyrosine residues in astrocytic proteins through nitration in the 3-position of the aromatic ring. Protein tyrosine nitration (PTN) in astrocytes is also found *in vivo* in ammonia-intoxicated or portocaval-shunted rats [181]. Astrocytes located near the blood–brain barrier exhibit especially high levels of PTN. Peroxynitrite is involved in ammonia- and swelling-induced PTN [182], whereas benzodiazepine-induced PTN involves activation of the peripheral, but not the central, benzodiazepine receptor (PBR) [183]. Ammonia, benzodiazepines, inflammatory cytokines and swelling synergistically promote PTN in astrocytes [133]. PTN does not appear to be an unselective process, because only distinct proteins undergo PTN. Among these, glutamine synthetase, PBR, glyceraldehyde-3 phosphate dehydrogenase and the extracellular signal-regulated kinase Erk-1 were identified [181]. 3-Nitrotyrosines in proteins are poor substrates for tyrosine phosphorylation reactions with impairment of signal transduction cascades that depend on reversible tyrosine phosphorylation [188–90]. PTN of glutamine synthetase involves the catalytic centre of the enzyme [191] and is associated with its inactivation [181]. Although PTN interferes with enzyme activities and signal transduction, its role in the pathogenesis of hepatic encephalopathy is unclear, although inhibition of ammonia-induced PTN by NMDA receptor antagonists, inhibitors of glutamine synthetase or NOS is associated with an amelioration of ammonia toxicity in animals.

Also, a diminished oxidant defence may contribute to the ammonia-induced oxidative stress. Astrocyte swelling leads to the release of taurine, and ammonia downregulates Cu/Zn-dependent, but upregulates Mn-dependent, superoxide dismutase and haemoxygenase-1 [171,172].

Energy metabolism

Metabolic diseases can alter the level of consciousness as a result of brain energy failure, as exemplified by the encephalopathy that accompanies hypoglycaemia, where the lack of substrate results in a loss of the energy required to maintain transmembrane ionic gradients. Alterations in brain energy metabolism have been detected in patients with severe hepatic encephalopathy [192]. Recent studies measuring glucose utilization in rats after portocaval anastomosis using autoradiographic techniques have yielded conflicting results as both an increase and a reduction in this parameter have been noted in several brain regions [48,49]. Measurements of human glucose consumption with PET scanning have also yielded conflicting results (reviewed in [193]). In one study with special attention to statistical analysis, only a selective loss of glucose consumption was noted, specifically in the area of the cingulate gyrus [194]. This observation would be in line with a diminished blood oxygen level-dependent (BOLD) activation in this area in patients with

cirrhosis who underwent examination with functional MRI [195]. Using ^{31}P-MRS, a reduction in the ratio of phosphomonoesters to adenosine triphosphate (ATP) was noted in human brain, a decrease that could reflect less breakdown of ATP to adenosine monophosphate (AMP) [196,197]; however, changes in other chemical compounds (such as choline) may explain these findings. Studies in animal models, in which a reduction in brain ATP was demonstrated [198], were performed at a late stage of the neurological picture. While newer technology may shed further light on this issue, a consensus has emerged that energy failure, although possibly present at the end of the clinical course, is not a primary pathogenic mechanism in hepatic encephalopathy [14].

Alterations in neurotransmission

Multiple neurotransmitter systems are altered in hepatic encephalopathy. This multiplicity is shared with other metabolic disorders of the brain and raises the question as to which changes are primarily responsible for symptoms and which are secondary to earlier modifications. In order to study this complex rearrangement, neurochemical measurements and behavioural testing are tools to probe such systems in the experimental animal. Recent technological advances, such as brain microdialysis, for example, have allowed measurements of transmitters in the extracellular space [199,200]. Improved methods for monitoring behaviour in small rodents are also becoming available [201]. A recent study on portocaval-shunted rats, which employed electrophysiological and behavioural approaches in the individual animal, showed deficits in cortico-striatal synaptic plasticity, which could be related to a disturbed processing of novel information and memory [202]. Correlations between synaptic plasticity and a variety of activity parameters in the open field were opposite for control and portocaval-shunted animals, indicating a disintegration of the relationship between synaptic plasticity and behaviour. The resulting habituation deficit in these animals may correspond to the cognitive and memory defects in patients with hepatic encephalopathy [203].

GABAergic neurotransmission

Several observations suggest that alterations in GABAergic neurotransmission may be present in hepatic encephalopathy. These include an excessive sedative response of cirrhotic patients to benzodiazepines [204] and the fact that the mental state improves in a subset of patients with hepatic encephalopathy after administration of flumazenil, a benzodiazepine receptor antagonist [205]. The lack of correlation between plasma levels of benzodiazepine receptor ligands and the clinical response to flumazenil suggested that the drug may also be working through other mechanisms. Recent observations implicate the PBR in the pathogenesis of hepatic encephalopathy [13,14]. In contrast to the central receptor, which is part of the neuronal GABA$_A$

complex, the PBR is located on the outer mitochondrial membrane of astrocytes, but is also found in most peripheral cell types. It has been implicated in many cellular functions [206,207]. One of the best characterized is the regulation of the synthesis of neurosteroids, such as allopregnenolone and allotetrahydrodeoxycorticosterone, which have positive $GABA_A$ receptor-modulatory activity and were identified in the brains of patients with hepatic coma [86].

In astrocytes, ammonia upregulates the PBR, increases its affinity for ligands [208] and induces tyrosine nitration of the PBR [181]; the functional relevance of these changes is unknown. Increased numbers of peripheral benzodiazepine receptors have been reported in rats after portocaval anastomosis [209] and, post mortem, in brains from patients with cirrhosis [87]. Such changes are also observed in a rat model of acute liver failure [88] and in hyperammonaemic mice with congenital ornithine transcarbamylase deficiency [210]. Another agonist of the peripheral receptor is the neuropeptide, diazepam-binding inhibitor [211], the levels of which are elevated in hepatic encephalopathy, and which exhibits antagonist activity at the level of the GABA receptor. The role of neurosteroids in the pathogenesis of hepatic encephalopathy is currently being explored. However, one must keep in mind that the PBR is also a component of the mitochondrial permeability transition pore, and its stimulation can induce apoptosis in some peripheral cell types [212]. Tyrosine nitration is known to inactivate the CD95 (Fas) death receptor [194] and, likewise, ammonia-induced PBR nitration may be protective. Activation of the PBR by benzodiazepines and synthetic ligands such as PK11195 or Ro5-4864 triggers an oxidative stress response and increases protein tyrosine nitration [183].

Glutamatergic neurotransmission

Glutamate is a major excitatory neurotransmitter in the brain. Profound alterations have been observed at many sites involved in glutamatergic neurotransmission. Total levels of brain glutamate are decreased in several animal models and in the tissue of patients with cirrhosis [46]; this reduction reflects its consumption in the formation of glutamine. However, increased levels in the CSF [213] and extracellular space [199,214] have been observed in animal models. Such an increase could be explained by an increased release, suggested from experimental preparations [215,216], and/or a defect in glial reuptake (see above). It should be noted that glutamate belongs to the osmolytes that are released from astrocytes in response to cell swelling [132].

This increased extracellular glutamate may explain the alterations in receptor binding reported in several models. Glutamate binds to ionotropic [NMDA, α-amino-3-hydroxy-5-methyl-4-isoxazolepropionic acid (AMPA) and kainate subtypes] and metabotropic receptors in postsynaptic membranes [217]. NMDA receptors are present on astrocytes [183,218]. As discussed above, NMDA receptor activation in astrocytes

is a key trigger for the ammonia-, swelling-, benzodiazepine- and cytokine-induced oxidative stress response. A reduction in NMDA receptor number [219] and in the affinity of non-NMDA receptors [220] has been reported in animal models.

Dopaminergic neurotransmission

As in Parkinson's disease, the presence of extrapyramidal symptoms in patients with cirrhosis suggests that a dopamine deficiency may play a functional role. However, when dopamine levels in cirrhotic patients were increased by the administration of L-dopa, no clear improvement in clinical encephalopathy was noted [221].

Recent observations have rekindled interest in possible alterations in the dopaminergic system. Autopsied brain tissue has shown increased levels of homovanillic acid, a dopamine metabolite [222]. Levels of monoamine oxidase A, the enzyme responsible for dopamine degradation, were increased in the brains of individuals with cirrhosis [223]. The number of D_2 dopamine receptors was specifically decreased in human tissue [224]. Of even greater interest is the observation that manganese toxicity is exerted via its accumulation in the pallidum and neurodegenerative changes that result in a reduction in D_2 receptors [225].

Serotoninergic neurotransmission

In hepatic encephalopathy, cerebral levels of the stable metabolite of serotonin, 5-hydroxyindolacetic acid, are consistently elevated in animals [226] and human tissue [222]. This could reflect an increased turnover of serotonin metabolism [227]. More recent data have shown an increase in the activity of monoamine oxidase A, the enzyme that is involved in the degradation of serotonin [228], which would explain the increased levels of 5-hydroxyindolacetic acid. An increased number of HT_2 receptors has been noted in human postmortem tissue [229], a factor that could account for the precipitation of overt hepatic encephalopathy by ketanserin, an HT_2 receptor antagonist [230]. However, nothing is known about other HT receptor subtypes. Methysergide, a non-specific receptor antagonist, had some beneficial effects on behavioural parameters in an animal model (reviewed in ref. 231). More work is needed to assess the pathogenic implications of an altered serotoninergic system.

Histaminergic neurotransmission

There is a high prevalence of sleep disturbances and abnormalities in circadian rhythmicity in patients with liver cirrhosis [232,233]. The histaminergic hypothalamic tuberomammillary nucleus is a major waking system of the brain that can elicit synaptic plasticity [234]. Histamine inhibits glutamatergic corticostriatal synaptic transmission through presynaptic histamine H_3 receptors [235]. The histamine level in CSF in humans with hepatic encephalopathy is increased [236], and an increased density of histamine H_1 receptors was found in brains from patients with cirrhosis and portocaval-shunted rats [237], whereas H_3 receptors are downregulated in patients who died in hepatic coma [238]. These findings seem consistent with changes in the histaminergic system and disturbances of sleep–waking regulation. In line with this concept, the histamine H_1 receptor blocker pyrilamine improved the spontaneous locomotor activity of portocaval-shunted rats and restored altered circadian rhythmicity [239]. In portocaval-shunted rats, corticostriatal synaptic plasticity is significantly impaired and also involves histamine H_3 receptor-mediated long-term depression [202].

Other neurotransmitter systems

Alterations in opioidergic neurotransmission may be involved in the alcohol preference of rats after portocaval anastomosis [240], an alteration that is accompanied by region-selective alterations in μ and δ receptors and responds to treatment with the opioid antagonist, naloxone [241]. Its role in hepatic encephalopathy, proposed as a result of altered levels of enkephalins and endorphins, is uncertain [242,243].

Receptor autoradiography was employed on brain slices from patients who died with hepatic encephalopathy (see Zilles, reported in ref. 3). Despite high regional and intersubject variabilities, the striatum of patients with hepatic encephalopathy presented lower kainate, $GABA_B$, muscarinic M_2, nicotinic, 5-HT_{1A} and adenosine A_1 and A_{2A} receptor densities compared with control subjects. In the primary somatosensory cortex of patients with hepatic encephalopathy, NMDA and 5-HT_{1A}

receptors were upregulated, whereas benzodiazepine binding sites, nicotinic and adenosine A_1 receptors were downregulated. These findings support the view that multiple receptor systems are affected in hepatic encephalopathy.

Disturbances of oscillatory networks in the brain

Magnetoencephalography (MEG) allows for non-invasive assessment of information processing in the human brain with high spatial and temporal resolution [244,245]. This technique was employed together with simultaneous electromyography (EMG) in patients with cirrhosis and hepatic encephalopathy in order to obtain insight into the neurophysiological basis of mini-asterixis, i.e. a postural tremor of varying frequency (6–12 Hz), which is observed in patients with low-grade hepatic encephalopathy [246,247]. MEG analysis by dynamic imaging of coherent sources [248] was used to identify brain sources coherent to the EMG and for cerebrocerebral coherence. Patients with hepatic encephalopathy exhibited a stronger corticomuscular coherence with a shift to lower frequencies when compared with control subjects [246], indicating a pathologically slowed and synchronized motor cortical drive (Fig. 5). The extent of these changes correlated with the severity of hepatic encephalopathy. This pathological motor cortical drive in hepatic encephalopathy results from altered thalamocortical

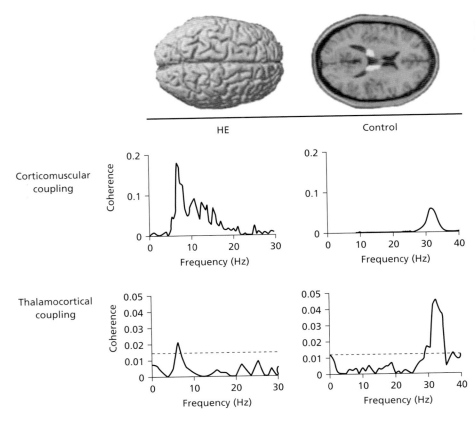

Fig. 5 Mini-asterixis in hepatic encephalopathy (HE) is induced by a pathologic thalamo–motorcortical coupling. Pathological oscillatory coupling in the motor system of a cirrhotic patient with HE. Cortical and muscular activities were recorded simultaneously by magnetencephalography and electromyography (EMG) (right extensor digitorum muscle) during forearm elevation with the right hand outstretched. Identification of brain sources coherent to each other or the peripheral EMG was performed by dynamic imaging of coherent sources. In both the healthy control subject and the cirrhotic HE patient with tremor (mini-asterixis), the M1 motor cortex is activated with electrical coupling to the thalamus (top). Corticomuscular coupling reveals a high-amplitude peak at the frequency of the tremor in the HE patient (centre), whereas coupling in the control patient is high frequency with a low amplitude. Thalamo-motor-cortical coupling in the HE patient occurs exactly at the individual tremor frequency, whereas in the control subject, thalamocortical coupling is at higher frequency, which also matches the frequency of corticomuscular coherence (bottom). Apparently, a pathologically rigid and slowed thalamocortical drive triggers mini-asterixis in HE (reproduced from ref. 247, with permission).

oscillatory coupling [247]. These findings point to a disturbance of cerebral oscillatory networks in hepatic encephalopathy that is triggered by possibly neurotoxin- and hydration-sensitive thalamic structures and results in an abnormally low frequency and rigid thalamocortical and corticomuscular coupling [249]. Such pathologically altered oscillatory networks may explain some motor and cognitive defects in patients with hepatic encephalopathy.

Current pathogenetic model

Based on the above considerations, a simplified pathogenetic model is presented (Fig. 6). In chronic liver disease, ammonia and other neurotoxins induce a low-grade cerebral oedema due to astrocyte swelling. This occurs without a clinically overt increase in intracranial pressure, but the hydration increase is sufficient to trigger multiple alterations in astrocyte function and gene expression and to induce oxidative/nitrosative stress with covalent protein modifications. An autoamplicatory loop between cell swelling and oxidative stress may be involved in these responses. In addition, there are direct, swelling-independent effects of neurotoxins on astrocyte and neuronal function. As a result of an altered astrocyte function, glioneuronal communication and multiple neurotransmitter systems become deranged, with an impact on synaptic plasticity and oscillatory cerebral networks. These changes may finally account for the

symptoms of hepatic encephalopathy. Not only ammonia, but also inflammatory cytokines, benzodiazepines and hyponatraemia, can induce astrocyte swelling and synergistically act on oxidative/nitrosative stress. This offers an explanation as to why rather heterogeneous conditions, such as bleeding, infections, electrolyte disturbances or drugs, can precipitate episodes of hepatic encephalopathy in patients with cirrhosis. Thus, multiple factors act synergistically on a common pathogenetic endpoint, i.e. glial swelling with its functional consequences. Patients without cirrhosis may tolerate such precipitating factors without developing hepatic encephalopathy symptoms, because their osmolyte systems for counteraction of cell swelling are not exhausted. In cirrhosis, however, organic osmolytes are largely depleted in order to compensate for glial glutamine accumulation, and there may be little room for the action of these volume-regulatory mechanisms against further challenges in cell volume. This labile situation may explain the rapid kinetics of hepatic encephalopathy episodes and why severe brain oedema with fatal outcome can occasionally develop in subjects with endstage cirrhosis.

Similarities may exist with respect to the pathogenesis of hepatic encephalopathy in cirrhosis and that of acute liver failure, but differences in the kinetics, extent and cell volume-regulatory mechanisms counteracting glial swelling may be responsible for differences in the clinical picture in both settings. In acute liver failure, astrocyte swelling appears to be too rapid to allow for

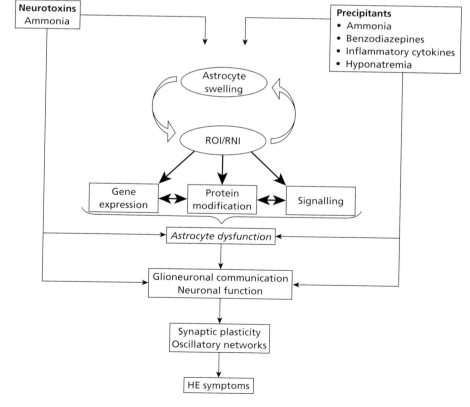

Fig. 6 Pathogenetic model for hepatic encephalopathy. Neurotoxins such as ammonia induce astrocyte swelling, which is aggravated synergistically by precipitants. Ammonia-induced osmolyte depletion reduces the volume-regulatory capacity and thus sensitizes astrocytes to swelling by precipitating factors. Astrocyte swelling involves NMDA receptor activation, Ca^{2+} and the generation of oxidative and nitrosative (ROI/RNI) stress. Swelling and oxidative stress are connected through an autoamplificatory loop. Sequelae of astrocyte swelling and oxidative/nitrosative stress are alterations in astrocyte function. Although astrocyte swelling is considered to be a major pathogenetic event, direct, swelling-independent effects of neurotoxins on astrocytes are also involved. Such alterations in astrocyte function involve gene expression and intracellular signal transduction as well as changes in transport, metabolism, neurotransmitter processing and the synthesis of neurosteroids. This astrocyte dysfunction is seen to reflect a major event, which affects glioneuronal communication. The latter is reflected by changes in synaptic plasticity and disturbances in oscillatory electrical networks in the brain as one basis for cerebral dysfunction in hepatic encephalopathy. This current model does not exclude direct neurotoxin effects on the neurons. ROI/RNI, reactive oxygen/nitrogen intermediates.

Table 2 Clinical features of HE in acute liver failure versus HE in chronic liver disease.

	Hepatic encephalopathy	
	Acute	Chronic
Overt brain oedema	Frequent	Very rare
Response to therapy	Poor	Acceptable
Agitation, seizures	20–30%	Very rare
Precipitating factors	Rare	Frequent
Short-term prognosis	Poor	Acceptable

efficient volume correction by volume-regulatory mechanisms, and clinical signs of increased intracranial pressure become evident.

Clinical manifestations

A wide range of symptoms and signs can be elicited in patients with hepatic encephalopathy. Some of them are seen throughout the spectrum of clinical syndromes; some are noted only in specific entities.

Encephalopathy of acute liver failure

The development of encephalopathy in a subject with an acutely failing liver is a serious prognostic sign. It can occur within 1 or 2 weeks after the onset of jaundice (hyperacute liver failure or fulminant hepatic failure) or after a more protracted time interval (subacute or subfulminant hepatic failure). The stages of encephalopathy have been well delineated, but some clinical manifestations are seldom seen in chronic liver disease (Tables 2 and 3). Periods of excitation and mania can be present in stage I, the prodromic phase of acute liver failure; this can be a difficult management problem, as pharmacological sedation obscures any spontaneous change in mental state. In stage II, coma is impending, with drowsiness and inability to maintain sphincter control; a flapping tremor can easily be elicited. Subclinical

seizure activity, myoclonic or focal, can be a feature of the late stages of acute hepatic failure and is rarely seen in chronic liver disease. The progression of changes in mental state can be very rapid, counted in hours, and in stages III (stupor) and IV (coma), brain oedema and intracranial hypertension can complicate the clinical course.

Brain oedema is clinically silent but, once a critical point is reached, the normal intracranial pressure (0–10 mmHg) begins to rise within the limits of the rigid skull. Once brain compliance has been critically reduced, intracranial pressure can increase swiftly and reduce the cerebral perfusion pressure (mean arterial pressure–intracranial pressure) to the point at which brain ischaemia develops. The clinical course culminates with the development of 'pressure waves' that elevate the pressure to critical levels and result in the displacement of brain structures (Fig. 7). Herniation of the temporal or uncal lobe can be life-threatening. Brain oedema and intracranial hypertension are a major cause of death in acute liver failure.

An increased intracranial pressure can be clinically silent until high pressure values are reached. Patients are deeply encephalopathic, and a sudden respiratory arrest can be a clinical presentation. Frequent monitoring of signs that indicate a high pressure, such as loss of the caloric or pupillary reflexes, is not an effective screening tool. Papilloedema is not detected. With this diagnostic difficulty, alternative methods for clinical monitoring have been examined (see below).

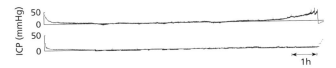

Fig. 7 Elevation of intracranial pressure (ICP) in a rat model of acute liver failure (ALF). Pressure is recorded continuously from the onset of ALF, and initial higher values stabilize 1 h after surgery in both ALF (top) and control (bottom) subjects. Within the last 2 h of the course, intracranial pressure progressively rises in ALF and, in the last 30 min, episodic elevations occur with values above 50 mmHg. These culminate in brain herniation and demise of the animal [reproduced from Webster (1991) *Hepatology* 14, 715, with permission].

Table 3 Grading of encephalopathy.

Grade	Level of consciousness	Intellectual function	Neurological abnormalities	EEG abnormalities
0	Normal	Normal	None	None
I	Lack of awareness Change in personality Day/night reversal	Short attention span Easy forgetfulness	Slight tremor Uncoordination Asterixis	Symmetric slowing
II	Lethargy Unsuitable behaviour	Loss of orientation	Asterixis Abnormal reflexes	Symmetric slowing Triphasic waves
III	Asleep but rousable Confused when awake	Loss of interpersonal communication	Abnormal reflexes	Triphasic waves
IV	Unarousable	Absent	Babinski/clonus Decerebrate	Delta (very slow)

Episodic encephalopathy in cirrhosis

This is the most common presentation in the hospital setting: a patient with known chronic liver disease develops an alteration in mental state as a result of a precipitating factor. Gastrointestinal haemorrhage, uraemia, infections and the use of sedatives are most commonly incriminated. Less frequent, but clinically relevant, precipitants include constipation, hypokalaemia and excessive protein consumption. Removal or antagonism of the precipitant factor will result in neurological improvement.

Exploration of mental status (Table 3)

Difficulties can arise in the diagnosis of early encephalopathy. Subtle alterations in behaviour are first detected by family members. Abnormalities of sleep, including insomnia, hypersomnia or inversion of sleep, can be an initial complaint. A shortened attention span, irritability or depression can be detected. In individuals with defined activities, abnormalities in handwriting or subtly impaired computations can become apparent. As encephalopathy progresses, intellectual function may show a loss of orientation to time, while an overt change in personality can occur in some individuals. A lethargic state of consciousness can evolve into confusion, stupor and coma; a detailed classification of coma is available (Table 4), although it is designed for traumatic head injury.

Physical signs

Several physical signs can be detected in such patients. Asterixis ('liver flap'), the most conspicuous, was first described in 1953 [52]. It represents an intermittency of sustained muscle contraction with arrhythmic lapses of sustained posture. Under normal circumstances, a very short myoelectrical silence can be detected

Table 4 Classification of coma (Glasgow coma scale).

Eyes open	
Spontaneously	4
To command	3
To pain	2
No response	1
Best motor response	
Obeys verbal command	6
Painful stimulus, localizes pain	5
Painful stimulus, flexion response	3
Painful stimulus, extension	2
No response	1
Best verbal response	
Oriented and conversant	5
Disoriented and conversant	4
Inappropriate words	3
Incomprehensible sounds	2
No response	1

Total score from 3 (worse) to 15 (best)

when maintaining a constant contraction of a muscle group; asterixis represents the prolongation of this myoelectrical silence, such that the contraction cannot be sustained. A mild form is probably the irregular postural tremor syndrome called 'mini-asterixis' [246,247]. It is most commonly elicited by asking the patient to extend his or her arm while retroflexing the wrist with separated digits. It is a feature of stages I and II encephalopathy; as the depth of encephalopathy progresses, the patient cannot cooperate with the request. In debilitated individuals, asterixis can also be elicited by asking the patient to extend the tongue or by having the examiner's fingers squeezed by the subject's hand; in both circumstances, the position cannot be maintained. Mini-asterixis and asterixis originate from derangements in central pathways rather than peripheral alterations, and reflect a pathologically slowed and synchronized motor cortical drive, which results from altered thalamocortical oscillatory coupling [246,247] (Fig. 5).

Asterixis is not a pathognomonic finding in hepatic encephalopathy; it can also be observed in other metabolic encephalopathies, such as uraemia, carbon dioxide narcosis, in hypomagnesaemia and with diphenylhydantoin intoxication. It can also be seen in focal neurological disease [250]. However, different mechanisms are involved in tremor generation in hepatic encephalopathy and Parkinson's disease [249].

Fetor hepaticus is a peculiar odour detected in the exhaled breath of patients with encephalopathy. It is difficult to define but, if sampled, it is easier to recognize in subsequent individuals. It is a pungent, somewhat sour, odour noted at all stages of encephalopathy. Volatile sulphur-containing compounds, such as mercaptans, may account for this finding [251].

A wide range of other neurological signs can be detected. Extrapyramidal abnormalities, including bradykinesia, dysarthria, rigidity and tremor, have been described in patients with cirrhosis [107]. Focal neurological findings can also be observed during the course of overt encephalopathy. Long-tract signs, such as Babinski and ankle clonus, can be unilateral or bilateral; they may be confusing in the individual who is stuporous or comatose but, in contrast to established neurological lesions, these focal signs characteristically wax and wane. Transient cortical blindness [252] and alternating gaze deviation [253] have been reported. It should be remembered that metabolic encephalopathies, such as hepatic encephalopathy, can result in the clinical expression of previously silent small focal lesions.

Diagnosis (Table 5)

Detection of a precipitating event is a critical initial step, which may require examinations to exclude gastrointestinal bleeding or infection; encephalopathy can be a presenting symptom of spontaneous bacterial peritonitis.

There are two clinical circumstances that pose difficulties in diagnosis. The first is the rare circumstance in which encephalopathy is the presenting symptom of liver disease. As in other cases of a new abnormal mental state, a thorough physical and laboratory examination should provide diagnostic clues. In

Table 5 Diagnostic approach to overt encephalopathy in cirrhosis.

1. Exclude other causes of encephalopathy

With fever and ↑WBC	Consider lumbar puncture
In active alcoholism	Consider subarachnoid haemorrhage
Alcoholism and confusion	Consider Wernicke's encephalopathy
	Obtain drug screen
Encephalopathy with asterixis	Rule out uraemia, CO_2 narcosis, ↓Mg
Decerebrate posturing	Consider brainstem lesions, but neuro-ophthalmological examination is normal in liver cases
Exclude dementia	Normal consciousness + global cognitive defect
	Long duration; insidious onset
Exclude psychosis	Normal consciousness + selective cognitive defect
	Short duration; acute onset

2. Search for precipitating factor of hepatic encephalopathy

Most common	Gastrointestinal haemorrhage, uraemia, use of sedatives, diuretics, dehydration
Other causes	Dietary indiscretion, infection, constipation, hypokalaemia
Also consider	Hypoxia, anaemia, hyponatraemia and hypophosphataemia
	Large spontaneous portal–systemic collaterals
When none found	Acute deterioration of liver function

3. Obtain diagnostic tests

Arterial ammonia	For diagnostic uncertainty, not needed for follow-up
EEG	For diagnostic uncertainty
Search for precipitant	Blood count and chemistry, blood/urine/ascites culture
	Rectal/nasogastric examination for occult blood
	Drug screen
Imaging	Brain CT for exclusion of other pathology

EEG, electroencephalogram.

this setting, measurement of plasma ammonia is useful; except for sedative-induced encephalopathy, many precipitating causes of encephalopathy are associated with an elevated ammonia level. Arterial blood provides a more accurate determination, as venous ammonia samples are influenced by the variable degree of peripheral metabolism. More recently, arterial and 'arterialized' samples (where the hand is warmed and the venous sample is drawn in a distal direction) or samples from the earlobe capillary [254] have been proposed, but their value has been questioned [57,255]. Immediate analysis and good laboratory practice are critical, as contamination should be rigorously avoided. Once the patient has been diagnosed as having hepatic encephalopathy, serial measurements of ammonia are unnecessary, as clinical examination is adequate to assess the evolution. In fact, as already discussed, mean blood ammonia levels correlate with stages of encephalopathy, but have poor predictive value in the individual case. Only in acute liver failure have arterial ammonia levels proved to potentially change management, as values > 200 mg/dL are associated with cerebral herniation [256].

The second diagnostic challenge is the exclusion of other causes of encephalopathy in patients with known liver disease. Alcoholic subjects may develop Wernicke's encephalopathy, in which a confusional state is associated with dysconjugate gaze. Fever and/or leucocytosis are not features of hepatic encephalopathy, and a lumbar puncture may be necessary to exclude meningitis; such patients may already exhibit a coagulopathy, and the procedure should be done by an experienced individual. If available, determination of glutamine in the CSF can assist in the diagnosis of hepatic encephalopathy. The presence of focal neurological signs may prompt neuroimaging with CT or MR. Brain atrophy may be seen, especially in alcoholic subjects [257], but its clinical relevance is questionable. A hyper-resonant globus pallidus is not diagnostic of hepatic encephalopathy [258]. Agitation and tremulousness, features of alcohol withdrawal, are seldom signs of hepatic encephalopathy. In other patients, extrapyramidal symptoms can be prominent; resistance to passive movements may increase with the velocity of limb displacement (*gegenhalten*). Parkinsonian features can be detected in up to 89% of subjects with advanced liver disease [120].

Persistent (chronic) encephalopathy

This category includes patients with recurrent episodes of encephalopathy as well as those in whom a persistent alteration in mental state can be detected clinically. In those with recurrent episodes, dietary indiscretion and constipation are more conspicuous precipitants than gastrointestinal haemorrhage and uraemia. In patients with cirrhosis and persistent abnormalities of mental state or in whom spontaneous episodes of encephalopathy recur, extensive spontaneous large-diameter portal–systemic shunts (e.g. splenorenal) can be detected [259–261]. Such cases may explain how, occasionally, patients can be discovered in psychiatric or neurological wards.

Individuals subjected to surgical portal–systemic anastomoses are especially prone to chronic encephalopathy that can vary according to the type of anastomosis and the nature of liver function [262,263]. Patients may develop an acute hypomanic or paranoid–schizophrenic reaction in the first months after the operation, but persistent changes tend to develop 1 year after surgery. Approximately 30% of patients in whom endoscopic and/or pharmacological techniques have failed to control portal hypertension-related bleeding and who receive an emergency surgical anastomosis, or in whom a TIPS is placed [264], develop episodes of encephalopathy. TIPS-induced hepatic encephalopathy is usually mild [265], but shunt-narrowing/occlusion techniques are required in severe cases [266]. In non-alcoholic cirrhosis, persistent encephalopathy is more often seen with non-selective central shunts (end-to-side and side-to-side portocaval anastomoses, mesocaval shunt) than with selective derivations (distal splenorenal shunts) [267]. No single hepatic or neurological test has emerged as a clear predictor of encephalopathy after shunt surgery [268,269]. In the case of TIPS, the procedure is employed in older subjects, and this has emerged as a risk factor [264,270]. The role of a previous episode of encephalopathy in predicting post-TIPS encephalopathy may depend on whether it occurred spontaneously or as a result of a precipitant factor [271]. As expected, the risk of hepatic encephalopathy increases with the diameter of the TIPS shunt [272]. Interestingly, patients with cirrhosis and loss of portal perfusion before TIPS were protected against post-TIPS chronic hepatic encephalopathy [273].

Hepatocerebral degeneration will develop many years after the surgical anastomosis or in patients with large portal–systemic shunts [274]. Patients develop a variety of extrapyramidal symptoms, including disturbances of gait, tremor, chorea and ataxia [275]. Muscle rigidity can be conspicuous. The patients can appear as somewhat jovial in spite of their severe limitations. If spastic paraparesis develops, movement may be severely limited [105]; loss of bladder control can be prominent.

Minimal (subclinical) encephalopathy

A variable number of patients with cirrhosis, who appear to be clinically normal and whose neurological examination at the bedside appears unremarkable, exhibit cognitive deficits on neuropsychological examination [276–279]. The prevalence of these abnormalities is variable and, in the absence of a 'gold standard', a true prevalence may be difficult to define; up to 70% of patients have been reported to exhibit such changes. The relevance of minimal hepatic encephalopathy is derived from the findings that it may impair daily life [280–282] and is of prognostic relevance [283–285].

There is agreement that minimal hepatic encephalopathy is not a distinct pathogenetic entity but describes one end of the continuous symptom spectrum of hepatic encephalopathy [7]. Thus, minimal hepatic encephalopathy describes a poorly defined syndrome found in the 'grey zone' between normality and overt hepatic encephalopathy. In line with this concept, minimal hepatic encephalopathy can predict the development of overt hepatic encephalopathy [286]. Subcortical alterations were described as a possible anatomical site responsible for minimal changes, with involvement of basal ganglia [111,287,288]. However, these structures are also involved in overt hepatic encephalopathy [247]. A selective reduction in glucose consumption in the area of the cingulate gyrus, a nucleus involved in the attention process [289], was reported. However, as shown in recent functional MRI studies, judgement-related blood oxygen level-dependent (BOLD) activation was not only decreased in the cingulate cortex in minimal hepatic encephalopathy [195], but progressively decreased with severity of hepatic encephalopathy (see Kircheis in ref. 3). Also, the relation of subclinical changes to protein and amino acid metabolism [276], data from quantitative water mapping (see Shah in ref. 3), the reports of global reduction in cerebral blood flow noted in these patients [290], coupled with the response of neuropsychological tests to therapeutic manipulations which are applied in overt encephalopathy, suggest a global impact of the liver disease on brain function, as seen in cases of clinical encephalopathy.

Minimal encephalopathy probably has an impact on the daily life of patients. Proscription of automobile driving was recommended to patients who exhibit abnormal visual reaction times [278]. Subsequent studies confirmed an impaired fitness to drive [291,292], whereas a prior pilot study, in which the quality of automobile driving was assessed blindly in patients without prior episodes of overt encephalopathy, did not reveal differences between patients with and without abnormal neuropsychological tests or in their comparison with carefully matched control subjects [293]. In the absence of clear guidelines, it would appear prudent to fully evaluate patients who depend on driving or operating heavy machinery for their livelihood, and to examine the effects of therapy on their performance. If patients have already exhibited overt episodes of encephalopathy, limitation of driving may be necessary.

Sleep abnormalities are frequent in unselected patients with cirrhosis [232,294]. They may be related to alterations in circadian function [295], but could also reflect elements of anxiety and depression that may arise as a result of living with chronic disease. They are not necessarily related to abnormal neuropsychological test results [232].

Quantifying hepatic encephalopathy

With the variability that characterizes the clinical expression of hepatic encephalopathy, it is not surprising that many tools are available for patient follow-up. In subjects with overt changes in mental state, no test supersedes a clinical assessment. It is in the diagnosis of the earlier stages, such as minimal encephalopathy, that a large number of tests have been developed. Low grades of encephalopathy can be viewed as a continuum and, ideally, tests will cover the spectrum of abnormalities currently divided into minimal, stage I and II encephalopathy.

Encephalopathy of acute liver failure

The development of brain oedema and intracranial hypertension poses diagnostic difficulties and influences the timing of liver transplantation. Brain swelling is not amenable to bedside clinical measurement as radiological techniques are imprecise and are not conducive to repeated measurements in these critically ill patients. Most of the effort is directed at measuring intracranial pressure. In the past few years, alternative non-invasive methods have been proposed, although none has emerged as a viable alternative.

Intracranial pressure monitoring

Patients with acute liver failure exhibit a severe coagulopathy, and placement of an intracranial pressure monitor may be associated with complications. A survey of clinical practice in the United States revealed a much lower incidence of haemorrhagic complications with the use of epidural transducers, while those monitors with which the dura mater was pierced (such as subdural bolts or intraventricular catheters) were associated with considerably more bleeding and even death [296]. Epidural monitors are less precise, and calibration can be problematic. The use of very thin transducers applied to the brain's surface has been suggested as an alternative, although complications do occur. Familiarity with the equipment and experience with such patients are important in reducing the complications. The procedure is mainly utilized in patients in whom liver transplantation is being considered, as evidence of increased survival by measurement of intracranial pressure has not been demonstrated [297]. Recent studies from the US Acute Liver Failure group indicate a 10% incidence of bleeding complications, including death [298]. Use of recombinant factor VII may decrease the incidence of complications [299].

Measurement of cerebral blood flow

Cerebral perfusion is decreased in the majority of patients with acute liver failure [300]. However, cerebral blood flow can increase prior to the development of intracranial hypertension [301] and, in the experimental animal, the signal for cerebral hyperaemia arises from the brain itself [302]. As mentioned, activation of haem oxygenase-1, as a result of oxidative stress, with generation of vasodilating carbon monoxide, is a leading candidate for the effect [173]. Furthermore, measurements of blood flow using radioactive xenon have shown that a subset of patients with acute liver failure may actually exhibit higher flows than would be expected for their cerebral metabolic rate, calculated as the product of cerebral blood flow and arteriovenous oxygen difference (the latter is estimated from measurements in a peripheral artery and in the jugular bulb). The term 'luxury perfusion' can describe this phenomenon [300], a change that

can increase cerebral blood volume and facilitate the development of intracranial hypertension. In addition, these patients lose the capacity to autoregulate their cerebral blood flow in the face of variations in arterial pressure [303]. In this setting, an increase in arterial pressure may result in cerebral hyperaemia. These abnormalities in autoregulation appear to regress after liver transplantation and are not seen in the majority of patients with cirrhosis [304]. Cerebral vasodilatation *per se* may aggravate brain swelling, as shown recently with terlipressin [305].

Tools are being developed to monitor cerebral perfusion. Repeated measurements using radioactive xenon are not a practical alternative. Use of Doppler insonation of the middle cerebral artery may provide a non-invasive measurement [300], but it requires further validation. The sole measurement of the arteriovenous oxygen difference across the brain (arterial and jugular vein samples) is theoretically insufficient, as changes in perfusion and in cerebral metabolism can independently affect its value. Elevated jugular venous lactate has been demonstrated in some patients, raising the possibility that these individuals may be suffering from brain ischaemia [306]. Whether any of these measurements could replace intracranial pressure monitoring remains to be proven; they are more likely to provide complementary information.

Auditory evoked potentials and other approaches

In one study, serial recording of sensory evoked potentials in patients with acute liver failure provided prognostic information. Disappearance of the N70 wave was associated with the patient's demise or the lack of spontaneous recovery [307]. This experience awaits confirmation from other centres. Limited experience with the determination of critical flicker frequency in patients with acute liver failure suggests that this approach may be helpful for follow-up of the evolution of hepatic encephalopathy [308]. However, the technique is applicable to cooperative patients only.

Encephalopathy in cirrhosis

The PSE index

Many studies examining both precipitant-induced and persistent encephalopathy have utilized the portal–systemic encephalopathy (PSE) index (described in ref. [309]). This method combines clinical features with objective data, scored in a semi-quantitative fashion. For scoring, greater weight is given to mental state (factor of 3) than to arterial ammonia, asterixis, electroencephalogram (EEG) findings and score in the trailmaking test (factor of 1), each with scores of 1+ to 4+. Adding the contribution of these five parameters results in a PSE index value. The index has shortcomings, as separation into grades for some of its parameters (asterixis, trailmaking, ammonia) may be artificial; furthermore, repeated EEGs may not be readily available. A recent consensus statement has not supported its use for clinical trials in hepatic encephalopathy [7].

EEG

The EEG shows characteristic changes in hepatic encephalopathy [310]. These include the replacement of the normal background waves of 9–12 cycles/s by progressively slower waves, including φ waves, triphasic and δ waves (the last exhibit 2–3 cycles/s). These changes are not specific, as other metabolic encephalopathies and psychotropic agents can induce similar alterations. Quantitative and automated electroencephalographic analysis integrates the tracing and delineates the dominant signals [311]. Abnormalities have been associated with a poor prognosis. However, the use of the EEG has fallen behind other neurophysiological tools, mainly because of its low sensitivity. It still plays a role in patients in whom the diagnosis of the cause of encephalopathy is unclear.

Critical flicker frequency (CFF)

Recent data suggest that determination of the critical flicker frequency threshold could be an objective and reproducible technique for assessment of the severity of low-grade hepatic encephalopathy [308]. With this technique, which requires cooperation from the patient, a high-frequency flickering light is presented to the patient, which gives the impression of a steady light. After stepwise reduction in the frequency of the flickering light, the frequency is determined at which the flickering nature of the intrafoveally presented light is recognized by the patient. Healthy control subjects and patients with cirrhosis without evidence of encephalopathy in computer psychometric testing exhibit flicker frequencies (CFF) above 39 Hz, whereas those with manifest hepatic encephalopathy have values consistently below this threshold. The technique is largely free from training effects, does depend on the patient's educational status and can be performed rapidly as a bedside test, but is not applicable in patients with colour blindness, other severe ophthalmological disease and patients who are unable to fix the presented light. Functional MRI (fMRI) studies and correlations with psychometric tests have revealed that CFF determinations engage several brain areas [195] and integrate a broad variety of neuropsychological qualities [308]. CFF can also be used for follow-up of hepatic encephalopathy evolution and efficacy of treatment. However, up to now, experience with CFF measurements has been restricted to a few centres and the relation between CFF and quality of life is unclear.

Other neurophysiological testing

The integrated electrical response to visual, auditory or somatosensory stimuli is the rationale for the use of evoked potentials [312]. Several parameters can be determined, including peaks and latencies; as a result, the function of afferent pathways and of the cerebral cortex can be evaluated. Results are expressed as time (in milliseconds) to positive (P) or negative (N) deflections. They have been used to detect minimal encephalopathy as well as to follow subjects with overt changes in mental state. For the latter, their sensitivity and specificity are questionable [311,313]. Assessment of visual evoked potentials

has been the tool most often evaluated, but differences in the type of light stimulus as well as in the liberal use of waves other than the P100 latency (100 ms between stimulation and peak) makes comparison between studies difficult.

For patients in whom minimal encephalopathy is suspected, endogenous event-related potentials may exhibit a greater sensitivity. In this test, two aspects are combined: visual or acoustic signals are presented but, in addition, the patient is asked to identify a predefined stimulus (such as a high-frequency sound). A prolongation of the P300 latency to acoustic stimuli was observed in patients with early encephalopathy [314,315]. Visual event-related potentials appeared to be superior to neuropsychological testing in detecting abnormalities in such individuals [316,317].

Neuropsychological testing

A large number of tests have been used in the diagnosis of minimal encephalopathy. The test most often utilized has been the number connection test (NCT). Although initially thought to reflect abnormalities corresponding to visuospatial perception, other neuropsychological areas appear to be involved in an abnormal result, including that of attention. The test is influenced by age and educational background, as well as being subject to the effects of repeated learning [319,320]. This may explain, in part, why single psychometric paper/pencil tests, such as NCT, digit symbol test and the line tracing test, are insufficiently sensitive to diagnose minimal hepatic encephalopathy [308]. Psychometric test batteries, as either paper/pencil tests or computer psychometry, were reported to be an accurate tool to diagnose subclinical encephalopathy [277,284]. One such battery, the psychometric hepatic encephalopathy score (PHES), simple to administer [320], is undergoing scrutiny at the present time. Other developments focus on the comparison between different neuropsychological domains as a useful diagnostic approach. However, in the absence of a 'gold standard', all these batteries require validation in the same patient over a period of time.

An important question is whether patients with alcoholic cirrhosis exhibit abnormalities as a result of the long-term neurological effects of alcohol. On a variety of neuropsychological tests, abstinent subjects with alcoholic cirrhosis perform comparably to their non-alcoholic counterparts [321]. After transplantation, the abnormalities in the alcohol group also improve [322].

Treatment of hepatic encephalopathy – general aspects

Several reviews on therapy have been published in recent years [323–326]. A rational therapeutic scheme for hepatic encephalopathy targets five possible non-mutually exclusive sites (Fig. 8):

1 the gut, decreasing the access of toxins to the systemic circulation;

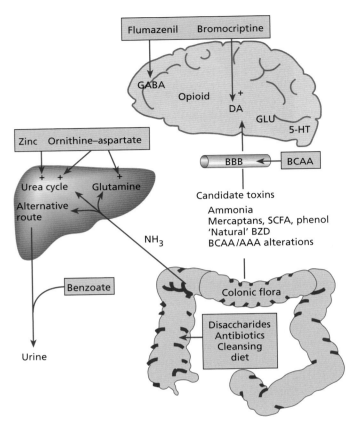

Fig. 8 Schematic diagram of therapeutic strategies in hepatic encephalopathy. Treatments reported to be successful are shaded. However, most effective therapy has been directed to the gut, where several options are available. The ability to increase urea and glutamine synthesis in a cirrhotic liver, as well as the activation of alternative pathways of nitrogen excretion (via the administration of benzoate), has not been fully evaluated. Branched-chain amino acids (BCAA) may work at the level of the blood–brain barrier (BBB), but their effectiveness is still a matter of conjecture. Two neurotransmitter systems have been manipulated pharmacologically, with limited results.

2 the liver, increasing the elimination of such toxins;

3 the muscle, as a possible alternative site for toxin disposal;

4 the blood–brain barrier, by interfering with toxin entry into the brain;

5 the brain itself, by attempting to restore the abnormalities of neurotransmission.

The gut

The therapeutic goal at this site is interference with the formation and/or absorption of nitrogenous compounds arising from bacterial metabolism in the colon, especially ammonia. Restriction of protein intake is one common approach to fulfilling this goal. However, malnutrition may arise from excessive protein restriction, and a recent study demonstrated no beneficial effect of protein restriction in episodic hepatic encephalopathy [327]. A positive nitrogen balance may actually benefit subjects with encephalopathy by increasing the ability of liver and muscle to carry out detoxification functions [328]. In the catabolic state of cirrhosis, a high protein intake, ~ 1.2 g/kg/day, may be necessary to accomplish this objective [329]. In addition, the type of ingested protein is important. Vegetable [330] and dairy-based protein [331] are better tolerated than animal-derived protein, as the high calorie to nitrogen ratio seen in the former reduces gluconeogenesis and has anabolic effects on the utilization of dietary proteins [332]. Vegetable-based diets have a high fibre content, which increases the elimination of nitrogen products in the stool [333]. For those intolerant of vegetable-based diets, administration of soluble forms of fibre can be added to a therapeutic regimen [324]. Protein-intolerant patients may benefit from oral supplements enriched with branched-chain amino acids [334–336] in order to reach a protein intake of at least 1 g/kg/day. The enteral route of nutrition is always preferred.

Bowel cleansing is another mainstay of therapy. Colonic cleansing reduces the luminal content of ammonia, decreases bacterial counts and lowers blood ammonia in cirrhotic patients. Although different laxatives could accomplish this effect, non-absorbable disaccharides have additional benefits and are widely used for this effect.

Since their original description, non-absorbable disaccharides have been widely used [337]. They include lactulose (β-galactosido-fructose) and lactitol (β-galactosido-sorbitol). When administered orally, they are not broken down by intestinal disaccharidases and thus reach the caecum, where enteric bacteria cleave the molecules and metabolize them, mainly to acetate; as a result, caecal pH drops [338,339]. In fact, acidification of the stool (pH < 6) can be used to monitor therapy, albeit it is not a very practical tool. The acidification results in a cathartic effect and favours non-ionic diffusion of ammonia into the lumen, where it is assimilated for bacterial metabolism. As a result, faecal nitrogen excretion is increased while plasma levels of ammonia and the total body pool of urea decrease [340].

Oral dosing (15–30 mL four times a day) is titrated to result in two or three soft bowel movements/day. In comatose patients, a more rapid onset of action may occur by administration via enema [341], with the patient in the Trendelenburg position to favour passage of the enema into the right colon. Complaints with oral administration include an excessively sweet taste, abdominal cramping and flatulence; these improve with continued administration. Excessive stool depositions as a result of overdosing can lead to loss of hypotonic colonic fluid with a resultant hypertonic dehydration with hypernatraemia, a factor that can by itself alter mental state.

Comparisons of lactitol with lactulose indicate similar effects but better palatability of the former agent [342]. The use of crystalline lactulose has been proposed to reduce potential contamination with other saccharides. In patients with known intestinal lactase deficiency, oral lactose will have similar effects [343].

Although lactulose is frequently used for the treatment of hepatic encephalopathy, its efficacy has not been shown unequivocally. The study design of many trials has been criticized [344]. Most studies conducted so far have compared lactulose with non-absorbable antibiotics and found therapeutic equivalence of both treatments. A meta-analysis of studies that compared lactulose with placebo or no intervention gave insufficient evidence to support or refute the use of non-absorbable disaccharides in hepatic encephalopathy [344]. In this analysis, antibiotics were found to be somewhat superior to disaccharides, although the clinical relevance of this finding was questioned.

Antibiotics affect the intestinal flora that generate the putative toxins. In the case of neomycin, the most widely used antibiotic [345], non-bacterial effects may also be present at the level of the intestinal mucosa [346]. Although poorly absorbed, oto- and nephrotoxicity can develop (as with the use of other aminoglycosides), especially after chronic use. Thus, it is less commonly administered as a first line of therapy. The starting dose is 3–6 g/day, in divided doses, which is reduced to 1–2 g/day for maintenance. Other antibiotics have also been evaluated. Metronidazole, 800 mg/day in divided doses, has been shown to have similar effects to neomycin, although its bacterial spectrum of action is dissimilar [347]. Metronidazole is metabolized in the liver, and reduction of the dose is necessary with liver failure [348]. Growing experience with other poorly absorbable antibiotics, such as vancomycin [349] and rifaximin [350], also suggests beneficial effects.

Patients with cirrhosis frequently exhibit overgrowth of the colonic flora with potentially pathogenic *Escherichia coli* and staphylococcal species. Therapeutic modulation of the gut flora by probiotics enriched with non-urease-producing lactobacilli or fermentable fibre was reported to improve minimal hepatic encephalopathy in cirrhosis [352] and to reduce endotoxinaemia. Further studies are required to settle this issue.

Helicobacter pylori is a urease-producing pathogen and could theoretically contribute to intestinal/gastric ammonia production. However, no correlation was found between *H. pylori* infection and plasma ammonia concentration or hepatic encephalopathy in patients with cirrhosis [352]. Eradication of *H. pylori* did not result in improvement in neuropsychological or neurophysiological parameters in stable patients [353].

The liver and muscle

The potential of the diseased liver to increase its metabolic capacity is limited, as a reduction in hepatic mass, intrahepatic shunting and alterations in the sinusoidal architecture impose fixed restrictions. Nonetheless, improvement in the capacity of the liver to clear ammonia has been sought. Zinc is a cofactor for many enzymes in the urea cycle, and a deficiency may exist in cirrhosis as a result of malnutrition and increased urinary excre-

tion. An improvement in the capacity to synthesize urea and in clinical status has been reported after administration of zinc acetate or sulphate, 600 mg/day in divided doses [354,355]. This has not been confirmed in other studies [356,357]. However, overt hepatic encephalopathy can be precipitated by overt zinc deficiency [358].

Ornithine–aspartate provides substrates for both urea and glutamine synthesis. It appears to prevent the rise of blood ammonia after a nitrogenous load [359], and therapeutic efficacy in patients with cirrhosis and hepatic encephalopathy has been shown [360,361]. Experimental studies have shown activity of the drug in the absence of a liver, indicating an effect on ammonia disposal by muscle [362]. Muscle is an important site for ammonia removal, where it is converted to glutamine via glutamine synthetase activity [24].

Children with urea cycle enzyme deficiencies are treated with drugs that allow an alternative pathway for nitrogen excretion. In the case of sodium benzoate, conjugation of one molecule of benzoyl-CoA with glycine results in one atom of nitrogen being excreted in the urine as hippurate. In one clinical trial, the drug was equally as effective as lactulose in the treatment of episodic encephalopathy in cirrhosis [363]. A second drug is phenylbutyrate; it is a precursor for the malodorous phenylacetate, which is conjugated in the liver with glutamine, and the product, phenylacetylglutamine, is excreted in the urine, resulting in the loss of two nitrogen atoms per molecule. Preliminary results are difficult to evaluate as patients were being treated with other medications [364]. The effectiveness of the hepatic conjugation process for both drugs in patients with advanced cirrhosis remains to be established.

The blood–brain barrier

Based on the (meanwhile abandoned) false neurotransmitter hypothesis, the effects of branched-chain amino acids, in both oral and intravenous forms, were tested. Numerous trials have been published in both precipitant-induced encephalopathy as well as in persistent encephalopathy [365]. Meta-analyses have yielded conflicting results [366,367]. Critical review of these studies did not find convincing evidence that branched-chain amino acids had a significant beneficial effect on patients with hepatic encephalopathy [368] but, given on a long-term basis, they may improve encephalopathy by increasing protein body stores [369]. They may provide a source of protein in patients with dietary protein intolerance. Even if beneficial for minimal encephalopathy, as suggested recently [335], their use is not justified in most patients on account of their relatively high cost.

The brain

As discussed above, multiple neurotransmitter systems are deranged in hepatic encephalopathy, and central effects of agonists/antagonists of these different systems could provide new therapeutic options as well as clues to the pathogenesis of encephalopathy. However, only a few have received extensive evaluation.

Flumazenil is a selective antagonist of the benzodiazepine receptor. In several controlled studies in patients with moderate and severe encephalopathy, the mental state of a subset of individuals, about 40%, was improved with a bolus of intravenous flumazenil, albeit transiently [370–372]. The beneficial effect of flumazenil was confirmed in a meta-analysis including six randomized controlled trials (RCTs) [373]. A source of controversy is whether such patients had received exogenous benzodiazepines (a common occurrence in hospitalized patients) but, in some, no detectable benzodiazepines could be found in their serum. A favourable response typically occurs within a few minutes of administration, and a repeat injection is possible. An oral preparation is as yet unavailable. The drug undergoes hepatic clearance, and its elimination half-life is doubled in cirrhotics [374].

Enhancement of dopaminergic neurotransmission by increasing dopamine levels has been sought with the use of L-dopa and bromocriptine. With the latter and when used to improve consciousness, no major benefits were seen [375,376]. However, bromocriptine, in association with non-absorbable disaccharides, at a dose of 10 mg twice a day, resulted in an improvement in extrapyramidal symptoms [377]. Manipulation of glutamatergic and serotoninergic neurotransmission and of neurosteroid synthesis has been tried in experimental models of hepatic encephalopathy but, as yet, has not reached the stage of clinical testing. The same holds true for memantine, a non-competitive NMDA receptor antagonist, which improves hyperammonaemia-induced encephalopathy in rats [378].

Treatment of hepatic encephalopathy – specific strategies (Table 6)

Encephalopathy of acute liver failure

Many of the measures used in the episode of encephalopathy in cirrhosis are also applied in this setting, such as protein restriction and bowel cleansing with non-absorbable disaccharides. Their effectiveness, never tested in a controlled trial, may be marginal at best. Correction of other factors that may affect mental state, such as hypoglycaemia, pharmacological sedation or infection, is mandatory.

Tracheal intubation is recommended at the onset of grade III coma to minimize the risk of sudden respiratory arrest. Intracranial hypertension, defined as a persistent elevation in intracranial pressure above 25 mmHg for more than 5 min or the appearance of sudden elevations in pressure (the so-called 'pressure waves'), is treated with mannitol, 0.5–1 g/kg intravenously [379,380]. The drug should not be readministered at fixed doses, but bolused again when needed. In patients with renal failure, hyperosmolarity is a risk, and the patients may require dialysis. Recent studies indicate benefits of increasing

Table 6 Therapeutic strategy in hepatic encephalopathy.

Episodic encephalopathy in cirrhosis

Identify, remove and treat precipitating event
  Removal of blood from the gastrointestinal tract
  Reversal of azotaemia
  Specific antagonists for sedative-induced encephalopathy
  Antibiotics for spontaneous bacterial peritonitis or other infections
  Correct electrolyte disturbances
Bowel cleansing
  Disaccharide enemas may be better than tap water enemas
Start oral non-absorbable disaccharides
  Lactulose or lactitol 30 mL every 1–2 h until bowel evacuation
  Then 15–45 mL every 6 h titrated to 2–3 soft bowel movements/day
Dietary management
  Provide calories as intravenous glucose on the first day
  Advance protein from 20 g/day to maximal tolerated

Persistant encephalopathy in cirrhosis

Search for precipitants
  Dietary indiscretion and constipation more prominent than in episodic encephalopathy
Oral medications
  If intolerance or ineffectiveness of non-absorbable disaccharides:
  Replace with neomycin (2–6 g/day); monitor for toxicity
  Replace with metronidazole (up to 800 mg/day); monitor for toxicity
  Consider the addition of zinc sulphate or zinc acetate 600 mg/day
  Consider the addition of neomycin to non-absorbable disaccharides
Dietary manipulation
  Increase consumption of vegetable and dairy sources of protein
  Feeding at bedtime (to decrease nocturnal gluconeogenesis)
  For those intolerant to protein, consider branched-chain amino acid supplements
For problematic encephalopathy
  Consider occlusion of large spontaneous portal–systemic shunt
  Reduction of lumen of TIPS or portal–systemic shunt
  Consider colonic exclusion in patient with reasonable liver function who is not a transplant candidate

serum osmolarity with hypertonic saline [381]. Emergency liver transplantation should be considered in the appropriate candidate. As a last resort, the patient can be treated with a barbiturate infusion, such as thiopental 180–500 mg administered intravenously over 15 min [382]. However, barbiturate coma is associated with arterial hypotension and requires EEG monitoring.

When liver transplantation is planned, moderate hypothermia (32°C) [383] may be an option in those patients with increased intracranial pressure that is resistant to standard medical therapy. The mechanisms by which hypothermia reduces the intracranial pressure are complex and may involve effects on cerebral blood flow, glutamate and lactate production [384]. Also, the methods of fractionated plasma separation and adsorption [385] as well as albumin dialysis [386] offer extracorporeal liver support devices, which were used successfully in preliminary studies to bridge patients with acute (on chronic) liver failure to transplantation.

Precipitant-induced (acute) encephalopathy in cirrhosis

Establishing the nature of the precipitating factor is critical, as removal or correction of the inciting cause is the most important therapeutic aspect. This point cannot be emphasized enough. Dietary protein intake is withheld for a few days only, and carbohydrates are administered intravenously. Oral protein is reintroduced once the mental state is improved, and enteral feeding provided for those patients in whom encephalopathy persists; oral supplements enriched in branched-chain amino acids are useful in highly protein-intolerant patients. Liver transplantation may be the ultimate solution of the problem, and the indications for this option have to be evaluated.

Regarding medical treatment, only a few approaches can be assumed to be effective on the basis of controlled randomized clinical trials, such as ornithine–aspartate and flumazenil (see above). Proof of treatment efficacy in most other cases is hampered by several problems. First, treatment of the precipitating factor leads to improvement in encephalopathy, making the efficacy of an additional medical treatment difficult to assess. Second, most previous clinical studies used endpoints such as mental state or results of paper/pencil tests, which do not allow (on account of inherent problems) accurate description of the evolution or resolution of hepatic encephalopathy. Neurophysiological tests of flicker frequency or evoked potentials are better suited to assess responses over short periods. Third, many previous trials were of insufficient quality or relied on case reports. Owing to the heterogeneous nature of the pathogenesis of hepatic encephalopathy and the many precipitants, only subgroups of patients may benefit from a given medical treatment. Finally, previous studies frequently used oral lactulose as a therapeutic gold standard and comparator for other treatment modalities, although the efficacy of oral lactulose is not really settled. There are only a few controlled studies comparing oral lactulose with placebo for this type of encephalopathy. As mentioned above, the ones that are available, especially those fulfilling the required quality standards, do not indicate a striking drug effect. Lactulose was as efficient as neomycin, but a combined treatment with lactulose and neomycin was not superior to placebo in the management of such episodes, with removal of the precipitating factor common to both groups [387].

It is difficult to interpret results in such patients, as allocation of precipitating factors during randomization cannot be fully controlled. Still, they highlight the importance of control of the precipitating factor as a key therapeutic step. Lactitol or lactose enemas appear to improve encephalopathy at a faster rate than cleansing enemas, as seen in a small group of 20 patients [341]. Nonetheless, clinical experience suggests that oral lactulose can be effective when given as 30–60 mL of syrup every 1–2 h until stooling occurs, at which time the dose is adjusted to 15–30 mL three or four times a day.

Flumazenil, 1 mg intravenous bolus, is certainly indicated for patients in whom benzodiazepines are identified or suspected as a precipitating factor. In a recent study, 6 of 13 patients in deep encephalopathy transiently improved their mental state with flumazenil, in contrast to none with placebo [370]. Similar results have been reported by other groups [388]. The effect is prompt but transient and, at 24 h, the two groups were indistinguishable. The impact of multiple dosing has not been evaluated. More information is needed on this type of agent.

Persistent (chronic) encephalopathy

Restriction of animal protein may be necessary to manage this type of patient, although high protein requirements may be needed for these catabolic patients. Consultation with a dietician should be considered in order to provide alternative sources, such as vegetable or casein-based protein or oral supplements enriched with branched-chain amino acids, in cases of severe protein intolerance. Non-absorbable disaccharides are also utilized. Although neither efficacy nor inefficacy has been shown in well-performed, randomized, placebo-controlled trials, these compounds are widely used. In crossover studies, reinstitution or switch to lactulose/lactitol is associated with an improvement in mental status. Results in this group are more easily interpretable, as the role of a precipitating factor is not as marked as in the acute precipitant-induced episode. However, neither disaccharides nor rifaximin were effective in the prophylaxis of hepatic encephalopathy during the first month after TIPS [389].

Oral, poorly absorbable antibiotics are seldom used as a first line of therapy, as concerns with long-term toxicity and bacterial resistance arise. If chronic neomycin is used, periodic auditory examinations and renal function testing are mandatory. For patients with difficulties in symptom control, zinc supplementation can be entertained, which also improves night-blindness, which can be observed in patients with cirrhosis. For those with prominent extrapyramidal symptoms, a trial of bromocriptine may be considered. Embolization of large spontaneous collaterals can be performed in patients with recurrent encephalopathy and good liver function [390,391].

Encephalopathy after portocaval anastomosis can be crippling and requires tight dietary control as well as the use of many drugs (preferably acting at different sites). Revision of the shunt [392], or narrowing or occlusion of the TIPS [393,394] are recommended for intractable cases. In suitable candidates, persistent encephalopathy is a clear indication for hepatic transplantation, although the procedure carries a greater mortality in patients with altered mental status at the time of the transplant. There are a few reports of improvement in the picture of hepatocerebral degeneration after the transplant procedure [395,396]. In non-transplant candidates with acceptable liver function, a surgical exclusion of the colon, preferably a colonic bypass, can provide relief from intractable encephalopathy [397].

Minimal hepatic encephalopathy

The indications to treat minimal encephalopathy would be clearer if the natural history of this condition was better defined. The indication for therapy should primarily take into account individual demands on the professional and daily life of the patient. Further, it may be prudent to separate patients according to a past history of an overt episode of encephalopathy. Consideration of the risk of driving an automobile may be more important if encephalopathy has been diagnosed previously. Sleep abnormalities, which cause considerable distress to patients, seldom respond, in the author's experience, to the usual measures employed to treat hepatic encephalopathy; general hygienic measures can be considered [398].

Neuropsychological tests do improve with many of the treatments that have been reviewed. These include protein restriction [399], non-absorbable disaccharides [400–402] and branched-chain amino acids [335,403]. The case of flumazenil is controversial, as one study showed benefit [404] while the other did not [405]; in the latter, patients with alcoholic cirrhosis developed more anxiety. Interpretation of these data is difficult, as techniques used to monitor the evolution of low-grade encephalopathy are not sensitive and objective enough. It is hoped that a recently suggested simplified grading system for the severity of hepatic encephalopathy (see Häussinger in ref. 3), which distinguishes only low- from high-grade encephalopathy and characterizes low-grade encephalopathy by means of an objective physical measure, such as critical flicker frequency, will provide a more reliable tool for future clinical studies assessing therapeutic options.

References

1 Conn HO, Lieberthal MM (1978) *The Hepatic Coma Syndromes and Lactulose*. Baltimore: Williams and Wilkins.

2 Conn HO, Bircher J (eds) (1994) *Hepatic Encephalopathy, Syndromes and Therapies*. Bloomington: Med-Ed Press.

3 Haussinger D, Kircheis G, Schliess F (eds) (2006) *Hepatic Encephalopathy and Nitrogen Metabolism*. Dordrecht: Springer Verlag.

4 Durand F, Valla D (2005) Assessment of the prognosis of cirrhosis: Child–Pugh vs MELD. *J Hepatol* 42 (Suppl. 1), S100–S107.

5 Coy DL, Srivastava A, Gottstein J et al. (1991) Postoperative course after portacaval anastomosis in rats is determined by the portacaval pressure gradient. *Am J Physiol* 261, G1072–G1078.

6 Nomura F, Ohnishi K, Terabayashi H et al. (1994) Effect of intrahepatic portal–systemic shunting on hepatic ammonia extraction in patients with cirrhosis. *Hepatology* 20, 1478–1481.

7 Ferenci P, Lockwood AR, Mullen K et al. (2002) Hepatic encephalopathy – definition, nomenclature, diagnosis, and quantification: Final Report of the Working Party at the 11th World Congress of Gastroenterology, Vienna 1998. *Hepatology* 35, 716–721.

8 Sherlock S, Sumerskill WH, White LP et al. (1954) Portal–systemic encephalopathy; neurological complication of liver disease. *Lancet* 267, 454–457.

9 McDermott WV Jr, Adams RD (1954) Episodic stupor associated with an Eck fistula in the human with particular reference to the metabolism of ammonia. *J Clin Invest* 33, 1–9.

10 Crespin J, Nemeck A, Rehkemper G et al. (2000) Intrahepatic portal-hepatic venous anastomosis: a portal–systemic shunt with neurological repercussions. *Am J Gastroenterol* 95, 1568–1571.

11 Ortiz M, Cordoba J, Alonso J et al. (2004) Oral glutamine challenge and magnetic resonance spectroscopy in three patients with congenital portosystemic shunts. *J Hepatol* 40, 552–557.

12 Ferenci P, Puspok A, Steindl P (1992) Current concepts in the pathophysiology of hepatic encephalopathy. *Eur J Clin Invest* 22, 573–581.

13 Mousseau DD, Butterworth RF (1994) Current theories on the pathogenesis of hepatic encephalopathy. *Proc Soc Exp Biol Med* 206, 329–344.

14 Butterworth RF (1996) The neurobiology of hepatic encephalopathy. *Semin Liver Dis* 16, 235.

15 Norenberg MD (1996) Astrocytic–ammonia interactions in hepatic encephalopathy. *Semin Liver Dis* 16, 245.

16 Fischer JE, Baldessarini RJ (1971) False neurotransmitters and hepatic failure. *Lancet* 2, 75–80.

17 Baraldi M, Zeneroli ZL (1982) Experimental hepatic encephalopathy: changes in the binding of gamma-aminobutyric acid. *Science* 216, 427–429.

18 Schafer DF, Jones EA (1982) Hepatic encephalopathy and the gamma-aminobutyric-acid neurotransmitter system. *Lancet* 1, 18–20.

19 Blei AT, Omary R, Butterworth RF (1992) Animal models of hepatic encephalopathies. In: Boulton AA, Baker GB, Butterworth RF (eds) *Animal Models of Neurological Disease, Neuromethods 22*. Clifton: Humana, pp. 183–222.

20 Geiger A, Magnes J, Taylor RM et al. (1954) Effect of blood constituents on uptake of glucose and on metabolic rate of the brain in perfusion experiments. *Am J Physiol* 177, 138–149.

21 Roche-Sicot J, Sicot C, Peignoux M et al. (1974) Acute hepatic encephalopathy in the rat: the effect of cross-circulation. *Clin Sci Mol Med* 47, 609–615.

22 Phillips GB, Schwartz R, Gabuzda GJ Jr et al. (1952) The syndrome of impending hepatic coma in patients with cirrhosis of the liver given certain nitrogenous substances. *N Engl J Med* 247, 239–246.

23 van Coulaert C, Deviller C, Halff M (1933) Troubles provoque par l'ingestion de sels ammoniacaux chez l'homme atteint de cirrhose de laennec. *CR Sci Soc Biol Ses Fil* 111, 739–740.

24 Olde-Damink SWM, Deutz NEP, Dejong CHC et al. (2002) Interorgan ammonia metabolism in liver failure. *Neurochem Int* 41, 177–188.

25 Haussinger D (1990) Nitrogen metabolism in liver: structural and functional organization and physiological relevance. *Biochem J* 267, 281–290.

26 Haussinger D, Stehle T (1988) Hepatocyte heterogeneity in response to icosanoids. The perivenous scavenger cell hypothesis. *Eur J Biochem* 175, 395–403.

27 Haussinger D, Gerok W (1984) Hepatocyte heterogeneity in ammonia metabolism: impairment of glutamine synthesis in CC14 induced liver cell necrosis with no effect on urea synthesis. *Chem Biol Interact* 48, 191–194.

28 Rikkers LF (1983) Portal hemodynamics, intestinal absorption, and postshunt encephalopathy. *Surgery* 94, 126–133.

29 Rudman D, DiFulco TJ, Galambos JT *et al.* (1973) Maximal rates of excretion and synthesis of urea in normal and cirrhotic subjects. *J Clin Invest* 52, 2241–2249.

30 Haussinger D, Lamers WH, Moorman AF (1992) Hepatocyte heterogeneity in the metabolism of amino acids and ammonia. *Enzyme* 46, 72–93.

31 Lockwood AH, McDonald JM, Reiman RE *et al.* (1979) The dynamics of ammonia metabolism in man. Effects of liver disease and hyperammonemia. *J Clin Invest* 63, 449–460.

32 Lustik SJ, Chhibber AK, Kolano JW *et al.* (1997) The hyperventilation of cirrhosis: progesterone and estradiol effects. *Hepatology* 25, 55–58.

33 Baertt JM, Sancetta SM, Gobuzda GJ (1964) Relation of acute potassium depletion to the renal ammonium metabolism in patients with cirrhosis. *N Engl J Med* 271, 1229–1235.

34 Lockwood AH, Yap EWH, Wong WH (1991) Cerebral ammonia metabolism in patients with severe liver disease and minimal encephalopathy. *J Cereb Blood Flow Metab* 11, 337–341.

35 Gunnarson E, Zelenina M, Aperia A (2004) Regulation of brain aquaporins. *Neuroscience* 129, 947–955.

36 Holm LM, Jahn TP, Moller AL *et al.* (2005) NH_3 and NH_4+ permeability in aquaporin-expressing *Xenopus* oocytes. *Pflugers Arch* 450, 415–428.

37 Kreis R, Ross BD, Farrow NA *et al.* (1992) Metabolic disorders of the brain in chronic hepatic encephalopathy detected with H-1 MR spectroscopy. *Radiology* 182, 19–27.

38 Häussinger D, Laubenberger J, vom Dahl S *et al.* (1994) Proton magnetic resonance spectroscopy on human brain myo-inositol in hypoosmolarity and hepatic encephalopathy. *Gastroenterology* 107, 1475–1480.

39 Laubenberger J, Haussinger D, Bayer S *et al.* (1997) Proton magnetic resonance spectroscopy of the brain in symptomatic and asymptomatic patients with liver cirrhosis. *Gastroenterology* 112, 1610–1616.

40 Bosman DK, Deutz NE, De Graaf AA *et al.* (1990) Changes in brain metabolism during hyperammonemia and acute liver failure: results of a comparative 1H-NMR spectroscopy and biochemical investigation. *Hepatology* 12, 281–290.

41 McConnell JR, Antonson DL, Ong CS *et al.* (1995) Proton spectroscopy of brain glutamine in acute liver failure. *Hepatology* 22, 69–74.

42 Cordoba J, Blei AT (1996) Brain edema and hepatic encephalopathy. *Semin Liver Dis* 16, 271.

43 Häussinger D, Kircheis G, Fischer R *et al.* (2000) Hepatic encephalopathy in chronic liver disease: a clinical manifestation of astrocyte swelling and low-grade cerebral edema. *J Hepatol* 32, 1035–1038.

44 Hourani BT, Hamilin EM, Reynolds TB (1971) Cerebrospinal fluid glutamine as a measure of hepatic encephalopathy. *Arch Intern Med* 127, 1033–1036.

45 Cooper AJL, Plum F (1987) Biochemistry and physiology of brain ammonia. *Physiol Rev* 2, 440–519.

46 Felipo V, Butterworth RF (2002) Neurobiology of ammonia. *Prog Neurobiol* 67, 259–279.

47 Hindfelt B, Plum F, Duffy TE (1977) Effect of acute ammonia intoxication on cerebral metabolism in rats with portacaval shunts. *J Clin Invest* 59, 386–396.

48 Lockwood AH, Ginsberg MD, Rhoades HM *et al.* (1986) Cerebral glucose metabolism after portacaval shunting in the rat. Patterns of metabolism and implications for the pathogenesis of hepatic encephalopathy. *J Clin Invest* 78, 86–95.

49 Hawkins RA, Mans AM (1993) Brain metabolism in hepatic encephalopathy and hyperammonemia. *Adv Exp Med Biol* 341, 13–19.

50 Lockwood AH (2002) Positron emission tomography in the study of hepatic encephalopathy. *Metab Brain Dis* 17, 431–435.

51 Barbiroli B, Gaiani S, Lodi R *et al.* (2002) Abnormal brain energy metabolism shown by *in vivo* phosphorus magnetic resonance spectroscopy in patients with chronic liver disease. *Brain Res Bull* 59, 75–82.

52 Adams RD, Foley JM (1953) The neurological disorder associated with liver disease. *Assoc Res Nerv Mental Dis Proc* 32, 198–237.

53 Bachmann C (2002) Mechanisms of hyperammonemia. *Clin Chem Lab Med* 40, 653–662.

54 Szerb JC, Butterworth RF (1992) Effect of ammonium ions on synaptic transmission in the mammalian central nervous system. *Prog Neurobiol* 39, 135–153.

55 Lai JC, Cooper AJ (1986) Brain alpha-ketoglutarate dehydrogenase complex: kinetic properties, regional distribution, and effects of inhibitors. *J Neurochem* 47, 1376–1386.

56 Kramer L, Tribl B, Gendo A *et al.* (2000) Partial pressure of ammonia versus ammonia in hepatic encephalopathy. *Hepatology* 31, 30–34.

57 Nicolao F, Efrati C, Masini A *et al.* (2003) Role of determination of partial pressure of ammonia in cirrhotic patients with and without hepatic encephalopathy. *J Hepatol* 38, 441–446.

58 Zieve L, Doizaki WM, Zieve J (1974) Synergism between mercaptans and ammonia or fatty acids in the production of coma: a possible role for mercaptans in the pathogenesis of hepatic coma. *J Lab Clin Med* 83, 16–28.

59 Blom HJ, Chamuleau RA, Rothuizen J *et al.* (1990) Methanethiol metabolism and its role in the pathogenesis of hepatic encephalopathy in rats and dogs. *Hepatology* 11, 682–689.

60 Phear EA, Ruebner B, Sherlock S *et al.* (1956) Methionine toxicity in liver disease and its prevention by chlortetracycline. *Clin Sci (Lond)* 15, 93–117.

61 Windus-Podehl G, Fyftogt C, Zieve L *et al.* (1983) Encephalopathic effect of phenol in rats. *J Lab Clin Med* 101, 586–592.

62 Mannaioni G, Carpenedo R, Pugliese AM *et al.* (1998) Electrophysiological studies on oxindole, a neurodepressant tryptophan metabolite. *Br J Pharmacol* 125, 1751–1760.

63 Carpenedo R, Mannaioni G, Moroni F (1998) Oxindole, a sedative tryptophan metabolite, accumulates in blood and brain of rats with acute hepatic failure. *J Neurochem* 70, 1998–2003.

64 Zieve L (1987) Pathogenesis of hepatic encephalopathy. *Metab Brain Dis* 2, 147–165.

65 Mortensen PB, Holtug K, Bonnen H *et al.* (1990) The degradation of amino acids, proteins, and blood to short-chain fatty acids in colon is prevented by lactulose. *Gastroenterology* 98, 353–360.

66 Shawcross DL, Davies NA, Williams R *et al.* (2004) Systemic inflammatory response exacerbates the neuropsychological effects of induced hyperammonemia in cirrhosis. *J Hepatol* 40, 247–254.

67 Blei AT (2004) Infection, inflammation and hepatic encephalopathy, synergism redefined. *J Hepatol* 40, 327–330.

68 Wilson JX, Young GB (2003) Progress in clinical neurosciences: sepsis-associated encephalopathy: evolving concepts. *Can J Neurol Sci* 30, 98–105.

69 Odeh M, Sabo E, Srugo I *et al.* (2004) Serum levels of tumor necrosis factor-alpha correlate with severity of hepatic encephalopathy due to chronic liver failure. *Liver Int* 24, 110–226.

70 Mans AM, Biebuyck JF, Shelly K et al. (1982) Regional blood–brain barrier permeability to amino acids after portacaval anastomosis. J Neurochem 38, 705–717.

71 Cangiano C, Cardelli-Cangiano P, James JH et al. (1983) Brain microvessels take up large neutral amino acids in exchange for glutamine. Cooperative role of Na⁺-dependent and Na⁺-independent systems. J Biol Chem 258, 894–954.

72 Morgan MY, Milsom JP, Sherlock S (1978) Plasma ratio of valine, leucine and isoleucine to tyrosine in liver disease. Gut 19, 1068–1073.

73 Fischer JE, Funovics JM, Aguirre A et al. (1975) The role of plasma amino acids in hepatic encephalopathy. Surgery 78, 276–290.

74 Cuilleret G, Pomier-Layargues G, Pons F et al. (1980) Changes in brain catecholamine levels in human cirrhotic hepatic encephalopathy. Gut 21, 565–569.

75 Knudsen GM, Schmidt J, Almdal T et al. (1993) Passage of amino acids and glucose across the blood-brain barrier in patients with hepatic encephalopathy. Hepatology 17, 987–992.

76 Rossle M, Mullen KD, Jones EA (1989) Cortical benzodiazepine receptor binding in a rabbit model of hepatic encephalopathy: the effect of Triton X-100 on receptor solubilization. Metab Brain Dis 4, 203–212.

77 Ferenci P, Ebner J, Zimmermann C et al. (1988) Overestimation of serum concentrations of gamma-aminobutyric acid in patients with hepatic encephalopathy by the gamma-aminobutyric acid-radioreceptor assay. Hepatology 8, 69–72.

78 Knudsen GM, Poulsen HE, Paulson OB (1988) Blood–brain barrier permeability in galactosamine-induced hepatic encephalopathy. No evidence for increased GABA-transport. J Hepatol 6, 187–192.

79 Lavoie J, Giguere JF, Layargues GP et al. (1987) Amino acid changes in autopsied brain tissue from cirrhotic patients with hepatic encephalopathy. J Neurochem 49, 692–697.

80 Butterworth RF, Lavoie J, Giguere JF et al. (1988) Affinities and densities of high-affinity [3H] muscimol (GABA-A) binding sites and of central benzodiazepine receptors are unchanged in autopsied brain tissue from cirrhotic patients with hepatic encephalopathy. Hepatology 8, 1084–1088.

81 Basile AS, Jones EA, Skolnick P (1991) The pathogenesis and treatment of hepatic encephalopathy: evidence for the involvement of benzodiazepine receptor ligands. Pharmacol Rev 43, 27–71.

82 Basile AS, Gammal SH, Jones EA et al. (1989) GABAA receptor complex in an experimental model of hepatic encephalopathy: evidence for elevated levels of an endogenous benzodiazepine receptor ligand. J Neurochem 53, 1057–1063.

83 Olesmaa M, Rothstein JD, Guidotti A et al. (1990) Endogenous benzodiazepine receptor ligands in human and animal encephalopathy. J Neurochem 55, 2015–2023.

84 Basile AS, Hughes RD, Harrison PM et al. (1991) Elevated brain concentrations of 1,4-benzodiazepines in fulminant hepatic failure. N Engl J Med 325, 473–478.

85 Yurdaydin C, Walsh TJ, Engler HD et al. (1995) Gut bacteria provide precursors of benzodiazepine receptor ligands in a rat model of hepatic encephalopathy. Brain Res 679, 42–48.

86 Ahboucha S, Pomier-Layargues G, Butterworth RF (2004) Increased brain concentrations of endogenous (non-benzodiazepine) GABA-A receptor ligands in human hepatic encephalopathy. Metab Brain Dis 19, 241–251.

87 Lavoie J, Layrargues GP, Butterworth RF (1990) Increased densities of peripheral-type benzodiazepine receptors in brain autopsy samples from cirrhotic patients with hepatic encephalopathy. Hepatology 11, 874–878.

88 Itzhak Y, Roig-Cantisano A, Dombro RS et al. (1995) Acute liver failure and hyperammonemia increase peripheral-type benzodiazepine receptor binding and pregnenolone synthesis in mouse brain. Brain Res 705, 345–348.

89 Jones EA (2002) Ammonia, the GABA neurotransmitter system, and hepatic encephalopathy. Metab Brain Dis 17, 275–281.

90 Livingstone AS, Potvin M, Goresky CA et al. (1977) Changes in the blood–brain barrier in hepatic coma after hepatectomy in the rat. Gastroenterology 73, 697–704.

91 Traber PG, Dal Canto M, Ganger DR et al. (1987) Electron microscopic evaluation of brain edema in rabbits with galactosamine-induced fulminant hepatic failure: ultrastructure and integrity of the blood–brain barrier. Hepatology 7, 1272–1277.

92 Martin H, Voss K, Hufnagl P et al. (1987) Morphometric and densitometric investigations of protoplasmic astrocytes and neurons in human hepatic encephalopathy. Exp Pathol 32, 241–250.

93 Hösslin CV, Alzheimer A (1912) Ein Betrag zur Klinik und patologischen Anatomie der Westphal-Strumpellachen Pseudosklerose. Z Gesamte Neurol Psychiat 8, 183–209.

94 Reichenbach A, Fuchs U, Kasper M et al. (1995) Hepatic retinopathy: morphological features of retinal glial (Muller) cells accompanying hepatic failure. Acta Neuropathol (Berl) 90, 273–281.

95 Cavanagh JB, Kyu MH (1971) Type II Alzheimer change experimentally produced in astrocytes in the rat. J Neurol Sci 12, 63–75.

96 Gutierrez JA, Norenberg MD (1975) Alzheimer II astrocytosis following methionine sulfoximine. Arch Neurol 32, 123–126.

97 Bruton CJ, Corsellis JA, Russell A (1970) Hereditary hyperammonaemia. Brain 93, 423–434.

98 Sobel RA, DeArmond SJ, Forno LS et al. (1981) Glial fibrillary acidic protein in hepatic encephalopathy. An immunohistochemical study. J Neuropathol Exp Neurol 40, 625–632.

99 Kretzschmar HA, DeArmond SJ, Forno LS (1985) Measurement of GFAP in hepatic encephalopathy by ELISA and transblots. J Neuropathol Exp Neurol 44, 459–471.

100 Norenberg MD (1995) Hepatic encephalopathy. In: Ketterman H, Ransom BR (eds) Neuroglia. New York: Oxford University Press, pp. 950–963.

101 Tarter RE, Hays AL, Sandford SS et al. (1986) Cerebral morphological abnormalities associated with non-alcoholic cirrhosis. Lancet 2, 893–895.

102 Zeneroli ML, Cioni G, Vezzelli C et al. (1987) Prevalence of brain atrophy in liver cirrhosis patients with chronic persistent encephalopathy. Evaluation by computed tomography. J Hepatol 4, 283–292.

103 Victor M, Adams RD, Cole M (1965) The acquired (non-Wilsonian) type of chronic hepatocerebral degeneration. Medicine (Baltimore) 44, 345–396.

104 Finlayson MH, Superville B (1981) Distribution of cerebral lesions in acquired hepatocerebral degeneration. Brain 104, 79–95.

105 Zieve L, Mendelson DF, Goepfert M (1960) Shunt encephalopathy. II. Occurrence of permanent myelopathy. Ann Intern Med 53, 53–63.

106 Pujol A, Graus F, Peri J et al. (1991) Hyperintensity in the globus pallidus on T1-weighted and inversion-recovery MRI: a possible marker of advanced liver disease. Neurology 41, 1526–1527.

107 Krieger S, Jauss M, Jansen O et al. (1996) Neuropsychiatric profile and hyperintense globus pallidus on T1-weighted magnetic resonance images in liver cirrhosis. Gastroenterology 111, 147–155.

108 Kulisevsky J, Pujol J, Balanzo J *et al.* (1992) Pallidal hyperintensity on magnetic resonance imaging in cirrhotic patients: clinical correlations. *Hepatology* 16, 1382–1388.

109 Pujol A, Pujol J, Graus F *et al.* (1993) Hyperintense globus pallidus on T1-weighted MRI in cirrhotic patients is associated with severity of liver failure. *Neurology* 43, 65–69.

110 Rose C, Butterworth FR, Zayed J *et al.* (1999) Manganese deposition in basal ganglia structures results from both portal-systemic shunting and liver dysfunction. *Gastroenterology* 117, 640–644.

111 Kulisevsky J, Pujol J, Deus J *et al.* (1995) Persistence of MRI hyperintensity of the globus pallidus in cirrhotic patients: a 2-year follow-up study. *Neurology* 45, 995–997.

112 Shah NJ, Neeb H, Zaitsev M *et al.* (2003) Quantitative T1 mapping of hepatic encephalopathy using magnetic resonance imaging. *Hepatology* 38, 1219–1226.

113 Pomier-Layargues G, Spahr L, Butterworth RF (1995) Increased manganese concentration in pallidum of cirrhotic patients. *Lancet* 345, 735.

114 Krieger D, Krieger G, Jansen O *et al.* (1995) Manganese and chronic hepatic encephalopathy. *Lancet* 346, 270–274.

115 Shinotoh H, Snow BJ, Hewitt KA *et al.* (1995) MRI and PET studies of manganese-intoxicated monkeys. *Neurology* 45, 1199–1204.

116 Brouillet EP, Shinobu L, McGarvey U *et al.* (1993) Manganese injection into the rat striatum produces excitotoxic lesions by impairing energy metabolism. *Exp Neurol* 120, 89–94.

117 Chen CJ, Liao SL (2002) Oxidative stress involves in astrocytic alterations induced by manganese. *Exp Neurol* 175, 216–225.

118 Hazell AS, Norenberg MD (1997) Manganese decreases glutamate uptake in cultured astrocytes. *Neurochem Res* 22, 1443–1447.

119 Hazell AS, Desjardins P, Butterworth RF (1999) Chronic exposure of rat primary astrocyte cultures to manganese results in increased binding sites for the 'peripheral-type' benzodiazepine receptor ligand 3H-PK 11195. *Neurosci Lett* 271, 5–8.

120 Spahr L, Butterworth RF, Fontaine S *et al.* (1996) Increased blood manganese in cirrhotic patients: relationship to pallidal magnetic resonance signal hyperintensity and neurological symptoms. *Hepatology* 24, 1116–1120.

121 Norton NS, McConnell JR, Zetterman RK *et al.* (1994) A quantitative evaluation of magnetic resonance image signal changes of the brain in chronic hepatic encephalopathy. *J Hepatol* 21, 764–770.

122 Blei AT, Larsen FS (1999) Pathophysiology of cerebral edema in fulminant hepatic failure. *J Hepatol* 31, 771–776.

123 Donovan JP, Schafer DF, Shaw BW Jr *et al.* (1998) Cerebral edema and increased intracranial pressure in chronic liver disease. *Lancet* 351, 719–721.

124 Kreis R, Farrow N, Ross BD (1990) Diagnosis of hepatic encephalopathy by proton magnetic resonance spectroscopy. *Lancet* 336, 635–636.

125 Ross BD, Jacobson S, Villamil F *et al.* (1994) Subclinical hepatic encephalopathy: proton MR spectroscopic abnormalities. *Radiology* 193, 457–463.

126 Shawcross DL, Balata S, Olde Daminck SW *et al.* (2004) Low myo-inositol and high glutamine levels in brain are associated with neuropsychological deterioration after induced hyperammonemia. *Am J Physiol Gastrointest Liver Physiol* 287, G503–G509. Epub May 6 2004.

127 Zwingmann C, Brand A, Richter-Landsberg C *et al.* (1998) Multinuclear NMR spectroscopy studies on NH4Cl-induced metabolic alteration and detoxification processes in primary astrocytes and glioma cells. *Dev Neurosci* 20, 417–426.

128 Paredes A, McManus M, Kwon HM *et al.* (1992) Osmoregulation of Na(+)-inositol cotransporter activity and mRNA levels in brain glial cells. *Am J Physiol* 263, 1282–1288.

129 Cordoba J, Gottstein J, Blei AT (1996) Glutamine, myo-inositol, and organic brain osmolytes after portocaval anastomosis in the rat: implications for ammonia-induced brain edema. *Hepatology* 24, 919–923.

130 Bluml S, Zuckerman E, Tan J *et al.* (1998) Proton-decoupled 31P magnetic resonance spectroscopy reveals osmotic and metabolic disturbances in human hepatic encephalopathy. *J Neurochem* 71, 1564–1576.

131 Norenberg MD, Baker L, Norenberg LO *et al.* (1991) Ammonia-induced astrocyte swelling in primary culture. *Neurochem Res* 16, 833–836.

132 Schliess F, Sinning R, Rischer R *et al.* (1996) Calcium-dependent activation of Erk-1 and Erk-2 after hypo-osmotic astrocyte swelling. *Biochem J* 320, 167–171.

133 Haussinger D, Schliess F (2005) Astrocyte swelling and protein tyrosine nitration in hepatic encephalopathy. *Neurochem Int* 47, 64–70.

134 Kimelberg HK (1995) Receptors on astrocytes – what possible functions? *Neurochem Int* 26, 27–40.

135 Kimelberg HK (1995) Current concepts of brain edema. Review of laboratory investigations. *J Neurosurg* 83, 1051–1059.

136 Bender AS, River IV, Norenberg MD (1992) Tumor necrosis factor alpha induces astrocyte swelling. *Trans Am J Neurochem*, 113.

137 Bender AS, Norenberg MD (1998) Effect of benzodiazepines and neurosteroids on ammonia-induced swelling in cultured astrocytes. *J Neurosci Res* 54, 673–680.

138 Moats RA, Lien YH, Filippi D *et al.* (1993) Decrease in cerebral inositols in rats and humans. *Biochem J* 295, 15–18.

139 Ross BD, Danielsen ER, Bluml S (1996) Proton magnetic resonance spectroscopy: the new gold standard for diagnosis of clinical and subclinical hepatic encephalopathy. *Dig Dis* 14, 30–39.

140 Cordoba J, Alonso J, Rovira A *et al.* (2001) The development of low grade cerebral edema in cirrhosis is supported by the evolution of (1) H-magnetic resonant abnormalities alter liver transplantation. *J Hepatol* 35, 598–604.

141 Miese F, Kircheis G, Wittsack HJ *et al.* (2006) [1]H-MR spectroscopy, magnetization transfer and diffusion-weighted imaging in alcoholic and nonalcoholic cirrhotic subjects with hepatic encephalopathy. *Am J Neuroradiol* 27, 1019–1026.

142 Sede HW, Gore CD, Hughes RD *et al.* (1984) Inhibition of rat brain Na+, K+-ATPase activity by serum from patients with fulminant hepatic failure. *Hepatology* 4, 74–79.

143 Record CO, Buxton B, Chase RA *et al.* (1976) Plasma and brain amino acids in fulminant hepatic failure and their relationship to hepatic encephalopathy. *Eur J Clin Invest* 6, 387–394.

144 Takahashi H, Koehler RC, Brusilow SW *et al.* (1991) Inhibition of brain glutamine accumulation prevents cerebral edema in hyperammonemic rats. *Am J Physiol* 261, H825–829.

145 Blei AT, Olafsson S, Therrien G *et al.* (1994) Ammonia-induced brain edema and intracranial hypertension in rats after portacaval anastomosis. *Hepatology* 19, 1437–1444.

146 Watson AJ, Chambers T, Karp JE *et al.* (1985) Transient idiopathic hyperammonemia in adults. *Lancet* 2, 1271–1274.

147 Munoz SJ, Robinson M, Northrup B *et al.* (1991) Elevated intracranial pressure and computed tomography of the brain in fulminant hepatocellular failure. *Hepatology* 13, 209–212.

148 Wijdicks EF, Plevak DJ, Rakela J et al. (1995) Clinical and radiological features of cerebral edema in fulminant hepatic failure. Mayo Clin Proc 70, 119–124.

149 Kato M, Hughes RD, Keays RT et al. (1992) Electron microscopic study of brain capillaries in cerebral edema from fulminant hepatic failure. Hepatology 15, 1060–1066.

150 Murphy S (ed.) (1995) Astrocytes: Pharmacology and Function. San Diego: Academic Press.

151 Kimelberg H, Ransom BR (eds) (1995) Neuroglia. New York: Oxford University Press.

152 Walz W (1989) Role of glial cells in the regulation of the brain ion microenvironment. Prog Neurobiol 33, 309–333.

153 Ransom BR, Sontheimer H (1992) The neurophysiology of glial cells. J Clin Neurophysiol 9, 224–251.

154 Sarna GS, Bradbury MW, Cavanagh J (1977) Permeability of the blood–brain barrier after portocaval anastomosis in the rat. Brain Res 138, 550–54.

155 Janzer RC, Raff MC (1987) Astrocytes induce blood–brain barrier properties in endothelial cells. Nature 325, 253–257.

156 Martinez-Hernandez A, Bell KP, Norenberg MD (1977) Glutamine synthetase: glial localization in brain. Science 195, 1356–1358.

157 Häussinger D (1996) The role of cellular hydration in the regulation of cell function. Biochem J 313, 697–710.

158 Lang F, Busch GL, Ritter M et al. (1998) Functional significance of cell volume regulatory mechanisms. Physiol Rev 78, 247–306.

159 Itzhak Y, Bender AS, Norenberg MD (1994) Effect of hypoosmotic stress on peripheral-type benzodiazepine receptors in cultured astrocytes. Brain Res 644, 221–225.

160 Fischer R, Schliess F, Haussinger D (1997) Characterization of the hypo-osmolarity-induced Ca^{2+} response in cultured rat astrocytes. Glia 20, 51–58.

161 Isaacks RE, Bender AS, Kim CY et al. (1999) Effect of osmolality and anion channel inhibitors on myo-inositol efflux in cultured astrocytes. J Neurosci Res 57, 866–871.

162 Busch GL, Wiesinger H, Gulbins E et al. (1996) Effect of astroglial cell swelling on pH of acidic intracellular compartments. Biochim Biophys Acta 1285, 212–218.

163 Dombro RS, Bender AS, Norenberg MD (2000) Association between cell swelling and glycogen content in cultured astrocytes. Int J Dev Neurosci 18, 161–169.

164 Jessy J, DeJoseph MR, Hawkins RA (1991) Hyperammonaemia depresses glucose consumption throughout the brain. Biochem J 277, 693–696.

165 Hawkins RA, Jessy J (1991) Hyperammonaemia does not impair brain function in the absence of net glutamine synthesis. Biochem J 277, 697–703.

166 Hawkins RA, Jessy J, Mans AM et al. (1993) Effect of reducing brain glutamine synthesis on metabolic symptoms of hepatic encephalopathy. J Neurochem 60, 1000–1006.

167 Häussinger D, Jungermann K (eds) (1998) Liver and Nervous System. Lancaster: Kluwer Academic Publishers.

168 Chepkova AN, Doreulee N, Yanovsky Y et al. (2002) Long-lasting enhancement of corticostriatal neurotransmission by taurine. Eur J Neurosci 16, 523–530.

169 Sergeeva OA, Chepkova AN, Doreulee N et al. (2003) Taurine induced long-lasting enhancement of synaptic transmission in mice: role of transporters. J Physiol 55, 911–919.

170 Oermann E, Warskulat U, Heller-Stilb B et al. (2005) Taurine-transporter gene knockout-induced changes in GABA (A), kainate and AMPA but not NMDA receptor binding in mouse brain. Anat Embryol (Berl) 210, 363–372.

171 Warskulat U, Görg B, Bidmon HJ et al. (2002) Ammonia-induced heme oxygenase-1 expression in cultured rat astrocytes and rat brain in vivo. Glia 40, 324–336.

172 Song G, Dhodda VK, Blei AT et al. (2002) Genechip analysis shows altered mRNA expression of transcripts of neurotransmitter and signal transduction pathways in the cerebral cortex of portocaval shunted rats. J Neurosci Res 68, 730–737

173 Vaquero J, Chung C, Blei AT (2004) Cerebral blood flow in acute liver failure: a finding in search of a mechanism. Metab Brain Dis 19, 177–194.

174 Zhou BG, Norenberg MD (1999) Ammonia downregulates GLAST mRNA glutamate transporter in rat astrocyte cultures. Neurosci Lett 276, 145–148.

175 Butterworth RF (2002) Glutamate transporters in hyperammonemia. Neurochem Int 41, 81–85.

176 Chan H, Zwingmann C, Pannunzio M et al. (2003) Effects of ammonia on high affinity glutamate uptake and glutamate transporter EAAT3 expression in cultured rat cerebellar granule cells. Neurochem Int 43, 137–146.

177 Braissant O, Henry H, Villard AM et al. (2002) Ammonium-induced impairment of axonal growth is prevented through glial creatine. J Neurosci 22, 9810–9820.

178 Bachmann C, Braissant O, Villard AM et al. (2004) Ammonia toxicity to the brain and creatine. Mol Genet Metab 81, S52–57.

179 Norenberg MD, Jayakumar AR, Rama Rao KV (2004) Oxidative stress in the pathogenesis of hepatic encephalopathy. Metab Brain Dis 19, 313–329.

180 Murthy CR, Rama Rao KV, Bai G et al. (2001) Ammonia-induced production of free radicals in primary cultures of rat astrocytes. J Neurosci Res 66, 282–288.

181 Schliess F, Görg B, Fischer R et al. (2002) Ammonia induces MK-801-sensitive nitration and phosphorylation of protein tyrosine residues in rat astrocytes. FASEB J 16, 739–741.

182 Schliess F, Foster N, Gorg B et al. (2004) Hyposmotic swelling increases protein tyrosine nitration in cultured rat astrocytes. Glia 47, 21–29.

183 Gorg B, Foster N, Reinehr R et al. (2003) Benzodiazepine-induced protein tyrosine nitration in rat astrocytes. Hepatology 37, 334–342.

184 Bender AS, Schousboe A, Reichelt W et al. (1998) Ionic mechanisms in glutamate-induced astrocyte swelling: role of K^+ influx. J Neurosci Res 52, 307–321.

185 Hermenegildo C, Marcaida G, Montoliu C et al. (1996) NMDA receptor antagonists prevent acute ammonia toxicity in mice. Neurochem Res 21, 1237–1244.

186 Vogels BA, Maas MA, Daalhuisen J et al. (1997) Memantine, a non-competitive NMDA receptor antagonist improves hyperammonemia-induced encephalopathy and acute hepatic encephalopathy in rats. Hepatology 25, 820–827.

187 Kosenko E, Kaminsky Y, Lopata O et al. (1998) Nitroarginine, an inhibitor of nitric oxide synthase, prevents changes in superoxide radical and antioxidant enzymes induced by ammonia intoxication. Metab Brain Dis 13, 29–41.

188 Klotz LO, Schroeder P, Sies H (2002) Peroxynitrite signaling: receptor tyrosine kinases and activation of stress-responsive pathways. Free Radic Biol Med 33, 737–743.

189 Saeki M, Maeda S (1999) p130cas is a cellular target protein for tyrosine nitration induced by peroxynitrite. Neurosci Res 33, 325–328.

190 Reinehr R, Gorg B, Hongen A *et al.* (2004) CD95-tyrosine nitration inhibits hyperosmotic and CD95 ligand-induced CD95 activation in rat hepatocytes. *J Biol Chem* 279, 10364–10373.

191 Gorg B, Wettstein M, Metzger S *et al.* (2005) LPS-induced tyrosine nitration of hepatic glutamine synthetase. *Hepatology* 42, 499.

192 Alman RW, Ehrmantraut WR, Fazekas JF *et al.* (1956) Cerebral metabolism in hepatic insufficiency. *Am J Med* 21, 843–849.

193 Morgan MY (1996) Non-invasive neuroinvestigation in liver disease. *Semin Liver Dis* 16, 293.

194 Lockwood AH, Yap EWH, Rhoades HM *et al.* (1991) Altered cerebral blood flow and glucose metabolism in patients with liver disease and minimal encephalopathy. *J Cerebr Blood Flow Metab* 11, 331–336.

195 Zafiris O, Kircheis G, Rood HA *et al.* (2004) Neural mechanism underlying impaired visual judgement in the dysmetabolic brain: an fMRI study. *Neuroimage* 22, 541–552.

196 Taylor-Robinson SD, Sargentoni J, Mallalieu RJ *et al.* (1994) Cerebral phosphorus-31 magnetic resonance spectroscopy in patients with chronic hepatic encephalopathy. *Hepatology* 20, 1173–1178.

197 Barbiroli B, Gaiani S, Lodi R *et al.* (2002) Abnormal brain energy metabolism shown by *in vivo* phosphorus magnetic resonance spectroscopy in patients with chronic liver disease. *Brain Res Bull* 59, 75–82.

198 Hindfelt B, Plum F, Duffy TE (1977) Effect of acute ammonia intoxication on cerebral metabolism in rats with portocaval shunts. *J Clin Invest* 59, 386–406.

199 deKnegt RJ, Schalm SW, van der Rijt CC *et al.* (1994) Extracellular brain glutamate during acute liver failure and during acute hyperammonemia simulating acute liver failure: an experimental study based on *in vivo* brain dialysis. *J Hepatol* 20, 19–26.

200 Rao VL, Audet RM, Butterworth RF (1995) Selective alterations of extracellular brain amino acids in relation to function in experimental portal-systemic encephalopathy: results of an *in vivo* microdialysis study. *J Neurochem* 65, 1221–1228.

201 Steindl PE, Coy DL, Finn B *et al.* (1996) A low-protein diet ameliorates disrupted locomotor activity in rats after portacaval anastomosis. *Am J Physiol* 271, G555–560.

202 Sergeeva OA, Schulz D, Doreulee N *et al.* (2005) Deficits in corticostriatal synaptic plasticity and behavioral habituation in rats with portocaval anastomosis. *Neuroscience* 134, 1091–1098.

203 Weissenborn K, Heidenreich S, Giewekemeyer K *et al.* (2003) Memory function in early hepatic encephalopathy. *J Hepatol* 39, 320–325.

204 Bakti G, Fisch HU, Karlaganis G *et al.* (1987) Mechanism of the excessive sedative response of cirrhotics to benzodiazepines: model experiments with triazolam. *Hepatology* 7, 629–638.

205 Pomier-Layrargues G, Giguere JF, Lavoie J *et al.* (1994) Flumazenil in cirrhotic patients in hepatic coma: a randomized double-blind placebo-controlled crossover trial. *Hepatology* 19, 32–37.

206 Zisterer DM, Williams DC (1997) Peripheral-type benzodiazepine receptors. *Genet Pharmacol* 29, 305–314.

207 Papadopoulos V (1993) Peripheral-type benzodiazepin/diazepam binding inhibitor receptor: biological role in steroidogenic cell function. *Endocrinol Rev* 12, 222–240.

208 Ducis I, Norenberg LO, Norenberg MD (1989) Effect of ammonium chloride on the astrocyte benzodiazepine receptor. *Brain Res* 493, 362–365.

209 Giguere JF, Hamel E, Butterworth RF (1992) Increased densities of binding sites for the peripheral-type benzodiazepine receptor ligand. [3H]PK 11195 in rat brain following portocaval anastomosis. *Brain Res* 585, 295–298.

210 Rao VL, Qureshi IA, Butterworth RF (1993) Increased densities of binding sites for the peripheral-type benzodiazepine receptor ligand [3H]PK 11195 in congenital ornithine transcarbamylase-deficient sparse fur mouse. *Pediatr Res* 34, 777–780.

211 Korneyev A, Pan BS, Polo A *et al.* (1993) Stimulation of brain pregnenolone synthesis by mitochondrial diazepam binding inhibitor receptor ligands *in vivo*. *J Neurochem* 61, 1515–1524.

212 Fischer R, Schmitt M, Bode JG *et al.* (2001) Expression of the peripheral-type benzodiazepine receptor and apoptosis induction in hepatic stellate cells. *Gastroenterology* 120, 1212–1226.

213 Swain MS, Bergeron M, Audet R *et al.* (1992) Monitoring of neurotransmitter amino acids by means of an indwelling cisterna magna catheter: a comparison of two rodent models of fulminant liver failure. *Hepatology* 16, 1028–1035.

214 Michalak A, Rose C, Butterworth J *et al.* (1996) Neuroactive amino acids and glutamate (NMDA) receptors in frontal cortex of rats with experimental acute liver failure. *Hepatology* 24, 908–913.

215 Moroni F, Lombardi G, Moneti G *et al.* (1983) The release and neosynthesis of glutamic acid are increased in experimental models of hepatic encephalopathy. *J Neurochem* 40, 850–854.

216 Tossman U, Delin A, Eriksson LS *et al.* (1987) Brain cortical amino acids measured by intracerebral dialysis in portacaval shunted rats. *Neurochem Res* 12, 265–269.

217 Cooper J, Bloom F, Roth RH (1996) *The Biochemical Basis of Neuropharmacology.* New York: Oxford University Press.

218 Schipke CG, Ohlemeyer C, Matyash M *et al.* (2001) Astrocytes of the mouse neocortex express functional N-methyl-D-aspartate receptors. *FASEB J* 15, 1270–1272.

219 Peterson C, Giguere JF, Cotman CW *et al.* (1990) Selective loss of N-methyl-D-aspartate-sensitive L-[3H] glutamate binding sites in rat brain following portacaval anastomosis. *J Neurochem* 55, 386–390.

220 Maddison JE, Watson WE, Dodd PR *et al.* (1991) Alterations in cortical [3H] kainate and alpha-[3H] amino-3-hydroxy-5-methyl-4-isoxazolepropionic acid binding in a spontaneous canine model of chronic hepatic encephalopathy. *J Neurochem* 56, 1881–1888.

221 Michel H, Solere M, Granier P *et al.* (1980) Treatment of cirrhotic hepatic encephalopathy with L-dopa. A controlled trial. *Gastroenterology* 79, 207–211.

222 Bergeron M, Reader TA, Layargues GP *et al.* (1989) Monoamines and metabolites in autopsied brain tissue from cirrhotic patients with hepatic encephalopathy. *Neurochem Res* 14, 853–859.

223 Rao VL, Giguere JF, Layargues GP *et al.* (1993) Increased activities of MAOA and MAOB in autopsied brain tissue from cirrhotic patients with hepatic encephalopathy. *Brain Res* 621, 349–352.

224 Mousseau DD, Perney P, Layargues GP *et al.* (1993) Selective loss of pallidal dopamine D2 receptor density in hepatic encephalopathy. *Neurosci Lett* 162, 192–196.

225 Butterworth RF, Spahr L, Fontaine S *et al.* (1995) Manganese toxicity, dopaminergic dysfunction and hepatic encephalopathy. *Metab Brain Dis* 10, 259–267.

226 Bengtsson F, Bugge M, Johansen KH *et al.* (1991) Brain tryptophan hydroxylation in the portacaval shunted rat: a hypothesis for the regulation of serotonin turnover *in vivo*. *J Neurochem* 56, 1069–1074.

227 Bugge M, Bengtsson F, Nobin A *et al.* (1987) The turnover of brain monoamines after total hepatectomy in rats infused with branched chain amino acids. *World J Surg* 11, 810–817.

228 Rao VL, Giguere JF, Layrargues GP *et al.* (1993) Increased activities of MAOA and MAOB in autopsied brain tissue from cirrhotic patients with hepatic encephalopathy. *Brain Res* 621, 349–352.

229 Rao VL, Butterworth RF (1994) Alterations of [3H]8-OH-DPAT and [3H] ketanserin binding sites in autopsied brain tissue from cirrhotic patients with hepatic encephalopathy. *Neurosci Lett* 182, 69–72.

230 Vorobioff J, Garcia-Tsao G, Groszmann R *et al.* (1989) Long-term hemodynamic effects of ketanserin, a 5-hydroxytryptamine blocker, in portal hypertensive patients. *Hepatology* 9, 88–91.

231 Ferenci P, Herneth A, Steindl P (1996) Newer approaches to therapy of hepatic encephalopathy. *Semin Liver Dis* 16, 329.

232 Cordoba J, Cabrera J, Lataif L *et al.* (1998) High prevalence of sleep disturbance in cirrhosis. *Hepatology* 27, 339–345.

233 Blei AT, Zee P (1998) Abnormalities of circadian rhythmicity in liver disease. *J Hepatol* 29, 832–835.

234 Haas H, Panula P (2003) The role of histamine and the tuberomammillary nucleus in the nervous system. *Nature Rev Neurosci* 4, 121–130.

235 Doreulee N, Yanovsky Y, Flagmeyer I *et al.* (2001) Histamine H(3) receptors depress synaptic transmission in the corticostriatal pathway. *Neuropharmacology* 40, 106–113.

236 Borg J, Warter JM, Schlienger JL *et al.* (1982) Neurotransmitter modifications in human cerebrospinal fluid and serum during hepatic encephalopathy. *J Neurol Sci* 57, 343–356.

237 Lozeva V, Tuomisto L, Sola D *et al.* (2001) Increased density of brain histamine H(1) receptors in rats with portacaval anastomosis and in cirrhotic patients with chronic hepatic encephalopathy. *Hepatology* 33, 1370–1376.

238 Lozeva V, Tuomisto L, Tarhanen J *et al.* (2003) Increased concentrations of histamine and its metabolite, tele-methylhistamine and down-regulation of histamine H3 receptor sites in autopsied brain tissue from cirrhotic patients who died in hepatic coma. *J Hepatol* 39, 522–527.

239 Lozeva V, Valjakka A, Lecklin A *et al.* (2000) Effects of the histamine H(1) receptor blocker, pyrilamine, on spontaneous locomotor activity of rats with long-term portacaval anastomosis. *Hepatology* 31, 336–344.

240 Martin JR, Porchet H, Buhler R *et al.* (1985) Increased ethanol consumption and blood ethanol levels in rats with portacaval shunts. *Am J Physiol* 248, G287–292.

241 de Waele JP, Audet RM, Leong DK *et al.* (1996) Portacaval anastomosis induces region-selective alterations of the endogenous opioid system in the rat brain. *Hepatology* 24, 895–901.

242 Panerai AE, Salerno F, Baldissera F *et al.* (1982) Brain beta-endorphin concentrations in experimental chronic liver disease. *Brain Res* 247, 188–190.

243 Yurdaydin C, Karavelioglu D, Onaran O *et al.* (1998) Opioid receptor ligands in human hepatic encephalopathy. *J Hepatol* 29, 796–801.

244 Lounasmaa OV, Hamalainen M, Hari R *et al.* (1996) Information processing in the human brain: magnetoencephalographic approach. *Proc Natl Acad Sci USA* 93, 8809–8815.

245 Schnitzler A, Gross J (2005) Normal and pathological oscillatory communication in the brain. *Nature Rev Neurosci* 6, 285–296.

246 Timmermann L, Gross J, Kircheis G *et al.* (2002) Cortical origin of mini-asterixis in hepatic encephalopathy. *Neurology* 58, 295–299.

247 Timmermann L, Gross J, Butz M *et al.* (2003) Mini-asterixis in hepatic encephalopathy induced by pathologic thalamo-motorcortical coupling. *Neurology* 61, 689–692.

248 Gross J, Kujala J, Hamalainen M *et al.* (2001) Dynamic imaging of coherent sources: studying neural interactions in the human brain. *Proc Natl Acad Sci USA* 98, 694–699.

249 Timmermann L, Gross J, Butz M *et al.* (2004) Pathological oscillatory coupling within the human motor system in different tremor

syndromes as revealed by magnetoencephalography. *Neurol Clin Neurophysiol* 30, 2004–2026.

250 Rio J, Montalban J, Pujadas F *et al.* (1995) Asterixis associated with anatomic cerebral lesions: a study of 45 cases. *Acta Neurol Scand* 91, 377–381.

251 Chen S, Zieve L, Mahadevan V (1970) Mercaptans and dimethyl sulfide in the breath of patients with cirrhosis of the liver. Effect of feeding methionine. *J Lab Clin Med* 75, 628–635.

252 Miyata Y, Motomura S, Tsuji Y *et al.* (1988) Hepatic encephalopathy and reversible cortical blindness. *Am J Gastroenterol* 83, 780–782.

253 Averbuch-Heller L, Meiner Z (1995) Reversible periodic alternating gaze deviation in hepatic encephalopathy. *Neurology* 45, 191–192.

254 Huizenga JR, Gips CH, Conn HO *et al.* (1995) Determination of ammonia in ear-lobe capillary blood is an alternative to arterial blood ammonia. *Clin Chim Acta* 239, 65–70.

255 Ong JP, Aggarwal A, Krieger D *et al.* (2003) Correlation between ammonia levels and the severity of hepatic encephalopathy. *Am J Med* 114, 188–193.

256 Clemmesen JO, Larsen FS, Kondrup J *et al.* (1999) Cerebral herniation in patients with acute liver failure is correlated with arterial ammonia concentration. *Hepatology* 29, 648–653.

257 Barthauer L, Tarter R, Hirsch W *et al.* (1992) Brain morphologic characteristics of cirrhotic alcoholics and cirrhotic nonalcoholics: an MRI study. *Alcohol Clin Exp Res* 16, 982–985.

258 Thuluvath PJ, Edwin D, Yue NC *et al.* (1995) Increased signals seen in globus pallidus in T1-weighted magnetic resonance imaging in cirrhotics are not suggestive of chronic hepatic encephalopathy. *Hepatology* 21, 440–442.

259 Takashi M, Igarashi M, Hino S *et al.* (1985) Portal hemodynamics in chronic portal-systemic encephalopathy. Angiographic study in seven cases. *J Hepatol* 1, 467–476.

260 Ohnishi K, Sato S, Saito M *et al.* (1986) Clinical and portal hemodynamic features in cirrhotic patients having a large spontaneous splenorenal and/or gastrorenal shunt. *Am J Gastroenterol* 81, 450–455.

261 Riggio O, Efrati C, Catalano C *et al.* (2005) High prevalence of spontaneous portal-systemic shunts in persistent hepatic encephalopathy: a case–control study. *Hepatology* 42, 1158–1165.

262 Mutchnick MG, Lerner E, Conn HO (1974) Portal-systemic encephalopathy and portacaval anastomosis: a prospective, controlled investigation. *Gastroenterology* 66, 1005–1019.

263 Langer B, Taylor BR, Mackenzie DR *et al.* (1985) Further report of prospective randomized trial comparing distal splenorenal shunt with end-to-side portacaval shunt. An analysis of encephalopathy, survival, and quality of life. *Gastroenterology* 88, 424–429.

264 Sanyal AJ, Freedman AM, Shiffman ML *et al.* (1994) Portosystemic encephalopathy after transjugular intrahepatic portosystemic shunt: results of a prospective controlled study. *Hepatology* 20, 46–55.

265 Mamiya Y, Kanazawa H, Kimura Y *et al.* (2004) Hepatic encephalopathy alter transjugular intrahepatic portosystemic shunt. *Hepatol Res* 30, 162–168.

266 Madoff DC, Wallace MJ, Ahrar K *et al.* (2004) TIPS-related hepatic encephalopathy: management options with novel endovascular techniques. *Radiographics* 24, 21–36.

267 Langer B, Taylor BR, Greig PD (1990) Selective or total shunts for variceal bleeding. *Am J Surg* 160, 75–79.

268 Pomier-Layargues G, Huet PM, Infante-Rivard C *et al.* (1988) Prognostic value of indocyanine green and lidocaine kinetics for survival and chronic hepatic encephalopathy in cirrhotic patients

following elective end-to-side portocaval shunt. *Hepatology* 8, 1506–1510.

269 Planas R, Gomes-Vieira MC, Cabre E *et al.* (1992) Prognostic factors of hepatic encephalopathy alter portacaval anastomosis, a multivariate analysis in 50 patients. *Am J Gastroenterol* 87, 1792–1796.

270 Somberg KA, Riegler JL, LaBerge JM *et al.* (1995) Hepatic encephalopathy after transjugular intrahepatic portosystemic shunts: incidence and risk factors. *Am J Gastroenterol* 90, 549–555.

271 Blei, AT (1994) Hepatic encephalopathy in the age of TIPS. *Hepatology* 20, 249–252.

272 Rossle M, Piotraschke J (1996) Transjugular intrahepatic portosystemic shunt and hepatic encephalopathy. *Dig Dis* 1, 12–19.

273 Hassoun Z, Dechenes M, Lafortune M *et al.* (2001) Relationship between pre-TIPS liver perfusion by the portal vein and the incidence of post-TIPS chronic hepatic encephalopathy. *Am J Gastroenterol* 96, 1205–1209.

274 Summerskill WH, Davidson EA, Sherlock S *et al.* (1956) The neuropsychiatric syndrome associated with hepatic cirrhosis and an extensive portal collateral circulation. *Q J Med* 25, 245–266.

275 Mendoza G, Marti-Fabregas J, Kulisevsky J *et al.* (1994) Hepatic myelopathy: a rare complication of portacaval shunt. *Eur Neurol* 34, 209–212.

276 Rikkers L, Jenko P, Rudman D *et al.* (1978) Subclinical hepatic encephalopathy: detection, prevalence and relationship to nitrogen metabolism. *Gastroenterology* 75, 462–469.

277 Gitlin N, Lewis DC, Hinkley L (1986) The diagnosis and prevalence of subclinical hepatic encephalopathy in apparent healthy, ambulant, nonshunted patients with cirrhosis. *J Hepatol* 3, 75–82.

278 Schomerus H, Hamster W, Blunck H *et al.* (1981) Latent portasystemic encephalopathy. *Dig Dis Sci* 26, 622–660.

279 Ortiz M, Jacas C, Cordoba J (2005) Minimal hepatic encephalopathy: diagnosis, clinical significance and recommendations. *J Hepatol* 42, S45–53.

280 Groeneweg M, Quero JC, DeBruijn I *et al.* (1998) Subclinical hepatic encephalopathy impairs daily functioning. *Hepatology* 28, 45–49.

281 Marchesini G, Bianchi G, Amodio P *et al.* (2001) Italian Study Group for quality of life in cirrhosis. Factors associated with poor health-related quality of life of patients with cirrhosis. *Gastroenterology* 120, 170–178.

282 Arguedas MR, DeLawrence TG, McGuire BM (2003) Influence of hepatic encephalopathy on health-related quality of life in patients with cirrhosis. *Dig Dis Sci* 48, 1622–1626.

283 Bustamante J, Rimola A, Ventura PJ *et al.* (1999) Prognostic significance of hepatic encephalopathy in patients with cirrhosis. *J Hepatol* 30, 890–895.

284 Amodio P, Del Piccolo F, Marchetti P *et al.* (1999) Clinical features and survival of cirrhotic patients with subclinical cognitive alterations detected by the number connection test and computerized psychometric tests. *Hepatology* 29, 1662–1667.

285 Hartmann IJ, Groeneweg M, Quero JC *et al.* (2000) The prognostic significance of subclinical hepatic encephalopathy. *Am J Gastroenterol* 95, 2029–2034.

286 Romero-Gomez M, Boza F, Garcia-Valdecasas MS *et al.* (2001) Subclinical hepatic encephalopathy predicts the development of overt hepatic encephalopathy. *Am J Gastroenterol* 96, 2718–2723.

287 Kono I, Ueda Y, Nakajima K *et al.* (1994) Subcortical impairment in subclinical hepatic encephalopathy. *J Neurol Sci* 126, 162–167.

288 McCrea M, Cordoba J, Vessey G *et al.* (1996) Neuropsychological characterization and detection of subclinical hepatic encephalopathy. *Arch Neurol* 53, 758–763.

289 Lockwood AH, Murphy BW, Donnelly KZ *et al.* (1993) Positron-emission tomographic localization of abnormalities of brain metabolism in patients wit minimal hepatic encephalopathy. *Hepatology* 18, 1061–1068.

290 Rodriguez G, Testa R, Celle G *et al.* (1987) Reduction of cerebral blood flow in subclinical hepatic encephalopathy and its correlation with plasma-free tryptophan. *J Cerebr Blood Flow Metab* 7, 768–772.

291 Watanabe A, Tuchida T, Yata Y *et al.* (1995) Evaluation of neuropsychological function in patients with liver cirrhosis with special reference to their driving ability. *Metab Brain Dis* 10, 239–248.

292 Wein C, Koch H, Popp B *et al.* (2004) Minimal hepatic encephalopathy impairs fitness to drive. *Hepatology* 39, 739–745.

293 Srivastava A, Mehta R, Rothke SP *et al.* (1994) Fitness to drive in patients with cirrhosis and portal-systemic shunting: a pilot study evaluating driving performance. *J Hepatol* 21, 1023–1028.

294 Tarter RE, Hegedus AM, Van Thiel DH *et al.* (1984) Nonalcoholic cirrhosis associated with neuropsychological dysfunction in the absence of overt evidence of hepatic encephalopathy. *Gastroenterology* 86, 1421–1427.

295 Steindl PE, Finn B, Bendok B *et al.* (1995) Disruption of the diurnal rhythm of plasma melatonin in cirrhosis. *Ann Intern Med* 123, 274–277.

296 Blei AT, Olafsson S, Webster S *et al.* (1993) Complications of intracranial pressure monitoring in fulminant hepatic failure. *Lancet* 341, 157–158.

297 Keays RT, Alexander GJ, Williams R (1993) The safety and value of extradural intracranial pressure monitors in fulminant hepatic failure. *J Hepatol* 18, 205–209.

298 Vaquero J, Fontana RJ, Larson AM *et al.* (2005) Complications and use of intracranial pressure monitoring in patients with acute liver failure and severe encephalopathy. *Liver Transpl* 11, 1581–1589.

299 Shami VM, Caldwell SH, Hespenheide EE *et al.* (2003) Recombinant activated factor VII for coagulopathy in fulminant hepatic failure compared with conventional therapy. *Liver Transpl* 9, 138–143.

300 Larsen FS (1996) Cerebral circulation in liver failure: Ohm's law in force. *Semin Liver Dis* 16, 281.

301 Aggarwal S, Obrist W, Yonas H *et al.* (2005) Cerebral hemodynamic and metabolic profiles in fulminant hepatic failure: Relationship to outcome. *Liver Transpl* 11, 1353–1360.

302 Master S, Gottstein J, Blei AT (1999) Cerebral blood flow and the development of ammonia-induced brain edema in rats after portacaval anastomosis. *Hepatology* 30, 876–880.

303 Larsen FS, Ejlersen E, Hansen BA *et al.* (1995) Functional loss of cerebral blood flow autoregulation in patients with fulminant hepatic failure. *J Hepatol* 23, 212–217.

304 Strauss GI, Hansen BA, Herzog T *et al.* (2000) Cerebral autoregulation in patients with end-stage liver disease. *Eur J Gastroenterol Hepatol* 12, 767–771.

305 Shawcross DL, Davies NA, Mookerjee RP *et al.* (2004) Worsening of cerebral hyperemia by the administration of terlipressin in acute liver failure with severe encephalopathy. *Hepatology* 39, 471–475.

306 Wendon JA, Harrison PM, Keays R *et al.* (1994) Cerebral blood flow and metabolism in fulminant liver failure. *Hepatology* 19, 1407–1413.

307 Madl C, Grimm G, Ferenci P *et al.* (1994) Serial recording of sensory evoked potentials: a noninvasive prognostic indicator in fulminant liver failure. *Hepatology* 20, 1487–1494.

308 Kircheis G, Wettstein M, Timmermann L *et al.* (2002) Critical flicker frequency for quantification of low grade hepatic encephalopathy. *Hepatology* 35, 357–366.

309 Horst D, Grace ND, Conn HO et al. (1984) Comparison of dietary protein with an oral, branched chain-enriched amino acid supplement in chronic portal-systemic encephalopathy: a randomized controlled trial. Hepatology 4(2), 279–287.

310 Parsons-Smith B, Sumerskill W, Dawson AM et al. (1957) The electroencephalograph in liver disease. Lancet 2, 866–871.

311 van der Rijt CC, Schalm SW (1992) Quantitative EEG analysis and evoked potentials to measure (latent) hepatic encephalopathy. J Hepatol 14, 141–142.

312 Kullmann F, Hollerbach S, Holstege A et al. (1995) Subclinical hepatic encephalopathy: the diagnostic value of evoked potentials. J Hepatol 22, 101–110.

313 Sandford NL, Saul RE (1988) Assessment of hepatic encephalopathy with visual evoked potentials compared with conventional methods. Hepatology 8, 1094–1098.

314 Davies MG, Rowan MJ, MacMathuna P et al. (1990) The auditory P300 event-related potential: an objective marker of the encephalopathy of chronic liver disease. Hepatology 12, 688–694.

315 Weissenborn K, Scholz M, Hinrichs H et al. (1990) Neurophysiological assessment of early hepatic encephalopathy. Electroencephalogr Clin Neurophysiol 75, 289–295.

316 Kugler CF, Petter J, Taghavy A et al. (1994) Dynamics of cognitive brain dysfunction in patients with cirrhotic liver disease: an event-related P300 potential perspective. Electroencephalogr Clin Neurophysiol 91(1), 33–41.

317 Kugler CF, Lotterer E, Petter J et al. (1992) Visual event-related P300 potentials in early portosystemic encephalopathy. Gastroenterology 103, 302–310.

318 Zeneroli ML, Cioni G, Ventura P et al. (1992) Interindividual variability of the number connection test. J Hepatol 15, 263–264.

319 Weissenborn K, Ruckert N, Hecker H et al. (1998) The number connection tests A and B: interindividual variability and use for the assessment of early hepatic encephalopathy. J Hepatol 28, 646–653.

320 Weissenborn K, Ennen JC, Schomerus H et al. (2001) Neuropsychological characterization of hepatic encephalopathy. J Hepatol 34, 768–773.

321 Tarter RE, Van Thiel DH, Arria AM et al. (1988) Impact of cirrhosis on the neuropsychological test performance of alcoholics. Alcohol Clin Exp Res 12, 619–621.

322 Arria AM, Tarter RE, Starzl TE et al. (1991) Improvement in cognitive functioning of alcoholics following orthotopic liver transplantation. Alcohol Clin Exp Res 15, 956–962.

323 Córdoba J, Blei AT (1997) Treatment of hepatic encephalopathy. Am J Gastroenterol 92, 1429–1439.

324 Mullen KD, Weber FL Jr (1991) Role of nutrition in hepatic encephalopathy. Semin Liver Dis 11, 292–304.

325 Ferenci P, Müller C (1999) Hepatic encephalopathy treatment. In: McDonald J, Burroughs AK, Feagan BG (eds) Evidence-based Gastroenterology and Hepatology. London: BMJ Publisher, pp. 3–15.

326 Riordan SM, Williams R (1997) Treatment of hepatic encephalopathy. N Engl J Med 337, 473–479.

327 Cordoba J, Lopez-Hellin J, Planas M et al. (2004) Normal protein diet for episodic hepatic encephalopathy: results of a randomized study. J Hepatol 41, 38–43.

328 Morgan TR, Moritz TE, Mendenhall CL et al. (1995) Protein consumption and hepatic encephalopathy in alcoholic hepatitis. VA Cooperative Study Group #275. J Am Coll Nutr 14, 152–158.

329 Plauth M, Merli M, Kondrup J et al. (1997) ESPEN guidelines for nutrition in liver disease and transplantation. Clin Nutr 16, 43–55.

330 Uribe M, Marquez MA, Garcia Ramos G et al. (1982) Treatment of chronic portal–systemic encephalopathy with vegetable and animal protein diets. A controlled crossover study. Dig Dis Sci 27, 1109–1116.

331 Fenton JC, Knight EJ, Humpherson PL (1966) Milk-and-cheese diet in portal-systemic encephalopathy. Lancet 1, 164–166.

332 Zieve L, Zieve FJ (1987) The dietary prevention of hepatic coma in Eck fistula dogs. Ammonia and the carbohydrate to protein ration. Hepatology 7, 196–198.

333 Weber FL Jr, Minco D, Fresard KM et al. (1985) Effects of vegetable diets on nitrogen metabolism in cirrhotic subjects. Gastroenterology 89, 538–544.

334 Horst D, Grace ND, Conn HO et al. (1984) Comparison of dietary protein with an oral, branched-chain-enriched amino acid supplement in chronic portal-systemic encephalopathy: a randomized controlled trial. Hepatology 4, 279–287.

335 Plauth M, Egberts EH, Hamster W et al. (1993) Long-term treatment of latent portosystemic encephalopathy with branched-chain amino acids. A double-blind placebo-controlled crossover study. J Hepatol 17, 308–314.

336 Marchesini G, Bianchi G, Merli M et al. (2003) Italian BCAA Study Group. Nutritional supplementation with branched-chain amino acids in advanced cirrhosis: a double-blind, randomized trial. Gastroenterology 124, 1792–1801.

337 Bircher J, Muller J, Guggenheim P et al. (1966) Treatment of chronic portal-systemic encephalopathy with lactulose. Lancet 1, 890–892.

338 Florent C, Flourie B, Leblond A et al. (1985) Influence of chronic lactulose ingestion on the colonic metabolism of lactulose in man (an in vivo study). J Clin Invest 75, 608–613.

339 Mortensen PB (1992) The effect of oral-administered lactulose on colonic nitrogen metabolism and excretion. Hepatology 16, 1350–1356.

340 Weber FL Jr, Fresard KM, Lally BR (1982) Effects of lactulose and neomycin on urea metabolism in cirrhotic subjects. Gastroenterology 82, 213–217.

341 Uribe M, Campollo O, Vargas F et al. (1987) Acidifying enemas (lactitol and lactose) vs. nonacidifying enemas (tap water) to treat acute portal-systemic encephalopathy: a double-blind, randomized clinical trial. Hepatology 7, 639–643.

342 Blanc P, Daures JP, Rouillon JM et al. (1992) Lactitol or lactulose in the treatment of chronic hepatic encephalopathy: results of a meta-analysis. Hepatology 15, 222–228.

343 Uribe M, Dibildox M, Malpica S et al. (1980) Treatment of chronic portal-systemic encephalopathy with lactose in lactase-deficient patients. Dig Dis Sci 25, 924–928.

344 Als-Nielsen B, Gluud LL, Gluud C (2004) Non-absorbable disaccharides for hepatic encephalopathy: systematic review of randomised trials. Br Med J 328, 1046.

345 Fisher CJ, Faloon WW (1957) Blood ammonia levels in hepatic cirrhosis: their control by the oral administration of neomycin. N Engl J Med 256, 1030–1035.

346 van Berlo CL, van Leeuwen PA, Soeters PB (1988) Porcine intestinal ammonia liberation. Influence of food intake, lactulose and neomycin treatment. J Hepatol 7, 250–257.

347 Morgan MH, Read AE, Speller DC (1982) Treatment of hepatic encephalopathy with metronidazole. Gut 23, 1–7.

348 Loft S, Sonne J, Dossing M et al. (1987) Metronidazole pharmacokinetics in patients with hepatic encephalopathy. Scand J Gastroenterol 22, 117–123.

349 Tarao K, Ikeda T, Hayashi K *et al.* (1990) Successful use of vancomycin hydrochloride in the treatment of lactulose resistant chronic hepatic encephalopathy. *Gut* 31, 702–706.

350 Mas A, Rodes J, Sunyer L *et al.* (2003) Spanish Association for the Study of the Liver Hepatic Encephalopathy Cooperative Group. Comparison of rifaximin and lactitol in the treatment of acute hepatic encephalopathy: results of a randomized, double-blind, double-dummy, controlled clinical trial. *J Hepatol* 38, 51–58.

351 Liu Q, Duan ZP, Ha da K *et al.* (2004) Symbiotic modulation of gut flora: effect on minimal hepatic encephalopathy in patients with cirrhosis. *Hepatology* 39, 1441–1449.

352 Huber M, Rossle M, Siegerstetter V *et al.* (2001) *Helicobacter pylori* infection does not correlate with plasma ammonia concentration and hepatic encephalopathy in patients with cirrhosis. *Hepatogastroenterology* 48, 541–544.

353 Vasconez C, Elizalde JI, Llach J *et al.* (1999) *Helicobacter pylori*, hyperammonemia and subclinical portosystemic encephalopathy: effects of eradication. *J Hepatol*, 260–264.

354 Reding P, Duchateau J, Bataille C (1984) Oral zinc supplementation improves hepatic encephalopathy. Results of a randomised controlled trial. *Lancet* 2, 493–495.

355 Marchesini G, Fabbri A, Bianchi G *et al.* (1996) Zinc supplementation and amino acid-nitrogen metabolism in patients with advanced cirrhosis. *Hepatology* 23, 1084–1092.

356 Riggio O, Ariosto F, Merli M *et al.* (1991) Short-term oral zinc supplementation does not improve chronic hepatic encephalopathy. Results of a double-blind crossover trial. *Dig Dis Sci* 36, 1204–1208.

357 Bresci G, Parisi G, Banti S (1993) Management of hepatic encephalopathy with oral zinc supplementation: a long-term treatment. *Eur J Med* 2, 414–416.

358 Van der Rijt CC, Schalm SW, Schat H *et al.* (1991) Overt hepatic encephalopathy precipitated by zinc deficiency. *Gastroenterology* 100, 1114–1118.

359 Staedt U, Leweling H, Gladisch R *et al.* (1993) Effects of ornithine aspartate on plasma ammonia and plasma amino acids in patients with cirrhosis. A double-blind, randomized study using a four-fold crossover design. *J Hepatol* 19, 424–430.

360 Kircheis G, Nilius R, Held C *et al.* (1997) Therapeutic efficacy of L-ornithine-L-aspartate infusions in patients with cirrhosis and hepatic encephalopathy: results of a placebo-controlled, double-blind study. *Hepatology* 25, 1351–1360.

361 Stauch S, Kircheis G, Adler G *et al.* (1998) Oral L-ornithine-L-aspartate therapy of chronic hepatic encephalopathy: results of a placebo-controlled double-blind study. *J Hepatol* 28, 856–864.

362 Rose C, Michalak A, Rao KV *et al.* (1999) L-ornithine-L-aspartate lowers plasma and cerebrospinal fluid ammonia and prevents brain edema in rats with acute liver failure. *Hepatology* 30, 636–640.

363 Sushma S, Dasarathy S, Tandon RK *et al.* (1992) Sodium benzoate in the treatment of acute hepatic encephalopathy: a double-blind randomized trial. *Hepatology* 16, 138–144.

364 Mendenhall CL, Rouster S, Marshall L *et al.* (1986) A new therapy for portal systemic encephalopathy. *Am J Gastroenterol* 81, 540–543.

365 Morgan MY (1990) Branched chain amino acids in the management of chronic liver disease. Facts and fantasies. *J Hepatol* 11, 133–141.

366 Eriksson LS, Conn HO (1989) Branched-chain amino acids in the management of hepatic encephalopathy: an analysis of variants. *Hepatology* 10, 228–246.

367 Naylor CD, O'Rourke K, Detsky AS *et al.* (1989) Parenteral nutrition with branched-chain amino acids in hepatic encephalopathy. A meta-analysis. *Gastroenterology* 97, 1033–1042.

368 Als-Nielsen B, Koretz RL, Kjaergard LL *et al.* (2003) Branched-chain amino acids for hepatic encephalopathy. *Cochrane Database Syst Rev* 2, CD001939.

369 Marchesini G, Dioguardi FS, Bianchi GP *et al.* (1990) Long-term oral branched-chain amino acid treatment in chronic hepatic encephalopathy. A randomized double-blind case-controlled trial. The Italian multicenter Study Group. *J Hepatol* 11, 92–101.

370 Pomier-Layrargues G, Giguere JF, Lavoie J *et al.* (1994) Flumazenil in cirrhotic patients in hepatic coma: a randomized double-blind placebo-controlled crossover trial. *Hepatology* 19, 32–37.

371 Barbaro G, Di Lorenzo G, Soldini M *et al.* (1998) Flumazenil for hepatic encephalopathy grade III and IVa in patients with cirrhosis: an Italian multicenter double-blind, placebo-controlled, cross-over study. *Hepatology* 28, 374–378.

372 Gyr K, Meier R, Haussler J *et al.* (1996) Evaluation of the efficacy and safety of flumazenil in the treatment of portal systemic encephalopathy: a double blind, randomised, placebo controlled multicentre study. *Gut* 39, 319–324.

373 Goulenok C, Bernard B, Cadranel JF *et al.* (2002) Flumazenil vs. placebo in hepatic encephalopathy in patients with cirrhosis: a meta-analysis. *Aliment Pharmacol Ther* 16, 361–372.

374 Pomier-Layrargues G, Giguere JF, Lavoie J *et al.* (1989) Pharmacokinetics of benzodiazepine antagonist Ro 15-1788 in cirrhotic patients with moderate or severe liver dysfunction. *Hepatology* 10(6), 969–972.

375 Uribe M, Farca A, Marquez MA *et al.* (1979) Treatment of chronic portal systemic encephalopathy with bromocriptine: a double-blind controlled trial. *Gastroenterology* 76, 1347–1351.

376 Als-Nielsen B, Gluud LL, Gluud C (2004) Dopaminergic agonists for hepatic encephalopathy. *Cochrane Database Syst Rev* 4, CD003047.

377 Morgan MY, Jakobovits AW, James IM *et al.* (1980) Successful use of bromocriptine in the treatment of chronic hepatic encephalopathy. *Gastroenterology* 78, 663–670.

378 Vogels BA, Maas MA, Daalhuisen J *et al.* (1997) Memantine, a noncompetitive NMDA receptor antagonist improves hyperammonemia-induced encephalopathy and acute hepatic encephalopathy in rats. *Hepatology* 25, 820–827.

379 Córdoba J, Blei AT (1995) Cerebral edema and intracranial pressure monitoring. *Liver Transpl Surg* 1, 187–194.

380 Muñoz SJ (1993) Difficult management problems in fulminant hepatic failure. *Semin Liver Dis* 13, 395–413.

381 Murphy N, Auzinger G, Bernel W *et al.* (2004) The effect of hypertonic sodium chloride on intracranial pressure in patients with acute liver failure. *Hepatology* 39, 464–470.

382 Forbes A, Alexander GJ, O'Grady JG *et al.* (1989) Thiopental infusion in the treatment of intracranial hypertension complicating fulminant hepatic failure. *Hepatology* 10, 306–310.

383 Jalan R, Olde Damink SW, Deutz NE *et al.* (2004) Moderate hypothermia in patients with acute liver failure and uncontrolled intracranial hypertension. *Gastroenterology* 127, 1338–1346.

384 Vaquero J, Blei AT (2005) Mild hypothermia for acute liver failure: a review of mechanisms of action. *J Clin Gastroenterol* 39 (Suppl. 2), S147–157.

385 Rifai K, Ernst T, Kretschmer U *et al.* (2003) Prometheus – a new extracorporeal system for the treatment of liver failure. *J Hepatol* 39, 984–990.

386 Heemann U, Treichel U, Loock J *et al.* (2002) Albumin dialysis in cirrhosis with superimposed acute liver injury: a prospective, controlled study. *Hepatology* 36, 949–958.

387 Blanc P, Daures JP, Liautard J *et al.* (1994) [Lactulose–neomycin combination versus placebo in the treatment of acute hepatic encephalopathy. Results of a randomized controlled trial] *Gastroenterol Clin Biol* 18, 1063–1068.

388 Cadranel JF, el Younsi M, Pidoux B *et al.* (1995) Flumazenil therapy for hepatic encephalopathy in cirrhotic patients: a double-blind pragmatic randomized, placebo study. *Eur J Gastroenterol Hepatol* 7, 325–329.

389 Riggio O, Masini A, Efrati C *et al.* (2005) Pharmacological prophylaxis of hepatic encephalopathy after transjugular intrahepatic portosystemic shunt: a randomized controlled study. *J Hepatol* 42, 674–679.

390 Uflacker R, Silva Ade O, d'Albuquerque LA *et al.* (1987) Chronic portosystemic encephalopathy: embolization of portosystemic shunts. *Radiology* 165, 721–725.

391 Vavasseur D, Duvoux C, Cherqui D *et al.* (1994) Chronic hepatic encephalopathy due to spontaneous splenorenal shunt: successful treatment by transhepatic shunt embolization. *Cardiovasc Intervent Radiol* 17, 298–300.

392 Dagenais MH, Bernard D, Marleau D *et al.* (1991) Surgical treatment of severe postshunt hepatic encephalopathy. *World J Surg* 15, 109–113.

393 Hauenstein KH, Haag K, Ochs A *et al.* (1995) The reducing stent: treatment for transjugular intrahepatic portosystemic shunt-induced refractory hepatic encephalopathy and liver failure. *Radiology* 194, 175–179.

394 Madoff DC, Wallace MJ, Ahrar K *et al.* (2004) TIPS-related hepatic encephalopathy: management options with novel endovascular techniques. *Radiographics* 24, 21–36; discussion 36–37. Erratum in *Radiographics* (2004) 24, 418.

395 Powell EE, Pender MP, Chalk JB *et al.* (1990) Improvement in chronic hepatocerebral degeneration following liver transplantation. *Gastroenterology* 98, 1079–1082.

396 Weissenborn K, Tietge UJ, Bokemeyer M *et al.* (2003) Liver transplantation improves hepatic myelopathy: evidence by three cases. *Gastroenterology* 124, 346–351.

397 Resnick RH, Ishihara A, Chalmers TC *et al.* (1968) A controlled trial of colon bypass in chronic hepatic encephalopathy. *Gastroenterology* 54, 1057–1069.

398 van Someren EJ, Mirmiran M, Swaab DF (1993) Non-pharmacological treatment of sleep and wake disturbances in aging and Alzheimer's disease: chronobiological perspectives. *Behav Brain Res* 57, 235–253.

399 de Bruijn KM, Blendis LM, Zilm DH *et al.* (1983) Effect of dietary protein manipulation in subclinical portal-systemic encephalopathy. *Gut* 24, 53–60.

400 McClain CJ, Potter TJ, Kromhout JP *et al.* (1984) The effect of lactulose on psychomotor performance tests in alcoholic cirrhotics without overt hepatic encephalopathy. *J Clin Gastroenterol* 6, 325–329.

401 Morgan MY, Alonso M, Stanger LC (1989) Lactitol and lactulose for the treatment of subclinical hepatic encephalopathy in cirrhotic patients. A randomised, cross-over study. *J Hepatol* 8, 208–217.

402 Salerno F, Moser P, Maggi A *et al.* (1994) Effects of long-term administration of low-dose lactitol in patients with cirrhosis but without overt encephalopathy. *J Hepatol* 21(6), 1092–1096.

403 Egberts EH, Schomerus H, Hamster W *et al.* (1985) Branched chain amino acids in the treatment of latent portosystemic encephalopathy. A double-blind placebo-controlled crossover study. *Gastroenterology* 88, 887–895.

404 Gooday R, Hayes PC, Bzeizi K *et al.* (1995) Benzodiazepine receptor antagonism improves reaction time in latent hepatic encephalopathy. *Psychopharmacology (Berl)* 119, 295–298.

405 Kapczinski F, Sherman D, Williams R *et al.* (1995) Differential effects of flumazenil in alcoholic and nonalcoholic cirrhotic patients. *Psychopharmacology (Berl)* 120, 220–226.

406 Görg B, Bidmon HJ, Foster N *et al.* (2006) Inflammatory cytokines induce protein-tyrosine nitration in rat astrocytes. *Arch Biochem Biophys* 449, 104–114.

7.9 Bacterial infections in portal hypertension

Javier Fernández and Miguel Navasa

Spontaneous bacterial peritonitis, urinary tract infections, respiratory infections and bacteraemia are the most frequent infective complications in cirrhosis. These infections are due to the concomitant presence of different facilitating mechanisms including changes in the intestinal flora and in the intestinal barrier, depression of activity of the reticuloendothelial system, decreased opsonic activity of the ascitic fluid, neutrophil leukocyte dysfunction and iatrogenic factors among others. Portal hypertensive patients with a high risk of developing bacterial infections are those with gastrointestinal haemorrhage, a past history of spontaneous bacterial peritonitis and low protein content in ascites fluid together with a poor hepatocellular function. Pathophysiology, treatment and prophylaxis of bacterial infections in these patients will be discussed in this chapter.

Spontaneous bacterial peritonitis

Spontaneous bacterial peritonitis (SBP) is defined as the infection of a previously sterile ascitic fluid, without any apparent intra-abdominal source of infection [1]. The prevalence of SBP in unselected cirrhotic patients with ascites admitted to a hospital ranges between 10% and 30% [2]. Diagnosis of SBP is established by a polymorphonuclear cell count in ascitic fluid equal to or higher than 250 cells/μL. In approximately 40–60% of cases, the organism responsible is isolated in ascitic fluid culture or in blood cultures [2,3]. The remaining cases are considered as a variant of SBP and are treated in the same way as those with a positive culture [4]. The outcome of cirrhotic patients with SBP has improved dramatically during the last 20 years. At present, the SBP resolution rate is approximately 90%, and hospital survival ranges between 70% and 90% [1–3]. An early diagnosis of SBP and especially the use of more adequate antibiotic therapy are the most likely reasons for the improvement in SBP prognosis. However, despite the resolution of the infection, the mortality rate of SBP is still high (10–30%), mainly due to the development of some complications such as renal impairment, gastrointestinal bleeding and progressive liver failure. Cirrhotic patients recovering from an episode of SBP should be considered as potential candidates for liver transplantation as the survival expectancy after this bacterial infection is very short.

Pathogenesis

Colonization of the ascitic fluid from an episode of bacteraemia is nowadays the most accepted hypothesis for the pathogenesis of SBP [2,4]. Although the passage of microorganisms from the bloodstream to ascites has never been documented, it can be assumed that bacteria present in the circulation may easily pass to the ascites because of the constant fluid exchange between these two compartments. Once bacteria have reached the ascites, the development of SBP depends on the antimicrobial capacity of the ascitic fluid. Patients with a decreased defensive capacity of ascitic fluid develop SBP.

As most organisms causing SBP are Gram-negative bacteria of enteric origin [2,4], several pathogenic mechanisms have been proposed to explain the passage of enteric organisms from the intestinal lumen to the systemic circulation:

1 Bacterial translocation, or the process by which enteric bacteria normally present in the gastrointestinal lumen can cross the mucosa, colonize the mesenteric lymph nodes and reach the bloodstream through the intestinal lymphatic circulation. Bacterial translocation could be the consequence of the intestinal bacterial overgrowth that leads to an increase in aerobic Gram-negative bacilli in the intestinal flora in cirrhosis and of the alteration in gut permeability due to portal hypertension or to circumstances decreasing mucosal blood flow (e.g. acute hypovolaemia or splanchnic vasoconstrictor drugs).

2 The depression of the hepatic reticuloendothelial system, which allows the free passage of microorganisms from the bowel lumen to the systemic circulation via the portal vein and prolongs bacteraemia. The skin and the urinary and upper respiratory tracts may be the sites by which non-enteric bacteria enter the circulation and cause SBP. This pathogenic mechanism is enhanced in many cases by diagnostic or therapeutic procedures that break the natural mucocutaneous barriers.

Whatever the source of the bacteria reaching the bloodstream, a bacteraemic event is more prolonged and, therefore, may more readily become clinically significant in cirrhotic than in non-cirrhotic patients, because of the marked depression of the ret-iculendothelial system in the former. As indicated above, once microorganisms have colonized the ascites, the development of SBP depends on the defensive capacity of the ascitic fluid.

Bacterial translocation

It has been shown that, in CCl_4-induced cirrhotic rats with ascites, there is an increased passage of bacteria from the intest-inal lumen to extraintestinal sites, including regional lymph nodes and the systemic circulation [5–10]. Causes for bacterial translocation are a disruption of the intestinal permeability barrier, bacterial overgrowth (IBO) and/or a decrease in host immune defences. The simultaneous presence of IBO and a severe disturbance in the intestinal barrier seem to be required for bacterial translocation to mesenteric lymph nodes (MLN) [6,7]. The alteration in gut permeability could be partially due to portal hypertension that causes marked oedema and inflamma-tion in the submucosa of the caecum in cirrhotic rats with ascites, thus facilitating bacterial translocation [10]. Increased permeability of the intestinal mucosa has also been observed after haemorrhagic shock, sepsis, injury or administration of endotoxin. In portal hypertensive rats [10,11], it has been shown that haemorrhagic shock is followed by increased bacterial translocation to MLN, suggesting that haemorrhagic shock [11], a not infrequent event in cirrhotic patients, could alter the intestinal barrier in these animals. Gram-negative bacilli over-growth has been demonstrated in the jejunal flora of cirrhotic patients [6,7]. The intestinal hypomotility caused by the sympa-thetic overactivity of cirrhotic patients could, at least partly, explain this fact [7]. The change in the intestinal flora may increase the chance of aerobic Gram-negative bacteria invading the bloodstream and causing infections of enteric origin in patients with cirrhosis. In patients with cirrhosis, bacterial translocation to MLN seems to be related to the presence of ascites and to the degree of hepatic insufficiency as it is significantly increased in Child C patients [12].

Depression of activity of the reticuloendothelial system

Although the reticuloendothelial system is widely distributed throughout the body, approximately 90% of this defensive sys-tem is in the liver, where Kupffer cells and endothelial sinusoidal cells are the major components [13]. Cirrhotic patients may have marked depression of reticuloendothelial system function. In addition, it has been shown that survival and the risk of acquiring bacteraemia and SBP in cirrhosis are directly related to the degree of dysfunction of the reticuloendothelial system in these patients [14,15].

Several mechanisms have been proposed to explain the impairment of the phagocytic activity of the reticuloendothelial system in cirrhosis including intrahepatic shunting, a reduction in the phagocytic capacity of monocytes, which are considered as the Kupffer cell precursors, and an impaired function of

macrophage Fc gamma receptors in alcoholic cirrhosis [13,16,17]. Moreover, serum opsonic activity has been found to be markedly reduced in most cirrhotic patients, probably as a consequence of a decreased serum concentration of comple-ment and fibronectin, substances that normally stimulate the phagocytosis of microorganisms by enhancing their adhesive-ness to the reticuloendothelial cell surface.

Decreased opsonic activity of ascitic fluid

The non-specific antimicrobial capacity of ascitic fluid in cirrho-sis varies greatly from patient to patient, and this variability may be involved in the pathogenesis of SBP. There is a highly inverse significant correlation between the opsonic activity of ascitic fluid and the risk of developing SBP in patients admitted to hospital with ascites [18].

The opsonic activity of ascitic fluid in cirrhosis is directly correlated with the total protein level in ascites and with the con-centration of defensive substances, such as immunoglobulins, complement and fibronectin [18–23]. Interestingly, several investigators have found that the concentration of total protein in ascitic fluid, a very easy measurement in clinical practice, correlates directly with the risk of SBP in cirrhosis with ascites. Patients with protein concentrations in ascitic fluid below 10 g/L develop peritonitis during their hospital stay with a significantly higher frequency than those with a higher protein content in ascites (15% vs. 2% respectively) [19], and the cumulative 1-year probability of developing peritonitis during long-term follow-up is significantly greater in this subgroup of cirrhotic patients than in those with an ascitic protein concentration over 10 g/L (20% vs. 2% respectively) [21,22]. Finally, the probability of developing the first episode of SBP in cirrhotic patients with ascites is significantly influenced by the antimicrobial capacity of ascitic fluid and by hepatic function, with ascitic fluid protein levels, platelet count and serum bilirubin levels being the most useful indicators of high risk of SBP [23].

The variation in the antimicrobial properties could be related to: (i) the serum levels of the defensive proteins involved in antibacterial mechanisms of ascitic fluid; (ii) the degree of portal hypertension and hepatic insufficiency; and (iii) the volume of water diluting ascitic fluid solutes. This last possibility is sup-ported by the finding that diuretic-induced reduction of water in ascitic fluid increases the total protein concentration and the antibacterial capacity of ascites, and by the common observation in clinical practice that SBP occurs predominantly in cirrhotic patients with large-volume ascites.

Neutrophil leukocyte dysfunction

A high proportion of cirrhotic patients show altered neutrophil leukocyte function at different levels. The most frequent distur-bance is a marked reduction in chemotaxis, probably caused by the presence of chemotactic inhibitory substances in the serum. The nature of these substances has not yet been determined. Furthermore, the phagocytic and bacterial killing capacity of neutrophils has been found to be reduced in cirrhosis [24].

However, as infections developed by patients with congenital or acquired neutrophil function abnormalities, mainly chronic granulomatous diseases and recurrent staphylococcal and fungal infections, are very different from those developed by cirrhotic patients, it seems very unlikely that leukocyte dysfunction plays a major role in the susceptibility of cirrhosis to bacterial infections.

Iatrogenic factors

In addition to procedures well known to predispose to infection, such as intravenous or urethral catheters and tracheal intubation, cirrhotic patients are frequently subjected to other diagnostic or therapeutic manoeuvres that may alter the natural defence barriers and, therefore, increase the risk of bacterial infection. In that sense, a recent study by our group showed an increasing frequency of infections caused by Gram-positive cocci related to invasive procedures in recent years in cirrhosis [3]. Endoscopic sclerotherapy for bleeding oesophageal varices, particularly emergency sclerotherapy, is associated with bacteraemia, with an incidence ranging from 5% to 30% [25]. Although, in some cases, sclerotherapy has been implicated in the development of serious infectious complications such as purulent meningitis and bacterial peritonitis, bacteraemia is usually a transient phenomenon, and the use of prophylactic antibiotics is not recommended. Finally, there is a very low risk of clinically relevant infections with other invasive techniques often performed in these patients, such as diagnostic or therapeutic paracentesis, variceal band ligation, percutaneous ethanol injection or transcatheter arterial embolization, but the use of antibiotic prophylaxis in these procedures is not supported. In order to reduce nosocomial infections in patients with cirrhosis, urinary and central venous catheters should be used only when necessary and removed as soon as possible. In addition, measures to avoid colonization of venous lines should be strictly applied. At present, antibiotic prophylaxis with first- or second-generation cephalosporins is only advised prior to transjugular intrahepatic portosystemic shunt (TIPS) insertions and surgical interventions.

Diagnosis

Clinical characteristics

The clinical presentation of SBP probably depends on the stage at which the infection is diagnosed. Most patients present signs or symptoms clearly suggestive of peritoneal infection, although SBP may be asymptomatic, especially in the initial stages. Abdominal pain and fever are the most characteristic symptoms. Other signs and symptoms such as alterations in gastrointestinal motility (vomiting, ileus and diarrhoea), hepatic encephalopathy, gastrointestinal bleeding, renal impairment, septic shock and hypothermia may be present in a large number of patients [1,2]. Diagnostic paracentesis should be performed at hospital admission in all cirrhotic patients with ascites to investigate the presence of SBP, and in hospitalized patients with ascites whenever they present with any of the following: (i) abdominal pain, vomiting, diarrhoea, ileus or rebound tenderness; (ii) systemic

signs of infection such as fever, leucocytosis, leucopenia or septic shock; and (iii) hepatic encephalopathy or impairment in renal function [1].

Laboratory and microbiological data

The diagnosis of SBP is based on clinical suspicion and on ascitic fluid analysis. An ascitic fluid polymorphonuclear (PMN) count $\geq$ 250 cells/μL is nowadays considered diagnostic of SBP and constitutes an indication to empirically initiate antibiotic treatment. In patients with haemorrhagic ascites, a subtraction of one PMN per 250 red blood cells should be made to adjust for the presence of blood in ascites [1].

The measurement of lactic dehydrogenase concentration, glucose levels and total protein concentration in ascitic fluid is important to establish a differential diagnosis between spontaneous and secondary peritonitis. A secondary peritonitis should be suspected when at least two of the following features are present in ascitic fluid: glucose levels < 50 mg/dL, protein concentration > 10 g/L, lactic dehydrogenase concentration > normal serum levels. Gram's stain of a smear of sediment obtained after centrifugation of ascitic fluid is frequently negative in SBP, as the concentration of bacteria is usually low (1 organism/mL or less). Nevertheless, it may be helpful in identifying patients with gut perforation in whom multiple types of bacteria can be seen [1].

Culture of ascitic fluid directly into blood culture bottles (aerobic and anaerobic media) at the bedside is positive in between 40% and 80% of cases. Moreover, blood cultures are positive in a significant proportion of patients with SBP. Table 1 shows the most common organisms isolated from patients with SBP.

Alterations in systemic laboratory parameters such as leucocytosis or leucopenia, azotaemia and acidosis can be seen in cirrhotic patients with SBP.

Treatment

Antibiotic therapy must be started once the diagnosis of SBP is established. Empirical treatment should cover all potential organisms responsible for SBP without causing adverse effects.

Table 1 Bacteria responsible for spontaneous bacterial peritonitis.

Culture-positive SBP	39–67%
Gram-negative bacilli	31–50%
Escherichia coli	25–37%
Klebsiella spp.	2–6%
Enterobacter spp.	1–2%
Others	3–7%
Gram-positive cocci	8–17%
Streptococcus pneumoniae	1–10%
Other streptococci	6%
Staphylococcus aureus	1%
Culture-negative SBP	33–61%

Table 2 Spontaneous bacterial peritonitis outcome depending on the different antibiotic therapy employed.

Antibiotic	Resolution rate (%)	Superinfection (%)	Hospital survival (%)
Cefotaxime (i.v.)			73
2 g/4 h	86	0	69
2 g/6 h	77	1	79
2 g/12 h	79	1	67
2 g/8 h/5 days	93	0	58
2 g/8 h/10 days	91	0	70
Ceftriaxone (i.v.)	91	0	63
Cefonicid (i.v.)	94	0	63
Amoxicillin–clavulanic acid (i.v.)	85	7	57
Aztreonam (i.v.)	71	14	81
Ofloxacin (oral)	84	1	

i.v. intravenously.

At present, third-generation cephalosporins are considered the gold standard in the treatment of SBP in cirrhosis. However, other antibiotics such as amoxicillin–clavulanic acid are also effective in the treatment of this infective complication [26–35]. Table 2 shows the SBP outcome depending on the antibiotic employed. At present, monotherapy with aztreonam is not recommended in the treatment of SBP as this antibiotic is only active against Gram-negative bacilli. Moreover, ofloxacin should not be employed in the treatment of SBP in patients submitted to long-term norfloxacin prophylaxis.

Intravenous albumin infusion in SBP

A randomized, multicentre, controlled trial has demonstrated that, in patients with SBP, treatment with intravenous albumin in addition to an antibiotic reduces the incidence of renal impairment and improves hospital survival [36]. The study included 126 patients with SBP, who were randomly assigned to treatment with intravenous cefotaxime (63 patients) or cefotaxime and intravenous albumin (63 patients). Albumin was given at a dose of 1.5 g/kg body weight at the time of diagnosis, followed by 1 g/kg body weight on day 3. Renal impairment developed in 21 patients in the cefotaxime group (33%) and in six in the cefotaxime plus albumin group (10%). The hospital mortality rate was 29% in the cefotaxime group compared with 10% in the cefotaxime plus albumin group. The results of this study suggest that cirrhotic patients with SBP should be expanded with albumin. However, it is important to identify those patients with SBP who may benefit from albumin infusion. In that sense, it should be noted that the incidence of

renal impairment among patients with a baseline bilirubin level of less than 4 mg/dL and a creatinine level of less than 1 mg/dL was very low in both treatment groups (7% and 0% in the cefotaxime and cefotaxime + albumin groups respectively). Therefore, patients with abnormal renal function [blood urea nitrogen (BUN) > 30 mg/dL and/or creatinine > 1 mg/dL] and/or high bilirubin levels (> 4 mg/dL) appear to be the subgroup of patients with SBP who derive the most benefit from volume expansion with albumin. Further studies are needed to determine whether lower doses of albumin have the same effects on renal function and survival. A recent study by our group suggests that albumin cannot be substituted by artificial plasma expanders in SBP [37].

As renal dysfunction is a result of an aggravation in vasodilatation and a decrease in effective arterial blood volume [38], procedures that lead to a decreased effective blood volume should be avoided, such as the use of diuretics and large-volume paracentesis.

Prophylaxis

Current indications for selective intestinal decontamination in SBP prevention are summarized in Table 3. Cirrhotic patients with gastrointestinal haemorrhage are predisposed to develop severe bacterial infections during or immediately after the bleeding episode. Short-term intestinal decontamination is effective in preventing SBP in cirrhotic patients with gastrointestinal haemorrhage [39,40]. The usefulness of systemic antibiotics in cirrhotic patients with gastrointestinal haemorrhage has also

Table 3 Indications and duration of selective intestinal decontamination for the prevention of SBP in cirrhotic patients.

Indication	Duration of prophylaxis
Cirrhotic patients recovering from a previous episode of SBP (secondary prophylaxis)	Indefinitely or until liver transplantation
Cirrhotic patients with gastrointestinal bleeding	Seven days
Cirrhotic patients with ascites and low ascitic fluid protein levels (≤ 10 g/L)	During hospitalization (no consensus)

been investigated in four controlled studies. In these studies, the treated groups received ofloxacin (initially intravenously and then orally), ofloxacin (initially intravenously and then orally) plus amoxicillin–clavulanic acid (before each endoscopy), ciprofloxacin plus amoxicillin–clavulanic acid (first intravenously and then orally once the bleeding was controlled) and oral ciprofloxacin [41–44]. The incidence of bacterial infections was significantly lower in the treated groups (10–20%) than in the corresponding control groups (45–66%). A relative limitation in these studies was the inability to assess the effect of antibiotic prophylaxis specifically on SBP as the incidence of both SBP and bacteraemia was analysed together. Nevertheless, the marked decrease in the rate of overall infections and the improvement in survival in the groups receiving antibiotic prophylaxis support such prophylaxis [45], with it being strongly recommended in cirrhotic patients with gastrointestinal haemorrhage independently of their specific risk of SBP [1]. Furthermore, a meta-analysis including all the above-mentioned studies showed a significant benefit in the subgroup of cirrhotic patients with ascites and gastrointestinal haemorrhage: 95% of patients were free of SBP in the treated group vs. 87% in the control group [45].

Cases with low ascitic fluid total protein concentration may be a second group of cirrhotic patients who may benefit from selective intestinal decontamination. In 63 patients admitted to hospital for the treatment of an episode of ascites with an ascitic fluid total protein concentration lower than 15 g/L, some of whom had had a previous episode of SBP, the continuous administration of norfloxacin, 400 mg/day, throughout the hospitalization period (32 patients), decreased the in-hospital incidence of SBP from 22% in the control group to 0% in the treated group [46]. In cirrhotic patients with ascitic fluid protein concentrations < 15 g/L and no previous episodes of SBP, the 6-month incidence of SBP was 0% in the group of patients prophylactically treated with norfloxacin, 400 mg/day for 6 months, compared with 9% in patients treated with placebo. Nevertheless, the incidence of SBP caused by Gram-negative organisms (the only one that can theoretically be prevented by norfloxacin prophylaxis) in the two groups was not statistically significant: 0% in the norfloxacin-treated group and 5% in the placebo-treated group [47].

Other antibiotic regimes have been evaluated in the prevention of SBP in high-risk patients. A placebo-controlled study demonstrated that 6-month prophylaxis with ciprofloxacin, 750 mg weekly, was effective in reducing the incidence of SBP in cirrhotic patients with low protein concentrations in ascitic fluid: 4% in the treated group and 22% in the placebo control group [48]. In this study, patients with and without a prior history of SBP were included together, and no attempt was made to evaluate the development of SBP in these two subgroups of patients separately. Trimethoprim–sulphamethoxazole (one double-strength tablet 5 days a week) is also effective in the prevention of SBP in cirrhotic patients with ascites [49]. In a randomized controlled trial with a median follow-up of only

90 days, the incidence of SBP was 26.7% in the control group and 3.3% in the group of patients receiving trimethoprim–sulphamethoxazole prophylaxis. Again, patients with different risks for SBP were analysed together: patients with low and high ascitic fluid protein and patients who had and who had not had previous SBP episodes.

Patients recovering from an episode of SBP represent a unique population in which to assess the effect of long-term intestinal decontamination in the prophylaxis of SBP. In a double-blind, placebo-controlled trial including 80 cirrhotic patients who had recovered from an episode of SBP, the overall probability of SBP recurrence at 1 year of follow-up was 20% in the norfloxacin group and 68% in the placebo group, and the probability of SBP caused by aerobic Gram-negative bacilli at 1 year of follow-up was 3% and 60% respectively. Only one patient treated with norfloxacin experienced side-effects related to treatment (oral and oesophageal candidiasis) [50]. Therefore, long-term selective intestinal decontamination dramatically decreases the rate of SBP recurrence in patients with SBP. Three recent economic analyses have calculated that long-term antibiotic prophylaxis in cirrhotic patients is associated with a reduced cost compared with the 'diagnosis and treat' strategy, suggesting that prophylaxis is cost-effective when applied to patients at high risk of developing SBP [51–53].

Taking into account all these prophylactic studies, it can be assumed that antibiotic prophylaxis in cirrhotic patients with ascites is indicated in patients who have had a previous episode of SBP because they are at high risk of SBP recurrence and because prophylaxis is cost-effective. In patients with low protein content in ascitic fluid who have never had SBP, the recommendation is difficult to establish due to the heterogeneity of the published studies, which included patients with low and high risk of SBP together. This is the main reason for the lack of consensus because, despite the positive results of all the studies investigating different antibiotics in the prophylaxis of SBP in patients with cirrhosis, they have been unable to identify subsets of patients who clearly benefit from this therapy. In that sense, it should be noted that three studies have been performed assessing the incidence and predictive factors of the first episode of SBP in cirrhotic patients with ascites, and they may help in deciding whether a patient should initiate antibiotic prophylaxis. In a series of 127 patients admitted to hospital for the treatment of an episode of ascites, the probability of the appearance of the first episode of SBP was 11% at 1 year and 15% at 3 years of follow-up [21]. Five variables obtained at admission were significantly associated with a higher risk of SBP appearance during follow-up [poor nutritional status, increased serum bilirubin levels, decreased prothrombin activity, increased serum aspartate aminotransferase (AST) levels and low ascitic fluid protein concentration], but only one (low ascitic fluid protein concentration) showed an independent predictive value. The 1-year and 3-year probabilities of the first episode of SBP in patients with ascitic fluid protein content lower than 10 g/L were 20% and 24%, respectively, whereas in those with ascitic fluid protein content equal to or greater than 10 g/L, they were 0% and 4% respectively. A clear conclusion from this study is that long-term prophylactic administration of antibiotics is not necessary in patients with high protein content in ascitic fluid, in whom the risk of developing SBP is negligible. In a similar study performed in 110 consecutive cirrhotic patients hospitalized for the treatment of an episode of ascites [22], six variables associated with a higher risk of first SBP appearance during follow-up (serum bilirubin > 2.5 mg/dL, prothrombin activity < 60%, ascitic fluid total protein concentration < 10 g/L, serum sodium concentration < 130 mEq/L, platelet count < 116 000/μL and serum albumin concentration < 26 g/L) were identified, but only two (ascitic fluid protein concentration and serum bilirubin) showed an independent predictive value. In a recent study, cirrhotic patients with low ascitic fluid protein levels (≤ 10 g/L) and high serum bilirubin level (> 3.2 mg/dL) and/or low platelet count (< 98 000/μL) presented a 1-year probability of developing a first SBP of 55% in comparison with 24% of patients with only low ascitic fluid protein levels [23]. Three studies, therefore, indicate that cirrhotic patients with ascites who are at risk of developing a first episode of SBP can be identified using routine biochemical parameters and might benefit from selective intestinal decontamination. However, the efficacy of antibiotic prophylaxis in these high-risk patients should be adequately investigated in prospective randomized trials.

A second reason for the lack of consensus in the prophylaxis of SBP, particularly in those patients who have never had a previous episode of SBP, is the problem of the development of quinolone-resistant enterobacteria. A review of the published data indicates that, from an initial stage when norfloxacin prophylaxis was considered effective and not associated with the development of quinolone-resistant bacteria, we have moved to a final stage in which quinolone-resistant bacteria may cause severe infections in these patients. Initial studies suggested that the risk of developing SBP or other infections caused by quinolone-resistant strains of Gram-negative bacilli was low, as the majority of SBP recurrences in patients on norfloxacin

prophylaxis were caused by Gram-positive cocci, mainly streptococci [50,54,55]. Thereafter, a high incidence of quinolone-resistant strains of *Escherichia coli* in the stools of cirrhotic patients undergoing long-term quinolone prophylaxis was reported in several studies, although none of these studies reported any infection due to quinolone-resistant *E. coli* [56,57]. In 1997, the first study on long-term norfloxacin prophylaxis in SBP was published, showing a relevant emergence of infections, mainly mild urinary infections, caused by Gram-negative bacilli resistant to quinolones (90% of *E. coli* isolated were resistant to quinolones) [58]. More recently, it has been shown that 39 out of 106 infections caused by *E. coli* in hospitalized cirrhotic patients were quinolone resistant, with long-term norfloxacin prophylaxis being significantly associated with the development of infections (mainly urinary tract infections) caused by quinolone-resistant *E. coli*. However, the development of SBP due to quinolone-resistant *E. coli* in decontaminated patients was scarcely reported [59].

Data from a study performed in our liver unit, which prospectively evaluated all bacterial infections occurring in a 2-year period, show a clear relationship between the development of SBP caused by quinolone-resistant Gram-negative bacilli and long-term treatment with norfloxacin (Table 4). In patients on long-term norfloxacin prophylaxis, 50% of culture-positive SBP were caused by quinolone-resistant Gram-negative bacilli, whereas only 16% of culture-positive SBP in patients not receiving this prophylaxis were caused by these resistant bacteria. Although SBP caused by quinolone-resistant Gram-negative bacilli represented only 26% of the culture-positive SBP in this study, quinolone-resistant SBP seem to be emerging for the first time as a real problem in hepatology, and this will probably increase in the near future [3]. This study also showed a high rate of culture-positive SBP caused by trimethoprim–sulphamethoxazole-resistant Gram-negative bacteria in patients on long-term treatment with norfloxacin (44%), suggesting that this antibiotic is not an alternative to norfloxacin. These results suggest that the effectiveness of norfloxacin is decreasing in

	Long-term norfloxacin	None
Total isolated GNB		
Quinolone-resistant strains	65%	29%
Trimethoprim–sulphamethoxazole-resistant strains	68%	44%
Cephalosporin-resistant strains	19%	16%
GNB isolated in SBP		
Quinolone-resistant strains	57%	21%
Trimethoprim–sulphamethoxazole-resistant strains	50%	24%
Cephalosporin-resistant strains	0	7%
GNB isolated in urinary infections		
Quinolone-resistant strains	92%	33%
Trimethoprim-sulphamethoxazole-resistant strains	92%	40%
Cephalosporin-resistant strains	8%	5%

Table 4 Antibiotic susceptibility of Gram-negative bacilli (GNB) isolated in cirrhotic patients submitted or not to long-term norfloxacin prophylaxis.

the prevention of SBP in cirrhotic patients and, therefore, this should be considered as an alarm signal.

Our study also showed no significant differences in the resolution rate of infections caused by *E. coli* resistant to quinolones in comparison with the resolution rate of those due to sensitive strains. The absence of cross-resistance between quinolones and other antibiotics commonly used to treat these bacterial infections, such as third-generation cephalosporins, could explain this finding (SBP resolution rate 92% vs. 91%). The fact that none of the *E. coli* isolated in patients undergoing long-term quinolone prophylaxis was resistant to third-generation cephalosporins reinforces the idea that this antibiotic constitutes the elective treatment for bacterial infections not only in non-decontaminated cirrhotic patients but also in those undergoing selective intestinal decontamination with quinolones. On the other hand, the high incidence of quinolone- and trimethoprim–sulphamethoxazole-resistant strains of *E. coli* isolated in decontaminated cirrhotic patients underlines the necessity of restricting the administration of prophylactic antibiotics only to those patients at the greatest risk of SBP. The increasing emergence of infections caused by quinolone- and trimethoprim–sulphamethoxazole-resistant strains of Gram-negative bacilli also suggests that the effectiveness of these antibiotics may decrease with time on account of their widespread use. Thus, further studies are needed to evaluate alternative prophylactic measures such as other antibiotic regimes and non-antibiotic procedures in SBP prophylaxis. Finally, it should be kept in mind that SBP carries a poor prognosis. The 1-year and 2-year probabilities of survival after an episode of SBP are 30–50% and 25–30% respectively [2]. Therefore, patients recovering from an episode of SBP should be considered as potential candidates for liver transplantation.

Other bacterial infections

Urinary tract infections

Several predisposing factors have been recognized for urinary tract infections (UTIs) in cirrhosis: the presence of urethral catheters, ascites and female sex [60]. Most cases are oligo or asymptomatic, and bacteriuria alone can be present in 40% of cases [61]. The microorganisms usually responsible for UTI in cirrhosis are Gram-negative bacilli and enterococci in cases of urinary manipulation [2,3]. The empirical treatment should include third-generation cephalosporins or amoxicillin–clavulanic acid [62,63]. In cases of treatment failure, add ampicillin if urinary catheterization is present and perform ultrasonography to rule out other facilitating pathologies in the urinary tract.

Pneumonia

The distinction between community- and hospital-acquired (nosocomial) pneumonia is very useful. The causative organisms

in cases of community-acquired pneumonia are the same as we can see in the general population: *Streptococcus pneumoniae*, *Haemophilus influenzae*, *Mycoplasma pneumoniae* or *Legionella* spp., and in addition Gram-negative bacilli, particularly *Klebsiella pneumoniae*, and anaerobic bacteria [3,64–66]. Empirical treatment should cover all these possibilities. The empirical use of third-generation cephalosporins or amoxicillin–clavulanic acid plus a macrolide (clarithromycin or azithromycin) or levofloxacin is at present recommended [66]. In case of treatment failure, the possibility of infection by *Staphylococcus aureus* and *Pseudomonas* spp. has to be considered.

Predisposing factors for nosocomial pneumonia are tracheal intubation, hepatic encephalopathy and oesophageal tamponade [67,68], with Gram-negative bacilli (*Pseudomonas* spp.) and *Staphylococcus* spp. being the bacteria most frequently responsible for infection in these cases [69–70]. Therefore, empirical treatment in patients with predisposing factors should include antipseudomonic antibiotics (i.e. ceftazidime or cefepime + ciprofloxacin), adding vancomycin in cases of tracheal intubation. In patients without predisposing factors for *Pseudomonas* spp. or Staphylococcus spp., third-generation cephalosporins are very effective and do not have significant adverse effects.

Spontaneous bacteraemia

The causative organisms are the same as those found in SBP because, in theory, spontaneous bacteraemia is a previous step in the colonization of ascitic fluid [3]. Therefore, the empirical treatment should cover Gram-negative bacilli and non-enterococcal streptococci, with third-generation cephalosporins being the most effective and safe treatment. Amoxicillin–clavulanic acid is another option. In case of treatment failure, blood cultures are very important to know the susceptibility of the bacteria. A secondary origin of the bacteraemia has to be excluded.

Secondary bacteraemia

The causative bacteria should be considered according to the origin of the bacteraemia. Catheter sepsis is usually caused by *Staphylococcus aureus* and *Staphylococcus epidermidis* [3]. Anaerobic facultative streptococci are usually involved in infectious complications after transcatheter arterial embolization [71]. Infections after TIPS insertion or revision are usually caused by Gram-positive cocci or enterobacteria [72]. Finally, both Gram-positive cocci and Gram-negative bacilli can cause infections after variceal sclerotherapy [25].

The recommended empirical treatment for catheter sepsis is vancomycin and removal of the catheter. Fever after transcatheter arterial embolization is frequent and does not necessarily mean infection. In case of bacteraemia, amoxicillin–clavulanic acid is a good antibiotic choice. Bacteraemia after TIPS insertion or revision should be treated with a third-generation cephalosporin plus vancomycin.

Endocarditis

Despite the initial suggestion of a high frequency of endocarditis in cirrhosis according to the observations in postmortem studies [73–75], this infection is rare in the absence of predisposing factors such as the presence of prosthetic valves and invasive procedures [3]. As a consequence, the most common causative organisms are Gram-positive cocci: *Staphylococcus aureus*, *S. epidermidis* and streptococci [75]. The 'classic' empirical treatment with ampicillin + gentamicin is very effective although, in the presence of prosthetic valves, ampicillin must be substituted by vancomycin.

Cellulitis and lymphangitis

Several predisposing factors have been implicated in these infections such as deficient hygienic standards, unapparent skin injuries and oedema [76]. The empirical treatment should cover Gram-positive cocci (*Staphylococcus aureus*, streptococci) and enterobacteria. Amoxicillin–clavulanic acid, a third-generation cephalosporin plus cloxacillin or ofloxacin are good options as empirical treatment.

Summary

Spontaneous bacterial peritonitis is a frequent and severe complication of cirrhotic patients with ascites. Its diagnosis is established on the basis of a polymorphonuclear cell count in ascitic fluid equal to or higher than 250 cells/µL. The routine use of diagnostic paracentesis whenever a cirrhotic patient with ascites is admitted to hospital usually allows early diagnosis of the infection. At present, third-generation cephalosporins are considered the gold standard in the treatment of SBP. Because of the high incidence of quinolone-resistant Gram-negative bacilli isolated in cirrhotic patients on long-term norfloxacin prophylaxis, SBP in these patients should not be treated with quinolones as empirical therapy. Although SBP prognosis has improved in recent years, the mortality rate associated with this bacterial infection is still high. The development of severe complications such as renal impairment and gastrointestinal bleeding is responsible for this poor prognosis. The mechanisms involved in the pathogenesis of these complications are under evaluation. Selective intestinal decontamination with quinolones has been demonstrated to be effective in SBP prophylaxis in patients who have recovered from a previous episode of SBP and in patients with gastrointestinal bleeding. The increasing emergence of quinolone-resistant organisms clearly establishes the necessity of restricting the primary prophylaxis to those subsets of patients at high risk of developing a first episode of SBP. The identification of these patients and the evaluation of alternative prophylactic measures such as other antibiotic regimes and no antibiotic procedures are still under investigation. Because of the poor survival expectancy after this bacterial infection, cirrhotic patients recovering from an episode of SBP should be considered as potential candidates for liver transplantation. Finally, other bacterial infections in cirrhosis and their most frequent causative organisms and empirical treatment are summarized.

References

1 Rimola A, Garcia-Tsao G, Navasa M *et al.* (2000) Diagnosis, treatment and prophylaxis of spontaneous bacterial peritonitis: a consensus document. *J Hepatol* 32, 142–153.

2 Navasa M, Rodés J (2004) Bacterial infections in cirrhosis. *Liver Int* 24, 277–280.

3 Fernández J, Navasa M, Gomez J *et al.* (2002) Bacterial infections in cirrhosis: epidemiological changes with invasive procedures and norfloxacin prophylaxis. *Hepatology* 35, 140–148.

4 Runyon BA, Hoefs JC (1984) Culture-negative neutrocytic ascites: a variant of spontaneous bacterial peritonitis. *Hepatology* 4, 1209–1211.

5 Runyon BA, Squier S, Borzio M (1994) Translocation of gut bacteria in rats with cirrhosis to mesenteric lymph nodes partially explains the pathogenesis of spontaneous bacterial peritonitis. *J Hepatol* 21, 792–796.

6 Casafont Morencos F, de las Heras Castaño G, Martín Ramos L *et al.* (1995) Small bowel bacterial overgrowth in patients with alcoholic cirrhosis. *Dig Dis Sci* 40, 1252–1256.

7 Perez-Paramo MP, Muñoz J, Albillos A *et al.* (2000) Effect of propranolol on the factors promoting bacterial translocation in cirrhotic rats with ascites. *Hepatology* 31, 43–48.

8 Sorell WT, Quigley EMM, Jin G *et al.* (1993) Bacterial translocation in the portal-hypertensive rat: studies in basal conditions and on exposure to haemorrhagic shock. *Gastroenterology* 104, 1722–1726.

9 Llovet JM, Bartoli R, Planas R *et al.* (1994) Bacterial translocation in cirrhotic rats. Its role in the development of spontaneous bacterial peritonitis. *Gut* 35, 1648–1652.

10 Garcia-Tsao G, Lee FY, Barden GE *et al.* (1995) Bacterial translocation to mesenteric lymph nodes is increased in cirrhotic rats with ascites. *Gastroenterology* 108, 1835–1841.

11 Llovet JM, Bartoli R, Planas R *et al.* (1996) Selective intestinal decontamination with norfloxacin reduces bacterial translocation in ascitic cirrhotic rats exposed to haemorrhagic shock. *Hepatology* 23, 781–787.

12 Cirera I, Bauer TM, Navasa M *et al.* (2001) Bacterial translocation of enteric organisms in patients with cirrhosis. *J Hepatol* 34, 32–37.

13 Jones EA, Summerfield JA (1988) Kupffer cells. In: Arias IM, Jakoby WB, Popper H *et al.* (eds) *The Liver: Biology and Pathobiology*, 2nd edn. New York: Raven Press, pp. 683–704.

14 Rimola A, Soto R, Bory F *et al.* (1984) Reticuloendothelial system phagocytic activity in cirrhosis and its relation to bacterial infections and prognosis. *Hepatology* 4, 53–58.

15 Bolognesi M, Merkel C, Bianco S *et al.* (1994) Clinical significance of the evaluation of hepatic reticuloendothelial removal capacity in patients with cirrhosis. *Hepatology* 19, 628–634.

16 Guarner C, Runyon BA (1995) Macrophage function in cirrhosis and the risk of bacterial infection. *Hepatology* 22, 367–369.

17 Gomez F, Ruiz P, Schreiber AD (1994) Impaired function of macrophage Fc gamma receptors and bacterial infection in alcoholic cirrhosis. *N Engl J Med* 331, 1122–1128.

18 Runyon BA (1988) Patients with deficient ascitic fluid opsonic activity are predisposed to spontaneous bacterial peritonitis. *Hepatology* 8, 632–635.

19 Runyon BA (1986) Low-protein-concentration ascitic fluid is predisposed to spontaneous bacterial peritonitis. *Gastroenterology* 91, 1343–1346.

20 Tito Ll, Rimola A, Gines P *et al.* (1988) Recurrence of spontaneous bacterial peritonitis in cirrhosis: frequency and predictive factors. *Hepatology* 8, 27–31.

21 Llach J, Rimola A, Navasa M *et al.* (1992) Incidence and predictive factors of first episode of spontaneous bacterial peritonitis in cirrhosis with ascites: relevance of ascitic fluid protein concentration. *Hepatology* 16, 724–727.

22 Andreu M, Solá R, Sitges-Serra A *et al.* (1993) Risk factors for spontaneous bacterial peritonitis. *Gastroenterology* 104, 1133–1138.

23 Guarner C, Sola R, Soriano G *et al.* (1999) Risk of a first community-acquired spontaneous bacterial peritonitis in cirrhotics with low ascitic protein levels. *Gastroenterology* 117, 414–419.

24 Garcia-Gonzalez M, Boixeda D, Herrero D *et al.* (1993) Effect of granulocyte–macrophage colony-stimulating factor on leukocyte function in cirrhosis. *Gastroenterology* 105, 527–531.

25 Rolando N, Gimson A, Philpott-Howard J *et al.* (1993) Infectious sequel after endoscopic sclerotherapy of oesophageal varices: role of antibiotic prophylaxis. *J Hepatol* 18, 290–294.

26 Felisart J, Rimola A, Arroyo V *et al.* (1985) Cefotaxime is more effective than is ampicillin–tobramycin in cirrhotics with severe infections. *Hepatology* 5, 457–462.

27 Runyon BA, McHutchison JG, Antillon MR *et al.* (1991) Short-course versus long-course antibiotic treatment of spontaneous bacterial peritonitis. A randomized controlled study of 100 patients. *Gastroenterology* 100, 1737–1742.

28 Rimola A, Salmeron JM, Clemente G *et al.* (1995) Two different dosages of cefotaxime in the treatment of spontaneous bacterial peritonitis in cirrhosis: results of a prospective, randomized, multicenter study. *Hepatology* 21, 674–679.

29 Mercader J, Gómez J, Ruiz J *et al.* (1989) Use of ceftriaxone in the treatment of bacterial infections in cirrhotic patients. *Chemotherapy* 35(Suppl. 2), 23–26.

30 Gómez-Jimenez J, Ribera E, Gasser I *et al.* (1993) Randomized trial comparing ceftriaxone with cefonicid for treatment of spontaneous bacterial peritonitis in cirrhotic patients. *Antimicrob Agents Chemother* 37, 1587–1592.

31 Ariza J, Xiol X, Esteve M *et al.* (1991) Aztreonam vs. cefotaxime in the treatment of gram-negative spontaneous peritonitis in cirrhotic patients. *Hepatology* 14, 91–98.

32 Grange JD, Amiot X, Grange V *et al.* (1990) Amoxicillin–clavulanic acid therapy of spontaneous bacterial peritonitis: a prospective study of twenty-seven cases in cirrhotic patients. *Hepatology* 11, 360–364.

33 Ricart E, Soriano G, Novella MT *et al.* (2000) Amoxicillin–clavulanic acid versus cefotaxime in the therapy of bacterial infections in cirrhotic patients. *J Hepatol* 32, 596–602.

34 Silvain C, Breux JP, Grollier G *et al.* (1989) Les septicémies et les infections du liquide d'ascite du cirrhotique peuvent-elles être traitées exclusivement par voie orale? *Gastroenterol Clin Biol* 13, 335–339.

35 Navasa M, Follo A, Llovet JM *et al.* (1996) Randomized, comparative study of oral ofloxacin versus intravenous cefotaxime in spontaneous bacterial peritonitis. *Gastroenterology* 111, 1011–1017.

36 Sort P, Navasa M, Arroyo V *et al.* (1999) Effect of intravenous albumin on renal impairment and mortality in patients with cirrhosis and spontaneous bacterial peritonitis. *N Engl J Med* 5, 403–409.

37 Fernández J, Monteagudo J, Bargalló X *et al.* (2005) A randomized unblinded pilot study comparing albumin versus hydroxyethyl starch in spontaneous bacterial peritonitis. *Hepatology* 42, 627–634.

38 Ruiz del Arbol L, Urman J, Fernández J *et al.* (2003) Cardiovascular, renal and hepatic hemodynamic derangement in cirrhotic patients with spontaneous bacterial peritonitis. *Hepatology* 38, 1210–1218.

39 Rimola A, Bory F, Terés J *et al.* (1985) Oral non-absorbable antibiotics prevent infection in cirrhosis with gastrointestinal haemorrhage. *Hepatology* 5, 463–467.

40 Soriano G, Guarner C, Tomás A *et al.* (1992) Norfloxacin prevents bacterial infection in cirrhotics with gastrointestinal haemorrhage. *Gastroenterology* 103, 1267–1272.

41 Blaise M, Pateron D, Trinchet J-C *et al.* (1994) Systemic antibiotic therapy prevents bacterial infection in cirrhotic patients with gastrointestinal haemorrhage. *Hepatology* 20, 34–38.

42 Pauwels A, Mostefa-Kara N, Debenes B *et al.* (1996) Systemic antibiotic prophylaxis after gastrointestinal haemorrhage in cirrhotic patients with a high risk of infection. *Hepatology* 24, 802–806.

43 Hsieh W-J, Lin H-C, Hwang S-J *et al.* (1998) The effect of ciprofloxacin in the prevention of bacterial infections in patients with cirrhosis after upper gastrointestinal bleeding. *Am J Gastroenterol* 93, 962–966.

44 Hou MC, Lin HC, Liu TT *et al.* (2004) Antibiotic prophylaxis after endoscopic therapy prevents rebleeding in acute variceal hemorrhage: a randomized trial. *Hepatology* 39, 746–753.

45 Bernard B, Grange JD, Khac EN *et al.* (1999) Antibiotic prophylaxis for the prevention of bacterial infections in cirrhotic patients with gastrointestinal bleeding: a meta-analysis. *Hepatology* 29, 1655–1661.

46 Soriano G, Guarner C, Teixidó M *et al.* (1991) Selective intestinal decontamination prevents spontaneous bacterial peritonitis. *Gastroenterology* 100, 477–481.

47 Grange J-D, Roulot D, Pelletier G *et al.* (1998) Norfloxacin primary prophylaxis of bacterial infections in cirrhotic patients with ascites: a double-blind randomised trial. *J Hepatol* 29, 430–436.

48 Rolanchon A, Cordier L, Bacq Y *et al.* (1995) Ciprofloxacin and long-term prevention of spontaneous bacterial peritonitis: results of a prospective controlled trial. *Hepatology* 22, 1171–1174.

49 Singh N, Gayowski T, Yu VL *et al.* (1995) Trimethoprim–sulfamethoxazole for the prevention of spontaneous bacterial peritonitis in cirrhosis: a randomized trial. *Ann Intern Med* 122, 595–598.

50 Ginès P, Rimola A, Planas R *et al.* (1990) Norfloxacin prevents spontaneous bacterial peritonitis recurrence in cirrhosis: results of a double-blind, placebo-controlled trial. *Hepatology* 12, 716–724.

51 Inadomi J, Sonnenberg A (1997) Cost-analysis of prophylactic antibiotics in spontaneous bacterial peritonitis. *Gastroenterology* 113, 1289–1294.

52 Younossi ZM, McHutchison JG, Ganiats TG (1997) An economic analysis of norfloxacin prophylaxis against spontaneous bacterial peritonitis. *J Hepatol* 27, 295–298.

53 Das A (1998) A cost analysis of long-term antibiotic prophylaxis for spontaneous bacterial peritonitis in cirrhosis. *Am J Gastroenterol* 93, 1895–1900.

54 Llovet JM, Rodríguez-Iglesias P, Moitinho E *et al.* (1997) Spontaneous bacterial peritonitis in patients with cirrhosis undergoing selective intestinal decontamination. *J Hepatol* 26, 88–95.

55 Campillo B, Dupeyron C, Richardet J-P *et al.* (1998) Epidemiology of severe hospital-acquired infections in patients with liver cirrhosis: effect of long-term administration of norfloxacin. *Clin Infect Dis* 26, 1066–1070.

56 Dupeyron C, Mangeney N, Sedrati L *et al.* (1994) Rapid emergence of quinolone resistance in cirrhotic patients treated with norfloxacin to prevent spontaneous bacterial peritonitis. *Antimicrob Agents Chemother* 38, 340–344.

57 Aparicio JR, Such J, Pascual S *et al.* (1999) Development of quinolone-resistant strains of *Escherichia coli* in stools of patients with cirrhosis undergoing norfloxacin prophylaxis: clinical consequences. *J Hepatol* 31, 277–283.

58 Novella M, Solà R, Soriano G *et al.* (1997) Continuous versus inpatient prophylaxis of the first episode of spontaneous bacterial peritonitis with norfloxacin. *Hepatology* 25, 532–536.

59 Ortiz J, Vila MC, Soriano G *et al.* (1999) Infections caused by *Escherichia coli* resistant to norfloxacin in hospitalized cirrhotic patients. *Hepatology* 29, 1064–1069.

60 Rabinivitz M, Prieto M, Gavaler JS *et al.* (1992) Bacteriuria in patients with cirrhosis. *J Hepatol* 16, 73–76.

61 Burroughs AK, Rosenstein IJ, Epstein O *et al.* (1984) Bacteriuria and primary biliary cirrhosis. *Gut* 25, 133–137.

62 Lipsky BA (1989) Urinary tract infections in men. Epidemiology, pathophysiology, diagnosis and treatment. *Ann Intern Med* 110, 138–150.

63 Westphal J-F, Jehl F, Vetter D (1994) Pharmacological, toxicologic, and microbiological considerations in the choice of initial antibiotic therapy for serious infections in patients with cirrhosis of the liver. *Clin Infect Dis* 18, 324–335.

64 Adams HG, Jordan C (1984) Infections in the alcoholic. *Med Clin North Am* 68, 179–200.

65 Bradsher RW (1983) Overwhelming pneumonia. *Med Clin North Am* 67, 1233–1250.

66 Levy M, Dromer F, Brion N *et al.* (1988) Community-acquired pneumonia. *Chest* 92, 43–48.

67 Panés J, Terés J, Bosch J *et al.* (1988) Efficacy of balloon tamponade in treatment of bleeding gastric and esophageal varices. Results in 151 consecutive patients. *Dig Dis Sci* 33, 454–459.

68 American Thoracic Society (1996) Hospital-acquired pneumonia in adults: diagnosis, assessment, initial severity and prevention. A consensus statement. *Am J Respir Crit Care Med* 153, 1711–1725.

69 Bodmann KF (2005) Current guidelines for the treatment of severe pneumonia and sepsis. *Chemotherapy* 51, 227–233.

70 Craven DE, De Rosa FG, Thornton D (2002) Nosocomial pneumonia: emerging concepts in diagnosis, management, and prophylaxis. *Curr Opin Crit Care* 8, 421–429.

71 Chen C, Chen PJ, Yang PM *et al.* (1997) Clinical and microbiological features of liver abscess after transarterial embolization for hepatocellular carcinoma. *Am J Gastroenterol* 92, 2257–2259.

72 Bouza E, Muñoz P, Rodriguez C *et al.* (2004) Endotipsitis: an emerging prosthetic-related infection in patients with portal hypertension. *Diagn Microbiol Infect Dis* 49, 77–82.

73 Snyder N, Atterbury CE, Correia JP *et al.* (1977) Increased occurrence of cirrhosis and bacterial endocarditis. A clinical and postmortem study. *Gastroenterology* 73, 1107–1113.

74 Denton JH, Rubio C, Velázquez J *et al.* (1981) Bacterial endocarditis in cirrhosis. *Dig Dis Sci* 26, 935–937.

75 Hsu RB, Chen RJ, Chu SH (2004) Infective endocarditis in patients with liver cirrhosis. *J Formos Med Assoc* 103, 355–358.

76 Swartz MN (1995) Cellulitis and subcutaneous tissue infections. In: Mandel GL, Bennett JE, Dolin R (eds) *Principles and Practice of Infectious Diseases*, 4th edn. New York: Churchill Livingstone, pp. 909–928.

7.10 Hypersplenism

P. Aiden McCormick

The spleen in liver disease

Splenomegaly is a frequent finding in patients with liver disease. The incidence of splenomegaly in cirrhotics varies from 36% to 92% in different series [1]. The cause of the liver disease influences the frequency of splenomegaly. Patients with idiopathic portal hypertension typically have large spleens, and it has been reported that patients with non-alcoholic cirrhosis tend to have larger spleens than patients with alcoholic cirrhosis [2]. A variable proportion of patients with liver disease and splenomegaly exhibit thrombocytopenia, anaemia and/or leucopenia (hypersplenism). Severe hypersplenism in cirrhotics is associated with a worsening of prognosis (see below). While passive venous congestion is believed to be the major cause of splenomegaly in portal hypertension, there is a poor correlation between portal venous pressure and spleen size [3]. The presence of splenomegaly, with an associated increase in splenic venous flow, may contribute to the maintenance of portal hypertension, particularly in idiopathic portal hypertension. If intrahepatic resistance is high enough to reverse blood flow in the splenic vein, prognosis is poor. In a prospective study of 50 patients with biopsy-proven severe alcoholic liver disease, survival at 1 year was significantly lower in patients with hepatofugal splenic blood flow than in those with hepatopetal blood flow in the splenic vein (41.7% vs. 82.4%; $P = 0.34$) [4]. The spleen may also contribute to increased intrahepatic resistance. Endothelin-1 is a potent vasoconstrictor, circulating levels of which are increased in cirrhotic patients, with higher levels in the superior mesenteric and splenic veins compared with the systemic circulation [5]. Immunostaining on surgically removed spleens in portal hypertensive patients has shown that endothelin-1 is produced by endothelial cells of the splenic sinus and lymphocytes in the marginal zones and germinal centres of the lymphoid sheaths and follicles.

Structure and functions of the spleen

The spleen is the largest lymphoid organ in the body and has important immunological and filtering functions. Resting splenic blood flow in animal studies is approximately 40–100 mL/min/100 g tissue [6]. This represents between 1% and 10% of cardiac output. In many species, the spleen is contractile and acts as a reservoir for blood cells. The human spleen is non-contractile, suggesting that this reservoir function is less important in man. The normal adult spleen weighs between 100 g and 174 g and becomes smaller in old age. It reaches its maximum size in late adolescence and may be palpable in up to 3% of apparently healthy young adults [7]. The spleen must double in size before it becomes palpable below the costal margin. It enlarges caudally and medially, and the spleen tip may be felt at the level of the 9th or 10th costal cartilage. In some patients with liver disease, it lies more posteriorly and may be missed unless palpation is performed in the left flank.

The spleen receives its arterial supply from the splenic artery and drains via the splenic vein into the portal vein. The spleen is divided into a variable number (3–7) of well-defined segments, each with its own blood supply and separated from each other by avascular planes [8]. Both splenic artery and vein lie close to the pancreas over much of their course and may be affected in conditions such as pancreatitis or pancreatic carcinoma. The cut surface of the spleen is characterized by red and white pulp. White pulp is visible as tiny white or grey spots (Malpighian corpuscles) seen against the dark background of the red pulp. The white pulp is lymphatic tissue which surrounds the splenic arterioles as a periarterial lymphatic sheath. It contains lymphocytes, monocytes and lymphoid follicles. The red pulp consists of a reticular meshwork, containing phagocytic reticular cells and endothelial macrophages, that lies between the splenic arterioles and the venous sinuses.

Microcirculation of the spleen

The microcirculation of the spleen is complex [6]. Microcirculatory studies suggest that there are two parallel functional blood flow pathways. Ninety per cent of blood flows through the fast pathway. Splenic arterioles lead to capillaries which, instead of leading into venules, empty into a reticular meshwork. The reticular network is not homogeneous. An area called the marginal zone or marginal sinus at the junction of the red and white pulp appears to receive the majority of the blood flow. Open-ended venous sinuses exist in this area that drain rapidly into the venous circulation. Blood in the remaining red pulp exits the spleen through the walls of venous sinuses, which have a structure similar to blind-ending sacs. Formed blood elements must pass through openings in the sinus walls called interendothelial slits (IESs). *In vivo* microscopy studies in the rat spleen suggest that these slits are contractile, and only approximately 20% are open during any particular 5-min observation period with a calculated flow rate of approximately three red blood cells/IES/min. It is believed that the red pulp provides the filtration function in the spleen. In contrast, blood flow through the marginal zone is believed to facilitate traffic of lymphocytes and macrophages into the lymphatic structures, as part of the immunological function of the spleen.

Functions of the spleen

The spleen has important immunological and filtration functions [9]. Splenectomized patients are particularly at risk of overwhelming infection from encapsulated bacteria such as pneumococcus, *Haemophilus influenzae* and meningococcus. The spleen functions as both a particulate filter and a lymphoid organ that can mount an adaptive immune response. In contrast to the hepatic Kupffer cells, splenic phagocytosis is effective even with poorly opsonized particles. There appears to be a distinct subset of mature peripheral B cells in the spleen, which respond rapidly to antigen and polyclonal activators, termed marginal zone (MZ) B cells [10]. These cells appear to bridge the gap between the innate immune system and the classic adaptive follicular B cells. The spleen is important in host defence against protozoal infections. More severe and frequent infections with malaria and babesiosis have been reported following splenectomy, although it should be noted that most splenectomized patients survive these infections [11].

Hypersplenism

It is believed that the term hypersplenism was first introduced by Chauffard in 1907 but was not precisely defined [12]. A clinical definition of hypersplenism has been suggested by Bowdler [13]: 'Hypersplenism is a syndrome in which there is enlargement of the spleen, accompanied by a deficit in one or more of the circulating cell lines of the peripheral blood (anaemic, thrombocytopenia, and granulopenia), together with demonstrated active haematopoiesis of the affected cell line(s) in the bone marrow. Retrospectively, the syndrome is justified by correction of the deficit by splenectomy.' This definition implies that a bone marrow examination is necessary to make the diagnosis. This is rarely done in practice unless there is doubt about the diagnosis. A more practical definition was suggested by Liangpunsakul *et al.* [14]. They defined hypersplenism as 'the presence of platelet count < 150 000/μL and/or white blood cell count

(WBC) < 3500/μL in conjunction with splenomegaly' [14]. Severe hypersplenism was defined as the presence of a platelet count of ≤ 75 000/μL and/or white cell count ≤ 2000/μL in conjunction with splenomegaly.

Incidence of hypersplenism

The reported incidence of hypersplenism in liver disease varies widely. Using the definitions shown above, Liangpunsakul *et al.* assessed the incidence of hypersplenism in 419 consecutive patients referred for liver transplantation [14]. Hypersplenism was present in 215 (51%) and severe hypersplenism in 108 (33%) patients. Decompensated liver disease and a history of excess alcohol consumption were independent risk factors. Interestingly, another 81 patients had either leucopenia or thrombocytopenia in the absence of splenomegaly. The incidence of hypersplenism may depend on the aetiology of the liver disease. Hypersplenism was present in 13/18 (72%) patients with cystic fibrosis-related cirrhosis [15]. In a study of 235 patients with non-alcoholic chronic liver disease, 64% of patients with severe fibrosis/cirrhosis had a platelet count of < 150 000/μL and 5% had leucopenia, with a circulating white cell count < 3500/μL [16]. In a retrospective study of 563 patients who had shunt surgery, El-Khishen *et al.* [17] found that 33 (6%) had a preoperative platelet count of < 50 000 μL and 30 (5%) had a white blood cell count < 2500 μL.

Mechanisms of hypersplenism

Thrombocytopenia in hypersplenism

The normal spleen stores between 30% and 45% of the circulating platelet pool, and this figure may rise of over 90% in patients with splenomegaly. There is a significant inverse correlation between the size of the spleen and the platelet count, although the relationship is very variable between individual patients (Fig. 1) [17]. Platelets are not irreversibly confined to the enlarged spleen, and a proportion may be released under conditions of stress or during an intravenous infusion of adrenaline (epinephrine) [18]. Thrombocytopenia in hypersplenism differs from idiopathic thrombocytopenia (ITP). In the former, it appears that the spleen contains the youngest and most haemostatically active platelets, which may be released at times of stress. Circulating platelets in ITP are larger, suggesting that the newly formed platelets are circulating in this condition [19]. Platelets transfused from asplenic donors appear to have a longer lifespan (~ 2 days) than those from normal donors, suggesting that young platelets are sequestered in the spleen before release into the circulation [20]. Exogenous platelets are also rapidly sequestered in the spleen. Approximately 20% of infused platelets are still present in the circulation 2 hours after infusion, compared with 60% in normal subjects (Fig. 2) [18].

In addition to increased sequestration of platelets, survival time appears to be decreased in cirrhotic patients. In one study,

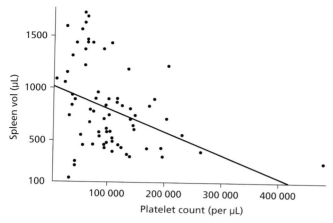

Fig. 1 Platelet count compared with spleen size. The platelet count is inversely related to spleen size, although the relationship is very variable between different patients. Reproduced from ref. 17: El-Khishen MA *et al.* (1985) Splenectomy is contraindicated for thrombocytopenia secondary to portal hypertension. *Surg Gynecol Obstet* (now *J Am Coll Surg*) 160, 233–238, with permission from the American College of Surgeons.

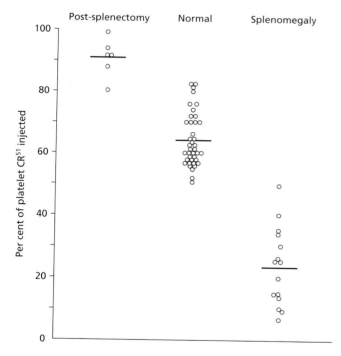

Fig. 2 Percentage of platelets remaining in the general circulation 2 hours after infusion. Reproduced from ref. 18: Aster RH (1966) Pooling of platelets in the spleen: role in the pathogenesis of 'hypersplenic' thrombocytopenia. *J Clin Invest* 45, 645, with permission from the American Society for Clinical Investigation.

mean survival was 5.8 days in cirrhotics compared with 9.5 days in normal control subjects [21]. The decreased survival time may be partially related to increased immune-related destruction. Platelet-associated immunoglobulin (PAIgG) is believed to render platelets more susceptible to immune-related destruction in the reticuloendothelial system. PAIgG is increased in

cirrhotic patients with portal hypertension, and the level appears to correlate with shortened platelet survival time [22].

Platelet production may also be impaired in cirrhosis. Thrombopoietin is a 353-amino-acid peptide produced at a constant rate mainly in the liver. Platelets have receptors for thrombopoietin, and bound thrombopoietin is not active in the bone marrow. In thrombocytopenia, free circulating thrombopoietin increases and stimulates platelet production. In idiopathic thrombocytopenic purpura, there is thrombocytopenia, an increase in thrombopoietin levels and an increased proportion of reticulated (young) platelets in the circulation. In contrast, patients with aplasia have thrombocytopenia, decreased reticulated platelets and high thrombopoietin levels. Cirrhotics appear to have normal or low thrombopoietin levels and normal or low circulating reticulated platelets [23]. The relatively low thrombopoietin levels could be because of binding to platelets in the spleen and/or reduced production in the failing liver. Certainly, liver transplantation generally increases both platelet counts and thrombopoietin levels, suggesting that there is a significant production deficit in cirrhosis [24]. The relative importance of sequestration, decreased production and increased production in cirrhotic thrombocytopenia is still a matter of some debate [25,26]. In patients with relatively well-preserved liver function and hypersplenism, e.g. schistosomiasis, decreased thrombopoietin production is less likely to be a significant contributory factor to thrombocytopenia [27].

Granulocytopenia in hypersplenism

Granulocytopenia is less common than thrombocytopenia in patients with hypersplenism, and there is a relatively poor correlation between spleen size and neutrophil counts (Fig. 3) [17].

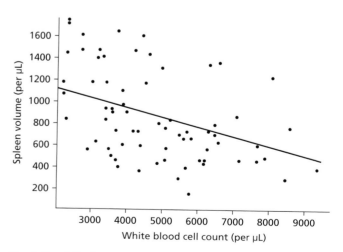

Fig. 3 Correlation between peripheral white blood cell count and spleen size. Reproduced from ref. 17: El-Khishen MA *et al.* (1985) Splenectomy is contraindicated for thrombocytopenia secondary to portal hypertension. *Surg Gynecol Obstet* (now *J Am Coll Surg*) 160, 233–238, with permission from the American College of Surgeons.

Radiolabelled studies suggest that there is a splenic pool of granulocytes that may be released under conditions of physiological stress, e.g. exercise [28]. Plasma myeloperoxidase levels are increased in cirrhotic patients compared with normal control subjects [29]. Myeloperoxidase is contained in the primary granules of neutrophils and released on activation or degradation. The high levels in cirrhosis are believed to be due to increased destruction or consumption of neutrophils along with decreased hepatic clearance. Levels are higher in patients with splenomegaly and correlate inversely with circulating neutrophil and platelet counts. This is indirect evidence that increased destruction along with splenic pooling may contribute to neutropenia in these patients. It has been suggested that plasma myeloperoxidase levels may be a possible marker of hypersplenism [30]. As well as splenic sequestration, neutropenia in cirrhosis may result from increased apoptosis in circulating polymorphonuclear leukocytes (PMNs). Ramirez *et al.* [31] demonstrated decreased viability on culture of PMNs from patients with decompensated liver disease compared with control subjects. These cells had morphological features of apoptosis and increased activity of caspase-3, an important transduction factor of apoptosis.

Anaemia in hypersplenism

Minor forms of anaemia are frequently seen in patients with liver disease and splenomegaly. The cause is often multifactorial and may include iron deficiency due to gastrointestinal bleeding, vitamin deficiencies, e.g. folate in alcoholic liver disease, haemolytic anaemia or the effects of toxins such as alcohol on the bone marrow. There is red cell pooling in the spleen, which may account for between 5% and 40% of the total red cell mass. The size of the splenic pool increases with spleen size, but the correlation is not close [32]. An additional factor contributing to anaemia is expansion of the plasma volume seen in cirrhosis. This expansion is probably secondary to the haemodynamic effects of cirrhosis and does not appear to be correlated with spleen size [33]. Increased red cell fragility may cause haemolysis in the spleen. Examples would be spur cell anaemia or the recently described haemolytic anaemia associated with a soluble variant of asialoglycoprotein receptor in the serum [34]. Both are usually seen in patients with alcoholic liver disease.

Clinical consequences of hypersplenism

Patients with severe hypersplenism (platelet count < 75 000/μL and/or white blood cell count < 2000/μL) appear to be at increased risk of variceal bleeding, spontaneous bacterial peritonitis and death compared with cirrhotic patients without severe hypersplenism [14]. In a study including 108 patients with and 221 patients without hypersplenism, the relevant figures for variceal bleeding were 19% vs. 5% ($P = 0.001$) (Fig. 4) and 16% vs. 3% for spontaneous bacterial peritonitis. The median survival was 32 months in the patients with severe

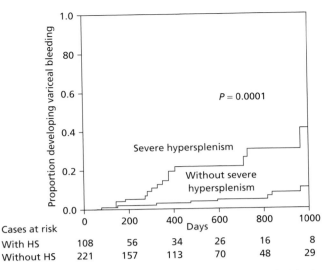

Cases at risk					
With HS	108	56	34	26	16	8
Without HS	221	157	113	70	48	29

Fig. 4 Cumulative probability of variceal bleeding in patients with cirrhosis and severe hypersplenism compared with cirrhotics without hypersplenism (HS). Reproduced from ref. 14: Liangpunsakul S *et al.* (2003) Predictors and implications of severe hypersplenism in patients with cirrhosis. *Am J Med Sci* 326, 111–116, with permission from the Southern Society for Clinical Invesitagtion.

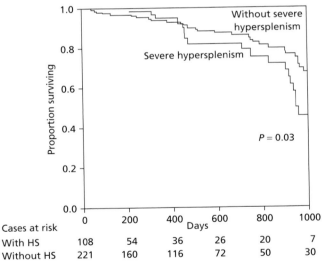

Cases at risk					
With HS	108	54	36	26	20	7
Without HS	221	160	116	72	50	30

Fig. 5 Cumulative probability of survival in cirrhotic patients with severe hypersplenism compared with cirrhotics without severe hypersplenism (HS). Reproduced from ref. 14: Liangpunsakul S *et al.* (2003) Predictors and implications of severe hypersplenism in patients with cirrhosis. *Am J Med Sci* 326, 111–116, with permission from the Southern Society for Clinical Invesitagtion.

hypersplenism compared with 47 months in those without ($P = 0.03$) (Fig. 5). It is likely that patients with more advanced liver disease will have an increased incidence of hypersplenism and increased risk of liver-related complications and mortality. However, severe hypersplenism remained an independent predictor in multivariate analysis. For mortality, the relationship

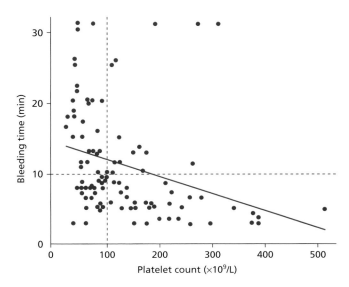

Fig. 6 Bleeding time compared with platelet count in cirrhotic patients. Overall, there is a weak but significant correlation between platelet count and bleeding time (RS = –0.048; $P < 0.001$). Reproduced from ref. 29: Blake JC *et al.* (1990) Bleeding time in patients with hepatic cirrhosis. *Br Med J* 301, 12–15, with permission from the BMJ Publishing Group.

between severe hypersplenism and mortality persisted even after controlling for Child–Pugh class [14].

It is easy to see that a low platelet count may increase the risk of variceal bleeding. In cirrhotics with thrombocytopenia, the bleeding time is prolonged and is significantly correlated with platelet count (Fig. 6) [29]. It is likely that bleeding may also be more severe or prolonged in patients with severe thrombocytopenia. In a large series of 695 cirrhotic patients admitted with variceal bleeding, platelet count was an independent predictor of early rebleeding [35]. Interestingly, platelet count was not an independent predictor of mortality in this study, although failure to control bleeding or early rebleeding was associated with higher mortality. Hypersplenism may also limit treatment options, particularly in patients with hepatitis C. A platelet count of $< 50/mm^3$ is regarded as a relative contraindication to treatment. Leucopenia is a frequent side-effect of treatment but may be effectively managed with granulocyte colony-stimulating factor (G-CSF).

Treatment of hypersplenism

It is important to realize that hypersplenism itself rarely requires specific treatment. The anaemia is seldom troublesome and, despite low granulocyte or platelet counts in the peripheral blood, cirrhotics with splenomegaly can usually mobilize granulocytes to deal with infection and platelets in the face of bleeding. If neutrophil counts are very low, therapy with G-CSF is often effective (see below). Thrombocytopenia is often more troublesome. Many patients with hypersplenism and thrombocytopenia receive platelet transfusions to cover surgery and invasive

procedures or as part of the treatment of variceal haemorrhage. In a study by the American College of Gastroenterology GI bleeding registry, data on 725 patients with bleeding oesophageal varices was gathered. A median of 1.5 units of platelets was transfused per episode of variceal bleeding [36]. Infused platelets are rapidly sequestered in the enlarged spleen with only about 20% still present in the circulation at 2 hours compared with 60% in normal subjects (Fig. 2) [18]. This suggests that prophylactic platelet transfusions should be administered during or shortly before invasive elective procedures to maximize their effectiveness. Unfortunately, there has been little study of the efficacy of platelet transfusion in patients with cirrhosis and hypersplenism. Platelet transfusions are a relatively scarce resource, and new strategies to maximize their effectiveness in this situation would be helpful. Many situations in which thrombocytopenia is a problem are short term or self-limiting, e.g. elective surgical procedures or biopsies. In other situations, e.g. recurrent variceal haemorrhage or severe epistaxis, thrombocytopenia may be a significant precipitant. Even in these situations, treatment directed at the site of bleeding, e.g. banding of varices or transjugular intrahepatic portosystemic shunts (TIPS), may solve the problem rather than therapy directed specifically at hypersplenism.

Granulocyte colony-stimulating factor (G-CSF)

G-CSF has been used to increase neutrophil counts in patients with hypersplenism. It appears to be effective in the majority of patients but has little effect on platelet numbers [37]. G-CSF appears to be well tolerated after liver transplantation and may be particularly useful in patients with cytomegalovirus (CMV) disease [38]. One large randomized controlled trial looked at the effect of routine G-CSF for the first 21 days after liver transplantation irrespective of neutrophil count. There were significant increases in neutrophil counts in the treatment group but no beneficial effects on infection rates or survival. Interestingly, there was a non-significant increase in the incidence of biopsy-proven rejection and nosocomial pneumonia in the treatment group [39].

Neutropenia and thrombocytopenia are frequent side-effects during antiviral treatment for hepatitis C virus [40]. Interferon causes a 10–50% reduction in peripheral platelet count, which may be clinically important in patients with hypersplenism and pre-existing thrombocytopenia. A reduction in dose is recommended if total neutrophil counts fall below 750/µL. An alternative strategy is to use G-CSF to increase neutrophil counts and maintain antiviral treatment doses.

Erythropoietin

Erythropoietin has been used extensively in renal patients with anaemia. It appears to have a modest effect in increasing platelet number. In a small randomized study, including patients with alcoholic cirrhosis and platelet counts < 120/μL, erythropoietin increased mean platelet count by about 25% [41].

Thrombopoietin

Thrombocytopenia causes most clinical problems in patients with cirrhosis and hypersplenism. The identification and purification of thrombopoietin in 1994 raised hopes that effective therapy might be at hand. To date, two forms have undergone extensive clinical testing, recombinant human thrombopoietin (rhTPO) and pegylated recombinant human megakaryocyte growth and development factor (PEG-rHuMGDF), mainly in oncology and haematology patients [42]. Both have been shown to stimulate megakaryocyte growth and platelet production and to ameliorate drug-induced thrombocytopenia. Results to date suggest that the peak response is delayed a few days and pretreatment is required. However, administration of multiple subcutaneous doses of PEG-rHuMGDF resulted in prolonged thrombocytopenia in 8–10% of patients. This appears to be due to the development of neutralizing antibodies that cross-react with native thrombopoietin. As a result, PEG-rHuMGDF was withdrawn from clinical trials. This effect has not been seen with rhTPO, which is given intravenously. In an analogous situation, cases of antibody-mediated pure red cell aplasia have been reported in renal patients following erythropoietin treatment [43]. They were attributed to subcutaneous rather than intravenous administration and to changes in stabilizers and storage methods. These problems were identified and resolved followed by the virtual disappearance of the clinical problem with erythropoietin. It is hoped that the similar problems with thrombopoietin will also be overcome. For the present, peptide thrombopoietin mimetics are being developed, designed to bind to and activate the thrombopoietin receptor. Thrombopoietin or thrombopoietin analogues would clearly be useful in patients with liver disease and thrombocytopenia, particularly for elective surgery or liver biopsy. Because of the delayed onset of action, they would be of limited value in emergency situations such as variceal haemorrhage.

Splenectomy

Splenectomy should cure hypersplenism. However, in patients with advanced liver disease, the procedure may be technically difficult and associated with considerable morbidity and mortality. Specific concerns include the risk of decompensation associated with surgery, postoperative portal vein thrombosis, increasing difficulty of subsequent liver transplantation and the increased risk of sepsis with encapsulated organisms such as pneumococcus. Splenectomy may be performed as part of the Sigiura procedure for patients with bleeding varices. This is now rarely performed in western countries as TIPS has superseded shunt surgery in many centres. Devascularization and splenectomy is still a major treatment option for patients with

schistosomal portal hypertension and bleeding varices [44]. Splenectomy may also be indicated in the rare patient with 'sinistral' or left-sided portal hypertension complicated by variceal bleeding [45]. This is characterized by splenic vein thrombosis and gastric varices.

While splenectomy is generally not recommended in cirrhotic patients, there is a suggestion that it may be useful in patients with cirrhosis and hepatoma. Wu et al. [46] reported a series of 41 patients treated in this way in a cohort of 526 hepatoma resections. These patients had preoperative platelet counts of < 80 000/μL. Morbidity and mortality rates were similar in patients treated with and without splenectomy. The authors claimed that this technique allowed them to increase the patients suitable for surgical resection in this situation [46]. Another Chinese group reported on 94 hepatoma patients treated with partial hepatectomy and splenectomy compared with partial hepatectomy alone in 110 patients [47]. They reported significantly improved 5-year disease-free survival in the splenectomy group (37% vs. 27.3%; $P = 0.003$), although overall survival was similar. However, all patients in the splenectomy group completed adjuvant chemotherapy compared with 15% in the hepatectomy alone group, which may have contributed to the observed differences. Clearly, controlled data will be required to confirm the role of splenectomy in this patient group.

Laparoscopic splenectomy has now been described in patients with cirrhosis and hypersplenism. A recent report described 11 patients with hepatitis C and thrombocytopenia which limited interferon treatment [48]. Laparoscopic splenectomy was successful in all, with no major complications. Mean spleen weight was 1043 g, and mean platelet count increased from 55/μL to 439/μL following surgery. It is important to note that all patients in this study had Child's class A liver disease. Partial splenectomy may be possible particularly in patients with schistosomal or non-cirrhotic portal hypertension. In a long-term (1–12 years) follow-up study of 32 patients, increases in circulating white cell counts and platelets were seen in 31% and 22% respectively [49].

Partial splenic embolization

Partial splenic embolization has been shown to produce significant increases in peripheral white cell and platelet counts. Interestingly, platelet survival time appears to improve after this procedure [22]. Initial enthusiasm was tempered by a high incidence of side-effects including pain, fever, splenic abscess, splenic rupture, acute pancreatitis and septicaemia. Side-effects may be reduced by careful aseptic technique, administration of prophylactic intravenous antibiotics and embolization of less than 70% of splenic volume. The place for this technique in the management of hypersplenism is still not clear. Reasonable long-term efficacy has been demonstrated in paediatric patients [50]. One cohort study suggested that the combination of variceal band ligation and partial splenic embolization reduced the risk of bleeding and improved prognosis in patients with varices and thrombocytopenia compared with band ligation alone [51]. Controlled studies will be required to confirm these findings. A recent variation on this technique is radiofrequency ablation of the spleen. A preliminary report of this technique in nine patients has appeared [52]. Improvement in hypersplenism and a low incidence of side-effects was described. There is an obvious potential for serious intraperitoneal haemorrhage with this technique, which may limit its applicability.

Transplantation

Successful liver transplantation replaces the failing liver, corrects portal hypertension and returns thrombopoietin production to normal. In the immediate post-transplant period, platelet levels may fall further as a result of consumption, immunosuppressive drugs or rejection. This can usually be managed conservatively with platelet transfusions as required. In very rare cases, severe symptomatic thrombocytopenia may persist following liver transplantation and require specific therapy, such as splenectomy [53]. Spleen size usually diminishes after transplantation, over time, but still remains somewhat enlarged in many patients. Platelet counts increase in the majority of patients, but many still have subnormal values on long-term follow-up [54].

Portosystemic shunts

Portosystemic shunt surgery and TIPS appear to have modest but somewhat unpredictably beneficial effects on hypersplenism. In two controlled studies of shunt surgery, splenomegaly diminished more often in the shunted patients [1,55]. However, only one study demonstrated an improvement in peripheral white cell and platelet counts [55]. The reported effect of TIPS on thrombocytopenia is also variable. An Austrian group noted a 19.7% increase in median platelet count over a 1-year period in 45 patients treated with TIPS [56]. There was a 17.1% drop in median platelet count in 110 control patients over the same time period. The percentage reduction in portosystemic gradient was not predictive of response. In contrast, an American group noted no significant change in platelet count in 60 patients treated with TIPS [57].

Venesection

An Italian group reported that phlebotomy caused increased platelet counts in cirrhotic patients with iron overload [58]. The aetiology of cirrhosis in this study was varied, including hepatitis C, alcohol and hereditary haemochromatosis. The increased platelet count was associated with improvements in alanine aminotransferase levels. Sixty-two patients were treated with an increase in mean platelet count from 110 to 168×10^9/L.

References

1 Mutchnick MG, Lerner E, Conn HO (1980) Effect of portocaval anastomosis on hypersplenism. *Dig Dis Sci* 25, 929–938.

2 Soper NJ, Rikkers LF (1982) Effect of operations for variceal hemorrhage on hypersplenism. *Am J Surg* 144, 700–703.

3 Shah SHA, Hayes PC, Allan PL *et al.* (1996) Measurement of spleen size and its relation to hypersplenism and portal hemodynamics in portal hypertension due to hepatic cirrhosis. *Am J Gastroenterol* 91, 2580–2583.

4 Duvoux C, Radier C, Roudot-Thoraval F *et al.* (2004) Low grade steatosis and major changes in portal flow as new prognostic factors in steroid-treated alcoholic hepatitis. *Hepatology* 40, 1370–1378.

5 Nagasue N, Dhar DK, Yamanoi A *et al.* (2000) Production and release of endothelin-1 from the gut and spleen in portal hypertension due to cirrhosis. *Hepatology* 31, 1107–1114.

6 Groom AC, MacDonald IC, Schmidt EE (2002) Splenic microcirculatory blood flow and function with respect to red blood cells. In: Bowdler AJ (ed.) *The Complete Spleen: Structure, Function and Clinical Disorders.* Totowa, NJ: Humana Press, pp. 23–50.

7 Ebaugh FG, McIntyre OR (1979) Palpable spleens: ten-year follow-up. *Ann Intern Med* 90, 130–131.

8 Redmond HP, Redmond JM, Rooney BP *et al.* (1989) Surgical anatomy of the human spleen. *Br J Surg* 76, 198–201.

9 Dailey MO (2002) The immune functions of the spleen. In: Bowdler AJ (ed.) *The Complete Spleen: Structure, Function and Clinical Disorders.* Totowa, NJ: Humana Press, pp. 51–69.

10 Lopes-Carvalho T, Kearney JF (2004) Development and selection of marginal zone B cells. *Immunol Rev* 197, 192–205.

11 Demar M, Legrand E, Hommel D *et al.* (2004) *Plasmodium falciparum* malaria in splenectomized patients: two case reports in French Guiana and a literature review. *Am J Trop Hyg* 71, 290–293.

12 Chauffard M (1907) Apropos de la communication de M Vaquez. *Bull Mem Soc Med Hop Paris* 24, 1201–1203.

13 Bowdler AJ (2002) The clinical significance of the spleen. In: Bowdler AJ (ed.) *The Complete Spleen.* Totowa, NJ: Humana Press, pp. 139–155.

14 Liangpunsakul S, Ulmer BJ, Chalasani N (2003) Predictors and implications of severe hypersplenism in patients with cirrhosis. *Am J Med Sci* 326, 111–116.

15 Psacharopolous HT, Howard ER, Portman B *et al.* (1981) Hepatic complications of cystic fibrosis. *Lancet* 2(8237), 78–80.

16 Bashour FN, Teran JC, Mullen KD (2000) Prevalence of peripheral blood cytopenias (hypersplenism) in patients with nonalcoholic chronic liver disease. *Am J Gastroenterol* 95, 2936–2939.

17 El-Khishen MA, Henderson JM, Millikan WJ *et al.* (1985) Splenectomy is contraindicated for thrombocytopenia secondary to portal hypertension. *Surg Gynecol Obstet* 160, 233–238.

18 Aster RH (1966) Pooling of platelets in the spleen: role in the pathogenesis of 'hypersplenic' thrombocytopenia. *J Clin Invest* 45, 645.

19 Karpatkin S, Freedman ML (1978) Hypersplenic thrombocytopenia differentiated from increased peripheral destruction by platelet volume. *Ann Intern Med* 89, 200–203.

20 Shulman NR, Watkins SP Jr, Itscoitz SB *et al.* (1968) Evidence that the spleen retains the youngest and hemostatically most effective platelets. *Trans Assoc Am Physiol* 81, 302–313.

21 Stein SF, Harker LA (1982) Kinetic and functional studies of platelets, fibrinogen and plasminogen in patients with hepatic cirrhosis. *J Lab Clin Med* 99, 217–230.

22 Noguchi H, Hirai K, Aoki Y *et al.* (1995) Changes in platelet kinetics after a partial splenic arterial embolization in cirrhotic patients with hypersplenism. *Hepatology* 22, 1682–1688.

23 Adinolfi LE, Giordano MG, Andreana A *et al.* (2001) Hepatic fibrosis plays a central role in the pathogenesis of thrombocytopenia in patients with chronic viral hepatitis. *Br J Haematol* 113, 590–595.

24 Haeh M, Hauser SP, Nydegger UE (2001) Transient thrombopoietin peak after liver transplantation for end-stage liver disease. *Br J Haematol* 112, 493–498.

25 Giannini E, Borro P, Botta F *et al.* (2002) Serum thrombopoietin levels are linked to liver function in untreated patients with hepatitis C virus-related chronic hepatitis. *J Hepatol* 37, 638–644.

26 Sanjo A, Satoi J, Ohnishi A *et al.* (2003) Role of elevated platelet-associated immunoglobulin G and hypersplenism in thrombocytopenia of chronic liver diseases. *J Gastroenterol Hepatol* 18, 638–644.

27 Souza MR, Aguiar L, Goto JM *et al.* (2002) Thrombopoietin serum levels do not correlate with thrombocytopenia in hepatic schistosomiasis. *Liver* 22, 127–129.

28 Allsop P, Peters AM, Arnot RN *et al.* (2005) Intrasplenic blood cell kinetics in man before and after brief maximal exercise. *Clin Sci* 83, 47–54.

29 Blake JC, Sprengers D, Grech P *et al.* (1990) Bleeding time in patients with hepatic cirrhosis. *Br Med J* 301, 12–15.

30 Nakamuta M, Ohashi M, Tanabe Y *et al.* (1993) High plasma concentration of myeloperoxidase in cirrhosis: a possible marker of hypersplenism. *Hepatology* 18, 1377–1383.

31 Ramirez MJ, Titos E, Claria J *et al.* (2004) Increased apoptosis dependent on caspase-3 activity in polymorphonuclear leukocytes from patients with cirrhosis and ascites. *J Hepatol* 41, 44–48.

32 Christensen BE (1975) Red blood cell kinetics. *Clin Haematol* 4, 393–405.

33 Blendis LM, Ramboer C, Williams R (1970) Studies on the haemodilution anaemia of splenomegaly. *Eur J Clin Invest* 1, 54–64.

34 Hilgard P, Schreiter T, Stockert RJ *et al.* (2004) Asialoglycoprotein receptor facilitates hemolysis in patients with alcoholic liver cirrhosis. *Hepatology* 39, 1398–1407.

35 Ben-Ari Z, Cardin F, McCormick PA *et al.* (1999) A predictive model for failure to control bleeding during acute variceal haemorrhage. *J Hepatol* 31, 443–450.

36 Sorbi D, Gostout CJ, Peura D *et al.* (2003) An assessment of the management of acute bleeding varices: a multicenter prospective member-based study. *Am J Gastroenterol* 98, 2424–2434.

37 Gurakar A, Fagiuoli S, Gavaler JS *et al.* (1994) The use of granulocyte–macrophage colony-stimulating factor to enhance hematologic parameters of patients with cirrhosis and hypersplenism. *J Hepatol* 21, 582–586.

38 Turgeon N, Hovingh GK, Fishman JA *et al.* (2000) Safety and efficacy of granulocyte colony-stimulating factor in kidney and liver transplant recipients. *Transpl Infect Dis* 2, 15–21.

39 Winston DJ, Foster PF, Somberg KA *et al.* (1999) Randomized, placebo-controlled, double-blind, multicenter trial of efficacy and safety of granulocyte colony-stimulating factor in liver transplant recipients. *Transplantation* 15(1298), 1304.

40 Russo MW, Fried MW (2003) Side effects of therapy for chronic hepatitis C. *Gastroenterology* 124, 1711–1719.

41 Homoncik M, Jilma-Stohlawetz P, Schmic M *et al.* (2004) Erythropoietin increases platelet reactivity and platelet counts in patients with alcoholic liver cirrhosis: a randomized double-blind, placebo-controlled study. *Aliment Pharmacol Ther* 20, 437–443.

42 Kuter DJ, Begley CG (2002) Recombinant human thrombopoietin: basic biology and evaluation of clinical studies. *Blood* 100, 3457–3469.

43 Casadevall N, Rossert J (2005) Importance of biologic follow-ons: experience with EPO. *Best Pract Res Clin Haematol* 18, 381–387.

44 Ferraz AA, Bacelar TS, Silveira MJ *et al.* (2001) Surgical treatment of schistosomal portal hypertension. *Int Surg* 86, 1–8.

45 Koklu S, Yuksel O, Arhan M *et al.* (2005) Report of 24 left-sided portal hypertension cases: a single-center prospective cohort study. *Dig Dis Sci* 50, 976–982.

46 Wu CC, Cheng SB, Ho WM *et al.* (2004) Appraisal of concomitant splenectomy in liver resection for hepatocellular carcinoma in cirrhotic patients with hypersplenic thrombocytopenia. *Surgery* 136, 660–668.

47 Chen XP, Wu ZD, Huang ZY *et al.* (2005) Use of hepatectomy and splenectomy to treat hepatocellular carcinoma with cirrhotic hypersplenism. *Br J Surg* 92, 334–339.

48 Kercher KW, Carbonell AM, Heniford BT *et al.* (2004) Laparoscopic splenectomy reverses thrombocytopenia in patients with hepatitis C cirrhosis and portal hypertension. *J Gastrointest Surg* 8, 120–126.

49 Petroianu A, da Silva RG, Simal CJ *et al.* (1997) Late postoperative follow-up of patients submitted to subtotal splenectomy. *Am Surg* 63, 735–740.

50 Nio M, Hayashi Y, Sano N *et al.* (2003) Long-term efficacy of partial splenic embolization in children. *J Pediatr Surg* 38, 1760–1762.

51 Ohmoto K, Yamamoto S (2003) Prevention of variceal recurrence, bleeding, and death in cirrhosis patients with hypersplenism, especially those with severe thrombocytopenia. *Hepatogastroenterology* 50, 1766–1769.

52 Liu Q, Ma K, He Z *et al.* (2005) Radiofrequency ablation for hypersplenism in patients with liver cirrhosis: a pilot study. *J Gastrointest Surg* 9, 648–657.

53 Altaca G, Scigliano E, Guy SR *et al.* (1997) Persistent hypersplenism early after liver transplant: the role of splenectomy. *Transplantation* 64, 1481–1483.

54 Yanaga K, Tzakis AG, Shimada M *et al.* (1989) Reversal of hypersplenism following orthotopic liver transplantation. *Ann Surg* 210, 180–183.

55 Felix WR Jr, Myerson RM, Sigel B *et al.* (1974) The effect of portocaval shunt on hypersplenism. *Surg Gynecol Obstet* 139, 899–904.

56 Gschwantler M, Vavrik J, Gebuer A *et al.* (1999) Course of platelet counts in cirrhotic patients after implantation of a transjugular intrahepatic portosystemic shunt – a prospective, controlled study. *J Hepatol* 30, 254–259.

57 Sanyal A, Freedman AM, Purdum PP *et al.* (1996) The hematologic consequences of transjugular intrahepatic portosystemic shunts. *Hepatology* 23, 32–39.

58 Franchini M (2003) Platelet count increase following phlebotomy in iron overloaded patients with liver cirrhosis. *Hematology* 8, 259–262.

8 Congenital hepatic fibrosis and non-parasitic cystic lesions of the liver and bile ducts

8.1 Congenital conditions

8.1.1. Congenital hepatic fibrosis

Jean-Pierre Benhamou

Congenital hepatic fibrosis is an inherited, congenital malformation characterized by portal spaces enlarged by fibrosis and multiple bile ductules, the main consequence of which is portal hypertension. The disease was described as fibrocystic disease of the liver by Grumbach [1]. The denomination of congenital hepatic fibrosis was introduced by Kerr [2].

Pathology and pathogenesis

The lesion of congenital hepatic fibrosis consists of portal spaces markedly increased in size because of abundant connective tissue and numerous bile ductules, more or less ectatic, communicating with the biliary tree. It must be emphasized that congenital hepatic fibrosis is not simply fibrosis and that bile ductular proliferation is an essential component of the lesion. A few portal spaces may remain normal, which explains why congenital hepatic fibrosis may be unrecognized by histological examination of a small specimen taken by liver biopsy. Some clusters of multiple bile ductules surrounded with fibrosis may be present within the lobules, apart from the portal spaces. Some bile ductules are so markedly dilated that they form microcysts: these microcysts communicate with the biliary tree. Separation between the fibrotic portal spaces and the rest of the liver parenchyma is sharp. Architecture of the liver remains normal. There is no regenerative nodule.

The primary disorder of congenital hepatic fibrosis is likely to be ductular proliferation, fibrosis being secondarily induced by the multiple bile ductules. The initial lesion might be clusters of multiple bile ductules, i.e. von Meyenburgh complexes, resembling the initial lesion of the liver cyst associated with adult polycystic kidney disease; however, in congenital hepatic fibrosis, the abnormal bile ductules maintain their communications with the biliary tree and, as a result, only microcysts are formed. In adult polycystic kidney disease, the abnormal bile ductules loose their communications with the biliary tree and, as a result, dilate markedly and form large cysts.

The mechanism for the development of multiple bile ductules in congenital hepatic fibrosis is unknown. It has been suggested that the abnormal abundance of bile ductules might result from a defect in the involution of the so-called ductular plate [3]. Normal involution would result in the obstruction of a large part of the ductular plate. The residual, undestroyed parts of the ductular plate would form intrahepatic bile duct. Congenital hepatic fibrosis would be due to the undestroyed parts of ductular plate. A similar disorder affecting the epithelium of the large bile ducts might account for Caroli's syndrome associated with congenital hepatic fibrosis. A similar mechanism might explain the dilatation of the renal collecting tubules and the dilatation of the pancreatic ducts, two extrahepatic malformations which may be associated with congenital hepatic fibrosis.

Aetiology

Congenital hepatic fibrosis is an inherited malformation, transmitted as an autosomal recessive trait [2,4]. The parents, presumably heterozygous, are phenotypically normal. Males and females are equally affected. Several siblings may be affected. Consanguinity increases the risk of congenital hepatic fibrosis.

The prevalence of congenital hepatic fibrosis is not established, but is certainly very low and might be of the same order of magnitude as that of another autosomal recessive liver disease, Wilson's disease, i.e. about 1:100 000 [5]. There is no ethnic predominance.

Manifestations and diagnosis

The main consequence of congenital hepatic fibrosis is portal hypertension, which is likely to be present from birth. The disease is recognized at the first episode of gastrointestinal bleeding resulting from ruptured oesophageal varices, which usually occurs between 5 and 20 years of age, but sometimes later. In a few patients, the disease is recognized before any gastrointestinal bleeding, because of blood disorders due to hypersplenism, abdominal discomfort resulting from an enlarged spleen, or the presence of abdominal collateral venous circulation.

At clinical examination, the liver is often, but not constantly, enlarged. Splenomegaly is present in most of the patients. Abdominal collateral venous circulation, Cruveilhier syndrome in some patients, is often visible. Ascites is absent. There is no symptom or sign indicating liver failure, in particular jaundice or spider naevi. The liver function tests are normal, except for moderately increased alkaline phosphatase and gammaglutamyl transpeptidase in a few patients. Endoscopic and/or radiographic examinations demonstrate oesophageal varices. Ultrasonography and/or computed tomography show that the liver is often enlarged, the portal vein is patent (which excludes extrahepatic portal hypertension), the spleen is enlarged, and portacaval collateral circulation is present; the venous phase of coeliac and mesenteric arteriography would provide similar information. Histological examination of an hepatic specimen taken by needle biopsy demonstrates the typical liver lesion in most patients; however, especially if the specimen is small, the lesion may be missed because, as mentioned above, some of the portal spaces may be normal.

Course and complications

The course of the disease is dominated by recurrent episodes of gastrointestinal bleeding, the frequency of which varies widely from patient to patient. The episodes of gastrointestinal bleeding are often well tolerated and are usually not followed by hepatic encephalopathy, ascites or jaundice. The patient's death is due to massive bleeding but not to liver failure. Thus, the course of congenital hepatic fibrosis resembles that of extrahepatic portal hypertension and differs from that of cirrhosis.

In a few patients, in the absence of Caroli's syndrome, congenital hepatic fibrosis is complicated by recurrent episodes of bacterial cholangitis. Uncontrolled, severe bacterial cholangitis may cause the death of such patients.

Thrombosis of the portal vein can complicate congenital hepatic fibrosis. This complication is often due to surgical operations on the portal vein or its branches, in particular splenectomy (which is unjustified in these patients).

Cholangiocellular carcinoma can complicate congenital hepatic fibrosis [6].

Associated malformations

Congenital hepatic fibrosis is often associated with Caroli's syndrome, either clinically silent or cholangitis determining (see below).

Congenital hepatic fibrosis is likewise often associated with a renal malformation consisting of ectatic collecting tubules resembling sponge kidney [7]; however, dilatation affects both the medullary and cortical portions of the collecting tubules in congenital hepatic fibrosis, whrereas dilatation is limited to the medullary portion in sponge kidney [8,9]. This renal malformation is clinically silent except for haematuria and/or urinary infection in a few patients. Dilatation of the collecting tubules can be demonstrated by intravenous pyelography showing enlarged kidneys and coarse striation of the medulla [7]. These radiological abnormalities are present in about two-thirds of the patients [4,7]; their presence is good evidence for, but their absence is not an argument against, the diagnosis of congenital hepatic fibrosis. In some patients with a normal intravenous pyelogram, histological examination of the kidneys may show ectatic collecting tubules [8].

In most patients, dilatation of collecting tubules remains stable. However, in some, the ectatic segments lose their communications with the urinary tract and transform into large renal cysts; the renal malformation then resembles adult polycystic kidney disease [10]. This transformation accounts for the large renal cysts detectable by intravenous pyelography or ultrasonography in a certain number of patients with congenital hepatic fibrosis [4]. This transformation may be rapid and take place in infancy or, more often, is more progressive, large renal cysts being formed only over 30 or 40 years. In patients with large renal cysts, the renal malformation may cause renal failure and/or arterial hypertension.

Other associated malformations are uncommon and include duplication of the intrahepatic portal vein branches [11], cystic dysplasia of the pancreas [2], intestinal lymphangectasia [12], pulmonary emphysema [13], cerebellar haemangioma [14], aneurysms of renal and cerebral arteries and cleft palate [2].

Treatment

Endoscopic sclerotherapy of oesophageal varices and/or non-selective beta blockers can be recommended for the prevention of recurrent bleeding, although these procedures have not been specifically evaluated in congenital hepatic fibrosis.

In patients in whom sclerotherapy and/or beta blockers are inefficient, a surgical portacaval shunt can be considered. Hepatic encephalopathy and liver failure after portacaval shunt is less common in patients with congenital hepatic fibrosis than in those with cirrhosis [4,15].

Splenectomy, which has been performed in a few patients in whom hypersplenism had not been related to congenital hepatic fibrosis, does not prevent occurrence or recurrence of gastrointestinal bleeding and may be followed by portal vein thrombosis, preventing subsequent surgical portacaval shunt (Benhamou, personal observation).

Operations or invasive investigations on the biliary tree, such as cholecystectomy, choledocotomy, T-tube drainage, intraoperative cholangiography or endoscopic retrograde cholangiography, must be avoided because of the risk of inducing bacterial cholangitis.

References

1 Grumbach R (1954) *Arch Anat Cytol Pathol* 30, 74–77.

2 Kerr DN, Harrison CV, Sherlock S *et al.* (1961) Congenital hepatic fibrosis. *Q J Med* 30, 91–117.

3 Desmet VJ (1992) Congenital diseases of intrahepatic bile ducts: variations on the theme 'ductal plate malformation'. *Hepatology* 16, 1069–1083.

4 Alvarez F, bernard O, Brunelle F *et al.* (1981) Congenital hepatic fibrosis in children. *J Pediatr* 99, 370–375.

5 Scheinberg IH (1984) *Wilson's Disease*. Philadelphia: Saunders, p. 71.

6 Yamoto (1998) *J Hepatol* 28, 717–722.

7 Kerr DN, Warrick CK, Hart-Mercer J (1962) A lesion resembling medullary sponge kidney in patients with congenital hepatic fibrosis. *Clin Radiol* 12, 85–91.

8 Clermont RJ, Maillard JN, Benhamou JP (1967) [Congenital hepatic fibrosis.] *Can Med Assoc J* 97, 1272–1278.

9 Fauvert R (1974) *The Liver and its Diseases*. New York: IMS, pp. 283–288.

10 Dupont HL (1978) Etiologic diagnosis of acute diarrhea. *Ann Intern Med* 88, 514–515.

11 Odièvre M, Chaumont P, Gautier M (1977) Transient hepatic peliosisin a child. *Radiology* 122, 427–430.

12 Chagnon (1982) [Primary biliary cirrhosis associated with digestive scleroderma without CRST syndrome or cutaneous involvement.] *Gastroenterol Clin Biol* 6, 326–332.

13 Williams R, Scheuer PJ, Heard BE (1964) Congenital hepatic fibrosis with an unusual pulmonary lesion. *J Clin Path* 17, 135–142.

14 Wagenvoort CA, Baggenstoss AH, Love JG (1962) Subarachnoid hemorrhage due to cerebellar hemangioma associated with congenital hepatic fibrosis and polycystic kidneys: report of a case. *Mayo Clin Proc* 37, 301–306.

15 Kerr DN, Okonkwo S, Choa RG (1978) Congenital hepatic fibrosis: the long-term prognosis. *Gut* 19, 514–520.

8.1.2. Simple cyst of the liver

Valérie Vilgrain

The simple cysts of the liver are cystic formations containing serous fluid, which do not communicate with the intrahepatic biliary tree. Numerous terms have been used: biliary cyst, non-parasitic cyst of the liver, benign hepatic cyst, congenital hepatic cyst, unilocular cyst of the liver, solitary cyst of the liver (this last designation is inappropriate because, as mentioned below, the simple cysts are often multiple). Although frequent in the general population, most simple cysts are less than 3 cm in diameter, easily identified at ultrasound and asymptomatic. Symptoms, when present, are usually related to intracystic

bleeding that changes the morphological appearance of the cyst and may mimic cystadenoma or hydatid disease.

Pathogenesis and pathology

Simple non-parasitic cysts of the liver are congenital. The pathogenesis of the simple cysts is still unclear, and it is usually considered that the pathogenesis is similar to that observed in polycystic diseases. During embryogenesis, abnormal or excessive numbers of intrahepatic ducts develop. These bile ducts fail to connect with the biliary tree and progressively dilate to form cysts. Despite this congenital origin, communication with the biliary tree is very rare. Liver cyst epithelial cells retain differentiated secretory function as they secrete fluid and generate a positive luminal pressure that may be greater than 30 cm H_2O. The composition of the fluid, which contains water and mineral electrolytes without bile acids and bilirubin, is close to that of the normal secretion of the epithelium of the bile ducts.

Macroscopically, simple cysts may be solitary or multiple, but are usually unilocular. Multilocular cysts are formed by the confluence of multiple adjacent cysts. They have a spherical or ovoid shape. The diameter ranges from a few millimetres to 20 cm or more. Up to five cysts can be observed, but the presence of multiple cysts should raise the possibility of adult polycystic kidney disease or adult polycystic liver disease. The presence of renal cysts or family history are key. The cystic fluid is usually clear yellow, but it may appear mucoid, bile stained or bloody because intracystic bleeding is relatively common. The inner surface is smooth. The small cysts are surrounded by normal hepatic tissue. The large cysts produce atrophy of the adjacent hepatic tissue: a huge cyst may result in complete atrophy of a hepatic lobe with compensatory hypertrophy of the other lobe. Atrophy respects the large bile ducts and blood vessels, which therefore appear to be abundant in the atrophic tissue in contact with the cyst. Large bile ducts and blood vessels persisting after atrophy may protrude and form folds over the inner surface of the cyst, which may mimic septae. Occasionally, von Meyenburg complexes can be present in the neighbouring liver.

Microscopically, the cystic epithelium is single cuboidal to columnar and resembles biliary epithelium. The cells are uniform, without any atypia. Epithelial cells contain small quantities of mucin and demonstrate weak immunostaining for epithelial antigen and carcinoembryonic antigen (CEA) [1].

Prevalence

Simple cysts have long been considered rare: up to 1971, only 350 cases had been reported [2,3], and early estimates of incidence from autopsy studies were less than 1% [4]. However, the development of imaging techniques has revealed that simple cysts are in fact much more frequent. Prevalence in ultrasonography studies is between 3% and 5% [5,6] and was as high as 18% in a recent spiral computerized tomography (CT) study of an adult population [7]. These discrepancies are explained by the usually small size of most cysts that are only discovered with accurate imaging techniques.

The prevalence of simple cysts is age and gender related. Simple cysts are uncommon before the age of 40 years, and their prevalence increases sharply thereafter. Simple cysts are also larger in adults over 50 years than in younger individuals [4]. Most studies show a higher prevalence in women (1.5 to four times higher) [5,6,8], and the female-to-male ratio rises to 9:1 in symptomatic or complicated simple cysts [3]. Huge cysts almost exclusively affect women over 50 years of age. An association between simple hepatic cysts and simple renal cysts has been documented [7], but is unexplained yet.

Manifestations

In the vast majority of cases, simple cysts – all the small cysts, but also most of the large cysts – are asymptomatic and fortuitously demonstrated by ultrasonography or CT. Symptoms are usually due to space occupation by the cysts and pressure on the adjacent structures; therefore, only some of the large cysts produce symptoms, but the severity of the symptoms does not correlate with the size of the cyst. Symptoms generally include abdominal pain (right upper quadrant or epigastric), discomfort, abdominal fullness, early satiety, dyspnoea, increasing abdominal girth or vomiting [9]. Sharp pain is not observed unless intracystic haemorrhage has occurred. Rarely, patients present with obstructive jaundice or oedema of the lower extremities. Because of the high prevalence of simple cysts in adults, and the vague symptomatology, the causal relationship between symptoms and a simple cyst of the liver should only be accepted if the cyst is large or complicated and if other possible causes of the symptoms have been excluded.

At clinical examination, only the large cysts can be palpated as spherical tumours. The condition of individuals with a simple cyst of the liver is good. Liver function tests are normal; abnormal liver function tests in a patient with a simple cyst of the liver are not related to the cyst and are caused by another liver disease, except when the cysts compress bile ducts.

Imaging

Ultrasonography is the best procedure for recognizing cysts. All cysts are characterized by anechoic or hypoechoic content. But other criteria have to be found to characterize the cystic lesion as a simple cyst (Fig. 1): round or oval shape; totally anechoic lesion; sharp and smooth borders with thin walls; strong acoustic posterior enhancement, which reflects an accentuation of the echoes beyond the cyst compared with echoes at a similar depth transmitted through normal adjacent liver tissue [10].

The posterior enhancement is observed only when the deep tissue transmits ultrasound and is not seen when a total reflector, such as gas or bone, lies behind the cyst. In some

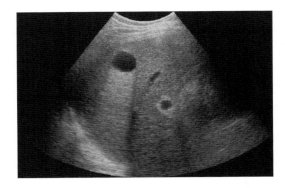

Fig. 1 Typical simple hepatic cyst at sonography. The lesion is strictly anechoic, with thin walls. Strong acoustic posterior enhancement is seen beyond the cyst.

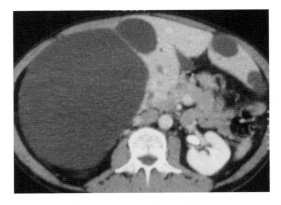

Fig. 2 Typical simple hepatic cysts on enhanced CT: homogeneous and hypoattenuating lesions that do not enhance after administration of contrast medium.

patients, because of intracystic bleeding, intracystic echoes can be detected. Focal thickening and nodularity are absent in simple cysts. Calcifications rarely occur and, if present, are localized and not circumferential. True septations are not seen in simple cysts, but the interface of several adjacent cysts may mimic septae; in such cases, the lobulated circumference of a cluster of multiple cysts allows distinction.

The other imaging procedures are generally unnecessary in uncomplicated cysts. A simple cyst appears as a homogeneous and hypoattenuating lesion on non-enhanced CT scans, with no enhancement of its wall or content after the administration of contrast material [11] (Fig. 2). Cysts are round or oval, and are thin-walled. In small cysts, recognition of water density may be difficult (the average density of the cyst being obscured by the density of the adjacent liver tissue). At magnetic resonance imaging (MRI), simple cysts have homogeneous very low signal intensity on T1-weighted images and homogeneous very high signal intensity on T2-weighted images. Strong hyperintensity persists on heavily T2-weighted images, and this feature allows differentiation from metastatic lesions [11]. No enhancement is seen after administration of gadolinium chelates.

When the diagnosis remains uncertain after complete non-invasive examination including MRI, aspiration may be useful for confirming the diagnosis by showing a clear fluid and by demonstrating the absence of communication with the biliary tree after intracystic injection of contrast medium [12]. It may also be used to rule out the presence of scolex if hydatid disease is suspected. The adjunctive use of measurements of cyst fluid CEA and CA19-9 levels has been reported. CEA measurements on the supernatant by enzyme immunoassay show negative levels (< 5 ng/mL) in fluids from benign cysts and elevated levels (> 600 ng/mL) in fluids from biliary cystadenoma/cystadeno-carcinoma and cystic metastases [13]. Only one case report of a simple cyst with markedly elevated CEA has been reported [14]. Because of the biliary epithelium, CA19-9 activity is very high in simple cysts, and this measurement may also be used to assess the effect of ethanol injection on a liver cyst [15].

Course and complications

In most cases, simple cysts remain silent; repeated ultrasonography usually shows no significant changes over years. In some patients, the cysts grow slowly (Fig. 3a and b). Why some simple cysts grow and others remain stable is not known. In a small number of patients, the size of the cysts increases rapidly: such a course, which may be associated with severe pain and

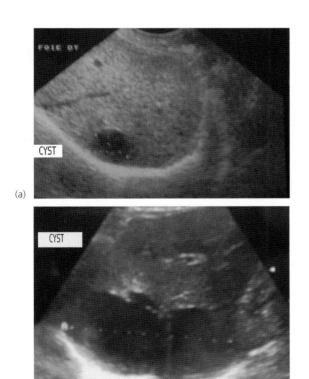

(a)

(b)

Fig. 3 Ultrasonography of a typical simple hepatic cyst which grew over a 10-year period: (a) first sonography; (b) sonography 10 years later.

discomfort, is observed almost exclusively in women over 50 years of age.

Complications are uncommon. Intracystic bleeding is by far the most frequent [3,16]. It is presumed to result from the erosion of an artery adjacent to the cyst. The clinical manifestations consist of sudden, severe pain and increase in the size of the cyst. The pain resolves in a few days. There is no evidence of anaemia, and the liver tests can only show a moderate elevation of γ-glutamyltransferase. At ultrasonography, echoic and mobile material, corresponding to clots, is present in the dependent part of the cyst, but thin and mobile septations may also be observed in haemorrhagic cysts (Fig. 4a). CT is usually unable to detect intracystic bleeding. MRI is very specific (Figs 4b–d). The complicated cysts are hyperintense on both T1- and T2-weighted sequences [17]. In most cases, the signal is heterogeneous on T1-weighted sequences (Fig. 4b). Thickened wall and fluid level may be seen (Fig. 4d).

Other complications are very uncommon. Spontaneous rupture may occur in the peritoneal cavity [18] or, more rarely, in the pleural cavity or the duodenum [19]. Rupture may also result from trauma [20] (Fig. 5). Unlike hydatid cysts, peritoneal perforation of simple cysts is exceptional and self-limited. Severe haemoperitoneum has only been described in patients with polycystic liver disease undergoing dialysis. Bacterial infection, although rare, has been reported. Simple cysts can induce compression of the bile ducts [3,21–23]. Large size and proximity to the main bile ducts are predisposing factors. Patients present with rising alkaline phosphatase and abdominal pain, but jaundice is observed in some patients. At imaging, the cyst responsible for biliary abnormalities is usually centrally located and leads to bile duct dilatation (Fig. 6). Other structures may be compressed by simple cysts: the inferior vena cava [16], which could result in clot formation and pulmonary embolism [24], and the portal vein with portal hypertension [25]. Communication with an intrahepatic duct [26], cholestasis due to haemobilia and torsion [27] have also been reported.

Squamous cell carcinoma of the liver originating from simple cysts has been reported several times in the literature [28]. It is hypothesized that the squamous epithelium arises from chronic inflammation and metaplasia. Ultrasonography and CT show large and complex cystic masses containing a solid component. Calcifications may be seen in the solid components [28].

Differential diagnosis

Simple cysts are easily distinguishable from liver abscess, necrotic malignant tumour, large haemangioma and haematoma. The clinical background of these lesions is different. At ultrasonography and CT, these lesions rarely appear as purely fluid-filled with sharply defined areas. However, some cystic metastases of endocrine origin or secondary to sarcomas can sometimes be difficult to distinguish from liver cysts because these tumours can be purely cystic. Careful analysis of the cystic wall usually demonstrates wall thickening or wall enhancement.

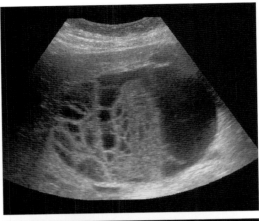

(a)

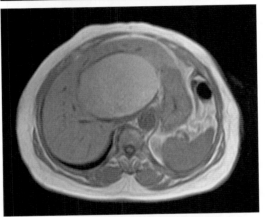

(b)

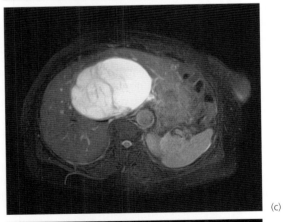

(c)

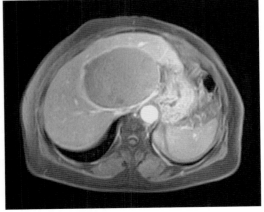

(d)

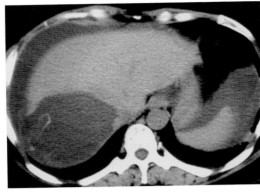

Fig. 5 Spontaneous rupture of a simple cyst on unenhanced CT. The cyst is ill-defined and communicates with peritoneal effusion.

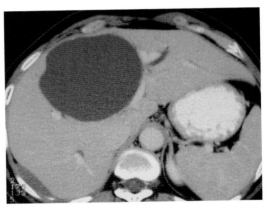

Fig. 6 Large simple hepatic cyst causing intrahepatic bile duct dilatation on enhanced CT. Large size and central location are the main predisposing factors.

The distinction between simple cyst and hydatid disease can be more difficult. Several characteristics of the simple cyst and hydatid disease, listed in Table 1, usually allow a clear distinction between the two diseases. However, difficulties may result from the following: (i) hydatid disease may have been contracted in an area where this parasitic infection is not endemic; (ii) calcifications, septations and split walls may be absent in hydatid cysts; (iii) septations may be observed in complicated cysts with intracystic haemorrhage or caused by contiguous simple cysts; (iv) serological tests for hydatid disease may be negative in some patients with hydatid cyst. In doubtful cases, serological tests for

Fig. 4 (*opposite*) Haemorrhagic cyst. The cyst has a complex appearance mainly at ultrasonography and MRI. (a) Ultrasonography shows echoic and mobile material within a cystic lesion. (b–d) MRI. The cyst is strongly hyperintense on T1- (b) and T2-weighted images (c). Septations are often seen. In contrast to non-complicated cysts, the wall may enhance after administration of chelates of gadolinium (d).

Table 1 Distinctive characteristics of simple hepatic cyst, hydatid cyst of the liver and biliary cystadenoma.

	Simple cyst	Hydatid cyst	Biliary cystadenoma
Septations	Absent	Common	Common
Calcifications	Absent	Common	Possible
Split wall	Absent	Possible	Absent
Papillary projections	Absent	Absent	Common
Communication with the biliary tree	Absent	Possible	Rare
Serological tests for hydatid disease	Negative	Positive[a]	Negative

[a] In most, but not in all, patients with hydatid disease.

this parasitic infection must be performed as well as microscopic examination of cystic fluid obtained by aspiration [29].

Distinction between a haemorrhagic cyst and a cystadenoma may be difficult too. The presence of associated typical hepatic cysts and the lack of enhancement of the septations after contrast injection in haemorrhagic cyst are helpful in suggesting the diagnosis of simple cyst (Table 1) [30].

Treatment

Asymptomatic liver cysts, even when large, need no treatment. When symptoms are present, treatment is indicated only if these symptoms are clearly related to the cyst. One should be very cautious before advocating any form of treatment in patients with cysts that are smaller than 8 cm and that do not protrude outside the liver surface. In case of doubt, an initial ultrasound-guided aspiration of the cyst is warranted to confirm that subsequent definitive treatment will resolve symptoms: if aspiration has no influence on the symptoms, an alternative source of symptoms should be investigated. Importantly, simple aspiration should never be used as definitive treatment because cyst recurrence is almost certain [31]. The treatment of simple cysts has changed over the last decades because of interventional procedures and the development of laparoscopy. Treatments include aspiration and sclerosis, laparoscopy and laparotomy for either resection or open fenestration. The choice depends on the cyst location, number and the complications. For instance, cysts in the dome of the liver can pose technical problems if the laparoscopic approach is used.

Percutaneous aspiration and sclerotherapy

This treatment is based on injection of a sclerosing agent into the cyst cavity, which aims at the destruction of the epithelium lining. The most frequently used sclerosing agent is ethanol. The cyst is punctured under ultrasound guidance. Cyst contents are aspirated, and biochemical analysis is performed in uncertain cases. A pigtail catheter is inserted into the cyst by a Seldinger technique. The volume of the aspiration is measured, and a cystogram is performed to check any vascular or biliary communication or perforation into the peritoneal cavity. After complete aspiration of the contrast medium, sterile absolute alcohol is

injected depending on the cyst volume, but not exceeding a total amount of 100 mL. The posture of the patient varies to ensure complete exposure of the sclerosing agent to the cyst wall (a total of 40 min exposure is the rule). Then, the ethanol is aspirated and the catheter is removed. Complications include severe abdominal pain during intracystic injection (generally due to extravasation of alcohol into the peritoneal cavity; this explains why this procedure should be done under complete sedation), alcohol intoxication, hypotension, pleural effusion, peritoneal extravasation, infection and inflammatory changes of the cysts. Overall, morbidity is less than 10%. Minocycline hydrochloride has been used as an alternative to ethanol and seems to be associated with fewer side-effects, although it may require multiple injections [32]. Although sclerotherapy has been used for almost 15 years, there are few large studies with prolonged follow-up [32–36]. The success rates range between 70% and 95%. Repeat aspiration and sclerotherapy may be required. Large cysts could have two sessions of sclerotherapy with a 24-h interval with the catheter left in the cyst between the sessions. Contraindication to this treatment is the presence of bile in the cyst cavity or leakage of contrast media injected in the cyst into the bile duct.

Laparoscopy

The laparoscopic technique has evolved recently and is the preferred treatment for some authors [37–42]. The laparoscopic approach permits both partial excision (including fenestration) and total excision. The goal of the fenestration is to establish a large communication between the cyst and the peritoneal cavity. Fluid continues to be produced by the epithelium lining but is reabsorbed by the peritoneum. Laparoscopic management has some advantages: it is less invasive than laparotomy and involves a shorter hospital stay. However, it has drawbacks: limited access to deep-seated or posteriorly situated cysts, in patients with a history of previous abdominal surgery (because of adhesions), when haemorrhage or infection within a liver cyst results in changes that mimic a liver tumour or a parasitic cyst, and in patients with multiple cysts unless a large accessible cyst is symptomatic. Similar to the experience of percutaneous aspiration and sclerosis, the reported number of patients treated is small, and the duration of follow-up is short. Success ranges from 75% to 100%. Conversion to an open laparotomy for treatment in these select patients may be required. The need for careful patient selection seems crucial [39,42–44]. Complications occur in 0–15% of patients and include shoulder pain, dyspnoea, pleural effusion, ascites (especially when the cyst is very large because fluid secretion may overflow the resorption capacity of the peritoneum), haemorrhage, infection and subhepatic bile collection. No mortality has been reported. Recurrence rate is less than 17% [42,43]. In patients with multiple cysts, the long-term outcome is similar to that in patients with single cysts [45].

Laparotomy

This was the treatment of choice for simple cysts before the percutaneous and laparoscopic techniques became widespread. The surgical technique was either partial or total cystectomy, and rarely hepatic resection. In contrast to total cystectomy or hepatic resection, partial cystectomy is associated with a risk of recurrence [9].

References

1 Terada T, Nakanuma Y, Ohta T et al. (1991) Mucin-histochemical and immunohistochemical profiles of epithelial cells of several types of hepatic cysts. *Virchows Arch A Pathol Anat Histopathol* 419, 499–504.

2 Flagg RS, Robinson DW (1967) Solitary non parasitic hepatic cysts. Report of oldest known case and review of the literature. *Arch Surg* 95, 964–973.

3 Moreaux J, Bloch P (1971) Les kystes biliaires solitaires du foie. *Arch Franç Mal Appar Dig* 60, 203–224.

4 Larsen KA (1961) Benign lesions affecting the bile ducts in the postmortem cholangiogram. *Acta Pathol Microbiol Immunol Scand* 51, 47–62.

5 Gaines PA, Sampson MA (1989) The prevalence and characterization of simple hepatic cysts by ultrasound examination. *Br J Radiol* 62, 335–337.

6 Caremani M, Vincenti A, Benci A et al. (1993) Echographic epidemiology of non-parasitic hepatic cysts. *J Clin Ultrasound* 21, 115–118.

7 Carrim ZI, Murchison JT (2003) The prevalence of simple renal and hepatic cysts detected by spiral computed tomography. *Clin Radiol* 58, 626–629.

8 Hadad AR, Westbrook KC, Graham GG et al. (1977) Symptomatic non parasitic liver cysts. *Am J Surg* 134, 739–744.

9 Karavias DD, Tsamandas AC, Payatake AH (2000) Simple (non-parasitic) liver cysts: clinical presentation and outcome. *Hepato-Gastroenterology* 47, 1439–1443.

10 Spiegel RM, King DL, Green WM (1978) Ultrasonography of primary cysts of the liver. *Am J Roentgenol* 131, 235–238.

11 Mortele KJ, Ros PR (2001) Cystic focal liver lesions in the adult: differential CT and MR imaging features. *Radiographics* 21, 895–910.

12 Roemer CE, Ferrucci JT, Mueller PR et al. (1981) Hepatic cysts: diagnosis and therapy by sonographic needle aspiration. *Am J Roentgenol* 136, 1065–1070.

13 Pinto MM, Kaye AD (1988) Fine needle aspiration of cystic liver lesions. Cytologic examination and carcinoembryonic antigen assay of cyst contents. *Acta Cytol* 33, 852–856.

14 Sato T, Kokudo N, Seki M et al. (1999) A case of simple liver cyst with markedly elevated CEA level in the cystic fluid. *Nippon Shokakibyo Gakkai Zasshi* 96, 530–534.

15 Ikeda Y, Kawasaki K, Uchida H et al. (1996) Treatment of large cyst evaluated with CA 19-9 In the cystic fluid. *HepatoPancreatoBil Surg* 9, 179–182.

16 Frisell J, Röjdmark S, Arvidsson H et al. (1979) Compression of the inferior caval vein. A rare complication of a large non-parasitic liver cyst. *Acta Med Scand* 205, 541–542.

17 Vilgrain V, Silbermann O, Benhamou JP et al. (1993) MR imaging in intracystic hemorrhage of simple hepatic cysts. *Abdom Imaging* 18, 164–167.

18 Akriviadis EA, Steindel H, Ralls P et al. (1989) Spontaneous rupture of nonparasitic cyst of the liver. *Gastroenterology* 97, 213–215.

19 Williamson RCN, Ramus NI, Shorey BA (1978) Congenital solitary cysts of the liver and spleen. *Br J Surg* 65, 871–876.

20 Yamaguchi M, Kuzume M, Matsumoto T et al. (1999) Spontaneous rupture of a nonparasitic liver cyst complicated by intracystic hemorrhage. *J Gastroenterol* 34, 645–648.

21 Santman FW, Thijs LG, Van der Veen EA et al. (1977) Intermittent jaundice: a rare complication of solitary nonparasitic liver cyst. *Gastroenterology* 72, 325–328.

22 Clinkscales NB, Trigg LP, Poklepovic J (1985) Obstructive jaundice secondary to benign hepatic cyst. *Radiology* 154, 643–644.

23 Cappell MS (1988) Obstructive jaundice from benign, nonparasitic hepatic cysts: identification of risk factors and percutaneous aspiration for diagnosis and treatment. *Am J Gastroenterol* 83, 93–96.

24 Buyse S, Asselah T, Vilgrain V et al. (2004) Acute pulmonary embolism: a rare complication of a large non-parasitic hepatic cyst. *Eur J Gastroenterol Hepatol* 16, 1241–1244.

25 Lebon J, Bourgeon R, Claude R (1955) Kyste solitaire du foie. *Arch Franç Mal Appar Dig* 44, 1274–1277.

26 Perreau P, Guntz M, Renier JC (1965) Kyste solitaire non parasitaire du foie. Considérations anatomo-cliniques, diagnostiques et thérapeutiques. *Arch Franç Mal Appar Dig* 54, 881–888.

27 Soud SC, Watson A (1974) Solitary cyst of the liver presenting as an abdominal emergency. *Postgrad Med J* 50, 48–50.

28 Yagi H, Ueda M, Kawachi S et al. (2004) Squamous cell carcinoma of the liver originating from non-parasitic cysts after a 15 year follow-up. *Eur J Gastroenterol Hepatol* 16, 1051–1056.

29 Giuliante F, D'Acapito F, Vellone M et al. (2003) Risk for laparoscopic fenestration of liver cysts. *Surg Endosc* 1, 1735–1738.

30 Vuillemin-Bodaghi V, Zins M, Vullierme MP et al. (1997) Imaging of atypical cysts of the liver. Study of 26 surgically treated cases. *Gastroenterol Clin Biol* 21, 394–399.

31 Saini S, Mueller PR, Ferrucci JT, Jr et al. (1983) Percutaneous aspiration of hepatic cysts does not provide definitive therapy. *Am J Roentgenol* 141, 559–560.

32 Yamada N, Shinzawa H, Ukai K et al. (1994) Treatment of symptomatic hepatic cysts by percutaneous instillation of minocycline hydrochloride. *Dig Dis Sci* 39, 2503–2509.

33 Simonetti G, Profili S, Sergiocomi GL et al. (1993) Percutaneous treatment of hepatic cysts by aspiration and sclerotherapy. *Cardiovasc Intervent Radiol* 16, 81–84.

34 Montorsi M, Torzilli G, Fumagalli U et al. Percutaneous alcohol sclerotherapy of simple hepatic cysts. Results from a multicentre survey in Italy. *HPB-Surgery* (1994) 8, 89–94.

35 Tanaka Y, Ogino M, Tokuda H et al. (1996) Examination of percutaneous minocycline hydrochloride injection therapy for hepatic cyst by one puncture method. *Nippon Shokakibyo Gakkai Sasshi* 93, 828–836.

36 Tikkakoski T, Mäkelä JT, Leinonen S, *et al.* (1996) Treatment of symptomatic congenital hepatic cysts with single-session percutaneous drainage and ethanol sclerosis: technique and outcome. *J Vasc Interv Radiol* 7, 235–239.

37 Morino M, De Guili M, Festa V *et al.* (1994) Laparoscopic management of symptomatic nonparasitic cysts of the liver. Indications and results. *Ann Surg* 219, 157–164.

38 Gigot JF, Jadoul P, Que F *et al.* (1997) Adult polycystic liver disease: is fenestration the most adequate operation for long-term management? *Ann Surg* 225, 286–294.

39 Emmermann A, Zornig C, Lloyd DM *et al.* (1997) Laparoscopic treatment of nonparasitic cysts of the liver with omental transposition flap. *Surg Endosc* 11, 734–736.

40 Fabiani P, Mazzsa D, Toouli J *et al.* (1997) Laparoscopic fenestration of symptomatic non-parasitic cysts of the liver. *Br J Surg (London)* 84, 321–322.

41 Klingler PJ, Gadenstätter M, Schmid T *et al.* (1997) Treatment of hepatic cysts in the era of laparoscopic surgery (review). *Br J Surg* 84, 438–444.

42 Martin IJ, McKinley AJ, Currie EJ *et al.* (1998) Tailoring the management of nonparasitic liver cysts. *Ann Surg* 228, 167–172.

43 Gigot JF, Legrand M, Hubens G *et al.* (1996) Laparoscopic treatment of nonparasitic liver cysts: adequate selection of patients and surgical technique. *World J Surg* 20, 556–561.

44 Marks J, Mouiel J, Katkhouda N *et al.* (1998) Laparoscopic liver surgery: a report of 28 patients. *Surg Endosc* 12, 331–334.

45 Farges O, Bismuth H (1995) Fenestration in the management of polycystic liver disease. *World J Surg* 19, 25–30.

8.1.3. Polycystic kidney disease

Valérie Vilgrain

Autosomal dominant polycystic disease is a frequent inherited disorder involving the liver. It is genetically heterogeneous and most commonly predisposes to the development of renal and cystic cysts.

Pathology and pathogenesis

The liver cysts in patients with adult autosomal dominant polycystic kidney disease (ADPKD) are macroscopically and microscopically similar to simple cysts of the liver. The main difference between these two entities concerns the number of liver cysts: the liver cysts, when present, are multiple in all patients with ADPKD; in contrast, numerous cysts are found only in a few patients with simple cysts of the liver.

Grossly, the liver in ADPKD is enlarged and diffusely cystic, the cysts varying from < 1 mm to 12 cm or more in diameter (Fig. 1). Occasionally, one lobe, usually the left, is affected. Diffuse dilatation of the intra- and extrahepatic bile ducts has been reported in some cases. The cysts contain a clear, colourless or yellow fluid. Analysis of the cyst fluid discloses similarities to the 'bile salt-independent' fraction of human bile, suggesting that such cysts are lined by a functioning bile duct epithelium.

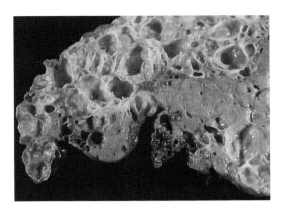

Fig. 1 Macroscopic view of multiple liver cysts in a patient with ADPKD.

Microscopically, the cysts are lined by columnar or cuboidal epithelium, but the larger cysts have a flat epithelium. Collapsed cysts resemble corpora atretica of the ovary. The supporting connective tissue is scanty except in relation to von Meyenburg complexes, a frequently associated lesion, where it may be dense and hyalinized. Inflammatory cells may infiltrate the stroma. Infected cysts contain pus and may rupture. Calcification of the wall of hepatic cysts in ADPKD has been reported.

Von Meyenburg complexes are considered to be part of the spectrum of ADPKD, and it is hypothesized that polycystic disease develops over the years by gradual cystic dilatation of these complexes [1]. It has also been suggested that the cystic dilatation of peribiliary glands may lead to the formation of the cysts in ADPKD.

Despite the large number and the large size of liver cysts, the hepatic parenchymal volume is preserved [2], which explains why normal hepatic function and normal intrahepatic circulation are maintained in most of these patients.

Genetics and molecular biology

The most common forms of ADPKD are linked to mutations in either *PKD1* or *PKD2* genes. *PKD1* [3] is localized on the short arm of chromosome 16. Transcription and translation of the *PKD1* gene produces polycystin-1, an integral membrane protein that may serve as an extracellular receptor. There are over 230 distinct mutations of the *PKD1* gene. The majority are missense or nonsense mutations, but splicing mutations and gene rearrangements have also been reported. Approximately 60% of all mutations introduce premature stop codons that result in truncated proteins [4]. It has been suggested that the type or position of mutations may predict the patient phenotype. Certain mutations are linked to intracranial aneurysms and more severe polycystic disease within individual ADPKD families [5]. Location of a mutation in the 5′ end of the gene predicts more rapid progression and greater severity of endstage renal disease [4]. *PKD1* mutations account for up to 90% of mutations in ADPKD families.

Most of the remaining are related to mutations in *PKD2* [6], localized on chromosome 4. The *PKD2* gene product, polycystin-2, is an integral membrane protein with molecular characteristics of a calcium-permeant cation channel. There are over 60 identified mutations of the *PKD2* gene, and mutations occur throughout the gene; severity of disease may vary with site of mutation in *PKD2* and the functional consequence on the resultant polycystin-2 protein. ADPKD at the cellular level is likely to be a 'molecular recessive' disease, requiring a second somatic mutation: the 'two-hit' model.

Molecular genetic testing may be considered in young (age < 30 years), presymptomatic individuals at risk of ADPKD, because ultrasonography may lack sensitivity and linkage analysis is impractical. The identification of a *PKD1* or *PKD2* mutation could affect family planning, monitoring and screening for associated conditions such as cerebral aneurysm or mitral valve prolapse.

Features of the cysts and their natural history are comparable whatever the mutation, although patients with *PKD2* mutations tend to have later onset of their disease than patients with *PKD1* mutations and approximately 16 years of increased life expectancy compared with patients who have mutations in *PKD1*. Two unrelated families have been described who, by genetic linkage analysis, lack mutations in either *PKD1* or *PKD2* [7,8]. These findings are controversial but suggest that mutations in at least a third gene may be responsible for ADPKD.

Natural history and risk factors for development and progression

Hepatic cysts, as for simple cysts, are rarely observed prior to puberty, and their prevalence increases thereafter. Kidney cysts in patients with ADKPD always precede the development of hepatic cysts. By the fifth decade of life, approximately 80% of patients with renal cysts have liver cysts [9] (Table 1). The number and size of the liver cysts are greater in females than in males, increase with the age of the patient, and are greater in patients with large renal cysts and severe kidney dysfunction than in patients with small renal cysts and mild renal insufficiency. As for simple cysts, men and women have an equal lifetime risk of developing hepatic cysts, but women experience greater numbers and larger sizes of hepatic cysts. Pregnancy and the use of female steroid hormones further increase the risk of severe hepatic cystic disease. One longitudinal study of anovulatory women with ADPKD treated with hormone replacement has suggested that estrogens may selectively increase the severity of hepatic cystic disease [10]. The pathological expansion of the liver cysts could be related to specific growth factors and cytokines contained in liver cyst fluid. Nichols *et al.* [11] have suggested an autocrine and paracrine model for ADPKD liver cyst growth. Local hypoxia induces the synthesis and release of cytokines and growth factors across the apical and basal membranes to signal to epithelial cells via apical domain receptors, endothelial cells and stellate and fibroblast cells [11].

Clinical features

Most patients with polycystic liver are asymptomatic or may note only a protuberant abdomen. Patients with ADPKD can be arbitrarily divided into two groups, massive or minimal, based on a definition of mass of total liver cyst/parenchymal volume ratio > 1 [2]. Most symptomatic cases are restricted to patients with massive hepatic cystic disease, with abdominal pain and discomfort and shortness of breath correlating with severity of hepatic cystic disease. Early postprandial fullness is mainly observed in patients with severe involvement of the left liver that compresses the stomach.

At clinical examination of patients with large cysts, the liver is enlarged, sometimes enormous; the cysts may be so tense that they can be confused with solid tumours. Usually, there are no signs or symptoms suggesting cholestasis, liver failure or portal hypertension. Liver tests are usually normal or show only a slight elevation in gamma-glutamyltransferase.

Imaging findings

Ultrasonography shows round, smooth-walled anechoic areas with marked distal echo enhancement. ADPKD typically appears as multiple homogeneous and hypoattenuating cystic lesions with a regular outline on non-enhanced computerized tomography (CT) with no wall or content enhancement on

| Age (years) | Series of Milutinovic *et al.* [48] | | Series of Thomsen and Thaysen [49] | |
	No. of patients studied	Percentage of patients with liver cysts	No. of patients studied	Percentage of patients with liver cysts
10–19	12	0	0	
20–29	47	11	1	0
30–39	31	32	15	40
40–49	30	37	17	53
50–59	25	40	20	65
>60	13	77	13	87
Total/mean	158	29	66	59

Table 1 Age and prevalence of liver cysts demonstrated by liver scintiscan [48] and by computerized tomography [49] in patients with adult polycystic kidney disease.

contrast-enhanced images (Figs 2a and b). Coalescence of cysts produces bizarre appearances. Coalescence of large cysts causes distortion of the shape of an individual cyst and may give a false appearance of a multiloculated or septated cystic lesion. Remaining hepatic parenchyma between the cysts may resemble mural nodules or thickened internal septa [12]. Calcification of the cysts has been reported, but is very rare [13,14] (Fig. 3a). On magnetic resonance imaging (MRI), hepatic cysts in ADPKD are homogeneously and strongly hyperintense on T2-weighted MR images owing to their pure fluid content (Fig. 3e) and strongly hypointense on T1-weighted images except when they are complicated by haemorrhage when they appear hyperintense on T1-weighted sequences. They do not enhance after administration of gadolinium contrast material.

In a series of 44 patients with ADPKD, CT showed many large liver cysts in 31.8% of patients, small liver cysts in 25% and no liver cysts in 43.2% [15]. Patients with many large cysts often showed increased liver volumes [2,15]. Splenic volumes did not differ significantly in patients with and without liver cysts, suggesting that portal hypertension is rarely associated with cystic liver disease. There was no correlation between severity of liver involvement and extent of renal cystic disease, as determined from urea nitrogen and creatinine levels and renal volumes.

In another series of 24 patients with ADPKD, an attempt was made to categorize these cysts into peribiliary cysts (located adjacent to larger portal triads or in the hepatic hilum) and intrahepatic cysts (within the liver parenchyma but not in

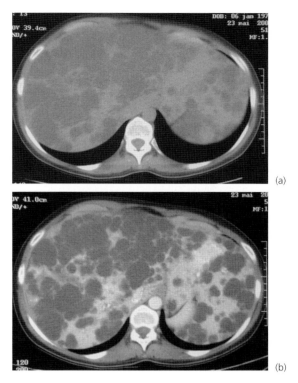

(a)

(b)

Fig. 2 Unenhanced (a) and enhanced (b) CT images of an ADPKD patient. CT shows multiple small cysts that do not enhance after the administration of contrast medium.

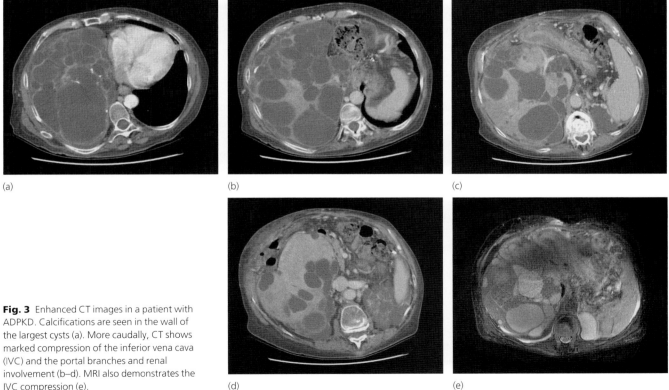

(a)

(b)

(c)

(d)

(e)

Fig. 3 Enhanced CT images in a patient with ADPKD. Calcifications are seen in the wall of the largest cysts (a). More caudally, CT shows marked compression of the inferior vena cava (IVC) and the portal branches and renal involvement (b–d). MRI also demonstrates the IVC compression (e).

contact with larger portal triads). Liver cysts were seen in 13 (54%) patients. Intrahepatic cysts were seen in 12 patients and were mainly peripheral in location with sizes ranging from less than 10 mm to 8 cm. Peribiliary cysts were seen in all 13 patients and were usually less than 10 mm in size. These cysts were seen as discrete cysts (eight patients), a string of cysts (10 patients) or as a tubular structure paralleling the portal vessels, mimicking biliary dilatation (11 patients). Twelve patients also showed indeterminate cysts, which defied definite categorization into either type; two common causes of confusion included large (more than 10 mm) discrete cysts in the hilar region and the presence of a vessel adjacent to peripheral cysts [16].

Although the diagnosis of polycystic disease is easily made with both CT and MRI, MRI is more sensitive for the detection of complicated cysts.

Complications

Liver cysts grow slowly. In some patients whose life has been prolonged by haemodialysis or renal transplantation, the size of liver cysts may become enormous.

The most common, clinically relevant complications arising from hepatic cysts are intracystic haemorrhage, infection or posttraumatic rupture (Table 2). Cystadenocarcinoma, biliary obstruction, Budd–Chiari syndrome, portal hypertension or hepatic failure are rarely reported.

Patients with haemorrhagic hepatic cysts usually present with a recent history of abdominal pain, but intracystic haemorrhage may also be detected fortuitously at imaging. CT is often unremarkable, whereas ultrasonography reveals heterogeneous content appearing as intracystic echogenic deposits or thin and mobile septations. In contrast to the septations observed in other tumours such as cystadenocarcinomas, these septations are not seen on CT images. MRI is key, demonstrating a hyperintensity on T1-weighted sequences (Fig. 4a) and a normal appearance on T2-weighted sequences (Fig. 4b) [17]. Theoretically, hyperintensity in cystic lesions on T1-weighted

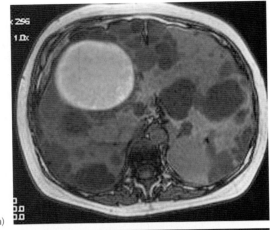

(a)

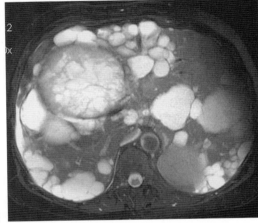

(b)

Fig. 4 MRI of an intracystic haemorrhage in an ADPKD patient. The complicated cyst has a signal intensity different from that of the non-complicated cysts: hyperintense on T1- (a) and hyperintense and heterogeneous on T2-weighted images (b).

images could also suggest mucin, high protein content or fat, but the diagnosis of haemorrhagic hepatic cyst is easy because of the clinical context.

Bacterial infection of a cyst [18,19] may be facilitated by immunosuppressive drugs administered to renal transplant recipients [20]. The clinical manifestations of patients with hepatic cyst infection are an acute (58%) or subacute (42%) febrile illness, typically associated with tenderness in the right upper quadrant, leucocytosis, a very high erythrocyte sedimentation rate, but minor abnormalities in liver function tests [19]. Bacteraemia is often present. Complex cysts are observed whatever the imaging modality: ultrasonography, CT and MRI. On CT scanning, the finding of fluid levels within cysts, cyst wall thickening, intracystic gas bubbles, cyst wall calcification and heterogeneous or increased density have all been correlated with infection of a hepatic cyst. Ultrasound imaging may show changes such as indistinct cyst margins or cystic wall changes as well as echogenic fluid. [111]In leukocyte scans are positive. An unfavourable outcome may be observed in patients

Table 2 Clinical complications of hepatic cysts in ADPKD.

Complications	Diagnostic tests
Cyst infection	Ultrasound
	Puncture
Cyst haemorrhage	Ultrasound
	MRI
Cyst rupture	Ultrasound
	CT
Portal hypertension	CT
	Endoscopy
Hepatic venous outflow obstruction	Ultrasound
	MRI
	Hepatic venous pressure
Biliary obstruction	MR cholangiography

treated only with antibiotics, therefore the treatment of choice is a combination of percutaneous drainage and antimicrobial therapy.

Cystic rupture is rare, and patients usually present with an acute history of abdominal pain. Imaging findings show an irregular subcapsular cyst with liver capsule disruption and the presence of ascites, which is very infrequent in ADPKD patients.

Obstructive jaundice due to polycystic liver disease is rare [21,22]. Immense size and porta hepatis proximity are major risk factors for developing jaundice. Abdominal pain of recent onset and rising alkaline phosphatase levels are warning signs that this complication is developing. In these situations, treatment prior to developing jaundice is recommended, and relief of jaundice may be obtained by percutaneous cyst aspiration, sclerosis or resection [23,24].

Jaundice due to malignant obstruction from cholangiocarcinoma has been described rarely with a total of 10 cases in the English literature, although whether the abnormal biliary epithelium of the hepatic cysts predisposes to the development of cholangiocarcinoma is unknown [25]. A potential association between ADPKD and ampulla of Vater adenomas may exist given the report of two sisters diagnosed with symptomatic biliary obstruction due to ampullary adenomas. A more recent case of ampullary adenoma in the setting of ADPKD has also been reported [26]. These few cases notwithstanding, it would seem that an ampullary adenoma in the setting of ADPKD is more likely to be the case of a rare finding superimposed on a common genetic disorder such as ADPKD.

Hepatic venous outflow obstruction is a rare but major complication of polycystic liver disease. All patients present with severe exudative ascites [27]. Some possible predisposing factors may be identified such as recent abdominal surgery. All patients have extrinsic compression of the hepatic veins and the inferior vena cava by hepatic cysts (Fig. 3b and e), and some have proven thrombosis of the inferior vena cava and/or hepatic veins [28]. Ultrasound and MRI are helpful in determining the level of obstruction in the inferior vena cava and the patency of the hepatic and portal veins. The outcome is worse in patients with thrombosis but, in patients without thrombosis, recovery is observed after alcohol sclerosis of a large dominant cyst or after hepatic resection and cyst fenestration. Hepatic venous outflow obstruction has probably been under-recognized as a cause of portal hypertension, ascites and liver dysfunction in polycystic liver disease.

The other complications, which are less common, include portal hypertension by compression of the portal branches causing gastrointestinal bleeding (Fig. 3c) [29] or refractory ascites [30], right atrium compression causing hypotension and leg oedema [31], denutrition by compression of the stomach and cholangiocellular carcinoma [15].

Associated conditions may include cerebral aneurysm and mitral valve prolapse. Cerebral aneurysms may be linked to the *PKD1* mutation [4]. Most of these aneurysms are small and do not appear to be at increased risk of growth or rupture [32].

Differential diagnosis

Liver cysts associated with ADPKD must be distinguished from multiple simple cysts of the liver. First, as ADPKD is transmitted as an autosomal dominant trait, it is usual for one parent or sibling to have been recognized as suffering from the disease. In the case of simple cysts of the liver, which are non-inherited malformations, parents and siblings are not affected by the disease. However, the presentation of ADPKD varies, and affected individuals may be asymptomatic and therefore unrecognized. Secondly, multiple renal cysts are constantly associated with liver cysts in ADPKD (Fig. 3d), whereas renal cysts are absent in multiple simple cysts of the liver. However, as mentioned above, one or a few simple renal cysts may be fortuitously associated with simple cysts of the liver. Patients with this fortuitous association must not be regarded as affected with ADPKD.

Treatment

Medical treatment

There are no effective medical therapies for polycystic liver disease. Although secretin triggers secretion by normal intrahepatic bile duct cells, somatostatin analogues have failed to reduce hepatic cyst growth or size [33]. There is no strong evidence that estrogen replacement therapy should be avoided, when indicated.

Cyst aspiration and sclerosis

Symptomatic patients with one or a few dominant cysts may be considered for cyst aspiration and sclerosis. Most patients with polycystic disease either have too many cysts or their cysts are of insufficient size to warrant this approach. Cyst sclerotherapy requires ultrasonographic or CT-guided percutaneous puncture of the targeted cyst and placement of an intracystic drainage catheter. For large cysts (> 100 mL or a diameter of ≥ 6 cm), the catheter may be left in place for 24 h, and a second treatment may be performed the following day. Success in obliterating individual cysts in polycystic patients is approximately 70–90% [34].

Surgical treatments

Symptoms in polycystic liver disease are mainly related to the volume of the liver rather than to a specific cyst, and the aim of treatment is to decompress the whole liver or remove as many cysts as possible. These objectives can be achieved in highly symptomatic patients by open fenestration, liver resection or liver transplantation. The aim of fenestration is to unroof as many cysts as possible, starting from the superficial cyst followed by stepwise opening of the deeper cysts. The laparoscopic approach is debated. For some authors, it is an alternative surgical technique [35]. Advantages of laparoscopic surgery include less morbidity, reduced hospital stay and the potential for outpatient surgical management. However, symptoms recur in approximately half of those cases. For others, the laparoscopic approach is contraindicated [36,37]. The vascular structures that are compressed by the cysts may be injured inadvertently.

Partial liver resection in combination with fenestration of the remnant liver has been proposed [38–40] in order to increase the regeneration of the non-cystic liver. Hepatic resection with cyst fenestration takes advantage of both operative techniques by removing diffusely cystic liver that cannot be adequately fenestrated and fenestrating cysts in relatively spared liver to preserve liver function.

Liver transplantation should be considered in patients in whom the above procedures have been unsuccessful, but it has only been performed in a very few patients [41–45]. Orthotopic liver transplantation for ADPKD is clearly indicated for patients with progressive ADPKD after resection/fenestration, in patients with concurrent liver dysfunction and renal failure and in those patients with diffuse ADPKD without segmental sparing. Operative mortality for orthotopic liver transplantation for ADPKD has approached 12%. Risk is increased by prior intervention, especially with open abdominal procedures. Orthotopic liver transplantation is particularly challenging in ADPKD. The massive size of the liver makes the access to the suprahepatic inferior vena cava extremely difficult.

All these treatments lack consensus on their respective indications. Available data indicate that: (i) open fenestration of the maximum number of cysts is associated with significant morbidity but provides long-term relief of symptoms in patients who do not have diffuse replacement of their liver by cysts [40,46,47]; (ii) liver resection, which often proves possible as a result of an asymmetry in cyst distribution, is a demanding procedure, associated with high morbidity rates, but achieves better results than fenestration alone; long-term sustained reduction in symptoms is observed in more than 90% of patients [39]; (iii) liver transplantation cures patients [45] but has its inherent mortality with 5-year survival of 69% (US scientific registry of transplant recipients). Despite its risk, transplantation is the only option in patients with kidney failure resulting from ADPKD or denutrition resulting from massive hepatomegaly. If liver transplantation is indicated *per se*, simultaneous renal transplantation should be considered if renal function is impaired. The rationale for a combined liver–kidney transplant using the grafts from the same donor are: (i) immunosuppression is difficult to manage in patients with renal failure; (ii) renal function may deteriorate further after liver transplantation because of the nephrotoxicity of immunosuppressive agents and/or progression of the kidney disease; (iii) rejection episodes seem to be fewer in patients receiving both organs from the same donor than from two donors.

Asymptomatic or paucisymptomatic patients should not be operated on. If kidney transplantation is indicated *per se*, simultaneous liver transplantation should be performed if liver cysts determine incapacitating manifestations. As immunosuppression following kidney transplantation is similar to that after liver transplantation, the additional risk of simultaneous liver transplantation is only related to surgical complications and not to immunosuppression.

References

1 Melnick PJ (1975) Polycystic liver. Analysis of seventy cases. *Arch Pathol Lab Med* 59, 162–172.

2 Everson GT, Scherzinger A, Berger-Leff N *et al.* (1988) Polycystic liver disease: quantitation of parenchymal and cyst volumes from computed tomography images and clinical correlates of hepatic cysts. *Hepatology* 8, 1627–1634.

3 Ward CJ, Turley H, Ong AC *et al.* (1996) Polycystin, the polycystic kidney disease 1 protein, is expressed by epithelial cells in fetal, adult, and polycystic kidney. *Proc Natl Acad Sci USA* 93, 1524–1528.

4 Rossetti S, Chauveau D, Kubly V *et al.* (2003) Association of mutation position in polycystic kidney disease 1 (PKD1) gene and development of a vascular phenotype. *Lancet* 361, 2196–2201.

5 Watnick TJ, Phakdeekitcharoen B, Johnson A *et al.* (1999) Mutation detection of PKD1 identifies a novel mutation common to three families with aneurysms and/or very-early-onset disease. *Am J Hum Genet* 65, 1561–1571.

6 Mochizuki T, Wu G, Hayashi T *et al.* (1996) PKD2, a gene for polycystic kidney disease that encodes an integral membrane protein. *Science* 272, 1339–1342.

7 deAlmeida S, deAlmeida E, Peters D *et al.* (1995) ADPKD: evidence for the existence of a third locus in a Portuguese family. *Hum Genet* 96, 83–88.

8 Ariza M, Alvarez V, Marin R *et al.* (1997) 96A family with a milder form of ADPKD is not linked to PKD1(16p) or PKD2(4q) genes. *J Med Genet* 34, 587–589.

9 Gabow PA, Johnson AM, Kaehny WD *et al.* (1990) Risk factors for the development of hepatic cysts in autosomal dominant polycystic kidney disease. *Hepatology* 11, 1033–1037.

10 Shrestha R, McKinley C, Russ P *et al.* (1997) Postmenopausal estrogen therapy selectively stimulates hepatic enlargement in women with autosomal dominant polycystic kidney disease. *Hepatology* 26, 1282–1286.

11 Nichols MT, Gidey E, Matzakos T *et al.* (2004) Secretion of cytokines and growth factors into autosomal dominant polycystic kidney disease liver cyst fluid. *Hepatology* 40, 836–846.

12 Wan SKH, Cochlin DL (1990) Sonographic and computed tomographic features of polycystic disease of the liver. *Gastrointest Radiol* 15, 310–312.

13 Kutcher R, Schneider M, Gordon DH (1977) Calcification in polycystic disease. *Radiology* 122, 77–80.

14 Coffin B, Hadengue A, Degos F *et al.* (1990) Calcified hepatic and renal cysts in adult dominant polycystic kidney disease. *Dig Dis Sci* 35, 1172–1175.

15 Levine E, Cook LT, Grantham JJ (1985) Liver cysts in autosomal-dominant polycystic kidney disease: clinical and computed tomographic study. *Am J Roentgenol* 145, 229–233.

16 Gupta S, Seith A, Dhiman RK *et al.* (1999) CT of liver cysts in patients with autosomal dominant polycystic kidney disease. *Acta Radiol* 40, 444–448.

17 Wilcox DM, Weinreb JC, Lesh P (1985) MR imaging of a hemorrhagic hepatic cyst in a patient with polycystic liver disease. *J Comput Assist Tomogr* 9, 183–185.

18 Robson GB, Fenster F (1964) Fatal liver abscess developing in a polycystic liver. *Gastroenterology* 47, 82.

19 Telenti A, Torres VE, Gross JB Jr et al. (1990) Hepatic cyst infection in autosomal dominant polycystic kidney disease. *Mayo Clin Proc* 65, 933–942.

20 Bourgeois M, Kinneart P, Vereerstraeten P et al. (1983) Infection of hepatic cysts following kidney transplantation in polycystic disease. *World J Surg* 7, 629–631.

21 Howard RJ, Hanson RF, Delaney JP (1976) Jaundice associated with polycystic liver disease. Relief by surgical decompression of the cysts. *Arch Surg* 111, 816–817.

22 Ergün H, Wolf BH, Hissung SL (1980) Obstructive jaundice caused by polycystic liver disease. *Radiology* 136, 435–436.

23 Garber S, Mathieson J, Cooperberg PL (1993) Percutaneous sclerosis of hepatic cysts to treat obstructive jaundice in a patient with polycystic liver disease. *Am J Roentgenol* 161, 77–78.

24 Lerner ME, Roshkow JE, Smithline A et al. (1992) Polycystic liver disease with obstructive jaundice: treatment with ultrasound-guided cyst aspiration. *Gastrointest Radiol* 17, 46–48.

25 Arnold HL, Harrison SA (2005) New advances in evaluation and management of patients with polycystic liver disease. *Am J Gastroenterol* 100, 1–14.

26 Serafini FM, Carey LC (1999) Adenoma of the ampulla of Vater: a genetic condition? *HPB Surg* 11, 191–193.

27 Uddin W, Ramage JK, Portmann B et al. (1995) Hepatic venous outflow obstruction in patients with polycystic liver disease: pathogenesis and treatment. *Gut* 36, 142–145.

28 Torres VE, Rastogi S, King BF et al. (1994) Hepatic venous outflow obstruction in autosomal dominant polycystic kidney disease. *J Am Soc Nephrol* 5, 1186–1192.

29 Ratcliffe PJ, Reeders S, Theaker JM (1984) Bleeding oesophageal varices and hepatic dysfunction in adult polycystic kidney disease. *Br Med J* 288, 1330–1331.

30 McGarrity TJ, Koch KL, Rasbach DA (1986) Refractory ascites associated with polycystic liver disease. Treatment with peritoneovenous shunt. *Dig Dis Sci* 31, 217–220.

31 Lasic LB, DeVita MV, Spiegel PJ et al. (2004) Refractory hypotension and edema caused by right atrial compression in a woman with polycystic kidney disease. *Am J Kidney Dis* 43, 13–17.

32 Gibbs GF, Huston J 3rd, Qian Q et al. (2004) Follow-up of intracranial aneurysms in autosomal-dominant polycystic kidney disease. *Kidney Int* 65, 1621–1627.

33 Chauveau D, Martinez F, Grunfeld JP (1993) Evaluation of octreotide in massive polycystic liver disease. 12th International Congress of Nephrology Conference Program 487A.

34 Van Sonnenberg E, Wroblicka JT, D'Agostino HB et al. (1994) Symptomatic hepatic cysts: percutaneous drainage and sclerosis. *Radiology* 190, 387–392.

35 Everson GT, Taylor MRG, Doctor RG (2004) Polycystic disease of the liver. *Hepatology* 40, 774–782.

36 Morino M, De Guili M, Festa V et al. (1994) Laparoscopic management of symptomatic nonparasitic cysts of the liver. Indications and results. *Ann Surg* 219, 157–164.

37 Kabbej M, Sauvanet A, Chauveau D et al. (1996) Laparoscopic fenestration in polycystic liver disease. *Br J Surg* 83, 1697–1701.

38 Soravia C, Mentha G, Giostra E et al. (1995) Surgery for adult polycystic liver disease. *Surgery* 117, 272–275.

39 Que F, Nagorney DM, Gross JB et al. (1995) Liver resection and cyst fenestration in the treatment of severe polycystic liver disease. *Gastroenterology* 108, 487–494.

40 Vons C, Chauveau D, Martinod E et al. (1998) Résection hépatique chez les malades atteints de polykystose hépatique. *Gastroentérol Clin Biol* 22, 50–54.

41 Starzl TE, Reyes J, Tzakis A et al. (1990) Liver transplantation for polycystic liver disease. *Arch Surg* 125, 575–577.

42 Washburn WK, Johnson LB, Lewis WD et al. (1996) Liver transplantation for adult polycystic liver disease. *Liver Transpl Surg* 2, 17–22.

43 Swenson K, Seu P, Kinkhabwala M et al. (1998) Liver transplantation for adult polycystic liver disease. *Hepatology* 28, 412–415.

44 Jeyarajah DR, Gonwa TA, Testa G et al. (1998) Liver and kidney transplantation for polycystic liver disease. *Transplantation* 66, 529–544.

45 Pirenne J, Aerts R, Yoong K et al. (2001) Liver transplantation for polycystic liver disease. *Liver Transplant* 7, 238–245.

46 Farges O, Bismuth H (1995) Fenestration in the management of polycystic liver disease. *World J Surg* 19, 25–30.

47 Gigot JF, Jadoul P, Que F et al. (1997) Adult polycystic liver disease: is fenestration the most adequate operation for long-term management? *Ann Surg* 225, 286–294.

48 Milutinovic J, Fialkow PJ, Rudd TG et al. (1980) Liver cysts in patients with autosomal dominant polycystic kidney disease. *Am J Med* 68, 741–744.

49 Thomsen HS, Thaysen JH (1988) Frequency of hepatic cysts in adult polycystic kidney disease. *Acta Med Scand* 224, 381–384.

8.1.4. Polycystic liver disease

Valérie Vilgrain

Polycystic liver disease (PCLD) may also be observed in the absence of renal cystic disease and is a rare autosomal dominant human disorder that has been described in less than 50 families of Finnish, Dutch, American, Belgian and Spanish Belgian ancestry. The pathology is characterized by the presence of multiple scattered cysts of biliary origin in the liver parenchyma. The occurrence of PCLD independently from polycystic kidney disease has been known for a long time. Autopsy or surgical series of PCLD have shown that polycystic kidney disease was observed in 50–60% of cases) [1]. However, it has been difficult to separate PCLD and autosomal dominant polycystic kidney disease (ADPKD) because cystic liver is also found in about 30% of ADPKD patients, and the liver pathology is indistinguishable between PCLD and ADPKD. A large autopsy study from Finland has identified 22 cases with either PCLD or polycystic kidney disease, but macrocystic cysts in both organs were seen in only one case, supporting the idea that PCLD and polycystic kidney disease are separate entities [2]. There are still no exact epidemiological data regarding the incidence of PCLD in any population. More recently, studies have demonstrated that isolated familial PCLD was unlinked to the *PKD1* and *PKD2* loci. Manifestations and complications (and management) are the same whether PCLD is isolated or associated with ADPKD [3].

Pathology and pathogenesis

The gross appearance of the resected liver is indistinguishable from that of those resected in patients with severe polycystic disease associated with ADPKD. All the specimens contain variable numbers of von Meyenburg complexes characterized by clusters of dilated bile ducts lined by a layer of cuboidal cells surrounded by a fibrous stroma. The epithelium of the complexes and most of the cysts is cytokeratin-7 positive, consistent with its origin from intrahepatic bile ducts. Small cysts often seem to arise from von Meyenburg complexes. Large cysts are lined by flattened epithelium. Peribiliary glands may be seen as well. The surrounding hepatic parenchyma is normal in most cases, but focal fibrosis may be seen near larger cysts [3]. Because both types of cysts (von Meyenburg complexes and peribiliary glands) are seen in ADPKD and PCLD, it suggests that both diseases have the same pathogenesis.

Genetics and molecular biology

The gene mutated in PCLD, known as protein kinase C (PKC) substrate 80K-H (*PRKCSH*), has been identified recently [4,5]. The PCLD gene locus has been mapped to chromosome 19p13.2–13.1. The *PRKCSH* gene encodes hepatocystin, a protein that moderates glycosylation and fibroblast growth factor receptor signalling [4]. Mutations that affect messenger RNA splicing or truncate hepatocystin have been reported in PCLD families. However, the distribution of mutations within the gene as well as genotype–phenotype relationships remain speculative [6]. Most PCLD families are linked to chromosome 19p13.2–13.1, but there exists a second PCLD locus yet to be found [7]. Mutations in *SEC63*, another gene encoding products involved in intracellular protein transport, have also been found in association with PCLD [8].

Diagnosis

Surgical reviews have attempted to distinguish multicystic liver (> five cysts) from simple cystic liver disease (< five cysts) [9], whereas other authors have described PCLD as having six or more cysts per liver [10] or as cystic involvement of more than 50% of the hepatic parenchyma [11,12]. The age of the individual is also crucial.

This is why some authors have proposed clinical criteria which allow the diagnosis of PCLD: subjects with more than 20 liver cysts who do not fulfil the criteria for ADPKD; at-risk individuals aged 40 years or younger with any liver cysts; and at-risk individuals older than 40 years with four or more liver cysts [3].

The sensitivity and specificity of these criteria are 70% and 100%, respectively, in individuals younger than 40 years. Therefore, the presence of any cysts in at-risk individuals aged 40 years or younger is diagnostic of the disease; however, negative findings on ultrasonography are insufficient to exclude the diagnosis in this age group. The sensitivity and specificity of these criteria are 78.3% and 100%, respectively, in individuals older than 40 years. Therefore, other criteria have been proposed in those older than 40 years as follows: at-risk individuals between the ages of 40 and 65 years with more than one liver cyst; and at-risk individuals older than 65 years with more than three liver cysts [3].

Natural history and risk factors for development and progression

Isolated polycystic liver disease seems to be less penetrant in the liver than ADPKD, and the development of liver cysts in PCLD may not occur until late in life. As in ADPKD, PCLD is more severe in women than in men, and there is a positive correlation between the severity of the disease and the number of pregnancies.

Clinical features and complications

PCLD is most often asymptomatic and is frequently diagnosed incidentally during the workup of other clinical problems or complaints. This is the case even in the families of patients with highly symptomatic disease, in which relatives are more likely to be aware of the symptoms and to undergo diagnostic testing [3]. When symptoms develop in PCLD, the spectrum is similar to that observed in ADPKD patients.

Patients with PCLD have minimal elevations in serum alkaline phosphatase and total bilirubin levels and lower serum levels of total cholesterol and triglycerides compared with their unaffected relatives [3]. This could suggest that the hepatic lipid metabolism may be altered in patients with PCLD [13].

Whether patients with PCLD are at increased risk of intracranial aneurysms and valvular heart disease is not known. Qian *et al.* [3] noted a trend towards increased risk of intracranial aneurysms, with almost 6% of patients with linkage analysis-confirmed PCLD being found to have either intracranial aneurysm or dissection. The paucity of data prevents more definitive recommendations from being made on screening the PCLD patient for aneurysmal disease.

The higher prevalence of mitral valve abnormalities in patients with PCLD compared with their unaffected relatives indicates that PCLD, like ADPKD, is a systemic disorder [3].

Treatment

Most patients with PCLD require no treatment, but percutaneous cyst aspiration and sclerosis, cyst fenestration, partial hepatectomy and liver transplantation, depending on the extent, distribution and anatomy of the cysts, may be indicated in highly symptomatic patients.

References

1 Melnick PJ (1954) Polycystic liver. Analysis of seventy cases. *Arch Pathol Lab Med* 59, 162–172.

2 Karhunen PJ, Tenhu M (1986) Adult polycystic liver and kidney diseases are separate entities. *Clin Genet* 30, 29–37.

3 Qian Q, Li A, King BF *et al.* (2003) Clinical profile of autosomal dominant polycystic liver disease. *Hepatology* 37, 164–171.

4 Drenth JP, Te Morsche RH, Smink R *et al.* (2003) Germline mutations in PRKCSH are associated with autosomal dominant polycystic liver disease. *Nature Genet* 33, 345–347.

5 Drenth JP, Martina JA, Te Morsche RH *et al.* (2004) Molecular characterization of hepatocystin, the protein that is defective in autosomal dominant polycystic liver disease. *Gastroenterology* 126, 1819–1827.

6 Everson GT, Taylor MRG, Doctor RG (2004) Polycystic disease of the liver. *Hepatology* 40, 774–782.

7 Tahvanianen P, Tahvanianen E, Reijonen H *et al.* (2003) Polycystic liver disease is genetically heterogeneous: clinical and linkage studies in eight Finnish families. *J Hepatol* 38, 39–43.

8 Davila S, Furu L, Gharavi AG *et al.* (2004) Mutations in SEC63 cause autosomal dominant polycystic liver disease. *Nature Genet* 36, 575–577.

9 Gigot JF, Metairie S, Etienne J *et al.* (2001) The surgical management of congenital liver cysts. *Surg Endosc* 15, 357–363.

10 Katkhouda N, Hurwitz M, Gugenheim J *et al.* (1999) Laparoscopic management of benign solid and cystic lesions of the liver. *Ann Surg* 229, 460–466.

11 Hansman MF, Ryan JA Jr, Holmes JH *et al.* (2001) Management and long-term follow-up of hepatic cysts. *Am J Surg* 181, 404–410.

12 Martin IJ, McKinley AJ, Currie EJ *et al.* (1998) Tailoring the management of nonparasitic liver cysts. *Ann Surg* 228, 167–172.

13 Luoma PV, Sotaniemi EA, Ehnholm C (1980) Low high-density lipoprotein and reduced antipyrine metabolism in members of a family with polycystic liver disease. *Scand J Gastroenterol* 15, 869–873.

8.1.5. Biliary hamartomas

Valérie Vilgrain

Biliary hamartomas, also called von Meyenburg complexes, are considered to be part of the spectrum of ductal plate abnormalities [1]. Multiple bile duct hamartomas are usually detected by pathologists as incidental findings, and have recently been better described in the radiological literature. They were first reported by Moschowitz in 1906 as aberrant intrahepatic bile ducts. Later, they were defined as hamartomatous lesions of bile ducts by Meyenburg in 1918. They may occur in an otherwise normal liver or in association with Caroli's disease, congenital hepatic fibrosis and autosomal dominant polycystic kidney or liver disease. Recognition of this entity is crucial because they often mimic liver metastases [2,3].

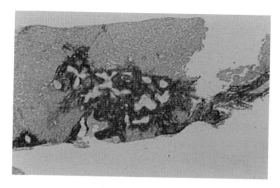

Fig. 1 Microscopic view of a biliary hamartoma showing dilated bile ducts embedded in a fibrous, sometimes hyalinized, stroma.

Pathology and pathogenesis

Biliary hamartomas are small (< 0.5 cm in diameter), greyish-white or green and are usually scattered in both lobes. Microscopically, the lesions are discrete, round to irregular in shape and typically paraportal in location. They comprise a variable number of dilated bile ducts embedded in a fibrous, sometimes hyalinized, stroma (Fig. 1). They are lined by low columnar or cuboidal epithelium and contain pink amorphous material that may be bile-stained or actual bile. On serial section examination, the bile duct lumina within a complex have been shown to be interconnecting [1]. Some of the duct structures may show polypoid projections in the lumen; others show, on section, a central island of connective tissue covered with the same type of epithelium as that lining the wall of the dilated duct. Rarely, in some biliary hamartomas, the bile duct profiles are involutive and seem to disappear in a hyalinized, scarring stroma. Classically, it is considered that the dilated ducts of the biliary hamartomas do not communicate with the rest of the biliary tree, but the presence of bile casts in the lumen of some cavities strongly supports the idea of a communication. Furthermore, a detailed serial reconstruction of a biliary hamartoma has demonstrated the communicating nature of these bile duct abnormalities [4].

The morphology of the biliary hamartoma suggests that the lesion represents a partially fibrosing and, on occasion, slowly involutive remnant of ductal plate malformation of the smaller, more peripheral, interlobular bile ducts. Owing to the embryology of intrahepatic bile ducts, which develop from the hilum of the liver to distal parts over time, it seems that the factor arresting or perturbing the remodelling of the ductal plates occurs in the later phases of embryological development of intrahepatic bile ducts [1]. Also, biliary hamartomas are often associated with other ductal plate abnormalities such as Caroli's disease, congenital hepatic fibrosis and polycystic diseases. Redston and Wanless examined the liver slides from 2843 autopsies in order to assess the prevalence of biliary hamartomas in both the general population and patients with adult polycystic kidney disease [5]. Biliary hamartomas were found in 5.6% of adults and in

0.9% of children. Among adults with adult polycystic kidney disease, biliary hamartomas were found in 97% and hepatic cysts in 88%. Because adult polycystic kidney disease could account for only 11% of the patients with biliary hamartomas, these authors suggest that biliary hamartomas, in the absence of adult polycystic kidney disease, are a manifestation of a different disease, which could be genetic or secondary to inflammation or ischaemia [5]. Then, biliary hamartomas seem to be at the origin of the development of adult polycystic kidney and liver disease by their progressive dilatation and fluid filling of the original clusters of bile duct structures [6].

The prevalence of biliary hamartomas varies according to the method of reference. In a study including 2000 liver needle biopsies, Thommesen examined the liver for the occurrence of biliary hamartomas and found 12 positive biopsies corresponding to 0.6% of the liver biopsies [7]. The prevalence is higher in autopsy studies, and the same author has reported biliary hamartomas in 2.8% of cases.

Sometimes, large numbers of duct profiles are in a biliary hamartoma, which may appear as a conglomerate of approximated ductal plate remnants, associated with an abnormal arborization pattern of the peripheral branches of the portal vein similar to that observed in early severe extrahepatic bile duct atresia and congenital hepatic fibrosis [6]. In our experience, biliary hamartomas were found at imaging in three of 18 adult patients with congenital hepatic fibrosis [8]. The paraportal location of some biliary hamartomas, fused to normal-appearing portal tracts, suggests that one of the branches may give rise to a normal portal tract with normal duct development, whereas the rest evolve into hypoplastic vein branches with fusion of adjacent portal tracts and clustering of their ductal plates.

Natural history and risk factors for development and progression

In patients with adult autosomal dominant polycystic kidney and liver disease, biliary hamartomas and peribiliary cysts are thought to be at the origin of the development of liver cysts. In patients with no history of fibrocystic disease, the natural history of biliary hamartomas is not known. Some cases of malignant transformation have been reported. The increased risk of malignancy has been attributed to the bile stasis and prolonged exposure of the parenchyma to potential carcinogens present in the bile [9]. Fewer than 15 cases have been reported in the literature [9,10–13]. The malignant transformation may be discovered fortuitously or revealed by biochemical or clinical abnormalities. Patients ranged in age from 35 to 80 years with a sex ratio of 1:1 [14]. Few patients had cirrhosis or genetic haemochromatosis [9,14,15]. Macroscopically, the liver contains biliary hamartomas and cholangiocarcinoma. Microscopically, there is evidence that the carcinoma evolves from biliary hamartoma through the intermediate stage of hyperplasia or adenomatous transformation and in situ carcinoma [9]. The adenomatous transformation may be seen in two forms: the

formation of distinct nodules of proliferating biliary hamartoma-like glandular structures; or marked tumour-like concentric or eccentric proliferation of ductular structures surrounding hepatic nodules [9].

In addition, some specimens show poorly differentiated areas that could be interpreted as hepatocellular carcinoma. Immunohistochemical staining shows positivity for epithelial membrane antigen, carcinoembryonic antigen and keratins in tumour cells consistent with cholangiocarcinoma [9].

Clinical features

Patients with biliary hamartomas are generally asymptomatic, and diagnosis of the liver lesions is usually made fortuitously or in the management of patients with other ductal plate malformations. However, a case report has described a patient who suffered from fever, jaundice and right upper quadrant pain due to bile duct hamartomas with microabscess formation associated with biliary stones and biliary tract infection [16]. The blood liver tests are usually normal, but association with other ductal plate malformations may explain blood liver test abnormalities in some patients.

Imaging findings

Imaging manifestations of biliary hamartomas are various. The number of lesions varies from one or two circumscribed lesions to multiple lesions and innumerable lesions with a size ranging from 2 to 10 mm in diameter [3]. Although there have been numerous case reports, the number of studies evaluating the imaging features is low [3,17–20].

Ultrasound (US) findings have been described as hypoechoic, hyperechoic or mixed heterogenic echoic structures [19,21]. These variations might reflect the histological features of biliary hamartomas, including dilated bile ducts and fibrocollagenous stroma. Luo et al. [18] described the sign of multiple comet-tail echoes, and speculated that it might be a specific US finding. Zheng et al. [19] have found multiple small comet-tail echoes in all but one case, which manifested as posterior echo enhancement of the lesions. This artefact might be due to the cystic feature of dilated bile duct and therefore resulted in good transmission of the sound beam. This suggests that the presence of multiple small comet-tail echoes is a unique US feature of biliary hamartomas and may have a high diagnostic value [19]. Anechoic lesions suggesting typical cysts up to 20 mm in diameter are often observed [18]. In patients with microbiliary hamartomas, US may be normal [18].

On plain computerized tomography (CT) images, almost all biliary hamartomas that have been reported were demonstrated to be multiple small hypodense lesions, usually measuring between 0.5 and 1 cm in diameter (Fig. 2a), whereas on enhanced CT images, although homogeneous enhancement of the lesions has been noted, no enhancement of the lesions is observed in most of the reported cases after intravenous

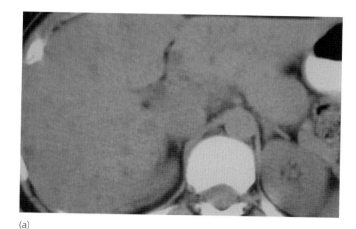

(a)

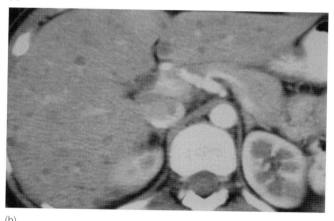

(b)

Fig. 2 Unenhanced (a) and enhanced (b) CT of biliary hamartomas. The lesions are much more conspicuous after administration of contrast medium.

administration of contrast medium [2,3,18–21] (Fig. 2b). The lesions usually increase in number on enhanced CT [18], meaning that, on unenhanced CT, approximately half the lesions are of isodensity or of far lesser conspicuity [18]. On enhanced CT, some lesions are noted to be located adjacent to the medium-sized portal veins (portal tracts, over fourth-order branches), but are to be found less frequently along the hepatic veins of similar size.

On magnetic resonance imaging (MRI), biliary hamartomas are hypointense on T1-weighted images and strongly hyperintense on T2-weighted images when compared with surrounding liver parenchyma [17–19,22,23] (Figs 3a and 4a and b). Usually, on account of the high lesion signal intensity, many more nodules are depicted on T2-weighted images than on T1-weighted images. On heavily T2-weighted images, the signal increases further, nearly reaching the signal of fluid [17]. Magnetic resonance cholangiopancreatography (MRCP) is considered to be highly sensitive in depicting intra- and extra-hepatic bile duct anomalies and cystic lesions of the liver, and often displays the biliary hamartomas more clearly than CT and MRI in relation to both the lesion number and shape [19] (Fig. 3b). This may result in part from the relatively large slice thickness in CT and MRI, resulting in the overlooking of lesions smaller than the slice thickness. MRCP also shows that the lesions do not communicate with intrahepatic bile ducts and are not associated with bile duct abnormalities except in Caroli's disease patients (Fig. 4c). Absence of communication between biliary hamartomas and intrahepatic bile ducts may be confirmed after intravenous injection of hepatospecific contrast agents such as Mn-DPDP. The presence and type of biliary hamartoma enhancement is still debated in the literature. While some authors did not find any enhancement following gadolinium administration [17] (Fig. 3c), others have described a homogeneous enhancement or a rim enhancement on early and

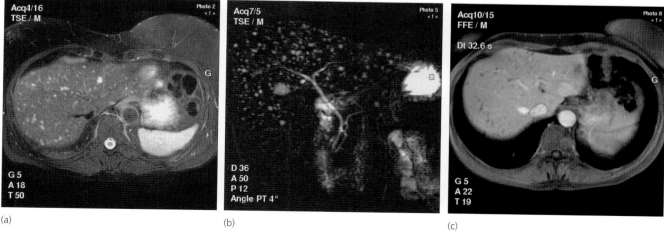

(a) (b) (c)

Fig. 3 MRI of biliary hamartomas. The lesions are strongly hyperintense on T2-weighted imaging (a) and even more intense on heavily T2-weighted sequences such as MRCP images (b). On T1-weighted images (c), after administration of chelates of gadolinium, the enhancement varies and is absent in this example.

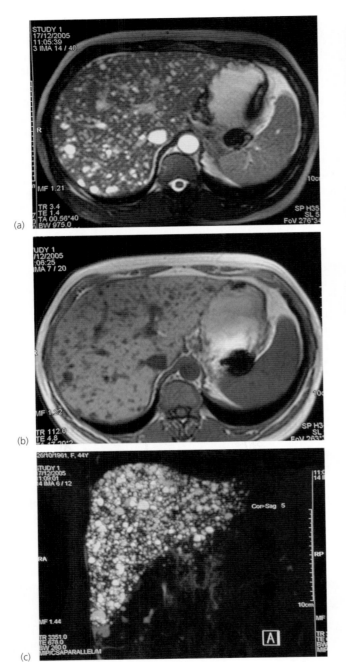

Fig. 4 MRI of multiple biliary hamartomas. The lesions are hypointense on T1- (a) and hyperintense on T2-weighted (b) images. Thick slab MRCP image shows innumerable lesions that do not communicate with the bile ducts (c).

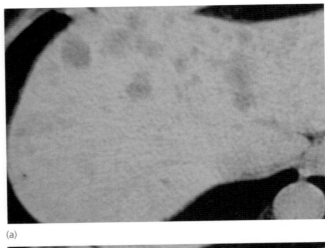

(a)

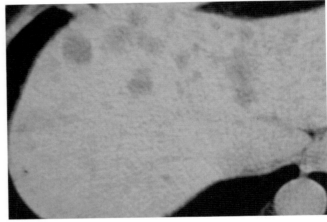

(b)

Fig. 5 Mural nodules in biliary hamartomas. Unenhanced (a) and enhanced (b) CT images demonstrating a mural nodule in the largest hamartoma, which enhances after the administration of contrast medium.

late postcontrast images [20,23]. On histopathology, the rim enhancement correlates with the compressed liver parenchyma surrounding the lesions [20]. Sometimes, biliary hamartomas exhibit mural nodules that have an intermediate signal on T2-weighted images and could be enhanced on portal and delayed-phase imaging [24] (Figs 5a and b). Interestingly, although angiography is not performed any more to characterize these lesions, a previous study has shown that biliary hamartomas appear as multiple areas of abnormal vascularity, which persist in the venous phase, but there is no evidence of tumour vessels leaking or arteriovenous shunting [25]. This difference in lesion enhancement may vary according to the lesion size, the connective tissue and the presence of an abnormal portal branch.

Diagnosis

Some authors claim that the imaging findings of biliary hamartomas are not specific and that liver biopsy is needed for a definitive diagnosis [3,26]. This is true with ultrasound even if multiple small comet-tail echoes could evoke the diagnosis. This is also true with CT because multiple tiny hypodense lesions scattered throughout the liver are not specific. However, with the use of advanced imaging modalities, especially MRI with heavily T2-weighted sequences and MRCP, it is possible to make a correct diagnosis of biliary hamartomas by imaging [17,19,20]. When typical imaging findings appear, such as subcentimetric multiple lesions high signal intensity on T2-weighted images and a mural nodule with normal intrahepatic bile ducts on MRI and MRCP, a diagnosis of biliary hamartomas can be considered. Liver biopsy may have limitations such as sample errors and performance difficulties due to the very small size of the lesions. Furthermore, fine needle aspiration is not diagnostic.

Differential diagnosis

The spectrum of differential diagnosis of biliary hamartomas is fairly wide. However, the most important one is liver metastasis especially in patients with extrahepatic malignant tumours [3,20]. Usually, multiple small metastases are ill-defined on plain CT and show various degrees of enhancement (such as rim enhancement) after intravenous administration of contrast medium. Even if some biliary hamartomas display rim enhancement, the rim enhancement is thin and uniform, may persist on delayed images but does not progress centripetally, and these lesions have a fluid content. However, for patients who are difficult to diagnose, final exclusion of metastatic lesions should still depend on liver biopsy or follow-up imaging studies.

Simple hepatic cysts are variable in number, size and location, and usually round in shape. As biliary hamartomas may coexist with simple hepatic cysts or polycystic liver and kidney diseases, it is sometimes difficult to make a definitive differentiation especially from polycystic liver disease on imaging. Simple hepatic cysts should be considered when the lesions are larger than 10 mm in diameter and round in shape, as most biliary hamartomas are reported to be less than 10 mm in diameter.

Peribiliary cysts are multiple, small, cystic dilatations of the intrahepatic extramural peribiliary glands and should also be included in the differential diagnoses of biliary hamartomas. Both lesions could coexist in patients with adult autosomal dominant polycystic kidney or liver disease. However, they are located exclusively in the hepatic hilum and along the larger portal tract, in contrast to the biliary hamartomas, which have a scattered distribution and predominate near the liver capsule.

Bile duct adenoma may be confused with biliary hamartomas. The bile duct adenoma is usually subcapsular and presents as a solitary, white and fibrous nodule. The histological appearance consists of small ducts that are lined by a single layer of cuboidal cells that may secrete mucin. Bile is not seen in the lumen.

Microabscesses of the liver can be differentiated from biliary hamartomas by means of clinical and radiological data. Imaging features are more heterogeneous.

Intrahepatic bile duct anomalies such as dilated bile ducts and Caroli's disease can be readily distinguished from biliary hamartomas by imaging, especially with MRCP.

Follow-up and treatment

Follow-up of these lesions with imaging modalities shows no remarkable change in the lesions [18]. When the diagnosis of biliary hamartomas is firmly established, because of the benign condition and the very low risk of malignant transformation, no recommendation based on a follow-up can be made. Follow-up study is necessary when the diagnosis is doubtful at imaging or at pathology, especially for the patient with malignant disease elsewhere in the body.

References

1 Desmet VJ (1998) Pathogenesis of ductal plate abnormalities. *Mayo Clin Proc* 73, 80–89.

2 Iha H, Nakashima Y, Fukukura Y *et al.* (1996) Biliary hamartomas simulating multiple hepatic metastasis on imaging findings. *Kurume Med J* 43, 231–235.

3 Lev-Toaff AS, Bach AM, Wechsler RJ *et al.* (1995) The radiologic and pathologic spectrum of biliary hamartomas. *Am J Roentgenol* 165, 309–313.

4 Otha W, Ushio H (1984) Histological reconstruction of a von Meyenburg's complex on the liver surface. *Endoscopy* 16, 71–74.

5 Redston MS, Wanless IR (1996) The hepatic von Meyenburg complex with hepatic and renal cysts. *Mod Pathol* 9, 233–237.

6 Desmet VJ (1992) Congenital diseases of intrahepatic bile ducts: variations on the theme 'ductal plate malformation'. *Hepatology* 16, 1069–1083.

7 Thommesen N (1978) Biliary hamartomas (von Meyenburg complexes) in liver needle biopsies. *Acta Pathol Microbiol Scand (Sect A)* 86, 93–99.

8 Zeitoun D, Brancatelli G, Colombat M *et al.* (2004) Congenital hepatic fibrosis: CT findings in 18 adults. *Radiology* 231, 109–116.

9 Jain D, Sarode VR, Abdul-Karim F *et al.* (2000) Evidence for the neoplastic transformation of Von-Meyenburg complexes. *Am J Surg Pathol* 24, 1131–1139.

10 Burns CD, Kuhns JG, Wieman TJ (1990) Cholangiocarcinoma in association with multiple biliary microhamartomas. *Arch Pathol Lab Med* 114, 1287–1289.

11 Homer LW, White HJ, Read RC (1968) Neoplastic transformation of Von Meyenburg complexes of the liver. *J Pathol Bacteriol* 96, 499–502.

12 Dekker A, Ten Kate FJW, Terpstra OT (1989) Cholangiocarcinoma associated with multiple bile-duct hamartomas of the liver. *Dig Dis Sci* 34, 952–958.

13 Hasebe T, Sakamoto M, Mukai K *et al.* (1995) Cholangiocarcinoma arising in bile duct adenoma with focal area of bile duct hamartoma. *Virchows Archiv* 426, 209–213.

14 Yaziji N, Martin L, Hillon P *et al.* (1997) Cholangiocarcinome développé sur micro-hamartomes biliaires chez un malade atteint d'hémochromatose. *Ann Pathol* 17, 346–349.

15 Wiesniewski B, Tordjman G, Tran Van Nhieu J *et al.* (2002) Cholangiocarcinome sur complexes de von Meyenburg au cours d'une hémochromatose génétique. *Gastroenterol Clin Biol* 26, 922–924.

16 Chen YC, Chien RN, Chen MF *et al.* (2000) Biliary hamartomas associated with biliary stones presenting as multiple microabscesses. *Chang Gung Med J* 23, 560–565.

17 Mortelé B, Mortelé K, Seynaeve P *et al.* (2002) Hepatic bile duct hamartomas (von Meyenburg complexes): MR and MR cholangiography findings. *J Comput Assist Tomogr* 26, 438–443.

18 Luo T-Y, Itai Y, Eguchi N *et al.* (1998) von Meyenburg complexes of the liver: imaging findings. *J Comput Assist Tomogr* 22, 372–378.

19 Zheng RQ, Zhang B, Kudo M *et al.* (2005) Imaging findings of biliary hamartomas. *World J Gastroenterol* 11, 6354–6359.

20 Semelka RC, Hussain SM, Marcos HB *et al.* (1999) Biliary hamartomas: solitary and multiple lesions shown on current MR techniques including gadolinium enhancement. *J Magn Res Imag* 10, 196–201.

21 Eisenberg D, Hurwitz L, Yu AC (1986) CT and sonography of multiple bile duct hamartomas simulating malignant liver disease (case report). *Am J Roentgenol* 147, 279–280.

22 Slone HW, Bennett WF, Bova JG (1993) MR findings of multiple biliary hamartomas. *Am J Roentgenol* 161, 581–583.

23 Maher MM, Dervan P, Keogh B *et al.* (1999) Bile duct hamartomas (von Meyenburg complexes): value of MR imaging in diagnosis. *Abdom Imag* 24, 171–173.

24 Cheung YC, Tan CF, Wan YL *et al.* (1997) MRI of multiple biliary hamartomas. *Br J Radiol* 70, 527–529.

25 McLoughlin MJ, Phillips MJ (1975) Angiographic findings in multiple bile-duct hamartomas of the liver. *Radiology* 116, 41–43.

26 Cooke JC, Cooke DAP (1987) The appearances of multiple biliary hamartomas of the liver (von Meyenburg complexes) on computed tomography. *Clin Radiol* 38, 101–102.

8.1.6. Peribiliary cysts

Valérie Vilgrain

There are glands within and around the walls of the extrahepatic bile ducts in humans, and these glands have been described as tubuloalveolar glands [1]. Under some circumstances, these glands may become cystic. Recognition of this entity is important because this abnormality often mimics intrahepatic bile duct disease.

Pathology

Peribiliary glands

The glandular structures can be classified into two types: one is located within the bile duct wall, the so-called 'intramural glands', and the glands are small in number and random in distribution; the other is found within the periductal connective tissue in the form of a lobule [1]. These glands are termed 'extramural glands' and are located at both sides of the bile ducts and parallel to the hepatic parenchyma. The patterns of distribution of these glands along the biliary tracts are divided into three forms: only at the common bile duct, and left and right hepatic duct; at the common bile duct, left and right hepatic duct and in smaller ducts such as segmental ducts; between the two patterns mentioned above.

There is a greater extension of glandular distribution in the left side than in the right side [1].

Histologically, the lobules of the extramural glands consist of several acini, serous (72%), mucous (17%), or mixed (11%). The epithelium of serous acini is low columnar or cuboidal in

shape with dark cytoplasm, while that of the mucous acini is columnar in shape with a clear cytoplasm. These lobules have their own excretory ducts, through which they communicate with the neighbouring bile duct lumen. The periductal glands are speculated to function as follows: the glandular mucus acts as a lubricant for the bile stream; the glands renew cells when epithelial loss occurs in the bile ducts; the glands concentrate the bile; the glandular mucus protects the mucosal surface from the bile and bacteria.

Heterotopic pancreas is found in 4.1% of the liver and is usually intermingled with intrahepatic peribiliary glands. It is situated exclusively in the large and medium-sized portal tracts [2].

Cystic dilatation

Some glands dilate to a grossly recognizable size, these markedly dilated glands being preferentially found along the edge of portal tracts. The cysts are usually unilocular, expanded, round, thin-walled and multiple, and contain serous fluid [3]. The largest cysts measure 2 cm in diameter.

Histologically, dilated cysts are lined by a cuboidal to columnar epithelia surrounded by thin fibrous tissue. These cysts are admixed with non-dilated or mildly dilated extramural glands. Inflammatory changes are seen in half the cases.

Pathogenesis

Most of the patients with peribiliary cysts have severe liver disease.

• Chronic liver disease and portal hypertension [4]. Nakanuma *et al.* [5] reported eight patients with peribiliary cysts and, among them, seven had oesophageal varices, five portal vein thrombosis, four had cirrhosis and three had hepatocellular carcinoma. Similarly, Wanless *et al.* [4] have described three cases. All three patients had portal vein thrombosis including two with alcoholic cirrhosis.

• Polycystic liver disease and polycystic kidney disease are also known to be associated with cystic dilatation of these glands to varying degrees, and these cystic changes in peribiliary glands may constitute part of the polycystic changes of the liver [3]. Peribiliary cysts seem to occur quite frequently in polycystic liver or kidney disease. In a series reported by Itai *et al.* [6], peribiliary cysts were definitely seen on computerized tomographic (CT) scans of 22/64 patients with autosomal dominant polycystic kidney disease and probably seen in 19 other patients, representing a total of 73% of all polycystic patients with hepatobiliary cysts.

• Other conditions have been described such as systemic infection and metastatic malignancy with or without obstructive jaundice.

• Hepatolithiasis. Terada *et al.* [7] reported a case of cholesterol hepatolithiasis with peribiliary cysts. In this observation, the peribiliary cysts were present around the intrahepatic large bile ducts.

• Peribiliary cysts have been reported recently as a rare post-transplant biliary tract complication, occurring in 2.6% of 493 consecutive liver transplants, including three patients with obstructive jaundice. Two types were identified: large and unilocular cavities probably secondary to sequestered remnants of the cystic duct and cystically dilated peribiliary glands similar to those described [8].

Although peribiliary cysts are usually observed in patients with chronic liver disease, their pathogenesis is still unknown. These chronic liver diseases are various and could provide a bias for detection of peribiliary cysts; however, despite many liver abnormalities or tumours that are discovered fortuitously, this does not seem to happen with peribiliary cysts.

Several mechanisms have been suggested for cystic dilatation of intrahepatic peribiliary glands:

• It might be due to ischaemic changes because some cases are associated with portal hypertension and/or portal thrombo-embolism [5].

• It might be congenital, especially in patients with polycystic liver disease or polycystic kidney disease.

• It might be related to obstruction of ducts of the intrahepatic peribiliary glands due to cholangitis (retention cysts) and/or local peribiliary ischaemia resulting from pressure from stone impaction [8].

Clinical presentation

In most reported patients with peribiliary cysts, patients have severe liver disease, but the cysts are usually asymptomatic. Wanless *et al.* [4] have reported the case of a patient with peribiliary cysts presenting as obstructive jaundice. In this case, the jaundice was secondary to obstruction of the hepatic ducts by periductal cysts. To our knowledge, malignant transformation of these cysts has never been described.

Imaging

Whatever imaging modalities are used, peribiliary cysts are characterized by their peculiar distribution (predominantly perihilar and on both sides of the bile ducts) and small size [9]. They may appear as discrete cysts, as a tubular structure paralleling the portal structures and as a string of cysts that simulate abnormal bile ducts [10].

On ultrasound, the cysts are detected within the echogenic larger portal tract or seem to appear as anechoic areas adjacent to or connecting with the portal vein [9] (Fig. 1a). Sonography appears to be sensitive for detecting the thin septa [10].

CT demonstrates more clearly the distribution of hepatic peribiliary cysts and their relationship with the bile ducts. On unenhanced CT scans, the peribiliary cysts may mimic the periportal collar or appear as cysts along the larger portal tract. They are best depicted after administration of contrast medium

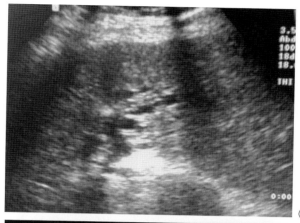

(a)

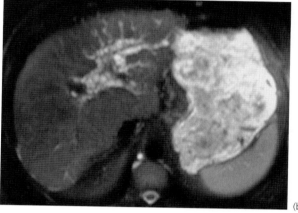

(b)

Fig. 1 Cystic dilatation of peribiliary glands. (a) Ultrasonography shows anechoic tubular structures paralleling the portal structures. (b) At MRI, they are strongly hyperintense on T2-weighted images and located on both sides of the bile ducts.

because they do not enhance (Fig. 2a). The size of the cysts ranges from a millimetre to > 10 mm [9]. They do not enhance after administration of cholangiographic contrast agent.

On MRI, the peribiliary cysts are hypointense on T1- (Figs 2b and 3b) and strongly hyperintense on T2-weighted imaging (Figs 1b, 2c, 3a) as well as on magnetic resonance cholangiopan-creato-graphy (MRCP) images [10] (Fig. 2d). They can mimic intrahepatic bile duct dilatation, but they arise predominantly around the hilum and are not associated with dilatation of small intrahepatic ducts. Similarly, they do not enhance after administration of hepatospecific contrast agents such as Mn-DPDP.

Differential diagnosis

The differential diagnosis is mainly represented by diffuse or local dilatation of the intrahepatic bile ducts. An important feature is that dilatation of intrahepatic bile ducts always appears on one side of the portal vein, conversely to the peribiliary cysts. Caroli's disease is also a common differential diagnosis because

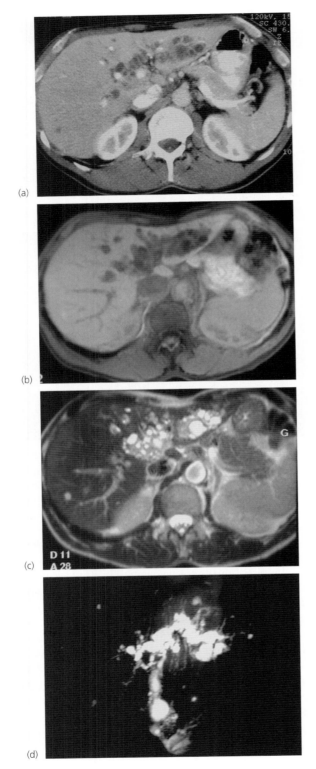

Fig. 2 Cystic dilatation of peribiliary glands. (a) Enhanced CT demonstrates multiple low-attenuation cysts along the left portal tract. The size of the cysts varies from a few millimetres to 1 cm. These cysts are hypointense on T1- (b) and strongly hyperintense on T2-weighted images (c). On MRCP images (d), the peribiliary cysts could mimic intrahepatic bile duct dilatation.

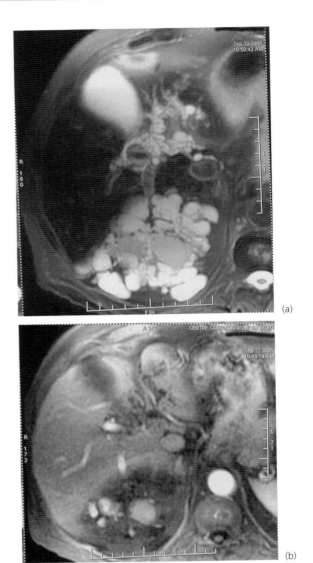

Fig. 3 Cystic dilatation of peribiliary glands in a patient with adult autosomal dominant polycystic kidney disease. T2- (a) and postcontrast T1-weighted (b) images demonstrate the peribiliary cysts, which do not enhance after administration of chelates of gadolinium. Multiple renal cysts are clearly seen; some of them are haemorrhagic. Interestingly, this patient had no liver cyst.

Caroli's disease may be localized. However, localized biliary dilatation that is limited to the larger ducts is rarely observed in Caroli's disease. Furthermore, the central dot sign, which is a key finding in Caroli's disease, is not described in peribiliary cysts [9]. Other differentials include von Meyenburg complexes (see Chapter 8.1.5), cholangitis and periportal collar. Cystic appearance and absence of communication with the bile ducts at imaging favour a diagnosis of peribiliary cysts.

In conclusion, hepatic peribiliary cysts are caused by the dilatation of the extramural peribiliary glands and are characterized by the presence of multiple tiny cysts seen exclusively within the larger portal tracts or hepatic hilum. Imaging is highly characteristic. Because these lesions are benign, no treatment or follow-up is recommended.

References

1   Tedara T, Nakanuma Y, Ohta G (1987) Glandular elements around the intrahepatic bile ducts in man: their morphology and distribution in normal livers. *Liver* 7, 1–8.

2   Terada T, Nakanuma Y, Kakita A (1990) Pathologic observations of intrahepatic peribiliary glands in 1000 consecutive autopsy livers. Heterotopic pancreas in the liver. *Gastroenterology* 98, 1333–1337.

3   Nakanuma Y, Sasaki M, Terada T *et al.* (1994) Intrahepatic peribiliary glands of humans. II. Pathological spectrum. *J Gastroenterol Hepatol* 9, 80–86.

4   Wanless IR, Zahradnik J, Heathcote EJ (1987) Hepatic cysts of periductal gland origin presenting as obstructive jaundice. *Gastroenterology* 93, 894–898.

5   Nakanuma Y, Kurumaya H, Ohta G (1984) Multiple cysts in the hepatic hilum and their pathogenesis. *Virchows Arch (Pathol Anat)* 404, 341–350.

6   Itai Y, Ebihara R, Eguchi N *et al.* (1995) Hepatobiliary cysts in patients with autosomal dominant polycystic kidney disease. *Am J Roentgenol* 164, 339–342.

7   Terada T, Matsushita H, Tashiro J *et al.* (2003) Cholesterol hepatolithiasis with peribiliary cysts. *Pathol Int* 53, 716–720.

8   Colina F, Castellano VM, Gonzalez-Pinto I *et al.* (1998) Hilar biliary cysts in hepatic transplantation. Report of three symptomatic cases and occurrence in resected liver grafts. *Transpl Int* 11, 110–116.

9   Itai Y, Ebihara R, Tohno E *et al.* (1994) Hepatic peribiliary cysts: multiple tiny cysts within the larger portal tract, hepatic hilum, or both. *Radiology* 191, 107–110.

10 Baron RL, Campbell WL, Dodd III GD (1994) Peribiliary cysts associated with severe liver diseases: imaging-pathologic correlation. *Am J Roentgenol* 162, 631–636.

8.1.7. Caroli syndrome

Jean-Pierre Benhamou

Caroli syndrome is a congenital malformation characterized by multifocal dilatation of the segmental bile ducts. The main consequence of this malformation is recurrent bacterial cholangitis.

Pathology, classification and aetiology

The lesion of Caroli syndrome consists of multifocal dilatation of the segmental bile ducts. The ectatic portions form cysts of various sizes, separated by portions of bile ducts which are normal or regularly dilated. The multifocal dilatation may be diffuse, affecting the whole intrahepatic biliary tree (although it may be more marked in a part of the liver), or it may be confined to a part of the liver, often the left lobe or a segment of the left lobe [1]. The number of cysts is large in the diffuse form and limited, usually less than 10, in the localized form.

Multifocal dilatation of the segmental bile ducts is not a single entity. In the majority of cases, it is associated with congenital hepatic fibrosis [2].

Manifestations and diagnosis

Caroli syndrome, which is likely to be present at birth, usually remains asymptomatic for the first 5 to 20 years of the patient's life, and in a few cases for the patient's whole life. Asymptomatic Caroli syndrome is unrecognized, except in patients in whom congenital hepatic fibrosis has been diagnosed and multifocal dilatation of the segmental bile ducts has been suspected and demonstrated by ultrasonography or computed tomography.

In most patients, the first episode of cholangitis occurs in the absence of any apparent cause. In a few, the first episode of cholangitis is the consequence of a surgical operation or an invasive investigation on the biliary tree, such as cholecystectomy, choledochotomy, T-tube drainage, intraoperative cholangiography, or endoscopic retrograde cholangiography (Benhamou, personal observation; see also refs 3–5).

The main and often the only symptom of cholangitis due to Caroli syndrome is fever, in contrast to cholangitis complicating common bile duct stones in which fever is usually accompanied by pain and/or jaundice. As a consequence, the first episodes of fever may not be attributed to cholangitis.

At clinical examination, the liver is usually enlarged. There is no sign or symptom indicating liver failure. In patients with Caroli syndrome associated with congenital hepatic fibrosis, manifestations of portal hypertension are present. Liver function tests are normal except for alkaline phosphatase and gammaglutamyl transpeptidase which may be moderately increased.

The best procedures for the diagnosis of Caroli syndrome are ultrasonography, computerized tomography and magnetic resonance cholangiography which show cystic formations of various size, diffuse or limited to a part of the liver, associated or not associated with tubular dilatation of segmental bile ducts. Ultrasonography and computerized tomography show tiny dots within dilated intrahepatic bile ducts (the central dot sign); these intraluminal dots correspond to intraluminal portal vein; this finding indicates that the portal radicles are surrounded by dilated intrahepatic bile ducts [6]. Computerized tomography after intravenous injection of biliary contrast may show opacification of cysts and dilated segmental bile ducts. Cystic formations, communicating with intrahepatic biliary tract, may be demonstrated by intraoperative cholangiography, postoperative cholangiography through a T-tube or endoscopic retrograde cholangiography; these three procedures must not be used in patients with asymptomatic Caroli syndrome, but can be employed in patients with Caroli syndrome already complicated by cholangitis.

The other imaging procedures have less interest for the diagnosis of Caroli syndrome. Radiocolloid liver scans show cold areas corresponding to the large cysts. Hepatobiliary scans shows cold areas in the early phase which become hot at a late phase of imaging [7].

Course and complications

The course of Caroli syndrome is dominated by recurrent episodes of cholangitis, the frequency of which varies widely: some patients experience 10 to 20 episodes a year, whereas others suffer only one or two episodes a year. In patients with frequent episodes of cholangitis, the prognosis is poor: generally, five to 10 years after the onset of recurrent cholangitis, such patients die from uncontrolled biliary bacterial infection.

Cholangitis may be complicated by liver abscesses, septicaemia, extrahepatic abscesses and secondary amyloidosis [8].

Cholangitis often induces the formation of intracystic stones [9], which are usually recognized at ultrasonography or endoscopic retrograde cholangiography but may be missed by computed tomography when not calcified. These stones can migrate from the cysts into the common bile duct and cause biliary pain and/or cholestasis and/or acute pancreatitis [10]. Cholangiocarcinoma develops in some patients with Caroli syndrome [11].

Associated malformations

In patients with Caroli syndrome and congenital hepatic fibrosis, the malformations associated with congenital hepatic fibrosis alone may obviously be present. In patients affected by Caroli syndrome with or, more often, without congenital hepatic fibrosis, associated choledocal cyst is relatively common [11]. Exceptionally, Caroli syndrome is associated with Laurence–Moon–Biedl syndrome [12].

Treatment

The treatment of the episodes of bacterial cholangitis is with appropriate antibiotics.

The prevention of recurrences of bacterial cholangitis is difficult. Periodic administration of antibiotics seems efficacious in some patients but completely inefficient in others. T-tube drainage is not effective and may be dangerous in patients with associated congenital hepatic fibrosis; large amounts of water and electrolytes, secreted by the multiple bile ductules, may be lost through the T-tube, which may result in severe dehydration [13]. Administration of ursodesoxycholic acid may be used for the prevention and treatment of intracystic stones [14] and has been recommended to be administered to all patients with Caroli syndrome [15]. Transhepatic intubation and drainage of the biliary tree have been used successfully in a small number of patients [16]. Surgical biliointestinal anastomoses or endoscopic papillotomy may facilitate the passage of stones into the intestine, but cannot be recommended because these procedures may increase the frequency and severity of the episodes of cholangitis [17]. In the localized form of Caroli syndrome, partial hepatectomy is indicated and excellent results can be expected [18]. In the diffuse form, if the cysts clearly predominate in a part of the liver, partial hepatectomy can also be envisaged; however, in such patients, partial hepatectomy is difficult because of associated congenital hepatic fibrosis and portal hypertension, and the long-term results may be compromised because multifocal dilatation affecting the remaining liver may be the source of recurrent cholangitis [18]. In the diffuse form without predominance of the cysts in any part of the liver and complicated by severe recurrent cholangitis, liver transplantation might be considered.

References

1 Caroli J, Couinaud C, Soupault R *et al.* (1958) [A new disease, undoubtedly congenital, of the bile ducts: unilobar cystic dilation of the hepatic ducts.] *Semin Hôp Paris* 34, 488–495.

2 Fauvert R (1974) *The Liver and its Diseases.* New York: IMS, pp. 283–288.

3 Clermont RJ, Maillard JN, Benhamou JP (1967) [Congenital hepatic fibrosis.] *Can Med Assoc J* 97, 1272–1278.

4 Erlinger (1969) [The angiocholitic forms of the congenital hepatic fibrosis.] *Presse Med* 77, 1189–1191.

5 Grumbach R (1954) *Arch Anat Cytol Pathol* 30, 74–77.

6 Choi IP, Berenstein A, Kagetsu NJ (1990) Irrigation device for neuroangiographic procedures. *Radiology* 174, 161–163.

7 Stillman AE (1981) *Gastroenterology* 80, 1295 (abstr.)

8 Fevery (1972) Congenital dilatation of the intrahepatic bile ducts associated with the development of amyloidosis. *Gut* 13, 604–609.

9 Mathias CG (1978) *Acta Hepatogastroenterol Belg* 25, 30–34.

10 Sahel (1976) [Caroli's disease with acute pancreatitis and angiocholitis. Diagnostic and therapeutic value of endoscopic choledochowirsungography.] *Nouv Presse Med* 5, 2067–2069.

11 Dayton MT, Longmire WP Jr, Tompkins RP (1983) Caroli's disease: a premalignant condition? *Am J Surg* 145, 41–48.

12 Tsuchiya R, Nishimur R, Ito T (1977) Congenital cystic dilation of the bile duct associated with Laurence–Moon–Biedl–Bardet syndrome. *Arch Surg* 112, 82–84.

13 Turnberg (1968) Biliary secretion in a patient with cystic dilation of the intrahepatic biliary tree. *Gastroenterology* 54, 1155.

14 Kutz K, Miederer SE, Paumgartner G (1978) Case report: chenodeoxycholic acid therapy of intrahepatic radiolucent gallstones in a patient with Caroli's syndrome. *Acta Hepatogastroenterol Stuttg.* 25, 398.

15 Ros E, Navarro S, Bruc *et al.* (1993) Ursodeoxycholic acid treatment of primary hepatolithiasis in Caroli's syndrome. *Lancet* 342, 404.

16 Witlin LT, Gadacz TR, Zuidema GD *et al.* (1982) Transhepatic decompression of the biliary tree in Caroli's disease. *Surgery* 91, 205–209.

17 Watts DR, Lorenzo GA, Beal JM (1974) Proceedings: congenital dilatation of the intrahepatic biliary ducts. *Arch Surg* 108, 592.

18 Ramond MJ, Huguet C, Danan G *et al.* (1984) Partial hepatectomy in the treatment of Caroli's disease. Report of a case and review of the literature. *Dig Dis Sci* 29, 367–370.

8.1.8. Choledocal cyst

Jean-Pierre Benhamou

Choledocal cyst is a rare congenital condition that is characterized by a cystic dilatation of a segment of the biliary ductal system. The disease should be termed 'bile duct cyst' rather than 'choledocal cyst'. The prevalence is higher in Asia than in western countries. The disease is four times more common in females than in males. Most surgeons accept the Todani modification of the Alonso–Lej classification [1]. In this schema, patients with type 1 cyst (the most common) have an extrahepatic biliary dilatation that can be divided into three groups: (A) cystic dilatation of the entire common bile duct; (B) focal segmental dilatation of the common bile duct; and (C) fusiform dilatation of the extrahepatic biliary tree. Type 2 cyst consists of a diverticulum of the common bile duct. Type 3 cyst, also known as 'choledococoele', represents cystic dilatation of the intraduodenal portion of the biliary tree. Type 4 cyst is divided into two subtypes: type 4-A has multiple intrahepatic and extrahepatic cysts; type 4-B has multiple extrahepatic cysts. Type 5, also known as Caroli's disease, is isolated to intrahepatic bile ducts.

The pathogenesis is unknown. However, in most cases, an anomalous pancreaticobiliary ductal junction is present, which has suggested that reflux of pancreatic juice into the common bile duct could play a role in the pathogenesis of choledocal cyst.

Classically, the patient with a choledocal cyst type 1 is a female infant of Asian descent who has a palpable mass, abdominal pain and jaundice. In fact, in currently reported series, an increasing number of patients are adults, and the classical triad is absent. The diagnosis is established by ultrasound, magnetic resonance cholangiography, computerized tomographic scan and endoscopic retrograde cholangiopancreatography.

Many complications have been reported including cholangitis, cholelithiasis, jaundice, acute pancreatitis and rupture. Carcinoma of the biliary tree is the most serious complication of choledocal cyst; it mainly affects adults over 50 years.

Prior to the two most recent decades, cyst drainage was considered to be the appropriate treatment of choledocal cyst. In fact, cyst drainage is associated with two problems: first, there is a very high incidence of stricture, probably related to the often severe inflammation of the cyst epithelium; secondly, there is a risk of malignancy in the dilated cyst segment.

Resection of the choledocal cyst with reconstruction of the biliary tree is the treatment of choice. The entire cyst must be excised; incomplete excision exposes to the risk of carcinoma on the remaining portion of the cyst.

Reference

1 Lipsett PA, Cameron JL (1996) Choledocal cyst disease: a review. *J Hep Bil Pancr Surg* 3, 389–395.

8.1.9 Ciliated hepatic foregut cyst

Jean-François Cadranel

Wheeler and Edmonson first used the term ciliated hepatic foregut cyst (CHFC) to describe a benign liver lesion that apparently arises from the embryologic foregut [1]. CHFC is an uncommon entity. Fewer than 70 cases have been reported in the English, French and Japanese language literature [1–27]. The majority of CHFC cases have been reported in the last 20 years [2]. The increase in reported cases over the last two decades has coincided with the increased used of abdominal imaging techniques [2,11].

Pathology

Histologically [1,11,12,24], the CHFC is lined with a pseudostratified cylindrical epithelium with ciliated and mucin-secreting cells. It is surrounded by connective tissue and a band of smooth muscle fibres [1,11,12,24]. The cyst wall consists of the following four layers: (i) a pseudostratified, columnar ciliated epithelium; (ii) a subepithelial connective tissue; (iii) a layer composed of smooth muscle bundles; and (iv) a fibrous capsule (Fig. 1). Small bile ductules can occasionally be observed in the cyst wall, lined by columnar non-ciliated epithelium [18,25].

The cyst epithelium contains ciliated cells, the cilia of which are strongly labelled with tubulin [23,24]. Goblet cells of the cyst epithelium contain neutral, carboxylated and sulphated mucins, like the mucin-secreting cells of the respiratory epithelium [23,24]. Goblet cells stain with periodic acid–Schiff (PAS), Alcian blue and high-iron diamine [12].

Immunohistochemical studies showed that the cyst epithelium contained endocrine cells immunoreactive for chromogranin,

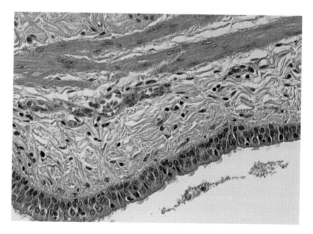

Fig. 1 Foregut ciliated cyst. Gross magnification. Note the four layers: (a) pseudostratified columnar ciliated epithelium; (b) subepithelial connective tissue: (c) smooth muscle bundles; (d) fibrous capsule (courtesy of Dr Valérie Paradis, Hôpital Beaujon, Clichy, France).

synaptophysin, calcitonin and bombesin [12]. This pattern is similar to that of endocrine cells present in the respiratory epithelium [14]. In contrast, endocrine cells were negative for serotonin, somatostatin, glucagon, insulin, gastrin and pancreatic polypeptide [12]. Immunoreactivity of some cells for CC10 strongly suggested the presence of Clara cells [12,23]. Ultrastructural observations revealed definite cilia arranged in a 9 + 2 pattern, as well as mucous cells [24].

Pathogenesis

The overall cellular features and architecture are similar to those of the respiratory bronchi and indicate that these cysts arise from abnormally developing ventral endoderm within the liver [1,12,24]. Mouse embryo studies have demonstrated that the ventral endoderm gives rise to the adult foregut structures, including the oropharynx down to the hepatic diverticulum [28]. CHFCs probably originated from embryogenic foregut remnants that persisted in the liver and differentiated towards bronchial structures [23,24].

Clinical presentation

Patients with CHFC average 52 years at presentation (range 5–82 years). The male to female ratio is 1.2:1. In two-thirds of patients, CHFC are found incidentally on imaging studies [11,12,17–19,23,24,27], at surgery or incidentally during autopsy [11]. About 25–30% of patients presented with abdominal pain [11,12,16,21–25,27] and abnormal liver function tests, but it is unclear how the cysts were discovered or whether they were responsible for the presenting signs and symptoms [11].

In one case, the cyst caused compression of the portal vein with resulting portal hypertension and splenomegaly [14]. One case has been reported in a cirrhotic patient [17]; we have also observed such a case (personal communication).

Imaging pattern

CFHC are more often located in the left lobe, especially in the medial segment (segment IV) [11,14,17,18,21,22,25,27]. A case has been reported in the left hepatic vein [4] and a few cases in the gallbladder wall [22]; one CHFC communicated with the gallbladder [3]. Most of the lesions were less than 4 cm (median 3 cm; range 0.4–9 cm) [1–27].

A larger size should raise suspicion of a malignant transformation. Indeed, three cases of squamous cell carcinoma arising in a CFHC were reported between 1999 and 2002 [29–31]. The sizes of the CFHC were 10 cm, 10 cm and 12 cm in these three cases [29–31]. CFHC appeared as well-delineated solitary, unilocular, hypoechoic small masses with or without posterior enhancement on ultrasonography [10,27]. Less frequently, CFHC are anechoic. They may occasionally have a pseudosolid pattern [13,25]. On computerized tomography (CT), CFHC appeared as well-defined, unilocular, isolated masses located beneath the

hepatic surface in the subcapsular areas [10,21,26,27]. Calcifications of the cyst wall are rare [27]. On CT scan, because they contain various elements ranging from clear serous material to milky white to brown mucoid material, and have variable viscosities, the different CT attenuation numbers can be shown [26]. On enhanced CT, CFHC appeared with low density and can be hypoattenuating or isoattenuating relative to the surrounding liver parenchyma; these lesions remained with low density after contrast enhancement [10,21,26,27]. Occasionally, CFHC may appear with slightly higher density before contrast enhancement, mimicking a solid tumour [25]. On magnetic resonance imaging (MRI), lesions are hyperintense on T2-weighted spin images [13,21,26,27]. On T1-weighted spin image MRIs, CFHC are usually hyperintense [13,21,26,27]. However, they are sometimes isointense [16,21] or hypointense [26,27] on T1 sequences. These different imaging features depend on the fluid composition of the cyst, related to viscosity, mucin density and the presence of calcium or cholesterol crystals [25,26]. There is no contrast enhancement after gadolinium injection [26]. According to the imaging pattern, several diagnoses may be discussed: solitary non-parasitic cyst in cases of anechoic patterns on ultrasonography, solid tumour in cases of pseudosolid patterns [13,25] or cystadenoma when mucoid material is rich. Comparison of ultrasound, CT scan and MRI may help in achieving a precise diagnosis [32]. Guided fine needle aspiration [18,19] may be helpful by showing columnar cells with basally oriented nuclei and prominent apical terminal plates with cilia [18,19].

Treatment

Four to five per cent of CHFC may have malignant transformation [2,29–31]. As discussed, the major risk factor for malignant transformation appears to be the size of the cyst. Because of this potential risk, total surgical excision is necessary in patients who have a cyst greater than 4–5 cm, a symptomatic cyst, an enlarging cyst or when imaging studies show abnormalities in the cyst wall [29–31]. Vick et al. [29] recommend surgical excision even for asymptomatic patients.

References

1 Wheeler DA, Edmondson HA (1984) Ciliated hepatic foregut cyst. *Am J Surg Pathol* 8, 467–470.
2 Jakowski JD, Lucas JG, Seth S et al. (2004) Ciliated hepatic foregut cyst: a rare but increasingly reported liver cyst. *Ann Diagn Pathol* 8, 342–346.
3 Koletsa T, Tzioufa V, Michalopoulos A et al. (2005) Ciliated hepatic foregut cyst communicating with the gallbladder. *Virchows Arch* 446, 200–201.
4 Momin TA, Milner R, Sarmiento JM (2004) Ciliated hepatic foregut cyst of the left hepatic vein. *J Gastrointest Surg* 8, 601–603.
5 Cai XJ, Huang DY, Liang X et al. (2004) Ciliated hepatic foregut cyst: report of first case in China and review of literature. *J Zhejiang Univ Sci* 5, 483–485.

6 Del Poggio P, Jamoletti C, Mattiello M *et al.* (2003) Images in hepatology. Ciliated hepatic foregut cyst. *J Hepatol* 39, 1090.

7 Balducci G, Bellagamba R, De Siena T *et al.* (2003) Ciliated hepatic foregut cysts: a case report. *G Chir* 24, 189–192.

8 Horii T, Ohta M, Mori T *et al.* (2003) Ciliated hepatic foregut cyst. A report of one case and a review of the literature. *Hepatol Res* 26, 243–248.

9 Bogner B, Hegedus G (2002) Ciliated hepatic foregut cyst. *Pathol Oncol Res* 8, 278–279.

10 Hirata M, Ishida H, Konno K *et al.* (2001) Ciliated hepatic foregut cyst: case report with an emphasis on US findings. *Abdom Imaging* 26, 594–596.

11 Vick DJ, Goodman ZD, Deavers MT *et al.* (1999) Ciliated hepatic foregut cyst: a study of six cases and review of the literature. *Am J Surg Pathol* 23, 671–677.

12 Chatelain D, Chailley-Heu B, Terris B *et al.* (2000) The ciliated hepatic foregut cyst, an unusual bronchiolar foregut malformation: a histological, histochemical, and immunohistochemical study of 7 cases. *Hum Pathol* 31, 241–246.

13 Wu ML, Abecassis MM, Rao MS (1998) Ciliated hepatic foregut cyst mimicking neoplasm. *Am J Gastroenterol* 93, 2212–2214.

14 Harty MP, Hebra A, Ruchelli ED *et al.* (1998) Ciliated hepatic foregut cyst causing portal hypertension in an adolescent. *Am J Roentgenol* 170, 688–690.

15 Kajiya Y, Nakajo M, Ichinari N *et al.* (1997) Retroperitoneal foregut cyst. *Abdom Imaging* 22, 111–113.

16 Carnicer J, Duran C, Donoso L *et al.* (1996) Ciliated hepatic foregut cyst. *J Pediatr Gastroenterol Nutr* 23, 191–193.

17 Murakami T, Imai A, Nakamura H *et al.* (1996) Ciliated foregut cyst in cirrhotic liver. *J Gastroenterol* 31, 446–449.

18 Hornstein A, Batts KP, Linz IJ *et al.* (1996) Fine needle aspiration diagnosis of ciliated hepatic foregut cysts: a report of three cases. *Acta Cytol* 40, 576–580.

19 Zaman SS, Langer JE, Gupta PK (1995) Ciliated hepatic foregut cyst. Report of a case with findings on fine needle aspiration. *Acta Cytol* 39, 781–784.

20 Kakita A, Kimura T, Takahashi T (1995) Ciliated hepatic foregut cyst and hepatic foregut cyst. *Ryoikibetsu Shokogun Shirizu* 8, 128–131.

21 Shoenut JP, Semelka RC, Levi C *et al.* (1994) Ciliated hepatic foregut cysts: US, CT, and contrast-enhanced MR imaging. *Abdom Imaging* 19, 150–152.

22 Peltier E, Leger-Ravet MB, Franco D *et al.* (1993) Ciliated cysts of the liver. 2 cases. *Gastroenterol Clin Biol* 17, 859–862.

23 Terada T, Nakanuma Y, Ohta T *et al.* (1991) Mucin-histochemical and immunohistochemical profiles of epithelial cells of several types of hepatic cysts. *Virchows Arch A Pathol Anat Histopathol* 419, 499–504.

24 Terada T, Nakanuma Y, Kono N *et al.* (1990) Ciliated hepatic foregut cyst. A mucus histochemical, immunohistochemical, and ultrastructural study in three cases in comparison with normal bronchi and intrahepatic bile ducts. *Am J Surg Pathol* 14, 356–363.

25 Kimura A, Makuuchi M, Takayasu K *et al.* (1990) Ciliated hepatic foregut cyst with solid tumor appearance on CT. *J Comput Assist Tomogr* 14, 1016–1018.

26 Kadoya M, Matsui O, Nakanuma Y *et al.* (1990) Ciliated hepatic foregut cyst: radiologic features. *Radiology* 175, 475–477.

27 Benlolo D, Vilgrain V, Terris B *et al.* (1996) Imagerie des kystes ciliés hépatiques ou biliaires à revêtement cilié. *Gastroenterol Clin Biol* 20, 497–504.

28 Zaret KS (2002) Regulatory phases of early liver development: paradigms of organogenesis. *Nature Rev Genet* 3, 449–512.

29 Vick DJ, Goodman ZD, Ishak KG (1999) Squamous cell carcinoma arising in a ciliated hepatic foregut cyst. *Arch Pathol Lab Med* 123, 1115–1117.

30 De Lajarte-Thirouard AS, Rioux-Leclercq N, Boudjema K *et al.* (2002) Squamous cell carcinoma arising in a hepatic foregut cyst. *Pathol Res Pract* 198, 697–700.

31 Furlanetto A, Deil Tos AP (2002) Squamous cell carcinoma arising in a ciliated hepatic foregut cyst. *Virchows Arch* 441, 296–298.

32 Vuillemin-Bodaghi V, Zins M, Vullierme MP *et al.* (1997) Imaging of atypical cysts of the liver. Study of 26 surgically treated cases. *Gastroenterol Clin Biol* 21, 394–399.

8.2 Acquired conditions

8.2.1 Inflammatory cystic diseases

Jean-François Cadranel

Endometrial cysts of the liver

Endometriosis is characterized by the presence of functioning endometrial tissue outside the uterine cavity [1]. Ectopic endometrium has been described in almost every location, but is most frequently located in the pelvic organs. Unusual sites of involvement include the umbilicus, laparotomy or incisional scars, arms, legs, kidney, diaphragm, gastrointestinal tract, bladder wall, lung, pleura, pancreas, heart and bone [2]. The only organ in the abdominal cavity that is apparently refractory to the disease is the spleen [2].

Hepatic endometriosis is extremely rare [1,3]. The first case was reported by Finkel *et al.* in a 21-year-old woman who complained of epigastric pain, nausea and vomiting. She was found to have an endometrial cyst (EC) measuring 13 cm in the left lobe of the liver [4]. To date, fewer than 20 cases have been reported [1,3,4,12].

EC of the liver occurred in women with an age ranging from 21 to 62 years [1]. One-third of the patients had a history of abdominal endometriosis, whereas the other two-thirds showed no evidence of endometrial implants other than in the liver [1]. However, some of the women without a history of pelvic-associated endometriosis had difficulty in conceiving, suggesting possible Fallopian tube lesions [1]. Two-thirds of the women presented with acyclic gastric or right upper abdominal tenderness or pain [1,3]. Right upper abdominal mass can be noted when EC are large. EC of the liver are located in either the left or the right lobe of the liver [1,3]. In two cases, pleural endometriosis was associated with EC of the liver [12]. EC range in size from 3 to 24 cm and average 10 cm. EC were solitary in all but one of the reported cases [1,3]. One 62-year-old woman [9] who presented with right upper abdominal tenderness had two EC of 3.1 cm and 2.8 cm located in the right lobe and the

falciform ligament respectively. The latter lesion was complicated by malignant transformation with moderately differentiated endometrioid adenosquamous carcinoma [9]. EC of the liver are either unilocular or multilocular and present with septations that are better seen during ultrasonography examination than during tomodensitometry examination [4,8]. Abdominal ultrasonography, computerized tomography (CT) scan and magnetic resonance imaging (MRI) showed cystic tumours that may be indistinguishable from a simple cyst. In some instances, however, irregularity of the cyst wall and septation led to a preoperative diagnosis of cystadenoma [8]. Large EC of the right lobe may be accompanied by a reactive enlargement of the left lobe [7]. Calcifications of the cyst wall have been reported occasionally [6,10]. Choledochal compression and communication with the biliary tract have been reported in one case each [7,8]. The content of EC is usually chocolate coloured and haemorrhagic-like, typical of endometriosis [1]; it may occasionally be clear [4]. Histologically, the cyst wall is lined by a single layer of cuboidal cells with occasional formation of endometrial glands. These glands are admixed with a well-vascularized mesenchymal stroma [8]. When performed, immunostaining is positive for estrogen and progesterone receptors [3]. The liver adjacent to EC is either normal or shows focal haemosiderin deposition [1]. A case of adenosarcoma arising in hepatic endometriosis has been reported. It presented as a huge heterogeneous mass containing septated thick-walled cystic lesions [11]; the patient was asymptomatic with no abnormalities on liver and abdominal CT scan after enlarged right hepatectomy at a 2-year follow-up. The treatment of EC of the liver is surgery; the median term results (when available) are good with no symptoms of recurrence after follow-up ranging from 10 to 22 months [1,5,6].

The pathogenesis of extra-abdominal endometriosis remains uncertain [3]. Many theories have been proposed, including coelomic metaplasia, retrograde menstruation, iatrogenic injury and haematogenous or lymphatic dissemination [13]. Metaplasia or differentiation from coelomic epithelium, triggered by many stimuli, has been observed frequently. Transportation of endometrial fragments by one means or another is important to the histogenesis and has been described after surgical procedures that involve the endometrium. Endometrial fragments have been observed in the oviduct and in the peritoneal cavity. Regurgitated menstrual fluid is not rare and may be responsible for the development of pelvic endometriosis. Endometrial tissue has been observed in lymphatic and blood vessels; vascular dissemination probably occurs more frequently after surgical trauma than spontaneously [3,13,14].

Pancreatic pseudocysts of the liver

Although pancreatic pseudocysts can form anywhere in the abdomen, intrahepatic occurrence is rare [15,16]. Hepatic extrapancreatic pseudocysts have been reported in the setting of acute alcoholic [15,17] or biliary pancreatitis [18], chronic pancreatitis [19] or pancreatic injury [16,20]. Pancreatic pseudocyst is a collection of pancreatic juice confined by a non-epithelialized wall of granulation tissue [21] and requires a least 4 weeks to form [21]. Unusual location of pancreatic pseudocysts has been reported in 22.4% of patients in one study [22]. The first two cases of hepatic pancreatic pseudocysts were reported by Siegelman *et al.* in 1980 [23]. In a literature review, we found 26 reported cases of pancreatic pseudocysts of the liver up to 2000 [24]. Occasional case reports have been reported after 2000 [18,25]. Intrahepatic location of the pseudocyst has been document by ultrasonography, CT scan, MRI or surgical exploration [21,24,26,27]. Clinical symptoms are usually related to the underlying inflammatory pancreatic disease. Elevated serum lipase and/or elevated serum and urinary amylase levels should arouse suspicion of this condition [16]. Continuous epigastric pain after acute pancreatitis [28] or recurrence of abdominal pain after initial clinical resolution of pancreatitis may be observed [24]. A palpable upper abdominal mass has been reported rarely [28–30]. Hepatomegaly has been reported occasionally [15,17,26]. Jaundice is rarely observed [24,30]. Results of liver function tests are usually within the normal range [24]. Serum aminotransferase activities are usually not elevated despite digestion of liver cells [16]. Correct diagnosis is not difficult with imaging when other signs of acute pancreatitis are present [16]. On CT, a mature intrahepatic pseudocyst appears as a well-defined, subcapsular, homogeneous, hypoattenuating mass surrounded by a thin fibrous capsule [31]. In the setting of acute pancreatitis, the attenuation of the fluid within the cyst may be high as a result of haemorrhage and necrotic debris, and the lesion may be less distinctly defined [31,32]. On MRI [21], a pancreatic pseudocyst appears as a well-circumscribed subcapsular lesion with low signal intensity on T1-weighted images (T1 WI) and markedly high signal intensity on T2-weighted images (T2 WI) [21]. In mature cysts, an enhancing capsule is observed following intravenous administration of gadolinium chelates [31]. When performed for diagnostic purposes, puncture shows a yellowish fluid with high lipase and amylase activity.

MRI is superior to CT for the prediction of drainability [21], allowing better visualization (on T2-weighted sequences) of fluid and solid components. Pancreatic pseudocyst percutaneous drainage has been reported to be an effective treatment method with a 90% cure rate [27], limiting the risks of major intra-abdominal surgery. Percutaneous drainage, when possible according to imaging results, permits treatment to be initiated rapidly [16,24,27], avoiding a wait of several weeks for cyst maturation prior to surgery. In addition, percutaneous catheter techniques may lower morbidity and mortality compared with surgical drainage [33]. Different hypotheses have been suggested to explain the extension of pancreatic pseudocysts in the liver, due to the proteolytic effect of pancreatic enzymes that reach the lesser sac and then the liver either directly through the liver capsule [20,34] or indirectly through the hepatic hilum vessels, the hepatogastric ligament [16,29,34] or, rarely, via the hepatoduodenal ligament [25]. These hypotheses account for the location of pancreatic pseudocysts in the left lobe. Ancel *et al.* [18] suggest that pancreatic enzymes could cause liver damage, through the pararenal anterior space, often infiltrated during acute pancreatitis, reaching the right hepatic lobe through the area nuda. This hypothesis may account for pseudocysts located in the right lobe.

Miscellaneous

Epidermoid cysts of the liver

Epidermoid cysts of the liver are extremely rare [35–40]. The origin of these cysts is unknown. It is postulated that they derive from accessory foregut buds [35]. They occur in children or young adults. They may be responsible for right upper quadrant abdominal pain or mass [35]. Liver tests may be normal or exhibit an increase in aminotransferase and alkaline phosphatase activities. Ultrasonography shows large solitary cystic lesions that may simulate a hydatid cyst [36]. Total enucleation is warranted as subtotal cystectomy may be followed by relapse [36]. Pathological examination of the cyst wall shows its epidermoid nature lined by stratified squamous epithelium. Occasional reports of squamous cell liver cancer arising from an epidermoid cyst have been noted [37,39,40]. Because of their malignant potential and tendency to reoccur, total excision should be performed.

Cystic hepatic peliosis

Peliosis hepatis is an uncommon condition characterized by numerous blood-filled cavities or cystic spaces. Although the cause is unknown, it has been reported in association with several disease states such as tuberculosis, malignancy, diabetes, sprue, postrenal and cardiac transplantation and medication, particularly androgenic steroids [41].

Peliosis hepatis may occasionally present a cystic appearance [42–45]; abdominal ultrasonography may demonstrate diffuse mixed echogenic masses, some with cystic cavities [42]. MRI findings are the following [43]: heterogeneic signal intensity on T1 WI with areas of high–intermediate and low signal intensity; a cystic round mass with a slim hyperintensity has been noted on T1 WI images [42]; heterogeneic signal on T2 WI with the presence of numerous intralesional 'cystic' hyperintense areas with a hypointense border [43]; after intravenous administration of gadolinium, enhancement is observed in the portovenous and late phases [43].

Cystic inflammatory pseudotumour of the liver

Inflammatory pseudotumours (IPT) of the liver are uncommon begin lesions that have been reported to occur in various organs and tissues [46]. Causes and pathogenesis of the lesion remain unknown. The term 'pseudotumour' arises from the discrepancy between the macroscopic appearance, indicative of a malignant tumour, and the histological picture, which reveals its inflammatory nature [46,47]. IPT has been reported increasingly in the liver, in both children and adults, usually presenting with systemic symptoms and fever [46,47].

Cystic appearance of IPT of the liver that masquerades as either a malignant cystic tumour of the liver [48] or a complicated hydatid cyst [47] has been reported rarely.

Cystic hepatic lymphangiomatosis

Hepatic lymphangiomatosis is a rare disorder characterized by cystic dilatation of the lymphatic vessels in the hepatic parenchyma [49]. It can occur in the liver alone, in the liver and spleen or in multiple organs [49,52]. Isolated case reports have focused on the cystic form of hepatic lymphangiomatosis [49–52] that can mimic polycystic liver disease [49] or hydatid cyst [50]. Some of the cysts contained caseous material [52].

References

1 Tuech JJ, Rousselet MC, Boyer J et al. (2003) Endometrial cyst of the liver: case report and review. Fertil Steril 79, 1234–1236.
2 Markham SM, Carpenter SE, Rock JA (1989) Extrapelvic endometriosis. Obstet Gynecol Clin North Am 16, 193–219.
3 Huang WT, Chen WJ, Chen CL et al. (2002) Endometrial cyst of the liver: a case report and review of the literature. J Clin Pathol 55, 715–717.
4 Finkel L, Marchevsky A, Cohen B (1986) Endometrial cyst of the liver. Am J Gastroenterol 7, 576–578.
5 Rovati V, Faleschini E, Vercellini P et al. (1990) Endometrioma of the liver. Am J Obstet Gynecol 163, 1490–1492.
6 Cravello L, D'Erenle C, Le Treut YP et al. (1996) Hepatic endometriosis a case report. Fertil Steril 66, 657–659.
7 Verbeke C, Härle M, Sturm J (1996) Cystic endometriosis of the upper abdominal organs. Report of three cases and review of the literature. Pathol Res Pract 192, 300–301.
8 Chung CC, Liew CT, Hewitt PM et al. (1998) Endometriosis of the liver. Surgery 123, 106–108.
9 Weinfeld RM, Johnson SC, Lucas CE et al. (1998) CT diagnosis of perihepatic endometriosis complicated by malignant transformation. Abdom Imaging 23, 183–184.
10 Inal M, Bicabei K, Soyupak S et al. (2000) Hepatic endometrioma: a case report and review of the literature. Eur Radiol 10, 431–434.
11 N'Senda P, Wendum D, Balladur P et al. (2000) Adenosarcoma arising in hepatic endometriosis. Eur Radiol 10, 1287–1289.
12 Bhaumik J, Hefni MA (2002) Endometriosis of liver and diaphragm: is the diagnosis often missed? Gynaecol Endosc 11, 155.
13 Jenkins S, Olive DL, Haney AF (1986) Endometriosis: pathogenetic implications of the anatomic distribution. Obstet Gynecol 76, 335–338.
14 Marik JJ, Jenkins S (1997) Endometrious etiology. J Reprod Med 19, 301–302.
15 Aiza I, Barkin JS, Casillas VJ et al. (1993) Pancreatic pseudocysts involving both hepatic lobes. Am J Gastroenterol 8, 1450–1452.
16 Okuda K, Sugita S, Tsukada E et al. (1991) Pancreatic pseudocyst in the left hepatic lobe: a review of two cases. Hepatology 13, 359–363.
17 Lederman E, Cajot O, Canva-Delcambre V et al. (1997) Pseudocysts in the left hepatic lobe: an unusual complication of acute pancreatitis. Gastroenterol Clin Biol 2, 340–341.
18 Ancel D, Lefebvre M, Peyrin-Biroulet L et al. (2005) Pancreatic pseudocysts of the right lobe during acute biliary pancreatitis. Gastroenterol Clin Biol 29, 743–745.
19 Roche J, Frairot A, Volle L et al. (1987) Intrahepatic localization of pancreatic pseudocyst. Treatment by simple puncture under ultrasonography. Presse Med 16, 2230.
20 Epstein BM, Conidaris C (1982) Pseudocysts involving the left lobe of the liver. CT demonstration. Br J Radiol 55, 928–930.
21 Baron TH, Morgan DE (1997) The diagnosis and management of fluid collections associated with pancreatitis. Am J Med 102, 555–563.
22 Hamm VB, Franzen N (1993) Atypically located pancreatic pseudocysts in liver, spleen, stomach wall and mediastinum: their CT diagnosis. Fortschr Rontgenstr 159, 522–527.
23 Siegelman SS, Copeland BE, Saba GP et al. (1980) CT of fluid collections associated with pancreatitis. Am J Roentgenol 134, 1121–1132.
24 Mofredj A, Cadranel JF, Dautreaux M et al. (2000) Pancreatic pseudocyst located in the liver. J Clin Gastroenterol 30, 81–83.
25 Shibasaki M, Bandai Y, Ukai T (2002) Pancreatic pseudocyst extending into the liver via the hepatoduodenal ligament: a case report. Hepatogastroenterology 49, 1719–1721.
26 Atienza P, Couturier D, Grandjouan S et al. (1987) Intrahepatic liquid collection of pancreatic origin. One case and a review of the literature. Presse Med 16, 1195–1198.
27 Boyd-Kranis RL, Bonn J (1997) Transhepatic transduodenal drainage of a pancreatic pseudocyst. J Vasc Interv Radiol 8, 659–662.
28 Gautier-Benoit C, Luez J, Cecile JP (1974) Pseudocyst of the pancreas with intrahepatic development. Semin Hôp Paris 50, 1235–1237.
29 Wang SJ, Chen JJ, Changchien CS et al. (1993) Sequential invasions of pancreatic pseudocysts in pancreatic tail, hepatic left lobe, caudate lobe, and spleen. Pancreas 8, 133–136.
30 Hospitel S, Guinot B, Teyssou H et al. (1983) Intrahepatic false cysts of the pancreas. J Radiol 64, 355–358.

31 Murphy BJ, Cassillas J, Ros PR *et al.* (1989) The CT appearance of cystic masses of the liver. *Radiographics* 9, 307–322.

32 Lantink JA, Heggelman BGF, Geerdink RA (1989) Intrahepatic rupture of a pancreatic pseudocyst: sonographic and CT demonstration. *Am J Roentgenol* 152, 1129.

33 Gumaste VV, Dave PB (1991) Pancreatic pseudocyst drainage: the needle or the scalpel? *J Clin Gastroenterol* 13, 500–505.

34 Okuda K, Sugita S (1998) Hepatobiliary images pancreatic pseudocysts in the liver. *J Gastroenterol Hepatol* 13, 433–436.

35 Schullinger JN, Wigger HJ, Price JB *et al.* (1983) Epidermoid cysts of the liver. *J Pediatr Surg* 18, 240–243.

36 Fernandez-Castroagudin J, Bustamante Montalvo M, Delgado Blanco M *et al.* (2001) Epidermoid cyst: a rare cause of cystic liver disease. *Gastroenterol Hepatol* 24, 247–249.

37 Yagi H, Ueda M, Kawachi S *et al.* (2004) Squamous cell carcinoma of the liver originating from non-parasitic cysts after a 15 year follow-up. *Eur J Gastroenterol Hepatol* 16, 1051–1056.

38 Ganti AL, Sardi A, Gordon J (2002) Laparoscopic treatment of large true cysts of the liver and spleen is ineffective. *Am Surg* 68, 1012–1017.

39 Caratozzolo E, Massani M, Recordare A *et al.* (2001) Squamous cell liver cancer arising from an epidermoid cyst. *J Hepatobiliary Pancreat Surg* 8, 490–493.

40 Lombardo FP, Hertford DE, Tan LK *et al.* (1995) Epidermoid cyst of the liver complicated by microscopic squamous cell carcinoma: CT, ultrasound, and pathology. *J Comput Assist Tomogr* 19, 131–134.

41 De Leve LD (2003) Vascular liver diseases. *Curr Gastroenterol Rep* 5, 63–70.

42 Saatci I, Coskun M, Boyvat F *et al.* (1995) MR findings in peliosis hepatis. *Pediatr Radiol* 25, 31–33.

43 Verswijvel G, Janssens F, Colla P *et al.* (2003) Peliosis hepatis presenting as a multifocal hepatic pseudotumor: MR findings in two cases. *Eur Radiol* 13, 40–44.

44 Shim SG, Paik SW, Hyun JG *et al.* (2001) Lipiodol accumulation in focal peliosis hepatis with sinusoidal dilatation. *J Clin Gastroenterol* 32, 356–358.

45 Staub PG, Leibowitz CB (1996) Peliosis hepatis associated with oral contraceptive use. *Australas Radiol* 40, 172–174.

46 Chen KT (1984) Inflammatory pseudotumor of the liver. *Hum Pathol* 15, 694–696.

47 Uccheddu A, Faa G, Cois A *et al.* (1995) Inflammatory pseudotumor of the liver. A report of two cases with unusual histologic picture. *Tumori* 81, 151–156.

48 Akiyama T, Saito H, Kiriyama M *et al.* (1995) A case of gallbladder cancer associated with a common bile duct neuroma, and a cystic lesion of the liver with histologic findings similar to those of an inflammatory pseudotumor. *J Gastroenterol* 30, 408–412.

49 O'Sullivan DA, Torres VA, de Groen PC *et al.* (1998) Hepatic lymphangiomatosis mimicking polycystic liver disease. *Mayo Clin Proc* 73, 1188–1192.

50 Clerici D, Griffa B, Ceppi M *et al.* (1989) Cystic lymphangioma of the liver. Presentation of a clinical case. *Minerva Chir* 44, 1139–1141.

51 Haratake J, Koide O, Takeshita H (1992) Hepatic lymphangiomatosis: report of two cases, with an immunohistochemical study. *Am J Gastroenterol* 87, 906–909.

52 McQuown DS, Fishbein MC, Moran ET *et al.* (1975) Abdominal cystic lymphangiomatosis: report of a case involving the liver and spleen and illustration of two cases with origin in the greater omentum and root of the mesentery. *J Clin Ultrasound* 3, 291–296.

8.2.2 Neoplasms including cystadenoma

Peter Starkel and André P. Geubel

Cystadenoma and cystadenocarcinoma

Prevalence

Biliary cystadenomas are rare multiloculated cystic tumours that represent less than 5% of cystic lesions of the liver [1]. They are 100 to 200 times less frequent than simple cysts of the liver and represent 1/10 000 to 1/20 000 hepatic tumours. They occur predominantly in middle-aged women (mean age 38 years) and are considered premalignant lesions [1,2].

Aetiology, pathogenesis and pathology

Aetiology and pathogenesis are unknown. A congenital origin from abnormal intrahepatic bile ducts or from misplaced germ cells has generally been suspected. Alternatively, a pseudo-ovarian origin would better account for the mucinous epithelium that delineates the cysts. Macroscopically, a large multiloculated-appearing tumour limited by a thin wall is found (Fig. 1a). The lesions are predominantly intrahepatic, but extrahepatic localizations have been reported [3]. The tumour generally contains a mucinous fluid. At microscopy, a single layer of mucin-secreting cuboidal epithelial cells with round or oval nuclei delineates the inner space of the cysts. The epithelium is

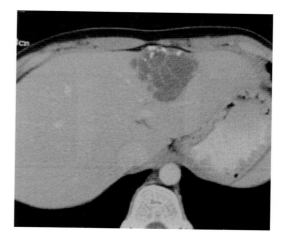

Fig. 1 Cystadenoma: tomodensitometry showing a multiloculated cystic lesion of the left lobe of the liver partly calcified in its anterior periphery. Morphological appearance of the columnar mucinous epithelium surrounded by a highly cellular mesenchymal tissue resembling ovarian stroma. Periodic acid–Schiff (PAS) mucus staining is shown in the lower right corner (see Plate 8.2.2.1, facing p. 72).

supported by a thick, cellular-rich, ovarian-like mesenchymal stroma (see Plate 8.2.2.1, facing p. 72) [4].

Clinical manifestations

Symptoms are usually related to the mass effect of the lesion and consist of intermittent abdominal discomfort, pain or swelling. Dyspepsia-like symptoms with nausea and anorexia may be encountered. A large hepatic mass can seldom be felt at abdominal examination. Signs of biliary tract obstruction may also be present.

Diagnosis

Liver function tests are usually normal. Diagnosis of cystadenoma relies on ultrasonography (US), computerized tomography (CT; Fig. 1a) and magnetic resonance imaging (MRI). At US, a large anechoic, fluid-filled globular area with irregular margins and internal echoes is seen corresponding to internal septa or papillary growths originating from the cystic wall [5]. CT shows a solitary cystic mass with a well-defined thick fibrous capsule, internal septa and mural nodules [2]. At MRI, a fluid-containing, multiloculated, septated mass is seen. Signal intensity of the content of the cysts is homogeneously low on T1-weighted images and high on T2-weighted images. Variable signal intensities on both T1- and T2-weighted images depend on the presence of solid components, haemorrhage or protein content. The portal–venous phase gadolinium-enhanced T1-weighted image shows enhancement of the capsule and septa [2]. Further imaging procedures [endoscopic retrograde cholangiopancreatography (ERCP), angiography, etc.] do not provide additional or useful information over the standard imaging techniques.

Course and complications

Cystadenomas are slow-growing tumours. Complications might result from various mass effects of the cyst that include compression of parts of the biliary tree leading to cholestasis. Intracystic haemorrhage, rupture or bacterial infections may also occur.

Cystadenomas have a clear malignant potential, and the most feared complication is transformation into cystadenocarcinoma. Malignant tumours almost exclusively arise in pre-existing cystadenomas, although rare cases of unusual origin have been reported [6,7]. Malignancy may affect the entire cyst but, more frequently, focal neoplastic transformation of the epithelium is observed. Intracystic haemorrhage in the absence of trauma, large projections protruding into the lumina of the lobules and calcification of the septa on imaging are arguments in favour of malignancy (Fig. 2a and b) [8,9]. Diagnosis of malignancy may require ultrasound-guided biopsy. Histologically, the malignant epithelium is multilayered with numerous papillary projections and dysmorphic epithelial cells invading the stroma. Cystadenocarcinoma's extension arises locally into the liver, with extrahepatic metastasis also being observed [10].

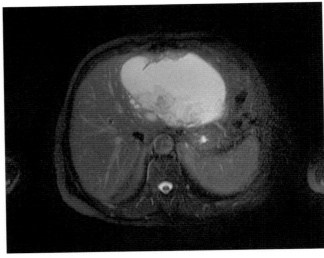

(a)

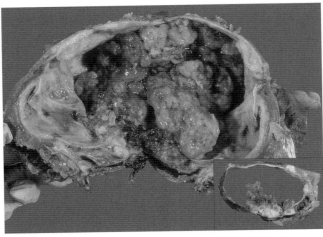

(b)

Fig. 2 Cystadenocarcinoma: T2-weighted MR image with fat suppression showing a voluminous cystic lesion in the left lobe with a heterogeneous signal at the posterior side of the lesion and a thickening of the anterior wall (a). Macroscopic appearance of the lesion together with a cut section seen in the lower right corner (b).

Differential diagnosis

Distinction between cystadenomas, simple liver cysts complicated by intracystic haemorrhage (Fig. 3) or even hydatid cysts, albeit important on clinical grounds, might be difficult. The presence of calcifications together with positive serology is a strong argument for hydatid disease. High levels of CA19-9 in a mucinous fluid obtained by percutaneous or echoendoscopic fine-needle aspiration seem to be suggestive of cystadenoma or cystadenocarcinoma and might be of help in distinguishing them from simple cysts [11,12]. The characteristics of other cystic neoplasms that may be relevant for the differential diagnosis will be discussed below.

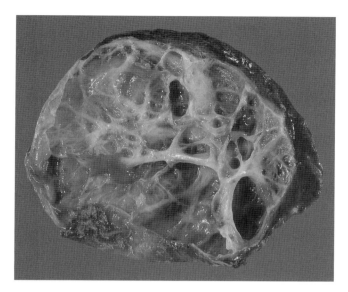

Fig. 3 Macroscopic aspect of a biliary cyst complicated by recurrent haemorrhagic episodes. Luminal scarring has the potential to induce a multiloculated appearance mimicking that of a cystadenoma (courtesy of Professor J.F. Gigot).

Treatment

When feasible, complete surgical excision, even in asymptomatic patients, is mandatory given the risk of recurrence after partial removal of the lesion and its potential for malignant transformation [13,14].

Cystic subtypes of primary liver neoplasms

Most of the primary liver neoplasms are solid lesions, and their cystic-like appearance is usually related to internal haemorrhage or necrosis following disproportionate growth.

Internal haemorrhage is the most frequent cause of a partially cystic appearance in hepatocellular adenoma. Rarely, cystic degeneration of adenomas has been reported [15].

Hepatocellular carcinoma may manifest as a partially cystic mass due to internal necrosis in large tumours or following locoregional treatment. Even in predominantly cystic tumours, the diagnosis of hepatocellular carcinoma may be suspected if CT or MRI shows features or complications suggestive of underlying liver cirrhosis. In addition, the presence of an encapsulated tumour with hypervascular solid parts on CT or MRI reinforces the diagnosis of hepatocellular carcinoma [2], especially when associated with elevated serum α-fetoprotein levels. Central cystic degeneration or extensive necrosis may result in a cyst-like presentation of giant cavernous haemangioma, the nature of which is generally easily recognized on CT and/or MRI. On contrast-enhanced imaging, their characteristic peripheral nodular enhancement together with a non-enhancing central cystic area is suggestive of the diagnosis [16,17].

Cystic metastases

Metastases to the liver are common, and some may exhibit a complete or partial cystic appearance. Rapid growth of hypervascular metastatic tumours leading to necrosis and cystic degeneration is frequently implicated in the cystic pattern of liver metastases from sarcoma, melanoma, lung and breast carcinoma. Contrast-enhanced CT and MRI usually demonstrate multiple, irregularly defined lesions with a strong enhancement of the peripheral viable tissue [18]. As the radiological picture is not specific for a particular primary tumour, the clinical circumstances and the determination of serum tumour markers such as carcinoembryonic antigen (CEA), CA15-3 and neuron-specific enolase (NSE) are useful in guiding additional diagnostic procedures.

The same pathophysiological mechanism and radiological appearances apply to cystic neuroendocrine tumours, particularly those of large size. However, in some instances, neoplasms may mimic benign cysts by their clinical and radiological appearances. In this particular situation, the various imaging modalities are rarely helpful in distinguishing between benign or neoplastic cysts [19]. If malignancy can be neither confirmed nor invalidated by standard diagnostic procedures including the neuroendocrine tumour markers chromogranin and NSE, a biopsy of the cyst wall for histological examination may be required to obtain a definite diagnosis.

Metastatic colorectal adenocarcinomas spread preferentially into the liver through the bloodstream and may present as intra-parenchymal cystic metastases as a result of their mucinous secretions (Fig. 4) [20]. Their radiological appearances are similar to those of other cystic metastases. In contrast, cystic metastases originating from ovarian adenocarcinoma usually present as cystic serosal implants on both the peritoneal surface of the liver and the parietal peritoneum, as they spread predominantly by peritoneal seeding [2,21].

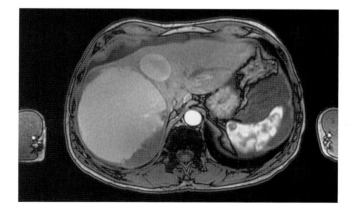

Fig. 4 Cystic metastases of the liver (adenocarcinoma of the colon): T1-weighted MR image with contrast injection showing two cystic lesions of the right lobe with a spontaneous hyperintense signal resulting from their high mucinous content. There is parietal thickening of the posterior wall of the largest lesion (courtesy of Professor B. Van Beers).

Miscellaneous and rare conditions

Neoplastic degeneration to squamous cell carcinoma has been described for solitary benign hepatic cysts. The tumour usually arises from metaplastic foci in pre-existing liver cysts that subsequently undergo neoplastic transformation [22].

Some rare forms of cholangiocarcinoma may present with a cyst-like appearance. Mucinous cholangiocarcinoma results from mucin production by adenocarcinoma cells that leads to the formation of multiple microcysts assembled in a honeycomb-like pattern [23]. Coexistence of solid cholangiocarcinoma with developmental liver cysts has also been reported. Whether this tumour arises directly from initially non-neoplastic cysts with atrophic epithelium and dysplastic changes remains unclear [24].

Although Von Meyenburg complexes are generally considered to be innocuous, their neoplastic transformation into cholangiocarcinoma has been described. Pathophysiology might involve a progressive transition through hyperplasia or adenomatous transformation. Several case reports in the literature describe a profoundly disturbed hepatic environment with extensive liver fibrosis and portal hypertension that might have contributed to neoplastic transformation [25].

Undifferentiated embryonal sarcoma is a rare malignant hepatic tumour that develops in older children, adolescents and, exceptionally, in young adults. At imaging, a large, solitary cystic mass is found with well-defined borders and, occasionally, a pseudocapsule. Given the high water content of the myxoid stroma of this tumour, hypointense signal on T1- and hyperintense signal on T2-weighted images are demonstrated in large portions of the tumoral tissue on MRI. Signs of intratumoral haemorrhage and a heterogeneous enhancement of the peripheral, solid parts of the mass may be present on contrast-enhanced CT or MRI [2].

References

1 Buetow PC, Midkiff RB (1997) Primary malignant neoplasms in the adult. *Magn Reson Imaging Clin N Am* 5, 289–318.
2 Mortelé KJ, Ros PR (2001) Cystic focal lesions in the adult: differential CT and MR imaging features. *Radiographics* 21, 895–910.
3 Palacios E, Shannon M, Solomon C et al. (1990) Biliary cystadenoma: ultrasound, CT and MRI. *Gastrointest Radiol* 15, 313–316.
4 Devaney K, Goodman ZD, Ishak KG (1994) Hepatobiliary cystadenoma and cystadenocarcinoma. A light microscopic and immunohistochemical study of 70 patients. *Am J Surg Pathol* 18, 1078–1091.
5 Forrest ME, Cho KJ, Shields JJ et al. (1980) Biliary cystadenomas: sonographic-angiographic-pathologic correlations. *Am J Roentgenol* 135, 723–727.
6 Devine P, Ucci AA (1985) Biliary cystadenocarcinoma arising in a congenital cyst. *Hum Pathol* 16, 92–94.
7 Horsmans Y, Laka A, van Beers BE et al. (1997) Hepatobiliary cystadenocarcinoma without ovarian stroma and normal CA19-9 levels. Unusually prolonged evolution. *Dig Dis Sci* 42, 1406–1408.
8 Stanley J, Vujic I, Schabel SI et al. (1983) Evaluation of biliary cystadenoma and cystadenocarcinoma. *Gastrointest Radiol* 8, 245–248.

9 Korobkin M, Stephen DH, Lee JK et al. (1989) Biliary cystadenoma and cystadenocarcinoma: CT and sonographic findings *Am J Roentgenol* 153, 507–511.
10 Iemoto Y, Kondo Y, Nakano T et al. (1983) Biliary cystadenocarcinoma diagnosed by liver biopsy performed under ultrasonographic guidance. *Gastroenterology* 84, 399–403.
11 Horsmans Y, Laka A, Gigot JF et al. (1996) Serum and cystic fluid CA19-9 determinations as a diagnostic help in liver cysts of uncertain nature. *Liver* 16, 255–257.
12 Bonnet S, Béchade D, Palazzo L et al. (2005) Ponction sous échoendoscopie d'un cystadénome hépatique. *Gastroenterol Clin Biol* 29, 607–609.
13 Lewis WD, Jenkins RL, Rossi RL et al. (1988) Surgical treatment of biliary cystadenoma. A report of 15 cases. *Arch Surg* 123, 563–568.
14 Kim J, Choi J, Park Y et al. (1998) Biliary cystadenoma of the liver. *Hepatobiliary Pancreat Surg* 5, 348–352.
15 Kobayashi M, Enzan H, Araki K et al. (1999) Spontaneous hepatocellular adenoma with marked cystic degeneration. *Hepatogastroenterology* 46, 2955–2958.
16 Vilgrain V, Boulos L, Vullierme MP et al. (2000) Imaging of atypical hemangiomas of the liver with pathologic correlation. *Radiographics* 20, 379–397.
17 Semelka RC, Sofka CM (1997) Hepatic hemangiomas. *Magn Reson Imaging Clin N Am* 5, 241–253.
18 Lewis KH, Chezmar JL (1997) Hepatic metastases. *Magn Reson Imaging Clin N Am* 5, 319–330.
19 Thompson NW, Eckhauser FE, Vinik AI et al. (1984) Cystic neuroendocrine neoplasms of the pancreas and liver. *Ann Surg* 199, 158–164.
20 Sugawara Y, Yamamoto J, Yamasaki S et al. (2000) Cystic liver metastases from colorectal cancer. *J Surg Oncol* 74, 148–152.
21 Lundstedt C, Holmin T, Thorvinger B (1992) Peritoneal ovarian metastases simulating liver parenchymal masses. *Gastrointest Radiol* 17, 250–252.
22 Monteagudo M, Vidal G, Moreno M et al. (1998) Squamous cell carcinoma and infection in a solitary hepatic cyst. *Eur J Gastroenterol Hepatol* 10, 1051–1053.
23 Sonobe H, Enzan H, Ido E et al. (1995) Mucinous cholangiocarcinoma featuring a unique microcystic appearance. *Pathol Int* 45, 292–296.
24 Azizah N, Paradinas FJ (1980) Cholangiocarcinoma coexisting with developmental liver cysts: a distinct entity different from liver cystadenocarcinoma. *Histopathology* 4, 391–400.
25 Jain D, Sarode VR, Abdul-Karim FW et al. (2000) Evidence for the neoplastic transformation of von-Meyenburg complexes. *Am J Surg Pathol* 24, 1131–1139.

8.2.3 Posttraumatic cystic diseases

Jean-François Cadranel

Biloma

Biloma is an abnormal fluid collection that can be intrahepatic or perihepatic [1,2]. Biloma results from rupture of the biliary system, which can be spontaneous, iatrogenic following surgery or interventional procedures or traumatic [1–3]. Extravasation of bile into the liver parenchyma generates an intense inflammatory reaction, thus inducing the formation of a well-defined pseudocapsule [1–3]. Clinical manifestations depend on the location and size of the biloma [2,3]. Ultrasonography revealed an anechoic well-defined collection [1]. It is usually located in the right hypochondrium near the hepatic pedicle or gallbladder [1]. On both computerized tomography (CT) and magnetic resonance imaging (MRI), a biloma appears as a well-defined or slightly irregular cystic mass without septa or calcifications [2,3]. Also, the pseudocapsule is usually not readily identifiable [2,3]. This imaging appearance, in combination with the clinical history and location, should enable a correct diagnosis [2]. Puncture of the collection showed a high level of bilirubin concentration allowing for the biliary nature of the collection [3]. Owing to potential injury to the peritoneum, biloma should be evacuated [1].

Haematoma

Posttraumatic haematoma are unusual sequelae of hepatic trauma [2,4–6]. Symptomatic manifestations depend on the severity of the bleeding, the location and the time frame during which the haemorrhage occurred [2].

Cystic transformation of hepatic haematoma is usual after hepatic trauma. It can be located either subcapsulac or in the parenchyma [1]. Imaging pattern depends on the cause of the bleeding and the lag time [1,2]. In an acute or subacute setting, haematic collection is heterogeneous on ultrasonography and is followed by an anechoic pattern [1]. On CT, during the acute or subacute phases, haemorrhage has a higher attenuation value than pure fluid due to the presence of aggregated fibrin components [7]. In the chronic phase, a haematoma has attenuation identical to that of pure fluid [2]. On MRI, the aspect is variable according to the lag time between the traumatic event and the imaging procedure.

High signal intensity on T1-weighted images is highly suggestive of the haematic nature of the collection [1]. Margins are usually irregular [1]. Coexistent features such as hepatic lacerations, rib fractures or perihepatic fluid may be present [2]. Owing to the paramagnetic effect of methaemoglobin, MRI is even more suitable than CT for the detection and characterization of haemorrhage [2]. Diagnosis of hepatic haematoma is based on the history of trauma, surgery or radiological intervention [1,6].

References

1 Vilgrain V (2001) Cystic lesions of the liver. *Gastroenterol Clin Biol* 25, B167–B177.
2 Mortele KJ, Ros PR (2001) Cystic focal liver lesions in the adult: differential CT and MR imaging features. *Radiographics* 21, 895–910.
3 Murphy BJ, Cassillas J, Ros PR *et al.* (1989) The CT appearance of cystic masses of the liver. *Radiographics* 9, 307–322.
4 Ratan SK, Bhandar I, Grover S *et al.* (1999) Post-traumatic hepatic cyst. *Ind Pediatr* 36, 1048–1051.
5 Sugimoto T, Yoshioko T, Sawada Y *et al.* (1982) Post traumatic cyst of the liver found on CT-scan. A new concept. *J Trauma* 22, 797–800.
6 Chuang JH, Huang SC (1996) Post traumatic hepatic cyst. An unusual sequel of liver injury in the era of imaging. *J Pediatr Surg* 31:272–274.
7 Merrine D, Fishman EK, Zerhoumi EA (1988) Spontaneous hepatic hemorrhage: clinical and CT findings. *J Comput Assist Tomogr* 12, 397–400.

9 Viral infections of the liver

9.1 Viral hepatitis

9.1.1 Viral hepatitis

Mario Rizzetto and Fabien Zoulim

Although many viruses can affect liver function and morphology indirectly as a result of systemic infections, only a minority are truly hepatotropic, that is infectious to the liver itself, producing hepatitis as the major clinical manifestation. The term 'viral hepatitis' refers to disease caused by this subgroup.

Historical background and nomenclature

Although viral hepatitis is a disease of antiquity, and epidemic jaundice is mentioned in the Talmud, the infectious nature of the disease was not recognized until the end of the nineteenth century.

The first description of 'hepatitis B' dates back to 1885 when Lürman, a public health officer in Bremen, Germany, gave a detailed report of an outbreak of jaundice that developed among workers at a local company vaccinated against smallpox with glycerinized human serum [1].

Transmission studies in human volunteers in the late 1930s and during the Second World War provided the first information about the infectivity, mode of transmission and properties of the hepatitis agents; they suggested that two distinct viral agents, lacking cross-immunity, were responsible for military outbreaks, and MacCallum introduced the classic terminology of hepatitis A virus (HAV) and hepatitis B virus (HBV) [2].

Faeces were shown to induce hepatitis A (infectious hepatitis) by the oral route; the incubation period was 15–30 days. Acute-phase serum was shown to induce hepatitis B (serum hepatitis), after several months, when given by the parenteral route.

Transmission studies in humans by Krugman and associates in the late 1950s and early 1960s, using the newly discovered assays for serum transaminases, contributed significantly to the understanding of the characteristics of the two hepatitis 'viruses' (identified by Krugman as the MS1 strain, causing hepatitis A, and the MS2 strain, causing hepatitis B) [3].

The discovery of the Australia antigen, now called hepatitis B surface antigen (HBsAg), by Blumberg and his associates in the mid-1960s [4], and the recognition by Prince [5] of its specific relation to hepatitis B, started the contemporary era in the field of hepatitis. Intensive research quickly led to the identification of the hepatitis B virion [6], to the recognition of its antigenic and genomic complexity [7] and oncogenic potential and, later, to the development of a safe and effective vaccine [8]. The lessons learned from work on hepatitis B helped in the rapid discovery of HAV. Using an immunoelectron microscopic technique, previously applied to reveal the nucleocapsid of HBV, Feinstone and associates identified the HAV in 1973 in immunocomplexes from faeces to which serum of a patient convalescent from hepatitis A had been added [9]. Then, in 1977, a discrepancy in immunofluorescence testing for HBV antigens in the liver led Rizzetto and associates to the discovery of the delta antigen [10], which was subsequently shown to be related to a new RNA virus designated the hepatitis delta virus (HDV).

When testing for hepatitis A and B was made generally available, it became clear that the two viruses did not explain all causes of viral hepatitis, as many patients lacked markers of either infection. Thus, the concept emerged in the 1980s of a new variant of viral hepatitis, which was called 'non-A, non-B hepatitis' to highlight the fact that the diagnosis was based on exclusion criteria, not on specific positive evidence [11]. The magnitude of the problem was best seen in relation to blood transfusion: in the wake of the widespread and increasing application of blood transfusion and plasma substitution, hepatitis continued to occur in 5–10% of the recipients of blood products, despite almost total control of HBV.

However, efforts to identify the major aetiological agent of endemic non-A, non-B hepatitis met with failure or with spurious results until 1989. The breakthrough resulted from exhaustive research involving the use of sophisticated technological methods. Several thousand clones of genetic material from a serum containing a putative agent of non-A, non-B hepatitis were systematically analysed by Houghton and associates [12], who ultimately identified a clone that met the criteria for being a new viral genome and provided the key to the characterization of the hepatitis C virus (HCV), alias transfusion-transmitted non-A, non-B virus. Meanwhile, a novel agent responsible for enterically transmitted outbreaks of epidemic non-A, non-B hepatitis in tropical and subtropical areas and named the hepatitis E virus (HEV) had been identified in the early 1980s by epidemiological analysis and human transmission studies [13].

The five viruses recognized by the end of the 1980s account for the great majority of viral hepatitides occurring at temperate latitudes. Since then, several new viruses, named the F, GB/HG, TT and SEN viruses, have been proposed as hepatitides agents, raising the hope that they might fill the remaining nosological gap. However, extensive scrutiny has failed to demonstrate that these agents play a causal role in acute or chronic liver disease, and they have not entered the differential diagnosis of viral liver disorders.

The enterically transmitted hepatitis F virus (HFV), described in 1994 [14] and thought to be responsible for sporadic non-A, non-E hepatitis, was probably a ubiquitous non-pathogenic intestinal resident that colonizes stools during liver injury.

The GB virus [15] C subtype and hepatitis G virus (HGV) [16] are a similar RNA flavivirus that is transmitted by blood transfusions; its prevalence is therefore high among groups with frequent parenteral exposures.

The TT virus (TTV) belongs to a large and heterogeneous DNA virus family classified as Circoviridae [17]; it shares a commensal non-pathogenic relationship with humans, is transmitted by parenteral routes and is prevalent in multiply-transfused subjects and in populations in Africa and South America.

The SEN virus (SENV), of which A–H variants have been described, was discovered using degenerate TTV primers; it shares properties with the latter, but is classified separately within the Circoviridae. It is transmitted by transfusion and probably by non-parenteral routes; its prevalence is high (20%) in healthy persons in Japan.

While the puzzle of the existence, if any, of other hepatitis viruses remains unresolved, the perspectives for the treatment of HBV and HCV disease have greatly increased in recent years. The advent of interferon in the mid-1980s [19] has provided the first valid, although limited, therapeutic panacea for all forms of chronic viral hepatitis. At the beginning of the third millennium, the combination of ribavirin with interferon and the advent of slow-release pegylated interferons have led to a significant improvement in the rate of HCV cure, while the tumultuous discovery of new synthetic antivirals is leading to better control of hepatitis B with better tolerance and less long-term resistance to the drugs. In parallel, the worldwide expansion of liver transplantation is offering a valid option for endstage cirrhotic disease with a risk of reinfection that has dramatically diminished for hepatitis B.

Further hope rests with the development of new treatments for hepatitis C based on protease and polymerase inhibitors, several of which are currently under clinical study.

While treatment strategies evolve and therapy is progressing from primarily treating a liver disease to the targeting of the viral disease via direct antiviral therapy, the worldwide implementation of the HBV vaccine represents the cornerstone for the global control of hepatitis B, and the development of a HCV vaccine remains the challenge for the next decade.

References

1 Lurman A (1885) Eine Icterusepidemie. *Berliner Klin Wochensch* 22, 20–23.

2 MacCallum FO (1947) Homologous serum jaundice. *Lancet* 2, 691–692.

3 Krugman S, Giles JP, Hammond J (1967) Infectious hepatitis: evidence for two distinctive clinical, epidemiological and immunological types of infection. *JAMA* 200, 365–373.

4 Blumberg BS, Gerstley BJS, Hungerford DA *et al.* (1967) A serum antigen (Australia antigen) in Down's syndrome, leukemia, and hepatitis. *Ann Intern Med* 66, 924–931.

5 Prince AM (1968) An antigen detected in the blood during the incubation period of serum hepatitis. *Proc Natl Acad Sci USA* 60, 814–821.

6 Dane DS, Cameron CH, Briggs M (1970) Virus-like particles in serum of patients with Australia-antigen-associated hepatitis. *Lancet* 1, 695–698.

7 Tiollais P, Charnay P, Vyas GN (1981) Biology of hepatitis B virus. *Science* 213, 406–411.

8 Szmuness W, Stevens CE, Harley EJ *et al.* (1980) Hepatitis B vaccine: demonstration of efficacy in a controlled clinical trial in a high-risk population in the United States. *N Engl J Med* 303, 833–841.

9 Feinstone SM, Kapikian AZ, Purcell RH (1973) Hepatitis A: detection by immune electron microscopy of a viruslike antigen associated with acute illness. *Science* 182, 1026–1028.

10 Rizzetto M, Canese MG, Aricò S *et al.* (1977) Immunofluorescence detection of new antigen-antibody system (delta/anti-delta) associated to hepatitis B virus in liver and in serum of HBsAg carriers. *Gut* 18, 997–1003.

11 Alter HJ, Purcell RH, Holland PV *et al.* (1975) Clinical and serological analysis of transfusion-associated hepatitis. *Lancet* 2, 838–841.

12 Choo Q-L, Kuo G, Weiner AJ *et al.* (1989) Isolation of a cDNA clone derived from a blood-borne non-A, non-B viral hepatitis genome. *Science* 244, 359–362.

13 Khuroo MS (1980) Study of an epidemic of non-A, non-B hepatitis. Possibility of another human hepatitis virus distinct from post-transfusion non-A, non-B type. *Am J Med* 68, 818–824.

14 Pillot J, Meng J, Maillard P *et al.* (1997) The "presumed" hepatitis F virus. In: Rizzetto M, Purcell RH, Gerin JL *et al.* (eds) *Viral Hepatitis and Liver Diseases*. Turin: Minerva Medica, pp. 399–401.

15 Simons JN, Leary TP, Dawson GJ *et al.* (1995) Isolation of novel virus-like sequences associated with human hepatitis. *Nature Med* 1, 564–569.

16 Linnen J, Wages J Jr, Zhang-Keck ZY *et al.* (1996) Molecular cloning and disease association of hepatitis G virus: a transfusion-transmissible agent. *Science* 271, 505–508.

17 Mushahwar IK, Erker JC, Muerhoff AS *et al.* (1999) Molecular and biophysical characterization of TT virus: evidence for a new virus family infecting humans. *Proc Natl Acad Sci USA* 96, 3177–3182.

18 Tanaka Y, Primi D, Wang RYH *et al.* (2001) Genomic and molecular evolutionary analysis of a newly identified infectious agent (SEN virus) and its relationship to the TT virus family. *J Infect Dis* 183, 359–367.

19 Hoofnagle JH, Mullen KD, Jones DB *et al.* (1986) Treatment of chronic non-A, non-B hepatitis with recombinant human alpha interferon. A preliminary report. *N Engl J Med* 315, 1575–1578.

9.1.2 The viruses of hepatitis

9.1.2.i Structure, replication and laboratory diagnosis of hepatitis B virus and hepatitis D virus

Stephan Schaefer and Wolfram H. Gerlich

Introduction

The stepwise discovery of hepatitis B virus (HBV) began with a serum antigen that was first detected in an Australian aborigine during genetic studies on serum protein polymorphisms. 'Australia antigen' was located on 20-nm large spherical lipoprotein particles. After several years, it was recognized that Australia antigen was not a genetic marker but an antigen acquired after infection with hepatitis type B. Australia antigen particles did not contain nucleic acid and were thus considered for a while to be an unconventional infectious agent like prions. However, in addition to the 20-nm particles, 42-nm large, double-shelled particles, known as Dane particles, were detected in sera from hepatitis B patients that carried Australia antigen on their surface and resembled viruses (Fig. 1). Soon afterwards, Robinson and coworkers detected an endogenous DNA polymerase within the Dane particles and, finally, a small circular DNA. Almeida and coworkers [1] released the core particles from the Dane particles using detergent, and were able to form immune complexes of these particles with antibodies from hepatitis B convalescents. These findings showed that Dane particles were the agent of hepatitis B with two antigen moieties: Australia antigen, which was renamed hepatitis B surface antigen (HBsAg), and hepatitis B core antigen (HBcAg). A third, non-structural HBV antigen in the serum of highly viraemic virus carriers was named HBeAg, in which 'e' has no specific meaning. Cloning, sequencing and expression of the DNA extracted from Dane particles allowed the identification of the viral genes. Since the early 1970s, the development of serological assays for the HBsAg helped to diagnose hepatitis B reliably and to screen for asymptomatic, but infectious, HBV carriers among blood and organ donors. Antibodies against HBcAg (anti-HBc) are present during the acute phase of hepatitis B and thereafter, but they do not protect against HBV. Antibodies against HBsAg (anti-HBs) are formed at resolution of acute hepatitis B and protect against infection. This observation opened the way to use HBsAg from virus carrier plasma as a vaccine against HBV. Later, the HBsAg was produced safely and in unlimited amounts in yeast cells transformed with the HBsAg gene. As HBV is the major cause of hepatocellular carcinoma, purified HBsAg serves as the first human antitumour vaccine with proven efficacy.

Two other hepatitis viruses (HCV and HDV) are also transmitted parenterally. Hepatitis D virus (HDV) was identified as an infectious agent that encoded delta antigen before the discovery of hepatitis C virus (HCV). Delta antigen was initially considered to be a new variant of HBV antigens, but it is the nucleoprotein of a completely different defective RNA virus that depends on envelopment by the HBV surface proteins.

Structure of HBV (Fig. 2)

HBV is enveloped and contains within its icosahedral core the viral DNA genome with a length varying from 3185 to 3248 basepairs (bp) depending on the HBV genotype (Table 1). Electron microscopy of negatively stained virions shows particles with a diameter of 42 nm but, in the hydrated state, the outer diameter is about 50 nm. The envelope of the virus is made up of an estimated 370–400 molecules of membrane-spanning HBV surface proteins, 160–200 of which show surface projections [2,3].

Taxonomy

HBV belongs to the family of Hepadnaviridae, which is made up of two genera [4,5]. The genus Avihepadnavirus is found

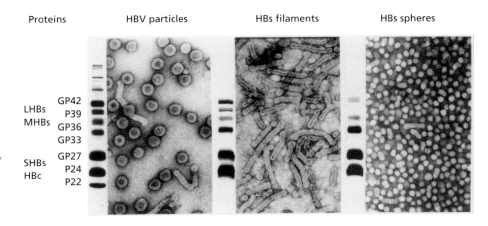

Fig. 1 HBV-associated particles purified from the plasma of a highly viraemic persistent HBV carrier. Electron micrographs and protein patterns in silver-stained gels after separation by denaturing sodium dodecyl sulphate (SDS) gel electrophoresis.

Proteins   HBV particles   HBs filaments   HBs spheres

LHBs   GP42 / P39
MHBs   GP36 / GP33
SHBs   GP27 / P24
HBc   P22

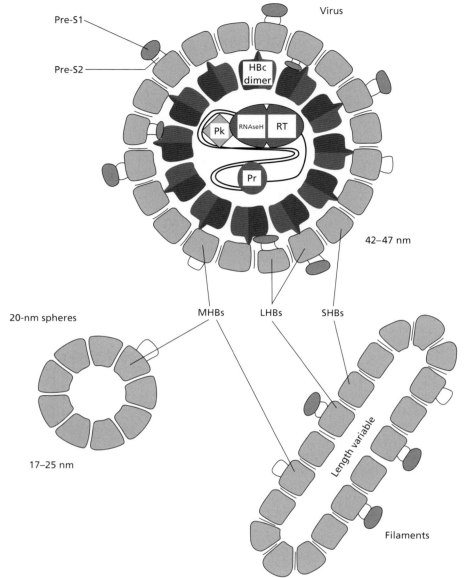

Fig. 2 Schematic model of HBV particles and subviral HBsAg particles. Pk, protein kinase; RT, reverse transcriptase; Pr, priming (or terminal) domain of the polymerase; L-, M-, SHBs, large, middle and small HBs protein with their domains, pre-S1, pre-S2.

in birds, and Orthohepadnavirus (Fig. 3) in mammals. Orthohepadnaviruses have been detected in rodents, the new world woolly monkey, in apes and in man [6,7].

Human HBV is subdivided into eight genotypes, called A–H, that differ by more than 8% from each other [8–10] (Fig. 3). HBV isolates found in apes form additional HBV genotypes in phylogenetic analyses and have been named HBVcpz, -oru, -gor and -gbn for their respective hosts chimpanzee, orang-utan, gorilla and gibbon (Fig. 3) [11].

HBV genotypes can be further subdivided into subgenotypes (Table 2), which differ by at least 4% from each other [12,13]. In HBV genotypes A, B and C, epidemiological data show that the respective subgenotype pairs A1/A2, B1/B2 [14] and C1/C2 [15–17] differ substantially in many virological, and probably

some clinical, parameters. Subgenotypes also show distinct geographic distribution (Fig. 4).

Hepadnaviruses replicate their genome via reverse transcription of a pregenomic (pg) RNA. Thus, in spite of being DNA viruses, they share many features with retroviruses, including sensitivity to certain human immunodeficiency virus (HIV) drugs.

HBV DNA

The DNA encapsidated in the mature virion has an unusual structure (Fig. 5a). The two DNA strands are linear but, because of 5′ terminal overlaps of 234 bases, the genomic DNA acquires a relaxed circular (rc) form. The strand encoding the viral

Table 1 Genotype, genome length and differences of HBV genotypes.

Genotype	Genome length (bp)	ORF differences
A	3221	Insertion of aa 153 and 154 in HBc
B	3215	
C	3215	
D	3182	Deletion of aa 1–11 in pre-S1
E	3212	Deletion of aa 11 in pre-S1
F	3215	
G	3248	Insertion of 12 aa in HBc Deletion of aa 11 in pre-S1
H	3215	

Bp, basepair; ORF, open reading frame; aa, amino acid.
The normal length of the HBV genome seems to be 3215 bp. Differences in genome length arise from deletions of 33 nucleotides (nt) (genotype D) or insertions of 6 nt (genotype A) or 33 nt (genotype G) in different parts of the genome.

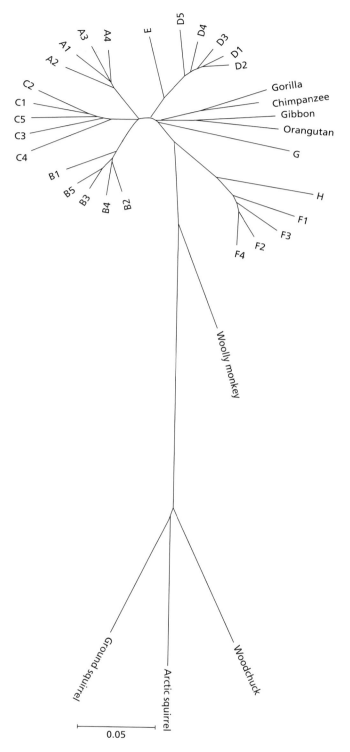

Fig. 3 Phylogenetic tree of complete orthohepadnaviral genomes. For human HBV sequences, only the designation of the subgenotype, e.g. A1, is indicated. For hepadnaviral genomes obtained from rodents or apes, the name of the host is given. The alignment of complete sequences was performed with Clustal W in the program DNAstar. The alignment was further analysed by bootstrapping using the neighbourhood-joining method contained in MEGA version 2.1 [153].

proteins is termed the minus strand because the mRNA transcribed from it is, by definition, plus stranded. The 5′ end of the minus strand is covalently linked via a phosphodiester bridge to the hydroxyl group of tyrosine 63 in the terminal protein domain of the polymerase protein. The 5′ end of the DNA plus strand is formed by the residual 18 bases of the pg RNA. In contrast to the minus strand, the plus strand is incomplete, leaving a single-stranded gap of several hundred up to 1500 bases. The rc DNA contains various elements required for replication, such as direct repeats DR1 and DR2, a short 3′ and 5′ terminal 9-bp redundancy r in the minus strand and sequence elements 5E, 3E and M for circularization. The covalently closed form of the DNA (Fig. 5b) is the template for transcription of the viral mRNAs. It encodes four conserved open reading frames: core (C), surface (pre-S1, pre-S2, S), X and pol. There are two enhancers (Enh I and II), four promoters (P), a negative regulatory element (NRE) and a glucocorticoid-responsive element (GRE).

Hepatitis B virus core protein

Most HBV genotypes code for a core protein (HBc) with 183 amino acids (aa) (185 aa for genotype A) [18]. The four C-terminal arginine-rich clusters bind the encapsidated viral nucleic acids. HBc forms dimers that are linked by cystine bridges after release from the reducing environment of the cytosol. During replication, core particles package a complex containing the viral pg RNA, the viral DNA polymerase, a cellular protein kinase and cellular chaperones. The interaction of the pg RNA with the basic arginine-rich clusters of HBc enhances assembly. However, HBc dimers may combine at high concentrations into trimers and assemble spontaneously into capsids even in the absence of other viral components [19]. Capsids are found in two populations of icosahedral particles with a T = 3

Table 2 HBV subgenotypes and geographical prevalence.

	Subgenotype	Synonyms	Geographical origin	References
A	A1	Aa, A′	Africa, (Asia, South America)	[122,154]
	A2	Ae, A–A′	Europe	
	A3	Ac	Gabon, Cameroon	[155,156]
	A4		Mali	[157]
	(A5)[a]		Nigeria	[157]
B	B1	Bj	Japan	[24,128]
	B2	Ba	Asia without Japan	
	B3		Indonesia, Philippines	[12]
	B4		Vietnam	[12]
	B5		Philippines	[158,159]
C	C1	Cs	South-east Asia (Vietnam, Myanmar, Thailand, southern China)	[15–17]
	C2	Ce	Far East (Korea, Japan, northern China)	
	C3		Micronesia	[12]
	C4		Australia	[160]
	C5		Philippines, Vietnam	[159,161]
D	D1		Mongolia, Europe	
	D2		India	
	D3		South Africa, East India, Europe, Serbia	[154,162]
	D4		Australia	[160]
	D5		East India	[162]
F	F1		South and Central America	[163,164]
	F2		South America	
	F3		Bolivia	[165,166]
	F4		Argentina	[165,166]

[a]No complete sequence available.

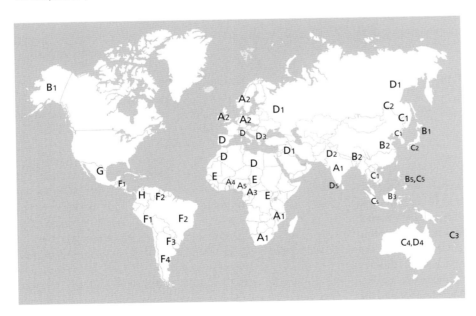

Fig. 4 Geographical distribution of HBV genotypes and subgenotypes. Modified from ref. 5.

and/or a T = 4 symmetry, having 180 or 240 subunits and a diameter of 32 or 36 nm respectively.

The immunodominant epitope of HBc has been mapped to residues 78–83 and requires the conformation of native core particles. Residues 78–83 are on the tip of the spikes that protrude from the capsid shell [20]. These spikes are four-helix bundles formed by the pairing of helix–turn–helix motifs from two subunits of the HBc dimer. Using monoclonal antibodies,

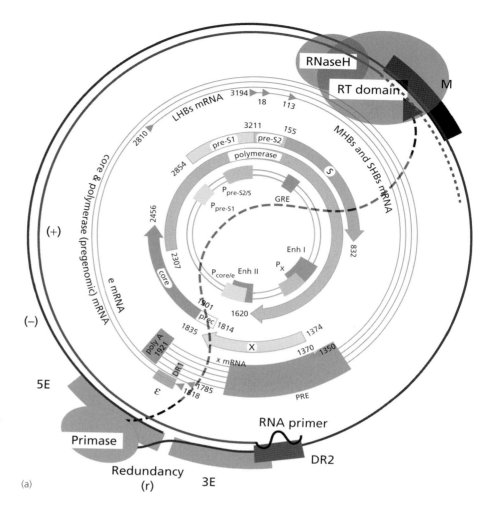

Fig. 5 Genome elements of HBV. (a) Virion-encapsidated DNA structure. M, 5E and 3E are sequence elements required for circularization of the genome. The priming (or terminal) domain of the polymerase is linked with the reverse transcription domain by the tether domain (broken line).

(a)

four or more possible epitopes were mapped on HBc capsids [21].

HBe protein

The nature of HBe protein remained enigmatic until 1982 when recombinant HBc particles, devoid of any other viral component, were converted into HBeAg by treatment with protease and ionic detergents. The reading frames and, hence, the immunological epitopes at T-cell level of HBc and HBeAg are almost identical. However, HBcAg and HBeAg are recognized distinctly by antibodies. An in-frame start codon upstream of the HBc start site results in a version of HBc with an extra 29 N-terminal amino acids. This additional 'precore' sequence serves as a signal peptide that directs the nascent peptide into the secretory pathway. After N-terminal cleavage by the signal peptidase at amino acid 19 [22], 10 amino acids of the precore sequence remain and interfere with the assembly of the core protein [23]. C-terminal cleavage at position 149 results in mature HBe, which is secreted into the bloodstream.

The function of HBeAg is not completely clear. The HBV genomes of many chronic HBV carriers harbour variants that prevent expression of HBeAg. HBe-negative HBV is infectious and has been associated with a fulminant course of hepatitis. While HBe-negative genomes replicate about 10-fold faster *in vitro*, patients with HBe-negative hepatitis B usually have lower concentrations of HBV DNA in serum compared with wild-type (wt) infections.

Evidence for the importance of HBeAg comes from HBV genotype G infection. Only HBV genotype G wt is unable to express HBeAg. But this may be compensated by the fact that genotype G is usually found together with other HBeAg-expressing HBV genotypes [24], although one case of transient low-level monoinfection has been described [25].

Apart from HBV genotype G, HBeAg is conserved in all hepadnaviruses including the avihepadnaviruses. This suggests that it provides an advantage for the survival and spread of the virus. Experimental infection of newborn woodchucks with an HBeAg-negative mutant led to acute but not chronic infection. Thus, HBeAg may suppress immune elimination of HBV and

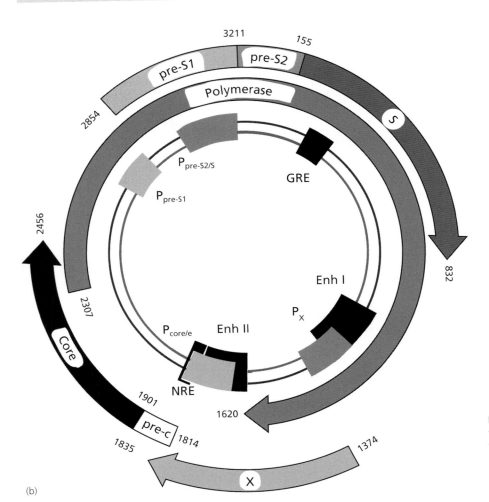

Fig. 5 (b) Open reading frames and transcription regulating elements in the ccc form of HBV DNA. P, promoter; NRE, negative regulatory element active in non-hepatic cells; GRE, glucocorticoid-responsive element. Numbering starts at the *Eco*RI site.

(b)

contribute to the development of the carrier state in newborns [26]. HBeAg accomplishes this by downregulating the host T-cell response to the nucleocapsid antigens via a variety of tolerance-inducing mechanisms [27].

Hepatitis B virus X protein

Hepatitis B virus X protein (HBx) is a viral regulatory protein with pleiotropic biochemical actions [28–34]. The HBx open reading frame (ORF) is conserved in all hepadnaviral species including avihepadnaviruses [35]. HBx protein is translated into a protein of 154 aa, with a short half-life of 30–120 min [36]. The concentration of X protein is low with $4–8 \times 10^4$ molecules per cell in the livers of infected woodchucks. Quantitative expression data for HBx in natural human infection are not available. However, the detection of HBx with a mainly cytoplasmic localization is possible by immunofluorescence in all stages of chronic HBV infection [37]. HBx has also been found in the nucleus of transfected cells.

HBx functions *in vitro* are:

- transactivation of a plethora of cellular and viral promoters;
- promiscuous binding to a multitude of cellular and viral proteins;
- interference with cellular DNA repair;
- inhibition of the cellular proteasome complex;
- positive and negative enhancement of regulated cell death;
- cofactor in tumour formation in HBx transgenic mice;
- malignant transformation of several cell lines.

In vitro, HBx is not essential, but increases virus production about 10-fold [38–40]. However, X-deficient genomes from the woodchuck HBV did not induce infection in animal experiments. Other studies showed that X-deficient genomes were not totally incapable of replication in woodchucks, but induced protective immunity against challenge with wt virus after low-level replication [41].

The activation of viral and cellular promoters by HBx as well as activation of viral replication appears to be mediated by an increased activity of cellular signalling cascades in the cytoplasm (for reviews, see refs 30,32). Activation of ras–raf signalling cascades [42] by tyrosine kinases, such as src or FAK (focal adhesion kinase) [30,43], with or without calcium release seems to

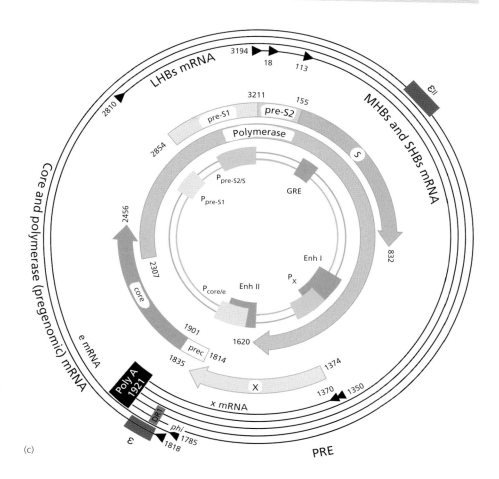

Fig. 5 (c) Elements of HBV mRNAs governing processing and reverse transcription. ε, encapsidation signal; ε II, phi, cofactors required for genome maturation; DR1, direct repeat 1; PRE, posttranscriptional regulatory element; poly A, polyadenylation site.

(c)

play a key role (for reviews, see refs 30,32). An important finding is that HBx regulates the phosphorylation of HBV capsids during replication [44]. Depending on the cell type, HBx has both proapoptotic and antiapoptotic activities [29,33] that are largely mediated by the transcription activation domains of HBx [45,46]. HBx-associated apoptosis and transcription activation is probably mediated by molecular mechanisms similar to calcium signalling [47].

HBx protein has been reported to bind to at least 28 cellular proteins with diverse functions in the cell. Only two of these proteins or protein complexes have been found by more than one group, and these two proteins give some insight into the molecular effects of HBx:

1 The HBx protein binds to proteasome subunits [48–50], which inhibits proteasomal activity *in vitro* [51] and *in vivo* [52,53] and enhances HBV replication [54]. In addition, the altered half-life of short-lived proteins, many of them proto-oncogenes or cell cycle regulators, may lead to disturbances of growth regulation.

2 The UV-damaged DNA binding protein 1 (DDB1) binds to HBx of HBV and WHV [55]. Binding of HBx to DDB1 seems to be necessary for transactivation [56,57], induction of apoptosis [58,59], infection [56] and stability of HBx [60]. The interaction of HBx with a subunit of the cellular DNA repair complex

may explain the reduced DNA repair activity in HBx-expressing cells and may be a cofactor in HBV-associated carcinogenesis [33,40].

HBx, expressed alone or in the context of the viral genome, behaves like an oncogene in cell culture and in transgenic mice (for reviews, see refs 28,29,31,34). The amino-terminus of HBx is sufficient for transformation [61]. However, the oncogenic effect of HBx is weak and needs additional cocarcinogenic factors. HBx protein is expressed in certain, but not all, hepatocellular carcinomas (HCC) [37]. The coding region of HBx is often integrated in the chromosomes of hepatocytes from patients with chronic hepatitis or HCC [62,63].

HBV polymerase

The HBV polymerase is a multifunctional protein that consists of four domains (Fig. 6) with defined functions [64]:
• the terminal protein (TP) that serves as a primer for the DNA minus strand;
• a spacer or tether region with undefined function;
• the reverse transcriptase (RT) domain for RNA- and DNA-dependent DNA synthesis;
• the ribonuclease (RNaseH) that degrades hybrid DNA/RNA strands.

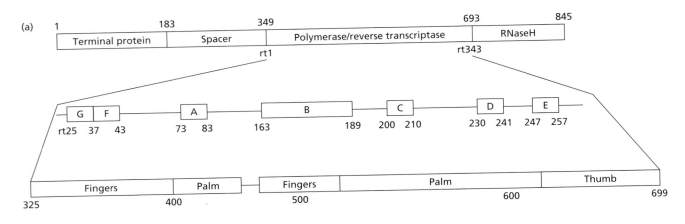

Fig. 6 Schematic representation of the HBV multifunctional polymerase protein (numbering for HBV genotype A). (a) Top: functional domains of the HBV polymerase. The numbering above delimits the borders of the domains with the methionine of the multifunctional protein set as 1. Below the scheme, the numbering following the new nomenclature [64] for the reverse transcriptase (RT) domain is indicated. Middle: domains A to G, numbered according to Sheldon *et al.* [135] and Stuyver *et al.* [64]. Bottom: domains involved in making up the three-dimensional conformation of the HBV polymerase, with amino acid coding according to Das *et al.* [70]. (b) Limits of the functional domains of the HBV polymerase of the eight HBV genotypes (modified from Stuyver *et al.* [64]).

Functional TP, RT [65] and RNaseH [66] domains can be expressed independently. TP and RT form a complex that is functional *in vitro* [65]. For the RT domain to function, most of the RNaseH domain is required [65], while RNaseH retains high activity when expressed independently [66].

The HBV RT domain is the prime target for antiviral therapy. Owing to differences in the length of the RT ORF between HBV genotypes, a nomenclature for drug-resistant HBV variants has been proposed [64], in which the first amino acid of the RT domain is a conserved E (glutamic acid) (Fig. 6b).

The structure of the HIV RT has been resolved by X-ray crystallography [67]. Based on the sequence homology of retroviral transcriptases, a three-dimensional model of the HBV RT domain has been derived [68–70]. The model assumes a right-handed conformation with thumb, palm and finger domains. The finger domains correspond structurally to deoxynucleoside triphosphate (dNTP) binding and catalysis sites (domains A, C and D). Thumb and palm domains most probably interact with the RNA template and the 3′ end (domains B and E) [71]. The C domain of the HBV RT contains the rt203YMDD motif, which is highly conserved in RTs. HBV RT is further divided into five subdomains, A–E, with additional domains F and G for RTs [72].

Crystallographic data show that the primary mechanism of resistance appears to be steric hindrance within the dNTP bind-

ing pocket [71]. Replacement of methionine in the YMDD motif with valine, isoleucine or serine leads to projections of the new amino acid side-chain into the dNTP binding site.

Other factors leading to resistance are caused by suboptimal nucleophilic attack geometry [73]. For the elongation of the DNA strand by incoming dNTP, a precise spatial arrangement of the 5′ phosphate and the 3′ hydroxyl group is important. Altered three-dimensional structures can reduce the efficiency of catalysis.

Hepatitis B virus surface proteins

Three HBs proteins, [L(arge), M(iddle) and S(mall)], are translated from one ORF using three in-frame start codons. Differences in size come from the amino-terminal domains added to the smallest protein SHBs. MHBs contains the pre-S2 region in addition to SHBs, whereas LHBs consists of the pre-S1 domain and the MHBs sequence. The pre-S (= pre-S1 + pre-S2) domain of LHBs exists in two orientations, facing either the outside or the interior of the viral particle [74,75]. About 50% of SHBs, 30% of MHBs and 90% of LHBs carry a complex glycan at position Asn146 of the S domain. The pre-S2 domain of MHBs contains a complex glycan at Asn4, whereas the same residue is glycan free in LHBs [76,77]. Thus, a very typical pattern of the

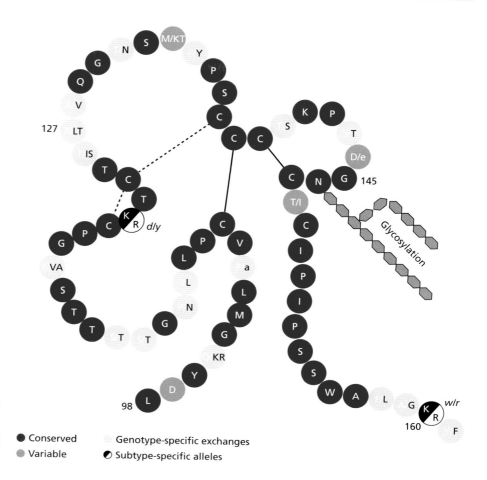

Fig. 7 Hypothetical model of the *a* determinant formed by the small surface protein. Residues 122 and 160, which confer subtype changes from *d/y* and *w/r*, respectively, are indicated in black and white. *w2* reactivity is determined by P127, *w3* by T127, *w4* by L/I127; I126 abolishes reactivity with *w* antisera and is linked to the *r* subdeterminant.

● Conserved
● Variable
○ Genotype-specific exchanges
◐ Subtype-specific alleles

six different proteins can be distinguished in sodium dodecyl sulphate (SDS) gel electrophoresis (Fig. 1).

Infected hepatocytes secrete subviral HBsAg particles in large excess in addition to infectious HBV. Particles with low content of LHBs form spherical particles with a size of ca. 20 nm, whereas a higher content of LHBs induces the formation of filaments with varying length (Figs 1 and 2). In serum samples from highly viraemic individuals, these particles can be found in up to 1000-fold excess over virions.

LHBs with a cytosolic pre-S domain is essential for envelopment of mature DNA-containing core particles [78]. For secretion of virus or subviral HBsAg particles, an excess of SHBs over LHBs is required because LHBs alone are retained in the endoplasmic reticulum (ER) where it can lead to the ground glass-like appearance of hepatocytes. MHBs seem to be non-essential but are conserved in all orthohepadnaviruses. Hypoglycosylation of MHBs inhibits secretion of virus and HBs particles [79]. The surface exposure of the pre-S domain is necessary for infectivity of the virus. The translocation from the interior to the surface of the virus or subviral particles occurs posttranslationally [74], possibly in a Golgi compartment [77]. The pre-S domain is largely hydrophilic, probably unstructured and highly sensitive to proteases. In contrast, the S domain or

SHBs is highly resistant against proteases and has at least two, possibly four, hydrophobic transmembrane domains creating an internal and an external hydrophilic loop. The external loop from amino acid 99 to about amino acid 170 carries the HBsAg epitopes. Most of these epitopes are conformational and require disulphide bridges (Fig. 7). All HBV strains are believed to share a set of common epitopes called determinant *a*, but they also express mutually exclusive subtype determinants *d* or *y* (K or R at amino acid 122) and *w* or *r* (K or R at amino acid 160). *w* may be further distinguished into *w1*, *w2* (P127), *w3*, (T127) and *w4* (L/I127). These determinants may be expressed in various combinations by the HBV genotypes.

The viral life cycle (Fig. 8)

For a long time, it was difficult to study the early steps in the viral life cycle *in vitro* because the available cell lines were not susceptible to HBV. Only primary hepatocyte cultures obtained from freshly excised human or primate liver could be infected with HBV and, even then, the efficiency of infection was low, and very little progeny virus could be obtained. Thus, most studies were done with rodent or avian hepadnaviruses. The late steps in the life cycle were easier to study because hepatoma cell lines could

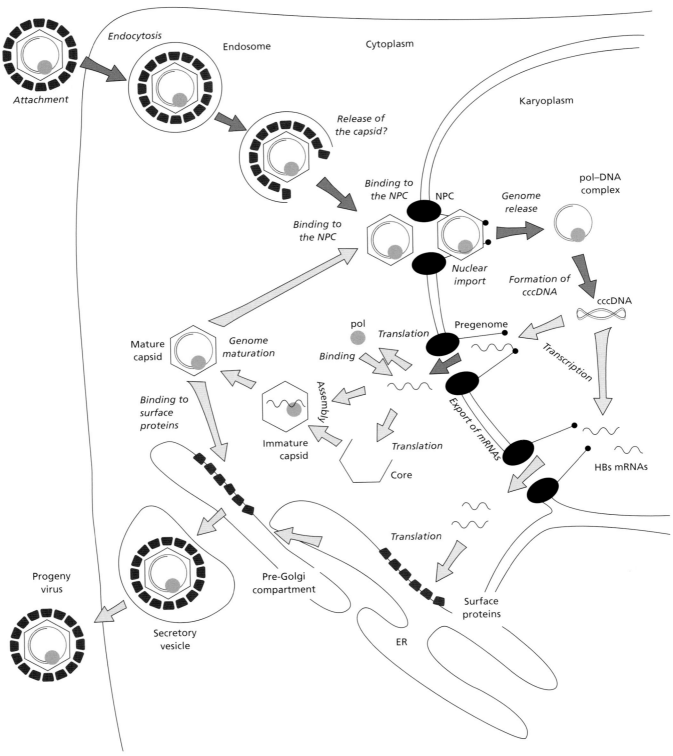

Fig. 8 Intracellular life cycle of HBV. NPC, nuclear pore complex. mRNAs are shown as wavy lines. Expression of X, subviral HBsAg and HBeAg is deleted for simplicity.

be transfected with cloned HBV DNA and were permissive for HBV production. Recently, two systems have become available for the study of the early steps in HBV replication: the redifferentiated hepatoma cell line Hepa RG [80] and cultures of primary tupaia hepatocytes [81]. Tupaias are small squirrel-like animals phylogenetically placed between primates and rodents.

Attachment and entry

HBV attaches via the amino-terminal sequence of the pre-S1 domain (9–48 in genotype D) first to sulphated glycosaminoglycans (D. Glebe, unpublished observations), and then via the same sequence to an unknown high-affinity receptor [82,83]. Thereafter, the S domain of LHBs mediates the uptake of virus and the release of core particles. Reductive cleavage of the disulphide bridges in the S domain prior to attachment destroys infectivity (D. Glebe, unpublished observations). The cysteines 121 and 124 are essential for infectivity [84]. In the duck hepatitis B virus (DHBV) system, the fusion peptide in the first transmembrane sequence of the large surface protein causes fusion of the viral envelope with the membrane of late endosomes [85]. A similar sequence is present in human HBV [86]. Surprisingly, the release of cores from the endosomes seems to be pH independent [87]. Attachment and entry limit the efficiency of infection and take 18 h.

Transport of the virus to endosomes [88] and of cores to the nucleus [89] requires microtubules but not actin filaments. Cytosolic core particles are rapidly transported within 1 h to the basket of the nuclear pore complex using the importing alpha-dependent pathway [90]. The cores are arrested there by the nuclear porin nup153, and finally release the viral genome to the nucleoplasma (Schmitz and Kann, unpublished observations). Ubiquitous cellular DNA repair enzymes (present even in *Escherichia coli*) remove the covalently bound polymerase, the RNA fragment, close the single-stranded gap and the nick, and thus convert the rc form into cccDNA. This is the first stable molecule generated during the life cycle and is, therefore, often taken as proof of infection.

Transcription and translation

The cccDNA is the template for the viral mRNAs. Liver enriched transcription factors are necessary for efficient and accurate transcription of mRNAs encoding core and LHBs, whereas transcription of M/SHBs and X also occurs efficiently in nonhepatic cells. Besides the promoters and enhancers, various activator or silencer elements are present on the DNA [91], e.g. the GRE (Fig. 5b). Transcription is regulated and seems to support viral expression optimally in resting, fully differentiated hepatocytes. Owing to the common polyadenylation site, four groups of mRNAs are generated that have an identical 3′ terminus (Fig. 5c). These encode HBeAg/core/pol, LHBs, M/SHBs and X. The mRNAs encoding core, small surface and X protein have heterogeneous 5′ ends. Thus, some of the largest mRNAs

of 3.5 kb start upstream of the precore sequence and encode HBeAg, whereas others start downstream of the HBeAg start codon and encode core and pol. The expression of both RNAs is tightly coupled [91]; however, natural variants and point mutations [92] located in this transcriptional element can uncouple the transcription of the RNAs. Fine tuning of the core promoter and enhancer determines the ratio of HBeAg- to core/pol-encoding mRNAs. A similar situation occurs with the middle-sized 2.1-kb RNA, in which a part encodes MHBs and another part SHBs. No splicing is required for expression of the known essential viral proteins, but splicing is known to occur to a limited extent, (e.g. [93]) and generates proteins of unknown significance [94,95]. The transport and stability of the mRNAs is regulated by the posttranscriptional regulatory element (PRE) [96] (Fig. 5c). Cellular factors interacting with the PRE also seem to regulate the extent of splicing [97].

The expression of core, pol and X protein occurs at cytosolic polyribosomes, whereas HBeAg and the HBs protein are translated at the rough ER and directed to membrane compartments. The polymerase does not have its own mRNA but is translated by internal initiation in the core mRNA. Core protein assembles into core particles, which encapsidate their own mRNA together with the polymerase. The suboptimal sequence context of the MHBs start codon favours translation initiation at the SHBs sequence even in those mRNAs that contain the MHBs start codon. Thus, MHBs is usually a minor protein, whereas SHBs is the major surface protein. The three surface proteins insert into the ER membrane, aggregate and bud as subviral particles to the ER. The X protein is very unstable [36] and difficult to detect [37].

Replication and morphogenesis

The elements steering reverse transcription and circularization of the genome [98] are shown in Figure 9. The mRNA for the core and pol protein is truly multifunctional and also functions as the precursor for the viral genome within core particles (pregenomic RNA or pg RNA). pg RNA forms a secondary structure at the 5′ end, ε (epsilon), which interacts with the primase (or terminal) domain of pol after binding and activation by the cellular chaperones Hsc70 and Hsp40. This complex initiates encapsidation by the core protein. For priming of DNA synthesis, the first nucleotide of the minus strand DNA is linked to the hydroxyl of tyrosine 63 in the primase domain (tyrosine 96 in DHBV). After the addition of four nucleotides, the nascent DNA strand is shifted to a sequence element in the 3′ terminal copy of DR1 of the pg RNA. From there, the polymerase elongates the minus strand until the 5′ end of the pg RNA is reached, generating a short terminal redundancy r of 8–10 bases. The RNaseH of pol concomitantly degrades the already transcribed pg RNA, leaving only the 18 5′ terminal bases of pg RNA at DR1 uncleaved. This short RNA segment is shifted to the DR2 element in the minus strand DNA and serves as a primer for the plus strand DNA. The nick in the minus-strand template is

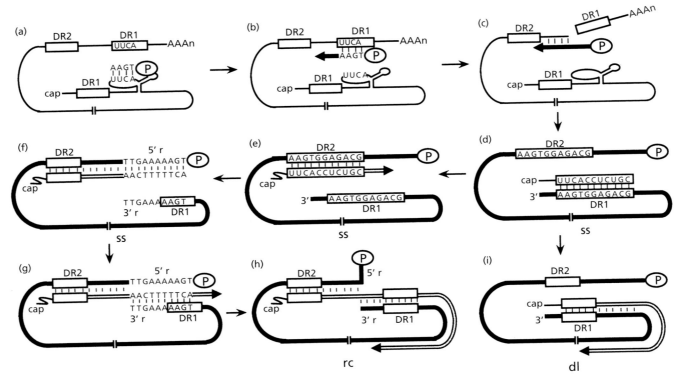

Fig. 9 Steps of genome maturation beginning (in a) with pregenome recognition by the priming domain (P) and ending (in h) with the relaxed circular (rc) form of HBV DNA. DR1, DR2, direct repeats 1 and 2; ss, single-stranded DNA; (i) shows double-stranded linear DNA (dl), which is a side-product of replication. From ref. 98 with permission.

bridged during plus strand synthesis with the aid of the redundancy r. The plus strand usually remains incomplete leaving a large gap. The entire replication occurs within the core particles. During this process, a series of phosphorylations modify the serines in the arginine-rich carboxy-terminal domain of the core protein. The nucleotide triphosphates necessary for replication and phosphorylation can enter the lumen of the cores via 2-nm large holes in the protein shell.

After completion of DNA synthesis (genome maturation), the core particles assume a different structure [99], and the C-terminal core domain becomes partially accessible at the surface. It contains a nuclear localization signal that mediates the transport of mature cores to the nuclear pore complex and the release of the viral DNA to the nucleus. In the early phase of infection, this reimport of viral genomes leads to the accumulation of cccDNA and establishes persistent infection of a cell. The generation and secretion of enveloped virus particles is regulated by the availability of LHBs with a cytosolic pre-S domain. The sequence between Arg103 and Ser124 of pre-S at the junction of pre-S1 and pre-S2 is essential for the interaction with mature cores. The interaction site on the core particles is formed by a ring-like groove around the spikes and by amino acids at the transition to the nucleic acid binding domain. Budding and secretion of enveloped virions requires an excess of SHBs over LHBs. Partial translocation of the pre-S domain to the surface of virions may

occur before secretion in a mildly acidic cell compartment because low pH favours this process. Envelopment and egress of virus particles involves the ubiquitin ligase Nedd4 and a putative endosomal sorting adaptor, gamma2 adaptin [100]. Possibly, secretion of the virus follows an endosomal pathway, whereas the subviral HBsAg particle follows the Golgi pathway.

Immunopathogenesis and clinical course of infection

The entire biology and clinical course of HBV infections can be understood only by the variable interaction of the virus with the immune system. Depending on the strength and timing of the immune response of the host, clinical courses from asymptomatic to fulminant hepatitis and from self-limiting to chronic infection are possible (Fig. 10). This section describes briefly the pathogenesis of HBV. Several reviews have been published recently [101–103].

Acute hepatitis B

The existence of a weeks- or months-long incubation phase with increasing and finally very high viraemia but without clinical or biochemical signs of liver damage shows that replication and persistance of HBV is not cytopathic *per se*. Analysis of the hepatic cellular expression patterns in acutely HBV-infected

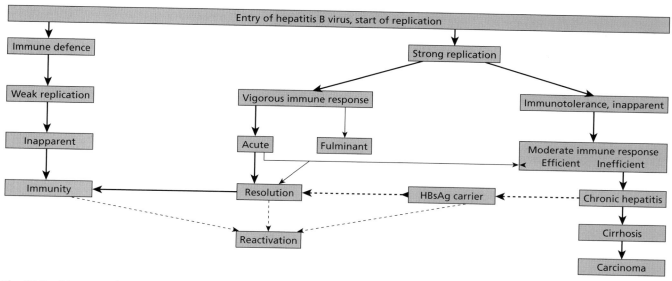

Fig. 10 Possible courses of HBV infection.

chimpanzees showed that no host response to viral replication occurred during the incubation phase. HBV behaved like a 'stealth virus' and did not stimulate the innate immune system which recognises pathogen-associated molecular patterns [104]. In contrast, later in the infection period, most of the effector molecules associated with the adaptive cellular immune response are induced, followed by HBV antibodies. HBV elimination starts several weeks before onset of the disease with T-cell-dependent noncytolytic mechanisms, but later cytolytic immune responses follow and generate the symptoms of acute hepatitis [105]. IFN-induced mechanisms seem to inhibit the maturation of pgRNA to cccDNA and to mediate its degradation both in the early and in the late phase [106]. During the acute disease, high numbers of cytolytic CD8+ T cells are present in the liver and these react with a multitude of HBV epitopes and eliminate the virus by destroying infected cells. High disease activity usually leads to clinical and serological resolution. However, even after serological resolution, small amounts of cccDNA persist in the liver for years, decades and possibly for life. T-cell immunity suppresses viral replication originating from these cccDNA copies to very low levels [107].

Anti-HBc appears with the onset of the disease as the first anti-HBV antibody, then anti-HBe, anti-pre-S and finally anti-SHBs. These antibodies probably contribute neither to virus elimination from the liver nor to the pathogenesis of hepatitis. However, anti-HBs formed during convalescence and later may enhance opsonisation of HBsAg and block *de novo* infection of hepatocytes by released HBV. In contrast to the other HBV antibodies, anti-HBc induction is partially T-cell independent. This explains the presence of anti-HBc even in those patients who do not build up an efficient immune response. Serological resolution is defined by disappearance of HBsAg which may take months after onset.

Inapparent transient infection

Most HBV infections worldwide remain asymptomatic and result in immmunity, as indicated by the presence of anti-HBs and anti-HBc. It is likely that the course of virus replication and elimination is similar to acute hepatitis B but that the immune reaction starts earlier at much lower levels of infection, thus resulting in minimal clinically asymptomatic liver damage. Factors favouring an unobtrusive course are a low dose of infecting virus, mucocutaneous entry and a mature, competent immune system. Viraemia and HBs antigenaemia are often short lived and may often go unnoticed, unless the person donates blood or organs. The benign course does, however, not exclude establishment of low-level persistence with small numbers of cccDNA in the liver that have the potential to activate under immune suppression. The term occult HBV infection has been coined for this condition.

Chronic HBV infection

HBV has the ability to persist in the liver in spite of effective elimination by the immune system. In contrast to this type of immune-controlled low-level persistence, frank chronicity is characterised by persistent HBs antigenaemia, indicating that T-cell activity and anti-HBs production were insufficient to overcome the expression of HBsAg. The inability of the immune system to cope with HBsAg may be based on the fact that it is produced to such great excess that it may induce a high dose tolerance. Furthermore, the antigen-presenting cells encounter HBsAg normally in the form of subviral particles without viral RNA or other danger signals. This may result in immunotolerance. These two and other factors may apply also to HBeAg as the secreted T-cell tolerance inducer for HBcAg. Furthermore, anti-HBV antibodies, particularly anti-HBc, may impair the T-cell response to the corresponding antigen. The state of immune inertia and/or tolerance can be maintained for years, allowing high replication and viraemia in the absence of disease. The absence of immune selection is confirmed by the highly conserved HBV DNA sequences within immunotolerant long-term carriers and within an infection chain. A rare complication of the highly viraemic carrier state is extrahepatic immune complex disease causing periarteriitis nodosa or glomerulonephritis.

T-cell tolerance to HBe/c is much less stable than that to HBsAg and breaks down after years or decades in the majority of chronic HBV carriers, resulting in immune elimination and pathogenesis. This event is often associated with a significant decrease in viraemia, a transiently enhanced liver damage, disappearance of HBeAg and appearance of anti-HBe. Finally, the sufferer reaches the stable state of an almost healthy HBsAg carrier with low or absent infectivity.

Less fortunate patients develop a labile equilibrium between virus and immune defence, which results in chronic disease. Patients with chronic infection have detectable but small numbers of HBV-specific T cells targeted against a small number of epitopes. Episodes of active disease may alternate with sometimes long episodes without recognisable disease. The inflammation is maintained by active HBV replication and causes hepatocellular damage and fibrosis. HBeAg may be present, but very often expression of HBeAg is abolished by the selection of HBe-negative mutants. The constant immune pressure enhances mutations in many regions of the HBV genome. Hotspots of functionally important mutations are the precore region, the core promoter overlapping with the X gene, the aminoterminal part of pre-S2 and various regulatory elements. The resulting imbalanced expression of HBV proteins may contribute directly to pathogenicity: some HBe-negative variants replicate more strongly and express more HBcAg which cannot be exported and may exert direct cytotoxicity. An excess of LHBs over SHBs causes storage disease and enhanced sensitivity to apoptosis. Patients with advanced liver disease harbour often defective interfering virus particles with deletions in the core gene or spliced genomes. In summary, three types of chronic HBV carriers can be distinguished:

1 immunotolerant HBV carriers, HBeAg positive, asymptomatic, highly viremic and infectious;

2 chronic hepatitis patients with variable levels of replication and immune response (active infection);

3 healthy HBsAg carriers without HBeAg and with low viremia (inactive infection).

Intermediate forms and transitions between these types are possible (see Chapter 9.1.2.iv).

Integration of HBV DNA to the host genome

In contrast to orthoretroviruses, integration is not a necessary step in the life cycle of HBV. However, the incompletely double-stranded DNA intermediates, which are generated during genome maturation and released in the nucleus before formation of cccDNA, are prone to illegitimate recombination events with themselves and with cellular DNA. Integrated HBV DNA has been identified in most HBV-associated hepatocellular carcinomas (HCC) but it can also be found in seemingly normal hepatocytes. Virtually all integrated HBV DNA fragments are incomplete and often rearranged. Thus, integrated HBV DNA is not a source of viral replication, but complementation of defective replicons in trans by integrated HBV genes cannot be excluded. Viral integration points are frequently around the DR1 region at the nick in the minus strand. The core gene is usually absent, whereas the surface gene is often present. It appears possible that in HBsAg carriers without detectable HBV DNA in the serum, a portion or all of the HBsAg in the serum is expressed from integrated DNA. This presumption is supported by the fact that HBsAg carriers often have large amounts of non-secreted LHBs protein but no core protein in the hepatocytes (ground-glass cells). Clonal integrates from HCC encode often truncated pre-S/S proteins which gain transactivating and potentially oncogenic properties. The X gene is usually also present in integrated HBV DNA and is often mutated. It has been suggested that these mutations enhance the weak oncogenicity of HBx protein.

Integration occurs often within cellular transcription units but there is no other preference for integration sites except a limited sequence homology with the viral insertion site. In HCC, the integrated HBV DNA can act as a transcriptional enhancer element and may support malignant growth by activation of various cellular growth-promoting genes. Details have been reviewed [108].

Laboratory diagnosis

Diagnosis of acute or chronic HBV infection is complex on account of the wide spectrum of clinical outcomes ranging from inapparent transient infection as the most benign form to fulminant acute hepatitis. As pointed out above, two forms of asymptomatic infection are possible: (i) transient or persistent low-level infection with low or no viraemia; and (ii) immunotolerance to HBV with very high persistent viraemia. Chronic hepatitis B and its sequelae develop if the immune defence is active but unable sufficiently to suppress viral activity. Episodes of active disease may interchange with long episodes without recognizable disease. Healthy adults usually resolve the infection with or without apparent disease, whereas infants and immunosuppressed patients usually develop chronic infection. A battery of laboratory tests allows for the accurate diagnosis and prognosis if used and interpreted properly (Table 3 and Fig. 11).

HBsAg

Detection of HBsAg in the serum of patients corresponds to ongoing HBV infection with two exceptions: (i) after vaccination, HBsAg can be detected in serum for up to 1 week; (ii) rare case reports have shown that HBsAg can be expressed independently from viral replication from HBV DNA integrated into chromosomal DNA even after resolved infection. However,

Table 3 Selection of the HBV test programme according to the medical question.

Immune?	
Prior to vaccination	Anti-HBc
After vaccination	Anti-HBs
Acute hepatitis, type?	HBsAg
	Anti-HBc IgM
Previous exposure?	Anti-HBc
Potential of reactivation?	HBsAg, anti-HBc
Chronic hepatitis, type?	HBsAg, anti-HBc
Chronic hepatitis B, activity?	HBV DNA, qPCR
	HBeAg
Infectivity	
HBsAg carrier	HBV DNA, qPCR
Blood donor	HBsAg, anti-HBc[a], HBV DNA[a]
Organ donors	HBsAg, anti-HBc

[a]Optional in some countries. qPCR, quantitative polymerase chain reaction.

integrated HBV DNA will usually be accompanied by episomal, replication-competent DNA.

The high clinical sensitivity of HBsAg is due to the fact that it is secreted into the serum in about 100-fold or higher excess compared with viral particles. In serum from immune-tolerant carriers, up to 1 000 000 ng/mL HBsAg can be found; typical concentrations are 30 000–150 000 ng/mL. These high concentrations of HBsAg pose several problems. Today's immune assays have a detection limit of 0.1 ng/mL. Thus, contamination of 1 mL of negative serum with 0.1 nL of carrier serum can give false-positive results. Furthermore, the high concentrations found in early acute infections and immune-tolerant carriers are far beyond the linear range of today's commercial immune assays, which usually end at 10 ng/mL. Accurate quantification of HBsAg is possible with well-calibrated assays and is useful as a prognostic factor for successful interferon (IFN) therapy. High HBsAg concentrations above 30 000 ng/mL correlate with poor response to IFN therapy [109]. One accurately assayed ng of HBsAg corresponds to 1 Paul-Ehrlich unit or 2 international units (IU).

In acute infections, HBsAg concentrations rise logarithmically for weeks to months from undetectable to typical final concentrations of 10 000–100 000 ng/mL with 2–4 days of doubling time [110]. If the acute HBV infection is resolved, HBsAg decreases with an initial half-life of 8 days until it has been removed completely from serum after weeks to months. In about 25% of acute resolving hepatitis B cases, the elimination of HBsAg proceeds much faster, with the consequence that samples taken in the late acute phase may be HBsAg negative [111].

A decrease in HBsAg concentration by more than 50% within the first 4 weeks indicates resolving acute infection in > 95% of cases [112]. Hence, quantitative analysis of highly concentrated HBsAg is an excellent prognostic marker, indicating progression to chronicity if the values remain stable or increase.

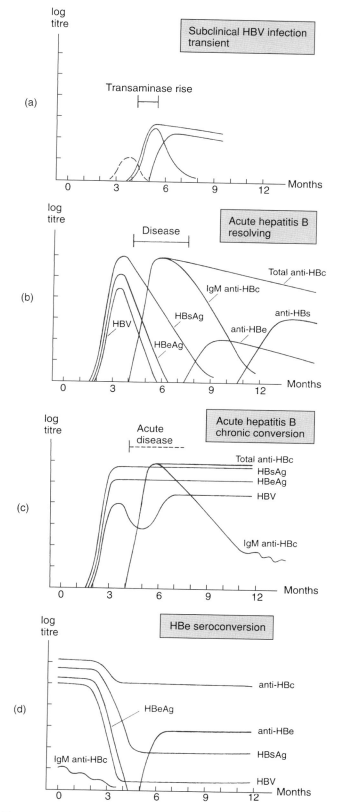

Fig. 11 Schematic serological profiles of various courses of HBV infections.

False-negative HBsAg results may be generated by natural variability, immune selection of variants or antiviral therapy [113]. As a consequence, the manufacturers have improved their assays with the inclusion of antibodies against assumed conserved epitopes from the *a* determinant of HBsAg. Nevertheless, new variants showing amino acid exchanges in the *a* determinant (Fig. 7) could not be detected by one or more commercial assays [113]. If false-negative HBsAg results are suspected, an analysis with the assay from another manufacture may give a correct positive result. Serologically undetectable HBsAg variants can usually be detected by amplification of the viral DNA with conserved primers.

Positive HBsAg screening results, e.g. at blood transfusion, should be reproduced by repetition in duplicate and, if reproduced, confirmed by assaying additional HBV markers, in particular anti-HBc and HBV DNA. If these markers are negative, the specificity should be tested by preincubation with anti-HBs and/or a second HBsAg assay.

HBeAg and anti-HBe

Testing for HBeAg is indicated only if HBsAg is positive in an immune assay. HBeAg is a marker of high replication activity and viral immune modulation. HBeAg-positive HBsAg carriers with mild or no liver disease often have higher viraemia than those with active hepatitis, because the immune reaction causing inflammation also suppresses virus replication [114]. HBeAg is an important marker for therapy monitoring. Loss of HBeAg suggests that a sustained resolution of disease has been achieved, and is one of the therapeutic targets in HBeAg-positive patients. Loss of HBeAg during acute hepatitis B is a good prognostic marker.

The absence of HBeAg does not exclude significant viraemia, particularly in HBsAg-positive patients with chronic hepatitis.

Testing for anti-HBe is useful to confirm a stable HBsAg carrier state with low viraemia and no inflammation. In subjects with anti-HBc, but without HBsAg and anti-HBs, a positive anti-HBe result supports the specificity of the anti-HBc result. During resolving acute hepatitis B, anti-HBe appears after anti-HBc but before anti-HBs. It usually disappears earlier than anti-HBs.

HBV DNA

Detection of HBV DNA is a central part of HBV diagnostics. In many instances, measurement of HBV DNA is a prerequisite for proper diagnosis and decision-making in chronic and, to a lesser extent, acute hepatitis B.

Highly sensitive (< 12.5 IU/mL) qualitative detection of HBV DNA is indispensable for:
- controlling the specificity of serological assays in patients with isolated anti-HBc or isolated HBsAg positivity without additional serological HBV signals;
- detection of the very early stages or occult forms of HBV infection.

Quantitative determination is necessary for:
- controlling antiviral treatment;
- estimating the infectivity of HBV-infected medical personnel.

These applications require DNA assays that reach a sensitivity of one genome per assay. However, available assays vary significantly in sensitivity (Table 4). With timely nucleic acid amplification techniques (NAT), the overall sensitivity of the assay is largely limited by the sample volume and the extraction method. Qualitative and quantitative detection of HBV DNA is preferably performed with the real-time polymerase chain reaction (PCR), in which the signal is generated *in situ* and measured after each amplification step [quantitative PCR (qPCR)]. qPCR offers the possibility of quantification over a very wide range of concentrations from < 100 to 10^{12} copies/mL. The risk of contamination by amplified DNA is reduced because amplification is carried out in closed systems. Furthermore, the specificity of the signal is obtained by interaction with HBV-specific probes, and the product is available for direct sequencing and cloning. Amplification of the S/RT region provides DNA that can be used simultaneously for genotyping and resistance analysis [115].

Standardized quantification of HBV DNA requires a standard sample with known concentration. The World Health Organization (WHO) has approved an international standard with a defined quantitative amount of HBV DNA [116]. The use of this standard for the quantification/standardization of in-house and commercial assays is encouraged.

Owing to variable results obtained with different methods of detection, the WHO has defined the amount of HBV DNA in international units (IU) and not in genome equivalents (g.e.)/mL or copies/mL. The observed variability in results comes mainly from losses during extraction. The HBV polymerase is covalently bound to the HBV DNA, and this protein alters the extraction properties of the DNA. Thus, for the standardization of HBV DNA assays, HB virion-derived DNA and not cloned DNA should be used. Furthermore, not all HBV genotypes may be amplified equally well.

With adequate extraction and calibration, 1 IU corresponds to 5 g.e./mL HBV DNA of genotype A2 [117]. One picogram (pg) of HBV DNA is 280 000 g.e./mL.

Antibody to the HB core antigen (anti-HBc)

Anti-HBc is present during ongoing or after previous HBV infection; it is therefore useful as a marker of HBV prevalence. Most assays use recombinant HBcAg as reagent and an inhibition format for detection. Both sensitivity and specificity are suboptimal. Most chronic HBsAg carriers are anti-HBc positive but, in perinatally infected carriers or immunodeficient patients, anti-HBc may be undetectable by less sensitive assays. Transient inapparent or previous infections may generate low levels of anti-HBc. On the other hand, anti-HBc assays may generate non-specific anti-HBc results.

The serological pattern 'anti-HBc only' is seen with varying prevalence in different countries [118]. In Germany, a country

Table 4 Commercially available quantitative HBV DNA assays (modified from ref. 167).

Assay	Manufacturer	Principle	Procedure	LDL (copies/mL)	Linearity	Genotypes detected
HBV Digene Hybrid Capture I	Digene Diagnostics	Hybridization	Manual	7×10^5	$7 \times 10^5 – 6 \times 10^8$	A–D
HBV Digene Hybrid Capture I	Digene Diagnostics	Hybridization with signal amplification	Manual	1×10^5	$1 \times 10^5 – 2 \times 10^9$	A–D
Ultra-sensitive HBV Digene Hybrid Capture II	Digene Diagnostics	Hybridization with signal amplification after centrifugation	Manual	5×10^3	$5 \times 10^3 – 6 \times 10^7$	A–D
VERSANT HBV DNA 1.0 assay	Bayer Diagnostics	Hybridization with signal amplification, bDNA	Manual	7×10^5	$7 \times 10^5 – 5 \times 10^9$	?
VERSANT HBV DNA 3.0 assay	Bayer Diagnostics	Hybridization with signal amplification, bDNA	Semi-automated	2×10^3	$2 \times 10^3 – 1 \times 10^8$	A–F
Amplicor HBV Monitor	Roche Diagnostics	PCR	Semi-automated	1×10^3	$1 \times 10^3 – 4 \times 10^7$	A–G
COBAS Amplicor HBV Monitor	Roche Diagnostics	PCR	Automated	2×10^2	$2 \times 10^2 – 2 \times 10^5$	A–F
TaqMan	Roche Diagnostics	PCR (real time)	Automated	2×10^1	$2 \times 10^2 – 1 \times 10^{10}$	A–F
RealArt HBV PCR	Artus	PCR (real time)	Automated	1	$1 – 4 \times 10^8$	A–G

with relatively low prevalence of HBV, 1.4–2.2% of patients have only anti-HBc [118,119]. Demographic factors associated with an anti-HBc-only pattern are male sex and higher age [118,119]. Some 20% of anti-HBc-only patients in Germany [112] and up to 50% of intravenous drug abusers [118] are HCV-positive. Possible explanations for this serological status are:

- window phase, early after infection;
- resolved HBV infection;
- false-positive anti-HBc test;
- false-negative or absent anti-HBs or HBsAg.

Currently, non-specific results of anti-HBc seem to be rare. Anti-HBc-only patients showed a high concordance of test results with three different assays [120]. Thus, anti-HBc only is usually associated with HBV infections that resolved a long time ago, and the anti-HBs concentration has decreased below the detection limit. In patients with proven resolved infection, HBV DNA can be detected in the serum, and this is also true for about 10% of anti-HBc-only patients, 36% of whom have HBV DNA in liver biopsies [120]. Thus, these patients are a possible source of HBV transmission by blood transfusion or liver transplantation (for reviews, see [118,121]).

False-negative HBsAg results are a concern in HBV diagnostics. Some isolated anti-HBc-positive individuals may be low-level carriers of HBsAg, where the HBsAg concentration is below the detection limit of current tests. A further explanation for missing HBsAg detection may be variants of HBsAg undetected by one or more tests [113]. Anti-HBs testing may also produce false-negative results. Up to 14.4% of anti-HBc-only individuals showed discrepant results when comparing two different anti-HBs tests [122].

Anti-HBc immunoglobulin (Ig)M

This marker may be useful in two situations:
1 to distinguish an acute hepatitis caused by HBV from a hepatitis of different aetiology in a HBV carrier;
2 to identify an acute hepatitis in some hepatitis B patients, particularly those with fulminant hepatitis B or HDV coinfection, where HBsAg may have been eliminated very rapidly.

Tests should be quantitative because anti-HBc IgM is also positive in chronic active hepatitis B and during convalescence. Levels > 600 Paul-Ehrlich units/mL suggest an acute HBV infection with high inflammatory activity. In all other situations, concentrations are lower or undetectable. Inactive HBsAg carriers are usually negative [123].

Antibody to the HBsAg (anti-HBs)

The meaning of the term anti-HBs is somewhat ambiguous. Some understand it to mean antibodies only against the small HBsAg protein (SHBs), others the entire antibody spectrum against all three surface proteins including pre-S1 and pre-S2. During acute infection, anti-pre-S antibodies appear before anti-SHBs, and they often coexist with HBsAg.

Anti-HBs indicates previous contact with HBsAg and, if no HB vaccine was given, it suggests previous HBV infection as a rule. In this case, anti-HBc should also be positive but, in rare cases, anti-HBc may appear later and/or disappear earlier than anti-HBs. Furthermore, the possibility of non-specific anti-HBs results must be considered.

Some HBsAg-positive persons are also anti-HBs positive. In this case, the HBsAg result is more relevant if its specificity is confirmed. Thus, screening for immunity against HBV by anti-HBs without prior anti-HBc and HBsAg testing may be misleading.

Anti-HBs protects against HBV infection. Persons who are found to be positive for anti-HBs need not be vaccinated, and vaccinated persons should be tested 4 weeks after the last dose to prove reliable protection. After active vaccination, 10 IU/L anti-HBs is considered to be the minimal protective level. For passive protection by hepatitis B immune globulin (HBIG), higher serum levels > 100 IU/L are necessary. One IU of anti-HBs binds about 900 ng of HBsAg. When a positive anti-HBs result is obtained, it should be documented even if it is < 10 IU/L.

Modern HB vaccines contain only small HBs protein of the European/US genotype A2. The anti-HBs induced by these vaccines does not contain anti-pre-S or HBsAg subtype-specific antibodies other than anti-HBs/adw2. Ninety-nine per cent of the HBV carriers worldwide have other HBsAg subtypes; the antibodies against the HBs subtype determinants are often present in larger amounts than the anti-*a* antibodies.

Different anti-HBs test kits use different types of HBsAg as reagent. Complete quantitative agreement between these assays should not be expected [124], but discordance is usually within a factor of 2.

Anti-HBs and particularly anti-pre-S1 neutralizes HBV infectivity *in vitro* and *in vivo*. However, it cannot suppress intracellular replication and spread of HBsAg escape mutants. Postexposure prophylaxis favours the selection of escape mutants.

Occult infection and reactivation

This term has been coined recently for HBV infections that are HBsAg negative for various reasons [121]. Very often, they are asymptomatic, of low replication activity and normally clinically irrelevant. However, there are three situations in which this condition is important:

1 The small amount of HBV present in these persons is sufficient to transmit full-blown HBV infection in recipients of blood or organ donations. Persistent occult infection is usually detectable by anti-HBc. Thus, liver donors and, in some countries, blood donors have to be screened for anti-HBc. HBV DNA assays, even if very sensitive, may be insufficient to detect such infections.

2 An occult HBV infection may reactivate in patients experiencing severe immunosuppression, e.g. during bone marrow or stem cell transplantation or aggressive leukaemia/lymphoma therapy. The reactivated virus may be wt or an escape mutant. In the latter case, HBsAg results may be false negative. Thus, monitoring of such patients is preferably done by HBV DNA assays.

3 Occult infections may represent the persistence of viral DNA after the serological cure and may be associated with liver cirrhosis and the development of hepatocellular carcinoma.

HBV genotypes, variants and mutants

HBV genotypes are important for the prognosis of interferon therapy [125–129], whereas therapy with RT inhibitors shows no clear genotype influence (for reviews, see [10,130]). Long-term prognosis of chronic HBV infection may be dependent on the genotypes. Furthermore, the genotypes give a hint to the origin of the infection. Genotyping methods based on various PCR techniques have been described, and test kits are available [11]. The most reliable method is sequencing. However, direct sequencing usually misses coinfections with two or more HBV genotypes [11]. Because coinfections with two genotypes have recently been reported to be of importance for the prognosis of the disease [131], hybridization-based [132] or multiplex PCR methods [133,134] appear to be advantageous. Recombinants of two genotypes have been described in some regions, but they are not predominant in Europe or the USA.

More important than genotypes and genosubtypes are probably the mutants that have been selected by the host's immune defence [135]. The primary target is expression of HBeAg, which may be suppressed by core promoter mutations, a stop codon in the precore region and/or other mutations affecting translation or processing of the HBe protein [114].

Another important target is MHBs, the start codon of which may be mutated. Alternatively, the pre-S1/S2 sequence around the amino acid 120 region may show small deletions [136]. Truncations of the S domain are often found in integrated HBV DNA fragments from hepatocellular carcinomas. X protein may be truncated by mutations/deletions in the core promoter. Deletions and truncations of the core protein have also been found in defective interfering genomes from kidney transplant recipients with terminal liver disease [137]. Such mutants are typically found in severely ill patients.

Escape mutations in the HBsAg loop may arise either on the background of profoundly altered genomes or in otherwise normal genomes [113]. Active or passive vaccination favours mutations in the SHBs region 120–145, with G145R being the most prominent. Naturally induced anti-HBs selects for a wider variety of mutations between amino acid 100 and 170. Detection of all these mutations is best accomplished by PCR and sequencing of the corresponding gene. Owing to morphogenesis and secretion defects, the genomes detected in the serum may not reflect the intrahepatic pattern of mutation.

A special case are resistance mutations under antiviral therapy [138]. If there is no decline or an increase in HBV DNA levels during therapy, this suggests that the therapy is ineffective; a genotypical resistance assay may help to find the polymerase gene mutation and allow the adaptation of antiviral therapy according to the known sensitivity of this mutant to antivirals. Hybridization of PCR products with selected probes is more sensitive than direct sequencing, but sequencing is able to detect new mutants as well.

Hepatitis D virus (HDV)

Taxonomy

HDV consists of an HBsAg envelope, an HDAg core and a small 1.7-kb RNA. After cloning and sequencing of the HDV RNA, a similarity of HDV with viroids and virusoids (plant pathogens) was recognized. Formally, HDV is now classified among negative-strand viruses as genus deltavirus without its own virus family [139]. However, it does not have much in common with other negative-strand viruses.

Virus structure (Fig. 12)

The structure and replication has been reviewed recently [140,141]. A nucleocapsid-like structure is formed by approximately 70 HD protein subunits together with the small RNA genome, but a (icosahedral) symmetry of this complex has not been identified and may in fact be absent. The HD protein exists in two forms: a small HD protein (SHD) with 195 amino acids and a collinear large form (LHD) with a carboxy-terminal extension of 19 amino acids. The envelope consists of SHBs, MHBs and LHBs. As with HBV, SHBs is the major component and MHBs a minor component. Assembled HDV particles have a size of 36–43 nm and a density in caesium chloride of 1.24–1.25 g/mL. HDAg can be released from HDV by treatment with non-ionic detergents. As the HBsAg envelope is required for infectivity, the stability of HDV is probably comparable to that of HBV.

Genome structure (Fig. 13)

HDV has a unique genome structure among the animal viruses. Its RNA forms a covalently closed single-stranded circle with

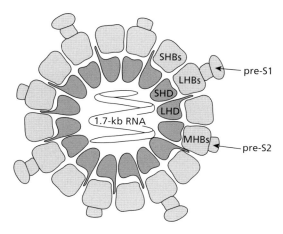

Fig. 12 Schematic model of hepatitis delta virus. The circular RNA genome is highly self-complementary and forms double-stranded rods. SHBs, MHBs, LHBs, small, middle and large hepatitis B surface protein; SHD, LHD, small and large hepatitis delta protein; pre-S1, pre-S2, domains of HBs proteins.

1670–1685 nucleotides depending on the isolate. On account of 70% self-complementarity within the RNA sequence, the circle folds to a double-stranded rod with covalently closed ends at base numbers 795 and 1638. In electron microscopy, the HDV genome appears as a short rod about 280 nm in length, which opens to a circle under denaturing conditions [142]. The minus-strand genome encodes the mRNA with one ORF for the two coterminal HD proteins.

RNA editing

In order to encode the two forms of HD protein, HDV has evolved a unique strategy. The replication-competent form of the HDV genome encodes the SHD protein because SHD is required for HDV genome replication. This SHD genome carries a U at position 1015 and, in the antigenome or the mRNA, an A as part of a UAG (amber) stop codon for the 195-amino acid SHD protein. For envelopment and secretion of the HDV, LHD protein is required. In order to encode LHD, the SHD antigenome is mutated (edited) by the cellular enzyme, double-stranded RNA adenosine deaminase (ADAR1), at position 1015 from A to inosine [143]. This unusual base is transcribed during RNA replication to C in the genome strand and to G in the newly produced mRNA and antigenome sequence. Thus, codon 196 of HD protein is no longer a stop codon, but encodes tryptophan and allows for an extension of 19 amino acids until the next stop codon occurs [144]. As SHD protein is required for genome replication, an HDV infection can only be established by the SHD genome, but spread of HDV and establishment of HD viraemia require partial conversion of SHD to LHD genomes.

Ribozyme activity

Similar to viroids, the genome and the antigenome contain a ribozyme structure that is able to self-cleave and self-ligate its own sequence (i.e. *in cis*). The delta-type ribozymes have four short double helices and a similar space structure to viroids [145]. The self-cleavage of the viral RNA phosphodiester backbone requires both divalent cations and a cytidine nucleotide. The ribozyme structures in the pre- and post-cleavage states reveal conformational changes after cleavage [146]. The self-cleavage occurs at the 5' end of this structure and may cleave off any sequence upstream. This property of the delta ribozyme has been used as a molecular tool to generate RNAs with exactly defined 3' ends that are necessary for the generation of replication-competent minus-strand RNA viruses (e.g. measles virus or influenza virus).

Properties of HD proteins

A schematic presentation of their various identified functions is shown in Figure 14. A region between amino acid 31 and 52 forms coils that can interact with each other and mediate oligomerization of HD proteins. HD proteins contain a bipartite nuclear localization signal. Thus, HD proteins are predominantly

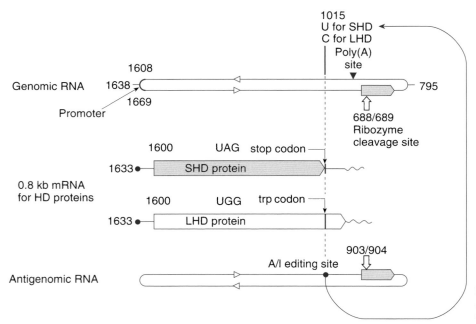

Fig. 13 Genome structure, RNA editing and expression products of HDV. U, uridine; C, cytidine; A, adenine; I, inosine.

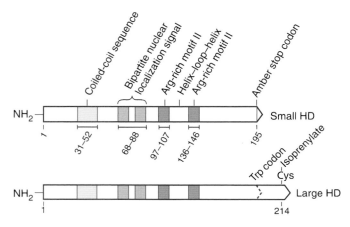

Fig. 14 Functions and motifs of the two HD proteins.

found in the nucleus. Two arginine-rich motifs support binding of RNA. They are specific for rod-like RNA structures with closed ends as in the HDV genome. All these features of SHD contribute to the replication of the HDV genome. LHD has an additional 19 amino acids, the sequence of which may be quite variable. A Cys-Arg-Pro-Glu motif is conserved at the carboxy end, which is a target for a linkage between the Cys and a 15-carbon farnesyl isoprenoid. This modification is required for the secretion of HD protein within the HBs envelope. LHD has a transdominant negative effect on the functions of SHD protein, which is mediated by the coil–coil interaction. LHD is possibly partially retained by the isoprenylate at the ER, whereas SHD functions only in the nucleus. Mature virions always contain

a mixture of SHD and LHD. *In vivo*, the small and large delta antigens assemble as antiparallel coiled-coil dimers and assume an octameric quaternary structure *in vivo* [147]. Both HD proteins are phosphorylated by casein kinase II. In addition, SHD gets phosphorylated by protein kinase C (PKC) and PKR [148]. PKC activates SHD functions, but LHD is six times more phosphorylated and inhibits SHD functions.

HD proteins are moderately immunogenic. Antibodies react with the nuclear localization signal and the C-terminal sequences of SHD- and LHDAg [149]. Patients' antibodies react well with the HD nucleoprotein complex and with denatured HD proteins in Western blots.

Genotypes and variability

The major part of the HDV genome is variable with the exception of essential motifs. Initially, three genotypes, I–III, were identified, which differ as much as 40% in nucleotide sequence. Later studies found four further clades (or genotypes) in Africa suggesting an African origin of HDV [150]. Today, HDV is divided into eight major clades [151]. Recombinations between two genotypes/clades have been found *in vivo* and *in vitro* [152].

Genotypes seem to influence the course of disease. Genotype I is most frequent worldwide and has variable pathogenicity. In a recent study, patients infected with genotype I HDV had a lower remission rate and more adverse outcomes [153] than those with genotype II HDV. Genotypes II and IV have been found in East Asia causing relatively mild disease [154], whereas genotype III is associated with HBV genotype F and fulminant hepatitis in South America [155].

Replication

Host and organ tropism

HDV can infect humans and primates if HBV is also present. Infection of woodchuck hepatitis virus (WHV)-carrying woodchucks with HDV of human origin is also possible [156]. The envelope of WHV is acquired in this case. If brought into cells by transfection (e.g. of cloned cDNA), HDV RNA can replicate in various mammalian cells, provided HD protein is present to initiate the replication cycle. Spread from cell to cell and secretion is only possible in the presence of SHBs and LHBs. In transgenic mice, the HDV genome is best expressed in muscle cells [157]. Thus, the natural organ specificity is most probably due to the attachment and penetration mediated by the HBs envelope proteins [82].

Genome expression

After penetration, the HDV genome reaches the nucleoplasm, possibly guided by the nuclear localization signal of the HD ribonucleoprotein complex. As with viroids, the cellular RNA polymerase II (against all the rules of normal gene expression) is believed to accept the HDV RNA genome as a template [140,141]. The RNA-encoded promoter is formed by sequence 1608–1669, which forms a stem–loop region with two bulges. This secondary structure is required for HDV genome expression and replication [158]. Proximal to the 3′ end of the HD gene, the genome contains a leaky signal for termination of transcription and polyadenylation. Thus, a 0.8-kb mRNA encoding either SHD or LHD depending on base 1015 is generated.

Genome replication (Fig. 15)

In the presence of increasing amounts of SHD protein, the poly-A site is suppressed, and the entire circular genome is transcribed to a linear more-than-genome length antigenomic intermediate. The nascent antigenomic RNA strand has the ability to fold first into the ribozyme structure and to clip the continuously growing intermediate into genome-long units. This molecule folds back to the rod-like structure and undergoes self-ligation. Host factor(s) prevent first folding of the rod structure and stabilize the ribozyme. After generation of the circular structure, the ribozyme is inactivated by RNA sequences *in cis*, which prevent further self-cleavage of the genome. The clipping and self-ligation is (*in vitro*) reversible and independent of any protein and, thus, a true ribozyme reaction. The energy of the phosphodiester bond is conserved in the cleaved state by transesterification of the phosphate from the 5′ group to a 2′,3′cyclic monophosphate terminus. The same process now starts with the antigenome, thus generating progeny genomes. Interaction with SHD stabilizes the RNA and facilitates further cycles of replication. The basepaired region around base 1015 of the antigenome is subject to RNA editing, and a certain proportion of the genome will finally encode LHD and no longer contribute to replication, but to envelopment and secretion.

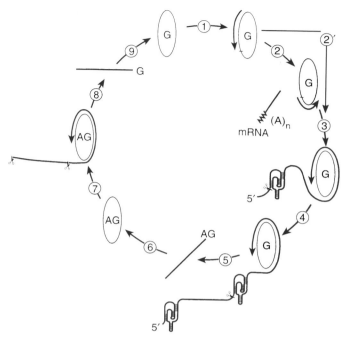

Fig. 15 HDV RNA replication cycle. The genomic (G) strand is transcribed (1) by RNA polymerase II to a short mRNA (2) and a long continuously growing strand (3), which cleaves itself by its ribozyme first at the 5′ end (4) and thereafter a second time resulting in a genome-long linear RNA (5). This antigenome (AG) is able to recircularize (6) and to repeat the cycle now with the genomic transcript (7–9). Courtesy of M.M.C. Lai.

Assembly

SHD has an affinity for the RNA rods of HDV, and it can also form mixed complexes with LHD. LHD interacts in the ER with SHBs. Isoprenylation is required for envelopment of LHD, but the oligomerization is dispensable for this function [159]. In contrast to HBV, LHBs is not required for envelopment of HDV nucleoprotein. However, mixed assembly of SHBs with LHBs is required for infectivity of HDV, whereas MHBs is dispensable (as is the case with HBV). The structure and function of the HBsAg envelope in HDV is different from that in the HBV envelope, because the host specificity of HDV is obviously not so narrow as for HBV and primary cell cultures can be infected more easily than with HBV.

Diagnosis of HDV infection

Course of the disease

Transmission occurs mainly by percutaneous contact with infectious blood and, less frequently than with HBV, by mucocutaneous contact. Two situations must be distinguished:

1 Coinfection in which the infectious material contains both HBV and HDV. HDV suppresses replication of HBV by unknown mechanisms; the course of infection is usually self-limiting, but the acute phase is of variable severity. The

infectivity titre of the inoculum is determined by either HBV or HDV, whichever is lower.

2 In superinfection, HDV infects an HBV carrier. Owing to the established colonization by HBV, HDV can replicate much more vigorously. Superinfection of HBV carriers usually leads to chronic HDV infection, and may cause fulminant hepatitis. The infectivity titre of the inoculum is determined only by HDV.

In both situations, the HD protein appears first in the liver after an incubation period of weeks or months. HDV is secreted to the blood before the onset of clinical disease, and starts to decrease during acute hepatitis. Infectivity titres of HDV may reach 10^{11}/mL of serum during the early acute phase, but are as a rule lower in persistent infection. Anti-HD antibodies appear during the acute phase, and may disappear within a few months after recovery. In persistent infection, titres remain high, as is also true for IgM anti-HD.

Anti-HD and HDAg

HDV infection occurs together with HBV infection. Thus, detection of HDV and anti-HD antibodies is normally indicated only for subjects with markers of ongoing HBV infection. HDV-infected patients who have received a liver transplant are exceptions. In such cases, the new liver can be infected in spite of seemingly absent HBV. As a general recommendation, an assay of anti-HD should be done as a screening test in all HBsAg-positive persons and in cases of HBsAg-negative acute hepatitis where no other agent can be identified. Owing to suppression of HBV by HDV, HBsAg may indeed be absent in some patients during acute HDV infection; usually, these patients have anti-HBc IgM. In drug abusers and recipients of blood products, testing for anti-HD may also be informative, even when HBsAg is absent.

During early acute hepatitis D as well as during the incubation period, anti-HD may still be negative; in this phase, HDAg may be detectable in detergent-treated serum samples. When anti-HD appears, direct testing for HDAg by immune assay is no longer useful unless HDV proteins are separated from anti-HD and detected by immunoblotting.

Disease activity and infectivity cannot be deduced from the presence of anti-HD, but only from the determination of HD protein in serum and liver or, preferably, from an assay of HDV RNA.

HDAg and anti-HD were first detected by immunofluorescence using liver biopsies from chronic HDV carriers as antigen and serum from the carriers as antibody. Currently, HDAg in serum is detected by sandwich immunoassays using high-titre IgG anti-HD as the capturing antibody and labelled anti-HD as the tracer. The inhibition of tracer binding to HDAg fixed on a solid phase indicates the presence of anti-HD in the serum sample. Several test kits for anti-HD and HDAg are available on the market. As with all inhibition assays, the analytical sensitivity is not high for anti-HD, but is sufficient to detect the great majority of productive HDV infections.

IgM anti-HD

The standard anti-μ capture assay is used for the detection of this antibody. The assay may be applied to diagnose acute infection, but patients with both acute and chronic disease have high titres of IgM anti-HD. IgM anti-HD may be considered as an indirect marker of active HDV infection and HDV-associated disease.

HDV RNA

No commercial assay is available for the detection of HDV RNA, but various methods have been published from specialized laboratories. Because of the high variability of the HDV genome, the choice of primers from a conserved site of the genome is crucial to avoid false-negative results.

At present, qPCR is the method of choice because it is sensitive and allows for quantification over a wide range [125]. The assay is indicated for confirmation and follow-up of a positive anti-HD result, and for monitoring chronic patients, especially when antiviral therapies are undertaken. In addition, the concentration of HDV RNA seems to be of prognostic significance because levels of HDV RNA in the serum of patients with chronic hepatitis or liver cirrhosis were reported to be higher than those in asymptomatic carriers [160].

References

1 Almeida JD, Rubenstein D, Stott EJ (1971) New antigen-antibody system in Australia-antigen-positive hepatitis. *Lancet* 2, 1225–1227.

2 Dryden KA, Wieland SF, Whitten-Bauer C *et al.* (2006) Native hepatitis B virions and capsids visualized by electron cryomicroscopy. *Mol Cell* 22, 843–850.

3 Kann M, Gerlich WH (2005) Hepatitis B virus and other Hepadnaviridae. Structure and molecular virology. In: Thomas H, Lemon S, Zuckerman A (eds) *Viral Hepatitis*, 3rd edn. Oxford: Blackwell, pp. 140–180.

4 Guo H, Mason WS, Aldrich CE *et al.* (2005) Identification and characterization of avihepadnaviruses isolated from exotic anseriformes maintained in captivity. *J Virol* 79, 2729–2742.

5 Schaefer S (2006) Hepatitis B virus taxonomy and hepatitis B virus genotypes. *World J Gastroenterol* 13, 14–21.

6 Dandri M, Burda H, Will H *et al.* (2000) Animal models of Hepadnavirus infection. A review. *J Viral Hepatitis Rev* 6, 29–45.

7 Schaefer S, Tolle T, Lottmann S *et al.* (1998) Animal models and experimental systems in hepatitis B virus research. In: Koshy R, Caselmann W (eds) *Hepatitis B Virus: Molecular Mechanisms in Disease and Novel Strategies for Therapy*. London: Imperial College Press, pp. 51–74.

8 Chu CJ, Lok AS (2002) Clinical significance of hepatitis B virus genotypes. *Hepatology* 35, 1274–1276.

9 Miyakawa Y, Okamoto H, Mayumi M (1997) The molecular basis of hepatitis B e antigen (HBeAg)-negative infections. *J Viral Hepat* 4, 1–8.

10 Schaefer S (2005) Hepatitis B virus – significance of genotypes. *J Viral Hepat* 12, 111–124.

11 Bartholomeusz A, Schaefer S (2004) Hepatitis B virus genotypes: comparison of genotyping methods. *Rev Med Virol* 14, 3–16.

12 Norder H, Couroucé A-M, Coursaget P *et al.* (2004) Genetic diversity of hepatitis B Virus strains derived worldwide: genotypes, subgenotypes, and HBsAg subtypes. *Intervirology* 47, 289–309.

13 Kramvis A, Kew M, Francois G (2005) Hepatitis B virus genotypes. *Vaccine* 23, 2409–2423.

14 Sugauchi F, Kumada H, Acharya SA *et al.* (2004) Epidemiological and sequence differences between two subtypes (Ae and Aa) of hepatitis B virus genotype A. *J Gen Virol* 85, 811–820.

15 Chan HL, Tsui SK, Tse CH *et al.* (2005) Epidemiological and virological characteristics of 2 subgroups of hepatitis B virus genotype C. *J Infect Dis* 191, 2022–2032.

16 Huy TT, Ushijima H, Quang VX *et al.* (2004) Genotype C of hepatitis B virus can be classified into at least two subgroups. *J Gen Virol* 85, 283–292.

17 Tanaka Y, Orito E, Yuen MF *et al.* (2005) Two subtypes (subgenotypes) of hepatitis B virus genotype C: A novel subtyping assay based on restriction fragment length polymorphism. *Hepatol Res* 33, 216–224.

18 Steven AC, Conway JF, Cheng N *et al.* (2005) Structure, assembly, and antigenicity of hepatitis B virus capsid proteins. *Adv Virus Res* 64, 125–164.

19 Zlotnick A, Johnson JM, Wingfield PW *et al.* (1999) A theoretical model successfully identifies features of hepatitis B virus capsid assembly. *Biochemistry* 38, 14644–14652.

20 Conway JF, Cheng N, Zlotnick A *et al.* (1998) Hepatitis B virus capsid: localization of the putative immunodominant loop (residues 78 to 83) on the capsid surface, and implications for the distinction between c and e-antigens. *J Mol Biol* 279, 1111–1121.

21 Belnap DM, Watts NR, Conway JF *et al.* (2003) Diversity of core antigen epitopes of hepatitis B virus. *Proc Natl Acad Sci USA* 100, 10884–10889.

22 Standring DN, Ou JH, Masiarz FR *et al.* (1988) A signal peptide encoded within the precore region of hepatitis B virus directs the secretion of a heterogeneous population of e antigens in Xenopus oocytes. *Proc Natl Acad Sci USA* 85, 8405–8409.

23 Wasenauer G, Köck J, Schlicht HJ (1992) A cysteine and a hydrophobic sequence in the noncleaved portion of the pre-C leader peptide determine the biophysical properties of the secretory core protein (HBe protein) of human hepatitis B virus. *J Virol* 66, 5338–5346.

24 Kato H, Orito E, Gish RG *et al.* (2002) Characteristics of hepatitis B virus isolates of genotype G and their phylogenetic differences from the other six genotypes (A through F) *J Virol* 76, 6131–6137.

25 Chudy M, Schmidt M, Czudai V *et al.* (2006) Hepatitis B virus genotype G monoinfection and its transmission by blood components. *Hepatology* 44, 99–107.

26 Milich D, Liang TJ (2003) Exploring the biological basis of hepatitis B e antigen in hepatitis B virus infection. *Hepatology* 38, 1075–1086.

27 Chen M, Sallberg M, Hughes J *et al.* (2005) Immune tolerance split between hepatitis B virus precore and core proteins. *J Virol* 79, 3016–3027.

28 Andrisani OM, Barnabas S (1999) The transcriptional function of the hepatitis B virus X protein and its role in hepatocarcinogenesis (review). *Int J Oncol* 15, 373–379.

29 Arbuthnot P, Capovilla A, Kew M (2000) Putative role of hepatitis B virus X protein in hepatocarcinogenesis: effects on apoptosis, DNA repair, mitogen-activated protein kinase and JAK/STAT pathways. *J Gastroenterol Hepatol* 15, 357–368.

30 Bouchard MJ, Schneider RJ (2004) The enigmatic X gene of hepatitis B virus. *J Virol* 78, 12725–12734.

31 Buendia MA (1998) Hepatitis B viruses and cancerogenesis. *Biomed Pharmacother* 52, 34–43.

32 Murakami S (1999) Hepatitis B virus X protein: structure, function and biology. *Intervirology* 42, 81–99.

33 Murakami S (2001) Hepatitis B virus X protein: a multifunctional viral regulator. *J Gastroenterol* 36, 651–660.

34 Schaefer S (2001) Hepatitis B virus in experimental carcinogenesis. In: Grand RJA (ed.) *Viruses, Cell Transformation and Cancer.* Amsterdam: Greenwich, Elsevier, pp. 193–228.

35 Chang SF, Netter HJ, Hildt E *et al.* (2001) Duck hepatitis B virus expresses a regulatory HBx-like protein from a hidden open reading frame. *J Virol* 75, 161–170.

36 Dandri M, Petersen J, Stockert RJ *et al.* (1998) Metabolic labeling of woodchuck hepatitis virus X protein in naturally infected hepatocytes reveals a bimodal half-life and association with the nuclear framework. *J Virol* 72, 9359–9364.

37 Su Q, Schröder CH, Hofmann WJ *et al.* (1998) Expression of hepatitis B virus X protein in HBV-infected human livers and hepatocellular carcinomas. *Hepatology* 27, 1109–1120.

38 Bouchard MJ, Wang LH, Schneider RJ (2001) Calcium signaling by HBx protein in hepatitis B virus DNA replication. *Science* 294, 2376–2378.

39 Hafner A, Brandenburg B, Hildt E (2003) Reconstitution of gene expression from a regulatory-protein-deficient hepatitis B virus genome by cell-permeable HBx protein. *EMBO Rep* 4, 767–773.

40 Tang H, Delgermaa L, Huang F *et al.* (2005) The transcriptional transactivation function of HBx protein is important for its augmentation role in hepatitis B virus replication. *J Virol* 79, 5548–5556.

41 Zhang Z, Torii N, Hu Z *et al.* (2001) X-deficient woodchuck hepatitis virus mutants behave like attenuated viruses and induce protective immunity in vivo. *J Clin Invest* 108, 1523–1531.

42 Benn J, Schneider RJ (1994) Hepatitis B virus HBx protein activates Ras–GTP complex formation and establishes a Ras, Raf, MAP kinase signaling cascade. *Proc Natl Acad Sci USA* 91, 10350–10354.

43 Bouchard MJ, Wang L, Schneider RJ (2006) Activation of focal adhesion kinase by hepatitis B virus HBx protein: multiple functions in viral replication. *J Virol* 80, 4406–4414.

44 Melegari M, Wolf SK, Schneider RJ (2005) Hepatitis B virus DNA replication is coordinated by core protein serine phosphorylation and HBx expression. *J Virol* 79, 9810–9820.

45 Bergametti F, Prigent S, Luber B *et al.* (1999) The proapoptotic effect of hepatitis B virus HBx protein correlates with its transactivation activity in stably transfected cell lines. *Oncogene* 18, 2860–2871.

46 Schuster R, Gerlich WH, Schaefer S (2000) Induction of apoptosis by the transactivating domains of the hepatitis B virus X gene leads to suppression of oncogenic transformation of primary rat embryo fibroblasts. *Oncogene* 19, 1173–1180.

47 Chami M, Ferrari D, Nicotera P *et al.* (2003) Caspase-dependent alterations of Ca2+ signaling in the induction of apoptosis by hepatitis B virus X protein. *J Biol Chem* 278, 31745–31755.

48 Fischer M, Runkel L, Schaller H (1995) HBx protein of hepatitis B virus interacts with the C-terminal portion of a novel human proteasome alpha-subunit. *Virus Genes* 10, 99–102.

49 Huang J, Kwong J, Sun EC *et al.* (1996) Proteasome complex as a potential cellular target of hepatitis B virus X protein. *J Virol* 70, 5582–5591.

50 Seeger C (1997) The hepatitis B virus X protein: the quest for a role in viral replication and pathogenesis. *Hepatology* 25, 496–498.

51 Hu Z, Zhang Z, Doo E *et al.* (1999) Hepatitis B virus X protein is both a substrate and a potential inhibitor of the proteasome complex. *J Virol* 73, 7231–7240.

52 Cui F, Wang Y, Wang J *et al.* (2006) The up-regulation of proteasome subunits and lysosomal proteases in hepatocellular carcinomas of the HBx gene knockin transgenic mice. *Proteomics* 6, 498–504.

53 Hu Z, Zhang Z, Kim JW *et al.* (2006) Altered proteolysis and global gene expression in hepatitis B virus X transgenic mouse liver. *J Virol* 80, 1405–1413.

54 Zhang Z, Protzer U, Hu Z *et al.* (2004) Inhibition of cellular proteasome activities enhances hepadnavirus replication in an HBX-dependent manner. *J Virol* 78, 4566–4572.

55 Sitterlin D, Lee TH, Prigent S *et al.* (1997) Interaction of the UV-damaged DNA-binding protein with hepatitis B virus X protein is conserved among mammalian hepadnaviruses and restricted to transactivation-proficient X-insertion mutants. *J Virol* 71, 6194–6199.

56 Sitterlin D, Bergametti F, Tiollais P *et al.* (2000) Correct binding of viral X protein to UVDDB-p127 cellular protein is critical for efficient infection by hepatitis B viruses. *Oncogene* 19, 4427–4431.

57 Wentz MJ, Becker SA, Slagle BL (2000) Dissociation of DDB1-binding and transactivation properties of the hepatitis B virus X protein. *Virus Res* 68, 87–92.

58 Bontron S, Lin-Marq N, Strubin M (2002) Hepatitis B virus X protein associated with UV-DDB1 induces cell death in the nucleus and is functionally antagonized by UV-DDB2. *J Biol Chem* 277, 38847–38854.

59 Lin-Marq N, Bontron S, Leupin O *et al.* (2001) Hepatitis B virus X protein interferes with cell viability through interaction with the p127-kDa UV-damaged DNA-binding protein. *Virology* 287, 266–274.

60 Bergametti F, Sitterlin D, Transy C (2002) Turnover of hepatitis B virus X protein is regulated by damaged DNA-binding complex. *J Virol* 76, 6495–6501.

61 Gottlob K, Pagano S, Levrero M *et al.* (1998) Hepatitis B virus X protein transcription activation domains are neither required nor sufficient for cell transformation. *Cancer Res* 58, 3566–3570.

62 Peng Z, Zhang Y, Gu W *et al.* (2005) Integration of the hepatitis B virus X fragment in hepatocellular carcinoma and its effects on the expression of multiple molecules: a key to the cell cycle and apoptosis. *Int J Oncol* 26, 467–473.

63 Schlüter V, Meyer M, Hofschneider PH *et al.* (1994) Integrated hepatitis B virus X and 3′ truncated preS/S sequences derived from human hepatomas encode functionally active transactivators. *Oncogene* 9, 3335–3344.

64 Stuyver L, Locarnini S, Lok A *et al.* (2001) Nomenclature for antiviral-resistant human hepatitis B virus mutations in the polymerase region. *Hepatology* 33, 751–757.

65 Lanford RE, Kim YH, Lee H *et al* (1999) Mapping of the hepatitis B virus reverse transcriptase TP and RT domains by transcomplementation for nucleotide priming and by protein–protein interaction. *J Virol* 73, 1885–1893.

66 Wei X, Peterson DL (1996) Expression, purification, and characterization of an active RNase H domain of the hepatitis B viral polymerase. *J Biol Chem* 271, 32617–32622.

67 Huang H, Chopra R, Verdine GL *et al.* (1998) Structure of a covalently trapped catalytic complex of HIV-1 reverse transcriptase: implications for drug resistance. *Science* 282, 1669–1675.

68 Allen MI, Deslauriers M, Andrews CW *et al.* (1998) Identification and characterization of mutations in hepatitis B virus resistant to lamivudine. Lamivudine Clinical Investigation Group. *Hepatology* 27, 1670–1677.

69 Bartholomeusz A, Groenen LC, Locarnini SA (1997) Clinical experience with famciclovir against hepatitis B virus. *Intervirology* 40, 337–342.

70 Das K, Xiong X, Yang H *et al.* (2001) Molecular modeling and biochemical characterization reveal the mechanism of hepatitis B virus polymerase resistance to lamivudine (3TC) and emtricitabine (FTC). *J Virol* 75, 4771–4779.

71 Gao HQ, Boyer PL, Sarafianos SG *et al.* (2000) The role of steric hindrance in 3TC resistance of human immunodeficiency virus type-1 reverse transcriptase. *J Mol Biol* 300, 403–418.

72 Bartholomeusz A, Tehan BG, Chalmers DK (2004) Comparisons of the HBV and HIV polymerase, and antiviral resistance mutations. *Antivir Ther* 9, 149–160.

73 Doo E, Liang TJ (2001) Molecular anatomy and pathophysiologic implications of drug resistance in hepatitis B virus infection. *Gastroenterology* 120, 1000–1008.

74 Bruss V, Lu X, Thomssen R *et al.* (1994) Post-translational alterations in transmembrane topology of the hepatitis B virus large envelope protein. *EMBO J* 13, 2273–2279.

75 Lambert C, Prange R (2001) Dual topology of the hepatitis B virus large envelope protein: determinants influencing post-translational pre-S translocation. *J Biol Chem* 276, 22265–22272.

76 Schmitt S, Glebe D, Alving K *et al.* (1999) Analysis of the pre-S2 N- and O-linked glycans of the M surface protein from human hepatitis B virus. *J Biol Chem* 274, 11945–11957.

77 Schmitt S, Glebe D, Tolle TK *et al.* (2004) Structure of pre-S2 N- and O-linked glycans in surface proteins from different genotypes of hepatitis B virus. *J Gen Virol* 85, 2045–2053.

78 Gerelsaikhan T, Tavis JE, Bruss V (1996) Hepatitis B virus nucleocapsid envelopment does not occur without genomic DNA synthesis. *J Virol* 70, 4269–4274.

79 Block TM, Lu X, Mehta AS *et al.* (1998) Treatment of chronic hepadnavirus infection in a woodchuck animal model with an inhibitor of protein folding and trafficking. *Nature Med* 4, 610–614.

80 Gripon P, Rumin S, Urban S *et al.* (2002) Infection of a human hepatoma cell line by hepatitis B virus. *Proc Natl Acad Sci USA* 99, 15655–15660.

81 Köck J, Nassal M, MacNelly S *et al.* (2001) Efficient infection of primary tupaia hepatocytes with purified human and woolly monkey hepatitis B virus. *J Virol* 75, 5084–5089.

82 Engelke M, Mills K, Seitz S *et al.* (2006) Characterization of a hepatitis B and hepatitis delta virus receptor binding site. *Hepatology* 43, 750–760.

83 Glebe D, Urban S, Knoop EV *et al.* (2005) Mapping of the hepatitis B virus attachment site by use of infection-inhibiting preS1 lipopeptides and tupaia hepatocytes. *Gastroenterology* 129, 234–245.

84 Jaoude GA, Sureau C (2005) Role of the antigenic loop of the hepatitis B virus envelope proteins in infectivity of hepatitis delta virus. *J Virol* 79, 10460–10466.

85 Chojnacki J, Anderson DA, Grgacic EV (2005) A hydrophobic domain in the large envelope protein is essential for fusion of duck hepatitis B virus at the late endosome. *J Virol* 79, 14945–14955.

86 Berting A, Fischer C, Schaefer S *et al.* (2000) Hemifusion activity of a chimeric influenza virus hemagglutinin with a putative fusion peptide from hepatitis B virus. *Virus Res* 68, 35–49.

87 Funk A, Mhamdi M, Hohenberg H *et al.* (2006) pH-independent entry and sequential endosomal sorting are major determinants of hepadnaviral infection in primary hepatocytes. *Hepatology* 44, 685–693.

88 Funk A, Hohenberg H, Mhamdi M *et al.* (2004) Spread of hepatitis B viruses in vitro requires extracellular progeny and may be codetermined by polarized egress. *J Virol* 78, 3977–3983.

89 Rabe B, Glebe D, Kann M (2006) Lipid-mediated introduction of hepatitis B virus capsids into nonsusceptible cells allows highly efficient replication and facilitates the study of early infection events. *J Virol* 80, 5465–5473.

90 Rabe B, Vlachou A, Pante N *et al.* (2003) Nuclear import of hepatitis B virus capsids and release of the viral genome. *Proc Natl Acad Sci USA* 100, 9849–9854.

91 Moolla N, Kew M, Arbuthnot P (2002) Regulatory elements of hepatitis B virus transcription. *J Viral Hepat* 9, 323–331.

92 Yu X, Mertz JE (1997) Differential regulation of the pre-C and pregenomic promoters of human hepatitis B virus by members of the nuclear receptor superfamily. *J Virol* 71, 9366–9374.

93 Sommer G, van Bommel F, Will H (2000) Genotype-specific synthesis and secretion of spliced hepatitis B virus genomes in hepatoma cells. *Virology* 271, 371–381.

94 Soussan P, Garreau F, Zylberberg H *et al.* (2000) In vivo expression of a new hepatitis B virus protein encoded by a spliced RNA. *J Clin Invest* 105, 55–60.

95 Soussan P, Tuveri R, Nalpas B *et al.* (2003) The expression of hepatitis B spliced protein (HBSP) encoded by a spliced hepatitis B virus RNA is associated with viral replication and liver fibrosis. *J Hepatol* 38, 343–348.

96 Huang J, Liang TJ (1993) A novel hepatitis B virus (HBV) genetic element with Rev response element-like properties that is essential for expression of HBV gene products. *Mol Cell Biol* 13, 7476–7486.

97 Heise T, Sommer G, Reumann K *et al.* (2006) The hepatitis B virus PRE contains a splicing regulatory element. *Nucleic Acids Res* 34, 353–363.

98 Liu N, Ji L, Maguire ML *et al.* (2004) cis-Acting sequences that contribute to the synthesis of relaxed-circular DNA of human hepatitis B virus. *J Virol* 78, 642–649.

99 Roseman AM, Berriman JA, Wynne SA *et al.* (2005) A structural model for maturation of the hepatitis B virus core. *Proc Natl Acad Sci USA* 102, 15821–15826.

100 Rost M, Mann S, Lambert C *et al.* (2006) {gamma}2-adaptin, a novel ubiquitin-interacting adaptor, and Nedd4 ubiquitin ligase control hepatitis B virus maturation. *J Biol Chem* 281, 29297–29308.

101 Thursz M (2004) Pros and cons of genetic association studies in hepatitis B. *Hepatology* 40, 284–286.

102 Visvanathan K, Lewin SR (2006) Immunopathogenesis: role of innate and adaptive immune responses. *Semin Liver Dis* 26, 104–115.

103 Wieland SF, Chisari F (2005) Stealth and cunning: hepatitis B and hepatitis C viruses. *J Virol* 79, 9369–9380.

104 Wieland S, Thimme R, Purcell RH *et al.* (2004) Genomic analysis of the host response to hepatitis B virus infection. *Proc Natl Acad Sci USA* 101, 6669–6674.

105 Murray JM, Wieland SF, Purcell RH *et al.* (2005) Dynamics of hepatitis B virus clearance in chimpanzees. *Proc Natl Acad Sci USA* 102, 17780–17785.

106 Wieland SF, Spangenberg HC, Thimme R *et al.* (2004) Expansion and contraction of the hepatitis B virus transcriptional template in infected chimpanzees. *Proc Natl Acad Sci USA* 101, 2129–2134.

107 Rehermann B, Ferrari C, Pasquinelli C *et al.* (1996) The hepatitis B virus persists for decades after patients' recovery from acute viral hepatitis despite active maintenance of a cytotoxic T-lymphocyte response. *Nat Med* 2, 1104–1108.

108 Cougot D, Neuveut C, Buendia MA (2005) HBV induced carcinogenesis. *J Clin Virol* 34(Suppl. 1), S75–S78.

109 Burczynska B, Madalinski K, Pawlowska J *et al.* (1994) The value of quantitative measurement of HBeAg and HBsAg before interferon-alpha treatment of chronic hepatitis B in children. *J Hepatol* 21, 1097–1102.

110 Whalley SA, Murray JM, Brown D *et al.* (2001) Kinetics of acute hepatitis B virus infection in humans. *J Exp Med* 193, 847–854.

111 Chulanov VP, Shipulin GA, Schaefer S *et al.* (2003) Kinetics of HBV DNA and HBsAg in acute hepatitis B patients with and without coinfection by other hepatitis viruses. *J Med Virol* 69, 313–323.

112 Gerlich W, Stamm B, Thomssen R (1977) [Prognostic significance of quantitative HBsAg determination in acute hepatitis B. Partial report of a cooperative clinical study of the DFG-focus of "virus hepatitis"]. *Verh Dtsch Ges Inn Med* 83, 554–557.

113 Gerlich WH (2004) Diagnostic problems caused by HBsAg mutants: a consensus report of an expert meeting. *Intervirology* 47, 310–313.

114 Funk ML, Rosenberg DM, Lok AS (2002) World-wide epidemiology of HBeAg-negative chronic hepatitis B and associated precore and core promoter variants. *J Viral Hepat* 9, 52–61.

115 Schildgen O, Sirma H, Funk A *et al.* (2006) Variant of hepatitis B virus with primary resistance to adefovir. *N Engl J Med* 354, 1807–1812.

116 Saldanha J (2001) Validation and standardisation of nucleic acid amplification technology (NAT) assays for the detection of viral contamination of blood and blood products. *J Clin Virol* 20, 7–13.

117 Heermann KH, Gerlich WH, Chudy M *et al.* (1999) Quantitative determination of hepatitis B virus DNA in two international reference plasmas. *J Clin Microbiol* 37, 68–73.

118 Grob P, Jilg W, Bornhak H *et al.* (2000) Serological pattern 'anti-HBc alone': report on a workshop. *J Med Virol* 62, 450–455.

119 Jilg W, Hottentrager B, Weinberger K *et al.* (2001) Prevalence of markers of hepatitis B in the adult German population. *J Med Virol* 63, 96–102.

120 Knoll A, Hartmann A, Hamoshi H *et al.* (2006) Serological pattern 'anti-HBc alone': characterization of 552 individuals and clinical significance. *World J Gastroenterol* 12, 1255–1260.

121 Allain JP (2004) Occult hepatitis B virus infection: implications in transfusion. *Vox Sang* 86, 83–91.

122 Weber B, Melchior W, Gehrke R *et al.* (2001) Hepatitis B virus markers in anti-HBc only positive individuals. *J Med Virol* 64, 312–319.

123 Gerlich WH, Uy A, Lambrecht F *et al.* (1986) Cutoff levels of immunoglobulin M antibody against viral core antigen for differentiation of acute, chronic, and past hepatitis B virus infections. *J Clin Microbiol* 24, 288–293.

124 Weber B (2006) Diagnostic impact of the genetic variability of the hepatitis B virus surface antigen gene. *J Med Virol* 78(Suppl. 1), S59–65.

125 Erhardt A, Gerlich W, Starke C *et al.* (2006) Treatment of chronic hepatitis delta with pegylated interferon-alpha2b. *Liver Int* 26, 805–810.

126 Flink HJ, van Zonneveld M, Hansen BE *et al.* (2006) Treatment with Peg-interferon alpha-2b for HBeAg-positive chronic hepatitis B: HBsAg loss is associated with HBV genotype. *Am J Gastroenterol* 101, 297–303.

127 Janssen HL, van Zonneveld M, Senturk H *et al.* (2005) Pegylated interferon alfa-2b alone or in combination with lamivudine for HBeApositive chronic hepatitis B: a randomised trial. *Lancet* 365, 123–129.

128 Kao JH, Wu NH, Chen PJ *et al.* (2000) Hepatitis B genotypes and the response to interferon therapy. *J Hepatol* 33, 998–1002.

129 Wai CT, Chu CJ, Hussain M *et al.* (2002) HBV genotype B is associated with better response to interferon therapy in HBeAg(+) chronic hepatitis than genotype C. *Hepatology* 36, 1425–1430.

130 Kramvis A, Weitzmann L, Owiredu WK *et al.* (2002) Analysis of the complete genome of subgroup A′ hepatitis B virus isolates from South Africa. *J Gen Virol* 83, 835–839.

131 Toan NL, Song le H, Kremsner PG *et al.* (2006) Impact of the hepatitis B virus genotype and genotype mixtures on the course of liver disease in Vietnam. *Hepatology* 43, 1375–1384.

132 Grandjacques C, Pradat P, Stuyver L *et al.* (2000) Rapid detection of genotypes and mutations in the pre-core promoter and the pre-core region of hepatitis B virus genome: correlation with viral persistence and disease severity. *J Hepatol* 33, 430–439.

133 Kirschberg O, Schuttler C, Repp R *et al.* (2004) A multiplex-PCR to identify hepatitis B virus-genotypes A–F. *J Clin Virol* 29, 39–43.

134 Naito H, Hayashi S, Abe K (2001) Rapid and specific genotyping system for hepatitis B virus corresponding to six major genotypes by PCR using type-specific primers. *J Clin Microbiol* 39, 362–364.

135 Sheldon J, Rodes B, Zoulim F *et al.* (2006) Mutations affecting the replication capacity of the hepatitis B virus. *J Viral Hepat* 13, 427–434.

136 Sugauchi F, Ohno T, Orito E *et al.* (2003) Influence of hepatitis B virus genotypes on the development of preS deletions and advanced liver disease. *J Med Virol* 70, 537–544.

137 Marschenz S, Endres AS, Brinckmann A *et al.* (2006) Functional analysis of complex hepatitis B virus variants associated with development of liver cirrhosis. *Gastroenterology* 131, 765–780.

138 Bartholomeusz A, Locarnini S (2006) Hepatitis B virus mutations associated with antiviral therapy. *J Med Virol* 78(Suppl. 1), S52–55.

139 Mason WS, Burrell CJ, Casey J *et al.* (2005) Hepadnaviridae. In: Fauquet CM, Mayo MA, Maniloff J *et al.* (eds) *Virus Taxonomy*, 8th Report of the International Committee on Taxonomy of Viruses. Philadelphia, PA: Elsevier.

140 Macnaughton TB, Lai MM (2006) HDV RNA replication: ancient relic or primer? *Curr Topics Microbiol Immunol* 307, 25–45.

141 Taylor JM (2006) Structure and replication of hepatitis delta virus RNA. *Curr Topics Microbiol Immunol* 307, 1–23.

142 Kos A, Dijkema R, Arnberg C *et al.* (1986) The hepatitis delta (delta) virus possesses a circular RNA. *Nature* 323, 558–560.

143 Wong SK, Lazinski DW (2002) Replicating hepatitis delta virus RNA is edited in the nucleus by the small form of ADAR1. *Proc Natl Acad Sci USA* 99, 15118–15123.

144 Polson AG, Bass BL, Casey JL (1996) RNA editing of hepatitis delta virus antigenome by dsRNA-adenosine deaminase. *Nature* 380, 454–456.

145 Ferre-D'Amare AR, Zhou K, Doudna JA (1998) Crystal structure of a hepatitis delta virus ribozyme. *Nature* 395, 567–574.

146 Ke A, Zhou K, Ding F *et al.* (2004) A conformational switch controls hepatitis delta virus ribozyme catalysis. *Nature* 429, 201–205.

147 Cornillez-Ty CT, Lazinski DW (2003) Determination of the multimerization state of the hepatitis delta virus antigens in vivo. *J Virol* 77, 10314–10326.

148 Chen CW, Tsay YG, Wu HL *et al.* (2002) The double-stranded RNA-activated kinase, PKR, can phosphorylate hepatitis D virus small delta antigen at functional serine and threonine residues. *J Biol Chem* 277, 33058–33067.

149 Bichko VV, Lemon SM, Wang JG *et al.* (1996) Epitopes exposed on hepatitis delta virus ribonucleoproteins. *J Virol* 70, 5807–5811.

150 Radjef N, Gordien E, Ivaniushina V *et al.* (2004) Molecular phylogenetic analyses indicate a wide and ancient radiation of African hepatitis delta virus, suggesting a deltavirus genus of at least seven major clades. *J Virol* 78, 2537–2544.

151 Deny P (2006) Hepatitis delta virus genetic variability: from genotypes I, II, III to eight major clades? *Curr Topics Microbiol Immunol* 307, 151–171.

152 Wang TC, Chao M (2005) RNA recombination of hepatitis delta virus in natural mixed-genotype infection and transfected cultured cells. *J Virol* 79, 2221–2229.

153 Su CW, Huang YH, Huo TI *et al.* (2006) Genotypes and viremia of hepatitis B and D viruses are associated with outcomes of chronic hepatitis D patients. *Gastroenterology* 130, 1625–1635.

154 Wu JC (2006) Functional and clinical significance of hepatitis D virus genotype II infection. *Curr Topics Microbiol Immunol* 307, 173–186.

155 Casey JL, Niro GA, Engle RE *et al.* (1996) Hepatitis B virus (HBV)/hepatitis D virus (HDV) coinfection in outbreaks of acute hepatitis in the Peruvian Amazon basin: the roles of HDV genotype III and HBV genotype F. *J Infect Dis* 174, 920–926.

156 Casey JL, Gerin JL (2006) The woodchuck model of HDV infection. *Curr Topics Microbiol Immunol* 307, 211–225.

157 Polo JM, Jeng KS, Lim B *et al.* (1995) Transgenic mice support replication of hepatitis delta virus RNA in multiple tissues, particularly in skeletal muscle. *J Virol* 69, 4880–4887.

158 Beard MR, MacNaughton TB, Gowans EJ (1996) Identification and characterization of a hepatitis delta virus RNA transcriptional promoter. *J Virol* 70, 4986–4995.

159 Sheu SY, Chen KL, Lee YW *et al.* (1996) No intermolecular interaction between the large hepatitis delta antigens is required for the secretion with hepatitis B surface antigen: a model of empty HDV particle. *Virology* 218, 275–278.

160 Yamashiro T, Nagayama K, Enomoto N *et al.* (2004) Quantitation of the level of hepatitis delta virus RNA in serum, by real-time polymerase chain reaction—and its possible correlation with the clinical stage of liver disease. *J Infect Dis* 189, 1151–1157.

153 Nei M, Kumar S (2000) *Molecular Evolution and Phylogenetics*. Oxford: Oxford University Press.

154 Kimbi GC, Kramvis A, Kew MC (2004) Distinctive sequence characteristics of subgenotype A1 isolates of hepatitis B virus from South Africa. *J Gen Virol* 85, 1211–1220.

155 Kurbanov F, Tanaka Y, Fujiwara K *et al.* (2005) A new subtype (subgenotype) Ac (A3) of hepatitis B virus and recombination between genotypes A and E in Cameroon. *J Gen Virol* 86, 2047–2056.

156 Makuwa M, Souquiere S, Telfer P *et al.* (2006) Identification of hepatitis B virus subgenotype A3 in rural Gabon. *J Med Virol* 78, 1175–1184.

157 Olinger CM, Venard V, Njayou M *et al.* (2006) Phylogenetic analysis of the precore/core gene of hepatitis B virus genotypes E and A in West Africa: new subtypes, mixed infections and recombinations. *J Gen Virol* 87, 1163–1173.

158 Nagasaki F, Niitsuma H, Cervantes JG *et al.* (2006) Analysis of the entire nucleotide sequence of hepatitis B virus genotype B in the Philippines reveals a new subgenotype of genotype B. *J Gen Virol* 87, 1175–1180.

159 Sakamoto T, Tanaka Y, Orito E *et al.* (2006) Novel subtypes (subgenotypes) of hepatitis B virus genotypes B and C among chronic liver disease patients in the Philippines. *J Gen Virol* 87, 1873–1882.

160 Sugauchi F, Mizokami M, Orito E *et al.* (2001) A novel variant genotype C of hepatitis B virus identified in isolates from Australian Aborigines: complete genome sequence and phylogenetic relatedness. *J Gen Virol* 82, 883–892.

161 Cavinta L, Sun J, Zarnekow M *et al.* (submitted) New hepatitis B virus subgenotype C5 from the Philippines.

162 Banerjee A, Kurbanov F, Datta S *et al.* (2006) Phylogenetic relatedness and genetic diversity of hepatitis B virus isolates in Eastern India. *J Med Virol* 78, 1164–1174.

163 Kato H, Fujiwara K, Gish RG *et al.* (2005) Classifying genotype F of hepatitis B virus into F1 and F2 subtypes. *World J Gastroenterol* 11, 6295–6304.

164 Norder H, Arauz-Ruiz P, Blitz L *et al.* (2003) The T(1858) variant predisposing to the precore stop mutation correlates with one of two major genotype F hepatitis B virus clades. *J Gen Virol* 84, 2083–2087.

165 Devesa M, Rodriguez C, Leon G *et al.* (2004) Clade analysis and surface antigen polymorphism of hepatitis B virus American genotypes. *J Med Virol* 72, 377–384.

166 Huy TT, Ushijima H, Sata T *et al.* (2006) Genomic characterization of HBV genotype F in Bolivia: genotype F subgenotypes correlate with geographic distribution and T(1858) variant. *Arch Virol* 151, 589–597.

167 Weber B (2005) Recent developments in the diagnosis and monitoring of HBV infection and role of the genetic variability of the S gene. *Expert Rev Mol Diagn* 5, 75–91.

9.1.2.ii Structure, replication and laboratory diagnosis of hepatitis C virus

Ralf Bartenschlager

Introduction

Persistent infection with the hepatitis C virus (HCV) is a major risk factor for the development of chronic liver disease. Although it was already known in the late 1970s that a non-A, non-B hepatitis virus must exist that frequently causes chronic liver disease after blood transfusion, it was not until 1988 that the genome of this virus could be cloned [1]. The availability of the cloned genome allowed the implementation of diagnostic tests to exclude HCV-contaminated blood products, resulting in a rapid and profound decline in the number of new infections [2]. One of the main routes of transmission is the use of HCV-contaminated needles; it is assumed that inadequately sterilized needles used during treatment of schistosomiasis from the 1960s to the 1980s account for the high prevalence of about 30% of HCV infections in Egypt [3].

Based on nucleotide sequence diversity of HCV genomes, six major genotypes and more than 100 subtypes have been defined. Viruses belonging to genotype 1 are distributed throughout the world, whereas other genotypes are primarily restricted to distinct geographical regions [4]. Apart from steatosis, which seems to be linked primarily to genotype 3 virus infections [5], no clear associations can be made between a distinct genotype and pathogenesis. However, sustained viral response rates are clearly associated with the genotype of the infecting virus because success of interferon (IFN)/ribavirin combination therapy with patients infected with genotype 2 and 3 viruses is in the range of 80% but only about 50% in genotype 1 and 4 virus infections [5]. The molecular details underlying this striking correlation are not yet understood, but it argues for viral determinants of IFN-α resistance (see below).

Clinical course of hepatitis C

The course and outcome of HCV infection are very variable [6,7]. In acute hepatitis C, only 30–35% of adults develop symptoms and these are fatal in less than 1%. The average incubation period of acute hepatitis C is about 50 days (Fig. 1). During this period, HCV RNA becomes detectable in serum with virus titres increasing to an average value of about 10^5 genome equivalents per mL (see below). Serum aminotransferase values typically rise 2–4 weeks after the appearance of viral RNA followed by rather non-specific symptoms such as malaise, weakness, nausea, poor appetite or muscle aches. In a fraction of patients, a typical icteric phase follows that may last 4–6 weeks. Concomitant with symptoms, HCV-specific antibodies become detectable and rise in titre during the following weeks. About 30% of patients mount an immune response that is sufficient to clear viral infection, accompanied by a resolution of symptoms. However, the majority of patients with an acute infection, in particular those who are asymptomatic, do not resolve the infection but, rather, develop chronic hepatitis C. In fact, about 75% of infected adults and 55% of infected children acquire a persistent infection. It is characterized by prolonged (usually 6 months and more) detection of viral RNA in the serum and, in about 50% of patients, elevated serum aminotransferases. However, there is significant fluctuation in both parameters, and persistently infected patients may have phases of normal serum aminotransferases and no detectable HCV RNA. Therefore, single time point measurements do not allow discrimination between acute resolved and chronic hepatitis C.

HCV genome organization and functions of the viral proteins

In silico analysis of the first HCV genome sequence revealed a genomic organization that is very similar to that of flaviviruses. Therefore, HCV was grouped in the family Flaviviridae to which the flaviviruses and the pestiviruses belong. These viruses have in common a single-stranded RNA genome of positive polarity

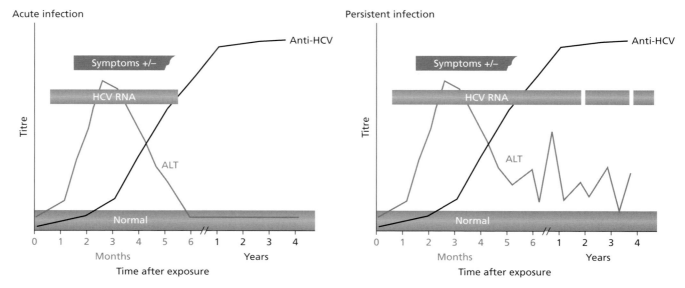

Fig. 1 Serological patterns of acute self-limiting HCV infection (left) or acute HCV infection leading to a persistent state (right). For details, see text. ALT, alanine aminotransferase.

that, in the case of HCV, has a length of about 9600 nucleotides (Fig. 2). It carries one long open reading frame (ORF) that is flanked at both ends by short non-translated regions (NTRs) that are essential for RNA translation and replication (reviewed in [8]). This ORF encodes an ~ 3000-amino-acid-long polyprotein that is cleaved co- and posttranslationally into at least 10 different products to which distinct functions could be ascribed (Fig. 2). The structural core proteins (core, E1 and E2) are the major constituents of the virus particle, and they reside in the amino (N)-terminal region of the polyprotein. p7 is a small hydrophobic protein that may act as a viroporin. It is essential for infectivity *in vivo*, can form oligomeric complexes in lipid membranes and is thought to form an ion channel. It was shown recently that p7 is required for assembly and release of virus particles from infected cells (E. Steinmann, R. Bartenschlager and T. Pietschmann, unpublished). NS2 is a bifunctional molecule. Its largely hydrophobic N-terminal domain that anchors this protein to intracellular membranes is involved in virus formation (N. Appel, T. Pietschmann and R. Bartenschlager, unpublished). In contrast, the NS2 carboxy (C)-terminal domain is part of the NS2/3 protease that is formed by this NS2 domain and the N-terminal NS3 domain. The NS2/3 protease catalyses cleavage at the NS2/3 site (reviewed in [8]). The protease is essential for RNA replication in cell culture and for infectivity *in vivo*. The N-terminal NS3 domain carries a serine-type protease that forms a tight complex with NS4A. The latter acts as a cofactor that, upon binding, activates the enzyme, which mediates cleavage at four sites at least (Fig. 2). The C-terminal NS3 domain binds to RNA and carries a nucleoside triphosphatase and a helicase activity. It is thought to catalyse unwinding of double-stranded (ds) RNA during replication and may also be involved in RNA translation. NS4B is a highly hydrophobic

protein that can induce membrane alterations important for the formation of the viral replication complex. The highly phosphorylated NS5A is also crucially involved in RNA replication, but its exact role is not yet defined (reviewed in [9]). NS5A binds to RNA [10,11] and may control the transition from RNA replication to virus assembly. In addition, NS5A appears to be involved in IFN-α resistance [9]. NS5B is the RNA-dependent RNA polymerase (RdRp), which is the core enzyme of the viral RNA amplification machinery. An 11th protein is generated in low amounts by a ribosomal frameshift event or by internal translation initiation [8]. The resulting product(s) designated F or ARF protein(s) is an unstable and barely detectable protein. However, both a humoral and a cellular immune response against this protein was found in a fraction of infected patients, arguing that F/ARF-P is expressed *in vivo*. Its role in the viral life cycle is not known, but it is dispensable for HCV RNA replication in cell culture.

Translation of the HCV genome is mediated by the 5′ NTR which folds into a complex higher order RNA structure [12] (Fig. 2). It serves as an internal ribosome entry site (IRES) that allows translation of the HCV genome in the absence of a 5′ terminal cap structure. The cap is usually added to the 5′ end of cellular mRNAs by enzymes residing in the nucleus; as HCV replicates in the cytoplasm and does not encode the enzymes required for cap formation, its viral genome must be translated by some alternative strategy. Apart from serving as an IRES, the first about 130 nucleotides of the genome are required for RNA replication and most likely serve as a 'core promoter' for the synthesis of positive strand RNA [13].

The 3′ end of the HCV genome is also formed by an NTR (Fig. 2). It has a tripartite structure composed of a variable region, a poly U/UC tract and a highly conserved, 98-nucleotide-long

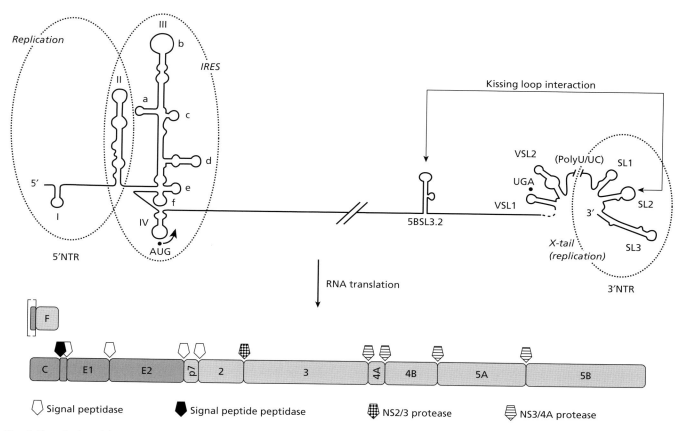

Fig. 2 Organization of the HCV genome and essential *cis*-acting RNA elements. The viral RNA with the secondary structures of the non-translated regions (NTRs) as well as 5BSL3.2 is given at the top. RNA elements in the NTRs required for translation and replication are encircled by dotted lines. The start and stop codons of the polyprotein are indicated by dots. The organization of the polyprotein with the individual cleavage products is drawn below. The F proteins generated by ribosomal frameshifting a few codons downstream of the core gene AUG start codon or by internal translation initiation are drawn above. Proteases responsible for polyprotein cleavage are given at the bottom. SL, stem–loop; VSL, stem–loop in the variable region; IRES, internal ribosome entry site.

sequence designated the X-tail [14,15]. Most of the 3′ NTR is essential for RNA replication and serves as a promoter for the synthesis of negative strand RNA.

A third RNA element that is essential for HCV replication was identified in the 3′ terminal coding region of NS5B [16] (Fig. 2). This element, designated 5BSL3.2, forms a stable stem–loop structure with the top loop sequence forming a basepairing interaction with the top loop region of SL2 in the 3′ NTR [17] (Fig. 2). It was found that 5BSL3.2 binds the NS5B RdRp with some specificity [18]. It is therefore plausible to speculate that, via binding of NS5B to this RNA structure, the polymerase is 'captured' and transferred to the 3′ NTR (for which the RNA–RNA interaction between the two stem–loops may be required) in order to initiate synthesis of negative strand viral RNA.

Structure of the virus particle

Owing to limiting amounts of HCV particles in infected tissues and, until very recently, the lack of efficient *in vitro* propagation systems, the molecular composition and structure of the virus particle could not be analysed in detail. Based on analogy with

the well-solved structures of the envelope proteins of the flaviviruses, tick-borne encephalitis virus and Dengue virus, and intensive biochemical studies of the HCV glycoproteins, a model was proposed (reviewed in [19]) (Fig. 3). E1 and E2 are tethered to the viral envelope via their hydrophobic transmembrane domains residing in the C-termini of the proteins. The same domains are also required for the formation of heterodimeric E1/E2 complexes that may form higher order oligomers. It is assumed that the ectodomain of E2 (and probably also of E1) lies rather flat on the surface of the envelope that surrounds the nucleocapsid. So far, it remains unclear whether the capsid has a regular symmetry or forms some rather unstructured ribonucleoprotein complex.

By using a novel system that allows the production of infectious HCV particles in cell culture, a first characterization of the virions could be made [20–22] (Fig. 3). HCV particles are spherical with an average diameter of about 55 nm and an inner spherical structure of about 30 nm that may represent the nucleocapsid (Fig. 3). Cell culture-grown HCV particles are rather heterogeneous in density, but the majority of particles sediment to a density of about 1.10 g/mL, which is similar to what was

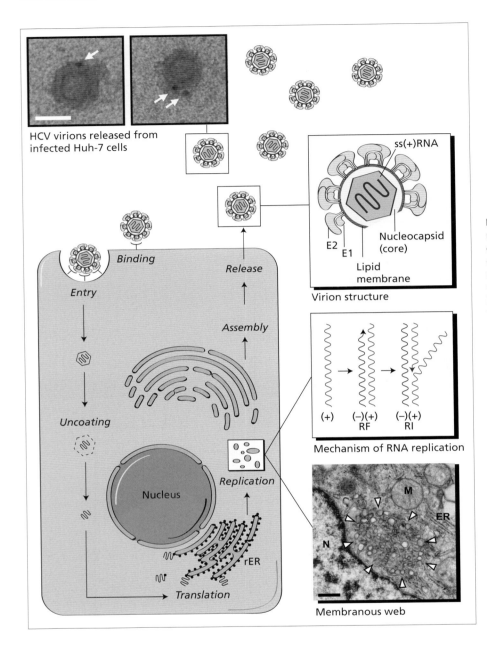

HCV virions released from infected Huh-7 cells

Virion structure

Mechanism of RNA replication

Membranous web

Fig. 3 Schematic diagram of the HCV replication cycle. Virus particles enter the host cell most likely by receptor-mediated endocytosis (binding and entry). The viral genome is liberated from the nucleocapsid (uncoating) and translated at the rough ER. Newly synthesized viral proteins induce the formation of membranous vesicles forming a membranous web, the site of HCV RNA replication (see electron micrograph at lower right; the arrowheads indicate the position of the web; note the close proximity of the web and ER membranes; N, nucleus; ER, endoplasmic reticulum, M, mitochondrium. bar = 500 nm). After genome amplification and further viral protein accumulation, progeny virions are assembled and released. The centre right part of the figure shows a model for the synthesis of negative (–) and positive (+) strand RNA via a replicative form (RF) and a replicative intermediate (RI). The upper right part shows a schematic representation of an HCV particle. The envelope proteins E1 and E2 are drawn according to the structure and orientation of the tick-borne encephalitis virus envelope proteins M and E respectively [46]. The two electron micrographs at the upper left corner of the figure show infectious HCV particles produced in the hepatoma cell line Huh-7 (arrows point to E2-specific immunogold particles; bar = 50 nm) (adapted from ref. 8 with permission from the publisher).

described for HCV in patient and chimpanzee sera. The heterogeneity is probably due to association of the viral particles with host cell components, most notably lipoproteins and antibodies.

The HCV replication cycle

HCV replicates primarily in hepatocytes, but there is convincing evidence that replication also occurs in lymphocytes, at least under laboratory conditions (reviewed in [8]). However, the importance of this extrahepatic reservoir for HCV persistence and success or failure of antiviral therapy is not clear. The recent demonstration of viral RNA in lymphocytes isolated from patients with spontaneous virus clearance or sustained viral

response suggests that HCV can persist in lymphatic cells [23,24]. It is questionable whether the residual viral RNA detected in these patients is of clinical and epidemiological relevance, as relapses are very rare in patients with sustained response induced by therapy and the amounts of viral RNA detected in lymphatic cells are very low.

Infection of the host cell starts with HCV binding to one or more cell surface molecules. Candidate receptors are CD81, scavenger receptor BI (SR-BI), low-density lipoprotein receptor and dendritic cell-specific ICAM-3-grabbing non-integrin (DC-SIGN) and L-SIGN (reviewed in [8]) receptors. However, none of these molecules is sufficient on its own to mediate productive infection. It is therefore assumed that some as yet unidentified molecule expressed preferentially on the surface of hepatocytes is also required for uptake of HCV into the host cell. The virus probably enters the cell by receptor-mediated endocytosis and, upon release of the RNA genome into the cytoplasm, the RNA is translated at the rough endoplasmic reticulum (ER) where processing of the structural proteins occurs (Fig. 3). It is assumed that NS4B, presumably in conjunction with some other viral and cellular protein(s), induces the formation of a distinct membranous compartment within the cytoplasm that has been designated the membranous web [25]. It carries most, if not all, viral proteins and is probably the site of HCV RNA replication. The positive strand RNA genome is amplified via a negative strand copy that may basepair with the positive strand RNA and form a double-stranded intermediate designated the 'replicative form' (RF) (Fig. 3). This RF would serve as a template for the production of excess amounts of positive strand RNA copies that can be used for translation (i.e. polyprotein synthesis), serve as a template for the production of new negative strand RNAs or become encapsidated into viral particles. The exact site of virus assembly and the underlying mechanisms are not known, but it is assumed that virus particles are formed at or in close proximity to the ER or ER-derived membranes. Interestingly, within a transfected or infected cell, the majority of the HCV core protein is associated with lipid droplets, raising the possibility that they play an important role in particle formation.

Recent achievements in cell-based HCV replication systems

With the availability of the first molecularly cloned HCV genome, initial progress was rapid and led to the elucidation of the viral genome structure and the characterization of several HCV proteins, most notably those enzymes that are prime targets for selective therapy (NS3 protease, NS3 helicase and NS5B RdRp). However, attempts to propagate HCV in cultured cells were of limited success and only in the past few years could this hurdle be overcome in a step-by-step process (reviewed in [26]). The first important achievement was the development of the HCV replicon system [27]. It is based on the self-replication of genetically engineered HCV 'minivariants' in which the region encoding core to NS2 is replaced by a selectable marker and a heterologous IRES (Fig. 4a). Synthetic RNAs produced from the cloned replicons were transfected into cells of the human hepatoma cell line Huh-7 and, after appropriate selection of the cells

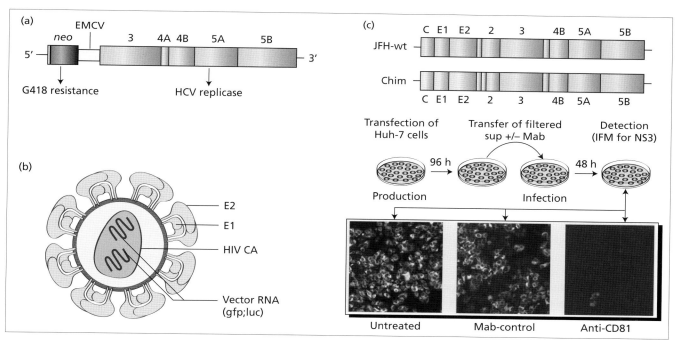

Fig. 4 Model systems for the study of HCV replication in cell culture. (a) Design of a selectable subgenomic HCV replicon carrying the selectable marker *neo* that confers resistance to the cytotoxic drug G418. The *neo* gene is translated via the HCV IRES, whereas the HCV replication factors NS3 to NS5B are translated from the EMCV IRES. (b) Structure of an HCVpp that is composed of a lipid envelope carrying the E1–E2 glycoprotein complexes, the HIV nucleocapsid (CA) and two copies of the HIV vector RNA, into which a marker gene has been inserted (most often the green fluorescent protein (gfp) or the luciferase (luc) gene). (c) Production of infectious HCV in cell culture. Huh-7 cells are transfected with genomic HCV RNA obtained by *in vitro* transcription from the cloned JFH-1 genome (top) or a JFH-1 chimera in which the region from core up to the N-terminus of NS2 (indicated by red) stems from another isolate of the same or a different genotype. Four days later, culture supernatant is harvested and used to inoculate naive Huh-7 cells. Forty-eight hours after inoculation, cells are analysed for infection using a NS3-specific immunofluorescence assay (bottom). Infection was performed directly with supernatant (left) or with supernatant containing either a CD81-specific antibody or a control antibody (right and centre respectively). Infection can be neutralized by CD81-specific antibodies, demonstrating that CD81 plays an important role in infection by HCV. Mab, monoclonal antibody.

(e.g. with G418 in the case of replicons carrying the *neo* gene), drug-resistant colonies were obtained that contained high amounts of self-replicating HCV RNAs. Subsequent studies confirmed and extended this observation, and it was found that the high level of HCV RNA replication in this system is due to cell culture adaptive mutations and the selection for cells that are highly permissive for HCV RNA replication (reviewed in [26]). The replicon system is in wide use nowadays both for basic research and for the development of antiviral compounds.

The next important achievement was the HCV pseudoparticle (pp) system [28,29]. HCVpps are composed of retroviral nucleocapsids (e.g. derived from HIV) that are surrounded by a lipid envelope into which native HCV glycoproteins are embedded (Fig. 4b). As infection [binding to the receptor(s), uptake into the cell and uncoating] is orchestrated primarily by the envelope glycoproteins, HCVpps are an ideal tool for the study of the early steps in the HCV replication cycle. In addition, they are also an important tool for characterizing the neutralizing capacity of antibodies directed against the HCV glycoproteins or cell surface molecules assumed to be required for infection. In fact, it was shown that antibodies directed against CD81, SR-B1 and LDL receptor interfere with infection by HCVpps, arguing that these cell surface molecules are critical for infection (reviewed in [8]). Moreover, it was shown that sera from hepatitis C patients contain (partially) neutralizing and even cross-neutralizing antibodies. However, the role of these antibodies in controlling an HCV infection is not clear.

Very recently, the first system for the production of infectious HCV in cell culture was established [20–22] (Fig. 4c). It is based on a distinct HCV genotype 2a isolate (designated JFH-1 because it was isolated from a Japanese patient with fulminant hepatitis) that, for unknown reasons, replicates to an unprecedentedly high level in Huh-7 cells and does not require cell culture adaptive mutations [30]. Upon transfection of these cells with RNA derived from the cloned JFH-1 genome, virus particles are released that are infectious for naive Huh-7 cells as well as for chimpanzees [20]. The latter observation confirms that cell culture-grown JFH-1 particles are authentic. Infectivity could be neutralized by CD81-specific antisera, antibodies against E2 and immunoglobulins isolated from chronically infected hepatitis C patients [20–22].

Apart from using the authentic JFH-1 genome, virus production could also be achieved using chimeric genomes in which the region from core to NS2 of JFH-1 is replaced by the analogous region from isolates of the same [21] or even a different genotype [31] (Fig. 4c). The production of such chimeras will greatly expand our arsenal of tools for studying the early steps of the viral life cycle, evaluating neutralizing and cross-neutralizing antibodies on a broad scale and developing compounds that interfere with the entry of most HCV genotypes into host cells.

HCV and innate immunity

Given the clear correlation between sustained viral response after IFN-α/ribavirin combination therapy and the genotype of the infecting HCV, it was assumed that viral factors contribute to IFN resistance. Based on comparative sequence analyses of HCV genomes isolated from IFN-α responders and non-responders as well as several biochemical and cell-based assays, the two viral proteins NS5A and E2 were identified as potential antagonists of the IFN-induced dsRNA-activated protein kinase PKR (reviewed in [32]). However, the results obtained in several follow-up studies were controversial, and it is still unclear whether and to what extent these viral factors contribute to IFN-α resistance.

Apart from a direct inhibition of a distinct effector molecule contributing to the IFN-induced antiviral state, there is increasing evidence that HCV interferes with signal transduction. One pathway that may be targeted by the HCV core protein is the Jak-STAT signalling pathway responsible for relaying the signal from the IFN-α receptor to the transcriptional activation of IFN-α-induced genes (reviewed in [8]).

The key player in blocking the induction of the early innate antiviral defence appears to be the NS3/4A protease that can interfere with the dsRNA-induced activation of IFN regulatory factor 3 (IRF-3) [33]. Within a cell, dsRNA is perceived by at least three different molecules: Toll-like receptor 3 (TLR3) and the RNA helicases retinoic acid-inducible gene I (RIG-I) and mda5 (also called Helicard) (reviewed in [34]). Upon activation by dsRNA binding, these molecules recruit adapter proteins, which are TRIF (also called TICAM-1) in the case of TLR3, and Cardif (also called IPS-1, MAVS or VISA) in the case of RIG-I. These adapter molecules relay their activation signal via induction of a kinase complex and phosphorylation of IRF-3, resulting in the transcriptional activation of IFN-β [34]. It was shown that both TRIF and Cardif can be cleaved by the NS3/4A protease, at least under various experimental conditions [35,36]. Although final proof for *in vivo* relevance is not yet available, Cardif is also cleaved by the NS3/4A protease in HCV-infected Huh-7 cells [35], suggesting that interference at least with the RIG-I pathway also occurs *in vivo*. This interference may contribute to the establishment of a persistent HCV infection.

HCV and adaptive immunity

As can be inferred from the high rate of persistent infections, HCV not only escapes innate immunity but also has the means to undermine adaptive immunity without globally affecting immune response to other infectious agents. It is generally accepted that the vigour and the breadth of the immune response mounted upon HCV infection determine the outcome of infection (reviewed in [37]). Therefore, a successful immune response targets multiple major histocompatibility complex (MHC) class I-restricted epitopes in the HCV polyprotein and induces rather large numbers of HCV-specific CD8+ T cells. In addition, a strong CD8+ T-cell response is usually accompanied by a strong and multispecific CD4+ T-cell proliferative response, and permanent loss of this response is a strong predictor of persistence [38,39]. Resolved infections usually leave a durable memory response, lowering the chance of persistence upon reinfection [40]. This appears to be brought about mainly by CD4+ T cells [41].

Given the high frequency of persistence, in most cases T-cell responses either are rather poor or decline rapidly after an initially strong response. The underlying reasons are not well understood, but it should be kept in mind that HCV infection does not lead to a general immune suppression as is the case, for example, with HIV but, rather, induces a defect in cellular immunity that is HCV specific. It is assumed that an HCV-specific loss of T-cell help is the key event by which the virus escapes adaptive immunity [41]. One could imagine that the interference of HCV with the innate immunity (e.g. TLR3, RIG-I) results in a series of consecutive events that lead to CD4+ T-cell impairment. As T-cell help is important for CD8+ T cells, the degree of helper cell impairment would be a critical determinant of virus elimination or persistence. A weak T-cell response would also facilitate the emergence of T-cell escape variants in HCV epitopes and may lead to functional impairment (anergy) of CD8+ T cells.

Thus far, it is uncertain to what extent B-cell responses contribute to viral clearance. On the one hand, immune escape mutants in B-cell epitopes have been described, arguing that HCV adapts to immune selection pressure exerted by antibodies. On the other hand, antibodies developed during self-limited infection do not prevent reinfection, indicating that they are of limited efficacy. Moreover, HCV infection can be terminated in the absence of antibodies [42]. It is therefore assumed that T-cell immunity is the primary determinant in controlling HCV infection.

Laboratory diagnosis

Two types of laboratory tests are used for detection and monitoring of HCV infection: virological assays measuring viral components (RNA and core protein) and serological assays measuring HCV-specific antibodies (Fig. 1). First-generation assays developed for the detection of HCV-contaminated blood and blood products were based on an antibody-specific enzyme-linked immunosorbent assay (ELISA) using a recombinant HCV antigen derived from the NS3 to 4B coding region [2]. Later on, this assay was steadily improved by the inclusion of antigens derived from core and NS5. Current ELISAs have a specificity of more than 99%, and they are positive in more than 99% of immunocompetent patients with detectable HCV RNA [43]. However, antibody detection is problematic in immuno-compromised and haemodialysis patients. RNA testing has therefore been recommended because of potentially false-negative antibody diagnosis in these individuals.

Anti-HCV antibodies can be detected in serum 2–4 months after infection, but seroconversion may take up to 6 months (Fig. 1). Given this large serological window (time from infection until the development of detectable antibodies), assays to detect anti-HCV IgM have been developed, but they do not narrow down the serological window significantly. Therefore, nucleic acid-based testing is used. To exclude false-positive ELISA results, confirmatory assays have been developed. The most commonly used is the recombinant immunoblot assay RIBA (Chiron Corporation, Emeryville, CA, USA), in which several recombinant peptide antigens are immobilized on a strip that is probed with a patient serum. This assay allows the detection of antibodies directed against individual HCV antigens.

Qualitative assays for RNA detection are based on target amplification using polymerase chain reaction (PCR) or transcription-mediated amplification (TMA) (reviewed in [44]). Two commercial kits are available: first, the PCR-based assay which has a detection cutoff of 50 international units (IU) of HCV RNA/mL (based on the HCV RNA IU as defined by WHO for standardization of HCV RNA quantification units); second, the TMA-based assay that is slightly more sensitive (~ 10 IU of HCV RNA/mL). Both assays have a specificity of about 99% and, because of their high sensitivity, are the gold standards for the detection of HCV. Qualitative RNA detection assays have been implemented in blood banks of, for example, the EU and the US in order to reduce the risk of transfusion-associated hepatitis C that arises as a result of the long serological window. Because of this rigorous screening, the risk of HCV transmission by this route has been reduced to less than 1 in 1 million blood donations.

Quantitative HCV RNA assays are based on branched (b)DNA technology, competitive reverse transcription (RT)-PCR or real-time RT-PCR. The broadest dynamic range of quantification is achieved with the last, which can cover a range from 30 to 2×10^8 IU/mL (Cobas TaqMan 48 HCV; Roche Molecular Systems, USA). The specificity of these assays is up to 99%, and they allow quantification of viral load independent of the genotype of the virus. The advantage of the bDNA assay is that no amplification of the target sequence is required, which reduces the risk of false-positive results, e.g. resulting from contamination, and false-negative results, e.g. on account of polymerase inhibitors present in the patient sample. The disadvantage of bDNA over RT-PCR-based methods is its lower sensitivity.

An alternative to qualitative and quantitative RNA detection methods is the detection of viral antigens, which is technically less challenging and less demanding for the instrumentation of the diagnostic laboratory. A core antigen-specific ELISA has been developed (Ortho-Clinical Diagnostics, USA), and it was shown that the core antigen titre correlates well with the HCV RNA level [45]. Core titres can therefore be used as a marker for viral RNA replication. However, given the lower sensitivity of this antigen ELISA compared with RNA detection methods, its clinical use is somewhat limited.

Determination of the genotype of the infecting virus is an important parameter for the design of antiviral combination therapy. Several commercial assays for genotyping are available that, with one exception (Murex HCV serotyping 1–6 assay; Murex Diagnostics, UK), are based on analysing viral RNA. One assay uses hybridization of amplicons with genotype-specific oligonucleotides immobilized on strips and colorimetric detection (InnoLIPA or Versant genotyping assay; Innogenetics, Belgium). Other assays are based on direct sequence analysis of amplicons derived from the 5′ NTR and subsequent alignment with an HCV genotype sequence database (Truegene HCV 5′ NC genotyping kit; Bayer, USA). Finally, a genotyping system based on multiple real-time PCR amplifications of the 5′ NTR and part of the NS5B coding region using genotype-specific primers is commercially available (HCV Geno ASR; Abbott, USA). All assays can discriminate between the six major genotypes but not, or only insufficiently, differentiate between subtypes. This is, however, not of clinical relevance, because decisions for therapy are based on genotypes and not subtypes.

References

1 Choo QL, Kuo G, Weiner AJ et al. (1989) Isolation of a cDNA clone derived from a blood-borne non-A, non-B viral hepatitis genome. Science 244, 359–362.

2 Kuo G, Choo QL, Alter HJ et al. (1989) An assay for circulating antibodies to a major etiologic virus of human non-A, non-B hepatitis. Science 244, 362–364.

3 Rao MR, Naficy AB, Darwish MA et al. (2002) Further evidence for association of hepatitis C infection with parenteral schistosomiasis treatment in Egypt. BMC Infect Dis 2, 29.

4 Simmonds P (1998) Variability of the hepatitis C virus genome. Curr Stud Haematol Blood Transfus 62, 38–63.

5 Pawlotsky JM (2003) Hepatitis C virus genetic variability: pathogenic and clinical implications. Clin Liver Dis 7, 45–66.

6 Hoofnagle JH (1997) Hepatitis C: the clinical spectrum of disease. Hepatology 26, 15S–20S.

7 Seeff LB (2002) Natural history of chronic hepatitis C. Hepatology 36, S35–S46.

8 Bartenschlager R, Frese M, Pietschmann T (2004) Novel insights into hepatitis C virus replication and persistence. Adv Virus Res 63, 71–180.

9 Macdonald A, Harris M (2004) Hepatitis C virus NS5A: tales of a promiscuous protein. J Gen Virol 85, 2485–2502.

10 Tellinghuisen TL, Marcotrigiano J, Rice CM (2005) Structure of the zinc-binding domain of an essential component of the hepatitis C virus replicase. Nature 435, 374–379.

11 Huang L, Hwang J, Sharma SD et al. (2005) Hepatitis C virus nonstructural protein 5A (NS5A) is a RNA-binding protein. J Biol Chem. 280, 36417–36428.

12 Honda M, Beard MR, Ping LH et al. (1999) A phylogenetically conserved stem–loop structure at the 5′ border of the internal ribosome entry site of hepatitis C virus is required for cap-independent viral translation. J Virol 73, 1165–1174.

13 Friebe P, Lohmann V, Krieger N et al. (2001) Sequences in the 5′ non-translated region of hepatitis C virus required for RNA replication. J Virol 75, 12047–12057.

14 Kolykhalov AA, Feinstone SM, Rice CM (1996) Identification of a highly conserved sequence element at the 3′ terminus of hepatitis C virus genome RNA. J Virol 70, 3363–3371.

15 Tanaka T, Kato N, Cho MJ et al. (1995) A novel sequence found at the 3′ terminus of hepatitis C virus genome. Biochem Biophys Res Commun 215, 744–749.

16 You S, Stump DD, Branch AD et al. (2004) A cis-acting replication element in the sequence encoding the NS5B RNA-dependent RNA polymerase is required for hepatitis C virus RNA replication. J Virol 78, 1352–1366.

17 Friebe P, Boudet J, Simorre JP et al. (2005) Kissing-loop interaction in the 3′ end of the hepatitis C virus genome essential for RNA replication. J Virol 79, 380–392.

18 Lee H, Shin H, Wimmer E et al. (2004) Cis-acting RNA signals in the NS5B C-terminal coding sequence of the hepatitis C virus genome. J Virol 78, 10865–10877.

19 Dubuisson J (2000) Folding, assembly and subcellular localization of hepatitis C virus glycoproteins. Curr Topics Microbiol Immunol 242, 135–148.

20 Wakita T, Pietschmann T, Kato T et al. (2005) Production of infectious hepatitis C virus in tissue culture from a cloned viral genome. Nature Med 11, 791–796.

21 Lindenbach BD, Evans MJ, Syder AJ et al. (2005) Complete replication of hepatitis C virus in cell culture. Science 309, 623–626.

22 Zhong J, Gastaminza P, Cheng G et al. (2005) Robust hepatitis C virus infection in vitro. Proc Natl Acad Sci USA 102, 9294–9299.

23 Pham TN, MacParland SA, Mulrooney PM et al. (2004) Hepatitis C virus persistence after spontaneous or treatment-induced resolution of hepatitis C. J Virol 78, 5867–5874.

24 Pham TN, MacParland SA, Coffin CS et al. (2005) Mitogen-induced upregulation of hepatitis C virus expression in human lymphoid cells. J Gen Virol 86, 657–666.

25 Gosert R, Egger D, Lohmann V et al. (2003) Identification of the hepatitis C virus RNA replication complex in huh-7 cells harboring subgenomic replicons. J Virol 77, 5487–5492.

26 Bartenschlager R, Kaul A, Sparacio S (2003) Replication of the hepatitis C virus in cell culture. Antiviral Res 60, 91–102.

27 Lohmann V, Körner F, Koch JO et al. (1999) Replication of subgenomic hepatitis C virus RNAs in a hepatoma cell line. Science 285, 110–113.

28 Bartosch B, Dubuisson J, Cosset FL (2003) Infectious hepatitis C virus pseudo-particles containing functional E1-E2 envelope protein complexes. J Exp Med 197, 633–642.

29 Hsu M, Zhang J, Flint M et al. (2003) Hepatitis C virus glycoproteins mediate pH-dependent cell entry of pseudotyped retroviral particles. Proc Natl Acad Sci USA 100, 7271–7276.

30 Kato T, Date T, Miyamoto M et al. (2003) Efficient replication of the genotype 2a hepatitis C virus subgenomic replicon. Gastroenterology 125, 1808–1817.

31 Pietschmann T, Kaul A, Koutsoudakis G et al. (2006) Construction and characterization of infectious intragenotypic and intergenotypic hepatitis C virus chimeras. Proc Natl Acad Sci USA 103, 7408–7413. Epub 1 May 2006.

32 Tan S-L, Katze MG (2001) How hepatitis C virus counteracts the interferon response: the jury is still out on NS5A. Virology 284, 1–12.

33 Foy E, Li K, Wang C et al. (2003) Regulation of interferon regulatory factor-3 by the hepatitis C virus serine protease. Science 300, 1145–1148.

34 Haller O, Kochs G, Weber F (2005) The interferon response circuit: induction and suppression by pathogenic viruses. Virology, 344, 119–130.

35 Meylan E, Curran J, Hofmann K et al. (2005) Cardif is an adaptor protein in the RIG-I antiviral pathway and is targeted by hepatitis C virus. Nature 437, 1167–1172

36 Li K, Foy E, Ferreon JC *et al.* (2005) Immune evasion by hepatitis C virus NS3/4A protease-mediated cleavage of the Toll-like receptor 3 adaptor protein TRIF. *Proc Natl Acad Sci USA* 102, 2992–2997.

37 Bowen DG, Walker CM (2005) Adaptive immune responses in acute and chronic hepatitis C virus infection. *Nature* 436, 946–952.

38 Diepolder HM, Zachoval R, Hoffmann RM *et al.* (1995) Possible mechanism involving T-lymphocyte response to non-structural protein 3 in viral clearance in acute hepatitis C virus infection. *Lancet* 346, 1006–1007.

39 Gerlach JT, Diepolder HM, Jung MC *et al.* (1999) Recurrence of hepatitis C virus after loss of virus-specific CD4(+) T-cell response in acute hepatitis C. *Gastroenterology* 117, 933–941.

40 Mehta SH, Cox A, Hoover DR *et al.* (2002) Protection against persistence of hepatitis C. *Lancet* 359, 1478–1483.

41 Grakoui A, Shoukry NH, Woollard DJ *et al.* (2003) HCV persistence and immune evasion in the absence of memory T cell help. *Science* 302, 659–662.

42 Post JJ, Pan Y, Freeman AJ *et al.* (2004) Clearance of hepatitis C viremia associated with cellular immunity in the absence of seroconversion in the hepatitis C incidence and transmission in prisons study cohort. *J Infect Dis* 189, 1846–1855.

43 Colin C, Lanoir D, Touzet S *et al.* (2001) Sensitivity and specificity of third-generation hepatitis C virus antibody detection assays: an analysis of the literature. *J Viral Hepatol* 8, 87–95.

44 Pawlotsky JM (2002) Molecular diagnosis of viral hepatitis. *Gastroenterology* 122, 1554–1568.

45 Bouvier-Alias M, Patel K, Dahari H *et al.* (2002) Clinical utility of total HCV core antigen quantification: a new indirect marker of HCV replication. *Hepatology* 36, 211–218.

46 Yagnik AT, Lahm A, Meola A *et al.* (2000) A model for the hepatitis C virus envelope glycoprotein E2. *Proteins* 40, 355–366.

9.1.2.iii Hepatitis A

Loriana Di Giammarino and Jules L. Dienstag

Definition and virology

Hepatitis A is an acute, self-limited, necroinflammatory disease of the liver resulting from infection with the enterically transmitted hepatitis A virus (HAV). HAV is a positive-stranded, non-enveloped, icosahedral, 27-nm RNA virus [1] now classified as a hepatovirus within the picornavirus family [2]. Unusually resistant to heat, ether and acid, HAV has an RNA genome of approximately 7500 nucleotides, the protein product of which is cleaved posttranslationally to yield three protein precursors of four capsid viral polypeptides, VP1–VP4. Nonstructural proteins include a viral polymerase and proteases. Although genomic heterogeneity of up to 25% exists among virus strains, and although at least seven genotypes have been identified, all isolates appear to be immunologically indistinguishable, i.e. only a single serotype exists [3]. Unlike most of the human hepatitis viruses, HAV can be cultivated in cell culture [4]; however, most strains replicate slowly and, unlike many picornaviruses, HAV is not cytopathic in culture [5]. The entire genome has been cloned and characterized [6,7].

Although HAV can be detected in stools within 10 days to 2 weeks after infection, the clinical incubation period, measured to the onset of symptoms, is approximately 4 (range 2–6) weeks. During the late incubation period (10–14 days before the onset of clinically apparent illness), the virus is excreted in the stool, but faecal excretion wanes rapidly and rarely lasts beyond the first few days of clinical or subclinical illness [8]; viraemia is very limited, detectable for a few days towards the end of the incubation period. The consensus is that HAV replication is limited to the liver; from the liver, the virus is excreted through the bile into the intestine and shed in the stool.

Although HAV can be detected in the liver for weeks, and although circulating HAV antigen can be detected in serum by sensitive immunoassays for longer than a week after the onset of clinical illness, infectivity does not extend beyond the first few days of illness (except when it recurs in 'relapsing' cases – see below). A potential exception to such brief faecal shedding of HAV has been reported in a neonatal intensive care unit, in which neonates with hepatitis A were infectious, presumably shedding faecal virus, for 6 months [9]. Faecal shedding of HAV persisting for months has also been documented in patients undergoing liver transplantation for fulminant hepatitis A [10]. Protracted hepatitis A and faecal shedding have not been documented in immunocompetent persons.

The primary antibody response to HAV, which is of the immunoglobulin (Ig)M class (IgM anti-HAV), lasts only a few months and is replaced ultimately by anti-HAV of the IgG class (IgG anti-HAV). After infection with HAV, IgG antibody remains detectable indefinitely and correlates with lasting immunity.

History

The illness we categorize today as hepatitis A was probably recognized during antiquity, but its link to viral infection was not established until the 1940s [11]. Epidemiological and volunteer studies during and after the Second World War differentiated between 'infectious hepatitis' and 'serum hepatitis' [12] and established that infectious hepatitis was caused by a filterable agent, presumably a virus, that had a short incubation period and was spread predominantly by the faecal–oral route.

Volunteer studies were continued in the 1950s and 1960s [13,14] and were supplemented by studies suggesting successful transmission of a viral agent in marmoset monkeys (tamarins) [15,16]. Ultimately, clinical specimens generated in volunteer and experimental animal studies provided the reagents that were used to identify HAV.

In 1973, investigators at the National Institutes of Health, using immune electron microscopy, found 27-nm virus-like particles that were aggregated by convalescent but not by preinfection serum in the stools of volunteers infected with HAV [1]. This discovery was followed rapidly by the development of serological tests, confirmation of the marmoset model and

Table 1 Epidemiology of hepatitis A virus.

Transmission in nature almost exclusively by the faecal–oral route
    Percutaneous transmission very rare
    Perinatal transmission unlikely
Endemic in developing countries (where infection is predominant in childhood)
Declining in developed countries
Mean age of exposure increasing
Frequency of clinically apparent disease increasing

establishment of the chimpanzee as an experimental model, the cultivation of HAV *in vitro* in 1979 [4] and the cloning [17] and sequencing [18,19] of the viral genome [20].

Epidemiology (Table 1)

Mode of transmission

Hepatitis A virus is transmitted in nature almost exclusively by the faecal–oral route. Although viraemia occurs, it is transient and does not contribute to transmission of HAV infection except in very unusual circumstances. As an enteric agent, hepatitis A is spread from person to person or is acquired when a susceptible person ingests food, water, milk, bivalve shellfish, etc. that has been contaminated with faecal material from an infected person, occasionally in the context of a food-borne outbreak traced to a foodhandler. Indeed, a massive shellfish-associated outbreak, involving more than 310 000 persons, occurred in Shanghai in 1988 [21].

Most recently, in 2003, HAV-contaminated green onions, imported from Mexico to a Pennsylvania restaurant, were the source of the largest outbreak of food-borne hepatitis A ever reported in the United States, involving at least 600 persons [22]; this report is an example of a series of recent food-borne outbreaks linked to ingestion in developed countries (where immunity is limited) of produce contaminated during harvest in developing countries (where water supplies are often contaminated with enteric agents).

Poor personal and environmental hygiene foster the spread of enteric agents such as HAV; both sporadic cases and outbreaks are common, and efficient intrafamilial spread accounts for secondary cases within the household of an infected person. Because infectivity peaks during the late incubation period, the risk of transmission is highest for those in contact with a patient just before clinically apparent illness, rather than for those exposed to the patient during or after the onset of clinical illness. Because HAV does not cause chronic infection and is not associated with a carrier state, perpetuation of infection within populations relies upon person-to-person transmission or environmental contamination; certainly, HAV has been shown to remain stable in the environment for many months [23]. In temperate climates, hepatitis A tended to occur in seasonal waves, concentrated in the late autumn and early winter, and

in epidemic waves cycling every 5–20 years, relying on the emergence of new susceptible populations; however, in developed countries, the frequency of hepatitis A declined regularly during the second half of the twentieth century, and these seasonal and generational cycles are not as apparent. Unexpected outbreaks, however, continue to emerge in developed countries, as noted above, fostered by a global economy in which food items that cannot be heat inactivated are imported from HAV-endemic countries [24].

Groups traditionally recognized as being at high risk of HAV infection include travellers from non-endemic to endemic areas, whose risk has been estimated to be three cases per 1000 travellers per month [25]; military personnel stationed in endemic areas; persons working with non-human primates; children, employees and parents of children in daycare centres; and clients and employees of institutions for the developmentally disabled [26,27]. Persons who work as foodhandlers are not considered to be at increased risk of occupationally acquired hepatitis A [28], despite the key role that they may have played in the recent outbreaks associated with food [29,30]. In daycare centres, hepatitis A in the children is so mild that clinical recognition is rare; outbreaks become apparent when adults exposed to the children, daycare centre employees and parents become clinically ill [31]. Although the role of sexual transmission is not known, men who have sex with men have an increased risk of HAV infection [32], probably through faecal exposure. Similarly, injection drug users have been found to have an increased risk of HAV infection, not as a result of percutaneous exposure to contaminated needles but rather related to poor hygiene. Outbreaks have been reported in the past among staff of neonatal intensive care units, presumably infected by exposure to faecal material from infected neonates [9], and among recipients of clotting factors [33]. An outbreak of hepatitis A in oncology patients treated with interleukin-2 and lymphokine-activated killer (LAK) cells was attributed to contaminated plasma used to dilute the LAK cells [34]. Such rare cases in blood-product recipients notwithstanding, hepatitis A is rarely transmitted by transfusion. Hepatitis A is rarely, if ever, transmitted perinatally from mother to offspring, one case report [35] notwithstanding, and health workers do not have a higher prevalence of infection than that of the general population [36].

Distribution within populations

In the United States and other developed countries, HAV accounts for approximately a quarter of all reported cases of acute viral hepatitis. Indeed, in the United States, approximately 26 000 cases of acute hepatitis A were reported annually to the Centers for Disease Control and Prevention during the 1980s and 1990s. After adjusting for under-reporting and asymptomatic cases, the number of new cases per year during those decades was estimated to be in excess of 270 000 [37]. During the last 10 years, however, the rate of hepatitis A declined substantially and, in 2003, the annual frequency of hepatitis A in the United States fell to the lowest ever recorded, 2.7 cases per 100 000 persons [38]. Exposure is inversely proportional to socioeconomic status, and seroprevalence surveys show an increase in anti-HAV frequencies with advancing age. The most compelling trend in the prevalence of HAV infection (reflected by anti-HAV frequencies) has been the regular decline in the frequency of infection in developed countries. When populations in the United States, western Europe and Australia are evaluated at intervals a decade apart, overall prevalences and age-specific prevalences have been documented to fall with each progressive decade.

In the United States, the most recent survey (Third National Health and Nutrition Examination Survey, NHANES-III, conducted between 1988 and 1994) revealed an anti-HAV prevalence of 33% [28], which is 5% lower than the 38% prevalence detected during the 1976–1980 NHANES-II survey [39] and 12% lower than the 45% prevalence reported in a serological survey of New York blood donors in 1976 [40]. In Europe, a north-to-south gradient exists in relative endemicity of hepatitis A, from negligible in northern Scandinavian countries to more common in southern Mediterranean countries.

In the United States, the frequency of acute hepatitis A was higher in western states as well as in certain populations, including Alaskan natives and native Americans [28]; however, following the 1999 recommendations for childhood vaccination, the frequency of hepatitis A declined steadily in these regions/populations to levels approximately equal to those in other regions and the general population of the US. An increasing proportion of cases now occur among high-risk populations. For example, the number of cases among men who have sex with men has increased from 1.5% in 1992 to 8.4% in 2002. Similarly, the proportion of hepatitis A cases attributed to travel rose from 1.3% (1992) to 9.4% (2002) [27].

Hepatitis A is primarily an infection of childhood, but the mean age of exposure increases with improvement in the levels of hygiene and sanitation. Thus, in developing countries, where HAV is endemic, e.g. Africa, Central and South America, Central Asia, Southeast Asia and Mediterranean countries, childhood exposure to HAV is almost universal, and almost all infections, and consequently immunity, are acquired by the age of 10 years. In highly developed countries, the overall prevalence of anti-HAV in the general population may be lower than 20% and the age of acquisition higher.

As infections in childhood decline, a population of adults emerges that, having escaped HAV infection in childhood, remains susceptible into adulthood. As this susceptible population matures into adulthood and becomes sufficiently affluent to travel, imported cases of acute hepatitis A begin to emerge in non-endemic areas.

Moreover, as infection with HAV becomes less frequent in a population, and as cases are shifted from younger to older segments of the population, a shift also occurs in clinical presentation. Because infections in young children tend to be subclinical (< 30% jaundiced), whereas infections in adults tend to

Table 2 Clinical features of HAV infection.

An acute, self-limited illness, with modest morbidity and negligible mortality
Incubation period 2–6 weeks, with a mean of 4 weeks
Occasional variants include cholestatic and relapsing hepatitis
Clinical severity and the likelihood of jaundice increase with age
Fatality rate (fulminant hepatitis) < 1/1000
No long-term sequelae, no chronic hepatitis A, no chronic carrier state

be clinically apparent and even severe (> 70% jaundiced), paradoxically, as the frequency of hepatitis A infections decreases in a population, the occurrence of clinically apparent and severe cases increases [41,42]. Therefore, in developed countries, cases of acute hepatitis A sufficiently severe to require hospitalization, even fulminant cases, are more common today than they were several decades ago.

Clinical and laboratory features

Clinical features (Table 2)

Infection with HAV may be asymptomatic or may result in acute hepatitis of variable severity, including fulminant hepatitis. Although the severity and duration of acute hepatitis A may vary, hepatitis A does not cause chronic hepatitis, and no hepatitis A carrier state exists.

The symptoms and signs of acute hepatitis A are similar to those for the other types of viral hepatitis. After a clinical incubation period of approximately 4 weeks (range 2–6 weeks), patients may experience prodromal, non-specific, systemic symptoms, such as fatigue, malaise, headache, low-grade fever, myalgias, arthralgias, nausea and vomiting, loss of appetite, alteration in gustatory and olfactory senses and weight loss. Hepatitis-specific symptoms, such as right upper quadrant pain, dark urine, jaundice and acholic stools, occur later, as the clinical illness peaks. When jaundice is severe, pruritus may occur. Physical examination usually reveals mildly tender hepatomegaly and, in icteric cases, scleral icterus and jaundice. Signs of chronic liver disease, such as spider angiomata and splenomegaly, are rare but can be seen transiently.

Except in fulminant cases, which are very rare (in the order of 1:1000 cases), symptoms and signs subside within several weeks, after which recovery is complete and without sequelae. Clinical and laboratory recovery occurs in approximately half of otherwise healthy young adults within 3 weeks, and the remainder recover thereafter; rarely, laboratory abnormalities may persist for months to a year. In a small proportion of cases, fatigue may be prolonged and outlast all other symptoms, signs and laboratory abnormalities.

Laboratory features

Levels of alanine aminotransferase (ALT) tend to exceed those of aspartate aminotransferase (AST). Values of several hundred

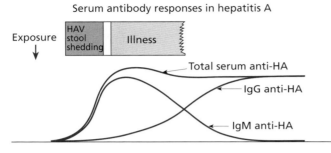

Fig. 1 Diagrammatic representation of the clinical, serological, and virological events that occur in HAV infection.

units are common but, occasionally, ALT and AST levels exceed 1000–2000 units. Elevations in aminotransferase activity tend to precede elevations in bilirubin, which may continue to climb even as aminotransferase levels decline.

Elevations in prothrombin time and reductions in serum albumin are rare, and alkaline phosphatase levels are normal or minimally elevated. Transient neutropenia and atypical lymphocytosis can occur, and an elevation in non-virus-specific serum IgM is a common feature, in addition to a mild increase in total gammaglobulin levels.

Diagnosis

Technically, a diagnosis of acute HAV infection can be made by demonstrating virus in stools or serum during the late incubation period; however, faecal shedding and viraemia have usually subsided by the time a patient presents clinically. In the same vein, diagnosis by cultivation of HAV *in vitro* is impractical because of the long latency of the virus in culture.

Therefore, a diagnosis is made by relying on serological detection of antibodies to HAV (anti-HAV) (Fig. 1). Antibodies to HAV appear early during acute illness, even while faecal shedding of virus is still occurring and while serum aminotransferase levels are elevated. The early antibody response is of the IgM class, and the presence of IgM anti-HAV establishes the diagnosis with 100% sensitivity and a specificity nearly as good, marred only by rare, confounding, non-specific immunoassay binding in the presence of rheumatoid factor. As tests for IgM anti-HAV are configured, this primary humoral immune response remains detectable for approximately 3 months in most patients, rarely lasting longer. Thereafter, beginning during convalescence and persisting indefinitely, IgG anti-HAV predominates and is associated with lifelong immunity to reinfection. In patients presenting with acute hepatitis whose serum contains IgG anti-HAV rather than IgM anti-HAV, the current acute hepatitis is not related to hepatitis A.

Because IgM anti-HAV persists for several months after acute infection, IgM anti-HAV testing can be used to make a retrospective diagnosis, for example in a person suspected as the source of a food-borne outbreak or in a traveller returning after recovery from acute illness.

Pathology

Liver biopsies are almost never indicated in patients with acute hepatitis A, a self-limited disease. Still, the histological hallmarks of acute hepatitis A have been described and share the typical features of all forms of acute viral hepatitis: ballooning of hepatocytes, coagulative necrosis, focal necrosis, portal expansion by a mononuclear infiltrate, periportal inflammation and Kupffer cell hyperplasia.

Cholestasis may be present and, in more severe cases, piecemeal necrosis or interface hepatitis (erosion of the limiting plate of periportal hepatocytes) and/or bridging necrosis (cell dropout that spans lobules) may be observed. Although periportal fibrosis may be seen in protracted cases, progression to cirrhosis has not been documented. When liver tissue is available, HAV can be localized by immunohistochemical staining to the hepatocyte cytoplasm [43].

Pathogenesis

HAV replicates predominantly in the liver; although the virus has been detected by some investigators in extrahepatic sites such as the gut [44,45] and, although virus replication has been identified in orally infected monkeys [46], the relative magnitude of intestinal HAV replication and its importance in the life cycle of the virus is not known.

HAV is not a cytopathic agent, and the virus is not cytolytic in cell culture, having no effect on the rate of host protein RNA synthesis [47]. Liver injury is almost certainly mediated by cellular immune responses to virus-infected hepatocytes. Cytolytic T-cell responses have been documented in acute hepatitis A [48–50], and T-cell epitopes, potential targets for cytolytic T cells, have been identified on HAV structural proteins [51].

A reasonable hypothesis is that CD8+ cytolytic T cells recognize HAV antigens complexed with hepatocyte cell surface host histocompatibility antigens and participate in the immunopathogenesis of hepatitis A by attacking and injuring HAV-infected hepatocytes.

Determinants of severity in acute hepatitis A are not well characterized. The size of the virus inoculum varies inversely with the length of the incubation period and does not affect the severity of acute hepatitis A. Age of infection is an important factor in the clinical expression of illness; the frequency of clinically apparent hepatitis increases with age [23]. Studies of candidate HAV vaccine strains after serial passage in cell culture have shown that the pathogenicity of the virus can be attenuated, and such attenuation has been linked to changes at the genome level [52–54]. Immune complex-mediated extrahepatic manifestations of acute hepatitis, such as rash (cutaneous vasculitis) and arthralgias/arthritis, have been reported only rarely in patients with acute hepatitis A [55,56]. Such manifestations have also been reported in patients with relapsing hepatitis A (see below) [55,57].

Complications

Patients with acute hepatitis A recover completely without any lasting sequelae. Neither chronic hepatitis A nor a chronic hepatitis A carrier state has been demonstrated to exist. In addition, recovery from acute hepatitis A is followed by lifelong immunity to reinfection. Fulminant hepatitis A, which occurs rarely, in approximately 1:1000 cases of acute hepatitis A can lead to death; based on an estimated (not the reported) number of deaths per year in the United States, the Centers for Disease Control and Prevention estimate a case fatality rate of 0.3% [27]. In patients older than 50 years, the case fatality rate is higher, 1.8% according to the Centers for Disease Control estimate and, in patients with underlying chronic liver disease, the risk of fulminant hepatitis A is increased [58].

Two variants of acute hepatitis A merit special attention, cholestatic hepatitis A and relapsing hepatitis A. Cholestatic hepatitis A, characterized by persistent jaundice and pruritus, with marked elevation of bilirubin levels, occurs rarely and can be misconstrued for extrahepatic biliary obstruction or chronic cholestatic liver disease. Although symptoms and biochemical abnormalities may persist for many months and even up to a year, cholestatic hepatitis A invariably resolves and is followed by complete recovery. Generally, liver biopsy is not required in this setting but, when obtained, liver tissue demonstrates profound centrolobular cholestasis as well as more typical portal inflammation [59].

Relapsing hepatitis A can occur in as many as 5–10% of patients with acute hepatitis A, usually reflected by an asymptomatic elevation in aminotransferases within weeks to months after apparent biochemical recovery [57,60–64]. In a proportion of cases, symptoms and jaundice recur during relapse, and resumption of faecal HAV excretion has been documented during relapse [65]. This variant, too, invariably resolves without any chronic sequelae.

Other complications during acute hepatitis A are rare, although a host of miscellaneous case reports link hepatitis A in rare instances to Guillain–Barré syndrome [66], pancreatitis [67], cholecystitis [68], aplastic anaemia, renal failure [69], encephalitis [70] and haemophagocytic syndrome [71].

Isolated cases have been described in which autoimmune hepatitis (with autoantibodies and substantial hyperglobulinaemia) followed acute hepatitis A [72–74].

Management

No specific therapy is required for acute hepatitis A or for its variants, cholestatic hepatitis A or relapsing hepatitis A. Because the disease is self-limited, specific antiviral therapy is not required, nor have any antiviral agents been shown to be clinically effective in hepatitis A. Management remains supportive, and hospitalization is rarely required, except for patients with other concurrent, serious medical problems, those who cannot maintain oral intake or those with incipient liver failure (e.g. coagulopathy, mental status changes).

Bedrest, restriction of physical activity or dietary restrictions are of no benefit [75], but abstaining from alcohol is a reasonable, common-sense approach, albeit one that has not been proven in clinical trials. Corticosteroids are not helpful and should be avoided. For the systemic symptoms of acute hepatitis A, patients may be instructed to take paracetamol or non-steroidal anti-inflammatory drugs in moderation; rarely, cholestyramine is required to manage severe pruritus. In patients with fulminant hepatitis A, meticulous, intensive supportive care is the only available intervention, short of liver transplantation. In a case report involving four patients with fulminant hepatitis A, interferon-β was administered and followed by recovery [76], but up to 80% of patients with fulminant hepatitis A managed with supportive care have been reported to survive. Both management of fulminant hepatitis and liver transplantation are addressed in other chapters in this volume.

Prevention

In areas of the world where hepatitis A is endemic, control of hepatitis A requires societal improvements in environmental hygiene, including a clean, safe water supply, adequate disposal of waste and improvements in living conditions. Although hepatitis A vaccines are now available in developed countries, simple, common sense hygienic measures such as handwashing, special training for foodhandlers, etc. play a role in limiting the spread of hepatitis A. Because HAV is spread by close person-to-person contact, no special precautions are required for classmates and co-workers of patients with acute hepatitis A.

Similarly, universal precautions currently practised in hospitals, clinics and physicians' offices are sufficient to prevent nosocomial hepatitis A; therefore, additional, cumbersome isolation in a private room as well as the use of gowns and gloves are not required. Travellers to endemic areas should avoid tap water and uncooked food and drinks potentially contaminated with water (salads, ice in drinks).

Currently, both passive immunization with immune globulin and active immunization with inactivated vaccines are available for prophylaxis against HAV infection. Active immunization with hepatitis A vaccine is discussed in Chapter 9.1.3.i.

Passive immunization

Before hepatitis A vaccines were developed, prophylaxis against hepatitis A relied upon passive immunization with immune globulin, prepared from large plasma pools, inactivated by cold ethanol fractionation and invariably containing anti-HAV. Cold alcohol fractionation has been shown to yield a safe product, free of infectious agents, including human immunodeficiency virus (HIV). Although the minimum protective concentration of anti-HAV in immune globulin is not known, all contemporary lots of immune globulin contain sufficient anti-HAV (at least 100 IU/mL) to be protective. The efficacy of immune globulin was first demonstrated in an outbreak at a summer camp in 1944 [77] and confirmed in large-scale studies among American soldiers serving in Europe during the Second World War [78], as well as in persons residing in institutions for the mentally handicapped [79].

Now that hepatitis A vaccine has widely replaced immune globulin for pre-exposure prophylaxis, the role of immune globulin has been confined to postexposure prophylaxis or for passive pre-exposure immunization in pregnant or lactating women and immunosuppressed persons.

Until very recently, in the United States, immune globulin was also recommended for protection against hepatitis A in children younger than 2 years; since October 2005, the Advisory Committee on Immunization Practices (ACIP) of the United States Public Health Service has recommended that all children between the ages of 1 and 2 years receive a two-dose vaccination against hepatitis A virus [80].

In some settings (e.g. in a traveller who does not have sufficient time before embarking to complete a course of hepatitis A vaccine and who expects to travel for an extended period or to travel frequently in the future), a combination of passive immunization with immune globulin plus active immunization with hepatitis A vaccine, at different sites of administration, is suggested [19]. Although levels of anti-HAV following combination passive and active immunization may be lower than those achieved after vaccination alone [81], for all practical purposes, the two types of immunization do not interfere with the efficacy of the other. Immune globulin is not known to interfere with any other killed vaccines either but can interfere with immune responses to live, attenuated vaccines; therefore, administration of such live, attenuated vaccines should be delayed for 5 months or longer after immune globulin administration [28]. When given pre-exposure, immune globulin is administered intramuscularly at a dose of 0.02 mL/kg for brief expected exposures (1–2 months, such as for recreational travel) or 0.06 mL/kg for longer exposures (3–5 months). For prolonged exposure, repeat injections of immune globulin at 5- to 6-month intervals were recommended; however, the need for repeat immune globulin injections has been supplanted by the availability of hepatitis A vaccine. When administered within 2 weeks of exposure, immune globulin has been shown to be at least 85% effective in preventing acute hepatitis A [25]. Levels of measurable anti-HAV are low or undetectable after passive immunization, and protection lasts for several months [82].

The earlier after exposure that immune globulin can be given, the more effective it is likely to be. When administered sufficiently early after exposure, immune globulin prevents HAV infection entirely; however, if administration is delayed into the late incubation period, immune globulin may not abort infection entirely but, instead, attenuate it and render the infection clinically inapparent. Consequently, longlasting immunity resulting from subclinical infection occurs, rather than transient

Table 3 Postexposure prophylaxis against HAV infection with immune globulin.

Indications:	Close personal contacts
	Household contacts
	Sexual contacts
	Daycare centres with recognized cases of hepatitis A
	Staff
	Children attending the centre
	Household members of children attending the centre
	Common-source exposure
	Other foodhandlers besides index case
	Patrons – prophylaxis unlikely to be of benefit unless administered within 2 weeks after exposure
	Schools, factories, offices, hospitals – not routinely recommended
Regimen:	0.02 mL/kg, intramuscularly, as soon after exposure as possible, not beyond 2 weeks of exposure

protection resulting from passive immunization, i.e. 'passive–active' immunity. Such postexposure prophylaxis should be given as soon after the exposure as possible (without prior anti-HAV testing, which would delay immunization unnecessarily and would add substantial expense) to household, sexual and institutional contacts of patients with acute hepatitis A; however, prophylaxis is not necessary for casual contacts (e.g. classmates, office and factory co-workers, hospital employees). Immune globulin has been given routinely to persons exposed to HAV in common-source (e.g. food-borne) outbreaks; however, by the time such outbreaks are recognized, a full incubation period has elapsed, and prophylaxis may be too late to prevent infection. On the other hand, prophylaxis this late may attenuate clinical illness in some recipients and/or potentially limit the number of secondary cases (Table 3).

References

1 Feinstone SM, Kapikian AZ, Purceli RH (1973) Hepatitis A: detection by immune electron microscopy of a viruslike antigen associated with acute illness. *Science* 182(116), 1026–1028.

2 Melnick JL (1992) Properties and classification of hepatitis A virus. *Vaccine* 10(Suppl. 1), S24–26.

3 Robertson BH, Jansen RW, Khanna B *et al.* (1992) Genetic relatedness of hepatitis A virus strains recovered from different geographical regions. *J Gen Virol* 73(Pt 6), 1365–1377.

4 Provost PJ, Hilleman MR (1979) Propagation of human hepatitis A virus in cell culture *in vitro*. *Proc Soc Exp Biol Med* 160(2), 213–221.

5 Lemon SM (1985) Type A viral hepatitis. New developments in an old disease. *N Engl J Med* 313(17), 1059–1067.

6 Ticehurst JR (1986) Hepatitis A virus: clones, cultures, and vaccines. *Semin Liver Dis* 6(1), 46–55.

7 Cohen JI (1989) Hepatitis A virus: insights from molecular biology. *Hepatology* 9(6), 889–895.

8 Dienstag JL, Feinstone SM, Kapikian AZ *et al.* (1975) Faecal shedding of hepatitis-A antigen. *Lancet* 1(7910), 765–767.

9 Rosenblum LS, Villarino ME, Nainan OV *et al.* (1991) Hepatitis A outbreak in a neonatal intensive care unit: risk factors for transmission and evidence of prolonged viral excretion among preterm infants. *J Infect Dis* 164(3), 476–482.

10 Fagan E, Yousef G, Brahm J *et al.* (1990) Persistence of hepatitis A virus in fulminant hepatitis and after liver transplantation. *J Med Virol* 30(2), 131–136.

11 Feinstone SM, Gust ID (1997) Hepatitis A virus. In: Livingstone C (ed.) *Clinical Virology*. New York, pp. 1049–1072.

12 MacCallum FO (1972) Early studies of viral hepatitis. *Br Med Bull* 28(2), 105–108.

13 Krugman S, Ward R, Giles JP (1962) The natural history of infectious hepatitis. *Am J Med* 32, 717–728.

14 Krugman S, Giles JP, Hammond J (1967) Infectious hepatitis. Evidence for two distinctive clinical, epidemiological, and immunological types of infection. *JAMA* 200(5), 365–373.

15 Deinhardt F, Holmes AW, Capps RB *et al.* (1967) Studies on the transmission of human viral hepatitis to marmoset monkeys. I. Transmission of disease, serial passages, and description of liver lesions. *J Exp Med* 125(4), 673–688.

16 Holmes AW, Wolfe L, Rosenblate H *et al.* (1969) Hepatitis in marmosets: induction of disease with coded specimens from a human volunteer study. *Science* 165(895), 816–817.

17 Ticehurst JR, Racaniello VR, Baroudy BM *et al.* (1983) Molecular cloning and characterization of hepatitis A virus cDNA. *Proc Natl Acad Sci USA* 80(19), 5885–5889.

18 Baroudy BM, Ticehurst JR, Miele TA *et al.* (1985) Sequence analysis of hepatitis A virus cDNA coding for capsid proteins and RNA polymerase. *Proc Natl Acad Sci USA* 82(7), 2143–2147.

19 Najarian R, Caput D, Gee W *et al.* (1985) Primary structure and gene organization of human hepatitis A virus. *Proc Natl Acad Sci USA* 82(9), 2627–2631.

20 Hollinger FB, Ticehurst JR (1996) Hepatitis A virus. In: Fields BN, Knipe DM, Howley PM *et al.* (eds) *Fields Virology*. Philadelphia: Lippincott-Raven, pp. 735–782.

21 Halliday ML, Kang LY, Zhou TK *et al.* (1991) An epidemic of hepatitis A attributable to the ingestion of raw clams in Shanghai, China. *J Infect Dis* 164(5), 852–859.

22 Anon (2003) Hepatitis A outbreak associated with green onions at a restaurant – Monaca, Pennsylvania, 2003. *MMWR Morb Mortal Wkly Rep* 52(47), 1155–1157.

23 Lednar WM, Lemon SM, Kirkpatrick JW *et al.* (1985) Frequency of illness associated with epidemic hepatitis A virus infections in adults. *Am J Epidemiol* 122(2), 226–233.

24 Di Giammarino L, Dienstag JL (2005) Hepatitis A – the price of progress. *N Engl J Med* 353(9), 944–946.

25 Steffen R, Kane MA, Shapiro CN *et al.* (1994) Epidemiology and prevention of hepatitis A in travelers. *JAMA* 272(11), 885–889.

26 Szmuness W, Purcell RH, Dienstag JL *et al.* (1977) Antibody to hepatitis A antigen in institutionalized mentally retarded patients. *JAMA* 237(16), 1702–1705.

27 Centers for Disease Control and Prevention (2004) *Hepatitis Surveillance Report No. 59*. Atlanta, GA: US Department of Health and Human Services. Centers for Disease Control and Prevention.

28 Anon (1999) Prevention of hepatitis A through active or passive immunization: Recommendations of the Advisory Committee on Immunization Practices (ACIP). *MMWR Recomm Rep* 48(RR-12), 1–37.

29 Hutin YJ, Pool V, Cramer EH *et al.* (1999) A multistate, foodborne outbreak of hepatitis A. National Hepatitis A Investigation Team. *N Engl J Med* 340(8), 595–602.

30 Wheeler C, Vogt T, Armstrong GL *et al.* (2005) An outbreak of hepatitis A associated with green onions. *N Engl J Med* 353, 890–897.

31 Hadler SC, Erben JJ, Francis DP *et al.* (1982) Risk factors for hepatitis A in day-care centers. *J Infect Dis* 145(2), 255–261.

32 Corey L, Holmes KK (1980) Sexual transmission of hepatitis A in homosexual men: incidence and mechanism. *N Engl J Med* 302(8), 435–438.

33 Soucie JM, Robertson BH, Bell BP *et al.* (1998) Hepatitis A virus infections associated with clotting factor concentrate in the United States. *Transfusion* 38(6), 573–579.

34 Weisfuse IB, Graham DJ, Will M *et al.* (1990) An outbreak of hepatitis A among cancer patients treated with interleukin-2 and lymphokine-activated killer cells. *J Infect Dis* 161(4), 647–652.

35 Watson JC, Fleming DW, Borella AJ *et al.* (1993) Vertical transmission of hepatitis A resulting in an outbreak in a neonatal intensive care unit. *J Infect Dis* 167(3), 567–571.

36 Gibas A, Blewett DR, Schoenfeld DA *et al.* (1992) Prevalence and incidence of viral hepatitis in health workers in the prehepatitis B vaccination era. *Am J Epidemiol* 136(5), 603–610.

37 Armstrong GL, Bell BP (2002) Hepatitis A virus infections in the United States: model-based estimates and implications for childhood immunization. *Pediatrics* 109(5), 839–845.

38 Centers for Disease Control and Prevention (2005) Summary of Notifiable Disease – United States, 2003. Report No. 54. *Morbidity and Mortality Weekly Report* 52, 1–88.

39 Shapiro CN, Coleman PJ, McQuillan GM *et al.* (1992) Epidemiology of hepatitis A: seroepidemiology and risk groups in the USA. *Vaccine* 10(Suppl. 1), S59–62.

40 Szmuness W, Dienstag JL, Purcell RH *et al.* (1976) Distribution of antibody to hepatitis a antigen in urban adult populations. *N Engl J Med* 295(14), 755–759.

41 Purcell RH (1994) Hepatitis viruses: changing patterns of human disease. *Proc Natl Acad Sci USA* 91(7), 2401–2406.

42 Shapiro CN, Margolis HS (1993) Worldwide epidemiology of hepatitis A virus infection. *J Hepatol* 18(Suppl. 2), S11–14.

43 Shimizu YK, Mathiesen LR, Lorenz D *et al.* (1978) Localization of hepatitis A antigen in liver tissue by peroxidase-conjugated antibody method: light and electron microscopic studies. *J Immunol* 121(5), 1671–1679.

44 Mathiesen LR, Feinstone SM, Purcell RH *et al.* (1977) Detection of hepatitis A antigen by immunofluorescence. *Infect Immun* 18(2), 524–530.

45 Karayiannis P, Jowett T, Enticott M *et al.* (1986) Hepatitis A virus replication in tamarins and host immune response in relation to pathogenesis of liver cell damage. *J Med Virol* 18(3), 261–276.

46 Asher LV, Binn LN, Mensing TL *et al.* (1995) Pathogenesis of hepatitis A in orally inoculated owl monkeys (*Aotus trivirgatus*). *J Med Virol* 47(3), 260–268.

47 Locarnini SA, Coulepis AG, Westaway EG *et al.* (1981) Restricted replication of human hepatitis A virus in cell culture: intracellular biochemical studies. *J Virol* 37(1), 216–225.

48 Vallbracht A, Gabriel P, Maier K *et al.* (1986) Cell-mediated cytotoxicity in hepatitis A virus infection. *Hepatology* 6(6), 1308–1314.

49 Vallbracht A, Maier K, Stierhof YD *et al.* (1989) Liver-derived cytotoxic T cells in hepatitis A virus infection. *J Infect Dis* 160(2), 209–217.

50 Fleischer B, Fleischer S, Maier K et al. (1990) Clonal analysis of infiltrating T lymphocytes in liver tissue in viral hepatitis A. Immunology 69(1), 14–19.

51 Wunschmann S, Vallbracht A, Flehmig B et al. (1997) Cytolytic T lymphocyte epitopes are present on hepatitis A virus structural proteins. In: Rizzetto M, Purcell RH, Gerin JL et al. (eds) Viral Hepatitis and Liver Disease. Turin: Edizione Minerva Medica, pp. 51–54.

52 Cohen JI, Rosenblum B, Feinstone SM et al. (1989) Attenuation and cell culture adaptation of hepatitis A virus (HAV): a genetic analysis with HAV cDNA. J Virol 63(12), 5364–5370.

53 Emerson SU, Huang YK, McRill C et al. (1992) Mutations in both the 2B and 2C genes of hepatitis A virus are involved in adaptation to growth in cell culture. J Virol 66(2), 650–654.

54 Zhang H, Chao SF, Ping LH et al. (1995) An infectious cDNA clone of a cytopathic hepatitis A virus: genomic regions associated with rapid replication and cytopathic effect. Virology 212(2), 686–697.

55 Inman RD, Hodge M, Johnston ME et al. (1986) Arthritis, vasculitis, and cryoglobulinemia associated with relapsing hepatitis A virus infection. Ann Intern Med 105(5), 700–703.

56 Scully LJ, Ryan AE (1993) Urticaria and acute hepatitis A virus infection. Am J Gastroenterol 88(2), 277–278.

57 Glikson M, Galun E, Oren R et al. (1992) Relapsing hepatitis A. Review of 14 cases and literature survey. Medicine (Baltimore) 71(1), 14–23.

58 Reiss G, Keeffe EB (2004) Review article: hepatitis vaccination in patients with chronic liver disease. Aliment Pharmacol Ther 19(7), 715–727.

59 Gordon SC, Reddy KR, Schiff L et al. (1984) Prolonged intrahepatic cholestasis secondary to acute hepatitis A. Ann Intern Med 101(5), 635–637.

60 Bamber M, Thomas HC, Bannister B et al. (1983) Acute type A, B, and non-A, non-B hepatitis in a hospital population in London: clinical and epidemiological features. Gut 24(6), 561–564.

61 Gruer LD, McKendrick MW, Beeching NJ et al. (1982) Relapsing hepatitis associated with hepatitis A virus. Lancet 2(8290), 163.

62 Jacobson IM, Nath BJ, Dienstag JL (1985) Relapsing viral hepatitis type A. J Med Virol 16(2), 163–169.

63 Chiriaco P, Guadalupi C, Armigliato M et al. (1986) Polyphasic course of hepatitis type A in children. J Infect Dis 153(2), 378–379.

64 Raimondo G, Longo G, Caredda F et al. (1986) Prolonged, polyphasic infection with hepatitis A. J Infect Dis 153(1), 172–173.

65 Sjogren MH, Tanno H, Fay O et al. (1987) Hepatitis A virus in stool during clinical relapse. Ann Intern Med 106(2), 221–226.

66 Tabor E (1987) Guillain–Barre syndrome and other neurologic syndromes in hepatitis A, B, and non-A, non-B. J Med Virol 21(3), 207–216.

67 Davis TV, Keeffe EB (1992) Acute pancreatitis associated with acute hepatitis A. Am J Gastroenterol 87(11), 1648–1650.

68 Mourani S, Dobbs SM, Genta RM et al. (1994) Hepatitis A virus-associated cholecystitis. Ann Intern Med 120(5), 398–400.

69 Geltner D, Naot Y, Zimhoni O et al. (1992) Acute oliguric renal failure complicating type A nonfulminant viral hepatitis. A case presentation and review of the literature. J Clin Gastroenterol 14(2), 160–162.

70 Thomas WJ, Bruno P, Holtzmuller K (1993) Hepatitis A virus anicteric encephalitis coexistent with hepatitis C virus infection. Am J Gastroenterol 88(2), 279–281.

71 Watanabe M, Shibuya A, Okuno J et al. (2002) Hepatitis A virus infection associated with hemophagocytic syndrome: report of two cases. Intern Med 41(12), 1188–1192.

72 Vento S, Garofano T, Di Perri G et al. (1991) Identification of hepatitis A virus as a trigger for autoimmune chronic hepatitis type 1 in susceptible individuals. Lancet 337(8751), 1183–1187.

73 Rahaman SM, Chira P, Koff RS (1994) Idiopathic autoimmune chronic hepatitis triggered by hepatitis A. Am J Gastroenterol 89(1), 106–108.

74 Huppertz HI, Treichel U, Gassel AM et al. (1995) Autoimmune hepatitis following hepatitis A virus infection. J Hepatol 23(2), 204–208.

75 Chalmers TC, Eckhardt RD, Reynolds WE et al. (1955) The treatment of acute infectious hepatitis. Controlled studies of the effects of diet, rest, and physical reconditioning on the acute course of the disease and on the incidence of relapses and residual abnormalities. J Clin Invest 34(7, Pt II), 1163–1235.

76 Yoshiba M, Inoue K, Sekiyama K (1994) Interferon for hepatitis A. Lancet 343(8892), 288–289.

77 Stokes J, Neefe JH (1945) The prevention and attenuation of infectious hepatitis by gamma-globulin. JAMA 127, 144–145.

78 Gellis SS, Stokes J, Brother GM et al. (1945) The use of human immune serum globulin (gamma-globulin) in infectious (epidemic) hepatitis in the Mediterranean theater of operations. I. Studies on prophylaxis in two epidemics of infectious hepatitis. JAMA 128, 1062–1023.

79 Krugman S (1976) Effect of human immune serum globulin on infectivity of hepatitis A virus. J Infect Dis 134(1), 70–74.

80 Charatan F (2005) US panel recommends young children receive hepatitis A vaccination. Br Med J 331(7525), 1102.

81 Wagner G, Lavanchy D, Darioli R et al. (1993) Simultaneous active and passive immunization against hepatitis A studied in a population of travellers. Vaccine 11(10), 1027–1032.

82 Fujiyama S, Iino S, Odoh K et al. (1992) Time course of hepatitis A virus antibody titer after active and passive immunization. Hepatology 15(6), 983–938.

83 World Health Organization. Department of Communicable Disease Surveillance and Response (2000) Hepatitis A. Bull World Health Org WHO/CDS/CSR/EDC/2000.7, 1–39.

84 Craig AS, Schaffner W (2004) Prevention of hepatitis A with the hepatitis A vaccine. N Engl J Med 350(5), 476–481.

85 Clemens R, Safary A, Hepburn A et al. (1995) Clinical experience with an inactivated hepatitis A vaccine. J Infect Dis 171(Suppl. 1), S44–49.

86 Tsai IJ, Chang MH, Chen HL et al. (2000) Immunogenicity and reactogenicity of the combined hepatitis A and B vaccine in young adults. Vaccine 19(4–5), 437–441.

87 Rothstein KD (2002) Hepatitis A vaccination in patients with chronic liver disease: to screen or not to screen? Am J Gastroenterol 97(7), 1590–1593.

88 Wasley A, Samandari T, Bell BP (2005) Incidence of hepatitis A in the United States in the era of vaccination. JAMA 294(2), 194–201.

89 Nainan OV, Armstrong GL, Han XH et al. (2005) Hepatitis A molecular epidemiology in the United States, 1996–1997: sources of infection and implications of vaccination policy. J Infect Dis 191(6), 957–963.

90 Dagan R, Leventhal A, Anis E et al. (2005) Incidence of hepatitis A in Israel following universal immunization of toddlers. JAMA 294(2), 202–210.

91 Connor BA (2005) Hepatitis A vaccine in the last-minute traveler. Am J Med 118(Suppl. 10A), 58S–62S.

92 Robertson BH, D'Hondt EH, Spelbring J et al. (1994) Effect of post-exposure vaccination in a chimpanzee model of hepatitis A virus infection. J Med Virol 43(3), 249–251.

93 D'Hondt E, Purcell RH, Emerson SU *et al.* (1995) Efficacy of an inactivated hepatitis A vaccine in pre- and postexposure conditions in marmosets. *J Infect Dis* 171(Suppl. 1), S40–43.

94 Bonanni P, Franzin A, Staderini C *et al.* (2005) Vaccination against hepatitis A during outbreaks starting in schools: what can we learn from experiences in central Italy? *Vaccine* 23(17–18), 2176–2180.

9.1.2.iv Hepatitis B

Geoffrey M. Dusheiko

Definition

Type B hepatitis is caused by the hepatitis B virus (HBV), a small, enveloped DNA virus that infects the liver causing hepatocellular necrosis and inflammation [1]. HBV infection can be either acute or chronic, and can range in severity from being asymptomatic to severe and symptomatic with progressive and even fatal illness.

Acute hepatitis B is defined as a self-limiting disease marked by acute inflammation and hepatocellular necrosis in association with a transient HBV infection. Chronic hepatitis B is defined as persistent HBV infection accompanied by evidence of hepatocellular injury and inflammation; the diagnosis is based upon the finding of abnormal concentrations of serum aminotransferases and hepatitis B surface antigen (HBsAg) in serum for 6 months or more. Chronic hepatitis B can enter a phase of remission with an improvement in serum aminotransferases despite the persistence of HBsAg [2]. However, these patients are at risk of reactivation of active hepatitis. Patients may ultimately develop cirrhosis, portal hypertension and hepatocellular failure. A proportion also develop hepatocellular carcinoma as a result of chronic HBV infection.

Introduction

After the identification of HBsAg, hepatitis B was clearly linked to the development of cirrhosis and hepatocellular carcinoma. Subtypes of HBsAg were described [3], the virus and subviral particles were identified in serum, a nucleocapsid core protein (HBcAg) and an associated DNA polymerase activity were described, and the genome of the virus was isolated and characterized as a small, circular molecule of DNA [4]. The identification of HBV led to the development of vaccines using HBsAg isolated from the serum of chronic carriers [5].

By 1978, the genome of the HBV had been cloned, and four open reading frames delineating the four gene products of HBV were identified [6]. Furthermore, identification of animal viruses resembling human HBV [7] led to the characterization of the replication cycle of this family of viruses, the so-called hepadnaviruses.

The virus exists as a 42-nm, double-shelled particle found in serum (see Chapter 9.1.2.i). HBV has an outer envelope component of HBsAg and an inner nucleocapsid component of HBcAg. In addition to actual virions, incomplete viral particles, 20-nm spheres and tubules, which consist entirely of HBsAg without HBcAg or nucleic acid, are present in serum and outnumber virions. HBsAg can also be detected in the liver. The nucleocapsid HBcAg is not found free in serum, but inside HBV virions. HBV DNA can be detected in serum and can be used to monitor viral replication. Hepatitis Be antigen (HBeAg), unlike HBsAg and HBcAg, is not particulate, but rather is detectable as a soluble, 17-kDa protein in serum. HBV replicates largely in the liver (see Chapter 9.1.2.i).

Transmission

Infection with HBV is a common problem worldwide [8]. Chronic hepatitis B is relatively uncommon in industrialized nations, affecting 1% or less of persons. In contrast, in undeveloped nations, HBV infection is an almost universal infection of childhood, and the HBsAg carrier state affects 5–15% of adults. Worldwide, approximately 5% of the population has chronic HBV infection, an estimated 300 million individuals. The ratio of males to females is usually between 1.5 and 2:1. The source of most HBV infection is probably exposure to blood secretions from chronic carriers. HBsAg carriers vary in their infectivity from less than 10 to more than 10^8 virions/mL of plasma. Patients with HBeAg in addition to HBsAg generally have 10^6 virions/mL and higher infectivity. However, anti-HBe-positive persons have virus in lower titre so that a larger volume exposure is necessary.

HBV has been transmitted by transfusion with HBsAg-negative, anti-HBc-positive blood, representing low levels of infection below the level of detection of HBsAg. HBV DNA has been detected in patients after clearance of HBsAg after the resolution of acute or chronic hepatitis B [9]. While HBsAg can occasionally be found in urine, breast milk, vaginal secretions, cerebrospinal fluid, sweat, tears, bile and faeces, the amounts are low.

The usual mode of transmission of hepatitis B is parenteral or percutaneous exposure such as blood transfusions, the use of unpasteurized plasma products, needlestick accidents and injections with unsterilized instruments such as in tattooing, acupuncture, ear piercing or dentistry. Outbreaks of nosocomial HBV infection have been ascribed to gynaecological surgery or dentistry. Recently, transmission from HBeAg-negative, HBV DNA-positive surgeons has also been reported. Hepatitis B from transfusion has become rare since the introduction of routine screening of blood donors for HBsAg. Routine nucleic acid testing of blood for anti-HBc (which was introduced as an indirect means of eliminating non-A, non-B hepatitis) may further decrease post-transfusion hepatitis B, but many countries have chosen not to include anti-HBc screening. Intravenous drug abuse is an increasing cause of hepatitis B in many areas of the world. Contaminated drug paraphernalia is often shared.

Careful investigation of cases of acute or chronic hepatitis B does not always uncover a potential parenteral source of transmission. In most developed countries of the world, the major mode of spread is probably sexual. This accounts for the very high rate of hepatitis B among male homosexuals and in promiscuous heterosexuals. Sexual spread of hepatitis B among heterosexuals also appears to occur, both female to male and male to female. Non-sexual intrafamilial spread is best described as inapparent parenteral spread, the vehicle perhaps being saliva, blood-tinged fluid and fluid from open sores, skin lesions or scratches. Thus, the non-sexual spread of hepatitis B in families, and particularly among small children, as appears to occur in underdeveloped areas of the world, is partially unexplained. The possible role of biting insects cannot be dismissed. Other cultural practices, such as tribal and witch doctor scarification and acupuncture, may spread hepatitis B. A splash of blood in the eye may also transmit the infection.

Perinatal spread is an important mode of transmission of hepatitis B. Newborns of mothers who are HBeAg positive are likely to develop HBV infection. The onset of infection is usually 3 months after birth. The acute phase of infection is typically mild, not associated with apparent illness and accompanied by minimal abnormalities in aminotransferases. However, infection during the neonatal period almost always leads to chronic infection. Maternal–infant spread is an important means by which this virus infection was sustained in populations prior to vaccination. Mothers with HBeAg in addition to HBsAg are the most infectious and, without vaccination, spread the chronic infection to their newborns in over 90% of cases.

Epidemiology

Low- (less than 2% of the population infected), intermediate- (2–8%) and high-prevalence (more than 8%) areas of hepatitis B infection are recognized. The disease is endemic in several regions: these include the Far East, more than 40 countries in the Pacific region and also large parts of Asia and sub-Saharan Africa. The disease is also prevalent in South America and in a number of foci in other regions, for example eastern Europe and the Arctic.

Some areas have an intermediate endemicity and appear to be in a state of transition from high to low. In some countries, such as Japan, countries of eastern Europe and in South America, the carrier rate among adults is 1–5%, and infections occur in both adults and children. In southern Europe, the incidence of HBV infections has consistently declined in the last decade.

The two extremes of endemicity could probably be accounted for in a prevaccination era by two separate major patterns of HBV transmission. In highly endemic areas, without vaccination, HBV was spread first by maternal–infant transmission, creating a cohort of children with chronic hepatitis B who were highly infectious. In turn, this pattern of childhood infection determined a high rate of chronic infection. Because infection occurred in childhood, the carrier rate was high, and the pool

of infected individuals was sustained to the next generation. Because disease complications occur only after decades of chronic infection, the infectious carriers had offspring and continued the cycle of infection. Horizontal transmission, that is child–child, was equally important. In endemic areas in Africa, the prevalence in children is quite low at 1 year of age but increases rapidly thereafter and, in many countries in this region, the prevalence reaches a peak in children of 7–14 years of age.

Infection of neonates at birth from their infected mothers was common in the Far East and China, whereas horizontal transmission from child to child was more common in Africa [10,11]. The patterns of transmission are related to the higher prevalence of HBeAg and, hence, higher infectivity in Chinese (40%) compared with African mothers (15%).

In areas of low endemicity, hepatitis B is a disease of adults, typically those who are in high-risk occupations or have high-risk habits such as drug abuse or sexual promiscuity. Hepatitis B in adults more frequently leads to acute, icteric hepatitis and rarely causes chronic hepatitis. Epidemiological characterization of cases suggests that most are attributable to drug abuse, heterosexual contact, transfusion and occupational exposure. These percentages have been changing over time, probably due to the initiation of vaccination programmes, the growth of drug abuse as a social problem and changes in high-risk sexual practices by homosexual men. These rates will begin to change now that HBV vaccine is available and recommended for these groups. Behavioural changes because of concerns about acquired immunodeficiency syndrome (AIDS) have been influential. Epidemiological studies of the last decade indicate that the reported rates of hepatitis B infection have significantly declined or are declining in western and northern Europe and the United States; the decline is the result of a number of factors, including safer sexual practices, behavioural changes, safe needle practices and vaccination but not as a result of widespread adoption of immunization, blood-screening refinements and the use of viral-inactivated blood components. Treatment may have reduced the infectivity of a proportion of carriers. Universal rather than selective vaccination has been more advantageous [12].

Changing patterns of HBV infection

In parallel with the decline in the prevalence of HBV, the virological pattern of chronic hepatitis B is changing in the developed world and in parts of the developing world. A few decades ago the disease was characterized primarily by the wildtype HBV virus prototype, capable of secreting HBeAg. However, in recent years the prevalence of HBeAg-positive relative to HBeAg-negative infection has diminished and a substantial proportion of HBV infections are now characterized by HBV mutants unable to secrete HBeAg. The predominant mutation in HBeAg-defective HBV in the Mediterranean area is a point mutation at nucleotide 1896 in the pre-core region that converts codon 28 from a tryptophan residue to a stop codon (so called pre-core mutants) [13,14]. The most frequent mutation in the basic core-promoter region is a double T to A and an A to G substitution at nucleotides 1762 and 1764, respectively, which reduces pre-core mRNA levels [15,16]. The two types of mutation can occur separately or together and can independently prevent the expression of HBeAg, through transcriptional inhibition in the case of basic core-promoter mutations or through translational inhibition in the case of pre-core mutations.

The 1896 stop codon mutant is associated with HBV genotypes harbouring a T at position 1858 (genotypes B, D, E and some of the genotype C and F strains); within these genotypes, the generation of the G to A mutation at nucleotide 1896 stabilizes the secondary structure of the encapsidation signal loop and the resulting mutants are viable [17]. In contrast, in genotypes A and some of genotype C and F strains, the presence of C at nucleotide 1858 would significantly reduce the possibility for G to A 1896 variants to be selected, because of lower replication fitness.

In the Asian Pacific area, the Mediterranean basin and North America/northern Europe, 15%, 33% and 14%, respectively, of HBsAg-positive infections currently exhibit the HBeAg-negative phenotype and, among HBeAg-negative HBV carriers from these areas (whether or not positive for anti-HBe), 36%, 24% and 22%, respectively, suffer from chronic hepatitis B [18]. These estimates would suggest that at least one-fifth of the HBsAg-positive population is HBeAg-negative in the various areas of the world [18].

Studies from clinical centres have shown that, in the Asian Pacific region, about 50% of chronic hepatitis B cases are infected with HBeAg-negative HBV, with a prevalence ranging from 45% in mainland China to 69% in Hong Kong [18,19]. Prevalence rates are distinctly higher in the Mediterranean basin, ranging from 63% in Spain to as high as 86% and 90.5% in Greece and Italy respectively [20,21]. Data are more variable in the few clinical series examined in northern Europe and North America, with only 9% and 22% of chronic hepatitis B cases being HBeAg-negative in the US, but with as many as 67% and 84% in Sweden and Germany respectively [21]; in France, the prevalence of HBeAg-negative chronic hepatitis B has increased from 22% in 1994 to 72% in 2005 [22].

Studies in Japan found the prevalence of mutant HBV in patients with chronic hepatitis B to range from 58% [23] to 83% [24], and in Korea [25] to be 38%. In that country, mutants were detectable in 86% of the patients with chronic hepatitis B-related hepatocellular carcinoma for whom DNA sequencing was possible. In India, 15% of chronic hepatitis B carriers were found to have mutant infection [26].

The median prevalence of pre-core variants in HBeAg-negative chronic hepatitis B was 50% (range 19–100%), 92% (range 67–100%) and 24% (range 0–53%), respectively, among patients in the Asian Pacific, Mediterranean and US/northern Europe regions and the median prevalence of basic core-promoter variants was 77% (range 59–98%) in the Asian Pacific.

Classification of HBV infections

The clinical outcome of HBV infection is the result of the level of replication attained by HBV and the efficacy of the host immune response against it. Upon exposure to HBV, individuals with a vigorous and broad immune response to the virus develop an acute self-limited infection which may result in acute hepatitis; an aberrant response can lead to fulminant hepatitis. Individuals who do not mount a broad and vigorous immune response do not clear the virus but develop persistent infection and become carriers of HBsAg. Chronic HBsAg carriers exhibit three clinical patterns (Fig. 1) [27–29]. A minority are immune tolerant and have subclinical or mild disease despite high replication of the virus; HBV DNA levels are elevated, typically $> 10^5$ copies/mL and alanine aminotransferase (ALT) levels are normal. The second pattern is that of active infection, i.e. sustained high replication of HBV, to which the host mounts an unsuccessful immune response. This response is unable to clear the virus but sustains its partial clearance with continuing inflammatory activity; HBV DNA levels are above 10^5 copies/mL, ALT levels are abnormal and liver disease is present on histological

	Immune tolerant	'Active'	'Inactive'
HBsAg	+	+/+	+
HBeAg	+	+/−	−
Anti-HBe	−	−/+	+
ALT	Normal	↑	Normal
HBV DNA (copies/mL)	$>10^5$	$>10^5/>10^{4a}$	$<10^{3-4}$
Histology	Normal/mild	Active	Normal

Fig. 1 Classification of HBV infections.
[a]Expert opinions on this value vary.

investigation. Active infections can be due either to infection in which wild-type HBeAg-positive HBV is predominant (chronic HBeAg-positive hepatitis B) or to infections in which mutant forms of HBV unable to secrete the HBeAg are predominant (chronic HBeAg-negative hepatitis B). Because the molecular identification of disease-specific mutations requires laborious genotyping, in practice, the lack of HBeAg together with the finding of HBV DNA > 10^4 copies/mL has become synonymous with mutant HBV infection without the need for further determining the precise viral sequence. The third pattern is that of inactive HBV infection, i.e. diminished HBV replication. Levels of HBV DNA are below 10^{3-4} copies/mL; the low level of viremia may denote immunological control; these individuals have normal levels of ALT.

These three phases are not static and can change one into the other; immunotolerant subjects may apparently develop a break in tolerance and develop active disease, carriers with inactive disease may develop active disease and high ALT levels, and vice versa, active disease may revert to inactive quiescent disease with no or minor disease upon therapy or spontaneously.

A fourth profile, of yet uncertain clinical significance, is occult HBV infection [30–34]. It is characterized by the persistence of HBV DNA in the liver tissue (± serum) of HBsAg-negative individuals. Recent evidence indicates that this particular form of HBV infection may be present not only in individuals with circulating anti-HBs and/or anti-HBc, but also in subjects negative for all HBV markers [35–37]; it may sometimes be associated with mutant viruses undetectable by commercial HBsAg assays [38]. The molecular bases of occult HBV infection appear to be related to the long-lasting persistence in the nuclei of the hepatocytes of the HBV cccDNA, an intermediate form of the virus life cycle that serves as template for gene transcription [39–41].

Occult HBV infection may have several clinical impacts. It is probably the main mechanism for the rare cases of transfusion-transmitted type B hepatitis that are still occasionally reported [42] and it may provoke HBV infection in recipients in cases of liver or other organ transplantation [43]. The development of an immunosuppressive status (for instance, chemotherapeutic treatments or HIV infection) may induce reactivation of occult HBV with the development of an acute hepatitis B that may have a fulminant course [44,45]. It is not certain whether occult HBV infection may by itself induce clinically significant chronic liver disease. Some studies have indicated its possible association also with cryptogenic liver disease [46] and with cirrhosis in chronic HCV carriers, suggesting that it might favour or accelerate the progression of the chronic hepatitis C [41]. There are data suggesting that occult HBV infection may also be a major risk factor for the development of hepatocellular carcinoma [47,48].

Pathogenesis

Hepatitis B is marked by necrosis of hepatocytes and an accompanying lymphocytic infiltrate. In acute hepatitis, the injury is diffuse, necrosis of individual cells is prominent, there is general cellular unrest, and inflammatory cells are found in the parenchyma and portal areas. Although serious or even fatal hepatitis may occur as a result of acute hepatitis B, the optimal outcome is eradication of infected hepatocytes, curtailment of viral replication and rapid hepatic regeneration. This process may occur in the absence of jaundice and symptoms. However, a proportion of patients exposed to HBV do not clear HBsAg but progress to chronic hepatitis. In chronic hepatitis, the cell injury and unrest are less severe, tend to be periportal, and focal and inflammatory cells are predominantly portal.

While acute and chronic infection are undoubtedly due to the viral infection, the nature and pattern of infection suggest that immunological factors are important [49,50].

In acute hepatitis B the cellular immune response is complex [49,50].

After acute hepatitis, low virus levels persist for decades after resolution of disease. Viral persistence is associated with the long-term persistence of CTL activation markers that maintain CTL response for life [51–54].

Recovery from acute hepatitis is thought to involve destruction of infected cells by CTL and NK cells, and apoptosis [55]. This killing is a T cell-dependent process.

Experiments to ascertain the relative contribution of CD4 and CD8 lymphocytes suggest that in CD8-depleted chimpanzees that CD8 T lymphocytes are the main effectors of viral clearance [56,57]. CTL recognition triggers apoptosis by physical engagement of CTL. Activated cells may produce inflammatory cytokines, especially interferon gamma, alpha, beta and TNF, to activate intracellular antiviral events that interrupt HBV infection. The inhibitory action of these cytokines implicates a non-cytolytic mechanism by which antigen-nonspecific immune responses in part regulate HBV replication in infected hepatocytes [58–60].

The elimination of virus-infected hepatocytes is dependent on the recognition of viral determinants in association with HLA proteins on the infected cells by cytotoxic T cells. In acute disease, a polyclonal and vigorous cytolytic T-cell response can occur [61]. HLA-restricted epitopes from the core, envelope and polymerase and, in particular, several HLA-A2-restricted, cytotoxic T-cell epitopes have been defined [51,62] The HBcAg epitope located between core amino acids 50–69 is most commonly recognised by class II-restricted lymphocytes in patients with acute hepatitis B [63]. Patients with acute, self-limiting hepatitis B also develop a polyclonal, HLA class I-restricted, cytotoxic T-cell response against numerous epitopes in the HBV envelope, nucleocapsid and polymerase proteins [49,64].

HBV-specific T-cell responses are very weak or totally undetectable in the peripheral blood of patients with long-lasting chronic hepatitis B [65–67]. The persisting ineffective immune response appears to be responsible for liver damage. Chronic HBeAg-positive disease is not infrequently accompanied by acute exacerbations that lead to downregulation of HBV DNA, a decline in HBV DNA and seroconversion to anti-HBe. The trigger to these exacerbations could conceivably involve a significant alteration in T-cell responsiveness to HBV. Available data suggest, therefore, that clonal deletion of T cells does not occur, albeit that antigen-specific T-cell responsiveness is difficult to discern in HBeAg-positive patients.

Varying levels of HBV replication may be found during chronic infection, but there is a spectrum of disease in patients, ranging from minimal hepatitis to rapidly progressive liver injury and cirrhosis. Patients with the highest concentrations of virus in liver and serum may have the mildest disease. These findings suggest that HBV is not cytopathic and that failure of clearance (establishment of chronic infection) is due to a failure of an adequate immune response. Chronic disease is unusual in patients with acute icteric hepatitis B, whereas the majority of cases of chronic hepatitis will not have been preceded by an episode of clinically apparent, icteric hepatitis, suggesting that the clearance of HBV requires a hepatitic illness.

The propensity to cause chronic infection is a property of hepadnaviral infections, particularly in those mammalian or avian hosts affected early in life. There is an inverse relation between age at infection and the probability of chronic disease.

In neonates, specific suppression of the cell-mediated immune response may favour infection, perhaps because of exposure to HBeAg inducing tolerance to epitopes that are usually the target of the cytotoxic T-cell response at a time when the immune system is ontogenically 'immature'. Clonal deletion of HBV-specific T cells may occur as as a consequence of transplacental infection of the developing fetus or transplacental passage of viral antigens. In murine transgenic experiments, non-transgenic progeny of HBeAg-positive transgenic mothers are known to be tolerant to both HBeAg and HBcAg at the T-cell level, perhaps owing to the thymic deletion of major histocompatibility complex (MHC) class II-restricted, HBV nucleocapsid-specific, helper T cells as a result of transplacental exposure to HBeAg [68].

In contrast with the vigorous, polyclonal, class I- and class II-restricted T-cell response that can be identified in patients with acute icteric hepatitis B, in chronic disease the HLA class II-restricted response in peripheral blood is relatively weak and focused (oligoclonal), and insufficient to clear replicating virus.

Mutations abrogating recognition of wild-type hepatitis B in patients infected by variants have been recognised. Natural variants of the HBcAg 18–27 core epitope that interfere with recognition of the wild-type epitope and act as T cell-receptor antagonists have been identified in two patients with chronic hepatitis [69]. This antagonism could lead, in theory, to an active inhibition of epitope recognition at T cell-receptor contact sites.

The mechanism of the immunological defect in otherwise healthy adult carriers is imprecisely understood. A B-lymphocyte defect may explain an impaired synthesis of anti-HBs after induction by non-specific mitogens; *in vitro* synthesis of anti-HBc and immunoglobulin remain normal in chronic carriers [70]. The high concentrations of HBsAg in the serum may lead to a state of tolerance.

Although the frequency of occurrence of HBV-specific, cytotoxic T-lymphocyte precursors is greatly diminished in the peripheral blood of chronically infected patients, such cells are nonetheless present at very low concentrations in the periphery and in the infected liver [67, 71–73]. This could explain both the continuing, indolent liver injury and exacerbations of the disease.

Acute hepatitis B

Acute hepatitis B resembles other forms of acute hepatitis clinically and cannot be distinguished by history, physical examination or routine serum biochemical tests. The course is divided into the incubation period, preicteric, icteric and convalescence phases. From the incubation period to the onset of symptoms or jaundice it averages 75 days (range 40–140 days).

The onset of hepatitis B is typically insidious, with non-specific symptoms of malaise, poor appetite, nausea and pain in the right upper quadrant. With the onset of the icteric phase, symptoms of fatigue and anorexia typically worsen. Jaundice can last from a few days to several months, the average being 2–3 weeks. Itching and pale stools may occur. Weight loss of 2–10 kg is typical. The convalescent phase of hepatitis B begins with the resolution of jaundice. Fatigue is generally the last symptom to abate and may persist for many months into convalescence.

The physical signs of typical acute hepatitis B are not prominent. Variable degrees of jaundice are present. The only other common physical finding in acute hepatitis B is a mild and slightly tender hepatomegaly. Mild enlargement of spleen or lymph nodes occurs uncommonly. Wasting, ascites, oedema, palmar erythema and prominent spider angiomas should suggest the presence of chronic liver disease.

As in other forms of acute hepatitis, the serum alanine and aspartate aminotransferases are usually markedly elevated and to the same extent (10- to 50-fold). The serum alkaline phosphatase and lactic dehydrogenase are usually only mildly elevated (less than threefold). The bilirubin is variably increased, in both direct and indirect fractions. Serum albumin rarely falls except with protracted severe disease. The prothrombin time can increase and is the most reliable marker of severity of injury. Blood counts do not usually change unless the disease is prolonged or fulminant. Various autoantibodies can appear during the course of acute hepatitis B, most typically to smooth muscle.

The results of serological testing provide the means for diagnosis of hepatitis B. The course of a 'typical' case of acute hepatitis B is shown in Figure 2. Tests for HBV DNA in serum are the most direct markers for assessing viral replication. The polymerase chain reaction technique for the detection of DNA has been adapted to the detection of HBV DNA in serum and liver. This technique is capable of detecting as few as 50–100 viral genomes per sample. In a number of patients with acute hepatitis B, the serological course may be atypical; these patients clear HBsAg rapidly and are negative for this viral marker when first seen by the physician. The diagnosis of acute hepatitis B can

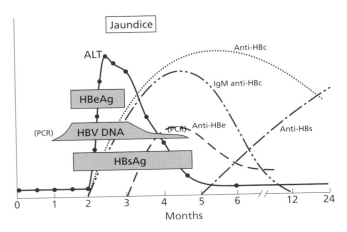

Fig. 2 Serological course of acute hepatitis B. ALT, alanine aminotransferase; PCR, polymerase chain reaction.

be made in these circumstances by detection of IgM anti-HBc, which is present in high titres.

In a small proportion of patients with acute hepatitis B, the disease may worsen over 1–3 months, with increasing jaundice, deteriorating coagulation, ascites, bleeding and encephalopathy. The serum aminotransferases may paradoxically improve as the disease worsens. Submassive hepatic necrosis, as the disease is also known, is more common in patients older than 40 years. Histopathological examination may reveal bridging or massive hepatic necrosis. The prognosis is poor.

Fulminant hepatitis refers to a clinical condition with rapid onset and development of acute hepatic failure, with encephalopathy, coma and death in more than 70% of cases. Fulminant hepatitis B is also an atypical course for this infection, occurring in less than 1% of icteric cases. Hepatitis D coinfection may predispose to fulminant hepatitis. The prevalence is approximately 2/1000 icteric cases. The mortality varies with the age of the patient. The onset of symptoms may also be insidious. Morphologically, the liver shows massive multilobular or bridging necrosis. The development of hepatic encephalopathy is the clinical criterion used for diagnosis of fulminant hepatitis. Encephalopathy may first be manifested by a subtle change in personality, abusive or violent behaviour, confusion or extreme lassitude. With progressive disease, stuporousness and then coma develop. Jaundice deepens progressively. With protracted disease, ascites may appear. Serum aminotransferases, while high at the onset of disease, may fall as the patient deteriorates. Serum bilirubin rises and albumin falls progressively. Most ominous, however, is a progressive rise in the prothrombin time, reflecting decreases in coagulation factors synthesized by the liver, particularly factors V and VII. Typically, in fulminant disease, HBV DNA and HBeAg become undetectable as hepatic failure supervenes. The pattern of serological markers during the course of fulminant hepatitis B suggests that this outcome is due to a sudden and extreme immunological response to HBV infection.

Chronic hepatitis B

The persistence of abnormal ALT activity for more than 6 months after the onset of acute hepatitis B is indicative of disease progression, and is usually accompanied by serological evidence of continued infection.

Prospective studies conducted by several groups have observed that 5–10% of adults exposed to the HBV may develop chronic type B viral liver disease [74]. The proportion of symptomatic patients who develop chronic liver disease after acute hepatitis B may be lower than this. In contrast, 90% of neonates infected perinatally will develop chronic hepatitis B. The incidence in children is inversely related to the age of onset. Males are more likely to become chronic carriers than females. Chronic hepatitis B is rather variable in its clinical course, presentation, progression and outcome. Two forms can be distinguished.

HBeAg-positive chronic hepatitis B

HBeAg-positive disease is typically associated with high levels of HBV replication for a prolonged period of time. The disease is found in young individuals with chronic hepatitis B, who have high levels of HBV DNA (usually $> 10^7$ copies/mL) in serum. Early on they may have been 'immunotolerant' of the disease, with normal serum aminotransferases (ALT), and have developed the ALT increase disease ('active infection') at a later stage. Spontaneous seroconversion rates are higher in patients with raised levels of ALT and genotype B (vs. C) and genotype D (vs. A) of HBV. The disease is not infrequently acquired in early childhood or the neonatal period in endemic areas. Patients may have normal or near normal ALT levels for decades, with little necroinflammatory disease. Importantly, patients with normal serum ALT levels and high circulating concentrations of HBV DNA display profound peripheral immunological tolerance. It is difficult to discern antigen-specific T cells in blood or in the liver. Treatment of these patients remains difficult, probably for this reason. These individuals are poor responders to interferon therapy and poor short-term responders to nucleoside or nucleotide antiviral drugs. Spontaneous seroconversion rates remain low in this group.

HBeAg-negative, anti-HBe-positive disease

This form of chronic hepatitis B is characterized by the absence of HBeAg in serum as a result of genotypic changes preventing expression of HBeAg. Viral replication continues and patients show an active disease course characterized typically by fluctuations in levels of HBV replication and, not infrequently, fluctuations in levels of serum ALT. These patients are HBsAg-positive and anti-HBe positive. HBV DNA concentrations are typically $> 10^5$ copies/mL but $< 10^7$ copies/mL. Liver biopsy shows necroinflammation and varying stages of fibrosis. Sustained antiviral responses are difficult to achieve with this group after both interferon and nucleoside analogue therapy.

Only a small percentage of patients with chronic infection give a history of acute hepatitis or jaundice. Thus, for the majority of patients with chronic hepatitis B, the time of onset is unknown, a circumstance that is typical of perinatal and childhood infection in endemic areas.

Most patients with uncomplicated chronic hepatitis B have no symptoms of liver disease. If symptoms are present, they are usually non-specific and mild. The most common symptom is fatigue. Myalgias, arthralgias and transient skin rashes are common extrahepatic manifestations of chronic hepatitis B, which may be due to immune complex deposition and occur more frequently in women than in men. With the development of cirrhosis, weight loss, weakness, wasting, abdominal swelling, oedema, dark urine and jaundice may become progressive problems. Many carriers may be detected through routine screening for HBsAg or through the presence of hepatomegaly and abnormal liver function tests. Older patients may present with complications of chronic active hepatitis and cirrhosis, or even with hepatocellular carcinoma, as typically occurs in Africa. A proportion of patients may present with an extrahepatic manifestation of HBV infection, for example glomerulonephritis, vasculitis or polyarteritis. HBV is an important cause of glomerulonephritis in tropical areas. Immunoelectron microscopy has been used to localize 'membrane attack complexes' and HBeAg to subepithelial deposits. With more severe disease, there may be spider angiomas and hepatomegaly. Wasting, ascites, peripheral oedema, palmar erythema, pale nails and bruising suggest advanced disease with cirrhosis. In patients with extrahepatic manifestations, there may be oedema from glomerulonephritis and hypoproteinaemia, fleeting urticarial or maculopapular rashes from mucocutaneous vasculitis, or mild tenderness, redness and synovial thickening from hepatitis B-related arthritis. The features of portal hypertension, such as ascites and bleeding oesophageal varices, are late features of a chronic active hepatitis accompanying cirrhosis.

Laboratory test results in typical, uncomplicated chronic hepatitis B are characteristic, demonstrating increases in alanine and aspartate aminotransferases with little or no increase in alkaline phosphatase, γ-glutamyltransferase or lactic dehydrogenase. The aminotransferases fluctuate over time, generally ranging from just above normal to between five- and eightfold elevated. Multiple ALT flares, accompanied by peaks of HBV viremia alternating with prolonged periods of biochemical and viral quiescence, are typical of chronic HBeAg-negative hepatitis B, occurring in as many as 60% of these patients.

Aspartate aminotransferase is usually lower than alanine aminotransferases. Serum bilirubin and albumin, the prothrombin time and the sedimentation rate are normal unless the disease is particularly severe. Serum immunoglobulins may demonstrate mild increases in IgG.

More emphasis is now placed on grading the degree of inflammation and staging the extent of fibrosis. Numerical assessments of liver biopsy findings have been developed as a tool for studying the course of chronic hepatitis B and for judging the efficacy of drugs in clinical therapeutic trials. There is consensus that scoring of the microinflammatory lesions should be separated from scoring of the architectural changes in the liver.

With progressive disease and the development of cirrhosis from chronic hepatitis B, the laboratory test results will change, becoming progressively more abnormal. By and large, the severity of the current injury and hepatitic disease activity is best reflected in the aminotransferase abnormalities, particularly aspartate. As cirrhosis develops, the ratio of aspartate aminotransferase:alanine aminotransferase will gradually increase; the finding of aspartate greater than alanine aminotransferase therefore suggests the presence of cirrhosis. In addition, alkaline phosphatase and γ-glutamyltransferase will increase, serum albumin will fall, and the prothrombin time will become prolonged with the onset of cirrhosis and worsening hepatocellular function. Autoantibodies, particularly smooth muscle autoantibodies and rheumatoid factor, may become detectable, and the immunoglobulins will increase in concentration, a raised IgA being particularly suggestive of cirrhosis. Hyperbilirubinaemia with depressed albumin and prolonged prothrombin time are poor prognostic findings.

A varying immune responsiveness plays a critical role in determining the outcome and pathogenesis of acute and chronic hepatitis B. It is likely that immune responses induced by antiviral therapy play a similar pivotal role. However, critical differences may occur in the two major forms of active chronic hepatitis B that usually require treatment: wild-type or HBeAg-positive chronic HBV infection and anti-HBe-positive or pre-core mutant disease. HBeAg seroconversion during antiviral therapy in HBeAg-positive disease may require an appropriate host T-cell response, which unfortunately is abrogated or dysfunctional in most patients.

Patients with an active infection and disease may revert to an inactive carrier state with remission of disease activity either spontaneously or after antiviral therapy. These patients are HBeAg-negative, anti-HBe-positive with lower HBV DNA levels ($\leq 10^4$ copies/mL) and little or no necroinflammation or fibrosis, depending on the timing of seroconversion. The disease may be a retrospective–prospective diagnosis as inactive carriers show some propensity to reactivation.

The subsequent course of chronic hepatitis B is variable (Fig. 3). Patients with chronic infection may have a relatively benign outcome. Probably only 15–20% of patients who acquire this infection in adulthood ultimately develop cirrhosis and any chronic disability. Furthermore, the development of cirrhosis is usually slow, occurring over 5–20 years. Infection in childhood may have a different prognosis, with a higher percentage of persons ultimately developing cirrhosis and hepatocellular carcinoma. Typically, the infection is mild in childhood and associated with few symptoms and minimal elevations of the aminotransferases. However, the disease may change once adulthood is reached, with marked fluctuations in its activity and the development of cirrhosis in up to 40% of patients.

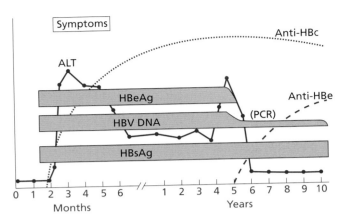

Fig. 3 Serological course of chronic hepatitis B. ALT, alanine aminotransferase; PCR, polymerase chain reaction.

Observations on large numbers of patients with chronic hepatitis B indicate that its course and outcome correlate with serological markers of viral replication. In a European analysis, 366 Caucasian HBsAg-positive patients with cirrhosis who had never had clinical manifestations of hepatic decompensation were enrolled and followed for a mean period of 72 months. Death occurred in 23%, mainly from liver failure or hepatocellular carcinoma. The probability of survival was 84% and 68% at 5 and 10 years respectively. The worst survival was in HBeAg- and HBV DNA-positive individuals (at diagnosis) [75]. Thus, progressive disease is associated with persistence of viral replication, and remission is associated with loss of active viral replication. The exacerbations associated with the decline in viral replication, or the reactivation of viral replication causing a recurrence of disease, can be severe and life-threatening. Indeed, the pattern of recurrent reactivation with multiple remissions and recurrences is a particularly severe form of this chronic infection, frequently leading to cirrhosis and, ultimately, hepatic failure.

Chronic hepatitis B can lead to hepatocellular carcinoma, which is a common form of cancer in many areas of the world where chronic hepatitis B is also common. Furthermore, a large percentage of patients with hepatocellular carcinoma have chronic HBV infection. Epidemiological and clinical studies suggest that hepatocellular carcinoma is a complication of prolonged HBV infection, most patients having had the disease for several decades before diagnosis of the carcinoma. Indeed, the majority of patients with this cancer also have cirrhosis, although it is often mild and inactive.

In a large European study, hepatocellular carcinoma developed during a mean follow-up of 6 years in 9% of 317 patients with compensated hepatic cirrhosis. Five years after diagnosis, the probability of hepatocellular carcinoma appearing was 6% (and that of decompensation 28%). After the first episode of decompensation, the 5-year probability of survival (35%) was poor [76].

Hepatocellular carcinoma is more common in men than in women and appears to be most common in patients who acquire HBV infection in childhood rather than in adulthood. Hepatocellular carcinoma is discussed elsewhere. In endemic areas of HBV infection, HBV carriers frequently have silent disease until the development of advanced hepatocellular carcinoma. For these reasons, ultrasonographic examinations and regular determinations of α-fetoprotein can be used to screen for hepatocellular carcinoma in high-risk populations. The populations at highest risk are men over the age of 40 years who acquired HBV infection during childhood and who have cirrhosis.

Although a large body of scientific evidence has confirmed a relation between chronic HBV infection and hepatocellular carcinoma, the mechanism of oncogenesis is not known. Exogenous factors may speed the process of oncogenesis, but chronic HBV infection must be considered as an important independent risk factor. The pathogenesis of HBV-associated hepatocellular carcinoma is unknown, however, and may be related to the phasic necrosis, regeneration and cirrhosis induced as a result of HBsAg infection. Although the molecular mechanism of HBV-associated carcinogenesis is unknown, HBV may have a direct cytogenetic role. Integration of the HBV genome into the hepatocyte DNA may be an important initiating factor. It is postulated that the development of hepatocellular carcinoma could be by insertional mutagenesis, or by the production of novel fusion genes, chromosomal deletions and translocations associated with HBV integration, or by loss of tumour-suppressor alleles or, as in woodchucks, by c-*myc* oncogene amplification. A retinoic acid receptor is expressed at high concentration in human hepatocellular carcinoma, in association with HBV integration [77]. Recent evidence has suggested that the translational product of the X gene, a 17-kDa protein, is a transactivating factor for viral enhancers and that, in cotransfection experiments, the X gene encodes a protein with the ability to stimulate transcription. The X-gene product does not bind DNA directly, but a number of effects of HBx on cell growth and cell cycle progression have been reported. Exposure to aflatoxin may be important in some geographical regions. A genetic susceptibility to hepatocellular carcinoma associated with genetic variation in enzymatic detoxification of aflatoxin has been reported.

In some parts of the world, codon 249 mutations in p53 are associated with aflatoxin exposure. The increased formation of carcinogen–DNA adducts may represent one mechanism adding to the association between chronic hepatitis B infection and the development of hepatocellular carcinoma [78,79].

References

1 Tiollais P, Pourcel C, Dejean A (1985) The hepatitis B virus. *Nature* 317, 489–495.

2 Hoofnagle JH, Shafritz DA, Popper H (1987) Chronic type B hepatitis and the 'healthy' HBsAg carrier state. *Hepatology* 7, 758–763.

3 Le Bouvier GL (1971) The heterogeneity of Australia antigen. *J Infect Dis* 123, 671–675.

4 Summers J, O'Connell A, Millman I (1975) Genome of hepatitis B virus: restriction of enzyme cleavage and structure of DNA extracted from Dane particles. *Proc Natl Acad Sci USA* 72, 4597–4601.

5 Szmuness W, Stevens CE, Harley EJ *et al.* (1980) Hepatitis B vaccine. Demonstration of efficacy in a controlled clinical trial in a high-risk population in the United States. *N Engl J Med* 303, 833–841.

6 Galibert F, Mandart E, Fitoussi F *et al.* (1979) Nucleotide sequence of the hepatitis B virus genome (subtype ayw) cloned in *E. coli. Nature* 281, 646–650.

7 Summers J, Smolec J, Snyder R (1978) A virus similar to human hepatitis B virus associated with hepatitis and hepatoma in woodchucks. *Proc Natl Acad Sci USA* 75, 4533–4537.

8 Alter MJ, Margolis HS (1990) The emergence of hepatitis B as a sexually transmitted disease. *Med Clin North Am* 74, 1529–1542.

9 Kaneko S, Miller RH, Feinstone SM *et al.* (1989) Detection of serum hepatitis B virus DNA in patients with chronic hepatitis using the polymerase chain reaction assay. *Proc Natl Acad Sci USA* 86, 312–316.

10 Botha JF, Ritchie MJ, Dusheiko GM *et al.* (1984) Hepatitis B virus carrier state in black children in Ovamboland: role of perinatal and horizontal infection. *Lancet* 1(8388), 1210–1212.

11 Dusheiko GM, Bowyer SM, Sjogren MH *et al.* (1985) Replication of hepatitis B virus in adult carriers in an endemic area. *J Infect Dis* 152, 566–571.

12 Anderson B, Bodsworth NJ, Rohrsheim RA *et al.* (1994) Hepatitis B virus infection and vaccination status of high risk people in Sydney: 1982 and 1991. *Med J Aust* 161, 368–371.

13 Carman WF, Jacyna MR, Hadziyannis S *et al.* (1989) Mutation preventing formation of hepatitis B e antigen in patients with chronic hepatitis B infection. *Lancet* 2, 588–591.

14 Brunetto MR, Stemler M, Shodell F *et al.* (1989) Identification of HBV variants which cannot produce pre-core derived HBeAg and may be responsible for severe hepatitis. *Ital J Gastroenterol* 21, 151–154.

15 Buckwold VE, Xu ZC, Chen M *et al.* (1996) Effects of a naturally occurring mutation in the hepatitis B virus basal core promoter on precore gene expression and viral replication. *J Virol* 70, 5845–5851.

16 Moriyama K, Okamoto H, Tsuda F *et al.* (1996) Reduced precore transcription and enhanced core-pregenome transcription of hepatitis B virus DNA after replacement of the precore-core promoter with sequences associated with e antigen-seronegative persistent infections. *Virology* 226, 269–280.

17 Lok ASF, Akarca U, Greene S (1994) Mutations in the pre-core region of hepatitis B virus serve to enhance the stability of the secondary structure of the pre-genome encapsidation signal. *Proc Natl Acad Sci USA* 91, 4077–4081.

18 Funk ML, Rosenberg DM, Lok AS (2002) World-wide epidemiology of HBeAg-negative chronic hepatitis B and associated precore and core promoter variants. *J Viral Hepat* 9, 52–61.

19 Yap I, Wee A, Guan R (1991) Chronic hepatitis B infection in Singapore. *Sing Med J* 32, 352–355.

20 Laras A, Koskinas J, Avgidis K *et al.* (1998) Incidence and clinical significance of hepatitis B virus precore gene translation initiation mutations in e antigen-negative patients. *J Viral Hepat* 5, 241–248.

21 Rizzetto M, Gaeta GB (2004) The expanding territory of HBeAg negative chronic hepatitis B. In: Jilbert AR (ed.) *Proceedings of the 11th International Symposium on Viral Hepatitis and Liver Disease.* Australian Centre for Hepatitis Virology, pp. 66–71.

22 Zazski JP, Marcellin P, Leroy V *et al.* (2006) Characteristics of patients with chronic hepatitis B in France: predominant frequency of HBe antigen negative cases. *J Hepatol* 45, 355–360.

23 Karasawa T, Shirasawa T, Okawa Y *et al.* (1997) Association between frequency of amino acid changes in core region of hepatitis B virus (HBV) and the presence of precore mutation in Japanese HBV carriers. *J Gastroenterol* 32, 611–622.

24 Nakahori S, Yokosuka O, Ehata T *et al.* (1995) Detection of hepatitis B virus precore stop codon mutants by selective amplification method: frequent detection of precore mutants in hepatitis B e antigen positive healthy carriers. *J Gastroenterol Hepatol* 10, 419–425.

25 Kim WH, Kim KH, Chung JP *et al.* (1993) Mutations in the pre-core region of hepatitis B virus DNA in patients with chronic liver diseases. *Yonsei Med J* 34, 158–165.

26 Guptan RC, Thakur V, Sarin SK *et al.* (1996) Frequency and clinical profile of precore and surface hepatitis B mutants in Asian–Indian patients with chronic liver disease. *Am J Gastroenterology* 91, 1312–1317.

27 Lai CL, Ratziu V, Yuen MF *et al.* (2003) Viral hepatitis B. *Lancet* 362(9401), 2089–2094.

28 Keeffe EB, Dieterich DT, Han SH *et al.* (2004) A treatment algorithm for the management of chronic hepatitis B virus infection in the United States. *Clin Gastroenterol Hepatol* 2, 87–106.

29 Lok AS, McMahon BJ (2004) Chronic hepatitis B: update of recommendations. *Hepatology* 39, 857–861.

30 Raimondo G, Balsano C, Craxi A *et al.* (2000) Occult hepatitis B virus infection. *Dig Liver Dis* 32, 822–826.

31 Brechot C, Thiers V, Kremsdorf D *et al.* (2001) Persistent hepatitis B virus infection in subjects without hepatitis B surface antigen: clinically significant or purely 'occult'? *Hepatology* 34, 194–203.

32 Hu KQ (2002) Occult hepatitis B virus infection and its clinical implications. *J Viral Hepat* 9, 243–257.

33 Torbenson M, Thomas DL (2002) Occult hepatitis B. *Lancet Infect Dis* 2, 479–486.

34 Liang TJ, Baruch Y, Ben-Porath E *et al.* (1991) Hepatitis B virus infection in patients with idiopathic liver disease. *Hepatology* 13, 1044–1051.

35 Cacciola I, Pollicino T, Squadrito G *et al.* (1999) Occult hepatitis B virus infection in patients with chronic hepatitis C liver disease. *N Engl J Med* 341, 22–26.

36 Zhang YY, Hansson BG, Kuo LS *et al.* (1993) Hepatitis B virus DNA in serum and liver is commonly found in Chinese patients with chronic liver disease despite the presence of antibodies to HBsAg. *Hepatology* 17, 538–544.

37 Carman W, Thomas H, Domingo E (1993) Viral genetic variation: Hepatitis B virus as a clinical example. *Lancet* 341, 349–353.

38 Pollicino T, Squadrito G, Cerenzia G *et al.* (2004) Hepatitis B virus maintains its pro-oncogenic properties in the case of occult HBV infection. *Gastroenterology* 126, 102–110.

39 Wieland SF, Spangenberg HC, Thimme R *et al.* (2004) Expansion and contraction of the hepatitis B virus transcriptional template in infected chimpanzees. *Proc Natl Acad Sci USA* 101, 2129–2134.

40 Werle-Lapostolle B, Bowden S, Locarnini S *et al.* (2004) Persistence of cccDNA during the natural history of chronic hepatitis B and decline during adefovir dipivoxil therapy. *Gastroenterology* 126, 1750–1758.

41 Raimondo G, Pollicino T, Squadrito G (2005) What is the clinical impact of occult hepatitis B virus infection? *Lancet* 365(9460), 638–640.

42 Allain JP (2004) Occult hepatitis B virus infection: implications in transfusion. *Vox Sang* 86, 83–91.

43 Chazouilleres O, Mamish D, Kim M *et al.* (1994) 'Occult' hepatitis B virus as source of infection in liver transplant recipients. *Lancet* 343(8890), 142–146.

44 Waite J, Gilson RJ, Weller IV *et al.* (1988) Hepatitis B virus reactivation or reinfection associated with HIV-1 infection. *AIDS* 2, 443–448.

45 Grumayer ER, Panzer S, Ferenci P *et al.* (1989) Recurrence of hepatitis B in children with serologic evidence of past hepatitis B virus infection undergoing antileukemic chemotherapy. *J Hepatol* 8, 232–235.

46 Chemin I, Zoulim F, Merle P *et al.* (2001) High incidence of hepatitis B infections among chronic hepatitis cases of unknown aetiology. *J Hepatol* 34, 447–454.

47 Brechot C, Gozuacik D, Murakami Y *et al.* (2000) Molecular bases for the development of hepatitis B virus (HBV)-related hepatocellular carcinoma (HCC). *Semin Cancer Biol* 10, 211–231.

48 Squadrito G, Pollicino T, Cacciola I *et al.* (2006) Occult hepatitis B virus infection is associated with the development of hepatocellular carcinoma in chronic hepatitis C patients. *Cancer* 106, 1326–1330.

49 Chisari FV, Ferrari C (1995) Hepatitis B virus immunopathogenesis. *Annu Rev Immunol* 13, 29–60.

50 Webster GJ, Reignat S, Maini MK *et al.* (2000) Incubation phase of acute hepatitis B in man: dynamic of cellular immune mechanisms. *Hepatology* 32, 1117–1124.

51 Rehermann B, Fowler P, Sidney J *et al.* (1995) The cytotoxic T lymphocyte response to multiple hepatitis B virus polymerase epitopes during and after acute viral hepatitis. *J Exp Med* 181, 1047–1058.

52 Rehermann B, Ferrari C, Pasquinelli C *et al.* (1996) The hepatitis B virus persists for decades after patients' recovery from acute viral hepatitis despite active maintenance of a cytotoxic T-lymphocyte response. *Nat Med* 2, 1104–1108.

53 Rehermann B (2003) Immune responses in hepatitis B virus infection. *Semin Liver Dis* 23, 21–38.

54 Rehermann B, Nascimbeni M (2005) Immunology of hepatitis B virus and hepatitis C virus infection. *Nat Rev Immunol* 5, 215–229.

55 Whalley SA, Murray JM, Brown D *et al.* (2001) Kinetics of acute hepatitis B virus infection in humans. Journal of Experimental Medicine 2001; 193, 847–853.

56 Guidotti LG, Ando K, Hobbs MV *et al.* (1994) Cytotoxic T lymphocytes inhibit hepatitis B virus gene expression by a noncytolytic mechanism in transgenic mice. *Proc Natl Acad Sci USA* 91, 3764–3768.

57 Guidotti LG, Rochford R, Chung J *et al.* (1999) Viral clearance without destruction of infected cells during acute HBV infection. *Science* 284, 825–829.

58 Romero R, Lavine JE (1996) Cytokine inhibition of the hepatitis B virus core promoter. *Hepatology* 23, 17–23.

59 Koziel MJ (1999) What once was lost, now is found: restoration of hepatitis B-specific immunity after treatment of chronic hepatitis B (Comments). *Hepatology* 29, 1331–1333.

60 Koziel MJ (1999) Cytokines in viral hepatitis. *Semin Liver Dis* 19, 157–169.

61 Van Hecke E, Paradijs J, Molitor C *et al.* (1994) Hepatitis B virus-specific cytotoxic T lymphocyte responses in patients with acute and chronic hepatitis B virus infection. *J Hepatol* 20, 514–523.

62 Rehermann B, Pasquinelli C, Mosier SM *et al.* (1995) Hepatitis B virus (HBV) sequence variation in cytotoxic T lymphocyte epitopes is not common in patients with chronic HBV infection. *J Clin Invest* 96, 1527–1534.

63 Ferrari C, Penna A, Bertoletti A *et al.* (1990) Cellular immune response to hepatitis B virus-encoded antigens in acute and chronic hepatitis B virus infection. *J Immunol* 145, 3442–3449.

64 Penna A, Chisari FV, Bertoletti A *et al.* (1991) Cytotoxic T lymphocytes recognize an HLA-A2-restricted epitope within the hepatitis B virus nucleocapsid antigen. *J Exp Med* 174, 1565–1570.

65 Jung MC, Pape GR (2002) Immunology of hepatitis B infection. *Lancet Infect Dis* 2, 43–50.

66 Ferrari C, Penna A, Bertoletti A *et al.* (1998) Antiviral cell-mediated immune responses during hepatitis B and hepatitis C virus infections. Recent Results Cancer Res 154, 330–336.

67 Webster GJ, Reignat S, Brown D *et al.* (2004) Longitudinal analysis of CD8+ T cells specific for structural and nonstructural hepatitis B virus proteins in patients with chronic hepatitis B: implications for immunotherapy. *J Virol* 78, 5707–5719.

68 Milich DR, Jones JE, Hughes JL (1990) Is a function of the secreted hepatitis B e antigen to induce immunologic tolerance *in utero*? *Proc Natl Acad Sci USA* 87, 6599–6603.

69 Bertoletti A, Costanzo A, Chisari FV *et al.* (1994) Cytotoxic T lymphocyte response to a wild type hepatitis B virus epitope in patients chronically infected by variant viruses carrying substitutions within the epitope. *J Exp Med* 180, 933–943.

70 Dusheiko GM, Hoofnagle JH, Cooksley WG *et al.* (1983) Synthesis of antibodies to hepatitis B virus by cultured lymphocytes from chronic hepatitis B surface antigen carriers. *J Clin Invest* 71, 1104–1113.

71 Barnaba V, Franco A, Alberti A *et al.* (1989) Recognition of hepatitis B virus envelope proteins by liver-infiltrating T lymphocytes in chronic HBV infection. *J Immunol* 143, 2650–2655.

72 Bertoletti A, Chisari FV, Penna A *et al.* (1993) Definition of a minimal optimal cytotoxic T-cell epitope within the hepatitis B virus nucleo-capsid protein. *J Virol* 67, 2376–2380.

73 Maini MK, Boni C, Ogg GS *et al.* (1999) Direct *ex vivo* analysis of hepatitis B virus-specific CD8+ T cells associated with the control of infection. Gastroenterology 117, 1386–1396.

74 Shah N, Ostrow D, Altman N *et al.* (1985) Evolution of acute hepatitis B in homosexual men to chronic hepatitis B. Prospective study of placebo recipients in a hepatitis B vaccine trial. *Arch Intern Med* 145, 881–882.

75 Realdi G, Fattovich G, Hadziyannis S *et al.* (1994) Survival and prognostic factors in 366 patients with compensated cirrhosis type B: a multicenter study. *J Hepatol* 21, 656–666.

76 Fattovich G, Giustina G, Schalm SW *et al.* (1995) Occurrence of hepatocellular carcinoma and decompensation in Western European patients with cirrhosis type B. *Hepatology* 21, 77–82.

77 Benbrook D, Lernhardt E, Pfahl M (1988) A new retinoic acid receptor identified from a hepatocellular carcinoma. *Nature* 333(6174), 669–672.

78 Kirk GD, Turner PC, Gong Y *et al.* (2005) Hepatocellular carcinoma and polymorphisms in carcinogen-metabolizing and DNA repair enzymes in a population with aflatoxin exposure and hepatitis B virus endemicity. *Cancer Epidemiol Biomarkers Prev* 14, 373–379.

79 Kirk GD, Camus-Randon AM, Mendy M *et al.* (2000) Ser-249 p53 mutations in plasma DNA of patients with hepatocellular carcinoma from the Gambia. *J Natl Cancer Inst* 92, 148–153.

9.1.2.v Hepatitis D

Antonella Smedile and Mario Rizzetto

Definition

Hepatitis D, also named hepatitis delta [1], is a disease caused by the hepatitis delta (D) virus (HDV), a unique hepatotropic human pathogen requiring obligatory helper functions provided by the hepatitis B virus (HBV) for *in vivo* infection. The virion of HDV is a particle of 36 nm diameter coated by the HB surface antigen (HBsAg), inside which are sequestered the RNA genome and the HD antigen (HDAg). The deltavirus genus includes at least eight major clades [2]. The three major genotypes, designated I, II and III, differ by as much as 40% over the entire genome and have different geographical prevalences [3,4]; two subgroups have been identified within genotypes I and II, named genotype IA and IB and genotype IIA and IIB.

Natural history

HDV can establish infection only in patients simultaneously infected by HBV [5]. It usually modifies the natural history of the underlying HBV infections upon which it thrives, aggravating pre-existent hepatitis B by adding HDV damage or creating hepatitis D in healthy carriers of HBV. Hepatitis D is a distinct medical entity that, as a rule, is more severe than disease caused by HBV alone [6–8]. Persons susceptible to HBV or already infected by it are susceptible to HDV and, therefore, hepatitis D occurs in two settings: in a normal person simultaneously infected by HDV–HBV (coinfection) or in a carrier of HBsAg superinfected by HDV (superinfection). Persons protected from HBV by the acquisition of antibody to HBsAg (anti-HBs) are protected from HDV.

Coinfection

In this setting, transmission of HDV is attained by infectious inocula containing both HBV and HDV (Fig. 1). Infection with HDV demands that the helper HBV be activated first, thus providing the functions (mainly the HBsAg) necessary for the activation of HDV [6–8].

As HDV cannot replicate until HBV has infected hepatocytes, the expression of the defective virus depends on (and is limited by) the virulence of the associated HBV. Slow spread of HBV to hepatocytes either fails to support HDV or supports only an abortive infection; rapid spread provides enough vulnerable hepatocytes for the defective virus to be activated to a clinically significant degree.

Because of the complex interactions between the two viruses, the expression of HDV is variable, ranging from incomplete to very virulent. However, as in normal individuals who are coinfected with the two viruses the background HBV infection

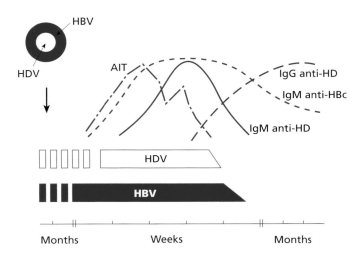

Fig. 1 Course of typical HBV–HDV coinfection; AIT, alanine aminotransferase. IgG anti-HD, IgG antibody to HDV; IgM anti-HD, IgM antibody to HDV; IgM anti-HBC, IgM antibody to hepatitis B core antigen.

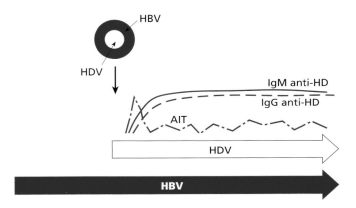

Fig. 2 Course of typical HDV superinfection in HBsAg carriers; AIT, alanine aminotransferase.

is usually self-limiting and HDV cannot outlive the elimination of its helper virus, acute HBV–HDV coinfections are rarely progressive and cause chronic liver disease in only about 2% of cases.

Superinfection

A pre-existing HBV infection (with production of HBsAg) provides the ideal background for the activation of the superinfecting HDV, affording a highly susceptible substrate that permits the rapid amplification of the defective pathogen (Fig. 2). In this setting, HDV establishes infection independently of the virulence of the HBV with which it was associated in the original inoculum; the helper function necessary for HDV replication is provided by the HBV colonizing the host. A pre-existing HBsAg state may rescue minimal amounts of HDV, and biological material containing HDV that is not infectious to the normal person (because the accompanying HBV is unable to establish its own helper infection) can nevertheless transmit hepatitis D to the carrier of HBsAg [6–8].

With superinfection, HDV transcapsidates from the HBsAg coat worn in the original inoculum to the coat made available by the HBV of the superinfected host, a process that also takes place with interspecies passage of HDV to animals infected with hepadnaviruses different from HBV [9].

Although superinfection can be self-limiting, it most often results in chronic HDV infection. As continuing production of HBsAg secures the indefinite survival of HDV, providing the biological niche in which it can replicate and from which it can seed continuously, the chronic carrier of HBsAg/HDV represents the main epidemiological reservoir and source of the virus [10].

Diagnosis

Screening for HDV relies primarily on indirect antibody testing; this is the first step in diagnosing hepatitis D [11]. The immunoglobulin (Ig)M antibody to HDV (IgM anti-HD) is detected transiently in acute hepatitis D with a mean delay of 7–15 days from admission [12]. It may be the only serum marker of acute HDV infection and persists, increasing in titre as hepatitis D progresses to chronicity.

During primary infections, the IgM antibody consists of pentameric 19S molecules [13]; in chronic infections, monomeric 7S molecules become prevalent. The IgM antibody was considered to be an indicator of HDV-related liver damage, but this role has been questioned.

The IgG antibody to HDV (anti-HD) is not protective; in immunocompetent patients with ongoing HDV infection, it coexists with concurrent replication of HDV. It may also be present as a serological 'scar' in patients whose double HBV–HDV infection has resolved. It is raised in acute hepatitis D and increases to high titres as HDV infection progresses to chronicity [6].

The finding in serum or liver of HDV RNA or of hepatitis D antigen (HDAg) establishes the presence of active HDV infection. The intrahepatic antigen can be demonstrated by immunohistological techniques in frozen and in fixed liver specimens [11,14]; fixed material must be predigested with protease. HDV genotypes can also be determined in liver tissue by immunohistochemistry [15]. The intrahepatic expression of HDAg decreases as the disease progresses, thus increasing the probability of a false-negative result caused by sampling variation in needle liver biopsies.

The HDV genome can be detected in formalin-fixed, paraffin-embedded liver sections by radioactive and non-radioactive *in situ* hybridization techniques [16].

Solid-phase immunosorbent tests for the measurement of HDAg in serum can detect antigen only during the early stage of primary infection, before the development of anti-HD; when the antibody appears in blood, HDAg is masked in immune complexes that render it unavailable to the assay.

The introduction of reverse transcriptase and polymerase chain reaction (PCR)-based assays for the detection of HDV RNA has increased the limit of sensitivity to less than 10 genome molecules per assay [17]. The use of PCR assays has shown that virtually all HBsAg carriers with chronic hepatitis D have continuing HDV replication. The PCR assay is also useful in early diagnosis and in monitoring the effect of therapy with interferon [18]. The choice of suitable primers for the amplification of HDV RNA is difficult because of the extensive sequence heterogeneity of the different viral isolates; only a few conserved regions exist in the HDV genome, and secondary and tertiary constraints may further reduce the efficiency of reverse transcription. Amplification of the C-terminal half of the HDAg coding region ensures the highest degree of efficiency. A reverse transcription PCR and a quantitative PCR have been developed recently [19]. The HDV genotype may be determined in serum by restriction fragment length polymorphism analysis of PCR amplification products or by sequencing.

Epidemiology

HDV is maintained by transmission through superinfection from carrier to carrier of the HBsAg; secondary extension of the virus to normal, HBsAg-negative individuals occurs in direct proportion to the rate of HDV-infected HBsAg carriers in the population and in reverse proportion to the rate of HBV immunity (presence of anti-HBs) in contacts. Spread to non-carriers has no long-term epidemiological consequences as it results in self-limiting forms of HBV–HDV infection.

HDV infection is acquired by the parenteral route, either overt or covert, in the same way as HBV infection. However, the relative efficiency of HDV transmission differs from that of HBV. Direct inoculation of HDV by infected paraphernalia is the most efficient route of transmission, and the highest rates of hepatitis D were reported in HBsAg-positive drug addicts; in chimpanzees carrying the HBsAg, HDV has been transmitted by inoculation of HDV-positive human serum diluted 10^{-11} [20]. Transmission is efficient both by sexual [5,6,21] and household contacts [22,23], but vertical transmission is rarely documented, and spread of HDV has been inconspicuous among homosexual men [5]. The contemporary control of blood for HBsAg eliminates virtually all blood containing HDV.

Hepatitis D occurs worldwide, the most important factor influencing its spread being the rate of HBV infection within the population. Surveys in the 1980s [6] had shown that the prevalence of HDV was high among HBsAg carriers in tropical and subtropical areas of the African and South American continents and intermediate in the Mediterranean area, in correlation with high and intermediate local rates of HBV infection; however, rates of HDV were low in the Far East despite locally high rates of HBV. Genetic analysis of HDV worldwide has likewise shown wide geographical variations [2,3,24]. Genotype I predominates in Italy [25], USA, Europe, Russia [26], Turkey [27], the Middle East and Mongolia; genotype IA predominates in Asia, IB in the USA, both are common in the Mediterranean basin and a subgroup of genotype I has been isolated in Africa [28]. Genotype II was found in Japan [29,30], Taiwan [31] and in Yakutia in Russia [32]. Genotype III has been identified in northern South America [33].

In northern Europe and North America, where the rates of HBV were low, HDV infection in the 1980s was confined to parenteral drug addicts and to immigrants from endemic areas [19]. In countries in the Mediterranean basin [34,35] and in Taiwan [36], the epidemiological pattern of infection was composite, resulting from endemic infection in the general populations and from epidemic outbreaks among drug addicts in urban areas. The infection peaked around the third to fourth decade of life, and endemic spreading occurred mainly in the household, facilitated by overcrowding and promiscuity. High rates of hepatitis D were found in Taiwanese and Greek HBsAg-positive prostitutes and in HBsAg-positive haemophiliacs [5].

Drug addicts are often also infected by the hepatitis C virus (HCV) and, in this setting, HDV infection was associated with high morbidity; clustered epidemics of fulminant hepatitis B were reported in drug-abusing communities of the United States and western Europe [6].

Important epidemiological changes have occurred in the last two decades in countries where HBV infection has been brought under control through better public health standards, universal HBV vaccination and measures to contain the spread of HIV, which is transmitted in the same way as HBV/HDV.

Paradigmatic are the changes that have occurred in Italy. In a baseline study performed in the country in the years 1978–1981, the prevalence of HDV infection in HBsAg carriers with liver disease, determined from the prevalence of anti-HD, was 24% [37]; it remained stable up to the second half of the 1980s [38] but, by the early 1990s, it had diminished to 14% [37] and, in nationwide surveys performed in the late 1990s, it has declined further to 7–8% [40,41].

In Spain, the rate of anti-HD in HBsAg carriers with chronic hepatitis diminished from 15% in 1975–1985 to 7.1% in 1986–1992 [42], and a significant decrease in the prevalence of HDV superinfection has been observed in Taiwan in both the general population and high-risk groups [43,44].

Information on the recent epidemiological trends in HDV infection from other countries is limited. However, it is unlikely that the pattern of HDV infection has changed in endemic areas of the developing world, unless the factors determining transmission and circulation of the helper HBV have been significantly modified in the last decades. Outbreaks of severe HDV hepatitis have continued to occur in the Amazon basin, extending from the Brazilian to the Peruvian and Ecuadorean areas [45]. The prevalence of HDV infection remains high in Turkey (33–59.4% prevalence of anti-HD in chronic HBsAg liver disease in Eastern Anatolia [46]) and in Albania [47]. Anti-HD has been detected in 8.6% of the HBsAg-positive chronic hepatitis patients in a recent large survey in Saudi Arabia [48]. Endemic HDV foci were reported from west Greenland and Mongolia [49], Tunisia [10] and Okinawa [10], and markers of HDV were found in a consistent proportion (18.35%) of

HBsAg-positive pregnant women in Moldova as well as in 13.15% of hepatitis B patients in the Shandong province in China [10]. In contrast, from 1991 to 1997, the prevalence of anti-HD in patients with HBsAg-positive cirrhosis in Belarus [10] has decreased from 47.6% to 15.4%.

Hepatitis D is rare in Poland [50], apparently absent in the high Andean plateau [10] and Nigeria [10], low in patients with HBsAg-positive liver disease in sub-Saharan Africa and in HBsAg carriers in north-west Mexico (6.5% and 4% respectively) [10]. In Korea [51], the prevalence of anti-HD was 4%; the antibody was found mainly in HBsAg-positive patients with hepatocellular carcinoma. Conflicting data were reported from India: anti-HD was found in 21.4% of HBsAg-positive liver disease in Northern India [52], and HDV was implicated as a major risk factor for fulminant hepatitis in the country [53], but anti-HD was rarely found in hospital patients and mixed clinical HBsAg-positive populations in Calcutta [54]. HDV infection was observed among inhabitants of the Nicobar Islands but not in those inhabiting the Andaman Islands [55].

The infection has also declined among risk groups in developed countries. In Taiwan, the rate of anti-HD in HBsAg-positive drug addicts diminished from 79% in 1985 to 14% in 2004; in this population, the average rate of decrease in the prevalence of HDV infection was 4.7% per year [44,56]. No HDV case was found in intravenous drug users in Rio de Janeiro, Brazil, despite a 7.8% prevalence of serum HBsAg in this community [10], and a 14.7% prevalence rate was found in HBsAg-positive drug users in Jeddah, Saudi Arabia [10].

Disease

Although viral and host immune response are likely to interact in the pathogenesis of the liver damage associated with HDV, the mechanisms conducive to HDV liver damage in humans remain unknown. Early hypotheses suggesting that viral cytotoxicity could be caused directly by intrahepatic expression of the HDAg or by a disturbance of cell function induced by HDV RNA base-pairing to corresponding RNA regions of the signal recognition particle, a structure involved in the targeting of secretory and membrane proteins to the membrane of the endoplasmic reticulum, have not been substantiated [57]. It was suggested that the pathogenicity of HDV may be modulated by the degree of replication of the helper HBV and/or by the genotype of HDV [58]; genotype III was associated with outbreaks of fulminant hepatitis in South America [33], and Japanese patients with genotype IIB showed greater progression of chronic hepatitis to cirrhosis than those with genotype II [4].

Course of coinfection and superinfection hepatitis D

The clinical and histological features of acute and chronic hepatitis D are not specific and are non-distinctive from ordinary hepatitis B, and recognition of the disease is based on specific serological testing [5,8,59]. In coinfections, the serological picture shows the features of acute HBV infection, including the IgM antibody to the hepatitis B core antigen (IgM anti-HBc) with superimposed markers of HDV. HD viraemia is usually transient and may be detected by PCR. Occasionally, HBV/HDV hepatitis acquired by coinfection may be severe; these forms exhibit a full serological response consisting of early HD antigenaemia followed by seroconversion to anti-HD, initially of the IgM and then of the IgG class.

The clinical presentation of HDV superinfection in patients chronically infected by HBV depends on whether they were asymptomatic carriers of HBsAg, or whether clinical features of type B hepatitis were present [5–8]. In the asymptomatic carrier, superinfection appears as an intercurrent hepatitis; in the patient with chronic type B hepatitis, it may be mistaken for an exacerbation of the underlying HBV disease. In asymptomatic carriers unaware of their HBsAg state, superinfection may mimic acute hepatitis B as a positive HBsAg test suggests this diagnosis if it is first performed after infection with HDV. Clues to the nature of the disease are a positive HDV serology and an incomplete or atypical HBV profile (superinfected carriers, unlike patients with acute hepatitis B, usually lack the IgM anti-HBc).

In superinfection, the antibody response is more uniform and consistent than in coinfection. There is a relatively brisk IgM and IgG anti-HD response; when superinfection progresses to chronicity, both antibodies increase rapidly in a few weeks, and persist in high titres as hepatitis D continues. In patients whose chronic hepatitis D resolves, the IgM antibody disappears, whereas IgG anti-HD declines slowly.

Whether acquired by coinfection with HBV or superinfection in a chronic HBsAg carrier, HDV can precipitate an episode of fulminant hepatitis [6]. In cases of fulminant hepatitis D in tropical areas, microscopic features of microvesicular steatosis and foamy degeneration were often observed; these aspects have rarely been observed in fulminant hepatitis D in developed countries [6].

Atypical acute hepatitis D

The course of HDV infection may be confounded by the inhibitory effect exerted by HDV on the replication of HBV. In coinfection, early repression of HBV can occasionally produce a picture of HBsAg-negative hepatitis resembling a non-B hepatitis. Sequential expression of HBV and HDV may result in a biphasic hepatitis.

HDV superinfection can occasionally terminate the HBsAg state with clearance of HBV and HDV. Clearance of the HBsAg occurs more frequently over the years in chronic HDV patients than in ordinary HBV patients [60], and prior delta infection may result in effective suppression of residual HBV infection [61].

Rarely, transient suppression of pre-existing HB viraemia can create diagnostic confusion because, with disappearance of HBsAg from serum caused by marked inhibition of HBV at the time of superinfection, anti-HBs may temporarily appear in these patients, simulating the resolution of an acute HBV hepatitis; the HBsAg, however, returns at the termination of florid HDV infection [5].

Chronic hepatitis D

Patients with chronic hepatitis D suffer from a disease that is more serious and progressive than ordinary hepatitis B. Studies conducted in the 1970s and 1980s in Europe and the United States have shown that markers of HDV were more prevalent in HBsAg carriers with chronic hepatitis than in apparently healthy carriers; in HBsAg carriers with liver damage, the prevalence of HDV was higher in those with chronic active hepatitis or cirrhosis than in those with chronic persistent hepatitis [5–8,59].

Superinfection hepatitis D often ran a rapidly progressive course to liver failure (within 2 years from exposure to HDV) in drug addicts with HBeAg-positive (wild-type) HBV infection. Triple HBV–HDV–HCV infection also occurred often in drug addicts; in studies from Europe and the USA, HDV [62–65] was the dominant virus inhibiting the other two; in a study from Taiwan [66], HCV was the dominant virus.

A survey of 148 Italian patients with chronic hepatitis from 1977 to 1994 [67] has shown two patterns of disease. In about 10%, the disease was mild, non-progressive and characterized at histology by portal inflammation only. In the other 90%, the disease was progressive and characterized by chronic active hepatitis or active cirrhosis. Progression to extensive fibrosis and cirrhosis was usually rapid, with about 30–40% of the patients with non-cirrhotic disease at baseline developing cirrhosis within 5 years of follow-up. However, the cirrhotic stage has often remained clinically stable for decades, and the course of cirrhosis has been asymptomatic over many years; these patients may exhibit a marked enlargement of the spleen. In Italian patients, infection with HDV increased the risk of hepatocellular carcinoma threefold and of mortality twofold in those with HBsAg-positive cirrhosis [68].

In oriental patients, the virological profile of progressive chronic hepatitis D consisted of an early phase following superinfection characterized by elevated alanine aminotransferase, active HDV replication and suppression of HBV, an intermediate phase characterized by moderately elevated alanine aminotransferase, decreasing HDV synthesis and reactivation of HBV, and a late cirrhotic phase characterized by marked reduction in the synthesis of both HBV and HDV [69].

In Mediterranean patients, the underlying HBV infection was most often inactive (HBV DNA negative by conventional hybridization assays or positive at low titre by PCR; HBeAg negative and anti-HBe positive in serum) [5–8], and a proportion of patients with early and florid disease raised a variety of autoantibodies, the most frequent of which was a liver–kidney microsomal antibody (LKM) similar in its immunofluorescence pattern to LKM of autoimmune type 2 hepatitis and directed against UDP glucuronyltransferase [70]. In children, the course of chronic hepatitis D was also severe and progressive. In view of the young age of acquisition and the accelerated course of disease, hepatitis D was an important cause of juvenile cirrhosis in the Mediterranean area in the 1970s to 1980s [8,59].

HDV coinfection remains an important problem in patients with human immunodeficiency virus (HIV) infection. HDV-coinfected immunocompromised patients with acquired immune deficiency syndrome (AIDS) may have blunted antibody responses to HDV [5,8] and may exhibit persistent HD antigenaemia. Studies on the mutual clinical influence of HIV and HDV, performed before the era of highly active antiretroviral therapy (HAART), were contradictory; early studies reported that HIV coinfection worsened liver damage by HDV [71,72], but other studies [73–75] showed that the course of chronic hepatitis D was not influenced by concomitant HIV infection.

In the last 15 years, the clinical scenario of HDV infections has changed significantly in the developed world, in parallel with the control of HBV fostered by universal vaccination, improvement in sanitation measures and efforts to contain the HIV epidemic. Along with the decline in the circulation of HDV in southern Europe, clinical changes have been most impressive in this area. The majority of hepatitis D patients collected in Italy in the 1980s had a florid chronic active hepatitis, and inactive cirrhosis residual to burnt-out inflammation was seen in fewer than 20% of cases; in contrast, by the end of the 1990s [63], the proportion of cirrhotic patients has increased in Italy to 70%. These patients represent the survivors of the epidemic of hepatitis D in the 1970s to 1980s; a minority have a long-standing indolent infection, the majority have advanced cirrhosis for which there is no specific medical therapy and only liver transplantation offers a therapeutical perspective.

References

1 Rizzetto M, Canese MG, Arico S et al. (1977) Immunofluorescence detection of new antigen-antibody system (delta/anti-delta) associated to hepatitis B virus in liver and in serum of HBsAg carriers. *Gut* 18, 997–1003.

2 Deny P (2006) Hepatitis delta virus genetic variability; from genotypes I, II, III to eight major clades? *Curr Topics Microbiol Immunol* 307, 151–171.

3 Casey JL, Polson AG, Bass BL et al. (1997) Molecular biology of HDV: analysis of RNA editing and genotype variations. In: Rizzetto M, Purcell RH, Gerin JL et al. (eds) *Viral Hepatitis and Liver Disease*. Turin: Minerva Medica Torino, pp. 290–294.

4 Watanabe H, Nagayama K, Enomoto N et al. (2003) Chronic hepatitis delta virus infection with genotype IIb variant is correlated with progressive liver disease. *J Gen Virol* 84, 3275–3289.

5 Rizzetto M, Ponzetto A, Bonino F et al. (1988) Hepatitis delta virus infection: clinical and epidemiological aspects. In: Zuckerman AJ (ed.) *Viral Hepatitis and Liver Disease*. New York: Alan R. Liss, pp. 389–394.

6 Smedile A, Rizzetto M, Gerin JL (1994) Advances in hepatitis D virus biology and disease. In: Boyer JL, Ockner RK (eds) *Progress in Liver Disease*, Vol. 12. Philadelphia: W.B. Saunders, pp. 157–175.

7 Hadziyannis SJ (1997) Hepatitis delta: an overview. In: Rizzetto M,

Purcell RH, Gerin JL (eds) *Viral Hepatitis and Liver Disease*. Turin: Minerva Medica pp. 283–289.

8 Farci P (2003) Delta hepatitis: an update. *J Hepatol* 39, S212–S219.

9 Ponzetto A, Cote PJ, Popper H et al. (1984) Transmission of the hepatitis B virus-associated delta agent to the eastern woodchuck. *Proc Natl Acad Sci USA* 81, 2208–2212.

10 Ciancio A, Rizzetto M (2002) Clinical patterns, epidemiology and disease burden of hepatitis D virus chronic liver disease. In: Margolis HS, Alter MJ, Liang TJ et al. (eds) *Proceedings of the 10th International Symposium on Viral Hepatitis and Liver Disease*. Atlanta, GA: International Medical Press, pp. 271–275.

11 Negro F, Rizzetto M (1995) Diagnosis of hepatitis delta virus infection. *J Hepatol* 22 (Suppl 1), 136–139.

12 Aragona M, Macagno S, Caredda F et al. (1987) Serologic response to the hepatitis Delta Virus in acute hepatitis D. *Lancet* 1, 478–480.

13 Macagno S, Smedile A, Caredda F et al. (1990) Monomeric (7S) immunoglobulin M antibodies to hepatitis delta virus in hepatitis type D. *Gastroenterology* 98, 1582–1586.

14 Abid K, Negro F (2004) Immunohistochemical detection of hepatitis delta antigen. In: *Methods in Molecular Medicine 95. Hepatitis B and D Protocols*, Vol. 1. *Detection, Genotypes and Characterization*. Humana Press, pp. 107–112.

15 Hsu SC, Syu WJ, Ting LT et al. (2000) Immunohistochemical differentiation of hepatitis D virus genotypes. *Hepatology* 32, 1111–1116.

16 Negro F (2004) Nonradioisotopic *in situ* hybridization for HDV RNA. In: *Methods in Molecular Medicine 95. Hepatitis B and D Protocols*, Vol. 1. *Detection, Genotypes and Characterization*. Humana Press, pp. 95–98.

17 Smedile A, Niro MG, Rizzetto M (2004) Detection of serum HDV-RNA by RT-PCR. In: *Methods in Molecular Medicine 95*, Vol. 1. *Detection, Genotypes and Characterization*. Humana Press, pp. 85–94.

18 Le Gal F, Gordien E, Affolabi D et al. (2005) Quantification of hepatitis delta virus RNA in serum by consensus real-time PCR indicates different patterns of virological response to interferon therapy in chronically infected patients. *J Clin Microbiol* 43, 2363–2369.

19 Yamashiro T, Nagayama K, Enomoto N et al. (2004) Quantitation of the level of hepatitis delta virus RNA in serum, by real-time polymerase chain reaction-and its possible correlation with the clinical stage of liver disease. *J Infect Dis* 189, 1151–1157.

20 Ponzetto A, Negro F, Popper H et al. (1988) Serial passage of hepatitis delta virus in chronic hepatitis B virus carrier chimpanzees. *Hepatology* 8, 1655–1661.

21 Wu JC, Chen CM, Sheen IJ et al. (1995) Evidence of transmission of hepatitis D virus to spouses from sequence analysis of the viral genome. *Hepatology* 22, 1656–1660.

22 Stroffolini T, Ferrigno L, Cialdea L et al. (1994) Incidence and risk factors of acute Delta hepatitis in Italy: results from a national surveillance system. SEIEVA Collaborating Group. *J Hepatol* 21, 1123–1126.

23 Niro GA, Casey JL, Gravinese E et al. (1999) Intrafamilial transmission of hepatitis delta virus: molecular evidence. *J Hepatol* 30, 564–569.

24 Shakil AO, Hadziyannis S, Hoofnagle JH et al. (1997) Geographic distribution and genetic variability of hepatitis delta virus genotype I. *Virology* 234, 160–167.

25 Niro GA, Smedile A, Andriulli A et al. (1997) The predominance of hepatitis delta virus genotype I among chronically infected Italian patients. *Hepatology* 25, 728–734.

26 Flodgren E, Bengtsson S, Knutsson M et al. (2000) Recent high incidence of fulminant hepatitis in Samara, Russia: molecular analysis of prevailing hepatitis B and D virus strains. *J Clin Microbiol* 38, 3311–3316.

27 Bozday AM, Aslan N, Bozday G et al. (2004) Molecular epidemiology of hepatitis B, C and D viruses in Turkish patients. *Arch Virol* 149, 2115–2129.

28 Zhang YY, Tsega E, Hansson BG (1996) Phylogenetic analysis of hepatitis D viruses indicating a new genotype I subgroup among African isolates. *J Clin Microbiol* 34, 3023–3030.

29 Sakugawa H, Nakasone H, Nakayoshi T et al. (1999) Hepatitis delta virus genotype IIb predominates in an endemic area, Okinawa, Japan. *J Med Virol* 58, 366–372.

30 Moriyama M, Taira M, Matsumura H et al. (2005) Full genomic analysis of hepatitis delta virus prevalent on Miyako Island, Japan. *Intervirology* 48, 246–254.

31 Kao JH, Chen PJ, Lai MY et al. (2002) Hepatitis D virus genotypes in intravenous drug users in Taiwan: decreasing prevalence and lack of correlation with hepatitis B virus genotypes. *J Clin Microbiol* 40, 3047–3049.

32 Ivaniushina V, Radjef N, Alexeeva M et al. (2001) Hepatitis delta virus genotypes I and II cocirculate in an endemic area of Yakutia, Russia. *J Gen Virol* 82, 2709–2718.

33 Nakano T, Shapiro CN, Hadler SC et al. (2001) Characterization of hepatitis D virus genotype III among Yucpa Indians in Venezuela. *J Gen Virol* 82, 2183–2189.

34 Rizzetto M, Hadziyannis S, Hansson BG et al. (1992) Hepatitis delta virus infection in the world, epidemiological patterns and clinical expression. *Gastroenterol Int* 5, 18–32.

35 Sagnelli E, Stroffolini T, Ascione A et al. (1992) The epidemiology of hepatitis delta infection in Italy. *Hepatology* 15, 211–215.

36 Liaw YF, Chiu KW, Chu CM et al. (1990) Heterosexual transmission of hepatitis delta virus in the general population of an area endemic for hepatitis B virus infection: a prospective study. *J Infect Dis* 162, 1170–1172.

37 Smedile A, Lavarini C, Aricò S et al. (1983) Epidemiological patterns of infection with the hepatitis B virus associated delta agent in Italy. *Am J Epidemiol* 117, 223–229.

38 Sagnelli E, Stroffolini T, Ascione A et al. (1993) The epidemiology of hepatitis delta infection in Italy over the last 18 years. *Prog Clin Biol Res* 382, 287–294.

39 Sagnelli E, Stroffolini T, Ascione A et al. (1997) Decrease in HDV endemicity in Italy. *J Hepatol* 26, 20–24.

40 Gaeta GB, Stroffolini T, Chiaramonte M et al. (2000) Chronic hepatitis D: a vanishing disease? An Italian multicenter study. *Hepatology* 32, 824–827.

41 Stroffolini T, Sagnelli E, Mele A et al. (2004) The aetiology of chronic hepatitis in Italy: results from a multicentre national study. *Dig Liver Dis* 36, 829–833.

42 Navascues CA, Rodriguez M, Sotorrio NG et al. (1995) Epidemiology of hepatitis D virus infection: changes in the last 14 years. *Am J Gastroenterol* 90, 1981–1984.

43 Huo TI, Wu JC, Lin RY et al. (1997) Decreasing hepatitis D virus infection in Taiwan: an analysis of contributory factors. *Gastroenterol Hepatol* 12, 745–746.

44 Huo TI, Wu JC, Wu SI et al. (2004) Changing seroepidemiology of hepatitis B, C, and D virus infections in high-risk populations. *J Med Virol* 72, 41–45.

45 Manock SR, Kelley PM, Hyams KC et al. (2000) An outbreak of fulminant hepatitis delta in the Waorani, an indigenous people of the Amazon basin of Ecuador. *Am J Trop Med Hyg* 63, 209–213.

46 Degertekin H, Yalcin K, Yakut M (2006) The prevalence of hepatitis delta virus infection in acute and chronic liver diseases in Turkey: an analysis of clinical studies. *Turk J Gastroenterol* 17, 25–34.

47 Dalekos GN, Zervou E, Karabini F et al. (1995) Prevalence of viral markers among refugees from southern Albania: increased incidence of infection with hepatitis A, B and D viruses. *Eur J Gastroenterol Hepatol* 7, 553–558.

48 Al-Traif I, Ali A, Dafalla M et al. (2004) Prevalence of hepatitis delta antibody among HBsAg carriers in Saudi Arabia. *Ann Saudi Med* 24, 343–344.

49 Inoue J, Takahashi M, Nishizawa T et al. (2005) High prevalence of hepatitis delta virus infection detectable by enzyme immunoassay among apparently healthy individuals in Mongolia. *J Med Virol* 76, 333–340.

50 Chlabicz S, Grzeszczuk A, Lapinski TW et al. (2003) Search for hepatitis delta virus (HDV) infection in hepatitis C patients in north-eastern Poland. Comparison with anti-HDV prevalence in chronic hepatitis B. *Eur J Epidemiol* 18, 559–561.

51 Jeong SH, Kim JM, Ahn HJ et al. (2005) The prevalence and clinical characteristics of hepatitis-delta infection in Korea. *Kor J Hepatol* 11, 43–50.

52 Singh V, Goenka MK, Bhasin DK et al. (1995) A study of hepatitis delta virus infection in patients with acute and chronic liver disease from northern India. *J Viral Hepat* 2, 151–154.

53 Narang A, Gupta P, Kar P et al. (1996) A prospective study of delta infection in fulminant hepatic failure. *J Assoc Phys India* 44, 246–247.

54 Bhattacharyya S, Dalal BS, Lahiri A (1998) Hepatitis D infectivity profile among hepatitis B infected hospitalised patients in Calcutta. *Ind J Public Health* 42, 108–112.

55 Murhekar MV, Murhekar KM, Arankalle VA et al. (2005) Hepatitis delta virus infection among the tribes of the Andaman and Nicobar Islands, India. *Trans R Soc Trop Med Hyg* 99, 483–484.

56 Kao J-H, Chen PV, Lai M-Y et al. (2002) Hepatitis D virus genotypes in intravenous drug users in Taiwan: decreasing prevalence and lack of correlation with hepatitis B virus genotypes. *J Clin Microbiol* 40, 3047–3049.

57 Negro F, Rizzetto M (1991) Pathobiology of hepatitis delta virus. In: Blaine Hollinger F, Lemon S, Margolis HS (eds) *Viral Hepatitis and Liver Disease*. Philadelphia, PA: Williams and Wilkins, pp. 477–480.

58 Smedile A, Rosina F, Saracco G et al. (1991) Hepatitis B virus replication modulates pathogenesis of hepatitis D virus in chronic hepatitis D. *Hepatology* 13, 413–416.

59 Smedile A, Ciancio A, Rizzetto M (2002) Hepatitis D, Hepatitis D virus. In: Richman DD, Whitley RJ, Hayden FG (eds) *Clinical Virology*. Washington, DC: ASM Press, pp. 1227–1240.

60 Niro GA, Gravinese E, Martini E et al. (2001) Clearance of hepatitis B surface antigen in chronic carriers of hepatitis delta antibodies. *Liver* 21, 254–259.

61 Chen PJ, Chen DS, Chen CR et al. (1988) Delta infection in asymptomatic carriers of hepatitis B surface antigen: low prevalence of delta activity and effective suppression of hepatitis B virus replication. *Hepatology* 8, 1121–1124.

62 Jardi R, Rodriguez F, Buti M et al. (2001) Role of hepatitis B, C, and D viruses in dual and triple infection: influence of viral genotypes and hepatitis B precore and basal core promoter mutations on viral replicative interference. *Hepatology* 34, 404–410.

63 Mathurin P, Thibault V, Kadidja K et al. (2000) Replication status and histological features of patients with triple (B, C, D) and dual (B, C) hepatic infections. *J Viral Hepat* 7, 15–22.

64 Raimondo G, Brunetto MR, Pontisso P *et al.* (2006) Longitudinal evaluation reveals a complex spectrum of virological profiles in hepatitis B virus/hepatitis C virus-coinfected patients. *Hepatology* 43, 100–107.

65 Eyster ME, Sanders JC, Battegay M *et al.* (1995) Suppression of hepatitis C virus (HCV) replication by hepatitis D virus (HDV) in HIV-infected hemophiliacs with chronic hepatitis B and C. *Dig Dis Sci* 40, 1583–1588.

66 Lu SN, Chen TM, Lee CM *et al.* (2003) Molecular epidemiological and clinical aspects of hepatitis D virus in a unique triple hepatitis viruses (B, C, D) endemic community in Taiwan. *J Med Virol* 70, 74–80.

67 Rosina F, Conoscitore P, Cuppone R *et al.* (1999) Changing pattern of chronic hepatitis D in Southern Europe. *Gastroenterology* 117, 161–166.

68 Fattovich G, Giustina G, Christensen E *et al.* (2000) Influence of hepatitis delta virus infection on morbidity and mortality in compensated cirrhosis type B. The European Concerted Action on Viral Hepatitis (Eurohep). *Gut* 46, 420–426.

69 Wu JC, Chen TZ, Huang YS *et al.* (1995) Natural history of hepatitis D viral superinfection: significance of viremia detected by polymerase chain reaction. *Gastroenterology* 108, 796–802.

70 Philip T, Durazzo M, Trautwein C *et al.* (1994) Recognition of uridine diphosphate glucuronosyl transferases by LKM-3 antibodies in chronic hepatitis D. *Lancet* 344, 578–581.

71 Novick DM, Farci P, Croxson TS *et al.* (1988) Hepatitis D virus and human immunodeficiency virus antibodies in parenteral drug abusers who are hepatitis B surface antigen positive. *J Infect Dis* 158, 795–803.

72 Housset C, Pol S, Camot F *et al.* (1992) Interactions between human immunodeficiency virus-1, hepatitis delta virus and hepatitis B virus infections in 260 chronic carriers of hepatitis B virus. *Hepatology* 15, 578–583.

73 Caredda F, Antinori S, Coppin P *et al.* (1991) The influence of human immunodeficiency virus infection on acute and chronic HBsAg-positive hepatitis. *Prog Clin Biol Res* 364, 365–375.

74 Pol S, Wesenfelder L, Dubois F *et al.* (1994) Influence of human immunodeficiency virus infection on hepatitis delta virus superinfection in chronic HBsAg carriers. *J Viral Hepat* 1, 131–137.

75 Buti M, Jardi R, Allende H *et al.* (1996) Chronic delta hepatitis: is the prognosis worse when associated with hepatitis C virus and human immunodeficiency virus infections? *J Med Virol* 49, 66–69.

9.1.2.vi Hepatitis C

Alfredo Alberti and Luisa Benvegnù

Definition

Hepatitis C is caused by the hepatitis C virus (HCV), an RNA virus that shares genomic similarities with the pestiviruses and has been classified within the Flaviviridae family [1].

Significant heterogeneity has been observed between different HCV isolates, leading to the classification of HCV into distinct genotypes, designated by Arabic numerals (i.e. HCV-1, HCV-2, HCV-3, etc), and subtypes, identified by lower case letters (i.e. HCV-1a, HCV-1b, HCV-1c, etc) [2]. HCV is a bloodborne agent that is transmitted parenterally. Before the discovery of HCV in 1989, blood transfusion was a frequent cause of hepatitis

C transmission. With the implementation of screening of blood donations for HCV, the risk of post-transfusion hepatitis C has been dramatically reduced; however, infection continues to occur via other modes of apparent and inapparent parenteral transmission.

Hepatitis C has a global distribution. Infection with HCV often results in chronicity because of the high propensity of this virus to persist by evading control by the immune system. The incidence of new cases is declining in most countries of the civilized world, but the prevalence of chronically infected individuals is still high, with at least 170 million carriers of the HCV worldwide. Chronic HCV infection is particularly frequent in a number of risk groups, including intravenous drug users, patients with haemophilia who received clotting factors before 1990–92, those who received blood transfusions before 1992 and patients on haemodialysis.

The diagnosis of hepatitis C rests upon detection of a set of antiviral antibodies (anti-HCV) and viral genomic sequences (HCV RNA) in serum.

HCV causes acute and chronic hepatocellular damage of variable severity and evolution, and is the leading cause of cirrhosis and hepatocellular carcinoma and the main reason for liver transplantation in many western countries. Infection may also occur in extrahepatic cells and tissues, leading to a spectrum of extrahepatic disorders, including immunological abnormalities, autoimmune phenomena, production of autoantibodies, cryoglobulinaemia, vasculitis and other types of immunocomplex disease. A cause–effect relationship of HCV to other disorders, such as porphyria cutanea tarda, thyroiditis, sialadenitis, psoriasis and B-cell non-Hodgkin's lymphoma, is also suspected but not yet clearly proven. More recently, HCV has also been linked to the development of insulin resistance and type 2 diabetes.

Acute HCV infection is defined as an infection of less than 6 months duration. Most often, acute infections are asymptomatic and remain clinically unrecognized and, for this reason, it has been problematic to define the precise incidence of hepatitis C. Severe and fulminant hepatitis C is extremely rare in the immunocompetent host but may occur under immunosuppression. Only a minority of cases of acute hepatitis C recover completely, with spontaneous virus eradication; in most cases, the acute infection progresses to chronicity. Chronic HCV infection is defined as an infection that persists for more than 6 months, with or without clinical manifestations of hepatic or extrahepatic disease. Around 35–45% of HCV carriers in the general population have no overt signs or symptoms of liver disease and persistently normal levels of serum alanine aminotransferase (ALT), although many of them have some underlying chronic liver lesions on liver biopsy. The remaining carriers have varying profiles of ALT abnormalities. Liver biopsy in compensated chronic hepatitis C shows a wide range of histological lesions, from minimal–mild to severe–advanced necroinflammatory changes and fibrosis. Progression to cirrhosis occurs slowly and in an unpredictable way in a subgroup of patients who may ultimately die of portal hypertension, hepatic failure or

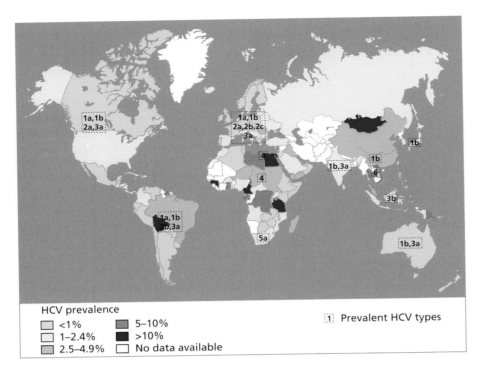

HCV prevalence

☐ <1%   ◼ 5–10%
☐ 1–2.4%   ◼ >10%
◼ 2.5–4.9% ☐ No data available

[1] Prevalent HCV types

Fig. 1 Prevalence of HCV infection and HCV genotypes/subtypes in different geographical regions.

hepatocellular carcinoma. The downhill course of chronic liver disease is accelerated by a number of aetiological cofactors, including coinfection with the hepatitis B virus (HBV) and the human immunodeficiency virus (HIV), excess alcohol consumption and the presence of a number of metabolic abnormalities, such as obesity, insulin resistance, liver steatosis, diabetes and iron overload. Race, gender and age at infection also play a role in determining the course and outcome of chronic HCV infection. The management of chronic HCV infection needs to be individualized based on a number of virus and host parameters that result in the heterogeneous clinical features and outcome of hepatitis C.

Epidemiology

Prevalence in the general population and in risk groups

The World Health Organization (WHO) estimates that at least 3% of the world's population is chronically infected with HCV [3]. The prevalence of chronic HCV carriers varies greatly depending on geographical location and the characteristics of the population analysed (Fig. 1 and Table 1) [4]. Low rates are found in the general adult population in North America and western Europe, intermediate rates in Japan and higher rates in some areas of eastern Europe, the Middle East and South America [5,6]. The number of infected individuals is particularly high in Egypt. High rates have also been found in the elderly population in some Mediterranean areas, including southern

Table 1 Reported prevalence of HCV infection in risk groups.

Risk group	Anti-HCV positive (%)
Intravenous drug users	35–90
Haemophiliacs treated before 1990	50–90
Thalassaemics	42–83
Haemodialysis patients	10–45
Prisoners	15–46
Alcoholics	15–25
HIV-positive individuals	20–65
Patients with history of blood transfusion received before 1992	15–25
Tattooed individuals	11
Heath-care professionals (exposed by needlestick)	0–10 (3–12)
People with disabilities/institutionalized individuals	4–7
Prostitutes	0.7–6
Homosexuals	3–18
Heterosexual partners of HCV carriers	0–18
Household non-sexual contacts of HCV carriers	0–11
Children born to HCV-infected mothers	0–6

Italy. In the general population, there is evidence for an age-related distribution of HCV infection, with prevalences that are minimal in childhood and progressively higher with increasing age. The prevalence of HCV infection is increased in several risk groups, which are listed in Table 1.

Incidence and prevalence in patients with liver disease

The incidence of acute symptomatic hepatitis C, which represents an underestimation of all cases of acute HCV infection as many cases remain asymptomatic, has been decreasing progressively since 1990 in most industrialized countries. HCV is the recognized cause of about 33% of cases of symptomatic acute hepatitis in the western world and 10% of cases in the Far East [7]. The prevalence of chronic HCV infection in patients with chronic hepatitis, cirrhosis and hepatocellular carcinoma is very high in southern Europe and Japan (60–90%), intermediate in other part of Europe, the United States, Australia and Africa (30–60%) and lower in China and other countries of the Far East (10–39%). HCV is the major cause, either alone or with other cofactors, of chronic liver disease, cirrhosis and hepatocellular carcinoma, and the main reason for liver transplantation in most countries of the western world, second only to alcohol-related diseases in a few geographical locations [8,9]. The prevalence of HCV infection is highest in patients who develop chronic liver disease after blood transfusion or who have a well-recognized risk for parenteral contamination in their previous history. The prevalence of HCV infection in patients with chronic liver disease or hepatocellular carcinoma varies around the world depending on the HBV endemicity. In areas of high HBV endemicity, HCV is relatively uncommon, whereas in areas of intermediate or low HBV endemicity, the prevalence of hepatitis C increases significantly. In areas of intermediate HBV endemicity, concurrent HBV and HCV infection is seen in patients with chronic liver disease and this association increases in frequency with the severity and stage of liver damage.

Transmission

HCV is efficiently transmitted in blood and blood products [10]. Currently, unsafe intravenous drug use is the main mode of transmission in most parts of the western world, whereas unscreened contaminated blood transfusion and folk-medicine practices still represent an important source of infection in underdeveloped countries [5,6]. Transmission of HCV between monogamous partners is thought to be rare; transmission increases significantly with multiple sexual partners [11]. Other documented sources of infection are needlestick exposure in health-care workers [12], sharing a razor or toothbrush with an infected individual [13], unsafe body piercing and tattooing [14]. There is also solid evidence of nosocomial transmission of HCV during invasive procedures. Major gynaecological and cardiovascular surgery carries a high risk; however, microsurgery, in particular, ophthalmic, has also been implicated. HCV is transmitted vertically to newborns by 3–5% of HCV-monoinfected mothers, but the risk increases significantly in the presence of HIV coinfection [15]. On the basis of these epidemiological data, recommendations for the prevention and control of HCV infection have been made (Table 2) [16,17]

Table 2 Recommendations for prevention and control of HCV infection.

HCV testing is highly recommended in:
Individuals with a risk factor (see list in Table 1)
Individuals with unexplained abnormalities of transaminases and/or other liver function tests
Individuals with signs or symptoms of liver disease

HCV-infected individuals should be counselled to:
Avoid sharing anything that might be contaminated by their own blood or body fluid
Not donate blood, body organs, other tissues or semen
Consider the risk of sexual transmission to be low but not absent

Diagnosis

Infection with HCV can be identified and staged with a variety of diagnostic tools that include (i) detection of antiviral antibodies (anti-HCV), a marker of past or ongoing infection; (ii) direct detection and quantification of the viral genome (HCV RNA) in serum, a marker of ongoing HCV infection and replicative activity; and (iii) analysis of the genomic sequences of the virus to define the genotype and subtype of the infecting HCV, an intrinsic characteristic of HCV genomic variability.

Detection of antiviral antibodies

Testing for anti-HCV antibodies is the primary tool to screen for HCV infection and to diagnose past or ongoing infection [18]. Anti-HCV antibodies can be detected by third-generation enzyme immunoassays (EIAs). These assays detect mixtures of antibodies directed against different HCV epitopes of the core and non-structural NS3, NS4 and NS5 proteins. The specificity of currently available commercial assays for anti-HCV antibodies is > 99%. In acute infection, detection of anti-HCV antibodies may be delayed compared with the appearance of HCV-RNA viraemia. In chronic infection, the sensitivity of anti-HCV antibody tests is excellent in immunocompetent individuals, whereas it is reduced in immunocompromized hosts, who may remain anti-HCV negative despite the presence of ongoing HCV replication. The interpretation of anti-HCV antibody results depends on the clinical setting (see below).

In clinical practice, the usual approach is to test initially for anti-HCV antibodies and, if the results are positive, assess for the presence of HCV RNA using a sensitive qualitative assay, to document viraemia and distinguish between ongoing and resolved infection.

Detection of serum HCV RNA

HCV replicates at low levels and, therefore, HCV RNA needs to be amplified to enable it to be detected in serum [19]. Two types of diagnostic assay are available for serum HCV-RNA testing: qualitative and quantitative. Qualitative assays are carried out using the classical polymerase chain reaction (PCR), real-time PCR or transcriptase-mediated amplification (TMA). Several commercial assays are available, with a lower limit of detection in the range of 5 IU/mL (real-time PCR), 5–10 IU/mL (TMA-based assays) and 30–100 IU/mL (classic PCR). These qualitative assays represent the gold standard for the diagnosis of ongoing HCV infection. They are essential for the diagnosis of hepatitis C in immunocompromized individuals who do not produce significant levels of anti-HCV antibodies and in the early phase of acute hepatitis C before anti-HCV seroconversion. Quantitative serum HCV-RNA assays are based on target amplification techniques (competitive PCR or real-time PCR) or signal amplification [branched DNA (bDNA) assay]. These assays measure viral load in viraemic patients and provide tools to monitor antiviral therapy.

Determination of HCV genotype

The six major HCV genotypes can be detected using commercial assays [20]. They have different geographical distributions (Fig. 1) and their prevalence also varies according to the epidemiological setting; HCV-3 is often associated with intravenous drug usage. HCV genotyping is of clinical utility in patients who are candidates for antiviral therapy, to enable the dose and duration of treatment to be determined and to predict the probability of achieving a sustained virological response. In many parts of the world, the prevalence of the different HCV genotypes within the HCV-infected population has changed over the last decade. Most studies report a progressive reduction in the prevalence of HCV-1b-infected individuals, which is counterbalanced by an increase in HCV-1a- and HCV-3-infected individuals [21–23]; this trend has also been recently observed in HCV-infected children [24]. Other studies indicate a rapid increase in the spread of HCV-4 in many European countries [25, 26].

Clinical use of HCV markers and diagnostic algorithms [27]

Patients with acute hepatitis
When acute hepatitis C is suspected, patients should be tested for serum HCV RNA with a sensitive qualitative assay and for anti-HCV antibodies using an EIA. Serum HCV RNA is the first marker to become detectable during the acute phase; it can be demonstrated by sensitive PCR as early as 1 week after exposure [7]. Viraemia then persists without an antibody response for a period of a few weeks to months (window phase). Anti-HCV seroconversion usually occurs 4–8 weeks after exposure but may be delayed by up to several weeks or months, with large individual variations. Immunoglobulin (Ig)M anti-HCV tests have not shown adequate specificity and sensitivity for the identification of acute hepatitis C and their use is not recommended. Serum HCV RNA, but not anti-HCV antibodies, is eventually cleared in the minority of patients whose hepatitis

Table 3 Interpretation of HCV marker profiles in patients with acute hepatitis.

Anti-HCV	HCV-RNA	Interpretation and follow-up
Negative	Negative	Acute hepatitis C excluded
Negative	Positive	Acute hepatitis C confirmed, follow-up for anti-HCV seroconversion
Positive	Negative	Acute hepatitis C unlikely (unless late testing)
Positive	Positive	Impossible to differentiate acute from reactivated chronic hepatitis C (follow-up and retesting needed)

C resolves; it persists, often with fluctuations, in patients who progress to chronic infection. The interpretation of different patterns of HCV serum markers in patients with acute hepatitis is described in Table 3.

Patients with chronic liver disease
The diagnosis of HCV infection in patients with overt evidence of chronic liver damage is initially based on anti-HCV antibody testing and confirmed by detection of serum HCV RNA by qualitative testing. However, serum HCV RNA should be tested in all immunocompromized or immunosuppressed patients with liver disease of unknown aetiology, even if negative for anti-HCV antibodies. This includes patients on chronic haemodialysis, those with HIV infection and recipients of organ transplants [27].

Detection of anti-HCV at occasional screening
Low-risk individuals with normal ALT levels and no evidence of liver disease, who are found to be anti-HCV antibody positive by EIA at occasional screening or at blood donation, should have serum HCV-RNA levels tested by sensitive qualitative assay to distinguish between ongoing and resolved infection. Repeated HCV-RNA testing (2–3 times at monthly intervals) is recommended for those individuals that are initially found to be HCV-RNA negative, to exclude intermittent viraemia.

Figure 2 describes the diagnostic algorithms that are used in clinical practice in anti-HCV-positive individuals to distinguish between (i) resolved HCV infection, (ii) chronic HCV infection with normal ALT and (iii) biochemically active chronic hepatitis C.

Natural history and clinical outcomes

The current knowledge of the natural history of acute and chronic hepatitis C infection is still incomplete because of the silent nature of many infections, which often impedes detection of the disease in its earliest stages, and also the slow, unpredictable and often discontinuous progression of liver damage, which takes at least one decade, but more frequently several decades, to produce serious chronic sequelae [28]. The outcome of HCV infection is influenced by many variables and cofactors that may significantly accelerate the natural course of liver

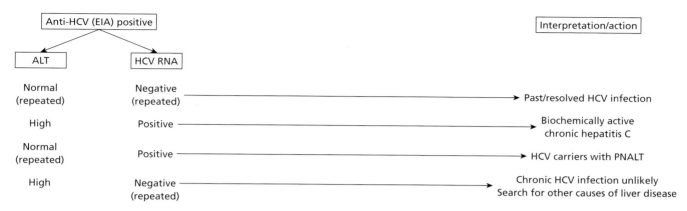

Fig. 2 Diagnostic algorithms in hepatitis C and interpretation of combined testing of viral markers and ALT. PNALT, persistently normal ALT levels.

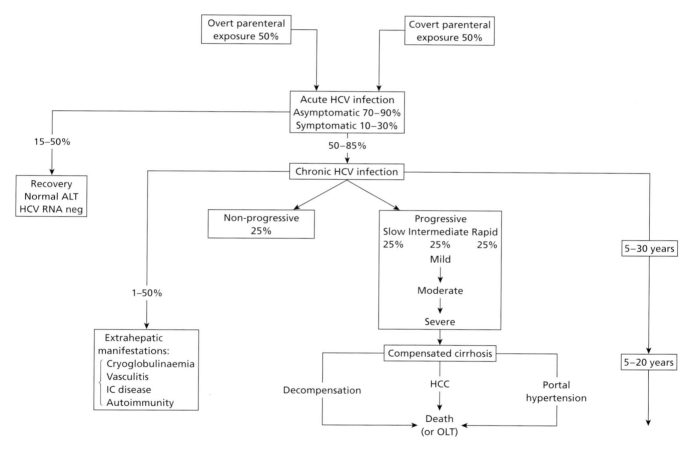

Fig. 3 Clinical spectrum and natural history of hepatitis C. Percentages indicate average prevalence/incidence of events. Wide variability of outcomes depends on many cofactors.

disease. For these reasons, the clinical course of hepatitis C is highly variable and the long-term prognostic assessment is problematic in the individual patient. Figure 3 describes the clinical spectrum of hepatitis C and the different stages and rates of progression.

Acute infection

The average incubation period of acute hepatitis C, as determined in prospective studies of post-transfusion hepatitis, is 7–8 weeks, but the range varies widely (from 2 to 26 weeks or more) [29]. Shorter incubation periods have been reported in experimental infections and in haemophiliacs treated with factor VIII. HCV viraemia is the first marker to become detectable during acute hepatitis C; it is demonstrable by sensitive PCR as early as 1 week after exposure. Viraemia then persists without an antibody response for a variable window period before anti-HCV seroconversion [30,31].

The onset of liver damage, marked by variable ALT elevations, is always delayed with respect to the appearance of viraemia and may either precede or follow seroconversion to anti-HCV. Patients rarely have prodromic symptoms or fever. The acute phase of hepatitis C is often mild and usually less severe than hepatitis A and B; more than two-thirds of cases are asymptomatic and anicteric. A severe or fulminant course of acute hepatitis C rarely occurs, except in patients with immunodeficiency, pre-existing liver disease or the presence of other cofactors, such as hepatitis A or B or intravenous drug use. The clinical profile of symptomatic acute hepatitis C is the same as that of any type of viral hepatitis and is often indistinguishable from hepatitis A and B. Symptomatic cases present with malaise, dark urine, nausea (with or without vomiting), abdominal discomfort and/or jaundice.

Hepatitis C exhibits several patterns of ALT elevation. The most typical is polyphasic, with significant fluctuations in enzyme levels that may last for a few weeks or several months. Sometimes, periods of biochemical abnormality are separated by periods of ALT normality. Chronic hepatitis develops frequently in patients with a polyphasic ALT pattern [32].

The histological features of acute hepatitis C include a few peculiar morphological changes, in addition to the classic features that are common to viral hepatitis in general. Liver biopsy may show eosinophilic clamping of the cytoplasm, macrovesicular steatosis, marked activation of sinusoidal cells, peeling up of bile ductular cells in the lumen and a large number of acidophilic bodies. A liver biopsy is not recommended for routine diagnosis of acute hepatitis C, as none of the histological lesions is specific, and it is not essential for identifying progression to chronicity. This can be diagnosed by monitoring ALT levels and serum HCV-RNA levels in the months after the onset of acute disease. By definition, patients who have abnormal ALT values for more than 6–12 months are progressing to chronic hepatitis C [7]. These patients have evidence of chronic hepatitis of variable activity and severity on liver biopsy. Likewise, patients who remain serum positive for HCV RNA, despite the return of ALT levels to normal, often exhibit evidence of chronic hepatitis in the liver biopsy, usually with mild activity. A subacute course of hepatitis C with progressive hepatic failure is exceptional and should prompt a search for other causes of liver damage. The most frequent course seen after acute HCV infection is chronic evolution, with fluctuating ALT levels and persistently- or intermittently-positive serum HCV-RNA levels. The outcome of acute hepatitis C varies, depending on virus and host factors and on the size of the infecting inoculum. Minimal exposure may result in transient infection with recovery and development of some kind of T-cell immunity, even in the absence of anti-HCV seroconversion.

Three main outcome profiles can be seen after acute HCV infection:

1 Recovery with virus eradication: this occurs in 20–50% of cases, more frequently with smaller inocula. It is characterized by persistent ALT normalization and a repeatedly-confirmed negative HCV-RNA test in the presence of persistent anti-HCV reactivity, which remains positive in the serum for many years.

2 Evolution into a biochemically active chronic hepatitis C, with elevated and often fluctuating ALT levels.

3 Evolution into the asymptomatic HCV carrier state, with persistently normal ALT (PNALT) levels.

The different clinical outcomes seen in acute hepatitis C, their serological and biochemical profiles and the main determinants of HCV clearance versus persistence are described in Fig. 4.

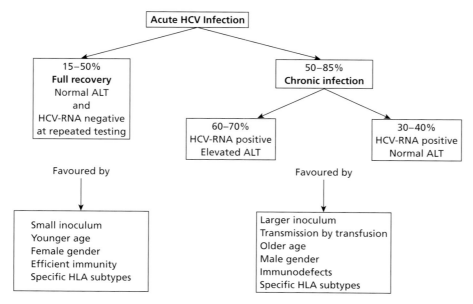

Fig. 4 Outcomes of acute HCV infection and predisposing variables. HLA, human leukocyte antigen.

Compensated phase of chronic HCV infection

Chronic HCV infection is defined as the persistence of serum HCV RNA for more than 6 months. It is usually not preceded by an overt acute onset. For this reason, patients with chronic HCV infection are usually diagnosed at different phases of the infection and may present at different stages of liver disease [9]. The main biochemical and clinical profiles are: (i) the typical form of chronic hepatitis C, with abnormal ALT levels and a wide spectrum of liver damage and progression rates; (ii) the HCV carrier state, with PNALT; and (iii) patients with extrahepatic manifestations of hepatitis C.

Biochemically active chronic hepatitis

The course of chronic hepatitis C with ALT elevations is often unpredictable in the individual patient. In a number of cases, it progresses slowly to more severe and active liver disease, with increasing fibrosis and, ultimately, transition to cirrhosis. Progression to cirrhosis may take years or decades. In other patients, the liver disease is minimal or mild and remains stable for decades, without significant worsening. The long-term outcomes of chronic HCV infection are schematically described in Fig. 3.

From chronic hepatitis C to compensated cirrhosis

Patients with biochemically active chronic hepatitis C have a persistently positive serum HCV-RNA test, and persistently or intermittently elevated ALT levels. Most are asymptomatic or have only mild and aspecific symptoms, such as chronic or parossistic fatigue, dyspepsia and myalgia. Chronic hepatitis C may be stable or progressive over time. Progression is marked by the worsening of liver fibrosis, a consequence of continuing necroinflammation and associated fibrogenesis [33,34]. Staging of liver fibrosis on liver biopsy is carried out using semiquantitative scoring systems: fibrosis is graded from 0 to 4 (METAVIR scoring system) [35] or from 0 to 6 (Ishak scoring system) [36]. Patients with chronic hepatitis C can be classified as being non-progressors, having stable disease, or being slow, intermediate or rapid progressors, with an estimated time interval between infection and development of cirrhosis of more than 50 years, 15–30 years or 3–10 years, respectively, and with about 25% of patients falling within each subgroup [37]. The risk of progression is dependent on a number of variables and cofactors, which are often interrelated. The stage of disease at presentation is obviously relevant for prognosis, and progression to cirrhosis is more frequent and imminent in those with more advanced liver disease [38]. The ALT levels and profile do correlate to some extent with disease activity and progression rate [39–41]. The age of the patient and mode of acquisition of HCV infection are important prognostic factors: older patients often have more rapid progression, although chronic HCV infection may also be benign and non-progressive in the elderly. Patients infected via a blood transfusion have more severe and progressive liver disease than those who acquire HCV by an inapparent source, possibly as a consequence of a larger virus inoculum, leading to higher virus spread and replication [42–46]. The role of HCV genotypes in determining disease outcomes is controversial. All HCV subtypes may be associated with mild, non-progressive, or severe and rapidly progressive liver disease. The actual viral loads are poorly correlated with disease severity and the measurement of serum HCV-RNA levels is not particularly useful in assessing disease outcomes in untreated patients. Alcohol [47], coinfection with HBV or HIV [38,48,49], impairment of the immune system and a coexisting malignancy have all been repeatedly and convincingly shown to aggravate the course of chronic hepatitis C. Metabolic factors are also important; obesity, insulin resistance and liver steatosis are associated with more rapid progression of liver fibrosis in hepatitis C [50–52].

Liver steatosis and metabolic abnormalities in hepatitis C

Liver steatosis is particularly frequent in hepatitis C; it is seen in more than 50% of cases and in more than 75% of those infected with HCV-3. The pathogenesis of liver steatosis in hepatitis C is multifactorial, being related to metabolic cofactors (insulin resistance) in some and to a more direct effect of HCV in others. The direct steatogenic effect of HCV has been attributed to the interference of the HCV core protein with mitochondrial function and apolipoprotein B-100 very-low-density lipoprotein (VLDL) secretion [53–55]; this results in the accumulation of triglycerides in hepatocytes, the induction of fatty acid oxidation and the release of cytokines, leading to steatosis and steatohepatitis [56,57]. In patients infected with HCV-3, the degree of fat infiltration appears to correlate with the level of HCV replication and protein expression, both in serum and in liver tissue [58], but not with liver fibrosis; in a recent study of over 3000 patients with HCV-related chronic hepatitis, the association between steatosis and fibrosis was confirmed in HCV-1-infected subjects but not in HCV-3-infected subjects [59]. Liver steatosis of the metabolic type should be corrected as it is more frequently associated with disease worsening and poor response to antiviral therapy. For this reason, hepatitis C is often more severe and progressive in overweight patients with type 2 diabetes. Liver iron overload is also associated with more advanced and progressive hepatitis C [60]. Other cofactors that have been associated with fibrosis progression in hepatitis C, including specific human leukocyte antigen (HLA) polymorphisms [61], are listed in Table 4.

HCV carrier state with persistently normal ALT

ALT levels may remain normal despite chronic HCV infection with ongoing HCV replication in the liver and a positive HCV-RNA serum test. This profile is characteristic of HCV carriers with PNALT. The number of HCV patients in this subgroup is consistent, representing around 20–45% of chronically infected individuals in the general population [62]. Many patients

Table 4 Cofactors and variables associated with more rapid evolution of chronic hepatitis C.

Larger inoculum
Acquisition by transfusion
Male gender
Older age at infection
Older age at diagnosis
Alcohol abuse
HBV coinfection
HIV coinfection
Obesity
Liver steatosis
Insulin resistance
Type 2 diabetes
Iron overload
Smoking
Malignancy
Immunosuppression/immunodefects
Organ transplantation
Some genetic polymorphisms
Some HLA subtypes

maintain PNALT levels over long-term follow-up, but a significant subgroup (around 20–25% over 3–5 years) develop biochemical reactivation, which may be transient or persistent and may be associated with disease worsening [63]. Most HCV carriers with PNALT have some degree of liver damage on liver biopsy, with the majority showing mild to moderate chronic hepatitis and fibrosis [64,65]. Liver disease is stable or progresses very slowly in these patients and the development of cirrhosis and endstage complications is rare. However, around 10–15% have advanced fibrosis or cirrhosis in the absence of biochemical (ALT) activity. Recently, the definition of ALT 'normality' has been challenged in patients with HCV, as the currently used upper limits of normality of ALT may underestimate a 'minimal' degree of liver cell necrosis. Therefore, liver biopsy remains the only tool to exactly define the degree and stage of liver disease in these patients. The indication to carry out a liver biopsy in HCV carriers with PNALT needs to be individualized, depending on the patient's age, life expectancy and motivation [63,66]. Currently, most international and national guidelines include liver biopsy in the clinical assessment of HCV carriers with normal ALT, particularly when a decision has to be made whether to treat with antiviral therapy. All patients presenting with chronic HCV infection and normal ALT should be monitored regularly (every 6–12 months) because of the possibility of ALT reactivation and liver disease worsening. Counselling regarding lifestyle and infectivity should be the same for these patients as it is for HCV-infected patients with elevated ALT.

The role of liver biopsy in assessing patients with chronic HCV infection

As in many other chronic liver diseases, liver biopsy is the gold standard for fibrosis staging in chronic hepatitis C. However,

biopsy interpretation may be limited by sampling errors, resulting in underestimation of fibrosis stage, particularly when the size of the liver sample is small or inadequate [67–69]; laparoscopic studies have shown that cirrhosis is missed in up to 10–20% of percutaneous biopsies obtained from the same patients. For this reason, in practice, it may be more reasonable to distinguish patients with no or minimal fibrosis from those with significant and advanced fibrosis, as this simple separation has important prognostic value. Because liver biopsy is invasive and costly and requires hospitalization, non-invasive surrogate methods to predict liver fibrosis would be useful. A number of potential tools are currently under evaluation and include biochemical makers and panels of biochemical tests, and methods to measure liver stiffness by elastography. It is expected that some of these approaches will be used in the near future in the clinic to reduce the number of liver biopsies needed to correctly stage liver fibrosis in patients with chronic hepatitis C, as well as other forms of chronic liver disease [70,71].

From HCV-related compensated cirrhosis to endstage liver disease

When patients with chronic hepatitis C reach the stage of cirrhosis, the risk of developing severe and endstage complications becomes significant. The progressive impairment of liver function and the development of portal hypertension are responsible for most complications, which include ascites, variceal bleeding and hepatic encephalopathy. Several prospective studies have indicated that hepatic decompensation, defined as an episode of ascites, jaundice, variceal bleeding or hepatic encephalopathy, occurs relatively late in the natural course of HCV-related cirrhosis, with an estimated annual decompensation rate of around 3–4% and a 5-year cumulative incidence of 15–18% [72]. The same studies demonstrated that, in western countries and Japan, cirrhosis caused by chronic HCV infection is a major risk factor for hepatocellular carcinoma. In these areas, the prevalence of HCV infection ranges from 50% to 70% among patients with hepatocellular carcinoma. In chronic HCV infection, hepatocellular carcinoma occurs almost invariably with cirrhosis or advanced fibrosis. The annual incidence of hepatocellular carcinoma in HCV-related cirrhosis is estimated to be 1–6%, with a 5-year cumulative incidence ranging from 7% to 30%. Because hepatocellular carcinoma rarely develops in the absence of cirrhosis, this condition represents the major risk factor for hepatocellular carcinoma in chronic HCV infection. Older age and long-lasting liver disease, as well as the presence of active liver disease and regeneration shown by high ALT and alpha-fetoprotein (AFP) levels, represent high-risk conditions for hepatocellular carcinoma development. Several cofactors increase the risk of hepatocellular carcinoma in HCV-related cirrhosis, including HBV coinfection, heavy alcohol intake (above 50–80 g/day), iron overload and the presence of the metabolic syndrome and liver steatosis [73]. Complications of cirrhosis are the primary cause of death in patients with chronic HCV infection. In patients with compensated cirrhosis, the 5-year survival rate is around 85–90%, whereas, after the first episode of decompensation, the 5-year survival rate is only 45–55%. In cohort studies, hepatocellular carcinoma was the primary cause of death in 47–72% of patients, followed by liver failure in 23–44% of cases and bleeding in 5–8% [74,75].

Extrahepatic manifestations of hepatitis C

Chronic HCV infection has been associated with a variety of extrahepatic manifestations (Table 5). These conditions may occur in the presence or absence of accompanying liver disease, which, if present, may be of variable severity. A direct cause–effect relationship is well established for mixed cryoglobulinaemia (MC) [76], vasculitis, membranoproliferative glomerulonephritis and a number of immune complex-associated disorders and some forms of low-grade malignant B-cell lymphoma. A relationship is suspected for porphyria cutanea tarda and some forms of autoimmune thyroiditis and diabetes mellitus; however, the association with HCV is weak or doubtful for the other conditions [77]. The association of HCV infection with an overt cryoglobulinaemic syndrome has clear geographical segregation (southern and eastern Europe), suggesting that genetic factors might be involved. The observation that the syndrome is more frequent in patients with long-standing infection suggests a role for chronic immune stimulation of B cells by HCV; this could also explain the production of autoantibodies and the risk of progression towards low-grade non-Hodgkin's B-cell lymphoma, which is reported in patients with chronic HCV. Many patients with chronic hepatitis C have detectable cryoglobulins in their serum but only small subgroups develop symptoms. Symptoms of HCV–MC are related to systemic vasculitis in small- and, less frequently, medium-sized vessels. Disease expression most often involves the skin and joints and, less frequently, the nerves and kidneys [78]. The main symptom is palpable purpura, which is reported in up to 90% of HCV–MC symptomatic patients;

purpura begins in the lower extremities [79] and may extend to the abdomen and trunk and, less frequently, to the upper extremities. It subsides after 3–10 days, leaving a brownish discoloration that is particularly marked in the lower limbs. Purpura may be accompanied by Raynauds syndrome and acrocyanosis. Bilateral symmetrical arthralgias involving the great joints are reported in 60–90% of patients. Neither arthritis nor joint destruction is a feature. Distal sensory or sensory–motor asymmetrical polyneuropathies and multiple mononeuropathies develop in 40% of cases. Renal disease, usually membranoproliferative glomerulonephritis, accompanied by proteinuria and microscopic haematuria, occurs in 25% of patients. There is no clinical indication to search for cryoglobulins in the serum of HCV patients who have no signs or symptoms that are suggestive of the clinical syndrome.

Clinical course of hepatitis C in special subgroups

The course of acute and chronic hepatitis C is influenced by the immunocompetence of the host and by several cofactors. In the immunocompromized host, hepatitis C often runs a more severe course; this is the case in renal transplant recipients in whom HCV is an important cause of liver disease, which may significantly reduce survival [80]. Patients with HIV are frequently coinfected with HCV (at a rate of about 30% in Europe) and exhibit an accelerated progression to cirrhosis and endstage liver disease, particularly in the presence of low CD4 counts. With the improved therapeutic control of HIV infection and reduced mortality rates from acquired immune deficiency syndrome (AIDS), the endstage complications of hepatitis C have become a leading cause of mortality among HIV–HCV coinfected individuals. Coinfection with HCV and HBV is also common, particularly when both virus infections have significant prevalence in the population; coinfection is often associated with more severe histological liver lesions and a more

Table 5 Extrahepatic manifestations caused by or associated with chronic HCV infection.

Syndrome	Link to HCV infection
Mixed cryoglobulinaemia Vasculitis Membranoproliferative glomerulonephritis	Proven (HCV has a pathogenetic role)
Porphyria cutanea tarda Low-grade non-Hodgkin's lymphoma	Most likely (HCV may act as cofactor)
Autoimmune thyroiditis Type 2 diabetes Lichen planus	Possible (more data needed)
Sjogren syndrome Idiopathic pulmonary fibrosis Aplastic anaemia Polyarteritis nodosa Erythema nodosum	Weak (etiological role of HCV is unlikely)

rapid progression to cirrhosis and liver failure. In a study of bone marrow transplant recipients [81], the long-term outcome of chronic HCV infection was described as being particularly severe, with a cumulative rate of progression to cirrhosis of 10% and 25% at 15 and 20 years after bone marrow transplant respectively.

Chronic hepatitis C in children

HCV infection is uncommon in children because vertical transmission, which is responsible for most cases of paediatric infection in the western world, occurs in only about 3–5% of cases. Blood transfusions were a major route of infection of children before the implementation of HCV screening of blood donors. Intravenous drug use and high-risk sexual behaviour are currently maintaining the reservoir of infection in adolescents, particularly in large urban areas. Chronic hepatitis C in childhood has been characterized by an asymptomatic presentation, a variable biochemical pattern and mild liver lesions at histology [82]. Nevertheless, the spontaneous clearance of HCV and definitive ALT normalization were infrequently observed throughout childhood and adolescence, and increasing rates of fibrosis were documented in the liver in a proportion of cases that were followed prospectively with sequential liver biopsies [83]. As a consequence, there was an increased risk of developing cirrhosis and hepatocellular carcinoma in adult life, although the frequency and timing of these complications remain undefined.

Management of chronic HCV infection in clinical practice

Once chronic HCV infection has been identified by serological testing (the presence of anti-HCV antibodies and HCV RNA in serum), patients should be evaluated for the presence and stage of liver disease. This is best achieved by liver histology. Liver biopsy is not necessary if clinical and/or biochemical/haematological signs of overt cirrhosis are present. On the basis of histological findings, chronic hepatitis C is classified as minimal/mild (with no fibrosis or only minimal/mild fibrosis limited to the portal tracts or few and incomplete septa) or moderate/severe (with many septa or bridging necrosis). This broad distinction is clinically useful in terms of prognostic assessment. Patients who are not considered for antiviral therapy and those who fail treatment need to be monitored periodically for disease progression; they are usually monitored at 6- to 12-month intervals for biochemical markers of liver function and disease activity. Periodical ultrasound examination of the upper abdomen is recommended for those with moderate/severe liver disease. Histological re-evaluation is usually recommended after 5–6 years for patients who initially present with minimal/mild disease, and after 2–3 years for those with moderate/severe disease. Monitoring for liver fibrosis with non-invasive markers may enter clinical practice in the future, if better standardization can be achieved. All patients with chronic HCV infection should be evaluated for disease cofactors, particularly those that can be modified by intervention. Because a 'metabolic type' of liver steatosis may aggravate the course of hepatitis C, this condition should be investigated and, when detected, patients should be appropriately counseled to reduce the grade of fatty changes in the liver (by diet, exercise or reduction of body weight; see Chapter 13 for the clinical management of non-alcoholic fatty liver disease). Abstinence or avoidance of excess alcohol is also recommended in patients with chronic HCV, particularly when liver disease is active or advanced. Patients with chronic HCV should be encouraged to undergo testing for HBV and HIV markers, particularly when specific risk factors are identified. HBV vaccination should be recommended to HCV carriers who are negative for all HBV markers, including antibodies to hepatitis B surface antigen (anti-HBs). Hepatitis A virus vaccination is also recommended for non-immune individuals. Adequate counseling to reduce the risk of HCV transmission is mandatory for all HCV carriers, regardless of the viraemic load, HCV genotype and grade and stage of liver disease.

Because of the major role of direct percutaneous exposure in the transmission of HCV, educational programs and ensuring access to sterile needles and syringes for intravenous drug users are of paramount importance. Because of the low risk of HCV transmission, monogamous couples do not need to use barrier protection (condoms), although they should be advised that condoms may reduce the risk of transmission. On the other hand, HCV-infected individuals with multiple sexual partners should be advised to use barrier protection. Sharing common household items that may be contaminated with blood, such as razors and toothbrushes, should be avoided. The risk of HCV infection from a needlestick injury, an accident that frequently occurs in the health-care setting, is estimated to be around 2% and, at present, immunoglobulin prophylaxis is not recommended. Whenever possible, the source should be tested for HCV and the exposed individual followed for seroconversion to obtain early identification of HCV infection, which may be treated when appropriate. The risk of perinatal transmission is approximately 2–5% for infants of anti-HCV-positive mothers. High HCV-RNA levels at delivery, and HIV coinfection, significantly increase this risk. Elective caesarean section has not been shown to reduce the risk. Invasive fetal monitoring and prolonged labour after rupture of membranes should be avoided. Breastfeeding does not appear to transmit HCV [84].

References

1 Choo QL, Kuo G, Weiner AJ et al. (1989) Isolation of a cDNA clone derived from a blood-born non-A, non-B viral hepatitis genome. Science 244, 359–362.

2 Simmonds P (2001) The origin and evolution of hepatitis viruses in humans. J Gen Virol 82, 693–712.

3 Anonymous (1999) Global surveillance and control of hepatitis C. Report of a WHO consultation organized in collaboration with the Viral Hepatitis Prevention Board. J Viral Hepat 6, 35–47.

4 Memon MI, Memon MA (2002) Hepatitis C: an epidemiological review. *J Viral Hepat* 9, 84–100.

5 Alter MJ (1995) Epidemiology of hepatitis C in the West. *Semin Liver Dis* 15, 5–14.

6 Mansell CJ, Locarnini SA (1995) Epidemiology of hepatitis C in the East. *Semin Liver Dis* 15, 15–32.

7 Orland JR, Wright TL, Cooper S (2001) Acute hepatitis C. *Hepatology* 33, 321–327.

8 Kim WR (2002) The burden of hepatitis C in the United States. *Hepatology* 36(5 Suppl 1), S30–34.

9 Hoofnagle JH (2002) Course and outcome of hepatitis C. *Hepatology* 36(5 Suppl 1), S21–29.

10 Schreiber GB, Busch MP, Kleinman SH *et al.* (1996) The risk of transfusion-transmitted viral infections. The Retrovirus Epidemiology Donor Study. *N Engl J Med* 334(26), 1685–1690.

11 Terrault NA (2002) Sexual activity as a risk factor for hepatitis C. *Hepatology* 36(5 Suppl 1), S99–105.

12 Puro V, Petrosillo N, Ippolito G (1995) Risk of hepatitis C seroconversion after occupational exposures in health careworkers. Italian Study Group on occupational risk of HIV and other bloodborne infections. *Am J Infect Control* 23, 273–277.

13 Tumminelli F, Marcellin P, Rizzo S *et al.* (1995) Shaving as potential source of hepatitis C virus infection. *Lancet* 345, 658.

14 Sun DX, Zhang FG, Geng YQ *et al.* (1996) Hepatitis C transmission by cosmetic tattooing in women. *Lancet* 347, 541.

15 Jonas MM (2002) Children with hepatitis C. *Hepatology* 36(5 Suppl 1), S173–178.

16 Alter MJ (2002) Prevention of spread of hepatitis C. *Hepatology* 36(5 Suppl 1), S93–98.

17 Recommendations for prevention and control of hepatitis C virus (HCV) infection and HCV-related chronic disease. Centers for Disease Control and Prevention (1998). *MMWR Recomm Rep* 47(RR-19), 1–39.

18 Pawlotsky JM (2002) Use and interpretation of virological tests for hepatitis C. *Hepatology* 36(5 Suppl 1), S65–73.

19 Pawlotsky JM (2002) Molecular diagnosis of viral hepatitis. *Gastroenterology* 122, 1554–1568.

20 Nolte FS, Green AM, Fiebelkorn KR *et al.* (2003) Clinical evaluation of two methods for genotyping hepatitis C virus based on analysis of the 5′ noncoding region. *J Clin Microbiol* 41, 1558–1564.

21 van Soest H, Boland GJ, van Erpecum KJ (2006) Hepatitis C: changing genotype distribution with important implications for patient management. *Neth J Med* 64, 96–99.

22 Dal Molin G, Ansaldi F, Biagi C *et al.* (2002) Changing molecular epidemiology of hepatitis C virus infection in Northeast Italy. *J Med Virol* 68, 352–356.

23 Ross RS, Viazov S, Renzing-Kohler K *et al.* (2000) Changes in the epidemiology of hepatitis C infection in Germany: shift in the predominance of hepatitis C subtypes. *J Med Virol* 60, 122–125.

24 Bortolotti F, Resti M, Marcellini M *et al.* (2005) Hepatitis C virus (HCV) genotypes in 373 Italian children with HCV infection: changing distribution and correlation with clinical features and outcome. *Gut* 54, 852–857.

25 Matera G, Lamberti A, Quirino A *et al.* (2002) Changes in the prevalence of hepatitis C virus (HCV) genotype 4 in Calabria, Southern Italy. *Diagn Microbiol Infect Dis* 42, 169–173.

26 Echevarria JM, Leon P, Pozo F *et al.* (2006) Follow-up of the prevalence of hepatitis C virus genotypes in Spain during a nine-year period (1996–2004). *Enferm Infecc Microbiol Clin* 24, 20–25.

27 Pawlotsky JM, Lonjon I, Hezode C *et al.* (1998) What strategy should be used for diagnosis of hepatitis C virus infection in clinical laboratories? *Hepatology* 27, 1700–1702.

28 Seeff LB, Hoofnagle JH (2002) National Institutes of Health Consensus Development Conference: management of hepatitis C: 2002. *Hepatology* 36(5 Suppl 1), S1–2.

29 Barrera JM, Bruguera M, Ercilla MG *et al.* (1995) Persistent hepatitis C viremia after acute self-limiting post transfusion hepatitis C. *Hepatology* 21, 639–644.

30 Farci P, Alter HJ, Wong D *et al.* (1991) A long-term study of hepatitis C virus replication in non-A, non-B hepatitis. *N Engl J Med* 325, 98–104.

31 Alter MJ, Margolis HS, Krawczynski K *et al.* (1992) The natural history of community-acquired hepatitis C in the United States. The Sentinel Counties Chronic Non-A, Non-B Hepatitis Study Team. *N Engl J Med* 327, 1899–1905.

32 Villano SA, Vlahov D, Nelson KE *et al.* (1999) Persistence of viremia and the importance of long-term follow-up after acute hepatitis C infection. *Hepatology* 29, 908–914.

33 Marcellin P, Asselah T, Boyer N (2002) Fibrosis and disease progression in hepatitis C. *Hepatology* 36(5 Suppl 1), S47–56.

34 Yano M, Kumada H, Kage M *et al.* (1996) The long-term pathological evolution of chronic hepatitis C. *Hepatology* 23, 1334–1340.

35 Bedossa P, Poynard T (1996) An algorithm for the grading of activity in chronic hepatitis C. The METAVIR Cooperative Study Group. *Hepatology* 24, 289–293.

36 Ishak K, Baptista A, Bianchi L *et al.* (1995) Histological grading and staging of chronic hepatitis. *J Hepatol* 22, 696–699.

37 Poynard T, Bedossa P, Opolon P (1997) Natural history of liver fibrosis progression in patients with chronic hepatitis C. The OBSVIRC, METAVIR, CLINIVIR, and DOSVIRC groups. *Lancet* 349, 825–832.

38 Alberti A, Benvegnù L (2003) Management of hepatitis C. *J Hepatol* 38(Suppl 1), S104–118.

39 Boccato S, Pistis R, Noventa F *et al.* (2006) Fibrosis progression in initially mild chronic hepatitis C. *J Viral Hepat* 13, 297–302.

40 Pradat P, Alberti A, Poynard T *et al.* (2002) Predictive value of ALT levels for histologic findings in chronic hepatitis C: a European collaborative study. *Hepatology* 36, 973–977.

41 Hui CK, Belaye T, Montegrande K *et al.* (2003) A comparison in the progression of liver fibrosis in chronic hepatitis C between persistently normal and elevated transaminase. *J Hepatol* 38, 511–517.

42 Seeff LB (2002) Natural history of chronic hepatitis C. *Hepatology* 36(5 Suppl 1), S35–46.

43 Casiraghi MA, De Paschale M, Romano L *et al.* (2004) Long-term outcome (35 years) of hepatitis C after acquisition of infection through mini transfusions of blood given at birth. *Hepatology* 39, 90–96.

44 Kenny-Walsh E (1999) Clinical outcomes after hepatitis C infection from contaminated anti-D immune globulin. Irish Hepatology Research Group. *N Engl J Med* 340, 1228–1233.

45 Alter HJ, Seeff LB (2000) Recovery, persistence, and sequelae in hepatitis C virus infection: a perspective on long-term outcome. *Semin Liver Dis* 20, 17–35.

46 Wiese M, Berr F, Lafrenz M *et al.* (2000) Low frequency of cirrhosis in a hepatitis C (genotype 1b) single-source outbreak in Germany: a 20-year multicenter study. *Hepatology* 32, 91–96.

47 Harris DR, Gonin R, Alter HJ *et al.*, National Heart, Lung, and Blood Institute Study Group (2001) The relationship of acute transfusion-associated hepatitis to the development of cirrhosis in the presence of alcohol abuse. *Ann Intern Med* 134, 120–124.

48 Monga HK, Rodriguez-Barradas MC, Breaux K *et al.* (2001) Hepatitis C virus infection-related morbidity and mortality among patients with human immunodeficiency virus infection. *Clin Infect Dis* 33, 240–247. Epub 2001 Jun 15.

49 Graham CS, Baden LR, Yu E *et al.* (2001) Influence of human immunodeficiency virus infection on the course of hepatitis C virus infection: a meta-analysis. *Clin Infect Dis* 33, 562–569.

50 Adinolfi LE, Gambardella M, Andreana A *et al.* (2001) Steatosis accelerates the progression of liver damage of chronic hepatitis C patients and correlates with specific HCV genotype and visceral obesity. *Hepatology* 33, 1358–1364.

51 Ortiz V, Berenguer M, Rayon JM *et al.* (2002) Contribution of obesity to hepatitis C-related fibrosis progression. *Am J Gastroenterol* 97, 2408–2414.

52 Monto A, Alonzo J, Watson JJ *et al.* (2002) Steatosis in chronic hepatitis C: relative contributions of obesity, diabetes mellitus, and alcohol. *Hepatology* 36, 729–736.

53 Sabile A, Perlemuter G, Bono F *et al.* (1999) Hepatitis C virus core protein binds to apolipoprotein AII and its secretion is modulated by fibrates. *Hepatology* 30, 1064–1076.

54 Perlemuter G, Sabile A, Letteron P *et al.* (2002) Hepatitis C virus core protein inhibits microsomal triglyceride transfer protein activity and very low density lipoprotein secretion: a model of viral-related steatosis. *FASEB J* 16, 185–194.

55 Mirandola S, Realdon S, Iqbal J *et al.* (2006) Liver microsomal triglyceride transfer protein is involved in hepatitis C liver steatosis. *Gastroenterology* 130, 1661–1669. Epub 2006 Mar 6.

56 Barba G, Harper F, Harada T *et al.* (1997) Hepatitis C virus core protein shows a cytoplasmic localization and associates to cellular lipid storage droplets. *Proc Natl Acad Sci USA* 94, 1200–1205.

57 Moriya K, Yotsuyanagi H, Shintani Y *et al.* (1997) Hepatitis C virus core protein induces hepatic steatosis in transgenic mice. *J Gen Virol* 78, 1527–1531.

58 Kumar D, Farrell GC, Fung C *et al.* (2002) Hepatitis C virus genotype 3 is cytopathic to hepatocytes: reversal of hepatic steatosis after sustained therapeutic response. *Hepatology* 36, 1266–1272.

59 Leandro G, Mangia A, Hui J *et al.* (2006) Steatosis is independently associated with fibrosis in chronic hepatitis C: a meta-analysis of individual patient data. *Gastroenterology* 130, 1636–1642.

60 Smith BC, Gorve J, Guzail MA *et al.* (1998) Heterozygosity for hereditary hemochromatosis is associated with more fibrosis in chronic hepatitis C. *Hepatology* 27, 1695–1699.

61 Thursz M, Yallop R, Goldin R *et al.* (1999) Influence of MHC class II genotype on outcome of infection with hepatitis C virus. The HENCORE group. Hepatitis C European Network for Cooperative Research. *Lancet* 354, 2119–2124.

62 Alberti A (2005) Towards more individualised management of hepatitis C virus patients with initially or persistently normal alanine aminotransferase levels. *J Hepatol* 42, 266–274.

63 Alberti A, Noventa F, Benvegnù L *et al.* (2002) Prevalence of liver disease in a population of asymptomatic persons with hepatitis C virus infection. *Ann Intern Med* 137(12), 961–964. Summary for patients in *Ann Intern Med* (2002) 137(12), I36.

64 Alberti A, Morsica G, Chemello L *et al.* (1992) Hepatitis C viraemia and liver disease in symptom-free individuals with anti-HCV. *Lancet* 340, 697–698.

65 Gholson CF, Morgan K, Catinis G *et al.* (1997) Chronic hepatitis C with normal aminotransferase levels: a clinical histologic study. *Am J Gastroenterol* 92, 1788–1792.

66 National Institutes of Health (2002) National Institutes of Health Consensus Development Conference Statement: management of hepatitis C: 2002. *Hepatology* 36(5 Suppl 1), S3–20.

67 Garcia G, Keeffe EB (2001) Liver biopsy in chronic hepatitis C: routine or selective. *Am J Gastroenterology* 96, 3053–3055.

68 Dienstag JL, McHutchison JG (2006) American Gastroenterological Association Medical Position Statement on the Management of Hepatitis C. *Gastroenterology* 130, 225–230.

69 Regev A, Berho M, Jeffers LJ *et al.* (2002) Sampling error and intraobserver variation in liver biopsy in patients with chronic HCV infection *Am J Gastroenterol* 97, 2614–2618.

70 Afdhal NH, Nunes D (2004) Evaluation of liver fibrosis: a concise review. *Am J Gastroenterol* 99, 1160–1174.

71 Sebastiani G, Alberti A (2006) Non invasive fibrosis biomarkers reduce but not substitute the need for liver biopsy. *World J Gastroenterol* 12, 3682–3694.

72 Fattovich G, Giustina G, Degos F *et al.* (1997) Morbidity and mortality in compensated cirrhosis type C: a retrospective follow-up study of 384 patients. *Gastroenterology* 112, 463–472.

73 Benvegnù L, Fattovich G, Noventa F *et al.* (1994) Concurrent hepatitis B and C virus infection and risk of hepatocellular carcinoma in cirrhosis. A prospective study. *Cancer* 74, 2442–2448.

74 Niederau C, Lange S, Heintges T *et al.* (1998) Prognosis of chronic hepatitis C: results of a large, prospective cohort study. *Hepatology* 28, 1687–1695.

75 Benvegnù L, Gios M, Boccato S *et al.* (2004) Natural history of compensated viral cirrhosis: a prospective study on the incidence and hierarchy of major complications. *Gut* 53, 744–749.

76 Agnello V, Chung RT, Kaplan LM (1992) A role for hepatitis C virus infection in type II cryoglobulinemia. *N Engl J Med* 327, 1490–1495.

77 Zignego AL, Brechot C (1999) Extrahepatic manifestations of HCV infection: facts and controversies. *J Hepatol* 31, 369–376.

78 Cacoub P, Renou C, Rosenthal E *et al.* (2000) Extrahepatic manifestations associated with hepatitis C virus infection. A prospective multicenter study of 321 patients. *Medicine (Baltimore)* 79, 47–56.

79 Monti G, Galli M, Invernizzi F *et al.* (1995) Cryoglobulinaemias: a multi-centre study of the early clinical and laboratory manifestations of primary and secondary disease. GISC Italian Group for the study of cryoglobulinaemias. *QJ Med* 88, 115–126.

80 Mathurin P, Mouquet T, Poynard T *et al.* (1999) Impact of hepatitis B and C virus on kidney transplantation outcome. *Hepatology* 29, 257–263.

81 Peffault de Latour R, Levy V, Asselah T *et al.* (2004) Long term outcome of hepatitis C infection after bone marrow transplantation. *Blood* 103, 1618–1624.

82 Shepard CW, Finelli L, Alter MJ (2005) Global epidemiology of hepatitis C virus infection. *Lancet Infect Dis* 5, 558–567.

83 McHutchinson JG (2004) Understanding hepatitis C. *Am J Manag Care* 10, S21–29.

84 NIH Consensus Statement on management of hepatitis C: 2002 (2002) *NIH Consens State Sci Statements* 19, 1–46.

9.1.2.vii Hepatitis E

Rakesh Aggarwal and Krzysztof Krawczynski

Definition

Hepatitis E is a form of acute viral hepatitis aetiologically related to hepatitis E virus (HEV) infection. The disease is endemic in developing countries in the Indian subcontinent, central and south-east Asia, Africa and the Middle East, where it is a cause of significant morbidity and mortality.

Virology

Morphology and genomic organization

HEV is a small RNA virus, 32–34 nm in diameter, non-enveloped, icosahedral in symmetry, with indentations and spikes on its surface. The virus is currently classified in a separate genus *Hepevirus* in the family Hepeviridae. The HEV genome is a single-stranded, positive-sense and polyadenylated RNA of approximately 7200 bases [1]. The genome carries a 7-methylguanosine (m^7G) nucleotide cap [2] and is composed of discontinuous and partially overlapping open reading frames (ORFs) flanked by a 5′ untranslated region and a 3′ poly-A tail (Fig. 1) [1]. ORF1 encodes non-structural proteins (RNA-dependent RNA polymerase, helicase and methyl transferase) that are used in viral replication. ORF2 codes for the major structural (capsid) protein which contains a signal sequence at the 5′ end and three glycosylation sites. ORF3 overlaps ORF1 and ORF2 by 1 and 328 nucleotides, respectively, and encodes a small phosphoprotein that associates with the cytoskeleton in *in vitro*

experiments. ORF3 may be involved in intracellular signal transduction and is associated with the assembly of virions. Details of HEV attachment and entry into hepatocytes, the primary target cells for the virus, HEV replication and release of mature virions remain unknown. Hypothetically, non-structural gene products are expressed from the full-length, positive-sense genome. Newly generated, negative-strand RNA may act as a template for the production of full-length genomic RNA that is packed into progeny virions or used for further expression of non-structural proteins. It is possible that host-derived proteins are involved in viral replication. Recently, infectious cDNA clones of HEV and a subgenomic replicon system were developed that allow the study of viral replication strategies [3], which had been hindered by the absence of a reliable tissue culture system for HEV and a small animal model of HEV infection.

Genotypes and genetic epidemiology

Various geographically distinct isolates of HEV have been classified into at least four genotypes, based on the phylogenetic relationship of their genomic sequences (Table 1) [4]. The various isolates included in genotype 1 ('Asian strain') have a nucleotide sequence homology of 92–99% (amino acid sequence homology 95–99%) with each other, but only a 75% nucleotide homology (86% amino acid homology) with the isolate included in genotype 2 ('Mexico strain'). Isolates from sporadic cases in the United States, a non-endemic region, classified as genotype 3, are 92% identical to each other but only 73.5–74.5% identical to isolates from genotypes 1 and 2. Genotype 4 comprises isolates from some parts of China and Taiwan. HEV isolates from Africa (Chad, Algeria, Egypt) are more closely related to the Burmese strain than to the Mexican strain; however a Nigerian isolate appears to be closer to the

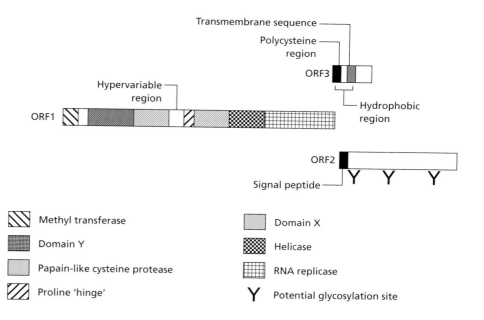

Fig. 1 A schematic diagram showing genomic organization of hepatitis E virus RNA, including its three open reading frames.

Table 1 Proposed genotype classification system for hepatitis E virus based on phylogenetic analysis of nucleotide sequences.

Genotype	Geographical origin of isolates
1	Asia
1A	India, Burma (Myanmar), Nepal
1B	China, Pakistan, former USSR
1C	Africa
1D	An isolate from a patient with fulminant hepatic failure and a few Indian isolates
2	Mexico and some African (Nigerian) strains
3	United States
4	China/Taiwan
5	Italy
6	Greece 1
7	Greece 2
8	Argentina (Argentina 1 and 2)

Based on ref. 4.

Mexican strain. Separate genotypes have been proposed for recently described single isolates from other non-endemic regions, such as Italy, Greece and Spain (genotypes 5–8). Despite significant genomic variability, all genotypes share at least one major serologically cross-reactive epitope.

Swine HEV, an HEV-like virus, was first identified in pigs in the midwestern United States [5], and later in other countries. It naturally infects pigs, inducing transient viraemia and antibodies that react with the capsid protein of human HEV strains. It has approximately 90.2–91.7% and 78.9–82.9% identity at the amino acid level with the Burmese and Mexican isolates of human HEV in the ORF2 and ORF3 regions respectively. In comparison, the US isolates of HEV share 92% identity with swine HEV and are more closely related to it than to the Burmese and Mexican strains. Similarly, swine HEV strains in Taiwan and Spain are more similar genetically to human HEV strains from these regions than to swine and human HEV isolates from other parts of the world. However, swine HEV identified in India, an HEV-endemic region, is genetically different from the HEV in patients from the same geographical region. Recently, an HEV-like virus was recovered from chickens; partial sequencing of its genome showed that it is genetically more diverse than isolates from mammalian species [6].

Clinical characteristics, pathology and pathogenesis

Clinical features

Clinical signs and symptoms in patients with symptomatic HEV infection are similar to those in persons with acute hepatitis A or B. Acute-phase symptoms include abdominal pain, anorexia, arthralgia, asthenia, malaise, flu-like symptoms, clay-coloured stools, dark or tea-coloured urine, diarrhoea, fever, jaundice,

nausea, vomiting, aversion to smoking, pruritus and skin rash [7–9]. The most commonly reported symptoms have been jaundice (90–100%), malaise (95–100%), anorexia (66–100%), nausea/vomiting (29–100%), fever (23–97%) and itching (14–59%) [7–9]. Common clinical findings include jaundice, hepatomegaly (10–85%) and, at times, splenomegaly. Laboratory findings are also similar to those in patients with other forms of viral hepatitis and include elevated levels of serum bilirubin, alanine aminotransferase (ALT), aspartate aminotransferase, alkaline phosphatase and γ-glutamyltransferase.

The incubation period in human volunteers after oral exposure was 4–5 weeks; incubation periods of 15–60 days have been reported during hepatitis E outbreaks. Acute-phase symptoms are preceded by a prodromal phase characterized by fever and nausea that diminish with the onset of jaundice (icteric phase). Most patients with acute hepatitis E have a self-limited course, and resolution of hyperbilirubinaemia and elevated aminotransferase levels generally occurs within 3 weeks (range 1–6 weeks) after illness onset. A subset of patients has a prolonged illness with prominent cholestasis, which usually resolves spontaneously. A few patients have a particularly severe disease and develop liver failure. The overall case–fatality ratio for the general population in disease-endemic countries has been from 0.1% to 4% [10]. Case–fatality rates are much higher (up to 25%) among pregnant women infected with HEV, especially during the third trimester [11]. The reason for the particularly high disease severity and mortality among pregnant women is not yet known.

The ratio of clinical to subclinical infections has not been determined; however, lower disease rates reported in younger age groups during several outbreaks may be the result of anicteric and/or subclinical HEV infections. In most hepatitis E outbreaks, the highest rates of symptomatic disease (jaundice) have been in young to middle-aged adults. No evidence of chronic hepatitis or liver cirrhosis has been detected among patients followed up clinically and among those who had liver biopsies after acute hepatitis E [12]. HEV infection in patients with pre-existing liver cirrhosis has been associated with the occurrence of acute-on-chronic liver failure. These patients may have a particularly poor outcome, although a subset improves to an asymptomatic state with compensated liver function [13].

Treatment for hepatitis E is essentially supportive. No data are available to evaluate the efficacy of antiviral agents or other specific therapies. The role of termination of pregnancy in pregnant patients with hepatitis E and fulminant hepatic failure has not been studied.

Pathology

Two histopathological patterns were observed in specimens obtained from an outbreak in Delhi, India: an obstructive or cholestatic pattern in 58% of examined cases, and a pattern similar to other forms of acute viral hepatitis in 42% of cases [14]. The cholestatic type was characterized by bile stasis in canaliculi and parenchymal cells, which were arranged in a gland-like fashion. Degenerative changes in liver cells (including acidophilic bodies) and focal necrosis were seen less frequently in the cholestatic type of hepatitis E. Polymorphonuclear leukocytes were observed in both intralobular infiltrate and portal tracts in larger amounts than those seen in classic acute viral hepatitis, although lymphomononuclear cells were the predominant cell type in portal tracts. Among the 'standard' changes typically observed in cases of viral hepatitis, ballooned hepatocytes, acidophilic degeneration of hepatocytes and acidophilic body formation were the most frequently encountered. The acidophilic type of hepatocytic degeneration was also a characteristic morphological feature of experimentally induced hepatitis E in cynomolgus macaques. Focal hepatocyte necrosis was observed in both patients and infected primates, with prominent accumulations of mononuclear macrophages and activated Kupffer cells and a much less striking presence of lymphocytes, which prevailed in portal infiltrates.

Elements of pathogenesis

Clinical and pathological features of HEV infection have been characterized based on surveys of patients involved in outbreaks of hepatitis E, studies of human volunteers and experimental models of infection in non-human primates. Data on virus replication in the liver, humoral immune response and liver pathology related to HEV infection were collected from these studies and used to develop a composite picture of the pathogenetic events of HEV infection (Fig. 2).

The pathogenic features associated with HEV infection have been characterized in rare volunteer studies [15]. In surveys of patients involved in outbreaks of acute hepatitis E, genomic sequences of HEV were identified in stools, bile and sera. HEV RNA has been detected in the faeces of most patients for about 2

weeks [16]; however, faecal HEV excretion for as long as 52 days has been reported. The relationship between HEV RNA detection and infectivity in stools has not been demonstrated. HEV RNA has been found in serum in virtually all patients within 2 weeks after illness onset [16]. Prolonged periods of HEV RNA positivity in serum ranging from 4 to 16 weeks have also been reported. Both immunoglobulin (Ig) M and IgG anti-HEV are generally detectable at the time of onset of illness, but the exact time course for the development of an antibody response is not known. It appears that the anti-HEV IgM response begins to develop just before the maximal ALT activity and disappears about 5 months into the convalescent phase of the disease [17,18]. The IgG response begins to develop shortly after the IgM response, and its titre increases throughout the acute phase and into the convalescent phase, remaining high from 1 to 4.5 years after the acute phase of the disease [17,18]. Virtually all patients have detectable IgG anti-HEV for at least 20 months after acute infection. In one study, nearly 50% of persons had detectable antibody approximately 14 years after infection [19], whereas the other half no longer had serological evidence of HEV infection. Recent data show that cellular immune responses are also activated during acute hepatitis E [20].

The experimental model of HEV infection is reproduced best in cynomolgus macaques and chimpanzees, although other non-human primates (rhesus, owl monkeys, tamarins) have been shown to be susceptible to HEV infection [21–23]. In macaques inoculated intravenously with HEV, expression of HEV antigen (HEVAg) in hepatocytes, indicative of viral replication, is first seen at about day 7 after infection [21]. HEVAg has been detected in 70–90% of hepatocytes at the peak of HEV replication, and decreases rapidly after the maximum ALT activity. HEVAg has been detected simultaneously in hepatocyte cytoplasm, bile and faeces during the second or third week after inoculation, and before and concurrently with the onset of ALT

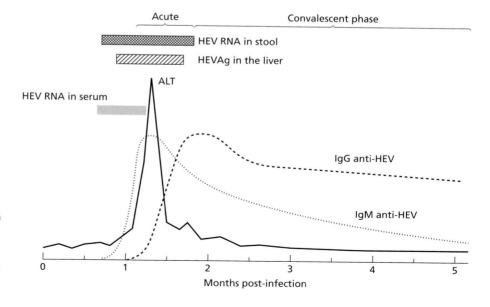

Fig. 2 Pathogenesis and clinical course of hepatitis E. A hypothetical graphical summary showing the course of events during HEV infection based on data from studies in human subjects and experimentally infected primates. The separation between the acute and convalescent phases of disease is arbitrary and is based on the alanine aminotransferase (ALT) levels.

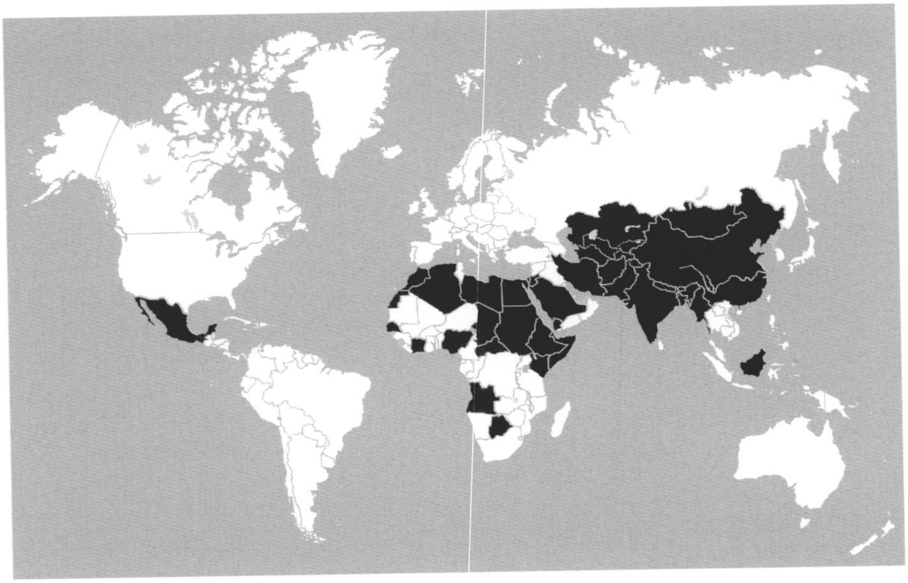

Fig. 3 Geographical distribution of HEV. The shaded areas represent disease-endemic regions.

elevation and histopathological changes in the liver [23]. These findings suggest that HEV may be released from hepatocytes into bile and, consequently, into faeces, before the peak morphological changes in the liver. The humoral immune response in infected animals resembles the pattern observed in humans. Both IgM and IgG anti-HEV are detected in serum in assays using immunoreactive epitopes of ORF2 and ORF3. As in humans, the IgM antibody level decreases rather precipitously, reaching negligible levels in the early convalescent phase. High titres of IgG anti-HEV are detected during convalescence. Anti-HEV has been observed as long as 10 years after inoculation and onset of liver injury in chimpanzees experimentally infected with serum specimens derived from HEV-infected patients in Tashkent, Pakistan and Mexico. In a challenge experiment that followed immunization of cynomolgus macaques with recombinant capsid proteins, the profile of the anti-ORF3 antibody response suggested that the presence of this antibody may be indicative of HEV replication. The mechanism responsible for the destruction of hepatocytes during HEV infection remains unknown. However, the onset of ALT elevation and histopathological changes in the liver generally corresponds with the detection of anti-HEV in serum and with decreasing levels of HEVAg in hepatocytes. In one study, infiltrating lymphocytes in the liver of HEV-infected cynomolgus macaques were found to have a cytotoxic/suppression immunophenotype [24], suggesting that liver injury may be immune mediated.

Inoculum titration experiments in cynomolgus macaques suggest that the size of the infectious dose may be related to the virological, immunological and pathological sequelae of infection [23,25]. Virus replication, anti-HEV immune response and acute hepatitis were all observed only after the administration of a high-titre inoculum. With decreasing amounts of inoculated HEV, biochemical and pathological evidence of liver injury and

Table 2 Epidemiology of hepatitis E outbreaks.

Occurrence in HEV-endemic regions	Large outbreaks involving thousands of cases, sporadic cases[a]
Mode of transmission	Faecal–oral
Vehicle of transmission in outbreaks	Faecally contaminated water
Peak of epidemic	6–7 weeks after primary exposure

Low secondary attack rate among exposed household members
Highest attack rate among individuals between 15 and 40 years of age
High case–fatality ratio among infected pregnant women (20%)

[a]Sporadic cases are also observed in non-endemic regions, primarily in travellers to HEV-endemic regions.

expression of HEVAg were absent; however, the subclinically infected animals excreted large amounts of viable HEV, capable of transmitting disease to naive animals, in their faeces [25]. The infection resulting from the endpoint dilution of the infectious inoculum (HEV Mexico strain) was marked only by seroconversion to anti-HEV.

Epidemiology

Epidemiology in HEV-endemic regions

Figure 3 shows the areas of the world where HEV infection is endemic. The characteristic epidemiological features of hepatitis E are summarized in Table 2. HEV is transmitted primarily by the faecal–oral route, and faecally contaminated drinking water has been identified as the likely vehicle of transmission in most reported outbreaks. Recurrent hepatitis E epidemics, with a periodicity of 5–10 years, have been observed in several parts of the world, including India, north-west China, Indonesia and the Central Asian republics of the former Soviet Union [8,10,26–28]. Reasons for this periodicity have not been determined; however, several outbreaks have occurred in a seasonal pattern after heavy rains. Person-to-person transmission of HEV appears to be uncommon, even in settings with poor environmental sanitation such as refugee camps [26,29]. Reported secondary attack rates for households with hepatitis E cases have ranged from 0.7% to 2.2% compared with 50–75% among susceptible contacts in households with hepatitis A cases. Vertical transmission of HEV infection from mother to infant has been shown to occur frequently [30]. A recent study showed that HEV infection can be transmitted through blood transfusions in HEV-endemic regions [31]; the significance of this route in the epidemiology of the disease has not been determined.

Areas of the world can be classified as HEV endemic based on the occurrence of hepatitis E outbreaks, which have been reported throughout Asia, Africa, the Middle East and Central America. The first extensively studied outbreak of waterborne hepatitis, which involved 29 000 cases of icteric hepatitis, was observed in Delhi, India, in 1955–1956 [26] and was serologically documented as non-A, non-B hepatitis several years later. Subsequent outbreaks of epidemic and sporadic hepatitis E in this region occurred in Kashmir [8], Kanpur [29] and Nepal. Many hepatitis E outbreaks have consisted of several thousand cases; the largest outbreak reported to date, involving more than 100 000 cases, occurred in north-western China between 1986 and 1988 [28]. Finally, small outbreaks of hepatitis E have been reported from the North American continent in two villages located south of Mexico City [32]. During outbreaks, disease attack rates are much higher among pregnant women than among men and non-pregnant women.

In many areas in which hepatitis E outbreaks have been reported, HEV infection accounts for a substantial proportion of acute sporadic hepatitis in both children and adults. In seroprevalence studies conducted in HEV-endemic countries, anti-HEV has been detected in as many as 5% of children aged < 10 years and in 10–40% of adults aged > 25 years [10]. These rates appear to be somewhat low in view of the frequent occurrence of outbreaks and nearly ubiquitous opportunities for infection, and may reflect the disappearance of antibodies with time. Hepatitis E may also be endemic in several countries where outbreaks have not been reported, including Hong Kong, Turkey and Egypt, based on a high incidence of sporadic hepatitis E cases in these countries. Recent data suggest that a proportion of healthy persons in these regions has detectable IgM anti-HEV and HEV RNA in their blood [31]; the exact significance of these findings is not yet clear.

Epidemiology in HEV non-endemic regions

In most countries where hepatitis E is not endemic, the disease accounts for fewer than 1% of reported cases of acute viral hepatitis. Most cases of acute hepatitis E reported in these countries have been associated with travel to HEV-endemic regions [33].

However, cases of acute hepatitis E have also been reported among persons with no history of travel to disease-endemic countries. In recent years, a few small outbreaks of acute hepatitis E related to the consumption of undercooked boar or deer meat have been recognized in Japan [34].

Seroprevalence studies among blood donors in some non-endemic countries have found an anti-HEV prevalence of 1–5%, which is relatively high compared with the low rate of clinically evident disease associated with HEV in these areas. Possible reasons for these findings include subclinical and/or anicteric HEV infection, serological cross-reactivity with other agents and false-positive test results. The higher antibody prevalence rates observed among swine handlers and sewage workers in these regions may reflect true positivity related to occupational exposure.

Reservoirs of HEV

It is possible that an environmental reservoir exists in disease-endemic geographical regions due to the continuous presence of conditions that allow faecal contamination of water sources and the environment. Another potential reservoir for HEV in these regions may be serial transmission of infection among susceptible individuals. Sporadic cases of hepatitis E account for a substantial proportion of acute viral hepatitis in countries where hepatitis E outbreaks have been reported, and these infections may maintain transmission of the virus during interepidemic periods. Consequently, serial transmission could be in the form of subclinical infection. Finally, HEV-like viruses have been detected in the faeces of wild-caught pigs, and anti-HEV has been detected in the serum of pigs, cattle and sheep in disease-endemic regions, suggesting the possibility of a zoonotic reservoir [35]. Although the close genetic relationship of human and swine HEV isolates from non-endemic regions supports the zoonotic hypothesis, differences in human and animal isolates in HEV-endemic regions counter this possibility.

Prevention

Development of an inactivated or live attenuated virus vaccine is not currently possible because of the lack of an efficient culture system. Neither pre-exposure nor postexposure use of immunoglobulin manufactured in hepatitis E-endemic areas has been found to be effective. Moreover, the natural history of protective immunity after acute HEV infection has not been fully determined, although the presence of pre-existing IgG anti-HEV was found to prevent hepatitis E in young adults. In two separate studies, neutralization epitopes have been identified and shown to span amino acids 452–617 and 458–607, respectively, of the HEV capsid protein [36,37]. Importantly, different HEV genotypes showed serological cross-reactivity and cross-neutralization in these subregions of the capsid protein. Recombinant HEV proteins evaluated in experimental studies as potential candidates for a prototype hepatitis E vaccine have been shown to attenuate HEV infection. In these studies, primates immunized with recombinant HEV proteins derived from HEV capsid protein and challenged either with the same strain of HEV or with a heterologous HEV strain divergent from the vaccine source were protected against liver injury, although faecal excretion of the virus was not prevented [38]. An experimental HEV DNA vaccine tested in cynomolgus macaques has been shown to induce levels of anti-HEV that are protective against heterologous HEV strain challenge [39]. One of the candidate vaccines has been shown to be safe and immunogenic in human subjects, but the results of efficacy trials are not yet available [40]. Modifications of the recombinant immunogen, the use of more efficient adjuvants and optimization of immunization schedules may help to induce higher levels of neutralizing antibodies and prolong the duration of protection. Further studies on HEV vaccines are needed because even short-term protection may be useful for travellers and pregnant women.

Given the lack of products to prevent hepatitis E, prevention relies primarily on the provision of clean drinking water. Limited data are available regarding the efficacy of chlorination of water in inactivating HEV, and studies are needed to identify other appropriate environmental control measures. Until such prevention measures are determined, the only prophylactic measures against HEV infection that can currently be recommended and applied are improved sanitation and sanitary handling of food and water. The best prophylaxis in disease-endemic areas is to drink water from safe sources, eat cooked vegetables and practise adequate personal hygiene.

References

1 Tsarev SA, Emerson SU, Reyes GR et al. (1992) Characterization of a prototype strain of hepatitis E virus. Proc Natl Acad Sci USA 89, 559–563.

2 Kabrane-Lazizi Y, Meng XJ, Purcell RH et al. (1999) Evidence that the genomic RNA of hepatitis E virus is capped. J Virol 73, 8848–8850.

3 Emerson SU, Nguyen H, Graff J et al. (2004) In vitro replication of hepatitis E virus (HEV) genomes and of an HEV replicon expressing green fluorescent protein. J Virol 78, 4838–4846.

4 Schlauder GG, Frider B, Sookoian S et al. (2000) Identification of 2 novel isolates of hepatitis E virus in Argentina. J Infect Dis 182, 294–297.

5 Meng XJ, Purcell RH, Halbur PG et al. (1997) A novel virus in swine is closely related to the human hepatitis E virus. Proc Natl Acad Sci USA 94, 9860–9865.

6 Haqshenas G, Shivaprasad HL, Woolcock PR et al. (2001) Genetic identification and characterization of a novel virus related to human hepatitis E virus from chickens with hepatitis-splenomegaly syndrome in the United States. J Gen Virol 82, 2449–2462.

7 Vishwanathan R, Sidhu AS (1957) Infectious hepatitis: clinical findings. Indian J Med Res 45 (Suppl.), 49–58.

8 Khuroo MS (1980) Study of an epidemic of non-A, non-B hepatitis: possibility of another human hepatitis virus distinct from post-transfusion non-A, non-B type. Am J Med 68, 818–823.

9 Tsega E, Krawczynski K, Hansson BG et al. (1991) Outbreak of acute hepatitis E virus infection among military personnel in northern Ethiopia. J Med Virol 34, 232–236.

10 Aggarwal R, Krawczynski K (2000) Hepatitis E: an overview and recent advances in clinical and laboratory research. J Gastroenterol Hepatol 15, 9–20.

11 Khuroo MS, Teli MR, Skidmore S et al. (1981) Incidence and severity of viral hepatitis in pregnancy. Am J Med 70, 252–255.

12 Khuroo MS, Saleem M, Teli MR et al. (1980) Failure to detect chronic liver disease after epidemic non-A, non-B hepatitis. Lancet ii, 97–98.

13 Kumar A, Aggarwal R, Saraswat V et al. (2004) Hepatitis E virus is responsible for decompensation of chronic liver disease in an endemic region. Indian J Gastroenterol 23, 59–62.

14 Gupta DN, Smetana HF (1957) The histopathology of viral hepatitis as seen in the Delhi epidemic (1955–56). Indian J Med Res 45 (Suppl.), 101–113.

15 Balayan MS, Andjaparidze AG, Savinskaya SS et al. (1983) Evidence for a virus in non-A, non-B hepatitis transmitted via the fecal–oral route. Intervirology 20, 23–31.

16 Aggarwal R, Kini D, Sofat S et al. (2000) Duration of viraemia and faecal viral excretion in acute hepatitis E. Lancet 356, 1081–1082.

17 Favorov MO, Fields HA, Purdy MA et al. (1992) Serologic identification of hepatitis E virus infections in epidemic and endemic settings. J Med Virol 36, 246–250.

18 Dawson GJ, Chau KH, Cabal CM et al. (1992) Solid-phase enzyme-linked immunosorbent assay for hepatitis E virus IgG and IgM antibodies utilizing recombinant antigens and synthetic peptides. J Virol Methods 38, 175–186.

19 Khuroo MS, Kamili S, Dar MY et al. (1993) Hepatitis E and long-term antibody status. Lancet 341, 1355.

20 Naik S, Aggarwal R, Naik SR et al. (2002) Evidence for activation of cellular immune responses in patients with acute hepatitis E. Indian J Gastroenterol 21, 149–152.

21 Krawczynski K, Bradley DW (1989) Enterically transmitted non-A, non-B hepatitis: identification of virus-associated antigen in experimentally infected cynomolgus macaques. J Infect Dis 159, 1042–1049.

22 Bradley DW, Krawczynski K, Cook EH et al. (1987) Enterically transmitted non-A, non-B hepatitis: serial passage of disease in cynomolgus macaques and tamarins and recovery of disease-associated 27–34 nm viruslike particles. Proc Natl Acad Sci USA 84, 6277–6281.

23 Tsarev SA, Emerson SU, Tsareva TS et al. (1993) Variation in course of hepatitis E in experimentally infected cynomolgus monkeys. J Infect Dis 167, 1302–1306.

24 Soe S, Uchida T, Suzuki K et al. (1989) Enterically transmitted non-A, non-B hepatitis in cynomolgus monkeys: morphology and probable mechanism of hepatocellular necrosis. Liver 9, 135–145.

25 Aggarwal R, Kamili S, Spelbring J et al. (2001) Experimental studies on subclinical hepatitis E virus infection in cynomolgus macaques. J Infect Dis 184, 1380–1385.

26 Vishwanathan R (1957) Infectious hepatitis in Delhi (1955–56): a critical study: epidemiology. Indian J Med Res 45 (Suppl. 1), 1–29.

27 Naik SR, Aggarwal R, Salunke PN et al. (1992) A large waterborne viral hepatitis E epidemic in Kanpur, India. Bull WHO 70, 597–604.

28 Zhuang H, Cao X-Y, Liu C-B et al. (1991) Enterically transmitted non-A, non-B hepatitis in China. In: Shikata T, Purcell RH, Uchida T (eds) Viral Hepatitis C, D and E. Amsterdam: Excerpta Medica, pp. 277–285.

29 Aggarwal R, Naik SR (1994) Hepatitis E: intrafamilial transmission versus waterborne spread. J Hepatol 21, 718–723.

30 Khuroo MS, Kamili S, Jameel S (1995) Vertical transmission of hepatitis E virus. *Lancet* 345, 1025–1026.

31 Khuroo MS, Kamili S, Yattoo GN (2004) Hepatitis E virus infection may be transmitted through blood transfusions in an endemic area. *J Gastroenterol Hepatol* 19, 778–784.

32 Valazquez O, Stetler HC, Avila C *et al.* (1990) Epidemic transmission of enterically transmitted non-A, non-B hepatitis in Mexico, 1986–1987. *JAMA* 263, 3281–3285.

33 Centers for Disease Control and Prevention (1993) Hepatitis E among US travelers, 1989–1992. *MMWR – Morb Mort Wkly Rep* 42, 1–4.

34 Tei S, Kitajima N, Takahashi K *et al.* (2003) Zoonotic transmission of hepatitis E virus from deer to human beings. *Lancet* 362, 371–373.

35 Meng XJ (2000) Novel strains of hepatitis E virus identified from humans and other animal species: is hepatitis E a zoonosis? *J Hepatol* 33, 842–845.

36 Meng J, Dai X, Chang JC *et al.* (2001) Identification and characterization of the neutralization epitope(s) of the hepatitis E virus. *Virology* 288, 203–211.

37 Zhou YH, Purcell RH, Emerson SU (2004) An ELISA for putative neutralizing antibodies to hepatitis E virus detects antibodies to genotypes 1, 2, 3, and 4. *Vaccine* 22, 2578–2585.

38 Zhang M, Emerson SU, Nguyen H *et al.* (2001) Immunogenicity and protective efficacy of a vaccine prepared from 53 kDa truncated hepatitis E virus capsid protein expressed in insect cells. *Vaccine* 20, 853–857.

39 Kamili S, Spelbring J, Carson D *et al.* (2004) Protective efficacy of hepatitis E virus DNA vaccine administered by gene gun in the cynomolgus macaque model of infection. *J Infect Dis* 189, 258–264.

40 Purcell RH, Nguyen H, Shapiro M *et al.* (2003) Pre-clinical immunogenicity and efficacy trial of a recombinant hepatitis E vaccine. *Vaccine* 21, 2607–2615.

9.1.3 Prevention and treatment of viral hepatitis

9.1.3.i Vaccines against hepatitis A

Pierre Van Damme, Koen Van Herck and Philippe Beutels

Introduction

Hepatitis A is one of the most common vaccine-preventable infectious diseases causing significant morbidity and mortality, with 1.5 million documented cases worldwide each year.

While no effective treatment is available against hepatitis A, vaccination of individuals implemented for more than 10 years according to selected strategies at international and national levels, together with improved sanitary conditions, have contributed to a substantial reduction in the economic burden associated with disease management. A selected number of countries with intermediate hepatitis A virus (HAV) endemicity are currently considering universal hepatitis A vaccination for their younger age population.

Currently available hepatitis A vaccines: composition, method of production, route of administration, dosage and schedule

Several inactivated and live attenuated vaccines against hepatitis A were developed in the 1980s and licensed for use in the early 1990s. These vaccines are safe and well tolerated, they are highly immunogenic, and they provide longlasting protection against hepatitis A disease in children and adults. Four formalin-inactivated, cell culture-produced, whole-virus vaccines are available internationally: Havrix (HM 175 strain, GlaxoSmithKline Biologicals, Rixensart, Belgium) [1,2], Vaqta (CR326F strain, Merck & Co., West Point, PA, USA) [3–5], Epaxal (RG SB strain, Berna Biotech Ltd, Bern, Switzerland) [6–8] and Avaxim (GBM strain, Sanofi Pasteur, Lyon, France) [9,10]. These have been approved for use in most parts of the world, and Havrix and Vaqta are also licensed in the US.

Other hepatitis A vaccines are produced with limited distribution. These include a Chinese live attenuated vaccine (H2 strain, Zhejiang Academy of Medical Sciences, Hangzhou, People's Republic of China) [11], a vaccine manufactured by Vaccine and Bio-product Company 1 in Vietnam since 2004 [12] and Nothav, an inactivated vaccine manufactured by Chiron Behring GmbH and distributed in Italy only [13].

Several types of combination vaccines containing an inactivated hepatitis A vaccine have been developed in order to protect individuals against more than one infectious disease when travelling to endemic countries. Such vaccines include Twinrix [14] (GlaxoSmithKline Biologicals, Rixensart, Belgium), the only combined vaccine against both hepatitis A and hepatitis B infections, licensed since 1996; other combined vaccines include Hepatyrix [15] (GlaxoSmithKline Biologicals, Rixensart, Belgium) and Viatim [9] (Sanofi Pasteur, Lyon, France), both protecting against hepatitis A and typhoid fever.

Inactivated hepatitis A vaccines all contain HAV antigen, but the content per vaccine dose is expressed in different units by manufacturers (Table 1). Recommended vaccination schedules, ages for which the vaccine is licensed and whether there is a paediatric and adult formulation also vary. All vaccines are licensed from 1 year of age in most countries, including the United States since September 2005 [16,17], except in Australia [18,19], where vaccines are licensed from 2 years, and in China where Epaxal is licensed from 6 months onwards. The inactivated vaccines are produced according to similar manufacturing processes involving whole-virus preparations of HAV strains growing in human MRC-5 diploid cell cultures, with subsequent virus purification and inactivation with formaldehyde. Havrix (HM 175 strain), Vaqta (CR326F strain) and Avaxim (GBM strain) are adjuvanted with alum, whereas Epaxal (RG SB strain) contains a liposome adjuvant in the form of immunopotentiating reconstituted influenza virosomes (IRIV). Havrix and Avaxim contain 2-phenoxyethanol as a preservative, while the other vaccines are preservative-free formulations [2,3,6,10]. All vaccines are

Table 1 Dosage and schedule for inactivated monovalent hepatitis A vaccines (in chronological order).

Vaccine	Antigen content (HAV strain)	Volume (mL)	Two-dose schedule (months)
Havrix 720 Junior	720 El.U (HM 175)	0.5	0, 6–12
Havrix 1440 Adult	1440 El.U (HM 175)	1	0, 6–12
Vaqta	25 U (CR326 F)	0.5	0, 6–18
Vaqta	50 U (CR326 F)	1	0, 6–18
Epaxal Junior	12 IU (RG SB)	0.25	0, 6–12
Epaxal	24 IU (RG SB)	0.5	0, 6–12
Avaxim 80U Paediatric	80 antigen units (GBM)	0.5	0, 6–12
Avaxim 160U	160 antigen units (GBM)	0.5	0, 6–12

administered via intramuscular injection, according to varying dosages and schedules, as described in Table 1.

If medically indicated, such as in haemophiliacs or in patients under anticoagulation, all four vaccines can be given subcutaneously [20–23].

Vaccine tolerability

To date, several million doses of hepatitis A vaccines have been administered to children and adults worldwide, with no serious adverse event ever statistically linked to their use [24]. The safety profile of inactivated hepatitis A vaccines has been reviewed extensively, and results from clinical trials, as well as postmarketing surveillance studies, have demonstrated that the vaccines are all safe and well tolerated [2,25–27]. The most commonly reported adverse events have included mild and transient local site reactions, such as pain, swelling and redness (21% in children and 52% in adults); Epaxal has a two to three times lower rate of local reactions in comparison with alum-adsorbed hepatitis A vaccines [27,28]. General reactions such as fever, fatigue, diarrhoea, vomiting and headache were reported in less than 5% of subjects [19,29].

Vaccine immunogenicity and protective efficacy

The absolute minimum level of anti-HAV antibodies required to prevent HAV infection has not been defined. Experimental studies in chimpanzees have shown that low levels of passively transferred antibody (< 10 mIU/mL) obtained from vaccinated persons do not protect against infection but do prevent clinical hepatitis and virus shedding [30].

In the absence of an absolute lower protective level of antibody required to prevent HAV infection, the lower limit of detection of the specific assay used in a study is generally considered as an accepted correlate of protection, i.e. 20 or 33 mIU/mL by enzyme-linked immunosorbent assay (ELISA) in clinical studies with Havrix; 20 mIU/mL by ELISA with Avaxim and Epaxal, and 10 mIU/mL by ELISA for Vaqta [2,4,6,9].

Currently licensed inactivated hepatitis A vaccines have proved highly immunogenic in extensive clinical studies, conferring protective immunity against the disease 2–4 weeks after first dose administration. Recent data have shown that a vast majority of individuals seroconvert within 2–4 weeks of vaccination, with rates ranging from 95% to 100% in children and adults. Administration of the second dose of the primary schedule (6–18 months after the first dose) ensures long-term protection [7,31]. Review of the immunogenicity data for each vaccine as well as results from several comparative clinical trials demonstrate the equally high immunogenicity and interchangeability of hepatitis A vaccines [1,9,27,32].

The protective efficacy of inactivated hepatitis A vaccines against clinical disease has been documented in several controlled clinical efficacy trials. The cumulative protective efficacy of the vaccination course with Havrix in more than 40 000 Thai children aged 1–16 years was 95% [33]. The observed protective efficacy of Vaqta was 100% after one vaccine dose in a trial involving more than 1000 children aged 2–16 years from a highly endemic community in the United States [3]. In a recent trial involving 274 Nicaraguan children aged 1.5–6 years, the protective efficacy of a single dose of Epaxal was also 100% [34].

The presence of passively transferred antibodies from previous maternal HAV infection has been shown to result in reduced antibody response to hepatitis A vaccination in infants [35–37]. However, in spite of lower antibody concentrations observed after primary vaccination of infants born to anti-HAV seropositive mothers, several studies have indicated that priming and immune memory were induced, as demonstrated by the anamnestic response at the time of booster [35–41]. This was the case after a second vaccine dose administered at 12 months to 300 infants born to either anti-HAV seronegative or seropositive mothers in a study conducted in Israel [38]. Similarly, in a study conducted in Turkey with children who had received primary vaccination at 2, 4 and 6 months of age, all subjects showed anamnestic response after booster vaccination at 4 years of age [39]. At 15 months, protective levels of antibody were also present in 93% of American Indian infants born to anti-HAV-positive mothers, who had received primary immunization at 2, 4 and 6 months or at 8 and 10 months of age [35]. Effective hepatitis A vaccination was also demonstrated in a study with 30 infants aged 6–7 months – half of them with maternal antibodies – and 30 children aged 6–7 years who were all seroprotected at month 1 and month 12 postvaccination and also showed a strong antibody response to booster vaccination [41].

Such findings relating to hepatitis A vaccine immunogenicity in children younger than 2 years of age, as well as studies that have shown that hepatitis A vaccine may be effectively and safely coadministered with other paediatric vaccines, such as diphtheria–tetanus–acellular pertussis, inactivated and oral polio, *Haemophilus influenzae* type b vaccine and hepatitis B vaccines [36,37], are of particular importance in the implementation of prevention strategies involving routine childhood vaccination programmes. Other studies in adults have demonstrated effective and safe coadministration of hepatitis A vaccine with traveller vaccines, including hepatitis B, polio, diphtheria, tetanus, typhoid fever, yellow fever, rabies, cholera and Japanese encephalitis [42–45].

In spite of an initially slower immune response observed in subjects over 40 years following administration of hepatitis A vaccines, response rates were similar to those observed in younger individuals on completion of the full vaccination course [46–48]. These data are confirmed by anti-HAV seroconversion rates of at least 98% in retrospective analyses of subjects ≥ 40 years of age who received a combined vaccine against hepatitis A and B [49,50].

Other conditions that may result in a lower immune response to hepatitis A vaccination include human immunodeficiency virus (HIV) infection and chronic liver disease. Limited data reported from studies conducted with HIV-infected male individuals have indicated that they had lower antibody concentrations than HIV-negative individuals and that approximately 75% had protective antibody levels on completion of the vaccination course [19]. Results from several trials evaluating the safety and immunogenicity of hepatitis A vaccine in chronic liver disease patients in the United States, Europe and Asia, including data collected in children, have been extensively reviewed and discussed elsewhere [2,19]. Mainly, these data indicate that hepatitis A vaccine was generally well tolerated and that the proportions of subjects with protective antibody levels were similar to those obtained in healthy individuals on completion of the vaccination course, while final antibody concentrations were substantially lower.

A few studies in transplant recipients also indicate a lower immune response following hepatitis A vaccination. While one study reported an acceptable 97% seropositivity in vaccinated liver transplant patients after two doses of hepatitis A vaccine on a 0- to 6 month schedule, compared with 100% in the control group, a third group of renal transplant recipients showed only 72% seropositivity. Moreover, seropositivity after the first dose was obtained in only 41% of liver transplant patients and 24% of

renal transplant patients, compared with 90% in the control group. Therefore, the authors concluded that transplant recipients should receive a full vaccination course before potential exposure to hepatitis A virus [51]. Two years later, only 59% and 26% of the seroconverters maintained anti-HAV seropositivity in the groups of liver transplant and renal transplant patients respectively. The rate of antibody loss in transplant patients therefore seems to be substantially higher [52].

Another study in liver transplant patients reached only 26% seropositivity after a full hepatitis A vaccination schedule [53]. These data reveal a lower hepatitis A vaccine efficacy in transplant patients, especially in those with stronger immunosuppressive regimens.

Hepatitis A vaccine has a recommended two-dose schedule, with the second dose being administered at 6–12 months in the case of Havrix, Avaxim and Epaxal, and at 6–18 months in the case of Vaqta. However, timing of the second dose is flexible as an anamnestic response has been shown to be triggered by a second dose when administered several years after the first vaccine dose in children and adults [54–58]. Flexible two-dose vaccination schedules with a 'delayed' second dose are of critical importance because travellers often miss the second dose and present themselves some years later with a new/repeated indication for hepatitis A vaccination. In addition, a flexible schedule might help in introducing hepatitis A vaccines into established childhood routine vaccination programmes. For example, a vaccination schedule for infants/children with the first dose administered during the second year of life and a second dose given at school entry at the age of 5–6 years seems to be worth investigating. Also, additional long-term follow-up studies of individuals who have received a single vaccine dose should help to formulate future recommendations in terms of dosing schedule.

Early protection and duration of protection

Hepatitis A vaccines confer early protection, as confirmed by recent data showing that a majority of individuals seroconvert within 2 weeks of vaccination, well within the 28-day incubation period of the virus. Travellers receiving the vaccine any time before departure may thus be expected to be protected against the disease [7,9,31].

With regards to duration of immunity, long-term follow-up studies have shown persistence of protective anti-HAV antibodies for at least 5 years in children and up to more than 12 years in adults postvaccination [8,40,59–61]. The kinetics of antibody persistence 10 years after primary immunization of 313 seronegative healthy adults with a two-dose inactivated hepatitis A vaccine administered either on a 0–6 or 0–12 schedule is presented in Figure 1 [62].

A robust immune response was also demonstrated in 31 vaccinated adults challenged with a paediatric dose of hepatitis A vaccine antigen 12 years after primary vaccination, while

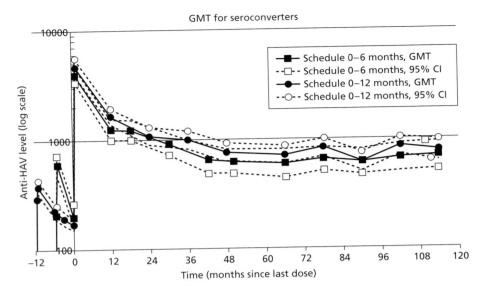

Fig. 1 Anti-HAV geometric mean titre (GMT) for the 0–6 and the 0–12-month schedules within their respective 95% confidence intervals (CI).

geometric mean anti-HAV antibody concentration was ≥ 15 IU/L before booster administration [63].

Mathematical models using data from vaccinated adults have estimated protective antibodies to persist for at least 25 years in more than 95% of vaccinees [8,9,64].

The role of immune memory in conferring protection for individuals vaccinated against hepatitis A was reviewed in 2002 by an International Consensus Group on HAV immunity [65]. The group concluded that evidence is accumulating that hepatitis A vaccines elicit immune memory persisting even after loss of detectable antibody. It recommended that reliance be placed on immune memory rather than booster doses to protect healthy individuals who received a full vaccination course. Based on the demonstrated persistence of protective antibodies for more than 10 years postvaccination, their estimated mathematical persistence for more than 25 years postvaccination and the presence of immune memory considered to confer protection even beyond detectable circulating antibodies, hepatitis A booster vaccination has been considered to be unnecessary in the healthy individual. Additional long-term follow-up studies should validate this expert consensus.

Field effectiveness of routine vaccination programmes

Hepatitis A routine immunization of young children has proved effective in rapidly reducing disease incidence and maintaining very low incidence levels among vaccine recipients as well as across all other age groups, thus demonstrating the development of herd immunity, in a number of settings. In the United States, the introduction of immunization programmes for children, with a primary focus on preschool children (i.e. 2–5 years), living in communities with the highest incidence rates, has resulted in a decrease in disease incidence to rates that are similar to the national average or even lower. In 2003, the overall

incidence rate of hepatitis A disease in the United States was 2.6 cases per 100 000, representing an overall decline of 76%, while targeted states had a reduction of 88% (even with levels of vaccination coverage not exceeding 50%), and a 53% decrease was observed in non-targeted states [66–68]. A national toddler immunization programme in place in Israel since 1999 has also demonstrated vaccine effectiveness, with a decrease in the annual incidence rate of hepatitis A disease from 50.4 cases per 100 000 (1993–1998) to 2.2–2.5 per 100 000 (2002–2004), representing more than a 95% reduction. This marked decline was seen in targeted vaccine recipients (85–90% coverage), as well as in all other age groups, thus demonstrating the effectiveness of hepatitis A vaccination, as well as the development of herd immunity [69]. Mass vaccination programmes also proved effective in localized regions of intermediate to high HAV endemicity in industrialized nations with otherwise low endemicity levels, such as the Puglia region of Italy, the Catalonia region of Spain and in North Queensland, Australia [18,70–72].

The real impact and added value of such mass vaccination programmes will need to be confirmed by continued disease surveillance. Indeed, although vaccination was a major contributer to the marked declines observed in the incidence of hepatitis A disease in Israel and the United States, it is difficult to evaluate to what extent this reduction could be partly due to improved sanitation and hygiene or to the epidemic cycles that have characterized the hepatitis A virus in the past [66,69,73]. Furthermore, the long-term effects of herd immunity are yet to be observed. As widespread vaccination continues, the accumulation of susceptible persons [in unvaccinated (age) groups] due to reductions in natural exposure may, in the long run, for instance, influence the frequency and size of outbreaks [outbreaks were observed to become less frequent and smaller in size in the short run in some settings (e.g. see [18])]. The associated increase in the average age at infection may also increase the occurrence of severe and fatal hepatitis A in adults and the elderly. These long-term effects ultimately depend on vaccine uptake, the duration of vaccine-induced protection (and therefore the realization of expectations regarding immunological memory) and concomitant improvements in safe water and sanitation in specific settings.

Field effectiveness of postexposure administration and in outbreak control situation

Studies in chimpanzees [74], further supported by randomized trials in humans [75,76], have shown that hepatitis A vaccine is effective in preventing HAV infection when administered post-exposure. Although the postexposure window for successful vaccination has yet to be defined, there is increasing evidence of the efficacy of hepatitis A as a valid alternative to passive postexposure prophylaxis with immune globulin, allowing, in particular, for a better control of outbreak situations.

Results from studies conducted in chimpanzees have also shown that vaccinated animals did not shed hepatitis A virus once exposed to the wild-type virus, thus demonstrating that the use of vaccines is effective in controlling spread in the case of outbreak [30].

The effectiveness of hepatitis A vaccination in controlling outbreak situations has been reported in various settings in the United States, including rural communities from Alaska, and Europe, including Slovakia, Croatia, the UK and Italy [1,19]. Recent data have reported the successful use of hepatitis A vaccine to control an outbreak among intravenous drug users in Bristol, UK, in 2000 [77], while the duration of two outbreaks was also substantially shortened in a maternal school and a daycare centre in Tuscany, Italy, at the end of 2002 [78].

Indications for vaccination and current recommendations

Inactivated hepatitis A vaccine is indicated for active immunization of susceptible infants ≥ 1 or ≥ 2 years of age at risk of hepatitis A and, in regions of low to intermediate endemicity, it is particularly recommended in individuals at increased risk of infection, at increased risk of spreading infection or at risk of complications in case of infection (see Table 2). On the basis of these indications, hepatitis A vaccination is currently recommended by both national and international authorities. Official recommendations made by the Advisory Committee on Immunization Practices (ACIP) of the US Public Health Service, World Health Organization (WHO) and the Viral Hepatitis Prevention Board (VHPB) are summarized in Table 2.

Next, to recommendations of 'at risk' groups, both the WHO and the VHPB [80,81] recommend the implementation of universal hepatitis A vaccination programmes in order to prevent and control hepatitis A epidemics in countries with intermediate endemicity level.

Table 2 Summary of current ACIP, WHO and VHPB recommendations for hepatitis A vaccination.

Persons at increased risk for HAV who should be routinely vaccinated

Persons travelling to or working in countries that have high or intermediate endemicity of infection

Men who have sex with men

Intravenous drug users

Persons who have occupational risk for infection

Persons who have clotting factor disorders

Daycare centre children and staff

Persons in residential institutions

Food handlers

Health-care workers

Persons who have chronic liver disease

Susceptible persons who have chronic liver disease or who are either awaiting or have received liver transplants

During outbreaks

Vaccination for outbreak control should take into consideration the characteristics of hepatitis A epidemiology in the community and existing hepatitis A vaccination programmes

From refs 79–81.

Of note, although studies of age-specific seroprevalence have distinguished different possible infection patterns, there is currently no global consensus on a definition of low, intermediate and high endemicity [82–84]. The key characteristics of HAV infection, including disease incidence, usual ages of infection and pathways of disease transmission, can be described within endemicity patterns presented in Table 3.

Both the WHO and the VHPB recommend that the decision of a moderate endemicity country to include hepatitis A vaccine in routine childhood immunization programmes should take into consideration the prevalence and incidence of hepatitis A disease, frequency of outbreaks, health impact of hepatitis A compared with other health priorities, feasibility of hepatitis A vaccination programmes and an economic evaluation of the different hepatitis A prevention strategies [80,81]. In addition, the VHPB recommends that childhood hepatitis A vaccination programmes currently implemented in some regions of European countries should be followed up and evaluated.

Official recommendations for the use of hepatitis A vaccine in the USA were first issued by the ACIP in 1996 and were updated in 1999 [79]. They are articulated as a regional strategy according to which children living in states, countries and communities with an annual HAV incidence rate ≥ 20 cases per 100 000 population during the period 1987–1997 should be routinely vaccinated while children living in states, countries and communities with an annual HAV incidence rate ≥ 10 cases (but < 20 cases) per 100 000 population should be considered for routine vaccination. On 26 October 2005, the ACIP voted to recommend that all children in the US receive hepatitis A vaccination between 12 and 23 months of age [85].

HAV endemicity	Reported disease incidence (per 10⁵/year)	Usual age of patients (years)	Risk groups
Very high	1–40	< 9	–
High	15–150	5–14	
Moderate	15–150	5–24	
Low	5–15	5–39	Many
Very low	< 5	> 20	Travellers, drug abusers

Table 3 Pattern of hepatitis A infection in Europe and the United States.

Adapted from ref. 82.

The future use of hepatitis A vaccines

Existing hepatitis A vaccines have an excellent safety profile, they are highly immunogenic and offer longlasting protection to individuals against all strains of HAV found in the community. Anti-HAV antibodies have been shown to persist for more than 12 years in vaccinated adults, and mathematical modelling has predicted their persistence in over 95% of vaccinees more than 25 years after immunization. Also, several studies have demonstrated the presence of longlasting immune memory induced by hepatitis A vaccination.

The field effectiveness of hepatitis A vaccines has been demonstrated in countries where routine vaccination programmes have been implemented. In addition to reinforcement of preventive measures including educational programmes, improved sanitation in countries of high HAV endemicity levels and improved surveillance systems in regions of low and intermediate endemicity, a review of current vaccination policy and strategies might be warranted by the global epidemiological shift towards lower endemicity experienced over the last decades, resulting in a growing pool of susceptible unprotected children, adolescents and adults, as well as an increased risk of epidemics and outbreaks.

Recommended universal vaccination programmes of children and adolescents in areas of HAV intermediate endemicity might be best implemented by the introduction of hepatitis A vaccine into existing programmes, with the first vaccine dose possibly administered at 1–2 years of age and the second at the first school health visit, at 5–6 years, in order to take advantage of existing childhood vaccination calendars.

The implementation of future hepatitis A prevention strategies, in particular universal vaccination programmes, warrants further investigations on co-administration of hepatitis A vaccines and flexibility of dosing schedules. Long-term protection studies should also be conducted, and vaccinated individuals should be followed up in order to assess the need for booster vaccinations and confirm the presence of immune memory, protecting individuals against the circulation of virus which could shift and allow infection to occur at an older age, causing intervention to convert an otherwise asymptomatic childhood infection into a symptomatic disease upon exposure later in life.

Continued disease surveillance will confirm the real impact of mass vaccination programmes on reduced hepatitis A incidence rates, as well as the indirect effect on non-vaccinated age groups, developing herd immunity.

Cost-effectiveness of hepatitis A vaccination

Model-based economic analyses assessing the cost-effectiveness of hepatitis A vaccination vary according to endemicity area, target group and model used (i.e. 'dynamic' models reflecting the disease transmission process and taking into account herd immunity vs. 'static' models which do not) [86].

In low and very low endemic regions, targeted hepatitis A vaccination has been shown to be cost-effective, depending on prophylaxis cost, previous exposure (mainly determined by age) and specific characteristics of the target group [87–91]. Postexposure prophylaxis and other outbreak control measures might prove potentially cost-effective in these areas too [89] (which is unlikely for universal childhood hepatitis A vaccination, from the perspective of both the health-care payer and society [86]). Cost-effectiveness of universal vaccination in low endemicity areas would be best assessed using a dynamic transmission model accounting for herd immunity effects (leading to reduced incidence in unvaccinated individuals and increased average age at infection). In areas of low and very low endemicity, there may be relatively small communities with an elevated incidence and disease burden from hepatitis A, such as immigrant families holidaying in their country of origin [92] or indigenous communities in Australia and Canada [93]. Childhood vaccination in such communities could have knock-on effects on the wider society, enhancing the cost-effectiveness of this option and yielding attractive results [92,93].

In areas of intermediate and high endemicity, the cost-effectiveness of universal childhood vaccination largely depends on the duration of vaccine-induced immunity, expected vaccine uptake and improvements in safe water and sanitation. The potential age shift caused by vaccination could have a more important impact on the cost-effectiveness than in low endemicity areas as the prevaccination average age at infection is very low when most infection is asymptomatic. In order to assess the cost-effectiveness in such areas, the use of dynamic models of infectious disease transmission is therefore recommended [86].

Summary

Experience over more than 10 years has shown that hepatitis A vaccines are safe, highly immunogenic and that they induce life-long protection, with no need for booster immunizations in healthy individuals. HAV vaccination has proved effective for prophylaxis and postexposure control of outbreaks, as well as in routine vaccination programmes. Many countries (in particular those with intermediate endemicity) have experienced a global epidemiological shift towards lower endemicity over the last decades. As a consequence, more adults and adolescents are put at risk of clinically severe disease, whereas the risk of epidemics and outbreaks has increased as a result of a growing number of susceptible individuals. For these reasons, universal vaccination programmes of children and adolescents are recommended in areas of intermediate endemicity, in addition to specific risk group vaccination. While completing the two-dose schedule within 6–18 months remains recommended, administering a delayed second dose a few years after the first one can be considered sufficient to complete the vaccination course.

References

1 Van Herck K, Van Damme P (2005) Prevention of hepatitis A by Havrix: a review. *Expert Rev Vaccines* 4(4), 459–471.

2 André F, Van Damme P, Safary A *et al.* (2002) Inactivated hepatitis A vaccine: immunogenicity, efficacy, safety and review of official recommendations for use. *Expert Rev Vaccines* 1, 9–23.

3 Werzberger A, Mensch B, Kuter B *et al.* (1992) A controlled trial of a formalin-inactivated hepatitis A vaccine in healthy children. *N Engl J Med* 327 (7), 453–457.

4 Werzberger A, Mensch B, Nalin DR *et al.* (2002) Effectiveness of hepatitis A vaccine in a former frequently affected community: 9 years' follow-up after the Monroe field trial of VAQTA®. *Vaccine* 20, 1699–1701.

5 Nalin DR, Kuter BJ, Brown L *et al.* (1993) Worldwide experience with the CR326F-derived inactivated hepatitis A virus vaccine in pediatric and adult populations: an overview. *J Hepatol* 18 (Suppl 2), S51–55.

6 Loutan L, Bovier P, Althaus B *et al.* (1994) Inactivated virosome hepatitis A vaccine. *Lancet* 343, 322–334.

7 Ambrosch F, Finkel B, Herzog C *et al.* (2004) Rapid antibody response after vaccination with a virosomal hepatitis A vaccine. *Infection* 32, 149–152.

8 Bovier PA, Bock J, Loutan L *et al.* (2002) Long-term immunogenicity of an inactivated virosome hepatitis A vaccine. *J Med Virol* 68, 489–493.

9 Vidor E, Dumas R, Porteret V *et al.* (2004) Aventis Pasteur vaccines containing inactivated hepatitis A virus: a compilation of immunogenicity data. *Eur J Clin Microbiol Infect Dis* 23 (4), 300–309.

10 Dagan R, Greenberg D, Goldenbertg-Gehtman P *et al.* (1999) Safety and immunogenicity of a new formulation of an inactivated hepatitis A vaccine. *Vaccine* 17 (15–16), 1919–1925.

11 Mao JS, Chai SA, Xie RY *et al.* (1997) Further evaluation of the safety and protective efficacy of live attenuated hepatitis A vaccine (H2-strain) in humans. *Vaccine* 15 (9), 944–947.

12 Rader RA (2005) Hepatitis A vaccine products. In: Rader RA (ed.) *Biopharmaceutical Products in the US and European Markets*, 4th edn. Rockville, MD: BioPlan Associates, 557 pp.

13 Minutello M, Zotti C, Orecchia S *et al.* (2000) Dose range evaluation of a new inactivated hepatitis A vaccine administered as a single dose followed by a booster. *Vaccine* 19 (1), 10–15.

14 Van Damme P, Van Herck K (2004) A review of the efficacy, immunogenicity and tolerability of a combined hepatitis A and B vaccine. *Expert Rev Vaccines* 3 (3), 249–267.

15 Beran J, Beutels M, Levie K *et al.* (2001) A single dose, combined vaccine against typhoid fever and hepatitis A: consistency, immunogenicity and reactogenicity. *J Travel Med* 7 (5), 246–252.

16 Merck (Press release, 15 August 2005) FDA Approves Expanded Age Indication for VAQTA® (Hepatitis A Vaccine, Inactivated), Merck's Hepatitis A Vaccine, to Children as Young as 12 Months of Age. Accessed at http://www.merck.com/newsroom/press_releases/product/2005_0815.html, 8 November 2005.

17 GlaxoSmithKline (2005) Havrix® (Hepatitis A vaccine, inactivated). Prescribing Information. Accessed at http://us.gsk.com/products/assets/us_havrix.pdf, 8 November 2005.

18 Hanna JN, Hills SL, Humphreys JL (2004) Impact of hepatitis A vaccination of indigenous children on notifications of hepatitis A in north Queensland. *Med J Aust* 181 (9), 482–485.

19 Bell BP, Feinstone SM (2004) Hepatitis A vaccine. In: Plotkin SA, Orenstein WA (eds) *Vaccines*, 4th edn. Philadelphia: W.B. Saunders, pp. 269–297.

20 Tilzey AJ, Palmer SJ, Harrington C *et al.* (1996) Hepatitis A vaccine responses in HIV-positive persons with haemophilia. *Vaccine* 14, 1039–1041.

21 Linglöf T, Van Hattum J, Kaplan KM *et al.* (2001) An open study of subcutaneous administration of inactivated hepatitis A vaccine (VAQTA) in adults: safety, tolerability, and immunogenicity. *Vaccine* 19, 3968–3971.

22 Steffen R, Lücking FP, Ciuera A *et al.* (2000) Subcutaneous versus intramuscular administration of a virosome formulated hepatitis A vaccine. Abstracts 10th Eur Congr Clin Microbiol Infect Dis (ECCMID), Stockholm; Abstract no. WeP307.

23 Fisch A, Cadilhac P, Vidor E *et al.* (1996) Immunogenicity and safety of a new inactivated hepatitis A vaccine: a clinical trial with comparison of administration route. *Vaccine* 14, 1132–1136.

24 World Health Organization (2000) Hepatitis A vaccines. WHO position paper. *Weekly Epidemiol Rec* 75, 38–44.

25 Black S, Shinefield H, Hansen J *et al.* (2004) A post-licensure evaluation of the safety of inactivated hepatitis A vaccine (VAQTA®, Merck) in children and adults. *Vaccine* 22, 766–772.

26 Zuckerman J, Peyron F, Wallon M *et al.* (1997) Comparison of the safety and immunogenicity of two inactivated hepatitis A vaccines. *Adv Ther* 14, 116–124.

27 Bovier PA, Farinelli T, Loutan L (2005) Interchangeability and tolerability of a virosomal and an aluminum-adsorbed hepatitis A vaccine. *Vaccine* 23, 2422–2427.

28 Clarke PD, Adams P, Ibanez R *et al.* (2005) Rate, intensity, and duration of local reactions to a virosome-adjuvanted versus an aluminium-adsorbed hepatitis A vaccine in UK travellers. Abstracts 9th Conference of the International Society of Travel Medicine (9th CISTM), Lisbon; Abstract no. PO 02.09.

29 Huang DB, Wu JJ, Tyring SK (2004) A review of licensed viral vaccines, some of their safety concerns, and the advances in the development of investigational viral vaccines. *J Infect* 49, 179–209.

30 Purcell RH, Dhondt E, Bradbury R *et al.* (1992) Inactivated hepatitis-A vaccine–active and passive immunoprophylaxis in chimpanzees. *Vaccine* 10 (Suppl 1), S148–S151.

31 Connor BA, Van Herck K, Van Damme P (2003) Rapid protection and vaccination against hepatitis A for travellers. *Biodrugs* 17 (Suppl 1), 19–21.

32 Bryan JP, Henry CH, Hoffman AG *et al.* (2001) Randomized, crossover, controlled comparison of two inactivated hepatitis A vaccines. *Vaccine* 19, 743–750.

33 Innis BL, Snitbhan R, Kunasol P *et al.* (1994) Protection against hepatitis A by an inactivated vaccine. *J Am Med Assoc* 271, 1328–1334.

34 Pérez OM, Herzog C, Zellmeyer M *et al.* (2003) Efficacy of virosome hepatitis A vaccine in young children in Nicaragua: randomized placebo-controlled trial. *J Infect Dis* 188, 671–677.

35 Letson GW, Shapiro CN, Kuehn D *et al.* (2004) Effect of maternal antibody on immunogenicity of hepatitis A vaccine in infants. *J Pediatr* 144, 327–332.

36 Kanra G, Yalcin SS, Ceyhan M *et al.* (2000) Clinical trial to evaluate immunogenicity and safety of inactivated hepatitis A vaccination starting at 2-month-old children. *Turk J Pediatr* 42 (2), 105–108.

37 Piazza M, Safary A, Vegnente A (1999) Safety and immunogenicity of hepatitis A vaccine in infants: a candidate for inclusion in the childhood vaccination programme. *Vaccine* 17, 585–588.

38 Dagan R, Amir J, Mijalovsky A *et al.* (2000) Immunization against hepatitis A in the first year of life: priming despite the presence of maternal antibody. *Pediatr Infect Dis* 19, 1045–1052.

39 Kanra G, Yalcin SS, Kara A *et al.* (2002) Hepatitis A booster vaccine in children after infant immunization. *Pediatr Infect Dis J* 21 (8), 727–730.

40 Fiore AE, Shapiro CN, Sabin K *et al.* (2003) Hepatitis vaccination of infants: effect of maternal antibody status on antibody persistence and response to a booster dose. *Pediatr Infect Dis J* 22 (4), 354–359.

41 Usonis V, Bakasénas V, Valentelis R *et al.* (2003) Antibody titres after primary and booster vaccination of infants and young children with a virosomal hepatitis A vaccine (Epaxal®). *Vaccine* 21, 4588–4592.

42 Bock HL, Kruppenbacher JP, Bienzle U *et al.* (2000) Does the concurrent administration of an inactivated hepatitis A vaccine influence the immune response to other travelers vaccines? *J Travel Med* 7 (2) 74–78.

43 Jong EC, Kaplan KM, Eves KA *et al.* (2002) An open randomized study of inactivated hepatitis A vaccine administered concomitantly with typhoid fever and yellow fever vaccines. *J Travel Med* 9 (2), 66–70.

44 Bovier PA, Althaus B, Glück R *et al.* (1999) Tolerance and immunogenicity of the simultaneous administration of virosome hepatitis A and yellow fever vaccines. *J Travel Med* 6 (4), 228–233.

45 Dumas R, Forrat R, Lang J *et al.* (1997) Safety and immunogenicity of a new inactivated hepatitis A vaccine in concurrent administration with a typhoid fever vaccine or a typhoid fever + yellow fever vaccine. *Adv Ther* 14 (4), 160–167.

46 Briem H, Safary A (1994) Immunogenicity and safety in adults of hepatitis A virus vaccine administered as a single dose with a booster 6 months later. *J Med Virol* 44, 443–445.

47 Reuman PD, Kubilis P, Hurni W *et al.* (1997) The effect of age and weight on the response to formalin inactivated, alum-adjuvanted hepatitis A vaccine in healthy adults. *Vaccine* 15 (10), 1157–1161.

48 D'Acremont V, Herzog C, Genton B (2006) Immunogenicity and safety of a virosomal hepatitis A vaccine (Epaxal) in the elderly. *J Travel Med* 13(2), 78–83.

49 Stoffel M, Lievens M, Dieussaert I *et al.* (2003) Immunogenicity of Twinrix in older adults: a critical analysis. *Expert Rev Vaccines* 2, 9–14.

50 Nothdurft HD (2004) Letter to the editor. *Vaccine* 22, 592–593.

51 Stark K, Gunther M, Neuhaus R *et al.* (1999) Immunogenicity and safety of hepatitis A vaccine in liver and renal transplant recipients. *J Infect Dis* 180, 2014–2017.

52 Gunther M, Stark K, Neuhaus R (2001) Rapid decline of antibodies after hepatitis A immunization in liver and renal transplant recipients. *Transplantation* 71, 477–479.

53 Arslan M, Wiesner RH, Poterucha JJ *et al.* (2001) Safety and efficacy of hepatitis A vaccination in liver transplantation recipients. *Transplantation* 72, 272–276.

54 Landry P, Tremblay S, Darioli R *et al.* (2001) Inactivated hepatitis A vaccine booster given ≥ 24 months after the primary dose. *Vaccine* 19, 399–402.

55 Iwarson S, Lindh M, Widerstrom L (2004) Excellent booster response 4 to 8 years after a single primary dose of an inactivated hepatitis A vaccine. *J Travel Med* 11, 120–121.

56 Williams JL, Bruden DA, Cagle HH *et al.* (2003) Hepatitis A vaccine: immunogenicity following administration of a delayed immunization schedule in infants, children and adults. *Vaccine* 21, 3208–3211.

57 Beck BR, Hatz C, Brönnimann R *et al.* (2003) Successful booster antibody response up to 54 months after single primary vaccination with virosome-formulated, aluminum-free hepatitis A vaccine. *Clin Infect Dis* 37, 126–128.

58 Beck BR, Hatz CF, Loutan L *et al.* (2004) Immunogenicity of booster vaccination with a virosomal hepatitis A vaccine after primary immunization with an aluminum-adsorbed hepatitis A vaccine. *J Travel Med* 11, 201–207.

59 Van Damme P, Thoelen S, Cramm M *et al.* (1994) Inactivated hepatitis A vaccine: reactogenicity, immunogenicity, and long-term antibody persistence. *J Virol Med* 44 (4), 446–451.

60 Wiens B, Bohidar N, Pigeon J *et al.* (1996) Duration of protection from clinical hepatitis A disease after vaccination with VAQTA. *J Med Virol* 49, 235–241.

61 Fan PC, Chang MH, Lee PI *et al.* (1998) Follow-up immunogenicity of an inactivated hepatitis A virus vaccine in healthy children: results after 5 years. *Vaccine* 16, 232–235.

62 Van Herck K, Van Damme P, Dieussaert I *et al.* (2004) Antibody persistence 10 years after immunisation with a two-dose inactivated hepatitis A vaccine. *11th International Congress on Infectious Diseases.* Cancun, Mexico. Poster 64.012:S225.

63 Van Herck K, Van Damme P, Lievens M *et al.* (2004) Hepatitis A vaccine: indirect evidence of immune memory 12 years after the primary course. *J Med Virol* 72, 194–196.

64 Van Herck K, Beutels P, Van Damme P *et al.* (2000) Mathematical models for assessment of long-term persistence of antibodies after vaccination with two inactivated hepatitis A vaccines. *J Med Virol* 60, 1–7.

65 Van Damme P, Banatvala J, Fay O *et al.* (2003) Consensus statement: hepatitis A booster vaccination: is there a need? *Lancet* 362, 1065–1071.

66 Wasley A, Samandari T, Bell B (2005) Incidence of hepatitis A in the United States in the era of vaccination. *J Am Med Assoc* 294, 194–201.

67 Averhoff F, Shapiro CN, Bell BP *et al.* (2001) Control of hepatitis A through routine vaccination of children. *J Am Med Assoc* 286, 2968–2973.

68 Bialek SR, Thoroughman DA, Hu D *et al.* (2004) Hepatitis A incidence and hepatitis A vaccination among American Indians and Alaska natives, 1990–2001. *Am J Public Health* 94 (6), 996–1001.

69 Dagan R, Leventhal A, Anis E *et al.* (2005) Incidence of hepatitis A in Israel following universal immunization of toddlers. *J Am Med Assoc* 294, 202–210.

70 MacIntyre CR, Burgess MA, Hull B *et al.* (2003) Hepatitis A vaccination options for Australia: review article. *J Paediatr Child Health* 39, 83–87.

71 Lopalco PL, Salleras L, Barbuti S *et al.* (2001) Hepatitis A and B in children and adolescents – what can we learn from Puglia (Italy) and Catalonia (Spain)? *Vaccine* 19, 470–474.

72 Dominguez A, Salleras L, Carmona G *et al.* (2003) Effectiveness of a mass hepatitis A vaccination program in preadolescents. *Vaccine* 21, 698–701.

73 Van Damme P, Van Herck K (2005) Effect of hepatitis A vaccination programs. *J Am Med Assoc* 294, 246–248.

74 Robertson BH, Dhondt EH, Spelbring J *et al.* (1994) Effect of postexposure vaccination in a chimpanzee model of hepatitis-A virus-infection. *J Med Virol* 43 (3), 249–251.

75 Sagliocca L, Amoroso P, Stroffolini T *et al.* (1999) Efficacy of hepatitis A vaccine in prevention of secondary hepatitis A infection: a randomized trial. *Lancet* 353, 1136–1139.

76 Furesz J, Scheifele DW, Palkonyay L (1995) Safety and effectiveness of the new inactivated hepatitis A virus vaccine. *Can Med Assoc J* 152 (3), 343–348.

77 Syed NA, Hearing SD, Shaw IS *et al.* (2003) Outbreak of hepatitis A in the injecting drug user and homeless populations in Bristol: control by a targeted vaccination programme and possible parenteral transmission. *Eur J Gastroenterol Hepatol* 15 (8), 901–906.

78 Bonanni P, Franzin A, Staderini C *et al.* (2005) Vaccination against hepatitis A during outbreaks starting in schools: what can we learn from experiences in central Italy? *Vaccine* 23, 2176–2180.

79 Centers for Disease Control and Prevention (1999) Prevention of hepatitis A through active or passive immunization: recommendations of the Advisory Committee on Immunization Practices (ACIP). *MMWR Recomm Rep* 48 (no. RR-12).

80 World Health Organization (1995) Public health control of hepatitis A: memorandum from a WHO meeting. *Bull WHO* 73 (1), 15–20.

81 Viral Hepatitis Prevention Board (1997) Hepatitis A: disease and epidemiology. Hepatitis A update. *Viral Hepatitis* 6, 5–14.

82 Hadler SC (1991) Global impact of hepatitis A virus infection: changing patterns. In: Hollinger FB, Lemon SM, Margolis HS (eds) *Viral Hepatitis and Liver Diseases*. Baltimore, MD: Williams & Wilkins, pp. 14–20.

83 Jacobsen KH, Koopman JS (2004) Declining hepatitis A seroprevalence: a global review and analysis. *Epidemiol Infect* 132, 1005–1022.

84 Jacobsen KH, Koopman JS (2005) The effects of socioeconomic development on worldwide hepatitis A virus seroprevalence patterns. *Int J Epidemiol* 34, 600–609.

85 ACIP (Press release, 28 October 2005). CDC's Advisory Committee on Immunization Practices Expands Hepatitis A Vaccination for Children: The recommendation for vaccination of children, between 1–2 years of age will be integrated into the routine childhood vaccination schedule. Accessed at http://www.cdc.gov/od/oc/media/pressrel/r051028.htm, 8 November 2005.

86 Beutels P, Edmunds WJ, Antoñanzas F *et al.* (2002) Economic evaluation of vaccination programmes: A consensus statement focusing on viral hepatitis. *PharmacoEconomics* 20 (1), 1–7.

87 Tormans G, Van Damme P, Van Doorslaer E (1992) Cost-effectiveness analysis of hepatitis A prevention in travellers. *Vaccine* 10 (Suppl 1), S88–S92.

88 Chodick G, Lerman Y, Wood F *et al.* (2002) Cost-utility analysis of hepatitis A prevention among health-care workers in Israel. *J Occup Environ Med* 44 (2), 109–115.

89 Péchevis M, Khoshnood B, Buteau L *et al.* (2003) Cost-effectiveness of hepatitis A vaccine in prevention of secondary hepatitis A infection. *Vaccine* 21 (25–26), 3556–3564.

90 Jacobs RJ, Rosenthal P, Meyerhoff AS (2004) Cost effectiveness of hepatitis A/B versus hepatitis B vaccination for US prison inmates. *Vaccine* 22 (9–10), 1241–1248.

91 Arguedas MR, Heudebert GR, Fallon MB *et al.* (2002) The cost-effectiveness of hepatitis A vaccination in patients with chronic hepatitis C viral infection in the United States. *Am J Gastroenterol* 97 (3), 721–728.

92 Postma MJ, Bos JM, Beutels P *et al.* (2004) Pharmaco-economic evaluation of targeted hepatitis A vaccination for children of ethnic minorities in Amsterdam (The Netherlands). *Vaccine* 22, 1862–1867.

93 Beutels P, MacIntyre R, McIntyre P (2005) Cost-effectiveness of childhood hepatitis A vaccination in Australia. 5th World Congress of the International Health Economics Association, Barcelona, Spain. Abstract no. 40.254 #1.

9.1.3.ii Hepatitis B vaccines and immunization

Daniel Lavanchy

Hepatitis B vaccines provide the best protection against HBV infection and its clinical sequelae, i.e. cirrhosis and hepatocellular carcinoma (HCC) [1–3]. They are therefore the first vaccines against cancer ever licensed [4].

Control and the eventual elimination of transmission of HBV infection is possible with the appropriate use of hepatitis B vaccines.

Vaccine preparations

Hepatitis B vaccines are highly purified preparations of the 22-nm spherical particles of hepatitis B surface antigen (HBsAg), containing aluminium salts as an adjuvant. Guiding principles for the public health purchase and use of vaccines have been published by the World Health Organization in *Vaccines and Biologicals. Ensuring the Quality of Vaccines at Country Level* (http://www.who.int/vaccinesdocuments/DocsPDF02/www693.pdf).

Plasma-derived vaccines

In the 1960s, it was shown that boiled serum from patients with 'serum hepatitis' could protect against clinical disease [5]. This led to the development of vaccines from highly purified preparations of HBsAg from the plasma of HBV carriers using various methods of purification and inactivation. These vaccines proved to be safe, highly immunogenic and effective in preventing disease. Plasma-derived vaccines became commercially available in 1982 and have been used extensively worldwide [6–8]. Today, they have been replaced by recombinant DNA vaccines.

Recombinant DNA vaccines

DNA recombinant vaccines were developed in the 1980s by inserting plasmids containing the HBV gene coding for HBsAg (with or without the pre-S1 and pre-S2 components) into yeast or mammalian cells. These cells then produce self-assembling, immunogenic HBsAg particles, almost identical to those found in the plasma of chronic HBV carriers [9,10].

Combination vaccines

Today, hepatitis B vaccines are not only available in monovalent formulations that protect only against hepatitis B, but also in combination formulations that protect against hepatitis B and other diseases [e.g. diphtheria–tetanus–pertussis (DTP)–HepB; DTP–HepB + *Haemophilus* influenza B (Hib); Hib–HepB] [11–15]. Table 1 shows the formulations of hepatitis B vaccine currently available. The most obvious benefits of combination vaccines are the immunization of all children receiving DTP with an additional antigen, but without an additional injection, resulting in increased injection safety and fewer vaccine-related costs and waste.

As the DTP and Hib antigens have reduced immunogenicity when given before the age of 6 weeks, a combination vaccine with a hepatitis B component cannot be used for newborns and, therefore, the monovalent hepatitis B vaccine must be used for vaccination at birth.

Vaccine schedules

The main objective of hepatitis B immunization is to prevent chronic HBV infection and its serious consequences, including liver cirrhosis and hepatocellular cancer (HCC). Routine vaccination of all infants against HBV infection should become an integral part of national immunization strategies. A high coverage of the primary vaccine series among infants will have the greatest overall impact on the prevalence of chronic HBV infection in children and should be given the highest priority.

A variety of schedules may be used for hepatitis B immunization in national programmes, depending on the local epidemiological situation. However, in countries where a high proportion of HBV infections are acquired perinatally, the first dose of hepatitis B vaccine should be given as soon as possible (< 24 hours) after birth. In countries where a lower proportion of HBV infections are acquired perinatally, the relative contribution of perinatal HBV infection to the overall disease burden, and the feasibility and cost-effectiveness of providing vaccination at birth, should be carefully considered before a decision is made on the optimal vaccination schedule.

Catch-up strategies targeted at older age groups or groups with risk factors for acquiring HBV infection should be considered as a supplement to routine infant vaccination in countries of intermediate or low hepatitis B endemicity. In such settings, a substantial proportion of the disease burden may be attributable to infections acquired by older children, adolescents and adults. In countries of high endemicity, large-scale routine vaccination of infants rapidly will rapidly reduce the transmission of HBV. In these circumstances, catch-up vaccination of older children and adults has relatively little impact on chronic disease because most of them have already been infected.

There are multiple options for incorporating the hepatitis B vaccine into national immunization programmes (Table 2) The minimum recommended interval between doses is 4 weeks. Longer intervals may increase the final anti-HBs titres but not the seroconversion rates. More than three doses of the vaccine are not required, regardless of duration (> 4 weeks) of the interval between them.

Table 1 Formulations of hepatitis B vaccine.

Monovalent	Hepatitis B
DTwP–HepB	Diphtheria + tetanus + whole-cell pertussis + hepatitis B
DTwP–Hib–HepB	Diphtheria + tetanus + whole-cell pertussis + *Haemophilus* influenza type B + hepatitis B
DTaP–Hib–IPV–HepB	Diphtheria + tetanus + acellular pertussis + *Haemophilus* influenza type B + inactivated polio vaccine + hepatitis B
DTaP–IPV–HepB	Diphtheria + tetanus + acellular pertussis + inactivated polio vaccine + hepatitis B
Hib–HepB	*Haemophilus* influenza type B + hepatitis B
HepA–HepB	Hepatitis A + hepatitis B

Hepatitis B vaccine is available as monovalent formulations or in fixed combination with other vaccines, including DTwP, DTaP, Hib, hepatitis A and IPV. When immunizing against HBV at birth, only monovalent hepatitis B vaccine should be used: the other antigens found in combination vaccines are currently not approved for use at birth.

A heptavalent EPI vaccine (DTwP, HepB, Hib, meningo A/C) is currently under development.

Table 2 Hepatitis B vaccine schedules.

Newborn

Visit	Age	Other antigens				Hepatitis B vaccine options		
						No birth dose	With birth dose	
						I	II	III
0	Birth	BCG OPV0[a]					HepB1[b]	HepB1[b]
1	6 weeks		OPV1	DTP1		HepB1[c]	HepB2[b]	HepB2[c]
2	10 weeks		OPV2	DTP2		HepB2[c]	NA	HepB3[c]
3	14 weeks		OPV3	DTP3		HepB3[c]	HepB3[b]	HepB4[c]
4	9–12 months		NA	NA	Measles	NA	NA	NA

Adult

Visit	Schedule			Hepatitis B vaccine
	Standard	Accelerated		
		I[e]	II[e]	
1	0	0	0	HepB[c]
2	1 month	1 month	7 days	HepB[c]
3	6–12 months	2 months	21 days	HepB[c]
4[d]		6–12 months	6–12 months	HepB[c]

NA, not applicable; BCG, bacillus Calmette–Guérin (vaccine); OPV, oral polio vaccine.
[a]Given only given in highly polio-endemic countries.
[b]Monovalent vaccine.
[c]Monovalent or combination vaccine.
[d]A fourth dose of vaccine is recommended after an accelerated schedule.
[e]Not licensed in all countries.

Recommended schedules for vaccination can be divided into those that include a birth dose and those that do not. Schedules with a birth-dose call for the first vaccination at birth, followed by a second and third dose at the time of the first and third DTP vaccination, respectively (Table 2, column II). Alternatively, a four-dose schedule may be employed, whereby the dose at birth is followed by three additional doses; these doses may be given either as monovalent vaccine or as a combination (e.g. with DTP and/or Hib) following the schedules commonly used for those vaccines (Table 2, column III). These schedules will prevent most perinatally acquired infection.

Experimental vaccines

Although HBsAg vaccine is effective in preventing HBV infection, it is poorly immunogenic (if not adjuvanted). While most recipients of three doses of currently available hepatitis B vaccines produce a strong and longlasting anti-HBs response, 5–10% of healthy adults do not produce protective levels of anti-HBs and can be considered non-responders [16,17]. Therefore, strategies to overcome non- or poor responsiveness to hepatitis B vaccines have been devised.

One such strategy is to *add pre-S epitopes to HBsAg (S-only) vaccine* [18,19]. Early trials demonstrated that pre-S2-containing vaccines are safe and immunogenic but failed to show an advantage over the existing S-only vaccines [20]. Other trials, using pre-S1- and pre-S2-containing recombinant HBsAg vaccines, suggested that pre-S sequences do confer increased immuno-

genicity in proven non-responders [21–24 and recent reference 119]. These conflicting results may result from the incorporation of different pre-S1 and pre-S2 epitopes, the protease sensitivity and resulting instability of certain products or the cell line used for the production. These issues need to be clarified before definitive statements can be made on the usefulness of vaccines containing pre-S sequences.

Immunization using *DNA vaccines* encoding for HBsAg is another area currently under investigation [25–27]. It still remains to be determined whether DNA-based immunization will prove to be more effective, less expensive or safer than recombinant proteins.

Hepatitis B core antigen (HBcAg) is far more immunogenic than HBsAg, making it extremely attractive for use as a carrier of heterologous B-cell epitopes. As a result, chimeric particles containing recombinant HBcAg and HBsAg sequences have been constructed. These constructs have shown enhanced immunogenicity for the inserted HBsAg. Further research is needed before such a vaccine can be recommended for public health use [28,29].

Enhanced immunogenicity of vaccines can also be achieved by *changing the adjuvant* used for delivery rather than the protein composition. For currently licensed vaccines, the only adjuvants approved for use are aluminium salts and MF59 [30,31]. HBV envelope proteins formulated in several adjuvant systems turned out to be more immunogenic than their non-adjuvanted or aluminium-adjuvanted counterparts [31–38]. It is conceivable that a two-dose hepatitis B vaccine schedule could be achieved using vaccines with enhanced immunogenicity, and eventually lead to reduced vaccine administration costs and improved compliance.

Vaccine efficacy

Immune response to vaccine

Hepatitis B vaccine schedules are flexible; there are various options for adding the vaccine to established national immunization schedules without requiring additional visits for vaccination. The most widely used vaccination schedule is 0, 1 and 6–12 months. Among immunocompetent infants, children and adults, a protective antibody response develops in 90–95% of vaccine recipients [16,17,39]. Protection lasts for as long as 15 years and outlasts the presence of detectable antibodies [40–42] because long-term protection relies on a T cell-based immunological memory, which provides an anamnestic response after exposure to HBV.

Studies in Alaska [16,50] have shown that titres of anti-HBs higher than 10 mIU/L persist in 75% and 65% of vaccinated individuals 10 and 15 years after vaccination respectively. Likewise 64% of Italians vaccinated at birth and 87% of those vaccinated at 12 years of age had titres of anti-HBs higher than 10 mIU/L 11 years aften vaccination; a booster dose in vaccinees that had lower antibody titres induced in all but 6% of individuals vaccinated at birth an ameliorative effect.

Booster doses

No data support the use of booster doses of hepatitis B vaccine among immunocompetent individuals who have responded to a complete primary vaccination series. Therefore, booster doses of vaccine are *not* recommended [42–45]. However, additional information is required to establish whether booster injections are needed for adults beyond 15 years after hepatitis B vaccination, for children immunized at birth (to determine whether the immunological memory persists into adolescence and adulthood) and for population groups at higher risk of infection with HBV. Booster doses are recommended for immunocompromised individuals.

Breakthrough infections after successful hepatitis B vaccination

A limited number of children have been infected with HBV after completing a full vaccination course [44]. These cases were attributed to HBV vaccine escape mutant strains carrying mutations on the antigenic *a* determinant of HBsAg [46–48]. The same phenomenon was also observed in almost 4% of babies born to HBsAg-positive mothers who received active and passive immunization at birth; some of the infected babies developed chronic hepatitis [49]. The risk of hepatitis B infection is inversely related to the titres of the anti-HBs generated by

vaccination [50]. Almost all infections occurring in successfully vaccinated individuals are clinically silent [39,51]. Although long-term follow-up studies are needed to determine the impact of disease from breakthrough infections, current hepatitis B vaccines have been shown to effectively protect whole populations [41,52–54].

Postvaccination testing for anti-HBs

Monitoring of anti-HBs titres is recommended for vaccinated immunocompromised persons considered at risk of HBV infection (e.g. haemodialysis patients). Adult vaccinees with ≤ 10 mIU/mL anti-HBs after a full hepatitis B vaccination course, measured 1–3 months following vaccination, should be considered for revaccination [43].

Vaccine safety issues

Contraindications to vaccination

There are few contraindications to hepatitis B vaccination: (i) severe reactions to previous doses; (ii) hypersensitivity to one of the vaccine components; and (iii) fever above 38.5°C [39,47].

Multiple sclerosis (MS), acute lymphoblastic leukaemia (ALL), macrophagal myofasciitis (MMF) or other autoimmune diseases potentially associated with HBV vaccination

The issue of a possible association between hepatitis B vaccination and the development of MS, first raised in France, has not been confirmed by convincing scientific data [39,55–59].

Likewise, the hypothetical link between vaccination and ALL in children has not been confirmed [56,57].

In 1993, MMF was investigated through biopsies of the deltoid muscle in patients with general systemic complaints (myalgia, fatigue, arthralgia, muscle weakness, fever, asthenia) [56,57]. The conclusions of a recently performed case–control study noted that there is no basis to reports that aluminium-containing vaccines pose a serious health risk [57].

Although the prevalence of autoimmune disease (AID) is generally quite low, the incidence has increased in industrialized countries during recent years, affecting approximately 5% of the population [60]. However, no scientific data support the existence of a causal link or triggering association between the administration of hepatitis B vaccine and the onset of an autoimmune disease [57]. Considering the high levels of vaccination coverage resulting from immunization programmes worldwide, and given that more than 1 billion doses of vaccine have been used since 1982, the most likely explanation for the occurrence of MS, ALL, MMF or other autoimmune diseases linked to a vaccination against hepatitis B is a coincidental temporal association. There is currently enough evidence to conclude that people suffering from autoimmune diseases can be vaccinated [57].

Thiomersal, also known as thimerosal, contains small amounts of ethyl mercury and has been used as a preservative in vaccines. Although the Institute of Medicine [61] found no evidence of a causal relationship between exposure to thiomersal and the development of autism, attention deficit hyperactivity disorder and speech or language delay, it has been eliminated from many preparations [56,62].

Addressing vaccine safety concerns

In a rapidly changing global environment, and as successful immunization programmes have led to less visible disease threats, many communities have lost the knowledge of the natural consequences of vaccine-preventable diseases that have disappeared (e.g. measles, diphtheria, acute viral hepatitis). In the absence of disease, the misconception arises that vaccination is no longer needed. Thus, interests may increasingly focus on vaccine adverse events rather than on the prevention and control of diseases, resulting in lower vaccine coverage and subsequent disease outbreaks.

Loss of public confidence in vaccination is one of the greatest threats to public health and needs to be addressed. Recent studies have indicated that the proven benefits of vaccination in general and, more specifically, those of hepatitis B vaccination are overwhelming and far outweigh any suggested risk. Consequently, immunization programmes should not stop while each hypothesis is investigated [63].

Injection safety issues

A real issue, unsafe injection practices, has aroused little interest and, therefore, its consequences are largely unknown to the public and to many health-care professionals. With approximately 16 billion injections administered worldwide each year (only 10% of them related to vaccination), it is estimated that 33% of injections in developing countries are unsafe, contributing annually to approximately 20 million new HBV infections (and also to 2 million hepatitis C virus (HCV) infections and 260 000 human immunodeficiency virus (HIV) infections). Promoting safer injection practices through education and the provision of autodisposable syringes is a global task [57,64,65].

Immunization strategies

For population-based immunizations, two strategies have been used [66,67]:
1 High-risk group targeting. Strategies aimed at vaccinating and changing behaviour in these high-risk groups (see Table 3) should be pursued. However, the targeted immunization of high-risk groups has failed to control hepatitis B infection in the general population [17,68–73].

Table 3 Groups at high risk of hepatitis B infection.

Injecting drug users
Persons engaging in unsafe sexual behaviour
Inmates and staff of prisons
Household contacts, other social contacts and sexual partners of persons with acute or chronic HBV infection
Babies born to mothers either with persistent HBV infection or suffering acute hepatitis B during pregnancy
Families adopting children originating from regions of intermediate or high hepatitis B endemicity
Immigrants or refugees from countries of intermediate or high hepatitis B endemicity
Workers whose occupation potentially involves exposure to blood and other body materials (e.g. health care workers and public safety workers)
Patients receiving frequently blood or blood products (e.g. haemophiliacs, haemodialysis patients, transplant patients and chronic liver disease patients)
Unimmunized or uninfected persons who travel to areas of intermediate or high hepatitis B endemicity

2 Universal vaccination programmes. Universal vaccination programmes are needed to eliminate hepatitis B infection, even in areas of low endemicity.

Targeted vaccination of risk groups

Persons with occupational risk

HBV infection is an occupational hazard for health-care workers and for public safety workers exposed to blood in the workplace. The risk of acquiring HBV infections depends on the frequency of percutaneous and permucosal exposure to blood or blood-contaminated body fluids. Therefore, workers who perform tasks involving contact with blood or blood-contaminated body fluid should be vaccinated, and vaccination should be completed during training in schools of medicine, dentistry, nursing, laboratory technology and other allied health professions before trainees have their first contact with blood [74–76].

Haemodialysis patients

Seroconversion rates and anti-HBs titres are lower (50–60%) in haemodialysis patients [77,78]. Vaccination of haemodialysis patients early in the course of renal disease is recommended because those who are vaccinated before entering dialysis are more likely to respond to the vaccine. Booster doses are necessary to maintain protective titres of anti-HBs [79–82].

Recipients of blood products

Patients receiving clotting factor concentrates, such as haemophiliacs or patients with β-thalassaemia major, are at greater risk of HBV infection, and they should be vaccinated as soon as their specific clotting disorder is identified [83,84].

Prevention of perinatal HBV transmission

Control of perinatal transmission can be achieved by delivering the first dose of vaccine at birth. This prophylactic strategy is very efficient in preventing chronic infection, bearing in mind that 70–90% of infants born to HBsAg-positive mothers become infected, 90% of whom remain chronically infected [41,85–90].

The prevention of perinatal HBV transmission (from mother to neonate) by universal antenatal screening for HBV markers in pregnant women should be encouraged where possible. Women who present for delivery without having been screened for HBsAg should be tested immediately. Newborns from HBsAg-positive mothers should be vaccinated within 12 h of birth. In cases where hepatitis B immune globulin (HBIG, 0.06 mL/kg, not available in all countries) is given, it should be administered concurrently with hepatitis B vaccine, but at a different site. Recent evidence suggests that vaccine alone may be just as effective [91]. HBsAg-positive mothers should not be discouraged from breastfeeding [92–95].

Household contacts and sexual partners of persons with hepatitis B virus infection

Hepatitis B vaccine is indicated in infants if the mother or primary caregiver has acute HBV infection. Prophylaxis for other household contacts of persons with acute HBV infection is not indicated unless they have had identifiable blood exposure to the index case. All household and sexual contacts of persons identified as chronically HBsAg positive should receive hepatitis B vaccine after performing a screening for serum HBV markers. The vaccine is not recommended for persons who have casual contact with chronic carriers at schools and offices as they have little risk of catching HBV.

Susceptible sexually active homosexual and bisexual men should be vaccinated, as vaccination remains the most effective tool for preventing hepatitis B in homosexual men [96,97]. Vaccination is also recommended for men and women with other recently acquired sexually transmitted diseases, for prostitutes and for persons who have a history of high sexual promiscuity [98]. Administering the vaccine with HBIG may improve the efficacy of postexposure prophylaxis.

Adopted or fostered orphans or unaccompanied minors originating from countries where HBV infection is endemic should be screened for HBsAg and, if the children are HBsAg positive, the other family members should be vaccinated [99,100].

International travellers

Hepatitis B is less common than hepatitis A and particularly affects those who engage in sexual activity abroad or who are exposed occupationally. Vaccination should be considered for persons who plan to spend more than 6 months in areas with high rates of HBV infection or who will have close contact with the local population. Vaccination should begin at least 6 months before travel to allow for completion of the full vaccine schedule, although a partial schedule will offer some protection. Rapid schedules can also be considered for last-minute travellers (0, 7, 21 and 360 days) [101].

Injecting illicit substance users

All injecting substance users who are susceptible to HBV should be vaccinated as soon as their drug use begins. Because of the high rate of HBV infection in this population, prevaccination screening should be considered. Drug users who do not respond to vaccination should be counselled [99].

Long-term prisoners

In many facilities the rates of HBV and HCV infection among prison inmates are high [102]. Prison officials should consider undertaking screening and vaccination programmes directed at inmates with histories of high-risk behaviour [99,103]. It may be appropriate to use the accelerated vaccination schedules, which provide protective levels of anti-HBs relatively quickly.

Universal immunization

Selected vaccination strategies targeted to identifiable high-risk groups failed to control transmission in the population and to reduce the incidence and prevalence of hepatitis B. This stimulated the recommendation for universal immunization programmes. Universal vaccination of infants is the best option because vaccines can be delivered to babies with a very high coverage and it is more acceptable to parents [104]. The World Health Organization (WHO) recommended in 1992 that all countries should introduce universal hepatitis B vaccination for the immunization of infants and adolescents into their national immunization programmes by December 1997 [68].

The impact of mass hepatitis B immunization on the chronic consequences of infection was first demonstrated in Taiwan. The HBsAg prevalence in the population of < 15-year-olds decreased from 9.8% (1984) to 0.7% (1999) [105], and, in children aged 6–14 years, the incidence of primary liver cancer declined from 0.7/100 000 in the period 1981–1986 to 0.57/100 000 in 1986–1990 and to 0.36/100 000 in 1990–1996 [53].

Proof of the decreasing incidence of acute hepatitis B after vaccination is also available from Italy, the first industrialized country to introduce routine immunization in a double cohort of subjects, i.e. infants and 12-year-old adolescents, leading to an all-time low for acute hepatitis B infection [54].

Similar successes induced by the universal vaccination of neonates were reported from Bulgaria [106] and Alaska (an area of traditionally high endemicity) [16].

As of today, 151 (WHO 2005) countries have implemented universal infant and/or adolescent vaccination against hepatitis B. However, many low-income countries do not yet use the vaccine, because the price of the hepatitis B vaccine is too expensive. The Global Alliance for Vaccines and Immunization (GAVI) was created in 1999. GAVI is helping 74 low-income countries to reinforce their national vaccine programmes and introduce hepatitis B vaccines into their national immunization programmes.

Some industrialized countries administer the vaccine to adolescents as their primary immunization strategy [84,107–

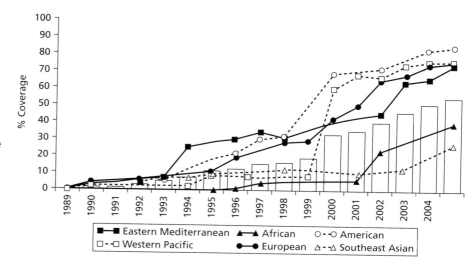

Fig. 1 Global and regional immunization at the third dose of hepatitis B vaccine in infants, 1989–2005. Bars show global coverage, symbols regional coverage as follows: Eastern Mediterranean (closed squares); Western Pacific (open squares); Europe (closed circles); the Americas (open circles); Africa (closed triangles); Southeast Asia (open triangles). Data courtesy of WHO and UNICEF.

109], either in addition to the universal infant immunization programme or as a catch-up vaccination for adolescents aged 9–18 years; combined universal early adolescent and infant vaccination programmes were shown to have the fastest impact on reducing levels of hepatitis B infection [110].

Combination vaccines serve as a vehicle to meet the goal of accelerating new vaccine use, although the process should be carefully managed to ensure affordability without jeopardizing the existing vaccination polices [11].

Immunization programme sustainability

To ensure that vaccine programmes are sustained over time, hepatitis B prevention programmes must be monitored, evaluated and updated. Efforts must focus on monitoring vaccination coverage and checking the incidence of acute disease [112,113].

Economic considerations

In industrialized countries, various economic evaluations have been performed in order to support decision-making; practically all evaluations have used models to predict the cost-effectiveness of immunization against hepatitis B. The complexity of HBV disease outcomes not only leads to a wide range of divergent cost-effectiveness ratios, but it also emphasizes unresolved methodological issues in economic evaluation, with discounting of health gains being one of the main factors of divergent opinions. These controversial results have raised suspicion about the validity and usefulness of economic evaluations among a number of policy-makers. However, the more frequent use of expensive therapies (including liver transplantation) and the sharp decrease in vaccination costs have made universal HBV vaccination strategies cost-effective when compared with other interventions in health care throughout most of the world [114–117].

In countries of very low HBV endemicity, doubts about universal immunization persist because of contradictory results

from cost-effectiveness evaluations. Nevertheless, the decision to implement universal immunization should not just be based on economic considerations, particularly in the light of the insufficient credibility of economic evaluations.

Little academic research has been carried out on the economics of combined vaccines [118].

The current status of hepatitis B immunization

To date 158 countries have followed the WHO recommendation to incorporate hepatitis B vaccine as an integral part of their national infant immunization programmes. Figure 1 presents global and regional summaries based on official data from member states. In recent years, the significantly reduced price of hepatitis B vaccine in developing countries has facilitated its introduction into many HBV-endemic areas, to the extent that global immunization coverage in infants reached 55% in 2005. HepB3 coverage has steadily increased since 1990 as a result of the increasing number of countries introducing the vaccine into their routine immunization services, as well as increasing coverage in these countries. Despite this steady progress, there is still room for improvement. The cost-effectiveness of large-scale vaccination against hepatitis B has also been clearly demonstrated, except in countries of very low endemicity, where economic evaluations have given contradictory results, depending on the model used.

References

1 Lavanchy D (2005) Worldwide epidemiology of HBV infection, disease burden, and vaccine prevention. *J Clin Virol* 34, S1–S3.
2 Gay N, Edmunds W, Bah E *et al.* (2001) *Estimating the Global Burden of Hepatitis B.* Geneva: World Health Organization Department of Vaccines and Biologicals.

3 Parkin DM, Bray F, Ferlay J *et al.* (2001) Estimating the world cancer burden: Globocan 2000. *Int J Cancer* 94, 153–156.

4 Hall A (1998) We have a cancer vaccine – why don't we use it? *Trop Med Int Health* 3, 337–338.

5 Krugman S, Giles JP, Hammond J (1971) Viral hepatitis, type B (MS-2 strain). Studies on active immunization. *J Am Med Assoc* 217, 41–45.

6 Maupas P, Goudeau A, Coursaget P *et al.* (1976) Immunisation against hepatitis B in man. *Lancet* 1, 1367–1370.

7 Purcell RH, Gerin JL (1975) Hepatitis B subunit vaccine: a preliminary report of safety and efficacy tests in chimpanzees. *Am J Med Sci* 270, 395–399.

8 Hilleman MR, Buynak EB, Roehm RR *et al.* (1976) Purified and inactivated human hepatitis B vaccine. *Am J Med Sci* 270, 401–404.

9 Valenzuela P, Medina A, Rutter WJ *et al.* (1982) Synthesis and assembly of hepatitis B surface antigen particles in yeast. *Nature* 298, 347–350.

10 Andre FE, Safary A (1988) Clinical experience with a yeast derived hepatitis B vaccine. In: Zuckerman AJ (ed.) *Viral Hepatitis and Liver Disease*. New York: Alan R. Liss.

11 VHPB (Viral Hepatitis Prevention Board) (2002) Combined hepatitis B vaccines. *Viral Hepat* 10, 1–20.

12 Chunsuttiwat S, Biggs BA, Maynard JE *et al.* (2002) Comparative evaluation of a combined DTP-HB vaccine in the EPI in Chiangrai Province, Thailand. *Vaccine* 21, 188–193.

13 Ramkissoon A, Coovadia HM, Jugnundan P *et al.* (2001) A new combined DTP-HBV-Hib vaccine – strategy for incorporation of Hib vaccination into childhood immunisation programmes. *S Afr Med J* 91, 864–869.

14 Nolan T, Hogg G, Darcy MA *et al.* (2001) A combined liquid Hib (PRP-OMPC), hepatitis B, diphtheria, tetanus and whole-cell pertussis vaccine: controlled studies of immunogenicity and reactogenicity. *Vaccine* 19, 2127–2137.

15 Papaevangelou G (1998) Current combined vaccines with hepatitis B. *Vaccine* 16 (Suppl), 69–72.

16 Harpaz R, McMahon BJ, Margolis HS *et al.* (2000) Elimination of new chronic hepatitis B virus infections: results of the Alaska immunization program. *J Infect Dis* 181, 413–418.

17 Hsu HM, Chen DS, Chuang CH *et al.* (1988) Efficacy of a mass hepatitis B vaccination program in Taiwan. Studies on 3464 infants of hepatitis B surface antigen-carrier mothers. *J Am Med Assoc* 260, 2231–2235.

18 Heerman KH, Goldmann U, Schwartz W *et al.* (1984) Large surface proteins of hepatitis B virus containing the pre-S sequence. *J Virol* 52, 396–402.

19 Neurath AR, Kent SBH, Strick N *et al.* (1985) Hepatitis B virus contains pre-S gene-encoded domains. *Nature* 315, 154–156.

20 Milich DR, Thornton GB, Neurath AR *et al.* (1985) Enhanced immunogenicity of the pre-S region of hepatitis B surface antigen. *Science* 228, 1195–1199.

21 Suzuki H, Iino S, Shiraki K *et al.* (1994) Safety and efficacy of a recombinant yeast-derived pre-S2 + S-containing hepatitis B vaccine (TGP-943): phase 1, 2 and 3 clinical testing. *Vaccine* 12, 1090–1096.

22 Kuroda S, Fujisawa Y, Iino S *et al.* (1991) Induction of protection level of anti-pre-S2 antibodies in humans immunized with a novel hepatitis B vaccine consisting of M (pre-S2 + S) protein particles (a third generation vaccine). *Vaccine* 9, 163–169.

23 Yamada K, Kotani M, Eguchi T *et al.* (1998) Efficacy of hepatitis B vaccines with and without preS2-region product in Sumo wrestlers in Japan. *Hepatol Res* 12, 3–11.

24 Shapira MY, Zeira E, Adler R *et al.* (2001) Rapid seroprotection against hepatitis B following the first dose of a Pre-S1/Pre-S2/S vaccine. *J Hepatol* 34, 123–127.

25 Mancini-Bourgine M, Fontaine H, Scott-Algara D *et al.* (2004) Induction or expansion of T-cell responses by a hepatitis B DNA vaccine administered to chronic HBV carriers. *Hepatology* 40, 874–882.

26 Tacket CO, Roy MJ, Widera G *et al.* (1999) Phase 1 safety and immune response studies of a DNA vaccine encoding hepatitis B surface antigen delivered by a gene delivery device. *Vaccine* 17, 2826–2829.

27 Davis HL, McCluskie MJ, Gerin JL *et al.* (1996) DNA vaccine for hepatitis B: evidence for immunogenicity in chimpanzees and comparison with other vaccines. *Proc Natl Acad Sci USA* 93, 7213–7218.

28 Chen X, Li M, Le X *et al.* (2004) Recombinant hepatitis B core antigen carrying preS1 epitopes induce immune response against chronic HBV infection. *Vaccine* 22, 439–446.

29 Yang HJ, Chen M, Cheng T *et al.* (2005) Expression and immuno-activity of chimeric particulate antigens of receptor binding site-core antigen of hepatitis B virus. *World J Gastroenterol* 11, 492–497.

30 Podda A, Del Giudice G (2003) MF59-adjuvanted vaccines: increased immunogenicity with an optimal safety profile. *Expert Rev Vaccines* 2, 197–203.

31 Heineman TC, Clements-Mann ML, Poland GA *et al.* (1999) A randomized, controlled study in adults of the immunogenicity of a novel hepatitis B vaccine containing MF59 adjuvant. *Vaccine* 17, 2769–2778.

32 Yang HZ, Xu S, Liao XY *et al.* (2005) A novel immunostimulator, N-[alpha-O-benzyl-N-(acetylmuramyl)-L-alanyl-D-isoglutaminyl]-N6-trans-(m-nitrocinnamoyl)-L-lysine, and its adjuvancy on the hepatitis B surface antigen. *J Med Chem* 48, 5112–5122.

33 Elias F, Flo J, Rodriguez JM *et al.* (2005) PyNTTTTGT prototype oligonucleotide IMT504 is a potent adjuvant for the recombinant hepatitis B vaccine that enhances the Th1 response. *Vaccine* 23, 3597–3603.

34 Vandepapeliere P, Rehermann B, Koutsoukos M *et al.* (2005) Potent enhancement of cellular and humoral immune responses against recombinant hepatitis B antigens using AS02A adjuvant in healthy adults. *Vaccine* 23, 2591–2601.

35 Cooper CL, Davis HL, Morris ML *et al.* (2004) CPG 7909, an immunostimulatory TLR9 agonist oligodeoxynucleotide, as adjuvant to Engerix-B HBV vaccine in healthy adults: a double-blind phase I/II study. *J Clin Immunol* 24, 693–701.

36 Boland G, Beran J, Lievens M *et al.* (2004) Safety and immunogenicity profile of an experimental hepatitis B vaccine adjuvanted with AS04. *Vaccine* 23, 316–320.

37 Joseph A, Louria-Hayon I, Plis-Finarov A *et al.* (2002) Liposomal immunostimulatory DNA sequence (ISS-ODN): an efficient parenteral and mucosal adjuvant for influenza and hepatitis B vaccines. *Vaccine* 20, 3342–3354.

38 Thoelen S, De Clercq N, Tornieporth N (2001) A prophylactic hepatitis B vaccine with a novel adjuvant system. *Vaccine* 19, 2400–2403.

39 Mahoney F, Kane M (1999) Hepatitis B vaccine. In: Plotkin SA, Orenstein WA (eds) *Vaccines*, 3rd edn. Philadelphia: W.B. Saunders Co., pp. 158–182.

40 Liao SS, Li RC, Li H *et al.* (1999) Long-term efficacy of plasma-derived hepatitis B vaccine: a 15-year follow-up study among Chinese children. *Vaccine* 17, 2661–2666.

41 Chen HL, Chang MH, Ni YH *et al.* (1996) Seroepidemiology of hepatitis B virus infection in children: Ten years of mass vaccination in Taiwan. *J Am Med Assoc* 276, 906–908.

42 Zanetti AR, Mariano A, Romano L *et al.* (2005) Long-term immunogenicity of hepatitis B vaccination and policy for booster: an Italian multicentre study. *Lancet* 366, 1379–1384.

43 European Consensus Group on Hepatitis B Immunity (2000) Are booster immunisations needed for lifelong hepatitis B immunity? *Lancet* 355, 561–565.

44 FitzSimons D, Francois G, Hall A *et al.* (2005) Long-term efficacy of hepatitis B vaccine, booster policy, and impact of hepatitis B virus mutants. *Vaccine* 23, 4158–4166.

45 John TJ, Cooksley G (2005) Hepatitis B vaccine boosters: is there a clinical need in high endemicity populations? *J Gastroenterol Hepatol* 20, 5–10.

46 Harrison TJ, Hopes EA, Oon CJ *et al.* (1991) Independent emergence of a vaccine-induced escape mutant of hepatitis B virus. *J Hepatol* 13, S105–107.

47 Hollinger FB, Liang TJ (2001) Hepatitis B virus. In: Knipe DM, Hawley PM (eds) *Fields Virology*. Philadelphia, PA: Lippincott Williams & Wilkins, pp. 2971–3036.

48 Zuckerman AJ (2000) Effect of hepatitis B virus mutants on efficacy of vaccination. *Lancet* 355, 1382–1384.

49 Whittle H, Jaffar S, Wansbrough M *et al.* (2002) Observational study of vaccine efficacy 14 years after trial of hepatitis B vaccination in Gambian children. *Br Med J* 325, 569.

50 McMahon BJ, Bruden DL, Petersen KM *et al.* (2005) Antibody levels and protection after hepatitis B vaccination: results of a 15-year follow-up. *Ann Intern Med* 142, 333–341.

51 Yuen MF, Lim WL, Chan AO *et al.* (2004) 18-year follow-up study of a prospective randomized trial of hepatitis B vaccinations without booster doses in children. *Clin Gastroenterol Hepatol* 2, 941–945.

52 Mele A, Tancredi F, Romano L *et al.* (2001) Effectiveness of hepatitis B vaccination in babies born to hepatitis B surface antigen-positive mothers in Italy. *J Infect Dis* 184, 905–908.

53 Chang MH, Chen CJ, Lai MS *et al.* (1997) Universal hepatitis B vaccination in Taiwan and the incidence of hepatocellular carcinoma in children. Taiwan Childhood Hepatoma Study Group. *N Engl J Med* 336, 1855–1859.

54 Stroffolini T, Mele A, Tosti ME *et al.* (2000) The impact of the hepatitis B mass immunisation campaign on the incidence and risk factors of acute hepatitis B in Italy. *J Hepatol* 33, 980–985.

55 Marwick C, Mitka M (1999) Debate revived on hepatitis B vaccine value. *J Am Med Assoc* 282, 15–17.

56 Anon (2002) Global advisory committee on vaccine safety. *Weekly Epidemiol Rec* 77, 389–404.

57 VHPB (2003) Hepatitis B vaccination: safety issues. *Viral Hepat* 12, 1–14.

58 WHO (1997) Expanded programme on immunization (EPI). Lack of evidence that hepatitis B vaccine causes multiple sclerosis. *Weekly Epidemiol Rec* 72, 149–152.

59 Ascherio A, Zhang SM, Hernan MA *et al.* (2001) Hepatitis B vaccination and the risk of multiple sclerosis. *N Engl J Med* 344, 327–332.

60 Jacobson DL, Gange SJ, Rose NR *et al.* (1997) Epidemiology and estimated population burden of selected autoimmune diseases in the United States. *Clin Immunol Immunopathol* 84, 223–243.

61 Committee Board of Health Promotion and Disease Prevention (2001) Thimerosol-containing vaccines and neurodevelopmental disorders. In: National Academy Press (ed.) *Immunization Safety Review*. Washington, DC: Institute of Medicine.

62 Clements CJ (2004) The evidence for the safety of thiomersal in newborn and infant vaccines. *Vaccine* 22, 1854–1861.

63 WHO position paper (1998) Hepatitis B immunization. *Weekly Epidemiol Rec* 73, 329.

64 Kane A, Lloyd J, Zaffran M *et al.* (1999) Transmission of hepatitis B, hepatitis C and human immunodeficiency viruses through unsafe injections in the developing world: model-based regional estimates. *Bull WHO* 77, 801–807.

65 WHO (2005) Global status of immunization safety: report based on the WHO/UNICEF Joint Reporting. *Weekly Epidemiol Rec* 80, 361–368.

66 Kane M (1995) Global programme for control of hepatitis B infection. *Vaccine* 13, S47–S49.

67 Grosheide P, van Damme P (1996) Prevention and control of hepatitis B in the community. *Commun Dis Ser* 1, 1–60.

68 Scientific Advisory Group of Experts (SAGE) (1996) Hepatitis B control through immunization. *WHO Global Programme for Vaccines and Immunization*, GPV/SAGE.96/WP.02.

69 Prince AM (1990) Control of hepatitis B virus infection in Third-World countries. *Transfus Med Rev* 4, 187–190.

70 Mahoney FJ (1999) Update on diagnosis, management, and prevention of hepatitis B virus infection. *Clin Microbiol Rev* 12, 351–366.

71 Bonanni P, Pesavento G, Bechini A *et al.* (2003) Impact of universal vaccination programmes on the epidemiology of hepatitis B: 10 years of experience in Italy. *Vaccine* 21, 685–691.

72 van Steenbergen JE (2002) Results of an enhanced-outreach programme of hepatitis B vaccination in the Netherlands (1998–2000) among men who have sex with men, hard drug users, sex workers and heterosexual persons with multiple partners. *J Hepatol* 37, 507–513.

73 Zanetti AR, Tanzi E, Romano L *et al.* (1993) Vaccination against hepatitis B: the Italian strategy. *Vaccine* 11, 521–524.

74 Bonanni P, Bonaccorsi G (2001) Vaccination against hepatitis B in health care workers. *Vaccine* 19, 2389–2394.

75 Mast EE, Alter MJ (1992) Prevention of hepatitis B virus infection among healthcare workers. In: Ellis RS (ed.) *Hepatitis B Vaccines in Clinical Practice*. New York: Marcel Dekker, pp. 295–307.

76 Roggendorf M, Viazov S (2003) Health care workers and hepatitis B. *J Hepatol* 39, S89–92.

77 Mannucci PM, Zanetti AR, Gringeri A *et al.* (1989) Long-term immunogenicity of a plasma-derived hepatitis B vaccine in HIV seropositive and HIV seronegative hemophiliacs. *Arch Intern Med* 149, 1333–1337.

78 Stevens CE, Alter HJ, Taylor PE *et al.* (1984) Hepatitis B vaccine in patients receiving hemodialysis. Immunogenicity and efficacy. *N Engl J Med* 311, 496–501.

79 Busek SU, Baba EH, Tavares Filho HA *et al.* (2002) Hepatitis C and hepatitis B virus infection in different hemodialysis units in Belo Horizonte, Minas Gerais, Brazil. *Mem Inst Oswaldo Cruz* 97, 775–778.

80 Hutin YJ, Goldstein ST, Varma JK *et al.* (1999) An outbreak of hospital-acquired hepatitis B virus infection among patients receiving chronic hemodialysis. *Infect Control Hosp Epidemiol* 20, 731–735.

81 Alter MJ, Favero MS, Francis DP (1983) Cost benefit of vaccination for hepatitis B in hemodialysis centers. *J Infect Dis* 148, 770–771.

82 Zoulim F (1999) Hepatitis C virus infection in special groups. *J Hepatol* 31, 130–135.

83 Schreiber GB, Busch MP, Kleinman SH *et al.* (1996) The risk of transfusion-transmitted viral infections. *N Engl J Med* 334, 1685–1690.

84 Alter MJ (2003) Epidemiology and prevention of hepatitis B. *Semin Liver Dis* 23, 39–46.

85 Mast EE, Alter MJ, Margolis HS (1999) Strategies to prevent and control hepatitis B and C virus infections: a global perspective. *Vaccine* 17, 1730–1733.

86 Edmunds WJ, Medley GF, Nokes DJ (1996) The transmission dynamics and control of hepatitis B virus in The Gambia. *Stat Med* 15, 2215–2233.

87 Beasley RP, Hwang LY, Lee GC *et al.* (1983) Prevention of perinatally transmitted hepatitis B virus infections with hepatitis B virus infections with hepatitis B immune globulin and hepatitis B vaccine. *Lancet* 2, 1099–1102.

88 Zanetti AR, Dentico P, Del Vecchio Blanco C *et al.* (1986) Multicenter trial on the efficacy of HBIG and vaccine in preventing perinatal hepatitis B. Final report. *J Med Virol* 18, 327–334.

89 VHPB (1998) VHPB recommendations on prevention of perinatal HBV transmission. *Viral Hepat* 7, 1–12.

90 Tsebe KV, Burnett RJ, Hlungwani NP *et al.* (2001) The first five years of universal hepatitis B vaccination in South Africa: evidence for elimination of HBsAg carriage in under 5-year-olds. *Vaccine* 19, 3919–3926.

91 Yang YJ, Liu CC, Chen TJ *et al.* (2003) Role of hepatitis B immunoglobulin in infants born to hepatitis B e antigen-negative carrier mothers in Taiwan. *Pediatr Infect Dis J* 22, 584–588.

92 Burke J (2005) Breastfeeding. *Am J Nurs* 105, 15.

93 Hill JB, Sheffield JS, Kim MJ *et al.* (2002) Risk of hepatitis B transmission in breast-fed infants of chronic hepatitis B carriers. *Obstet Gynecol* 99, 1049–1052.

94 Wang JS, Zhu QR, Wang XH (2003) Breastfeeding does not pose any additional risk of immunoprophylaxis failure on infants of HBV carrier mothers. *Int J Clin Pract* 57, 100–102.

95 World Health Organization (1998) Hepatitis B and breastfeeding. *J Int Assoc Phys AIDS Care* 4, 20–21.

96 Gerbase AC, Rowley JT, Heymann DH *et al.* (1998) Global prevalence and incidence estimates of selected curable STDs. *Sex Transm Infect* 74, S12–16.

97 Piot P, Goilav C, Kegels E (1990) Hepatitis B: transmission by sexual contact and needle sharing. *Vaccine* 8, S37–40; discussion S41–33.

98 Alter MJ, Hadler SC, Margolis HS *et al.* (1990) The changing epidemiology of hepatitis B in the United States. Need for alternative vaccination strategies. *J Am Med Assoc* 263, 1218–1222.

99 Recommendations of the Immunization Practices Advisory Committee (ACIP) (1991) Hepatitis B virus: a comprehensive strategy for eliminating transmission in the United States through universal childhood vaccination:. *Morbidity Mortality Weekly Rep* 40, 1–19.

100 Hershow RC, Hadler SC, Kane MA (1987) Adoption of children from countries with endemic hepatitis B: transmission risks and medical issues. *Pediatr Infect Dis J* 6, 431–437.

101 Bock HL, Loscher T, Scheiermann N *et al.* (1995) Accelerated schedule for hepatitis B immunization. *J Travel Med* 2, 213–217.

102 Butler TG, Dolan KA, Ferson MJ *et al.* (1997) Hepatitis B and C in New South Wales prisons: prevalence and risk factors. *Med J Aust* 166, 127–130.

103 Spaulding AC, Lally M, Rich JD *et al.* (1999) Hepatitis B and C in the context of HIV disease: implications for incarcerated populations. *AIDS Read* 9, 481–491.

104 Zuckerman AJ (1996) Hepatitis viruses. In: Baron S. (ed.) *Medical Microbiology*, 4th edn. Galveston, TX: The University of Texas Medical Branch at Galveston, pp. 849–863.

105 Ni YH, Chang MH, Huang LM *et al.* (2001) Hepatitis B virus infection in children and adolescents in a hyperendemic area: 15 years after mass hepatitis B vaccination. *Ann Intern Med* 135, 796–800.

106 Gatcheva N, Vladimirova N, Kourtchatova A (1995) Implementing universal vaccination programmes: Bulgaria. *Vaccine* 13 (Suppl 1), S82–83.

107 Kammerlander R, Vaudaux B, Bourquin C *et al.* (1998) Vaccination contre l'hépatite B en Suisse: vers une stratégie globale. *Rev Med Suisse Romande* 118, 335–339.

108 Bonanni P (1998) Universal hepatitis B immunization: infant, and infant plus adolescent immunization. *Vaccine* 16, S17–22.

109 Tepper ML (1998) Universal hepatitis B immunization: young adolescent immunization. *Vaccine* 16, S23–26.

110 WHO (2001) Hepatitis B immunization. Introducing hepatitis B into national immunization services. *Fact sheet* WHO/V&B/01.

111 Stroffolini T, Cialdea L, Tosti ME *et al.* (1997) Vaccination campaign against hepatitis B for 12-year-old subjects in Italy. *Vaccine* 15, 583–585.

112 Henderson DA (1999) Lessons from the eradication campaigns. *Vaccine* 17 (Suppl 3), 53–55.

113 Bonanni P, Colombai R, Gasparini R *et al.* (1999) Impact of routine infant and adolescent hepatitis B vaccination in Tuscany, Central Italy. *Pediatr Infect Dis J* 18, 677–682.

114 Beutels P (2001) Economic evaluations of hepatitis B immunization: a global review of recent studies (1994–2000). *Health Econ* 10, 751–774.

115 Beutels P, Edmunds WJ, Antonanzas F *et al.* (2002) Economic evaluation of vaccination programs; a consensus statement focusing on viral hepatitis. *Pharmacoeconomics* 20, 1–7.

116 Da Villa G, Sepe A (1999) Immunization programme against hepatitis B virus infection in Italy: cost-effectiveness. *Vaccine* 17, 1734–1738.

117 Margolis HS, Coleman PJ, Brown RE *et al.* (1995) Prevention of hepatitis B virus transmission by immunization. An economic analysis of current recommendations. *J Am Med Assoc* 274, 1201–1208.

118 Lieu TA, Black SB, Ray GT *et al.* (2000) The hidden costs of infant vaccination. *Vaccine* 19, 33–41.

119 Rendi-Wagner P, Shouval D, Genton B *et al.* (2006) Comparative immunogenicity of a PreS/S hepatitis B vaccine in non- and low responders to conventional vaccine. *Vaccine* 24, 2781–2789.

9.1.3.iii Therapy of acute viral hepatitis

Markus Cornberg, Heiner Wedemeyer and Michael P. Manns

Introduction

Infection with the common hepatitis viruses A, B, C, D and E can cause acute inflammation in the liver. However, not all patients develop symptoms. For example, the typical symptom jaundice is present in less than one-third of patients with acute hepatitis C virus (HCV) infection. Fortunately, fulminant hepatitis is a rare event; however, acute hepatitis A virus (HAV) and hepatitis B virus (HBV) infection still represent frequent causes of acute liver failure in the US and Europe. While acute hepatitis D is a problem in the Mediterranean area, hepatitis E can cause severe disease, particularly in pregnant women. Two to five per cent of adult patients with acute HBV infection and 50–90% of patients with acute HCV infection develop a persistent infection. A good reason for submitting to antiviral treatment of acute viral hepatitis would be the potential prevention of a persistent infection. However, in this respect, there is no reason to treat acute hepatitis A, and treatment of acute hepatitis B may be questionable because the chance of developing a chronic HBV infection is rather low for immunocompetent adults. Another reason for antiviral therapy may be reduction in the severity of the acute disease. However, this only has a rationale if the available antiviral drug acts quickly and has few side-effects. As long as the role of antiviral therapies needs to be established, only the best supportive care is warranted for patients with acute viral hepatitis. The optimal management includes the timely referral of patients with impending liver failure to specialized centres that offer the option of emergency liver transplantation if fulminant hepatitis develops.

Supportive care for acute viral hepatitis

Patients with acute viral hepatitis need to be monitored to identify those who may develop fulminant hepatitis with the risk of liver failure. Severe acute viral hepatitis is more often caused by HAV and HBV than by HCV. Fulminant hepatitis develops in 0.4% of cases with HAV infection and in 1% of cases with HBV infection [1]. Acute liver failure is seen more often in patients with HBV and hepatitis D superinfection (2.5–6%). Hepatitis E can cause a dramatic course in the third trimester of pregnancy. Fulminant hepatitis due to an acute HCV infection is extremely rare and may only be seen in combination with additional factors (e.g. coinfection, drugs). Transaminases, bilirubin and liver synthesis markers [albumin, international normalized ratio (INR)] should be measured at least twice weekly during the first weeks of infection depending on the individual kinetics of the laboratory values. Patients with signs of severe flare of hepatitis or liver failure should be transferred to a hospital with the capability for liver transplantation. The mortality of fulminant hepatitis (thrombin time < 40%, encephalopathy) is up to 80%, and liver transplantation is the only curative option.

Antiviral therapy of acute hepatitis B

Antiviral therapy in acute hepatitis B can have two aims. First, it may reduce the severity of the disease. Second, treatment should prevent viral reinfection after liver transplantation in the case of fulminant hepatitis B. The course of disease is severe in about one-third of patients with acute hepatitis B infection. Many patients require hospitalization, and recovery is rather slow. Data on the treatment of acute hepatitis B are limited and, thus, recommendations for the treatment of acute hepatitis B vary. One might expect that the strong immune response that causes fulminant hepatitis should eradicate the virus efficiently. However, low levels of viraemia can be detected in most cases with fulminant hepatitis B with sensitive assays [2]. Tillmann and colleagues reported 37 patients with fulminant hepatitis who were treated with lamivudine in order to prevent reinfection after a potential liver transplantation; interestingly, most of the patients recovered in a short time, and only eight patients required liver transplantation (25%) [2]. This rate of terminal liver failure was lower compared with historical control subjects, among whom 70–100% of those with fulminant hepatitis B either died or were transplanted [2–4]. Treated patients had a rapid improvement in liver synthesis (INR) and inflammation (transaminases). The results of this study have led to the recommendation of the German consensus conference to treat fulminant hepatitis B with lamivudine [5]; this recommendation is further supported by several other reports [6,7].

Antiviral therapy of acute hepatitis C

The aim of acute hepatitis C treatment is the prevention of persistent HCV infection. Early therapy in order to reduce the severity of symptoms of acute hepatitis C infection has no justifiable rationale as severe symptoms occur infrequently, fulminant cases are extremely rare, and the only available therapy is based on interferon (IFN)-α and is therefore associated with significant side-effects. However, the reason to treat acute hepatitis C is the risk of progression to chronicity. The rate of chronic evolution is 50–90%, and chronic hepatitis C can progress to liver cirrhosis and hepatocellular carcinoma [8]. The social burden of the HCV infection can be high, particularly for health-care workers. Extrahepatic manifestations of HCV are often troublesome and may not be reversible with viral eradication later on [9]. As a specific vaccine is not yet available, the early treatment of acute HCV infection with IFN-α is the only option to prevent persistent HCV infection; however, the diagnosis of acute primary HCV infection may be difficult, and distinction from the exacerbation of an underlying unrecognized chronic HCV infection may be impossible [10].

Problems in the early treatment of acute hepatitis C

The overall impact of the early treatment of acute HCV infection to prevent chronic disease has limitations. A main problem is that primary HCV infection is usually asymptomatic, and most patients are not identified in the early stages of disease. Another reason is that a number of patients have medical contraindications for IFN or are not suitable for therapy because they frequently use intravenous (i.v.) drugs. There are two concerns in treating active drug addicts with IFN. One problem is the ongoing drug abuse. In cases of successful therapy, the risk of reinfection with HCV is high [11]. Another reason is the side-effect profile of IFN, especially the neuropsychiatric problems during therapy that may result in resuming the drug habit [12]; furthermore, it has been shown that the acceptance of and adherence to antiviral therapy by these patients is low because of side-effects such as depression [13] (Fig. 1).

Nevertheless, in certain circumstances (e.g. good compliance), early treatment may be a chance for a drug addict ultimately to get rid of both in the end, the HCV and the drugs.

Treatment modalities

Efficacy of therapy

Early therapy with IFN monotherapy can prevent chronic hepatitis C in about 90% of patients with symptomatic acute HCV infection. This was shown in many small single-centre studies (14). In an early study, 24 patients with acute HCV infection, most of them i.v. drug addicts, were treated with high daily doses of standard IFN until normalization of transaminases. Chronicity was prevented in 18 of 22 patients who completed therapy [15]. This gave the rationale for the first German multi-centre acute HCV study in which 44 patients with acute HCV infection were treated for 24 weeks with standard IFN (see Fig. 2). All patients responded and were HCV-RNA-negative at the end of treatment, and only one patient demonstrated a relapse [16]. The sustained virological response was longlasting in those patients who could be followed for 52–224 weeks [17]. Several studies have investigated the efficacy of pegylated (PEG)-IFN in patients with acute hepatitis C (see Table 1).

The second German multicentre acute HCV study [12], supported by the German competence network for viral hepatitis [19], recruited twice as many patients in the same time as the first study by Jaeckel *et al.* [16]. The overall sustained viral response (SVR) rates were only 71% in the intention-to-treat analysis. However, patients who were adherent to treatment had a SVR of 89% [12]. Although previous drug abuse did not significantly influence adherence in our study, 6 out of 13 patients who were lost to follow-up had a history of drug abuse. In conclusion, early therapy of patients with acute hepatitis C with IFN or PEG-IFN can be highly successful if the patients are compliant and adherent to therapy; close monitoring during both therapy and follow-up is required, especially in patients

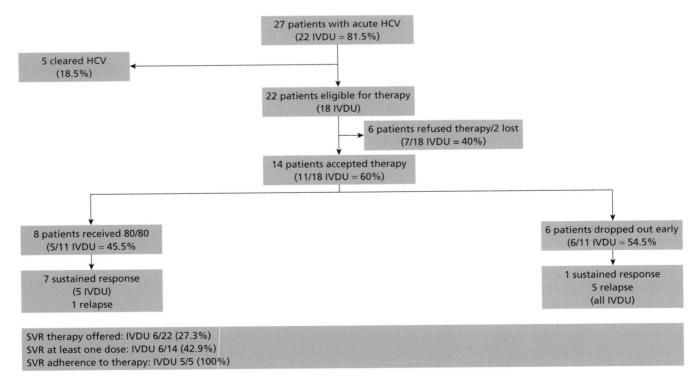

Fig. 1 Low acceptance of therapy and poor compliance of patients with a history of intravenous drug use (IVDU) limit the success of early treatment of acute HCV infection with PEG-IFN. Twenty-two patients with IVDU were eligible for acute HCV therapy: 40% refused therapy and, out of 14 who were treated, less than 50% were adherent to therapy. However, those patients who were compliant and adherent to therapy demonstrated a 100% sustained response.

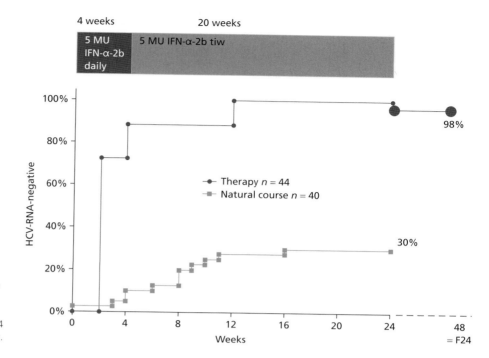

Fig. 2 Treatment schedule and cumulative incidence of undetectable serum HCV RNA during treatment (small circles) and follow-up (large circles). Natural-course patients (small squares) were not treated and demonstrated the expected rate of chronic evolution after 24 weeks of observation. tiw, three times a week.

Table 1 Results of three different studies with PEG-IFN.

Ref. no.	n	Treatment	Start of therapy	Duration	Efficacy
[18]	28	PEG-IFN-α-2b (1.5 µg/kg/week)	12 weeks after onset of disease (17/28 chronic, 16 were treated)	24 weeks	15/16 (94%)
[13]	27 (22 IVDU)	PEG-IFN-α-2b (1.5 µg/kg/week)	100 ± 82 days after onset of symptoms, 63 ± 82 days after diagnosis (asymptomatic) (22/27 chronic, 14 were treated)	24 weeks	8/14 (57%) 7/8 (88%) of adherent patients
[12]	89 recruited in 53 centres	PEG-IFN-α-2b (1.5 µg/kg/week)	76 days after infection (range 14–150 days), 27 days after onset of symptoms (range 5–131 days)	24 weeks	63/89 (71%) 58/65 (89%) of adherent patients

with a history of drug abuse [13]. For certain patients, e.g. those asymptomatic with low alanine aminotransferase (ALT) baseline levels, an induction as used in the Jaeckel study may be considered. The results of the major trials showed that there is no need for a combination with ribavirin [16,20]. Also, the only randomized trial so far demonstrated no further benefit of a ribavirin combination [21]. However, the recent studies with PEG-IFN showed that some patients experienced a relapse after the end of treatment. The question is whether we can avoid the relapse with ribavirin in those patients? Patients with baseline factors that are associated with a lower response (e.g. low ALT value) may require additional ribavirin.

Treatment duration

Most studies treated for 24 weeks [15,22,23]. As in chronic hepatitis C, viral kinetics may predict the response [24,25], and treatment duration can be individually tailored to the viral

kinetics; it may also be possible to treat acute HCV infection for less than 24 weeks in individual cases. However, the treatment of acute HCV infection requires a simple algorithm to avoid complicated management of these difficult to manage patients. Strategies to enhance the adherence to treatment may be more important than further optimizing the already highly efficacious treatment strategy.

Timing of treatment

A most important question is whether the initiation of treatment can wait until one is certain that the patients will not recover spontaneously. This strategy would avoid the unnecessary inconvenience of IFN side-effects and costs in patients recovering spontaneously. A study by Hofer and colleagues demonstrated a high chance of spontaneous recovery from acute HCV infection in symptomatic patients [26]. The time from infection to spontaneous viral clearance was 77 ± 25 days and

35 ± 22 days from the onset of symptoms. The authors suggested that early and frequent HCV-RNA measurements may discriminate patients with spontaneous recovery from those with chronically evolving HCV infection. It appeared that only patients who failed to clear the virus within the first 35 days after the onset of symptoms needed treatment [26]. This information raises the question whether it is wise to wait for about 12 weeks until a chronic course becomes likely and then treat only the patients who are likely to progress to chronic hepatitis C. A study that adopted the wait-and-see strategy demonstrated that treatment of these patients who remain HCV-RNA-positive for more than 12 weeks after the onset of symptoms resulted in an overall SVR (self-limited and treatment induced) in 91% of patients [27,28]. In the natural (untreated) course of acute symptomatic hepatitis C, spontaneous clearance was observed in 52%, usually within 12 weeks after the onset of symptoms, whereas all asymptomatic patients developed chronic hepatitis C. The SVR to the subsequent IFN or IFN/ribavirin treatment started beyond 12 weeks after the onset of acute hepatitis C in those who developed chronic hepatitis C was 80%, independent of the severity of the acute HCV infection. In conclusion, the wait-and-see strategy avoided unnecessary treatment in half the symptomatic patients, but may not be adequate for asymptomatic patients.

Of note, a study from Japan showed that treatment of acute HCV infection may not be as effective after waiting too long. Treatment within 8 weeks after the onset of acute hepatitis resulted in a 100% SVR compared with only 40% when treatment was initiated after 1 year [23].

The treatment of acute hepatitis C is effective regardless of the genotype [16], but the genotype must be taken into account in treatment decisions. The data indicate that patients with HCV genotype 3 may resolve acute HCV infection more frequently than patients with HCV genotype 1 [29]. Considering the high chance of successful treatment of chronic HCV genotype 3 infection with 12–24 weeks of treatment with PEG-IFN-α and ribavirin, it may be wise to avoid early treatment in acute HCV genotype 3 infection, but rather consider the wait-and-see strategy. This concept may be considered in particular for patients with more than one of the factors associated with spontaneous clearance (see Table 2).

The important open questions on the treatment of acute hepatitis C are listed in Table 3.

Postexposure prophylaxis

Postexposure prophylaxis after contact with HCV-contaminated blood (e.g. needlestick) is not necessary. First, the early therapy or the wait-and-see strategy is effective in more than 90% of cases. Second, the use of IFN after exposure to HCV has been shown not to be superior [32].

Concluding remarks

Early identification of patients with acute viral hepatitis infec-

Table 2 Factors potentially associated with spontaneous HCV clearance.

Factors associated with spontaneous clearance	Ref. no.
Symptomatic hepatitis C	[27]
Female gender	[27]
HCV kinetics early after infection	[26]
HCV genotype 3	[29]
HLA B27	[30]
Vigorous T-cell immunity	[31]

HLA, human leukocyte antigen.

Table 3 Questions and best possible answers regarding the therapy of acute HCV infection.

Question	Answer
Is early treatment with IFN effective?	≥ 90% sustained virological response possible
Which patients should be treated?	Asymptomatic > symptomatic? HCV genotype 1 > HCV genotype 2/3
When to start treatment?	Immediately in asymptomatic patients Symptomatic patients: immediate therapy vs. wait-and-see under investigation
Which drugs?	IFN-α (5 MU daily for first 4 weeks) or 1.5 µg/week PEG-IFN-α Ribavirin not necessary
Treatment duration?	24 weeks Shorter may be possible

tion is important for their optimal management. Early referral to a transplant centre is mandatory if patients develop fulminant hepatitis, and best supportive care may prevent further complications in some patients. Antiviral treatment of fulminant hepatitis B with lamivudine can prevent liver failure and reduces the need for liver transplantation. Early measurement of HCV RNA is mandatory in cases of suspicion of acute hepatitis C. Asymptomatic patients have the highest chance of developing chronic hepatitis C and may thus benefit from early (PEG)-IFN-α monotherapy. Symptomatic patients have a high chance of clearing the HCV virus spontaneously. A study is under way to test whether a wait-and-see strategy may be as effective as immediate treatment. Postexposure prophylaxis is not indicated. The future may bring highly effective antiviral drugs that may allow short-term treatment for all acute HCV patients. HCV polymerase and protease inhibitors are the most promising drugs. The first drugs have already been tested in phase I/II trials, and the proof of concept has been demonstrated (reviewed in [33]). The ultimate goal for preventing chronic hepatitis C is a protective vaccine. The first studies in chimpanzees give hope. However, it may not be possible to induce sterilizing immunity, but a less severe course and the prevention of chronic infection may be possible (reviewed in [34]).

References

1 Hoofnagle JH, Carithers RL Jr, Shapiro C et al. (1995) Fulminant hepatic failure: summary of a workshop. *Hepatology* 21(1), 240–252.

2 Tillmann HL, Hadem J, Leifeld L et al. (2006) Safety and efficacy of lamivudine in patients with severe acute or fulminant hepatitis B, a multicenter experience. *J Viral Hepat* 13(4), 256–263.

3 Garfein RS, Bower WA, Loney CM et al. (2004) Factors associated with fulminant liver failure during an outbreak among injection drug users with acute hepatitis B. *Hepatology* 40(4), 865–873.

4 Bernuau J, Goudeau A, Poynard T et al. (1986) Multivariate analysis of prognostic factors in fulminant hepatitis B. *Hepatology* 6(4), 648–651.

5 Manns MP, Wedemeyer H, Meyer S et al. (2004) [Diagnosis, progression and therapy of hepatitis-B-virus infection – results of an evidenced based consensus conference of the German Society for Alimentary Metabolic Disorders and in cooperation with the Hepatitis Competence Network]. *Z Gastroenterol* 42(8), 677–678.

6 Clark FL, Drummond MW, Chambers S et al. (1998) Successful treatment with lamivudine for fulminant reactivated hepatitis B infection following intensive therapy for high-grade non-Hodgkin's lymphoma. *Ann Oncol* 9(4), 385–387.

7 Santantonio T, Mazzola M, Pastore G (1999) Lamivudine is safe and effective in fulminant hepatitis B. *J Hepatol* 30(3), 551.

8 Hoofnagle JH (2002) Course and outcome of hepatitis C. *Hepatology* 36(5 Suppl. 1), S21–S29.

9 Manns MP, Rambusch EG (1999) Autoimmunity and extrahepatic manifestations in hepatitis C virus infection. *J Hepatol* 31(Suppl. 1), 39–42.

10 Pawlotsky JM (2002) Use and interpretation of virological tests for hepatitis C. *Hepatology* 36(5 Suppl. 1), S65–S73.

11 Davis GL, Rodrigue JR (2001) Treatment of chronic hepatitis C in active drug users. *N Engl J Med* 345(3), 215–217.

12 Wiegand J, Buggisch P, Boecher W et al. (2006) Early monotherapy with pegylated interferon alfa-2b for acute hepatitis C infection: The HEP-NET Acute-HCV-II Study. *Hepatology* 43(2), 250–256.

13 Broers B, Helbling B, Francois A et al. (2005) Barriers to interferon-alpha therapy are higher in intravenous drug users than in other patients with acute hepatitis C. *J Hepatol* 42(3), 323–328.

14 Poynard T, Regimbeau C, Myers RP et al. (2002) Interferon for acute hepatitis C. *Cochrane Database Syst Rev* 1, CD000369.

15 Vogel W, Graziadei I, Umlauft F et al. (1996) High-dose interferon-alpha2b treatment prevents chronicity in acute hepatitis C: a pilot study. *Dig Dis Sci* 41(12 Suppl.), 81S–85S.

16 Jaeckel E, Cornberg M, Wedemeyer H et al. (2001) Treatment of acute hepatitis C with interferon alfa-2b. *N Engl J Med* 345(20), 1452–1457.

17 Wiegand J, Jackel E, Cornberg M et al. (2004) Long-term follow-up after successful interferon therapy of acute hepatitis C. *Hepatology* 40(1), 98–107.

18 Santantonio T, Fasano M, Sinisi E et al. (2005) Efficacy of a 24-week course of PEG-interferon alpha-2b monotherapy in patients with acute hepatitis C after failure of spontaneous clearance. *J Hepatol* 42(3), 329–333.

19 Manns MP, Meyer S, Wedemeyer H (2003) The German network of excellence for viral hepatitis (Hep-Net). *Hepatology* 38(3), 543–544.

20 Wedemeyer H, Jackel E, Wiegand J et al. (2004) Whom? When? How? Another piece of evidence for early treatment of acute hepatitis C. *Hepatology* 39(5), 1201–1203.

21 Kamal SM, Ismail A, Graham CS et al. (2004) Pegylated interferon alpha therapy in acute hepatitis C: relation to hepatitis C virus-specific T cell response kinetics. *Hepatology* 39(6), 1721–1731.

22 Delwaide J, Bourgeois N, Gerard C et al. (2004) Treatment of acute hepatitis C with interferon alpha-2b: early initiation of treatment is the most effective predictive factor of sustained viral response. *Aliment Pharmacol Ther* 20(1), 15–22.

23 Nomura H, Sou S, Tanimoto H et al. (2004) Short-term interferon-alfa therapy for acute hepatitis C: a randomized controlled trial. *Hepatology* 39(5), 1213–1219.

24 von Wagner M, Huber M, Berg T et al. (2005) Peginterferon alfa-2a (40KD) and ribavirin for 16 or 24 weeks in patients with genotype 2 or 3 chronic hepatitis C. *Gastroenterology* ??, 000–000.

25 Mangia A, Santoro R, Minerva N et al. (2005) Peginterferon alfa-2b and ribavirin for 12 vs. 24 weeks in HCV genotype 2 or 3. *N Engl J Med* 352(25), 2609–2617.

26 Hofer H, Watkins-Riedel T, Janata O et al. (2003) Spontaneous viral clearance in patients with acute hepatitis C can be predicted by repeated measurements of serum viral load. *Hepatology* 37(1), 60–64.

27 Gerlach JT, Diepolder HM, Zachoval R et al. (2003) Acute hepatitis C: high rate of both spontaneous and treatment-induced viral clearance. *Gastroenterology* 125(1), 80–88.

28 Pimstone NR, Pimstone D, Saicheur T et al. (2004) 'Wait-and-see': an alternative approach to managing acute hepatitis C with high-dose interferon-alpha monotherapy. *Ann Intern Med* 141(6), W91–W92.

29 Lehmann M, Meyer MF, Monazahian M et al. (2004) High rate of spontaneous clearance of acute hepatitis C virus genotype 3 infection. *J Med Virol* 73(3), 387–391.

30 Neumann-Haefelin C, McKiernan S, Ward S et al. (2006) Dominant influence of an HLA-B27 restricted CD8+ T cell response in mediating HCV clearance and evolution. *Hepatology* 43(3), 563–572.

31 Rehermann B, Nascimbeni M (2005) Immunology of hepatitis B virus and hepatitis C virus infection. *Nature Rev Immunol* 5(3), 215–229.

32 Chung H, Kudo M, Kumada T et al. (2003) Risk of HCV transmission after needlestick injury, and the efficacy of short-duration interferon administration to prevent HCV transmission to medical personnel. *J Gastroenterol* 38(9), 877–879.

33 Cornberg M, Manns MP (2005) New approaches and therapeutic modalities for the treatment of patients with chronic hepatitis C. *Ann Hepatol* 4(3), 144–150.

34 Houghton M, Abrignani S (2005) Prospects for a vaccine against the hepatitis C virus. *Nature* 436(7053), 961–966.

9.1.3.iv Antiviral therapy of chronic hepatitis B

Fabien Zoulim and Mario Rizzetto

Pathobiology background

As hepatitis B virus (HBV) replication does not lead by itself to a cytopathic effect, chronic hepatitis B is the result of an ongoing liver injury mediated by the T-cell immune response targeting hepatocytes that harbour HBV replication [1,2]. Our knowledge of the pathobiology of HBV infection has come from clinical studies and from experimental investigations performed in animal models. Viral clearance requires the coordinated action of several components of the immune response [3–6]: (i) a cytotoxic T-helper 1 (Th1) response by CD8-positive cells recognizing infected hepatocytes expressing viral antigens; (ii) a non-cytolytic Th1 response whereby the CD8-positive cells produce Th1 cytokines such as interferon (IFN)-γ, tumour necrosis factor (TNF)α and interleukin (IL)-12, which exhibit a direct antiviral effect in the infected liver; (iii) the innate immune response mediated by natural killer (NK) and NKT cells; (iv) the production of neutralizing antibodies by B cells to prevent the infection of new hepatocytes by residual virions; (v) cell lysis and turnover to generate new uninfected cells that will repopulate the liver.

While there is a consensus on the role of these different effectors, the order of events is still debated. In transgenic mice and acutely infected chimpanzees, several studies have shown a major role for non-cytolytic processes in the immune-mediated clearance of viral infection. In contrast, in the woodchuck and duck models of acute infection, evidence has been obtained that cell lysis and hepatocyte turnover are required to clear infection.

In the setting of chronic infection, antivirals decrease viral production and thus prevent a new round of infection, but also restore the specific CD4- and CD8-mediated immune response following the decrease in viral load in the infected host [7,8]. An HBV load of 10^7 copies/mL appears to be a threshold below which circulating multispecific HBV-specific CD8+ T cells are consistently detected [9]. It is also possible that prolonged antiviral treatment may induce cell curing by inhibiting the intracellular recycling of viral cccDNA. It was also shown that viral persistence during long-term antiviral therapy in the duck and woodchuck models is linked to a long half-life of viral cccDNA [10,11]. Following the development of polymerase chain reaction (PCR)-based assays, the kinetics of viral cccDNA clearance from the liver have been studied in detail in chronically infected patients. The results suggest that viral cccDNA may persist over decades even after the serological clearance of viral infection and that resolution of infection may not occur via sterilizing immunity but by the continuous control of viral infection over time [12,13]. These data suggest that the reservoir of cccDNA may be the source of renewed viral replication and clinical reactivation in case of loss of immunological control, i.e. immunosuppression, organ transplantation, human immunodeficiency virus (HIV) coinfection. It also indicates that antiviral treatment should be maintained until the specific anti-HBV immune response controls the residual low levels of viral replication [13–15].

Unfortunately, long-term therapy exposes to the risk of selection of drug-resistant mutants [16]. Indeed, owing to the spontaneous viral genome variability, the pharmacological pressure may select for the viral species that exhibit the best replication capacity in this new treatment environment. The mutations conferring resistance to nucleoside analogues are located in the viral polymerase gene. The rapidity of selection of drug-resistant mutants depends on their replication capacity and fitness, their level of resistance and the free liver space available for infection by these mutants. This explains the differences in the rate of resistance for the different drugs that are clinically available.

Indication to antiviral therapy

Based on the present knowledge of the natural history of chronic HBV hepatitis and on the efficacy of antiviral drugs, treatment is indicated only in hepatitis B surface antigen (HBsAg) carriers with liver disease.

HBsAg carriers with chronic hepatitis B who should be treated

Antiviral therapy of chronic HBV infection is indicated in patients with chronic hepatitis B in the immunoactive phase. As this phase is characterized by high levels of viral replication and immunomediated damage of HBV-containing hepatocytes, these HBsAg-positive carriers usually have levels of viral DNA in serum higher than 10^4 copies/mL and exhibit elevated serum alanine aminotransferase (ALT) levels.

Liver histology usually shows inflammatory activity and variable degrees of liver fibrosis depending on the duration of the disease. As continuing HBV replication and elevation of ALT levels imply a significant risk of disease progression towards liver cirrhosis and hepatocellular carcinoma [17,18], antiviral therapy is indicated to decrease viral load, normalize ALT levels and induce a remission of the liver disease.

There are two main forms of chronic HBsAg-positive hepatitis [19]. The HBeAg-positive form is associated with a so-called wild-type virus infection, HBsAg and HBeAg positivity, high HBV DNA levels usually > 10^6 copies/mL and elevated ALT levels. The HBeAg-negative form is associated with precore mutant virus infection, HBsAg positivity and HBeAg negativity (most patients have anti-HBe antibody), HBV DNA levels that are fluctuating but usually > 10^4 copies/mL and elevated ALT levels that may also be fluctuating over time. Treatment endpoints differ depending on the form of chronic hepatitis B.

Chronic HBsAg carriers who should not be treated

Patients with chronic HBV infection who are in the immunotolerance phase should not be treated. These individuals represent a minority among chronic HBsAg carriers. They are defined serologically by HBsAg positivity, HBeAg positivity, high HBV DNA levels (usually higher than 10^8 copies/mL) and normal serum ALT levels. They usually have no liver damage or only minimal liver disease at liver biopsy examination, but they are highly infectious. The risk of disease progression is low as long as ALT levels remain within the normal range. The results of clinical trials of IFN-α or nucleoside analogues indicate that patients with high HBV DNA load and normal ALT levels have almost no chance of responding to therapy, i.e. HBeAg seroconversion. However, patients should be monitored carefully on a regular basis to diagnose a break in immune tolerance characterized by an elevation in ALT levels and a decline in viral load. These events reflect the onset of liver damage and may represent an indication for antiviral therapy, unless HBeAg seroconversion (which is the ultimate goal of therapy, see below) occurs spontaneously.

A 6-monthly analysis of ALT levels and HBV DNA is recommended in chronic carriers who are in the immunotolerance phase. Patients' relatives and household contacts should be screened for HBV markers and vaccinated against HBV if not protected.

The other category of patients with chronic HBV infection who should not be treated is the HBsAg inactive carriers. These individuals are the majority among HBsAg carriers. They are characterized by HBsAg positivity, HBeAg negativity, anti-HBe antibody positivity, low HBV DNA levels ($< 10^4$ copies/mL) and normal ALT levels. Liver histology usually shows no or minimal damage, and the risk of progressive liver disease is considered to be minimal as long as ALT levels remain normal and viraemia remains below 10^4 copies/mL. It is currently recommended that these patients should not be treated, but followed carefully to diagnose reactivation of viral replication and ALT exacerbations promptly, should these occur. A 6-monthly follow-up of ALT levels and HBV DNA is suitable to make sure that the inactive state is maintained over time.

Goals of antiviral therapy

The main goal of antiviral therapy is to suppress HBV replication to induce the remission of liver disease activity. In addition, the inhibition of HBV replication decreases patients' infectivity and the risk of HBV transmission. This is especially important in health-care workers. Recent studies suggest that lamivudine therapy of chronically HBV-infected pregnant women during the last trimester of pregnancy increases the protection of newborns who receive hepatitis B immune globulin (HBIG) and vaccine at birth.

In patients with wild-type virus infection, the primary goal of antiviral therapy is to achieve seroconversion from HBeAg to the homologous anti-HBe antibody (referred to hereafter as HBe seroconversion) as this immunological event is associated with a reduction in the risk of progression of the liver disease. Of note, a prior decline in viral load is mandatory to obtain HBe seroconversion, which is subsequently required to achieve seroconversion from HBsAg to the homologous anti-HBs antibody (referred to hereafter as HBs seroconversion).

In patients with an HBeAg-negative chronic hepatitis B, available antiviral agents are effective in suppressing HBV replication but, in most cases, are not capable of eradicating the virus. Therefore, the main objective of therapy is to control viral replication to prevent ALT flares and/or induce remission of disease. The only event marking a sustained response to therapy would be HBs seroconversion to anti-HBs, which unfortunately occurs only seldom.

Different types of responses have been defined during the European Consensus Conference in 2002 [20], i.e. the initial response, the on-treatment or maintained response and the sustained response when antiviral treatment has been stopped. The virological response is defined by the decline in HBV DNA below 10^4 or 10^3 copies/mL, the biochemical response by the normalization of ALT levels and the histological response by improvement in the histological activity or fibrosis indices (Knodell or Ishak or METAVIR scores). The combined response is defined by improvement in ALT levels and decrease in viral load, while the complete response is characterized by the combination of a decrease in viral load, normalization of ALT levels, occurrence of an HBe or HBs seroconversion and histological improvement in liver disease.

The treatment response is also defined depending on the timing during therapy. The initial response is characterized by a decrease in viral load at week 12 of therapy by at least 1 log10 copies/mL compared with the baseline value. The maintained response is defined by a low viral load during therapy (Fig. 1).

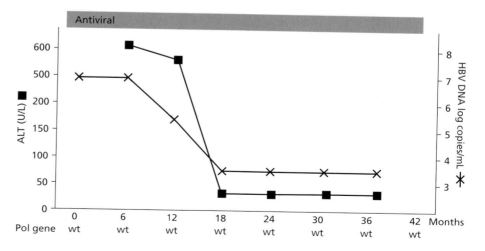

Fig. 1 Maintained antiviral response. wt, wild type HBV polymerase gene sequence.

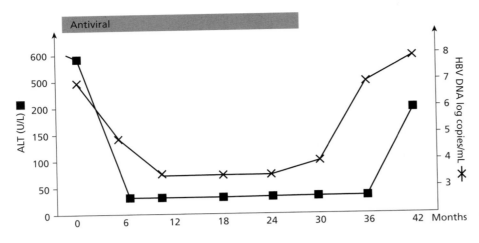

Fig. 2 Relapse after treatment cessation.

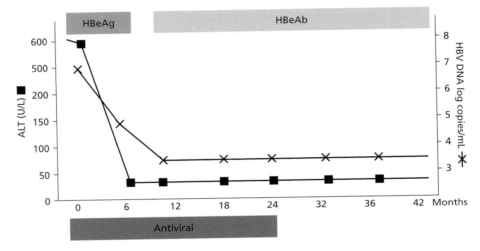

Fig. 3 Sustained antiviral response.

Depending on the use of nucleoside analogue or interferon, there is no agreed threshold to define the maintained response. Usually, a decrease in viral load below 10^4 copies/mL is associated with an improvement in liver histology. However, with nucleoside analogues, the lower the viral load, the less is the risk of developing viral drug resistance. For instance, it was shown that, during lamivudine therapy, the risk of further resistance to treatment was significantly lower when viral load was below 10^3 copies/mL. The end-of-treatment response is defined by the response observed at the end of therapy, if it was decided to stop treatment. A relapse is defined by the increase in viral load after treatment cessation (Fig. 2). The sustained response is defined conventionally by the maintenance of the response 6 months after drug withdrawal (Fig. 3).

Antiviral agents

IFN-α was introduced in clinical practice in the 1980s as initial therapy for chronic hepatitis B. In the 1990s, the advent of nucleoside analogues targeting specific viral functions has provided a therapeutic alternative. However, viral persistence and

the emergence of resistance remain a major challenge to the use of nucleoside analogues, and research continues in an attempt to discover new agents that are more efficacious and less prone to induce viral resistance.

Study models of anti-HBV agents

Antiviral agents have been studied extensively in experimental models, *in vitro* in tissue culture and *in vivo* in ducks and woodchucks [16]. Infection and complete replication including formation of the viral minichromosome (cccDNA), which plays an essential role in the persistence of infection and in the long-term resistance to treatment, can be obtained only in primary cultures of hepatocytes and in the HepaRG cells. Cell culture systems, useful for the screening of anti-HBV compounds and study of their mode of action, are (i) stably transfected hepatoma lines HepG2.2.15 or HepAD38, (ii) transiently transfected hepatoma cell lines [HepG2 or Huh-7 human cells for HBV and LMH avian cells for duck HBV (DHBV)], and (iii) hepatoma cell lines infected via recombinant HBV baculovirus that allow full viral replication including cccDNA formation. Determination of the mode of action has been investigated (i) in primary cultures of hepatocytes taken from the well-characterized animal models of HBV, the duck and the woodchuck, (ii) on endogenous viral DNA- and RNA-dependent DNA polymerase, which can be assayed in purified nucleocapsid or (iii) in a tube reconstituted assay for both priming and reverse transcription of the viral genome. The *in vivo* models allowed the study of the antiviral efficacy, the kinetics of viral clearance, the emergence of drug resistance, as well as the toxicity of the drugs [11,21–24]. All these *in vitro* and animal models contributed to the molecular characterization of the replication cycle of HBV and, consequently, to the identification of viral targets for antiviral therapy of HBV infection [25]: (i) neutralization of the virus–cell interaction with anti-envelope antibodies; (ii) cytokine and/or antisense inhibition of viral transcription and viral gene expression; (iii) packaging inhibition with peptides; (iv) RNA- or DNA-dependent DNA polymerase activity inhibition by nucleoside analogues or antisense; and (v) viral secretion with glucosidase inhibitors.

Immunomodulatory approaches

One strategy to eradicate viral infection consists of the enhancement of the specific immune response, using cytokines such as IFN-α, IFN-γ, TNFα, IL-12 or a viral recombinant protein or plasmid DNA-based vaccine approach. The combination of nucleoside analogues to inhibit viral production with immunomodulatory approaches to eradicate the residual infected hepatocytes (that may support the replication of escape mutants) warrants further evaluation in animal models of hepadnavirus infection and in clinical trials.

Interferon alpha and pegylated IFN

IFN-α belongs to a family of naturally occurring proteins that have antiviral and immunomodulatory actions. They bind to cellular receptors and activate secondary messengers in order to initiate the production of multiple proteins critical to the defence of the cell against viruses. The antiviral effects include degradation of viral mRNA, inhibition of viral protein synthesis and prevention of the viral infection of cells. The immunomodulating effects include enhancement of foreign antigen presentation by human leukocyte antigen (HLA) I and II to the immune system, activation of NK cells and other immune cells and increased cytokine production. IFN-α is obtained by two main methods. It can be either purified from human lymphoblastoid cells, which have been stimulated by Sendai virus, or produced using recombinant molecular biology in *Escherichia coli*. In the latter case, the gene encoding one of the human subtypes (α-2a or α-2b) of interferon is cloned into a bacterial expression vector and used for production. An important advance was the development of slow-release pegylated IFN-α-2a and -α-2b, which exhibit a better antiviral effect than standard interferon. Pegylated IFN is the result of a linkage between standard IFN and polyethylene glycol (PEG), which decreases the kidney

clearance of IFN and therefore increases its half-life, allowing a single injection weekly. The side-effects of pegylated IFN-α-2a and -α-2b are similar to those of standard IFNs and have been described in Chapter 9.1.3.v. It is noteworthy that the rate of depression seems to be lower in patients with chronic hepatitis B than in those with chronic hepatitis C who receive pegylated IFN-α-2a or -α-2b.

Vaccine therapy

A new concept has emerged with the use of HBV vaccine as a therapeutic tool to break immune tolerance. The first attempts were made with recombinant HBsAg vaccines alone or in combination therapy. Early studies suggested a trend towards an increased rate of HBeAg seroconversion and some level of restoration of immune responses against HBV [26]. More recently, the use of a DNA vaccine approach relying on the administration of a DNA plasmid encoding for the viral envelope gene has been evaluated, as it was shown that this strategy may be more effective in the stimulation of the immune response via antigen presentation by dendritic cells [27,28]. A phase I clinical trial has been performed and will be followed by phase II evaluation [29].

Nucleoside/nucleotide analogues

Lamivudine

Lamivudine (β-L-2′,3′-dideoxy-3′thiacytidine or 3TC) is a cytidine analogue that belongs to the L-nucleoside analogue family. After cellular penetration, it is transformed into its triphosphate form by cytidine kinase. Lamivudine triphosphate has a poor affinity for cellular polymerases (i.e. mitochondrial and nuclear polymerases) and is preferentially targeted to viral polymerases, explaining its very good selectivity index [30]. This explains why lamivudine is very well tolerated by the patients and has no significant side-effects. Elimination occurs mainly by kidney filtration, explaining why lamivudine dosage should be adapted to creatinine clearance.

Lamivudine is a potent *in vitro* inhibitor of both duck and human hepadnaviruses, acts as a chain terminator of reverse transcription and has no mitochondrial toxicity. Lamivudine is a very effective inhibitor of DHBV in ducks, and HBV in chimpanzees, but only a moderate inhibitor of the woodchuck hepatitis virus (WHV) in woodchucks. Consistent with the last observation, it was observed that a prolonged 3TC treatment of primary woodchuck hepatocytes infected by WHV does not allow viral eradication. Lamivudine treatment promotes viral resistance [31]. Variants emerging during lamivudine therapy display mutations in the viral polymerase, within the catalytic domain (C-domain), which includes the YMDD motif (e.g. M204V or M204I), and within the B-domain (e.g. L180M or V173L). These mutants have a reduced replicative capacity compared with the wild-type virus. To find an alternative treatment for lamivudine-resistant patients, the susceptibility of these mutants to other drugs has been studied. Two categories of drug have been characterized: those that present a cross-resistance pattern with lamivudine, such as the pyrimidine analogues, i.e. emtricitabine or clevudine, and those that are active against lamivudine-resistant mutants, such as the purine analogues, i.e. adefovir, tenofovir and entecavir. Details on these drugs follow.

Emtricitabine

Emtricitabine (β-L-2'3'-dideoxy-5'fluoro-3'thiacytidine or FTC) is a 5-fluoro-oxathiolane derivative, closely related to lamivudine [32]. Not surprisingly, it exhibits a similar potency as an inhibitor of HBV replication in vitro and in vivo. However, the same profile of resistance has been observed in vitro, as well as in patients treated with emtricitabine who select for the same drug-resistant mutants as those treated with lamivudine. The drug is currently in phase III trial for the treatment of chronic hepatitis B [33].

Clevudine

Clevudine (2'-fluoro-5-methyl-β-L-arabinofuranosyluracil or L-FMAU), a novel β-L-nucleoside analogue derived from deoxythymidine (TTP), is a potent inhibitor of HBV replication in HepG2.2.15 cells and has a low in vitro cytotoxicity [34]. In this cell line, L-FMAU inhibits HBV replication without affecting the host DNA synthetic machinery. In contrast to D-FMAU and D-FIAU, L-FMAU does not decrease mitochondrial DNA content and function and is not incorporated in cellular DNA. L-FMAU exhibits antiviral activity in vivo in the duck and woodchuck model. Interestingly, L-FMAU is a weak inhibitor of reverse transcriptase activity, but mainly an inhibitor of DNA-dependent DNA polymerase activity. Phase II clinical trials have been performed; the drug has been approved recently in Korea.

Adefovir dipivoxil

Adefovir dipivoxil [9-(2-phosphonolmethoxyethyl) adenine or PMEA] is an acyclic phosphonate nucleotide analogue of adenosine monophosphate. Unlike nucleoside analogues, it does not require the first of three phosphorylation steps for conversion to the active triphosphate form. Adefovir diphosphate, the active metabolite of adefovir, is a potent inhibitor of HBV polymerase activity and viral replication in human hepatoma cells lines stably transfected with HBV and in primary duck hepatocytes infected with DHBV [35]. The antihepadnaviral activity of adefovir dipivoxil was also demonstrated in vivo, in the duck model and in woodchucks chronically infected with WHV. Although adefovir dipivoxil is a more potent inhibitor of DHBV replication than lamivudine in experimentally infected ducklings and primary duck hepatocytes, it fails to prevent cccDNA synthesis and accumulation [36]. The most important feature of adefovir dipivoxil resides in its capacity to inhibit the replication of lamivudine-resistant mutants. However, with prolonged administration of the drug, resistant mutants may emerge: rtA181V and rtN236T in the polymerase gene [37,38].

Adefovir is also eliminated by the kidney. Clinical studies have shown a dose-dependent toxicity on kidney tubules, which causes hypophosphoraemia and increased blood creatinine level. Adefovir dipivoxil dosage should also be adapted to creatinine clearance.

Entecavir

Entecavir, also known as BMS-200475, is a cyclopentyl guanosine analogue. It is both a highly potent inhibitor of HBV replication in hepatoma cell lines and among the most potent antiviral agents against WHV [39]. In chronically infected woodchucks, long-term antiviral therapy with entecavir leading to control of viral replication allowed delay in the onset of hepatocellular carcinoma [40]. This compound inhibits the priming and elongation of minus strand DNA synthesis as well as DNA-dependent DNA polymerase by its incorporation in the DNA strand in exchange for the natural dGTP [41]. Cross-resistance testing in tissue culture showed that entecavir exhibits a reduced inhibitory activity against lamivudine-resistant mutants [42]. Furthermore, it was shown that the first cases of entecavir resistance occurred in patients who were treated for lamivudine failure, with the entecavir resistance mutations in the viral polymerase adding up on a background of lamivudine resistance [43].

Tenofovir

Tenofovir disoproxil fumarate is the prodrug of tenofovir (PMPA). Tenofovir is active in vitro and in vivo against both wild-type and lamivudine-resistant strains of HIV and HBV [44]. This antiviral profile makes its use very interesting in HIV–HBV coinfected patients.

Telbivudine

Telbivudine (β-L-2'-deoxythymidine) is an orally bioavailable L-nucleoside with potent anti-HBV activity in vitro and in the woodchuck hepadnavirus model, and a favourable preclinical toxicological profile [45,46].

Combination of drugs

The concept of combination therapy in chronic hepatitis B virus infection is becoming a critical issue to overcome the problem of persistence and selection of drug-resistant mutants [16,47]. To be suitable, combination of drugs must achieve at least an additive and, in the best case, a synergistic effect and prevent or delay the occurrence of drug resistance. The use of a combination should also allow reduction in the dosage of each drug, thus reducing the risk of toxicity. The combination of polymerase inhibitors is one of the potential approaches. To obtain a synergistic antiviral effect, a combination of nucleoside analogues exhibiting different mode of actions (antipriming, anti-elongation, purine analogues, pyrimidine analogues) is expected to be the best option. A few studies have shown that the combination of lamivudine with penciclovir and/or adefovir may synergistically inhibit DHBV replication in primary duck hepatocyte cultures. This should decrease on a statistical basis the risk of selection of polymerase mutants. The combination of compounds with different patterns of viral resistance will also be required to further decrease the risk of selecting multiple drug-resistant mutants [48,49].

Treatment of the clinical forms of chronic hepatitis B

Wild-type virus infection, i.e. HBeAg-positive chronic hepatitis B

In this setting, the goal is to achieve HBe seroconversion, which usually results in remission of the liver disease. There are currently two treatment options: the use of a finite course of standard or pegylated IFN or long-term therapy with nucleoside analogues. The choice should depend on the evaluation of factors predictive of treatment response, the past history of the patient (contraindications to IFN for instance), his/her lifestyle, the desire for a pregnancy, as well as the personal choice of the patient (Table 1).

Results of standard IFN-α

Administration of standard IFN induces a sustained response, defined by HBe seroconversion 24 weeks after treatment, in 20–40% of patients depending on patient characteristics, while only 5–10% of patients seroconvert in the placebo group [50,51]. Patients with high ALT levels, a high histology activity index (HAI) score and low HBV DNA levels have a higher chance of HBe seroconversion (> 40%). Response is marked by the clearance of serum HBV DNA and an increase in ALT levels during the second or third month of therapy, which reflects the immunological response leading to clearance of the virus. Clearance of HBsAg and seroconversion to anti-HBs is a late event; the percentage of patients who became HBsAg negative after seroconverting to anti-HBe has varied widely (7–65%) for follow-ups of 3–4 years [52,53]. Studies on survival and the cost–benefit of therapy, based on models predictive of the likely clinical outcome and related medical expenses, have also shown that interferon is able to prolong life in patients with chronic hepatitis B who have HBeAg in their serum. Furthermore, benefits exceed costs when an evaluation of life expectancy is included in the analysis [54,55]. The European consensus conference recommended using a regimen of 5 MU daily or 10 MU thrice weekly for 24 weeks [20]. However, because of the fre-

quency of side-effects at these high doses of IFN, 5–6 MU of IFN thrice weekly may be an optimal choice to allow the continuation of therapy. Several studies have suggested that, in patients who present a virological response with an HBV DNA level below 10^5 copies/mL, it is recommended to continue IFN therapy until HBe seroconversion. It was likewise suggested to continue therapy 2–3 months after seroconversion to limit the risk of reactivation after treatment withdrawal.

Side-effects are frequent and numerous, but usually mild and reversible after treatment withdrawal. The most frequent is a flu-like syndrome consisting of fever, arthralgia, headache and shivering; it is usually well controlled by paracetamol prescription. Other side-effects are asthenia, weight loss, alopecia, sleep disorders, mood disorders, concentration disorders and skin dryness. Psychiatric symptoms may be serious. Depression can occur in 10% of patients and should be treated as early as possible to avoid severe consequences (i.e. suicide attempt). Mental function may decompensate if the patient had a pre-existing psychosis. Thyroiditis with either hypo- or hyperthyroid syndrome may develop, although less frequently than in hepatitis C patients. Pregnancy is a contraindication for IFN therapy.

Results of pegylated IFN-α

In a phase II clinical trial, administration of pegylated IFN for 24 weeks was superior to that of standard IFN in terms of HBe seroconversion (37% vs. 25%) [56]. Subsequently, two other phase III trials have evaluated the antiviral effect of pegylated IFN-α-2a or -2b administration for 48 weeks and showed an HBe seroconversion rate of approximately 30% 6 months after treatment [57,58]. Interestingly, an HBs seroconversion rate of 3–5% was observed at the end of follow-up, while HBsAg negativity was observed in up to 7% of patients. Pretreatment predictive factors for HBe seroconversion were high ALT levels [> 5 × upper limit of normal (ULN)], low HBV DNA levels (< 10^7 copies/mL) and infection with HBV genotype A or genotype B.

Tolerance of pegylated IFN-α was generally similar to that of standard IFN, and side-effects were similar in nature and frequency. Flu-like syndrome, inflammatory skin reaction at the injection site and neutropenia were more frequent with pegylated IFN than with standard IFN. Depression appears to be less frequent in chronic hepatitis B patients than in hepatitis C patients receiving pegylated IFN.

Table 1 Treatment of HBeAg-positive chronic hepatitis B.

	PEG-IFN	Lamivudine	Adefovir	Entecavir
Viral suppression	4.5 log10 copies/mL	5–6 log10 copies/mL	3–4 log10 copies/mL	6–7 log10 copies/mL
HBe seroconversion	30%	15–20% at 1 year	10–15% at 1 year	20% at 1 year
		25–30% at 2 years		30% at 2 years
Predictive factors	High ALT levels	High ALT levels	High ALT levels	?
	Low HBV DNA levels			
Side-effects	+	−	−	−
Resistance	No resistance but non-response	20% per year	20% at 4 years	0% at 2 years

Results of lamivudine administration

Several phase III trials have evaluated the antiviral efficacy of lamivudine administration in patients with HBeAg-positive chronic hepatitis B [59–61]. Lamivudine presents several advantages: it is administered orally, associated with an excellent safety profile and rapid antiviral effect. Viral load declines by 3–5 log10 copies/mL after 1 year of therapy compared with baseline values. The antiviral effect is accompanied by a significant decrease in ALT levels and an improvement in the HAI. An improvement in liver fibrosis has also been observed during lamivudine therapy [62]. However, the primary goal of therapy, i.e. HBe seroconversion, is obtained in only approximately 20% of patients after 1 year of treatment. The rate of HBe seroconversion is significantly higher than in patients receiving placebo (5–10%).

Continuous lamivudine therapy is indicated in patients who do not seroconvert. It avoids rebounds of viral replication and exacerbations of liver disease. Prolonged lamivudine therapy is associated with an increased number of patients who undergo HBe seroconversion, reaching approximately 50% after 4 years of therapy [63]. In contrast to IFN, no ALT flares occur at HBe seroconversion induced by lamivudine. The durability of HBe seroconversion is tightly linked to the duration of lamivudine therapy after seroconversion. When lamivudine therapy is stopped just after seroconversion, most patients revert to HBeAg. In contrast, when lamivudine is continued for at least 6 months after seroconversion, viral reactivation and HBeAg reversion occur in only approximately 20% of the patients. The only predictive factor for HBe seroconversion at baseline is the level of serum ALT. In patients with ALT higher than 3 × ULN or even 5 × ULN, the likelihood of HBe seroconversion after 1 year of therapy is significantly increased [64].

The major problem with long-term lamivudine therapy is the occurrence of drug resistance. The spontaneous variability of the HBV genome and the slow kinetics of viral clearance are the biological basis for the selection of drug-resistant mutants. The main mutations conferring resistance are located within the YMDD motif in the C-domain of the viral polymerase: M204I or M204V mutants. These mutations can be accompanied by other mutations in the B-domain of the viral polymerase, i.e. V173L and L180M, named compensatory because they provide a higher replication capacity than the YMDD mutants [65]. The results of phase III clinical trials and of cohort studies have shown an incidence of lamivudine resistance of approximately 20% per year [66]. Lamivudine resistance develops in up to 70% of patients after 4 years of therapy [67]. Lamivudine resistance is associated with an increase in viral load (viral breakthrough), which is followed by an increase in ALT levels (biochemical breakthrough), a reduced HBe seroconversion rate and a progression of liver disease. The reactivation of HBV under therapy recapitulates disease; although the clinical/biochemical breakthrough is often delayed, ultimately, all patients who develop resistance exhibit a recrudescence of hepatitis within 24–32 months from the viral breakthrough. In some patients, especially those with liver cirrhosis or severe fibrosis, lamivudine resistance may be associated with a severe and acute exacerbation of liver disease, which may cause liver failure [67–69]. It is therefore necessary to make an early diagnosis of drug resistance to adapt antiviral therapy prior to the degradation of liver functions [69,70].

Results of adefovir dipivoxil administration

A large phase III trial has evaluated the antiviral efficacy of adefovir dipivoxil administration in 515 patients with HBeAg-positive chronic hepatitis B [71]. After 48 weeks of therapy, the median viral load decline was approximately 3.5 log10 copies/mL in comparison with pretreatment values. HBe seroconversion was achieved in only a minority of patients, i.e. 12% in the group of patients receiving adefovir dipivoxil 10 mg daily vs. 6% in the placebo group. Normalization of ALT levels was observed in 48% of patients receiving adefovir vs. 16% in the placebo group. An improvement in liver histology was observed in 53% of patients vs. 25% in the placebo group. With a daily dose of 10 mg, tolerance was comparable to placebo. After 48 weeks of therapy, no genotypical resistance was observed. Extended administration of adefovir dipivoxil showed an increased rate of HBe seroconversion over time, and an increasing number of patients showed a significant decline in viral load. However, a longer follow-up in patients with HBeAg-negative chronic hepatitis B has shown the occurrence of adefovir resistance starting from the second year of treatment (see below).

Recent data of adefovir administration for 5 years showed probabilities of HBeAg loss of 60% and HBe seroconversion of 48%. Four patients (2%) had an HBs seroconversion. HAI and fibrosis scores improved in 67% and 60% of patients, respectively. Adefovir resistance mutations developed in 20% of patients after 4 years.

Results of combination therapy

Several studies have evaluated the efficacy of a combination of PEG-IFN-α-2a or -2b with lamivudine in comparison with PEG-IFN alone and/or lamivudine alone [57,58]. Treatment was administered for 48 weeks, and endpoints were analysed 24 weeks after treatment. During therapy, there was a benefit in the combination by comparison with the single treatment in terms of viral load decline. The rate of lamivudine resistance was lower in patients who received the combination of lamivudine with PEG-IFN by comparison with lamivudine monotherapy. However, 24 weeks after therapy, the rate of HBe seroconversion was similar in patients who received PEG-IFN alone or the combination with lamivudine, i.e. approximately 30%. The HBe seroconversion rate was lower in patients who received lamivudine monotherapy, i.e. approximately 20%. These results are also in agreement with those of combination studies with standard IFN and lamivudine, which did not show an added benefit of the combination. New studies are clearly warranted to evaluate the combination of PEG-IFN and lamivudine or other antivirals with different schedules of administration.

The few published studies of the combination of lamivudine and adefovir dipivoxil in naive patients in comparison with lamivudine alone have analysed virological endpoints after a short-term treatment of 48 weeks. There was no significant difference in terms of viral load between the two groups. The rate of lamivudine resistance was lower in patients who received the combination of drugs. The major drawback of these studies is the absence of a comparative arm with adefovir dipivoxil monotherapy. Long-term combination studies are required to determine whether a combination of nucleoside analogues will show an added benefit in terms of prevention of drug resistance.

Results of new drugs: entecavir, telbivudine, tenofovir, emtricitabine

Entecavir

Entecavir was evaluated in phase II trials [73,74] and, more recently, in three controlled phase III trials involving 1633 patients with chronic HBV infection, detectable HBV DNA, persistently elevated ALT levels and chronic inflammation on liver biopsy. In two randomized studies involving nucleoside-naive patients, entecavir administered 0.5 mg orally once daily for 52 weeks was superior to lamivudine (100 mg orally once daily for 52 weeks) on the primary efficacy endpoint of histological improvement and on secondary endpoints, such as the reduction in viral load and normalization of ALT. After 2 years of treatment, 81% of patients receiving entecavir had a viral load below 300 copies/mL vs. only 39% of patients receiving lamivudine, 31% seroconverted to anti-HBe vs. 26% in the lamivudine group, and 5% showed a clearance of HBsAg vs. 3% in lamivudine-treated patients [75].

In lamivudine-refractory patients, entecavir administered at 1 mg once daily was superior to lamivudine in terms of viral load reduction and histological improvement. Entecavir was approved recently, first by the US Food and Drug Administration (FDA) and then in Europe, for the treatment of chronic HBV infection in adults with evidence of active viral replication and evidence of either persistent elevation in serum ALT or histologically active disease.

Entecavir resistance mutants have been rarely identified in treatment-naive patients; they have been described, mostly in patients with lamivudine resistance [43]. Approximately 9% of lamivudine-resistant patients treated with entecavir develop resistance to entecavir after 2 years of therapy. The resistant mutants are then resistant to both lamivudine and entecavir [76].

Telbivudine

Safety, antiviral activity and pharmacokinetics of telbivudine have been assessed in 43 adults with HBeAg-positive chronic hepatitis B [77]. This placebo-controlled, dose escalation trial investigated six telbivudine daily dosing levels (25, 50, 100, 200, 400 and 800 mg/day); treatment was given for 4 weeks. Telbivudine was well tolerated at all dosing levels, with no dose-related or treatment-related clinical or laboratory adverse events. Marked dose-related antiviral activity was evident, with a maximum at telbivudine doses of 400 mg/day or more. In the 800 mg/day cohort, the mean HBV DNA reduction was 3.75 log10 copies/mL at week 4, comprising a 99.98% reduction in serum viral load. Subsequently, large phase III studies have shown the superiority of telbivudine compared with lamivudine in the suppression of viral load (by 6.5 log10 vs. 5.5 log10) and improvement in liver histology [78]. Telbivudine resistance was observed in approximately 5% of patients after 1 year of therapy. The resistance mutations were the same as those responsible for lamivudine resistance, i.e. M204I mutation in the viral polymerase. Telbivudine has been approved in the US at the end of 2006.

Tenofovir

Tenofovir is already approved for the treatment of HIV infection. Its anti-HBV activity has been studied mainly in HIV–HBV coinfected patients. In this patient population, tenofovir administration significantly decreased HBV load in both lamivudine-naive and lamivudine-resistant patients [79–82]. Several non-randomized studies suggest that tenofovir may be more potent than adefovir in reducing HBV load [83]. Several phase III trials are ongoing to compare the anti-HBV activities of tenofovir and adefovir in HBV monoinfected patients and in HIV–HBV coinfected patients.

Emtricitabine

Emtricitabine was evaluated in phase II and phase III trials. Ninety-eight patients were randomized to receive emtricitabine at 25 mg, 100 mg or 200 mg daily for 48 weeks and then 200 mg until week 96. The dose of 200 mg daily gave the best results. After 2 years, 53% of patients had serum HBV DNA below 4700 copies/mL, 33% seroconverted to anti-HBe and 85% had normal ALT levels. Resistance mutations were observed in 18% of patients after 96 weeks of therapy [72].

Predictive factors of treatment response

Pretreatment factors predictive of therapy response have been identified. They may be useful for the decision to treat and the choice of drug to use. The results of clinical trials have shown that high ALT values ($> 3 \times$ ULN or $> 5 \times$ ULN) and low viral load ($< 10^7$ copies/mL) are predictive of a favourable response to standard or pegylated IFN. Recent studies suggested that HBV genotypes A (vs. D) and B (vs. C) are associated with a better response to IFN therapy. In patients treated with nucleoside analogues (lamivudine or adefovir), the only established baseline predictor of response is the level of ALT values. The chance of HBe seroconversion is significantly higher when ALT levels are greater than 3 or $5 \times$ ULN.

The collation of these predictive factors as well as the past history of the patient (previous non-response to IFN, side-effects to a previous course of IFN, contraindications to IFN, lifestyle of the patient and professional obligations, willingness for a pregnancy) are critical for decision-making. In young patients, a finite course with PEG-IFN may be proposed especially for those who have predictive factors for a favourable response. In patients who present a low chance of response to IFN, long-term therapy with a nucleos(t)ide analogue should be proposed.

Precore mutant infection, i.e. HBeAg-negative chronic hepatitis B

Standard IFN administration was the only treatment available until the end of the 1990s. Trials using 6–12 months of IFN therapy showed that, regardless of IFN dosage, there was a good response while on therapy (inhibition of HBV DNA, normalization of ALT), but relapses after therapy were common and observed in a majority of patients. These initial studies therefore indicated that therapy should not rely on courses of IFN shorter than 1 year. Long-term administration for at least 2 years showed clinical benefit in terms of viral suppression and ALT normalization. Approximately 30% of patients may present a sustained response after treatment withdrawal when the IFN course was sufficiently long to maintain the suppression of viral replication [84,85]. However, side-effects and poor tolerance of IFN administration limit its prolonged use in this form of chronic hepatitis B.

Lamivudine administration has been evaluated in patients with HBeAg-negative chronic hepatitis B in randomized trials and in cohort studies. Lamivudine given at a dose of 100–150 mg daily for 52 weeks induces a marked suppression of serum HBV DNA accompanied by normalization of ALT in approximately 80% of patients, together with liver histology improvement. However, most treated patients do not clear HBsAg and, therefore, show disease reactivation after discontinuing therapy [86]. Long-term therapy is therefore recommended. Unfortunately, prolonged lamivudine therapy is hampered by the emergence of drug resistance. Long-term lamivudine studies have shown that, after reaching a peak between 6 and 12 months of therapy, the response rate decreases because of virological breakthroughs associated with the emergence of lamivudine-resistant HBV mutants. Resistance occurs through mutations at the YMDD locus, as for HBeAg-positive patients. In a study, the virological response diminished from 68% at month 12 to 52% and 41.6%, respectively, at months 18 and 24 of therapy [68]. The virological breakthroughs were not uneventful, as ALT flares were observed in 6 of 11 patients who experienced a virological breakthrough, and one of these patients became jaundiced. Long-term studies showed that the antiviral efficacy and histological improvement are progressively lost with time, as the prevalence of resistance mutations increases [87]. After 3–4 years of therapy, lamivudine resistance outweighs the initial clinical benefit [88–91]. In a single-centre study in Greece, ALT levels increased progressively with the duration of infection with the lamivudine-resistant mutants: no patient with lamivudine resistance mutations for 24 months had normal ALT levels [90].

Likewise, in a multicentre study, only 5% of the patients with lamivudine-resistant mutants for 12–24 months had normal ALT levels compared with 72% of those without YMDD mutants [91]. In a retrospective nationwide analysis of lamivudine therapy in Italy, the development of clinically important events after virological breakthroughs depended on the severity of the underlying liver disease; severe hepatitis flares at the emergence of lamivudine-resistant mutants were noted in patients with Child B and C cirrhosis but not in patients with non-cirrhotic chronic hepatitis [89]. These studies confirmed that severe exacerbations of liver disease may occur in patients with precore mutant infection in whom lamivudine resistance develops, especially in those who had liver cirrhosis prior to therapy [68,69].

In HBeAg-negative chronic hepatitis, adefovir dipivoxil administration has shown similar results after 1 year of therapy compared with the treatment of HBeAg-positive patients [92]. At week 48, 64% of patients had improvement in histological liver abnormalities, compared with 33% of patients in the placebo group ($P < 0.001$). Serum HBV DNA levels were reduced to < 400 copies/mL in 51% of patients in the adefovir dipivoxil group (63 of 123) and in 0% in the placebo group ($P < 0.001$). The median decrease in log-transformed HBV DNA levels was greater with adefovir dipivoxil treatment than with placebo (3.91 vs. 1.35 log10 copies/mL , $P < 0.001$). ALT levels had normalized at week 48 in 72% of patients receiving adefovir dipivoxil (84 of 116), compared with 29% of those receiving placebo (17 of 59, $P < 0.001$) [93]. A longer duration study for 144 weeks showed a median decrease in serum HBV DNA of 3.47 log10 copies/mL at 96 weeks and 3.63 log10 copies/mL at week 144 [93]. HBV DNA was below 1000 copies/mL in 71% and 79% of patients after 96 and 144 weeks respectively. Interestingly, in the majority of patients who were switched from adefovir to placebo, the benefit of treatment was lost, indicating that antiviral therapy with nucleoside analogues has to be prolonged in this patient population to avoid viral reactivation and ALT flares. Resistance mutations rtN236T and rtA181V were identified in 3% and 5.9% of patients after 96 and 144 weeks respectively. Side-effects after 144 weeks were similar to those observed at week 48. Recent studies showed the clinical response after 5 years of therapy: 70% of patients have a suppression of viral load accompanied by ALT normalization and histology improvement, while 29% of patients developed adefovir-resistant mutations [94].

Among patients with HBeAg-negative chronic hepatitis B who were not previously treated with a nucleoside analogue, the rates of histological improvement, virological response and normalization of ALT levels were significantly higher at 48 weeks with entecavir than with lamivudine. The safety profile of the two agents was similar, and there was no evidence of viral resistance to entecavir during the study period [95].

One study has evaluated the efficacy of a combination of PEG-IFN-α-2a with lamivudine in comparison with PEG-IFN alone and lamivudine alone [96]. Treatment was administered for 48 weeks, and endpoints were analysed 24 weeks after treatment.

Table 2 Treatment of HBeAg-negative chronic hepatitis B.

	PEG-IFN	Lamivudine (100 mg/day)	Adefovir (10 mg/day)	Entecavir
Long-term therapy	+	+ (continuous)	+ (continuous)	+ (continuous)
Side-effects	+	–	–	–
Resistance	–	20% per year	–	–
Sustained response	≤ 30%	30–35% at 3 years	29% at 5 years	0% at 2 years
Clearance of HBsAg	+	–	> 70% at 5 years	> 90% at 2 years
Cost	++	±	–	–
			+	+

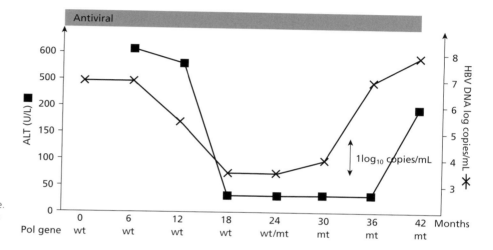

Fig. 4 Viral breakthrough and drug resistance. wt, wild-type HBV polymerase gene sequence; mt, drug-resistant HBV mutant.

During therapy, there was a benefit in the combination in comparison with the single treatment in terms of viral load decline. The rate of lamivudine resistance was lower in patients who received the combination of lamivudine with PEG-IFN in comparison with lamivudine monotherapy. However, 24 weeks after therapy, there was no difference in the rate of ALT normalization (approximately 60%) or virological response (approximately 20% of patients) between the groups who received PEG-IFN alone or in combination with lamivudine. The two groups of patients who received PEG-IFN had a better response rate 24 weeks after therapy than the group who received lamivudine alone. In view of the fluctuating nature of HBeAg-negative disease, long-term follow-up studies are necessary to determine whether sustained responses (maintained 6–12 months after therapy) herald permanent responses or represent spontaneous remissions of the disease.

A summary of treatment options in HBeAg-negative chronic hepatitis B is shown in Table 2.

Patients with drug resistance

The rescue treatment of patients with drug resistance has improved significantly in recent years. Indeed, new drugs are available, and the knowledge of the *in vitro* cross-resistance profile has provided the rationale for their use in patients with treatment failure. HBV resistance to antivirals can be defined at

different levels (Fig. 4): (i) genotypic resistance is the detection of polymerase gene mutations known to confer resistance to the drug; (ii) virological breakthrough is defined by an increase in HBV DNA of at least 1 log10 copies/mL compared with the lower value during treatment, associated with the presence of resistance mutations; it usually follows genotypic resistance; (iii) clinical failure is defined by viral breakthrough, increase in ALT levels and subsequent progression of liver disease.

Lamivudine resistance

Mutations conferring resistance to lamivudine are mainly located in the C-domain of reverse transcriptase within the YMDD motif, i.e. M204V or M204I, and may be associated with compensatory mutations in the C-domain, i.e. V173L or L180M (Fig. 5). After 1 year of treatment, lamivudine-resistant mutants emerged in 32% of patients, increasing to 38% after 2 years, 53% after 3 years and 66% after 4 years [67] (see also Fig. 6). *In vitro* studies showed that the main lamivudine resistance mutants remain sensitive to adefovir and tenofovir and have a reduced susceptibility to entecavir [16,47]. Adefovir has a proven clinical benefit in the treatment of lamivudine resistance with a significant inhibition of viral mutant replication and improvement in liver function after 1 year of therapy. Several studies compared the addition of adefovir to ongoing lamivudine with the switch from lamivudine to adefovir [97,98]. After 48 weeks of therapy, there was no difference in viral load decline in these

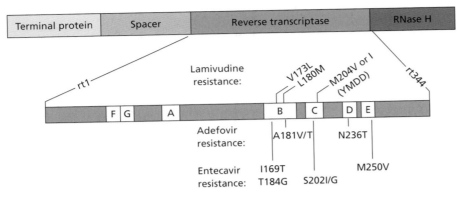

Fig. 5 Polymerase gene mutations conferring drug resistance.

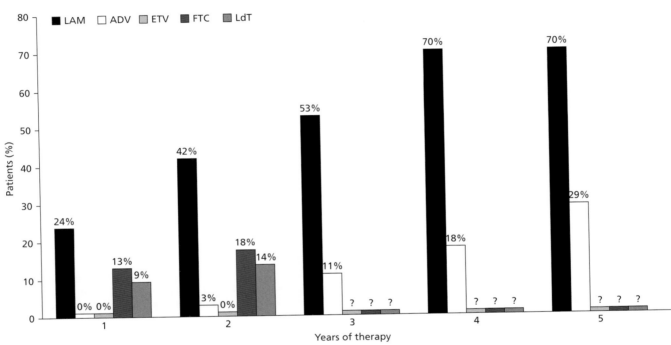

Fig. 6 Incidence of resistance in treatment-naive patients. LAM, lamivudine; ADV, adefovir; ETV, entecavir; FTC, emtricitabire; LdT, telbivudine.

two treatment groups. Indeed, in most clinical trials of adefovir administration for lamivudine failure, virogical endpoints were examined at week 48 of therapy, while adefovir resistance starts to occur during the second year. Because of the lack of cross-resistance between the two drugs, there is now a consensus among experts that adefovir should be added to lamivudine in patients with lamivudine failure to prevent or delay the subsequent selection of new resistant mutants.

Entecavir administration has also been evaluated in patients with lamivudine failure at a higher dose of 1 mg daily (compared with 0.5 mg in naive patients) because of the reduced susceptibility of the lamivudine resistance mutant to entecavir *in vitro*. Entecavir administration was associated with a significant decline in viral load in these lamivudine-refractory patients [98]. Of note, the only cases of entecavir resistance described so far have been observed in lamivudine-resistant patients, suggesting

a certain level of cross-resistance between these two drugs, leading to the selection of mutants resistant to both drugs. With the current knowledge, it is therefore questionable to use entecavir in patients with prior lamivudine resistance, as subsequent selection of entecavir-resistant mutants may occur in as many as 38% of these patients after 3 years of therapy.

Adefovir resistance

Adefovir 10 mg/day is associated with the emergence of drug-resistant mutants in less than 3% of patients after 2 years of therapy, 11% after 3 years, 18% after 4 years and 29% after 5 years (Fig. 6). Resistance to adefovir is conferred by the selection of a N236T mutation in the D-domain of the HBV polymerase or a A181V mutation in the B-domain of the polymerase [37,38,48] (Fig. 5). *In vitro*, the N236T mutation is sensitive to both lamivudine and entecavir; the A181V showed a decreased susceptibility to lamivudine. Few reports showed the benefit of lamivudine administration in patients with adefovir resistance.

Entecavir resistance

Entecavir resistance has so far been observed only during the therapy of lamivudine-refractory patients. The resistance rate appears to be approximately 10% per year in patients with lamivudine failure. The main resistance mutations are rtT184G, rtS202I and rtM250V on a background of lamivudine resistance mutations [43] (Fig. 5). These mutants are resistant to lamivudine. One *in vitro* study showed their susceptibility to adefovir and tenofovir. Clinical data are awaited to provide recommendations for the treatment of entecavir-resistant patients.

Monitoring of antiviral therapy

The risk of the emergence of drug resistance mandates the monitoring of antiviral therapy when patients are treated with nucleos(t)ides. The rationale for the timing of monitoring derives from the consideration that the biochemical breakthrough usually occurs with a delay of several weeks after the virological breakthrough and that the clinical impact is usually different in non-cirrhotic than in cirrhotic disease. In the former, the ALT breakthrough most usually has no major clinical consequences; in the latter, it may precipitate liver failure and death. Monitoring should be performed by measuring the viral load with quantitative HBV DNA testing whenever possible and affordable.

Early during therapy (week 8 or 12), viral load monitoring allows the assessment of the initial response, which may predict the treatment outcome. In HBeAg-positive patients treated with lamivudine or adefovir dipivoxil, the magnitude of HBV DNA decline early on during therapy is associated with a greater tendency towards HBe seroconversion [100]. The antiviral response at week 24 of therapy was also found to be a predictor of subsequent efficacy (HBeAg loss, HBV DNA < 200 copies/mL, ALT normalization and viral breakthrough) in patients treated with lamivudine or telbivudine [78]. In the 5-year study of adefovir dipivoxil administration in HBeAg-negative chronic hepatitis, patients with a viral load lower than 3 log10 copies/mL after 1 year of therapy had a significantly lower risk of developing resistance by year 3 of treatment (< 3%) compared with a risk of 26% and 66% for those having a viral load between 3 and 6 log10 copies and > 6 log10 copies/mL respectively [94].

During long-term treatment, a 3- or 6-monthly assessment of viral load and serological markers is required to monitor antiviral treatment efficacy and to determine whether the response is maintained or drug resistance is likely to occur. In patients with moderate liver disease, 6-monthly monitoring might be sufficient during the first 2 years of treatment when using drugs with a slow rate of resistance, but more frequent monitoring may be necessary thereafter when the risk of resistance increases significantly. In patients with advanced liver

disease, 3-monthly monitoring is required to detect incoming viral drug resistance and thus provide immediate rescue with alternative antiviral therapy prior to a potentially dangerous flare of ALT levels.

HBV drug resistance is defined by the confirmed increase in viral load by at least 1 log10 by comparison with the nadir value during therapy [65] (Fig. 4). It is important to assess drug compliance, as any drug interruption may lead to a rebound of viral replication and ALT flares. The detection of polymerase mutations by sequencing, line probe assay, DNA chip technologies or other tools will be important in the future to target new treatment to the profile of mutations in the polymerase gene [69,101]. Indeed, the cross-resistance profile is different from one mutant to another [102,103].

New tools may become available in the future to monitor the efficacy of antiviral therapy, such as the quantification of intrahepatic cccDNA or the quantification of serum HBsAg as a surrogate marker [13–15]. Furthermore, with the development of new drugs and the increasing complexity of the resistance profile, phenotypic assays to determine the drug susceptibility of the clinical isolates may prove useful to tailor antiviral therapy to the virological situation of the patient, as already shown in HIV [102,103].

Special forms of chronic hepatitis B

Liver cirrhosis

In patients with compensated cirrhosis, the risk of the development of complications including decompensation and development of hepatocellular carcinoma is significantly higher in those who maintain a high level of viral replication and ALT [18]. The advent of nucleos(t)ide analogues that control HBV replication has significantly changed the management of these patients. It was demonstrated recently in a phase III trial of lamivudine in cirrhotics that control of viral replication decreases the risk of liver disease progression, as assessed by the Child–Pugh score and compared with the placebo group [104]. Furthermore, in patients who developed lamivudine resistance, there was a higher risk of liver disease progression, although it remained lower than in the placebo group, at least during the study period. Tolerance of the drug was very good. The results of this study demonstrate the clinical benefit of viral replication suppression and advocate treatment strategies aiming at maintaining viral suppression in the context of liver cirrhosis.

In patients with decompensated liver cirrhosis, the use of IFN-α is limited by the risk of severe side-effects including severe neutropenia and infection, thrombopenia and the hazard of ALT flares upon HBe seroconversion induced by IFN, which may lead to rapid liver failure. The development of nucleoside analogues, whose mode of action is mainly to control viral replication, for the therapy of chronic HBV infection has changed the management of these patients. Several studies have shown that lamivudine therapy of patients with decompensated liver cirrhosis is associated with control of HBV replication, improvement in ALT levels and liver function tests (bilirubin, albumin and prothrombin time), as well as a significant clinical improvement assessed by the Child–Pugh score [105–107]. Tolerance was also very good in this setting. Many patients had a marked clinical improvement and, therefore, were withdrawn from the transplantation waiting list. However, it is important to note that lamivudine resistance may occur in the long term and may subsequently be associated with a new deterioration of liver functions. In these patients, it is therefore mandatory to monitor viral load closely and adapt antiviral therapy prior to the progression of the disease.

Adefovir dipivoxil administration was also evaluated in a large cohort of cirrhotic patients who were candidates for transplantation and had developed lamivudine resistance [108]. It was shown that adefovir dipivoxil therapy, by controlling viral replication, induces a significant improvement in liver function tests. Therefore, there is a large body of evidence that nucleos(t)ide analogues should be prescribed as early as possible in patients with decompensated HBV cirrhosis. First-line therapy in this group of patients may vary from country to country depending on administrative issues related to treatment reimbursement, but some centres favour the use of a combination of lamivudine and adefovir to reduce the risk of subsequent drug resistance. The place of entecavir in this population of patients remains to be determined.

Liver transplantation (see Chapter 25.1)

It is now recommended in patients with endstage liver cirrhosis who are candidates for liver transplantation to start nucleos(t)ide analogue administration prior to transplantation to lower viral load and thus decrease the risk of HBV recurrence after transplantation, and to maintain or improve liver function while the patient is on the waiting list [109,110]. Patients should be monitored closely to diagnose viral breakthrough and allow adefovir dipivoxil to be added as soon as possible to control viral replication and allow liver transplantation. Adefovir dipivoxil therapy may also be started as first-line treatment in the pretransplant setting as the risk of resistance is lower. However, some studies suggest a lag between the start of adefovir therapy and the control of viral replication and the subsequent clinical improvement. For this reason, several centres use a combination of lamivudine and adefovir dipivoxil to rapidly improve the clinical situation and delay the risk of drug resistance while the patient is on the waiting list.

After liver transplantation, administration of HBIG and the continuation of the nucleoside analogue is recommended. With such a prophylaxis regimen, the risk of HBV recurrence in the liver graft has decreased dramatically below 10% [111].

In patients with HBV recurrence after liver transplantation, liver disease may progress very rapidly. Antiviral therapy is recommended as soon as the diagnosis of recurrence has been made [112].

HIV–HBV coinfected patients

In these patients, HBV infection is becoming a major clinical problem, as the restoration of immune response induced by highly active antiretroviral therapy (HAART) may trigger liver damage. Furthermore, antivirals used in the HAART regimen may be hepatotoxic, and some of them exhibit both anti-HIV and anti-HBV activities. The increasing choice of drugs to treat coinfected patients will help to manage these patients especially when facing problems of HIV and/or HBV drug resistance. Several antivirals are effective against both HIV and HBV, such as lamivudine, emtricitabine and tenofovir. Other drugs such as adefovir and entecavir are active only against HBV. The decision of which drug to use for therapy of chronic HBV infeition depends also on the HIV status and the requirement or not of nucleoside RT inhibitors. A specific chapter is dedicated to HIV and the liver (see Chapter 9.3).

Coinfection with hepatitis delta virus

Interferon therapy

IFN-α has been most studied in this situation. In two controlled Italian therapeutic trials of chronic hepatitis D that have included a consistent number of patients [113,114], IFN-α induced biochemical responses (normalization of ALT) while the patients were on therapy but, in the majority of responders, there was a relapse after therapy discontinuation. There was no effect of therapy on the hepatitis D virus (HDV); in most patients, the level of HDV RNA was unaffected. Specifically, liver tests became normal or improved significantly after 4 months of therapy in 42% of the patients who received 5 MU/m^2 IFN-α-2b thrice weekly for 4 months followed by 3 MU/m^2 for 8 more months. However, only eight (25%) were in remission when IFN was discontinued, and there was a relapse in all but one (3%) during the post-therapy follow-up [114]. Better on-therapy results were obtained with a more aggressive therapeutic protocol [113]. ALT normalized in 10 of 14 (71%) patients receiving 9 MU of IFN-α-2a for 48 weeks compared with 4 of 14 (29%) treated with 3 MU and 1 of 13 untreated control subjects (8%). In patients treated with 9 MU, the normalization of ALT levels was associated with marked histological improvement, and no HDV RNA was detected while they where on therapy. In five patients, the biochemical response persisted for up to 4 years; however, there was no long-term effect on HDV as HDV RNA reappeared in the serum of all responders. Overall, the data from these studies and from other controlled and uncontrolled studies including limited numbers of patients have shown that liver chemistry ameliorates in about 50% of HDV patients while on therapy, but only a minority exhibits a sustained normalization of ALT levels with clearance of HDV; in these latter patients, IgM anti-HD disappears from serum and the HBsAg is cleared within months to years with seroconversion to anti-HBs [115]. Of note, there is no clear evidence that this minority benefited from a therapeutic advantage rather than from a more benign course of the disease; no statistically significant long-term effect of IFN on HDV has been shown by controlled study, and spontaneous long-term remissions are known to occur in the natural history of HDV disease. Indeed, in a follow-up study, the rate of spontaneous HBsAg clearance over the years was increased in HDV-positive compared with HDV-negative HBsAg carriers [115].

Nevertheless, after 2–14 years of follow-up, complete fibrosis regression and loss of HDV RNA were reported in some of the patients who had achieved a persistent biochemical response and lost IgM anti-HD with high-dose IFN therapy, all of whom had an initial diagnosis of active cirrhosis [116]. Likewise, in another study, resolution of chronic hepatitis D was reported up to 12 years after continuous IFN therapy [117]. Few data are available for the treatment of other categories of HDV carriers such as children [115] or HIV-positive patients [118].

Nucleoside analogue therapy

Famciclovir, lamivudine and adefovir, which are inactive on HDV replication but efficacious in inhibiting the helper HBV, have been tested with discouraging results. No patients with chronic hepatitis D responded to famciclovir administered at 500 mg three times a day for 6 months and then followed up for 6 months after treatment [119].

Several small trials of lamivudine have been performed in chronic hepatitis D. Five patients received oral lamivudine 100 mg daily for 12 months [120]. HBV DNA became undetectable in four patients and decreased by 5 log10 in the other but, in all, ALT levels remained abnormal, HDV RNA detectable and HBsAg positive.

In another study, a 12-month vs. a 24-month course of lamivudine 100 mg/day were compared [121]. Thirty-one patients were randomized to treatment, 11 to placebo and 20 to lamivudine for 12 months; thereafter, all were given lamivudine on an open-label basis for 12 months and followed up for a further 16 weeks. At the end of treatment, HDV RNA was negative and ALT levels normal in three patients, but only two patients remained virus free at the end of follow-up. In another study [122], eight patients with chronic hepatitis D were treated with lamivudine for at least 24 weeks, and then lamivudine was combined with high-dose IFN followed by 9 MU of IFN thrice weekly; the patients were followed up for 12 weeks after therapy. The HBsAg concentration in serum decreased in two patients. There was no significant decrease in serum HDV RNA during treatment. At the end of treatment, ALT levels had normalized in one patient and decreased in three other patients, but three of these four patients showed a biochemical rebound after withdrawal of therapy.

Recommendations for therapy of HBV–HDV coinfection

There is as yet no established therapy for chronic hepatitis D. However, as IFN-α appears to be capable of controlling inflammation in a proportion of patients, this cytokine may be used in order to slow disease progression. To achieve biochemical responses, high dosages of IFN (between 6 and 9 MU) given thrice weekly for prolonged periods (over 12 months) are recommended. Treatment should be maintained for 12 months after normalization of ALT levels.

Treated patients can lose HDV markers from serum while on therapy, but may relapse when treatment is discontinued if they remain HBsAg positive; therefore, therapy should not be discontinued prematurely on the basis of the clearance of HDV. Loss of HBsAg is a reliable marker of resolution of hepatitis D [115]. Pegylated IFNs appear to represent a logical therapeutic option for the long-term treatment required for chronic hepatitis D. Preliminary results are encouraging. In a recent study [132], a sustained clearance of HDV-RNA was obtained in 6 out of 14 (43%) patients with chronic hepatitis D treated with PEG-IFN-α-2b (1.5 µg/kg per week). Viral kinetics were predictive of the response; after 3 months of therapy, HDV-RNA was significantly lower in responders than in non-responders.

Ferenci et al. [124] reported the clearance of HDV RNA and a sustained clinical amelioration in a patient with HDV cirrhosis treated for 6 months with PEG-IFN-α-2a and lamivudine. However, confirmation of the efficacy of PEG-IFN in the setting of HDV infection requires larger prospective studies.

The factors determining a biochemical response are not known. The type of underlying HBV infection, whether HBeAg positive or HBeAg negative, does not influence response. Indeed, although HDV patients with concomitant HBeAg-positive HBV infection seroconverted to anti-HBe during IFN therapy, the control of HBV infection had no impact on HDV infection or disease activity [115]. Whether response may depend on the HBV or HDV genotype is unknown.

Of note, a major factor influencing the response to therapy in chronic hepatitis D, as in all forms of viral hepatitis, is the duration of the viral infection and disease, with patients with early disease responding better than those with longstanding fibrosis or cirrhosis. Therefore, the prospects of therapy for HDV infection appear to be even less encouraging in the Mediterranean area as, in this area, the spectacular decline in HDV infection fostered by the control of HBV has led to an increase in IFN-resistant fibrotic and cirrhotic forms (representing longstanding disease) over more therapy-susceptible recent forms of the disease.

Liver transplantation

Liver transplantation is a valid treatment option for endstage HDV liver disease. The risk of spontaneous reinfection is lower for HDV than for HBV. The prospect of an uneventful clinical course after transplantation was improved by the long-term administration of hyperimmune serum against HBsAg. The 5-year survival rate of 76 patients transplanted in Paris for terminal delta cirrhosis was 88%, with reappearance of HBsAg in only 9% under long-term anti-HBs prophylaxis [125]. The addition of lamivudine also helps to decrease the risk of viral recurrence in patients with replicating HBV prior to transplantation. In another series, none of 62 HDV patients transplanted experienced a viral recurrence, of whom 48 were given HBIG after transplantation and 14 were given lamivudine before transplantation and lamivudine together with HBIG after transplantation [126].

Extrahepatic manifestations of HBV infection

Extrahepatic manifestations of HBV infection, such as periarteritis nodosa (PAN), are due to immune complexes involving viral envelope proteins. As their formation is the consequence of active viral replication, treatment of HBV-associated PAN relies on the use of antiviral therapy. This may be combined initially, especially in patients with severe symptoms, with plasmapheresis and a short course of corticosteroids to decrease the effect of the deposit of immune complexes on the artery walls [127,128]. When the clinical situation is under control, prednisone and plasmapheresis can be stopped while antiviral therapy is continued until HBe or HBs seroconversion.

Several studies have shown the clinical benefit of anti-HBV agents, including vidarabine, IFN-α, lamivudine, famciclovir and adefovir [129–133]. Indeed, the control of viral replication is accompanied by a decrease in immune complex formation and improvement in the clinical signs of vasculitis. Clearance of HBsAg and cure of the vasculitis have been reported by several investigators.

Special cases

In health-care workers chronically infected with HBV, antiviral therapy may be indicated to suppress viral load and reduce the risk of nosocomial transmission to patients.

In pregnant women, the prevention of mother-to-baby transmission usually relies on HBIG and vaccine administration to newborns at birth. However, it was shown that, in highly viraemic mothers, this may not be sufficient to provide complete prophylaxis. One study showed that lamivudine administration during the last month of pregnancy, combined with vaccination of the newborn, prompted a significant decrease in the risk of vertical transmission [134].

In children, chronic hepatitis B is usually mild because of the immunotolerant status. This may explain the relatively poor rate of HBe seroconversion observed in children treated with lamivudine [135] or standard IFN [136,137]. However, in children with chronic active hepatitis and elevated ALT levels, both drugs have shown a beneficial effect.

Conclusions

A treatment algorithm is proposed in Figure 7. Currently, patients with minimal disease, whether in the immunotolerance phase or with inactive infection, should not be treated. In patients with chronic hepatitis proven by ALT elevation and abnormal liver histology, antiviral therapy is indicated because all studies have shown that antiviral therapy decreases the risk of liver disease progression compared with the natural history of the disease. In patients who are HBeAg positive, the primary goal of antiviral therapy is to obtain an HBe seroconversion. If the patient is young and has predictive factors of favourable response, a finite course of pegylated IFN should be tried as a first-line option. In other cases (including non-responders to IFN, patients intolerant to IFN and those with factors predictive of poor response to IFN), long-term therapy with nucleoside analogues is usually needed.

In patients who are HBeAg negative, long-term therapy is required. In this situation, nucleoside analogues are better tolerated than pegylated IFN, but the therapeutic choice has to take into account the risk of drug resistance. In patients with severe liver disease, i.e. decompensated liver cirrhosis or HBV recurrence on the liver graft, one might consider combining nucleoside analogues lacking cross-resistance to provide the best chance of long-term control of viral replication and disease progression. In the situation of treatment failure, knowledge of

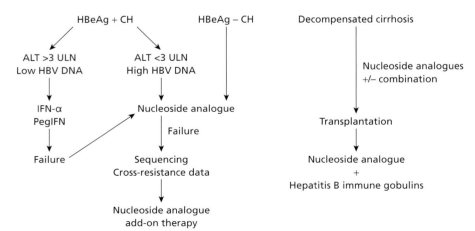

Fig. 7 Treatment algorithm. CH, chronic hepatitis.

the resistance profile is important to adapt antiviral therapy. One of the major questions in the future will be how to delay or prevent drug resistance. Combination therapy, although currently very expensive, will probably become part of the treatment paradigm.

Perspectives: can we prevent or delay drug resistance?

The rationale for combination therapy relies on experimental findings in the hepadnavirus models and on HIV therapy experience [138]: (i) simple mutants pre-exist as shown by longitudinal studies of viral polymerase gene sequence; (ii) genetic variants harbouring multiple mutations have less chance to pre-exist or to occur; (iii) retreatment leads to a rapid re-emergence of resistant mutants, although wild-type virus re-emerges after the first treatment interruption; the same applies to sequential treatment selecting for partially cross-resistant strains, i.e. lamivudine and entecavir; (iv) cccDNA represents a genetic archive for a more rapid reselection of resistance.

The optimal antiviral regimen may combine drugs with a different mechanism of action on viral replication, lacking cross-resistance and exhibiting antiviral synergy. These theoretical combinations should reduce the risk of the selection of drug-resistant mutants because of the inhibition of viral replication and the selective pressure exerted on the different viral strains that compose the quasi-species. For instance, it was shown that the combination of lamivudine and famciclovir accelerates the kinetics of viral clearance, although no long-term follow-up was available to determine its effect on the prevention of drug resistance [139].

With the development and evaluation of newer drugs acting at different steps in viral genome replication, it will be easier to choose the best combination relying on drugs with different mechanisms of action, for instance drugs with potent antipriming activity, drugs inhibiting viral minus strand DNA synthesis and others inhibiting plus strand DNA synthesis. The combination of such compounds was found to be either additive or, more rarely, synergistic in polymerase assays (reverse transcriptase activity) [147] as well as in tissue culture experiments (viral DNA synthesis) or in chronically infected woodchucks [140–144]. By more potently inhibiting viral DNA synthesis, such combinations may therefore delay the onset of viral resistance by limiting the chance of a given mutation occurring. Furthermore, results of cross-resistance studies on the main lamivudine-, adefovir- and entecavir-resistant strains are now becoming available [37,38,42,49,145–147]. This should allow the evaluation of rationale combinations, taking into account the mechanism of action of the drugs as well as their antiviral activity and cross-resistance profile, to better suppress viral replication and prevent the selection of resistant mutants within the viral quasi-species [47,148]. This should pave the way for future clinical trials and improved treatment of chronic hepatitis B.

References

1 Bertoletti A, Naoumov NV (2003) Translation of immunological knowledge into better treatments of chronic hepatitis B. *J Hepatol* 39, 115–124.

2 Ganem D, Prince AM (2004) Hepatitis B virus infection – natural history and clinical consequences. *N Engl J Med* 350, 1118–1129.

3 Guidotti LG, Rochford R, Chung J et al. (1999) Viral clearance without destruction of infected cells during acute HBV infection. *Science* 284, 825–829.

4 Summers J, Jilbert AR, Yang W et al. (2003) Hepatocyte turnover during resolution of a transient hepadnaviral infection. *Proc Natl Acad Sci USA* 100, 11652–11659.

5 Summers J, Mason WS (2004) Residual integrated viral DNA after hepadnavirus clearance by nucleoside analog therapy. *Proc Natl Acad Sci USA* 101, 638–640.

6 Wieland S, Thimme R, Purcell RH et al. (2004) Genomic analysis of the host response to hepatitis B virus infection. *Proc Natl Acad Sci USA* 101, 6669–6674.

7 Boni C, Bertoletti A, Penna A et al. (1998) Lamivudine treatment can restore T cell responsiveness in chronic hepatitis B. *J Clin Invest* 102, 968–975.

8 Boni C, Penna A, Ogg GS et al. (2001) Lamivudine treatment can overcome cytotoxic T-cell hyporesponsiveness in chronic hepatitis B: new perspectives for immune therapy. *Hepatology* 33, 963–971.

9 Webster GJ, Reignat S, Brown D et al. (2004) Longitudinal analysis of CD8+ T cells specific for structural and nonstructural hepatitis B virus proteins in patients with chronic hepatitis B: implications for immunotherapy. *J Virol* 78, 5707–5719.

10 Mason W, Cullen J, Saputelli J et al. (1994) Characterization of the antiviral activity of 2'carbodeoxyguanosine in ducks chronically infected with duck hepatitis B virus. *Hepatology* 19, 398–411.

11 Mason WS, Cullen J, Moraleda G et al. (1998) Lamivudine therapy of WHV-infected woodchucks. *Virology* 245, 18–32.

12 Maynard M, Parvaz P, Durantel S et al. (2005) Sustained HBs seroconversion during lamivudine and adefovir dipivoxil combination therapy for lamivudine failure. *J Hepatol* 42, 279–281.

13 Werle-Lapostolle B, Bowden S, Locarnini S et al. (2004) Persistence of cccDNA during the natural history of chronic hepatitis B and decline during adefovir dipivoxil therapy. *Gastroenterology* 126, 1750–1758.

14 Sung JJ, Wong ML, Bowden S et al. (2005) Intrahepatic hepatitis B virus covalently closed circular DNA can be a predictor of sustained response to therapy. *Gastroenterology* 128, 1890–1897.

15 Zoulim F (2005) New insight on hepatitis B virus persistence from the study of intrahepatic viral cccDNA. *J Hepatol* 42, 302–308.

16 Zoulim F (2004) Mechanism of viral persistence and resistance to nucleoside and nucleotide analogs in chronic Hepatitis B virus infection. *Antiviral Res* 64, 1–15.

17 Realdi G, Fattovich G, Hadzyiannis S et al. (1994) Survival and prognostic factors in 366 patients with compensated cirrhosis type B: a multicenter study. *J Hepatol* 21, 656–666.

18 Yang HI, Lu SN, Liaw YF et al. (2002) Hepatitis B e antigen and the risk of hepatocellular carcinoma. *N Engl J Med* 347, 168–174.

19 Lok AS, McMahon BJ (2001) Chronic hepatitis B. *Hepatology* 34, 1225–1241.

20 de Franchis R, Hadengue A, Lau G et al. (2003) EASL International Consensus Conference on Hepatitis B, 13–14 September, 2002,

Geneva, Switzerland. Consensus statement (long version). *J Hepatol* 39 (Suppl 1), S3–25.

21 Le Guerhier F, Pichoud C, Guerret S, *et al.* (2000) Characterization of the antiviral effect of 2′,3′-dideoxy-2′, 3′-didehydro-beta-L-5-fluorocytidine in the duck hepatitis B virus infection model. *Antimicrob Agents Chemother* 44, 111–122.

22 Le Guerhier F, Pichoud C, Jamard C *et al.* (2001) Antiviral activity of beta-L-2′,3′-dideoxy-2′,3′-didehydro-5-fluorocytidine in woodchucks chronically infected with woodchuck hepatitis virus. *Antimicrob Agents Chemother* 45, 1065–1077.

23 Zhou T, Saputelli J, Aldrich CE *et al.* (1999) Emergence of drug-resistant populations of woodchuck hepatitis virus in woodchucks treated with the antiviral nucleoside lamivudine. *Antimicrob Agents Chemother* 43, 1947–1954.

24 Zhu Y, Yamamoto T, Cullen J *et al.* (2001) Kinetics of hepadnavirus loss from the liver during inhibition of viral DNA synthesis. *J Virol* 75, 311–322.

25 Seeger C, Mason WS (2000) Hepatitis B virus biology. *Microbiol Mol Biol Rev* 64, 51–68.

26 Pol S, Nalpas B, Driss F *et al.* (2001) Efficacy and limitations of a specific immunotherapy in chronic hepatitis B. *J Hepatol* 34, 917–921.

27 Le Guerhier F, Thermet A, Guerret S *et al.* (2003) Antiviral effect of adefovir in combination with a DNA vaccine in the duck hepatitis B virus infection model. *J Hepatol* 38, 328–334.

28 Michel ML, Loirat D (2001) DNA Vaccines for prophylactic or therapeutic immunization against hepatitis B. *Intervirology* 44, 78–87.

29 Mancini-Bourgine M, Fontaine H, Scott-Algara D *et al.* (2004) Induction or expansion of T-cell responses by a hepatitis B DNA vaccine administered to chronic HBV carriers. *Hepatology* 40, 874–882.

30 Bridges E, Cheng Y (1995) Use of novel b-L(−)-nucleoside analogues for treatment and prevention of chronic hepatitis B virus infection and hepatocellular carcinoma. *Prog Liver Dis* 13, 231–245.

31 Allen MI, Deslauriers M, Andrews CW *et al.* (1998) Identification and characterization of mutations in hepatitis B virus resistant to lamivudine. *Hepatology* 27, 1670–1677.

32 Condreay L, Condreay J, Jansen R *et al.* (1996) (−)-cis-5-fluoro-1-(2-(hydroxymethyl)-1,3-oxathiolan-5-yl)cytosine (524W91) inhibits hepatitis B virus replication in primary human hepatocytes. *Antimicrob Agents Chemother* 40, 520–523.

33 Marcellin P, Mommeja-Marin H, Sacks SL *et al.* (2004) A phase II dose-escalating trial of clevudine in patients with chronic hepatitis B. *Hepatology* 40, 140–148.

34 Pai S, Liu S, Zhu Y *et al.* (1996) Inhibition of hepatitis B virus by a novel L-nucleoside, 2′-fluoro-5-methyl-b-L-arabinofuranosyl uracil. *Antimicrob Agents Chemother* 40, 380–386.

35 Xiong X, Flores C, Yang H *et al.* (1998) Mutations in hepatitis B DNA polymerase associated with resistance to lamivudine do not confer resistance to adefovir in vitro. *Hepatology* 28, 1669–1673.

36 Delmas J, Schorr O, Jamard C *et al.* (2002) Inhibitory effect of adefovir on viral DNA synthesis and covalently closed circular DNA formation in duck hepatitis B virus-infected hepatocytes in vivo and in vitro. *Antimicrob Agents Chemother* 46, 425–433.

37 Angus P, Vaughan R, Xiong S *et al.* (2003) Resistance to adefovir dipivoxil therapy associated with the selection of a novel mutation in the HBV polymerase. *Gastroenterology* 125, 292–297.

38 Villeneuve JP, Durantel D, Durantel S *et al.* (2003) Selection of a hepatitis B virus strain resistant to adefovir in a liver transplantation patient. *J Hepatol* 39, 1085–1089.

39 Innaimo SF, Seifer M, Bisacchi GS *et al.* (1997) Identification of BMS-200475 as a potent and selective inhibitor of hepatitis B virus. *Antimicrob Agents Chemother* 41, 1444–1448.

40 Colonno RJ, Genovesi EV, Medina I *et al.* (2001) Long-term entecavir treatment results in sustained antiviral efficacy and prolonged life span in the woodchuck model of chronic hepatitis infection. *J Infect Dis* 184, 1236–1245.

41 Seifer M, Hamatake RK, Colonno RJ *et al.* (1998) In vitro inhibition of hepadnavirus polymerases by the triphosphates of BMS-200475 and lobucavir. *Antimicrob Agents Chemother* 42, 3200–3208.

42 Levine S, Hernandez D, Yamanaka G *et al.* (2002) Efficacies of entecavir against lamivudine-resistant hepatitis B virus replication and recombinant polymerases in vitro. *Antimicrob Agents Chemother* 46, 2525–2532.

43 Tenney DJ, Levine SM, Rose RE *et al.* (2004) Clinical emergence of entecavir-resistant hepatitis B virus requires additional substitutions in virus already resistant to lamivudine. *Antimicrob Agents Chemother* 48, 3498–3507.

44 Ying C, De Clercq E, Neyts J (2000) Lamivudine, adefovir and tenofovir exhibit long-lasting anti-hepatitis B virus activity in cell culture. *J Viral Hepat* 7, 79–83.

45 Bryant ML, Bridges EG, Placidi L *et al.* (2001) Antiviral L-nucleosides specific for hepatitis B virus infection. *Antimicrob Agents Chemother* 45, 229–235.

46 Standring DN, Bridges EG, Placidi L *et al.* (2001) Antiviral beta-L-nucleosides specific for hepatitis B virus infection. *Antiviral Chem Chemother* 12 Suppl 1, 119–129.

47 Zoulim F (2004) Antiviral therapy of chronic hepatitis B: can we clear the virus and prevent drug resistance? *Antiviral Chem Chemother* 15, 299–305.

48 Brunelle MN, Jacquard AC, Pichoud C *et al.* (2005) Susceptibility to antivirals of a human HBV strain with mutations conferring resistance to both lamivudine and adefovir. *Hepatology* 41, 1391–1398.

49 Seigneres B, Pichoud C, Martin P *et al.* (2002) Inhibitory activity of dioxolane purine analogs on wild-type and lamivudine-resistant mutants of hepadnaviruses. *Hepatology* 36, 710–722.

50 Perillo, R, Schiff E, Davis G *et al.* (1990) A randomized, controlled trial of interferon alfa-2b alone and after prednisone withdrawal for the treatment of chronic hepatitis B. *N Engl J Med* 323, 295–301.

51 Wong DK, Cheung AM, O'Rourke K *et al.* (1993) Effect of alpha-interferon treatment in patients with hepatitis B e antigen-positive chronic hepatitis B. A meta-analysis (see comments). *Ann Intern Med* 119, 312–323.

52 Korenman J, Baker B, Waggoner J *et al.* (1991) Long-term remission of chronic hepatitis B after alpha-interferon therapy. *Ann Intern Med* 114, 629–634.

53 Lok AS, Chung HT, Liu VW *et al.* (1993) Long-term follow-up of chronic hepatitis B patients treated with interferon alfa. *Gastroenterology* 105, 1833–1838.

54 Dusheiko, GM, Roberts JA (1995) Treatment of chronic type B and C hepatitis with interferon alfa: an economic appraisal. *Hepatology* 22, 1863–1873.

55 Wong JB, Koff RS, Tine F *et al.* (1995) Cost-effectiveness of interferon-alpha 2b treatment for hepatitis B e antigen-positive chronic hepatitis B. *Ann Intern Med* 122, 664–675.

56 Cooksley WG, Piratvisuth T, Lee SD *et al.* (2003) Peginterferon alpha-2a (40 kDa): an advance in the treatment of hepatitis B e antigen-positive chronic hepatitis B. *J Viral Hepat* 10, 298–305.

57 Janssen HL, van Zonneveld M, Senturk H *et al.* (2005) Pegylated interferon alfa-2b alone or in combination with lamivudine for HBeAg-positive chronic hepatitis B: a randomised trial. *Lancet* 365, 123–129.

58 Lau GK, Piratvisuth T, Luo KX *et al.* (2005) Peginterferon Alfa-2a, lamivudine, and the combination for HBeAg-positive chronic hepatitis B. *N Engl J Med* 352, 2682–2695.

59 Dienstag JL, Schiff ER, Wright TL *et al.* (1999) Lamivudine as initial treatment for chronic hepatitis B in the United States. *N Engl J Med* 341, 1256–1263.

60 Lai CL, Chine RW, Leung NWY *et al.* (1998) A one year trial of lamivudine for chronic hepatitis B. *N Engl J Med* 339, 61–68.

61 Zoulim F (2002) A preliminary benefit-risk assessment of Lamivudine for the treatment of chronic hepatitis B virus infection. *Drug Safety* 25, 497–510.

62 Dienstag JL, Goldin RD, Heathcote EJ *et al.* (2003) Histological outcome during long-term lamivudine therapy. *Gastroenterology* 124, 105–117.

63 Leung NW, Lai CL, Chang TT *et al.* (2001) Extended lamivudine treatment in patients with chronic hepatitis B enhances hepatitis B e antigen seroconversion rates: results after 3 years of therapy. *Hepatology* 33, 1527–1532.

64 Chien RN, Liaw YF, Atkins M (1999) Pretherapy alanine transaminase level as a determinant for hepatitis B e antigen seroconversion during lamivudine therapy in patients with chronic hepatitis B. Asian Lamivudine Trial Group. *Hepatology* 30, 770–774.

65 Locarnini S, Hatzakis A, Heathcote J *et al.* (2004) Management of antiviral resistance in patients with chronic hepatitis B. *Antiviral Ther* 9, 679–963.

66 Zoulim F, Poynard T, Degos F *et al.* (2006) A prospective study of the evolution of lamivudine resistance mutations in patients with chronic hepatitis B treated with lamivudine. *J Viral Hepat* 13, 278–288.

67 Lai CL, Dienstag J, Schiff E *et al.* (2003) Prevalence and clinical correlates of YMDD variants during lamivudine therapy for patients with chronic hepatitis B. *Clin Infect Dis* 36, 687–696.

68 Hadziyannis SJ, Papatheodoridis GV, Dimou E *et al.* (2000) Efficacy of long-term lamivudine monotherapy in patients with hepatitis B e antigen-negative chronic hepatitis B. *Hepatology* 32, 847–851.

69 Nafa S, Ahmed S, Tavan D *et al.* (2000) Early detection of viral resistance by determination of hepatitis B virus polymerase mutations in patients treated by lamivudine for chronic hepatitis B. *Hepatology* 32, 1078–1088.

70 Lampertico P, Vigano M, Manenti E *et al.* (2005) Adefovir rapidly suppresses hepatitis B in HBeAg-negative patients developing genotypic resistance to lamivudine. *Hepatology* 42, 1414–1419.

71 Marcelli M, Chang TT, Lim SG *et al.* (2003) Adefovir dipivoxil for the treatment of hepatitis B e antigen-positive chronic hepatitis B. *N Engl J Med* 348, 808–816.

72 Gish RG, Trinh H, Leung N *et al.* (2005) Safety and antiviral activity of emtricitabine (FTC) for the treatment of chronic hepatitis B infection: a two-year study. *J Hepatol* 43, 60–66.

73 Lai CL, Rosmawati M, Lao J *et al.* (2002) Entecavir is superior to lamivudine in reducing hepatitis B virus DNA in patients with chronic hepatitis B infection. *Gastroenterology* 123, 1831–1838.

74 Wolters LM, Hansen BE, Niesters HG *et al.* (2002) Viral dynamics during and after entecavir therapy in patients with chronic hepatitis B. *J Hepatol* 37, 137–144.

75 Chang TT, Gish RG, de Man R *et al.* (2006) A comparison of entecavir and lamivudine for HBeAg-positive chronic hepatitis B. *N Engl J Med* 354, 1001–1010.

76 Colonno RJ, Rose R, Baldick CJ *et al.* (2006) Entecavir resistance is rare in nucleoside-naïve patients with hepatitis B. *Hepatology* 44, 1656–1665.

77 Lai C, Lim SG, Brown NA *et al.* (2004) A dose-finding study of once-daily oral telbivudine in HBeAg-positive patients with chronic hepatitis B virus infection. *Hepatology* 40, 719–726.

78 Lai CL, Gane E, Liaw Y-F *et al.* (2005) Telbivudine versus lamivudine for chronic hepatitis B: first year results from the international phase III globe trial (abstract LB01). *Hepatology* 42 (Suppl 1), 748A.

79 Bani-Sadr F, Palmer P, Scieux C *et al.* (2004) Ninety-six-week efficacy of combination therapy with lamivudine and tenofovir in patients coinfected with HIV-1 and wild-type hepatitis B virus. *Clin Infect Dis* 39, 1062–1064.

80 Benhamou Y, Tubiana R, Thibault V (2003) Tenofovir disoproxil fumarate in patients with HIV and lamivudine-resistant hepatitis B virus. *N Engl J Med* 348, 177–178.

81 Dore GJ, Cooper DA, Pozniak AL *et al.* (2004) Efficacy of tenofovir disoproxil fumarate in antiretroviral therapy-naive and -experienced patients coinfected with HIV-1 and hepatitis B virus. *J Infect Dis* 189, 1185–1192.

82 Lacombe K, Gozlan J, Boelle PY *et al.* (2005) Long-term hepatitis B virus dynamics in HIV-hepatitis B virus-co-infected patients treated with tenofovir disoproxil fumarate. *AIDS* 19, 907–915.

83 van Bommel F, Wunsche T, Mauss S *et al.* (2004) Comparison of adefovir and tenofovir in the treatment of lamivudine-resistant hepatitis B virus infection. *Hepatology* 40, 1421–1425.

84 Lampertico P, Del Ninno E, Manzin A *et al.* (1997) A randomized, controlled trial of a 24-month course of interferon alfa 2b in patients with chronic hepatitis B who had hepatitis B virus DNA without hepatitis B e antigen in serum. *Hepatology* 26, 1621–1625.

85 Manesis EK, Hadziyannis SJ (2001) Interferon alpha treatment and retreatment of hepatitis B e antigen-negative chronic hepatitis B. *Gastroenterology* 121, 101–109.

86 Tassopoulo, NC, Volpes R, Pastore G *et al.* (1999) Efficacy of lamivudine in patients with hepatitis B e antigen-negative/hepatitis B virus DNA-positive (precore mutant) chronic hepatitis B (in process citation). *Hepatology* 29, 889–896.

87 Rizzetto M, Tassopoulos NC, Goldin RD *et al.* (2005) Extended lamivudine treatment in patients with HBeAg-negative chronic hepatitis B. *J Hepatol* 42, 173–179.

88 Buti M, Cotrina M, Jardi R *et al.* (2001) Two years of lamivudine therapy in anti-HBe-positive patients with chronic hepatitis B. *J Viral Hepat* 8, 270–275.

89 Di Marco V, Marzano A, Lampertico P *et al.* (2004) Clinical outcome of HBeAg-negative chronic hepatitis B in relation to virological response to lamivudine. *Hepatology* 40, 883–891.

90 Papatheodoridis GV, Dimou E, Laras A *et al.* (2002) Course of virologic breakthroughs under long-term lamivudine in HBeAg-negative precore mutant HBV liver disease. *Hepatology* 36, 219–226.

91 Rizzetto M (2002) Efficacy of lamivudine in HBeAg-negative chronic hepatitis B. *J Med Virol* 66, 435–451.

92 Hadziyannis SJ, Tassopoulos NC, Heathcote EJ *et al.* (2003) Adefovir dipivoxil for the treatment of hepatitis B e antigen-negative chronic hepatitis B. *N Engl J Med* 348, 800–807.

93 Hadziyannis SJ, Tassopoulos NC, Heathcote EJ et al. (2005) Long-term therapy with adefovir dipivoxil for HBeAg-negative chronic hepatitis B. N Engl J Med 352, 2673–2681.

94 Hadziyannis S, Tassopoulos N, Chang TT et al. (2005) Long-term adefovir dipivoxil treatment induces regression of liver fibrosis in patients with HBeAg-negative chronic hepatitis B: results after 5 years of therapy (abstract LB14). Hepatology 42 (Suppl 1), 745A.

95 Lai CL, Shouval D, Lok AS et al. (2006) Entecavir versus lamivudine for patients with HBeAg-negative chronic hepatitis B. N Engl J Med 354, 1011–1020.

96 Marcellin P, Lau GK, Bonino F et al. (2004) Peginterferon alfa-2a alone, lamivudine alone, and the two in combination in patients with HBeAg-negative chronic hepatitis B. N Engl J Med 351, 1206–1217.

97 Perrillo R, Hann HW, Mutimer D et al. (2004) Adefovir dipivoxil added to ongoing lamivudine in chronic hepatitis B with YMDD mutant hepatitis B virus. Gastroenterology 126, 81–90.

98 Peters MG, Hann HW, Martin P et al. (2004) Adefovir dipivoxil alone or in combination with lamivudine in patients with lamivudine-resistant chronic hepatitis B. Gastroenterology 126, 91–101.

99 Sherman M, Yurdaydin C, Sollano J et al. (2006) Entecavir for treatment of lamivudine-refractory HBeAg-positive chronic hepatitis B. Gastroenterology 130, 2039–2049.

100 Werle B, Cinquin K, Marcellin P et al. (2004) Evolution of hepatitis B viral load and viral genome sequence during adefovir dipivoxil therapy. J Viral Hepat 11, 74–83.

101 Lok AS, Zoulim F, Locarnini S et al. (2002) Monitoring drug resistance in chronic hepatitis B virus (HBV)-infected patients during lamivudine therapy: evaluation of performance of INNO-LiPA HBV DR assay. J Clin Microbiol 40, 3729–3734.

102 Durantel D, Carrouee-Durantel S, Werle-Lapostolle B et al. (2004). A new strategy for studying in vitro the drug susceptibility of clinical isolates of human hepatitis B virus. Hepatology 40, 855–864.

103 Yang H, Westland C, Xiong S et al. (2004) In vitro antiviral susceptibility of full-length clinical hepatitis B virus isolates cloned with a novel expression vector. Antiviral Res 61, 27–36.

104 Liaw YF, Sung JJ, Chow WC et al. (2004) Lamivudine for patients with chronic hepatitis B and advanced liver disease. N Engl J Med 351, 1521–1531.

105 Villeneuve JP, Condreay LD, Willems B et al. (2000) Lamivudine treatment for decompensated cirrhosis resulting from chronic hepatitis B. Hepatology 31, 207–210.

106 Yao FY, Bass NM (2000) Lamivudine treatment in patients with severely decompensated cirrhosis due to replicating hepatitis B infection (in process citation). J Hepatol 33, 301–307.

107 Yao FY, Terrault NA, Freise C et al. (2001) Lamivudine treatment is beneficial in patients with severely decompensated cirrhosis and actively replicating hepatitis B infection awaiting liver transplantation: a comparative study using a matched, untreated cohort. Hepatology 34, 411–416.

108 Schiff ER, Lai CL, Hadziyannis S et al. (2003) Adefovir dipivoxil therapy for lamivudine-resistant hepatitis B in pre- and post-liver transplantation patients. Hepatology 38, 1419–1427.

109 Buti M, Mas A, Prieto M et al. (2003) A randomized study comparing lamivudine monotherapy after a short course of hepatitis B immune globulin (HBIg) and lamivudine with long-term lamivudine plus HBIg in the prevention of hepatitis B virus recurrence after liver transplantation. J Hepatol 38, 811–817.

110 Perrillo RP, Wright T, Rakela J et al. (2001) A multicenter United States-Canadian trial to assess lamivudine monotherapy before and after liver transplantation for chronic hepatitis B. Hepatology 33, 424–432.

111 Zoulim F (2003) Towards an improved and cost-saving prophylaxis of hepatitis B virus recurrence after liver transplantation? J Hepatol 38, 850–852.

112 Perrillo R, Rakela J, Dienstag J et al. (1999) Multicenter study of lamivudine therapy for hepatitis B after liver transplantation. Lamivudine Transplant Group. Hepatology 29, 1581–1586.

113 Farci P, Mandas A, Coiana A et al. (1994) Treatment of chronic hepatitis D with interferon alfa-2a. N Engl J Med 330, 88–94.

114 Rosina F, Pintus C, Meschievitz C et al. (1991) A randomized controlled trial of a 12-month course of recombinant human interferon-alpha in chronic delta (type D) hepatitis: a multicenter Italian study. Hepatology 13, 1052–1056.

115 Niro GA, Rosina F, Rizzetto M (2005). Treatment of hepatitis D. J Viral Hepat 12, 2–9.

116 Farci P, Roskams T, Chessa L et al. (2004) Long-term benefit of interferon alpha therapy of chronic hepatitis D: regression of advanced hepatic fibrosis. Gastroenterology 126, 1740–1749.

117 Lau DT, Kleiner DE, Park Y et al. (1999) Resolution of chronic delta hepatitis after 12 years of interferon alfa therapy. Gastroenterology 117, 1229–1233.

118 Puoti M, Rossi S, Forleo MA et al. (1998) Treatment of chronic hepatitis D with interferon alpha-2b in patients with human immunodeficiency virus infection. J Hepatol 29, 45–52.

119 Yurdaydin C, Bozkaya H, Gurel S et al. (2002) Famciclovir treatment of chronic delta hepatitis. J Hepatol 37, 266–271.

120 Lau DT, Doo E, Park Y et al. (1999) Lamivudine for chronic delta hepatitis (see comments). Hepatology 30, 546–549.

121 Niro GA, Ciancio A, Tillman HL et al. (2005) Lamivudine therapy in chronic delta hepatitis: a multicentre randomized-controlled pilot study. Aliment Pharmacol Ther 22, 227–232.

122 Wolters LM, van Nunen AB, Honkoop P et al. (2000) Lamivudine-high dose interferon combination therapy for chronic hepatitis B patients co-infected with the hepatitis D virus. J Viral Hepat 7, 428–434.

123 Castelnau C, LeGal F, Ripault MP et al. (2006) Efficacy of Peginterferon alpha 2-b in chronic hepatitis delta: relevance of quantitative RT-PCR for follow-up. Hepatology 44, 728–735.

124 Ferenci P, Formann E, Romeo R (2005) Successful treatment of chronic hepatitis D with a short course of peginterferon alfa-2a. Am J Gastroenterol 100, 1626–1627.

125 Samuel D, Zignego AL, Reynes M et al. (1995) Long-term clinical and virological outcome after liver transplantation for cirrhosis caused by chronic delta hepatitis. Hepatology 21, 333–339.

126 Marzano A, Lampertico P, Mazzaferro V et al. (2005) Prophylaxis of hepatitis B virus recurrence after liver transplantation in carriers of lamivudine-resistant mutants. Liver Transpl 11, 532–538.

127 Prince AM, Trepo C (1971) Role of immune complexes involving SH antigen in pathogenesis of chronic active hepatitis and polyarteritis nodosa. Lancet 1, 1309–1312.

128 Trepo C, Thivolet J (1970) Hepatitis associated antigen and periarteritis nodosa (PAN). Vox Sang 19, 410–411.

129 Erhardt A, Sagir A, Guillevin L et al. (2000) Successful treatment of hepatitis B virus associated polyarteritis nodosa with a combination

of prednisolone, alpha-interferon and lamivudine. *J Hepatol* 33, 677–683.

130 Krüger M, Böker KHW, Zeidler H *et al.* (1997) Treatment of hepatitis B-related polyarteritis nodosa with Famciclovir and interferon alfa-2b. *J Hepatol* 26, 935–939.

131 Maclachlan D, Battegay M, Jacob AL *et al.* (2000) Successful treatment of hepatitis B-associated polyarteritis nodosa with a combination of lamivudine and conventional immunosuppressive therapy: a case report (letter). *Rheumatology (Oxford)* 39, 106–108.

132 Wartelle-Bladou C, Lafon J, Trepo C *et al.* (2001) Successful combination therapy of polyarteritis nodosa associated with a pre-core promoter mutant hepatitis B virus infection. *J Hepatol* 34, 774–779.

133 Wicki J, Olivieri J, Pizzolato G *et al.* (1999) Successful treatment of polyarteritis nodosa related to hepatitis B virus with a combination of lamivudine and interferon alpha (letter). *Rheumatology (Oxford)* 38, 183–185.

134 van Zonneveld M, van Nunen AB, Niesters HG *et al.* (2003) Lamivudine treatment during pregnancy to prevent perinatal transmission of hepatitis B virus infection. *J Viral Hepat* 10, 294–297.

135 Jonas MM, Kelly DA, Mizerski J *et al.* (2002) Clinical trial of lamivudine in children with chronic hepatitis B. *N Engl J Med* 346, 1706–1713.

136 Bortolotti F, Jara P, Barbera C *et al.* (2000) Long term effect of alpha interferon in children with chronic hepatitis B. *Gut* 46, 715–718.

137 Lai CL, Lok AS, Lin HJ *et al.* (1987) Placebo-controlled trial of recombinant alpha 2-interferon in Chinese HBsAg-carrier children. *Lancet* 2, 877–880.

138 Richman DD (2000) The impact of drug resistance on the effectiveness of chemotherapy for chronic hepatitis B. *Hepatology* 32, 866–867.

139 Lau GK, Tsiang M, Hou J *et al.* (2000) Combination therapy with lamivudine and famciclovir for chronic hepatitis B-infected Chinese patients: a viral dynamics study (see comments). *Hepatology* 32, 394–399.

140 Seigneres B, Martin P, Werle B *et al.* (2003) Effects of pyrimidine and purine analog combinations in the duck hepatitis B virus infection model. *Antimicrob Agents Chemother* 47, 1842–1852.

141 Colledge D, Civitico G, Locarnini S *et al.* (2000) In vitro antihepadnaviral activities of combinations of penciclovir, lamivudine, and adefovir (in process citation). *Antimicrob Agents Chemother* 44, 551–560.

142 Colledge D, Locarnini S, Shaw T (1997) Synergistic inhibition of hepadnaviral replication by lamivudine in combination with penciclovir in vitro. *Hepatology* 26, 216–225.

143 Korba BE (1996) In vitro evaluation of combination therapies against hepatitis B virus replication. *Antiviral Res* 29, 49–51.

144 Korba BE, Cote P, Hornbuckle W *et al.* (2000) Enhanced antiviral benefit of combination therapy with lamivudine and famciclovir against WHV replication in chronic WHV carrier woodchucks. *Antiviral Res* 45, 19–32.

145 Delaney WET, Edwards R, Colledge D *et al.* (2001) Cross-resistance testing of antihepadnaviral compounds using novel recombinant baculoviruses which encode drug-resistant strains of hepatitis B virus. *Antimicrob Agents Chemother* 45, 1705–1713.

146 Fu L, Cheng YC (2000) Characterization of novel human hepatoma cell lines with stable hepatitis B virus secretion for evaluating new compounds against lamivudine- and penciclovir-resistant virus (in process citation). *Antimicrob Agents Chemother* 44, 3402–3407.

147 Menne S, Roneker CA, Korba BE *et al.* (2002) Immunization with surface antigen vaccine alone and after treatment with 1-(2-fluoro-5-methyl-beta-L-arabinofuranosyl)-uracil (L-FMAU) breaks humoral and cell-mediated immune tolerance in chronic woodchuck hepatitis virus infection. *J Virol* 76, 5305–5314.

148 Zoulim F (2003) Treatment of pre- and post-liver transplantation HBV infection: Should we aim at combination therapy? *Hepatology* 38, 1353–1355.

9.1.3.v Therapy for chronic hepatitis C

Giorgio Saracco, Fabien Zoulim and Mario Rizzetto

Introduction

Interferon (IFN) was introduced as monotherapy for chronic hepatitis C at the end of the 1980s [1,2]. Different types of α- and beta-IFNs initially shared the therapeutic arena, with the recommended duration of therapy 24 weeks; this was later extended to 48 weeks [3]. The rates of sustained responses were initially limited, in the range of 12–16% [4]. A therapeutic advance was made with the introduction of ribavirin (RBV) in association with IFN in 1998 [5,6]; in all of the different clinical subsets of hepatitis C virus (HCV)-infected patients, this combination virtually doubled the rate of cure that was achieved with IFN monotherapy. In parallel, recombinant α-IFNs have emerged as the most efficacious among the different types of IFNs.

At the end of the 1990s, the development of pegylated IFN led to further improvements [7–9]; currently, about 50% of HCV patients treated with the combination of pegylated IFN and RBV are expected to be cured of infection.

The interferons

The IFNs are a family of cytokines that are produced by eukaryotic cells in response to a variety of stimuli [10]. They are biologically multivalent, possessing antiproliferative, antiviral and immunomodulant properties. There are three types of natural IFN: IFN-α, produced mainly by leukocytes, IFN-β, produced mainly by fibroblasts, and IFN-γ, produced mainly by T lymphocytes. IFN-α and -β interact with the same cellular receptor, whereas IFN-γ interacts with different receptors.

There are two major types of IFN-α available for therapeutic use, both produced by recombinant technology: IFN-α-2a and IFN-α-2b. Standard IFN-α are dosed in million units (MU). A hybrid bioengineered 'consensus' molecule (IFN-alfacon-1) is also available for therapy [11]; it is composed of the amino acids that are most frequently conserved at each position of the α IFNs and shares 89%, 30% and 60% identity with IFN-α, IFN-β and IFN-γ respectively. The optimal dosing schedule is 9–15 μg daily; efficacy is similar to that of IFN-α-2b. In some European countries, leukocyte-derived IFN-α, produced by the stimulation of human leukocytes, is used in patients who are intolerant to recombinant IFN-α. IFN-beta is used in Japan; the use of lymphoblastoid-derived IFN-α has been dismissed.

The process of pegylation, by which an inert molecule of polyethylene glycol (PEG) is covalently linked to a protein, increases the molecular weight of IFN, thus inducing a slower absorption, reduced clearance and an increased serum half-life [12]. Two formulations of PEG-IFN are available: PEG-IFN-α-2b, in which IFN-α-2b is attached to a single 12 kDa PEG molecule, and PEG-IFN-α-2a, in which IFN-α-2a is attached to a branched 40 kDa methoxy-PEG moiety. Pegylated IFNs are dosed in micrograms (μg).

Both PEG-IFNs are administered subcutaneously at once-weekly intervals, and the serum concentrations of IFN are maintained throughout the dosing interval. PEG-IFN-α-2a is metabolized primarily in the liver by non-specific proteases; biodistribution is restricted predominantly to the blood and extracellular volume [13]. PEG-IFN-α-2b is eliminated primarily via the kidney and is widely distributed throughout body fluids and tissues, the volume distribution depending on body weight; weight-based dosing is recommended [13].

IFN-α-2b has also been fused with recombinant human serum albumin producing an 85.7 kDa protein (Albuferon). The more extended half-life of Albuferon permits dosing once every 2–4 weeks; the longer duration of therapeutic activity might improve the efficacy and tolerability compared with conventional IFNs and PEG-IFNs [14].

Ribavirin

RBV is a synthetic guanosine analogue that has been used for the treatment of respiratory syncytial virus infection in infants. It inhibits the RNA-dependent RNA polymerase of all six HCV subtypes as well as the subgenomic HCV replicon system *in vitro*, but has no clinically significant effect on viral replication [15]; although it exerts only an early, transient and moderate antiviral action *in vivo*, it may significantly decrease serum alanine aminotransferase (ALT) activity in approximately 50% of patients, with an improvement in liver histology [16,17]. Despite the lack of antiviral efficacy when used as monotherapy, in association with IFNs or PEG-IFNs, RBV significantly improves the rates of sustained virological responses, reducing virological relapses during follow-up. It is rapidly absorbed following oral administration and bioavailability is increased when it is administered with a fat meal. The drug accumulates with repeated administration; its concentration is several-fold higher in erythrocytes than in blood [15]. Excretion of RBV and its metabolites is by the renal route and it should not be used in patients with kidney failure.

RBV is currently used at dosages between 800 and 1200 mg/day, in two divided doses. Its mechanism of action remains unclear, but the lack of virological efficacy suggests that its beneficial effect may be immune-mediated [18]. Alternatively, it may act through the inhibition of HCV RNA-dependent RNA polymerase at the level of the catalytic site [19] or it may have mutagenic properties, leading to 'error catastrophe' and resulting in the generation of non-viable HCV quasi-species [20]. RBV may also inhibit inosine monophosphate dehydrogenase (IMPDH), resulting in depletion of the intracellular pool of dGTP, which may subsequently lead to decreased viral replication levels. RBV was also shown in mouse model experiments to modulate the immune response towards a T-helper 1 (Th1) response, which may account for its synergistic effect in combination with IFN-α.

Definition of response

The goal of therapy is the eradication of HCV. A biphasic HCV decay is seen with current antiviral therapies [21]. The HCV decline slopes differ among treated patients and can be distinguished as rapid, slow or flat. The type of slope correlates with the probability of a sustained virological response (SVR); patients with an initially rapid slope achieve the highest rate of sustained responses. In the rapid phase of the response, which occurs during the first 2 days of therapy, the serum titre of HCV declines quickly, reflecting the inhibition of virus replication by IFN and its degradation in serum. The decline of HCV titre starts 8–12 h after the first dose of IFN; the HCV-RNA serum titre diminishes by 0.5–1.5 logs within the next 48 h [22]. The slope pattern and viral decline depend on the type and dose of IFN. In the second slower phase, starting 2–3 days after therapy begins, the virus decline is slower, reflecting the clearance of infected cells; complete virus elimination requires several months of further therapy [23]. Usually, the clearance of the virus is accompanied by normalization of liver enzymes and an improvement of histology; if this does not occur despite virus elimination, a concomitant cause of liver damage other than HCV should be suspected. Occasionally, ALT may become normal in patients who remain viraemic, possibly because of a normalizing effect of RBV on ALT levels. Alternatively, ALT levels may remain elevated despite the clearance of viraemia and the lack of other risk factors for liver disease; this may particularly be the case in patients treated with PEG-IFN and in those with fibrosis and cirrhosis, and may be the result of a minor toxic effect of IFN [7,8]; the enzyme levels return to normal when therapy is terminated [6–8].

During therapy, the clearance of HCV follows defined time points that have prognostic significance and help to guide the management of the patient [24,25]. The end-of-therapy virological response (ETR) is defined as the clearance of HCV during therapy, which is maintained at the end of therapy. The achievement of a ETR is mandatory for the eradication of the virus. A virological relapse is defined as the reappearance of HCV RNA in serum during follow-up, after its apparent clearance following therapy. A virological breakthrough is defined as the early disappearance of HCV RNA during therapy, followed by the reappearance of the virus before the end of therapy. Effective therapy is confirmed by the achievement of a SVR. This is defined as the maintenance of virus clearance 6 months after termination of therapy.

Long-term post-treatment follow-up studies have shown that HCV RNA remains undetectable in more than 95% of patients who achieve a SVR [26–28], and that SVR results in long-term histological improvement [28–31]; therefore, SVR is adopted as a surrogate marker of cure. Of note, hepatocellular carcinoma (HCC) may still develop in patients who originally presented with cirrhosis or fibrosis and who had a SVR to antiviral therapy [32,33]; however, the incidence of HCC in sustained responders is lower than that in untreated or non-responding patients.

Two additional interim response points have attracted clinical interest, the early virological response (EVR) [34], defined by the clearance of HCV RNA or a decrease of at least 2 log10 in the viraemic titre compared with baseline, 12 weeks after starting therapy, and the rapid virological response (RVR), defined as the clearance of HCV RNA, 4 weeks after starting therapy [35]. A SVR can be predicted with more than 70% probability by an EVR, and the failure to achieve an EVR predicts a lack of SVR with almost 98% probability; similarly, it has been reported that a RVR predicts a SVR with almost 90% probability. Therefore, EVR appears to be a strong negative and RVR a strong positive predictor of a virological response.

Unfortunately, differences in the sensitivity and dynamic ranges of currently available assays used to measure HCV-RNA levels in serum limit the usefulness of quantitative HCV-RNA testing and comparisons [36]. Standardization of all HCV-RNA assays to a World Health Organization standard, and expression of results as a common international unit has been proposed [37]. Assays with a wide dynamic range should be used, with a lower detection limit of at least 50 IU/mL. The use of the ultrasensitive transcription-mediated amplification (TMA) assay (with a detection limit of 10 IU/mL) may further help to determine the optimal duration of treatment. In the HALT-C study [38], patients who were negative at week 48 of therapy, based on the Roche COBAS Amplicor 2.0 assay (sensitivity ≥ 100 IU/mL), but who remained TMA-positive, had an 89% chance of post-treatment relapse. Therefore, TMA testing during, or at the end of, antiviral therapy might help to identify patients who could benefit from extended antiviral treatment.

Therapeutic protocols

The combination of PEG-IFN with RBV (PEG-IFN/RBV) has become the standard of care for chronic hepatitis C [7–9]. PEG-IFN/RBV is more effective than standard IFN at doses between 3 and 6 MU with RBV (IFN/RBV) (overall SVR rate of 54% versus 47% respectively) [5–9,39] or PEG-IFN alone (overall SVR rate of 54% versus 39% respectively) [40]. PEG-IFN alone is significantly superior to standard IFN alone (overall

SVR rate of 39% versus 19%), particularly in cirrhotic patients (overall SVR rate of 30% versus 8%) [41].

The efficacy of PEG-IFN-α-2b was documented in a randomized controlled trial of 1530 patients [7]. The highest SVR rate (54%) was observed in patients treated with 1.5 μg/kg of PEG-IFN in combination with 800 mg daily of RBV. The SVR rate was 47% in patients treated with 0.5 μg/kg of PEG-IFN or standard IFN. The SVR rate among HCV-1-infected patients treated with PEG-IFN/RBV (42%) was significantly higher than that observed with standard IFN/RBV (33%) and significantly lower than the 80% SVR rate observed in patients with HCV-2 or -3 from all therapy groups.

The efficacy of PEG-IFN-α-2a/RBV was determined in two multicentre trials of 1121 [8] and 1311 [9] patients. In the first trial [8], a 56% SVR rate was obtained among patients treated with a 'flat' dose of PEG-IFN-α-2a (180 μg weekly) plus RBV (1000–1200 mg daily); the SVR rate was significantly higher in patients with HCV-2 or -3 (76%) than in those with HCV-1 (46%). In the second trial [9], among HCV-1 patients treated with 180 μg weekly of PEG-IFN-α-2a and 1000–1200 mg daily of RBV, the SVR rate was significantly higher in those treated for 48 weeks (52.2%) than in those treated for 24 weeks only (41%). Among HCV-2 and HCV-3 patients given PEG-IFN-α-2a at a dose of 180 μg weekly, those treated with a low dose (800 mg/day) of RBV for 24 weeks had the same SVR (80%) as those treated for 48 weeks or those treated for 24 weeks with higher RBV doses (1000–1200 mg/day).

There are few data available on the responsiveness of HCV-4 patients. A study that was targeted to these patients [42] found a SVR rate of 68%, with baseline predictive factors of response that were identical to those observed in HCV-1 patients. HCV-5 appears to be a relatively easy virus to treat, with response rates that are similar to those of HCV-2 and -3 after a 48-week course of therapy. Response rates in patients with HCV-6 may be intermediate between HCV-1 and HCV-2 or -3; the optimal duration of treatment (24 versus 48 weeks) for this genotype is unclear and under investigation [43].

The current treatment protocols recommended by the National Institutes of Health (NIH) consensus conference [44] are reported in Table 1. The dosage of PEG-IFN-α-2b should be tailored to the weight of the patient, i.e. 1.5 μg/kg/week; PEG-IFN-α-2a is administered at a fixed dose (180 μg/week). These recommendations may have to be revised according to the results of ongoing trials designed to assess whether 1 μg/kg/week of PEG-IFN-α-2b is as effective as 1.5 μg/kg/week [45]. A dose of PEG-IFN-α-2a of 135 μg/week may be as effective as 180 μg/week in HCV-2 and -3 patients [46].

In HCV-1-infected patients treated with PEG-IFN-α-2b, the dose of RBV should be adjusted according to weight (10.6 mg/kg). In contrast, in HCV-2 or -3 patients treated with both PEG-IFN-α-2b and PEG-IFN-α-2a, a flat RBV dose of 800 mg/day can be given [47]; preliminary data suggest that, in these patients, daily doses of 400 mg may be as effective [48]. Dosing may be determined by measuring RBV plasma

Treatment schedule	Dosage	
	Genotype 1 (48 weeks)	Genotypes 2 and 3 (24 weeks)
PEG-IFN-α-2a + RBV	IFN: 180 μg/week; RBV: 1000 mg/day (< 75 kg) or 1200 mg/day (> 75 kg)	IFN: 180 μg/week; RBV: 800 mg/day
PEG-IFN-α-2b + RBV	IFN: 1.5 μg/kg/week; RBV: > 10.6 mg/kg/day	IFN: 1.5 μg/kg/week; RBV: 800 mg/day[a]

Table 1 Current recommended treatment schedules for naive patients.

[a]Not proven by specific randomized trials.

concentrations using liquid chromatography; in one study [49], RBV plasma concentrations varied widely and were predictive of anaemia and early virological responses.

A more prolonged 72-week course of therapy may be of benefit in slow-responder patients who fail to clear HCV RNA early [50–54]. In one study [53], 326 patients who did not achieve a RVR were randomized to a 48- or a 78-week course of treatment; the SVR was significantly higher in the latter group (45% versus 32%, $P = 0.01$). In another study [54], the lack of an EVR appeared to be more critical in discriminating patients who might benefit from extended therapy; among patients who failed to achieve an EVR and who were randomized to a 48- or 72-week course of therapy, 29% (31 out of 106) of the latter group obtained a SVR compared with 17% (17 out of 100) of the former ($P = 0.04$).

Patients with the more favourable HCV-2 and -3 genotypes may respond to a short 12-week course of combination therapy, with SVR rates that are similar to those obtained after the standard 24-week course [55,56]; the efficacy of a short-term course appears to be higher in patients with a low viraemia titre before therapy ($\leq 800\ 000$ IU/mL). However, in a prospective study of 1469 patients [57], the overall 76% SVR rate in HCV-2 and -3 patients treated for 24 weeks with PEG-IFN-α-2a/RBV was significantly higher than the 65% rate achieved with 16 weeks of therapy; the difference was accounted for by the higher relapse rate in patients treated for the shorter time period. It is doubtful whether short treatment is efficacious in HCV-3 patients with a high viraemia titre ($\geq 800\ 000$ IU/mL) [58]; whether these patients should be treated for 24 weeks or even longer has to be addressed by further studies [59].

Similarly, a reduced 24-week course of combination therapy may be as effective as the standard 48-week course in HCV-1 patients with low baseline viraemia (< 600 000 IU/mL) [60] and in those who achieve a RVR at week 4 (HCV RNA < 50 IU/mL) [61].

Of note, although reduced therapy courses may be proposed to patients with the appropriate virological credentials who are at risk of side-effects or who are reluctant to undergo full therapy, neither the 12-week course for favourable genotypes nor the 24-week course for the difficult HCV-1 genotype has yet been recommended by consensus conferences.

Many other modified therapeutic protocols have been proposed over the years, including an early induction phase, with IFN given at a higher dosage and/or at more frequent intervals for the first 4–12 weeks [62], late IFN dose reductions after an initial full dose, or intermittent therapy or therapy targeted to the individual virological response [63]. Despite claims that some of these protocols are more efficacious or more cost-effective than the standard protocols, none has been recommended for general use.

Monitoring

Monitoring is important to assess the efficacy of therapy and the development of toxic drug effects. Baseline evaluation should include determinations of white and red blood cell counts, haemoglobin concentration, platelet counts, ALT levels, thyroid-stimulating hormone (TSH) levels, quantitative HCV viraemia and viral genotype. A serum sample should be frozen for possible further re-evaluation and comparison of HCV-RNA titres. Determinations of ALT, liver function tests, haemoglobin concentration, white blood cell count and platelet count should be performed every month to detect toxicity. TSH should be tested every 3 months in order to individuate hyper/hypothyroidism.

Monitoring of serum HCV-RNA levels should be performed at 12 and 24 weeks and at the end of therapy in patients treated for 48 weeks. No interim HCV-RNA monitoring during therapy is required for patients with HCV-2 or -3 who are treated for 6 months; in these patients, HCV-RNA levels should be determined at the end of therapy. A final HCV-RNA test is required at 6 months post-therapy to establish successful eradication of the virus.

Contraindications

Pregnancy

Pregnancy is an absolute contraindication to combination therapy. RBV was found to be teratogenic in animals [19] and fetal mortality was high in women who became pregnant during combination therapy. Patients of childbearing age are required to use stringent contraceptive methods during therapy and for 6 months after treatment suspension.

Ischaemic cardiac and cerebrovascular disease

Patients with ischaemic cardiac and cerebrovascular disease are unsuitable candidates for therapy because of the risk of acute ischaemia secondary to the sudden fall in haemoglobin levels induced by RBV [24,64–66]. Rarely, IFN may induce a reversible cardiac arrhythmia or cardiomyopathy.

Autoimmune disease

Because of the potential for IFN to enhance immune and autoimmune responses [66–69], combination therapy is not recommended for individuals with clinical autoimmune diseases. However, immune-mediated thyroiditis, diabetes, neuropathy and other autoimmune disorders develop in only 1% of treated patients. An increase in the level of autoantibodies during therapy does not imply that an autoimmune disease is developing [70]; in many patients, raised autoantibody levels disappear after therapy withdrawal.

Retinopathy

Ophthalmological side-effects have been reported during IFN therapy, particularly retinal lesions and neurovisual impairment. Patients with hepatitis C who have risk factors for retinopathy should undergo an ophthalmoscopical evaluation before starting treatment. In a study [71] of 156 patients with chronic viral hepatitis and without baseline risk factors for retinopathy who were treated with standard or PEG-IFN, signs of retinopathy and neurovisual impairment were common during therapy but were rarely symptomatic.

Dermatological diseases

Dryness, itching and a wide range of non-specific skin lesions, such as transient rashes, diffuse erythema and urticaria, have been reported during IFN/RBV therapy. Lichen planus and psoriasis may develop or worsen during therapy [72,73]. Both diseases may induce a premature discontinuation of therapy but do not represent an absolute contraindication to treatment.

Side-effects

The common and/or important side-effects of IFN/RBV therapy, their frequency and the methods used to control them are summarized in Table 2 [74–76]. Less common or rare adverse events caused by IFN/PEG-IFN and RBV are reported in Table 3. The 'flu-like' syndrome (fever, chills, headache, myalgias, arthralgia) occurs frequently during the first weeks of therapy, can be prevented by paracetamol and generally abates after the first month of therapy. Other IFN/PEG-IFN-induced symptoms are fatigue, loss of appetite, weight loss, diarrhoea, skin rash, hair loss and insomnia; erythema at the injection site occurs in about 40% of patients and is more frequent with PEG-IFN. Leukocyte IFN-α has been used for IFN retreatment in patients who are intolerant to other IFNs [77].

Haematological side-effects are frequent and may be important [78]. Anaemia usually complicates therapy, with an average

Table 2 Interferon and ribavirin therapy: frequent side-effects of combination therapy.

Side-effect	Frequency (%)	Solution
Flu-like symptoms	59	Paracetamol
Anaemia (> 10% decrease in baseline haemoglobin)	34	RBV dose reduction, epoetin
Alopecia	24	–
Dyspnoea	24	–
Rash	23	Antihistamines, topical steroids
Injection-site inflammation	23	Antihistamines
Dry skin	22	–
WBC count decrease (< 3000 cells/µL); platelet decrease (< 80 000 cells/µL)	21	PEG-IFN dose reduction, G-CSF, GM-CSF
Psychiatric symptoms	19	Antidepressants, diphenhydramine
Nausea	12	–
Anorexia	11	–
Vomiting	10	–
Diarrhoea	10	–
Abdominal pain	8	–
Thyroid disease	5	Substitution therapy
Pruritus	4	–
Cough	3	–

G-CSF, granulocyte colony-stimulating factor; GM-CSF, granulocyte–macrophage colony-stimulating factor; WBC, white blood cell.

Table 3 Interferon and ribavirin therapy: less common or rare adverse events.

Neuropsychiatric
Suicidal ideation or suicide attempt
Personality change
Confusion and coma
Memory loss
Substance-abuse relapse
Tinnitus
Hearing loss
Motor and sensory neuropathy
Seizures

Autoimmune
Type 1 diabetes mellitus
Addison's disease
Coeliac disease
Idiopathic thrombocytopenia
Myasthenia gravis
Autoimmune hepatitis

Pulmonary
Interstitial pneumonitis
Bronchiolitis obliterans organizing pneumonia
Sarcoidosis

Ocular
Retinal haemorrhage
Visual loss
Cotton wool spots
Retinal vein thrombosis

Dermatological
Photosensitivity
Psoriasis flare
Lichen planus

Cardiovascular
Arrhythmias
Congestive heart failure
Myocardial infarction
Angina
Transient ischaemic attack
Stroke

Miscellaneous
Acute renal failure
Exacerbation of hepatitis
Local abscess formation

haemoglobin drop of 2–3 g/dL; more pronounced anaemia (haemoglobin < 10 g/dL) occurs in 5–10% of patients. There is a gradual decline in haemoglobin levels during the first month of therapy, after which the haemoglobin level usually stabilizes. In one study [79], 54% of the patients on combination therapy experienced a haemoglobin decrease of > 3 g/dL. The cause is multifactorial, with RBV inducing a dose-dependent haemolytic anaemia [80,81] and IFN suppressing erythroid progenitor cells and red blood cell production [82]; the level of reticulocytes

markedly increases as a response to anaemia. RBV withdrawal or dose reductions are mandatory when haemoglobin levels fall below 10 g/dL. RBV may also cause nausea, dry skin, pruritus, cough and hyperuricaemia. It may also result in an increase in the level of ferritin during therapy because of haemolysis; however, there is usually no need to remove iron.

Anaemia can be treated with erythropoietin (epoetin) [83–85]. A dose of epoetin of 40 000 IU/week subcutaneously increased the level of haemoglobin by approximately 2 g/dL in patients who developed anaemia, allowing the full RBV dose to be continued in about 90% of patients and improving the quality of life [85]. Common adverse effects of epoetin are headache and nausea; the drug can also result in the formation of thrombi.

Leukocytopenia with granulocytopenia and thrombocytopenia are also common side-effects of therapy; granulocytopenia occurs more frequently with PEG-IFN than with standard IFN. In about 10–20% of treated patients, neutropenia requires a dose reduction of PEG-IFN; however, therapy suspension – mandatory when the neutrophil count decreases to less than 500/μl – is rarely needed. Granulocyte–macrophage colony-stimulating factor can be used to raise the granulocyte count [86,87]. Thrombocytopenia is common but rarely causes symptoms (purpura) or forces dose reductions. Nevertheless, it is the most common cause for excluding cirrhotics from therapy: the exclusion threshold is usually 40 000–50 000 platelets/μl. RBV attenuates thrombocytopenia by stimulating megakaryocytes and thrombocytosis as a reaction to anaemia; therefore, thrombocytopenia is more pronounced in patients given IFN alone.

Treatment may induce dysthyroidism [88,89]; however, there is no association between thyroid dysfunction and IFN dosage or efficacy of therapy [90]. Female gender and the presence of antithyroid microsomes or antithyroperoxidase antibodies before beginning antiviral therapy are predictive of dysthyroidism during therapy [91].

Although the finding of thyroid autoantibodies may help to identify patients who are at risk for thyroid disease during therapy, these patients should not be excluded from therapy because only a minority will develop abnormalities of thyroid function. Likewise, therapy should not be suspended in patients who develop thyroid autoantibodies during therapy but maintain a normal TSH level. Thyroid IFN-related dysfunction is reversible in most, but not all, patients after stopping therapy; hypothyroidism may ensue [92].

Patients with spontaneous or IFN-related stable hypothyroidism (treated with thyroid hormone replacement) can be safely given or regiven IFN. Treatment should be discontinued in patients who develop hyperthyroidism; however, in cases in which there is significant HCV liver disease, it can be continued in association with antithyrotoxic therapy and supervision by an endocrinologist. Of note, the development of fatigue, anxiety and tachycardia during therapy should alert the clinician to thyroid dysfunction as well as to RBV-induced anaemia.

Therapy with IFN tends to aggravate a depressive personality; therefore, treatment should only be offered to depressed patients who have severe liver disease, provided that psychiatric stabilization can be achieved [93–95]. Psychiatric side-effects during therapy may be severe, ranging from irritability and mood changes to profound depression and suicide attempts [96]. Side-effects occur more frequently during early than late therapy. Depression can be controlled by paroxetine (a serotonin reuptake inhibitor), initiated before and continued during treatment [97]. If IFN is absolutely contraindicated and liver disease is progressing, RBV monotherapy may be considered.

Epilepsy may be exacerbated by IFN therapy; however, epileptic patients who are undergoing drug treatment to achieve neurological control can be given antiviral therapy.

Rules for stopping treatment

The current recommendation is to discontinue treatment in patients who do not achieve a EVR or a reduction in HCV-RNA levels from baseline of at least 2 log10 by treatment week 12 (negative predictive value approaching 100%). In contrast, patients who achieve these endpoints have an increased probability (67–83%) of achieving a SVR and should be encouraged to continue treatment. However, the favourable prognostic significance of a viraemic decline that is short of complete virus clearance has been questioned; a recent analysis has shown that a distinct proportion of patients who had a reduced viraemic titre of lower than 2 log10 at 12 weeks of therapy failed to eradicate HCV and experienced viral rebounds during and after therapy [54].

Patients who achieve an EVR can complete therapy without further HCV-RNA testing, whereas those who remain HCV-RNA-positive (regardless of the 2 log10 reduction) should be retested for HCV RNA at 24 weeks. Patients who remain HCV-RNA-positive at 24 weeks should stop treatment, whereas those who are negative should complete the course of therapy.

These rules for stopping therapy do not apply to patients with HCV-2 or -3, who have a high probability of achieving a SVR and who do not require assessment of an EVR.

Factors predictive of a response to antiviral therapy

Both viral [65] and host [98] factors influence the probability of achieving a response to antiviral therapy; most factors are fixed, although a few may be correctable (Table 4). The most important factor is the HCV genotype; in each clinical category of hepatitis C patients, genotypes 2 and 3 are easier to treat, with SVR rates that are double those achieved with the difficult-to-treat genotype 1 [5,8,44,58,60,64,65,99]; genotype 1a may respond better than genotype 1b [100]. Genotypes 4, 5 and 6 appear to respond less well than genotypes 2 and 3, but better than 1a and 1b [42,43].

Patients with high serum viral loads respond less well than those with low viraemia [5,8]. However, what is considered a low or a high viral titre is arbitrary to a considerable degree;

Table 4 Baseline factors affecting the response to therapy.

Non-modifiable factors
Gender
Age
Ethnicity
Histology
Viral load
Genotype

Modifiable factors
Body mass index
Intrahepatic iron levels
Insulin resistance (?)

recent studies have individuated a cut-off of 600 000 IU/mL [58–60]. The prognostic impact of the viral load is currently considered marginal compared with the impact of the genotype.

Host factors affecting the antiviral response are age, gender and ethnicity. Younger patients and women respond better than older patients and men. Despite the lower rate of response with increasing age and the higher percentage of side-effects, treatment is often appropriate in older patients because hepatitis C tends to progress more rapidly with advancing age. The response in HCV genotype 1 patients of Afro-American descent is poorer than that in Caucasians [101,102]; however, the response appears to be similar in both genotype 2 and 3 patients from these two ethnic groups [103].

Overweight patients respond less well, even after the dosages of IFN and RBV are adjusted according to weight [104]. About 50% of patients with HCV genotype 1 are insulin resistant, and insulin resistance was shown to be an independent predictor of a diminished response to antiviral therapy [105]. Liver steatosis secondary to insulin resistance also diminishes the response to antiviral therapy [106]. Steatosis observed in patients infected with HCV genotype 3 appears to be related to a viral mechanism; in these patients, the response to therapy is associated with reductions in hepatic fat [107] and the recurrence of infection is generally accompanied by the recrudescence of steatosis. In 1428 naive patients, the presence of steatosis was associated with a lower SVR rate than that seen in non-steatotic patients but, in patients who achieved a SVR, steatosis was most improved in those with HCV genotype 3; low baseline serum cholesterol was also corrected by IFN treatment in genotype 3 responders [106].

Patients with intrahepatic iron overload have a lower response rate to IFN [108,109], and iron removal by phlebotomy improves responses in these patients [110]. Adjuvant iron reduction also appears to improve the therapeutic response in patients with normal baseline ferritin and transferrin saturation [111–113].

The extent of liver fibrosis also has an impact on treatment outcome and may be taken into account as a secondary predictive factor, together with the above-mentioned criteria.

Adherence to therapy

Adherence to therapy is an important determinant of a SVR. In one study, a 3×80 adherence rule, i.e. administration of at least 80% of the originally prescribed dose of IFN and RBV for at least 80% of the planned duration of therapy, was considered to define compliance, resulting in the expected rate of efficacy [114]. HCV genotype 1 patients who did not reduce therapy below the 80% rule had a significantly higher SVR rate than patients who were unable to adhere to the full dose. However, further analysis indicated that early low adherence (during the first 12–20 weeks of therapy) diminished the SVR rate more significantly than late (20–48 weeks) non-compliance and that, during early therapy, keeping the full dose of RBV was more important than keeping the full dose of IFN. In the HALT-C study [38], dose reductions of PEG-IFN from greater than 80% to less than 60% of the target dose within the first 20 weeks of therapy did not diminish SVR rates, whereas reductions of the target dose of RBV to less than 60% resulted in a significant reduction in the SVR; a reduction of either drug after 20 weeks, when HCV-RNA levels had become undetectable, did not significantly effect the SVR.

As dose reductions of IFN and RBV are usually forced by treatment-related adverse events, management of side-effects is important to ensure compliance and achieve the highest possible SVR. The control of RBV-induced anaemia with epoetin may improve compliance [88,90]. Granulocyte growth factors may also be administered to combat IFN-induced leukopenia.

Compliance is a major problem in drug addicts because of a poor rate of acceptance of or adherence to therapeutic regimens; treatment with PEG-IFN/RBV is safe and sufficiently effective in patients on methadone maintenance [115].

Which HCV subject to treat?

All patients with chronic hepatitis C are potential candidates for antiviral therapy [44]. However, treatment may be associated with important side-effects and the results of current antiviral therapy are variable, depending on viral and individual factors. Therefore, the decision whether to treat a patient should be based on: (i) the risk of the underlying liver disease evolving into cirrhosis and HCC in the lifetime of the patient, (ii) the possible impact of treatment-related adverse effects on the patient's general health, and (iii) the probability of achieving a response, taking into consideration the HCV genotype and viral load and the clinical features and comorbidities of the patient. Of note, the data on which current antiviral drugs and treatment protocols were licensed have been collected from selected clinically homogeneous HCV patients without significant comorbidities; results may be less favourable in field practice in the general HCV population, in whom the epidemiological and clinical scenario is more disparate [75].

These issues need to be exhaustively discussed with the patients. Patients must be fully aware of the pros and cons of therapy and must participate in the decision-making process, ultimately deciding themselves whether the risk-to-benefit ratio of therapy is acceptable. Patients with no evidence of progressive disease, with HCV genotype 1 and with comorbid conditions may reasonably decide to delay therapy until more efficient and tolerable treatments become available.

The presence of elevated ALT levels is the main determinant in the decision to start therapy, as there is a correlation between ALT abnormalities and liver disease activity and progression. There is a consensus that liver biopsy is not necessary in the treatment of HCV-2 and -3 patients. Given that the indication to treat now extends to the whole spectrum of histological lesions, from initial fibrosis to established compensated cirrhosis, and that histological scores may grossly underestimate the extent of fibrosis because of sampling errors, the need to take a confirmatory liver biopsy in HCV patients willing to submit to therapy is currently being debated; a biopsy should be recommended for HCV-1 patients who are unwilling to undergo therapy or who have comorbid conditions that increase the risk of side-effects, in order to motivate treatment or justify its withdrawal. The role of non-invasive markers of liver fibrosis (serum markers and/or elastogram) in the treatment decision-making process is still to be determined.

Individuals with persistently normal ALT

The issue of whether HCV-RNA-positive subjects with persistently normal ALT levels should be treated is evolving. These subjects appear to respond as well as, and according to the same prognostic factors as, patients with abnormal ALT levels [116,117]; SVR rates of 40% and 72% were obtained in genotype 1 and 2/3 patients, respectively, when PEG-IFN plus RBV was given for 48 and 24 weeks respectively [116].

The decision to treat should be individualized and based not only on the clinical suspicion of underlying liver disease but also on the age and motivation of the patient; a major determinant of treatment may be the negative perception of the chronic infection and the psychological impact of being a potential source of HCV transmission. The need for a liver biopsy is controversial; young motivated patients at no increased risk, in particular those with HCV-2 and -3, may be treated without a biopsy [118]. A confirmatory liver biopsy may be useful in patients who are older than 50 and who have relative contraindications to therapy and genotypes that are difficult to treat; in these patients, the decision to treat should be based on the finding of significant fibrosis [118]. Hopefully, the introduction of non-invasive methods such as the liver elastogram will help to differentiate patients with and without fibrosis and enable liver biopsies to be targeted to those with a stiff liver.

Cirrhosis

There is indication to treat patients with compensated cirrhosis [119–121]. Although fibrosis has been considered to be an important negative predictor of response to antiviral therapy, registrative PEG-IFN/RBV studies have shown that the rate of SVR in compensated patients with advanced fibrosis and cirrhosis is only marginally less than in patients without fibrosis (44% versus 54% [7]; 43% versus 56% [8]).

Although antiviral therapy is evolving in patients with decompensated cirrhosis, there is, as yet, no indication to treat such patients. The clinical status at the time of initiating antiviral therapy appears to be the major limiting factor; treatment must be avoided in patients with a Child–Turcotte–Pugh (CTP) score of > 11 or a model for endstage liver disease (MELD) score of > 25, as the risk of precipitating liver failure is high [122]. Published reports mostly describe patients undergoing liver transplantation. The series of patients included have been clinically heterogeneous and not comparable; most studies have considered a lack of HCV reinfection in the liver graft as evidence of treatment efficacy [123]. Treatment can be considered in patients with CTP scores of 8–11 (MELD scores 18–25); although SVR responses as high as 90% were reported in patients with HCV-2 and -3 and responses of 30% were reported in patients with HCV-1, treatment benefit was offset by severe complications related primarily to neutropenia, thrombocytopenia and anaemia [124–125]. Low initial escalating doses of IFN have been proposed for patients with blood cytopenia [120].

Children

In children, the course of chronic hepatitis C is usually benign and progression is slow; thus, in most paediatric patients, therapy is not necessary or can be delayed. Treatment may be considered in children who are viraemic and who have persistently abnormal ALT levels [126]. They are good candidates for therapy as the HCV infection is short-lived, they do not usually have advanced fibrosis and they appear to tolerate treatment well; however, therapy should be avoided in children of less than 3 years because it may adversely affect growth [127].

In various heterogeneous studies in which 336 children were treated with IFN monotherapy, the average SVR rate was 36% and, in several limited series in which children were treated with standard IFN/RBV, the SVR rate varied between 50% and 64% [128].

Among children treated with PEG-IFN-α-2b/RBV [129], a SVR was obtained in 47.8% of patients with HCV-1, 100% of patients with HCV-2 and -3, and 50% of patients with HCV-4. Treatment was generally well tolerated; however, three children required dose reductions and 10.3% developed thyroid autoantibodies and thyroid dysfunction.

Patients with autoantibodies

IFN therapy has occasionally been associated with hepatitic flares in patients with autoantibodies [130,131]. However, borderline antinuclear autoantibody (ANA) or smooth muscle autoantibody (SMA) reactivities often occur in hepatic as well as in all forms of liver disease, and their frequency increases with age and with the inflammatory activity of the underlying liver disease; in the absence of other signs of autoimmunity, these autoantibodies do not contraindicate the use of IFN or PEG-IFN. In patients with well-documented hepatitis C, the presence of liver–kidney microsomal (LKM) antibodies does not predict autoimmune hepatitis or hyporesponsiveness to IFN/RBV [132,133]. In patients with hepatitis C who have significant titres of autoantibodies, attention should be given to the presence of other autoimmune stigmata such as arthritis, haemolytic anaemia and a high level of immunoglobulin (Ig)G. In order to identify possible cases of autoimmune hepatitis, one can apply the International Autoimmune Hepatitis Group Scoring System [134], which was devised to identify autoimmune liver disease. If the aggregate score is non-diagnostic, therapy with IFN appears to be safe; if the score points to probable or definite autoimmune hepatitis, steroids should be considered.

Mixed cryoglobulinaemia

In a proportion of mixed cryoglobulinaemia (MC) patients, treatment with IFN monotherapy at doses of 3–6 MU three times a week for 6–12 months reduced the cryocrit, improved the cutaneous rash and joint symptoms and led to the clearance of HCV RNA [135,136]; in some studies, IFN was used in combination with low doses of steroids [137]. However, the virological and clinical response was lower and the relapse rate higher than in hepatitis C patients without MC. Variations in the biological markers of MC (cryocrit, rheumatoid factor, complement) may be independent of the virological or ALT response. In some patients with severe MC symptoms, long-term maintenance therapy is required because they respond well to IFN but promptly relapse at therapy withdrawal. The efficacy of IFN in treating MC-associated neuropathies is debated. Concomitant with HCV-RNA clearance, IFN therapy may lead to the disappearance of monoclonal B-cell infiltrates and to a lack of detection of circulating t(14:18) translocated B-cell clones; the latter reappear if serum HCV reactivates [138,139]. In a study of nine symptomatic and refractory HCV–MC patients, there was an improvement in the symptoms of the majority of the patients after treatment with standard IFN/RBV, even though HCV clearance was only obtained in a minority (22%) [140].

In two pilot studies of 9 and 18 MC patients [141,142], PEG-IFN-α-2b/RBV given for 12–13 months induced a virological and clinical response in the majority of patients (78%–83%) while on therapy; however, in one of the studies, the rate of relapse was high (44%) [142].

The persistence of MC despite the clearance of HCV RNA from serum may be associated with residual HCV infection in lymphocytes [143].

In patients who are non-responders to PEG-IFN/RBV combination therapy and who show clinically significant symptoms of

MC, administration of anti-CD20 monoclonal antibody (rituximab) against B-cell monoclonal proliferation may be considered.

Immunodepressed patients

Treatment of chronic hepatitis C in HIV and transplanted patients is discussed in Chapters 9.3 and 25.5 respectively.

HCV–HBV coinfected patients

Data on the long-term outcome for individuals coinfected with HCV and HBV suggest that these patients have higher rates of progressive liver disease and HCC; effective treatment for such individuals is, therefore, of particular importance. In general, in double infections such as these, one virus usually inhibits the other; therefore, it is essential to measure both HBV-DNA and HCV-RNA levels to determine which infection is dominant and treat accordingly. If both infections are active, initial therapy with IFN and RBV, according to the protocols used for the treatment of hepatitis C, may be the first option, as eradication of HCV is more likely than eradication of HBV, and IFN may also control HBV infection. To date, no specific randomized trials have addressed the issues of an optimal treatment protocol and therapeutic outcome in HCV–HBV coinfected patients.

Patients with comorbidities

Renal disorders

HCV infection is frequent in haemodialyzed patients with renal insufficiency [144]. The course of HCV disease in these patients is characterized by low or normal ALT values and viraemic levels that are lower than in non-uremic patients; viraemia may spontaneously become transiently negative.

The clearance of RBV is much reduced in patients with kidney failure and the drug is not removed by dialysis. Even a dosage of RBV of as low as 200 mg/day can precipitate serious anaemia [145–146] and, therefore, its use is contraindicated. The clearance of standard IFN is also reduced and dosages should be adapted to plasma creatinine values [147].

A review of 269 dialysis patients from 14 heterogeneous clinical trials showed that standard IFN monotherapy given for 4–12 months induced a SVR in 37% of patients, with a dropout rate of 17% [148]. The overall weighted estimate for a SVR in HCV-1 patients was 30.6%; a negative serum HCV-RNA test at 8–12 weeks correlated with a SVR. Tolerance was lower than in non-uremic patients and prolonged IFN monotherapy did not improve the SVR. In a further study of haemodialysis patients [149], the SVR was 34% in 29 patients who completed treatment (out of 46 who originally enrolled in the study). Finally, in a preliminary study [150], PEG-IFN-α-2b and low-dose RBV (target concentration of 10–15 mmol/L) were given to six haemodialysis patients; all patients became HCV-RNA-negative during therapy and three remained negative with extended follow-up.

Haematological disorders

Trials in hepatitis C patients with thalassemia have shown that treatment with IFN and RBV is safe and effective [151,152], as long as adequate haemoglobin levels can be maintained by transfusion.

Red blood cells of individuals with the Mediterranean form of glucose-6-phosphate dehydrogenase deficiency do not appear to be more susceptible to the haemolytic potential of RBV; 26 Sardinian HCV patients with severe glucose-6-phosphate dehydrogenase deficiency were safely treated with PEG-IFN/RBV, with responses that were similar to patients with HCV alone [153].

HCV patients with haemophilia have also been safely treated with standard IFN/RBV therapy [154]; the overall SVR rate was lower (29%) than in patients with HCV alone, but it was high among adolescents younger than 18 years (59%).

Diabetes

Although IFN may precipitate diabetic decompensation, particularly in patients with pancreatic autoantibodies [155–157], compensated diabetes is not a contraindication to therapy in chronic HCV hepatitis. In one study of a patient with pre-existing diabetes, the diabetes resolved after combination therapy [158].

Hepatitis C in liver transplants
(See Chapter 25.5)

Retreatment

Non-response to therapy is defined as the persistence of serum HCV RNA throughout, and at the end of, treatment. Relapse is defined as the recurrence of serum HCV RNA during the post-therapy follow-up, after apparent clearance of viraemia throughout therapy. As chronic hepatitis C is a curable disease, it is important to consider retreatment in patients who were previous non-responders or relapsers after a first course of antiviral therapy. In one study [159] of patients who previously relapsed after treatment with standard IFN monotherapy or standard IFN/RBV therapy, the overall SVR rate after retreatment with PEG-IFN/RBV was 60% and 53% respectively. Retreatment with combination therapy resulted in a SVR in about 25% of patients who were non-responders to IFN monotherapy but who had a partial biochemical or virological response during the monotherapy course [160–162].

New information is emerging from two large-scale studies whose aim is to retreat patients with advanced compensated liver disease (bridging fibrosis or cirrhosis) for 48 weeks with PEG-IFN/RBV (lead-in phase), and maintain long-term with low-dose PEG-IFN monotherapy those who fail to achieve a SVR with full antiviral therapy. Preliminary results from the lead-in phase of the HALT-C study [38] (designed to retreat non-responders to IFN monotherapy or standard IFN/RBV therapy with PEG-IFN-α-2a/RBV) have shown a 28% SVR rate in previous non-responders to IFN alone and a 12% SVR rate in non-responders to standard IFN/RBV. Similarly, preliminary results from the EPIC3 study (designed to retreat relapsers and non-responders to IFN/RBV therapy with PEG-IFN-α-2b/RBV) [163] have shown SVR rates of 41% in relapsers and 14% in non-responders. In both studies, HCV genotypes 2 and 3 responded significantly better than HCV genotype 1 (54–65% versus 14%).

In a recent study [164], 19% of the genotype 1 patients who were retreated with PEG-IFN-α-2b/RBV after failing to respond to standard IFN/RBV therapy achieved a SVR; independent predictors of response were low γ-glutamyltransferase levels and low viral load. In another PEG-IFN/RBV retreatment study [165], an overall SVR rate of 23% was obtained in patients who had not previously responded to IFN monotherapy or IFN/RBV therapy. Among standard α IFN/RBV non-responders retreated with daily consensus IFN and RBV, 22% achieved a SVR [166].

These data suggest that it is reasonable to retreat patients who relapse to IFN monotherapy or standard IFN/RBV combination therapy with PEG-IFN/RBV, and to retreat patients who do not respond to IFN monotherapy with PEG-IFN/RBV. Although it also seems reasonable to retreat HCV genotype 2 and 3 patients who do not respond to standard IFN/RBV therapy with PEG-IFN/RBV, current retreatment SVR rates in HCV genotype 1 patients who do not respond to standard IFN/RBV therapy are lower than 20% and, therefore, the efficacy of treating these patients, who account for the larger proportion of non-responders, is doubtful.

The addition of histamine in triple combination with PEG-IFN and RBV was of no benefit and the efficacy of the addition of amantadine is debated [167]; this triple combination is not generally used. Large-scale studies are in progress to evaluate the efficacy of retreatment with high doses of PEG-IFN/RBV [168] and with triple combinations including thymosin or protease inhibitors.

Long-term maintenance monotherapy with reduced weekly dosages of PEG-IFN has been proposed to prevent progression of disease in patients with advanced disease who fail or do not tolerate full antiviral therapy [169]. Three major long-term trials are ongoing to assess the efficacy of maintenance therapy (COPILOT, HALT-C, EPIC3); preliminary results have been encouraging [170].

New treatments in development

Approximately 50–60% of patients with chronic HCV infection do not achieve a SVR with current therapy. Treatment failures are often considered to be the result of the virus being 'resistant' to therapy, with antiviral resistance being commonly defined as the mechanisms that a virus develops to continue replication and escape the antiviral effects of treatment and/or the immune response of the host. However, it is not known whether the failure to achieve a SVR can be entirely considered as being 'true' resistance according to this definition. Non-responders to current therapy show little or no decrease in serum HCV-RNA

levels during therapy. In these patients, the lack of immune clearance of infected cells may be a key determinant in the lack of viral eradication [171]. In addition, the genetic heterogeneity or quasi-species nature of HCV raises important therapeutic implications, as the generation and selection of resistant variants can allow the virus to escape the antiviral pressure exerted by treatment [172].

New HCV inhibitors

With improved understanding of HCV molecular virology, new therapies that specifically target HCV replication are being developed. A number of protease or polymerase inhibitors directed against HCV genotype 1 enzymes have been identified. Several are now undergoing phase I/II clinical trials in monotherapy and in combination with pegylated IFN, in order to increase the virus clearance rate and decrease the resistance rate; amongst the most promising are the NS3 serine protease inhibitors [173] and the NS5B RNA-dependent RNA polymerase inhibitors.

New IFNs (Albuferon) are also being evaluated, as well as RBV derivatives (viramidine, etc.) that are less prone to induce haemolysis.

Drug resistance is a major consideration for novel direct antivirals

Because of the high mutation rate observed with HCV, it is likely that mutated viruses having a reduced sensitivity to antiviral therapies will emerge. In addition, the overall prevalence of individual mutations changes over time, indicating that the relative 'fitness' (ability to replicate) of a resistant variant will play a role in viral dynamics during treatment [174]. Potential resistance mutations in both the polymerase and protease enzymes have been identified. As the active site for protease inhibitors is a long shallow groove, a single point mutation in this enzyme may be sufficient to hinder the binding of antivirals, with different mutations conferring low-level or high-level resistance. There have been several studies reporting the selection of HCV mutants that are resistant against various protease inhibitors using the *in vitro* replicon system [174–180].

The active site of the NS5B RNA-dependent RNA polymerase is a highly conserved region in all HCV genotypes and any amino acid mutation in this region may inhibit the ability of the virus to replicate. This suggests that mutations in this enzyme, which could result in resistance to nucleoside polymerase inhibitors, may not readily develop. *In vitro* studies have shown that replicons carrying mutations showed decreased replication fitness [178–183]. The NS5B polymerase has also been targeted through the interaction of its thumb and palm structural domains with non-nucleoside analogues. *In vitro* resistance to this class of inhibitor arises through single mutations within the inhibitor binding site, which strongly reduces its affinity for the inhibitors [179,180]. The success of future HCV antiviral agents will be heavily influenced by their ability to inhibit viral variants and prevent the emergence of escape mutants. Agents with different mechanisms of action show limited cross-resistance in laboratory studies, suggesting that these therapies may be used in combination. Thus, the ultimate pharmacological control of HCV may be best achieved with a combination of agents that are specifically designed to inhibit different virus-specific targets through complimentary mechanisms of action, e.g. protease inhibitors with polymerase inhibitors or nucleoside with non-nucleoside polymerase inhibitors [184]. Clinical trials are ongoing to determine if these new inhibitors will improve the rate of SVR in chronic hepatitis C.

References

1 Davis GL, Balart LA, Schiff ER et al. (1989) Treatment of chronic hepatitis C with recombinant interferon alfa. A multicenter randomized controlled trial. N Engl J Med 321, 1501–1506.

2 Di Bisceglie AM, Martin P, Kassianides C et al. (1989) Recombinant interferon alfa therapy for chronic hepatitis C. A randomized, double-blind, placebo-controlled trial. N Engl J Med 321, 1506–1510.

3 Poynard T, Leroy V, Cohard M et al. (1996) Meta-analysis of interferon randomized trials in the treatment of viral hepatitis C: effects of dose and duration. Hepatology 24, 778–789.

4 Carithers RL, Emerson SS (1997) Therapy of hepatitis C: meta-analysis of interferon alfa-2b trials. Hepatology 26(Suppl), S83–88.

5 McHutchison JG, Gordon SC, Schiff ER et al. (1998) Interferon alfa-2b alone or in combination with ribavirin as initial treatment for chronic hepatitis C. N Engl J Med 339, 1485–1492.

6 Poynard T, Marcellin P, Lee SS et al. (1998) Randomised trial of interferon alpha2b plus ribavirin for 48 weeks or for 24 weeks versus interferon alpha2b plus placebo for 48 weeks for treatment of chronic infection with hepatitis C virus. Lancet 352, 1426–1432.

7 Manns M, McHutchison J, Gordon S et al. (2001) Peginterferon alfa-2b plus ribavirin compared with interferon alfa-2b plus ribavirin for initial treatment of chronic hepatitis C: a randomised trial. Lancet 358, 958–965.

8 Fried MW, Shiffman ML, Reddy KR et al. (2002) Peg-Interferon alfa2a plus ribavirin for chronic hepatitis C virus infection. N Engl J Med 347, 975–982.

9 Hadziyannis SJ, Sette H Jr, Morgan TR et al. (2004) Peginterferon-alpha2a and ribavirin combination therapy in chronic hepatitis C: a randomized study of treatment duration and ribavirin dose. Ann Intern Med 140, 346–355.

10 Baron S, Tyring SK, Fleischmann WR Jr et al. (1991) The interferons. Mechanisms of action and clinical applications. JAMA 266, 1375–1383.

11 Blatt LM, Davis JM, Klein SB et al. (1996) The biologic activity and molecular characterization of a novel synthetic interferon-alpha species, consensus interferon. J Interferon Cytokine Res 16, 489–499.

12 Glue P, Fang JW, Rouzier-Panis R et al. (2000) Pegylated interferon-alpha2b: pharmacokinetics, pharmacodynamics, safety, and preliminary efficacy data. Clin Pharmacol Ther 68, 556–567.

13 Zeuzem S, Welsch C, Herrmann E (2003) Pharmacokinetics of peginterferons. Semin Liver Dis 23(Suppl 1), 23–28.

14 Bain VG, Kaita KD, Yoshida EM et al. (2006) A phase 2 study to evaluate the antiviral activity, safety, and pharmacokinetics of recombinant human albumin-interferon alfa fusion protein in genotype 1 chronic hepatitis C patients. J Hepatol 44, 671–678.

15 Glue P (1999) The clinical pharmacology of ribavirin. Semin Liver Dis 19(Suppl 1), 17–24.

16 Zoulim F, Haem J, Ahmed SS et al. (1998) Ribavirin monotherapy in patients with chronic hepatitis C: a retrospective study of 95 patients. J Viral Hepat 5, 193–198.

17 Hoofnagle JH, Lau D, Conjeevaram H et al. (1996) Prolonged therapy of chronic hepatitis C with ribavirin. J Viral Hepat 3, 247–252.

18 Lau JY, Tam RC, Liang TJ et al. (2002) Mechanism of action of ribavirin in the combination treatment of chronic HCV infection. Hepatology 35, 1002–1009.

19 Pawlotsky JM, Dahari H, Neumann AU et al. (2004) Antiviral action of ribavirin in chronic hepatitis C. Gastroenterology 126, 703–714.

20 Crotty S, Cameron CE, Andino R (2001) RNA virus error catastrophe: direct molecular test by using ribavirin. Proc Natl Acad Sci USA 98, 6895–6900.

21 Layden JE, Layden TJ (2002) Viral kinetics of hepatitis C: new insights and remaining limitations. Hepatology 35, 967–970.

22 Zeuzem S, Herrmann E, Lee JH et al. (2001) Viral kinetics in patients with chronic hepatitis C treated with standard or peginterferon alpha2a. Gastroenterology 120, 1438–1447.

23 Herrmann E, Lee JH, Marinos G et al. (2003) Effect of ribavirin on hepatitis C viral kinetics in patients treated with pegylated interferon. Hepatology 37, 1351–1358.

24 Heathcote J (2000) Antiviral therapy for patients with chronic hepatitis C. Semin Liver Dis 20, 185–199.

25 Strader DB, Wright T, Thomas DL et al. (2004) Diagnosis, management, and treatment of hepatitis C. Hepatology 39, 1147–1471.

26 Reichard O, Glaumann H, Fryden A et al. (1999) Long-term follow-up of chronic hepatitis C patients with sustained virological response to alpha-interferon. J Hepatol 30, 783–787.

27 Veldt BJ, Saracco G, Boyer N et al. (2004) Long term clinical outcome of chronic hepatitis C patients with sustained virological response to interferon monotherapy. Gut 53, 1504–1508.

28 Barnes E, Webster G, Jacobs R et al. (1999) Long-term efficacy of treatment of chronic hepatitis C with alpha interferon or alpha interferon and ribavirin. J Hepatol 31(Suppl 1), 244–249.

29 Poynard T, McHutchison J, Manns M et al. (2002) Impact of pegylated interferon alfa-2b and ribavirin on liver fibrosis in patients with chronic hepatitis C. Gastroenterology 122, 1303–1313.

30 Camma C, Di Bona D, Schepis F et al. (2004) Effect of peginterferon alfa-2a on liver histology in chronic hepatitis C: a meta-analysis of individual patient data. Hepatology 39, 333–342.

31 Shiratori Y, Imazeki F, Moriyama M et al. (2000) Histologic improvement of fibrosis in patients with hepatitis C who have sustained response to interferon therapy. Ann Intern Med 132, 517–524.

32 Yoshida H, Shiratori Y, Moriyama M et al. (1999) Interferon therapy reduces the risk for hepatocellular carcinoma: national surveillance program of cirrhotic and noncirrhotic patients with chronic hepatitis C in Japan. Ann Intern Med 131, 174–181.

33 Ikeda K, Saitoh S, Arase Y et al. (1999) Effect of interferon therapy on hepatocellular carcinogenesis in patients with chronic hepatitis type C: a long-term observation study of 1,643 patients using statistical bias correction with proportional hazard analysis. Hepatology 29, 1124–1130.

34 Davis GL, Wong JB, McHutchison JG et al. (2003) Early virologic response to treatment with peginterferon alfa-2b plus ribavirin in patients with chronic hepatitis C. Hepatology 38, 645–652.

35 Jensen D, Morgan T, Marcellin P et al. (2005) Rapid virologic response at week 4 (RVR) of peginterferon alfa-2a (40 KD) (Pegasys)

plus ribavirin (RBV, Copegus) treatment predicts sustained virological response (SVR) after 24 weeks in genotype 1 patients. *Hepatology* 42(Suppl 1), 650A.

36 Pradat P, Chossegros P, Bailly F *et al.* (2000) Comparison between three quantitative assays in patients with chronic hepatitis C and their relevance in the prediction of response to therapy. *J Viral Hepat* 7, 203–210.

37 Pawlotsky JM, Bouvier-Alias M, Hezode C *et al.* (2000) Standardization of hepatitis C virus RNA quantification. *Hepatology* 32, 654–659.

38 Shiffman ML, Di Bisceglie AM, Lindsay KL *et al.* (2004) Peginterferon alfa-2a and ribavirin in patients with chronic hepatitis C who have failed prior treatment. *Gastroenterology* 126, 1015–1023.

39 Reichard O, Norkrans G, Fryden A *et al.* (1998) Randomised, double-blind, placebo-controlled trial of interferon alpha-2b with and without ribavirin for chronic hepatitis C. *Lancet* 351, 83–87.

40 Zeuzem S, Feinman SV, Rasenack J *et al.* (2000) Peginterferon alfa-2a in patients with chronic hepatitis C. *N Engl J Med* 343, 1666–1672.

41 Heathcote EJ, Shiffman ML, Cooksley WG *et al.* (2000) Peginterferon alfa-2a in patients with chronic hepatitis C and cirrhosis. *N Engl J Med* 343, 1673–1680.

42 Hasan F, Asker H, Al-Khaldi J *et al.* (2004) Peginterferon alfa-2b plus ribavirin for the treatment of chronic hepatitis C genotype 4. *Am J Gastroenterol* 99, 1733–1737.

43 Nguyen MH, Keefe EB (2005) Prevalence and treatment of hepatitis C virus genotypes 4,5, and 6. *Clin Gastroenterol Hepatol* 3(Suppl 2), S97–101.

44 NIH Consensus Statement (2002) Management of hepatitis C. *Hepatology* 19, 1–46.

45 Craxi A, Camma C (2006) Treating patients with HCV genotype 1 and low viraemia: more than meets the eye. *J Hepatol* 44, 4–7.

46 Weiland O, Schwarcz R, Mattsson L *et al.* (2006) 135 microg Peg-IFN alpha-2a in combination with weight-based ribavirin for genotype 2 and 3 is highly efficacious. *J Hepatol* 44(Suppl 2), S230.

47 Brown RS, Jacobson IM, Afdhal N *et al.* (2006) Differences in treatment outcome to antiviral therapy based on genotype and viral load in hepatitis C genotypes 2 and 3 in the WIN-R trial. *J Hepatol* 44(Suppl 2), S20.

48 Ferenci P, Brunner H, Laferl H *et al.* (2006) Further reduction of ribavirin dose in HCV genotype 2/3 patients receiving PegInterferon alpha-2a (40 kDa) (Pegasys) plus ribavirin (Copegus): interim results of a randomised controlled trial. *J Hepatol* 44(Suppl 2), S37.

49 Rendon A, Nunez M, Romero M *et al.* (2005) Early monitoring of ribavirin plasma concentrations may predict anemia and early virologic response in HIV/hepatitis C virus-coinfected patients. *J Acquir Immune Defic Syndr* 39, 401–405.

50 Fontana RJ (2006) Optimizing outcomes in hepatitis C: is treatment beyond 48 weeks ever justified? *Gastroenterology* 130, 1357–1362.

51 Drusano GL, Preston SL (2004) A 48-week duration of therapy with pegylated interferon alpha 2b plus ribavirin may be too short to maximize long-term response among patients infected with genotype-1 hepatitis C virus. *J Infect Dis* 189, 964–970.

52 Brouwer JT, Nevens F, Bekkering FC *et al.* (2004) Reduction of relapse rates by 18-month treatment in chronic hepatitis C. A Benelux randomized trial in 300 patients. *J Hepatol* 40, 689–695.

53 Sanchez-Tapias JM, Diago M, Escartin P *et al.* (2006) Peginterferon alfa-2a plus ribavirin for 48 weeks in patients with detectable hepatitis C virus RNA at week 4 of treatment. *Gastroenterology* 131, 451–460.

54 Berg T, von Wagner M, Nasser S *et al.* (2006) Extended treatment duration for hepatitis C virus type 1: comparing 48 versus 72 weeks of peginterferon-alfa-2a plus ribavirin. *Gastroenterology* 130, 1086–1097.

55 Mangia A, Santoro R, Minerva N *et al.* (2005) Peginterferon alfa-2b and ribavirin for 12 vs. 24 weeks in HCV genotype 2 or 3. *N Engl J Med* 352, 2609–2617.

56 Von Wagner, Huber M, Berg T *et al.* (2005) Peginterferon-alpha-2a (40KD) and ribavirin for 16 or 24 weeks in patients with genotype 2 or 3 chronic hepatitis C. *Gastroenterology* 129, 522–527.

57 Shiffman ML, Pappas S, Nyberg L *et al.* (2006) Peginterferon alpha-2a (Pegasys) plus ribavirin (Copegus) for 16 or 24 weeks in patients with genotype 2 or 3. *J Hepatol* 44(Suppl 2), S271.

58 Zeuzem S, Hultcrantz R, Bourliere M *et al.* (2004) Peginterferon alfa-2b plus ribavirin for treatment of chronic hepatitis C in previously untreated patients infected with HCV genotypes 2 or 3. *J Hepatol* 40, 993–999.

59 Alberti A (2004) Optimizing PEG-interferon and ribavirin combination therapy for patients infected with HCV-2 or HCV-3: is the puzzle completed? *J Hepatol* 40, 1032–1035.

60 Zeuzem S, Buti M, Ferenci P *et al.* (2006) Efficacy of 24 weeks treatment with peginterferon alfa-2b plus ribavirin in patients with chronic hepatitis C infected with genotype 1 and low pretreatment viraemia. *J Hepatol* 44, 97–103.

61 Ferenci P, Bergholz U, Laferl H *et al.* (2006) 24 weeks treatment regimen with peginterferon alpha-2a (40kD) (Pegasys) plus ribavirin (Copegus) in HCV genotype 1 or 4 'super-responders'. *J Hepatol* 44(Suppl 2), S6.

62 Ferenci P, Brunner H, Nachbaur K *et al.* (2001) Combination of interferon induction therapy and ribavirin in chronic hepatitis C. *Hepatology* 34, 1006–1011.

63 Neumann AU, Hagai E, Schalm SW *et al.* (2003) Early viral kinetics prediction of sustained virological response after 1 or 4 weeks of Peg-Interferon-alfa-2A and ribavirin therapy. *Hepatology* 38, 248A.

64 Booth JC, O'Grady J, Neuberger J (2001) Clinical guidelines on the management of hepatitis C. *Gut* 49(Suppl 1), 1–21.

65 Di Bisceglie AM, Hoofnagle JH (2002) Optimal therapy of hepatitis C. *Hepatology* 36(5 Suppl 1), S121–127.

66 Reddy KR, Wright TL, Pockros PJ *et al.* (2001) Efficacy and safety of pegylated (40-kd) interferon alpha-2a compared with interferon alpha-2a in noncirrhotic patients with chronic hepatitis C. *Hepatology* 33, 433–438.

67 Selmi C, Lleo A, Zuin M *et al.* (2006) Interferon alpha and its contribution to autoimmunity. *Curr Opin Investig Drugs* 7, 451–456.

68 Wilson LE, Widman D, Dikman SH *et al.* (2002) Autoimmune disease complicating antiviral therapy for hepatitis C virus infection. *Semin Arthritis Rheum* 32, 163–173.

69 Wesche B, Jaeckel E, Trautwein C *et al.* (2001) Induction of autoantibodies to the adrenal cortex and pancreatic islet cells by interferon alpha therapy for chronic hepatitis C. *Gut* 48, 378–383.

70 Muratori P, Muratori L, Guidi M *et al.* (2005) Clinical impact of non-organ-specific autoantibodies on the response to combined antiviral treatment in patients with hepatitis C. *Clin Infect Dis* 40, 501–507.

71 D'Alteroche L, Majzoub S, Lecuyer AI *et al.* (2006) Ophtalmologic side effects during alpha-interferon therapy for viral hepatitis. *J Hepatol* 44, 56–61.

72 Jubert C, Pawlotsky JM, Pouget F *et al.* (1994) Lichen planus and hepatitis C virus-related chronic active hepatitis. *Arch Dermatol* 130, 73–76.

73 Funk J, Langeland T, Schrumpf E *et al.* (1991) Psoriasis induced by interferon-alpha. *Br J Dermatol* 125, 463–465.

74 Fattovich G, Giustina G, Favarato S *et al.* (1996) A survey of adverse events in 11,241 patients with chronic viral hepatitis treated with alfa interferon. *J Hepatol* 24, 38–47.

75 Gaeta GB, Precone DF, Felaco FM *et al.* (2002) Premature discontinuation of interferon plus ribavirin for adverse effects: a multicentre survey in 'real world' patients with chronic hepatitis C. *Aliment Pharmacol Ther* 16, 1633–1639.

76 Russo MW, Fried MW (2003) Side effects of therapy for chronic hepatitis C. *Gastroenterology* 124, 1711–1719.

77 Cacopardo B, Benanti F, Brancati G *et al.* (1998) Leucocyte interferon-alpha retreatment for chronic hepatitis C patients previously intolerant to other interferons. *J Viral Hepat* 5, 333–339.

78 Maddrey WC (1999) Safety of combination interferon alfa-2b/ribavirin therapy in chronic hepatitis C-relapsed and treatment-naive patients. *Semin Liver Dis* 19(Suppl 1), 67–53.

79 Sulkowski MS, Wasserman R, Brooks L *et al.* (2004) Changes in haemoglobin during interferon alpha-2b plus ribavirin combination therapy for chronic hepatitis C virus infection. *J Viral Hepat* 11, 243–250.

80 Van Vlierbergh H, Delanghe JR, De Vos M *et al.* (2001) Factors influencing ribavirin-induced hemolysis. *J Hepatol* 34, 911–916.

81 De Franceschi L, Fattovich G, Turrini F *et al.* (2000) Hemolytic anemia induced by ribavirin therapy in patients with chronic hepatitis C virus infection: role of membrane oxidative damage. *Hepatology* 31, 997–1004.

82 Peck-Radosavljevic M, Wichlas M, Homoncik-Kraml M *et al.* (2002) Rapid suppression of hematopoiesis by standard or pegylated interferon-alpha. *Gastroenterology* 123, 141–151.

83 Brau N (2004) Epoetin alfa treatment for acute anaemia during interferon plus ribavirin combination therapy for chronic hepatitis C. *J Viral Hepat* 11, 191–197.

84 Di Fazio I, Motta M, Musumeci S *et al.* (2004) Efficacy of human recombinant erythropoietin plus IFN-alpha in patients affected by chronic hepatitis C. *J Interferon Cytokine Res* 24, 594–599.

85 Afdhal NH, Dieterich DT, Pockros PJ *et al.* (2004) Epoetin alfa maintains ribavirin dose in HCV-infected patients: a prospective, double-blind, randomized controlled study. *Gastroenterology* 126, 1302–1311.

86 Shiffman ML, Hofmann CM, Luketic VA *et al.* (1998) Use of granulocyte macrophage colony stimulating factor alone or in combination with interferon-alpha-2b for treatment of chronic hepatitis C. *J Hepatol* 28, 382–389.

87 Carreno V, Martin J, Pardo M *et al.* (2000) Randomized controlled trial of recombinant human granulocyte-macrophage colony-stimulating factor for the treatment of chronic hepatitis C. *Cytokine* 12, 165–170.

88 Kee KM, Lee CM, Wang JH *et al.* (2006) Thyroid dysfunction in patients with chronic hepatitis C receiving a combined therapy of interferon and ribavirin: incidence, associated factors and prognosis. *J Gastroenterol Hepatol* 21, 319–326.

89 Prummel MF, Laurberg P (2003) Interferon-alpha and autoimmune thyroid disease. *Thyroid* 13, 547–551.

90 Dalgard O, Bjoro K, Hellum K *et al.* (2002) Thyroid dysfunction during treatment of chronic hepatitis C with interferon alpha: no association with either interferon dosage or efficacy of therapy. *J Intern Med* 251, 400–406.

91 Moncoucy X, Leymarie F, Delemer B *et al.* (2005) Risk factors and long-term course of thyroid dysfunction during antiviral treatments in 221 patients with chronic hepatitis C. *Gastroenterol Clin Biol* 29, 339–345.

92 Doi F, Kakizaki S, Takagi H *et al.* (2005) Long-term outcome of interferon-alpha-induced autoimmune thyroid disorders in chronic hepatitis C. *Liver Int* 25, 242–246.

93 Zdilar D, Franco-Bronson K, Buchler N *et al.* (2000) Hepatitis C, interferon alfa, and depression. *Hepatology* 31, 1207–1211.

94 Hauser P, Khosla J, Aurora H *et al.* (2002) A prospective study of the incidence and open-label treatment of interferon-induced major depressive disorder in patients with hepatitis C. *Mol Psychiatry* 7, 942–947.

95 Asnis GM, De La Garza R (2006) Interferon-induced depression in chronic hepatitis C: a review of its prevalence, risk factors, biology, and treatment approaches. *J Clin Gastroenterol* 40, 322–335.

96 Schaefer M, Schmidt F, Folwaczny C *et al.* (2003) Adherence and mental side effects during hepatitis C treatment with interferon alfa and ribavirin in psychiatric risk groups. *Hepatology* 37, 443–451.

97 Musselman, Lawson DH, Gumnick JF *et al.* (2001) Paroxetine for the prevention of depression induced by high-dose interferon alfa. *N Engl J Med* 344, 961.

98 Gao B, Hong F, Radaeva S (2004) Host factors and failure of interferon-alpha treatment in hepatitis C virus. *Hepatology* 39, 880–890.

99 Craxì A, Cammà C (2006) Treating patients with HCV genotype 1 and low viraemia: more than meets the eye. *J Hepatol* 44, 4–7.

100 Alberti A, Colombo M, Craxi A *et al.* (2006) HCV-1 subtypes and response to pegylated interferon plus ribavirin therapy. *J Clin Virol* 36 (Suppl 2), S132.

101 McHutchison JG, Poynard T, Pianko S *et al.* (2000) The impact of interferon plus ribavirin on response of therapy in black patients with chronic hepatitis C. *Gastroenterology* 119, 1317–1323.

102 Muir AJ, Bornstein JD, Killenberg PG (2004) Peginterferon alfa-2b and ribavirin for the treatment of chronic hepatitis C in blacks and non-Hispanic whites. *N Engl J Med* 350, 2265–2271.

103 Brau N, Bini EJ, Currie S *et al.* (2006) Black patients with chronic hepatitis C have a lower sustained viral response rate than non-blacks with genotype 1, but the same with genotypes 2/3, and this is not explained by more frequent dose reductions of interferon and ribavirin. *J Viral Hepat* 13, 242–249.

104 Bressler BL, Guindi M, Tomlison G *et al.* (2003) High body mass index is an independent risk factor for nonresponse to antiviral treatment in chronic hepatitis C. *Hepatology* 38, 639–644.

105 Romero-Gomez M, Del Mar Viloria M, Andrade RJ *et al.* (2005) Insulin resistance impairs sustained response rate to peginterferon plus ribavirin in chronic hepatitis C patients. *Gastroenterology* 128, 636–641.

106 Poynard T, Ratziu V, McHutchison J *et al.* (2003) Effect of treatment with peginterferon or interferon alfa-2b and ribavirin on steatosis in patients infected with hepatitis C. *Hepatology* 38, 75–85.

107 Rubbia-Brandt L, Giostra E, Mentha G *et al.* (2001) Expression of liver steatosis in hepatitis C virus infection and pattern of response to alpha-interferon. *J Hepatol* 35, 307.

108 Bonkovsky HL (2002) Iron as a comorbid factor in chronic viral hepatitis. *Am J Gastroenterol* 97, 1–4.

109 Olynyk JK, Reddy KR, Di Bisceglie AM *et al.* (1995) Hepatic iron concentration as a predictor of response to interferon alfa therapy in chronic hepatitis C. *Gastroenterology* 108, 1104–1109.

110 Rulyak SJ, Eng SC, Patel K *et al.* (2005) Relationships between hepatic iron content and virologic response in chronic hepatitis C patients treated with interferon and ribavirin. *Am J Gastroenterol* 100, 332–337.

111 Di Bisceglie AM, Bonkovsky HL, Chopra S *et al.* (2000) Iron reduction as an adjuvant to interferon therapy in patients with chronic hepatitis C who have previously not responded to interferon: a

multicenter, prospective, randomized, controlled trial. *Hepatology* 32, 135–138.

112 Fontana RJ, Israel J, LeClair P *et al.* (2000) Iron reduction before and during interferon therapy of chronic hepatitis C: results of a multicenter, randomized, controlled trial. *Hepatology* 31, 730–736.

113 Fargion S, Fracanzani AL, Rossini A *et al.* (2002) Iron reduction and sustained response to interferon-alpha therapy in patients with chronic hepatitis C: results of an Italian multicenter randomized study. *Am J Gastroenterol* 97, 1204–1210.

114 McHutchison JG, Manns M, Patel K *et al.* (2002) Adherence to combination therapy enhances sustained response in genotype-1-infected patients with chronic hepatitis C. *Gastroenterology* 123, 1061–1069.

115 Mauss S, Berger F, Goelz J *et al.* (2004) A prospective controlled study of interferon-based therapy of chronic hepatitis C in patients on methadone maintenance. *Hepatology* 40, 120–124.

116 Zeuzem S, Diago M, Gane E *et al.* (2004) Peginterferon alfa-2a (40 kilodaltons) and ribavirin in patients with chronic hepatitis C and normal aminotransferase levels. *Gastroenterology* 127, 1724–1732.

117 Zehnter E, Mauss S, John C *et al.* (2006) Efficacy and safety of Peginterferon alpha-2a (40KD) [PEG] plus ribavirin (RBV) 1000/1200 mg/d in genotype 1 patients with chronic hepatitis C and 'normal' ALT levels. *J Hepatol* 44(Suppl 2), S622.

118 Alberti A (2005) Towards more individualised management of hepatitis C virus patients with initially or persistently normal alanineaminotransferase levels. *J Hepatol* 42, 266–274.

119 Arenas JI, Vargas HE (2004) Hepatitis C virus antiviral therapy in patients with cirrhosis. *Gastroenterol Clin North Am* 33, 549–562.

120 Everson GT, Trotter J, Forman L *et al.* (2005) Treatment of advanced hepatitis C with a low accelerating dosage regimen of antiviral therapy. *Hepatology* 42, 255–262.

121 Fontana RJ, Everson GT, Tuteja S *et al.* (2004) Controversies in the management of hepatitis C patients with advanced fibrosis and cirrhosis. *Clin Gastroenterol Hepatol* 2, 183–197.

122 Everson GT (2004) Treatment of chronic hepatitis C in patients with decompensated cirrhosis. *Rev Gastroenterol Disord* 4(Suppl 1), S31–38.

123 Forns X, Garcia-Retortillo M, Serrano T *et al.* (2003) Antiviral therapy of patients with decompensated cirrhosis to prevent recurrence of hepatitis C after liver transplantation. *J Hepatol* 39, 389–396.

124 Crippin JS, McCashland T, Terrault N *et al.* (2002) A pilot study of the tolerability and efficacy of antiviral therapy in hepatitis C virus-infected patients awaiting liver transplantation. *Liver Transpl* 8, 350–355.

125 Thomas RM, Brems JJ, Guzman-Hartman G *et al.* (2003) Infection with chronic hepatitis C virus and liver transplantation: a role for interferon therapy before transplantation. *Liver Transpl* 9, 905–915.

126 Elisofon SA, Jonas MM (2006) Hepatitis B and C in children: current treatment and future strategies. *Clin Liver Dis* 10, 133–148.

127 Pembrey L, Newell M, Tovo P (2005) The management of HCV infected pregnant women and their children. *J Hepatol* 43, 515–525.

128 Gonzalez-Peralta RP, Kelly DA, Haber B *et al.* (2005) Interferon alfa-2b in combination with ribavirin for the treatment of chronic hepatitis C in children: efficacy, safety, and pharmacokinetics. *Hepatology* 42, 1010–1018.

129 Wirth S, Pieper-Boustani H, Lang T *et al.* (2005) Peginterferon alfa-2b plus ribavirin treatment in children and adolescents with chronic hepatitis C. *Hepatology* 41, 1013–1018.

130 Papo T, Marcellin P, Bernau J *et al.* (1992) Autoimmune chronic hepatitis axacerbated by alpha interferon. *Ann Int Med* 116, 51–53.

131 Muratori L, Lenzi M, Cataleta M *et al.* (1994) Interferon therapy in liver/kidney microsomal antibody type 1-positive patients with chronic hepatitis C. *J Hepatol* 21, 199–203.

132 Todros L, Saracco G, Durazzo M *et al.* (1995) Efficacy and safety of interferon alfa therapy in chronic hepatitis C with autoantibodies to liver-kidney microsomes. *Hepatology* 22, 1374–1378.

133 Monti V, Aghemo A, Rumi MG *et al.* (2005) The prevalence, clinical features and response to antiviral therapy of patients with chronic hepatitis C who are seropositive for liver-kidney microsome type 1 antibodies. *Antivir Ther* 10, 715–720.

134 Alvarez F, Berg PA, Bianchi FB *et al.* (1999) International Auto-immune Hepatitis Group report: review of criteria for diagnosis of autoimmune hepatitis. *J Hepatol* 31, 929–938.

135 Ferri C, Marzo E, Longombardo G *et al.* (1993) Interferon-alpha in mixed cryoglobulinemia patients: a randomized, crossover-controlled trial. *Blood* 81, 1132–1136.

136 Misiani R, Bellavita P, Fenili D *et al.* (1994) Interferon alfa-2a therapy in cryoglobulinemia associated with hepatitis C virus. *N Engl J Med* 330, 751–756.

137 Casato M, Agnello V, Pucillo LP *et al.* (1997) Predictors of long-term response to high-dose interferon therapy in type II cryoglobulinemia associated with hepatitis C virus infection. *Blood* 90, 3865–3873.

138 Zuckerman E, Zuckerman T, Sahar D *et al.* (2001) The effect of antiviral therapy on t(14;18) translocation and immunoglobulin gene rearrangement in patients with chronic hepatitis C virus infection. *Blood* 97, 1555–1559.

139 Giannelli F, Moscarella S, Giannini C *et al.* (2003) Effect of antiviral treatment in patients with chronic HCV infection and t(14;18) translocation. *Blood* 102, 1196–1201.

140 Zuckerman E, Keren D, Slobodin G *et al.* (2000) Treatment of refractory, symptomatic, hepatitis C virus related mixed cryoglobulinemia with ribavirin and interferon-alpha. *J Rheumatol* 27, 2172–2178.

141 Cacoub P, Saadoun D, Limal N *et al.* (2005) PEGylated interferon alfa-2b and ribavirin treatment in patients with hepatitis C virus-related systemic vasculitis. *Arthritis Rheum* 52, 911–915.

142 Mazzaro C, Zorat F, Caizzi M *et al.* (2005) Treatment with peg-interferon alfa-2b and ribavirin of hepatitis C virus-associated mixed cryoglobulinemia: a pilot study. *J Hepatol* 42, 632–638.

143 Giannini C, Giannelli F, Zignego AL (2006) Association between mixed cryoglobulinemia, t(14;18) translocation, and persistence of occult HCV lymphoid infection after treatment. *Hepatology* 43, 1166–1167.

144 Meyers CM, Seeff LB, Stehman-Breen CO *et al.* (2003) Hepatitis C and renal disease: an update. *Am J Kidney Dis* 42, 631–657.

145 Bruchfeld A, Stahle L, Andersson J *et al.* (2001) Ribavirin treatment in dialysis patients with chronic hepatitis C virus infection – a pilot study. *J Viral Hepat* 8, 287–292.

146 Tan AC, Brouwer JT, Glue P *et al.* (2001) Safety of interferon and ribavirin therapy in haemodialysis patients with chronic hepatitis C: results of a pilot study. *Nephrol Dial Transplant* 16, 193–195.

147 Bruchfeld A, Lindahl K, Stahle L *et al.* (2003) Interferon and ribavirin treatment in patients with hepatitis C-associated renal disease and renal insufficiency. *Nephrol Dial Transplant* 18, 1573–1580.

148 Fabrizi F, Dulai G, Dixit V *et al.* (2003) Meta-analysis: interferon for the treatment of chronic hepatitis C in dialysis patients. *Aliment Pharmacol Ther* 18, 1071–1081.

149 Rocha CM, Perez RM, Ferreira AP *et al.* (2006) Efficacy and tolerance of interferon-alpha in the treatment of chronic hepatitis C in end-stage renal disease patients on hemodialysis. *Liver Int* 26, 305–310.

150 Bruchfeld A, Lindahl K, Reichard O et al. (2006) Pegylated interferon and ribavirin treatment for hepatitis C in haemodialysis patients. *J Viral Hepat* 13, 316–321.

151 Inati A, Taher A, Ghorra S et al. (2005) Efficacy and tolerability of peginterferon alpha-2a with or without ribavirin in thalassaemia major patients with chronic hepatitis C virus infection. *Br J Haematol* 130, 644–646.

152 Butensky E, Pakbaz Z, Foote D et al. (2005) Treatment of hepatitis C virus infection in thalassemia. *Ann NY Acad Sci* 1054, 290–299.

153 Demelia L (2007) Tolerability of Peg interferon (alpha) 2b and ribavirin therapy in patients with chronic hepatitis C and glucose-6-phosphate dehydrogenase deficiency. *J Hepatol*, 46, 171–173.

154 Fried MW, Peter J, Hoots K et al. (2002) Hepatitis C in adults and adolescents with hemophilia: a randomized, controlled trial of interferon alfa-2b and ribavirin. *Hepatology* 36, 967–972.

155 Fabris P, Betterle C, Fioreani A et al. (1992) Development of type 1 diabetes mellitus during interferon alpha therapy for chronic HCV hepatitis. *Lancet* 340, 548.

156 Cozzolongo R, Betterle C, Fabris P et al. (2006) Onset of type 1 diabetes mellitus during peginterferon alpha-2b plus ribavirin treatment for chronic hepatitis C. *Eur J Gastroenterol Hepatol* 18, 689–692.

157 Primo Vera J (2004) Pegylated-interferon-induced diabetes mellitus type 1 in two patients with chronic hepatitis C. *Gastroenterol Hepatol* 27, 69.

158 Tahrani A, Bowler L, Singh P et al. (2006) Resolution of diabetes in type 2 diabetic patient treated with IFN-alpha and ribavirin for hepatitis C. *Eur J Gastroenterol Hepatol* 18, 291–293.

159 Krawitt EL, Ashikaga T, Gordon SR et al. (2005) Peginterferon alfa-2b and ribavirin for treatment-refractory chronic hepatitis C. *J Hepatol* 43, 243–249.

160 Shiffman ML, Hofmann CM, Gabbay J et al. (2000) Treatment of chronic hepatitis C in patients who failed interferon monotherapy: effects of higher doses of interferon and ribavirin combination therapy. *Am J Gastroenterol* 95, 2928–2935.

161 Saracco G, Ciancio A, Olivero A et al. (2001) A randomized 4-arm multicenter study of interferon alfa-2b plus ribavirin in the treatment of patients with chronic hepatitis C not responding to interferon alone. *Hepatology* 34, 133–138.

162 Di Marco V, Vaccaro A, Ferraro D et al. (2001) High-dose prolonged combination therapy in non-responders to interferon monotherapy for chronic hepatitis C. *Aliment Pharmacol Ther* 15, 953–958.

163 Poynard T, Schiff E, Terg R et al. (2004) High early viral response (EVR) with Peg-Intron Rebetol (PR) weight based dosing (WBD) in previous interferon/ribavirin HCV treatment failures; early results of the epic trial. *Hepatology*, 40(Suppl 1), 170A.

164 Taliani G, Gemignani G, Ferrari C et al. (2006) Pegylated interferon alfa-2b plus ribavirin in the retreatment of interferon–ribavirin non-responder patients. *Gastroenterology* 130, 1098–1106.

165 Sherman M, Yoshida EM, Deschenes M et al. (2006) Peginterferon alfa-2a (40KD) plus ribavirin in chronic hepatitis C patients who failed previous interferon therapy. *Gut*, 55, 1631–1638.

166 Cornberg M, Hadem J, Herrmann E et al. (2006) Treatment with daily consensus interferon (CIFN) plus ribavirin in non-responder patients with chronic hepatitis C: a randomized open-label pilot study. *J Hepatol* 44, 291–301.

167 Maynard M, Pradat P, Bailly F et al. (2006) Amantadine triple therapy for non-responder hepatitis C patients. Clues for controversies. *J Hepatol* 44, 484–490.

168 Jensen DM, Marcellin P (2005) Rationale and design of the REPEAT study: a phase III, randomized, clinical trial of peginterferon alfa-2a (40 kDa) plus ribavirin in non-responders to peginterferon alfa-2b (12 kDa) plus ribavirin. *Eur J Gastroenterol Hepatol* 17, 899–904.

169 Kelleher TB, Afdhal N (2005) Maintenance therapy for chronic hepatitis C. *Curr Gastroenterol Rep* 7, 50–53.

170 Afdhal N, Freilich B, Levine R et al. (2004) Colchicine versus Peg-Intron long-term (COPILOT) trial: interim analysis of clinical outcomes at year 2. *Hepatology*, 40(Suppl 1), 180A.

171 Pawlotsky JM (2003) The nature of interferon-alpha resistance in hepatitis C virus infection. *Curr Opin Infect Dis* 16, 587–592.

172 Martell M, Esteban JI, Quer J et al. (1992) Hepatitis C virus (HCV) circulates as a population of different but closely related genomes: quasispecies nature of HCV genome distribution. *J Virol* 66, 3225–3229.

173 Reesink HW, Zeuzem S, Weegink CJ et al. (2006) Rapid decline of viral RNA in hepatitis C patients treated with VX-950: a phase Ib, placebo-controlled, randomized study. *Gastroenterology* 131, 997–1002.

174 Tong X, Chase R, Skelton A et al. (2006) Identification and analysis of fitness of resistance mutations against the HCV protease inhibitor SCH 503034. *Antivir Res* 70, 28–38.

175 Lin C, Lin K, Luong Y-PB et al. (2004) In vitro resistance studies of hepatitis C virus serine protease inhibitors, VX-950 and BILN 2061: structural analysis indicates different resistance mechanisms. *J Biol Chem* 279, 17508–17514.

176 Lin K, Perni RB, Kwong AD et al. (2006) VX-950, a novel hepatitis C virus (HCV) NS3–4A protease inhibitor, exhibits potent antiviral activities in HCV replicon cells. *Antimicrob Agents Chemother* 50, 1813–1822.

177 Lu L, Pilot-Matias TJ, Stweart KD et al. (2004) Mutations conferring resistance to a potent hepatitis C virus serine protease inhibitor *in vitro*. *Antimicrob Agents Chemother* 48, 2260–2266.

178 Trozzi C, Bartholomew L, Ceccacci A et al. (2003) In vitro selection and characterization of hepatitis C virus serine protease variants resistant to an active-site peptide inhibitor. *J Virol* 77, 3669–3679.

179 Tomei L, Altamura S, Paonessa G et al. (2005) HCV antiviral resistance: the impact of *in vitro* studies on the development of antiviral agents targeting the viral NS5B polymerase. *Antivir Chem Chemother* 16, 225–245.

180 De Francesco R, Migliaccio G (2005) Challenges and successes in developing new therapies for hepatitis C. *Nature* 436, 953–960.

181 Seiwert S, Andrews SW, Tan H et al. (2006) Generation and characterization of HCV replicons with reduced sensitivity to Itmn 191, a macrocyclic inhibitor of NS3/4a. *Gastroenterology* 130(Suppl 2), A195.

182 Migliaccio G, Tomassini JE, Carroll SS et al. (2003) Characterization of resistance to non-obligate chain-terminating ribonucleoside analogs that inhibit hepatitis C virus replication *in vitro*. *J Biol Chem* 278, 49164–49170.

183 Le Pogam S, Kang H, Harris SF et al. (2006) Selection and characterization of replicon variants dually resistant to thumb- and palm-binding non-nucleoside polymerase inhibitors of the hepatitis C virus. *J Virol* 80, 6146–6154.

184 Mo H, Lu L, Pilot-Matias T et al. (2005) Mutations conferring resistance to a hepatitis C virus (HCV) RNA-dependent RNA polymerase inhibitor alone or in combination with an HCV serine protease inhibitor *in vitro*. *Antimicrob Agents Chemother* 49, 4305–4314.

9.2 Systemic virosis producing hepatitis

Alberto Biglino and Mario Rizzetto

Introduction

Many viral agents may induce liver damage as part of a systemic infection or an infection primarily involving other organs. Although hepatic involvement with these agents is usually mild and the clinical picture is dominated by systemic complications or complications in other organs, severe hepatitis with acute liver failure or fulminant hepatitis may occur, either as part of disseminated disease or, less frequently, as the main clinical manifestation.

These viral agents include the herpesviruses (herpes simplex virus, varicella-zoster virus, Epstein–Barr virus, cytomegalovirus and the human herpesviruses types 6, 7 and 8), the adenoviruses, human parvovirus B19, the measles and rubella viruses, and the enteroviruses.

Herpesviruses

The herpesviruses are a family of about 150 large enveloped DNA-containing viruses that are infectious to a wide range of invertebrate and vertebrate hosts. The eight known human herpesviruses (HHV) are classified into three subfamilies (Alpha-, Beta- and Gammaherpesvirinae) according to genome homology, host range and cell tropism. Herpesviruses vary widely in their ability to infect different types of cells, including epithelial and nerve cells, fibroblasts and lymphocytes. Following primary infection, all herpesviruses undergo lifelong latency in their natural hosts, either as extrachromosomal or integrated DNA, or as slowly replicating forms. Latency is maintained in 'immunologically privileged' sites, such as sensory nerve ganglia, secretory glands or B and T lymphocytes, because of the capacity of the virus to interfere with major histocompatibility complex (MHC)-I-driven immune recognition and cytotoxic T-lymphocyte-mediated destruction of infected cells. Reactivation, leading to recurrent disease or invasive infection, may be induced by immune suppression or by other poorly defined stimuli. Herpesviruses may induce disease by direct tissue damage, immune-mediated cytolysis or neoplastic transformation.

Alphaherpesvirinae subfamily

In both primary and recurrent infections, tissue tropism in the immunocompetent host involves mucocutaneous epithelia and neuronal cells. Visceral infections, including hepatitis, pneumonia, encephalitis and retinitis, or disseminated disease may occur in neonates and immunocompromised hosts. Latency is established primarily, but not exclusively, in sensory ganglia.

Herpes simplex virus

Herpes simplex virus (HSV) types 1 and 2 (HSV-1 and HSV-2) are double-stranded DNA viruses belonging to the Alphaherpesvirinae subfamily. HSV has a worldwide distribution; the seroprevalence in the general population of Europe and the United States is about 13% and 22%, respectively, and rates between 25% and 64% are found in people attending clinics for sexually transmitted diseases [1]. Infection is spread through close contact with peripheral lesions on the skin or mucosae; however, asymptomatic shedding is common with both HSV-1 and HSV-2 [2], and so oropharyngeal and genital secretions are important sources of infection in the absence of typical lesions. The virus enters the human host through mucosal surfaces (oropharynx, cervix, conjunctivae) or the damaged epidermis and replicates within the nuclei of epithelial cells. Infection leads to the formation of typical vesicles, which may rupture leaving shallow or confluent ulcers. Primary HSV infection may be either subclinical or accompanied by significant systemic and local symptoms such as fever, headache, myalgias, irritability and wide local mucocutaneous involvement with satellite lymphadenopathy (both in orofacial and genital localizations). The virus is transported intra-axonally along peripheral sensory nerves to the nerve cell bodies in dorsal root ganglia, where it replicates and from where it spreads to the mucosal or skin surface by centrifugal migration through the same sensory nerves [3]. Latency is established in sensory nuclei; upon reactivation, the virus returns to the mucocutaneous surfaces by anterograde axonal movement [4].

Visceral HSV infection usually follows viraemia; multiple-organ involvement is common, including oesophagitis, pneumonitis, acute respiratory distress syndrome, adrenalitis and hepatitis with disseminated intravascular coagulation. Neonatal HSV-1 and HSV-2 infection, and primary infection in immunosuppressed subjects (particularly children), are associated with visceral infections. Prompt diagnosis of HSV-related liver damage is critical, as this is one of the very few treatable causes of acute hepatitis. The disease has a high mortality rate (41–79%); the liver lesions are severe and lead to rapid hepatic failure [5].

Neonatal HSV hepatitis occurs in the setting of disseminated infection; it affects 25% of HSV-infected neonates, with an incidence of one case per 2000–5000 deliveries per year [6], and is the most common of the infectious causes of neonatal acute liver failure [7]. Besides the liver, other organs that are involved include the central nervous system (CNS), lungs, adrenal glands, skin, eyes and/or mouth. Diagnosis may be difficult because 60–80% of women who deliver an HSV-infected infant have no evidence of genital HSV infection at delivery, or a past history of genital herpes or sexual partner(s) with genital HSV [8]. Without appropriate antiviral therapy and liver transplantation, the prognosis is poor.

HSV hepatitis in healthy adults is a rare, but potentially fatal, disease, occurring mainly during primary infection; no definite case of acute hepatitis has been reported during recurrent infection in immunocompetent hosts, although HSV may affect the liver in this setting [9]. Mortality rates in untreated patients with severe HSV hepatitis may be as high as 80% [10].

The clinical picture of acute HSV-related hepatitis includes fever, upper right abdominal quadrant tenderness, abrupt elevations of bilirubin and serum aminotransferase levels and leukopenia (< 4000 white blood cells/μL). Disseminated intravascular coagulation may also develop, rapidly followed by oliguria, encephalopathy and coma.

HSV hepatitis during pregnancy may result from primary or reactivated infections caused by both HSV-1 and HSV-2. The differential diagnosis includes severe preeclampsia, preeclampsia/haemolysis, elevated liver function and low platelets (HELLP syndrome) and acute fatty liver of pregnancy, as well as hepatitis caused by other viral pathogens or exposure to exogenous substances, such as drugs [11]. Mucocutaneous lesions are absent in nearly half of the cases [12]. Maternal and neonatal mortality rates from HSV hepatitis may be as high as 39% [13].

Diagnosis is difficult because disseminated HSV infection is rarely suspected in apparently immunocompetent, otherwise healthy, subjects. Initial symptoms are non-specific; mucocutaneous oral/genital lesions are evident in 40–70% of cases [9,14]. In a review of HSV hepatitis [15], herpes simplex was considered in the differential diagnosis in only 33% of patients, although the reported cases included 26 pregnant women and 15 patients receiving immunosuppression for a variety of diagnoses. Fatal HSV hepatitis has also been reported after corticosteroid treatment in a neoplastic patient [16].

A high index of suspicion is required in order to ask for more specific tests (HSV-DNA detection in blood or biopsy specimens). Given the potential for cure, the diagnostic workup should proceed even in the presence of severe liver failure with coagulopathy; prompt diagnosis via transjugular liver biopsy should be undertaken and empirical treatment with aciclovir also considered, even in the absence of typical cutaneous manifestations.

Immunocompromised hosts, such as bone marrow and solid-organ transplant patients, patients undergoing chemotherapy and those with extensive burns or who are severely malnourished, are at greater risk of severe HSV infection. In these subjects, HSV causes extensive mucocutaneous infections and may disseminate.

HSV-related disease in immunosuppressed patients is usually the consequence of the reactivation of a latent infection [17]. The majority of patients awaiting liver transplantation are HSV-antibody positive [18]. In the immediate postoperative period, the risk of HSV reactivation is high because of the induction of immunosuppression at the time of surgery. Most recipients of kidney, liver and bone marrow transplants excrete HSV-1 in saliva during the first 2–3 weeks after grafting. HSV-1-seropositive recipients of a bone marrow transplant from an HSV-seronegative donor are at higher risk for recurrence and are more likely to develop aciclovir-resistant strains of HSV than those who receive marrow from HSV-1-positive donors [19]. Mucocutaneous infection is the most common manifestation of HSV reactivation, but HSV pneumonia and fatal hepatitis have also been documented. Prophylaxis against HSV infection in liver transplant recipients is not performed routinely, possibly because data regarding the incidence and significance of HSV reactivation in this population are lacking. In one study, ganciclovir was shown to reduce the incidence of symptomatic HSV infections after liver transplantation to 3.5%, compared with 23.5% in transplant recipients given placebo [20].

Liver histology of fulminant HSV hepatitis reveals large areas of necrosis, with HSV-DNA-positive hepatocytes detected using in situ hybridization. Occasionally, Cowdry's type A intranuclear inclusions are seen, which disappear after starting antiviral treatment; numerous hepatocytes show DNA accumulation beneath the nuclear membrane [21]. Massive liver infiltration with mononuclear cells is not consistent with fulminant HSV hepatitis; in addition to necrosis, apoptosis may play a significant role in liver damage [22].

Diagnosis

Antibodies to purified HSV-1 and HSV-2 proteins are readily detectable in serum of HSV-infected individuals but are of no use for diagnosing acute infection; the presence of serum immunoglobulin (Ig)M antibodies, as well as fourfold increases in the IgG antibody titre, are not patognomonic of primary infection because they may arise during reactivation. Nevertheless, serology is an accurate tool for identifying subjects with longstanding HSV infection [23]. Type-specific IgG antibodies to the glycoproteins gG1 (HSV-1) and gG2 (HSV-2), which are antigenically distinct, may be detected in serum, and

HSV-2 screening is recommended in selected groups at risk [24]; Western blotting may distinguish HSV-1 from HSV-2 infections, with a sensitivity and specificity that is greater than 98% [25].

Herpes simplex should be considered in the differential diagnosis of acute hepatitis when other viral or toxic causes are ruled out. Patients should be asked about sore throat, odynophagia, dysuria or genital discharge to determine the most likely location of vesicles. Both exposed and unexposed skin surfaces should be examined, searching for mucocutaneous lesions; a pelvic examination may be necessary as vesicles on the cervix may not be accompanied by vulvar or vaginal vesicles. If lesions are identified, Giemsa or Wright staining of scrapings from their base (Tzanck test) allows a rapid microscopic diagnosis, with demonstrations of multinucleated giant cells with the characteristic ground-glass nuclear inclusion bodies (Cowdry's type A). Viral antigens may also be demonstrated on cytological preparations using fluorescent antibody staining [5]. HSV infection can be confirmed by viral culture or by polymerase chain reaction (PCR) detection of HSV DNA in blood and tissue specimens. Cultures should always be undertaken because they provide a virus isolate that can be typed. A scraping of skin vesicles should be taken from any skin lesions and transferred in appropriate virus transport media to a virology laboratory for inoculation onto a susceptible cell culture. A cytopathic effect usually develops 24–48 h after inoculation; antiviral treatment should not be delayed while awaiting cultural diagnosis [18].

Therapy

Aciclovir, a synthetic acyclic purine nucleoside analogue, is the standard first-line therapy for HSV infection. The precursor drugs valaciclovir and famciclovir have better oral bioavailability than their activated forms aciclovir and penciclovir respectively. Renal dysfunction can occur, especially with rapid intravenous infusion of large doses of aciclovir, but this is rare and usually reversible. The risk of nephrotoxicity can be reduced by slow infusion and by ensuring adequate hydration. The intravenous administration of aciclovir has also been linked to disturbances of the CNS (agitation, hallucinations, disorientation, tremors and myoclonus). Oral aciclovir has been associated with renal failure in elderly individuals [26]. Because aciclovir crosses the placenta and is concentrated in amniotic fluid, there is concern about potential fetal nephrotoxicity; however, none has been observed [27].

In immunocompromised patients, particularly after induction chemotherapy or transplantation, aciclovir prophylaxis reduces the rate of symptomatic HSV infection; famciclovir and valaciclovir have similar effects [6].

Resistance to aciclovir can develop and is often associated with clinical failure; this is an important issue in allogeneic bone marrow transplant recipients [28]. Resistance most often occurs via mutations in the gene for viral thymidine kinase (TK), which is required for phosphorylation of the drug; resistance was reported in 0.28–0.33% of HSV isolates recovered from normally immunocompetent subjects in the general population [29]. Higher resistance rates were observed in subjects with a depressed immune function (6–7.6%), in bone marrow graft recipients (7.0–15.4%) [28] and in subjects with human immunodeficiency virus (HIV) infection (4.2–7.1%) [30]. Factors that increase the development of aciclovir resistance include previous treatment with aciclovir, HIV-1 infection and graft-versus-host disease (GVHD).

Foscarnet and cidofovir retain activity against TK-deficient strains of HSV. Foscarnet is the treatment of choice for aciclovir-resistant HSV infection; mutations in the HSV-DNA polymerase occur less frequently but may confer resistance to either foscarnet or aciclovir [31]. Infections with HSV strains that are resistant to both aciclovir and foscarnet can be treated with cidofovir, a nucleotide analogue that is active against a wide range of DNA viruses, including HSV [32]. HSV resistance to cidofovir has also been reported [28].

Ganciclovir, a synthetic analogue of 2′-deoxyguanosine, inhibits the replication of HSV-1 and HSV-2 *in vitro*, but it has not been used in HSV infections in humans; HSV strains that are resistant to aciclovir appear to also be resistant to ganciclovir.

Varicella-zoster virus

Humans are the only host and reservoir of varicella-zoster virus (VZV). Primary infection is spread via the respiratory route; the virus replicates in the nasopharynx and is transferred to migrating T cells, with dissemination to the lymphoreticular organs and the skin, resulting in chickenpox with a rash (varicella). After primary infection, VZV becomes latent within the dorsal root ganglia; when latency is disrupted, the virus is transported along neuronal axons to the skin and this reactivaction leads to herpes zoster. VZV is endemic in the population but becomes epidemic among susceptible individuals during seasonal periods (late winter and early spring).

Clinical hepatitis is not observed in healthy children with uncomplicated primary varicella, although 28% of them may show abnormal aminotransferase levels [33]; however, in one study [34], only 1.4% of healthy children showed an increase in the alanine aminotransferase level that was at least two times greater than the upper limit of normality. In apparently immunocompetent infants of less than 12 months, primary varicella may result in high mortality rates [35] because of complications such as pneumonitis, encephalitis and haemorrhagic manifestations (but not severe hepatitis). Reye syndrome, an abrupt mitochondrial failure manifesting as acute encephalopathy and liver dysfunction with fatty infiltration, is often preceded by varicella.

Perinatal varicella is associated with mortality rates that are as high as 30% when maternal disease develops between 5 days before delivery and 48 h postpartum.

Primary varicella may run a severe course in apparently immunocompetent adults and may be complicated by pneumonia (occurring in about 1 in 400 cases), viral encephalitis, haemorrhagic conditions and secondary infections. However, even in these cases, severe hepatitis with liver failure is exceptional, although liver enzyme elevations of up to three times the upper normal level or higher are common (particularly in men) [36,37].

In immunocompromised children and adults, primary varicella may be life-threatening. Most cases of VZV-related hepatitis and acute liver failure were reported in patients who were immunocompromised because of acute leukaemia, [38,39], bone marrow [40–42] or solid-organ transplantation [43,44], or acquired immune deficiency syndrome (AIDS) [45].

The use of systemic corticosteroids greatly increases the risk of fatal primary varicella hepatitis, even in the absence of underlying pathological conditions [46,47].

VZV reactivation is common after haematopoietic stem cell transplantation (HSCT), as T-cell immunity against VZV, which is crucial for the re-establishment of latency, recovers slowly [48]. The incidence of herpes zoster in children following HSCT has been reported to be in the range of 23–67% in the 5 years post-HSCT [49].

The infection may be confined to the skin; however, visceral involvement, including hepatitis, pneumonitis and meningo-encephalitis, can also occur. Visceral involvement occurs in approximately 1% of adults [40] and in around 7% of paediatric bone marrow transplant recipients with VZV reactivation [50]; pneumonitis and hepatic failure are the most important causes of death. Visceral involvement is probably underdiagnosed, as immunosuppressed patients may fail to develop the skin rash in the early phase of the infection; nevertheless, aminotransferases are frequently slightly elevated before development of the rash in cases in which herpes zoster involves visceral abdominal organs [51]. Therefore, an otherwise unexplained aminotransferase elevation might serve as a potential marker for preclinical herpes zoster infection [52]. Visceral VZV infection often presents as poorly localized abdominal pain accompanying pancreatitis, hepatitis and paralytic ileus. In a series of patients [40], the pain was epigastric, occasionally involving the right upper quadrant or radiating to the back. Fever and skin rash may be initially absent and may develop up to 5 days or later after abdominal pain. [53]. VZV reactivation should be included in the differential diagnosis of the many causes of elevated alanine and aspartate aminotransferases post-HSCT; in one study [42], the majority of patients with elevated alanine aminotransferase levels preceding herpes zoster did not have concomitant GVHD, which can independently cause liver dysfunction.

The diagnosis of VZV hepatitis is based on PCR and immuno-histochemical analysis of liver tissue obtained by biopsy or post-mortem. PCR analysis of blood may be of diagnostic value in visceral VZV before the signs of infection appear on the skin, enabling early diagnosis and treatment [54].

Therapy
Prevention of VZV infection/reactivation has been attempted in immunocompromised (mostly transplanted) patients using both antiviral drugs and vaccines. Aciclovir, either at low (400 mg/day) or high (1600 mg/day) doses, taken for up to 6–12 months after bone marrow transplantation, was shown to delay, but not prevent, disseminated herpes zoster [55,56]; ganciclovir showed similar results [55].

Inactivated varicella vaccine is immunogenic; it significantly reduced the incidence of herpes zoster when four doses, the first given 30 days before transplant, were administered to patients with lymphoma who received an autologous HSCT [57].

Betaherpesvirinae subfamily

The Betaherpesvirinae subfamily includes human cytomegalovirus (CMV; HHV-5), HHV-6 and HHV-7.

Cytomegalovirus

Virology
CMV or HHV-5 is the largest known HHV, with a linear double-stranded DNA of about 230 kDa. The viral DNA is wrapped in a nucleoprotein core and is surrounded by a proteinaceous matrix and the pp65 antigen, which can be detected in host cells by immunofluorescence, immunoperoxidase and other antigen detection methods. The viral matrix is surrounded by a lipid bilayer containing viral glycoproteins. Glycoprotein B (gB) is the major envelope glycoprotein of CMV; it is implicated in host-cell entry, cell-to-cell virus transmission and fusion of infected cells and is also an important target for both humoral and cellular immune responses [58]. Latency of CMV depends on mechanisms that are still unknown; the downregulation of human leukocyte antigen (HLA)-1 expression at the cell surface may play a role by preventing immune recognition and destruction of infected cells. Disease most often follows the reactivation of CMV induced by HIV- or drug-mediated immunosuppression.

Diagnosis of CMV infection
Serology is useful only for the determination of a patient's serostatus, as in pretransplant workup; it is of limited value in the diagnosis of acute CMV infection, with the exception of infection in immunocompetent adults. The presence of IgM antibodies to CMV immediate-early and tegument proteins, as well as to membrane glycoproteins, is usually associated with acute infection in immunocompetent subjects [59]; however, they are also reported in about one-third of recurrent infections in transplanted patients. On the other hand, specific IgM antibodies may be absent in AIDS patients with generalized CMV infection. Primary acute infection in immunocompetent adults can be diagnosed by IgG antibody seroconversion (i.e. IgG serology changing from negative to positive) to both non-structural and structural CMV antigens. A low avidity of IgG antibodies is also significantly associated with recent primary infection.

In all other situations, only the direct demonstration of the virus or its components is of diagnostic value. This is particularly the case in immunocompromised patients, in whom the diagnosis of 'CMV infection' requires isolation of CMV or detection of viral proteins/nucleic acid in body fluids or tissue specimens. [60]. Traditional viral cultures on human fibroblast cells are too time-consuming and insensitive to be of diagnostic use in acute disease. Modern culture techniques using 'shell vial' cell monolayers and monoclonal antibodies to immediate-early CMV antigens can result in the detection of viral growth after overnight incubation. Virus may be grown from semen or cervical swabs from healthy subjects, as well as from throat swabs and urine from patients with asymptomatic infection or during recovery from acute primary infection. Viraemia, defined as the isolation of CMV from blood by standard or 'shell vial' rapid culture techniques, is highly suggestive of pathogenic infection in immunocompetent subjects. Rapid viral culture for diagnosing acute systemic infection is best carried out using tissue, bronchoalveolar lavage (BAL) fluid and urine; however, CMV growth from these specimens taken from immunocompromised subjects is often positive in the absence of invasive disease. In viraemic patients, viral antigens, such as the matrix phosphoprotein pp65, are detectable in peripheral blood granulocytes using a monoclonal antibody (CMV antigenaemia). As with viraemia, the presence of antigenaemia in an immunocompetent subject is suggestive of clinically relevant infection.

In immunocompromised patients, antigenaemia resulting from recurrent CMV infection is frequent, regardless of the clinical features, and cannot be used to diagnose end-organ disease. However, as the rate of antigen-carrying cells correlates with both viraemia and CMV mRNA levels in leukocytes, counts of pp65-positive cells exceeding six per 200 000 granulocytes are predictive of the development of clinical disease [61].

To assess the viral load in immunocompromised patients, many laboratories are now using molecular techniques based on the detection of CMV DNA by signal or DNA amplification or on the detection of late-CMV mRNA. Some of these techniques allow a true quantitative definition of the 'CMV viral load' (CMV DNAemia) in samples of plasma, whole blood or peripheral blood buffy-coat specimens. Viral load can be used as a predictor for the development of CMV end-organ disease in AIDS [62] and transplant patients [63,64]; trends are more useful than individual assay results, as the rate of rise of viral load and initial quantitative viral load assessment are independent indicators of CMV disease risk [65]. In liver transplant patients, the optimal cutoff for CMV viral load that can be used to predict disease is around 5000 copies/mL, with a sensitivity of 85.7% and a specificity of 86.8% [66]. Determination of the CMV viral load appears to be the key diagnostic tool for patient surveillance and management of CMV disease if pre-emptive approaches are used, i.e. the use of antiviral therapy to lower CMV-DNA levels to prevent end-organ disease. The detection of CMV pp65 mRNA in plasma, whole blood or buffy-coat specimens using nucleic acid sequence-based amplification (NASBA) or reverse transcriptase PCR ('RNAemia') has been found to be predictive for the development of symptomatic disease, although with a lower sensitivity [67].

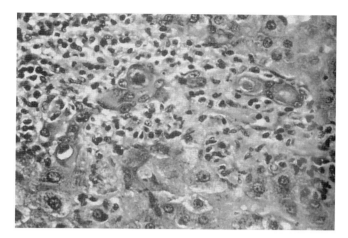

Fig. 1 CMV liver infection. 'Owl's eye' inclusions in bile duct cells within portal inflammation (× 400).

Histopathological examination of tissue is important in diagnosing invasive disease, as virus cultivation from tissue and body fluids may be the consequence of viraemia and not of tissue invasion. Single large intranuclear inclusions, which give the cell an 'owl's eye' appearance, may be found in lung, hepatocytes, Kupffer cells and biliary tract epithelium (Fig. 1). The use of immunohistochemistry with monoclonal antibodies and/or *in situ* hybridization to identify CMV-infected cells results in more sensitive morphological analysis.

Epidemiology and pathogenesis

Primary infection may be acquired at any age via saliva, sexual contact, placental transfer, breastfeeding, blood transfusion or solid-organ transplantation or HSCT. Congenital infection follows intrauterine transmission; this can occur in about 40–45% of pregnant women who acquire a primary CMV infection during the first trimester of gestation, and in about 8% of women who have preconceptional primary infections [68].

The rate of CMV infection increases steadily with age, resulting in a seroprevalence of 30–70% in young adults in developed countries, and of nearly 100% in some African regions. Primary infection is frequent during adolescence, and rates of congenital CMV infection are higher among infants born to mothers younger than 20 years of age [69]. In socially disadvantaged groups – particularly in developing countries – and homosexual men, seroprevalence rates may exceed 90% [70].

After a primary infection, the virus persists in the body and is harboured mainly in leukocytes, cells of the myeloid lineage and endothelial cells, from where recurrent infection may develop [71].

'Recurrent infection' is defined as the new detection of CMV infection in a patient with a previously documented infection, in whom the virus was not detected for an interval of at least 4 weeks during active surveillance. Recurrent infection may result from reactivation of the latent virus (endogenous) or reinfection (exogenous). 'Reinfection' is defined as the detection of a CMV strain which is different from the strain that caused the patient's original infection, and may be documented by sequencing specific regions of the viral genome. In immunocompetent subjects, primary infections, as well as reactivations and reinfections, are usually asymptomatic; however, there are rare reports of severe and even fatal CMV infections in previously healthy children and adults. In contrast, immunosuppressed patients and, particularly, organ transplant recipients have significant mortality and morbidity rates as a result of primary CMV infection from donated organs or blood products, as well as from reactivation [72] or reinfection.

CMV hepatitis

'CMV hepatitis' is defined by the presence of elevated liver enzyme and/or bilirubin levels, the absence of other causes of hepatitis and the detection of CMV in a liver biopsy specimen (by culture, immunohistochemical analysis or *in situ* hybridization). Detection of CMV by PCR analysis of serum is not sufficient, as it only implies the presence of viraemia; the finding of CMV within liver tissue is required.

In neonatal hepatitis, newborns may display hepatosplenomegaly, cholestatic jaundice, thrombocytopenia, petechiae and elevated liver enzymes in a setting of intrauterine growth retardation and severe neurological symptoms; the hepatitis tends to be self-limiting, although mortality may be as high as 10% and neurological sequelae persist [73].

Primary CMV infection in young adults may cause an infectious mononucleosis-like syndrome with fever, weakness, lymphadenopathy, pharyngitis and lymphocytosis. It is estimated that 79% of infectious mononucleosis is caused by the Epstein–Barr virus (EBV) and the other 21% by acute CMV infection. [73]. Patients with acute CMV are usually older than those with EBV mononucleosis (more than 30 years of age compared with 15–20 years) and have longer durations of fever and malaise (up to 32 weeks, with a mean duration of 7–8 weeks). Pharyngeal exudates, lymphadenopathy and peripheral leukocytosis are less common in CMV than in EBV infection; atypical lymphocytosis may be delayed by several weeks, but may persist for months. Although symptomatic hepatitis is rare in immunocompetent patients with CMV mononucleosis, liver function abnormalities are found in 69% of acute CMV infections [74]. Frank jaundice is seen in only about 10% of patients, with haemolytic anaemia sometimes contributing to the icterus [75,76].

A diagnosis of CMV hepatitis is very likely in this clinical setting; it is confirmed by high CMV IgM levels (> 300 U/mL) and IgG seroconversion [71]. CMV pp65 antigenaemia is of little help in diagnosis because it has poor sensitivity in immunocompetent patients (about 50%); in addition, the CMV-DNA viral load is usually low and does not correlate with the severity of clinical disease. Liver histology reveals mononuclear cells infiltrating the portal areas, along with giant cells, microscopic granulomas and few foci of necrosis. 'Owl's eye'

cells are rare or may be absent in hepatocytes but are more frequent in the bile duct epithelium. Acute hepatitis in the setting of acute primary CMV infection generally resolves.

CMV hepatitis in immunocompromised subjects is usually a manifestation of disseminated disease in AIDS patients or after transplantation. As recurrent infection is common, it may be difficult to distinguish between CMV reactivation with viraemia and end-organ disease.

In solid-organ transplantation, the risk of developing clinically significant CMV disease depends primarily on the CMV serostatus of both the donor and recipient. Seronegative recipients of an allograft from a seropositive donor are at greatest risk [77]; without effective prophylaxis, 50–75% will develop CMV disease [78]. If the donor is CMV-seronegative, CMV transmission – particularly in stem-cell transplantation – occurs mainly via blood products; the use of blood products from seronegative donors or of leukocyte-depleted blood products is recommended. The risk of CMV disease is also dependent on age, occurring in 5–16% of adult and 6% of paediatric transplant recipients, and on the type of organ transplanted. Steroids, the monoclonal antibody OKT-3 and polyclonal antilymphocyte globulins have been associated with an increased risk of disease, whereas ciclosporin and tacrolimus were not found to be of risk; conflicting data exist on the risk of mycophenolate mofetil. The risk associated with newer agents, such as sirolimus and the interleukin (IL)-2-receptor antibody, is unknown. The overall intensity of immunosuppression appears to be more important in determining risk than the use of any specific immunosuppressive agent [79]. Higher and more rapid increases in CMV viral load, as well as the presence of multiple CMV gB genotypes rather than a single gB genotype, are associated with an increased risk of CMV infection/disease [80] and with acute graft rejection (in renal transplantation) or chronic graft dysfunction.

Hepatitis is the most common organ-specific complication of CMV infection after liver transplantation. In a study of 253 liver transplantations, CMV hepatitis was diagnosed in 11% of patients; the incidence was higher among seronegative (26%) than seropositive recipients (9%), and most cases (70%) occurred during reactivation rather than primary infection. The histological alterations associated with CMV infection may cause problems in the differential diagnosis of acute rejection, in particular, mild forms of rejection. The ballooning of hepatocytes, a marked Kupffer cell reaction and the presence of microabscesses are typical of CMV hepatitis. Findings of portal lymphocytic infiltration, endotheliitis and cholestasis may not be distinguishable from findings in mild forms of acute rejection. Evidence of graft dysfunction, together with minor but confusing histological findings, may lead to unnecessary antirejection treatments, which may further aggravate CMV infection. Of note, it has been suggested that CMV infection may trigger a mild subclinical rejection [81]. CMV significantly increased the expression of ICAM-1/VCAM-1 adhesion molecules and their ligands (LFA-1, VLA-4), as well as MHC class II- and IL-2-receptor-positive lymphocytes in the graft. CMV hepatitis had no influence on the long-term outcome of the graft, but biliary complications were common [81].

CMV infection has been associated with cirrhosis and graft failure after liver transplantation, and with a more aggressive relapse of hepatitis C with rapid progression of fibrosis. CMV-induced immunosuppression may increase the risk of opportunistic (particularly fungal) infections, as well as EBV-related post-transplant lymphoproliferative disorders [82]. Infection is diagnosed by monitoring CMV pp65 antigenaemia; liver histology is required for definite diagnosis, including the demonstration of CMV antigens on immunohistochemistry and CMV DNA by *in situ* hybridization. CMV antigens are mainly located in the inflammatory cells of portal infiltrates, but can also be found within a few infected hepatocytes. No CMV-positive endothelial or bile duct epithelial cells have been recorded.

Therapy

Ganciclovir, foscarnet and cidofovir are the antiviral drugs that are currently used for the treatment of systemic CMV disease. Ganciclovir remains the preferred first-line agent; the other two drugs may be nephrotoxic when combined with ciclosporin. Appropriate drug dosing is important because subtherapeutic drug levels in the face of high viral loads promote resistance; however, the majority of documented cases of recurrent CMV disease have been caused by incomplete suppression of viral replication rather than drug resistance.

Symptomatic CMV disease is generally treated with a 2–4 week course of intravenous ganciclovir; the risk of relapse is estimated to be about 25–30% [83]. Factors such as pretransplant donor/recipient CMV serostatus, the presence of multisystem disease, treatment of rejection and intensity of immunosuppression (e.g. antilymphocyte therapy) may influence the risk of relapse. Patients who relapse have significantly higher initial CMV viral loads, lower rates of CMV clearance and are significantly more likely to have CMV viral loads that are detectable in peripheral blood or plasma at the end of therapy [84]. Thus, viral load kinetics (i.e. rate of change of viral load) seems to be an early predictor of both an increased risk of developing CMV disease, which is associated with a faster rate of viral load increase [65], and a good response to treatment, which is associated with a faster rate of viral load decrease (mean half-life of 3.17 days, compared with 8.8 days in non-responders).

Foscarnet and cidofovir are alternative treatments when drug-resistant strains emerge during ganciclovir therapy. Drug resistance may also appear during treatment with foscarnet or cidofovir; cidofovir cross-resistance can result from prolonged therapy with ganciclovir alone. CMV drug resistance mutations map to the UL97 phosphotransferase (kinase) sequence at codons 460, 520 and 591–607, which confer resistance only to ganciclovir, or to the DNA polymerase gene between codons 300 and 1000; resistance to each of the three drugs has been mapped within this codon range [85], and appears to be significantly associated with drug-resistant CMV with high peak virus loads.

The genotypic drug resistance assay is the test of choice for guiding treatment strategy, as rapid results may be obtained and many different mutations are detectable by automated sequencing of PCR products amplified from DNA extracted from viral cultures.

CMV-seronegative recipients of a liver graft from CMV-seropositive donors have the greatest risk for CMV disease. A prophylaxis trial of sequential intravenous and oral ganciclovir versus prolonged intravenous ganciclovir in high-risk CMV-seronegative liver transplant recipients with CMV-seropositive donors did not show significant differences between the two groups. All cases of CMV occurred more than 90 days after transplantation and there were no deaths from CMV in either study group. Both oral and intravenous ganciclovir were generally well tolerated. This study indicates that, after induction with 14 days of intravenous ganciclovir, oral treatment can be as effective as intravenous for the long-term prophylaxis of CMV disease [77].

Human herpesvirus types 6 and 7

HHV-6 and HHV-7 are lymphotropic viruses with high tropism for human CD4+ T lymphocytes; they may infect monocytes/macrophages and embryonic glial cells, as well as EBV-transformed B lymphocytes. About 64–83% of all humans are already infected with HHV-6 by 13 months of age, and more than 96% are infected by the age of 2 years [86]; HHV-7 infection is acquired later, over the first 5–6 years of life. After primary infection, both viruses persist for life and are shed in saliva, which is the major route of transmission [87]. Liver involvement was not observed in a large series of acutely ill, febrile children with culture-proven HHV-6 primary infection [88], but a few anecdotal cases of severe or fulminant hepatitis at the time of primary HHV-6 infection have been reported in newborns or infants [89,90], as well as in adults [91]. However, although HHV-6 infection appeared to be well-documented in these cases, the involvement of the virus in episodes of clinically relevant hepatitis remains questionable. As HHV-6 is ubiquitous, its long-lasting persistence or reactivation may be concomitant with an acute hepatitis episode but may not necessarily cause it; even the detection of viral DNA in tissue using PCR cannot be considered as definite proof of virus-related organ disease, as circulating lymphocytes carrying latent HHV-6 may be trapped within the liver in viraemic patients. More convincing data on the relationship between HHV-6 primary infection and severe acute hepatitis has arisen from recent studies employing real-time quantitative PCR analysis of liver tissue [92]. This technique, which allows a precise assessment of tissue viral HHV-6 DNA levels normalized for the number of hepatocytes examined [93], has led to the detection of liver viral loads exceeding 270 000 copies/10^5 hepatocytes, ruling out the possibility of 'incidental' lymphocytes or other mononuclear cells within the liver carrying the virus.

Virus reactivation with viraemia is common after transplantation, occurring in one-third of solid-organ and half of bone marrow recipients within 4 weeks of transplantation; however, no definite role of reactivation has been documented, so far, in organ disease (including post-transplant hepatitis) [94]. Symptomatic HHV-6 reactivation with fever or rash may be temporally associated with pneumonia, encephalitis and GVHD. These conditions are usually caused by reactivation of other, more overwhelming, opportunistic agents like CMV [95,96].

Treatment

The *in vitro* sensitivity of both HHV-6 and -7 to anti-herpetic drugs parallels that of CMV: cidofovir and foscarnet are inhibitory at pharmacologically suitable concentrations, ganciclovir activity is variable and aciclovir is inactive.

Both ganciclovir and foscarnet have been reported to be effective for prophylaxis or treatment of HHV-6 infections in transplanted patients [97].

Gammaherpesvirinae subfamily

The gammaherpesvirinae subfamily is characterized by a relatively restricted host range. Gamma-1 herpesviruses (lymphocryptoviruses) include EBV and EBV-like viruses, which infect humans and nonhuman primates respectively; gamma-2 herpesviruses (rhadinoviruses) may infect humans (Kaposi's sarcoma-associated herpesvirus; KSHV or HHV-8), as well as rodents and old- and new-world monkeys. Specific cell tropism, including B and T lymphocytes (*in vivo*) and lymphoblastoid cells (*in vitro*), latency in either B or T cells, and cell-transformation capabilities with frank oncogenic potentials, are typical of this subfamily.

Epstein–Barr virus

EBV (HHV-4) is a ubiquitous HHV; it is the causative agent of heterophile-positive infectious mononucleosis (whereas the heterophile-negative form is mainly caused by CMV). EBV is associated with the development of malignancies, including Burkitt's lymphoma, Hodgkin's lymphoma, nasopharyngeal carcinoma and immunosuppression-related lymphomas, such as post-transplant lymphoproliferative disease (PTLD) and the AIDS-related diffuse large-cell (B-cell) lymphoma, primary CNS lymphoma and primary effusion lymphoma of body cavities.

Virology and serology

EBV has a double-stranded DNA genome encased in a protein nucleocapsid, which is surrounded by a lipid envelope with embedded viral glycoproteins. Primary infection results from the exposure of susceptible individuals to oropharyngeal secretions of seropositive subjects through kissing, intimate contact or sharing of food; it is debated whether productive (lytic) replication in epithelial cells precedes virus spreading to the B-cell compartment [98]. B lymphocytes are driven to rapid and continuous proliferation by EBV, resulting in indefinite *in vitro* propagation (immortalization) [99]; *in vivo*, these cells are usually removed from the circulation in immunocompetent hosts as a result of a strong T-cell adaptive response [100].

Viral persistence is established by switching to latency, in which the genome circularizes in the nucleus and is replicated as an episome by the host-cell enzyme machinery. Although complete virions are not produced, this in not true latency; limited gene transcription continues, with the expression of different proteins such as the EBV nuclear antigens (EBNAs) and latent infection membrane proteins (LMP-1 and LMP-2) [101]. EBNAs promote the replication of the latent viral genome in the episomal state by host-cell machinery, ensure proper segregation of the EBV genome in daughter cells and activate expression of remaining nuclear proteins and of LMP-1 and LMP-2 [102]. LMP-1 is the major EBV oncogene, whose expression results in B-cell lymphomas [103]. EBV accounts for 1% of the global cancer burden and 5.6% of all infection-related malignancies [104]; most EBV-associated malignancies are associated with latent infection and latent gene expression.

Lytic infection, with active production of virions and cell death, may be the consequence of either primary infection or reactivation. Reactivation of latent infection is induced by different stimuli, particularly by antibodies to surface immunoglobulins (B-cell receptors) after antigenic stimulation. As a consequence, expression of immediate-early genes is induced, leading to production of early antigens (EAs) involved in viral replication (thymidine kinase, DNA polymerase), followed by expression of late genes encoding structural (capsid) antigens (viral capsid antigens, VCAs) [105].

The humoral immune response to EBV is characterized by the production of specific antibodies to the lytic infection-associated antigens (VCA and EA) and latency-associated nuclear antigens [EBNA-1, -2 and -3, and the EBV nuclear leader protein (EBNALP)], as well as to some antigens found on sheep, horse and beef red cells (heterophile antibodies).

Heterophile agglutinating antibodies (mostly IgM) to sheep and horse red cells are detectable in 90% of patients at some point during infectious mononucleosis, and persist for 1 year in 70–75% of cases. Heterophile antibodies may also be present in normal serum (naturally occurring Forssman's antibodies), leading to false-positive results. The differential absorption of serum with guinea pig kidney cells (which remove Forssman's and serum sickness-associated antibodies, but not mononucleosis-associated heterophile antibodies) and with beef red cells (which remove mononucleosis-associated but not Forssman's antibodies) increases the test specificity. Titres of 40 or more after guinea pig absorption are compatible with infectious mononucleosis, although false-positive results may be found in 7–12% of patients, and false-negative results are common in paediatric age groups or in the very early phase of disease, warranting later retesting in the course of the illness.

Specific antibodies to structural VCAs and nonstructural EAs expressed during the lytic cycle, as well as antibodies to latent EBNAs, are detectable by indirect immunofluorescence or enzyme immunoassays. Anti-VCA IgG antibody levels are usually close to peak at the time of presentation, so that a four-fold rise in titre, which is required to confirm acute infection, is detectable in only 10–20% of patients with mononucleosis or related complications. As IgG antibodies to VCAs persist for life, their detection is only useful for an assessment of serostatus. Conversely, IgM antibodies to VCAs at titres of 1/32 or greater are detectable in 90% of early acute infections, but are present in no more than 10% of patients after 4 months; their presence is therefore diagnostic of acute EBV infection. IgM antibodies to VCAs may be absent in 10–20% of acute infections. This diagnostic dilemma may be solved by measuring the avidity of IgG antibodies, i.e. the stability of binding to the antigen in the presence of urea; recent infection is characterized by low IgG avidity values.

Antibodies to EAs are found in about 70% of patients with acute infectious mononucleosis, peak at 3–4 weeks after disease onset and disappear after 3–6 months; in contrast, antibodies to EBNAs are not detectable until 3–4 weeks after disease onset, but persist for life in about 100% of infected patients. Thus, the appearance of antibodies to EBNAs in patients who were negative at the beginning of the illness is diagnostic of acute primary EBV infection.

In view of the high sensitivity and specificity of the serological tests, and the intermittent virus shedding by healthy seropositive subjects, virus detection by culture of oropharyngeal washings or circulating mononuclear cells is of little value in immunocompetent subjects with acute infection. The detection of virus in tissues by PCR amplification of viral DNA or by EBV-encoded RNA *in situ* hybridization (EBER-RISH) is also of limited clinical use when employed alone, because of the ubiquitous presence of virus-infected B lymphocytes trapped in peripheral organs [106]. When obtained in combination, serological data consistent with active infection and suggestive histopathological features and tissue detection of viral DNA by PCR may be useful.

Epidemiology and pathogenesis

Antibodies to EBV are detectable in more than 90% of the world's adult population, without predilection for sex, ethnicity and socioeconomic status. In the western world, only 50% of primary infections occur before the age of 5 years, with a second wave of infections occurring in the second decade of life. EBV is labile when exposed to the environment, and may be spread only by intimate contact with virus shedders (kissing in adolescents/young adults or transfer of saliva to susceptible children within families through shared objects or food).

Most signs and symptoms of acute primary EBV infection (infectious mononucleosis) in immunocompetent subjects are produced by immune activation, aimed at both EBNA-expressing B cells and EBV-transformed mononuclear cells, which represent 20% of circulating B cells and 0.5% of mononuclear cells respectively. Antigen-activated CD8+ cytotoxic T lymphocytes (CTLs) that are highly specfic for EBV lytic antigens or EBNA proteins are the major effectors of removal of proliferating or transformed mononuclear cells during acute infection and suppression of

EBV-infected B-lymphocyte growth during subsequent viral latency respectively [107].

EBV hepatitis

Typical infectious mononucleosis is characterized clinically by fever, sore throat, lymphadenopathy and splenomegaly, by the appearance of heterophile antibodies and by mononuclear leukocytosis with atypical lymphocytes. Transient and self-limited liver enzyme elevations are found in the majority of patients (80–90%) [108]. In adults over the age of 40, abdominal pain with fever and transaminase/akaline phosphatase alterations may predominate. Jaundice with a frank cholestatic picture may be present in 5–7% of cases [108–111]. Histopathology shows minimal swelling and vacuolization of hepatocytes and bile ducts, with pleomorphic lymphocyte and monocyte portal infiltration; biliary stasis is rare.

Severe hepatitis is rare in immunocompetent individuals with infectious mononucleosis and only a few lethal cases have been reported [112,113]. The majority of cases of severe and potentially lethal liver damage are observed in immunocompromised subjects with either X-linked (Duncan's) lymphoproliferative disease (frequently resulting in fulminant hepatitis at the time of primary EBV infection) or post-transplant lymphoproliferative disease, especially after liver transplantation (as a result of primary EBV infection or reactivation).

'Chronic' hepatitis has been tentatively linked to primary infection [114] or chronic EBV infection [115]; liver histology in these patients shows portal and intrasinusoidal mononuclear inflammatory cell infiltrates (mostly B and T lymphocytes, with rare plasma cells) and fatty changes, without significant hepatocyte necrosis or liver structure disarray.

Autoimmune chronic hepatitis triggered by EBV through the continuous proliferation of asialoglycoprotein receptor-specific B lymphocytes has been reported [116]. Histopathology reveals active lobular hepatitis with portal and sinusoidal mononuclear cell infiltration, piecemeal necrosis and portal or bridging fibrosis [117,118]. Anti-smooth muscle antibodies may be present [119].

In these patients, serology is generally consistent with latent EBV infection, with absent or low-level antibodies typical of lytic infection (IgG antibodies to EAs and IgM antibodies to VCAs), but with significant titres of IgG antibodies to both VCAs and EBNAs. Molecular techniques have revealed the presence of EBV in liver tissue; however, the specificity of these techniques may be weakened by the presence of circulating EBV-carrying B lymphocytes 'trapped' within the liver at the moment of biopsy. The paradox of viral latency in the lymphocytes infiltrating the liver but not in the hepatocytes, which lack the CD21 epithelial cell receptor for EBV and have not been found to contain EBV sequences, remains unexplained [120].

As the mechanisms underlying EBV-related hepatitis are poorly understood, reliable diagnostic criteria for EBV hepatitis are lacking. Recent data suggest that the diagnosis of acute and chronic EBV hepatitis should be based on the combination of four parameters: elevated liver enzymes, serology indicating active EBV infection, typical histopathological changes and demonstration of the viral genome in liver tissue by PCR or EBER-RISH [121]. None of these parameters alone is sufficient for a reliable diagnosis of EBV hepatitis outside infectious mononucleosis. In all other situations, quantification of EBV DNA should be carried out with highly standardized procedures, such as real-time PCR [122,123], to establish clinically significant thresholds for differentiating EBV-associated liver damage from non-specific amplification of viral genomes in circulating B cells trapped within the liver.

Treatment

Adenine arabinoside, aciclovir and ganciclovir inhibit EBV replication *in vitro*; these drugs are active only during lytic and not latent infection, as they target the EBV DNA polymerase. A decrease or suppression of viral excretion in pharyngeal secretions may be obtained in infectious mononucleosis, without affecting the course of disease. In fact, no significant benefit of aciclovir in the treatment of mild, moderate and severe infectious mononucleosis was demonstrated in a meta-analysis of five randomized controlled trials [124].

Severe post-transplant EBV-related hepatitis is treated with aciclovir or ganciclovir [125,126]. As the majority of cells in lymphoproliferative disease are latently infected and do not express the EBV DNA polymerase, they should not be sensitive to aciclovir and ganciclovir; however, these drugs may act on lytic EBV replication occurring in a small number of cells, limiting cell-to-cell spread of EBV and, thus, reducing the pool of infected B cells [127].

Human herpesvirus type 8

HHV-8 (KSHV) is the only known human gamma-2 herpesvirus (rhadinovirus). Transmission is via sexual and non-sexual routes; in adults from developed countries, 15–20% of HIV-negative and 40% of HIV-infected male homosexuals are HHV-8 seropositive, whereas 10–20% of children in the subendemic/endemic areas of the Mediterranean Basin [128] and up to 50% of the general population of sub-Saharan Africa are seropositive [129]. Saliva is likely to be the principal vehicle of transmission [130]. HHV-8 DNA is detectable in tissues and peripheral blood mononuclear cells from patients with HHV-8-related diseases. The virus induces both latent and lytic infection; latent infection is the basis for the lifelong persistence of the virus in human hosts, and latency-associated antigens induce tumorigenesis by promoting cell growth and inhibiting apoptosis [131].

HHV-8 is the cause of Kaposi's sarcoma (KS), a proliferation of virus-infected malignant dermal spindle cells with mononuclear cell infiltration. The classic form of KS typically affects elderly men of Mediterranean descent, with an indolent or slowly progressive course involving the skin of the lower limbs. The endemic KS of sub-Saharan Africa behaves similarly to the classic form in adults but, in children under 10 years of age, it may show an aggressive multifocal lymphadenopathic course, which is usually fatal. The AIDS-associated KS observed in HIV-infected adults predominates in homosexual men; it shows a rapidly progressive and wide dissemination involving the skin of the face and trunk, as well as the gastrointestinal and respiratory tract. Invasive manifestations in other organs are less frequent. The iatrogenic form of KS is reported with increasing frequency in transplanted patients and patients who are on immunosuppressive or cytostatic treatment for autoimmune and neoplastic diseases respectively. Primary HHV-8 infection in immunocompetent hosts is usually asymptomatic; however, a mild self-limited illness with fever and a maculopapular rash spreading from face to trunk and limbs may be seen in children [132], whereas fever, diarrhoea, localized rash and cervical lymphadenopathy may be seen in immunocompetent adults [133].

Primary infection in immunocompromised patients shows a different clinical picture and may have significant consequences. In HIV-positive subjects, HHV-8 seroconversion may be followed after some weeks by high fever, arthralgia, lymphadenopathy, splenomegaly and skin lesions showing foci of KS and angiolymphoid hyperplasia; lesions have not recurred after starting antiretroviral treatment. Disseminated KS with plasmacytosis and bone marrow failure or fatal HHV-8-positive lymphoproliferative disease has occurred in recipients a few weeks after transplant of renal [134] or liver allografts, respectively, from HHV-8 seropositive donors [135,136].

Significant liver involvement has not been reported in immunocompetent subjects with HHV-8 primary infection. In contrast, liver tissue may be involved in KS and other HHV-8-related malignancies in immunocompromised patients, particularly in the setting of primary acute disseminated infection – as in transplant recipients from an infected donor – or, less frequently, during HHV-8 reactivation in HIV-positive patients.

Treatment

Ganciclovir, cidofovir, foscarnet and adefovir, but not aciclovir, show significant activity *in vitro* against HHV-8 lytic replication but, similarly to other anti-herpetic drugs, not against latent viral forms, which predominate in all HHV-8-associated diseases; their use in this setting, therefore, seems unreasonable. Only anecdotal reports exist on the treatment of acute infections with disseminated disease following seroconversion in transplanted patients [137]; further studies are needed to elucidate the role of antivirals in this setting, as well as in the prophylaxis/pre-emptive treatment of graft recipients from HHV-8-positive donors.

Measles

Measles is an acute, highly contagious, febrile illness caused by the rubeola virus, a morbillivirus belonging to the family Paramyxoviridae.

Diagnosis is based on the demonstration of a serological response, virus isolation (particularly in immunosuppressed patients in whom the antibody response is impaired) and identification of viral antigens or RNA in tissue specimens. The current standard serological diagnosis is based on the enzyme-linked immunosorbent assay (ELISA) detection of specific IgM antibodies alongside the rash, or on a fourfold or higher IgG antibody titre increase in convalescent serum.

Clinically significant hepatitis in measles is rarely observed; overt jaundice has been reported in only a few cases [138], although increases in liver enzyme levels are seen in up to 80% of patients, particularly young adults [139]. In a small series of patients with uncomplicated measles and asymptomatic liver dysfunction, maximum alanine aminotransferase levels ranged from 46 to 2910 IU/L; liver histology showed small foci of hepatocyte necrosis, but no piecemeal necrosis, cellular infiltration or portal fibrosis were observed. Electron microscopy showed no virus particles, and immunohistochemistry was negative, although measles virus RNA was detectable in one case [140]. The pathogenesis of liver injury in measles is poorly understood; immune-mediated or antipyretic-induced damage have been hypothesized [141].

Secondary bacterial superinfections should be vigorously treated as they are correlated with the severity of liver damage. The efficacy of parenteral, as well as aerosolized, ribavirin in complicated measles remains unclear.

Rubella

Rubella (German measles) is a febrile exanthem of children and adults that is caused by a togavirus and is spread by droplets from respiratory secretions of infected patients.

Mild hepatitis has been reported as an unusual manifestation of postnatal rubella [142]. In the few cases reported in the literature, the age of the patients ranged from the second to the sixth decade; aminotransferases did not exceed 350 IU/mL, whereas lactate dehydogenase (LDH) levels were greatly increased [143]. Liver histology revealed focal hepatocellular necrosis, cellular swelling and mononuclear infiltration of portal spaces [144]; inflammatory cells within the liver were mainly CD8-positive/CD16-negative mononuclear cells (T-cytotoxic lymphocytes), suggesting that cell-mediated immune responses may play a role in liver injury [145]. Thrombocytopenic purpura, meningoencephalitis, hepatosplenomegaly, jaundice and hepatitis are transient manifestations that are observed at birth; type 1 diabetes may develop in late childhood. Cholestatic jaundice with high levels of alkaline phosphatase and bilirubin, and less significant alterations of aminotransferases, are observed immediately after birth; true hepatitis may occasionally occur, with focal hepatocyte necrosis, giant-cell hepatitis and viral colonization of the liver.

Enteroviruses

The non-poliovirus enteroviruses (coxsackieviruses and echoviruses) are responsible for febrile syndromes and exanthems in immunocompetent children and adults.

They commonly infect newborns, with consequences ranging from asymptomatic infection and benign illness to life-threatening generalized disease and death [146]; however, they are rarely associated with hepatitis in adults. Clinical manifestations of neonatal enteroviral infections include meningoencephalitis, pneumonia, myocarditis, coagulopathy and hepatitis.

Fulminant hepatitis may develop in disseminated coxsackievirus B infections in newborns and young infants, dominating the clinical picture. In a small series, coxsackievirus B1 infection was diagnosed in four patients with hepatitis and coxsackievirus B3 in one; hepatic involvement progressed rapidly to jaundice and coagulopathy [147]. Severe neonatal hepatitis has also been reported in association with coxsackievirus B5 [148], echovirus 11 [149] and echovirus 18 infection [150]. Echovirus 33, a relatively uncommon enterovirus, led to 75 virologically-confirmed cases of infection during the winter of 2000 in New Zealand; two infants died of systemic disease, including a neonate with fulminant hepatitis [151]. In a series of 61 neonatal echovirus infections, the mortality rate in infants with severe hepatitis was 83% [152].

Diagnosis

The mainstay of diagnosis has traditionally been viral isolation from tissue culture; however, PCR analysis is more sensitive than viral culture, highly specific and rapid [153]. Histology may show a syncytial giant-cell hepatitis with mixed lymphocytic and neutrophilic infiltrates; however, syncytial giant-cell hepatitis in the neonatal period has also been associated with CMV, rubella virus, HSV, HHV-6, varicella virus, reovirus 3, parvovirus B19 and paramyxovirus infections [154].

Treatment

Immunoglobulin has been used to treat neonates with enterovirus disease, but its efficacy is not proven. Specific antiviral therapy for enteroviruses is in development; pleconaril is an investigational agent that inhibits viral attachment to host cell receptors and uncoating of viral nucleic acid. Three newborns presenting at 4–5 days of age with neonatal echovirus infection, fulminant hepatic failure and severe coagulopathy were treated with 5 mg/kg of pleconaril every 8 h by nasogastric tube; two recovered fully [155]. A benefit of pleconaril was also shown in children and adults with enteroviral meningitis, and in adults with upper respiratory tract infections caused by picornaviruses (rhinoviruses or enteroviruses) [153].

Adenoviruses

The adenoviruses (ADV) include non-enveloped double-stranded DNA viruses that infect humans via the respiratory, faecal–oral or conjunctival routes [156]. Infection in immunocompetent hosts is usually subclinical (in about 50% of cases) or characterized by mild to moderate upper respiratory disease.

Manifestations are relatively common in paediatric age groups, in whom infection is endemic, causing 10% of respiratory infections [156].

Liver involvement in immunocompetent adults and children with primary ADV infection is unusual and characterized by mild enzyme abnormalities. Severe hepatic damage has been reported in a few paediatric cases, one of which presented with fulminant hepatic failure, pancreatitis and encephalopathy; this patient was treated with cidofovir and recovered without transplantation [157].

Invasive multiorgan disease, including hepatitis, is a frequent and often fatal complication of ADV infection in immuno-compromized individuals [158]. Definition of invasive disease requires the identification of positive viral cultures with the addition of either the finding of ADV at the corresponding site (definite case) or a compatible clinical picture (probable case) [159]. Invasive or disseminated (> two organ systems) disease is particularly frequent in immunocompromised paediatric patients, but has also been shown to occur in 1.1% of immuno-competent children during epidemics, particularly with serotypes 3, 5, 7 and 21 [160], and, exceptionally, in immuno-competent adults [161]. Since the 1960s, ADV infection in children with congenital immune deficiencies has been reported to result in severe hepatitis with a high mortality rate [162].

In acquired immunodeficiencies, severe ADV hepatitis with liver failure is rare as an initial manifestation, but is a deadly complication of disseminated disease [163].

ADV-related disease occurs in about 11% of all transplanted patients [164,165]. Invasive disease has been reported in 6–9.6% of paediatric bone marrow transplant/HSCT recipients [159,166,167], with evidence of severe hepatitis in 0.5–1.5%. Fulminant hepatitis as the sole manifestation of invasive disease after bone marrow transplant is rare [168]. Among adult bone marrow transplant recipients, the incidence of invasive disease was 2.6–4.2%, with evidence of hepatitis in 0.25% [169].

In solid-organ transplant recipients, the most common manifestation of invasive disease is pneumonia, although trans-planted organs – particularly liver and kidney – are often targets. The overall rate of ADV infection following liver transplantation is 5.8–11%, with higher rates in paediatric patients [163], and the incidence of hepatitis ranges from 1.9% to 4%; half of the patients die from massive liver necrosis [170]. Hepatitis may be caused either by reactivation of disease or by transmission from a seropositive donor liver; ADV-seropositive recipients have a better prognosis.

Induction chemotherapy used for the treatment of acute leukaemias has been rarely associated with fulminant ADV hepatitis [171,172].

Diagnosis

Direct fluorescent assays (DFA) of nasal washes have limited sensitivity. ADV isolation from cell culture is very sensitive but requires several days unless the shell vial technique is employed

[173]. Immunohistochemistry with type-specific monoclonal antibodies can be used to detect ADV in the cytoplasm of exfoli-ated cells from BAL fluid or urine sediment [174], as well as in tissue specimens [175]. ADV-DNA detection by PCR analysis of peripheral blood predicts disseminated disease, allowing earlier diagnosis and treatment [176]. A quantitative PCR technique, which measures the ADV viral load, has been developed [177].

Histopathology demonstrates multifocal or widespread hepa-tocyte necrosis involving both periportal and centrolobular areas [178], macrovesicular fat distributed in hepatocyte cytoplasm with minimal inflammation, and 'smudgy' cells containing eosinophilic nuclear inclusions.

Treatment

Vidarabine, ribavirin and cidofovir have been used to treat severe ADV diseases [175,179–184]. Cidofovir inhibits viral DNA polymerase and ADV replication in animal models [185], but its use may be limited by renal toxicity. Cidofovir has been employed with apparent benefit in stem-cell transplant recipients, at doses ranging from 1 mg/kg three times weekly to 5 mg/kg once weekly [186,187], and in solid-organ transplant recipients [188]. Recent data suggest that optimal therapeutic responses may be achieved by combining antiviral therapy with immunotherapeutic approaches [189].

Human parvovirus B19

Human parvovirus B19 (HPV-B19) is a small DNA virus that can induce the erythematous 'fifth disease' in children, arthritis in the presence of acute infections and a variety of blood dyscrasias in predisposed patients, such as those with chronic haemolytic anaemia and AIDS [190]. Diagnosis is based on the finding of the IgM antibody to HPV-B19 by immunoassay or of viral DNA by PCR [191]. Most infections are subclinical, benign and self-limited and result in lifelong immunity [190]; liver enzyme levels may transiently rise without signs of liver dysfunction.

The prevalence of infection increases with age; in the United Kingdom, up to 80% of subjects older than 70 have IgG antibod-ies to HPV-B19 [191]. Infection prevalence was reported to be higher in HCV-positive than in HCV-negative subjects [192].

HPV-B19 has been implicated in cases of fulminant hepatitis that are unrelated to the hepatitis A, B and C viruses [193,194]; many of these patients had aplastic anaemia and, in young children, the recovery from the HBV-B19-related severe liver disease was significantly more frequent and rapid than in patients with fulminant hepatitis of other origin [195].

References

1 Corey L, Wald A, Celum CL et al. (2004) The effects of herpes simplex virus-2 on HIV-1 acquisition and transmission: a review of two over-lapping epidemics. *J Acquir Immune Defic Syndr* 35, 435–445.

2 Wald A, Zeh J, Selke S *et al.* (2000) Reactivation of genital herpes simplex virus type 2 infection in asymptomatic seropositive persons. *N Engl J Med* 342, 844–850.

3 Sawtell NM (2003) Quantitative analysis of herpes simplex virus reactivation *in vivo* demonstrates that reactivation in the nervous system is not inhibited at early times postinoculation. *J Virol* 77, 4127–4138.

4 Whitley RJ, Kimberlin DW, Roizman B (1998) Herpes simplex viruses. *Clin Infect Dis* 26, 541–555.

5 Sharma S, Shobha S, Mosunjac M (2004) Herpes simplex hepatitis in adults: a search for muco-cutaneous clues. *J Clin Gastroenterol* 38, 697–704.

6 Whitley RJ, Roizman B (2001) Herpes simplex virus infections. *Lancet* 357, 1513–1518.

7 Squires RH Jr, Shneider BL, Bucuvalas J *et al.* (2006) Acute liver failure in children: the first 348 patients in the pediatric acute liver failure study group. *J Pediatr* 148, 652–658.

8 Verma A, Dhawan A, Zuckerman M *et al.* (2006) Neonatal herpes simplex virus infection presenting as acute liver failure: prevalent role of herpes simplex virus type I. *J Pediatr Gastroenterol Nutr* 42, 282–286.

9 Velasco M, Llamas E, Guijarro-Rojas M *et al.* (1999) Fulminant herpes hepatitis in a healthy adult: a treatable disorder? *J Clin Gastroenterol* 28, 386–389.

10 Farr RW, Short S, Weissman D (1997) Fulminant hepatitis during herpes simplex virus infection in apparently immunocompetent adults: report of two cases and review of the literature. *Clin Infect Dis* 24, 1191–1194.

11 Corey L (2005) Herpes simplex virus. In: Mandell GJ, Bennett JE, Dolin R (eds) *Mandell, Douglas and Bennett's Principles and Practice of Infectious Diseases*, 6th edn. Philadelphia, PA: Elsevier, p. 1771.

12 Allen RH, Tuomala RE (2005) Herpes simplex virus hepatitis causing acute liver dysfunction and thrombocytopenia in pregnancy. *Obstet Gynecol* 106, 1187–1189.

13 Kang AH, Graves CR (1999) Herpes simplex hepatitis in pregnancy: a case report and review of the literature. *Obstet Gynecol Surv* 54, 463–468.

14 Kaufman B, Gandhi SA, Louie E *et al.* (1997) Herpes simplex virus hepatitis: case report and review. *Clin Infect Dis* 24, 334–338.

15 Sharma S, Mosunjac M (2004) Herpes simplex hepatitis in adults: a search for muco-cutaneous clues. *J Clin Gastroenterol* 38, 697–704.

16 Mariani P, Paul MD, Vilenski LMD (2005) Fulminant hepatitis due to herpes simplex virus: a case report. *Infect Dis Clin Pract* 13, 274–276.

17 Griffiths WJH, William JH, Wreghitt TG *et al.* (2005) Reactivation of herpes simplex virus after liver transplantation. *Transplantation* 80, 1353–1354.

18 Peters DJ, Greene WH, Ruggiero F *et al.* (2000) Herpes simplex-induced fulminant hepatitis in adults: a call for empiric therapy. *Dig Dis Sci* 45, 2399–2404.

19 Nichols WG, Boeck M, Carter RA *et al.* (2003) Transferred herpes simplex virus immunity after stem-cell transplantation: clinical implications. *J Infect Dis* 187, 801–808.

20 Gane E, Faouzi S, Valdecasas GJC *et al.* (1997) Randomised trial of efficacy and safety of oral ganciclovir in the prevention of cytomegalovirus disease in liver-transplant recipients. *Lancet* 350, 1729–1733.

21 Jacques SM, Quresci F (1992) Herpes simplex virus hepatitis in pregnancy: a clinicopathologic study of three cases. *Hum Pathol* 23, 183–187.

22 Prétet JL, Pelletier L, Bernard B *et al.* (2003) Apoptosis participates to liver damage in HSV-induced fulminant hepatitis. *Apoptosis* 8, 655–663.

23 Cowan FM, French RS, Mayaud P *et al.* (2003) Seroepidemiological study of herpes simplex virus types 1 and 2 in Brazil, Estonia, India, Morocco, and Sri Lanka. *Sex Transm Infect* 79, 286–290.

24 Guerry SL, Bauer HM, Klausner JD *et al.* (2005) Recommendations for the selective use of herpes simplex virus type 2 serological tests. *Clin Infect Dis* 40, 38–45.

25 Golden MR, Ashley-Morrow R, Swenson P *et al.* (2005) Herpes simplex virus type 2 (HSV-2) Western blot confirmatory testing among men testing positive for HSV-2 using the focus enzyme-linked immunosorbent assay in a sexually transmitted disease clinic. *Sex Transm Dis* 32, 771–777.

26 Yavuz BB, Cankurtaran M, Halil M *et al.* (2005) Renal dysfunction after oral acyclovir treatment in a geriatric woman: a case report. *Scand J Infect Dis* 37, 611–613.

27 Stone KM, Reiff-Eldridge R, White AD *et al.* (2004) Pregnancy outcomes following systemic prenatal acyclovir exposure: conclusions from the international acyclovir pregnancy registry, 1984–1999. *Birth Defects Res A Clin Mol Teratol* 70, 201–207.

28 Chen Y, Schieux C, Garrait V *et al.* (2000) Resistant herpes simplex virus type 1 infection: an emerging concern after allogeneic stem cell transplantation. *Clin Infect Dis* 31, 927–935.

29 Danve-Szatanek C, Aymard M, Thouvenot D *et al.* (2004) Surveillance network for herpes simplex virus resistance to antiviral drugs: 3-year follow-up. *J Clin Microbiol* 42, 242–249.

30 Levin MJ, Bacon TH, Leary JJ (2004) Resistance of herpes simplex virus infections to nucleoside analogues in HIV-infected patients. *Clin Infect Dis* 39, S248–257.

31 Wyles DL, Patel A, Madinger N *et al.* (2005) Development of herpes simplex virus disease in patients who are receiving cidofovir. *Clin Infect Dis* 41, 676–680.

32 Martinez CM, Luks-Golger DB (1997) Cidofovir use in acyclovir-resistant herpes infection. *Ann Pharmacother* 31, 1519–1521.

33 Pitel PA, McCormick KL, Fitzgerald E *et al.* (1980) Subclinical hepatic changes in varicella infection. *Pediatrics* 65, 631–633.

34 Peterson CL, Mascola S, Chao SM *et al.* (1996) Children hospitalized for varicella: a prevaccine review. *J Pediatr* 129, 529–536.

35 Meyer PA, Seward JF, Jumaan AO *et al.* (2000) Varicella mortality: trends before vaccine licensure in the United States, 1970–1994. *J Infect Dis* 182, 383–390.

36 Anderson DR, Schwartz J, Hunter NJ *et al.* (1994) Varicella hepatitis: a fatal case in a previously healthy, immunocompetent adult. Report of a case, autopsy, and review of the literature. *Arch Intern Med* 154, 2101–2106.

37 Vartian CV (1999) Varicella-zoster virus infection associated with acute liver failure. *Clin Infect Dis* 28, 412–413.

38 Kavaliotis J, Loukou I, Trachana M *et al.* (1998) Outbreak of varicella in a pediatric oncology unit. *Med Pediatr Oncol* 31, 166–169.

39 Mantadakis E, Anagnostatou N, Danilatou V *et al.* (2005) Fulminant hepatitis due to varicella zoster virus in a girl with acute lymphoblastic leukemia in remission: report of a case and review. *J Pediatr Hematol Oncol* 27, 551–553.

40 David DS, Tegtmeier BR, O'Donnell MR *et al.* (1998) Visceral varicella zoster after bone marrow transplantation: report of a case series and review of the literature. *Am J Gastroenterology* 93, 810–813.

41 Kim SH, Haycox C (1999) Primary disseminated varicella presenting as an acute abdomen. *Pediatr Dermatol* 16, 208–210.

42 Grant RM, Weitzman SS, Sherman CG *et al.* (2002) Fulminant disseminated varicella zoster virus infection without skin involvement. *J Clin Virol* 24, 7–12.

43 Dits H, Frans E, Wilmer A *et al.* (1998) Varicella-zoster virus infection associated with acute liver failure. *Clin Infect Dis* 27, 209–210.

44 Os I, Strom EH, Stenehjem A *et al.* (2001) Varicella infection in a renal transplant recipient associated with abdominal pain, hepatitis, and glomerulonephritis. *Scand J Urol Nephrol* 35, 330–333.

45 Vafai A, Berger M (2001) Zoster in patients infected with HIV: a review. *Am J Med Sci* 321, 372–380.

46 Dowell SF, Bresee JS (1993) Severe varicella associated with steroid use. *Pediatrics* 92, 223–228.

47 Hyvernat H, Roger PM, Pereira C *et al.* (2005) Fatal varicella hepatitis in an asthmatic adult after short-term corticosteroid treatment. *Eur J Intern Med* 16, 361–362.

48 Redman RL, Nader S, Zerboni L *et al.* (1997) Early reconstitution of immunity and decreased severity of herpes zoster in bone marrow transplant recipients immunized with inactivated varicella vaccine. *J Infect Dis* 176, 578–585.

49 Koc Y, Miller KB, Schenkein DP *et al.* (2000) Varicella zoster virus infections following allogeneic bone marrow transplantation: frequency, risk factors, and clinical outcome. *Biol Bone Marrow Transplant* 6, 44–49.

50 Berman JN, Wang M, Berry W *et al.* (2006) Herpes zoster infection in the post-hematopoietic stem cell transplant pediatric population may be preceded by transaminitis: an institutional experience. *Bone Marrow Transplant* 37, 73–80.

51 Rogers SY, Irving W, Harris A *et al.* (1995) Visceral varicella zoster infection after bone marrow transplantation without skin involvement and the use of PCR for diagnosis. *Bone Marrow Transplant* 15, 805–807.

52 Leung TF, Chik KW, Li CK *et al.* (2000) Incidence, risk factors and outcome of varicella-zoster virus infection in children after haemapoietic stem cell transplantation. *Bone Marrow Transplant* 25, 167–172.

53 Leena M, Ville V, Veli-Jukka A (2006) Visceral varicella zoster virus infection after stem cell transplantation: a possible cause of severe abdominal pain. *Scand J Gastroenterol* 41, 242–244.

54 de Jong MD, Weel JF, van Oers MH *et al.* (2001) Molecular diagnosis of visceral herpes zoster. *Lancet* 357, 2101–2102.

55 Steer CB, Szer J, Sasadeusz J *et al.* (2000) Varicella-zoster infection after allogenic bone marrow transplantation: incidence, risk factors and prevention with low-dose acyclovir and ganciclovir. *Bone Marrow Transplant* 25, 657–664.

56 Thomson KJ, Hart DP, Banerjee L *et al.* (2005) The effects of low-dose acyclovir on reactivation of varicella-zoster virus after hematopoietic stem cell transplant. *Bone Marrow Transplant* 35, 1065–1069.

57 Hata A, Asanuma H, Rinki M *et al.* (2002) Use of an inactivated varicella vaccine in recipients of hematopoietic-cell transplants. *N Engl J Med* 347, 26–34.

58 Coaquette A, Bourgeois A, Dirand C *et al.* (2004) Mixed cytomegalovirus glycoprotein B genotypes in immunocompromised patients. *Clin Infect Dis* 39, 155–161. Available: http://

www.journals.uchicago.edu/CID/journal/issues/v39n2/32984/32984.text.html – fn1#fn1

59 Wreghitt TG, Teare EL, Sule O *et al.* (2003) Cytomegalovirus infection in immunocompetent patients. *Clin Infect Dis* 37, 1607–1608.

60 Ljungman P, Griffiths P, Paya C (2002) Definitions of cytomegalovirus infection and disease in transplant recipients. *Clin Infect Dis* 34, 1094–1097.

61 Humar A, Gregson D, Caliendo AM *et al.* (1999) Clinical utility of quantitative cytomegalovirus viral load determination for predicting cytomegalovirus disease in liver transplant recipients. *Transplantation* 68, 1305–1311.

62 Shinkai M, Bozzette SA, Powderly W *et al.* (1997) Utility of urine and leukocyte cultures and plasma DNA polymerase chain reaction for identification of AIDS patients at risk for developing human cytomegalovirus disease. *J Infect Dis* 175, 302–308.

63 Imbert-Marcille BM, Cantarovich D, Ferre-Aubineau V *et al.* (1997) Usefulness of DNA viral load quantification for cytomegalovirus disease monitoring in renal and pancreas/renal transplant recipients. *Transplantation* 63, 1476–1481.

64 Flexman J, Kay I, Fonte R *et al.* (2001) Differences between the quantitative antigenemia assay and the cobas amplicor monitor quantitative PCR assay for detecting CMV viraemia in bone marrow and solid organ transplant patients. *J Med Virol* 64, 275–282.

65 Emery VC, Sabin CA, Cope AV *et al.* (2000) Application of viral-load kinetics to identify patients who develop cytomegalovirus disease after transplantation. *Lancet* 355, 2032–2036.

66 Piiparinen H, Hockerstedt K, Lappalainen M *et al.* (2002) Monitoring of viral load by quantitative plasma PCR during active cytomegalovirus infection of individual liver transplant patients. *J Clin Microbiol* 40, 2945–2952.

67 Gerna G, Lilleri D, Baldanti F *et al.* (2003) Human cytomegalovirus immediate-early mRNAemia versus pp65 antigenemia for guiding pre-emptive therapy in children and young adults undergoing hematopoietic stem cell transplantation: a prospective, randomized, open-label trial. *Blood* 101, 5053–5060.

68 Revello MG, Zavattoni M, Furione M *et al.* (2006) Preconceptional primary human cytomegalovirus infection and risk of congenital infection. *J Infect Dis* 193, 783–787.

69 Pass RF (2004) A key role for adolescents in the epidemiology of cytomegalovirus and genital herpes infection. *Clin Infect Dis* 39, 1439–1440.

70 Stanberry LR, Rosenthal SL, Mills L *et al.* (2004) Longitudinal risk of herpes simplex virus (HSV) type 1, HSV type 2, and cytomegalovirus infections among young adolescent girls *Clin Infect Dis* 39, 1433–1438.

71 Gandhi MK, Khanna R (2004) Human cytomegalovirus: clinical aspects, immune regulation, and emerging treatments. *Lancet Infect Dis* 4, 725–738.

72 Kytö V, Vuorinen T, Saukko P *et al.* (2005) Cytomegalovirus infection of the heart is common in patients with fatal myocarditis. *Clin Infect Dis* 40, 683–688.

73 Crumpacker CS, Wadhwa S (2005) Cytomegalovirus. In: Mandell GJ, Bennett JE, Dolin R (eds) *Mandell, Douglas and Bennett's Principles and Practice of Infectious Diseases*, 6th edn. Philadelphia, PA: Elsevier, pp. 1786–1800.

74 Wreghitt TG, Teare EL, Sule O *et al.* (2003) Cytomegalovirus infection in immunocompetent patients. *Clin Infect Dis* 37, 1603–1606.

75 Revello MG, Zavattoni M, Sarasini A *et al.* (1998) Human cytomegalovirus in blood of immunocompetent persons during

primary infection: prognostic implications for pregnancy. *J Infect Dis* 177, 1170–1175.

76 Amory JK, Rosen H, Sukut C *et al.* (2006) Clinical problem-solving. A jaundiced eye. *N Engl J Med* 354, 1516–1520.

77 Winston DJ, Busuttil RW (2004) Randomized controlled trial of sequential intravenous and oral ganciclovir versus prolonged intravenous ganciclovir for long-term prophylaxis of cytomegalovirus disease in high-risk cytomegalovirus-seronegative liver transplant recipients with cytomegalovirus-seropositive donors. *Transplantation* 77, 305–308.

78 Paya CV (2001) Prevention of cytomegalovirus disease in recipients of solid-organ transplants. *Clin Infect Dis* 32, 596–603.

79 Preiksaitis JK, Brennan DC, Fishman J *et al.* (2005) Canadian society of transplantation consensus workshop on cytomegalovirus management in solid organ transplantation final report. *Am J Transplant* 5, 218–227.

80 Cope AV, Sabin C, Burroughs A *et al.* (1997) Interrelationships among quantity of human cytomegalovirus (HCMV) DNA in blood, donor-recipient serostatus, and administration of methylprednisolone as risk factors for HCMV disease following liver transplantation. *J Infect Dis* 176, 1484–1490.

81 Lautenschlager I, Halme L, Hockerstedt K *et al.* (2006) Cytomegalovirus infection of the liver transplant: virological, histological, immunological, and clinical observations. *Transpl Infect Dis* 8, 21–30.

82 Moutaftsi M, Mehl AM, Borysiewicz LK *et al.* (2002) Human cytomegalovirus inhibits maturation and impairs function of monocyte-derived dendritic cells. *Blood* 99, 2913–2921.

83 Falagas ME, Snydman DR, Griffith J *et al.* (1997) Clinical and epidemiological predictors of recurrent cytomegalovirus disease in orthotopic liver transplant recipients. Boston Center for Liver Transplantation CMVIG Study Group. *Clin Infect Dis* 25, 314–317.

84 Sia IG, Wilson JA, Groettum CM *et al.* (2000) Cytomegalovirus (CMV) DNA load predicts relapsing CMV infection after solid organ transplantation. *J Infect Dis* 181, 717–720.

85 Lurain NS, Bhorade SM, Pursell KJ *et al.* (2002) Analysis and characterization of antiviral drug-resistant cytomegalovirus isolates from solid organ transplant recipients. *Clin Infect Dis* 186, 760–768.

86 Huang LM, Lee CY, Chen JY *et al.* (1992) Primary human herpesvirus 6 infections in children: a prospective serologic study. *J Infect Dis* 165, 1163–1164.

87 Ward KN (2005) The natural history and laboratory diagnosis of human herpesviruses-6 and -7 infections in the immunocompetent. *J Clin Virol* 32, 183–193.

88 Hall CB, Long CE, Schnabel KC *et al.* (1994) Human herpesvirus-6 infection in children. A prospective study of complications and reactivation. *N Engl J Med* 331, 432–438.

89 Aita K, Jin Y, Irie H *et al.* (2001) Are there histopathologic characteristics particular to fulminant hepatic failure caused by human herpesvirus-6 infection? A case report and discussion. *Hum Pathol* 32, 887–889.

90 Ohashi M, Yoshikawa T, Asonuma K *et al.* (2004) Human herpesvirus-6 fulminant hepatic failure treated by living donor liver transplantation. *Pediatr Int* 46, 730–732.

91 Harma M, Hockerstedt K, Lautenschlager I (2003) Human herpesvirus-6 and acute liver failure. *Transplantation* 76, 536–539.

92 Safronetz D, Humar A, Tipples GA (2003) Differentiation and quantitation of human herpesviruses 6A, 6B and 7 by real-time PCR. *J Virol Methods* 112, 99–105.

93 Cacheux W, Carbonell N, Rosmorduc O *et al.* (2005) HHV-6-related acute liver failure in two immunocompetent adults: favourable outcome after liver transplantation and/or ganciclovir therapy. *J Intern Med* 258, 573–578.

94 Feldstein AE, Razonable RR, Boyce TG *et al.* (2003) Prevalence and clinical significance of human herpesviruses 6 and 7 active infection in pediatric liver transplant patients. *Pediatr Transplant* 7, 125–129.

95 Mendez JC, Dockrell DH, Espy MJ *et al.* (2001) Human beta-herpesvirus interactions in solid organ transplant recipients. *J Infect Dis* 183, 179–184.

96 Clark DA, Griffiths PD (2003) Human herpesvirus 6: relevance of infection in the immunocompromised host. *Br J Haematol* 120, 384–395.

97 Tokimasa S, Hara J, Osugi Y *et al.* (2002) Ganciclovir is effective for prophylaxis and treatment of human herpesvirus-6 in allogeneic stem cell transplantation. *Bone Marrow Transplant* 29, 595–598.

98 Tugizov SM, Berline JW, Palefsky JM (2003) Epstein-Barr virus infection of polarized tongue and nasopharyngeal epithelial cells. *Nat Med* 9, 307–314.

99 Cohen JI (2000) Epstein-Barr virus infection. *N Engl J Med* 343, 481–492.

100 Tsurumi T, Fujita, Kudoh A (2005) Latent and lytic Epstein-Barr virus replication strategies. *Rev Med Virol* 15, 3–15.

101 Kieff E, Rickinson AB (2001) Epstein-Barr virus and its replication. In: Knipe DM, Howley PM (eds) *Fields' Virology*, 4th edn. Philadelphia, PA: Lippincott Williams & Wilkins, pp. 2511–2574.

102 Harada S, Kieff E (1997) Epstein-Barr virus nuclear protein LP stimulates EBNA-2 acidic domain-mediated transcriptional activation. *J Virol* 71, 6611–6618.

103 Kulwichit W, Edwards RH, Davenport EM *et al.* (1998) Expression of the Epstein-Barr virus latent membrane protein 1 induces B cell lymphoma in transgenic mice. *Proc Natl Acad Sci USA* 95, 11963–11968.

104 Parkin DM (2002) The global health burden of infection-associated cancers in the year 2002. *Int J Cancer* 118, 3030–3044.

105 Ragoczy T, Heston L, Miller G (1998) The Epstein-Barr virus Rta protein activates lytic cycle genes and can disrupt latency in B lymphocytes. *J Virol* 72, 7978–7984.

106 Middeldorp JM, Brink AA, Van den Brule AJ *et al.* (2003) Pathogenic roles for Epstein-Barr virus (EBV) gene products in EBV-associated proliferative disorders. *Crit Rev Oncol Hematol* 45, 1–36.

107 Klenerman P, Hill A (2005) T cells and viral persistence: lessons from diverse infections. *Nat Immunol* 6, 873–879.

108 Markin RS (1994) Manifestations of Epstein-Barr virus-associated disorders in liver. *Liver* 14, 1–13.

109 Shaukat A, Tsai HT, Rutherforth R *et al.* (2005) Epstein-Barr virus induced hepatitis: An important cause of cholestasis. *Hepatol Res* 33, 24–26.

110 Kimura H, Nagasaka T, Hoshino Y *et al.* (2001) Severe hepatitis caused by Epstein-Barr virus without infection of hepatocytes. *Human Pathol* 32, 757–762.

111 Hinedi TB, Koff RS (2003) Cholestatic hepatitis induced by Epstein-Barr virus infection in an adult. *Dig Dis Sci* 48, 539–541.

112 Markin RS, Linder J, Zuerlein K *et al.* (1987) Hepatitis in fatal infectious mononucleosis. *Gastroenterology* 93, 1210–1217.

113 Jimenez-Saenz M, Perez-Pozo JM, Leal-Luna A *et al.* (2002) Lethal liver failure in an elderly patient with hepatitis B superinfected with Epstein-Barr virus. *Eur J Gastroenterol Hepatol* 14, 1283–1284.

114 Sakamoto T, Uemura M, Fukui K *et al.* (1992) Chronic active Epstein-Barr virus infection in an adult. *Intern Med* 31, 1190–1196.

115 Yuge A, Kinoshita E, Moriuchi M *et al.* (2004) Persistent hepatitis associated with chronic active Epstein-Barr virus infection. *Pediatr Infect Dis J* 23, 74–76.

116 Vento S, Guella L, Mirandola F *et al.* (1995) Epstein-Barr virus as a trigger for autoimmune hepatitis in susceptible individuals. *Lancet* 346, 608–606.

117 Chiba T, Goto S, Yokosuka O *et al.* (2004) Fatal chronic active Epstein-Barr virus infection mimicking autoimmune hepatitis. *Eur J Gastroenterol Hepatol* 16, 225–228.

118 Vento S, Cainelli F (2004) Is there a role for viruses in triggering autoimmune hepatitis? *Autoimmun Rev* 3, 61–69.

119 Nobili V, Comparcola D, Sartorelli MR *et al.* (2003) Autoimmune hepatitis type 1 after Epstein-Barr virus infection. *Pediatr Infect Dis J* 22, 387.

120 Negro F (2006) The paradox of Epstein-Barr virus-associated hepatitis. *J Hepatol* 44, 839–841.

121 Drebber U, Kasper HU, Krupacz J *et al.* (2006) The role of Epstein-Barr virus in acute and chronic hepatitis. *J Hepatol* 44, 879–885.

122 Ruiz G, Pena P, de Ory F *et al.* (2005) Comparison of commercial real-time PCR assays for quantification of Epstein-Barr virus DNA. *J Clin Microbiol* 43, 2053–2057.

123 Stevens SJ, Verkuijlen SA, Middeldorp JM (2005) Quantitative detection of Epstein-Barr virus DNA in clinical specimens by rapid real-time PCR targeting a highly conserved region of EBNA-1. *Methods Mol Biol* 292, 15–26.

124 Torre D, Tambini R (1999) Acyclovir for treatment of infectious mononucleosis: a meta-analysis. *Scand J Infect Dis* 31, 543–547.

125 Andreone P, Gramenzi A, Lorenzini S *et al.* (2003) Posttransplantation lymphoproliferative disorders. *Arch Intern Med* 163, 1997–2004.

126 Preiksaitis JK, Keay S (2001) Diagnosis and management of post-transplant lymphoproliferative disorder in solid-organ transplant recipients. *Clin Infect Dis* 33(Suppl 1), S38–46.

127 Gershburg E, Pagano JS (2005) Epstein-Barr virus infections: prospects for treatment. *J Antimicrob Chemother* 56, 277–281.

128 Ablashi DV, Chatlynne LG, Whitman JE Jr *et al.* (2002) Spectrum of Kaposi's sarcoma-associated herpesvirus, or human herpesvirus 8, diseases. *Clin Microbiol Rev* 15, 439–464.

129 Chatlynne LG, Ablashi DV (1999) Seroepidemiology of Kaposi's sarcoma-associated herpesvirus (KSHV). *Semin Cancer Biol* 9, 175–185.

130 Verna SC, Robertson ES (2003) Molecular biology and pathogenesis of Kaposi sarcoma-associated herpesvirus. *FEMS Microbiol Lett* 222, 155–163.

131 Dourmishev LA, Dourmishev AL, Palmieri D *et al.* (2003) Molecular genetics of Kaposi's sarcoma-associated herpesvirus (human herpesvirus-8) epidemiology and pathogenesis. *Microbiol Mol Biol Rev* 67, 175–212.

132 Andreoni M, Sarmati L, Nicastri E *et al.* (2002) Primary human herpesvirus 8 infection in immunocompetent children. *JAMA* 287, 1295–1300.

133 Wang QJ, Jenkins FJ, Jacobson LP *et al.* (2001) Primary human herpesvirus 8 infection generates a broadly specific CD8(+) T-cell response to viral lytic cycle proteins. *Blood* 9, 2366–2373.

134 Luppi M, Barozzi P, Schulz TF *et al.* (2000) Bone marrow failure associated with human herpesvirus 8 infection after transplantation. *N Engl J Med* 343, 1378–1385.

135 Verucchi G, Calza L, Trevisani F *et al.* (2005) Human herpesvirus-8-related Kaposi's sarcoma after liver transplantation successfully treated with cidofovir and liposomal daunorubicin. *Transpl Infect Dis* 7, 34–37.

136 Marcelin AG, Roque-Afonso AM, Hurtova M *et al.* (2004) Fatal disseminated Kaposi's sarcoma following human herpesvirus 8 primary infections in liver-transplant recipients. *Liver Transpl* 10, 295–300.

137 Boeckle E, Boesmuller C, Wiesmayr S *et al.* (2005) Kaposi sarcoma in solid organ transplant recipients: a single center report. *Transplant Proc* 37, 1905–1909.

138 Odeh M, Oliven A, Potasman I (1995) Hepatitis with overt jaundice in acute measles infection. *J Clin Gastroenterol* 20, 345–346.

139 Khatib R, Siddique M, Abbass M (1993) Measles associated hepatobiliary disease: an overview. *Infection* 21, 112–114.

140 Satoh A, Kobayashi H, Yoshida T *et al.* (1999) Clinicopathological study on liver dysfunction in measles. *Intern Med* 38, 454–457.

141 Ackerman Z, Flugelman MY, Wax Y *et al.* (1989) Hepatitis during measles in young adults: possible role of antipyretic drugs. *Hepatology* 10, 203–206.

142 Zeldis JB, Miller JD, Dienstag JL (1985) Hepatitis in an adult with rubella. *Am J Med* 79, 515–516.

143 Arai M, Wada N, Maruyama N *et al.* (1995) Acute hepatitis in an adult with acquired rubella infection. *J Gastroenterol* 30, 539–542.

144 Tameda Y, Kosaka Y, Shiraki K *et al.* (1993) Hepatitis in an adult with rubella. *Intern Med* 32, 580–583.

145 Gershon AA (2005) Rubella virus. In: Mandell GJ, Bennett JE, Dolin R (eds) *Mandell, Douglas and Bennett's Principles and Practice of Infectious Diseases*, 6th edn. Philadelphia, PA: Elsevier, pp. 1921–1926.

146 Verboon-Maciolek MA, Krediet TG, van Loon AM *et al.* (2002) Epidemiological survey of neonatal non-polio enterovirus infection in the Netherlands. *J Med Virol* 66, 241–245.

147 Wang SM, Liu CC, Yang YJ *et al.* (1998) Fatal coxsackievirus B infection in early infancy characterized by fulminant hepatitis. *J Infect* 37, 270–273.

148 Clavell M, Barkemeyer B, Martinez B *et al.* (1999) Severe hepatitis in a newborn with coxsackievirus B5 infection. *Clin Pediatr* 38, 739–741.

149 Hsiao CC, Tsao LY, Chen HN (2003) Echovirus 11 sepsis in a neonate: report of one case. *Acta Paediatr Taiwan* 44, 104–105.

150 Shah SS, Gallagher PG (1997) Neonatal sepsis due to echovirus 18 infection. *J Perinat Med* 25, 311–384.

151 Huang QS, Carr JM, Nix WA *et al.* (2003) An echovirus type 33 winter outbreak in New Zealand. *Clin Infect Dis* 37, 650–657.

152 Modlin JF (1986) Perinatal echovirus infection: insights from a literature review of 61 cases of serious infection and 16 outbreaks in nurseries. *Rev Infect Dis* 8, 918–926.

153 Abzug MJ (2004) Presentation, diagnosis, and management of enterovirus infections in neonates. *Paediatr Drugs* 6, 1–10.

154 Hicks J, Barrish J, Zhu SH (2001) Neonatal syncytial giant cell hepatitis with paramyxoviral-like inclusions. *Ultrastruct Pathol* 25, 65–71.

155 Aradottir E, Alonso EM, Schulman ST (2001) Severe neonatal enteroviral hepatitis treated with pleconaril. *Pediatr Infect Dis J* 20, 457–459.

156 Baum SG (2005) Adenovirus. In: Mandell GJ, Bennett JE, Dolin R (eds) *Mandell, Douglas and Bennett's Principles and Practice of Infectious Diseases*. 6th edn. Philadelphia, PA: Elsevier, 1835–1841.

157 Rocholl C, Gerber K, Daly J *et al.* (1992) Adenoviral infections in children: the impact of rapid diagnosis. *Pediatrics* 113, 51–56.

158 Hierholzer JC (1992) Adenoviruses in the immunocompromised host. *Clin Microbiol Rev* 5, 262–274.

159 Flomenberg P, Babbitt J, Drobyski WR *et al.* (1994) Increasing incidence of adenovirus disease in bone marrow transplant recipients. *J Infect Dis* 169, 775–781.

160 Munoz FM, Piedra PA, Demmler GJ (1998) Disseminated adenovirus disease in immunocompromised and immunocompetent children. *Clin Infect Dis* 27, 1194–1200.

161 Two fatal cases of adenovirus-related illness in previously healthy young adults–Illinois, 2000 (2001) *MMWR Morb Mortal Wkly Rep* 50, 553–555.

162 Wigger HJ, Blanc WA (1966) Fatal hepatic and bronchial necrosis in adenovirus infection with thymic alymphoplasia. *N Engl J Med* 275, 870–874.

163 Kojaoghlanian T, Flomenberg P, Horwitz MS (2003) The impact of adenovirus infection on the immunocompromised host. *Rev Med Virol* 13, 155–171.

164 Blanke C, Clark C, Broun ER *et al.* (1995) Evolving pathogens in allogeneic bone marrow transplantation: increased fatal adenoviral infections. *Am J Med* 99, 326–328.

165 Howard DS, Phillips II GL, Reece DE *et al.* (1999) Adenovirus infections in hematopoietic stem cell transplant recipients. *Clin Infect Dis* 29, 1494–1501.

166 Bordigoni P, Carret AS, Venard V *et al.* (2001) Treatment of adenovirus infections in patients undergoing allogeneic hematopoietic stem cell transplantation. *Clin Infect Dis* 32, 1290–1297.

167 Hale GA, Heslop HE, Krance RA *et al.* (1999) Adenovirus infection after pediatric bone marrow transplantation. *Bone Marrow Transplant* 23, 277–282.

168 Bertheau P, Parquet N, Ferchal F *et al.* (1996) Fulminant adenovirus hepatitis after allogeneic bone marrow transplantation. *Bone Marrow Transplant* 17, 295–298.

169 La Rosa AM, Champlin RE, Mirza N *et al.* (2001) Adenovirus infections in adult recipients of blood and marrow transplants. *Clin Infect Dis* 32, 371–376.

170 Michaels MG, Green M, Wald ER *et al.* (1992) Adenovirus infection in pediatric liver transplant recipients. *J Infect Dis* 165, 170–174.

171 Kaur B, Gottardo NG, Keil AD *et al.* (2002) A rare case of adenovirus fulminant hepatic necrosis after chemotherapy. *Pediatr Hematol Oncol* 19, 361–371.

172 Hough R, Chetwood A, Sinfield R *et al.* (2005) Fatal adenovirus hepatitis during standard chemotherapy for childhood acute lymphoblastic leukemia. *J Pediatr Hematol Oncol* 27, 67–72.

173 Shih SR, Tsao KC, Ning HC *et al.* (1999) Diagnosis of respiratory tract viruses in 24 h by immunofluorescent staining of shell vial cultures containing Madin-Darby Canine Kidney (MDCK) cells. *J Virol Methods* 81, 77–81.

174 Grandien M, Pettersson CA, Gardner PS *et al.* (1985) Rapid viral diagnosis of acute respiratory infections: comparison of enzyme-linked immunosorbent assay and the immunofluorescence technique for detection of viral antigens in nasopharyngeal secretions. *J Clin Microbiol* 22, 757–760.

175 Gavin P, Katz BZ (2002) Intravenous ribavirin treatment for severe adenovirus disease in immunocompromised children. *Pediatrics* 110, e9.

176 Echavarria M, Forman M, van Tol MJD *et al.* (2001) Prediction of severe disseminated adenovirus infection by serum PCR. *Lancet* 358, 384–385.

177 Lankester AC, van Tol MJ, Claas EC *et al.* (2002) Quantification of adenovirus DNA in plasma for management of infection in stem cell graft recipients. *Clin Infect Dis* 34, 864–867.

178 Charles AK, Caul EO, Porter HJ *et al.* (1995) Fatal adenovirus 32 infection in a bone marrow transplant recipient. *J Clin Pathol* 48, 779–781.

179 Kitabayashi A, Hirokawa M, Kuroki J *et al.* (1994) Successful vidarabine therapy for adenovirus type II-associated acute hemorrhagic cystitis after allogeneic bone marrow transplantation. *Bone Marrow Transplant* 14, 853–854.

180 La Rosa AM, Champlin RE, Mirza N *et al.* (2001) Adenovirus infections in adult recipients of blood and marrow transplants. *Clin Infect Dis* 32, 871–876.

181 Miyamura K, Hamaguchi M, Taji H *et al.* (2000) Successful ribavirin therapy for severe adenovirus hemorrhagic cystitis after allogeneic marrow transplant from close HLA donors rather than distant donors. *Bone Marrow Transplant* 25, 545–548.

182 Arav-Boger R, Echavarria M, Forman M *et al.* (2000) Clearance of adenoviral hepatitis with ribavirin therapy in a pediatric liver transplant recipient. *Pediatr Infect Dis J* 19, 1097–1100.

183 Aebi C, Hendrick CL, McCracken GH *et al.* (1997) Intravenous ribavirin therapy in a neonate with disseminated adenovirus infection undergoing extracorporeal oxygenation. *J Pediatr* 130, 612–615.

184 Wulffraat NM, Geelen SP, van Dijken PJ *et al.* (1995) Recovery from adenovirus pneumonia in a severe combined immunodeficiency patient treated with intravenous ribavirin. *Transplantation* 59, 927.

185 de Oliveira CB, Stevenson D, LaBree L *et al.* (1996) Evaluation of Cidofovir (HPMPC, GS-504) against adenovirus type 5 infection *in vitro* and in a New Zealand rabbit ocular model. *Antiviral Res* 31, 165–172.

186 Legrand F, Berrebi D, Houhou N *et al.* (2001) Early diagnosis of adenovirus infection and treatment with cidofovir after bone marrow transplantation in children. *Bone Marrow Transplant* 27, 621–626.

187 Hoffman JA, Shah AJ, Ross LA *et al.* (2001) Adenoviral infections and a prospective trial of cidofovir in pediatric hematopoietic stem cell transplantation. *Biol Blood Marrow Transplant* 7, 388–394.

188 Ison MG (2006) Adenovirus infections in transplant recipients. *Clin Infect Dis* 43, 331–339.

189 Lenaerts L, Naesens L (2006) Antiviral therapy for adenovirus infections. *Antiviral Res* 71, 172–180.

190 Clewley JP (2006) Polymerase chain reaction assay of parvovirus B19 DNA in clinical specimens. *J Clin Microbiol.* 27, 2647–2651.

191 Anderson LS (2002) Human parvovirus B19. In: Richman DD, Whitley RS, Hayden FG (eds) *Clinical Virology.* Washington, DC: American Society for Microbiology (ASM) Press, pp. 597–612.

192 Cacoub P, Boukli N, Hausfater P *et al.* (1998) Parvovirus B19 infection, hepatitis C virus infection, and mixed cryoglobulinaemia. *Ann Rheum Dis* 57, 422–424.

193 Langnas A, Markin RS, Cattral LS *et al.* (1995) Parvovirus B19 as a possible causative agent of fulminant liver failure and associated aplastic anemia. *Hepatology* 22, 1661–1665.

194 Karetnyi Y, Beck PR, Markin PR *et al.* (1999) Human parvovirus B19 infection in acute fulminant liver failure. *Arch Virol* 144, 1713–1724.

195 Sokal E, Melchior M, Comu C *et al.* (1998) Acute parvovirus B19 infection associated with fulminant hepatitis of favourable prognosis in young children. *Lancet*, 35, 1739–1741.

9.3 Human immunodeficiency virus and the liver

Vincent Soriano, Pablo Barreiro, Javier García-Samaniego, Luz Martín-Carbonero and Marina Nuñez

Liver damage in patients with human immunodeficiency virus (HIV) infection can result from multiple factors, including HIV itself, coinfection with hepatitis viruses, hepatic involvement during the course of systemic infections, drug toxicities and tumours (Table 1). Since the advent of highly active antiretroviral therapy (HAART), severe HIV-related immunodeficiency is only rarely seen in the developed world. Accordingly, the spectrum of liver complications in HIV+ persons has changed dramatically. Liver involvement due to opportunistic infections (i.e. cytomegalovirus, toxoplasmosis, tuberculosis, etc.) or neoplasms (i.e. Kaposi's sarcoma, lymphomas, etc.) is no longer an important issue. In contrast, chronic hepatitis B and C have emerged as one of the leading causes of hospital admission and death among HIV+ patients in the new millennium.

Hepatitis B

Introduction

The prevalence of chronic hepatitis B virus (HBV) infection among HIV+ individuals varies according to geography and risk category. In western countries, chronic hepatitis B is overall 10-fold more frequent among HIV+ individuals than in the general population [1]. Men infected through homosexual contacts tend to show the highest rates (6–10%); rates are slightly lower among intravenous drug users (IDUs) and much lower among persons infected through heterosexual contacts [1].

Table 1 Aetiology of liver damage in HIV-infected patients.

1 Chronic viral hepatitis: HBV and HCV
2 Other hepatitis viruses: A, E, G, EBV, CMV
3 Infections of the liver: tuberculosis, toxoplasmosis, cryptococcosis, others
4 Liver tumours: hepatocarcinoma, lymphomas, Kaposi's sarcoma
5 Drug-related liver toxicity: antiretrovirals, other medications
6 Biliary disease

HBV, hepatitis B virus; HCV, hepatitis C virus; EBV, Epstein–Barr virus; CMV, cytomegalovirus.

HIV infection has a deleterious effect on the outcome of chronic viral hepatitides, and complicates their management. Mortality is higher in HIV-positive individuals with chronic hepatitis, either B and/or C, than in those with HIV alone [1–3], with the highest rates being reported among those with multiple hepatitides [3]. In one study conducted before 2000, HBV co-infection was associated with a nearly 13-fold higher risk of liver-related mortality in HIV-positive patients, and this negative impact was more prominent in subjects with low CD4 counts [2]. There are scarce data on the outcome of HBV infection in the HAART era [1,4].

The reciprocal interferences between HIV and HBV infections result in specific problems in coinfected patients [4]. Poorer response to interferon alpha (IFN-α), and faster selection of lamivudine (3TC)-resistant HBV strains have been reported [4]. The higher risk of selecting drug-resistant HIV and/or HBV argues against monotherapy with nucleos(t)ide analogues in this population. Thus, the management of both infections should be carefully coordinated.

For a long time, 3TC has been the only available oral drug with dual activity against HIV and HBV. However, since the approval of tenofovir disoproxil fumarate (TDF) and emtricitabine (FTC) for the treatment of HIV infection, chronic HBV infection in HIV-coinfected patients may also benefit from using these new drugs, even though they have not yet been approved for the treatment of HBV monoinfection. In addition, the new pegylated IFN-αs, which may be administered subcutaneously once a week, have recently attracted attention, as they are more convenient and potent.

Efficacy of anti-HBV drugs in HIV-coinfected patients

Four drugs have been approved so far for the treatment of chronic hepatitis B: IFN-α, 3TC, adefovir dipivoxil (ADV) and entecavir (ETV). However, other compounds showing anti-HBV activity have already been approved as therapy against either HIV (i.e. TDF and FTC) or hepatitis C (i.e. pegylated IFN-α). Although not yet approved against HBV, these drugs

Table 2 HBV arsenal in HIV-infected patients.

Drug	Anti-HIV activity	Anti-HBV potency	Resistance barrier	Comments
Pegylated interferon	Yes	High	No	Weekly subcutaneous administration Contraindicated in ESLD
Lamivudine	Yes	Intermediate	Low	6–12 months' treatment duration > 30% resistance at 12 months Excellent tolerance
Emtricitabine	Yes	Intermediate	Low	Equivalent to lamivudine Co-formulated with tenofovir
Adefovir[a]	No	Intermediate	Intermediate	Useful in ESLD and 3TC failures 15% resistance at 4 years Good tolerance
Tenofovir	Yes	High	High	Useful in 3TC and adefovir failures
Entecavir	No	High	High	Useful but less potent in 3TC failures Good tolerance

[a]Adefovir at doses of 10 mg daily.
ESLD, endstage liver disease; 3TC, lamivudine.

are often used in HBV/HIV-coinfected patients. Table 2 summarizes the current therapeutic armamentarium against HBV [5].

IFN-α

While responses in HIV+ patients are superior compared with no treatment, they tend to be lower than in HIV-negative individuals. Higher CD4+ counts and higher baseline transaminase levels are predictors of IFN response. The therapeutic response to IFN-α in HBV is worse when HCV and/or HDV coinfections are present, a common situation in HIV+ IDUs. Therefore, several reasons may account for the lower response to IFN-α seen in HBV/HIV-coinfected patients, such as low CD4 counts, low transaminase levels and frequent HCV coinfection.

Lamivudine (3TC)

Although the inhibitory dosage for blocking HBV replication is lower (100 mg/day) than that needed for inhibiting HIV, 300 mg/day of the drug should be given when treating HBV/HIV-coinfected patients, and 3TC should always be combined with at least two other anti-HIV agents. Otherwise, 3TC monotherapy would rapidly select HIV resistance mutations [5].

Anti-HBe seroconversion occurs in only a minority of patients treated with 3TC, but many show improvements in liver histology; reversal of liver decompensations is common in those with advanced cirrhosis. However, the downside of 3TC monotherapy is the relatively high incidence of HBV resistance mutations over time (~20% per year) [6].

Emtricitabine (FTC)

This cytosine analogue, closely related to 3TC, has been approved for the treatment of HIV infection. FTC should not be used as monotherapy in this population due to the high risk of selecting HIV resistance mutations. FTC is not indicated after 3TC failure, as both drugs show cross-resistance.

Adefovir (ADV)

The dose recommended is 10 mg daily, which does not show clinical activity against HIV. In a study conducted in 35 HIV/HBV-coinfected patients with 3TC-resistant HBV strains, the addition of ADV to 3TC provided a significant reduction in serum HBV DNA, which was maintained for 192 weeks, along with normalization of transaminases in most cases [7]. ADV-resistant mutations were not selected in HBV or in HIV. However, in other studies, mutations rtN236T and rtA181V were shown to be selected in 29% of HBV-monoinfected individuals treated with ADV monotherapy for 5 years.

Tenofovir (TDF)

Lamivudine is no longer a protagonist in the treatment of HBV in HIV-coinfected patients since the approval of TDF for the treatment of HIV infection. TDF is a nucleotide analogue with both anti-HIV and anti-HBV activity; it is a very potent inhibitor of HBV replication *in vitro*, even in the presence of 3TC resistance. The results of retrospective studies assessing the efficacy of TDF against HBV in HIV-coinfected patients are shown in Table 3. Serum HBV DNA levels declined on average 4 log10, despite most patients carrying 3TC-resistant mutations [8–13].

Entecavir (ETV)

This is one of the most potent anti-HBV agents examined so far and shows a relatively good safety profile. It lacks any anti-HIV activity. Data have been released from a randomized and double-blind study performed on 68 HIV/HBV-coinfected patients failing 3TC. Either a 2 $\log_{10}$ reduction in viral load from baseline or undetectable HBV DNA (< 400 copies/mL) were achieved at 24 weeks by 84% of ETV-treated patients. Virological responses to ETV are seen in patients with 3TC-resistant HBV, although they tend to be lower than in 3TC-naive

Table 3 Efficacy of tenofovir against HBV in HIV-coinfected patients.

Author [ref.]	No.	YMDD mutants	Mean ↓HBV DNA (log10) at 24 weeks	Seroconversion Anti-HBe	Seroconversion Anti-HBs
Núñez et al. [8]	12	8	−3.8[a]	1/9	1/12
Van Bömmel et al. [9]	5	5	−4.5	0/4	0/5
Ristig et al. [10]	6	3	−4.3	0/6	0/6
Nelson et al. [11]	20	11	−4.0[a]	2/20	0/20
Benhamou et al. [12]	12	10	−3.8	0/?	0/12
Dore et al. [13]	12	7	−4.9	1/10	0/10

[a]Median.

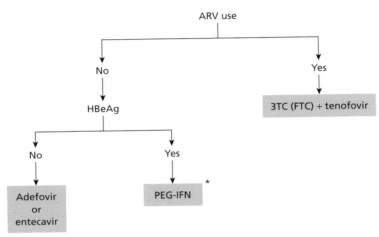

* With caution in cirrhotics

Fig. 1 Preferred anti-HBV agents in HBV/HIV-coinfected patients in distinct situations. ARV, antiretroviral.

patients. Resistance to ETV results from the accumulation of multiple changes in the HBV polymerase, including those linked to 3TC resistance. For this reason, ETV doses of 0.5 mg daily are recommended in drug-naive patients, but doses of 1.0 mg daily are preferred for patients with 3TC-resistant HBV strains. In HBV/HIV-coinfected patients, doses of 1.0 mg/day are preferred at first, given the overall higher HBV viraemia seen in this population [5].

HBV resistance to nucleos(t)ide analogues

On average, YMDD mutations develop at a rate of 15−20% per year of 3TC treatment, but are more rapidly selected in HBV/HIV-coinfected subjects, with incidences of 50% and 90% after 2 and 4 years of 3TC therapy, respectively [6]. Selection of HBV resistance to FTC seems to occur more slowly than with 3TC, with rates of 19% after 2 years of FTC treatment.

Hepatitis B surface antigen (HBsAg) should be screened in all HIV-infected individuals. If positive, full serological assessment of HBV infection should be performed, including testing for HBeAg and anti-HBe antibody and plasma HBV DNA measurement [5]. HBV treatment is generally indicated for those patients with active disease and viral replication.

The HIV/HBV-coinfected population is unique in the sense that some nucleos(t)ide analogues frequently used as antiretrovirals also have anti-HBV activity. If HIV needs to be treated, in the presence of an active HBV infection, drugs such as TDF and 3TC (FTC), preferentially in combination, should be considered as the best option (Fig. 1). The problem of when to treat HBV in HIV-coinfected patients becomes more relevant when there is no need to initiate antiretroviral therapy. Most recent guidelines do not support the requirement for a liver biopsy, relying more on serum markers such as alanine aminotransferase (ALT) levels, HBV DNA and HBeAg serostatus to decide whether HBV treatment should be initiated or may be delayed [5,14]. However, liver biopsy may be convenient in patients with no indication for antiretrovirals when ALT levels are normal but serum HBV DNA is greater than 10^4 copies/mL (Fig. 2) [5]. The advent of non-invasive techniques to assess liver fibrosis, such as serum biochemical markers and liver elastography, might be

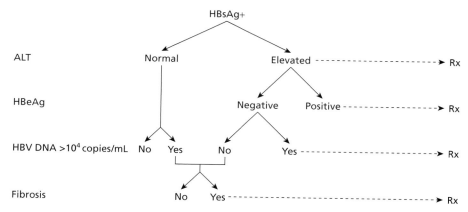

Fig. 2 HBV treatment (Rx) decision algorithm in HIV/HBV-coinfected patients.

useful to stage liver fibrosis in chronic hepatitis B, avoiding the performance of liver biopsy [15]. Liver biopsy could be left only for discordant cases.

While recent guidelines in HIV-negative individuals with chronic hepatitis B have recommended that treatment should be considered for patients with serum HBV DNA above 10^5 copies/mL in HBeAg-positive patients [16], a lower threshold could be appropriate for HBeAg-negative patients and those with decompensated cirrhosis (thresholds of 10^4 and 10^3 copies/mL respectively) [16]. At this time, the recommendations for treating HBV in the setting of HIV coinfection should be taken individually and based on the consideration of aspects related to the HIV situation [5]. The coexistence of HIV infection along with chronic hepatitis B makes an integrated approach necessary for the appropriate management of both infections.

Table 4 summarizes the treatment options for HIV-infected subjects with chronic hepatitis B. A major issue is the indication to give or not to give antiretroviral therapy. If HBV is the only virus to be treated, the pegylated forms of IFN-α could be a valid option [5]. The presence of HBeAg is one of the most important determinants in favour of IFN-α. The proportion of patients achieving HBeAg seroconversion using IFN-α is higher than with nucleos(t)ide analogues. An advantage of IFN-α is

that it is given for a limited period of time (6–12 months). However, IFN-α should not be used in patients with decompensated cirrhosis, as necroinflammatory flares accompanying HBeAg clearance may lead to liver decompensation. IFN-α appears to be safe in patients with compensated cirrhosis, although there is still a risk of hepatic decompensation with prolonged therapy [16]. Given the lack of data on the use of pegylated IFN-α in HBV/HIV-coinfected subjects, these patients should be treated within clinical trials.

The choice of oral anti-HBV drugs should be based on their efficacy in the clinical setting. ETV is a good choice in HBV/HIV-coinfected patients who do not need antiretroviral therapy and may be the best option for HBeAg-negative hepatitis B. ADV may be considered as a reasonable alternative choice, although the potential selection of resistance mutations in the HIV genome has been a matter of concern [5]; however, this does not seem to represent a major problem [17].

The use of 3TC, FTC or TDF in monotherapy should be avoided in HIV/HBV-coinfected patients, as it would favour the selection of HIV resistance mutations. Antiretroviral therapy including either 3TC (FTC) and TDF could be discontinued in patients who achieve a response, i.e. anti-HBe seroconversion, but it should be stopped no earlier than 6 months after the response in order to minimize the risk of relapses upon drug discontinuation [16].

In patients who meet the criteria for antiretroviral therapy as well as for HBV treatment, triple regimens containing 3TC (or FTC) and TDF should be the preferred option [5]. Although the role of combination therapy for HBV is unclear at this time, 3TC (FTC) along with TDF appears at present to be an appropriate backbone, and their combination appears therefore to be the first choice [5]. In cases of no clear indication for anti-HBV treatment, the inclusion of active drug(s) against HBV in the HAART regimen may be considered to avoid hepatic flares in the context of immune reconstitution [5].

HBV resistance should be suspected in patients with detectable HBV viraemia who have already received 3TC. FTC is not useful in this setting, and switching to or adding TDF is recommended. If HIV replication is already suppressed, adding ADV or ETV is a reasonable option.

Table 4 HBV treatment options in HIV/HBV-coinfected patients.

HBV treatment only	Pegylated interferon
HBeAg-positive	ETV
	ADV
HBeAg-negative	ETV
	ADV
HIV and HBV treatment	HAART including TDF ± (3TC or FTC)
	HAART + (ADV or ETV)
HIV treatment only	Consider including at least one anti-HBV drug in the HAART regimen to avoid flares due to immune reconstitution

ADV, adefovir; ETV, entecavir; HAART, highly active antiretroviral therapy; 3TC, lamivudine; FTC, emtricitabine; TDF, tenofovir.

Finally, HBV/HIV-coinfected patients not treated for HBV should regularly undergo biochemical and virological follow-up (every 3–6 months) to re-evaluate the need for anti-HBV treatment. Biannual α-fetoprotein and ultrasound are recommended in cirrhotics. There has been no agreement as to the time for repeating liver biopsies in patients with no or minimal activity in a first biopsy. However, the availability of the new non-invasive tools for assessing liver fibrosis may overcome this problem. Periodic monitoring with these techniques is particularly helpful in HBV/HIV-coinfected patients in whom progression to endstage liver disease may be accelerated [18].

Hepatitis C

Introduction

Chronic HCV infection has been the focus of particular attention in HIV-positive patients over the last few years. HCV-related liver disease is now a leading cause of morbidity and mortality among HIV-infected individuals in areas with a high prevalence of IDUs [19]. This increased rate of liver complications among HIV-infected patients is due to the dramatic decrease in opportunistic infections as a result of the widespread use of HAART, to the accelerated course of HCV-related liver disease in the HIV setting and to the enhanced risk of liver toxicity using antiretroviral agents in the presence of underlying chronic hepatitis C.

The bidirectional interferences between HCV and HIV infections have clinical consequences and make the management of coinfected individuals complex [14,20].

Epidemiology of HIV/HCV coinfection

Given that HIV and either hepatitis B and C viruses share similar routes of transmission, coinfection is relatively frequent (Fig. 3).

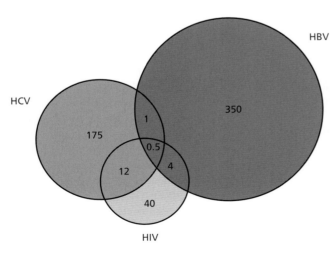

Fig. 3 Estimated number of individuals (in millions) with HIV, HBV and HCV worldwide.

In the United States and western Europe, around one-third of HIV-infected individuals are coinfected with HCV [21]. HCV and HIV are both transmitted by whole blood and blood products, with HCV being 10 times more infectious than HIV. Coinfection with HIV and HCV is therefore frequent in persons with increased blood exposure such as IDUs and haemophiliacs, who have a prevalence of coinfection > 75%. Sexual transmission of HCV is infrequent; this explains the low rate of HCV coinfection among homosexual HIV+ patients. Nevertheless, recent outbreaks of acute HCV infection have been described in association with some homosexual practices.

Laboratory markers and diagnosis of hepatitis C in the HIV setting

Current guidelines recommend that all HIV-infected individuals should be screened for HCV antibodies by enzyme-linked immunosorbent assay (ELISA) [14,20]. More than 85% of anti-HCV antibody-positive patients have detectable HCV RNA in the setting of HIV infection, whereas HCV RNA is detectable in only 75% of HIV-negative patients with HCV antibody. Patients with repeatedly elevated aminotransferases of unclear cause (HCV antibody negative) should also be tested for HCV RNA, given that rare cases of silent HCV infection have been reported, mainly among subjects with profound immunodeficiency [20].

In all HCV RNA-positive patients, the HCV genotype should be determined before making any therapeutic decision. Finally, around 20% of HIV+ patients with active HCV replication may show repeatedly normal transaminases. At present, the management of this subset of patients is unclear. HIV/HCV-coinfected patients should be vaccinated against hepatitis A virus if they have not been previously exposed or immunized, because acute hepatitis A may be more severe in the presence of underlying chronic hepatitis C. Likewise, HBV vaccination should not be forgotten in these patients, as up to 20% of HIV-infected individuals may lack markers of ongoing and/or past HBV infection.

Natural history of HIV/HCV coinfection

The coexistence of HIV and HCV in the same individual results in complex interactions between both infections, leading to changes in their respective natural histories. With HAART, HCV-related liver disease might progress less rapidly than in severely immunosuppressed individuals who have no control of HIV replication.

Influence of chronic hepatitis C on the course of HIV infection

Clinical studies of the influence of HCV on HIV disease progression are conflicting. In the Swiss cohort, HIV-positive individuals with HCV infection progressed faster to AIDS and death than HCV-negative patients [22] whereas, in an American cohort, the progression rates to AIDS and survival were similar in both groups [23].

Results are also conflicting on the possible negative influence of HCV infection in HIV patients who recover immunity using antiretroviral therapy. Although CD4 gains seem to be blunted in HCV/HIV-coinfected individuals recruited in some studies [22], similar gains in CD4 cell counts compared with HCV-negative patients have been seen by others [23]. If the deleterious effect exists, a successful treatment of HCV infection might contribute to higher CD4 gains using HAART in the coinfected population.

HCV may negatively influence HIV disease through indirect pathways, such as forcing antiretroviral treatment discontinuation more frequently because of an increased risk of liver toxicity. Up to one-quarter of coinfected patients who initiate HAART stop therapy on account of drug-related hepatotoxicity [24]; an increased risk ratio of 3.7 times for developing liver toxicity was found in one study [25]. This risk might be even more pronounced in patients carrying HCV genotype 3, given that baseline steatosis is associated with this HCV variant [26]. Liver toxicity is most often asymptomatic, but occasionally it may lead to acute liver failure [27].

Influence of HIV infection on the course of chronic hepatitis C

Acute HCV infection evolves more easily into chronic hepatitis in HIV-infected individuals, especially in those with a more advanced immune deficiency. HCV RNA levels are much higher in HIV-coinfected patients than in HCV-monoinfected individuals, both in plasma and in the liver. The reason for the higher level of HCV replication in HIV-coinfected patients seems to be the poorer control of HCV infection, mainly due to a decrease in anti-HCV-specific CD8 responses, which are more evident in patients with lower CD4 counts. Although the implications of these findings on the natural history of HCV infection are uncertain, patients with high levels of HCV replication may have lower chances of response to IFN-based treatments [28].

The progression of liver fibrosis is accelerated in HIV/HCV-coinfected patients, especially when immune deficiency is profound. In a recent multicentre European study that assessed liver biopsies from 914 patients coinfected with hepatitis C and HIV, the distribution of METAVIR liver fibrosis stages was F0 in 10% of patients, F1 in 33%, F2 in 22%, F3 in 22% and F4 in 13%, highlighting the high degree of liver fibrosis in this population [29]. Nearly half of patients had advanced liver fibrosis (F3–F4) after the age of 40 years. Clearly, progression to endstage liver disease occurs faster in the HIV/HCV-coinfected population, including the development of hepatocellular carcinoma at younger ages [30]. Overall, 25% of the HIV/HCV-coinfected patients will develop cirrhosis within 15 years after HCV exposure, whereas this occurs in only 5% of those without HIV infection [31].

HAART might be associated with better survival through decreasing HIV-related and also liver-related deaths [32]. The improved prognosis in HIV/HCV-coinfected patients conferred by HAART could be related to a slower progression of liver fibrosis. Several studies have reported significantly reduced fibrosis scores in patients on protease inhibitor (PI)-based HAART. HAART may reverse at least partially the negative effect of HIV infection on HCV-related liver disease, in particular when the immune deficiency is more profound.

Treatment of hepatitis C in the HIV setting

Until the advent of HAART, liver disease associated with HCV had minimal impact on the outcome of HIV+ individuals, and classical opportunistic illnesses were the main concern, particularly at advanced stages of immunosuppression. However, since 1996, potent antiretroviral therapy has permitted the reversal of the immune deficiency in most HIV-infected individuals and, therefore, the risk of developing opportunistic infections. As a consequence, other illnesses such as chronic viral hepatitis have become much more relevant.

Rationale

The treatment of hepatitis C in HIV+ patients has become a priority for two main reasons. First, progression to endstage liver disease due to HCV occurs more rapidly in the HIV setting. Second, the tolerance of antiretroviral agents is much poorer in the presence of underlying chronic hepatitis C, with a greater risk of developing hepatotoxicity [20].

Current results

Pegylated IFN (PEG-IFN) plus ribavirin (RBV) should be considered as the current treatment of choice in this population [14,20]. However, treatment responses are lower than in HCV-monoinfected patients. Because both PEG-IFN and RBV act, at least in part, as immunomodulatory agents, immune defects driven by HIV infection might negatively affect the performance of these drugs.

Most of the studies assessing the efficacy and safety of peg-IFN plus RBV in coinfected patients provided treatment for 12 months to all patients, irrespective of their HCV genotype [33–36]. Because of concerns about drug interactions and further toxicities, lower (800 mg daily) than recommended doses of RBV were prescribed. Only patients with a relatively good immunological status were recruited. Table 5 summarizes the treatment schedules and the results obtained in the main prospective randomized trials.

The high rate of HCV treatment discontinuation in some trials may reflect a higher frequency of serious adverse events in HIV-positive compared with HIV-negative patients; it might also reflect fears by some HIV physicians not familiar enough with the management of side-effects of anti-HCV therapy. Thus, efforts to minimize side-effects with symptomatic treatments and appropriate management of complications are critical to ensure completion of HCV therapy [20].

Table 5 Response to PEG-IFN plus ribavirin in HCV/HIV-coinfected patients in four studies.

	ACTG 5071 [33]	RIBAVIC [34]	APRICOT [35]	Laguno *et al.* [36]
No. of patients	66	205	289	52
Type of PEG-IFN	Roche	Schering-Plough	Roche	Schering-Plough
RBV dose	Escalating 600→1000 mg/day	800 mg/day	800 mg/day	800–1200 mg/day
IDU	80%	81%	62%	75%
Cirrhosis	11%	18%	15%	11%
Genotypes 1–4	77%	69%	67%	63%
Median CD4 count	492 cells/µL	525 cells/µL	520 cells/µL	624 cells/µL
With ARV	85%	82%	84%	94%
Premature stop	12%	36%	25%	25%
ETR (ITT)	41%	36%	49%	52%
SVR (ITT)	27%	27%	40%	44%

ETR, end-of-treatment response; SVR, sustained virological response; ARV, antiretroviral therapy; PEG-IFN, pegylated interferon; RBV, ribavirin; ITT, intention to treat; IDU, intravenous drug user.

Selection of candidates for HCV therapy

Histology

The value of liver biopsy before prescribing anti-HCV therapy has lost importance as anti-HCV therapy has become more efficacious. Outside academic purposes, many experts feel that it is no longer needed in most cases [20,37]. Liver histology allows staging of HCV hepatic damage and may predict the development of cirrhosis. It may also provide information to rule out other causes of liver damage. However, the reproducibility is quite low and largely affected by the size of the hepatic fragment and the expertise of the pathologist.

The controversy on the need for a liver biopsy may be even less justified in HCV/HIV-coinfected patients, in whom the fibrosis progression rate is faster than in HCV-monoinfected persons. Nearly half of coinfected patients may show cirrhosis or precirrhosis after 40 years of age [29]; it should be noted that the mean age of HCV/HIV-coinfected patients currently seen in clinics in the USA and western Europe is above 40 years of age.

CD4 counts

The efficacy of HCV therapy depends somewhat on the baseline CD4 cell count [28]. Candidates to receive HCV therapy should ideally have more than 200–350 CD4+ T cells/µL, a feasible threshold for most patients if antiretroviral therapy is used appropriately [20]. That figure is also currently the immunological threshold for initiating HAART in drug-naive patients.

In patients with CD4 counts below 200 cells/µL and already under HAART, the decision to treat HCV infection must take into account other factors, such as the estimated length of HCV infection, the severity of liver disease, the extent of HIV suppression and classical predictors of response to HCV therapy such as HCV genotype and viral load. Toxicities of IFN and/or RBV as well as poorer responses may be more frequent in this subset of patients. In general, HCV therapy should be deferred in individuals with less than 200 CD4+ T cells/µL, as the risk of toxicity is increased and the response may be poorer. IFN-based therapies cause a decline in the CD4 count, which may put patients at risk of developing opportunistic infections if baseline counts are low. Therefore, in drug-naive coinfected patients, antiretroviral therapy should be considered at first. Once the CD4 count has risen and plasma HIV RNA is under control, the prescription of HCV therapy should be reassessed [20].

Conversely, in antiretroviral-naive individuals with HCV/ HIV coinfection, hepatitis C should be treated first if the CD4 count does not warrant immediate antiretroviral therapy. It is debated whether, in patients with CD4 counts above 350 cells/ µL but with high plasma HIV RNA levels, suppression of HIV replication should be attempted first, deferring HCV therapy until undetectable HIV viraemia is attained [20]. Finally, the greater efficacy of HCV therapy in patients with higher CD4 counts should be balanced against a higher risk of interactions between antiretrovirals and anti-HCV drugs [14,20].

Contraindications and special populations

Contraindications to the use of IFN or RBV are the same as in HIV-negative patients (see Chapter 5.1.3.v).

Patients on methadone are acceptable candidates for anti-HCV therapy. However, up to one-third of them may need adjustments in methadone dosage. This is generally due to psychological demands rather than to pharmacological interactions between anti-HCV drugs and methadone. Ideally, a multidisciplinary team, including experts in addiction medicine and psychologists/psychiatrics, should take care of these patients.

Patients with repeated normal liver enzymes, particularly those infected with HCV genotypes 2 or 3, might benefit from anti-HCV therapy. However, more information on liver damage in this subset of HCV/HIV-coinfected patients is needed to balance the cost–benefit of HCV therapy in them [14,20]. In the RIBAVIC trial [33], significant liver fibrosis was recognized in a substantial proportion of coinfected patients with normal ALT levels, but treatment responses were lower in this population.

In summary, all HIV+ persons with chronic HCV infection should be considered as potential candidates for HCV therapy, given their higher risk of progression to endstage liver disease compared with HIV-negative patients and their increased risk of liver toxicity after beginning antiretroviral therapy. The timing for anti-HCV treatment should be decided on an individual basis. Severe neuropsychiatric disorders [38] and alcohol and drug abuse generally contraindicate current HCV treatment. However, methadone use and non-decompensated cirrhosis are not contraindications for therapy. Treatment of patients with CD4 counts below 200 cells/µL is risky and should generally not be advised.

Monitoring and duration of HCV therapy in coinfected patients

Despite a possible slower initial HCV RNA decay in HIV-coinfected patients, all patients who attain a sustained viral response (SVR) showed a decline greater than 2 logs at week 12 of therapy [32–34]. Therefore, the predictive roles of early virological response (EVR) also apply to HCV/HIV-coinfected patients (see Chapter 5.1.3.v). Furthermore, one recent report has demonstrated the negative predictive value of the 2 log rule at week 12 in coinfected patients [39], showing that the only difference between HIV-positive and HIV-negative patients with hepatitis C was the proportion of patients reaching virological responses at any given time point (lower in the coinfected population, although this could be due to the relatively low doses of RBV used in that study); using adequate RBV doses, HCV kinetics do not seem to differ much in HIV-positive and HIV-negative subjects, except that baseline HCV RNA is much higher in coinfected individuals and, therefore, it may take longer to reach undetectable viraemia [40,41]. Thus, the principles guiding anti-HCV therapy in HIV-negative patients may equally apply to HIV-coinfected patients.

Patients with high HCV loads may show a good EVR but may fail to clear viraemia at week 24, and may clear the virus later on. This subset of patients represents less than 3% of HCV-monoinfected individuals, but it is larger in HIV-coinfected patients, given their higher baseline HCV RNA levels and possible slower HCV RNA decays on therapy. Therefore, extending treatment beyond 6 months may be advisable in coinfected patients who showed more than 2 log HCV RNA falls at week 12 but are still HCV RNA positive at week 24. If HCV RNA is still detectable at month 9, therapy should be discontinued.

The second phase of clearance of HCV RNA on HCV therapy, which accounts for the steady destruction of infected liver cells, may also be delayed in HIV/HCV-coinfected patients, and could explain the more frequent relapse rate in early virological responders seen in HIV-coinfected patients [42]. Therefore, HIV/HCV-coinfected patients who carry genotypes 2 or 3 should be treated for 12 months.

The use of high doses of RBV seems to enhance substantially the virological response, and this may be even more apparent in the setting of HIV coinfection. Therefore, an effort to keep patients on adequate doses of the drug should be attempted. The administration of recombinant erythropoietin has been proposed as a useful strategy in the management of RBV-related anaemia.

Patients not achieving HCV eradication with treatment might benefit from long-term therapy with PEG-IFN alone. Maintenance therapy with PEG-IFN may provide histological improvement and even reduce the risk of hepatocellular carcinoma; this approach is currently being investigated as an alternative strategy in large trials (i.e. HALT-C and EPIC) in HCV-monoinfected patients. Whether this strategy may also be applicable to non-responding HIV/HCV-coinfected individuals with advanced liver fibrosis remains to be elucidated. However, the potential benefit of this approach should be balanced against the compromise in the quality of life and the reduced CD4+ T cell count caused by PEG-IFN [43].

Interactions between antiretroviral agents and HCV medications

HCV treatment in the presence of HIV infection may be complicated by the interactions between RBV and some antiretrovirals. The intracellular levels of some HIV nucleoside analogues may be decreased by RBV, but the interactions seem to have no clinical consequences. However, a higher toxicity was noted with the concomitant use of didanosine (ddI) and RBV; toxicity is further increased using stavudine (d4T) and ddI together with RBV due to the enhancement of mitochondrial toxicity. Hepatitis C, HIV, RBV and HIV nucleoside analogues may all cause mitochondrial dysfunction and act synergistically [44]. Hepatic decompensation, sometimes with fatal outcome [45], was described with the co-administration of these drugs in cirrhotic patients. Lactic acidosis and pancreatitis have also been reported with the combined use of RBV and ddI; therefore ddI should be avoided in patients receiving anti-HCV therapy [20].

It is also advisable to avoid zidovudine (AZT) when anti-HCV therapy is initiated, because anaemia is more frequent and severe in patients taking AZT along with RBV [46]. A recent study showed a correlation between RBV plasma levels and anaemia, with higher RBV concentrations in patients receiving AZT compared with other nucleoside analogues [46].

How to improve HCV treatment responses

Multiple factors may account for the lower response to HCV therapy seen in HIV-coinfected vs. HCV-monoinfected patients. In view of the low eligibility and applicability of HIV/HCV-coinfected subjects to receive anti-HCV treatment, the first effort needed is to increase the population of candidates for therapy. Poor compliance with follow-up visits was one of the most common causes for excluding HIV/HCV-coinfected patients from therapy. Drugs and alcohol abuse are also often reported as barriers to treating hepatitis C in this population. Special efforts should be made to follow very closely and to manage appropriately the side-effects derived from anti-HCV medications in coinfected patients to avoid unnecessary discontinuations.

Recent reports have shown the achievement of higher early and sustained responses in HIV/HCV-coinfected subjects with more elevated RBV plasma levels, suggesting that, in this setting, it is also important to maximize the exposure to RBV [40,46].

In contrast to HCV-monoinfected patients, treatment should be given for 48 weeks to HIV/HCV-coinfected patients with HCV genotype 3, as this schedule seems to decrease the number of relapsers after the initial response. Relapses in HIV-positive patients coinfected with HCV genotypes 1 or 4 treated for 12 months occur in 20–30% of patients. In this population, the benefit of prolonged periods of therapy, at least among early virological responders, should be investigated [47]. Tailoring the duration of treatment according to early kinetics might be another strategy to maximize the proportion of SVR. Thus, patients with slower declines during the first weeks of therapy could benefit from receiving more prolonged therapy than those showing a rapid decline in HCV RNA levels [48]. However, extending the duration of treatment in patients who had not attained an adequate virological response at week 12 (> 2 log10) did not increase SVR in HIV/HCV-coinfected subjects.

Management of endstage liver disease in HCV/HIV-coinfected patients

Owing to the accelerated progression of the histological liver damage in the HIV setting, the time to evolve to endstage liver disease (ESLD) is shortened in coinfected patients. Individuals with ESLD have a very poor prognosis, and liver transplant is the only change of survival for them. Results of studies evaluating the outcome of liver-transplanted HIV-infected subjects suggest that HIV should no longer be considered an absolute contraindication for orthotopic liver transplantation (OLT) in coinfected patients [49]. Early evaluation of candidates is critical in this population [50]. Patients with ESLD due to viral hepatitis are also at high risk of developing hepatocellular carcinoma.

Liver transplantation in HCV/HIV-coinfected patients

Given the improved survival and quality of life achieved with HAART, OLT is currently being proposed for HIV/HCV-coinfected patients with ESLD. The first OLT attempts, before the introduction of HAART, provided very poor results, with only a small percentage of transplanted HIV+ recipients achieving a satisfactory outcome. However, more recently, short- and mid-term survival has improved significantly in HIV-infected OLT recipients, although the management of liver transplant entails major difficulties in HIV/HCV-coinfected patients.

The criteria used for OLT are relatively similar worldwide, including CD4 counts above 100 cells/μL, undetectable plasma HIV RNA on HAART or available antiretrovirals for the post-OLT period if the HIV load is detectable, and absence of prior history of AIDS-defining conditions other than pulmonary tuberculosis. The risk of opportunistic infections in the post-transplant period is low as long as HIV replication is well controlled with antiretrovirals. Furthermore, CD4 cell counts remain stable or even increase after transplantation. Therefore, the use of standard immunosuppressive therapy in patients with well-controlled HIV infection seems to be safe and does not increase the risk of developing opportunistic infections.

There are, however, a number of issues involved in both the pre- and post-transplant period that make it more difficult to achieve satisfactory OLT outcomes in the HIV population. First, the selection of HIV-infected candidates for transplantation, because patients with ESLD often present a poor profile (alcohol abuse, drug addiction, prior AIDS-defining conditions, etc.). Second, the priority of organ allocation, as most HIV-infected patients, because of their rapid clinical deterioration, will not survive sufficiently long to receive a liver transplant if they are not prioritized. Therefore, new approaches to make liver transplantation available sooner after the assignment of HIV patients to the waiting list should be assessed [50].

Intolerance to HAART and drug-to-drug interactions between antiretrovirals and immunosuppressive agents create further difficulties. Some antiretrovirals may produce liver toxicity, which makes the interpretation of liver enzyme elevations more complicated. Low doses of ritonavir (RTV) or non-nucleoside analogues (nevirapine or efavirenz) should be used with caution because of their effects on cytochrome P-450 and P-glycoprotein, which may cause important pharmacokinetic interactions with immunosuppressive agents, such as ciclosporin A and tacrolimus. Administration of lower doses of calcineurin inhibitors and/or ciclosporin are needed in patients on protease inhibitors (PIs), and their plasma levels should be closely monitored. Episodes of acute rejection have been reported in patients who stopped PIs without adapting doses of calcineurin inhibitors. Patients taking HIV non-nucleoside reverse transcriptase inhibitors may show reduced plasma levels of immunosuppressive drugs, which may make them prone to graft rejection. The use of higher levels of immunosuppressive drugs may favour fibrocholestatic hepatitis C and rapid progression to ESLD in patients with HCV relapse after transplantation. Therapeutic drug monitoring of immunosuppressive agents is mandatory when taking antiretrovirals.

HIV coinfection and hepatitis A, D and G viruses

Hepatitis A virus (HAV) vaccine should be recommended to all HIV-infected adults who have no HAV antibodies. The safety and efficacy has already been proven in this population; immunogenicity is only slightly reduced in subjects with very low CD4 counts [51].

As in HIV-negative subjects, hepatitis D may be acquired coincident with exposure to HBV or, in HIV-positive patients, appear as a superinfection in a patient with chronic hepatitis B.

Progression of liver fibrosis occurs rapidly in chronic hepatitis D, and response to IFN therapy is low, even using high doses of IFN, such as 9 MU t.i.w, particularly in the setting of HIV coinfection [52]. In patients with advanced HIV immunosuppression, the Delta antigen can be recognized in the serum and not only in the liver.

A study suggested that the course of HIV infection is less progressive in HIV patients coinfected with the hepatitis G virus or GB virus (a lymphotropic virus replicating in B and T lymphocytes) than in HIV-monoinfected patients [53]; this issue has also raised debate as to whether IFN therapy of hepatitis C in HIV/HCV/hepatitis G-coinfected patients might accelerate progression of HIV disease due to the clearance of the hepatitis G virus that is sensitive to IFN. Neither assumption has been confirmed.

Other infections of the liver

Cytomegalovirus

All herpesviruses and particularly cytomegalovirus (CMV) cause disseminated disease in severely immunosuppressed patients. Although chorioretinitis is the most frequent CMV-related complication in HIV-infected individuals with less than 100 CD4+ T cells/μL, lung, gastrointestinal and liver involvement is also frequent in these patients.

Tuberculosis

Infection with *Mycobacterium tuberculosis* is one of the most frequent illnesses in HIV-infected patients in developing regions and among IDUs in North America and western Europe. It may develop in subjects without severe immunodeficiency as pulmonary tuberculosis (TB), although it tends to present as disseminated TB in patients with low CD4 counts. In the latter situation, hepatic involvement is frequent. It complicates treatment management as most anti-TB drugs are hepatotoxic to some degree (mainly rifampin, isoniazid and pirazinamid). Characteristic large and multiple hepatosplenic abscesses have been reported in association with intra-abdominal lymphadenopathies in HIV-infected immunosuppressed patients, mimicking lymphomas [55]. They may also develop as a result of an immune reconstitution syndrome following initiation of HAART. Hepatic TB may be part of miliary disease, featuring granulomatous hepatitis in the liver biopsy and fever of apparently unknown origin.

Mycobacterium avium complex (MAC)

Atypical mycobacteria of the *M. avium–intracellulare* complex are among the most common opportunistic organisms identified in the liver biopsy of severely immunosuppressed HIV-infected patients. Their presence is usually associated with fever, night sweats and weight loss, as well as elevated serum alkaline phosphatase and transaminases [56]. Infection is usually disseminated, and examination and culture of bone marrow, lymph node aspirates or blood will often give the diagnosis, avoiding the need for liver biopsy. Granuloma formation is often scanty, and the examination of smears and culture of biopsy tissue are essential. Response to treatment, particularly in patients with advanced disease, is often poor, and maintenance therapy is required to prevent relapse. However, since the advent of HAART, the improvement in the immune status in most patients on therapy has dramatically reduced the incidence of this complication. Conversely, immune reconstitution syndromes with lymph node enlargement and fever have been described following initiation of HAART in subjects with subclinical atypical mycobacterial infections.

Toxoplasmosis

Symptomatic infection with *Toxoplasma gondii* in HIV-positive patients generally manifests as cerebral toxoplasmosis. However, in severely immunosuppressed individuals, disseminated toxoplasmosis may appear with lung and/or hepatic involvement [57].

Drug-related liver toxicity

Background

Liver enzyme elevations are often seen following initiation of antiretroviral therapy. Liver toxicity is an important cause of morbidity, mortality and treatment discontinuation in HIV-infected patients. Drug liver toxicity has affected the recommendations for antiretroviral therapy in certain scenarios, as in the case of nevirapine in post-exposure prophylaxis [58], which should be avoided in women with CD4 counts > 250 cells/μL.

Definition of hepatotoxicity

There is a broad variability across studies in the criteria used to categorize the severity of hepatotoxicity. We propose as the most accepted, the AIDS Clinical Trials Group (ACTG) scale of liver toxicity. Accordingly, patients with transaminases within normal limits at baseline are considered to develop hepatotoxicity when ALT and/or aspartate aminotransferase (AST) rise above the upper limits of normal. Severe hepatic injury (the primary study outcome) is defined as grade 3 or 4, a > fivefold or > 10-fold change in AST and/or ALT levels during antiretroviral treatment respectively.

To avoid an over-representation of individuals with chronic hepatitis at baseline experiencing liver toxicity, changes in transaminase levels should be recorded based on baseline values. Therefore, transaminase level elevation is scored as grade 1 (1.25–2.5 × baseline), grade 2 (2.6–3.5 × baseline), grade 3 (3.6–5 × baseline) and grade 4 (> 5 × baseline) in subjects with abnormal liver enzyme values at baseline [24].

Incidence and risk factors

The reported incidence of severe liver toxicity after initiating HAART ranges from 2% to 18%. Differences in study populations, as well as in the methods used, account for this wide range. Liver toxicity is more frequent among subjects with chronic hepatitis C and/or B than in those without underlying liver disease. A higher risk of hepatotoxicity has been found in patients carrying HCV genotype 3 compared with other genotypes [26].

Among the PIs, full-dose RTV is more hepatotoxic than other drugs [25]; it has caused fatal acute hepatitis. The use of two PIs, often including RTV at low doses as a booster for the second PI, does not increase the risk of liver toxicity. The incidence of liver toxicity with lopinavir (LPV), which is given with fixed low doses of RTV (200 mg/day), is low. Atazanavir also has a good liver safety profile, even if used with low-dose RTV. In contrast, tipranavir, the last approved PI, appears to be more hepatotoxic, possibly because it is given with higher doses of RTV (400 mg/day) as a booster.

Some nucleoside reverse transcriptase inhibitors (NRTIs), such as 3TC and TDF, have a low incidence of hepatotoxicity. The mitochondrial damage is thought to be the mechanism involved in the development of liver injury by other NRTIs [24]. Cases of hepatic failure have been reported in patients taking AZT, although ddI and d4T are the most common agents causing severe hepatotoxicity. Abacavir (ABC) and TDF, which have a low potential for mitochondrial damage, have a safer liver profile.

Non-nucleoside reverse transcriptase inhibitors (NNRTIs) may cause liver toxicity by several mechanisms [24]. Cases of severe liver toxicity have been reported, some of them fatal, in subjects receiving nevirapine (NVP) as part of a post-exposure prophylaxis regimen [58]. Likewise, in a trial assessing the NRTI emtricitabine (FTC), a higher incidence of hepatotoxicity was observed among patients taking NVP [59]. Of interest, in both the post-exposure prophylaxis and the FTC trial, hepatotoxicity developed early following initiation of treatment and predominated among black African women in the FTC study. These data suggest a hypersensitivity reaction causing the liver abnormalities. However, in other reports, the hepatotoxicity of NVP-containing regimens had a later onset (beyond the fourth month), with an increase in the cumulative incidence over time [60,61]. Therefore, it is likely that NVP causes liver toxicity through a second mechanism, more common than the hypersensitivity syndrome. More importantly, while the allergic phenomenon might not be favoured by underlying hepatitis B or C, the toxic cumulative mechanism could be more frequent in patients with chronic viral hepatitis.

Several retrospective studies have evaluated the development of hepatotoxicity linked to the use of NNRTIs. In general, the incidence of liver toxicity is higher compared with other antiretrovirals, particularly in populations with a high prevalence of chronic HCV infection and with NVP rather than efavirenz.

Table 6 Mechanisms of liver toxicity of antiretroviral drugs.

Mitochondrial toxicity
Exclusive to NRTI, particularly d4T and ddI
Tends to occur after prolonged exposure
Hypersensitivity reaction
Associated with nevirapine and abacavir
Occurs early, often within the first 12 weeks
HLA-linked
Often associated with rash and fever
Not favoured by HCV or HBV
Direct damage
With PI and NNRTI
Favoured by HCV and/or HBV
Two modalities:
Intrinsic toxicity: dose-dependent, early onset
Idiosyncratic: not dose-dependent, latent period often long
Immune reconstitution
Mainly in patients with low CD4 counts and high viral load
Only in patients with HCV and/or HBV

HLA, human leukocyte antigen.

Mechanisms of liver toxicity

The possible mechanisms involved in the development of hepatotoxicity associated with the use of antiretrovirals are summarized in Table 6. Four main pathogenic mechanisms of hepatotoxicity of antiretrovirals exist, including direct drug toxicity, immune reconstitution in the presence of HCV and/or HBV coinfections, hypersensitivity reactions with liver involvement and mitochondrial toxicity. It is probable that multiple pathogenic pathways occur simultaneously in some patients. Other pathogenic mechanisms may also be involved, such as insulin resistance, which is favoured by several antiretrovirals and may contribute to the development of steatohepatitis [24].

Therapeutic management

The three main considerations necessary for the adequate management of transaminase elevations following the introduction of HAART are severity, clinical impact and aetiological mechanism. The suspicion of hypersensitivity reactions or lactic acidosis, and the development of liver decompensation, are all reasons for stopping treatment immediately [20]. Severe liver toxicity (grades 3–4), even in the absence of symptoms, similarly warrants discontinuation of antiretroviral therapy.

If fatty liver is present, the removal of factors predisposing to steatosis is indicated. If the patient is taking an antiretroviral with higher hepatotoxic potential (i.e. NVP), replacement of this drug is an option. The continuation of the same regimen, with spontaneous decrease in transaminase values, has been reported in immune reconstitution cases. Liver enzyme elevations may persist in some patients; the long-term consequences are unknown, yet sporadic cases of severe liver disease potentially linked to prolonged antiretroviral exposure have been reported recently.

Liver tumours

Neoplasias involving the liver are not uncommon in HIV-infected individuals. Primary tumours are mainly represented by hepatocellular carcinoma, lymphomas and Kaposi's sarcoma. Metastatic lesions are seen in subjects with colorectal cancer. While the incidence of hepatocellular carcinoma seems to be on the rise in HIV-infected patients with chronic hepatitis B and/or C, other hepatic tumours are declining since the introduction of HAART.

Hepatocarcinoma

Concurrent HIV infection may increase the incidence of hepatocellular carcinoma in cirrhotic patients with either HBV and/or HCV. In a study, six cases of hepatocellular carcinoma in a cohort of 2383 HIV-infected patients were identified, with an incidence ratio of 13.95, higher than expected in the general population [30]. A more aggressive course was also identified as a distinctive feature of chronic hepatitis C-associated hepatocellular carcinoma in the HIV setting.

HIV-infected cirrhotic patients should be screened for hepatocellular carcinoma at 6-month intervals using ultrasonography and measurement of alpha-fetoprotein levels [14,20]. Percutaneous ethanol injection can be indicated for small tumours in patients who are not candidates for surgery. Chemoembolization may improve survival in cases with late-stage hepatocellular carcinoma. In general, HIV-infected patients with hepatocellular carcinoma do not qualify for liver transplantation.

Lymphomas

The incidence of non-Hodgkin's lymphoma (NHL) is increased in HIV-infected individuals, but has declined significantly since the introduction of HAART. Hepatic involvement is frequently seen in NHL, but almost always as part of a systemic disease and very rarely as a primary tumour [62]. Hodgkin's disease is less frequent, but may likewise involve the liver at presentation or thereafter in the absence of response to chemotherapy.

Kaposi's sarcoma

Infection with human herpesvirus type 8 (HHV-8) is associated with three different clinical entities: (i) Kaposi's sarcoma (KS); (ii) primary effusive lymphomas; and (iii) multicentre Castleman's disease. Symptomatic HHV-8 infection was particularly frequent among homosexual men until the advent of HAART. Since then, the incidence of these neoplasias has declined dramatically. Vascular lesions of KS in the liver were common in subjects with visceral disease, and almost always accompanied cutaneous lesions.

HIV-associated biliary disease

The biliary tract may be involved in HIV disease as a result of infection with *Cryptosporidium*, *Microsporidium*, *Cyclospora*, MAC and tuberculosis. Chronic sclerosing cholangitis often results in cholestasis, jaundice and pruritus. In some HIV-infected subjects, the cholangiopathy has been limited to the distal choledochus, resulting in a dilated bile duct; resolution was obtained with endoscopic retrograde cholangiography followed by resection. As with other opportunistic infections, HAART has almost eliminated HIV-related cholangiopathy.

References

1 Konopnicki D, Mocroft A, de Wit S *et al.* (2005) Hepatitis B and HIV: prevalence, AIDS progression, response to HAART and increased mortality in the EuroSIDA cohort. *AIDS* 19, 593–602.

2 Thio C, Seaberg E, Skolasky RD *et al.* (2002) HIV-1, hepatitis B virus, and risk of liver-related mortality in the Multicenter AIDS Cohort Study (MACS). *Lancet* 360, 1921–1926.

3 Bonacini M, Bzowej N, Louie S *et al.* (2004) Survival in patients with HIV infection and viral hepatitis B or C. *AIDS* 18, 2039–2045.

4 Nuñez M, Puoti M, Camino N *et al.* (2003) Treatment of chronic hepatitis B in the HIV-infected patient: present and future. *Clin Infect Dis* 37, 1678–1685.

5 Soriano V, Puoti M, Bonacini M *et al.* (2005) Care of patients with chronic hepatitis B and HIV coinfection: recommendations from an international HBV/HIV Panel. *AIDS* 19, 221–240.

6 Benhamou Y, Bochet M, Thibault V *et al.* (1999) Long term incidence of hepatitis B virus resistance to lamivudine in HIV-infected patients. *Hepatology* 30, 1303–1306.

7 Benhamou Y, Thibault V, Vig P (2006) Long-term treatment with adefovir dipivoxil 10 mg in patients with lamivudine-resistant HBV and HIV co-infection results in significant and sustained clinical improvement. *J Hepatol* 44, 62–67.

8 Núñez M, Pérez-Olmeda M, Díaz B *et al.* (2002) Activity of tenofovir on hepatitis B virus replication in HIV-co-infected patients failing or partially responding to lamivudine. *AIDS* 16, 2352–2354.

9 Van Bömmel F, Wünsche T, Schürmann D *et al.* (2002) Tenofovir treatment in patients with lamivudine-resistant hepatitis B mutants strongly affects viral replication. *Hepatology* 36, 507–508.

10 Ristig MB, Crippin J, Aberg J *et al.* (2002) Tenofovir disoproxil fumarate therapy for chronic hepatitis B in HIV/hepatitis B virus-coinfected individuals for whom interferon-α and lamivudine therapy have failed. *J Infect Dis* 186, 1844–1847.

11 Nelson M, Portsmouth S, Stebbing J *et al.* (2003) An open-label study of tenofovir in HIV-1 and hepatitis B virus co-infected individuals. *AIDS* 17, F7–F10.

12 Benhamou Y, Tubiana R, Thibault V (2003) Tenofovir disoproxil fumarate in patients with HIV and lamivudine-resistant hepatitis B virus. *N Engl J Med* 348, 177–178.

13 Dore G, Cooper D, Pozniak A *et al.* for 903 and 907 Study Teams (2004) Efficacy of tenofovir disoproxil fumarate in antiretroviral therapy-naïve and -experienced patients coinfected with HIV-1 and hepatitis B virus. *J Infect Dis* 189, 1185–1192.

14 Alberti A, Clumeck N, Collins S *et al.* (2005) Short statement of the first European Consensus Conference on the treatment of chronic hepatitis B and C in HIV co-infected patients. *J Hepatol* 42, 615–624.

15 Castera L, Vergniol J, Foucher J et al. (2005) Prospective comparison of transient elastography, Fibrotest, APRI, and liver biopsy for the assessment of fibrosis in chronic hepatitis C. *Gastroenterology* 128, 343–350.

16 Keeffe E, Dieterich D, Han S-H, et al. (2004) A treatment algorithm for the management of chronic hepatitis B virus infection in the United States. *Clin Gastroenterol Hepatol* 2, 87–106.

17 Sheldon J, Corral A, Rodes B et al. (2005) Risk of selecting K65R in antiretroviral-naïve HIV-infected individuals with chronic hepatitis B treated with adefovir. *AIDS* 19, 2036–2038.

18 Colin J, Cazals-Hatem D, Loriot M (1999) Influence of HIV infection on chronic hepatitis B in homosexual men. *Hepatology* 29, 1306–1310.

19 Martín-Carbonero L, Soriano V, Valencia E et al. (2001) Increasing impact of chronic viral hepatitis on hospital admissions and mortality among HIV-infected patients. *AIDS Res Hum Retroviruses* 17, 1467–1472.

20 Soriano V, Puoti M, Sulkowski M et al. (2004) Care of patients with hepatitis C and HIV co-infection. Updated recommendations from the HIV-HCV International Panel. *AIDS* 18, 1–12.

21 Rockstroh J, Mocroft A, Soriano V et al. (2005) Influence of hepatitis C on HIV disease progression and response to antiretroviral therapy. *J Infect Dis* 192, 992–1002.

22 Greub G, Ledergerber B, Battegay M et al. (2000) Clinical progression, survival, and immune recovery during antiretroviral therapy in patients with HIV-1 and HCV coinfections. *Lancet* 356, 1800–1805.

23 Sulkowski M, Moore R, Mehta S et al. (2002) Hepatitis C and progression of HIV disease. *JAMA* 288, 199–206.

24 Nuñez M, Soriano V (2005) Hepatotoxicity of antiretrovirals: incidence, mechanisms and management. *Drug Safety* 28, 53–66.

25 Sulkowski M, Thomas D, Chaisson R et al. (2000) Hepatotoxicity associated with antiretroviral therapy in adults infected with HIV and the role of hepatitis C or B virus infection. *JAMA* 283, 74–80.

26 Núñez M, Ríos P, Martín-Carbonero L et al. (2002) Role of hepatitis C virus genotype in the development of severe transaminase elevation after the introduction of antiretroviral therapy. *J Acquir Immun Defic Syndr* 30, 65–68.

27 Nuñez M, Soriano V (2005) Risks and benefits of antiretroviral therapy in HIV-HCV co-infected patients. *J Hepatol* 42, 290–292.

28 Soriano V, García-Samaniego J, Bravo R et al. (1996) Interferon alpha for the treatment of chronic hepatitis C in patients infected with HIV. *Clin Infect Dis* 23, 585–591.

29 Martin-Cabonero L, Benhamou Y, Puoti M et al. (2004) Incidence and predictors of severe liver fibrosis in HIV infected patients with chronic hepatitis C – a European collaborative study. *Clin Infect Dis* 38, 128–133.

30 Puoti M, Bruno R, Soriano V et al. (2004) Hepatocellular carcinoma in HIV-infected patients: epidemiological features, clinical presentation and outcome. *AIDS* 18, 2285–2293.

31 Soto B, Sanchez-Quijano A, Rodrigo L et al. (1997) HIV infection modifies the natural history of chronic parenteral acquired hepatitis C with an unusually rapid progression to cirrhosis. *J Hepatol* 26, 1–5.

32 Qurishi N, Kreuzberg C, Lüchters G et al. (2003) Effect of antiretroviral therapy on liver-related mortality in patients with HIV and hepatitis C coinfection. *Lancet* 362, 1708–1713.

33 Chung R, Andersen J, Volberding P et al. (2004) Peginterferon Alfa-2a plus ribavirin versus interferon alfa-2a plus ribavirin for chronic hepatitis C in HIV-coinfected persons. *N Engl J Med* 351, 451–459.

34 Carrat F, Bani-Sadr F, Pol S et al. (2004) Pegylated interferon alfa-2b vs standard interferon alfa-2b, plus ribavirin, for chronic hepatitis C in HIV-infected patients. *JAMA* 292, 2839–2848.

35 Torriani F, Rodriguez-Torres M, Rockstroh J et al. (2004) Peginterferon Alfa-2a plus ribavirin for chronic hepatitis C virus infection in HIV-infected patients. *N Engl J Med* 351, 438–450.

36 Laguno M, Murillas J, Blanco JL et al. (2004) Peginterferon alfa-2b plus ribavirin compared with interferon alfa-2b plus ribavirin for treatment of HIV/HCV co-infected patients. *AIDS* 18, F27–36.

37 Soriano V, Martín-Carbonero L, García-Samaniego J (2003) Treatment of chronic hepatitis C virus infection: we must target the virus or liver fibrosis? *AIDS* 17, 751–753.

38 Soriano V, Maida I, Garcia-Samaniego J et al. (2004) Long-term follow-up of HIV-infected patients with chronic hepatitis C virus infection treated with interferon-based therapies. *Antivir Ther* 9, 987–992.

39 Soriano V, Nuñez M, Camino N et al. (2004) Hepatitis C virus-RNA clearance in HIV-coinfected patients with chronic hepatitis C treated with pegylated interferon plus ribavirin. *Antivir Ther* 9, 505–509.

40 Nuñez M, Camino N, Ramos B et al. (2005) Impact of ribavirin exposure on early virological response to hepatitis C therapy in HIV-infected patients with chronic hepatitis C. *Antivir Ther* 10, 657–662.

41 Sherman K, Shire N, Rouster S et al. (2005) Viral kinetics in hepatitis C or hepatitis C/HIV-infected patients. *Gastroenterology* 128, 313–327.

42 Soriano V, Pérez-Olmeda M, Ríos P et al. (2004) Hepatitis C virus (HCV) relapses after anti-HCV therapy are more frequent in HIV-infected patients. *AIDS Res Hum Retroviruses* 20, 351–354.

43 Soriano V, Bravo R, García-Samaniego J et al. (1994) CD4+ T lymphocytopenia in HIV-infected patients receiving interferon therapy for chronic hepatitis C. *AIDS* 8, 1621–1622.

44 De Mendoza C, Sánchez-Conde M, Timmermans E et al. (2005) Mitochondrial DNA depletion in HIV-infected patients is more pronounced with chronic hepatitis C and enhanced following treatment with pegylated interferon plus ribavirin. *Antivir Ther* 10, 557–561.

45 Mauss S, Valenti W, DePamphilis J et al. (2004) Risk factors for hepatic decompensation in patients with HIV/HCV coinfection and liver cirrhosis during interferon therapy. *AIDS* 18, F21–25.

46 Rendon A, Nuñez M, Romero M et al. (2005) Early monitoring of ribavirin plasma concentrations may predict anemia and early virological response in HIV/hepatitis C virus-coinfected patients. *J Acquir Immune Defic Syndr* 39, 401–405.

47 Brouwer J, Nevens F, Bekkering F et al. (2004) Reduction of relapse rates by 18-month treatment in chronic hepatitis C: a Benelux randomised trial in 300 patients. *J Hepatol* 40, 689–695.

48 Drusano G, Preston S (2004) A 48-week duration of therapy with pegylated interferon alpha 2b plus ribavirin may be too short to maximize long-term response among patients infected with genotype-1 hepatitis C virus. *J Infect Dis* 189, 964–970.

49 Neff G, Shire N, Rudich S (2005) Outcomes among patients with end-stage liver disease who are coinfected with HIV and hepatitis C virus. *Clin Infect Dis* 41(Suppl. 1), 50–55.

50 Maida I, Núñez M, González-Lahoz J et al. (2005) Liver transplantation in HIV-HCV coinfected candidates: what is the most appropriate time for evaluation? *AIDS Res Hum Retroviruses* 21, 599–601.

51 Wallace M, Brandt C, Earhart K et al. (2004) Safety and immunogenicity of an inactivated hepatitis A vaccine among HIV-infected subjects. *Clin Infect Dis* 39, 1207–1213.

52 Puoti M, Rossi S, Forleo M et al. (1998) Treatment of chronic hepatitis D with interferon alpha 2b in patients with HIV infection. *J Hepatol* 29, 45–52.

53 Tillmann H, Heiken H, Knapick-Botor A *et al.* (2001) Infection with GB virus C and reduced mortality among HIV-infected patients. *N Engl J Med* 345, 715–724.

54 Kaiser T, Tillmann H (2005) GB virus C infection: is there a clinical relevance for patients with the HIV? *AIDS Rev* 7, 3–12.

55 Soriano V, Tor J, Gabarre E *et al.* (1991) Multifocal splenic abscesses caused by *Mycobacterium tuberculosis* in HIV-infected drug users. *AIDS* 5, 901–902.

56 Poles M, Dieterich D, Schwarz E *et al.* (1996) Liver biopsy findings in 501 patients infected with HIV. *J Acquir Immun Defic Syndr* 11, 170–177.

57 Rabaud C, May T, Amiel C *et al.* (1994) Extracerebral toxoplasmosis inpatients infected with HIV: a French national survey. *Medicine (Baltimore)* 73, 306–314.

58 CDC (2001) Serious adverse events attributed to nevirapine regimens for post-exposure prophylaxis after HIV exposures-worldwide, 1997–2000. *Morb Mortal Wkly Rep* 49, 1153–1156.

59 Sanne I, Mommeja-Marin H, Hinkle J *et al.* (2005) Severe hepatotoxicity associated with nevirapine use in HIV-infected subjects. *J Infect Dis* 191, 825–829.

60 Martínez E, Blanco J, Arnáiz J *et al.* (2001) Hepatotoxicity in HIV-infected patients receiving nevirapine-containing antiretroviral therapy. *AIDS* 15, 1261–1268.

61 Gonzalez de Requena D, Nuñez M, Jimenez-Nacher I *et al.* (2002) Liver toxicity caused by nevirapine. *AIDS* 16, 290–291.

62 Antinori S, Ridolfo A, Esposito R *et al.* (1994) Liver involvement in AIDS-associated malignancies. *J Hepatol* 21, 1145–1146.

9.4 Exotic virus infections of the liver

Viral haemorrhagic fevers

Pierre E. Rollin and Thomas G. Ksiazek

Patients with viral haemorrhagic fevers frequently present with similar and non-specific clinical signs resembling malaria, typhoid fever and pharyngitis. A detailed travel history, coupled with a high index of suspicion and the availability of definitive virological tools, should facilitate a rapid diagnosis and the timely implementation of appropriate patient isolation, clinical management procedures and public health measures.

Lassa fever and other arenaviruses

Arenaviruses cause chronic infections of wild and peridomestic rodents indigenous to Europe, Africa and the Americas. When these asymptomatically infected animals come into contact with man, human disease may result. Arenavirus infections of humans are common and, in some cases, cause severe haemorrhagic fevers.

Aetiological agent and epidemiology

Arenaviruses are spherical enveloped viruses that have a sandy, granular appearance by thin-section electron microscopy. The lipid envelope of arenaviruses makes them susceptible to organic solvents and detergents. The arenavirus genome consists of two single-stranded RNA molecules, which are designated S (small) and L (large). Two genes are encoded in an ambisense orientation on each RNA. The family Arenaviridae is divided into two complexes [1]. The lymphocytic choriomeningitis (LCM) or Old World complex contains LCM virus and the Lassa viruses, and also includes a number of related and apparently benign viruses (Mopeia, Mobala and Ippy). All have been isolated from rodents of the family Muridae. The Tacaribe or New World complex includes several severe human pathogens (Junin, Machupo, Guanarito, Sabia, Flexal and Chapare viruses), some viruses that are responsible for mild laboratory infections (Pichinde, Tacaribe) and some that are not associated with human disease (Amapari, Bear Canyon, Cupixi, Latino, Parana, Oliveros, Pirital, Tamiami and Whitewater Arroyo viruses).

In nature, arenaviruses are maintained by association with specific rodent hosts, in whom they produce chronic viraemia and/or viruria; they are routinely isolated from blood and urine samples. Naturally occurring human disease can usually be traced to direct or indirect contact with infected rodents. Aerosol infectivity is thought to be an important natural route of human infection [1,2]. Attempts to implicate arthropod vectors have been unsuccessful, but ectoparasites taken from viraemic mammalian hosts have occasionally yielded arenavirus isolates. Rodents serve as a food source in Lassa fever-endemic regions and handling of these animals is a risk factor for Lassa virus infection.

Lassa fever is endemic in several countries of West Africa: Sierra Leone, Guinea, Liberia and Nigeria. The rodent reservoir, and certainly the virus, is also present in other West African countries. The natural host species of Lassa virus are African rodents of the genus *Mastomys* [1,2].

The Argentine haemorrhagic fever (AHF)-endemic region is limited to the Pampa area of Argentina, but has shown a continuing northward extension since the first description of the disease, now covering 150 000 square kilometers. The peak incidence occurs during harvesting in May and is correlated with the population density of the reservoir, the drylands vesper mouse (*Calomys musculinus*). Male rural workers were the population at risk; however, health education and recent intensive human vaccination have changed the epidemiological pattern. AHF, caused by the Junin virus, is not usually contagious, although person-to-person transmission by sexual contact has been described [1].

Bolivian haemorrhagic fever (BHF; caused by Machupo virus) has been described in the Beni department of Bolivia. The reservoir of the virus is *Calomys callosus*. BHF is a seasonal disease, with more cases occurring in the dry season. The cases are sporadic, with small clusters of cases caused by human-to-human transmission. In the past, large epidemics in towns have been described following unusually high rodent density levels [1].

Since its description in 1989, Venezuelan haemorrhagic fever (VHF; caused by Guanarito virus) has been restricted to the municipality of Guanarito, in the southern tip of Portuguesa state in Venezuela, with *Zygodontomys brevicauda* being the reservoir. As is often the case with arenaviral haemorrhagic fevers, the seasonal incidence and agricultural activity peaks coincide. Person-to-person transmission has not been observed [1].

The epidemiology of Sabia and Flexal viruses is not known, but severe, or even fatal, laboratory infections have been described for these two viruses.

Pathology and pathogenesis

Arenavirus pathogenesis is difficult to understand from pathological examination of tissues from animal models or humans. The observed lesions cannot explain the severity of the disease and arenaviruses are not highly cytopathic. In Lassa fever, the virus can be isolated from all organs and the liver is consistently affected, as confirmed by aspartate aminotransferase (AST) elevation and pathological examination of liver biopsies or post-mortem tissues [3]. Levels of coagulation factors are slightly decreased and functional disturbances have been found in platelets [4]. In Lassa fever patients, a fatal outcome correlates with low levels of circulating interleukin (IL)-8 and interferon-inducible protein (IP)-10. This down-regulation of the immune system is also associated with an impaired B-cell response: there is a low or absent antibody response in fatal cases. Proinflammatory cytokines are elevated and, in AHF, there is a correlation between mortality and the levels of tumour necrosis factor (TNF)-α and interferon (IFN). In arenavirus infections, haemorrhages result from the activation and dysregulation of infected macrophages, endothelial and inflammatory cells. The levels of virus replication are important and are indirectly correlated with the patient's outcome of infection via a pathophysiological cascade [1].

Clinical manifestations

Lassa fever patients usually present with fever, sore throat, severe lower back pain, cough and conjunctivitis. In tropical areas, this syndrome can easily be misdiagnosed and is very often labeled as malaria. During the second week of infection, digestive signs include nausea, vomiting, diarrhoea and abdominal pain. In most patients, the disease is self-limiting; however, in a small percentage, the disease is more severe and patients are hospitalized. A maculopapular rash, bleeding from the gums and the nose, haematemesis and oedema of the face may develop, but frank haemorrhage is seen in only a proportion of the most severe cases. Pleural and pericardial effusions are common and can be massive. Respiratory distress, hypovolemic shock and bleeding are usually associated with fatal cases, which is the outcome in 15–20% of patients with Lassa fever who are hospitalized. Central nervous system involvement (seizures and encephalopathy) is frequent [5]. Lassa fever is a particularly severe disease among pregnant women, and fetal loss occurs in more than 80% of cases [6]. Ataxia and deafness are not uncommon sequelae. In infants, swollen-baby syndrome, which is characterized by anasarca, abdominal distension and bleeding, is also typical [2].

The clinical pictures of AHF, BHF and VHF are similar. Incubation periods range from 7 to 14 days and the onset is generally gradual, with fever, anorexia and malaise occurring over several days. The disease is multisystemic, including the gastrointestinal, cardiovascular and central nervous systems. On initial examination, flushing of the face, neck and chest and bleeding from the gums with enanthem are common. Other complications include extensive petechial haemorrhages, oozing from puncture wounds, melena and haematemesis. In addition, among the 15% of patients who die from these conditions, hypotension and shock may develop. During the second week of illness, clinical improvement may begin or complications may develop. Neurological involvement ranges from mild irritability and lethargy to coma, delirium and convulsions in severely ill patients, with or without any haemorrhagic manifestations. Recovery is slow; weakness, fatigue and mental difficulties may last for weeks. In AHF, a significant proportion of patients relapse with a 'late neurological syndrome', which includes headache, cerebellar tremor and cranial nerve palsies; deafness has also been described as a sequela [1].

Laboratory findings

In Lassa fever, patients are frequently dehydrated and have high haematocrits. Proteinuria is usually present, and lymphopenia and relative or absolute neutrophilia is the rule. Platelet numbers are reduced but, most importantly, an inhibitor of platelet function (e.g. aggregation) is present [4,5]. A serum AST level of 150 units/mL or higher on admission is associated with a high risk of mortality [7]. The impact of infection on liver function is limited (glucose and bilirubin are normal) and cannot be responsible for the severity of the disease [8,9]. In contrast to Lassa fever, clinical laboratory studies in cases of Junin virus infection are frequently useful for diagnosis. Proteinuria is constant. Total leukocyte counts usually fall to 1000–2000 cells/μL, although the differential remains normal. Platelet counts fall precipitously, usually to between 25 000 and 100 000 cells/μL. Routine clotting parameters are usually normal or slightly abnormal; however, patients with severe cases of disease may show evidence of disseminated intravascular coagulation (DIC). Transaminases generally remain normal [1].

Diagnosis

The specific diagnosis of arenavirus haemorrhagic fever requires biological containment and is limited to only a few laboratories in the world. Acute human infections are associated with viraemia. Viral antigen, viral RNA or virus can easily be identified by antigen detection enzyme-linked immunosorbent assay (ELISA), reverse transcriptase-PCR (RT-PCR) or isolation respectively [10,11]. In the rapidly fatal forms of Lassa or Machupo haemorrhagic fevers, patients may often die without any detectable antibodies. Specific antibodies become detectable in the second week of the disease and can be detected using IgM capture ELISA and IgG ELISA tests. Immunohistochemical assays can be used to detect virus antigen in liver biopsies or tissues collected during post-mortem.

Treatment and prevention

Barrier nursing is very important in arenavirus haemorrhagic fever and should be implemented as early as possible. Numerous episodes of nosocomial infection have been described for Lassa and Machupo haemorrhagic fever. Specimens collected for diagnosis and management of the patient should also be handled with extreme precautions. Variable results have been observed in the treatment of Lassa fever with immune plasma. Convalescent immune plasma, selected on the basis of neutralizing antibody concentration, has been used with success for the treatment of AHF [1]. About 10% of the recipients developed a transient neurological syndrome. Intravenous ribavirin, a broad-spectrum antiviral, is the treatment of choice for Lassa fever [6,7]. Its efficacy is particularly evident when used early in the disease. Treatment starts with a loading dose of 30 mg/kg (with a maximum of 2 g), followed by 16 mg/kg every 6 h for 4 days and 8 mg/kg every 8 h for 6 days. Ribavirin is also likely to be an effective therapy for South American arenavirus infections.

No vaccine is currently available for Lassa fever. A Junin vaccine has been developed and is used in the endemic area. This vaccine also protects non-human primates against Machupo virus.

Rift Valley fever

The Rift Valley fever (RVF) virus is a mosquito-borne agent that is mainly responsible for disease in domestic ruminants (sheep, goats and cattle). The virus was though to be enzootic in East Africa only, but has been found in virtually all sub-Saharan countries. The virus was responsible for massive animal and human epidemics that occurred in 'virgin soil', including Egypt, and, more recently, Saudi Arabia and Yemen [3].

Aetiological agent and epidemiology

The RVF virus is a negative-sense, trisegmented, single-stranded RNA enveloped virus belonging to the family Bunyaviridae. The virus was first isolated in 1930 during an outbreak of disease in sheep in the Rift Valley of Kenya. For many years, heavy rainy seasons in this area were regularly followed by small epidemics in ruminants. The virus was also found to be present in other countries, but the human impact was very limited with a few cases of self-limiting febrile illness. However, in 1977, a massive epidemic occurred in Egypt, with more than 200 000 people infected and nearly 600 deaths. Because of the large number of cases, a more complete clinical spectrum of human disease was reported. Since the Egyptian outbreak, there have been several sites of considerable outbreaks in animals and humans, including Mauritania in 1987, Madagascar in 1990, and Saudi Arabia and Yemen in 2000 [12,13]. Although the enzootic maintenance and transmission cycle is not entirely understood, heavy rains and flooding, irrigated farming and water management (dams) have an obvious impact on the populations of *Culex* and *Aedes* mosquitoes before and during outbreaks. Susceptibility to the virus among breeds of animals is variable, but the abortion rate can reach 100% in afffected pregnant animals and mortality in young animals is also very high. Because of the lack of effective animal disease surveillance systems, severe human disease has very often been the initial indicator revealing epizootics.

Pathology and pathogenesis

A viraemic phase, corresponding to an initial febrile period, is the first step in infection and leads to dissemination of the virus, with secondary replication in endothelial cells and hepatocytes. RVF virus is very cytolytic and infection results in hepatocellular degeneration, necrosis that is mainly centrizonal and scattered lobular foci of necrosis [3]. Massive necrosis associated with the loss of hepatic architecture is seen in the severe form of disease, as demonstrated by immunohistochemistry of post-mortem specimens. Intrathecal replication of the virus is at the origin of RVF encephalitis. The pathogenesis of retinal lesions is not understood, but is coincidental with the onset of antibody circulation. In non-human primate models, the late onset of the IFN response is associated with more severe disease and DIC, suggesting that the early production of IFN is influential in limiting the severity of disease; in the same model, prophylactic administration of recombinant IFN-α limited viraemia, hepatocellular damage and haemostatic derangement [14].

Clinical manifestations

The most frequent clinical manifestations include the sudden onset of fever, myalgia, headache and anorexia of a week's duration, followed by a complete recovery. Three other clinical syndromes have been seen, particularly in large outbreaks of disease. Some patients develop an acute decrease in visual acuity about 5–15 days after the onset of disease. Retinal lesions can be uni- or bilateral and are characterized by macular lesions, edema, vasculitis and haemorrhage. Recovery is often not complete and half of these patients have some permanent loss of vision [12,15,16]. The other two severe complications have been described in approximately 1% of the total number of cases. In the haemorrhagic fever form of the disease, haemorrhagic manifestations become evident in the few days following onset of disease, with epistaxis, gingival bleeding, haematemesis and melena. The prognosis is very bad, frequently with DIC and hepatic and renal failure. A few other patients develop headache, meningismus and confusion, 7–10 days after onset. In this meningoencephalitic form of the disease, the mortality rate is high and residual sequelae are frequent. Human-to-human transmission has never been described, although laboratory infections commonly occur in individuals.

Laboratory findings

In acute uncomplicated RVF, clinical laboratory tests show leukopenia, but liver function tests and platelet counts are within the normal range. In the severe syndromes, half of the patients show anaemia with evidence of DIC. The most obvious abnormal findings are marked abnormal liver function tests [elevated alanine aminotransferase (ALT) and AST]; lactic dehydrogenase and creatine phosphokinase levels are also elevated [13,15,17,18]. Hepatic failure is frequent and may lead to fatal hepatic encephalopathy. Renal failure with high creatinine and urea levels is also common and may require haemodialysis [12]. In patients with encephalitis, the cerebrospinal fluid shows pleocytosis (mostly lymphocytes) and normal glucose and protein concentrations.

Diagnosis

At the very acute stage of RFV disease, viraemia is very significant and it is easy to detect viral antigen (by antigen capture ELISA), viral RNA (by RT-PCR) or virus (by isolation) [11,13]. After 1–2 days, the virus or antigen can no longer be detected because of the presence of detectable IgM and IgG antibodies. As for other diseases, it is best to use a combination of the available assays for diagnosis. The same tests can be applied to confirm a clinical suspicion of disease in animals. Specific immunohistochemical assays can detect viral antigen in post-mortem human and animal specimens (liver being the optimal specimen).

Treatment and prevention

There is no specific antiviral treatment for RVF disease. Most patients with severe disease should receive supportive care, including intravenous fluids and, when indicated, blood and freshly frozen plasma transfusions, mechanical ventilation, haemodialysis and antimicrobial therapy for secondary bacterial or fungal infections [12,13]. Ribavirin is effective against RVF virus in cell culture but, during one human trial, there was no suggestion of any benefit for patients and a suggestion of adverse effects. Very effective inactivated vaccines against RVF have been developed by the US Department of Defense, but they are not available for the general population. Proper vaccination of domestic animals in the endemic area is possible and important, as livestock usually serve as the amplificatory step.

Marburg and Ebola virus diseases

The Marburg and Ebola viruses, which are filoviruses, are responsible for severe disease in Central Africa. Although case fatality rates vary between the viruses, the symptomatology,

progression of disease, pathogenesis and epidemiology are very similar, and only specific laboratory testing allows a specific diagnosis to be made.

Aetiological agent and epidemiology

The viral genomes of the Marburg and Ebola viruses consist of nonsegmented, negative-sense, single-stranded RNAs. These viruses contain seven virus-specific structural proteins that are expressed from seven genes [19]. The Marburg and Ebola viruses are easy to identify by electron microscopy because of the characteristic combination of the size and shape of the virions: they have widely variable lengths, as well as branching circular or '6' shapes. Phylogenetic analysis clearly separates the Marburg and Ebola viruses into two genera, *Marburgvirus* and *Ebolavirus*, with one species for the Marburg virus and four for the Ebola virus: Zaire *Ebolavirus* (EBO-Z), Sudan *Ebolavirus* (EBO-S), Reston *Ebolavirus* (EBO-R) and Tai forest *Ebolavirus* (formerly known as Ivory Coast *Ebolavirus*) [19]. Heat, lipid solvents, β-propiolactone, formaldehyde, ultraviolet light and gamma radiation can be used to inactivate these viruses.

The Marburg virus was the first filovirus to be recognized: in 1967, 31 individuals in Germany and Yugoslavia became infected following contact with monkeys or their tissues or with other patients. In 1976, Ebola virus was responsible for two simultaneous outbreaks in Zaire and Sudan. Around 500 cases were reported, with case-fatality rates of 88% in Zaire and 53% in Sudan. Despite the simultaneous emergence, these viruses (EBO-Z and EBO-S) are distinct species by serological and sequence analysis criteria. More recently, two additional distinct Ebola virus species have been isolated. In 1989, a new strain of Ebola virus (EBO-R) was isolated from monkeys held in quarantine in Virginia (USA), following importation from the Philippines. No human disease was recorded, although several animal handlers at the quarantine facility seroconverted. EBO-R reappeared in monkeys exported from the same facility in the Philippines to Siena, Italy, in 1992 and to Alice, Texas, in 1996. In 1994, the fourth genetically distinct species of Ebola virus (Tai forest *Ebolavirus*) was associated with disease in a human and deaths among chimpanzees in West Africa.

In 1995, EBO-Z was responsible for a massive outbreak in Zaire and, subsequently (1996, 2001–2005), a number of outbreaks occurred in Gabon and adjacent areas of the Republic of Congo among apes and humans; several of the human cases were exposed to infected non-human primates. In 2000, EBO-S was responsible for a large outbreak of disease in Gulu, in the north-west of Uganda. More than 400 people were infected and 53% of them died. In 2004, in Yambio (Sudan), 17 individuals were infected with EBO-S and seven of them died. From 1999 to 2000, an outbreak of disease caused by the Marburg virus occurred in the eastern Democratic Republic of Congo. In the spring of 2005, a large outbreak of Marburg occurred in Uige, northern Angola, with a total of 252 cases and 227 deaths reported by the end of August of that year. Following every large outbreak, a search for the animal reservoirs of filoviruses have been made without success. Non-human primates, the source of many human infections, are not considered to be a likely reservoir. The real reservoirs have not yet been found, although recent data have implicated fruit bats [20].

Pathology and pathogenesis

The understanding of the pathogenesis of these diseases is derived from animal-model studies and from the very few human specimens, including tissues, collected during outbreaks. Extensive and disseminated infection and necrosis is obvious in major organs such as the liver, spleen, lung and kidney. Extensive hepatocellular necrosis is associated with the formation of characteristic intracytoplasmic viral inclusions; lymphoid depletion is particularly obvious in the spleen; and virus replication in endothelial cells and macrophages plays a role in vascular dysregulation and permeability, cytokine induction and haemostatic balance [19].

Clinical manifestations

Marburg and Ebola virus infections are clinically similar. The incubation period varies from 4 to 16 days. The onset is sudden and marked by a non-specific syndrome, including fever, chills, headache, anorexia, and myalgia. Digestive signs and symptoms follow: nausea, vomiting, sore throat, abdominal pain and diarrhoea. On examination, patients are usually dehydrated, apathetic and disoriented. Pharyngeal and conjunctival injection is usual. After 3–4 days, a characteristic maculopapular rash over the trunk, petechiae and mucous membrane haemorrhages appear; however, they may be difficult to see on dark-skinned patients. Gastrointestinal bleeding is common, accompanied by intense epigastric pain. Severe cases can develop petechiae and bleeding from puncture wounds and mucous membranes [21,22]. Multiorgan failure with shock usually precedes death, which occurs in 80–90% and 51% of cases of EBO-Z and EBO-S respectively. The case-mortality rates in Marburg virus infection have varied from 30% in the original outbreak to 90% in the recent outbreak in Angola.

Laboratory findings

Clinical laboratory studies usually reveal an early and profound leukopenia, which is sometimes moderately elevated at a later stage. Platelet counts decline to 50 000–100 000 cells/μL during the haemorrhagic phase. Elevated liver enzyme (AST and ALT) values reflect the gravity of the syndrome [21]. Abnormalities in coagulation parameters include fibrin split products and prolonged prothrombin and partial thromboplastin times, suggesting that DIC is a terminal event and usually associated with multiorgan failure. More recent studies have shown that D-dimers are detectable early in the disease. During the terminal stages, kidney failure is confirmed by high creatinine and blood urea nitrogen values. Ebola or Marburg viral antigens

are present at high levels in all tissues, including the skin, allowing a specific diagnosis to be made post-mortem by immunohistochemistry.

Diagnosis

The specific diagnosis of filovirus infection requires tests that are not usually available in the endemic areas of these viruses, or in any hospital in the western world. Diagnosis initially requires the elimination of a number of viral haemorrhagic fevers. In general, viraemia and antigenaemia are present during the acute phase of the disease. The best approach is to use a combination of tests, including antigen detection ELISA assay, RT-PCR (usually more sensitive but subject to artifacts and contamination) and IgM capture ELISA [11,23,24]. RT-PCR has the advantage of allowing genetic analysis of the products. Virus can be isolated, but this requires time and adequate levels of containment (BSL-4 level). During rapid fatal disease, patients may often die without any detectable antibodies; however, ELISA tests can be used to detect IgM antibodies, which may be present during illness and usually appear early in convalescence. IgG ELISA tests play little role in establishing acute diagnosis, but can be used for retrospective or epidemiological studies. Post-mortem diagnosis can be carried out using specific immunohistochemical analysis of tissues, including skin biopsies, collected after deaths that are suspected to be caused by filovirus infection; this is a distinct advantage in highly fatal diseases [25].

Treatment and prevention

Barrier nursing and the avoidance of parenteral exposure of hospital staff are important in the management of filovirus infections because of the frequency with which nosocomial transmission is seen. Symptomatic and supportive management, with careful maintenance of fluid balance, is the only available treatmtent option at this time. No antiviral drugs or vaccines are currently available for human use, but several candidate vaccines have shown potential in animal models.

Crimean–Congo haemorrhagic fever

Crimean–Congo haemorrhagic fever (CCHF) was first recognized in the Crimean peninsula (former USSR) at the end of the Second World War. In 1969, the causal virus was found to be identical to a virus isolated from a febrile child in 1956 in Stanleyville, a town in the former Belgian Congo [26,27]. Since then, the virus has been found from Africa to the western provinces of China.

Aetiological agent and epidemiology

The CCHF virus, a tick-borne virus found in Africa, eastern Europe and Asia, belongs to the genus *Nairovirus* of the family Bunyaviridae. The genome is composed of three segments of negative-sense, single-stranded RNA. Virions contain two envelope glycoproteins, a nucleocapsid protein and a RNA polymerase. The CCHF virus is an enveloped virus.

CCHF virus has been isolated from 30 species of ixodid ticks and, with the exception of Madagascar, the distribution of the virus overlaps with the distribution of *Hyalomma* ticks. These ticks feed on different hosts during their life-cycle, from rodents and birds to small ruminants and cattle. Transovarial transmission of virus from female ticks to progeny occurs [27]. Although several species of mammal can be infected, disease only develops in humans. The virus is usually contracted through the bite of an infected tick, or by contact with blood or tissue from a viraemic animal or a patient at home or in a hospital setting. The number of human cases during outbreaks is usually small and, frequently, those in contact with animals (farm or slaughterhouse workers) are at the origin of the infection; health-care personnel who take care of infected patients are involved secondarily in small clusters [13].

Pathology and pathogenesis

Because of the lack of an animal model, the occurrence of the disease in remote areas and the limited number of specialized laboratories, the pathogenesis of CCHF is poorly understood. Few tissues collected during necropsies have been made available for analysis. Pathological examination of liver tissue reveals hepatocellular necrosis with prominent Councilman bodies, hypertrophic Kupffer cells and lack of inflammatory mononuclear cell infiltrates. Abundant immunostaining of CCHF virus antigens reveals replication of the virus in hepatocytes, mononuclear phagocytes and endothelial cells [28]. The infection of endothelial cells plays an important role in the vascular leakage and haemostasis that are observed in the disease [13].

Clinical manifestations

The incubation period can be as short as 3 days but is usually around 7 days. Onset is characterized by the sudden appearance of headache, dizziness, fever, nausea, vomiting and abdominal pain. Behavioural changes, such as somnolence or depression, are frequent; some patients are confused or even aggressive [29,30]. During the clinical examination, conjunctival injection and enanthem are usually obvious and lymphadenopathies and hepatomegaly may be present, as well as tenderness of the right upper quadrant of the abdomen. A petechial rash on the trunk and limbs may be seen by the end of the first week of illness [27,30,31]. In some patients, large ecchymoses and bruises are indications of the haemorrhagic tendencies of CCHF infections. Epistaxis, haematemesis and melena are common. The most severely ill patients develop multiorgan failure, coma and DIC [27,29,31,32]. In mild forms of the disease, defervescence is observed during the second week, with progressive general improvement; convalescence is usually prolonged.

Laboratory findings

Leukopenia is only transient, but thrombocytopenia is an early and consistent feature of CCHF. Elevations of blood urea nitrogen and creatinine levels are accompagnied by proteinuria. All patients have abnormal liver functions, with elevated levels of serum AST, ALT and gamma-glutamyltransferase [18,29]. Most patients show a decline in haemoglobin levels [27,31,32]. During the course of fatal infections, elevations of the prothrombin ratio, activated partial thromboplastin time, fibrin degradation products and D-dimers, and low fibrinogen levels, are typical of DIC.

Diagnosis

Laboratory diagnosis of the infection at the early stage of the disease is carried out by detection of the CCHF virus, antigen or RNA. This is achieved using an antigen detection ELISA or by RT-PCR analysis of serum or blood [11,27,29]. Virus isolation from cell cultures or suckling mice is sensitive but requires several days and a laboratory with adequate levels of containment. Tissues collected during necropsies are also suitable for CCHF antigen, RNA or virus isolation [13,28]. In addition, immunohistochemical assays can specifically confirm the aetiological diagnosis [28]. IgM and IgG antibodies, detectable by ELISA, may often be absent in fatal cases and appear later in the disease process.

Treatment and prevention

Most of the facilities where CCHF patients are hospitalized have no diagnostic capabilities and the treatment is symptomatic. Good barrier-nursing practices should be initiated in areas where disease is present [13]. Ribavirin is effective against the CCHF virus in cell cultures and, although no rigorous clinical trials have been carried out, intravenous and oral ribavirin have been used in South Africa, Pakistan, Iran and Turkey with apparent success [31–33].

Disclaimer

The findings and conclusions in this report are those of the authors and do not necessarily represent the views of the funding agency.

References

1 Enria D, Mills JA, Flick R *et al.* (2006) Arenavirus infections. In: Guerrant RL, Walker DH, Weller PF (eds) *Tropical Infectious Diseases. Principles, Pathogens and Practice*, 2nd edn. Philadelphia, PA: Elsevier Churchill Livingstone, pp. 734–755.

2 Gunther S, Lenz O (2004) Lassa virus. *Crit Rev Clin Lab Sci* 41, 339–390.

3 Walker DH, McCormick JB, Johnson KM *et al.* (1982) Pathologic and virologic study of fatal Lassa fever in man. *Am J Pathol* 107, 349–356.

4 Cummins D, Fisher-Hoch SP, Walshe KJ et al. (1989) A plasma inhibitor of platelet aggregation in patients with Lassa fever. Br J Haematol 72, 543–548.

5 Cummins D (1992) Lassa fever encephalopathy: clinical and laboratory findings. J Trop Med Hyg 95, 197–201.

6 McCormick JB, King IJ, Webb PA et al. (1987) A case-control study of the clinical diagnosis and course of Lassa fever. J Infect Dis 155, 445–455.

7 Johnson KM, McCormick JB, Webb PA et al. (1987) Clinical virology of Lassa fever in hospitalized patients. J Infect Dis 155, 456–464.

8 McCormick JB, Walker DH, King IJ et al. (1986) Lassa virus hepatitis: a study of fatal Lassa fever in humans. Am J Trop Med Hyg 35, 401–407.

9 Schmitz H, Kohler B, Laue T et al. (2002) Monitoring of clinical and laboratory data in two cases of imported Lassa fever. Microbes Infect 4, 43–50.

10 Bausch DG, Rollin PE, Demby AH et al. (2000) Diagnosis and clinical virology of Lassa fever as evaluated by enzyme-linked immunosorbent assay, indirect fluorescent-antibody test, and virus isolation. J Clin Microbiol 38, 2670–2677.

11 Drosten C, Gottig S, Schilling S et al. (2002) Rapid detection and quantification of RNA of Ebola and Marburg viruses, Lassa virus, Crimean-Congo hemorrhagic fever virus, Rift Valley fever virus, Dengue virus, and Yellow fever virus by real-time reverse transcription-PCR. J Clin Microbiol 40, 2323–2330.

12 Madani TA, Al-Mazrou YY, Al-Jeffri MH et al. (2003) Rift Valley fever epidemic in Saudi Arabia: epidemiological, clinical, and laboratory characteristics. Clin Infect Dis 37, 1084–1092.

13 Watts DM, Flick R, Peters CJ et al. (2006) Bunyaviral fevers: Rift Valley fever and Crimean-Congo hemorrhagic fever. In: Guerrant RL, Walker DH, Weller PF (eds) Tropical Infectious Diseases. Principles, Pathogens and Practice. Philadelphia, PA: Elsevier Churchill Livingstone, pp. 756–761.

14 Morrill JC, Jennings JB, Johnson AL et al. (1990) Pathogenesis of Rift Valley fever in rhesus monkeys: role of interferon response. Arch Virol 110, 195–212.

15 van Velden DJ, Meyer JD, Olivier J et al. (1977) Rift Valley fever affecting humans in South Africa: a clinicopathological study. South African Med J 51, 867–871.

16 Al-Hazmi M, Ayoola EA, Abduraman M et al. (2003) Epidemic Rift Valley fever in Saudi Arabia: a clinical study of severe illness in humans. Clin Infect Dis 36, 245–252.

17 Adam F, Jouan A, Philippe B et al. (1992) Biological parameters of patients infected by the Rift Valley fever virus in Rosso (Mauritania). Presse Medicale – Paris 21, 1731.

18 Ayoola AE, Al-Hazmi MH, Michail NT et al. (2003) Liver involvement in patients with moderately severe Rift Valley fever. Am J Gastroenterol 98(9 Suppl), S92.

19 Sanchez A, Khan AS, Zaki SR et al. (2001) Filoviridae: Marburg and Ebola viruses. In: Fields' Virology, 4th edn. Philadelphia, PA: Lippincott Williams & Wilkins, pp. 1279–1304.

20 Leroy EM, Kumulungui B, Pourrut X et al. (2005) Fruit bats as reservoirs of Ebola virus. Nature 438, 575–576.

21 Martini GA (1971) Marburg virus disease. Clinical syndrome. In: Martini GA, Siegert R (eds) Marburg Virus Disease. New York: Springer-Verlag, pp. 1–9.

22 Bwaka M, Bonnet M-J, Calain P et al. (1999) Ebola hemorrhagic fever in Kikwit, Democratic Republic of Congo (former Zaire): clinical observations. J Infect Dis 179(Suppl 1), S1–7.

23 Ksiazek TG, Rollin PE, Williams AJ et al. (1999) Clinical virology of Ebola hemorrhagic fever (EHF) virus: virus, virus antigen, and IgG and IgM findings among EHF patients in Kikwit, Democratic Republic of Congo, 1995. J Infect Dis 179(Suppl), S177–187.

24 Towner JS, Rollin PE, Bausch DG et al. (2004) Rapid diagnosis of ebola hemorrhagic fever by reverse transcription-PCR in an outbreak setting and assessment of patient viral load as a predictor of outcome. J Virol 78, 4330–4341.

25 Zaki SR, Shieh W-J, Greer PW et al. (1999) A novel immunohistochemical assay for detection of Ebola virus in skin: implications for diagnosis, spread, and surveillance of Ebola hemorrhagic fever. J Infect Dis 177(Suppl 1), S36–47.

26 Casals J (1969) Antigenic similarity between the virus causing Crimean hemorrhagic fever and Congo virus. Proc Soc Exp Biol Med 131, 2333–2336.

27 Hoogstraal H (1979) The epidemiology of tick-borne Crimean-Congo hemorrhagic fever in Asia, Europe, and Africa. J Med Entomol 15, 307–417.

28 Burt FJ, Swanepoel R, Shieh W-J et al. (1997) Immunohistochemical and in situ localization of Crimean-Congo hemorrhagic fever (CCHF) virus in human tissues and implications for CCHF pathogenesis. Arch Pathol Lab Med 121, 839–846.

29 Swanepoel R, Gill DE, Shepherd AJ et al. (1989) The clinical pathology of Crimean-Congo hemorrhagic fever. Rev Infect Dis 11(Suppl 4), 794–800.

30 Athar MN, Baqai HZ, Ahmad M et al. (2003) Crimean-Congo hemorrhagic fever outbreak in Rawalpindi, Pakistan, February 2002. Am J Trop Med Hyg 69, 284–287.

31 Jamil B, Hasan RS, Sarwari AR et al. (2005) Crimean-Congo hemorrhagic fever: experience at a tertiary care hospital in Karachi, Pakistan. Trans Royal Soc Trop Med Hyg 99, 577–584.

32 Ozkurt Z, Kiki I, Erol S et al. (2006) Crimean-Congo hemorrhagic fever in Eastern Turkey: clinical features, risk factors and efficacy of ribavirin therapy. J Infect 52, 207–215.

33 Mardani M, Jahromi MK, Naieni KH et al. (2003) The efficacy of oral ribavirin in the treatment of Crimean-Congo hemorrhagic fever in Iran. Clin Infect Dis 36, 1613–1618.

Dengue and yellow fever

Alberto Queiroz Farias and Flair José Carrilho

Dengue

Aetiological agent and epidemiology

Dengue infection is currently ranked as the most important mosquito-borne viral disease worldwide. The disease is endemic in more than 100 countries and affects 100 million people, mainly in tropical and subtropical regions, with 450 000 annual cases of the haemorrhagic form of the disease. The vector is the day-biting mosquito of the genus *Aedes*, usually *Aedes aegypti*, although *A. albopictus* and *A. polynesensis* may also have epidemiological relevance depending on the geographical location.

A. aegypti breeds in small collections of water and the eggs are resistant to desiccation. Transovarial virus transmission may account for the maintenance of a reservoir without human participation. The dengue virus is a single-stranded RNA virus of the Flaviviridae family with a genome of 11 kb. The disease is caused by any of the four dengue virus serotypes (DEN-1 to DEN-4). The infection induces specific, but not cross-protective, immunity [1,2].

Pathology and pathogenesis

The dengue virus replicates within cells of the mononuclear phagocyte system and in mast, dendritic and endothelial cells. Bone marrow suppression occurs in dengue infection and contributes to low lymphocyte and platelet counts [3,4]. Occasionally, the dengue virus crosses the blood–brain barrier and causes encephalitis. The viraemic and infective phase lasts for up to 5 days after the onset of symptoms and is followed by the appearance of specific IgM antibodies around the sixth day [5]. Most of the patients recover, but a small percentage of cases progress to dengue haemorrhagic fever (DHF), which is characterized by plasma leakage. The risk of severe disease is highly increased in cases of sequential infection by a different serotype. Circulating cross-reacting non-neutralizing antibodies, either from previous dengue episodes or from acquired maternal IgG in the neonatal period, are implicated in DHF. During secondary infection, the Fc portion of those antibodies forms complexes with the dengue virus and enhances cell-surface binding and entry of the second virus serotype into macrophages, leading to DHF [6]. The underlying pathophysiological process in DHF is increased capillary permeability, producing plasma leakage; microscopically, there is no necrosis or inflammation of capillary vessels. Higher levels of cytokines and other markers of activated T cells support the role of these mediators in increasing capillary permeability.

The liver in dengue virus infection

Liver involvement is characterized by focal midzonal necrosis of varying degrees of severity and by microvesicular steatosis. Focal perivenular necrosis and dropout of hepatocytes are common findings. Low-grade inflammation is usually found and residual parenchymal calcification may occur. Plate 9.4.1 (facing p. 72) shows immunohistochemical staining of dengue virus antigen in liver tissue.

Clinical manifestations

The incubation period is 4–7 days. Dengue infection may be asymptomatic. According to the World Health Organization (WHO), symptomatic infections can be classified into three categories [1,7,8]:

1 Undifferentiated fever – usually seen in primary infection and indistinguishable from other acute viral disorders.

2 Dengue fever – characterized by sudden onset of high fever (40°C or 104°F) with a biphasic course and including two or more of the following manifestations: intense myalgia ('breakbone fever'), arthralgia, headache, retro-orbital pain, leukopenia and haemorrhagic diathesis. Manifestations such as flushing, coryza, rash and seizure may also occur. The tourniquet test may be positive in some subjects, presumably because of capillary fragility.

3 DHF – the WHO case definition must fulfill all of the following four criteria:
- acute sudden onset of high fever for 2–7 days;
- haemorrhagic manifestations demonstrated by spontaneous bleeding or positive tourniquet test;
- platelet count $< 100 \times 10^9$ cells/L;
- plasma leakage shown by a raised packed cell volume of $> 20\%$ in serial measurements or by the development of ascites or pleural effusions.

DHF is classified into four grades of severity based on the presence of spontaneous bleeding and the severity of plasma leakage. Dengue shock syndrome includes DHF grades III and IV. Although rare, DHF may be complicated by myocarditis, haemolytic uremic syndrome, acute renal failure, encephalopathy, encephalitis and fulminant liver failure.

Laboratory findings and diagnosis

Laboratory findings are variable and more conspicuous in DHF. The most common findings are a decreased platelet count, leukopenia, atypical lymphocytosis, an abnormal coagulation profile and reduced serum complement levels. Liver enzymes are elevated in most infected individuals. Infections with DEN-3 or DEN-4 serotypes are believed to induce a higher increase in liver enzymes than other genotypes. Other findings include low albumin levels and acid–base and electrolyte disturbances.

A definite diagnosis of dengue virus infection depends on the detection of specific circulating antibodies, viral isolation and detection of viral RNA in tissue or serum samples. The monoclonal antibody-based capture enzyme-linked immunosorbent assay (ELISA) is still the most commonly used serological test. However, antibodies are not detectable until at least 5 days after infection, and cross-reactivity with other flaviviruses is possible. Inoculation on mosquito cell cultures (mainly the C6/36 clone of *A. albopictus*) has become the standard technique for dengue virus isolation. Viral RNA detection by reverse transcriptase-polymerase chain reaction (RT-PCR) may be used; however, it still needs to be internationally standardized [9–11].

Treatment, prognosis and prevention

Most cases are self-limited and hospitalization is not required. Treatment is merely symptomatic. Antiviral drugs are not effective, but therapy with paracetamol has been proposed. Acetylsalicylic acid (aspirin) should be avoided because of the risks of bleeding episodes and the development of Reye syndrome. In the case of DHF or dengue shock syndrome, the life-threatening forms of the infection, therapy is aimed at adequate and prompt fluid replacement. Although dengue fever is self-limited, DHF is associated with high mortality rates. Adequate supportive therapy for DHF has been reported to successfully decrease fatalities from 40% to less than 1%. Currently, no effective vaccine is commercially available. The most effective strategy for prevention of infection is vector control, which may be achieved by removing stagnant pools of water around houses, treating stored water with larvicide, the biological control of vectors (with the use of larvivorous fish or endotoxin-producing bacteria) and education [1,12].

Yellow fever

Aetiological agent and epidemiology

Yellow fever (YF) is a systemic mosquito-borne viral infection that affects approximately 200 000 individuals annually in tropical regions of Africa and Central and South America. The disease probably originated in Africa and was brought to the New World during the period of the slave trade. The infectious agent is a flavivirus of 25–65 nm in size, and there are seven strains that are infectious to man. In Africa, YF is endemic in 29 countries and both rural and urban outbreaks have occurred. In the Americas, YF has not been reported in urban areas for the last 50 years and is now restricted to the tropical rain forests. There are two cycles of YF in endemic regions: the forest (jungle or sylvatic) cycle and the urban cycle. In America, the forest cycle is maintained in monkeys and, probably, in rodents. The vectors are *Haemagogus* spp. and *Sabethes* spp. forest-dwelling mosquitoes. The *Aedes aegypti* mosquito is responsible for urban outbreaks. In Africa, infection in monkeys, mainly Cercopithecus monkeys (vervet), accounts for the jungle cycle, and a number of *Aedes* spp. mosquitoes play a role in virus transmission. Infected hosts transmit the YF virus to mosquitoes during the period of fever. The intrinsic cycle in the mosquito is 4–18 days, depending on environmental conditions, and the infection is lifelong in mosquitoes. Transovarial viral transmission contributes to YF virus maintenance during the dry seasons. Individuals entering the forest are bitten by mosquitoes that have acquired infection from primates; these individuals then serve as reservoirs when they return to urban areas. The peridomiciliar *A. aegypti* may disseminate the YF virus, beginning the urban cycle [3,13,14]. Interhuman transmission is unimportant. YF virus has also been isolated from the tick *Amblyomma variegatum*, but the epidemiological significance of this finding is unclear [15].

Pathology and pathogenesis

Initial replication probably takes place in the draining lymph nodes. During the subsequent haematogenous dissemination, the liver becomes the principal focus of infection. Kupffer cells are infected first, followed by hepatocytes. Pathogenesis is mediated by direct viral injury to hepatocytes. Stroma cells are not involved, and typical lesions may not be found in biopsy specimens during the recovery phase. Liver involvement is conspicuous and characterized by extensive midzonal necrosis with minimal inflammation. The more intense immunostaining of YF antigens in the midzonal region suggests a specific viral tropism toward zone 2.

Lesions in other organs are variable. Myocarditis is characterized by degenerative and focal fatty changes and may result in circulatory dysfunction and arrhythmias. Fatty changes may be seen in the sinoatrial node and in the bundle of His and are related to the clinical finding of bradycardia. Encephalitis, cerebral edema and perivascular haemorrhages can also occur. In the kidneys, the most important pathological findings are in the renal tubules, which show acute tubular necrosis and fatty changes. Haemorrhagic diathesis is characterized by decreased synthesis of clotting factors and disseminated intravascular coagulation. Haemorrhages occur in the digestive system, eyes, lungs, uterus, liver, spleen and kidneys. The number of spleen and lymph node lymphocytes decrease and adrenal lesions may be found. Death results from hepatorenal failure, although heart dysfunction may also contribute [16,17].

The liver in yellow fever

In the liver, the characteristic histopathological changes are seen between the third and eighth day of illness. The hallmark of liver infection is the clear preferential involvement of zone 2, as seen by midzonal necrosis of the parenchyma with degenerated hepatocytes forming eosinophilic Councilman bodies. Nuclei are pyknotic and have enlarged nucleoli and sometimes nuclear inclusions (Torres bodies). Villela bodies are similar structures, but are restricted to the cytoplasm of hepatocytes. Microvesicular steatosis and Kupffer cell hyperplasia also occur. Hepatocytes around the portal and centrolobular veins are spared, inflammatory cells are not prominent and the reticulin framework is preserved [18]. The pattern of midzonal injury, initially thought to represent a characteristic histopathological finding of YF, is also observed with relative frequency in infections by other viral haemorrhagic fevers, such as dengue and Rift Valley fever viruses. Plate 9.4.2 (facing p. 72) shows the major histological findings in the liver that are associated with YF.

Clinical manifestations

The incubation period is 3–6 days. The spectrum of infection is variable; in the majority of cases, the disease is mild or subclinical. Severe classic YF accounts for 10–20% of cases. The typical presentation of severe forms of YF is characterized by three distinct periods (Fig. 1) [13]:

1 Period of infection – this early period corresponds to the viraemic stage and lasts for 3 days. Prodromal symptoms are

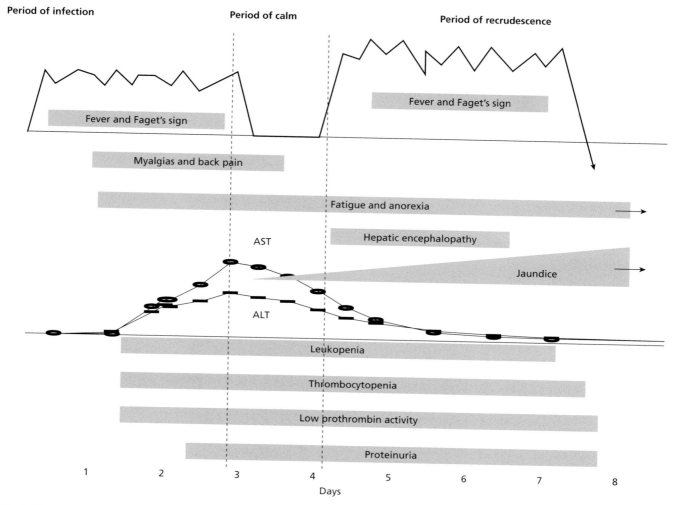

Period of infection

Period of calm

Period of recrudescence

Fever and Faget's sign

Fever and Faget's sign

Myalgias and back pain

Fatigue and anorexia

AST

Hepatic encephalopathy

Jaundice

ALT

Leukopenia

Thrombocytopenia

Low prothrombin activity

Proteinuria

1   2   3   4   5   6   7   8

Days

Fig. 1 Clinical course in a patient with yellow fever.

usually absent. There is an abrupt onset with a fever of up to 40°C, chills, headache, nausea, vomiting, abdominal pain, myalgia and lumbosacral pain. Conjunctival injection and hyperaemia along the edges of the tongue may be found. On the second day, despite a rising temperature, the pulse may decrease (Faget's sign). Nasal bleeding is a common finding.

2 Period of calm – this phase is characterized by the fall of fever; it lasts from several hours to a day, and the patient may enter clinical remission or progress to the following period.

3 Period of recrudescence – viraemia is no longer detectable and circulating antibodies may be present. The fever returns, Faget's sign reappears and the patient's condition deteriorates. Liver and kidney failure develop. Jaundice becomes evident but is never as deep as in viral hepatitis. As in other haemorrhagic fevers, bleeding from different organs may occur, in particular from the eyes, nose, mouth, bladder, uterus and digestive tract. The classical manifestation of coffee-ground haematemesis or

'black vomit' carries a dismal prognosis. In spite of severe proteinuria, ascites is rare. Myocardial dysfunctions are characterized by hypotension, heart failure, arrhythmias and ST segmental changes. Central nervous system involvement is suggested by signs of meningitis or encephalitis. Suppurative parotitis and pneumonia may complicate YF. Death usually occurs on the seventh to tenth day of illness, but the duration of the period of recrudescence is quite variable and may last for up to two weeks.

Laboratory findings and diagnosis

Clinical laboratory tests reveal leukopenia, thrombocytopenia and hypoglycaemia and elevated levels of conjugated bilirubin, serum aminotransferases [particularly aspartate aminotransferase (AST)], blood urea nitrogen and creatinine in endstage disease. Serological tests, such as haemaglutination inhibition, complement fixation, indirect immunofluorescence, ELISA and radioimmunoassay, have been used as a supplementary tool for diagnosis. However, cross-reactivity to other flavivirus is a concern. An elevation in the titre of IgM antibodies indicates recent infection; paired acute and convalescent sera should be tested, with rising antibody titres providing a confirmatory diagnosis. Inoculation onto mosquito cell cultures is the method of choice for virus isolation. YF antigen may be demonstrated in formalin-fixed tissue from the liver, kidney and heart by immunohistochemical staining [17]. However, histopathological examination of the liver is not recommended because of the high risk of life-threatening bleeding from the biopsy site. A PCR-based test is available to detect the YF virus.

Treatment, prognosis and prevention

During the acute phase of YF, the patient should be protected from mosquito bites to avoid the spread of infection. Treatment is supportive and symptomatic. Inhibitors of gastric acid secretion are advisable to decrease the risk of gastric bleeding. Dialysis may be required. Heparin therapy is controversial and should be reserved for selected patients with documented severe disseminated intravascular coagulation. No specific antiviral drug is available. The overall case fatality rate during outbreaks is between 5% and 10%. The prognosis for patients with jaundice is poor, with up to 50% dying between the seventh and tenth day after onset. YF is a preventable disease and vaccination is mandatory for populations at risk and travellers to endemic areas. The live attenuated 17D vaccine, produced from chicken embryos and delivered by a single subcutaneous dose, induces long-lasting immunity in more than 95% of people. Immunity is probably lifelong but, for travel certification, revaccination is recommended every 10 years. The vaccine must not be given to infants of less than 6 months of age because of the risk of post-vaccinal encephalitis; if possible, it is best to delay vaccination until 12 months of age. The rate of encephalitis is from 0.5 to 4.0 in 1000 in those younger than 9 months and one in eight million in those older than 9 months [19,20]. Immunization during pregnancy is contraindicated because of the fetal risk and poor maternal immune response. The YF vaccine is inexpensive and relatively safe. More than 400 million doses have been used since the implementation of the seed-lot system in 1945, and only 27 cases of postvaccinal encephalitis and 12 cases of viscerotropic complications have been reported. Six fatal vaccine-associated cases have been reported worldwide [21]. In Brazilian patients among these cases, the course resembled classic YF. [22]

The possibility of eradicating YF in endemic forest regions seems remote. The control of A. aegypti is the cornerstone strategy for the prevention of urban YF. This includes the removal of mosquito breeding sites in stagnant waters and the biological or chemical control of vectors.

References

1 Malavige GN, Fernando S, Fernando DJ et al. (2004) Dengue viral infections. Postgrad Med J 80, 588–601.

2 Pinheiro FP, Corber SJ (1997) Global situation of dengue and haemorrhagic fever, and its emergence in the Americas. World Health Stat Q 50, 161–169.

3 Solomon T, Mallewa M (2001) Dengue and other emerging flavivirus. J Infect 42, 104–115.

4 Ho LJ, Wang JJ, Shaio MF et al. (2001) Infection of human dendritic cells by dengue virus causes cell maturation and cytokine production. J Immunol 166, 1499–1506.

5 Vaughn DW, Green S, Kalayanarooj S et al. (2000) Dengue viremia titer, antibody response pattern, and virus serotype correlate with disease severity. J Infect Dis 181, 2–9.

6 Littaua R, Kurane I, Ennis FA (1990) Human IgG Fc receptor II mediates antibody-dependent enhancement of dengue virus infection. J Immunol 144, 3183–3186.

7 WHO (1997) Dengue Hemorrhagic Fever, Diagnosis, Treatment, Prevention and Control, 2nd edn. Geneva: World Health Organization.

8 Deen JL, Harris E, Wills B et al. (2006) The WHO dengue classification and case definition: time for a reassessment. Lancet 368, 170–173.

9 De Paula SO, Fonseca BAL (2004) Dengue: a review of the laboratory tests a clinician must know to achieve a correct diagnosis. Braz J Infect Dis 8, 390–398.

10 Telles FRR, Prazeres DMF, Lima-Filho JL (2005) Trends in dengue diagnosis. Rev Med Virol 15, 287–302.

11 Kao CL, King CC, Chao DY et al. (2005) Laboratory diagnosis of dengue virus infection: current and future perspectives in clinical diagnosis and public health. J Microbiol Immunol Infect 38, 5–16.

12 Kabra SK, Jain Y, Singhal T et al. (1999) Dengue hemorrhagic fever: clinical manifestations and management. Indian J Pediatr 66, 93–101.

13 Monath TP (2001) Yellow fever: an update. Lancet Infect Dis 1, 11–20.

14 Rogers DJ, Wilson AJ, Hay SI et al. (2006) The global distribution of yellow fever and dengue. Adv Parasitol 62, 181–220.

15 Cornet JP, Huard M, Camicas JL et al. (1982) Experimental transmission of the yellow fever virus by the tick Amblyoma variegatum. Bull Soc Pathol Exot Filiales 75, 136–140.

16 Monath TP, Barret AD (2003) Pathogenesis and pathophysiology of yellow fever. Adv Virus Res 60, 343–395.

17 De Brito T, Siqueira SAC, Santos RTM et al. (1992) Human fatal yellow fever. Immunohistochemical detection of viral antigens in the liver, kidney and heart. Path Res Pract 188, 177–181.

18 Vieira WT, Gayotto LC, de Lima CP et al. (1983) Histopathology of the human liver in yellow fever with special emphasis on the diagnostic role of the Councilman body. Histopathology 7, 195–208.

19 Monath TP (1999) Yellow fever. In: Protkin S, Orenstein W (eds) Vaccines. New York: WB Saunders, pp. 815–998.

20 Robertson SE (1993) The immunological basis for immunization. 8: yellow fever. Document WHO/EPI/GEN/93.18. Geneva: WHO.

21 Seligman SJ, Gould EA (2004) Live flavivirus vaccines: reasons for caution. Lancet 363, 2073–2075.

22 Vasconcelos PF, Luna EJ, Galler LJ et al, Brazilian Yellow Fever Vaccine Evaluation Group (2001) Serious adverse events associated with yellow fever 17DD vaccine in Brazil: a report of two cases. Lancet 358, 91–97.

10 Other infections of the liver

10.1 Bacterial, rickettsial and spirochaetal infections

José M. Sánchez-Tapias

Bacterial infection

Introduction

A large number of bacteria may affect the liver either as a result of parenchymal or biliary invasion or as a manifestation of bacteraemia or toxaemia. There is a wide spectrum of clinical manifestations, ranging from asymptomatic abnormalities of liver function tests to jaundice and, occasionally, severe liver failure.

Liver dysfunction in extrahepatic infection

Patients with extrahepatic infection often have clinical or biochemical signs of liver dysfunction [1]. Jaundice was described as early as 1836 in patients with pneumococcal pneumonia, but the overall prevalence of liver dysfunction in infected patients remains undefined. Liver disorder is more frequent in children than in adults, and its frequency increases with the severity of the underlying condition, being highest in patients with septic shock and multiple organ failure [2]. About half of patients with severe infection admitted to intensive care units may have bilirubin serum concentrations higher than 2 mg/dL. Liver dysfunction occurs mostly in patients with documented Gram-negative bacteraemia, especially *Escherichia coli* and *Klebsiella* spp., although Gram-positive organisms may be involved as well, especially *Streptococcus pneumoniae* and *Staphylococcus aureus*. The most common sources of bacteraemia in these patients are pneumonia, urinary tact infection and soft-tissue infection, although organisms may originate from other sources such as pelvic infection, diverticulitis, appendicitis, peritonitis, meningitis, lung abscess, septic abortion or others.

The severity of liver disorder is variable, ranging from subclinical evidence of cholestasis to deep jaundice. Pruritus is fairly uncommon. Symptoms are those of the underlying condition. Viral, drug-related and ischaemic hepatitis must be excluded. In severe infections, other complications may ensue, including renal failure, respiratory distress syndrome and coagulopathies. Prognosis is related to the underlying condition, and mortality seems to be related more closely to renal, neurological and coagulation complications than to hepatic impairment itself [3,4].

Pyogenic liver abscess

Pyogenic liver abscess results from bacterial infection of the liver parenchyma and subsequent infiltration of the area with neutrophils and other phagocytes to form a collection of pus. The wall of the abscess may be formed, for instance, by biliary epithelium or by the lining of a hydatid cyst, in cases secondary to infection of ectatic bile ducts or parasitic cyst respectively.

There have been changes in the epidemiology of pyogenic liver abscess in recent years. The age distribution now has a peak at around 60–70 years, and an increase in prevalence has been noted between 1977 and 2002 from 6 to 18 per one million, most probably as a result of using more sensitive diagnostic tools [5].

Biliary tract infection resulting from obstruction of the common bile duct accounts for about 40% of cases and is the most frequent of the known causes of pyogenic liver abscess, but no underlying cause can be identified in nearly one-third of cases [6,7]. Systemic bacteraemia is thought to be the most common cause in infants and young children and is responsible for 10–20% of cases in adults, sometimes by infection of pre-existing tumours or intrahepatic haematomas following blunt trauma. Portal bacteraemia caused by intra-abdominal infections, such as appendicitis, diverticulitis, abscesses, inflammatory bowel disease and others, may lead to liver abscess formation, but this is less frequent than in the pre-antibiotic era. Liver abscesses may also result from extension of septic processes in the vicinity of the liver, such as cholecystitis, pancreatitis or penetrating gastric or duodenal ulcers. Occasionally, treatment of liver tumours by transarterial embolization and, more rarely, by ethanol injection may cause abscess formation.

The causative organisms vary according to the primary site of infection. Abscesses following cholangitis or intra-abdominal sepsis are frequently polymicrobial and involve enteric Gram-negative organisms and anaerobes, whereas systemic bacteraemia causes abscesses with a single organism, such as *Staph. aureus*, streptococci or aerobic Gram-negative organisms. *Escherichia coli* is classically the organism most frequently involved, but *Klebsiella pneumoniae* has increasingly been recovered from cultures in recent years, particularly among Asian patients [8,9], and a genetically determined increased tissue invasiveness has recently been recognized in involved strains [10].

Patients typically present with slow onset of fever and pain or tenderness in the right upper quadrant, loss of appetite and body weight. These symptoms may last for weeks before the diagnosis is made, but there may be rapid deterioration with signs of sepsis, jaundice and septic shock, particularly in cases associated with biliary obstruction.

Laboratory abnormalities are not specific. Increased erythrocyte sedimentation rate (ESR), elevated alkaline phosphatase, increased leukocyte count with neutrophilia, and mild anaemia are usually found. Blood cultures are positive in about half the cases. On chest X-rays, there may be elevation of the right hemidiaphragm, pleural effusion or a basal infiltrate, but abdominal ultrasonography, computerized tomography (CT) or magnetic resonance imaging (MRI) are essential for diagnosis. Modern imaging techniques are important because they can provide relevant information regarding underlying biliary or abdominal disorders, and facilitate aspiration of pus for diagnostic or therapeutic purposes.

The prognosis of pyogenic liver abscess has very much improved in recent years. Early diagnosis and appropriate management have reduced overall mortality to about 10% or less, although it remains high in patients with subjacent malignancies [5,11].

Treatment is based on the administration of appropriate antibiotics and evacuation of pus. In selected patients, antibiotic therapy alone may be an option. In view of the wide range of possible organisms, microbiological diagnosis is important in choosing the most effective antibiotics. Empiric therapy should include antibiotics active against Gram-negative bacteria, streptococci, including enterococci, and anaerobes. Duration of therapy depends on the response but, in general, antibiotics should be given intravenously (i.v.) for 2 weeks and by mouth for a further 4 weeks. Evacuation of pus must be done surgically in patients with large abscesses [12]; otherwise, percutaneous, ultrasound-guided drainage is less aggressive and very effective [13]. Percutaneous evacuation of pus can be done by continuous drainage via an inserted catheter or by intermittent needle aspiration. A recent controlled trial suggests that needle aspiration may be the procedure of choice as a first option [14].

Liver dysfunction following infection with specific organisms

Staphylococcus aureus and the toxic shock syndrome

The toxic shock syndrome is a severe multisystem disorder that occurs in patients infected with a strain of *Staph. aureus* producing a specific toxin called TSST-1. This syndrome was initially described in adult females at the onset of menstruation and was related to the use of specific tampons. Following adequate preventive measures, the incidence of this syndrome has markedly decreased in this setting, but still occurs as a complication of surgical procedures, trauma, burns and other local infections [15].

Clinically, it is characterized by high fever, hypotension, erythematous rash and multiorgan involvement affecting the gastrointestinal tract, kidney, central nervous system and liver. Liver dysfunction is characterized by a transient, moderate increase in bilirubin, transaminases and alkaline phosphatase. Diagnosis is based on clinical criteria. *Staph. aureus* is rarely recovered from blood but may be isolated from vaginal swabs or from other sites. Differential diagnosis is that of multisystem disease with fever, hypotension and rash and includes scarlet fever, meningococcaemia, erythema multiforme, drug eruption, leptospirosis and others. Treatment is based on supportive measures, drainage of infected sites, appropriate antibiotics and, in severe cases, intravenous immunoglobulin, which contains anti-TSST-1 antibodies, may be considered.

Clostridium perfringens

Clostridium perfringens may directly affect the liver in the form of an abscess or, very rarely, by causing diffuse, necrotizing, massive gas gangrene of the liver, leading to fulminant hepatic failure [16]. Patients with gas gangrene elsewhere, following septic abortion or wound infection, may be jaundiced mostly as a consequence of massive haemolysis.

Listeria monocytogenes

Listeria monocytogenes, a Gram-positive, aerobic bacillus, is widely distributed in nature but rarely causes symptomatic infection, except in pregnant women, immunocompromised subjects and neonates. Hepatic involvement with *L. monocytogenes* may occur as a solitary liver abscess or may be more widespread and present as an acute hepatitis with high transaminases. High fever, neutrophilia and the presence of granulomas in the liver may be valuable for distinction from viral hepatitis [17,18]. This organism has been recognized as a cause of spontaneous bacterial peritonitis in patients with cirrhosis [19]. Diagnosis is confirmed by isolation of the organism from blood, tissue or organic fluid cultures. Ampicillin is the drug of choice.

Legionella pneumophila

Legionella pneumophila causes Legionnaire's disease, which is a pneumonia with multisystem involvement. This disease has its highest incidence in the 40- to 70-year-old age group and is more frequent in men. Alcoholics, smokers and subjects with chronic diseases are at highest risk. Abnormalities of liver function test are quite common, but frank jaundice is rarer [20]. Histological changes of the liver are non-specific. The diagnosis is mostly based on serology, and the differential diagnosis includes other bacterial pneumonias, *Mycoplasma* infection, psittacosis and Q fever. Oral azithromycin or clarithromycin is the treatment of choice in the immunocompetent host, whereas immunocompromised or patients with severe disease need i.v. therapy with azithromycin, levofloxacin or ciprofloxacin.

Brucella spp.

Brucellosis is a worldwide zoonosis that occasionally affects man. There are three important pathogenic species: Br. abortus, Br. melitensis and Br. suis, which have different geographic distributions and somewhat different clinical presentation [21]. Brucellosis is an occupational infection of farmers, veterinary surgeons, meat handlers and microbiology laboratory workers and is also transmitted by raw milk, particularly goat milk, and dairy products.

The presentation of the disease may be acute, subacute or chronic. Major features are fever, sweating, malaise, headache, rigors, arthralgia, myalgia and back pain. The liver, the spleen or both are enlarged in about one-third of cases, but significant liver damage with jaundice or liver abscess formation is infrequent, and chronic hepatosplenic suppurative brucellosis is rare [22,23]. Elevation of alkaline phosphatase, suggesting an infiltrative process within the liver, is the most prominent biochemical abnormality. Liver biopsy usually shows non-specific inflammation, reactive changes and small non-caseating granulomas, the last being found infrequently when the disease becomes chronic [24]. Large liver abscesses are rare, and symptoms are insidious, but imaging techniques characteristically show large, poorly defined, hypodense areas surrounding a patent central calcification [23,25]. Several serological tests [Bengala rose, Coombs, enzyme-linked immunosorbent assay (ELISA)] are available for diagnosis, but interpretation may be difficult, particularly in endemic areas or in chronic infection. Brucella can frequently be isolated from blood in the early stages of infection, but cultures are rarely positive at later stages, during non-febrile periods. Several days or weeks may be necessary for cultures to grow. Modified automated culture techniques and polymerase chain reaction (PCR)-based methods have increased sensitivity and are helpful in speeding diagnosis [26]. Therapy is based on prolonged administration of antibiotics, mostly doxycycline in combination with streptomycin or rifampicin. Surgical excision may be required for large liver abscesses.

Neisseria gonorrhoeae

Gonococcal perihepatitis, with the formation of violin-string fibrin adhesions between the liver capsule and the peritoneal wall, may result from direct spreading through the peritoneum of germs causing pelvic inflammatory disease in women or, rarely, by retroperitoneal lymphatic or haematogenous dissemination in men. Clinically, it is characterized by severe pain in the right upper quadrant and fever, and there may be a friction rub. Liver function tests are usually normal, although serum transaminases may be raised. CT scan or ultrasonography may show thickening of the peritoneum. Laparoscopy is useful to confirm the diagnosis and to relieve pain by section of the adhesions. This clinical picture (Fitz-Hugh and Curtis syndrome) may also be caused by Chlamydia trachomatis. Antibiotic

therapy is based on a combination of doxycycline and ceftriaxone.

Burkholderia pseudomallei

Burkholderia pseudomallei, a Gram-negative aerobic bacillus, is a soil saprophyte that can easily be recovered from water and wet soils in endemic areas. Melioidosis is a very important cause of sepsis during the rainy seasons in northeastern Thailand and has also been recognized in other Southeast Asian countries, the north of Australia and Central America. Melioidosis mostly affects people who have direct contact with wet soils and have a predisposition to infection, such as diabetes or other chronic diseases. The skin is the portal of entry. The disease may present as severe sepsis, often fatal, or a chronic debilitating condition with abscess formation mostly in the lung, although virtually any organ, including the liver, spleen, kidney, brain, skeletal muscle, skin and, in children, parotid gland, may be involved [27]. On ultrasound examination, liver abscesses may present as multiple hypoechoic areas or large, multiloculated lesions [28]. Melioidosis should be considered in severely septic patients living in or coming from endemic areas. Rapid diagnosis and immediate therapy are important. Serologic tests are of little help in endemic areas. B. pseudomallei can readily be cultured from infected sites or from blood within 48–72 h. Indirect immunofluorescence of sputum, urine or pus is very specific and provides much more rapid diagnostic information [29]. Immunoperoxidase staining of fixed specimens may be useful as well [30]. Rapid and specific PCR techniques have been described [31], but their applicability is probably low in endemic areas. Initial intensive care management, intravenous ceftazidime followed by prolonged oral administration of chloramphenicol, doxycycline and trimethoprim–sulphamethoxazole is the therapy of choice [27].

Hepatic involvement in infections with bacterial enteric pathogens

Salmonella spp.

Several Salmonella species may cause cholangitis, cholecystitis and liver abscesses. Salmonella typhi and S. paratyphi cause enteric fever. Liver involvement, as indicated by enlarged liver and abnormal liver function tests, is frequent in patients with typhoid fever. Histological findings are non-specific. Occasionally, typhoid nodules, which consist of aggregates of Kupffer cells, may be found [32]. More serious liver injury and clinical jaundice, the so-called typhoid hepatitis, is rare but may resemble viral hepatitis. High fever, bradycardia, lower peak serum aminotransferases level, high peak alkaline phosphatase and low alanine aminotransferase (ALT) to lactate dehydrogenase (LDH) ratio suggest typhoid hepatitis, but culture of salmonella from blood stool is important for diagnosis [33]. Salmonella is able to colonize the gallbladder, leading to a chronic carrier state that causes prolonged shedding of the organism. Chloramphenicol was traditionally the first-line antibiotic for the treatment of typhoid fever, but fluoro-quinolones are more effective, as these drugs provide a rapid cure in most patients, with a very low rate of both relapse or faecal carriage of the organism [34].

Other bacterial enteric pathogens

Abnormalities of liver function tests and an enlarged, tender liver may frequently be found in infections with *Shigella* spp. and *Campylobacter* spp., but clinical hepatitis or jaundice is rare. A few cases of spontaneous peritonitis caused by *Campylobacter* have been reported in patients with cirrhosis. Liver abscesses caused by *Yersinia*, although uncommon, have mostly been reported in patients with genetic haemochromatosis or secondary iron overload.

Tularaemia

Franciscella tularensis is a Gram-negative coccobacillus that causes tularaemia in wild rodents. Infection may be transmitted to man directly from infected animals, by insect bites or by drinking contaminated water. *F. tularensis* is distributed worldwide, but human disease is rare and occurs mainly in persons in contact with infected animals [35]. Clinical manifestations are variable and include fever, malaise, headache and a local reaction at the entry site, causing several types of illness: glandular, ulceroglandular, oculoglandular, pulmonary, oropharyngeal and typhoidal. Elevation of aminotransferases is frequent, but clinically apparent liver involvement is rare, although hepatic abscesses and hepatic granulomas have been reported. *F. tularensis* is difficult to culture, and the handling of this bacterium poses risks to laboratory workers. Microagglutination and ELISA tests and PCR-based methods are being used for diagnosis [36]. Streptomycin and aminoglycosides are the antibiotics of choice for treatment

Q fever

Q fever is a worldwide distributed zoonosis with protean clinical manifestations [37,38]. The responsible agent is *Coxiella burnetti*, a pleomorphic, Gram-negative, strictly intracellular coccobacillus. Recent phylogenetic studies showed that *C. burnetti* belongs to the order of Legionellales rather than Rickettsiales. A wide variety of animals can be infected, including domesticated and wild mammals, reptiles, amphibians, fish and ticks. Most human infections occur in persons in direct contact with infected animals such as cattle, sheep or goats, but may also occur by indirect exposure in rural or urban areas, mostly by inhalation of wind-spread infectious aerosol particles or consumption of unpasteurized dairy products.

Q fever usually presents as a febrile influenza-like illness with pneumonitis, hepatitis or both. Jaundice is rare, but elevation of liver enzymes and hepatomegaly are very common. Pericarditis, myocarditis, neurological manifestations, such as meningitis, meningoencephalitis or peripheral neuropathies, and dermatological lesions may be present. Bradycardia is common. Fever of unknown origin and abnormal liver enzymes are a frequent form of presentation. Liver histology shows parenchymal granulomas with a characteristic ring of fibrinoid necrosis, which is surrounded by histocytes and lymphocytes and centred by a fat vacuole. This 'doughnut' or lipogranuloma lesion is highly suggestive of Q fever, but not pathognomonic, as it may be found in other granulomatous diseases such as typhoid fever, lymphoma, vasculitis and Epstein–Barr virus and cytomegalovirus infection [39]. Q fever is often autolimited, but may very occasionally be fatal. Endocarditis is by far the best characterized consequence of chronic infection. It has also been suggested that the chronic fatigue syndrome may be associated with protracted infection in some patients.

In patients with acute disease, the diagnosis can be confirmed by serology, with detection of rising antibodies against phase II antigens, but significant titres may take 3 or 4 weeks to appear. The diagnostic value of PCR assays in serum samples is limited, but may be useful for earlier diagnosis in some cases, as PCR may be positive within the first 2 weeks from the onset, when conventional serology is still negative [40]. Patients with chronic infection have high titres of antibodies against phase I antigen.

Doxycycline is the treatment of choice, but macrolides and fluoroquinolones have also been used. Several types of vaccines have been developed and may be efficacious in persons at risk.

Chlamydia

Chlamydia trachomatis

Infection with *C. trachomatis* is virtually restricted to humans and distributed worldwide. This pathogen causes a wide variety of disorders, including trachoma and conjunctivitis, sexually transmitted diseases in adults and pneumonia in the newborn. In males with lymphogranuloma venereum, increased liver enzymes and hepatic granuloma formation have been described. However, perihepatitis is the most typical hepatic disorder caused by *C. trachomatis*. Perihepatitis occurs mostly in young females via peritoneal spread of germs from the genital tract, although cases have been described in men, via blood or lymphatic dissemination. The disease results from localized inflammation, which leads to the formation of adhesions between the parietal and visceral peritoneum overlying the liver. In most cases, perihepatitis is associated with salpingitis and presents with fever and severe pain in the right upper quadrant, which exacerbates with deep breathing and coughing. Laparoscopy shows the typical fibrin 'violin-string' adhesions (Fitz-Hugh and Curtis syndrome). Perihepatitis may be found incidentally in non-symptomatic patients who undergo laparoscopic examination for other reasons [41]. *C. trachomatis* may be grown in cell culture or demonstrated by immunofluorescence from vaginal, endocervical or ureteral swabs. More recently, molecular procedures for amplification and hybridization of specific nucleic acid fragments have been developed and are commercially available [42]. This condition must be distinguished from acute cholecystitis and appendicitis, and from perihepatitis caused by *N. gonorrhoeae*. Doxycycline and azithromycin are the antibiotics of choice.

Chlamydophila psittaci

Psittacosis is a worldwide distributed zoonosis that affects birds. *C. psittaci* is transmitted to man by the oral route, replicates in the liver and spleen and reaches the lung and other tissues following haematogenous dissemination. Symptoms are those of a non-specific atypical pneumonia: high fever, headache, malaise, dry cough; there may be some haemoptysis, but pleuritic pain is absent. Many patients have splenomegaly and enlarged liver, and a maculopapular rash may be present. Mild elevation of transaminases is frequent, but jaundice is rare, except in the most severe cases. Diagnosis is based on increasing titres of antibodies in sequential sera. Culture is difficult and hazardous for laboratory workers. PCR-based techniques are under development. Doxycycline is the antibiotic of choice, and macrolides and chloramphenicol may alternatively be used.

Chlamydophila pneumoniae

Chlamydophila pneumoniae has been recognized as an important aetiological agent in acute respiratory disorders and community-acquired pneumonia, mostly in young people. Over the past few years, there has been much debate about the possible role of this agent in atherosclerosis. Recently, *C. pneumoniae* antigen and RNA have been detected in explanted liver tissue from patients with primary biliary cirrhosis, and a controversy on its role in this disease has been opened [43].

Mycoplasma pneumoniae

Mycoplasma pneumoniae is a small Gram-negative eubacterium that does not have a cellular wall. It is distributed worldwide and produces pharyngitis and tracheobronchitis, and is a frequent cause of community-acquired pneumonia. Most infections are mild and do not require hospitalization. Symptoms are not specific. Some patients have a maculopapular rash or a bullous myringitis. Characteristically, respiratory physical signs are scarce, whereas chest X-ray shows prominent changes. Liver involvement is not frequent, but some patients may have elevated transaminases, and cholestatic hepatitis has been described in children. Cases of mild hepatitis in patients without pneumonia have also been reported [44]. Diagnosis is mostly based on serology. The antibiotic of choice is azithromycin.

Cat-scratch disease

Cat-scratch disease is an infection caused by *Bartonella henselae*, a small Gram-negative bacillus that infects cats, dogs and their fleas. Children and young adults are most frequently affected. In the majority of patients, cat-scratch disease is characterized by regional granulomatous lymphadenopathy following a cat scratch or bite. The site of inoculation is marked by a vanishing papular lesion. General symptoms such as low-grade fever or malaise may be present or not, and spontaneous, although slow, resolution is frequent. Liver involvement is rare. There are

atypical cases in which the characteristic regional lymphadenitis and inoculation papule are absent. Granulomatous hepatic and splenic involvement has been reported in a few cases [45]. Diagnosis is based on serology and PCR amplification of bacterial DNA from tissue specimens. Therapy may not be necessary in localized, typical forms. Otherwise, a wide variety of antibiotics including fluoroquinolones, new macrolides such as azithromycin and co-trimoxazole may be useful.

In immunocompromised patients, *B. henselae* may cause severe granulomatous hepatitis and peliosis hepatis [46]. These patients have an enlarged and tender liver and appear seriously ill. Imaging techniques show multiple focal nodular hypodense lesions that must be differentiated from malignancies and a number of other granulomatous or infectious diseases that may affect the liver.

Mycobacteria

Involvement of the liver is frequent in patients with mycobacterial infections. Until recently, the incidence of tuberculosis has been declining in developed countries, but there is a recrudescence of mycobacterial infection due to immigration from underdeveloped countries and to the emergency of the acquired immune deficiency syndrome (AIDS). In this setting, in addition to *Mycobacterium tuberculosis*, other species such as *M. avium intracellulare* or, more rarely, *M. genavense*, may be involved. In addition, due to immune suppression, organ-transplanted patients are also at increased risk of developing tuberculosis. Liver-transplanted patients are prone to develop significant hepatotoxicity from standard antituberculous therapy, and alternative regimens should be considered [47].

The clinical spectrum of liver disease due to *Mycobacterium* spp. ranges from the absence of symptoms to severe hepatic disease, including liver failure. Multiple small granuloma formation within the parenchyma is the most common lesion. However, granulomas may also coalesce and form large tuberculomas, may affect the intrahepatic or extrahepatic biliary tree or the lymph nodes at the porta hepatis and cause biliary obstruction. Furthermore, patients with extrahepatic tuberculosis may have drug-induced hepatitis, non-specific lesions such as fatty infiltration or reactive hepatitis. Granulomatous hepatitis has been reported in patients undergoing bacille Calmette-Guérin (BCG) systemic immunization or local instillation in patients with carcinoma of the urinary bladder.

Tuberculosis is a frequent cause of liver granulomatosis. The number of granulomas is variable, being greater in patients with disseminated miliary tuberculosis. Hepatic tuberculosis occasionally occurs in the absence of apparent tuberculosis elsewhere [48]. Granulomatous hepatic tuberculosis does not usually cause symptoms, and the clinical manifestations are those of non-hepatic disease. Hepatomegaly and abnormal liver function tests, particularly elevation of alkaline phosphatase, are incidental findings. Jaundice and ascites are rare, and related to involvement of the biliary tree or the peritoneum respectively. Cases of liver failure mimicking fulminant viral hepatitis have been reported. Suspicion of liver involvement arises from clinical symptoms or biochemical abnormalities. Plain X-ray may show multiple calcifications in the hepatic area. Imaging techniques do not provide specific data, but may be useful in ruling out other lesions. Liver biopsy demonstrates the presence of granulomas, which are formed by aggregates of epithelioid cells surrounded by mononuclear inflammatory cells and contain a few multinucleated giant cells. Caseation may be found in half the cases, but none of these features is specific. Acid-fast bacilli may be demonstrated by Ziehl–Nielsen staining in a minority of cases. *Mycobacteria* may be isolated in less than half the cases. Recently, several PCR-based assays have been developed for rapid and specific diagnosis of tuberculosis in clinical specimens, but the performance of these techniques in liver biopsies has not been fully evaluated in hepatic miliary tuberculosis.

Hepatic tuberculoma, tuberculous hepatic abscess, nodular or pseudotumoral hepatic tuberculosis are terms used to designate larger hepatic lesions resulting from the coalescence of tuberculous granulomas. They may be single or multiple and of variable size, although lesions greater than 3 cm in diameter are rare [49]. Abdominal pain, fever and weight loss are the most usual symptoms, but these may not be very apparent, and a tuberculous abscess may be discovered incidentally, when patients with abnormal liver function tests, particularly increased alkaline phosphatase, are investigated. Manifestations of pulmonary tuberculosis are often absent. Imaging techniques show a diversity of space-occupying lesions without specific features, which must be differentiated from primary or metastatic neoplasms or fungal infection. Histological examination of liver tissue obtained by percutaneous biopsy may show granulomas or non-specific inflammatory or fibrotic material. Staining for acid-fast bacilli, cultures and PCR-based DNA amplification are necessary for diagnosis. Most patients respond well to antituberculous regimens, but improvement may not be immediate and prolonged treatment is necessary.

Rickettsial infection

Rocky Mountain spotted fever

This condition is a tick-borne, multisystemic disease caused by *Rickettsia rickettsii* [50]. It is endemic in some areas in North, Central and South America, and has its highest incidence in children as they play outdoors and with dogs. Most patients have a mild or moderate illness, but the disease may be severe in some cases. High fever, malaise, headache, muscle aches, abdominal symptoms and an initially distal maculopapular rash are the first symptoms. A significant proportion of patients are not aware of having been bitten by a tick. Abnormal elevation of ALT is frequent, but clinical manifestations of liver involvement are rare. Prompt treatment is essential, as mortality in untreated patients may be high. Immunofluorescence assays and ELISA tests using specific antigens as well as PCR-based techniques are available, but treatment initiation must not await serological confirmation

when there is a reasonable degree of clinical suspicion. Doxycycline is the drug of choice.

Mediterranean spotted fever (tick typhus, 'fievre boutonneuse')

This acute febrile illness is caused by *Rickettsia connorii*, which is transmitted to man mostly by a dog tick. It is endemic in the Mediterranean basin, the Middle East, India and South Africa, but a number of cases have been reported recently from central Europe. Initial symptoms are high fever, headache, myalgia, photophobia and a distal papular rash, which later extends onto the trunk and face. A characteristic black eschar, which is the inoculation site and where the tick may still be found, can be observed in a large proportion of patients. Hepatic involvement is very common and is manifested by liver enlargement, elevated transaminases, alkaline phosphatase and γ-glutamyl transpeptidase, and hepatic granulomas may be found [51]. Diagnosis can be based on clinical data. Rickettsias may be detected by direct immunofluorescence of cutaneous lesions, by increased specific antibody titres or by a positive Weil–Felix reaction. The course of the disease is usually benign. Doxycycline is very effective, but co-trimoxazole and chloramphenicol may also be used. Clarythromycin and azithromycin are effective in children. No vaccines are available.

Ehrlichioses and anaplasmosis

Human monocytotropic ehrlichiosis and human granulocytotropic anaplasmosis, formerly known as human granulocytotropic ehrlichioses, are tick-borne zoonoses caused by *Ehrlichia chaffeensis* and *Anaplasma phagocytophilum* respectively [50,52,53]. These conditions are characterized by infection of leukocytes, where the agents may form microcolonies within cytoplasmic vacuoles called morulae, which may be found in conventional smears of peripheral blood. Most patients have a moderately severe febrile illness with flu-like symptoms, and a cutaneous rash may be present, especially in patients with ehrlichiosis. Severe complications such as respiratory or renal failure, gastrointestinal haemorrhage or neurological complications may occur, mostly in patients of advanced age. Leukopenia (40%), thrombocytopenia (70%) and mildly increased aminotransferase serum levels (70%) are frequently found, and a few patients may be jaundiced. As symptoms are non-specific, a high index of suspicion is essential for early diagnosis. The presence of morulae in leukocytes is highly suggestive, but blood smear is quite insensitive, as morulae are found in a minority of cases. Immunofluorescence and ELISA assays are available, but these tests do not allow for early diagnosis because specific antibody response does not occur until the second week. Demonstration of rising IgG or IgM titres in serum specimens taken 2 or 3 weeks apart is required to confirm acute infection. PCR techniques can detect specific DNA sequences earlier, mostly in whole blood specimens, but a negative test does not rule out the diagnosis.

Culture is difficult. Antibiotic therapy must be initiated as soon as the diagnosis is suspected. Doxycycline is the drug of choice.

Spirochaetal infections

Treponema pallidum (syphilis)

Syphilis is a multisystem, sexually transmitted infection, which evolves through several clinical stages when left untreated. It may be transmitted to the fetus during pregnancy. Liver involvement may occur at every stage of the infection.

Besides the characteristic mucocutaneous lesions, osteitis and osteochondritis, babies with congenital syphilis have hepatitis with hepatosplenomegaly and jaundice [54]. Serum transaminases may reach very high levels, and aspartate aminotransferase (AST) is typically higher than ALT. Liver biopsies show multiple epithelioid granulomas and portal and pericellular fibrosis. Spirochaetes are localized mostly at the space of Disse and may be demonstrated by silver staining or electronic microscopy of liver tissue. Granulomas may evolve silently over the years and become manifest later in infancy or during adolescence as a hepar lobatum or hepatic gummas. Serological diagnosis may be difficult in the early stages because of the presence of maternal antibodies.

A resurgence of syphilis is being observed, particularly among human immunodeficiency virus (HIV)-infected individuals [55]. Liver involvement is relatively frequent in patients with secondary syphilis, but recognition may be obscured by coincidental, sexually transmitted, viral hepatitis. Patients present with anorexia, loss of weight, weakness, hepatomegaly and pruritus, but jaundice is uncommon [56]. In HIV-infected patients, neurological involvement seems to be more prominent than cutaneous or hepatic involvement [57]. A cutaneous rash, but not the primary chancre, is still present. Liver function tests are abnormal, and alkaline phosphatase is disproportionately elevated. A variety of histological changes have been described, including portal inflammation, areas of hepatocellular necrosis, granuloma formation, pericholangiolar inflammation, vasculitis and cholestasis. Spirochaetes are rarely found, and the pathogenesis of these liver lesions is unclear. Diagnosis is based on serology and on the demonstration of treponemes in cutaneous and mucous membrane lesions. All abnormalities subside rapidly with penicillin therapy.

In untreated patients, the clinical manifestations of secondary syphilis resolve spontaneously within a few weeks, and the infection enters into a state of latency. Recurrent secondary eruptions may occur but are rare. Latency may last for years and produce a variety of lesions leading to neurological, ocular, cardiovascular, skeletal, cutaneous or hepatic manifestations. Hepatic involvement is very rare and consists of the formation of gummas, which are granulomatous formations with no specific features. Gummas are space-occupying lesions that do not usually cause symptoms, but may be confounded with malignant lesions, mostly metastatic cancer [58]. Cases with pain over the right

hypochondrium, loss of weight and presentation as a Budd–Chiari syndrome caused by compression of the inferior vena cava have been described. Percutaneous liver biopsy and specific treponemic tests are useful for diagnosis. Patients respond well to penicillin. Doxycycline has also been used successfully.

Borrelia burgdorferi (Lyme disease)

Lyme disease is a multisystem disorder caused by B. burgdorferi, a tick-borne microaerophilic spirochaete that is distributed worldwide. The distribution of the disease is related to the geographic prevalence of the tick vector. The disease follows three consecutive stages. Following inoculation, the organism multiplies locally and spreads into the regional lymph nodes and then to the organs and joints. The initial symptoms are those of a generalized infection, with fever, malaise, headache, lymphadenopathy, arthralgia, myalgia and a characteristic rash, named erythema chronicum migrans, a reddish macular or papular rash, which expands over time while fading centrally [59]. Neurological or cardiac abnormalities occur weeks or months later and may persist for several weeks. The late phase is characterized by the development of chronic erosive arthritis that may resemble rheumatoid arthritis. Hepatic involvement is very frequent in the early stage, when about half the patients have abnormal liver function tests resembling acute viral hepatitis. Liver lesions include portal inflammation, ballooning and microvesicular fatty degeneration of hepatocytes, abundant mitoses and infiltration of sinusoid with inflammatory cells [60,61]. Diagnosis is based on serological ELISA and immunofluorescence tests and, recently, on DNA amplification by PCR-based assays. Doxycycline is the drug of choice, but azithromycin is also effective.

Borrellia recurrentis

Relapsing fever is a louse-borne disease that is transmitted from man to man and occurs mostly in epidemics associated with very poor hygiene conditions. It is caused by B. recurrentis, a microaerophilic spirochaete that has no animal reservoir. The disease presents with rigors, high fever, arthralgia, myalgia, vomiting, photophobia and a cutaneous rash that may be petechial. Hepatosplenomegaly is present in most patients, jaundice is common, transaminasas are elevated, and there may be thrombocytopenia. Within less than 2 weeks, the initial episode abruptly subsides. At this time, death may occur as a consequence of cardiovascular collapse. Following an afebrile period that lasts several days, there is a relapse that resembles the initial episode [62]. Relapses are caused by the emergence of organisms able to evade protecting antibodies due to changing antigenicity. Diagnosis is made by direct demonstration of the organism in blood extension during a febrile episode. Tetracyclines and erythromycin are more effective than penicillin.

Leptospirosis

Leptospirosis results from infection with different serovars belonging to the species *Leptospira interrogans*, such as *L. icterohaemorrhagiae*, *L. canicola*, *L. pomona*, *L. andamana*, *L. autumnalis*, *L. copenhageni*, *L. gripptyphosa*, *L. hebdomadis* and others. Leptospirosis occurs worldwide, in rural and urban areas, but is more frequent in underdeveloped or developing countries and still remains an important public health problem [63]. There are many animal hosts, mostly rodents, which act as reservoirs and eliminate the leptospires in the urine. Stagnant water and warm temperature favour survival of the organisms. Humans are infected by contact of abraded skin with contaminated water or soil. Infection can also occur by penetration of the organisms through mucosal surfaces, including ingestion of contaminated food. The disease often results from occupational exposure in persons working in sewers, mines or rice and sugar cane plantations, as well as in persons who handle animal tissues or fluids.

The incubation period is 10 days on average. The severity of the illness varies widely, from asymptomatic cases to a severe disease with jaundice, renal failure and haemorrhages (Weil's disease). Most symptomatic patients have a biphasic disease. The first phase lasts several days and is characterized by sudden onset of high fever, rigors, severe headache, myalgia and abdominal complaints. There may be stiffness of the neck suggesting meningitis, and muscle pain is prominent. During this phase, leptospires are found in blood and in the cerebrospinal fluid. After a relatively asymptomatic interval lasting a few days, a second phase ensues, in which symptoms are variable, with a predominance of neurological manifestations, mostly meningitis and optical neuritis or iridocyclitis. Leptospires are excreted in the urine during this phase.

The manifestations of the second phase of leptospirosis may be severe. Weil's disease is characterized by marked jaundice, renal failure, haemorrhagic manifestation such as purpura or bleeding from the nose, gums or gastrointestinal tract, and neurological manifestations. Patients may have myocardial damage, which may cause arrythmias and heart failure. Typically, there is a moderate increase in serum transaminases in contrast to very high levels of bilirubin and γ-glutamyl transferase. Histology shows relatively little liver damage. Apart from prominent cholestatic features, the parenchyma appears well preserved, with some oedema and inflammation of the portal tracts, mitotic activity of the hepatocytes and hyperplasia of Kupffer cells.

Diagnosis should first be based on clinical and epidemiological suspicion. Leptospires can be isolated from blood or cerebrospinal fluid during the first phase and from urine during the second phase. Several methods are available for the detection of specific antibodies during the second phase, including macroscopic and microscopic agglutination, immunofluorescence and ELISA tests. Detection of leptospires in blood or urine by PCR amplification techniques allows early confirmation of the diagnosis during the initial phase of the illness [64].

Most patients with mild leptospirosis heal spontaneously. Doxycycline may reduce the duration of the illness in these patients, but there is no clear evidence that antibiotics are effective in modifying the illness in patients with severe disease, where doxycycline, cefotaxime and penicillin appear to be equally effective [65].

References

1 Gimson AES (1987) Hepatic dysfunction during bacterial sepsis. *Intensive Care Med* 13, 162–166.

2 Brienza N, Dalfino L, Cinnella G *et al.* (2006) Jaundice in critical illness: promoting factors of a concealed reality. *Intensive Care Med* 32, 267–274.

3 Russell JA, Singer J, Bernard GR (2000) Changing pattern of organ dysfunction in early human sepsis related to mortality. *Crit Care Med* 28, 3405–3411.

4 Gogos Lekkou A, Papageorgiou O *et al.* (2003) Clinical prognostic markers in patients with severe sepsis: a prospective analysis of 139 consecutive cases. *J Infect* 47, 300–306.

5 Jepsen P, Vilstrup H, Schonheyder HC *et al.* (2005) A nationwide study of the incidence and 30-day mortality of pyogenic liver abscess in Denmark, 1977–2002. *Aliment Pharmacol Ther* 15, 1185–1188.

6 Setto RK, Rockey DC (1996) Pyogenic liver abscess: changes in etiology, management and outcome. *Medicine (Baltimore)* 75, 99–113.

7 Johannsen EC, Sifri CD, Madoff LC (2000) Pyogenic liver abscesses: *Infect Dis Clin North Am* 14, 547–563.

8 Rahimian J, Wilson T, Oram V *et al.* (2004) Pyogenic liver abscess: recent trends in etiology and mortality. *Clin Infect Dis* 39, 1654–1659.

9 Lederman ER, Crum NF (2005) Pyogenic liver abscess with a focus on *Klebsiella pneumoniae* as a primary pathogen: an emerging disease with unique clinical characteristics. *Am J Gastroenterol* 100, 322–331.

10 Ma LC, Fang CT, Lee CZ *et al.* (2005) Genomic heterogeneity in *Klebsiella pneumoniae* strains is associated with primary pyogenic liver abscess and metastatic infection. *J Infect Dis* 192, 117–128.

11 Wong WM, Wong BC, Hui CK *et al.* (2002) Pyogenic liver abscess: retrospective analyses of 80 cases over 10-year period. *J Gastroenterol Hepatol* 17, 1001–1007.

12 Tan YM, Chung AY, Chow PK *et al.* (2005) An appraisal of surgical and percutaneous drainage for pyogenic liver abscesses larger than 5 cm. *Ann Surg* 241, 485–490.

13 Girogio A, Tarantino I, Mariniello N *et al.* (1995) Pyogenic liver abscesses: 13 years of experience in percutaneous needle aspiration with US guidance. *Radiology* 195, 122–124.

14 Yu SC, Ho SS, Lau WY *et al.* (2004) Treatment of pyogenic liver abscess: prospective randomized comparison of catheter drainage and needle aspiration. *Hepatology* 39, 932–938.

15 McCormick JK, Yarwood JM, Schlievert PM (2001) Toxic shock syndrome and bacterial superantigens: an update. *Annu Rev Microbiol* 55, 77–104.

16 Begert H, Illert T, Friedrich K *et al.* (2004) Fulminant liver failure following infection with *Clostridium perfringens*. *Surg Infect (Larchmt)* 5, 205–209.

17 Yu VL. Miller WP, Wing EJ *et al.* (1982) Disseminated listeriosis presenting as acute hepatitis. *Am J Med* 73, 773–777.

18 Vargas V, Aleman C, de Torres I *et al.* (1998) *Listeria monocytogenes*-associated acute hepatitis in a liver transplant recipient. *Liver* 18, 213–215.

19 Nolla-Salas J, Almela M, Gasser I et al. (2002) Spontaneous *Listeria monocytogenes* peritonitis. A population-based study of 13 cases collected in Spain. *Am J Gastroenterol* 97, 1507–1511.

20 Kirby BD, Snyder KM, Meyer RD et al. (1980) Legionnaire's disease: report of sixty-five nosocomially acquired cases and review of the literature. *Medicine* 59, 188–205.

21 Troy SB, Rickman LS, Davis CE (2005) Brucellosis in San Diego: epidemiology and species-related differences in acute clinical presentation. *Medicine (Baltimore)* 84, 174–187.

22 Colmenero JD, Reguera JM, Martos F et al. (1996) Complications associated with *Brucella melitensis* infection: a study of 530 cases. *Medicine (Baltimore)* 75, 195–211.

23 Ariza J, Pigrau C, Canas C et al. (2001) Current understanding and management of hepatosplenic suppurative brucellosis. *Clin Infect Dis* 32, 1024–1033.

24 Cervantes F, Bruguera M, Carbonell J et al. (1982) Liver disease in brucellosis. A clinical and pathological study of 40 cases. *Postgrad Med J* 58, 346–350.

25 Colmenero JD, Queipo-Ortuño MI, Reguera JM et al. (2002) Chronic hepatosplenic abscesses in brucellosis. Clinico-therapeutic features and molecular diagnostic approach. *Diagn Microbiol Infect Dis* 42, 159–167.

26 Queipo-Ortuño MI, Colmenero JD, Baeza G et al. (2005) Comparison between lightcycler real-time polymerase chain reaction (PCR) assay with serum and PCR-enzyme linked immunosorbent assay with whole blood samples for the diagnosis of human brucellosis. *Clin Infect Dis* 40, 260–264.

27 White NJ (2003) Melioidosis. *Lancet* 361, 1715–1722.

28 Vatcharapreechasakul T, Suputtamongkol Y, Dance DA et al. (1992) *Pseudomonas pseudomallei* liver abscess: a clinical, radiographic and ultrasonographic study. *Clin Infect Dis* 14, 412–417.

29 Walsh AL, Smith MD, Wuthiekanun V et al. (1994) Immunofluorescence microscopy for the rapid diagnosis of melioidosis. *J Clin Pathol* 47, 377–379.

30 Wong KT, Vadivelu J, Puthucheary SD et al. (1996) An immunohistochemical method for the diagnosis of melioidosis. *Pathology* 28, 188–191.

31 Ulrich MP, Norwood DA, Christensen DR et al. (2006) Using real-time PCR to specifically detect *Burkholderia pseudomallei*. *J Med Microbiol* 55, 551–559.

32 Koshla SN, Singh R, Singh GP et al. (1988) The spectrum of hepatic injury in enteric fever. *Am J Gastroenterol* 83, 413–416.

33 El-Newihi HM, Alamy ME, Reynolds TB (1999) Salmonella hepatitis: analysis of 27 cases and comparison with acute viral hepatitis. *Hepatology* 24, 516–519.

34 Bhan MK, Bahl R, Bhatnagar S (2005) Typhoid and para typhoid fever. *Lancet* 366, 749–762.

35 Eliasson H, Broman T, Forsman M et al. (2006) Tularemia: current epidemiology and disease management. *Infect Dis Clin North Am* 20, 289–311.

36 Ellis J, Oyston PC, Gree M et al. (2002) Tularemia. *Clin Microbiol Rev* 15, 631–646.

37 Raoult D, Tissot-Dupont H, Foucault C et al. (2000) Q fever 1985–1998: clinical and epidemiological features of 1383 infections. *Medicine (Baltimore)* 79, 109–123.

38 Parker NR, Barralet JH, Bell AM (2006) Q fever. *Lancet* 367, 679–688.

39 Bonilla MF, Kaul DR, Saint S et al. (2006) Ring around the diagnosis. *N Engl J Med* 354, 1937–1942.

40 Fournier PE, Raoult D (2003) Comparison of PCR and serology assay for early diagnosis of acute Q fever. *J Clin Microbiol* 41, 5094–5098.

41 Sharma JB, Malhotra M, Arora R (2002) Incidental Fitz-Hugh–Curtis syndrome at laparoscopy for benign gynecological conditions. *Int J Gynecol Obstet* 79, 237–240.

42 Johnson RE, Newhall WJ, Papp JR et al. (2002) Screening tests to detect *Chlamydia trachomatis* and *Neisseria gonorrhoeae* infections – 2002. *MMWR Recomm Rep* 51(RR-15), 1–38.

43 Abdulkarim AS, Petrovic LM, Kim WR et al. (2004) Primary biliary cirrhosis: an infectious disease caused by *Chlamydia pneumoniae*? *J Hepatol* 40, 380–384.

44 Romero Gómez M, Otero MA, Sánchez-Muñoz D et al. (2006) Acute hepatitis due to *Mycoplasma pneumoniae* without lung involvement in adult patients. *J Hepatol* 44, 827–828.

45 Le Tallec V, Abgueguen P, Pichard E et al. (2003) Localisations hépatospléniques de la maladie du griffe du chat chez l'adulte immunocompetent. Deux cas. *Gastroenterol Clin Biol* 27, 225–229.

46 Liston TE, Koehler JE (1996) Granulomatous hepatitis and necrotizing splenitis due to *Bartonella henselae* in a patient with cancer: case report and review of hepatosplenic manifestations of bartonella infection. *Clin Infect Dis* 22, 951–957.

47 Meyers BR, Papanicolau GA, Sheiner P et al. (2000) Tuberculosis in orthotopic liver transplant patients: increased toxicity of recommended agents: cure of disseminated infection with non conventional regimens. *Transplantation* 15, 64–69.

48 Mert A, Bilir M, Tabak-Ozaras R et al. (2001) Miliary tuberculosis: clinical manifestations, diagnosis and outcome in 38 adults. *Respirology* 6, 217–224.

49 Huang WT, Wang CC, Chen WJ et al. (2003) The nodular form of hepatic tuberculosis: a review with five additional cases. *J Clin Pathol* 56, 835–839.

50 Chapman AS, Bakken JS, Folk SM et al. (2006) Diagnosis and management of tickborne rickettsial diseases: Rocky Mountain spotted fever, ehrlichioses, and anaplasmosis, United States. A practical guide for physicians and other health-care and public health professionals. *MMWR Recomm Rep* 55(RR-4), 1–27.

51 Guardia J, Vilaseca J, Moragas A et al. (1981) Hepatitis in exanthematous Mediterranean fever. *Hepatogastroenterology* 28, 81–83.

52 Dumler JS (2005) *Anaplasma* and *Ehrlichia* infection. *Ann NY Acad Med Sci* 1063, 361–373.

53 Dumler JS, Choi KS, García-García JC et al. (2005) Human granulocytic anaplasmosis and *Anaplasma phagocytophilum*. *Emerg Infect Dis* 11, 1828–1834.

54 Woods CR (2005) Syphilis in children: congenital and acquired. *Semin Pediatr Infect Dis* 16, 245–257.

55 Mullick CJ, Liappis AP, Benator DA et al. (2004) Syphilitic hepatitis in HIV-infected patients: a report of 7 cases and review of the literature. *Clin Infect Dis* 39, 100–105.

56 Witkowski JA, Parish LC (2002) The great imitator: malignant syphilis with hepatitis. *Clin Dermatol* 20, 152–163.

57 Baughn RE, Musher DM (2005) Secondary syphilitic lesions. *Clin Microbiol Rev* 18, 205–216.

58 Maincent G, Labadie H, Fabre M et al. (1997) Tertiary hepatic syphilis: a treatable cause of multinodular liver. *Dig Dis Sci* 42, 447–450.

59 Wormser GP (2006) Early Lyme disease. *N Engl J Med* 354, 2794–2781.

60 Horowitz HW, Dworkin B, Forseter G et al. (1996) Liver function in early Lyme disease. *Hepatology* 23, 1412–1417.

61 Zaidi SA, Singer C (2002) Gastrointestinal and hepatic manifestations of tickborne diseases in the United States. *Clin Infect Dis* 34, 1206–1212.

62 Johnson WD, Golightly LM (2000) *Borrelia* species (relapsing fever). In: Mandell GL, Bennett JE, Dolin R (eds) *Mandell, Douglas and Bennett's Principles and Practice of Infectious Diseases*, 5th edn. Philadelphia: Churchill Livingstone, pp. 2502–2504.

63 Bharti AR, Nally JE, Ricaldi JN *et al.* (2003) Leptospirosis: a zoonotic disease of global importance. *Lancet Infect Dis* 3, 757–771.

64 Ahmad SN, Shah S, Ahmad FM (2005) Laboratory diagnosis of leptospirosis. *J Postgrad Med* 51, 195–200.

65 Suputtamongkol Y, Niwattayakul K, Suttinont C *et al.* (2004) An open, randomized, controlled trial of penicillin, doxycycline, and cefotaxime for patients with severe leptospirosis. *Clin Infect Dis* 39, 1417–1424.

10.2 Fungal infections affecting the liver

Roderick J. Hay

The liver becomes a target for infection in certain systemic fungal infections for several reasons. First, fungi of the appropriate size, such as *Histoplasma capsulatum*, are taken up by reticuloendothelial cells. Second, because of the volume of blood flow through the liver, fungi disseminated through the bloodstream commonly involve this organ. Third, certain fungi, notably *Candida albicans* and *Candida tropicalis*, are thought to penetrate the gastrointestinal mucosa in severely ill, neutropenic patients and spread directly to the liver via the portal vein before invading other organs. Despite this, the liver is not commonly reported as a site of fungal infection, possibly through simple oversight. It also reflects the fact that symptoms resulting from invasion of other sites such as the central nervous system or lung may dominate the clinical picture. The mycoses most frequently associated with invasion of the liver are shown in Table 1. They include the systemic fungal infections histoplasmosis, coccidioidomycosis penicillinosis due to *Penicillium marneffei*, paracoccidioidomycosis and, less frequently, blastomycosis. Of the opportunistic fungal pathogens, both *Aspergillus* and *Cryptococcus* may spread to this site, but liver infection is more often seen in disseminated candidosis as well as in rarer diseases such as trichosporonosis.

The other important way in which fungi may cause damage to hepatocytes is via mycotoxicosis produced by ingestion of fungal toxins. Many of the aflatoxins produced by a range of environmental fungi such as *Aspergillus* spp. may cause hepatic necrosis or cirrhosis. Other mycotoxins, such as patulin and ochratoxin A, affect the liver in laboratory animals, although the contribution made by these substances to human disease is largely unproven.

Candidosis

Definition

Infections caused by fungi of the genus *Candida*, known as candidosis or candidiasis, may be either superficial or systemic [1]. Liver involvement follows dissemination via the circulation, either after direct introduction of the organisms through a contaminated intravenous line or intravenous injection in a drug abuser, or after invasion via the gastrointestinal tract. While hepatic infection may pass virtually unrecognized among the other manifestations of fulminant systemic candidosis, in certain patients, *Candida* infection of the liver and spleen produces a characteristic syndrome called hepatosplenic candidosis (chronic disseminated candidosis).

Introduction

In the last 30 years, systemic *Candida* infections have become a relatively frequent occurrence in certain groups such as neutropenic cancer or postoperative or intensive therapy unit (ITU) patients. Infection of the liver has been a consistent finding in many autopsy surveys of systemic candidosis.

Epidemiology

Candidosis has a worldwide distribution [1]. The most common species that causes human infection is *Candida albicans*, although others such as *C. tropicalis*, *C. parapsilosis* and *C. glabrata* may also be implicated. *Candida krusei* and *C. glabrata* are usually resistant to the antifungal drug fluconazole. Overall, there has been a change in the distribution of different *Candida* species in systemic infections, with a higher proportion of infections occurring in ITU and neutropenic patients being caused by species other than *C. albicans* such as *C. glabrata* or *C. parapsilosis*.

Table 1 Liver involvement has been reported in the following deep fungal infections.

Opportunistic mycoses
Candidosis – includes hepatosplenic candidosis
Cryptococcosis
Less common: aspergillosis, mucormycosis, trichosporonosis

Pathogenic mycoses
Histoplasmosis – disseminated (classical) histoplasmosis
Paracoccidioidomycosis
Less common: coccidioidomycosis, African histoplasmosis, blastomycosis, penicillinosis

Candida spp. are common commensal organisms, being carried by a significant proportion of the healthy population in the mouth (25%), gastrointestinal tract (16%) and vagina (22%). The organisms become pathogenic under appropriate conditions, a change often associated with the development of hyphae. These conditions range from abnormalities of epithelial surfaces to physiological changes, endocrine or metabolic disease and primary or secondary immunodeficiency states.

Pathogenesis and pathology

Candida causes disease by invasion of tissue. There are various potential routes of systemic invasion. The organisms may be introduced directly into the bloodstream by injection, a form of disease seen in intravenous drug addicts, in whom fungi cause infection of the eyes, hair follicles and bones. *Candida* may also gain entry via an intravenous drip site by contamination of intravenous fluids or the skin. A major route of entry in neutropenic patients is via the gastrointestinal (probably jejunal) mucosa. This may follow invasion of the mucosa, or a process known as persorption in which particles such as *Candida* cells rapidly cross an intact mucosal wall. This is based on evidence in man that non-pathogenic yeasts can appear rapidly in the bloodstream after oral administration and, in neonatal mice, transfer of yeasts from the bowel lumen to the circulation appears to occur in the jejunum.

In tissue, *C. albicans* is normally found in both yeast and hyphal forms in small abscesses, and there are usually many organisms present. However, in patients with hepatosplenic candidosis, in whom the infection may persist for weeks despite a return of white cell counts to the normal range, few organisms are seen in the later stages of infection, and the tissue response may be granulomatous or mixed, with granulomas surrounding neutrophil abscesses. Hyphae are seldom produced in tissues by *Candida* spp. other than *C. albicans*. The pattern of disease associated with hepatosplenic candidosis has been described as an immunorestitution syndrome [not associated with human immunodeficiency virus (HIV)], a description that explains some of the features of the condition [2].

Clinical features and complications

Systemic candidosis usually has few clinical features that can be used to separate it from other septicaemic illnesses in severely ill patients. Patients present with pyrexia, usually after abdominal surgery or during neutropenia. Occasionally, there are helpful signs that may give a clue to the diagnosis, such as the appearance of multiple skin nodules, muscle pains or retinal deposits. The liver may be enlarged in such cases, but this is very variable. Hepatic lesions are usually found incidentally at autopsy. A number of risk factors have been associated with fungal liver infection in bone marrow transplant recipients. These include deep fungal infection after transplantation, colonization or superficial fungal infection after transplantation and severe liver dysfunction through veno-occlusive disease or graft-vs.-host disease [3].

Hepatosplenic candidosis

In recent years, increasing numbers of patients have been described with a syndrome whose principal feature is *Candida* infection of the liver and spleen [4]. The main characteristics of these patients were reviewed by Odds (Table 2) [1]. Most have leukaemia and have had a prolonged episode of neutropenia. The infection is most often caused by *C. albicans*. Unlike other forms of candidosis, the signs may appear after the patient appears to be in remission from the primary disease. The main clinical features are high, swinging pyrexia and chills, with right upper abdominal pain. Appetite is poor and patients show a variable degree of malaise. Progress is variable but, in untreated patients, the infection persists over weeks. It is also notoriously resistant to therapy [5–7]. The names hepatosplenic or chronic disseminated candidiasis have been used for this syndrome.

Diagnosis and differential diagnosis

Systemic candidosis may be difficult to diagnose, particularly in the immunocompromised patient. Blood cultures should be set up and repeated if necessary; cultures of intravenous line tips may also be helpful. Blood cultures are positive in a high proportion of patients after surgery, but in less than 20% of those with neutropenia. Other methods of diagnosis include serology, which is often only available in specialized centres. There are a few commercial kits available for the detection of *Candida* antibodies or antigen. These investigations may be contributory, but should not be regarded as diagnostic, particularly in the absence of any other evidence of *Candida* infection. The most reliable method of diagnosis is by biopsy and histopathological examination of appropriate lesions such as skin nodules. Percutaneous liver biopsy has not been widely used, except in hepatosplenic candidosis, where it is the definitive method of diagnosis [8].

Hepatosplenic candidosis

In this syndrome, a number of approaches to diagnosis in addition to biopsy may also be contributory. The most consistent results are seen with computerized tomography (CT) or magnetic resonance imaging (MRI) scans, which will show liver or spleen granulomas and abscesses [9,10]. The biphasic spiral liver CT technique shows specific patterns of enhancement, and the pattern is best seen in the arterial phase of perfusion [11]. MRI is a useful technique for following the course of infection. Ultrasonography has been less helpful, but is an alternative. Radionucleotide scanning with technetium-99 or gallium-67 has produced variable results. To prove the identity of the infection, it may be necessary to attempt liver biopsy with echo guidance or open biopsy at laparotomy. Serological tests may be positive in some of these patients and, in many such cases, antibody rather than antigen titres may be considerably elevated. The use of polymerase chain reaction (PCR) techniques can improve the diagnostic yield [12]. Liver enzymes are usually

Table 2 Clinical and pathological features of hepatosplenic candidosis.

Feature	Details	Percentage with feature
Sex distribution	Male:female	45.2:54.8
Age distribution (years)	<1	0
	1–9	25.0
	10–29	25.0
	30–49	34.1
	50–69	13.6
	>70	2.3
Underlying diseases	Acute leukaemia	86.3
	Aplastic anaemia	5.9
	Other	7.8
Diagnostic features	Fever	100.0
	Upper quadrant abdominal pain	96.3
	Raised alkaline phosphatase	100.0
	Blood leucocytosis	81.0
	CT scan abnormalities	93.8
	Ultrasound abnormalities	66.7
Sites affected	Liver alone	23.5
	Spleen alone	13.7
	Both liver and spleen	62.7
Causative organism	*Candida albicans*	88.2
	C. tropicalis	5.9
Outcome	Patient died	43.2

Data taken from Table 22.3 in Odds FC (1988) *Candida and Candidosis*. London: Baillière Tindall, pp. 196–205, with permission.

elevated, although the most consistent abnormality has been in alkaline phosphatase.

In hepatosplenic candidosis, the presence of a high, swinging pyrexia should alert the attending physician.

Treatment and prognosis

The mainstay of treatment for systemic *Candida* infections is intravenous amphotericin B (0.5–1.0 mg/kg body weight). Other choices include lipid-associated forms of amphotericin B [13], amphotericin B combined with flucytosine, itraconazole (oral), caspofungin and fluconazole (oral or intravenous). The range of treatment regimes employed suggests that these are difficult infections, possibly in keeping with their designation as part of an immune reconstitution syndrome. There is a high mortality in proven infections affecting neutropenic patients; therapy should be continued, where possible, until there is recovery of white cell numbers and, at any rate, for a minimum of 2–3 weeks. Treatment of hepatosplenic infections is also difficult, and many patients fail to respond to long courses of amphotericin B and flucytosine or fluconazole [5]. Some successes have been achieved with the lipid-associated forms of amphotericin B that are liposome based (AmBisome), a colloidal dispersion (ABCD or Amphocil) or a lipid complex (ABLC or Abelcet). Once again, there are few case reports on these compounds in hepatosplenic candidosis. Hepatosplenic candidosis is not necessarily a contraindication to bone marrow transplantation, provided that recipients are treated with antifungals both before and after engraftment until the graft is established [14]. There is little experience to date with voriconazole in this variety of candidosis.

Other opportunistic fungal infections

Invasive aspergillosis may be associated with solitary or multiple liver abscesses in 13–41% of cases [15]. The usual pattern of infection is the invasion of tissue, with scattered fungal hyphae penetrating necrotic liver parenchyma [16]. Occasionally, the fungus may form into a fungus ball, or aspergilloma, at this site [17]. Likewise, liver abscesses have been recorded with systemic infections caused by other fungi such as *Trichosporon beigelii* [18]. Mucormycosis, invasive zygomycosis and *Scedosporium* infections have only occasionally been recorded as causing liver disease, largely because they are often rapidly fatal even with localized infection of a distal site. All these infections are treated in much the same way as systemic candidosis, usually with amphotericin B in conventional or lipid-associated forms and/or flucytosine.

Cryptococcosis

Cryptococcosis is caused by *Cryptococcus neoformans*, a yeast that is found in the environment in association with pigeon excreta [19]. There are two varieties of the organism: *C. neoformans neoformans*, which causes disease in Europe and parts of the United States in otherwise healthy people and immunocompromised patients including those with acquired immunodeficiency virus (AIDS); and *C. neoformans gattii*, which is seen mainly in non-AIDS patients in Africa and the Far East. The former is associated with pigeon excreta, the latter with certain species of Eucalyptus. Infection usually follows inhalation. Previously healthy individuals may be infected, particularly in the tropics but, in many parts of the world, cryptococcosis is seen mainly in patients with defective T-lymphocyte function, including those with Hodgkin's disease, AIDS, systemic lupus erythematosus, and in patients on steroid therapy as well as those receiving immunosuppression after organ transplants.

The primary focus of infection is the lung, but the most common clinical manifestation of the disease is meningitis. Skin or bone lesions may also occur. About 10–15% of patients have some evidence of pulmonary involvement, indicating that the primary focus often heals, despite dissemination. Liver infiltration during disseminated cryptococcosis is not common, but has been reported, particularly in patients with AIDS, where enlargement of the liver is not infrequent [20]. Patients may present with apparent biliary obstruction due to liver infiltration [21,22].

In non-AIDS patients, other patterns of liver infiltration have been recorded rarely. These include focal granulomatous hepatitis, which may mimic viral hepatitis and, on occasion, widespread infiltrates resulting in hepatic failure [23].

Another rare method of presentation is with obstructive jaundice secondary to sclerosing cholangitis, where the yeasts can be identified in the common bile duct [24]. In at least one such case, there has been histological evidence of pre-existing cirrhosis. Extensive hepatic necrosis associated with cryptococcal infection leading to liver failure has been described [25].

The best method of laboratory diagnosis is direct microscopic examination of smears, sputum or cerebrospinal fluid. The samples can be stained with India ink or nigrosin, both of which emphasize the yeast capsule. Cultures can also be taken and are usually positive in infected cases. There is a rapid antigen detection test using the agglutination of latex particles coated with antibody or an enzyme-linked immunosorbent assay (ELISA) that can be performed on serum or cerebrospinal fluid.

In most patients, the most appropriate therapy is amphotericin B with or without flucytosine given in doses of 0.3–0.6 mg/kg daily and 150 mg/kg daily respectively. Therapy in patients with AIDS is associated with a high relapse rate (over 70%), and it is usually necessary to give long-term treatment at weekly intervals after the induction of remission, the length of suppressive treatment depending on the response to highly active antiretroviral therapy (HAART). Fluconazole produces significant remissions at a dose of 400 mg daily in comparison with amphotericin B, but there may be a somewhat higher frequency of early relapse with fluconazole. Higher doses of fluconazole (600–800 mg daily) appear to be more effective.

However, fluconazole is effective as a long-term treatment after initial remission.

Histoplasmosis

Definition

Histoplasmosis is a systemic infection caused by *Histoplasma capsulatum*, a dimorphic organism that can be found in the environment in soil or material contaminated with bird or bat excreta [19]. Infection follows inhalation and, in most people, this is asymptomatic. Occasionally, the infection may disseminate from the lungs to involve other organs, notably those rich in macrophages. The liver is affected in disseminated infections. This type of infection is known as classical or small-form histoplasmosis and is caused by a specific variant of the fungus, *H. capsulatum capsulatum*. The small-form disease is characterized by the presence of tiny yeasts (2–4 μm in diameter) in tissue macrophages; it has a worldwide distribution.

A second type of histoplasmosis, African or large-form histoplasmosis, caused by another variant of *H. capsulatum*, named *H. capsulatum* var. *duboisii*, is seen in central regions of Africa. Liver infection is not commonly recorded in this form of the disease. The tissue yeast forms in African histoplasmosis are large (10–12 μm in diameter) and are found in foreign-body giant cells; both forms of *H. capsulatum* are culturally indistinguishable. African histoplasmosis will be discussed separately.

Prevalence and epidemiology

Histoplasmosis (classical) has a well-defined endemic area, being found in the east and central regions of the United States as well as Central and South America, Africa, the Indian subcontinent and the Far East. Exposure, as assessed by conversion rates on the histoplasmin skin test, is highest in the United States and northern South America. In parts of the United States, over 90% of the healthy populace are skin test positive. A lower prevalence of positive skin test (under 20%) is seen in Africa and the Far East. These findings suggest that the infection is usually asymptomatic and self-healing. Infection follows inhalation of the organism, which is particularly associated with large accumulations of bird droppings in roosting sites and old buildings. In the tropics, important sites of potential exposure are bat-infested caves or buildings housing bat colonies.

Pathogenesis

Most of the systemic mycoses follow a common pattern of infection shown in Table 3. Subclinical infection is common, but the primary infection may be symptomatic where it is associated with massive exposure to a natural source of the fungus, for instance in a cave (cave fever). Chronic infection of the lungs may develop in those with pre-existing pulmonary disease, such as emphysema. The infection is a frequent, self-healing event,

Table 3 Scheme for clinical features of systemic mycoses due to endemic pathogenic fungi (histoplasmosis, blastomycosis, etc.).

Asymptomatic (sensitization)	Positive delayed-type hypersensitivity to fungal antigen
Acute pulmonary	Acute pulmonary infection after high-dose exposure
Chronic pulmonary	
Inactive	Asymptomatic pulmonary nodule(s)
Active	Chronic consolidation or cavitary lung disease
Disseminated[a]	
Acute	Widespread extrapulmonary dissemination
Chronic	Focal slowly progressive dissemination
Primary cutaneous	Skin lesion and lymphadenopathy following inoculation

[a]The progress and extent of dissemination in deep mycoses varies depending on the infection and the underlying condition of the patient.

even in subclinical cases because, in endemic areas, splenic or hepatic calcification of the site of healed metastatic lesions, some of which contain *H. capsulatum*, is common. In addition to this, dissemination may be progressive, particularly in patients with defective resistance. In rapidly disseminated forms of histoplasmosis, liver involvement may be more common, but it is also a feature of the indolent, chronic form of disseminated histoplasmosis in which the main clinical abnormalities are oral ulceration, hepatic enlargement or adrenal insufficiency [26].

Clinical features

The clinical features of histoplasmosis are largely determined by the site of infection. Acute and chronic pulmonary histoplasmosis are dominated by respiratory symptoms such as cough, weight loss, chest pain and fever. Disseminated disease is also associated with weight loss and fever but, in the chronic forms of infection, oral or laryngeal ulcers or adrenal insufficiency may appear [19].

Symptomatic hepatic involvement may be seen in the rapid-onset, disseminated form of *Histoplasma* infection. Studies indicate that as many as 66% of patients have hepatomegaly [27,28]. The enlarged liver may be tender, and the spleen is frequently enlarged also. Lesions are usually diffusely distributed through the liver, with multiple granulomas or parenchymal infiltration with many macrophages being stuffed with organisms [26]. Abnormalities of liver function may also occur. In patients with AIDS, liver enlargement has also been a common feature in those presenting with histoplasmosis [29–31].

The liver may also be involved in chronic disseminated forms of the infection. Here, there may be only slight hepatic enlargement. Interestingly, the most common pathological pattern is diffuse granuloma formation and, in many of these lesions, organisms cannot be found [32]. Infiltration of an allograft liver has also been reported [33].

Investigations

Histoplasma capsulatum is very small and difficult to demonstrate in pathological material without experience. Giemsa- or methenamine silver-stained sections or biopsies may show the organisms. *Histoplasma* can be cultured from such cases. Liver biopsies may also be a source of histopathological material [34]. Serological tests (immunodiffusion and complement fixation) are useful procedures for diagnosis and monitoring therapy. Two very specific precipitin bands, H and M, are found in histoplasmosis, the former being a more reliable indicator of active disease. Newer antigen detection tests are available and are particularly helpful for AIDS patients.

Therapy

The treatment of the patient with histoplasmosis affecting the liver is the same as that used for disseminated infections. Amphotericin B is the main treatment and is given in doses of 0.8–1.0 mg/kg daily. The duration of treatment varies, but it may need to be continued until a total dose of 2.0 g is achieved. Itraconazole is effective in some forms of histoplasmosis and is probably the treatment of choice in chronically disseminated forms of the disease; it is also effective in patients with AIDS both for initial therapy at 200–400 mg daily and for long-term suppressive therapy (cf. cryptococcosis) at 100–200 mg daily [35]. These regimens can be modified depending on the response to HAART.

African histoplasmosis

African histoplasmosis is an uncommon disease. Patients mainly present with disseminated lesions affecting the skin, bones and lymph nodes. Pulmonary involvement is rare. There are few reports of liver involvement in the course of African histoplasmosis [36].

Paracoccidioidomycosis

Definition

Paracoccidioidomycosis is a systemic fungal infection caused by the dimorphic fungus *Paracoccidioides brasiliensis* [37]. The infection is seen only in parts of South and Central America and Mexico. The organism causes either a widely disseminated infection or one localized to one or two sites, particularly the oral mucosa or lungs. Involvement of the liver is infrequently recognized, although it is probably common in widespread infections.

Epidemiology and pathogenesis

Paracoccidioidomycosis is a New World infection, although imported cases have been described outside this area in Japan and Europe. While it is believed that *P. brasiliensis* is found in nature, it has only been identified in the natural environment on a few occasions and, therefore, its true ecological niche is unknown.

Cases of the infection are not common, even in endemic areas, and are mainly seen in adult males. This is thought to be due to an unusual effect of human androgens on the conversion of the organism to the yeast phase. There have been several surveys which suggest that exposure to the organism is fairly widespread in the population of endemic areas, although only occasionally have more than 20–25% of the community been found to be skin test positive to intradermal antigens of *P. brasiliensis*. Infection follows inhalation.

Clinical features

Paracoccidioidomycosis is a multisystem disease involving the lungs and the lymphatic system. It is often classified, as with the other systemic mycoses, into pulmonary and disseminated forms, or by location into pulmonary, lymphatic, mucocutaneous and mixed depending on the predominant site(s) of clinical involvement. Like histoplasmosis, a proportion of those exposed to this organism appear to develop asymptomatic infection, and the process resolves with the only evidence of infection being a positive skin test. Respiratory disease may also coexist with extrapulmonary infection, particularly ulcerative lesions of the oral or genital mucosa as well as adjacent skin. Lymph node involvement is also common.

Evidence for hepatic involvement is largely based on autopsy surveys, in which between 24% and 56% of those who die with paracoccidioidomycosis are found to have liver involvement [38,39]. In some series, over 40% of those with disseminated forms of infection have had hepatomegaly. The liver in these cases is said to be enlarged diffusely with unchanged consistency. Jaundice is rare and is found in less than 6% of cases [40]. Biopsy shows lesions ranging from small granulomas to diffuse infiltration of yeast forms and fibrosis. The bile ducts are commonly involved. The earliest signs are changes in aminotransferase concentrations; changes in alkaline phosphatase or bilirubin tend to occur in late disease.

Investigations

The diagnosis is confirmed by the demonstration of the organism in tissue and its isolation in culture. *Paracoccidioides brasiliensis* characteristically produces multipolar buds around the circumference of a yeast cell, and these can be seen in direct examination of smears. The organisms grow well in primary culture. Serodiagnosis may be very helpful, and immunodiffusion and complement fixation tests are available for this disease.

Therapy

The most appropriate therapy available at present is itraconazole, which is given in doses of 100–200 mg daily for 3–6 months or longer if necessary. The older azole antifungal, ketoconazole, is also very active. Other methods include intravenous amphotericin B and sulphonamides. Relapse after using the latter is very common.

Coccidioidomycosis

Coccidioidomycosis is an infection caused by *Coccidioides immitis*, a soil organism found in the arid western parts of the United States in California, Arizona, Texas and New Mexico, as well as in certain areas in South and Central America (northern Argentina, Colombia, Uruguay) [41]. Infection follows inhalation of the fungus and, like histoplasmosis, many of those exposed simply become sensitized without infection. Like histoplasmosis, acute or chronic pulmonary infections may result, or the disease may spread from the primary lung focus to involve other sites including the liver.

The main features of infection are therefore respiratory, and patients present with acute or chronic cough, malaise and fever. Dissemination often occurs in immunocompromised patients and is also more frequently seen in certain ethnic groups such as Indians or African Americans. The principal sites for dissemination are the meninges, joints and skin. In severe and widely disseminated infections, involvement of the liver is common, and one autopsy survey suggested that hepatic foci could be found in at least half of those with this type of disease [42]. The pattern of liver involvement ranges from focal granuloma formation to diffuse inflammatory infiltration [42,43]. Liver enlargement can occur together with changes in liver enzymes. Liver involvement has also been reported in patients with AIDS who develop coccidioidomycosis [44].

This infection is diagnosed by culture or by finding the characteristic *Coccidioides* spherules in smears or histologically. The organism grows well in laboratory culture. Laboratory staff should be warned about a possible diagnosis of coccidioidomycosis if they are attempting cultures. Serology (immunodiffusion, enzyme immunoassay or counter-immunoelectrophoresis) is very helpful in both establishing the diagnosis and monitoring the course of disease. Liver biopsy has been reported as a diagnostic procedure in coccidioidomycosis [43].

Although the management of some forms of coccidioidomycosis may be relatively simple, disseminated infections are difficult to treat. Amphotericin B is the mainstay of therapy, although some patients with soft-tissue disease may respond to ketoconazole, itraconazole or fluconazole.

Other systemic mycoses

Blastomycosis due to the dimorphic fungus, *Blastomyces dermatitidis*, is occasionally associated with liver infiltration in disseminated forms [45]. The geographical range of this disease is fairly wide, with cases being found in north and central United States and Canada, Africa, the Middle East and occasionally elsewhere. It is uncommon and has only occasionally been reported in disseminated infections in immunocompromised patients [46]. In one study in such groups, two of six patients with chronic myeloid and chronic lymphocytic leukaemia, respectively, had diffuse infiltrations of leukaemic cells and *B. dermatitidis* in the liver at autopsy.

Penicillinosis due to *Penicillium marneffei* is a disease recently reported from Southeast Asia and in individuals who have visited that area. The organism naturally causes infection in bamboo rats. Its mode of transmission and pathogenesis is unknown, but widespread disseminated forms of the disease have been seen, with foci of infection in bone marrow, spleen, lung and liver [47]. The infection is generally associated with AIDS, and it is encountered regularly as an AIDS-related complication in endemic areas in Thailand, South China, Malaysia, Hong Kong and Myanmar. Patients generally present with disseminated disease in which there are widespread skin lesions and bone marrow infiltration with yeast cells. They are febrile and systemically unwell. Less frequently, patients may present without skin lesions and with tender hepatomegaly [48].

The organism can be recognized histologically and isolated in culture. In tissue, *P. marneffei* may resemble *Histoplasma* small forms, but it does not form buds and individual cells divide by transverse fission. Hepatic lesions are of one of three types: diffuse, granulomatous and mixed. The diffuse pattern showed a diffuse infiltration of foamy macrophages that contained numerous *P. marneffei*, whereas in the granulomatous pattern, true granulomas are seen with various degrees of inflammatory cell infiltration. The mixed pattern shows features of both forms. All show abnormal liver function, but there are no specific features that will distinguish the types, and there is usually a granulomatous response. This infection can be treated with itraconazole or amphotericin B.

Actinomycete infections

The actinomycetes are filamentous bacteria that may cause a variety of different diseases. By convention, two of these, actinomycosis and nocardiosis, are usually considered with the fungal infections.

Actinomycosis

Actinomycosis is an infection caused by actinomycetes of the genus *Actinomyces*, notably *A. israelii*, *A. bovis* and *A. naeslundii*. More rarely, other actinomycete species are involved. Infections often occur in specific sites such as the mouth (cervicofacial), abdomen, thorax or uterus (pelvic). In the pelvic site of infection, there has been an association with certain intrauterine contraceptive devices.

In many cases, it appears that aggregates of *Actinomyces* are associated with other bacteria such as coliforms. The part played by these bacteria in the pathogenesis of the infection is unknown. Actinomycosis is mainly seen in otherwise healthy patients. The hallmark of the infection is the formation of inflammatory masses containing granules. Such masses encroach on other structures, and multiple draining sinuses are formed. These may involve the jaw, the chest or the pelvis, and can be confused with a range of other conditions such as mycetoma or tumours. Infection of the liver is unusual but has been recorded.

In about 15% of cases of abdominal actinomycosis, itself a rare condition, the liver is affected [49]. The route of infection to this site is unknown, but it has been suggested that spread follows passage through the portal vein after appendicitis or surgery [50]. Most commonly, it presents as a solitary liver abscess and may spread to affect adjacent sites such as the bowel and the diaphragm. The liver may appear enlarged, but jaundice is rare [51]. The course of this infection may be very slow (over 2 years).

The diagnosis is made on the basis of cultures after needle aspiration or biopsy. CT scans show single or multiple, poorly defined areas of increased density [50]. The presumptive diagnosis is of liver abscess; aspirated material should be cultured. The main treatment is penicillin given parenterally ($2-12 \times 10^6$ units daily in adults), the dose depending on the site. Alternatives include erythromycin or tetracycline

Nocardiosis

Nocardia asteroides, *N. brasiliensis* and *N. caviae* are aerobic actinomycetes that may cause human disease [51]. There are two main clinical varieties: mycetoma, a subcutaneous infection resulting from implantation; and systemic nocardiosis, an invasive disease seen in both immunocompromised and healthy patients. Liver invasion is occasionally seen in disseminated nocardiosis. The primary portal of infection is thought to be the lung, and patients may present with primary lung disease and pulmonary infiltrates or with clinical lesions due to extrapulmonary dissemination, for instance to the brain or skin. The liver is a rare target in disseminated nocardiosis. In one survey of 230 cases of disseminated nocardiosis, only 3% of patients had proven hepatic lesions, either solitary or multiple abscesses. In one instance, the diagnosis was established by CT-guided needle aspiration of a subcapsular abscess [52]. Most patients with disseminated *Nocardia* infections have some form of underlying disease affecting T-lymphocyte function, such as lymphoma or AIDS, chronic granulomatous disease [53] or are receiving immunosuppressive regimens including corticosteroids.

The diagnosis is confirmed by culture, although the presence of partially acid-fast filaments in smears or histopathological sections is helpful. Nocardiosis often responds to treatment with co-trimoxazole. Alternative drugs include minocycline, ampicillin, amikacin and impipenem.

References

1 Odds FC (1988) *Candida and Candidosis*. London: Baillière Tindall, pp. 196–206.

2 Cheng VC, Yuen KY, Wong SS *et al.* (2001) Immunorestitution diseases in patients not infected with HIV. *Eur J Clin Microbiol Infect Dis* 20, 402–406.

3 Rossetti F, Brawner DL, Bowden R *et al.* (1995) Fungal liver infection in marrow transplant recipients: prevalence at autopsy, predisposing factors, and clinical features. *Clin Infect Dis* 20, 801–811.

4 Bodey GP, DeJongh D, Isassi A *et al.* (1969) Hypersplenism due to disseminated candidiasis in a patient with acute leukemia. *Cancer* 24, 417–420.

5 Tashjian LS, Abramson JS, Peacock JE Jr (1984) Focal hepatic candidiasis: a distinct clinical variant of candidiasis in immunocompromised patients. *Rev Infect Dis* 6, 689–703.

6 Linker CA, DeGregorio MW, Ries CA (1984) Computerized tomography in the diagnosis of systemic candidiasis in patients with acute leukemia. *Med Pediatr Oncol* 12, 380–385.

7 Sallah S, Semelka RC, Wehbie R *et al.* (1999) Hepatosplenic candidiasis in patients with acute leukaemia. *Br J Haematol* 106, 697–701.

8 Miller JH, Greenfield LD, Wald BR (1982) Candidiasis of the liver and spleen in childhood. *Radiology* 142, 375–380.

9 Bartley DL, Hughes WT, Parvey LS *et al.* (1982) Computed tomography of hepatic and splenic fungal abscesses in leukemic children. *Pediatr Infect Dis* 1, 317–321.

10 Linker CA, DeGregorio MW, Ries CA (1984) Computerized tomography in the diagnosis of systemic candidiasis in patients with acute leukemia. *Med Pediatr Oncol* 12, 380–385.

11 Rudolph J, Rodenwaldt J, Ruhnke M *et al.* (2004) Unusual enhancement pattern of liver lesions in hepatosplenic candidiasis. *Acta Radiologica* 45, 499–503.

12 Kirby A, Chapman C, Hassan C *et al.* (2004) The diagnosis of hepatosplenic candidiasis by DNA analysis of tissue biopsy and serum. *J Clin Pathol* 57, 764–765.

13 Sallah S, Semelka RC, Sallah W *et al.* (1999) Amphotericin B lipid complex for the treatment of patients with acute leukemia and hepatosplenic candidiasis. *Leukemia Research* 23, 995–999.

14 Bjerke JW, Meyers JD, Bowden RA (1994) Hepatosplenic candidiasis – a contraindication to marrow transplantation? *Blood* 84, 2811–2814.

15 Denning DW (1998) Invasive aspergillosis. *Clin Infect Dis* 26, 781–803.

16 Callister ME, Griffiths MJ, Nicholson AG *et al.* (2004) A fatal case of disseminated aspergillosis caused by a non-sporulating strain of *Aspergillus fumigatus*. *J Clin Pathol* 57, 991–992.

17 Baker RD (1962) Leukopenia and therapy in leukemia as factors predisposing to fatal mycoses. Mucormycosis, aspergillosis, and cryptococcosis. *Am J Clin Path* 37, 358–373.

18 Haupt HM, Merz WG, Beschorner WE *et al.* (1983) Colonization and infection with Trichosporon species in the immunosuppressed host. *J Infect Dis* 147, 199–203.

19 Perfect JR, Casadevall A (2002) Cryptococcosis. *Infect Dis Clin North Am* 16, 837–874.

20 Dismukes WE (1988) Cryptococcal meningitis in patients with AIDS. *J Infect Dis* 157, 624–628.

21 Goenka MK, Mehta S, Yachha SK *et al.* (1995) Hepatic involvement culminating in cirrhosis in a child with disseminated cryptococcosis. *J Clin Gastroenterol* 20, 57–60.

22 Kothari AA, Kothari KA (2004) Hepatobiliary dysfunction as initial manifestation of disseminated cryptococcosis. *Indian J Gastroenterol* 23, 145–146.

23 Sabesin SM, Fallon HJ, Andriole VT (1963) Hepatic failure as a manifestation of cryptococcosis. *Arch Intern Med* 111, 661–669.

24 Bucuvalas JC, Bove KE, Kaufman RA *et al.* (1985) Cholangitis associated with *Cryptococcus neoformans*. *Gastroenterology* 88, 1055–1059.

25 Lin JI, Kabir MA, Tseng HC *et al.* (1999) Hepatobiliary dysfunction as the initial manifestation of disseminated cryptococcosis. *J Clin Gastroenterol* 28, 273–275.

26 Sarosi GA, Voth DW, Dahl BA *et al.* (1971) Disseminated histoplasmosis: results of long-term follow-up. A Center for Disease Control cooperative mycoses study. *Ann Intern Med* 75, 511–516.

27 Schwarz J (1981) *Histoplasmosis*. New York: Praeger.

28 Deepe GS (2005) *Histoplasma capsulatum*. In: Mandell GL, Bennett JE, Dolin R (eds) *Principles and Practice of Infectious Diseases*. Philadelphia: Elsevier Churchill Livingstone, pp. 3013–3026.

29 Symmers WS (1972) Histoplasmosis in southern and south-eastern Asia. A syndrome associated with a peculiar tissue form of histoplasma: a study of 48 cases. *Ann Soc Belge Med Trop* 52, 435–452.

30 Mandell W, Goldberg DM, Neu HC (1986) Histoplasmosis in patients with the acquired immune deficiency syndrome. *Am J Med* 81, 974–978.

31 Huang CT, McGarry T, Cooper S *et al.* (1987) Disseminated histoplasmosis in the acquired immunodeficiency syndrome. Report of five cases from a nonendemic area. *Arch Intern Med* 147, 1181–1184.

32 Wheat LJ, Slama TG, Zeckel ML (1985) Histoplasmosis in the acquired immune deficiency syndrome. *Am J Med* 78, 203–210.

33 Sylvestre PB, Gonzalez-Koch AR, Ishitani MB (2000) *Liver Transpl* 6, 643.

34 Christian ER (1952) An evaluation of needle biopsy of the liver. *Am J Med* 13, 689–703.

35 Hecht FM, Wheat J, Korzun AH *et al.* (1997) Itraconazole maintenance treatment for histoplasmosis in AIDS: a prospective, multicenter trial. *J Acquir Immune Defic Syndr Hum Retrovirol* 16, 100–107.

36 Wheat J (2001) Laboratory diagnosis of histoplasmosis. Update 2000. *Semin Resp Infect* 16, 131–140.

37 Williams AO, Lawson EA, Lucas AO (1971) African histoplasmosis due to *Histoplasma duboisii*. *Arch Pathol* 92, 306–318.

38 Pinto HB (1961) La Paracoccidioidosis brasiliensis como enfermedad sistemica. *Mycopathologia* 15, 90–114 [in Portuguese].

39 Teixeira F, Gayotto LC, De Brito T (1978) Morphological patterns of the liver in South American blastomycosis. *Histopathology* 2, 231–237.

40 Raphael A, Campana AO, Waiman J (1964) [Hepatic coma in South America blastomycosis.] *Rev Assoc Med Bras* 10, 151–154 [in Portuguese].

41 Restrepo A (2003) Paracoccidioidomycosis. In: Dismukes WE, Pappas PG, Sobel JK (eds) *Clinical Mycology*. New York: Oxford University Press, pp. 328–345.

42 Stevens DA (ed.) (1981) *Coccidioidomycosis*. New York: Plenum.

43 Huntington RW, Waldman WJ, Sargent JA *et al.* (1967) Pathologic and clinical observations of fatal coccidioidomycosis with necropsy. In: Ajello L (ed.) *Coccidioidomycosis*. Tucson: University of Arizona Press, pp. 143–163.

44 Dodd LG, Nelson SD (1990) Disseminated coccidioidomycosis detected by percutaneous liver biopsy in a liver transplant recipient. *Am J Clin Pathol* 93, 141–144.

45 Galgiani JN (1999) Coccidioidomycosis: A regional disease of national importance. Rethinking approaches for control. *Ann Intern Med* 130, 293–300.

46 Recht LD, Davies SF, Eckman MR *et al.* (1982) Blastomycosis in immunosuppressed patients. *Am Rev Resp Dis* 125, 359–362.

47 Supparatpinyo K, Khamwan C, Baosoung V *et al.* (1994) Disseminated *Penicillium marneffei* infection in southeast Asia. *Lancet* 344(8915), 110–113.

48 Kantipong P, Panich V, Pongsurachet V *et al.* (1998) Hepatic penicilliosis in patients without skin lesions. *Clin Infect Dis* 26, 1215–1217.

49 Bradsher RW (2003) Blastomycosis. In: Dismukes WE, Pappas PG, Sobel JD (eds) *Clinical Mycology*. New York: Oxford University Press, pp. 299–310.

50 Yousukh A, Jutavijittum P, Pisetpongsa P *et al.* (2004) Clinicopathologic study of hepatic *Penicillium marneffei* in Northern Thailand. *Arch Pathol Lab Med* 128, 191–194.

51 Felekouras E, Menenakos C, Griniatsos J *et al.* (2004) Liver resection in cases of isolated hepatic actinomycosis: case report and review of the literature. *Scand J Infect Dis* 36, 535–538.

52 Cockerill FR III, Edson RS, Roberts GD *et al.* (1984) Trimethoprim/sulfamethoxazole-resistant *Nocardia asteroides* causing multiple hepatic abscesses. Successful treatment with ampicillin, amikacin, and limited computed tomography-guided needle aspiration. *Am J Med* 77, 558–560.

53 Sereti I, Holland SM (2001) Disseminated nocardiosis in a patient with X-linked chronic granulomatous disease and human immunodeficiency virus infection. *Clin Infect Dis* 33, 235–239.

10.3 Protozoal infections affecting the liver

10.3.1 Amoebiasis, giardiasis and cryptosporidiosis

David Kershenobich, Guillermo Robles Díaz and Juan Miguel Abdo

Introduction

Amoebae, *Giardia* and *Cryptosporidium* are among the most common protozoa that can infect humans, mainly in the tropics. By far the most favourable sites for intestinal parasites are the duodenum, ileum, caecum and large intestine. To survive and to reproduce in the gastrointestinal tract, the parasites have to adapt to continuous physiological changes relative to the feeding habits of the host, the battery of protein, fat and carbohydrate-splitting enzymes, pH changes and the almost oxygen-free environment [1,2]. These protozoa can gain access to the bloodstream and biliary tract and eventually disseminate to extraintestinal organs, mainly the liver, leading to variable clinical manifestations [3,4]. Hepatic involvement is a frequent clinical presentation for amoeba infection, whereas *Giardia* and *Cryptosporidium* are uncommon aetiological agents of hepatobiliary damage and affect mainly selected populations, such as immunocompromised individuals [5–10].

Epidemiology

Amoebae, *Giardia* and *Cryptosporidium* can be found worldwide but are still more prevalent in tropical and subtropical regions. They affect persons in all age groups, and one of the diseases caused, giardiasis, has been considered the most common protozoan infection in humans with a worldwide incidence ranging between 20–60% and 2–7% in industrialized countries [11]. The implications of invasive amoebiasis and its extension to the liver causing liver abscess continue to stand out as the most consequential protozoan infection in the liver. Most of the estimates regarding the global magnitude of amoebiasis were assessed before the identification of *Entamoeba dispar* as a

separate species that is non-invasive and does not cause disease (Fig. 1); however, among the estimated 500 million people infected each year with *Entamoeba histolytica*, there are approximately 48 million cases of colitis and liver abscess and 70 000 deaths [12–14] (Fig. 2).

About 200 million people have symptomatic giardiasis in Asia, Africa and Latin America with some 500 000 new cases reported each year [15]. Approximately 20 000 cases are reported annually in a Giardiasis surveillance programme in the United States [16]. In a meta-analysis conducted in the Nordic countries of Denmark, Finland, Norway and Sweden, which analysed the data from 13 clinically and methodologically non-heterogeneous studies published before 2004, the estimated prevalence of *Giardia* cases in an asymptomatic (i.e. no gastroenteric symptoms) population was 2.97% (2.64–3.31%) and in a symptomatic population 5.81% (5.34–6.30%) [17].

The proportion of the general population excreting *Cryptosporidium* oocysts is 1–3% in the developed countries and 10% in developing countries. Cryptosporidial infection

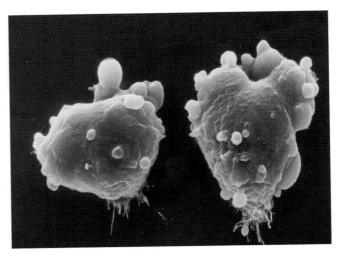

Fig. 1 *Entamoeba histolytica* and *Entamoeba dispar*. Both species are morphologically indistinguishable. Differentiation should be made by isoenzyme analysis, by monoclonal antibodies and by PCR.

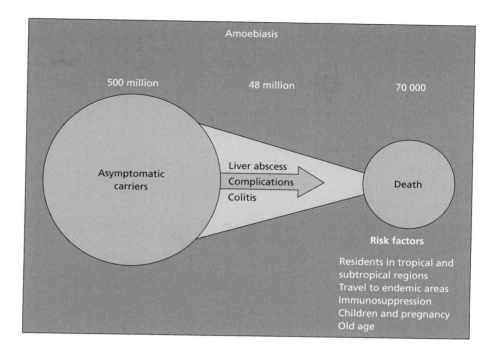

Fig. 2 Worldwide impact of amoebiasis.

accounts for 2.2% (0.26–22%) of cases of diarrhoea in immuno-competent persons in developed countries and 6.1% (1.4–4%) in immunocompetent persons in developing countries. In immunocompromised persons, cryptosporidiosis occurs in 14% (6–70%) of the population in developed countries and in 24% (8.7–48%) in developing countries [18].

Most giardiasis and cryptosporidiosis cases occur sporadi-cally, but outbreaks are well documented, mainly linked to infected recreational or drinking water and also food-borne outbreaks [11,16,19–21].

Demographic changes have modified susceptibility to proto-zoan infections. The impact of parasitic infections in the devel-oping countries is brought home to citizens of the developed countries when tourists, immigrants or soldiers returning or migrating from these less developed countries are infected with endemic parasites [22]. The clinical relevance of this phenomenon is exemplified in a study of 56 patients with an amoebic liver abscess (ALA) at two large San Francisco Hospitals from 1979 to 1994, in which the patients with a history of travel to an endemic area were a decade older and tended to have an insidious onset [23].

We have entered the twenty-first century with a new term introduced to our vocabulary, emergent risk factors, which include the increase in drug abusers, human immunodeficiency virus (HIV)-infected subjects, organ transplant recipients or drug-induced immunosuppressed patients (Table 1). The rapidly evolving context of host immune deficiency requires that biologists and health professionals maintain attentiveness and update their knowledge of the problem in the setting of parasitic infections. In the above-mentioned study of ALA in San Francisco [23], one-third of the patients studied had no associated travel history or endemic origin as risk factors. Of

Table 1 Risk factors for protozoan infections.

Travel history to an endemic area
Contamination of recreational or drinking water
Unsafe food-related habits
Drug abusers
HIV-infected patients
Organ transplant recipients
Drug-induced immunosuppression
Underlying systemic disease

these, 63% had a condition consistent with severe immuno-suppression, such as infection with HIV, malnourishment with severe hypoalbuminaemia or chronic infection. During the last 5 years of the study, one-third of all patients diagnosed with ALA were HIV positive. Also associated with a decrease in the immune system, sclerosing cholangitis due to cryptosporidiosis has been described in liver-transplanted children receiving immunosuppression with tacrolimus and prednisone [24]. Although *Cryptosporidium parvum*, in particular genotypes human type 1 and bovine type 2, are the most common species in humans, *C. felis*, *C. muris* and *C. meleagridis* have also been identified in immunocompromised persons [25,26].

Life cycle

Entamoeba histolytica

Humans are the primary reservoir for *E. histolytica*; the main source of transmission is the chronically infected human. Stools infected with the cysts from the parasites may contaminate food or water. Another common source of transmission is oral–anal sexual contacts. There may be some animal reservoirs of *E. histolytica* (dogs, monkeys and probably pigs), but they represent a very small source of human infection. As humans are infected by ingesting infected cysts, they travel through the gut lumen to the small intestine where they excyst to form trophozoites. The trophozoite of *E. histolytica* can convert to a precyst form with a nucleus and mature into a tetranucleated cyst, which migrates down and out of the colon where it becomes a mature and infectious cyst [27,28].

Giardia lamblia

Giardia is found in humans and in other animals such as cats, dogs, beavers and cattle. The *Giardia* life cycle involves two stages: the cyst, which is the infectious form and is ingested in contaminated water, food, direct oral–faecal contact in children and sexual practices that include oral–anal contact. Once ingested, the low pH in the stomach and pancreatic proteases found in the proximal small intestine promote rapid excitation, giving rise to the trophozoites that are responsible for symptomatic illness. The trophozoites attach to the mucosa of the duodenum and proximal jejunum, where they multiply rapidly via binary division. Responding to unknown stimuli, possibly bile salts, some trophozoites encyst in the ileum and are eliminated in the stools of infected hosts [29–33].

Cryptosporidium

Various domestic animals and cattle are potential sources of human infection. Transmission occurs by the faecal–oral route (person to person and animal to person) and via contaminated food and water [34]. The developmental stages of *Cryptosporidium* originate in an intracellular, extracytoplasmic location within parasitophorous vacuoles of host cell origin; these vacuoles are found at the microvillous surface of the host cell. Humans are infected when they ingest *Cryptosporidium* oocysts. Once ingested, oocysts excyst in the gastrointestinal tract and release infective sporozoites that affix to the apical membrane of the host epithelial cell. Such attachment induces reorganization of the host cell actin cytoskeleton and swelling of the host cell membrane around the sporozoite to form a vacuole in which the organism remains intracellular but extracytoplasmic. The internalized sporozoite then matures and undergoes asexual reproduction (schizogony) to produce merozoites. After release into the intestinal lumen, merozoites can either infect other epithelial cells or mature into gametocytes, the sexual form of the parasite. The life cycle is repeated after fertilization occurs in the intestinal tract, producing thin-walled oocysts that sporulate to release sporozoites again; this can lead to autoinfection and heavy, persistent infections, with massive shedding of oocysts in the faeces of an infected patient. The presence of a thin-walled autoinfective oocyst can cause an overwhelming infection in a susceptible host and explains the persistent, life-threatening infections in immunocompromised patients in the absence of repeated exposure to oocysts [35,36].

Pathophysiology

Protozoan infections are usually brought to a halt by different pathophysiological mechanisms occurring mainly at the level of the intestine. Disease processes intrinsic to host–parasite interactions may, however, lead to more severe and life-threatening complications that affect the liver and biliary tract. Among these pathophysiological mechanisms, some of the most relevant are tissue inflammation, neutrophil adherence to endothelium, endothelial disruption, release of cytokines, release of active oxidants, changes in the permeability of plasma membranes, lysosomal disruption, release of proteolytic enzymes and cell death. Abnormalities in intestinal function can alter the secretion of products that undergo enterohepatic circulation and increase the synthesis of bile acids by the liver. In addition, bile acids that enter the colon induce water secretion by the colonic mucosa and cause diarrhoea. Understanding the mechanisms involved in the relation of protozoan infections and the liver is still an open issue, with some insights coming from the analysis of each particular infection (Table 2).

E. histolytica

An important factor contributing to the pathogenesis of *E. histolytica* is its highly effective actomyosin cytoskeleton, which allows fast morphological changes associated with amoebic

Table 2 Pathophysiological mechanisms involved in protozoan infections in the intestine and the liver.

Amoebiasis
Parasite motility
Cell adhesion
Cytoskeletal re-arrangement
Signal transduction
Cytolysis
Migration in the liver
Release of proteases
Necrosis, apoptosis

Giardiasis
Attachment to intestinal epithelium
Altered brush border, crypt hyperplasia
Decreased disaccharidase activity
Giardia–bile salt interactions
Epithelial damage/increased permeability
Cytokine-induced liver damage?

Cryptosporidiosis
Intestinal epithelial damage
Humoral and cell-mediated immunity
Invasion of biliary epithelial cells
Morphofunctional changes in hepatocytes

motility and spatial reorganization of cellular components [37]. The earliest observations of this protozoa noted that their motility involved force generation through either the microtubule- or the microfilament-based cytoskeletal elements. The amoeba is a protozoa that crawls along a solid substratum in a fashion known as 'amoeboid movement'. Amoeba projects out a pseudopodium, or false foot, from the cell body. The pseudopodium then attaches to the substratum and pulls the rest of the cell body forward. The force involved in this movement is generated by another cytoskeletal system, which is composed of actin and myosin. Actin forms long filaments, also known as microfilaments, and myosin is a motor protein that moves along the microfilaments in an adenosine triphosphate (ATP)-dependent manner [38,39]. Its motility, cell adhesion properties and aggressive behaviour are however variable and may depend on the host immune system and on the localization in the host.

Contact-dependent cytolysis of host cells by *E. histolytica* is an important event in the pathogenesis of amoebic liver abscess [40]. *E. histolytica* may be viewed as a cytotoxic effector cell with an extraordinary capacity for killing various target cells and also as a primitive actively phagocytosing eukaryotic cell that uses bacteria as a major nutrient source [41].

The coordinated action of the *E. histolytica* cytoskeleton and surface adhesion molecules is a key factor in pathogenesis [42–44]. Some of the best characterized parasite surface molecules involved in amoeba binding to host cells are the Gal/GalNac lectin [45] and myosin II [46], which enables adhesion of the trophozoite to intestinal epithelial cells by high-affinity interactions with cell surface glycoproteins. Experimental studies in hamsters show that the disruption of Gal/GalNac and myosin II impairs the area of contact between *E. histolytica* and the enterocytes. Intraportal delivery of these parasites to the liver leads to the formation of small abscesses with disorganized morphology that are localized in the vicinity of blood vessels. Successful invasion of the liver parenchyma requires that the trophozoite binds strongly to the endothelium to counteract the pressure imposed by the bloodstream, extravasation and migration through the three-dimensional structure of the hepatic tissue. The trophozoite has to survive the host inflammatory response at each of these steps. Adhesion to the host cells modulates the distribution of trophozoites in the liver and their capacity to migrate in the hepatic tissue [38].

Initial steps in tissue invasion may be aided by the release of proteases from trophozoites that degrade extracellular matrix components such as fibronectin and laminin [47]. In patients with invasive amoebiasis, *E. histolytica* causes vast tissue damage that is believed to be a direct result of its ability to induce necrosis and host cell apoptosis (Fig. 3). *In vitro* trophozoites of *E. histolytica* induce apoptosis of host cells including neutrophils, T lymphocytes and macrophages [48]. Nuclei of hepatocytes of murine amoebic liver abscess are positive by terminal deoxynucleotidyl transferase-mediated dUTP-biotin end labelling (TUNEL) staining [49]; treatment of mice with a pan-caspase inhibitor blocks the formation of amoebic liver abscesses [50].

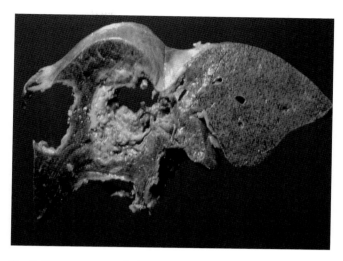

Fig. 3 Gross appearance of a huge amoebic liver abscess at autopsy.

Reactive oxygen species (ROS)-mediated activation of ERK1/2 is required for the entamoeba to induce neutrophil apoptosis [51]. In contrast to life in the anoxic colon, *E. histolytica* encounters a relatively high oxygen environment during invasive amoebiasis; ability to cope with this change is an important factor in determining its virulence. *E. histolytica* has four copies of flavoprotein E, which detoxifies nitric oxide and/or oxygen [52] and also contains rubrerythrin [53], which is protective against intracellular hydrogen peroxide in anaerobic bacteria. Taking all these observations together, it has been proposed that the regulatory mechanisms of redox signalling may be relevant in the amoebic-induced inflammatory response [51].

E. histolytica uses a complex mix of signal transduction systems in order to sense and interact with the different environments it encounters. The analysis of its genome has revealed almost 270 putative *E. histolytica* protein kinases representing members of all seven families of the eukaryotic protein kinase superfamily. These include tyrosine kinase with SH2 domains, tyrosine kinase-like protein kinases and 90 putative receptor SER/THR kinases. *E. histolytica* contains more than 100 protein phosphatases that dephosphorylate proteins. All these observations come from the analysis of the genome of *E. histolytica* [54], whose comparisons with other genomes will help to resolve fundamental issues relating to eukaryote and amoeba phylogeny.

Giardia

Giardia has a special disc located on its ventral surface, which is relevant to its attachment to the intestinal epithelium [55]. This process is mediated by specific lectins. During the process of attachment, intestinal damage can ensue. The brush border is altered, there is crypt hyperplasia and disaccharidase activity decreases [11]. In the small bowel, *Giardia* trophozoites harbouring peripheral bacterial endosymbionts are destroyed and lysed by the Paneth cells located at the base of the crypts of

Lieberkuhn, which leads to greater intestinal epithelial damage [56]. Bile specifically stimulates the growth of *Giardia* by unknown mechanisms, and it is avidly consumed by the parasite, leading to reduced intraluminal bile salt concentrations [57]. It seems that *Giardia* is unable to survive in the absence of bile acids, but it does not reside in the biliary tract where the pH and the absence of nutritional substrate do not allow its colonization [58]. The increase in intestinal epithelial permeability may allow the passage of toxic substances or cytokines that could eventually cause damage to the liver.

There is evidence for diversity in infectivity and host specificity of *Giardia* species. An ongoing genome project plans to obtain approximately 95% of the genome by a random approach, as well as a complete physical map using a bacterial artificial chromosome library. The *Giardia* genome project [59] promises to greatly increase our understanding of this interesting and enigmatic organism as well as its phylogenetic relationship to other primitive organisms. Also, an important role of variant-specific surface proteins (VSPs) in *Giardia lamblia*–host interactions has been demonstrated that exert both positive and negative selective pressures on the parasite, independent of the adaptive immune response [60].

Host defences against *Giardia* infection must act in the gut lumen in the absence of induction by classical inflammatory mediators. Secretory IgA antibodies have a major role in the control of infection [61], but other immunoglobulins and B cell-independent mechanisms also exist and can contribute to eradication of the parasite. Neither Th1 nor Th2 cells are strictly necessary for the clearance of *Giardia* infection, whereas mucosal T cells may have an important role, and T-cell cytokines may induce the production and release of anti-giardial defensins into the intestinal lumen [11,62].

Cryptosporidium

Cryptosporidium oocytes enter the brush border of intestinal epithelium, develop into merozoites and multiply, impairing absorption of glucose, electrolytes, water, fats and vitamin B12 [63]. There is a general consensus that the mechanisms responsible for clearing *Cryptosporidium* from the gastrointestinal tract involve a role for gamma interferon, although the mechanism by which this cytokine impairs resistance is unclear. After infection with *Cryptosporidium*, CD40 ligand and interferon gamma knockout mice develop a very aggressive type of liver damage [64], suggesting that the absence of the CD40–CD40 ligand interaction and/or the downregulation of interferon gamma may be related to the development of *Cryptosporidium*-associated sclerosing cholangitis, bile duct dysplasia and possibly neoplasms [65,66]. It is also clear that CD4 T lymphocytes are necessary for the resolution of both acute and chronic cryptosporidiosis [67]. The spectrum and severity of the disease in immunocompromised individuals with cryptosporidiosis reflect this importance, as individuals with a defect in T-cell response have more severe disease [68].

No difference has been found between cryptosporidiosis in normal and B cell-depleted neonatal mice, suggesting that antibody production may play a less important role in recovery from infection [69].

In an *in vitro* model of human biliary cryptosporidiosis during internalization of the parasite, numerous vacuoles covered by its plasma membrane are formed and cluster together to establish a preparasitophorous vacuole. This preparasitophorous vacuole comes into contact with host cell membrane to form a host cell–parasite membrane interface. Vacuole-like structures appear in the apical complex region of the attached sporozoite, which bud out into host cells. A tunnel directly connecting the parasite to the host cell cytoplasm forms during internalization and remains when the parasite is totally internalized [70].

C. parvum has the capacity to invade epithelial cells and induce survival signals. It activates the NFkappaB/I(kappa)B system in infected biliary epithelia, thus protecting infected cells from death and facilitating parasite survival and propagation [71]. *C. parvum* invasion of biliary epithelial cells requires host cell tyrosine phosphorylation of cortactin to induce actin polymerization at the attachment site, a process associated with microbial secretion but independent of host cell endocytosis [72].

In experimental animals, morphofunctional changes in hepatocytes have been demonstrated after infection with different doses of oocysts of *C. parvum*, which include an increase in multinuclear hepatocytes, a decrease in the quantity of glycogen and an increase in proteins and nuclear DNA [73].

Clinical manifestations

Amoebic liver abscess

This is the most common extraintestinal manifestation of amoebiasis. It occurs more frequently in tropical regions, in men between the ages of 20 and 40 years, although cases are found at both age extremes, the youngest patients having been described at 6 weeks of age. The characteristic clinical manifestations may vary in relation to the size, number and localization of the lesions as well as the development of possible complications secondary to rupture or communication of liver abscesses to neighbouring organs. Most frequently, patients with ALA present an abrupt onset of fever between 38°C and 40°C, accompanied by chills and profuse sweating, severe and progressive pain in the right upper abdominal quadrant radiating to the scapular region and right shoulder. The pain increases with movement, deep breathing or coughing. Patients usually refer with a history of malaise in the preceding days and weight loss. On physical examination, the liver is usually large and tender, ventilation in the right lung is restricted, and the respiratory sounds are reduced. Jaundice is present in less than 10% of the cases.

Although the colon is the portal of entry and colonic involvement is of considerable importance, there are surprisingly few studies of the colon with ALA. Colonic ulcers, when investigated, are found in approximately 55% of patients with ALA;

they are more likely to be present if the patient has diarrhoea as a presenting symptom or has had diarrhoea in the recent past. However, diarrhoea is observed in less than a third of patients with ALA [74]. It has been suggested that either the colon is involved minimally without symptoms or there is a considerable time interval between the colonic and liver involvement, allowing for healing of the colonic lesions, and presentation later with an ALA. Multiple, large and left-sided ulcers are more common in elderly patients and in those in whom diarrhoea is the presenting symptom [75].

Invasive amoebiasis as an emerging parasitic disease is being recognized more frequently among immunosuppressed patients. Investigators in Japan, Italy, Korea and Taiwan have found a higher prevalence of antibody to *E. histolytica* in homosexual men with or without HIV infection [5].

Giardiasis

In humans, clinical manifestations of giardiasis range from asymptomatic to symptoms such as chronic diarrhoea, weight loss, vomiting, abdominal distension and abdominal pain. The severity of symptoms may vary and has been found to be related to the number of cysts ingested, the age of the host and the state of the host immune system [76]. Malabsorption caused by disaccharidase deficiency has been described and is related to the parasite burden in the small intestine [77].

Overt involvement of the liver by *Giardia* is rare; however, when investigated intentionally, alterations in hepatic histology including steatosis, inflammatory lesions and data of chronic active hepatitis have been reported in patients with a diagnosis of giardiasis by duodenal intubation [8]. Cases of granulomatous hepatitis and cholangitis [78] or biliary giardiasis in HIV patients have been reported [79,80].

Cryptosporidiosis

Although *Cryptosporidium* has been described as causing a self-limited diarrhoeal illness in immunocompetent people, lasting between 2 and 4 weeks, it is a major problem in immunocompromised patients causing chronic debilitating diarrhoea [81].

Extraintestinal cryptosporidiosis may involve the respiratory system, middle ear, pancreas, stomach and biliary tract. Biliary cryptosporidiosis is the most common extraintestinal manifestation, causing gallbladder disease and sclerosing cholangitis [82–84]. Two distinct presentations are seen, papillary stenosis with extrahepatic ductal dilatation and sclerosing cholangitis or acalculous cholecystitis. These manifestations have also been described in patients with AIDS and intestinal cryptosporidiosis before retroviral treatment [85,86]. *C. parvum*-induced sclerosing cholangitis has been found in other immunodeficient states such as congenital immunodeficiency and X-linked immunodeficiency with hyper-IgM [87] and in renal or liver transplant recipients [82,83]. Besides diarrhoea, there is pain in the right upper quadrant, nausea, vomiting and fever.

Diagnosis

Imaging

Imaging plays a pivotal role in the workup of patients with suspected ALA and has reduced the delay in diagnosis. Studies include chest X-ray, liver ultrasound, computerized tomography (CT), magnetic resonance imaging (MRI) and ^{99}Tc liver scan. Ultrasonography is the first choice. A space-occupying lesion is seen in at least 75% of cases. The lesions tend to be round or oval, with well-defined margins. The lesions are primarily hypoechoic [88]. Within the lesion, there may be hyperechoic areas corresponding to necrotic conglomerates especially in the early phases; when this occurs, Doppler examination is useful as it fails to detect any signal in the interior of the abscess [89].

CT is indicated when the diagnosis has not been confirmed by other methods, when symptoms persist under medical treatment or when the need for differential diagnosis with other lesions arises. On contrast-enhanced CT, amoebic abscesses appear as lesions with attenuation values that indicate the presence of complex fluid (10–20 HU). An enhancing wall 3–15 mm in thickness and a peripheral zone of oedema around the abscess are common and somewhat characteristic. The central abscess cavity may show multiple septa or fluid debris levels and, rarely, air bubbles or haemorrhage [88,90].

On MRI, ALA has homogeneous low signal intensity and high signal intensity on T1- and T2-weighted images respectively. Perilesional oedema is seen on T2-weighted MR images in 50% of cases [91].

Chest X-ray abnormalities include atelectasis, pulmonary infiltrates and pleural effusion or elevated right diaphragm [92].

Ultrasonographic findings of biliary disease in cryptosporidiosis are the thickening of the biliary duct wall and/or dilatation of the gallbladder. Endoscopic retrograde cholangiopancreatography is indicated in these cases and can reveal papillary stenosis or long extrahepatic bile duct strictures [7]. Endoscopic ultrasonography can be useful in detecting papillary stenosis.

Laboratory findings

The majority of patients with ALA have an increased white blood cell count, with neutrophilia, elevated alkaline phosphatase, mild anaemia and increased erythrocyte sedimentation rate. Slight increases in bilirubin are seen in approximately one-third of patients.

Serological test methods for the detection of antiamoebic antibodies are useful for the diagnosis of ALA. Indirect haemagglutination (IHA) and enzyme-linked immunosorbent assay (ELISA) are the most often used. A cutoff value of 1:512 is considered diagnostic. Titres may persist after resolution of the amoebic abscess. Serology is often positive in areas of endemicity where circulating antibodies may reflect a past infection. In countries where amoebiasis is uncommon and its presence may be an emerging pathology, antiamoebic serology is usually correlated with disease.

In those patients in whom an aspirate is obtained, the material should be sent for Gram stain, determination of the presence of neutrophils and culture. Amoebic culture and visualization of trophozoites can be done using the last 5 mL of aspirate [93].

Diagnosis of *Giardia lamblia* infection is established by the microscopic examination of stool for the parasite [94,95]. Detection of anti-*Giardia* salivary IgA antibodies is an excellent tool for screening *G. lamblia* in patients with longstanding symptoms of more than 1 month duration [96].

Cryptosporidium stains intensely red by modified acid-fast techniques on microscopic examination of stool [97] Serological testing using EIA has been described. Serological tests are of limited value as antibodies to *Cryptosporidium* can be found in previously exposed persons.

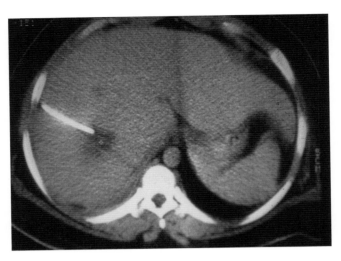

Fig. 4 Guided percutaneous aspiration of an amoebic liver abscess.

Treatment

Amoeba

The drugs of choice for invasive amoebiasis are tissue active agents, such as metronidazole, tinidazole and chloroquine, or the more toxic emetin derivatives, including dehydroemetine [98,99].

Metronidazole and tinidazole are derived from 5-nitroimidazole, which kills the trophozoites by alterations in the protoplasmic organelles of the amoeba [100]. Metronidazole is the drug of choice in the treatment of uncomplicated amoebic liver abscess. The oral dose is 1 g twice daily for 15 days in adults and 30–50 mg/kg daily for 10 days in three divided doses for children; intravenous metronidazole is given at a dose of 500 mg every 6 h in adults and 7.5 mg/kg every 6 h for children. Tinidazole is given orally 2 g daily for 15 days. While on treatment, patients should abstain from alcohol as these drugs have an antiabuse effect.

Chloroquine is derived from 4-aminoquinolines; it acts on the vegetative forms of the parasite and kills it by inhibiting DNA synthesis. Adults should receive 1 g/day orally for 2–5 days followed by 500 mg/day for 2–3 weeks; in children, the dose is 15 mg/kg orally, daily for 2–5 days followed by 5 mg/kg daily for 2 weeks [101].

Percutaneous aspiration/drainage can be used as a diagnostic or therapeutic tool and should be performed with imaging guidance (Fig. 4). Indications include the lack of clinical response to medical treatment, defined as no decrease in fever or pain, no reduction in the white cell count in a 5-day period following initiation of treatment. It is also indicated when less than 1 cm of rim liver tissue remains around a liquefied abscess or when it becomes necessary to rule out a pyogenic abscess.

Rupture of an abscess into the lungs, pleural space, pericardium or peritoneum has a severe rate of mortality and requires urgent surgical intervention.

Giardia

Therapy of diarrhoea caused by giardiasis includes a vast range of drugs, mainly nitroimidazoles, nitazoxanide, paromomycin, furazolidone, albendazole or quinacrine [102–104]. Of these, metronidazole has been the most thoroughly studied and also the most commonly used worldwide at a dose of 500 mg three times a day for 5 days [105]. Tinidazole at a single dose of 1.0–2.0 g has the advantage of compliance and has similar proven efficacy [106].

Resistance has been reported with all the different agents; strategies to overcome resistance are the use of higher doses of the original agent or using a different drug to avoid cross-resistance. Combination therapy may be necessary in immunosuppressed patients.

Cryptosporidium

Cryptosporidium carriage in liver-transplanted children with sclerosing cholangitis has been successfully treated with paromomycin, a non-absorbable aminoglycoside, while immunosuppression is decreased according to graft tolerance [107]. Paromomycin 500 mg three times daily for 2 weeks has been used to treat cryptosporidiosis in patients with AIDS, while these patients continue to receive antiretroviral therapy [108]. Recent reports suggest that, in the setting of *C. parvum* infection, sclerosing cholangitis may be completely reversible if the infection can be eradicated quickly. Protease inhibitors have a direct inhibitory effect on *Cryptosporidium* infection [109].

Nitazoxanide, paromomycin and azithromycin are commonly used to eradicate *Cryptosporidium* infection in both immunocompetent and immunosuppressed patients [110].

References

1 Cox FEG (2003) Taxonomy and classification of human parasites. In: Murray PR, Baron EJ, Jorgensen JH *et al.* (eds) *Manual of Clinical Microbiology*, 8th edn. Washington, DC: ASM Press, pp. 1897–1902.

2 Sleigh MA (1991) The nature of protozoa. In: Kreier JP (ed.) *Parasitic Protozoa*, 2nd edn, Vol. 1. San Diego, CA: Academic Press, pp. 1–53.

3 Bruckner DA (1992) Amebiasis. *Clin Microbiol Rev* 5, 356–369.

4 Barsoum RS (2004) Parasitic infections in organ transplantation. *Exp Clin Transplant* 2, 258–267.

5 Hung Ch Ch, Deng HY, Hsiao WH *et al.* (2005) Invasive amebiasis as an emerging parasitic disease in patients with human immunodeficiency virus type 1 infection in Taiwan. *Arch Intern Med* 165, 409–415.

6 Vakil NB, Schwartz SM, Buggy BP *et al.* (1996) Biliary cryptosporidiosis in HIV-infected people after the waterborne outbreak of cryptosporidiosis in Milwaukee. *N Engl J Med* 334, 19–23.

7 Schneiderman DJ, Cello JP, Laing FC (1987) Papillary stenosis and sclerosing cholangitis in the acquired immunodeficiency syndrome. *Ann Intern Med* 106, 546–549.

8 Sotto A, Gra B (1985) Hepatic manifestations in giardiasis. *Acta Gastroenterol Latinoam* 15, 89–94.

9 Roberts-Thomson IC, Anders RF, Bhathal PS (1982) Granulomatous hepatitis and cholangitis associated with giardiasis. *Gastroenterology* 83, 480–483.

10 Sotto A, Alvarez JL, Garcia B *et al.* (1990) Acute hepatic lesion caused by *Giardia lamblia. Rev Esp Enferm Dig* 77, 24–28.

11 Hawrelak J (2003) Giardiasis: pathophysiology and management. *Altern Med Rev* 8, 129–142.

12 Farthing MJG, Cevallos AM, Kelly P (2003) Intestinal protozoa. In: Cook GC, Zumla AL (eds). *Manson's Tropical Diseases*, 21st edn. Edinburgh: Elsevier Science, pp. 1373–1386.

13 World Health Organization (1998) *The World Health Report. Life in the 21st Century: A Vision for All.* Geneva: WHO.

14 World Health Organization (1997) Amoebiasis. *WHO Wkly Epidemiol Record* 72, 97–100.

15 World Health Organization (1996) *The World Health Report. Fighting Disease, Fostering Development.* Geneva: WHO.

16 Hlavsa MC, Watson JC, Beach MJ (2005) Giardiasis surveillance – United States, 1998–2002. *MMWR Surveill Summ* 54, 9–16.

17 Horman A, Korpela H, Sutinen J *et al.* (2004) Meta-analysis in assessment of the prevalence and annual incidence of *Giardia* spp. and *Cryptosporidium* spp. infections in humans in the Nordic countries. *Int J Parasitol* 34, 1337–1346.

18 Guerrant RL (1997) Cryptosporidiosis: an emerging, highly infectious threat. *Emerg Infect Dis* 3, 51–57.

19 Chen XM, Keithly JS, Paya CV *et al.* (2002) Cryptosporidiosis. *N Engl J Med* 346, 1723–1731.

20 Lavas MC, Watson JC, Beach MJ (2005) Cryptosporidiosis surveillance – United States 1999–2002. *MMWR Surveill Summ* 54, 1–8.

21 Cifuentes E, Suarez L, Espinosa M *et al.* (2004) Risk of *Giardia intestinalis* infection in children from an artificially recharged groundwater area in Mexico City. *Am J Trop Med Hyg* 71, 65–70.

22 Chistie JD, García LS (2004) Emerging parasitic infections. *Clin Lab Med* 24, 737–772.

23 Seeto RK, Rockey DC (1999) Amebic liver abscess: epidemiology, clinical features, and outcome. *West J Med* 170, 104–109.

24 Campos M, Jouzdani E, Sempoux C *et al.* (2000) Sclerosing cholangitis associated to cryptosporidiosis in liver-transplanted children. *Eur J Pediatr* 159, 113–115.

25 Coupe S, Sarfati C, Hamane S *et al.* (2005) Detection of *Cryptosporidium* and identification to the species level by nested PCR and restriction fragment length polymorphism. *J Clin Microbiol* 43, 1017–1023.

26 Carreno RA, Pokorny NJ, Lee H *et al.* (2001) Phenotypic and genotypic characterization of *Cryptosporidium* species isolates. *J Ind Microbiol Biotech* 26, 95–106.

27 Huston CHD, Haque R, William AP (1999) Molecular-based diagnosis of *Entamoeba histolytica* infection. *Expert Rev Mol Med* 1–11.

28 García LS (2001) *Diagnostic Medical Parasitology*, 4th edn. Washington, DC: ASM Press.

29 Rendtorff RC (1954) The experimental transmission of human intestinal protozoan parasites. II. *Giardia lamblia* cysts given in capsules. *Am J Hyg* 59, 209–220.

30 Rendtorff RC (1978) The experimental transmission of *Giardia lamblia* among volunteer subjects. In: Jacubowski W, Hoff JC (eds) *Waterborne Transmission of Giardiasis.* EPA 600/9-79-001. Washington, DC: US Environmental Protection Agency, pp. 64–81.

31 Rice EW, Schaefer FW (1981) Improved *in vitro* excystation procedure for *Giardia lamblia* cyst. *J Clin Microbiol* 14, 709–710.

32 Erlandsen SL, Macechko PT, Van Keulen H *et al.* (1996) Formation of the *Giardia* cyst wall: studies on extracellular assembly using immunogold labeling and high resolution field emission SEM. *J Eukaryot Microbiol* 43, 416–429.

33 Lujan HD, Mowatt MR, Nash TE (1997) Mechanism of *Giardia lamblia* differentiation into cysts. *Microbiol Mol Biol* 61, 294–304.

34 Tzipori S, Widmer G (2000) The biology of *Cryptosporidium. Contrib Microbiol* 6, 1–32.

35 O'Donoghue PJ (1995) *Cryptosporidium* and cryptosporidiosis in man and animals. *Int J Parasitol* 25, 139–195.

36 Ferreira MS, Borges AS (2002) Some aspects of protozoan infections in immunocompromised patients – a review. *Mem Inst Oswaldo Cruz* 97, 443–457.

37 Guillén, N (1996) Role of signaling and cytoskeletal rearrangements in the pathogenesis of *Entamoeba histolytica. Trends Microbiol* 4, 191–196.

38 Tavares P, Rigothier MCH, Khum H *et al.* (2005) Roles of cell adhesion and cytoskeleton activity in *Entamoeba histolytica* pathogenesis: a delicate balance. *Infect Immun* 73, 1771–1778.

39 Dominik M, Klopocka W, Pomorski P *et al.* (2005) Characterization of *Amoeba proteus* myosin VI immunoanalog. *Cell Motil Cytoskel* 61, 172–188.

40 Stanley SL Jr (2003) Amoebiasis. *Lancet* 361, 1025–1034.

41 Benkert C, Jacobs T, Berninghausen O *et al.* (1997) Molecular basis of aggressive and defensive functions of *Entamoeba histolytica. Arch Med Res* 28, S211–S213.

42 Wehrle-Haller B, Imhof B (2002) The inner lives of focal adhesions. *Trends Cell Biol* 12, 382–389.

43 Tsutsumi V, Mena-Lopez R, Anaya-Velásquez F *et al.* (1984) Cellular bases of experimental amebic liver abscess formation. *Am J Parasitol* 117, 81–91.

44 Tavares P, Sansonetti P, Guillen N (2000) Cell adhesion and polarization in a pathogenic protozoan: role of the *Entamoeba histolytica. Arch Med Res* 2, 643–649.

45 Rawal S, Majumdar S, Vohra H (2005) Activation of MAPK kinase pathway by Gal/GalNAc adherence lectin of *E. histolytica*: gateway to host response. *Mol Cell Biochem* 268, 93–101.

46 Arhets P, Olivo JC, Gounon P *et al.* (1998) Virulence and functions of myosin II are inhibited by overexpression of light meromyosin in *Entamoeba histolytica*. *Mol Biol Cell* 8, 1537–1547.

47 Stanley SL Jr (2001) Pathophysiology of amoebiasis. *Trends Parasitol* 17, 280–285.

48 Petri WA, Haque R, Mann BJ (2002) The bittersweet interface of parasite and host: lectin–carbohydrate interactions during human invasion by the parasite *Entamoeba histolytica*. *Annu Rev Microbiol* 56, 39–54.

49 Velázquez C, Shibayama-Sales M, Aguirre-García J *et al.* (1998) Role of neutrophils in innate resistance to *Entamoeba histolytica*. *Cell Microbiol* 20, 255–262.

50 Yan L, Stanley L (2001) Blockade of caspases inhibits amebic liver abscess formation in a mouse model of disease. *Infect Immun* 69, 7911–7914.

51 Sim S, Yong TS, Park SJ *et al.* (2005) NADPH oxidase-derived reactive oxygen species-mediated activation of ERL1/2 required for apoptosis of human neutrophils induced by *Entamoeba histolytica*. *J Immunol* 174, 4279–4288.

52 Gomes CM, Giuffre A, Forte E *et al.* (2002) A novel type of nitric-oxide reductase. *Escherichia coli* flavorubredoxin. *J Biol Chem* 277, 25273–25276.

53 Sztukowska M, Bugno M, Potempa J *et al.* (2002) Role of rubrerythrin in the oxidative stress response of *Porphyromonas gingivalis*. *Mol Microbiol* 44, 479–488.

54 Loftus B, Anderson I, Davies R *et al.* (2005) The genome of the protist parasite *Entamoeba histolytica*. *Nature* 433, 865–868.

55 Leber AL, Novak SM (2003) Intestinal and urogenital amebae, flagellates and ciliates. In: Murray PR, Baron EJ, Jorgensen JH *et al.* (eds) *Manual of Clinical Microbiology*, Vol. 2. Washington, DC: American Society for Microbiology, pp. 1990–2007.

56 El-Shewy KA, Eid RA (2005) In vivo killing of *Giardia* trophozoites harbouring bacterial endosymbionts by intestinal Paneth cells: an ultrastructural study. *Parasitology* 130, 269–274.

57 Halliday CE, Clark C, Farthing MJ (1988) *Giardia*–bile salt interactions *in vitro* and *in vivo*. *Trans R Soc Trop Med Hyg* 82, 428–432.

58 Vesy CJ, Peterson WL (1999) Review article: the management of giardiasis. *Aliment Pharmacol Ther* 13, 843–850.

59 McArthur AG, Morrison HG, Nixon JE *et al.* (2000) The *Giardia* genome project database. *FEMS Microbiol Lett* 189, 271–273.

60 Carranza PG, Feltes G, Ropolo A *et al.* (2002) Simultaneous expression of different variant-specific surface proteins in single *Giardia lamblia* trophozoites during encystation. *Infect Immun* 70, 5265–5268.

61 Tellez A, Palm D, Weiland M *et al.* (2005) Secretory antibodies against *Giardia intestinalis* in lactating Nicaraguan women. *Parasite Immunol* 27, 163–169.

62 Eckmann L (2003) Mucosal defences against *Giardia*. *Parasite Immunol* 25, 259–270.

63 Barbot L, Topouchian A, Capet C *et al.* (2001) *Cryptosporidium parvum*: functional study of the intestinal malabsorption syndrome. *Ann Pharm Fr* 59, 305–311.

64 Stephens J, Cosyns M, Jones M *et al.* (1999) Liver and bile duct pathology following *Cryptosporidium parvum* infection of immunodeficient mice. *Hepatology* 30, 27–35.

65 Stout RD, Suttles J, Xu J *et al.* (1996) Impaired T cell mediated macrophage activation in CD40 ligand deficient mice. *J Immunol* 156, 8–11.

66 Kline TJ, De las Morenas T, O'Brien M *et al.* (1993) Squamous metaplasia of extrahepatic biliary system in an AIDS patient with cryptosporidia and cholangitis. *Dig Dis Sci* 38, 960–962.

67 McDonald V, Smith R, Robinson H *et al.* (2000) Host immune responses against *Cryptosporidium*. *Contrib Microbiol* 6, 75–91.

68 Hunter PR, Nichols G (2002) Epidemiology and clinical features of *Cryptosporidium* infection in immunocompromised patients. *Clin Microbiol Rev* 15, 145–154.

69 Gomez Morales MA, Pozio E (2002) Humoral and cellular immunity against *Cryptosporidium* infection. *Curr Drug Targets Immune Endocr Metabol Disord* 2, 291–301.

70 Huang BQ, Chen XM, LaRusso NF (2004) *Cryptosporidium parvum* attachment to and internalization by human biliary epithelia *in vitro*: a morphologic study. *J Parasitol* 90, 212–221.

71 Chen XM, Levine SA, Splinter PL *et al.* (2001) *Cryptosporidium parvum* activates nuclear factor kappaB in biliary epithelia preventing epithelial cell apoptosis. *Gastroenterology* 120, 1774–1783.

72 Chen XM, Huang BQ, Splinter PL *et al.* (2003) *Cryptosporidium parvum* invasion of biliary epithelia requires host cell tyrosine phosphorylation of cortactin via c-Src. *Gastroenterology* 125, 216–228.

73 Beier TV, Anastskaia RAS, Sidorenko NV *et al.* (2002) Morphofunctional changes in hepatocytes during the early postnatal development of rats experimentally infected with the intestinal protozoan pathogen *Cryptosporidium parvum* (Coccidia, Sporozoa). *Tsitologiia* 44, 1046–1057.

74 Misra SP, Misra V, Dwivedi M *et al.* (2004) Factors influencing colonic involvement in patients with amebic liver abscess. *Gastrointest Endosc* 59, 512–516.

75 Sachdev GK, Dhol P (1997) Colonic involvement in patients with amebic liver abscess: endoscopic findings. *Gastrointest Endosc* 46, 37–39.

76 Farthing MJG (1996) Giardiasis. *Gastroenterol Clin North Am* 25, 493–515.

77 Jennings W, Rowl R, Hecker R *et al.* (1976) The significance of lowered jejunal disaccharidase levels. *Aust NZ J Med* 6, 556–560.

78 Roberts-Thomson IC, Anders RF, Bhathal PS (1982) Granulomatous hepatitis and cholangitis associated with giardiasis. *Gastroenterology* 83, 480–483.

79 Esfiandari A, Swartz J, Teklehaimanot S (1997) Clustering of giardiasis among AIDS patients in Los Angeles County. *Cell Mol Biol* 43, 1077–1083.

80 Aronson NF, Cheney C, Rholl V *et al.* (2001) Biliary giardiasis in a patient with human immunodeficiency virus. *J Clin Gastroenterol* 33, 167–170.

81 Current R, Bailey W, Heyman M *et al.* (1983) Human cryptosporidiosis in immunocompetent and immunodeficient persons. *N Engl J Med* 308, 1252–1257.

82 Abdo A, Klassen J, Urbansski S *et al.* (2003) Reversible sclerosing cholangitis secondary to cryptosporidiosis in a renal transplant patient. *J Hepatol* 38, 688–691.

83 Campos M, Jouzdani E, Sempoux C *et al.* (2000) Sclerosing cholangitis associated to cryptosporidiosis in liver transplanted children. *Eur J Pediatr* 159, 113–115.

84 Cordero E, Lopez Cortez LF, Belda O *et al.* (2001) Acquired immunodeficiency syndrome related cryptosporidial cholangitis: resolution with endobiliary prosthesis insertion. *Gastrointest Endosc* 53, 534–535.

85 Gross T, Wheat J, Bartlett M *et al.* (1986) AIDS and multiple system involvement with cryptosporidiosis. *Am J Gastroenterol* 81, 456–458.

86 Kaplan JE, Hanson D, Dworkin MS (2000) Epidemiology of human immunodeficiency virus associated opportunistic infections in the United States in the era of highly active retroviral therapy. *Clin Infect Dis* 30, S5–S14.

87 Levy J, Espanol-Boren T, Thomas C *et al.* (1997) Clinical spectrum of X-linked hyper-IgM syndrome. *J Pediatr* 131, 47–54.

88 Mortele KJ, Segatto E, Ros PR (2004) The infected liver: radiologic–pathologic correlation. *RadioGraphics* 24, 937–955.

89 Grant EG (1992) Liver. In: Mittelstaedt CA (ed.) *General Ultrasound.* New York: Churchill Livingstone, Ch. 5, pp. 208–211.

90 Radin DR, Ralls P, Coletti PM *et al.* (1988) CT of amebic liver abscess. *Am J Roentgenol* 150, 1297–1301.

91 Mortele KJ, Ross PR (2001) Cystic focal lesions in the adult: differential CT and MR imaging features. *RadioGraphics* 21, 895–910.

92 Shamsuzzaman SM, Hashiguchi Y (2002) Thoracic amebiasis. *Clin Chest Med* 23, 479–492.

93 Khanna D, Chaudhary D, Kumar A *et al.* (2005) Experience with aspiration in cases of amebic liver abscess in an endemic area. *Eur J Clin Microbiol Infect Dis* 24, 428–430.

94 Souza DS, Barreiros JT, Papp KM *et al.* (2003) Comparison between immunomagnetic separation, coupled with immunofluorescence, and the techniques of Faust *et al.* and of Lutz for the diagnosis of *Giardia lamblia* cysts in human feces. *Rev Inst Med Trop Sao Paulo* 45, 339–342.

95 Fedorko DP, Williams EC, Nelson NA *et al.* (2000) Performance of three enzyme immunoassays for detection of *Giardia lamblia* in stool specimens preserved in ECOFIX. *J Clin Microbiol* 38, 2781–2783.

96 Shatla HM, el-Hodhod MT, Mohsen DM *et al.* (2004) Potential diagnosis of *Giardia lamblia* infection through specific antibody detection in saliva. *J Egypt Soc Parasitol* 34, 621–630.

97 Didier ES, Orenstein JM, Aldra D *et al.* (1995) Comparison of three staining methods for detecting microsporidia in fluids. *J Clin Microbiol* 33, 3138–3145.

98 Hughes MA, Oetri WA Jr (2000) Amebic liver abscess. *Infect Dis Clin North Am* 14, 565–583.

99 Torre A, Kershenobich D (2002) Amebic liver abscess. *Ann Hepatol* 1, 45–47.

100 Rosenblatt JE, Edson RS (1987) Metronidazole. *Mayo Clin Proc* 62, 1013–1017.

101 Badalamenti S, Jameson JE, Reddy KR (1999) Amebiasis. *Curr Treat Options Gastroenterol* 2(2), 97–103.

102 Karabay O, Tamer A, Gunduz H *et al.* (2004) Albendazole versus metronidazole treatment for adult giardiasis: an open randomized clinical study. *World J Gastroenterol* 10, 1215–1217.

103 Wright JM, Dunn LA, Upcroft PJA (2003) Efficacy of antigiardial drugs. *Expert Opin Drug Safety* 2, 529–541.

104 Fox LM, Saravolatz LD (2005) Nitazoxanide: a new thiazolide antiparasitic agent. *Clin Infect Dis* 40, 1173–1180.

105 Petri WA (2005) Treatment of giardiasis. *Curr Treat Options Gastroenterol* 8, 13–17.

106 Gardner TB, Hill DR (2001) Treatment of giardiasis. *Clin Microbiol Rev* 14, 114–128.

107 Zardi EM, Picardi A, Afeltra A (2005) Treatment of cryptosporidiosis in immunocompromised hosts. *Chemotherapy* 51, 193–196.

108 Hommer V, Eichholz J, Petry F (2003) Effect of antiretroviral protease inhibitors alone, and in combination with paromomycin, on the excystation, invasion and *in vitro* development of *Cryptosporidium parvum. J Antimicrob Chemother* 52, 359–364.

109 Smith HV, Corcoran GD (2004) New drugs and treatment for cryptosporidiosis. *Curr Opin Infect Dis* 17, 557–564.

110 Giacometti A, Burzacchini F, Cirioni O *et al.* (1999) Efficacy of treatment with paromomycin, azithromycin, and nitazoxanide in a patient with disseminated cryptosporidiosis. *Eur J Clin Microbiol Infect Dis* 18, 885–889.

10.3.2 Malaria

Montse Renom and Pedro L. Alonso

Malaria, caused by *Plasmodium* protozoan parasites, represents a major global health problem [1]; it is the most important parasitic disease of man. Approximately 4% of the world's population is infected; the disease is endemic in more than 100 countries and 40% of the world's population is at risk. Every year, approximately 500 million people suffer the disease, of whom approximately 1–3 million die, 90% in sub-Saharan Africa and 75% of them children [1–3].

The disease is caused by an intracellular protozoan of the *Plasmodium* genus that is transmitted to humans by the bite of the female mosquito of the *Anopheles* genus. The infection can also be acquired by blood transfusion, through the placenta (congenital transmission) as well as by the use of contaminated needles or syringes.

In non-endemic areas, the disease should be suspected in all febrile patients with a travel history to endemic countries. Needless to say, malaria should be suspected in all febrile patients in endemic areas.

Four species of *Plasmodium* infect humans (*P. falciparum, P. vivax, P. ovale* and *P. malariae*). *P. falciparum* is encountered mainly in African countries and is responsible for the most severe forms of the disease. *P. vivax* and *P. ovale* are known to form resting stages in the liver (hypnozoites) that may reactivate and can cause clinical relapse many months after the initial clinical presentation [3].

Epidemiology

At present, malaria is found throughout the tropics in 103 countries in Africa, Latin America, Asia and Oceania. The epidemiology of the disease is complex and varies in different areas within the same geographical zone. The transmission depends on at least four interrelated factors: the vector (*Anopheles*), the parasite (*Plasmodium*), the human host and the environment [4,5].

In Africa, Papua Guinea and Haiti, *P. falciparum* is the predominant species; *P vivax* is more common in Central and South America, North Africa, the Middle East and the Indian subcontinent. The prevalence of both species is approximately equal in other parts of South America, East Asia and Oceania. *P. vivax* is rare in sub-Saharan Africa, whereas *P. ovale* is relatively uncommon outside West Africa. *P. malariae* is found in most areas, but is less common outside Africa. *P. vivax* strains may still be found in China and adjacent countries.

Malaria was endemic in some areas of Europe and northern Asia, and was introduced to North America, but has been eradicated from these areas since the mid-nineteenth century.

The epidemiology of malaria is described as endemic (stable transmission) when the incidence is relatively constant annually; transmission may be seasonal or perennial. It is defined as epidemic (unstable transmission) when marked differences exist between different years. Endemic areas were further classified (from low to high) as hypoendemic, mesoendemic, hyperendemic and holoendemic depending on the intensity of transmission and the effects on the population. Epidemics occur when one or several of the following factors appear: (i) increase in the number of susceptible individuals in the population; (ii) increase in the gametocyte reservoir of the population; (iii) increased contact between human and vector; and (iv) increased effectiveness in vector transmission.

Epidemics often occur in hypoendemic and mesoendemic areas and are characterized by an elevated mortality affecting all age groups. In areas of high endemicity, mortality is mainly seen in the most vulnerable groups such as children under 5 years of age. Malaria infection also poses substantial risks to pregnant women and their fetuses and may result in spontaneous abortion and stillbirth. Most cases diagnosed in Europe and the USA are imported. More than 15 000 and 1200 cases are declared annually in Europe and the USA respectively.

Aetiology

There are 120 *Plasmodium* species that affect animals (primates, birds and reptiles), only four of which affect humans. The genomic sequence of *P. falciparum* has been described recently. The *Plasmodium* life cycle is complex and similar in the four species infecting humans: (i) a sexual exogenous phase in certain *Anopheles* mosquitoes (sporogony); and (ii) an asexual endogenous phase in humans, which includes an exoerythrocytic phase and an erythrocytic phase.

Humans may be infected through the bite of a female *Anopheles* mosquito which inoculates the sporozoites (infective form) into the dermis and the bloodstream. The blood drives the sporozoites to the liver where they invade the hepatocytes. This phase is known as the exoerythrocytic or hepatic schizogony phase. The circumsporozoite protein and TRAP (organelle protein translocated to the sporozoite surface) bind to hepatocytes through the heparan sulphate glycosaminoglycans (GAGs) specifically expressed on the hepatocyte surface. Malaria sporozoites actively enter the Kupffer cells prior to hepatocyte invasion [6–10]. In the hepatocyte, the sporozoite becomes schizont through schizogony and divides into several thousand merozoites. Up to this stage, there is no obvious effect on liver function, nor are signs and symptoms of the disease observed. Infection with *P. vivax* and *P. ovale* may lead to the persistence

of pre-erythrocytic forms in the liver (hypnozoite), which can awake and mature into schizonts months after the initial infection. This is not seen with *P. falciparum* or *P. malariae* parasites.

After 6–16 days, depending on the species, merozoites are delivered into the bloodstream where they invade red blood cells (RBCs). At this point, the erythrocytic schizogony phase starts. In the initial stages, the parasite can be seen as annular rings or trophozoites and, in the following stages, the trophozoite absorbs haemoglobin resulting in the formation of haemozoin pigment. After a maturation period, the trophozoite undergoes multiple divisions forming the schizont. When the schizont becomes engorged with merozoites, the RBC is destroyed, and all merozoites are released into the bloodstream ready to infect other RBCs where the same process takes place. The duration of the erythrocytic phase varies between species being 48 h in *P. vivax*, *P. ovale* and *P. falciparum* and 72 h in *P. malariae*. Many generations after the initial merozoites, a few of them evolve into differentiated sexual forms (gametocytes).

When a female *Anopheles* mosquito feeds from an infected individual, parasites are delivered into its stomach, the asexual forms and RBCs are destroyed and gametocytes continue with the maturation process. Fecundation takes place, giving rise to a zygote which evolves into oocytes that contain sporozoites. Sporozoites will accumulate in the mosquito salivary gland and enter the human host through a bite. The sexual cycle in the mosquito lasts approximately 10–20 days, and the ideal temperature for it to happen is between 15 and 32°C. It does not take place at altitudes above 2000 m.

Clinical manifestations

Malaria has a wide range of clinical manifestations which depend mainly on the species of *Plasmodium* and the previous immune status of the host; children less than 5 years, pregnant women and travellers from non-endemic areas are most vulnerable and suffer more severe forms.

The pathogenetic effect is the result of erythrocyte destruction, liberation of the parasite and RBC degradation products into the bloodstream and host responses to these events. Known physiopathological phenomena that have been recognized so far to cause damage are: (i) cytokine toxicity; (ii) cytoadherence phenomena in the blood vessels and organs with microcirculation occlusion; (iii) rosetting, non-infected erythrocytes adhere to parasitized RBCs; (iv) deformability, parasitized RBCs become more rigid. The organs most affected during malaria infection are the brain, spleen, liver [11], kidney, lungs and placenta. The incubation period varies between 8 and 30 days depending on the species: shorter for *P. falciparum* and longer for *P. malariae*. Nevertheless, some *P. vivax* may have an incubation period of almost a year. The clinical features of uncomplicated malaria are common in the four species and consist of fever, headache, muscle aches, abdominal discomfort, lethargy and anaemia. Diarrhoea and respiratory symptoms may be present.

Severe malaria, mainly caused by *P. falciparum*, is often classified as: cerebral malaria (which includes a Blantyre coma score ≤ 2), severe malarial anaemia (including a haematocrit ≤ 15) or other forms of severe malaria (which may include multiorgan failure, severe hypoglycaemia, respiratory distress, acidosis or circulatory collapse) [12–15].

Malaria hepatic dysfunction

Jaundice in malaria

Although jaundice is considered to be a frequent sign in malaria, there is a wide variation in its reported incidence ranging from 2.58% to 62% [16]. Possible reasons for this wide variation could include the level of endemicity (endemic vs. epidemic), age, the *Plasmodium* species (*vivax* vs. *falciparum*) and case definition used (e.g. inclusion of complicated cases only where the incidence of jaundice is higher).

Jaundice in malaria is multifactorial and mostly due to one or several of the following:

1 intravascular haemolysis due to destruction of parasitized and non-parasitized RBCs;
2 coexistent malnutrition;
3 shock and disseminated intravascular coagulation leading to microangiopathic haemolysis;
4 hepatocyte dysfunction.

Malarial hepatitis

Hepatocellular dysfunction is observed in falciparum malaria. This clinical picture may range from different degrees of conjugated hyperbilirubinaemia with or without mild elevation of transaminases to fulminant hepatic failure [16–18].

Several mechanisms conducive to hepatic have been described dysfunction Organ damage, including the liver, is believed to be related to cytoadherence of parasitized red blood cells (pRBCs) to the vascular and sinusoidal endothelium, leading to stagnant anoxaemia. Reduction in portal venous flow has been described as a consequence of micro-occlusion of portal venous branches by pRBCs. Liver function abnormalities have been reported in severe systemic infections and endotoxaemia; this has also been described, with or without concomitant bacterial infections, in complicated malaria. An additional mechanism is the intrahepatic cholestasis secondary to reticuloendothelial blockage and disturbances of the hepatic microvilli. In many cases, the biochemical and histological evidence of hepatocellular injury is minimal.

The traditional view that, besides jaundice, signs of hepatic dysfunction are unusual, and clinical signs of liver failure such as asterixis or 'liver flap' are never seen unless there is concomitant viral hepatitis [19], has been challenged in recent years by a number of reports describing the occurrence of hepatic encephalopathy in infections caused by falciparum malaria [20,21]. Other reports have also inappropriately used the term fulminant hepatic failure in malaria patients with coma, without ruling out a neurological involvement by malaria (cerebral malaria) rather than hepatic encephalopathy.

Malarial hepatopathy has a wide range of presentations that are classified in two large groups:
• type A involves a fulminant illness with coma, jaundice, purpura and multiorgan failure [19];
• type B, a milder illness with fever, headache and vomiting, resolving in 10–15 days [22].

Jaundice is the commonest sign of hepatic dysfunction; according to some classifications, it can be considered as a sign of severe malaria.

Anatomopathological findings

In acute falciparum malaria, the liver is enlarged and can weigh approximately 2.5 kg. It is congested and pigmented dark brown. A wide variety of histological changes have been reported in malaria which are not consistently found in all studies. By electron microscopy, Kupffer cells are hypertrophied and contain haemozoin pigment. The sinusoids are dilated, and the portal tracts may be infiltrated with inflammatory cells. The parasites are rarely demonstrable (seen in less than half the cases). Additional changes include steatosis, focal hepatocyte swelling and necrosis and focal accumulation of histiocytes forming non-granulomatous lesions. Parasitized red blood cells are seen in Kupffer cells and endothelial cells. Characteristically rectangular, crystalline malaria pigment granules are seen in these cells. The hepatocytes contain lipofuchsin and haemosiderin as well as fat droplets. There are changes in the endoplasmic reticulum and mitochondria. The spaces of Disse can become narrow with loss of microvilli in the hepatocytes and the bile canaliculi. Centrizonal necrosis has also been described and, of the other non-specific changes, it is a strong indicator of hepatocellular damage [23]. It still needs to be resolved whether this is due to malaria infection itself or to terminal hypotension artifacts.

Diagnosis

Malaria

The diagnostic gold standard remains the microscopic examination of a thick and thin blood smear stained with Giemsa, Leishman or Romanowsky–eosin. Thick smears have a greater sensitivity because erythrocytes are haemolysed, and intraerythrocytic parasites are then liberated. It provides a simpler method of counting parasites that allows formulation of the relative parasite count and gives the results in a semi-quantitative scale (one to five crosses). Thin smears have a better specificity because they keep the parasite morphology allowing the identification of species and stage. They allow parasite counting per microlitre (μL); this is based on the number of parasites per μL of blood, counted in relation to a predetermined number of leukocytes. An average of 8000 leukocytes/μL is taken as the standard. Despite inaccuracies due to variations in ill persons, this standard permits reasonable comparisons.

Other diagnostic methods are QBC (quantified buffy coat), DNA probes, detection of monoclonal antibodies. They still do not have a role in clinical settings and are only used in epidemiological studies. Antibody determination is useless in acute episodes but may be useful in epidemiological studies to confirm past exposure.

Malarial hepatitis diagnosis

The diagnosis is made on clinical evidence of signs and symptoms of liver injury, confirmed by the appropriate laboratory tests of liver dysfunction. In 29 patients with malaria hepatitis [24], the ultrasound examination found hepatomegaly with low echogenicity and thick gallbladder similar to that seen in acute viral hepatitis. No data are available on the features of livers in malaria by computerized tomography or magnetic resonance imaging. It is therefore important to make the diagnosis of liver dysfunction in the context of an already made diagnosis of malaria, as well as to consider malaria as the cause of a suspected liver injury of varying degrees. In the context of malaria, unconjugated bilirubin is often elevated in association with intravascular haemolysis of multifactorial origin, but the finding of increased conjugated bilirubin with elevation in liver enzymes should lead to the diagnosis of malarial hepatopathy. Haemolysis alone does not cause severe jaundice or predominantly conjugated hyperbilirubinaemia. Therefore, major patients with serum bilirubin levels of more than 10 mg% and a are likely to suffer from proportion of conjugated bilirubin associated hepatocellular injury; these patients also have increased liver enzymes.

Malarial hepatitis: diagnostic criteria [16]
• Demonstration of *P. falciparum* infection by the detection of parasites in peripheral blood smear;
• Hyperbilirubinaemia > 10 mg% with elevated conjugated bilirubin;
• A minimum of a threefold rise in transaminases, especially alanine aminotransferase, on two consecutive blood samples taken 24 h apart with or without the presence of conjugated hyperbilirubinaemia;
• Absence of serological evidence suggesting viral infection;
• No intake of drugs that may affect liver function;
• Clinical response to antimalarials;

Malarial hepatitis differential diagnosis

Malaria must enter the differential diagnosis of patients with a history of travel to endemic areas who present with fever and jaundice or any sign of liver dysfunction. While the full-blown presentation with oligoanuria, disproportionate anaemia with normal and increased liver mass, as well as persistent fever and mild elevations in liver enzymes, should prompt consideration of malaria as a cause, it is important also to include malaria in the differential diagnosis of minor signs of liver dysfunction in travellers, as malarial disease is reversible if treated but may progress rapidly if unrecognized. In this regard, it should be noted that malarial hepatitis may mimic fulminant hepatic failure from whatever cause; it is vital to start antimalarial therapy

immediately as severe malarial hepatitis may very rapidly lead to death if untreated or treated with delay. Thinking about malaria is important in developed countries where travel to endemic areas is becoming frequent, and medical professionals are not yet accustomed to include parasitic and/or other tropical diseases in their differential diagnosis of liver disorders. Imported falciparum malaria in the USA is often misdiagnosed as hepatitis and gastroenteritis or, in the severe presentations, as fulminant hepatic failure.

Fulminant hepatic failure (FHF), defined as the onset of encephalopathy within 8 weeks from the first symptom of hepatic injury, is commonly due to viral hepatitis and drug use. Infectious diseases such as sepsis or typhoid fever may also rarely present with FHF. Altered consciousness in malarial hepatitis, although uncommon, may make the distinction between malarial hepatitis and viral FHF very difficult. Malaria is treatable with numerous drugs, and the outcome, when prompt treatment is started, is often good. Mortality was 24% in cases of malarial hepatitis compared with 76% in the viral FHF group [20,25].

Jaundice induced by antimalarial drugs
A minimal elevation of liver enzymes has been described after exposure to mefloquine, especially in previously damaged livers. The drug should, therefore, be prescribed with caution in patients with known liver disease. Fatal acute hepatitis has been reported secondary to amodiaquine and hepatitis has been reported with chloroquine prophylaxis. Combination therapies, which are recommended to delay the development of resistance to *P. falciparum*, were also associated with hepatic alterations. An episode of acute asymptomatic hepatitis was described in two healthy volunteers after two doses of amodiaquine plus artesunate as well as after the administration of pyrimethamine–sulphadoxine; a case of granulomatous hepatitis has been attributed to pyrimethamine–chloroquine administered for prophylaxis.

Coexisting acute viral hepatitis
In endemic areas, it is important to differentiate whether jaundice is secondary to malaria *per se* or to acute viral hepatitis. In the former, it is characteristic to see a disproportionate hyperbilirubinaemia with mild elevation of the liver enzymes. Acute hepatitis E and malaria can commonly coexist in tropical countries [26,27]. Hepatic failure is mostly associated with viral infection or with severe falciparum malaria. Hepatitis A has also been reported in association with malaria [28].

Underlying chronic hepatitis
The overall prevalence of HBsAg was found to be higher (23.77%) than previously described (9.8%) among adult Vietnamese patients admitted for severe falciparum malaria [29]. HBsAg was present in a slightly greater proportion in patients admitted for cerebral malaria. However, no association was found between the risk of death and the coexistence of

severe malaria and HBsAg. Chronic infection with hepatitis B virus (HBV) may nevertheless be a risk factor for severe malaria. It has been suggested that the immunoresponse-raising anti-RESA (antibody against *P. falciparum* ring-infected erythrocytes surface antigen) could be suppressed in chronic HBsAg carriers [30]. There have also been reports of an association between HBsAg carriage and severe malaria in Gambian children [31]; this association, which could be explained by a reduced level of HLA class I antigen expression on hepatocytes infected by HBV, impairing the clearance of liver parasites, has not been shown in other studies in different endemic areas.

Vice versa, malaria infection might influence the course and pathogenesis of HBV infection and modulate viraemia in chronic hepatitis B [32]. Interestingly, severe flares of HBV hepatitis B with liver cell failure were seen after discontinuation of chloroquine given for malaria prophylaxis [33]. The proposed mechanism is through chloroquine inhibiton of the association of the major histocompatibility complex (MHC) type 2 with HBV, therefore inhibiting T cell-mediated lysis of infected cells.

Malarial hepatitis simulating FHF vs. fulminant hepatic failure [25,34]

Severe malaria due to *P. falciparum* may masquerade as FHF. Simple clinical and laboratory parameters together with a high index of suspicion can easily distinguish these entities. A detailed and focused medical history, physical examination and pattern of liver test abnormalities may help to distinguish both entities. The presence of hepatomegaly and normal prothrombin time (PT) are characteristic of malarial hepatitis. In contrast, a decreased liver size and prolonged PT are the hallmarks of FHF. In patients presenting with FHF, clinical suspicion of malaria and, in a non-endemic area, history of recent travel to an endemic area should prompt a peripheral blood smear to rule out malaria.

Treatment

Uncomplicated malaria

During the last 50 years, treatment has been based on chloroquine, a safe, efficacious, easy to take and cheap drug. However, during the past two decades, development by the parasite of resistance to chloroquine has increased so much that this drug is no longer recommended as first-line treatment (although it is still used in some countries, particularly in West Africa). The emergence and spread of resistance to sulphadoxine–pyrimethamine is also rendering this drug of limited value as a first-line substitute. The artemisinine derivative, especially in combination with other antimalarial drugs, is showing promising results and is being introduced in many countries. Its availability and cost are the main limitations as well as the limited availability of safety data in certain groups such as pregnant women [35]. Other options are quinine, mefloquine, halofantrine, doxycycline and clindamycin.

Complicated malaria

Current recommendations are parenteral quinine salt 20 mg/kg body weight infused over a 4-h period followed by 10 mg/kg infused over a 4-h period every 8 h. Once patient consciousness improves, medication is switched to oral quinine 650 mg every 8 h for a total duration of 7 days. Oral doxycycline should be added for 7 days when possible.

Treatment of the intrahepatic forms (*P. vivax* and *P. ovale*)

Primaquin 15 mg base/day (0.25 mg/kg) for 2 weeks. Contraindicated in pregnant women, in the breastfeeding period and for those with glucose-6-phosphate dehydrogenase deficiency.

Malarial hepatitis treatment

Measures should be addressed to correct the hepatocellular dysfunction if needed, as well as to appropriately treat malaria. Hepatocellular jaundice is indicative of severe malaria and, therefore, appropriate intravenous antimalarial treatment is indicated (described above). As quinine elimination half-life is prolonged and clearance is lower, current dosage regimens may need to be adjusted or followed closely in patients with acute hepatitis and/or renal dysfunction and in those who had an acute hepatitis within the previous 3 months.

Mild cases of liver disorders have improved with antimalarial therapy, with amelioration of liver function tests [21].

Prevention

At present, the malaria prevention strategies are vector control, the reduction of human–vector contact and drugs for its prevention and treatment [36]. Treatment in developing areas is hindered by the lack of effective, safe and cheap drugs. Intermittent preventive treatment in infants and pregnant women is being developed. A malaria vaccine, RTS,S/ASO2A, has shown promising results in endemic areas but is still under investigation [37,38].

References

1 Snow RW, Hay SI (2006) Comparing methods of estimating the global morbidity burden from *Plasmodium falciparum* malaria. *Am J Trop Med Hyg* 74(2), 189–190.

2 Guinovart C, Navia MM, Tanner M *et al.* (2006) Malaria: burden of disease. *Curr Mol Med* 6(2), 137–140.

3 Greenwood BM, Bojang K, Whitty CJ *et al.* (2005) Malaria. *Lancet* 365(9469), 1487–1498.

4 White NJ (2003) Malaria. In: Cook GC (ed.) *Manson's Tropical Diseases*, Philadelphia, PA: W.B. Saunders, pp. 1207–1295.

5 Menendez Santos C (1997) Paludismo. I, 1836–1841. In: *Medicina Interna*. J. Rodés Teixidor.

6 Barnwell JW (2001) Hepatic Kupffer cells: the portal that permits infection of hepatocytes by malarial sporozoites? *Hepatology* 33(5), 1331–1333.

7 Sinnis P (1996) The malaria sporozoite's journey into the liver. *Infect Agents Dis* 5(3), 182–189.

8 Pradel G, Frevert U (2001) Malaria sporozoites actively enter and pass through rat Kupffer cells prior to hepatocyte invasion. *Hepatology* 33(5), 1154–1165.

9 Mota MM, Pradel G, Vanderberg JP *et al.* (2001) Migration of *Plasmodium* sporozoites through cells before infection. *Science* 291(5501), 141–144.

10 Pradel G, Wagner C, Mejia C *et al.* (2005) *Plasmodium falciparum*: co-dependent expression and co-localization of the PfCCp multi-adhesion domain proteins. *Exp Parasitol* 112, 263–268.

11 Molyneux ME, Looareesuwan S, Menzies IS *et al.* (1989) Reduced hepatic blood flow and intestinal malabsorption in severe falciparum malaria. *Am J Trop Med Hyg* 40(5), 470–476.

12 Mackintosh CL, Beeson JG, Marsh K (2004) Clinical features and pathogenesis of severe malaria. *Trends Parasitol* 20(12), 597–603.

13 Krishnan A, Karnad DR (2003) Severe falciparum malaria: an important cause of multiple organ failure in Indian intensive care unit patients. *Crit Care Med* 31(9), 2278–2284.

14 Harris VK, Richard VS, Mathai E *et al.* (2001) A study on clinical profile of falciparum malaria in a tertiary care hospital in south India. *Ind J Malariol* 38(1–2), 19–24.

15 World Health Organization, Communicable Diseases Cluster (2000) Severe falciparum malaria. *Trans R Soc Trop Med Hyg* 94(Suppl. 1), S1–90.

16 Anand AC, Puri P (2005) Jaundice in malaria. *J Gastroenterol Hepatol* 20(9), 1322–1332.

17 Kochar DK, Singh P, Agarwal P *et al.* (2003) Malarial hepatitis. *J Assoc Phys India* 51, 1069–1072.

18 Anand AC (2001) Liver in malaria. *Ind J Gastroenterol* 20(Suppl. 1), C37–C38.

19 Murthy GL, Sahay RK, Sreenivas DV *et al.* (1998) Hepatitis in falciparum malaria. *Trop Gastroenterol* 19(4), 152–154.

20 Kochar DK, Agarwal P, Kochar SK *et al.* (2003) Hepatocyte dysfunction and hepatic encephalopathy in *Plasmodium falciparum* malaria. *Q J Med* 96(7), 505–512.

21 Anand AC, Ramji C, Narula AS *et al.* (1992) Malarial hepatitis: a heterogeneous syndrome? *Natl Med J India* 5(2), 59–62.

22 Ghoda MK (2002) Falciparum hepatopathy: a reversible and transient involvement of liver in falciparum malaria. *Trop Gastroenterol* 23(2), 70–71.

23 Mishra SK, Mohanty S, Das BS *et al.* (1992) Hepatic changes in *P. falciparum* malaria. *Ind J Malariol* 29(3), 167–171.

24 Kachawaha S, Pokharana R, Rawat N *et al.* (2003) Ultrasonography in malarial hepatitis. *Ind J Gastroenterol* 22(3), 110.

25 Devarbhavi H, Alvares JF, Kumar KS (2005) Severe falciparum malaria simulating fulminant hepatic failure. *Mayo Clin Proc* 80(3), 355–358.

26 Ghoshal UC, Somani S, Chetri K *et al.* (2001) *Plasmodium falciparum* and hepatitis E virus co-infection in fulminant hepatic failure. *Ind J Gastroenterol* 20(3), 111.

27 Bansal R, Kadhiravan T, Aggarwal P *et al.* (2002) *Plasmodium vivax* and hepatitis E co-infection – a rare cause of malarial jaundice. *Ind J Gastroenterol* 21(5), 207–208.

28 Katou K, Nakamura C, Amano F *et al.* (1982) [Hepatitis A and *Salmonella enteritis* complicated with malaria]. *Kansenshogaku Zasshi* 56(10), 872–876.

29 Barcus MJ, Hien TT, White NJ *et al.* (2002) Short report: hepatitis b infection and severe *Plasmodium falciparum* malaria in Vietnamese adults. *Am J Trop Med Hyg* 66(2), 140–142.

30 Souto FJ, Fontes CJ, Gaspar AM (2002) Relation between hepatitis B carrier status and antibody against synthetic *Plasmodium falciparum* erythrocyte surface. *Mem Inst Oswaldo Cruz* 97(2), 197–198.

31 Thursz MR, Kwiatkowski D, Torok ME *et al.* (1995) Association of hepatitis B surface antigen carriage with severe malaria in Gambian children. *Nature Med* 1(4), 374–375.

32 Brown AE, Mongkolsirichaikul D, Innis B *et al.* (1992) Falciparum malaria modulates viremia in chronic hepatitis B virus infection. *J Infect Dis* 166(6), 1465–1466.

33 Helbling B, Reichen J (1994) [Reactivation of hepatitis B following withdrawal of chloroquine]. *Schweiz Med Wochenschr* 124(18), 759–762.

34 Ahsan T, Rab SM, Shekhani MS (1993) Falciparum malaria or fulminant hepatic failure? *J Pak Med Assoc* 43(10), 206–208.

35 Newman RD, Parise ME, Slutsker L *et al.* (2003) Safety, efficacy and determinants of effectiveness of antimalarial drugs during pregnancy: implications for prevention programmes in *Plasmodium falciparum*-endemic sub-Saharan Africa. *Trop Med Int Health* 8(6), 488–506.

36 Alonso PL, Guinovart C (2004) Malaria: situation, control tools, resources and solutions. *Ars Med Rev Hum* 2, 166–179.

37 Alonso PL, Sacarlal J, Aponte JJ *et al.* (2004) Efficacy of the RTS,S/AS02A vaccine against *Plasmodium falciparum* infection and disease in young African children: randomised controlled trial. *Lancet* 364(9443), 1411–1420.

38 Alonso PL, Sacarlal J, Aponte JJ *et al.* (2005) Duration of protection with RTS,S/AS02A malaria vaccine in prevention of *Plasmodium falciparum* disease in Mozambican children: single-blind extended follow-up of a randomised controlled trial. *Lancet* 366(9502), 2012–2018.

10.3.3 Visceral leishmaniasis

Manuel Corachan

Introduction

The protozoan parasite responsible for visceral leishmaniasis (VL) was morphologically described by Laveran and Mesnil in 1903; it was given the name of *Leishmania donovani* when, almost simultaneously, Leishman in Calcutta and Donovan in Madras published a sketch of the parasite in the spleens of patients with remittent types of fevers.

The epidemiology, diagnostic approach and therapy of VL have changed significantly in the last two decades, as a result primarily of the increase in *Leishmania* coinfection with the human immunodeficiency virus (HIV virus). Coinfection has been brought under partial control in some areas, such as the the EU Mediterranean, zone thanks to the new therapeutic possibilities and preventive efforts targeted against drug addiction; however, in other places, it is still on the rise, as in Brazil. Besides representing an emerging risk for HIV-immunocompromised subjects, *Leishmania* is also emerging as a risk for people who receive organ transplants.

Transmission occurs through phlebotomine arthropods with *Phlebotomus argentipes* in the Old World and *Lutzomia longipalpis* in the New World being the most prevalent among several hundred sandfly species described. The phlebotomines ingest the parasite from a human or canine reservoir which can be wild or domestic. The parasite inoculated by the sandfly colonizes the mononuclear phagocytic system throughout the body, stimulating a T-helper cell response that may contain disease despite the persistence of the infection. Infected people raise antibodies to *Leishmania*, but these are not protective. Infection includes a febrile illness that may result in marked organomegaly, cachexia and pancytopenia.

The overall annual incidence of infection by *Leishmania* species is estimated to be between 1.5 and 2 million; this includes the various types of clinical presentations (cutaneous, mucocutaneous or visceral). Visceral leishmaniasis is also known as 'kala-azar' from the Hindi language meaning dark fever.

Epidemiology

Leishmania infection is endemic in more than 60 countries with an estimated 500 000 new cases per year and around 41 000 deaths [1].

The sandflies have nocturnal feeding habits. Their precise breeding sites are still controversial, but it is known that they feed on several species of mammals including rodents, canines, marsupials and primates. In the Old World, the dog is the most important reservoir, and the animal itself may undergo a severe and often fatal disease.

Infection via blood transfusion or through neonatal transmission is extremely rare; however, the exchange of syringes among drug users has been responsible for the spread of *Leishmania* coinfection with HIV in Europe, especially in the Mediterranean basin. Infection can be transmitted by transplantation of infected organs.

In the last two decades, endemic areas have undergone considerable geographical extension for several reasons, among which war, famine, drought and economic migration were the most important [2].

A small outbreak of VL produced by *Leishmania tropica* (usually producing urban cutaneous leishmaniasis) affected the US troops during the Gulf War. The Indian subcontinent, Sudan and the northeast of Brazil register more than 80% of total cases. The epidemiology in India and Brazil shows a similar pattern in which the classical rural infection and the urban HIV pandemic are joining forces, thus resulting in significant numbers of coinfections. The spreading of coinfections produces a considerable increase in the human reservoir and complicates the diagnosis and therapy of the parasitic disease, which will be prone to frequent relapses [3]. In this setting therapeutic responses are poor, clinical manifestations atypical and *Leishmania* serology often negative, thus hampering the diagnostic approach.

Table 1 Visceral leishmaniasis.

Species	Geography	Reservoir
L. donovani	East Africa, India	Human
L. infantum	Mediterranean	Canine
L. chagasi[a]	Central and South America	Canine

[a]*L. chagasi* is currently considered as a synonym of *L. infantum*.

In East Africa and the Indian subcontinent humans are the reservoir of the parasite; most VL elsewhere are considered as zoonoses, and their geographical distribution coincides with that of the presence of the vector. The geographical distribution of the species and the nature of the reservoir are shown in Table 1 and Figure 1.

Clinical features

The incubation period ranges from a few weeks to several years (average 2–6 months).

Fever is the dominant feature, and the disease is classically considered in the differential diagnosis of pyrexia of unknown origin (PUO) syndrome. All types of fever have been described, bimodal being the most frequent; apyrexial periods are usually intercalated. There is progressive asthenia and weight loss accompanied by signs of anaemia, lymphadenopathy, occasional hepatomegaly and the almost constant finding of progressive splenomegaly that extends below the umbilicus producing a protuberant abdomen.

The size of the spleen correlates with the degree of pancytopenia and the duration of the illness. There is no convincing evidence that autoimmune haemolysis contributes to the severity of anaemia [4]. Liver laboratory abnormalities are not characteristic; aminotransferases and alkaline phosphatase may be increased, usually to a relatively minor degree. Overt ascites and liver failure occur rarely.

Pulmonary involvement and bleeding episodes can occur in advanced disease. The natural course of the chronic infection will be fatal in 90% of cases due to intercurrent infections or bleeding complications.

Clinical variants of these 'classical' features occur. Subclinical infections have been described in Kenya, Brazil and the Mediterranean. These subclinical cases may change to full-blown disease when the patient immune status changes. Immunosuppressive therapy or the development of acquired immunodeficiency syndrome (AIDS) may convert latent infections of long standing to overt VL. In the Mediterranean basin, the form of kala-azar caused by *Leishmania infantum* is predominant in the under 5-year age group compared with the adult form; however, at the peak of the AIDS epidemic in the European Mediterranean area, the prevalences of *L. infantum* infection became almost equal in children and adults. VL has

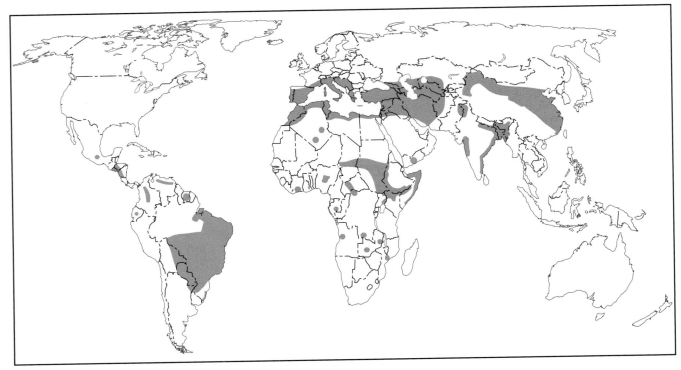

Fig. 1 Map showing geographical distribution of visceral leishmaniasis, showing the four main zones and sporadic human cases.

developed in patients who received liver, heart and kidney transplants.

Post-kala-azar dermal leishmaniasis (PKDL)

Between 5% and 60% (depending on the geographical area) of patients with VL develop PKDL during or years after receiving treatment. This complication was described many decades ago, but its importance and its epidemiological implications (especially in East Africa) have only recently been recognized. Usually, it appears during the first months after treatment of VL in East Africa but after 2–3 years in the Indian subcontinent and in Asia. PKDL is more severe, the shorter the interval between treatment and the development of the complication. Younger age is predictive of severity.

It presents as a macular, papular rash in a patient who is recovering from systemic illness, starting on the face and spreading over the rest of the body when severe. Biopsy of the lesions can show the parasites, although the clinical picture in a treated patient is the main diagnostic element. Serological tests and the leishmanin skin test are of no clinical value in this situation, but polymerase chain reaction (PCR) will detect the parasites in more than 80% of cases [5].

Laboratory parameters and diagnosis

Pancytopenia is accompanied by important changes in plasma proteins resulting in the classical profile of low albumin levels together with overproduction of polyclonal IgG; erythrocyte sedimentation rate (ESR) and C-reactive protein are increased due to the inflammatory syndrome.

Pancytopenia is a consequence of hypersplenism. Anaemia is the most visible sign. In chronic disease, neutropenia increases the risk of associated infections and thrombopenia is responsible for bleeding episodes if alteration of coagulation factors is also present.

The identification of the parasite through culture techniques or direct observation confirms the clinical suspicion. The parasite can be stained or cultured in aspirates of bone marrow, spleen, lymph node or liver. Most rewarding is the spleen aspirate used as a last measure in developed countries but as a routine diagnosis in field practice in Kenya and Sudan (Fig. 2).

In patients with *Leishmania*/HIV coinfection, the parasite can often be directly detected in peripheral blood. In immunocompromised patients, it is also possible to find parasites in unusual localizations such as the pleural fluid, cerebrospinal fluid and in the mucosa of the digestive tract.

The classical blood agar 3N medium is the most currently used, but other diphasic and liquid methods are also available; the strains involved in visceral leishmaniasis are less difficult to isolate and culture than the cutaneous strains, such as *Leishmania venezuelensis* or *Leishmania braziliensis*.

PCR evaluation is very sensitive, permitting the detection of very low levels of the parasite in the blood [6,7]. This technique is also useful in monitoring relapses of HIV coinfections, but

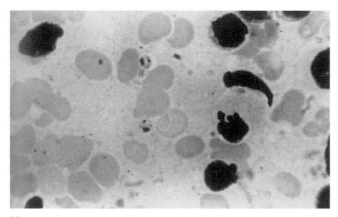

(a)

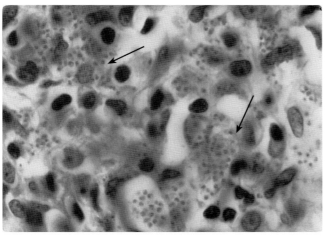

(b)

Fig. 2 (a) Two amastigotes of *L. donovani* in the spleen aspirate of a patient with visceral leishmaniasis. Parasites are usually extracellular in smears, because the macrophages that contain them rupture when the smear is made; they are intracellular in tissue sections. (b) *L. donovani* in Kupffer cells in the liver (× 1000).

it is still not available for fieldwork leishmaniasis in areas of high prevalence such as in the horn of Africa.

Serological techniques

Immunocompetent patients raise high levels of specific antibodies during active VL, but in immunocompromised patients, the antibody response is blunter. Direct and latex agglutination tests, Dot and fast enzyme-linked immunosorbent assay (ELISA) are usually available in most laboratories for the identification of antibodies. However, cross-reactions with other blood protozoa (malaria and trypanosomes) and helminths (schistosoma) do occur.

Research efforts are now devoted to the development of recombinant DNA-derived leishmania proteins of potential use in diagnosis and probably in future vaccines. A promising recombinant antigen is rK39, which is used to diagnose VL caused by *L. donovani*, *L. chagasi* or *L. infantum*. Serological testing showed that 98% of Brazilian and 100% of Sudanese VL patients have high levels of antibodies against this antigen, and this finding correlated with clinical disease [8,9].

High antibody titres of *L. donovani* hydrophilic acylated surface protein (HASPB1) and *L. major* gen B protein (GBP) are present in the serum of VL patients. Both can also induce antibodies that are detectable in patients with post-kala-azar dermal leishmaniasis (PKDL). Public health attention is also directed towards the identification of asymptomatic infected dogs (the main reservoir of the infection), as the control of the canine disease could have an impact in reducing transmission to humans.

Treatment

The earlier the treatment is started, the better is the response. It is worth remembering that there are many more subclinical than overt cases of VL [10]; generally speaking, the clinical response is slow whatever the drug used and often a second course of treatment is needed to complete the cure.

Antimonials (already in use for almost a century) are still the most widely used therapy in less developed countries because of economic constraints. An exception is northern India (Bihar state) where resistance to the antimonials has emerged. Table 2 shows the antileishmanial drugs currently utilized.

Antimonial therapy

Resistance to these widely used drugs (pentavalent anti-monials) is increasing, as suggested by studies in India [11] and Sudan. They have several disadvantages, mainly cardiotoxicity (at the repolarization conduction level) and other side-effects such as arthralgia, nausea and acute pancreatitis (the last is frequent in HIV coinfections). Relapses are frequent after inadequate or incomplete treatment with a single drug as monotherapy may select resistant mutants. Local pain at sites of injection due to the prolonged treatment diminishes acceptance of this drug in endemic areas. It has practically been abandoned in industrialized areas with fewer economic constraints.

Amphotericin B

Currently used for treating systemic fungal infections, it has become the first-line drug in areas of known resistance and in wealthy countries; the more expensive lipid-associated amphotericin B or the liposomal amphotericin are used as alternative treatments. Efficient plasma concentrations are achieved with its intravenous infusion. Fever, chills, thrombophlebitis, hypotension, vertigo and, exceptionally, cardiogenic shock are infusion related side-effects that can be lessened by a slow rate of infusion and the addition of corticosteroids at the infusion drip. The renal elimination is rather slow; nephrotoxicity is the most serious of the more frequent side-effects.

Table 2 Antileishmanial therapy.

Drug	Dose	Notes
Pentavalent antimonials Sodium stibogluconate (100-mL bottle: 100 mg Sb/mL) Meglumine antimoniate (5-mL ampoules: 85 mg Sb/mL	20 mg/kg/day for 3–6 weeks Depending on the geographical area, parenterally	Haematological and biochemistry controls as well as ECG controls are recommended during the period of treatment
Amphotericin B Formulated as a colloidal suspension	7–20 mg/kg as a total dose over 2–3 weeks	Slow (6–8 h) intravenous infusion Watch dose-limiting toxicity
Lipid-associated amphotericin B Liposomal Colloidal dispersion	10–20 mg/kg total dose. Given over 10 days (5–10 doses) i.v.	Retreatment of antimonial failures. First line in an HIV coinfection. First line in wealthy countries Optimum dosage needs to be defined
Miltefosine Alkyl phospholipid	100 mg/day over 4 weeks 2.5 mg/kg/day in children	First highly effective oral drug Most probably will need to be used in combination to avoid early development of resistance

In areas of India where it has become the drug of choice, amphotericin B achieved more than 97% cure rates with no evidence of resistance to date [12].

Lipid-associated amphotericin B

Liposomal amphotericin B is less toxic than the conventional amphotericin B and more efficient in immunocompetent as well as in immunocompromised patients; it has become first-line treatment in the developed countries.

A short course of treatment is currently used (see Table 2). For immunocompromised patients, the number of injections is increased to a total of 10.

Two other lipid-associated formulations, amphotericin B phospholipid complex and amphotericin B cholesterol dispersion, are not yet licensed for the treatment of visceral leishmaniasis.

Miltefosine

This alkyl phospholipid derives from oncology. Studies in India have shown a 100% cure rate with a dosage of 100 mg/day orally for 4 weeks. Gastrointestinal side-effects are frequent but do not usually interfere with treatment. Toxicity to male dog gonads has raised concern for teratogenicity, but in phase III trials in humans the drug did not affect male fertility [2].

The long half-life of this drug together with its narrow therapeutic index have a potential for the emergence of resistant mutants; combination therapy should be considered to delay this possibility.

Others

Paromomycin and aminosidine

These broad-spectrum aminoglycosides were used successfully in combination with pentavalent antimonials [13] in East Africa, India and in the UK in complicated cases. This valuable drug is at present undergoing a phase III clinical trial promoted by the Tropical Diseases Research (TDR) programme of the WHO as the traditional parenteral formulation is no longer available on the market.

Imidazoles

These have weak anti-leishmania activity when used as a single drug. In combination with allopurinol, isolated cases of cure have been reported, but there have been no formal clinical trials of the combination.

Allopurinol

This is another oral drug with weak anti-leishmania activity when used as monotherapy. Limited clinical trials have also shown a synergistic activity with pentavalent antimonials as well as with the imidazoles.

Interferon-γ

Because *Leishmania* infection depends on a defect in macrophage activation, the therapeutic use of this macrophage-activating cytokine has a rationale, but no convincing clinical studies have been carried out to date with this agent.

Treatment of PKDL

Most cases of PKDL undergo spontaneous healing, but this can take months. When treatment is required, the same drugs are used as for classical VL. Patients with mild clinical presentation can be left untreated. Patients with more severe forms, high serum antibody titres and a negative leishmanin skin test should receive treatment [5].

Cure rates of 62–90% were achieved with sodium stibogluconate at 20 mg/kg/day in India; this therapy needs to be administered for 3–4 months. Case reports are available on the efficacy of amphotericin B and liposomal amphotericin B; the latter is probably the best drug for the treatment of both VL and PKDL.

There is a need for testing of the new oral compound miltefosine. If proven beneficial, it could avoid the lengthy courses of daily parenteral treatment in countries where the amphotericin group of drugs are too expensive for the national health services.

References

1 WHO (2001) *The World Health Report 2001*. Geneva: WHO.

2 Guerin PhJ, Olliaro P, Sundar S *et al.* (2002) Visceral leishmaniasis: current status of control, diagnosis and treatment. *Lancet Infect Dis* 2, 494–501.

3 Pintado V, Lopez Velez R (2001) HIV-associated visceral leishmaniasis. *Clin Microbiol Infect* 7, 291–300.

4 Fleming AS, de Silva PS (2003) Haematological disease in the tropics. In: Cook GC, Zumla A (eds) *Manson's Tropical Diseases*, 21st edn. Philadelphia: Saunders, pp. 170–251.

5 Zijlstra EE, Musa AM, Khalil EAG *et al.* (2003) Post-kala-azar dermal leishmaniasis. *Lancet Infect Dis* 3, 87–98.

6 Salotra P, Sreenivas G, Pogue GP *et al.* (2001) Development of a species-specific PCR assay for detection of *Leishmania donovani* in clinical samples from patients with kala-azar and post kala-azar dermal leishmaniasis. *J Clin Microbiol* 39, 849–854.

7 Kubar J, Fragaki K (2005) Recombinant DNA-derived leishmania proteins: from the laboratory to the field. *Lancet Infect Dis* 5, 107–114.

8 Burns JM Jr, Shrefler WG, Benson DR *et al.* (1993) Molecular characterization of a kinesin-related antigen of *Leishmania chagasi* that detects specific antibody in African and American visceral leishmaniasis. *Proc Natl Acad Sci USA* 90, 775–779.

9 Ziljstra EE, Nur Y, Desjeux P *et al.* (2001) Diagnosing visceral leishmaniasis with the recombinant K39 strip test: experience from the Sudan. *Trop Med Int Health* 6, 108–113.

10 Ho M, Siongok TK, Lyerly WH *et al.* (1982) Prevalence and disease spectrum in a new focus of visceral leishmaniasis in Kenya. *Trans R Soc Trop Med Hyg* 76, 741–746.

11 Sundar S (2001) Drug resistance in Indian visceral leishmaniasis. *Trop Med Int Health* 6, 849–854.

12 Thakur CP, Sinha GP, Pandey AK (1996) Comparison of regimens of amphotericin B deoxycholate in kala-azar. *Ind J Med Res* 103, 259–263.

13 Thakur CP, Kanyok TP, Pandey AK (2000) A prospective randomised, comparative, open-label trial of the safety and efficacy of paromomycin (aminosidine) plus sodium stibogluconate versus sodium stibogluconate alone for the treatment of visceral leishmaniasis. *Trans R Soc Trop Med Hyg* 94, 429–431.

10.4 Helminthiasis

10.4.1 Blood flukes (schistosomes) and liver flukes

Flair Carrilho, Pedro Paulo Chieffi and Luiz Caetano Da Silva

Blood flukes

Blood flukes are trematode worms belonging to the genus *Schistosoma*, which inhabit either intestinal or vesical venous circulations in their definitive hosts. Among the five species of *Schistosoma* that infect humans, *Schistosoma mansoni*, *S. japonicum*, *S. intercalatum* and *S. mekongi* are found in the intestinal venous circulation, and *S. mansoni* and *S. japonicum* mainly affect the liver through the portal system, sometimes causing severe disease. *S. haematobium*, another important human parasite, inhabits the vesical venules and may damage the urinary bladder and the ureters.

The life cycle of *Schistosoma* species alternates between a sexual stage of adult schistosomes in the definitive vertebrate host and an asexual stage in a molluscan host. *S. mansoni* has snails of the genus *Biomphalaria* as intermediate hosts; *Oncomelania* and *Bulinus* are the molluscan intermediate hosts of *S. japonicum* and *S. haematobium*, respectively, and *S. intercalatum* and *S. mekongi* have the asexual stages in snails of the genus *Bulinus* and *Neotricula* respectively.

The life cycle of schistosomes begins with the shedding of eggs in the urine (*S. haematobium*) or stool (other *Schistosoma* species) of the vertebrate hosts. After reaching fresh water collections, the miracidium, a free-swimming stage, hatches from the egg and infects the snail intermediate host, giving rise to sporocysts that, at the end of 35–45 days, produce numerous free-swimming cercariae, the infective stage in vertebrate hosts. Both miracidium and cercariae are short-lived stages, keeping their infective properties for only 10–12 h.

Cercariae may actively enter human skin and give rise to schistosomulae, which mature to adult *Schistosoma*, reaching their normal habitat according to each species: the venous urinary system for *S. haematobium* and the mesenteric and portal venous systems for the other *Schistosoma* species. Approximately 45–60 days after infection, eggs are eliminated in either the urine or the stool of the infected vertebrate host.

Excluding *S. haematobium*, which infects humans almost exclusively, other *Schistosoma* species infecting man are zoonoses. *S. haematobium* has rarely been found to infect other vertebrates (primates or rodents), but this kind of infection is considered to be coincidental, without importance in the natural transmission to humans. *S. japonicum*, besides man, can infect several species of wild and domestic mammals; *S. mekongi* has only dogs as reservoir hosts. *S. mansoni* infects mainly humans, but it was frequently found to be a natural infection in several species of small rodents in Brazilian endemic areas.

Schistosomiasis mansoni

This section will discuss liver disease caused by *S. mansoni*, which is the most widely distributed schistosome in man and is found in both the Old and New Worlds. Mansonian schistosomiasis is endemic in the northeast of Brazil, where it affects around 2.5 million people [1]. The prevalence of *S. mansoni* is nowadays very low (below 1%) in some areas such as the Caribbean Islands, Venezuela and Suriname. This might be due, at least in part, to the predatory action of some snails (e.g. *Thiara granifera*) on the intermediate host *Biomphalaria glabrata* [2]. This hypothesis may be valid in restricted areas, but not where the *Biomphalaria* snails are distributed in vast territories. In Brazil, a big programme to control *S. mansoni* based on treatment with oxamniquine and snail control resulted in a sharp decrease in the hepatosplenic and other advanced forms of schistosomiasis [1].

Schistosomiasis is considered to be a 'man-made disease' because man is the victim and the source of infection at the same time. People's habits regarding defaecation in canal water and exposure to the polluted water by bathing, swimming for recreation and washing purposes characterize the endemic areas. Exposure starts as early as 6 months of age, and infection and its severity occur in early childhood (10–14 years) followed by progressive decrease with increasing age. The lower prevalence in adults may be explained by less exposure to contaminated water and the development of concomitant acquired immunity [1].

Environmental changes that result from the development of water resources and the growth and migration of populations can facilitate the spread of schistosomiasis. For example, the construction of the Diama Dam led to the introduction of *S. mansoni* into Mauritania and Senegal [3].

Clinical forms and pathogenesis

Liver disease in schistosomiasis results from the entrapment of eggs that are not excreted but instead lodge in portal venules that match the smallest diameter of the eggs, about 50 μm. Eggs in the liver remain viable for about 3 weeks and secrete products that initially elicit a characteristic response, the schistosome egg granuloma. In some persons with heavy infections, the final result of hepatic schistosomiasis is a severe portal fibrosis (Fig. 1). Advanced schistosomal hepatic fibrosis gives a gross appearance of greatly enlarged fibrotic portal tracts, described by Symmers in 1904 as resembling clay pipestems thrust through the liver, and now termed Symmers' pipestem fibrosis.

Schistosome infection can be divided into distinct stages. The prepatent stage begins with cercarial invasion and ends with

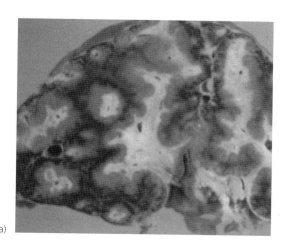
(a)

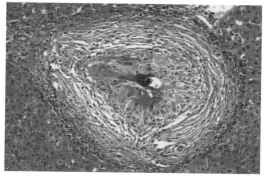
(b)

Fig. 1 Symmers' periportal fibrosis of the liver (a) with *Schistosoma mansoni* showing an egg at the centre of a granuloma (b).

initiation of egg laying. The patent (acute) stage coincides with schistosome egg production and can be further divided into acute and chronic schistosomiasis [1].

Acute form (Katayama fever)

Acute schistosomiasis results from a new fresh infection. Clinical manifestations may be absent, particularly in individuals living in an endemic area. Occasionally, some individuals may develop the syndrome after exposure to water contaminated by *S. mansoni* cercariae. The most common manifestations are fever, chills, weakness, headache, anorexia, nausea, vomiting and general malaise. Severe watery diarrhoea, sometimes bloody stools, non-productive cough and rapid weight loss may develop [1].

Occasionally, patients with acute schistosomiasis mansoni are misdiagnosed as having typhoid fever, hepatitis, pancreatitis, miliary tuberculosis, myelitis and appendicitis. Hepatomegaly is virtually constant and frequently accompanied by slight right upper quadrant tenderness. Transitory generalized lymphadenopathy and splenomegaly appear frequently, but there is no jaundice. Laboratory examinations show leucocytosis with eosinophilia, which can reach 70%, and slight changes in serum aminotransferase [1].

Ultrasonography studies are scarce in patients with acute schistosomiasis, and the ultrasound and computerized tomography (CT) features of this form are unknown.

Acute schistosomiasis usually progresses to an asymptomatic infection and eventually to the chronic forms. In patients with acute schistosomiasis admitted to hospital with severe symptoms, treatment should be started with corticosteroids, followed by schistosomicides. However, this situation is quite uncommon.

Chronic forms

The life cycle of the parasite in the host explains why *S. mansoni* can produce damage in organs other than the intestines and the liver [4]. However, these localizations are by far the most frequent.

Intestinal and hepatointestinal forms

Intestinal manifestations may be diarrhoea and colicky pain, but asymptomatic forms are more frequent.

Rearrangement of the egg granuloma is observed during the transition of the acute form to the chronic form; this results in a less pathogenic effect on the liver cells. According to some authors, in patients who fail to remodel the granuloma, the disease tends to evolve to the hepatosplenic form [5].

As the intestinal form is frequently asymptomatic, the diagnosis is based on the finding of *S. mansoni* eggs in the stools of the patients.

Schistosomotic intestinal poliposis is uncommon in Brazil, but is frequently observed in Egypt [1].

The subdivision into an intestinal form and a hepatointestinal form is not uniformly accepted, but enlargement of the liver, mainly of the left lobe, may be seen in schistosomotic individuals living in highly endemic areas, and this characterizes the hepatointestinal form. Recently, portal and splenic overflow was reported in both hepatointestinal and hepatosplenic forms of schistosomiasis by our group [1].

Hepatosplenic form and portal hypertension

Pathophysiology. Formation of the egg granuloma appears to be the main process responsible for the tissue damage in organs such as liver, intestines, lung and pancreas; however, immuno-complexes derived from parasite antigens are responsible for additional lesions such as glomerulopathy [4].

Hepatic granulomas initially form endovascularly in presinu-soidal areas, usually at inlet venules or terminal portal venules. Following an initial endothelial proliferation, the blood vessels rapidly become occluded with eventual obliteration of the lumen and displacement of hepatocytes by the developing granuloma. Symmers' fibrosis of the liver, which may result in portal hyper-tension and congestive splenomegaly, predominates in the 6- to 20-year age group and occurs 5–15 years after the onset of infection. It is the most severe form and the most common cause of morbidity or death. However, in heavily infected young patients, there is a 'non-congestive' phase of the disease with splenomegaly but without signs of portal hypertension. Data from Brazil show that, in such cases, the spleen may become non-palpable after adequate chemotherapy. In young patients, a strong correlation has been shown repeatedly between the hep-atosplenic form and the worm load. Furthermore, experimental studies suggest that massive infections during the initial expo-sure to cercariae may be important. The individual failure in the immunological modulation of the inflammatory reactions seems to play a role. These and other factors would explain the presence of hepatosplenic schistosomiasis (HSS) in only a small percentage of patients with heavy worm burden [4].

Hepatic periportal fibrosis is caused by the T cell-rich granu-loma that develops around schistosome eggs. Experimental models of infection have shown that granuloma and fibrosis are regulated by cytokines. However, it is unknown why advanced periportal fibrosis occurs only in certain subjects.

In some patients with heavy infection, chemotherapy may produce a peculiar type of pulmonary lesions, 'the dead worm' pneumonitis; this event has been attributed to a hyperergic pulmonary reaction to the products of dead worms.

Family-based studies have found a highly significant concen-tration of hepatosplenic forms among children from the same nuclear family, particularly when the mother was affected by the same form of the disease. Furthermore, hepatosplenic schistosomiasis occurs with higher frequency in whites than in blacks, despite the fact that Brazilian whites have better social and economic conditions. This evidence would point to an as yet undetermined genetic component.

It is generally accepted that *S. mansoni* infection alone does not lead to cirrhosis. Hepatitis B and C virus infections are im-portant pathogenic factors in causing progression of hepatic schistosomiasis to cirrhosis and decompensation.

Haemodynamic aspects. Intrahepatic angiographic changes sug-gestive of hepatosplenic schistosomiasis are the enlargement of the hepatic veins and a marked reduction in branching, along with a more pronounced arching of large branches [4]. In 50 patients studied by Mies *et al.* [6], the gradient between hepatic vein wedged and free pressures was at the upper limit of normal (9.1 ± 5.7 mmHg). In about 40% of cases, however, it was raised: the gradient ranged from 10.4 to 22.7 mmHg.

Contrast material injected into the portal system shows an intrahepatic pattern characterized by gross amputations of large branches, and by the appearance of a dense network of small-calibre vessels around portal branches. These aspects were described by Bogliolo in 1957 and are known as 'Bogliolo's sign'. Enlargement of splenic and portal veins is usually present. Portal pressure is raised to levels similar to those seen in liver cirrhosis.

Angiographic studies have shown a reduced diameter of the hepatic artery, with thin, arched branches outlining vascular gaps. The tortuous aspect characteristic of liver cirrhosis is not observed. These aspects suggest that the poor intrahepatic arterial vascularization demonstrated by selective arteriography in human hepatosplenic schistosomiasis is due to a 'functional deviation' of arterial blood to the splenic territory [4]. In advanced schistosomiasis, the hepatic artery may be hyper-trophic [1].

Total liver blood flow, measured by different methods, is normal; this suggests that the increased portal blood flow is accompanied by a reduction in the arterial blood flow, pointing to an interaction between portal and arterial blood flow.

Dynamic studies have demonstrated that a high splenic blood flow may be responsible for the increased portal blood flow. It seems that the splenic component and the abundant network around portal branches ('Bogliolo's sign') may be pre-ponderant (hyperflow component) over the obstruction of the intrahepatic portal branches produced by parasitosis (presinu-soidal block), at least in cases of severe splenomegaly. However, ultrasound studies show that an extensive periportal thickening of the liver may be found in some patients without a palpable spleen, probably as a consequence of spontaneous shunts. Furthermore, schistosomic portal hypertension is not restricted to patients with splenic hyperdynamic circulation. Mies *et al.* [7] showed that, despite small changes in sinusoidal pressure and liver function, schistosomotic patients present with high cardiac index and low systemic vascular resistance compatible with a systemic hyperdynamic circulatory status similar to cirrhosis.

Clinical and laboratory changes. Schistosomiasis mansoni exhibits a wide range of clinical manifestations, varying from asymptomatic to several symptomatic forms. Occasionally, the disease is discovered accidentally, either by a routine stool exam-ination or by enlargement of the liver or spleen on physical examination [4].

Hepatosplenic schistosomiasis can be divided clinically into compensated and decompensated forms. The latter is characterized by muscular wasting, low serum albumin and, occasionally, chronic ascites. However, other causes, such as alcoholism and hepatitis B and C virus infection, are frequently responsible for the decompensation of liver funetion.

The main symptoms of the hepatosplenic form are related to splenomegaly and haemorrhage. Spontaneous ascites is uncommon; it usually appears after episodes of bleeding or infection or when schistosomiasis is associated with other causes of liver damage.

Spontaneous neuropsychiatric symptoms are very rare in hepatosplenic schistosomiasis, even with abundant collateral circulation. These symptoms are seen only after precipitating factors, mainly haemorrhage or infection. Anaemia with delayed somatic and sexual development may be observed in young people. Spider naevi, gynaecomastia and palmar erythema are rare in uncomplicated schistosomiasis. Leucopenia and thrombocytopenia are found in most cases of hepatosplenic schistosomiasis [4].

In hepatosplenic schistosomiasis, clotting defects result from an impaired rate of protein synthesis by the liver or localized consumption coagulopathy, or both. The relative role of these two factors is not well established. Changes in the plasma coagulation systems may be partially corrected by subcutaneous heparinization but the most effective correction is by splenectomy [8].

Diagnosis

Direct methods of diagnosis are based on the demonstration of eggs or of miracidia. Eggs may be found in the stools by the Kato–Katz quantitative method. The hatching test provides a simple, cheap and useful method, without the need for microscopy and is especially useful for the diagnosis of *S. haematobium*, whose eggs are eliminated into the urine. Rectal biopsy is used in suspected cases with negative parasitological tests.

Immunological methods, indirect immunofluorescence, indirect haemagglutination and enzyme-linked immunosorbent assay (ELISA) give a high degree of positivity.

Antibody titres are usually higher in the hepatosplenic form than in the hepatointestinal form. Titres increase early and significantly after chemotherapy as a consequence of the death of the worms.

A major diagnostic problem is the demonstration of periportal fibrosis at histology, even with wedged liver biopsies. Ultrasonography has however become a reliable and sensitive method of demonstrating this type of lesion [9]. Ultrasonography can provide reliable information on the state of internal organs in schistosomiasis as well as on regression of pathological changes after treatment.

Periportal fibrosis, seen in ultrasonography as echodense areas along the portal vein (Fig. 2), is an important diagnostic feature, and also an indicator of the possible existence of portal hypertension. Until fibrosis becomes advanced and generalized, thickened patches are typically scattered throughout the liver;

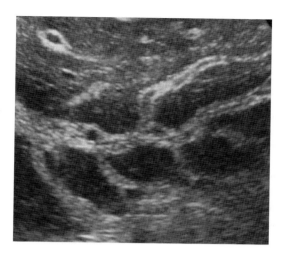

Fig. 2 Ultrasonographic features of periportal fibrosis in schistosomiasis mansoni.

the portal vein and the structures around it can best be visualized in the left liver lobule [9].

Variceal bleeding in patients with hepatosplenic schistosomiasis correlates with endoscopic (variceal size, red signs, congestive gastropathy and fundic varices) and ultrasonographic (portal vein diameter and periportal thickness) parameters [10].

By Doppler ultrasonography, hepatic left lobe hypertrophy and right lobe atrophy are commonly observed in hepatosplenic schistosomiasis [9,11]. In summary, our group showed that portal overflow may be found in both forms of schistosomiasis.

Course and prognosis

The prognosis for hepatic schistosomiasis is good in the acute and hepatointestinal forms. The prognosis for the hepatosplenic forms depends on whether the liver disease is compensated or decompensated. Fortunately, most cases remain compensated: the prognosis is better than for patients with cirrhosis. Recovery after haematemesis is rapid and the patients live longer [5]. Hepatic coma and ascites after haemorrhage are less frequent and easier to control [4].

Treatment

Treatment of helminthiasis

The treatment of helminthiasis is indicated in all stages and clinical forms of mansonian schistosomiasis, but some patients with a very advanced form or with concomitant non-hepatic disorders may not tolerate chemotherapy.

There are two highly effective chemotherapeutic drugs: oxamniquine, used at different doses in Latin America and Africa, and praziquantel; both are given by the oral route.

Praziquantel can also be safely given to patients with compensated hepatosplenic forms of the disease.

Treatment of portal hypertension

Non-surgical treatment of bleeding oesophageal varices

The management of patients with oesophageal and gastric varices remains a challenge, particularly when prophylactic procedures are considered.

Endoscopic changes indicative of a high risk of bleeding include the finding of large varices, cherry-red spots, varices on varices, erosions on varices [10] and hypertensive gastropathy. These and ultrasonographic changes should be used in the identification of patients for prophylactic procedures, including drug therapy, sclerotherapy and surgery.

The utility of β-blockers such as propranolol, which are efficacious in liver cirrhosis, is not well established in chronic schistosomiasis.

Propranolol seems to protect patients with schistosomiasis against gastrointestinal rebleeding during the short periods of time that precede definitive surgical treatment. A single oral 'blockade dose' may induce a significant decrease in the azygous blood flow [12].

In a retrospective study of sclerotherapy of bleeding oesophageal varices in schistosomiasis, the eradication of varices was obtained in nearly 70% of patients during a follow-up period lasting between 48 and 132 months. Sclerotherapy was effective in the control of rebleeding in 97% of the patients previously submitted to portal hypertension surgery and in 73% of the patients without previous portal hypertension surgery, with a smaller number of sessions of sclerotherapy per patient in the former group [13]. A prospective non-randomized trial comparing elective sclerotherapy with a control group during a 5-year follow-up showed that the incidence of rebleeding was 28% and 45%, respectively, a difference that was not significant; however, the mortality from rupture of oesophageal varices was 3% in the sclerotherapy group and 28% in the control group, which was a significant difference [14].

Surgical treatment of portal hypertension

Until 1986, three major types of operations were used in Brazil: oesophagogastric devascularization plus splenectomy (EGDS), splenectomy with splenorenal shunt, selective portal decompression (SPD) or distal splenorenal shunt (DSS).

In a prospective randomized trial [15] comparing the results of the three surgical techniques, the proximal splenorenal shunt (SRS) induced portosystemic encephalopathy with a high frequency (39%). Later on, a long-term follow-up study (85.7 ± 33.1 months) in the same patients showed that gastrointestinal bleeding occurred in 24.1% of the patients, with no significant differences among the three groups, but rebleeding because of varices was more frequent after oesophagogastric devascularization with splenectomy (EGDS). Hepatic encephalopathy was significantly higher after proximal SRS (39.3%) compared with distal splenorenal shunting (DSS, 14.8%) and EGDS (0%). Mortality was also significantly higher after SRS (42.9%) compared with DSS (14.8%) and EGDS

(7.1%). EGDS therefore appeared to be the best surgical option.

In our department, patients with schistosomiasis and bleeding oesophageal varices are treated with oesophagogastric devascularization with splenectomy and, if rebleeding occurs, by sclerosis of the varices [4].

Liver flukes

Definition

Liver flukes are trematode worms found in the bile ducts, where they may determine hepatic disease. Some species such as *Fasciola hepatica*, *F. gigantica*, *Opisthorchis felineus*, *O. viverrini* and *Clonorchis sinensis* can infect humans. Rarely, *Dicrocoelium dendriticum* and *Eurytreme pancreaticum* produce human infections.

Fasciola hepatica and Fasciola gigantica

The genus *Fasciola* comprises digenetic trematode parasites of herbivorous mammals such as livestock. Two species, *F. hepatica* and *F. gigantica*, are known, and the former is much more important as a human parasite because of its higher prevalence rate. *F. hepatica* infects sheep or cattle in Central and South America, some European countries, Australia, China and the Middle East. *F. gigantica* is endemic in Southeast Asia, some African countries and in the western Pacific [16].

The human infection by *F. hepatica* or *F. gigantica* depends on the ingestion of raw vegetables, especially common watercress (*Nasturtium officinale*), in the leaves of which the cercariae, having been eliminated by limnaeid snails of the genus *Lymnaea* or *Galba*, encyst as metacercariae. Less frequently, human infection may result from ingestion of contaminated water by floating metacercariae. In human bile ducts, adults of *Fasciola* can survive at least 10 years. Once in the duodenum, larvae emerge and burrow through the bowel wall into the peritoneal cavity. The larvae penetrate Glisson's capsule and migrate through the hepatic parenchyma to the bile ducts. The larvae mature into adult flukes within the larger intrahepatic bile ducts over 2–3 months and start producing eggs. The eggs are shed in the bile and enter the host intestinal tract through the ampulla of Vater. To complete the life cycle, the eggs must be shed into fresh water, hatch into miracidia and enter fresh water snails, where they develop into cercariae [16].

The pathogenesis of liver disease from fascioliasis results from the larval migration through the hepatic parenchyma and the chronic inflammatory changes induced within the biliary tract. As the larvae travel through the hepatic parenchyma, there is a marked local inflammatory reaction with eosinophilia, hepatocyte necrosis, haemorrhage and abscess formation, followed by fibrosis. The severity of the hepatic inflammation and damage is proportional to the parasite load; in Bolivia, approximately 17% of cases present with massive infestation. In the chronic biliary phase of infestation, the adult fluke incites hyperplasia and desquamation of the biliary epithelial layer, resulting in thickened, dilated and fibrotic bile ducts. The adult fasciola and its ova, in addition to causing chronic intermittent obstruction, are a nidus for recurrent cholelithiasis. Secondary biliary cirrhosis and sclerosing cholangitis have been reported. The adult fluke is thought to feed on host hepatocytes and biliary epithelial cells while residing in the large intrahepatic and extrahepatic bile ducts [16,17].

The clinical manifestations of fascioliasis are reflective of the parasite life cycle. In 50% of cases, the initial presentation is subclinical. The acute hepatic phase begins within 12 weeks of exposure and is characterized by low-grade fever, tender hepatomegaly, anorexia, nausea and pruritus. A mild to moderate peripheral eosinophilia is common, but can become marked during larval migration through the liver. Elevated levels of alkaline phosphatase and γ-glutamyl transpeptidase are typical, with high aminotransferase levels seen only with significant hepatocellular necrosis. Jaundice, urticaria, weight loss, ascites formation and haemobilia have been reported in children with massive infestations [16,17].

During the chronic biliary phase, patients may be asymptomatic or complain of non-specific symptoms such as dyspepsia, dull right upper quadrant discomfort or diarrhoea. If the biliary tract becomes obstructed (with either flukes or gallstones), patients may present with typical biliary colic, ascending cholangitis, acute pancreatitis or cholecystitis (adult flukes occasionally migrate into the gallbladder). As mentioned previously, chronic inflammation and obstructation have been reported to lead to marked biliary dilatation, sclerosing cholangitis and biliary cirrhosis. In the chronic phase of infestation, peripheral eosinophilia may be mild or absent [16].

Detection of eggs in the faeces, bile or duodenal aspirate is the definitive test. However, multiple stool specimens and concentration techniques are often necessary in light infestations because egg production and shedding may be low. In a patient with the proper clinical presentation and travel history, a negative stool examination does not rule out fascioliasis. ELISA-based tests aid in diagnosis because of their extremely high sensitivity (> 95%) and specificity (97–100%). Serological tests are also useful in the acute phase of disease prior to the larvae maturing into adult liver flukes. Antibody titres should decline after successful therapy and can therefore be used to monitor treatment response [16,17].

Imaging techniques are also helpful in establishing the diagnosis, particularly in the chronic biliary phase. Hepatic ultrasound may demonstrate adult flukes in the bile ducts or gallbladder as well as hyperechoic lesions corresponding to the migrating larvae. CT scanning may also reveal characteristic 1- to 10-mm hypodense linear lesions in a 'radiating' pattern that corresponds to the larval burrows in the hepatic parenchyma. In addition, CT may show small peripheral hypodense nodules, calcifications and a thickened liver capsule. Endoscopic retrograde cholangiopancreatography (ERCP) plays an important role in diagnosis and therapy when biliary obstruction from adult flukes or choledocholithiasis is suspected [16,17].

The current therapy of choice is triclabendazole, 10–12 mg/kg/day. However, this drug is not widely available. The alternative therapy is biothionol, 30–50 mg/kg/day for 10–15 days. Intramuscular dehydroemetine, 1 mg/kg/day for 14 days, is another alternative. Praziquantel is also used for liver flukes but, because *F. hepatica* does not respond to this agent, it is not recommended. In biliary obstruction, ERCP with endoscopic sphincterotomy and antihelminthic therapy are recommended. In light infestation, a dormia basket or biliary balloon can be used to clear the bile ducts of adult flukes. In patients with heavy burden and resistance to oral therapy, intraductal endoscopic treatment with a fasciolicidal agent has been successful; a 10% povidine iodine solution (mixed with contrast) is instilled into the biliary system and left in place by occluding the distal common bile duct with a biliary balloon (for 10 min), after which the ducts can be swept free of the dead liver flukes [16–19].

Clonorchis sinensis, Opisthorchis felineus and Opisthorchis viverrini

Clonorchis sinensis is a trematode endemic in many oriental countries such as Taiwan, continental China, Japan, South and North Korea and Vietnam. Anecdotal human infections have been noticed in western countries as a consequence of imported contaminated food from endemic areas. *C. sinensis* shows a zoonotic behaviour, infecting several mammal species besides man. Dogs, cats, pigs, rats, badgers, mink and camels can harbour natural infections. In humans, the adult worms can survive for a long time (approximately 20 years). Humans and other mammal species may be infected by *C. sinensis* by ingestion of either raw or undercooked freshwater fish of the family Cyprinidae, in which metacercariae can be encysted. The fish usually become infected by ingesting snails of the genus *Parafossarulus*; less frequently, fish infection is caused by ingestion of snails of the genus *Thiara* or *Melanoides* [16,20].

Opisthorchis viverrini is the most common liver fluke infestation in Southeast Asia. The World Health Organization estimates that 16 million people worldwide are infested with *O. felineus* and another 10 million with *O. viverrini*. These three liver flukes are found in close association with fish-eating mammals and the human consumption of raw or pickled fish. As in fascioliasis, these liver flukes can survive for decades in the host biliary system [16,20].

The pathogenesis of hepatic disease in *Clonorchis* and *Opisthorchis* human infections depends on alterations in the biliary tract induced by their infestation, which may either be acute or, most commonly, chronic. The severity of the disease is, in the majority of cases, a consequence of the worm burden. The acute phases of *Clonorchis* and *Opisthorchis* infections are usually asymptomatic but, in 10% of the patients, fever, malaise and abdominal pain may be present. Patients with chronic heavy infections by *C. sinensis* usually complain of weakness, weight loss, abdominal pain and diarrhoea. The development of intra-hepatic gallstones is common and, sometimes, cholangitis and cholecystitis occur. The rate of cholangiocarcinoma is higher in these patients. Mild infections by O. viverrini are usually asymptomatic. When the worm burden is higher, there is loss of appetite, abdominal pain, flatulence, moderate fever and, more rarely, jaundice. Eventually, hepatic cirrhosis and cholangiocarcinoma may develop. In patients infected by O. felineus symptoms were the same as those with O. viverrini; however, rates of cholangiocarcinoma were not higher [21–23].

Detection of eggs in the faeces, bile or duodenal aspirate is the definitive test. However, multiple stool specimens and concentration techniques are often necessary in light infestations because egg production may be low. Serological tests are available for Clonorchis (immunoblot antigen assay and ELISA) and O. viverrini (ELISA) but are not routinely used except as an adjunct to stool studies or cholangiography [16,20].

Transabdominal ultrasonography detects abnormalities in approximately 50% of patients with liver fluke infestation. The findings may be consistent with chronic cholecystitis, biliary sludge, hepatomegaly or hydropic gallbladder. Liver flukes appear as non-shadowing echogenic material within the bile ducts. CT scanning may also reveal dilated or thickened intrahepatic bile ducts that are not appreciated on liver ultrasonography. Cholangiography may reveal duct wall irregularities, multiple cystic dilations of the intrahepatic ducts with tapering at the periphery and an overall decrease in intrahepatic radicles. If visible, Clonorchis appears as a wavy, elliptiform filling defect [16,20].

The treatment of choice is praziquantel, 75 mg/kg divided into three doses a day. Single dose therapy (praziquantel, 40 mg/kg) is not advocated in Clonorchis species because of low cure rates. The recommended alternative treatment is albendazole, 10 mg/kg/day for 7 days. As an adjunct to medical therapy, endoscopic management of acute and chronic complications may be necessary. Biliary decompression is often needed in patients with ascending cholangitis on an emergency basis. Chronic complications include recurrent intrahepatic pigment stones, biliary strictures and cholangiocarcinoma, which can be managed endoscopically or surgically depending upon regional availability and local expertise [16,24].

Dicrocoelium and Eurytrema

Dicrocoeliasis and eurytremiasis are infections of the bile and pancreatic ducts of herbivorous mammals caused, respectively, by the trematodes Dicrocoelium dendriticum and Eurytrema pancreaticum. Human infections have been reported, but are rare. Sometimes, the finding of eggs in human stool represents a spurious infection, due to ingestion of infected animal livers. The two trematodes have similar life cycles, and both require two intermediate hosts: the first is a snail (genus Zebrina, Helicella, Cionella or Bradybaena for D. dendriticum and Ganesella for E. pancreaticum). The second intermediate hosts

for D. dendriticum are ants of the genus Formica; the grasshoppers (genus Conocephalus) or tree crickets (genus Oecanthus) are the second intermediate hosts for E. pancreaticum. Infection of the definitive hosts by these trematodes depends on the ingestion of metacercariae encysted on the insect second intermediate host tissues. The adults of both species produce and shed morphologically similar eggs, making specific diagnosis by faecal examination difficult. The definitive diagnosis depends on the recovery of adult worms at surgery or necropsy. Dicrocoeliasis and eurytremiasis usually cause mild symptoms in humans. However, heavy infections may produce biliary, pancreatic and gastrointestinal disturbances and, sometimes, jaundice. Occasionally, enlarged liver and systemic symptoms are found. Human infections by these trematodes should be treated with praziquantel; as second choice, the drug triclabendazole may be used [25,26].

References

1 Da Silva LC, Chieffi PP, Carrilho FJ (2005) Schistosomiasis mansoni – clinical features. *Gastroenterol Hepatol* 28, 30–39.

2 Giboda M, Malek EA, Correa R (1997) Human schistosomiasis in Puerto Rico: reduce prevalence rate and absence of *Biomphalaria glabrata*. *Am J Trop Med Hyg* 57, 564–568.

3 Ross AGP, Bartley PB, Sleigh AC et al. (2002) Schistosomiasis. *N Engl J Med* 346, 1212–1220.

4 Da Silva LC, Carrilho FJ (1992) Hepatosplenic schistosomiasis. Pathophysiology and treatment. *Gastroenterol Clin North Am* 21, 163–177.

5 Rezende SA, Lambertucci JR, Goes AM (1997) Role of immune complexes from patients with different clinical forms of schistosomiasis in the modulation of *in vitro* granuloma reaction. *Mem Inst Oswaldo Cruz* 92, 683–687.

6 Mies S, Mori T, Larsson E et al. (1980) A veia cava inferior e as veias supra-hepáticas na esquistossomose hepatoesplênica. Estudo angiográfico. *Rev Hosp Clin Fac Med São Paulo* 35, 136–142.

7 Mies S, Neto OB, Beer A Jr et al. (1997) Systemic and hepatic hemodynamics in hepatosplenic Manson's schistosomiasis with and without propranolol. *Dig Dis Sci* 42, 751–761.

8 Manoukian N, Borges DR (1984) Prealbumin, prekallikrein and prothrombin in hepatosplenic schistosomiasis: increased turnover of the clotting proteins? *Rev Inst Med Trop Sao Paulo* 26, 237–240.

9 Cerri GG, Alves VA, Magalhaes A (1984) Hepatosplenic schistosomiasis mansoni: ultrasound manifestations. *Radiology* 153, 777–780.

10 Martins RD, Szejnfeld J, Lima FG et al. (2000) Endoscopic, ultrasonographic, and US-Doppler parameters as indicators of variceal bleeding in patients with schistosomiasis. *Dig Dis Sci* 45, 1013–1018.

11 Paranagua-Vezozzo DC, Cerri GG (1992) Duplex hemodynamic evaluation of hepatosplenic mansoni schistosomiasis. *Mem Inst Oswaldo Cruz* 87(Suppl. 4), 149–151.

12 Neto OB, Beer A Jr, Baia CE et al. (1997) Systemic and hepatic hemodynamics in hepatosplenic manson's schistosomiasis with and without propranolol. *Dig Dis Sci* 42, 751–761.

13 Sakai P, Boaventura S, Ishioka S et al. (1990) Sclerotherapy of bleeding esophageal varices in schistosomiasis. Comparative study in patients with and without previous surgery for portal hypertension. *Endoscopy* 22, 5–7.

14 Cordeiro F (1990) Variceal sclerosis in schistosomotic patients: a five-year follow-up study. *Gastrointest Endosc* 36, 475–478.

15 Da Silva LC, Strauss E, Gayotto LCC *et al.* (1986) A randomized trial for the study of the elective surgical treatment of portal hypertension in mansonic schistosomiasis. *Ann Surg* 204, 148–153.

16 Pockros PJ, Capozza TA (2005) Helminthic infections of the liver. *Curr Infect Dis Rep* 7, 61–70.

17 Roig CV (2002) Hepatic fascioliasis in the Americas: a new challenge for therapeutic endoscopy. *Gastrointest Endosc* 56, 315–317.

18 Dowidar N, el Sayad M, Osman M *et al.* (1999) Endoscopic therapy of fascioliasis resistant to oral therapy. *Gastrointest Endosc* 50, 345–351.

19 Saba R, Korkmaz M, Inan D *et al.* (2004) Human fascioliasis. *Clin Microbiol Infect* 10, 385–387.

20 Bunnag D, Cross JH, Bunnag T (2000) Liver fluke infections. In: Strickland GT (ed.) *Hunter's Tropical Medicine and Emerging Infectious Disease*, 8th edn. Philadelphia: W.B. Saunders Co., pp. 840–847.

21 Acha PN, Szyfres B (2003) *Zoonosis y Enfermedades Transmisibles communes al Hombre ya a los Animales*, Vol. III, *Parasitosis*, 2nd edn. Publicación Científica y Técnica no. 580. Washington: Organización Mundial de la Salud.

22 Choi BI, Han JK, Hong ST *et al.* (2004) Clonorchiasis and cholangiocarcinoma: etiologic relationship and imaging diagnosis. *Clin Microbiol Rev* 17, 540–552.

23 Wang KX, Zhang RB, Cui YB *et al.* (2004) Clinical and epidemiological features of patients with clonorchiasis. *World J Gastroenterol* 10, 446–448.

24 Keiser J, Utzinger J (2004) Chemotherapy for major food-borne trematodes: a review. *Expert Opin Pharmacother* 5, 1711–1726.

25 Ishii Y, Koga M, Fujino T *et al.* (1983) Human infection with the pancreas fluke *Eurytrema pancreaticum*. *Am J Trop Med Hyg* 32, 1019–1022.

26 El-Shiekh-Mohamed AR, Mummery Y (1990) Human dicrocoeliasis. Report of 208 cases from Saudi Arabia. *Trop Geogr Med* 42, 1–7.

10.4.2 Echinococcosis of the liver

S. Bresson-Hadni, G.A. Mantion, J.P. Miguet and D.A. Vuitton

Cystic echinococcosis (CE, or hydatid disease) and alveolar echinococcosis (AE) are different in presentation, natural history and complications, and will be described separately; their immunodiagnosis and chemotherapy, which share many points, will be presented together [1].

Cystic echinococcosis

Epidemiology

Life cycle
The adult cestode develops in the small intestine of the definitive host, a carnivore. The last segments (proglottids) of this worm (3–5 mm long) contain eggs that are released into the intestine, and dispersed on the grass with the stools of the host. When eggs are eaten by the intermediate host (usually a mammal), the hexacanth embryo, released into the duodenum, passes through the intestinal wall and usually settles in the liver as 'cysts' ('hydatids'). Sheep, cattle, camels, swine or (accidentally) humans serve as intermediate hosts. Commonly, dogs are infected by eating raw infected offal containing hydatid larvae. Man becomes infected either by touching dogs with contaminated hair or by ingesting vegetables or water infected by dog stools [2]. Less commonly, the cycle involves a wild carnivore such as the wolf, jackal or coyote and a wild herbivore such as the elk, caribou or reindeer [3].

Prevalence
The disease is prominent in rural areas where humans, dogs and cattle coexist closely, with poor housing conditions and low levels of sanitation, and is most common in the regions of the world where raising livestock is a major industry: the entire Mediterranean littoral, the former USSR, China and parts of South America, particularly Uruguay, Argentina and Chile; New Zealand and Australia, highly endemic in the past, are now far less infected [2,4]. The highest prevalence is observed in western China (up to 5–10% of screened people) [4]. The disease remains frequent in Turkey and the Middle East countries, and is re-emerging in several countries where it had been partially controlled, especially in the endemic ex-USSR territories, e.g. Bulgaria and Romania, in Europe and the central Asian republics [5]. The diagnosis should thus be evoked for any suspect occupying lesion of the liver seen in immigrants from these countries.

Prevention and control
Control of *Echinococcus granulosus* is a realistic objective [2,4,5]; it has been achieved in islands where importation of animals was more easily controlled, such as Iceland, New Zealand and Tasmania. Eradication is much more difficult in continental areas, where reinfection of animals may occur easily from the surrounding regions. Cultural, economic and political factors may interfere with any control campaign, and these are the major pitfalls that preclude the theoretical 'easy control' of the disease [4–6].

Preventive measures include treatment of dogs with praziquantel and/or destruction of stray dogs, education campaigns, active measures to prevent access by dogs to infected offal and development of safe livestock slaughtering facilities [6]. Effective control must involve all approaches, including vaccination of animal intermediate hosts (mostly sheep) using the very efficient EG95 vaccine [7].

Pathogenesis
After ingestion of the eggs, the embryos of *E. granulosus* develop into a metacestode delimited by an inner, fertile membrane, the germinal layer, and an outer hyaline membrane, the laminated layer [1,2,8]. 'Brood capsules' containing numerous protoscolices (the future head of the adult cestode) develop by budding

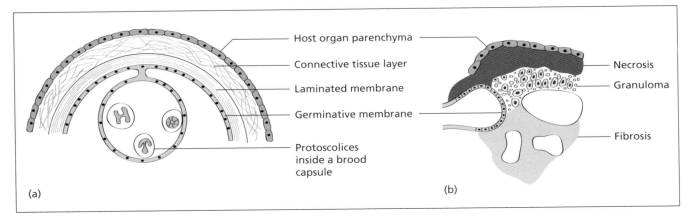

Fig. 1 (a and b) Diagrammatic structure of an *Echinococcus granulosus* cyst.

from the germinal layer. The laminated layer is surrounded by a fibrous wall, derived from host tissue, sometimes calcified, which limits the extension of the cyst. Outside this wall, the liver appears normal (Fig. 1a).

The cyst grows at a rate of about 0.3 cm/year. A significant proportion of cases either degenerate or never increase [9]. The cysts are filled with fluid under pressure and contain protoscolices (called 'hydatid sand' or 'granula', which gave the parasite the species name *granulosus*). Daughter cysts may develop inside or outside the germinal layer.

The cysts may be of any size, solitary or multiple, and located in any area of the liver. The right lobe is involved in 75% of cases; one-third of cysts are solitary [2]. Two-thirds of the lesions are located in the liver, a quarter in the lungs, 15% in muscle, 3% in bone, 2% in kidney, 1% each in spleen and brain [2]; multiple organs are involved in 20% of patients [2]. Bone, chest and brain localizations have been extensively studied; cysts may occur in the heart, biliary tract, thyroid and parotid gland, tongue, tooth, broad ligament, prostate, bladder, tonsil, pulmonary artery and inferior vena cava [1,8].

Clinical features and complications

The hydatid cyst remains clinically silent for a long time and is often discovered incidentally during routine abdominal ultrasound examination (US). The patient may complain of vague right upper quadrant pain, urticaria, episodes of itching or of a right upper quadrant tumoral mass. Clinical symptoms are usually absent until the cyst has reached 10 cm in diameter; a mass is rarely palpable until it reaches 20 cm. The diagnosis is usually made when a complication occurs, usually jaundice. In endemic areas, mass screening programmes using US and serology have shown that liver cysts, albeit far more numerous than lung cysts, were more frequently asymptomatic and remained so for a long period of time [9–13].

Physical examination of the liver may be normal or may disclose an enlarged and regular liver. If the cyst is located in the anterior liver, a round, painless tumour can be palpated with, exceptionally, a 'hydatid thrill' [1,8]. Compression of the common bile duct, portal or hepatic veins or inferior vena cava is uncommon. Rupture of the cyst (usually into the bile ducts) is more common: at diagnosis, 36–40% of cysts have ruptured or have become infected. Cysts can erode and perforate the diaphragm into the pleural and pericardial cavities, the lung or the bronchi, and the peritoneum into the peritoneal cavity or the duodenum, stomach, colon or right renal pelvis. This may lead to extrahepatic hydatic cysts, which favour the development of daughter cysts and may cause allergic symptoms (increase in blood eosinophils, itching urticaria and anaphylactic shock). More commonly, the rupture of hydatid cysts occurs into bile ducts and is revealed by cholestatic jaundice, cholangitis or biliary pain. Ruptures may be clinically silent, and are thus only disclosed during an operation.

Diagnosis

The two key procedures for diagnosis are US and serology.

Plain films of the abdomen and/or chest may show highly suggestive arc-shaped calcifications, characteristic deformation of the diaphragm and sometimes images in the lungs or mediastinum.

US can be used to recognize cysts as small as 1 cm in diameter. It can show one or several round masses with a well-defined contour, which may be empty or filled with echogenic structures corresponding to daughter cysts. It can be used to recognize the rupture of the germinative membrane by showing a folded, detached endocyst. When cysts become infected, they are diffusely hyperechogenic and no longer exhibit characteristic features. In 1981, a US classification was proposed by Gharbi *et al.* [10] based on a correlation between five US types and pathological findings. Several classifications have since been proposed with various aims and degrees of complexity. The WHO Informal Working Group on Echinococcosis (IWGE) has promoted a unified classification, shown in Table 1, which might be

Table 1 Ultrasonographic classification of hydatic cyst of the liver.

Gharbi *et al.* (1981) [10]	WHO classification [11]	Clinical correlation
–	CL	No pathognomonic signs of cystic echinococcosis
Type 1	CE1	Group 1: active lesions
		Evolutive cysts, usually fertile
Type 3	CE2	Group 2: transitional lesions
Type 2	CE3	Cysts becoming degenerated, but usual persistence of viable protoscolices with possible evolution to CE2 type
Type 4	CE4	Group 3: inactive lesions
Type 5	CE5	Degenerated cysts or partially/totally calcified. High probability of sterilization

CL, cystic lesion.

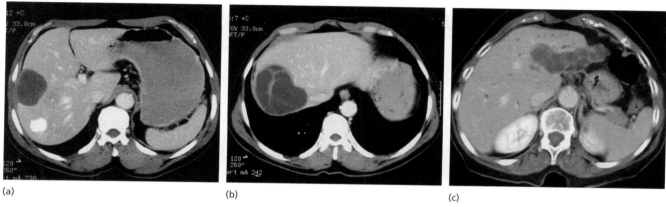

Fig. 2 CT images of cystic echinococcosis of the liver. (a) Two cysts located in the right lobe. The anterior one, corresponding to a type 1 (CE1), is characterized by a hypodense content and well-defined contour. The posterior one, totally calcified, corresponds to a type 5 (CE5). (b) Huge, well-delineated hydatid cyst in the top of the right liver classified as type 2 (CE3): detached membranes are well visualized inside the hydatid fluid. (c) Complicated cystic echinococcosis. The cyst in the left liver (containing multiple daughter cysts) has ruptured in the biliary duct and is responsible for a biliary obstruction (note the intrahepatic biliary duct dilatations).

used to compare data from mass screenings and therapeutic interventions as well [11]. This classification attempts to follow the natural history of the cyst; however, stage CE3 (Gharbi II), characterized by the detachment of membranes, may progress either to development of daughter cysts or to degeneration. When the classification is used to assess any therapeutic intervention, the diameter of cysts (in cm) rather than semi-quantitative values should be given [14].

On computerized tomography (CT) (Fig. 2a–c), the unilocular cyst with its spherical or oval structure of near water density is easily recognized [1,8]. Conversely, multilocular cysts may have several CT patterns depending on the space occupied by daughter cysts inside the mother cyst; however, the CT densities of viable daughter cysts are always lower than those of mother hydatid cysts. Abscesses or necrotic tumours may mimic hydatid cysts. In these cases, if serology is negative, only aspiration cytology can establish the diagnosis of hydatid cyst [15]. Hydatid cyst aspiration with a fine needle under US guidance is currently considered medically and ethically acceptable [15,16]. However, the procedure must be accompanied by appropriate precautions

aimed at preventing and/or treating any anaphylactic complication and protoscolex spillage, and must be systematically followed by the puncture, aspiration, injection and reaspiration (PAIR) technique if the diagnosis of hydatid cyst is confirmed.

Treatment

Surgery has long been considered the first choice treatment for all cases of hydatid cysts. Current availability of alternative therapies has made this statement obsolete. In 1996, treatment guidelines published by the WHO-IWGE stated that the therapeutic strategy should consider chemotherapy and PAIR [17]. Since then, the results of long-term evaluation of these treatments have been made available, and surgery should always be discussed regarding cyst location in the liver, number of cysts, presence of other cysts in other organs, anatomical/clinical complications, clinical status of the patient, but also surgical facilities, expertise of the surgical team and quality of follow-up. New guidelines are currently being discussed by the WHO-IWGE and should be published soon. A recent meta-analysis aimed at finding 'evidence-based' answers to the main questions about treatment strategy in cystic echinococcosis [18]. The main results, graded according the Cochrane system (level of evidence and grade of recommendation), were the following: (i) chemotherapy is not the ideal treatment for uncomplicated hydatid cysts of the liver when used alone; (ii) the level of evidence is too low to help in deciding between radical or conservative treatment; (iii) omentoplasty associated with radical or conservative treatment is efficient in preventing deep abscesses; (iv) the laparoscopic approach is safe; (v) drug treatment associated with surgery requires further studies; (vi) percutaneous drainage associated with albendazole therapy is safe and efficient in selected patients; the level of evidence is low concerning treatment of complicated cysts. This has led some authors to write this rather provocative statement: 'Surgery should be reserved for patients with hydatid cysts refractory to PAIR because of secondary bacterial infection or for those with difficult-to-manage cyst–biliary communication or obstruction' [19], whereas others still write: 'Although certain types of hydatid cysts are successfully treated by PAIR, surgery remains the treatment of choice' [20]. This discrepancy clearly indicates that further well-designed studies are in order.

Surgery

The goal of surgery is eradication, i.e. to remove all parasitic cysts and fluid completely; eradication achievable by surgery is a major advantage compared with other types of treatment. Controversies still exist about the best operative technique. The main surgical alternatives are cystectomy, with an appropriate management of the residual cavity, and hepatic resection. Despite the high number of hydatid cysts removed surgically worldwide, few large reviews of surgical cases with a significant follow-up are available. In a European non-endemic country, a recent retrospective study, in 84 patients followed up for a median of 8 years, showed that almost half the patients operated on for liver hydatid cysts had complicated disease [21]; after complete removal of cystic and pericystic tissue with simultaneous treatment of the fistulous tract, in 23% of the patients, there was postoperative morbidity, but no mortality and no recurrence of disease. In a highly endemic area in Kenya, among 663 patients managed with surgery, there was one intraoperative and one postoperative death, and 47 patients underwent repeated operations [22] for postoperative complications and/or recurrences. Recurrences are estimated to occur in 2–25% of cases, depending on the size, location, number or peroperative rupture of the original cysts, as well as on the expertise of the surgical team.

Various types of cystectomy permit the complete removal of the parasite without the risks of liver resection [1,8]. To avoid spillage of the contents of the hepatic cyst, the peritoneal cavity must be carefully protected during cyst evacuation. The contents of the cyst are first sterilized by the injection of scolicidal agents and then evacuated. Formalin and hypertonic saline should not be used because of the risk of caustic sclerosing

cholangitis. Chlorehexidine, H_2O_2, 80% alcohol or 0.5% cetrimide are safer. Their intracystic injection should not be used if there is any evidence of biliary communication. Pretreatment of patients with antiparasitic drugs may make scolicidal agents obsolete; however, there is as yet no long-term study that has evaluated the efficacy of chemotherapy in preventing recurrence. After the liver overlying the cyst has been incised, attempts should be made to excise the laminated membrane intact; this may be done by cleaving through the virtual gap existing between the inner and outer fibrous layer surrounding the cyst ('total subadventitial cystectomy') [23].

Hepatic resection is usually only recommended for central cysts of a left lateral segment. Liver transplantation (LT) has exceptionally been performed in patients with acute Budd–Chiari syndrome and secondary biliary cirrhosis related to toxic sclerosing cholangitis [24].

Instrumental treatment: puncture–aspiration–injection–reaspiration (PAIR)

Since 1986, PAIR has been proposed as an alternative to surgery [25]. After percutaneous puncture under US guidance, aspiration is performed; the residual cavity is then completely filled with a scolicidal agent, usually ethanol, which is reaspirated 10 min later. Detailed practical guidelines for a wider use of the PAIR technique have been published by the WHO-IWGE [16]. A long-term follow-up of patients is now available [26]; a meta-analysis has confirmed that PAIR is efficacious, safe and useful in selected indications [27]. A very limited number of anaphylactic shocks, nearly always reversible with appropriate resuscitation, and no secondary dissemination have been reported. Recurrence of the cysts in most series is lower than after surgery. PAIR can be proposed for type CE1 and selected cases with CE2 and CE3 cysts. It is contraindicated if there is a communication of the cyst with the biliary tree, assessed through puncture of the cyst with cystocholangiography or, in disadvantaged settings, by checking bilirubin in the cyst content. The duration of pre- and postinterventional benzimidazole therapy necessary to avoid parasitic spillage has not been properly evaluated. In experienced hands, PAIR represents the first choice of treatment [28]; drainage may be associated with PAIR in treating large cysts [28]. To treat cysts with numerous daughter cysts, a PAIR-like technique ('percutaneous puncture drainage and curettage') [29], which uses larger tubes and vacuum aspiration through a small surgical incision, was first described in western China; similar procedures have since been published in Europe [30,31].

Laparoscopic aspiration and sterilization of the cysts is also feasible; however, it is more frequently complicated by spillage and recurrence [32].

Treatment of complications

Cholangitis is usually treated by biliary surgical drainage. In some instances, papillotomy during endoscopy may be proposed. The rupture of a hepatic cyst into the peritoneal cavity remains difficult to cure. Despite the removal of cyst contents from the peritoneal cavity at surgery, residual protoscolices form daughter cysts that almost inevitably lead to recurrence. Benzimidazole–praziquantel combined therapy should be used in these situations.

Alveolar echinococcosis

Alveolar echinococcosis (AE) of the liver is an uncommon parasitic disease of the northern hemisphere which is due to the intrahepatic growth of the larva of *Echinococcus multilocularis* (*E.m.*). AE behaves as a liver cancer and is always fatal unless completely removed by surgery. The significant advances achieved in the management of AE during the past 20 years have led to a dramatic improvement in the prognosis of AE, even in inoperable cases.

Epidemiology

Life cycle

A cycle in wild animals allows the parasite to subsist in nature [33]. The adult cestode usually develops in the small intestine of the fox. The last segments (2–4 mm long) are released into the intestine, and their eggs are dispersed on the ground with the stools, contaminating the grass. Eggs are surrounded by an envelope that allows them to resist very low temperatures (down to −40°C); they die at +60°C. When eggs are eaten by the intermediate host, usually a wild rodent, the hexacanth embryo is released into the duodenum, enters the liver through the intestinal wall and can reach the lungs, brain and bones. In rodents, AE consists of a mass of small vesicles each lined by the germinal layer from which enormous numbers of protoscolices develop; lesions produced by several embryos may coalesce and can occupy a considerable part of the liver [2]. The life cycle is completed when the intermediate host, containing infected larvae, is eaten by foxes. Dogs are the most common definitive hosts in some areas, such as China. Less commonly, other carnivores including coyotes and cats can also serve as definitive hosts [33,34].

Prevalence

Humans become infected either by eating contaminated wild fruits or by touching infected foxes or pets. Risk factors for human AE in endemic regions include occupation in agriculture (or activity in gardening, foresting, hunting), a history of dog/cat ownership and residence in a rural upland landscape that favours high densities of small mammals, especially voles [35]. Because of immunogenetic (but also behavioural) factors, the wide distribution and generally high frequency of *E. multilocularis* in foxes is not reflected in disease prevalence in humans, which is low in most endemic areas [34,36]. Among European patients, 54% were female and 46% male with a median age at diagnosis of 56 years [37]; although AE was also disclosed in young children, a mean period of 15 years is usual between contamina-

tion and presenting symptoms. The average incidence, referred to the total population of a country, is rather low, ranging from 0.02 (Austria) to 0.10 (Switzerland) cases per 100 000 inhabitants per year in western Europe. However, because of the geographically focused epidemiology of the parasitic cycle, local incidence rates may be much higher. In a retrospective study of 559 European AE cases diagnosed between 1982 and 2000, 42% were in eastern France, 23.6% in southern Germany and 21% in northeast Switzerland [37]. The increase in fox populations and parasite prevalences and the increasing encroachment of foxes into urban areas, with spillover of *E. multilocularis* infection from wild carnivores to domestic dogs and cats, might point to the emergence of a new AE public health hazard in central Europe [34,37,38]. Neither human cases nor fox infection have ever been found in the British islands [39]. Other endemic regions for AE in humans are many areas of the former Soviet Union, eastern Turkey, northern Japan, China and Alaska. Reports of adult or larval cestodes in the wild fauna of north central America suggest that, in the United States, the parasite is still moving south and east [34]. In north and northwestern China, the prevalence of alveolar echinococcosis in humans can be as high as 16% in some villages [34,40].

Prevention and control

Mass surveys using US and serology are recommended in high-risk populations in endemic areas to monitor epidemiological trends and support health education [12,40,41]. Prevention measures are limited to educational programmes aimed at warning the population in endemic areas of the hazards of touching foxes and eating uncooked fruits and vegetables. It may be advisable to enclose a kitchen garden located near a forest. Extermination of foxes and/or rodents is not a realistic objective and could be deleterious. A third option consists of mass dosing of foxes with praziquantel-treated baits; pilot studies have been done to assess the feasibility and efficacy of this option in non-urban areas and are currently ongoing in urban areas [38,42]. Praziquantel provides a 100% elimination of the parasite from dogs when given at a dose of 5 mg/kg body weight; it should therefore be used for the deworming of domestic dogs in the endemic areas [2,5,38].

Pathogenesis

The hepatic lesions of humans generally consist of a unique mass of fibrous tissue that displays a multitude of cavities, ranging from a few millimetres to a few centimetres in size (Fig. 1b). *E. multilocularis* induces hepatic necrosis allowing the parasite to invade the liver step by step in a way similar to a liver carcinoma. The lesions are not limited by a fibrous shell. The parasitic tissue electively involves and destroys the bifurcation of intrahepatic bile ducts. It may also invade major hepatic vessels and the inferior vena cava [1,43,44]. The lesions are usually most prominent in the right lobe of the liver. Microscopically, they consist of numerous parasitic vesicles (1 mm to 1 cm in diameter) lined by an inner germinal layer and an outer laminated layer. Protoscolices are observed in only 15% of cases, and the germinal layer is usually absent in 'old' vesicles embedded in a dense fibrosis. The parasitic vesicles are surrounded by concentric layers of 'epithelioid cells' of the macrophagic lineage, by a macrophagic/fibroblastic infiltrate and collagen bundles, and by peripheral lymphocytes (mostly CD8 T-cell lymphocytes), arranged in a granuloma [36,45]. The parasitic granuloma (absent in cystic echinococcosis) leads to a fibrotic scar which compresses and then destroys the hepatic vessels and the bile ducts. The resulting necrotic process leads to the formation of large cavities containing parasitic and hepatic debris, blood, bile and sometimes pus; the migration of necrotic fragments is responsible for cholangitis and systemic bacteraemia. The migration of parasitic material through the hepatic vessels may result in distant metastases [46].

Clinical features and complications

AE was frequently diagnosed at an advanced stage and mimicked neoplasia. Jaundice was the most frequent presenting symptom before the 1980s; it was observed in 43% in our series [44], either as a gradual-onset jaundice with pruritus related to hilum involvement or as intermittent jaundice with pain and fever related to superimposed bacterial biliary infection. Hard and massive hepatomegaly was classically the revealing symptom in about 25% of cases.

During the past 20 years, the symptoms at presentation have changed with the earlier diagnosis of less severe and asymptomatic cases. In a series of patients diagnosed between 1983 and 1993, only 25% presented with jaundice, and hepatomegaly was observed in 16%. Vague abdominal right upper quadrant pain is a presenting symptom in about one-third of cases. The contrast between a huge hepatomegaly mimicking a liver carcinoma and a good clinical status should raise suspicion of AE in endemic areas. Currently, a significant number of patients with AE are asymptomatic: they may be diagnosed by chance (during surgery or an ultrasonographic examination for other reasons) or as a result of mass screening in an endemic area.

Complications are rarely the first manifestations of the disease. The most frequent are biliary infection with septicaemia and septic shock and liver abscesses resulting from bacterial or fungal infection of the central necrotic area. Owing to locoregional extension or haematogenous spread of parasitic tissue to distant metastases (in approximately 12% of cases, mainly in the lungs) [37], symptoms ranging from dyspnoea and bile sputum to seizures and stroke as well as skin nodules [43,47] or bone pain may be the presenting clinical manifestations. Anaphylactic reactions are exceptional as initial symptoms [46]. Earlier diagnosis and prophylaxis of variceal bleeding with β-blockers have diminished bleeding from oesophagogastric varices related to portal hypertension, secondary to biliary cirrhosis or to chronic parasitic Budd–Chiari syndrome or portal thrombosis.

Diagnosis

Laboratory findings

Lymphopenia is frequent. Total and conjugated bilirubin are increased in proportion to the degree of jaundice; γ-glutamyl transferase and alkaline phosphatase are markedly increased in jaundiced patients as well as in patients without jaundice. Conversely, serum transaminases are usually normal except for the few patients with a necrotic process in the liver, in whom a two- to fourfold increase is usual. Eosinophilia greater than 7% is found in 10% of patients. A high level of C-reactive protein is suggestive of a latent biliary infection [43]. Prothrombin time and factor V are usually normal. In 80% of patients, serum gammaglobulins are over 30 g/L; electrophoresis shows a polyclonal, and only exceptionally a monoclonal, gammopathy. All three classes of immunoglobulins (G, A, M) are increased.

Morphological findings

US and CT remain the basic morphological imaging techniques in AE [47]. US is the current screening method of choice for diagnosis and regular follow-up in AE [48,49]. A typical US aspect is observed in 70% of cases: the lesion is characterized by irregular limits and heterogeneous content with juxtaposition of hyperechogenic and hypoechogenic areas (Fig. 3a). The hyperechogenic fibrous tissue often contains scattered calcifications. Another US aspect typical of AE is a huge lesion with large central necrosis surrounded by a hyperechogenic ring. However, in endemic AE areas, the following atypical US aspects account for 30% of cases: (i) a small haemangioma-like hyperechogenic nodule which corresponds to an early homogeneous nodular lesion; (ii) a pseudocystic form in the case of a huge AE lesion with massive necrosis; the irregular lining suggests the diagnosis of AE; (iii) a small calcified lesion that corresponds to an abortive form of the disease or a small developing AE [41,48]. US can also provide information on the biliary and vascular involvement.

The typical CT aspect is a lesion with irregular linings and heterogeneous contents of various densities: hyperdense scattered calcifications and hypodense areas corresponding to necrosis and active parasitic tissue (Fig. 3b). No significant enhancement is observed within the lesion after the intravenous bolus administration of contrast medium. The dilatation of the intrahepatic bile ducts in the contralateral lobe of the liver is the hallmark of an infiltration of the hilum by the parasitic process.

Magnetic resonance imaging (MRI) may facilitate the diagnosis in uncertain cases with non-calcified lesions. It is the best technique to characterize the different components of the parasitic lesion and to study the extension to adjacent structures. Cholangio-MRI has now advantageously replaced the classical percutaneous cholangiography. It is an important part of the preoperative evaluation, as it provides information on the relationship between the AE lesion and the biliary tree. Positron emission tomography using [18F]fluorodeoxyglucose has recently been developed for the follow-up of inoperable AE patients

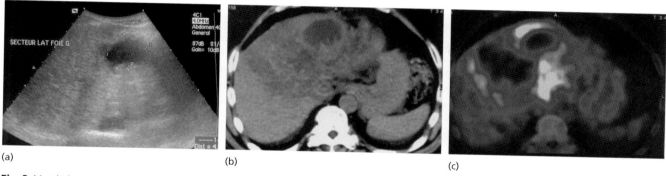

(a)   (b)   (c)

Fig. 3 Morphological aspects of alveolar echinococcosis (AE) of the liver. (a) Ultrasonic aspect of a huge AE lesion located in the left and the central part of the liver, characterized by irregular limits, a heterogeneous content with central hypoechogenic area (necrosis) surrounded by the hyperechogenic fibrous tissue containing scattered calcifications. (b) CT images of the same lesion: heterogeneous content with irregular border and hypodense central area. (c) Positron emission tomography using [18F]fluorodeoxyglucose in the same patient, before the introduction of albendazole therapy: very intense perilesional activity within the inflammatory reaction that indirectly traduces the parasitic viability.

under long-term benzimidazole therapy [50,51]. This approach seems to be promising in assessing inflammatory activity and thereby indirectly depicting parasitic activity (Fig. 3c).

Treatment

Modern treatment of AE clearly requires a multidisciplinary approach with benzimidazole therapy as a common denominator (see below). Depending on the size of the lesion, its location in the liver and vascular and biliary involvement, the option may be a curative resection, an interventional radiological procedure or, exceptionally, a liver transplant. Partial debulking resections followed by continuous administration of a benzimidazole must be avoided [52]. A classification system has been developed recently that could be useful in helping clinicians to choose the appropriate treatment [53].

The sole efficient treatment is partial hepatectomy when the lesions are sufficiently localized [53–55]. Because the intrahepatic common bile duct is usually involved, it is often necessary to remove the bifurcation and to reconstruct the biliary tract using a Roux-en-Y loop [56]. In our series from 1983 onwards, 35% of patients underwent a curative partial hepatectomy, compared with 10% before 1983.

For unresectable patients, palliative surgery is now advantageously replaced by instrumental treatment procedures [47,57,58], which consist of percutaneous radiological drainage of huge centroparasitic abscesses or a dilated intrahepatic bile duct above a hilar stenosis. The best option is to push the drain beyond the stenosis to obtain external/internal biliary drainage. Such drains may be maintained for years; with chemotherapy, they have allowed prolonged survival in initially very severe AE cases [59]. Biliary endoprosthesis could also be inserted, but the stent may become obstructed by necrotic plugs; it is far more difficult to change a stent than an external–internal drain.

A retrospective analysis of the results of LT for unresectable AE (45 cases from different European centres) has been pub-

lished recently [60]. From this experience, LT is indicated only for incurable symptomatic biliary AE with life-threatening cholangitis and/or symptomatic secondary biliary cirrhosis; despite this major procedure, only half the patients have actually been definitively cured by LT. In other patients, parasitic residues were observed with accelerated progression related to immunosuppressive therapy [60,61]. The actuarial survival rate was 58% at 5 years.

Immunological and molecular diagnosis

Numerous immunodiagnostic tests have been developed for CE and AE, but there is currently no standard, highly sensitive and specific as well as cheap test available for antibody detection in either disease. Cross-reactivity is observed between both cestodes, and most tests for CE can be used for the diagnosis of AE and vice versa. In some endemic countries, both diseases may be found in the same area (this is especially the case in China, but also in Turkey and most central Asian countries), and a differential diagnosis could theoretically be useful. Cellular tests are interesting for research but have no value in the diagnosis of these diseases [36]. The intradermal 'Casoni' test is no longer used because of its lack of sensitivity and specificity as well as safety.

Serological tests

Assays for specific antibodies in serum have used natural antigens obtained from both *Echinococcus granulosus* (hydatid fluid or hydatid sand) and *Echinococcus multilocularis* (protoscolices or parasitic extracts) and/or purified antigens or recombinant proteins from either *Echinococcus* sp. [62]. The following considerations apply to serological testing; (i) complement fixation tests are no longer used because of poor sensitivity and specificity; (ii) indirect haemagglutination and latex tests, with crude *Echinococcus* extracts, are both cheap and sensitive but poorly specific; (iii) immunoelectrophoresis or immunosyneresis is specific, but poorly sensitive and time-consuming; (iv) ELISA tests, using crude antigens from *E. granulosus* or *E. multilocularis*, are sensitive but poorly specific; (v) more specific are ELISA tests using purified antigenic fractions or recombinant antigens such as antigen 5 or antigen B of *Echinococcus granulosus*, the Em2 or the Em18 fractions of *Echinococcus multilocularis*, the specific alkaline phosphatase of *E. multilocularis*, the recombinant Em3/10 and Em18; (vi) Western blots use either crude extracts from *E. granulosus* or *E. multilocularis* (more sensitive) or purified fractions or recombinant antigens (more specific). The combination of antigens in a single test (such as the EM2+) or Western blot patterns have attempted to provide both the positive and the differential diagnosis. By comparing the 'best' serological tests with ultrasound- and/or CT-confirmed lesions, the overall sensitivity reaches 80% for liver hydatid cysts (it is lower for lung cysts, averaging 65%) and 90% for alveolar echinococcosis; specificity may reach 90% for both [62]. The diagnostic efficiency of serology is limited by the reduced capacity of some infected subjects to develop specific antibodies and the failure to release specific antigens by some hydatid cysts (decreased sensitivity) and the existence of infected non-diseased subjects in endemic areas (decreased specificity). Positive serological results in individuals account for at least five different situations: (i) 'patent', overt disease with symptoms; (ii) 'latent', non-apparent disease; (iii) calcified dead lesions in the liver; (iv) hydatid cyst in the lung or other organs and exceptional cases of isolated extrahepatic AE; and (v) no parasitic lesions at all [12,13,36,40,43,45]. Negative serology with patent CE or AE lesions has been found in all mass screenings and is the rule in all published hospital case series [13,40,43]. Serology should thus never be used as a 'first intent' test for mass screening; it should always be combined with ultrasound imaging, and used to confirm a diagnosis suspected on the basis of imaging techniques.

The predominant antibody response consists mainly of the IgG1 and IgG4 subclasses. Elevated total IgE and specific IgE against *Echinococcus* antigens, which may be found in the serum of CE patients, are significantly more elevated when a rupture or a fissuration of the cyst occurs; an increased eosinophil count may also be observed in these situations. Specific IgE antibodies against *E. multilocularis* antigens may be found in AE patients, and histamine release from circulating basophils stimulated with *Echinococcus* antigens is constant in AE patients [36].

In the post-surgery follow-up, after a temporary increase, antibody levels progressively decrease for 1–2 years before turning negative. The persistence of raised levels or a further increase is suggestive of residual disease or a recurrence; however, the long-term persistence of antibodies in some patients is not evidence against the eradication of the parasite. IgE, IgG4 and IgG2 antibodies seem to be associated with progressive and severe cases and are the first to disappear after surgery or efficient chemotherapy [62]. In AE patients with a recurrence

after LT, antibodies detected using crude antigens (e.g. crude hydatid fluid) were observed at an early stage in recurrence, and more specific antibodies (e.g. against the *E. multilocularis* specific Em2 antigen) could only be detected later [63]. Similar observations have been made at mass screenings: early lesions were associated with antibodies against crude extracts and could thus be missed using more specific antigens/recombinant proteins [64].

Molecular tests

Molecular identification of both *E. granulosus* and *E. multilocularis* is mostly based on polymerase chain reaction (PCR) using mitochondrial DNA probes [64]. It may be used on liver needle aspiration (for CE) and/or liver biopsy (for AE), if echinococcosis is suspected despite negative serology. In addition, it may be useful in epidemiological studies to identify the subspecies of *E. granulosus* involved in human contamination from the animal cycle: more than 10 subspecies have been described, the most frequently involved in humans being the G1 ('sheep') and G6 ('camel') subspecies. Recent reports have shown that the latter is also infectious to humans [65]. *E. multilocularis* is far less heterogeneous, and only minor differences in geographical isolates may be disclosed.

Medical treatments of echinococcosis

Although no well-designed clinical trials have been performed for any medical treatment modality in either form of echinococcosis, two benzimidazole compounds have proved efficacious against both alveolar and cystic echinococcosis: mebendazole (MBZ) (4.5 g/day) and albendazole (ABZ) (10–15 mg/kg/day). Because of limited toxicological data, ABZ was originally administered intermittently. More recent data suggest that continuous treatment achieves equivalent or improved efficacy with no increased adverse effects [66].

Benzimidazoles (BZM) in cystic echinococcosis

Three randomized controlled trials showed that ABZ alone had a better effect on hydatid cysts than placebo [67,68] or MBZ [69]. One prospective controlled trial compared ABZ in combination with praziquantel (25 mg/kg/day) vs. ABZ alone [70] and concluded that the combined treatment was more effective than ABZ alone. However, complete disappearance of all cysts was never reached. Therefore, chemotherapy is not the ideal treatment when used alone. This therapeutic option is indicated for patients with multiple cysts in two or more organs and for patients with peritoneal cysts. ABZ is poorly absorbed by the gastrointestinal tract. To improve absorption, ABZ should be taken with a fatty meal [71].

Pre- and postintervention chemotherapy with BZM may reduce the risk of recurrence and intraperitoneal seeding. There is no optimal scheme, but the current recommendation is to administer ABZ 3 weeks before and for 1–2 months after the intervention [18]. PAIR plus chemotherapy is associated with increased clinical and parasitological efficacy [27]. ABZ is to be given the day before and for 1 month after PAIR [72]; ABZ should not be administered when PAIR is performed during pregnancy.

Benzimidazoles in alveolar echinococcosis

MBZ and ABZ are the drugs of choice in the treatment of AE. However, these drugs only have a parasitostatic effect and do not kill the parasite in most cases. There are no comparative studies, but ABZ is currently preferred because it is > 40% less expensive, is easier to take and is now licensed for AE in many countries [73]. In case of extirpable AE lesions, it is recommended to initiate ABZ before the operation and to maintain ABZ for at least 2 years to avoid recurrence [17]. In inoperable cases, long-term chemotherapy may significantly prolong survival (10-year survival of approximately 80% in treated cases, compared with less than 25% in historical untreated control subjects) [74]. Recent reports emphasize the possibility of parasite death under long-term BZM therapy [74–76]. By assessing parasite viability, the combination of sequential PET-CT and new serological markers offers the prospect of a more personalized medical treatment of inoperable AE patients: discontinuation of BZM after many years of treatment could be feasible in selected cases using these new tools [51,74]. If LT is indicated, ABZ must be initiated before the operation and maintained after LT for at least 2 years (lifelong in case of metacestode remnants or new AE foci discovered during post-LT follow-up) [17].

Side-effects of BZM

Adverse events of BZM were reported in 5.8–20% of the patients treated. General complaints include headache, nausea, anorexia, vomiting, abdominal pain and itching. In the first weeks of treatment, a transient increase in liver enzymes may be observed; it usually appears to be the result of drug efficacy rather than evidence of drug toxicity [77]. Idiosyncratic reactions have been observed in a few cases [78]. Regular monitoring is therefore recommended: if aminotransferase levels rise to 200–300 IU/L, discontinuation of therapy should be considered. A significant but usually reversible alopecia occurs in about 5% of cases. In AE, this effect has been observed particularly in patients with portal hypertension and/or severe cholestasis. The risk, albeit small, of bone marrow depression (neutropenia or even rarely aplastic anaemia) should prompt regular checking of blood cell count [79]. ABZ has been shown to be teratogenic in rats and rabbits and, therefore, should be avoided, if possible, during pregnancy (in particular during the first trimester) and lactation [8]. Although they are closely related drugs, MBZ may be better tolerated by patients with ABZ side-effects and vice versa; a switch to the other drug can thus be tried before withdrawing chemotherapy definitively [43].

Future prospects in the treatment of echinococcosis of the liver

Research is in progress to increase the serum concentrations of ABZ. Studies with liposome-entrapped ABZ have given promising results [80,81]. Amphotericin B has been used as salvage treatment for AE patients with intolerance or resistance to BZM; although the drug is only parasitocidal [82], it effectively halted parasite progression in a small series of patients [83]. Nitazoxanide (NTX), a broad-spectrum antihelminthic agent, also used for enteric bacteria treatment, seems to be promising for AE treatment: a parasitocidal effect was demonstrated *in vitro* [84,85]. Immunomodulatory treatment with interferon-α might be a future treatment goal for AE [86,87]. Radiothermal ablation by radiofrequency is currently under investigation for cystic echinococcosis [88]. However, the best strategy to direct therapeutic options is to design controlled studies aimed at more clearly defining the respective place of surgery (and what type of surgery) and of PAIR [89,90].

References

1 Amman RW, Eckert J (1996) Cestodes. *Echinococcus.* In: *Parasitic Diseases of the Liver and Intestines. Gastroenterol Clin North Am* 25, 655–689.

2 Eckert JP, Deplazes PS, Craig M *et al.* (2001) Echinococcosis in animals: clinical aspects, diagnosis and treatment. In: Eckert J, Gemmell MA, Meslin F-X *et al.* (eds) *WHO/OIE Manual on Echinococcosis in Humans and Animals: a Public Health Problem of Global Concern.* Paris: World Organisation for Animal Health (OIE), pp. 72–99.

3 Jenkins DJ, Macpherson CN (2003) Transmission ecology of *Echinococcus* in wild-life in Australia and Africa. *Parasitology* 127, S63–72.

4 Torgerson PR, Budke C (2003) Echinococcosis – an international public health challenge. *Res Vet Sci* 74, 191–202.

5 Ito A, Urbani C, Jiamin Q *et al.* (2003) Control of echinococcosis and cysticercosis: a public health challenge to international cooperation in China. *Acta Trop* 86, 3–17.

6 Torgerson PR, Heath DD (2003) Transmission dynamics and control options for cystic echinococcosis. *Parasitology* 127, S143–S158.

7 Lightowlers MW, Heath DD (2004) Immunity and vaccine control of *Echinococcus granulosus* infection in animal intermediate hosts. *Parasitologia* 46, 27–31.

8 Kern P (2003) *Echinococcus granulosus* infection: clinical presentation, medical treatment and outcome. *Langenbecks Arch Surg* 388, 413–420.

9 Frider B, Larrieu E, Odriozola M (1999) Long-term outcome of asymptomatic liver hydatidosis. *J Hepatol* 30, 228–231.

10 Gharbi HA, Hassine W, Brauner MW *et al.* (1981) Ultrasound examination of the hydatic liver. *Radiology* 139, 459–463.

11 WHO Informal Working Group on Echinococcosis (2003) International classification of ultrasound images in cystic echinococcosis for application in clinical and field epidemiological settings. *Acta Trop* 85, 253–261

12 Macpherson CN, Bartholomot B, Frider B. (2003) Application of ultrasound in diagnosis, treatment, epidemiology, public health and control of *Echinococcus granulosus* and *E. multilocularis. Parasitology* 127, S21–35.

13 Larrieu EJ, Frider B (2001) Human cystic echinococcosis: contributions to the natural history of the disease. *Ann Trop Med Parasitol* 95, 679–687.

14 Wang Y, Zhang X, Bartholomot B *et al.* (2003) Classification, follow-up and recurrence of hepatic cystic echinococcosis using ultrasound images. *Trans R Soc Trop Med Hyg* 97, 203–211.

15 Hira PR, Lindberg LG, Francis I *et al.* (1988) Diagnosis of cystic hydatid disease: role of aspiration cytology. *Lancet* 2, 655–657.

16 WHO-Informal Working Group on Echinococcosis (2003) *PAIR: a New Option for the Treatment of Cystic Echinococcosis.* Geneva: WHO.

17 WHO-Informal Working Group on Echinococcosis (1996) Guidelines for treatment of cystic and alveolar echinococcosis in humans. *Bull World Health Org* 74, 231–242.

18 Dziri C, Haouet K, Fingerhut A (2004) Treatment of hydatid cyst of the liver: where is the evidence? *World J Surg* 28, 731–736.

19 Smego RA Jr, Sebanego P (2005) Treatment options for hepatic cystic echinococcosis. *Int J Infect Dis* 9, 69–76.

20 Sayek I, Tirnaksiz MB, Dogan R (2004) Cystic hydatid disease: current trends in diagnosis and management. *Surg Today* 34, 987–996.

21 Chautems R, Buhler LH, Gold B *et al.* (2005) Surgical management and long-term outcome of complicated liver hydatid cysts caused by *Echinococcus granulosus. Surgery* 137, 312–316.

22 Cooney RM, Flanagan KP, Zehyle E (2004) Review of surgical management of cystic hydatid disease in a resource limited setting: Turkana, Kenya. *Eur J Gastroenterol Hepatol* 16, 1233–1236.

23 Wu XW, Peng XY, Zhang SJ *et al.* (2004) Formation mechanisms of the fibrous capsule around hepatic and splenic hydatid cyst. *Zhongguo Ji Sheng Chong Xue Yu Ji Sheng Chong Bing Za Zhi* 22, 1–4 (in Chinese).

24 Moreno-Gonzalez E, Loinaz Segurola C, Garcia Urena MA *et al.* (1994) Liver transplantation for *Echinococcus granulosus* hydatid disease. *Transplantation* 58, 797–800.

25 Ben Amor N, Gargouri M, Gharbi HA *et al.* (1986) Trial therapy of inoperable abdominal hydatid cysts by puncture. *Ann Parasitol Hum Comp* 61, 689–692 (in French).

26 Akhan O, Ozmen MN, Dinçer A *et al.* (1996) Liver hydatid disease: long term results of percutaneous treatment. *Radiology* 198, 259–264.

27 Smego RA Jr, Bhatti S, Khaliq AA *et al.* (2003) Percutaneous aspiration-injection-reaspiration drainage plus albendazole or mebendazole for hepatic cystic echinococcosis: a meta-analysis. *Clin Infect Dis* 37, 1073–1083.

28 Felice C, Pirola F, Brunetti E *et al.* (1990) A new therapeutic approach for hydatid liver cysts. *Gastroenterology* 98, 1366–1368.

29 Wang XZ, Yongshou L, Sheng F *et al.* (1994) Clinical treatment of hepatic and abdominal hydatidosis with percutaneous puncture drainage and curettage (report of 869 cases). *Chin J Parasitol Parasitic Dis* 12, 285–287.

30 Schipper HG, Laméris JS, van Delden OM *et al.* (2002) Percutaneous evacuation (PEVAC) of multivesicular echinococcal cysts with or without cystobiliary fistulas which contain non-drainable material: first results of a modified PAIR method. *Gut* 50, 718–723.

31 Avtan L (2005) A new 'Perforator Grinder-Aspirator Apparatus (PGAA)' for the minimal access surgery of cystic liver hydatidosis. *Hepatogastroenterology* 52, 339–342.

32 Baskaran V, Patnaik PK (2004) Feasibility and safety of laparoscopic management of hydatid disease of the liver. *J Soc Laparoendosc Surgeons* 8, 359–363.

33 Craig P (2003) *Echinococcus multilocularis. Curr Opin Infect Dis* 16, 437–444.

34 Vuitton DA, Zhou H, Bresson-Hadni S *et al.* (2003) Epidemiology of alveolar echinococcosis with particular reference to China and Europe. *Parasitology* 127, S87–107.

35 Giraudoux P, Craig PS, Delattre P *et al.* (2003) Interactions between landscape changes and host communities can regulate *Echinococcus multilocularis* transmission. *Parasitology* 127, S121–131.

36 Vuitton DA (2003) The ambiguous role of immunity in echinococcosis: protection of the host or of the parasite? *Acta Trop* 85, 119–132.

37 Kern P, Bardonnet K, Renner E *et al.*; European Echinococcosis Registry (2003) European echinococcosis registry: human alveolar echinococcosis, Europe, 1982–2000. *Emerg Infect Dis* 9, 343–349.

38 Deplazes P, Hegglin D, Gloor S *et al.* (2004) Wilderness in the city: the urbanization of *Echinococcus multilocularis. Trends Parasitol* 20, 77–84.

39 Smith GC, Gangadharan B, Taylor Z *et al.* (2003) Prevalence of zoonotic important parasites in the red fox (*Vulpes vulpes*) in Great Britain. *Vet Parasitol* 118, 133–142.

40 Bartholomot B, Vuitton DA, Harraga S *et al.* (2002) Combined ultra-sound and serologic screening for hepatic alveolar echinococcosis in central China. *Am J Trop Med Hyg* 66, 23–29.

41 Bresson-Hadni S, Laplante JJ, Lenys D *et al.* (1994) Seroepidemiologic screening of *Echinococcus multilocularis* in a European area endemic for alveolar echinococcosis. *Am J Trop Med Hyg* 5, 837–846.

42 Ito A, Romig T, Takahashi K (2003) Perspective on control options for *Echinococcus multilocularis* with particular reference to Japan. *Parasitology* 127, S159–172.

43 Bresson-Hadni S, Vuitton DA, Bartholomot B *et al.* (2000) A twenty-year history of alveolar echinococcosis: analysis of a series of 117 patients from eastern France. *Eur J Gastroenterol Hepatol* 12, 327–336.

44 Kasai Y, Koshino I, Kawanishi N *et al.* (1980) Alveolar echinococcosis of the liver. Studies on 60 operated cases. *Ann Surg* 191, 145–152.

45 Vuitton DA, Zhang SL, Yang YR *et al.* (2006) Survival strategy of *Echinococcus multilocularis* in the human host. *Parasitol Int* 55(Suppl.), 551–555.

46 Bresson-Hadni S, Vuitton D, Didier D *et al.* (1989) Metastases pulmonaires de l'echinococcose alveolaire. Frequence et mecanismes de survenue. *Presse Med* 18, 83.

47 Bresson-Hadni S, Humbert P, Paintaud G *et al.* (1986) Skin localization of alveolar echinococcosis of the liver. *J Am Acad Dermatol* 34, 873–877.

48 Bresson-Hadni S, Delabrousse E, Blagosklonov O *et al.* (2006) Imaging aspects and non-surgical interventional treatment in human alveolar echinococcosis. *Parasitol Int* 55(Suppl.), S267–S272.

49 Craig PS, Giraudoux P, Shi D *et al.* (2000) An epidemiological and ecological study of human alveolar echinococcosis transmission in south Gansu, China. *Acta Trop* 77, 167–177.

50 Reuter S, Schirmeister H, Kratzer W *et al.* (1999) Pericystic metabolic activity in alveolar echinococcosis: assessment and follow-up by positron emission tomography. *Clin Infect Dis* 29, 1157–1163.

51 Reuter S, Buck A, Manfras S *et al.* (2004) Structured treatment interruption in patients with alveolar echinococcosis. *Hepatology* 39, 509–517.

52 Kadry Z, Renner EC, Bachmann LM *et al.* (2005) Evaluation of treatment and long-term follow-up in patients with hepatic alveolar echinococcosis. *Br J Surg* 92, 1110–1116.

53 Kern P, Gruener B, Sato N *et al.* (2006) WHO classification of alveolar echinococcosis: principles and application. *Parasitol Int* 55(Suppl.), 5283–5287.

54 Miguet JP, Bresson-Hadni S (1989) Alveolar echinococcosis of the liver. *J Hepatol* 8, 373–379.

55 Wilson JF, Rausch RL, Wilson FR (1995) Alveolar hydatid disease. Review of the surgical experience in 42 cases of active disease among Alaskan eskimos. *Ann Surg* 221, 315–323.

56 Gillet M, Bresson-Hadni S (1991) L'échinococcose alvéolaire hépatique. *Rev Prat* 41, 1805–1811.

57 Mosimann F (1980) Is alveolar hydatid disease of the liver incurable? *Ann Surg* 192, 118–123.

58 Bret PM, Paliard P, Partensky C *et al.* (1984) Le traitement de la cholestase par stenose des voies biliaires intrahepatiques au cours de l'echinococcose alveolaire. Essai de drainage biliaire par voie percutanée transhepatique. *Gastroenterol Clin Biol* 8, 308–313.

59 Bresson-Hadni S, Mantion GA, Vuitton DA *et al.* (2004) Echinococcose alvéolaire en région parisienne. *Gastroenterol Clin Biol* 28, 1147–2251.

60 Koch S, Bresson-Hadni S, Miguet JP *et al.* (2003) Experience of liver transplantation for incurable alveolar echinococcosis: a 45 case European collaborative report. *Transplantation* 75, 856–863.

61 Bresson-Hadni S, Koch S, Beurton I *et al.* (1999) Primary disease recurrence after liver transplantation for alveolar echinococcosis: long term evaluation in 15 patients. *Hepatology* 30, 857–864.

62 Craig PS, Rogan MT, Campos-Ponce M (2003) Echinococcosis: disease, detection and transmission. *Parasitology* 127, S5–20.

63 Bresson-Hadni S, Franza A, Miguet JP *et al.* (1991) Orthotopic liver transplantation for incurable alveolar echinococcosis of the liver: report of 17 cases. *Hepatology* 13, 1061–1070.

64 Ito A, Craig PS (2003) Immunodiagnostic and molecular approaches for the detection of taeniid cestode infections. *Trends Parasitol* 19, 377–381.

65 Bardonnet K, Piarroux R, Dia L *et al.* (2002) Combined eco-epidemiological and molecular biology approaches to assess *Echinococcus granulosus* transmission to humans in Mauritania: occurrence of the 'camel' strain and human cystic echinococcosis. *Trans R Soc Trop Med Hyg* 96, 383–386.

66 McManus D, Zhang W, Li J *et al.* (2003) Echinococcosis. *Lancet* 362, 1295–1304.

67 Gil-Grande LA, Rodriguez-Caabeiro F, Prieto JG *et al.* (1993) Randomized controlled trial of efficacy of albendazole in intra-abdominal hydatid disease. *Lancet* 342, 1269–1272.

68 Keshmiri M, Baharvahdat F, Fattahi SH *et al.* (2001) Albendazole versus placebo in the treatment of echinococcosis. *Trans R Soc Trop Med Hyg* 95, 190–191.

69 Franchi C, Di Vico B, Teggi A (1999) Long-term evaluation of patients with hydatidosis treated with benzimidazole. *Clin Infect Dis* 29, 304–309.

70 Mohamed AE, Yasawy MI, Al Karawi MA (1998) Combined albendazole and praziquantel versus albendazole alone in the treatment of hydatid disease. *Hepatogastroenterology* 45, 1690–1694.

71 Schipper HG, Kager PA (2004) Diagnosis and treatment of hepatic echinococcosis: an overview. *Scand J Gastroenterol* 39 (Suppl. 241), 50–55.

72 Vuitton DA, Bresson-Hadni S, Delabrousse E *et al.* (2004) Foie et maladies parasitaires. *Gastroenterol Clin Biol* 28, 1122–1137.

73 Reuter S, Jensen B, Buttenschoen K *et al.* (2000) Benzimidazoles in the treatment of alveolar echinococcosis: a comparative study and review of the literature. *J Antimicrob Chemother* 46, 451–456.

74 Ammann RW, Renner EC, Gottstein B *et al.* (2004) Immuno-surveillance of alveolar echinococcosis by specific humoral and cellular immune tests: long-term analysis of the Swiss chemotherapy trial (1976–2001). *J Hepatol* 41, 551–559.

75 Ammann RW, Fleiner-Hoffmann A, Grimm F *et al.* (1998) Long-term mebendazole therapy may be parasitocidal in alveolar echinococcosis. *J Hepatol* 29, 994–998.

76 Ammann RW, Ilitsch N, Marincek B *et al.* (1994) Effect of chemotherapy on the larval mass and the long-term course of alveolar echinococcosis. *Hepatology* 19, 735–742.

77 Horton RJ (1997) Albendazole in treatment of human cystic echinococcosis: 12 years of experience. *Acta Trop* 6, 79–93.

78 Horton J (2003) Albendazole for the treatment of echinococcosis. *Fund Clin Pharmacol* 17, 205–212.

79 Opatrny L, Prichard R, Snell L *et al.* (2005) Death related to albendazole-induced pancytopenia: case report and review. *Am J Trop Med Hyg* 72, 291–294.

80 Wen H, New RRC, Muhmut M *et al.* (1996) Pharmacology and efficacy of liposome-entrapped albendazole in experimental secondary alveolar echinococcosis and effect of co-administration with cimetidine. *Parasitology* 113: 111–121.

81 Chai J, Menghebat T, Wei J *et al.* (2004) Observations on clinical efficacy of albendazole emulsion in 264 cases of hepatic cystic echinococcosis. *Parasit Int* 53, 3–10.

82 Reuter S, Merkle M, Brehm K *et al.* (2003) Effect of amphotericin B on larval growth of *Echinococcus multilocularis*. *Antimicrob Agents Chemother* 47, 620–625.

83 Reuter S, Buck A, Grebe O *et al.* (2003) Salvage treatment with amphotericin B in progressive human alveolar echinococcosis. *Antimicrob Agents Chemother* 47, 3586–3591.

84 Stettler M, Fink R, Walker M *et al.* (2003) In vitro parasiticidal effect of nitazoxanide against *Echinococcus multilocularis* metacestodes. *Antimicrob Agents Chemother* 47, 467–474.

85 Stettler M, Rossignol JF, Fink R *et al.* (2004) Secondary and primary murine alveolar echinococcosis: combined albendazole/nitazoxanide chemotherapy exhibits profound anti-parasitic activity. *Int J Parasitol* 34, 615–624.

86 Harraga S, Godot V, Bresson-Hadni S *et al.* (1999) Clinical efficacy of and switch from T helper 2 to T helper 1 cytokine profile after interferon alpha2a monotherapy for human echinococcosis. *Clin Infect Dis* 29, 205–206.

87 Godot V, Harraga S, Podoprigora G *et al.* (2003) IFN alpha-2a protects mice against a helminth infection of the liver and modulates immune responses. *Gastroenterology* 124, 1441–1450.

88 Brunetti E, Filice C (2001) Radiofrequency thermal ablation of echinococcal liver cysts. *Lancet* 358, 1464.

89 Buttenschoen K, Carli Buttenschoen D (2003) *Echinococcus granulosus* infection: the challenge of surgical treatment. *Langenbecks Arch Surg* 388, 218–230.

90 Kjossev KT, Losanoff JE (2005) Classification of hydatid liver cysts. *J Gastroenterol Hepatol* 20, 352–359.

10.4.3 Ascariasis, visceral larva migrans, strongyloidiasis, capillariasis and pentastomiasis

Marcelo Simão Ferreira and Edna Strauss

Introduction

Parasitic diseases of the liver and the biliary system are frequent in tropical and subtropical regions of the world and cause important morbidity and mortality. In general, the clinical and laboratory findings are not specific enough to lead to suspicion of hepatobiliary parasitosis and, in most cases, the presence of infection can only be confirmed with modern imaging methods and parasitological tests. In this section, we describe infections caused by *Ascaris lumbricoides* including the visceral larva migrans, by strongyloidiasis and by two other relatively rare parasitoses, namely capillariasis and pentastomiasis.

Ascariasis

Introduction

Infection by *A. lumbricoides* is widespread throughout the world, and is particularly prevalent in developing countries. The worm has been known to be a parasite of man since Ancient Greek times. The adults are yellowish-pink, round helminths, ranging from 15 to 35 cm in size and occasionally reaching 50 cm in length; the females are generally larger than the males, and the latter have a characteristic curved posterior end. They live in the small intestine of humans and feed on its contents. The nematode is extremely mobile and does not attach itself permanently to the mucosa. The number of parasites that an individual can host varies and can reach as many as 500–600 adult worms in some cases. The females release about 200 000 eggs a day, and their uterus can contain as many as 27 million eggs. These are round or oval shaped and yellowish-brown in colour, measuring 60 μm in length. They are covered with a wrinkled or mammilliform albuminous layer, which has a brown colour as a result of the biliary pigments absorbed from the faeces. The eggs are eliminated before embryonation and are highly resistant to environmental factors [1,2].

Epidemiology

Ascariasis is the most widespread intestinal parasitosis in the world, and recent figures from the World Health Organization show that one billion people are infected by this helminth. The high temperature and humidity in tropical parts of the world favour maturation of the eggs. Children, particularly those in rural areas, appear to be most affected. Populations living in poor hygienic conditions where potable water is not readily available are highly susceptible. Eggs present in the soil can survive for long periods (45–55 days) even at low temperatures (16–18°C), most notably in clay soils, which retain water and prevent the eggs becoming desiccated. Under favourable conditions, the eggs become infective in around 2 weeks, embryonate with third-stage larvae and can be found in different environments, including objects for personal use, furniture, swimming pools, fruit, vegetables, coins, notes and also drinking water [1,3].

Life cycle

After being ingested and reaching the duodenum, the infective eggs release the third-stage larvae, which migrate to the caecum, where they penetrate the wall and enter the bloodstream or the lymphatic system, through which they reach the liver and right heart, and then the lungs. They remain in the lungs for several days, undergoing two moults. They then pass through the bronchioles, bronchi and trachea to reach the epiglottis, where they are eliminated by the saliva or swallowed. After being swallowed, and on reaching the stomach and small intestine, they undergo the fourth moult and, at this stage, they are 10 times larger than their original size (about 2 mm). Approximately 60 days after being ingested, the parasites become adults and start oviposition. Many third-stage larvae are destroyed in the liver during the beginning of the life cycle, and only a small percentage reach the right heart.

The swine ascarid, *Ascaris suum*, although morphologically similar to the human one, is unable to complete its life cycle in a human host. Its larvae, however, can produce symptoms of visceral larva migrans when migrating erratically through the liver and lungs.

Pathogenesis and pathology

The migratory larvae do not normally produce an inflammatory reaction in the liver in individuals with a primary infection, but an inflammatory process rich in neutrophils and eosinophils does occur in individuals who are re-exposed to infection. If the larvae die, as is very often the case, their fragments can elicit a granulomatous reaction. Helminths can obstruct the choledochum and other intrahepatic biliary branches, leading to acute periductal inflammation (Fig. 1). The walls of the choledochum thicken and its diameter increases; many ducts are amputated; the damage can be observed at cholangiography (Fig. 2). The hepatic parenchyma may be invaded, and many helminths perforate the Glisson's capsule and enter the subdiaphragmatic space. The papilla of Vater, which is the helminth's point of entry into the biliary system, may show signs of papillitis. In cases of massive infection, all the intra- and extrahepatic ducts are ectasic, and there is periductal fibrosis, oedema, degenerative change in the biliary epithelium, ulcerated areas, epithelial hyperplasia and, less commonly, intraductal papillomas (Fig. 3). When the helminths die in the hepatobiliary system, the body of the parasite disintegrates, a large number of eggs

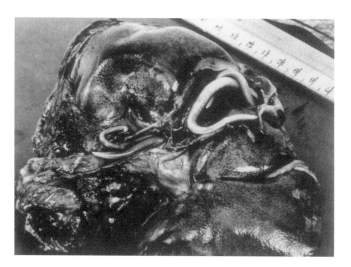

Fig. 1 Biliary ascariasis at autopsy. The bodies of adult worms are seen in the gallbladder and in the common bile duct (courtesy of Dr Luiz Carlos C. Gayotto).

are released, and suppurative cholangitis is produced. This very often involves the hepatic veins and circumadjacent hepatocytes. Multiple hepatic abscesses can be produced, and remnants of the parasites and their eggs are commonly found in the pus within the necrotic areas; in addition, enterobacteria and anaerobes may also be isolated from this material. Granulomas may occasionally be seen throughout the hepatic parenchyma and around the small intrahepatic biliary ducts, especially in areas where eggs and fragments of the worms are deposited and sometimes phagocytosed by large giant cells (Fig. 4). The presence of this material from degenerated nematodes appears to be essential for the formation of intrahepatic calculi (hepatolithiasis). This formation is facilitated by the high level of glycuronidase activity present in these helminths, which deconjugates bilirubin and contributes to the formation of pigmented calculi. The prolonged presence of *A. lumbricoides* in the biliary tree may cause ductal stenosis, chronic cholangitis, hepatolithiasis and secondary biliary cirrhosis [4–7].

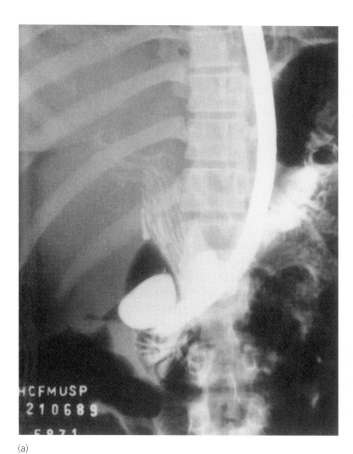

(a)

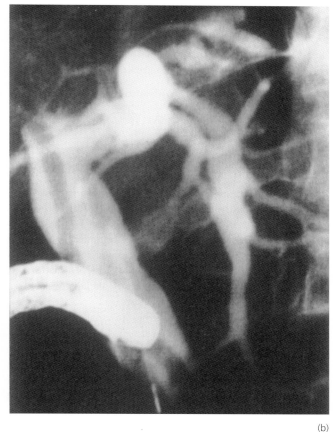

(b)

Fig. 2 Endoscopic retrograde cholangiopancreatography in a case of biliary ascariasis showing filling defects corresponding to adult worms in a dilated common bile duct. There is amputation of several branches of the biliary tree (courtesy of Dr Ernesto Damerau). (a) Endoscopic retrograde cholangiopancreatography in a case of biliary ascariasis. (b) In a markedly dilated common bile duct, filling defects show many bodies of adult worms. Seventy-six worms were removed from the biliary tree (courtesy of Dr Marcel C. Machado).

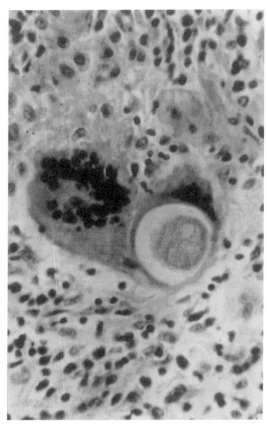

Fig. 3 Remnants of a dead worm mixed with cellular debris are tightly adherent to the hyperplastic epithelial lining of a bile duct. The portal tract shows fibrosis, inflammation and erosion of the limiting plate (Masson's trichrome) (courtesy of Dr Luiz Carlos C. Gayotto).

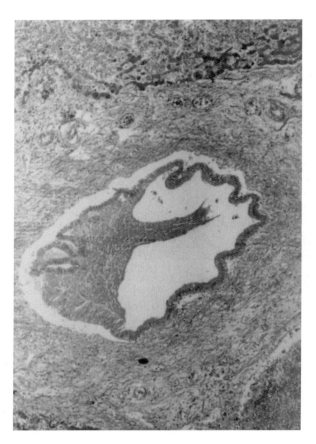

Fig. 4 An egg of *A. lumbricoides* is phagocytosed by a foreign body giant cell around which there is an eosinophilic infiltrate (haematoxylin and eosin) (courtesy of Dr Luiz Carlos C. Gayotto).

Clinical picture: hepatobiliary involvement

In the initial phase of ascariasis, the larvae may produce symptoms of asthmatiform bronchitis and pneumonitis as they pass through the lungs; symptoms are more severe during reinfections and massive infections. Blood eosinophilia is very often present during this phase. This set of symptoms is known as Loeffler syndrome; it can also be seen in infections caused by other nematodes with a pulmonary cycle (ancillostomides and *Strongyloides stercoralis*) [2,8].

The presence of adult worms in the small intestine may be asymptomatic, especially when few helminths are present. Some individuals, however, may complain of abdominal pain and intermittent cramps accompanied by nausea. The most common complication of the disease is obstruction of the intestine by an 'Ascaris' bolus. This is particularly common in undernourished children with a low standard of living, and can evolve in some cases to ischaemic necrosis of the intestinal wall, perforation and peritonitis [2,8].

Penetration of the biliary system may initially be asymptomatic. However, depending on the number of worms in the biliary system, abdominal pain in the upper right quadrant,

nausea and vomiting are present in most cases; fever with shivering and jaundice are present in up to 20–30% of patients and reflect concomitant acute suppurative cholangitis. At physical examination, hepatomegaly is the most important finding after jaundice [2]. Laboratory data show leucocytosis and eosinophilia, which can be very conspicuous in some cases (> 40%). It is not unusual in such cases for *Ascaris* to be eliminated orally or anally. Some authors recognize five clinical forms of hepatobiliary ascariasis: acute cholecystitis (sometimes with acute hepatitis), acute cholangitis, biliary colic, acute pancreatitis and hepatic abscess [2,5,8]. Another rare form of this liver parasitosis is the formation of a pseudotumour as a result of granulomas that coalesce around *A. lumbricoides* eggs [4,6]. The hepatic mass, simulating a malign tumour, can be detected with ultrasonography or computerized tomography (CT). The actual nature of the process can only be disclosed by histopathological examination [4,5,9,10].

Ascariasis-associated hepatolithiasis is very common in Asian countries and can lead to recurrent pyogenic cholangitis, multiple hepatic abscesses, secondary biliary cirrhosis and cholangiocarcinoma. The calculi are usually located in the intrahepatic biliary ducts close to the junction of the right and left liver. The clinical picture results from biliary stasis and bacterial infections which ascend from the intestinal lumen [5–7,9–11].

Diagnosis

Intestinal ascariasis is easily diagnosed by detecting the parasite's eggs in faeces [12], using suitable methods such as those of Lutz (Hoffman, Pons and Janner) and of Kato–Katz. Coproscopic examinations can be negative if infection is sustained by a single parasite or by males alone, or if carried out in the preoviposition period (60 days after infection). The haemogram may show eosinophilia, particularly in the larval phase of the disease [5,9,10].

Helminths in the biliary system can be detected by ultrasonography; with this technique, it is possible to observe their movements in the gallbladder or in the larger ducts. The parasites appear as long, linear or curved, strongly echogenic structures, very often with an acoustic shadow. The imaging can also show dilatation of the biliary system, and can confirm the presence of gallbladder oedema, single or multiple hepatic abscesses or oedematous pancreatitis [5,13].

CT and retrogade endoscopic cholangiography are also useful in diagnosing hepatobiliary ascariasis. Liver histology can occasionally reveal granulomas around the helminth's eggs.

Treatment

Intestinal ascariasis can be treated with various anthelminthic drugs:

1 Mebendazole – oral dose of 100 mg twice daily for 3 days or a single dose of 600 mg orally, independently of body weight.
2 Albendazole – single oral dose of 400 mg for adults and a 10 mg/kg dose for children.
3 Levamisole (or tetramisole) – single oral dose of 150 mg for adults and 80 mg for children.

Any treatment results in a high cure rate, generally above 90%. In cases of intestinal obstruction, piperazine salts (50–100 mg/kg/day) delivered by nasogastric probe should be used; they act on the myoneural junction of the helminths, producing paralysis and facilitating elimination of the bolus by peristaltic movements. Treatment of the hepatolithiasis associated with biliary ascariasis involves the endoscopic extraction of the helminths and the calculi from the larger biliary ducts with or without sphincterotomy. A partial hepatectomy is sometimes required in cases with serious complications. Of note, in hyperendemic regions, sphincterotomy has the disadvantage that it allows the helminths to reach the biliary system more easily in future reinfections. Anthelminthic therapy over a prolonged period (with albendazole, for example) is needed in most cases of hepatobiliary ascariasis.

Prevention and control

Measures for controlling ascariasis are primarily aimed at reducing the prevalence and severity of infection by means of basic sanitation, health education, disinfection and treatment of carriers, which is essential to eliminate sources of infection in the population. The last procedure appears to be the simplest and most efficient for interrupting the epidemiological chain of the parasitosis. Campaigns against the parasite endemia should promote treatment on a widespread scale, primarily in small communities. It is important to administer the anthelminthic agent in a single dose every 1 or 2 months for at least 1 year in order to reduce the prevalence of the disease to reasonably acceptable levels.

Visceral larva migrans

Introduction

The 'larva migrans' syndrome was first identified and proposed as a term in 1952 by Beaver *et al.* when they described the clinical picture in American children of hepatomegaly, pulmonary manifestations, severe eosinophilia and ascarid larvae at liver biopsy. This syndrome is caused by the erratic migration of nematode larvae across the organs of non-natural (paratenic) hosts such as man, where the parasite's normal cycle is not completed and is blocked at the larval stage. Various helminths may be responsible for this syndrome. The most common are ascarid parasites of dogs and cats that belong to the genera *Toxocara* (*T. canis*, *T. cati*) and *Toxascaris*. In addition, *Gnathostoma spinigerum*, *Ancylostoma caninum* and *Angyostrongylus costaricencis* can cause the 'larva migrans' syndrome by erratic migration in man. *T. canis* is the most important agent of this disease in Latin American countries, and the term toxocariasis has become synonymous with visceral 'larva migrans' in the literature [14].

Epidemiology

T. canis infects a large percentage of canids throughout the world, particularly in tropical and subtropical regions. The transmission to man is by ingestion of the nematode's eggs containing third-stage larvae. Development of disease in humans depends on a high concentration of *T. canis* eggs in the soil, a situation commonly found in areas with large numbers of dogs. Public places frequented by large numbers of people and animals favour transmission of the disease, with children being particularly at risk as they have frequent contact with the soil while playing games. The eggs must remain in the soil for 2–5 weeks to become infective. Habits such as geophagia and onychophagia increase the risk of contracting the disease. The incidence of anti-*Toxocara* antibodies is higher in individuals who keep dogs at home. Population studies using serology (ELISA) have shown a prevalence of 1–5% in the general population, with a distinctly higher prevalence among children and adolescents. The ingestion of raw or poorly cooked meat and/or offal from animals that are paratenic hosts to *T. canis* (poultry and rabbits) has been suspected as a means of transmission of the parasitosis to man [14].

Life cycle

The normal life cycle of the helminth is not completed in man. After ingestion, the larvae are released in the small intestine, penetrate the mucosa, enter the portal circulation, reach the liver and, from there, the lungs, heart, central nervous system and ocular globe. The eggs and larvae are not detectable in faeces [14,15].

Pathogenesis and pathology

The presence of the larvae causes local reactions of an immunoallergic nature in the different human organs, attributable mainly to their death. The parasites also stimulate a humoral and cellular immune response. The *Toxocara* antibodies appear at an early stage and belong to the IgM, IgG and IgE classes. Their appearance is accompanied by marked peripheral eosinophilia, reflecting a type Th$_2$ immunocellular response. Pathological changes are most common in the liver, although other organs can show significant changes as well. Macroscopically, the organ increases in volume, with sinuous lesions about 2–5 cm in size on the surface. Small nodules, spread throughout the liver, can sometimes be observed (Fig. 5). Microscopically, there is an extensive inflammatory process, with areas of necrosis and cellular infiltrate composed of eosinophils and Charcot–Leyden crystals; sometimes, real eosinophilic abscesses are formed.

An important inflammatory reaction also develops around the larvae, consisting of granulomas made up of histocytes, giant cells, lymphocytes, plasmocytes and eosinophils (Fig. 6). These lesions may occasionally progress to become fibrous nodules or even simulate neoplastic processes. Biliary ductopenia and cholestasis may be observed on rare occasions. The larvae (or their remnants) cannot easily be seen in ordinary histological preparations, and a large number of histological sections may be needed to detect their presence [11,14,16,17]. However, immunohistological techniques can reveal the presence of parasite antigens in liver cuts and can confirm the diagnosis.

Clinical picture: hepatobiliary involvement

The clinical picture of visceral 'larva migrans' varies depending on the parasitic load, length of infection and location of the larvae in the tissues. Most infections are asymptomatic and probably occur in all age groups. The symptomatology consists of fever, fatigue, pruriginous skin rash, abdominal pain, nausea, vomiting, diarrhoea, weight loss and hepatosplenomegaly [17]. Pulmonary symptoms such as coughing, dyspnoea and

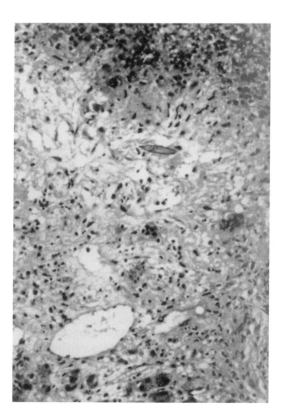

Fig. 6 Liver biopsy in a case of visceral larva migrans. Florid reaction made up of extensive necrosis of the liver parenchyma, an eosinophilic infiltrate and many fragments of larval bodies, some phagocytosed by foreign body giant cells (haematoxylin and eosin) (courtesy of Dr Luiz Carlos C. Gayotto).

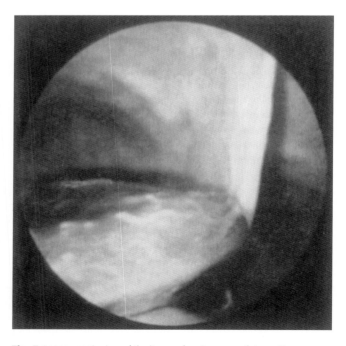

Fig. 5 Laparoscopic view of the liver surface in a case of visceral larva migrans. Typical serpiginous lesions (courtesy of Dr Raimundo Llanio).

expectoration are common and probably reflect migration of the larvae to the lungs. A picture of progressive cholestatic jaundice has been reported [16,18]. Less common manifestations include cardiac dysfunction, nephrotic syndrome and neurological manifestations (epilepsy, paresia and transverse myelitis). The association between visceral 'larva migrans' and deep abscesses has been confirmed in recent years in experimental and clinical studies. Hepatic, renal and muscular abscesses (tropical pyomyositis) have been attributed to toxocariasis in tropical areas where the parasitosis is common [16,19]. The lesions induced by the larvae can predispose to the appearance of staphylococcal infections. Larvae in the ocular globe can lead to loss of sight [11,14,17].

Laboratory findings include occasional anaemia, leucocytosis with intense eosinophilia, hypergammaglobulinaemia and an increase in hepatic enzymes, in particular alkaline phosphatase and γ-glutamyl-transferase [16]. Imaging methods can be used to demonstrate hepatic involvement [20]; ultrasonography shows single or multiple hypoechoic lesions in one or both lobes that can progress to hyperechoic lesions. On CT, these hepatic lesions appear as hypodense nodules and, in nuclear magnetic resonance, as lesions with a low-intensity signal on T1 and a high-intensity signal on T2. The differential diagnosis should include primary or secondary neoplastic lesions of the liver; other granulomatous diseases, such as tuberculosis and sarcoidosis, should also be considered [19,20].

Diagnosis

Visceral 'larva migrans' is not easy to diagnose. The larvae can be found in hepatic tissue obtained by biopsy, but it is often difficult to identify them. Immunohistochemical techniques applied to the tissue are extremely helpful in confirming the diagnosis [21].

Serological diagnosis is important, and enzyme-linked immunosorbent assay (ELISA) techniques using *Toxocara* larvae secretor/excretor antigens are widely used in clinical practice. In regions where ascariasis is endemic, sera must be treated with *Ascaris* antigens beforehand to increase the reaction's specificity [22,23].

Indirect haemagglutination and agar gel double diffusion have also been used to diagnose visceral 'larva migrans', but they have low sensitivity. Alternatively, the assay for *Toxocara* larva-specific IgE has good sensitivity. A Western blot technique has been developed and is a possible diagnostic option in daily clinical practice [22].

Treatment

One 50-mg/kg/day dose of thiabendazole taken orally for 10 days is the treatment of choice for visceral 'larva migrans'. This drug inhibits migration of the larvae through the tissues and contributes to an inflammatory reaction against the parasite. Symptomatic patients should be treated. There is controversy as to whether treatment should be given to patients with few or no symptoms. Other drugs such as diethylcarbamazine, albendazole, levamisole and ivermectin can also be used to kill or immobilize the helminth in the tissues [22]. Corticosteroids can be useful in serious cases involving the lungs, central nervous system or ocular globe. The signs and symptoms of disease usually disappear within a few weeks, but eosinophilia may persist for months after treatment. Deaths are rare and, in most patients, the course of the disease is benign [17].

Prevention and control

Prevention of visceral 'larva migrans' depends on the control of canine infection and contamination of the soil by *T. canis* eggs. Treatment of dogs and cats with imidazolic derivatives is very efficient; it should be carried out regularly in order to eradicate the adult parasites from animals. Puppies and kittens should also be treated from 3 weeks of age on. Various countries now adopt legislation which makes dog and cat owners responsible for removing and cleaning up pet wastes in public places. This step has been efficacious in reducing contamination of the soil with *T. canis* eggs. It is also important to eliminate stray dogs and cats from city streets and squares. Health education with information to the population of the risks of owning a dog carrying the nematodes in the house is fundamental in controlling this helminthiasis [17].

Strongyloidiasis

Introduction

Strongyloidiasis is a helminthiasis prevalent in some tropical areas of the world. Its importance, as an intestinal parasitosis, is related to the severity of its lesions and dissemination in multiple organs. Severe forms of the infection occur primarily in immunodepressed individuals.

Epidemiology

Strongyloidiasis is endemic in tropical areas of Africa, Asia and the Americas, in particular in populations from poor socioeconomic backgrounds. Strongyloidiasis is also endemic in some European countries and central areas of the United States, although the prevalence in these regions is low. Countries with the highest rates of parasitism in the Americas are Peru, Brazil, Chile and Colombia. Suitable environmental conditions, a temperature between 25°C and 30°C and sandy soil are essential for the development of the two different phases (free-living and parasitic stage) of the parasite life cycle.

Man plays an important role in transmitting the infection as he is the only host of *S. stercoralis*. Animals do not function as reservoirs of the human disease. Lack of sanitary facilities, defaecation in the peridomicile area, ingestion of contaminated food and water and the habit of not wearing shoes are essential factors in the transmission of this parasitosis [15].

Life cycle

The life cycle of this helminth has two different patterns. In the direct cycle, the filariform larvae, which are eliminated in the faeces of the carrier, penetrate the skin or mucosa, enter the circulatory system and cross the lungs, where they rupture into the pulmonary alveoli. They then ascend to the pharynx through the bronchi, are swallowed and subsequently mature into adult parthenogenetic females in the small intestine. Oviposition starts and rhabditoid larvae hatch from the eggs while in the intestinal lumen. The larvae are then eliminated in the faeces. They may sometimes transform into filariform larvae in the lumen of the small intestine, subsequently penetrating the mucosa and completing the pulmonary cycle. This type of life cycle is called internal autoinfection. In most cases, however, the rhabditoid larvae eliminated by the faeces to the soil develop into free-living males and females, which in turn produce rhabditoid larvae again. After two moults, rhabditoid larvae transform into filariform larvae which can infect man (indirect cycle). Filariform larvae that reach the perianal region when faeces are passed can cause autoinfection by penetrating the skin in this area [24].

Pathology

Autoinfection allows the parasitosis to persist for decades in the human body. Immunodepression can accelerate the life cycle of the parasite, increasing the parasitic load and disseminating filariform larvae to many organs. This 'hyperinfection' was reported in patients with severe malnutrition, those who use corticosteroids in large doses, transplant recipients, lymphoma and acquired immune deficiency syndrome (AIDS) patients. The presence of eggs and helminths in the mucosa and submucosa of the small intestine results in a significant inflammatory reaction, which may lead to extensive, usually superficial ulcerations. In massive infections, the stomach and colon can also be involved. Intestinal microorganisms may superinfect mucosal ulcerations and cause bacteraemia and remote infections.

In the liver, the larvae are found in the portal tracts, in the periportal areas and even inside the intrahepatic veins. They are generally surrounded by an eosinophilic infiltrate or by a granulomatous reaction rich in eosinophils. Miliary granulomas without the larva can also be found (Fig. 7). Although necrosis of hepatocytes is rare, areas of steatosis and discrete cholestasis are common. The larvae have a characteristic appearance, with double lateral alae, which is easily recognized at histology [24–26].

Clinical picture: hepatobiliary involvement

Most individuals infected by S. stercoralis are asymptomatic or oligosymptomatic. Passage of the larvae through the lungs may result in pneumonitis, with asthmatiform manifestations and peripheral eosinophilia. The duodenum and proximal jejunum are the segments of the small intestine preferred by the parasite;

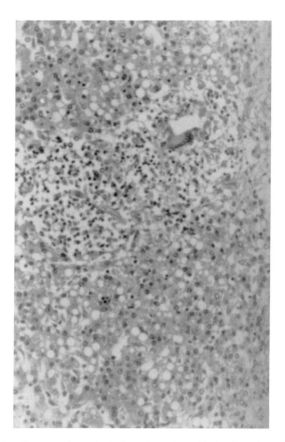

Fig. 7 Miliary granulomas in the liver of a patient with the disseminated form of strongyloidiasis: a giant cell, a few epithelioid cells, a dense eosinophilic infiltrate and fragments of the larva in a loose arrangement. There is fatty change in the parenchyma (haematoxylin and eosin) (courtesy of Dr Maria de Fatima Araujo).

it may also be found, sometimes in large numbers, in the terminal ileum and colon. Symptomatic patients complain of epigastric pain, anorexia, nausea, vomiting, abdominal distension and prolonged diarrhoea. In patients with a high parasitic load, diarrhoea may be intense, voluminous and malabsorptive in nature, with steatorrhoea and enteric protein loss. In the disseminated form of the disease ('hyperinfection syndrome'), bronchopulmonary symptoms and fever, the latter arising from the presence of larvae in multiple organs, can be observed in addition to gastrointestinal symptoms. Hepatobiliary manifestations include hepatomegaly and cholestatic jaundice. The latter can be the result of biliary obstruction due to papillary stenosis, which can resolve with specific treatment [25]. Usually, many larvae can be found in the bile. Laboratory tests demonstrate increases in alkaline phosphatase, γ-glutamyl-transferase and aminotransferases. Cross-infective hepatitis of bacterial origin and pyogenic hepatic abscesses can develop during disseminated strongyloidiasis because, on leaving the intestine, the larvae carry Gram-negative bacteria in their tegument that cause bacteraemia and severe sepsis [25,26].

Diagnosis

Strongyloidiasis can be diagnosed [27] by detecting the helminth larvae in the faeces using suitable methods such as the Baerman–Moraes or modified Rugai techniques. These techniques are very sensitive and are based on the thermotropism and hydrotropism of the parasite larvae. At least three samples of faeces are needed to achieve maximum sensitivity. Coproculture techniques are more sensitive and can be used to detect different phases of the helminth's life cycle. The best known are the Harada–Mori and agar plate techniques. Larvae can also be detected in other organic fluids such as the duodenal contents, obtained by endoscopy, and respiratory secretions collected during bronchoscopy procedures. Serology is rarely used and is useful only in epidemiological studies in endemic areas [23].

Treatment

Few drugs are available to treat strongyloidiasis. The most often used are:
1 thiabendazole – 50 mg/kg/day (maximum 3 g/day) for 3 days;
2 cambendazole – 5 mg/kg/single dose;
3 albendazole – 400 mg twice daily for 3–5 days;
4 ivermectin – 200 μg/kg/single dose.

These drugs have variable cure rates of between 85% and 95%. Patients with the disseminated form should take thiabendazole or albendazole for an extended period (up to 10 days). A 200 μg/kg dose of ivermectin on days 1, 2, 15 and 16 is recommended for patients with AIDS. Clinical and parasitological cure has been reported with this dosage in most cases. The therapeutic efficacy can be evaluated by parasitological examination on the 7th, 14th and 21st days after treatment.

In the systemic forms of the disease, broad-spectrum antibiotics (cephalosporins and quinolones) must be used in conjunction with anthelminthic agents to fight associated bacterial infections.

Capillariasis

Introduction

Hepatic capillariasis is caused by the nematode *Capillaria hepatica*. Another species of the genus, *Capillaria philippinensis*, is found in the small intestine of humans and can cause chronic and malabsorptive diarrhoea. The hepatic form of the disease is rare in humans, and few cases have been reported. The parasite can be found in the liver of rats, squirrels, dogs, beavers and some primates. Man is probably an accidental host.

Epidemiology

By the end of the twentieth century, only 32 cases of this disease had been published. This is somewhat surprising in view of the high prevalence of infection among domestic rodents, which are in close contact with human populations living in poor conditions. Many cases go undetected. Sometimes, the infection is discovered only at necropsy or biopsy of suspected cases. Cases of human infection have been described in different parts of the world, including Brazil [10].

Life cycle

The non-embryonated eggs of *C. hepatica* are released from the carcasses of infected animals; they may also be eliminated in the faeces of rodents or humans. The eggs embryonate in the environment and become infective to humans approximately 2–6 weeks later. Infection occurs mainly in small children, who occasionally practise geophagia. When the eggs reach the caecum, they release the larvae, which cross the intestinal mucosa, enter the portal system and lodge in the liver. They mature in this organ, become adults in around 3 weeks and start oviposition. When they die, they release a large number of eggs in the parenchyma [28–30].

Pathology

The liver is enlarged and its surface shows small 0.1–0.2 cm yellowish granulomatous nodules surrounded by an area of induration up to 3 cm in diameter. Granulomas made up of epithelioid and giant cells can be found surrounding the eggs and necrotic remains of the parasite [28]. Experimental studies in rodents indicate that the nematode can induce the formation of a long, thin, septal fibrosis in acinar zone III of the liver, starting about 30 days after the oral contamination with the embryonated eggs. The fibrosis increases progressively and can lead to cirrhosis. The presence of sequestered parasitic antigens, which are probably released slowly in the liver, appears to be the most important factor in the pathogenesis of septal fibrosis [29–31].

Clinical picture

Commonly observed clinical symptoms in hepatic capillariasis are persistent fever, hepatosplenomegaly and hypereosinophilia. Visceral larva migrans, acute schistosomiasis and the larval phase of some intestinal parasitoses (ascariasis, ancylostomiasis and strongyloidiasis) should be considered in the differential diagnosis. In most cases, liver function tests are altered, with pronounced increases in cholestatic enzymes (alkaline phosphatase and GGT) and aminotransferases [3,29,30].

Diagnosis and treatment

In exceptional cases, the diagnosis may be based on the identification of operculated and striated eggs of *C. hepatica* in faeces, but the vast majority are based on histopathology, on a liver biopsy. Granulomas surrounding the eggs and the remnants of the helminth, associated with extensive septal fibrosis, confirm the diagnosis [3,29–31].

There is no consensus regarding treatment because of the small number of cases published. Good results were described in Brazil and Germany with thiabendazole, albendazole and ivermectin. Adding corticosteroids can help to reduce the inflammatory reaction in the liver [3,29].

Pentastomiasis

Introduction

Pentastomiasis (or porocephalosis) is induced by hae-matophagous endoparasites of vermiform appearance that belong to the phylum Arthropoda. Two families are of medical interest: Linguatulidae, with the species *Linguatula serrata*, and Porocephalidae, with the species *Armillifer* (or *Porocephalus*) *armillatus* [32,33].

Epidemiology

The adult parasites live in the respiratory tract of carnivorous animals and snakes. The larval stage can occasionally be found in man. Human infection has been described in various countries. Cases have been confirmed in the Americas (the United States, Canada, Panama, Brazil, etc.), Europe (Switzerland and Germany), Southeast Asia and Africa (Zaire and Nigeria). Infestation can be found in up to 2.2% of autopsies in some areas of Malaysia and Africa [30–33].

Life cycle

Adult parasites attach with their hooks to the respiratory tract of the final host and feed on epithelial cells, blood, lymph and mucous. They are of different sex; males are smaller. The fertilized eggs are eliminated in the nasal secretions, saliva and faeces of carnivores and snakes, and may be ingested by various intermediate hosts, including man. The eggs release first-stage larvae in the intestine, which penetrate the bowel wall and reach the liver. There they undergo nine moults in 6 months and form third-stage larvae or infective nymphs which then become encysted. The larva grows progressively and can behave like a space-occupying lesion inside the parenchyma of the liver. The larva usually dies with time; occasionally, it can escape from the cyst and invade the peritoneal cavity [30,32,34].

Pathogenesis and pathology

The death of the larva may result in a prominent inflammatory reaction that subsequently undergoes calcification. The infection is usually discovered by chance during radiological investigations, surgery or autopsy. Nymphs may cause disease depending on their location, the number of parasites and where they have migrated to. The encysted nymph in the liver is surrounded by a dense fibrous tissue and is often calcified. Granulomas develop around the remnants of the disintegrated parasite and are generally necrotic. Pyogenic abscesses may occasionally form around the larvae [30,32,34].

Clinical picture

The clinical picture varies from subclinical to a serious illness presenting as pneumonitis, intestinal obstruction, biliary obstruction with cholestasis, hepatic abscess, meningitis and pericarditis. Calcifications are typically 5 mm in diameter, elongate or rounded; they may be found in several organs. Humans are highly tolerant to this infection. Peripheral eosinophilia is almost always present in all the clinical forms of the disease [33,34].

Diagnosis and treatment

Diagnosis of pentastomiasis is based on the detection of parasite nymphs in tissue during autopsy or surgery, or at biopsy. A serological test has been developed in France, but its role in diagnosis has yet to be determined [34,35].

Pentastomiasis does not need to be treated. Curative surgery can be carried out in cases where the lesions take up space in organ parenchymas. Antibiotics may be required for secondary pyogenic complications [32,35].

References

1 Crompton DW (2001) Ascaris and ascariasis. *Adv Parasitol* 48, 285–375.
2 Hsu FH (1962) Clinical observation on 110 cases of *Ascaris* invasion into the biliary tract. *Nagoya J Med Sci* 24, 215–233.
3 Pereira VG, França LCM (1983) Successful treatment of *Capillaria hepática* infection in an acutely ill adult. *Am J Trop Med Hyg* 32, 1272–1274.
4 Fogaça HS, Oliveira CS, Barbosa HT *et al.* (2000) Liver pseudotumor: a rare manifestation of hepatic granulomata caused by *Ascaris lumbricoides* ova. *Am J Gastroenterol* 95, 2099–2101.
5 Khuroo MS (2001) Hepatobiliary and pancreatic ascariasis. *Ind J Gastroenterol* 20, C 28–32.
6 Leung JW, Yu AS (1997) Hepatolithiasis and biliary parasites. *Baillières Clin Gastroenterol* 11, 681–706.
7 Pilankar KS, Amarapurkar AD, Joshi RM *et al.* (2003) Hepatolithiasis with biliary ascariasis – a case report. *BMC Gastroenterol* 3, 35–39.
8 Khuroo MS, Zargar SA (1985) Biliary ascariasis. A common cause of biliary and pancreatic disease in an endemic area. *Gastroenterology* 88, 418–423.
9 Khuroo MS, Zargar SA, Mahajan R *et al.* (1987) Sonographic appearances in biliary ascariasis. *Gastroenterology* 93, 267–272.
10 Khuroo MS, Zargar SA, Mahajan R (1990) Hepatobiliary and pancreatic ascariasis in India. *Lancet* 335, 1503–1506.
11 Ehrhard T, Kernbaum S (1979) *Toxocara canis* et toxocarose humaine. *Bull Inst Pasteur* 77, 225–287.
12 Hall A, Holland C (2000) Geographical variation of *Ascaris lumbricoides* fecundity and its implications for helminth control. *Parasitol Today* 16, 540–544.
13 Khuroo MS, Zargar SA, Yatoo GN *et al.* (1993) Worm extraction and

biliary drainage in hepatobiliary and pancreatic ascariasis. *Gastrointest Endosc* 39, 680–685.

14 Beaver PC (1969) The nature of visceral larva migrans. *J Parasitol* 55, 3–12.

15 Glickman LT, Schantz PM (1981) Epidemiology and pathogenesis of zoonotic toxocariasis. *Epidemiol Rev* 3, 230–250.

16 Gonzalez MT, Ibanez O, Balcarce N *et al.* (2000) Toxocariasis with liver involvement. *Acta Gastroenterol Latinoamer* 30, 187–190.

17 Zinkham WH (1978) Visceral larva migrans. A review and reassessment indicating two forms of clinical expression: visceral and ocular. *Am J Dis Child* 132, 627–633.

18 Hartleb M, Januszewski K (2001) Severe hepatic involvement in visceral larva migrans. *Eur J Gastroenterol Hepatol* 13, 1245–1249.

19 Rayes AA, Lambertucci JR (1999) The association between human toxocariasis and pyogenic abscesses. *Rev Soc Bras Med Trop* 32, 425–438.

20 Azuma K, Yashiro N, Kinoshita T *et al.* (2002) Hepatic involvement of visceral larva migrans due to *Toxocara canis*: a case report – CT and MR findings. *Radiat Med* 20, 89–92.

21 De Brito T, Chieffi PP, Peres BA *et al.* (1994) Immunohistochemical detection of toxocaral antigens in human liver biopsies. *Int J Surg Pathol* 2(2), 117–124.

22 Bahia V, Sarin SK (1994). Hepatic visceral larva migrans: evolution of the lesion, diagnosis and role of high-dose albendazole therapy. *Am J Gastroenterol* 89, 624–627.

23 Glickman L, Schantz P, Dombroske R *et al.* (1978) Evaluation of serodiagnostic tests for visceral larva migrans. *Am J Trop Med Hyg* 27, 492–498.

24 Haque AK, Schnadig V, Rubin SA *et al.* (1994) Pathogenesis of human strongyloidiasis: autopsy and quantitative parasitological analysis. *Mod Pathol* 7, 276–288.

25 Delaracque Astagnau E, Hadengue A *et al.* (1994) Biliary obstruction resulting from *Strongyloides stercoralis* infection: report of a case. *Gut* 35, 705–707.

26 Poltera AA, Katsimbura N (1974) Granulomatous hepatitis due to *Strongyloides stercoralis*. *J Pathol* 113, 241–245.

27 Siddigui AA, Berk SL (2002) Diagnosis of *Strongyloides stercoralis* infection. *Clin Infect Dis* 34, 1280–1281.

28 Galvão VA (1981) *Capillaria hepatica*: an evaluation of its pathogenic role in man. *Mem Inst Oswaldo Cruz* 76, 415–433.

29 Pannenbecker J, Miller TC, Muller J *et al.* (1990) Severe liver involvement by *Capillaria hepatica*. *Monastsschr Kinderheilkd* 138, 767–771.

30 Sawamura R, Fernandes MI, Peres LC *et al.* (1999) Hepatic capillariasis in children: report of 3 cases in Brazil. *Am J Trop Med Hyg* 61, 642–647.

31 Ferreira LA, Andrade ZA (1993) *Capillaria hepatica*: a cause of septal fibrosis of the liver. *Mem Inst Oswaldo Cruz* 88, 441–447.

32 Nzeh DA, Akinlemibola JK, Nzeh GC (1996) Incidence of *Armillifer armillatus* (pentastome) calcification in the abdomen. *Central Afr J Med* 42, 29–31.

33 Prathap K, Lau KS, Bolton JM (1969) Pentastomiasis: a common finding at autopsy among Malaysian aborigines. *Am J Trop Med Hyg* 18, 20–27.

34 Self JT, Hopps HC, Olufemi Williams A (1975) Pentastomiasis in Africans. *Trop Geogr Med* 27, 1–13.

35 Smith JA, Oladiran B, Lagundoye SB *et al.* (1975) Pentastomiasis and malignancy. *Ann Trop Med Parasitol* 69, 503–512.

Index

non-alcoholic steatohepatitis 1198
primary sclerosing cholangitis 1106,
1490
proteomics 414
simple cyst of the liver 784
Agilent Bioanalyser, RNA quality 402,
402f
agmatinase 182
agnogenic myeloid metaplasia (primary
myelofibrosis) 1665
AIDS
cholangitis 1546
cryptococcosis 1014
granulomas 1713
histoplasmosis 1015
penicillinosis 1017
vanishing bile duct syndrome 1115
see also HIV infection
ajmaline
acute hepatitis induction 1230
prolonged cholestasis induction
1254
Alagille syndrome 1387, 1805,
1848–1849, 2124–2125
clinical features 1805, 1848–1849
facial features 1848
growth hormone resistance 1741
management 1849
vanishing bile duct syndrome 1112,
1114t, 1115
AL amyloidosis
clinical manifestations 1704
hepatic involvement 1705
management 1707
pathogenesis 1702
systemic 1703–1704
alanine
ammonia production 181
glucogenic properties 145
alanine aminotransferase (ALT)
451–453
abnormal values
hepatobiliary diseases 452, 453f
nonhepatobiliary diseases 452–453
acalculous cholecystitis 1950
alcoholic cirrhosis 1166
alcoholic macrovesicular steatosis
1160
assays 451–452
Budd–Chiari syndrome 1406, 1407
cirrhosis 612
cocaine users 1232
distribution 451
drug-induced acute hepatitis 1216
hepatic *vs.* cholestatic disease 1900
hepatitis A 859–860
hepatitis C, acute 886
hepatitis E diagnosis 895
hyperbilirubinaemia, postoperative
1949
hypothyroidism 1685
ischaemic hepatitis 1610, 1949
localization 451
non-alcoholic fatty liver disease
1199
non-alcoholic steatohepatitis 1199
normal values 452
postoperative drug-induced liver
injury 1949
primary sclerosing cholangitis 1105
reactions 451
sepsis-induced cholestasis 1950
tacrine 1240

total parental nutrition-induced
cholestasis 1950
type 2 diabetes mellitus 1681
albendazole
alveolar echinococcosis 1055
ascariasis 1061
Clonorchis sinensis 1046
cystic echinococcosis 1055
strongyloidiasis 1065
Albuferon, chronic hepatitis C 942, 951
albumin 250–255, 454–455
alcoholic hepatitis 1163
assays 454
bilirubin binding 170
cirrhosis 454–455, 612, 674
cirrhotic ascites 667
clinical usefulness 455
conformational adaptation 251
conformational breathing 251
cortisol binding 1752
electrophoresis 454
endoderm hepatic specification 65
functions 454
oncotic 253
hepatobiliary disease 454–455
hepatorenal syndrome prevention 717
infusion
spontaneous bacterial peritonitis
764
volume expansion 1728
ligands bound 250–251, 251t
nonhepatobiliary disease 454
normal values 454
renal hypoperfusion 1725
sex hormone binding 1755
structure 251
synthesis, influencing factors 454
testosterone binding 1687
thyroid hormone binding 1684, 1747,
1747t
albumin dialysis
alcoholic hepatitis 1165
hepatorenal syndrome type 1 716
Albumin gene 65
alcohol
absorption 1135
abstinence 1179–1185
alcoholic cirrhosis 1167
chronic hepatitis C 890
cognitive behavioural treatment
1180–1181
controlled drinking *vs.* 1179–1180
maintenance, long-tern 1180–1182
pharmacological agents 1181–1182
combinations 1182
pre-surgery 1171
pre-transplant 1183
altered substrate utilization 1838
clearance, age-related changes 1873
consumption 1129–1130, 1129t
beverage type 1130
gamma-glutamyl transpeptidase
levels 464
retinoid depletion 217
dependence
definition 1179
diagnosis 1179
distribution 1135
dose, risk of liver disease 1142
estrogen receptors 1759
excretion 1135
fibrosis 1141, 1142t

hepatic blood flow 77
hepatocellular carcinoma 1438–1439
hepatotoxicity 413, 1379–1380
insulin secretion 1735
intestinal protein loss 1837
iron metabolism, effects on 1769
leucocyte abnormalities 1770
lipid storage disease induction 1246
liver injury 1135t
metabolism 1135–1136, 1837
alcoholic liver disease pathogenesis
1136–1139
altered redox state 1136–1137
antibodies to 1140–1141
chronic consumption and 1136
fatty liver 1136–1138, 1137f
oxidation sites 1135
oxidation to acetaldehyde
1135–1136
zero-order kinetics 1135
mitochondria, effects on 413,
1379–1380
nutrient malabsorption 1837
selenium deficiency 235
spermatogenesis 1756
testosterone production 1756
total plasma calcium levels 1750
units 1135
vitamin B12 absorption 1769
withdrawal 1179–1185
ambulatory 1180
elderly 1873
institutional setting 1180
Zieve syndrome 1770
alcohol dehydrogenase (ADH)
alcohol oxidation 1136
cirrhosis 681
polymorphism, alcoholic liver disease
and 358
stomach 1135
alcoholic cardiomyopathy 1185–1186,
1613
liver transplantation 1185–1186
alcoholic cirrhosis 1165–1167
abstinence 1167
alpha-1-antitrypsin 1153
bile secretion impairment 1153
clinical presentation 1165
extrahepatic manifestations 1162t,
1165
definition 1165
diagnosis 1166
elderly 1873
endocrine dysfunction 1165, 1758,
1820
feminization 1758
gastro-oesophageal reflux 1798
glomerulonephritis 1817t
haemodynamic studies 1166
hepatic venous pressures 568
hepatocellular carcinoma 1153
hepatorenal syndrome type 1 676
imaging 1166
laboratory values 1166
large-cell hepatocellular dysplasia
1153
leucocyte abnormalities 1771
liver biopsy 1166
liver transplantation 1183–1184
macronodular 1153, 1153f
malnutrition 1165–1166
pathogenesis 1165–1166
micronodular 1152–1153, 1152f

mixed micronodular and
macronodular 1153
mortality 1130–1132, 1130f, 1179
alcohol intake 1131–1132
beverage type 1131, 1132f
dose consumed 1132
natural history 1159, 1165
neurological manifestations 1824t
pathogenesis 1165
pathology 1152–1153
prognosis 1164t, 1166–1167
prostate 1820
regression 1153
renal tubular acidosis 1819–1820
renal tubular necrosis 702
resting energy expenditure 1837
small-cell hepatocellular dysplasia
1153
surgery 1171
thyroid hormones 1748t
treatment 1167
alcoholic clear cells 423
alcoholic fatty liver disease (AFLD) *see*
alcoholic liver disease (ALD)
alcoholic foamy degeneration 428,
1246
alcoholic hepatitis 1161–1165, 1195
alcohol abstinence 1164
anti-TNFα agents 1164–1165
clinical diagnosis 1163
clinical examination 1161–1162
clinical features 1161–1162
definition 1161
differential diagnosis 1163
enteral nutrition 1908
extrahepatic manifestations 1162,
1162t
haemodynamic studies 568, 569, 1163
hepatocellular lesions 1149–1150
hepatocyte apoptosis 341, 1149, 1150f
hepatorenal syndrome prevention 717
histology 430, 1152
imaging 1163
induced hepatocytes 1149f, 1150
inflammatory infiltration 1150–1152,
1151f
laboratory values 1162–1163
liver transplantation 1183
malnutrition 1906
clinical outcome 1907
management 1839
markedly active 1152
minimal 1152
moderately active 1152
natural history 1158–1159
non-alcoholic steatohepatitis *vs.* 1161
oxidative stress 1169
pathogenesis 1161
pathology 1148–1152, 1161
pericellular fibrosis 1151, 1151f
prognosis 1163–1164, 1164t
progression to cirrhosis 1152
scoring systems 436
surgery 1171
treatment 1164–1165
tumour necrosis factor 313
alcoholic hyaline *see* Mallory bodies
alcoholic liver disease (ALD) 1127–1190
alcoholic hepatitis *see* alcoholic
hepatitis
animal models
baboons 409–410
gene array data 411

cutaneous manifestations 1806
neurological signs 1362
type 3 (juvenile/norbottnian) 1362,
2135
type 3A 1362
type 3B 1362
type 3C 1362
GBE1 gene mutations 1374
Gc protein, acute liver failure 1302
gelatinases, extracellular matrix
degradation 270
gelophysic dysplasia 2136
gemcitabine, gallbladder carcinoma
1580
gemfibrozil, hepatotoxicity 1232
GenBank, proteome complexity and 412
GenBank human UniGene clusters 407
gender
alcoholic liver disease 1132–1133,
1142, 1159
cystic fibrosis 1338
drug-induced liver injury 1212–1213
gallstone disease 1523
hepatitis B infection 865
hepatocellular carcinoma 1437
liver cysts, ADPKD 790
primary biliary cirrhosis 1071
primary sclerosing cholangitis 1106
simple cyst of the liver 784
gene arrays 399–403, 400f
alcoholic liver disease 409–410
assumptions 412
autoimmune hepatitis 410
biases 406, 412
biliary atresia 410
cholangiocarcinoma 411
comparative hybridization 399f, 401,
403
cystic fibrosis 410
definition 399
experimental design 400–401, 400f
biological replicates 401, 401f
technical replicates 401, 401f
future directions 414
gene expression profile
('transcriptome') 398f, 399, 407
hepatitis B 409
hepatitis C 407–409, 408t
hepatocellular carcinoma 409,
410–411
in liver disease 407–411, 408t
MIAME guidelines 399–400, 402
multiplexing 415
non-alcoholic fatty liver disease 410
normal human liver 407, 408t
one-probe 399f, 403
platforms 403
primary biliary cirrhosis 410
primary sclerosing cholangitis 410
probe sources 403
proteomics *vs.* 403, 405
QTL analysis in inbred mice 379–380
hepatocellular carcinoma analysis
380
reproducibility/variability 399–400,
400f
sample preparation
labelling 403
pooling 401
RNA amplification 402–403
RNA isolation/quality 402, 402f
RNA quantities 402
SNP analysis 414
targeted 414

validation 401
see also bioinformatics
GeneChip™ 403
gene–environment interactions, liver
disease and 361, 371, 372
gene expression 90–91
analysis
high-throughput technologies *see*
gene arrays
'transcriptome' 398f
liver cell plate 90
compartmentalized expression
90–91
differential expression 90
posttranscriptional 191–195
translational control 195–196
gene–gene interactions, liver disease and
372
Gene Ontology (GO) Consortium 407
generalized pustular psoriasis 1642
gene targeting experiments, QTL
verification, mice 380
genetically modified animals
QTL analysis in inbred mice
functional testing using 380
HCC experiments 379
see also knockout animals
genetic instability, carcinogenesis
391–392
genetic polymorphism and liver disease
356–364
alcoholic liver disease 356, 357t, 358,
360t, 1142–1143, 1159
candidate gene approach 359
alcoholic liver disease 358
chronic hepatitis C
fibrosis risk and 357t, 358–359,
360t, 361, 381
IFN response and 357t, 358, 360t
drug-induced liver injury 1213
environmental interactions 361, 371,
372
genetic interactions 361
genome-wide association studies 359,
361–362, 361f
immune response genes *see*
immunogenetics, liver disease
inflammation and 369
linkage disequilibrium 360, 361
non-alcoholic fatty liver disease 356,
357t, 360t, 1198, 1201
non-alcoholic steatohepatitis 356, 1198
primary biliary cirrhosis 357t, 358,
360t, 1073–1074
quantitative trait locus and 379
see also quantitative trait locus
(QTL) analysis
study design and analysis 359–361
clinical endpoints 361, 362
controls 360
ethnicity and 360
follow-up genotyping 361
sample size 360
work flow 361–362, 361f
twin studies 358
validated markers 357t, 360t
definition 356, 362
selection 359
validation 359–360
see also individual markers
see also specific diseases
genetics and liver disease 356–383
complex (polygenic) diseases
371–383

approaches to study 372
diagnosis and 364
ethnicity/race and 360
goals of study 364
immune response genes *see*
immunogenetics, liver disease
management and 364
monogenic diseases 372
mouse models *see* mouse models of
human liver disease
pathology and 364
polymorphisms *see* genetic
polymorphism and liver disease
see also individual diseases/genes;
specific methods
genome-wide association studies 359
design 361–362, 361f
genome-wide haplotype analysis, QTL
analysis in inbred mice 377t, 378
genotyping
follow-up 361
Gaucher's disease 1363
germander (*Teucrium chamaedrys*),
hepatotoxicity 1282t, 1284,
2110–2111
ghrelin 1689
Gianotti–Crosti syndrome 1806
giant cell arteritis 1698
giant cell hepatitis, acute liver failure
1300
giant cells 1709
giant mitochondria, alcoholic hepatitis
1150, 1150f
Giardia 1020
genome project 1024
intestinal epithelium, attachment to
1023–1024
life cycle 1022
giardiasis 1020–1029
clinical manifestations 1025
diagnosis 1025–1026
epidemiology 1020–1022
host defences 1024
laboratory findings 1026
pathophysiology 1023–1024
risk factors 1021, 1021t
treatment 1026
Gilbert syndrome 460, 1355–1356
colorectal cancer risk 1356
diagnosis 1356
genetic defect 1354, 1355–1356
jaundice 1352
postoperative 1949
pregnancy 1886
Gjedde–Patlak calculation, simplified
562, 564
glafenine, acute hepatitis induction
1234
Glasgow coma scale 741t
glass beads, gene array platforms 403
glass slides, gene array platforms 403
Gleevac 596
glibenclamide
hepatotoxicity 1242
prolonged hyperglycaemia induction
1737
gliclazide 1737
gliotoxin, fibrosis 597
glipizide 1737
Glissonian territories, venous drainage 5
Glisson's capsule 9, 16
Global Alliance for Vaccines and
Immunization (GAVI), hepatitis
B vaccination programme 912

globulin
cirrhosis 612
cirrhotic ascites 667
globus pallidus, hepatic encephalopathy
732, 733f
glomerular abnormalities
cirrhosis 1817–1818
liver disease associated 1816–1820,
1817t
glomerular filtration rate
angiotensin II 677
cirrhotic ascites, post-peritoneovenous
shunting 695
hepatorenal syndrome 676, 712,
713–714
glomerulonephritis
chronic hepatitis B 871
liver disease associated 1816–1820,
1817t
glomerulus, immunoglobulin A deposits
329
glucagon
amino acid catabolism regulation 144
cirrhosis 1737–1738
glycogenolysis 130
hepatic blood flow regulation
76–77
insulin-like growth factor binding
proteins regulation 1743
liver disease 1737–1739
portal hypertension pathogenesis
634–635
secretion 129–130
cirrhotics 1738
splanchnic blood flow modulation
634–635
tumour-associated hypoglycaemia
1745
urea synthesis regulation 183
glucagon-like peptide 1735
1,4-glucan-6-glycosyl transferase
deficiency 1861
glucocorticoid receptor, hepatobiliary
transport regulation 388
glucocorticoids
insulin-like growth factor-I regulation
1742
lipid storage disease induction 1248
plasma transport 1752
thyroid stimulating hormone
suppression 1750
urea synthesis regulation 183
glucokinase (hexokinase IV) 91, 1370
gluconeogenesis (GNG) 130–131
across liver cell plate 91
cirrhosis 132
diabetes 131, 131f
insulin, effects of 129
measurement 130–131, 130f
post-overnight fast 131
regulation, efferent hepatic nerves
117–118
starvation 144
glucopalaeogenesis 145
glucose
blood concentration, across liver cell
plate 91
cholangiocyte reabsorption 53, 113
glycogen storage disease type I 1373
incretin effect 1735
intolerance
assessment 1732
cirrhosis 1732–1733
liver disease 1732–1737, 1733f

Larrea tridentata (chaparral),
    hepatotoxicity 1282t, 1285
Larsen syndrome 2143
larva
    Ascaris lumbricoides 1058
    Capillaria hepatica 1066
    Strongyloides stercoralis 1064
laryngeal cancer, alcohol consumption
    and 1186
laser capture microdissection, protein
    prefractionation and 404
laser lithotripsy, choledocholithiasis
    1531
Lassa fever 988–990
    clinical manifestations 989
    diagnosis 989–990
    epidemiology 988
    laboratory findings 989
    nosocomial infection 990
    pathogenesis 989
    pathology 989
    swollen-baby syndrome 989
    treatment 990
latent infection membrane proteins
    (LMPs), Epstein–Barr virus 964
lateral hypothalamic area
    liver function regulation 114
    parasympathetic hepatic nerves
        114–115
Laurence–Moon–Bardet–Biedl
    (Bardet–Biedl) syndrome
    2125–2126
Lawrence–Seip syndrome (Berardinelli
    syndrome) 2126
L-dopa, hepatic encephalopathy 748
lead 233t
    aminolaevulinic acid dehydrase 208
    deficiency 233t
    hepatotoxicity 1344, 2111
league tables, cost-effectiveness 2085
learning methods, unsupervised 406
lecithin 139
lecithin–cholesterol acyltransferase
    (LCAT) 139, 140f
leflunomide
    hepatotoxicity 1236, 1647–1648
    liver transplantation 2008
    mechanism of action 1647–1648
left gastric vein
    anatomy 623
    gastro-oesophageal varices inflow 627
left ventricular ejection fraction
    ascites 1722
    cirrhosis 1721
Legionella pneumophila 1002–1003
Legionnaire's disease 1002–1003, 1618
    allograft recipients 1618
    treatment 1002–1003
leiomyosarcoma 1460–1461
Leishmania chagasi 1035t
Leishmania donovani 1035, 1035t
Leishmania infantum 1035t, 1036
Leishmania tropica 1035
leptin
    non-alcoholic steatohepatitis 611
    stellate cell fibrogenesis 594
Leptospira interrogans 1008
leptospirosis 1007–1008
    animal hosts 1008
    clinical features 1008
    diagnosis 1008
    geographical distribution
        2100–2101t, 2104t

pregnancy 1888
treatment 1008
lesser omentum 4
Letterer–Siwe disease (Langerhans cell
    histiocytosis) 1618–1619, 1645
leucine
    macroautophagy regulation 148f, 149
    protein synthesis regulation 148, 148f
leucocytosis 1770
leuconychia (white nails), cirrhosis 611
leucopenia 1770
leukaemia, hepatic involvement
    1664–1665
leukocyte receptor complex (LRC)
    cluster 370
leukocytes
    abnormalities, liver disease and
        1770–1771
    periportal sinusoidal plugging 81
leukocytopenia, antiviral side-effects 946
leukotriene D4 682
leukotrienes C4 682
levamisole 1061
LeVeen shunts 695
L-γ-glutamyl-L-cysteinyl-glycine *see*
    glutathione
lichen planus 1642–1643
    hepatitis 1643
    hepatitis C 945, 1807
    primary biliary cirrhosis 1643
lifestyle
    alcoholic cirrhosis 1132
    non-alcoholic fatty liver disease
        prevention/management
        1203–1204
    non-alcoholic steatohepatitis
        prevention/management
        1203–1204
ligamentum teres hepatis (round
    ligament) 3
ligamentum venosum 3–4
ligandin *see* glutathione-*S*-transferases
    (GSTs)
ligase chain reaction (LCR) DNA
    amplification, *Mycobacterium
    tuberculosis* 670
light chain (deposit) disease 428
limit dextrinosis *see* glycogen storage
    disease (GSD), type 3
limited scleroderma 1697
limiting plate 10, 10f
Lind, James 572
linear regression analysis 2061
linear RNA amplification, gene array
    analysis 402–403
line tracing test, hepatic encephalopathy
    745
Linguatula serrata 1066
linkage analysis
    gallstone disease 1524
    mouse models of human liver disease
        372
    QTL and 375
    synteny and 377–378
linkage disequilibrium (LD), genetic
    polymorphism and liver disease
    360, 361
lipid(s)
    absorption 291
    composition in membranes 96
    digestion 291
    hepatic stellate cells 44, 45f
    metabolism

across liver cell plate 91–92
    neural modulation 117
    obstructive jaundice 1505
    natural killer T-cells 321
    as second messenger 103
    total parenteral nutrition-related liver
        disease 1636
lipidation 135
lipidosis
    extracellular 1360–1369
    intracellular 1360–1369
lipid peroxidation
    drug-induced 1220
    drug-induced steatohepatitis 1246
    extracellular matrix production 592
    non-alcoholic steatohepatitis 591–592
lipid peroxides, stellate cell activation
    591–592
lipid radicals 1220
lipid storage diseases
    drug-induced 1214t, 1242–1251,
        1243t
        drugs causing 1246–1251
    macrovacuolar steatosis 1243
lipocytes *see* hepatic stellate cell (HSC)
lipofuscin 12, 428, 1870
lipogenesis, across liver cell plate 91
lipogranulomas 428, 1709, 1710f
    macrovesicular steatosis 1148
LipoKinetix, hepatotoxicity 205, 1286
lipophilic vitamins, absorption in liver
    disease 1916
lipopolysaccharide
    alcoholic liver disease 40
    Kupffer cells 37
    liver injury induction
        gene array data 410
        proteomics 414
lipoprotein(s)
    characteristics 134t
    density 134
    disorders 1366–1367
    metabolism 91, 92, 133–142
    size 134
    structure 134–135, 134f
    see also individual types
lipoprotein lipase (LPL) 136–137
    expression, muscle *vs.* adipose tissue
        136
lipotoxicity, non-alcoholic
    steatohepatitis 1202
Listeria monocytogenes 1002
LITH gene/protein, gallstone disease
    1525
Lith loci 376
lithotripsy, haemobilia 1551
Liv.52, hepatotoxicity 1286
liver
    abnormalities, rare diseases with
        2122–2160
    age-related changes 1870–1871
        functional 1870–1871
        morphology 1870
    biliary drainage 5
    capsule stretching 443–444
    divisions 5–7
        1–2–20 principle 6–7, 6f
        Couinaud concept 6, 6f
        hemilivers 6
        portal segments 6, 6f
        vascular territories 6
    drug-induced damage *see* drug-
        induced liver injury

embryology 65–71
    cytokines 314t
external anatomy 3–4, 3f
extrahepatic infection 1001
functional organization 89–96
functional unit (lobule) 9–10, 9f, 11f,
    80, 80f
functions *see* liver function
as haematopoeitc organ 1767, 1767t
hilus (porta hepatitis) 3, 79
histological features 9–19, 9f,
    423–432
    hepatocellular changes 423
    inflammation 424–425
    necrosis 424–425
    regeneration 430
    storage phenomena 428–429
    vascular changes 427–428
imaging 500–548
innervation 5, 114–121
    extrinsic 16
    intrinsic 16–17, 16f
    nerve fibre types 16–17
internal anatomy 4–5, 4f
lobes 3, 3f, 5
    atrophy, simple cyst of the liver 783
    caudate (Spigelian) 3
    left 3
    quadrate 3
    right 3
lymphatics *see* lymphatics
macroscopic anatomy 3–8
morphology, functional aspects 17
neuropeptides 16–17
'nutmeg' appearance, congestive heart
    failure 1612
percussion 447–448
peritoneal attachments 4
prostatic cancer and 1658–1659
pulsatile 447–448
radiation injury 1277–1278
regeneration *see* regeneration
renal transplantation and 1657–1658
resection *see* hepatectomy
scarring *see* fibrosis
stress response, age-related changes
    1871
structure 89
synthetic function 250–273
'transcriptome' 407
transplant *see* liver transplantation
vascular development 69–70
volume, age-related changes 1870
liver adenomatosis
    definition 1430
    diagnosis 1431
    management 1432
liver biopsy 489–499
    acute fatty liver of pregnancy 1882,
        1883
    acute graft-*vs.*-host disease 1673, 1674f
    alcoholic cirrhosis 1166
    alcoholic hepatitis 1163
    alcoholic liver disease 491–492, 1154
    alpha-1-antitrypsin deficiency 1332,
        1333
    Amanita phalloides poisoning 1271
    angiosarcoma 1458
    bile duct injury, post-cholecystectomy
        1959
    biliary hamartomas 1574
    bleeding risk 1788t
    brucellosis 1003

Wilson's disease acute haemolytic
syndrome 1769–1770
window for immunological engagement
(WOFIE), immunosuppression
2003
Wnt-3a, hepatoblasts 66, 68
Wnt signalling cascade
hepatocellular carcinoma 1440
oncogenesis 392–393, 392t
HBx and 393
primary biliary cirrhosis and 410
target genes 392
Wolman disease 1365–1366, 2159
clinical presentation 1365
World Health Organization (WHO),
hepatitis B vaccine
recommendations 912
wound healing, obstructive jaundice
1505
WY14,643 1137

X

xanthelasma, primary biliary cirrhosis
1075
xanthine oxidase 238
xanthoma
familial hypercholesterolaemia
1367

glycogen storage disease type 1 1372
primary biliary cirrhosis 1075
xanthomatous biliary cirrhosis see
primary biliary cirrhosis (PBC)
xanthomatous cells 425
xenobiotics 1218, 1226–1227
excretion in bile 291
metabolism 92–93
toxicity investigations 122
xenogenic extracorporeal liver perfusion,
acute liver failure 1306
xenon, cerebral blood flow measurement
744
XIAP 227t, 228
X-linked glycogen storage disease
(Keating syndrome) 2143
X-linked liver phosphorylase kinase
deficiency (glycogen storage
disease type IXa) 1374
X-linked lymphoproliferative disease,
Epstein–Barr virus infection 965
X-rays
amoebic liver abscess 1025
cystic echinococcosis 1049
Gaucher's disease type 1 1361
granulomatous hepatic tuberculosis
1006
Mycoplasma pneumoniae 1005
osteoporosis 1831

primary sclerosing cholangitis 1105
pyogenic liver abscess 1002
X-ray venography, Budd–Chiari
syndrome 1408, 1409
xylene, hepatotoxicity 2120

Y

yeast two-hybrid system, proteomics
2092
yellow fever 996–998
aetiological agent 996
clinical manifestations 996–997, 997f
diagnosis 997
epidemiology 996
geographical distribution 2100t, 2101t
histology 996
laboratory findings 997
liver involvement 996
pathogenesis 996
pathology 996
prevention 997–998
treatment 997–998
vaccinations 998
Yersinia 1004
Y-protein see glutathione-S-transferases
(GSTs)
Yu-Cheng outbreaks (oil disease) 1273
Yusho outbreaks (oil disease) 1273

Z

zafirlukast, hepatotoxicity 1241
zalcitabine, hepatotoxicity 1248
zeiosis 335
Zellweger syndrome 176, 2159–2160
zidovudine see azidothymidine
(AZT)
Zieve syndrome 1770
Zimmermann–Laband syndrome
2160
zinc 233t, 237
antioxidant function 237
deficiency 233t
alcoholic cirrhosis 1166
excretion 237
Wilson's disease 1320
functions 233t
pregnancy 1886
supplementation 237
alcoholic cirrhosis 1166
cirrhosis 185, 237
hepatic encephalopathy 747, 749,
1839, 1908
uptake 237
Wilson's disease 1318–1319, 1320,
1855
zonula occludens see tight junctions
zygomycosis 1013